KU-740-087

Oxford Textbook of

Clinical Nephrology

Project Administration Newgen Imaging Systems (P) Ltd
Project Manager Kate Martin
Indexer Newgen Imaging Systems (P) Ltd
Design Manager Andrew Meaden
Publisher Helen Liepman

Editors

Alex M. Davison

Emeritus Professor of Renal Medicine, St James's University Hospital, Leeds, UK

J. Stewart Cameron

Emeritus Professor of Renal Medicine, Guy's, King's and St Thomas' School of Medicine, London, UK

Jean-Pierre Grünfeld

Professor of Nephrology, Hôpital Necker, Faculté de Médecine de Paris 5, Paris, France

Claudio Ponticelli

Professor and Director, Division of Nephrology and Dialysis, Istituto Scientifico Ospedale Maggiore Milano, Milan, Italy

Eberhard Ritz

Emeritus Professor of Nephrology, Department of Internal Medicine, Division of Nephrology, Heidelberg, Germany

Christopher G. Winearls

Consultant Nephrologist, Oxford Radcliffe Hospital, Oxford, UK

Charles van Ypersele

Professor of Medicine, Universite Catholique de Louvain, Cliniques Universitaires Saint-Luc, Brussels, Belgium

Subject Editors

Martin Barratt

Emeritus Professor of Paediatric Nephrology, Institute of Child Health, University College London, London, UK

James M. Ritter

Professor of Clinical Pharmacology, Guy's, King's and St Thomas' School of Medicine, London, UK

Jan Weening

Professor of Renal Pathology, University of Amsterdam, The Netherlands

volume **2**

Oxford Textbook of Clinical Nephrology

Third Edition

Edited by

Alex M. Davison
J. Stewart Cameron
Jean-Pierre Grünfeld
Claudio Ponticelli
Eberhard Ritz
Christopher G. Winearls
and Charles van Ypersele

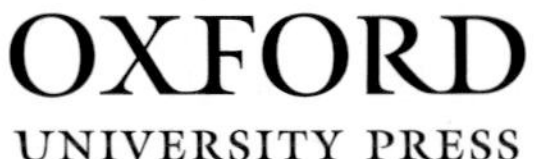

OXFORD
UNIVERSITY PRESS

OXFORD
UNIVERSITY PRESS

Great Clarendon Street, Oxford OX2 6DP

Oxford University Press is a department of the University of Oxford. It furthers the University's objective of excellence in research, scholarship, and education by publishing worldwide in

Oxford New York

Auckland Cape Town Dar es Salaam Hong Kong Karachi Kuala Lumpur Madrid Melbourne Mexico City Nairobi New Delhi Shanghai Taipei Toronto

With offices in

Argentina Austria Brazil Chile Czech Republic France Greece Guatemala Hungary Italy Japan South Korea Poland Portugal Singapore Switzerland Thailand Turkey Ukraine Vietnam

Published in the United States by Oxford University Press Inc., New York

First edition published 1992
Reprinted (with corrections) 1992
Second edition published 1998
Third edition published 2005

British Library Cataloguing in Publication Data

Data available

Library of Congress Cataloging in Publication Data

ISBN 0 19 856796 0 (volume 1)
0 19 856797 9 (volume 2)
0 19 856798 7 (volume 3)
0 19 850824 7 (set)
available as a set only

10 9 8 7 6 5 4 3 2 1

Typeset by Newgen Imaging Systems (P) Ltd, Chennai, India
Printed in Italy
on acid-free paper by Lego

Summary of contents

Contents

Volume 1

Section 1 Assessment of the patient with renal disease

Volume 3

Section 18 The patient with malignancy of the kidney and urinary tract

Section 19 Pharmacology and drug use in kidney patients

Index

Preface to the third edition

Seven years after the publication of the second edition of this clinical text many advances in clinical practice justify the publication of a third edition. The text remains primarily a reference for the practising clinician. The chapters of the second edition have been carefully and critically reviewed. The overall framework of the book has been retained. Several previous chapters have been changed and some additions have been made. In line with our previous policy, the Editors have also modified the authorship of several chapters so as to keep the text as fresh as possible. As with previous editions we have, wherever possible, limited authors to two for each chapter. It is not surprising that a new view on a subject brings a different approach but this maintains vitality. In addition, where new concepts develop and new information becomes available, we have included such material—as illustrated by the information about the influence of smoking on renal diseases.

In this edition we have encouraged authors to add appropriate illustrations and to include pathological illustrative material. Wherever possible we have tried to avoid duplication in text, tables, and figures in an effort to maintain a reasonable overall size to the text. Some repetitions are unavoidable, but they have been included to avoid unnecessary cross-references.

In the production of a text of this size there are a number of people to thank for their hard work and devotion. There has been a change in Editors in that Claudio Ponticelli and Charles van Ypersele have joined the Editorial Board in place of David Kerr who has retired. We would like to thank David Kerr most sincerely for his encouragement in the production of this third edition and his invaluable help with the first two editions. Once again thanks go to the Subject Editors who have provided much useful critical advice which has gone a long way in securing authority and currency. Finally our thanks to the production team at Oxford University Press for all they have done towards launching this third edition.

Alex M. Davison
J. Stewart Cameron
Jean-Pierre Grünfeld
Claudio Ponticelli
Eberhard Ritz
Christopher G. Winearls
Charles van Ypersele
October 2004

Preface to the second edition

We have been gratified by the sales and published reviews of the first edition of our clinical text, published in 1992. During the preparation of this second edition all chapters in the first edition were subjected to review by practising nephrologists who were given the specific task of critically commenting on the content and practical value of each chapter. The authors were asked to revise their chapters in the light of the comments and the advances in clinical science since the production of the first edition. In some areas, such as molecular medicine, there have been very significant advances in our understanding of renal disease while in other areas there have been few changes. The challenge was readily accepted by the contributors and we hope that the final result is a thoroughly revised and up-to-date text.

We have retained the prime aim of the first edition—to produce a text of value to those with clinical responsibility for patients with renal disease. The changes we have introduced have been made in order to keep the text fresh; as a matter of policy we have introduced some new chapters and some new authors for existing chapters. The overall structure is unchanged: each section is centred on the patient with a particular disease or syndrome but the order of the sections has been slightly changed to a more logical sequence.

A major change has been the introduction of colour illustrations throughout the text, wherever possible. We greatly appreciate the efforts of chapter authors in finding suitable clinical and pathological illustrative material. We hope that the clinical illustrations will be of particular value to those in training.

It is with great sadness that we record the deaths of four distinguished authors, Professor Claude Amiel of Paris, Dr Ross R. Bailey of Christchurch, New Zealand, Dr A. Gordon Leitch of Edinburgh, and Professor Tony Raine of London. Claude and Tony died after tragic illnesses borne with supreme courage, Ross while swimming, and Gordon suddenly by drowning while trying to save the life of a fellow holiday-maker. Their chapters are a fitting memorial to their lives. We are all diminished by their loss.

The revision of the text could not have been undertaken without the enthusiastic support of a number of people. We would like to record our thanks to our Subject Editors, Martin Barratt (paediatrics), Michael Dunnill (pathology), Rainer Greger (physiology), and James Ritter (pharmacology) and to our Associate Editors, Claudio Ponticelli, Andy Rees, and Charles van Ypersele de Strihou without whose help and expertise this revised text would not have been completed. In addition our thanks are due to Marion Davison for secretarial support and to the staff of Oxford University Press for their devotion in seeing this venture to conclusion.

Alex M. Davison
J. Stewart Cameron
Jean-Pierre Grünfeld
David N.S. Kerr
Eberhard Ritz
and Christopher Winearls
June 1997

Preface to the first edition

Why another large text of nephrology? Because this one is *different*. It begins not with the anatomy of the nephron, but with the approach to the renal patient. It is intended as a text on *clinical nephrology*, of primary use to those caring for patients with renal disease. Not that we do not value the science that underlies our clinical practice—far from it. In each section the basic science relevant to the problem under discussion will be found incorporated at the appropriate point in the text for the clinician. In this area we have had the assistance of one of the foremost renal physiologists.

We deal in this book with many of the rarer renal problems and renal manifestations of systematic disease that are not dealt with in other texts—as a glance at the index and that of other similar volumes will show. A unique feature of the book is that at the end we have provided a guide to the book from the point of view of other specialist physicians—gastroenterologists, rheumatologists, neurologists, and so on—so that both they and generalists can enter the complex world of nephrology more easily. We have paid special attention to the handling of drugs by the kidney, and to the effects of drugs upon the kidney and renal tract. In this we have been assisted by our distinguished editor in clinical pharmacology.

We have tried to look at nephrology in a global context, remembering that the great majority of patients with renal diseases live in the developing world. Several chapters deal specifically with nephrology as it is seen in the tropics. We have also included chapters which deal with renal disease at the extremes of life. Paediatric nephrology has been blended into the text throughout with the assistance of our able paediatric editor, and several chapters deal with the special problems of the growing number of elderly patients with renal disease.

Finally, we hope that these volumes will be, as well as for day-to-day use when needed, a useful and pleasurable source for browsing when the pressure is off. Above all we hope that these volumes will be a literate as well as a comprehensive guide to diseases of the kidney, and diseases affecting the kidney. We thank our Associate Editors Luis Hernando, Claudio Ponticelli, Andy Rees, Charles van Ypersele de Strihou, and C.J. Winearls without whom these volumes could never have been completed.

Stewart Cameron
Alex M. Davison
Jean-Pierre Grünfeld
David Kerr
Eberhard Ritz

Contributors

Daniel Abramowicz Departement Medico-Chirurgical de Nephrologie, Dialyse et Transplantation, Hopital Erasme, Brussels, Belgium
13.2.2 Immunosuppression for renal transplantation

Horacio J. Adrogué Chief, Renal Section, The Methodist Hospital, Professor of Medicine, Baylor College of Medicine, Houston, Texas, USA
2.1 Hypo–hypernatraemia: disorders of water balance
5.4 Renal tubular acidosis

Dwomoa Adu Department of Nephrology, University Hospital Birmingham, Birmingham, UK
4.9 The patient with rheumatoid arthritis, mixed connective tissue disease, or polymyositis
6.3 Non-steroidal anti-inflammatory drugs and the kidney

J.-R. Allenberg Department of Vascular Surgery, University of Heidelberg School of Medicine, Heidelberg, Germany
9.7 Renovascular hypertension

Alessandro Amore Professor of Nephrology, Nephrology Dialysis Transplantation Unit, Ospedale Regina Margherita, Turin, Italy
4.5.2 The nephritis of Henoch–Schönlein purpura
11.3.11 Effect on the immune response

Corinne Antignac INSERM U574 and Department of Genetics, Hôpital Necker—Enfants Malades, Paris, France
16.3 Nephronophthisis

Pierre Aucouturier INSERM E209, Hopital Saint-Antoine, Batiment Raoul Kourilsky 184, Paris, France
4.3 Kidney involvement in plasma cell dyscrasias

Manuel Urrutia Avisrror Professor of Urology, Department of Surgery, University of Salamanca, Salamanca, Spain
18.1 Renal carcinoma and other tumours

Giovanni Banfi Vice-Director, Division of Nephrology, Instituto Scientifico, Ospedale Maggiore di Milano, Milan, Italy
4.7.2 Systemic lupus erythematosus (clinical)

Rashad S. Barsoum Professor of Internal Medicine, Cairo Kidney Center, Antikhana, Bab-El-Louk, Cairo, Egypt
7.4 Schistosomiasis

Chris Baylis Professor of Physiology and Medicine, University of Florida, Gainsville, Florida, USA
15.1 The normal renal physiological changes which occur during pregnancy
15.3 Pregnancy in patients with underlying renal disease

Michel Beaufils Department of Internal Medicine, Hopital Tenon, Paris, France
10.7.2 Pregnancy

Gordon M. Bell Consultant Nephrologist and Clinical Director of Nephrology, Royal Liverpool University Hospital, Liverpool, UK
4.12.1 Substance misuse, organic solvents and kidney disease

Rinaldo Bellomo Department of Intensive Care, Austin & Repatriation Medical Centre, Heidelberg, Victoria, Australia
10.4 Renal replacement methods in acute renal failure

Jo H.M. Berden Professor of Nephrology, Department of Nephrology 545, University Medical Center St Radboud, Nijmegen, The Netherlands
1.8 Immunological investigation of the patient with renal disease

Jaap J. Beutler Consultant Nephrologist, Department of Nephrology and Hypertension, University Medical Centre Utrecht, Utrecht, The Netherlands
1.6.1.vii Isotope scanning

Daniel G. Bichet Professor of Medicine, Universite de Montreal, Canada Research Chair, Genetics in Renal Diseases, Director, Clinical Research Unit, Hospital du Sacre-Coeur de Montréal, Montréal, Québec, Canada
5.6 Nephrogenic diabetes insipidus

Carol M. Black Professor of Rheumatology, Centre for Rheumatology, Royal Free & University College London Medical School, Royal Free Campus, London, UK
4.8 The patient with scleroderma—systemic sclerosis

Guillaume Bobrie Unite d'hypertension arterielle, Hopital Europeen Georges Pompidou, Paris, France
16.4.3 Nail-patella syndrome and other rare inherited disorders with glomerular involvement

Paola Boccardo Mario Negri Institute for Pharmacological Research, Bergamo, Italy
11.3.12 Coagulation disorders

Jürgen Bommer Klinikum der Universitat Heidelberg, Sektion Nephrologie, Heidelberg, Germany
11.3.3 Sexual disorders

Michael Boulton-Jones Renal Unit, Walton Building, Royal Infirmary, Glasgow, UK
4.2.1 Amyloidosis

J. Douglas Briggs 48 Kingsborough Gardens, Glasgow, UK
13.3.3 Long-term medical complications

J. Trevor Brocklebank Reader in Paediatric Nephrology, Department of Paediatrics, Clinical Science Building, St James's University Hospital, Leeds, UK
10.7.1 Infants and children

Nilufer Broeders Hopital Erasme, Brussels, Belgium
13.2.2 Immunosuppression for renal transplantation

Alison L. Brown Consultant Nephrologist, Freeman Hospital, High Heaton, Newcastle-upon-Tyne, UK
9.2 Clinical approach to hypertension

Michael Broyer Group Hospitalier, Hopital Necker-Enfants Malades, Paris, France
16.5.1 Cystinosis

Vincenzo Cambi Cattedra di Nefrologia, Ospedale Maggiore, Parma, Italy
12.1 Dialysis strategies

J. Stewart Cameron Emeritus Professor of Renal Medicine, Guy's, King's, and St Thomas' School of Medicine, London, UK
1.5 The ageing kidney
3.3 The patient with proteinuria and/or haematuria
3.4 The nephrotic syndrome: management, complications, and pathophysiology
6.4 Uric acid and the kidney
14.2 Chronic renal failure in the elderly
16.5.3 Inherited disorders of purine metabolism and transport
16.7 Some rare syndromes with renal involvement
17.5 Medullary sponge kidney

José M. Campistol Renal Transplant Unit, Hospital Clinic, University of Barcelona, Barcelona, Spain
10.6.4 Acute renal failure in liver disease

Marco Cappelletti Radiologist, Viale Scarampo, Milan, Italy
1.6.2.v Living donor workup

Ruggero Caputo Director, Institute of Dermatological Sciences, University of Milan, IRCCS Osperdale Maggiore, Milan, Italy
11.3.13 Dermatological disorders

Andrés Cárdenas Instructor in Medicine, Division of Gastroenterology and Hepatology, Beth Israel Deaconess Medical Center, Harvard Medical School, Boston, Massachusetts, USA
10.6.4 Acute renal failure in liver disease

D.J.S. Carmichael Consultant Nephrologist, Southend General Hospital, Pricklewood Chase, Westcliff on Sea, Essex, UK
19.2 Handling of drugs in kidney disease

Ralph Caruana Professor of Medicine, Vice Dean for Clinical Affairs, Medical College of Georgia, Augusta, Georgia, USA
4.11 The patient with sickle-cell disease

Michael J.D. Cassidy Clinical Director, Renal and Transplant Unit, Nottingham City Hospital NHS Trust, Nottingham, UK
11.2 Assessment and initial management of the patient with failing renal function

W.R. Cattell 30 Tavistock Terrace, London, UK
7.1 Lower and upper urinary tract infections in the adult

Daniel Cattran University Health Network, Toronto General Hospital, Toronto, Ontario, Canada
3.7 Membranous nephropathy

Dominique Chauveau Service de Néphrologie, Hôpital Necker, Paris, France
16.2.2 Autosomal-dominant polycystic kidney disease

Paramit Chowdhury Department of Nephrology, King's College London, London, UK
9.5 Ischaemic nephropathy
10.6.5 Ischaemic renal disease

Y. Chrétien Radiotherapie, Hopital europeen Georges-Pompidou, Paris, France
1.6.1.iii Percutaneous nephrostomy and ureteral stenting

Kirpal S. Chugh Emeritus Professor of Nephrology, National Kidney Clinic and Research Centre, Chandigarh, India
3.14 Glomerular disease in the tropics
10.7.3 Acute renal failure in the tropical countries

Pierre Cochat Professor of Pediatrics/Head Renal Unit, Department of Pediatrics, Hopital Edouard Herriot, Universite Claude-Bernard, Lyon, France
16.5.2 The primary hyperoxalurias

Fredric L. Coe Professor of Medicine and Physiology, University of Chicago School of Medicine, Chicago, Illinois, USA
8.2 The medical management of stone disease

Eric P. Cohen Professor of Medicine, Nephrology Division, Medical College of Wisconsin, Milwaukee, Wisconsin, USA
6.6 Radiation nephropathy

Rosanna Coppo Ospedale Regina Margherita, Nefrologia, Dialisi e Trapianto, Turin, Italy
3.6 IgA nephropathies
4.5.2 The nephritis of Henoch–Schönlein purpura
11.3.11 Effect on the immune response

Catherine M. Corbishley Consultant Histopathologist, Department of Cellular Pathology, St George's Hospital, London, UK
7.3 Renal tuberculosis and other mycobacterial infections

François Cornud Consultant Radiologist, Hospital Cochin, Paris, France
1.6.1.iii Percutaneous nephrostomy and ureteral stenting

Jean-Michel Correas Vice Chairman, Service de Radiologie, Hôpital Necker, Paris, France
1.6.1.i Ultrasound
1.6.2.ii Hypertension and suspected renovascular disease
1.6.2.iv Renal masses
1.6.2.vi Transplant dysfunction

J.P. Cosyns Professor of Clinical Pathology, Department of Pathology, Medical School, Cliniques Universitaires Saint-Luc, Universite Catholque de Louvain, Brussels, Belgium
6.7 Balkan nephropathy
6.8 Chinese herbs (and other rare causes of interstitial nephropathy)

Malcolm G. Coulthard Department of Paediatric Nephrology, Royal Victoria Infirmary, Newcastle-upon-Tyne, UK
7.2 Urinary tract infections in infancy and childhood

Vincenzo D'Intini Divisione Nefrologia, Ospedale San Bortolo, Vicenza, Italy
10.4 Renal replacement methods in acute renal failure

André Noël Dardenne Associate Professor of Radiology, Universite Catholique de Louvain, Cliniques Universitaires Saint-Luc, Brussels, Belgium
1.6.1.v CT scanning and helical CT

Markus Daschner Pediatric Nephrologist, University Children's Hospital, Heidelberg, Germany
11.3.2 Endocrine disorders

Andrew Davenport Consultant Nephrologist/Honorary Senior Lecturer, Centre for Nephrology, Royal Free Campus, Royal Free and University College Medical School, London, UK
11.3.14 Neuropsychiatric disorders

Salvatore David Cattedra di Nefrologia, Ospedale Maggiore, Parma, Italy
12.1 Dialysis strategies

Alex M. Davison Emeritus Professor of Renal Medicine, St James's University Hospital, Leeds, UK
1.1 History and clinical examination of the patient with renal disease
3.12 Infection related glomerulonephritis
3.13 Malignancy-associated glomerular disease

John M. Davison School of Surgical and Reproductive Sciences, Department of Obstetrics & Gynaecology, Medical School, Newcastle-upon-Tyne, UK
15.1 The normal renal physiological changes which occur during pregnancy
15.2 Renal complications that may occur in pregnancy
15.3 Pregnancy in patients with underlying renal disease

Marc E. De Broe Department of Nephrology, University Hospital Antwerp, Edegem/Antwerp, Belgium
6.2 Analgesic nephropathy
6.5 Nephrotoxic metals
19.1 Drug-induced nephropathies

John M.H. De Klerk Consultant in Nuclear Medicine, Department of Nuclear Medicine, University Centre Utrecht, Utrecht, The Netherlands
1.6.1.vii Isotope scanning

Rita De Smet Department of Nephrology, University Hospital, Ghent, Belgium
11.3.1 Uraemic toxicity

Peter R.F. Dear Regional Neonatal Intensive Care Unit, St James's University Hospital, Leeds, UK
1.4 Renal function in the newborn infant

Christopher P. Denton Clinical Research Fellow, Academic Unit of Rheumatology, Royal Free Hospital School of Medicine, University of London, London, UK
4.8 The patient with scleroderma—systemic sclerosis

Robert J. Desnick Professor and Chairman, Department of Human Genetics, Mount Sinai School of Medicine, New York, USA
16.4.2 Fabry disease

Olivier Devuyst Division of Nephrology, UCL Medical School, (Universite Catholique de Louvain), Brussels, Belgium
16.2.2 Autosomal-dominant polycystic kidney disease

Ralf Dikow Sektion Nephrologie, Heidelberg, Germany
4.1 The patient with diabetes mellitus
9.6 Hypertension and unilateral renal parenchymal disease
9.8 Malignant hypertension
11.3.4 Hypertension
14.3 The diabetic patient with impaired renal function

John H. Dirks Chair, ISN COMGAN, President, The Gairdner Foundation, Senior Fellow, Massey College, University of Toronto, Toronto, Ontario, Canada
2.5 Hypo–hypermagnesaemia

Ciaran Doherty Regional Nephrology Unit, Belfast City Hospital, Belfast, UK
10.1 Epidemiology of acute renal failure
11.3.6 Gastrointestinal effects

Raymond A.M.G. Donckerwolcke Professor and Chairman, Department of Paediatrics, University Hospital Maastricht, Maastricht, The Netherlands
3.4 The nephrotic syndrome: management, complications, and pathophysiology

Sven Dorph Department of Radiology, Helsingor Hospital, Helsingor, Denmark
1.6.2.i Haematuria, infection, acute renal failure, and obstruction

Dominique Droz Service d'Anatomie Pathologique, Hopital Saint-Louis, Paris, France
10.6.2 Acute tubulointerstitial nephritis

Tilman B. Drüeke INSERM Unit 507 and Division of Nephrology, Hopital Necker, Paris, France
11.3.9 Skeletal disorders

I. Dulau-Florea Schwabing General Hospital, Ludwig Maximilians University, Munich, Germany
9.7 Renovascular hypertension

John B. Eastwood Consultant Renal Physician and Reader in Medicine, Department of Renal Medicine, and Transplantation, St George's Hospital, London, UK
7.3 Renal tuberculosis and other mycobacterial infections

Kai-Uwe Eckardt Department of Nephrology and Medical Intensive Care, Charité, Campus Virchow Klinikum, Berlin, Germany
11.3.8 Haematological disorders

Lisette El Hajj Hôpital de Rangueil, Service Central d Radiologie, Toulouse, France
1.6.1.iv Renal arteriography

A. Meguid El Nahas Professor of Nephrology, Sheffield Kidney Institute, Sheffield teaching Hospitals NHS Trust, Northern General Hospital, Sheffield, UK
11.1 Mechanisms of experimental and clinical renal scarring

Marlies Elger Abteilung Nephrologie, Forschungszentrum der Medizinischen Hochschule, am Oststadtkrankenhaus, Hannover, Germany
3.1 The renal glomerulus—the structural basis of ultrafiltration

Paul Emery ARC Professor of Rheumatology, Molecular Medicine Unit, School of Medicine, Leeds, UK
4.9 The patient with rheumatoid arthritis, mixed connective tissue disease, or polymyositis

Karlhans Endlich Assistant Professor, Department of Anatomy and Cell Biology, University of Heidelberg, Heidelberg, Germany
9.1 The structure and function of blood vessels in the kidney

John Feehally Department of Nephrology, Leicester General Hospital, Leicester, UK
3.2 Glomerular injury and glomerular response

Terry Feest The Richard Bright Renal Unit, Southmead Hospital, Westbury-on-Trym, Bristol, UK
1.9 The epidemiology of renal disease

J.D. Firth Consultant Physician and Nephrologist, Addenbrooke's Hospital, Cambridge, UK
10.3 The clinical approach to the patient with acute renal failure

Maggie Fitzpatrick Consultant Paediatric Nephrologist, Department of Paediatrics Nephrology, St James's Hospital, Leeds, UK
1.1 History and clinical examination of the patient with renal disease
10.7.1 Infants and children

Jürgen Floege Medizinische Klinik II der RWTH, Aachen, Germany
3.2 Glomerular injury and glomerular response

Giovanni B. Fogazzi Divisione di Nefrologia e Dialisi, Oespadele Maggiore, IRCCS, Milan, Italy
1.2 Urinalysis and microscopy

Robert N. Foley Department of Medicine, Hennepin County Medical Center, Minneapolis, Minnesota, USA
11.3.5 Cardiovascular risk factors

Gérard Friedlander Professor and Chief, INSERM U 426, Department of Physiology, Xavier Bichat Medical Faculty, Paris, France
1.3 The clinical assessment of renal function
2.4 Hypo–hyperphosphataemia

Marie-France Gagnadoux Pediatric Nephrologist, Necker-Enfants Malades, Paris, France
16.2.1 Polycystic kidney disease in children

Gillian Gaskin Renal Section, Division of Medicine, Faculty of Medicine, Imperial College, Hammersmith Hospital, London, UK
4.5.3 Systemic vasculitis

Pere Ginès Associate Professor of Medicine, Liver Unit, Institut de Malalties Digestives, Hospital Clinic, University of Barcelona, Barcelona, Spain
10.6.4 Acute renal failure in liver disease

Matthias Girndt Assistant Professor of Internal Medicine and Nephrology, Medical Department IV, University of Saarland, Homburg, Germany
11.3.7 Liver disorders

Sven Glaesker Department of Nephrology, Clinics of the Albert Freiburg University, Freiburg, Germany
16.6 Renal involvement in tuberous sclerosis and von Hippel–Lindau disease

Griet Glorieux Nephrology Department, University Hospital Ghent, Ghent, Belgium
11.3.1 Uraemic toxicity

Ram Gokal Consultant Nephrologist, Honorary Professor of Medicine, Manchester Royal Infirmary, Manchester, UK
12.4 Peritoneal dialysis and complications of technique

David S. Goldfarb Associate Professor of Medicine and Physiology, New York University School of Medicine, Nephrology/111G, NY Department of Veterans Affairs Medical Centre, New York, USA
8.2 The medical management of stone disease

John M. Grange Visiting Professor, Royal Free and University College Medical School, Windeyer Institute for Medical Science, London, UK
7.3 Renal tuberculosis and other mycobacterial infections

Ian A. Greer Deputy Dean—Faculty of Medicine, Regius Professor—Obstetrics and Gynaecology, University of Glasgow, Glasgow Royal Infirmary, Glasgow, UK
15.4 Pregnancy-induced hypertension

Rainer Greger Physiologisches Institut, Albert-Ludwigs-Universität, Freiburg, Germany
19.3 Action and clinical use of diuretics

Jean-Pierre Grünfeld Professor of Nephrology, Hôpital Necker, Faculté de Médecine de Paris 5, Paris, France
1.1 History and clinical examination of the patient with renal disease
16.4.1 Alport's syndrome
16.4.2 Fabry disease
16.4.3 Nail-patella syndrome and other rare inherited disorders with glomerular involvement
16.7 Some rare syndromes with renal involvement

Marie-Claire Gubler INSERM U574, Hôpital Necker—Enfants Malades, Paris, France
16.3 Nephronophthisis
16.5.1 Cystinosis

Sanjeev Gulati Department of Nephrology, Sanjay Gandhi Postgraduate Institute of Medical Sciences, Lucknow, India
3.8 Mesangiocapillary glomerulonephritis

Krishan Lal Gupta Additional Professor of Nephrology, Postgraduate Institute of Medical Education and Research, Chandigarh, India
7.5 Fungal infections and the kidney

Suresh K. Gupta 46 Glebe Avenue, Grappenhal, Warrington, UK
8.3 The surgical management of renal stones

Kenneth R. Hallows Assistant Professor, Renal-Electrolyte Division, Department of Medicine, University of Pittsburgh School of Medicine, Pittsburgh, Pennsylvania, USA
2.2 Hypo–hyperkalaemia

Neveen A.T. Hamdy Head Clinic Section, Department of Endocrinology & Metabolic Diseases, Leiden University Medical Center, Leiden, The Netherlands
2.3 Hypo–hypercalcaemia

Barrie Hartley Department of Pathology, St James's University Hospital, Leeds, UK
3.13 Malignancy-associated glomerular disease

George B. Haycock Consultant in Paediatrics, Guy's, King's, and St Thomas' Hospital, London, UK
5.2 Isolated defects of tubular function

August Heidland Department of Internal Medicine, University of Wurzburg, Kuratorium für Dialysis und Nierentransplantation, Wurzburg, Germany
19.3 Action and clinical use of diuretics

Olivier Hélénon Chairman, Service de Radiologie, Hôpital Necker, Paris, France
1.6.1.i Ultrasound
1.6.1.iii Percutaneous nephrostomy and ureteral stenting
1.6.2.ii Hypertension and suspected renovascular disease
1.6.2.iv Renal masses
1.6.2.vi Transplant dysfunction

Udo Helmchen Department of Pathology, Universitätsklinikum Hamburg-Eppendorf, Hamburg, Germany
9.4 The effects of hypertension on renal vasculature and structure

Elizabeth Petri Henske Fox Chase Cancer Center, 7701 Burholme Avenue, Philadelphia, Pennsylvania, USA
16.6 Renal involvement in tuberous sclerosis and von Hippel–Lindau disease

Lukas B. Hilbrands University Medical Centre Nymegen, Department of Nephrology, Nijmegen, The Netherlands
13.1 Selection and preparation of the recipient

Friedhelm Hildebrandt Professor of Pediatrics and Human Genetics, Huetwell Professor for the Cure and Prevention of Birth Defects, Department of Pediatrics, University of Michigan, Ann Arbor, Michigan, USA
16.1 Strategies for the investigation of inherited renal disease

Andries J. Hoitsma Division of Nephrology, University Medical Center St Radboud, Nijmegen, The Netherlands
13.1 Selection and preparation of the recipient

Christer Holmberg Hospital for Children and Adolescents, University of Helsinki, Helsinki, Finland
16.4.4 Congenital nephrotic syndrome

Matthew L.P. Howse Link 6C, Royal Liverpool University Hospital, Liverpool, UK
4.12.1 Substance misuse, organic solvents and kidney disease

Othon Iliopoulos MGH Cancer Center, Massachusetts General Hospital, Boston, Massachusetts, USA
16.6 Renal involvement in tuberous sclerosis and von Hippel–Lindau disease

Enrico Imbasciati Director, Division of Nephrology, Ospedale Maggiore di Lodi, Lodi, Italy
1.7 Renal biopsy: indications for and interpretation

David A. Isenberg Centre for Rheumatology, Royal Free and University College Hospital, London, UK
4.7.1 The pathogenesis of systemic lupus erythematosus

Claude Jacobs Groupe hospitalier Pitié-Salpêtrière, Service de nephrologie, Paris, France
12.6 Medical management of the dialysis patient

Michel Jadoul Cliniques Universitaires St Luc, Department of Nephrology, Brussels, Belgium
11.3.10 β2M Amyloidosis

Hannu Jalanko Hospital for Children and Adolescents, University of Helsinki, Helsinki, Finland
16.4.4 Congenital nephrotic syndrome

Vivekanand Jha Associate Professor, Department of Nephrology, Postgraduate Institute of Medical Education and Research, Chandigarh, India
3.14 Glomerular disease in the tropics
10.7.3 Acute renal failure in the tropical countries

Francis G. Joffre Hôpital de Rangueil, Service Central d Radiologie, Toulouse, France
1.6.1.iv Renal arteriography

Kate Verrier Jones KRUF Children's Kidney Centre for Wales, University of Wales, College of Medicine, Heath Park, Cardiff, UK
17.2 Vesicoureteric reflux and reflux nephropathy

Nicola Joss Renal Unit, Walton Building, Royal Infirmary, Glasgow, UK
4.2.1 Amyloidosis

Islam Junaid Consultant Urologist and Transplant Surgeon, Department of Renal Medicine & Transplantation, The Royal London Hospital, Whitechapel, London, UK
17.3 The patient with urinary tract obstruction

Brian Junor Consultant Nephrologist, Renal Unit, Western Infirmary, Glasgow, UK
13.3.5 Outcome of renal transplantation

Cees G.M. Kallenberg Department of Clinical Immunology, University Hospital Groningen, Groningen, The Netherlands
4.5.1 Pathogenesis of angiitis

John A. Kanis Sheffield Metabolic Bone Unit, Sheffield, UK
2.3 Hypo–hypercalcaemia

Alexandre Karras Service de Néphrologie et Transplantation Rénale, Hopital Saint-Louis, Paris, France
10.6.2 Acute tubulointerstitial nephritis

Akira Kawashima Professor of Radiology, Mayo Clinic College of Medicine, Department of Radiology, Mayo Clinic, Rochester, Minnesota, USA
1.6.1.ii Plain radiography, contrast radiography, and excretion radiography
1.6.1.vi Magnetic resonance imaging

Vijay Kher Department of Nephrology, Indraprastha Apollo Hospitals, New Delhi, India
3.8 Mesangiocapillary glomerulonephritis

Bernard F. King, Jr. Mayo School of Graduate Medical Education, Department of Radiology, Mayo Clinic, Rochester, Minnesota, USA
1.6.1.vi Magnetic resonance imaging

Bertrand Knebelmann Hôpital Necker, Paris, France
16.4.1 Alport's syndrome

Nine V.A.M. Knoers University Hospital Nijmegen, Nijmegen, The Netherlands
5.5 Hypokalaemic tubular disorders

Karl-Martin Koch Medizinische Hochschule Hannover, Zentrum Innere Medizin und Dermatologie, Abteilung Nephrologie, NHH, Hannover, Germany
12.3 Haemodialysis, haemofiltration, and complications of technique

Hans Köhler Universitätskliniken des Saarlandes, Medizinische Klinik und Poliklinik, Medical Department IV, University of Saarland, Homburg, Germany
11.3.7 Liver disorders

Hein A. Koomans Professor of Nephrology and Head of Department of Nephrology and Hypertension, Department of Nephrology, University Centre Utrecht, Utrecht, The Netherlands
1.6.1.vii Isotope scanning

Stephen M. Korbet Professor of Medicine, Rush University Medical Center, Chicago, Illinois, USA
4.2.2 Fibrillary and immunotactoid glomerulopathy

Wilhelm Kriz Professor and Chairman, Institute of Anatomy and Cell Biology, University of Heidelberg, Heidelberg, Germany
3.1 The renal glomerulus—the structural basis of ultrafiltration

B. Krumme Department of Nephrology, Deutsche Klinik fur Diagnostick, Wiesbaden, Germany
9.7 Renovascular hypertension

Heather J. Lambert Department of Paediatric Nephrology, Royal Victoria Infirmary, Newcastle-upon-Tyne, UK
7.2 Urinary tract infections in infancy and childhood

Norbert Hendrik Lameire Renal Division, University Hospital Ghent, Ghent, Belgium
10.2 Acute renal failure: pathophysiology and prevention
10.7.4 The elderly
11.3.1 Uraemic toxicity

Florian Lang Department of Physiology, University of Tubingen, Tubingen, Germany
19.3 Action and clinical use of diuretics

Andrew J. LeRoy Associate Professor of Radiology, Mayo Clinic College of Medicine, Department of Radiology, Mayo Clinic, Rochester, Minnesota, USA
1.6.1.ii Plain radiography, contrast radiography, and excretion radiography

Philippe Lesavre Service de Nephrologie, Hôpital Necker, Paris, France
3.12 Infection related glomerulonephritis

Jeremy Levy Consultant Nephrologist and Physician, Imperial College, Hammersmith Hospital, London, UK
3.10 Crescentic glomerulonephritis

Edmund J. Lewis Professor of Medicine, Rush University Medical Center, Chicago, Illinois, USA
4.2.2 Fibrillary and immunotactoid glomerulopathy

Gerhard Lonnemann Department of Nephrology, Medical School, Hannover, Germany
12.3 Haemodialysis, haemofiltration, and complications of technique

Iain C. Macdougall The Renal Unit, King's College Hospital, London, UK
11.3.8 Haematological disorders

Nicolaos E. Madias Chairman, Department of Medicine, Caritas St Elizabeth's Medical Center and Professor of Medicine, Tufts University School of Medicine, Boston, Massachusetts, USA
2.1 Hypo–hypernatraemia: disorders of water balance
5.4 Renal tubular acidosis

J.F.E. Mann Krankenhaus Monchen Schwabing, Munich, Germany
9.7 Renovascular hypertension

A.M. Marinaki Purine Research Unit, Guy's Hospital, London Bridge, London, UK
16.5.3 Inherited disorders of purine metabolism and transport

Frank Martinez Service de Néphrologie et Transplantation Rénale, Hopital Saint-Louis, Paris, France
10.6.2 Acute tubulointerstitial nephritis

Angelo Valerio Marzano Assistant Dermatologist, Institute of Dermatological Sciences, University of Milan, IRCCS Osperdale Maggiore, Milan, Italy
11.3.13 Dermatological disorders

L.J. Mason Research Assistant, Centre for Rheumatology, University College London, Windeyer Institute of Medical Sciences, London, UK
4.7.1 The pathogenesis of systemic lupus erythematosus

Philip D. Mason Consultant Nephrologist, Oxford Kidney Unit, Churchill Hospital, Headington, Oxford, UK
10.6.1 Glomerulonephritis, vasculitis, and the nephrotic syndrome

Arnaud Méjean Service d'Urologie, Paris, France
1.6.2.iv Renal masses
1.6.2.vi Transplant dysfunction

Jean-Philippe Méry 59 rue Madame, Paris, France
4.4 The patient with sarcoidosis

Alain Meyrier Hôpital Europeen Georges-Pompidou, Paris, France
3.5 Minimal change and focal–segmental glomerular sclerosis

Michael J. Mihatsch Director, Institute for Pathology, University of Basel, Basel, Switzerland
1.7 Renal biopsy: indications for and interpretation

Robert D. Mills Consultant Urologist, Norfolk & Norwich University Hospital, Norwich, UK
18.4 Tumours of the bladder

Christopher Mitchell Paediatric Haematology/Oncology Unit, The John Radcliffe Hospital, Headington, Oxford, UK
18.2 Wilms' tumour

Leo A.H. Monnens Department of Pediatrics, University Hospital Nijmegen, Nijmegen, The Netherlands
5.5 Hypokalaemic tubular disorders

Emmanuel Morelon Department on Transplantation, Hôpital Necker, Universite Paris V, Paris, France
1.6.2.vi Transplant dysfunction

Stephen H. Morgan Basildon Hospital, Nether Mayne, Basildon, UK
16.4.2 Fabry disease

Gabriella Moroni Assistant Nephrologist, Division of Nephrology, Instituto Scientifico, Ospedale Maggiore di Milano, Milan, Italy
4.7.2 Systemic lupus erythematosus (clinical)

Béatrice Mougenot Pathologist, Hôpital Tenon, Paris, France
4.3 Kidney involvement in plasma cell dyscrasias

Claudia A. Müller Section Transplantation Immunology, ZMF, Tubingen, Germany
6.1 Mechanisms of interstitial inflammation

Gerhard A. Müller Universitätsklinikum/Innere Medizin, Abteilung für Nephrologie und Rheumatologie, Göttingen, Germany
6.1 Mechanisms of interstitial inflammation

Robert G. Narins Director of Postgraduate Education, American Society of Nephrology, Washington, DC, USA
2.6 Clinical acid–base disorders

Guy H. Neild Institute of Urology and Nephrology, Middlesex Hospital, London, UK
10.6.3 Acute renal failure associated with microangiopathy (haemolytic–uraemic syndrome and thrombotic thrombocytopenic purpura)

Hartmut P.H. Neumann Medizinische Universitätsklinik, Freiburg im Breisgau, Germany
16.6 Renal involvement in tuberous sclerosis and von Hippel–Lindau disease

Simon J. Newell Regional Neonatal Intensive Care Unit, St James's University Hospital, Leeds, UK
1.4 Renal function in the newborn infant

Chas G. Newstead Department of Renal medicine, St James's University Hospital, Leeds, UK
13.3.4 Recurrent disease and de novo disease

Patrick Niaudet Nephrologie Paediatrique, Hospital Necker-Enfants Malades, Paris, France
3.5 Minimal change and focal–segmental glomerular sclerosis

Michael Nicholson Division of Transplant Surgery, Leicester General Hospital, Leicester, UK
13.3.1 Surgery and surgical complications

Juan F. Macías-Núñez Unidad de Hipertension, Hospital Universitario de Salamanca, Salamanca, Spain
1.5 The ageing kidney
14.2 Chronic renal failure in the elderly

Christopher Olbricht Klinik fur Nieren-und Hochdruckkrankheiten, Katharine Hospital, Stuttgart, Germany
12.3 Haemodialysis, haemofiltration, and complications of technique

Stephan R. Orth Dialysis Centre Schwandorf, Schwandorf, Germany
4.12.2 Smoking and the kidney

Kazuo Ota Director, Ota Medical Research Institute, Chouo-ku, Tokyo, Japan
12.2 Vascular access

Edgar Otto Research Investigator, Department of Pediatrics, University of Michigan, Ann Arbor, Michigan, USA
16.1 Strategies for the investigation of inherited renal disease

Biff F. Palmer Professor of Internal Medicine, Department of Internal Medicine, Division of Nephrology, University of Texas Southwestern Medical School, Dallas, Texas, USA
2.6 Clinical acid–base disorders

Vicente Arroyo Pérez Institute of Digestive Diseases, Hospital Clinic 1 Provincial de Barcelona, Barcelona, Spain
10.6.4 Acute renal failure in liver disease

Phuong-Chi T. Pham Assistant Clinical Professor of Medicine, Division of Nephrology, Department of Medicine, David Geffen School of Medicine at UCLA, Los Angeles, California, USA
13.3.2 The early management of the recipient

Phuong-Thu T. Pham Assistant Clinical Professor of Medicine, Division of Nephrology, Kidney Transplant Program, David Geffen School of Medicine at UCLA, Los Angeles, California, USA
13.3.2 The early management of the recipient

Yves Pirson Department of Nephrology, University of Louvain Medical School, Cliniques Universitaires St Luc, Faculté de médecine, Brussels, Belgium
16.2.2 Autosomal-dominant polycystic kidney disease

Wolfgang Pommer Director, Department of Internal Medicine—Nephrology, Vivantes Humboldt Klinikum, Berlin, Germany
6.2 Analgesic nephropathy

Claudio Ponticelli Professor and Director, Division of Nephrology and Dialysis, Istituto Scientifico Ospedale Maggiore Milano, Milan, Italy
1.6.2.iii Renal biopsy—procedure and complications
1.6.2.v Living donor workup
1.7 Renal biopsy: indications for and interpretation
4.7.2 Systemic lupus erythematosus (clinical)
11.3.13 Dermatological disorders

Dominique Prié Assistant Professor INSERM U 426, Department of Physiology, Xavier Bichat Medical Faculty, Paris, France
1.3 The clinical assessment of renal function

Charles D. Pusey Renal Section, Division of Medicine, Imperial College, Hammersmith Hospital, London, UK
3.10 Crescentic glomerulonephritis

Uwe Querfeld Director, Pediatric Nephrology, Department of Pediatric Nephrology, Charité Campus, Virchow Klinkum Children's Hospital, Berlin, Germany
14.1 Chronic renal failure in children

Wolfgang Rascher Professor of Pediatrics, Head and Chairman, Department of Pediatrics, Erlangen, Germany
9.9 The hypertensive child
17.4 Congenital abnormalities of the urinary tract

Andrew J. Rees Regius Professor of Medicine, University of Aberdeen, Institute of Medical Sciences, Foresterhill, Aberdeen, UK
3.11 Antiglomerular basement disease

Giuseppe Remuzzi Division of Nephrology and Dialysis, Ospedali Riuniti di Bergamo, Mario Negri Institute for Pharmacological Research, Bergamo, Italy
11.3.12 Coagulation disorders

Eberhard Ritz Emeritus Professor of Nephrology, Department of Internal Medicine, Division of Nephrology, Heidelberg, Germany
4.1 The patient with diabetes mellitus
9.8 Malignant hypertension
11.3.4 Hypertension
11.3.5 Cardiovascular risk factors
11.3.9 Skeletal disorders
14.3 The diabetic patient with impaired renal function

Paul J. Roderick Senior Lecturer in Public Health Medicine, Applied Clinical Epidemiology Group, Community Clinical Sciences Research Division, School of Medicine, University of Southampton, Southampton, UK
1.9 The epidemiology of renal disease

Bernardo Rodríguez-Iturbe Professor of Medicine and Chief of Nephrology, Hospital Universitario, Universidad del Zulia and Director, Instituto de Investigaciones Biomedicas, Maracaibo, Venezuela
3.9 Acute endocapillary glomerulonephritis

Marie-Odile Rolland Laboratoire de Biochimie Pediatrique, Hospitalk Debrousse, Lyon, France
16.5.2 The primary hyperoxalurias

Claudio Ronco Director, Department of Nephrology, St Bortolo Hospital, Vicenza, Italy
10.4 Renal replacement methods in acute renal failure

Pierre M. Ronco Renal Department and INSERM, Unité 489, Hôpital Tenon, Paris, France
4.3 Kidney involvement in plasma cell dyscrasias

Wolfgang H. Rösch Kinderurologische Abteilung der Universität Regensburg, In der Klinik St Hedwig, Regensburg, Germany
17.4 Congenital abnormalities of the urinary tract

Luis M. Ruilope Univdad de Hipertension, Hospital 12 de Octubre, Madrid, Spain
9.3 The kidney and control of blood pressure

Rémi Salomon INSERM U574 and Department of Pediatric Nephrology, Hôpital Necker—Enfants Malades, Paris, France
16.3 Nephronophthisis

John Savill Professor of Medicine, Vice Principal and Head of the College of Medicine & Veterinary Medicine, University of Edinburgh, Edinburgh, UK
3.2 Glomerular injury and glomerular response

Franz Schaefer Division of Pediatric Nephrology, University Children's Hospital, Heidelberg, Germany
11.3.2 Endocrine disorders

Francesco Paolo Schena University of Bari, Renal Unit, Policlinico, Bari, Italy
3.6 IgA nephropathies

Michael Schömig Sektion Nephrologie, Heidelberg, Germany
9.6 Hypertension and unilateral renal parenchymal disease

Melvin M. Schwartz Professor of Pathology, Rush University Medical Center, Chicago, Illinois, USA
4.2.2 Fibrillary and immunotactoid glomerulopathy

John E. Scoble Department of Renal Medicine and Transplantation, Guy's Hospital, London, UK
9.5 Ischaemic nephropathy
10.6.5 Ischaemic renal disease

Katarina Sebekova Institute of Preventive and Clinical Medicine, Bratislava, Slovakia
19.3 Action and clinical use of diuretics

Günter Seyffart Head, Dialysis Center, Bad Homburg, Germany
10.5 Dialysis and haemoperfusion treatment of acute poisoning

David G. Shirley Research Fellow and Honorary Reader, Royal Free & University College Medical School, London, UK
5.1 The structure and function of tubules

Caroline Silve Senior Investigator, INSERM U 426, Department of Physiology, Xavier Bichat Medical Faculty, Paris, France
2.4 Hypo–hyperphosphataemia

H. Anne Simmonds Purine Research Unit, Guy's Hospital, London Bridge, London, UK
6.4 Uric acid and the kidney
16.5.3 Inherited disorders of purine metabolism and transport

Visith Sitprija Director, Queen Saovabha Memorial Institute, Thai Red Cross Society, Patumwan, Bangkok, Thailand
10.7.3 Acute renal failure in the tropical countries

Philip H. Smith 2 Creskeld Lane, Bramhope LS16 9AW, UK
18.5 Tumours of the prostate

John S. Smyth Department of Renal Medicine, Guy's, St Thomas' NHS Trust, London, UK
10.6.5 Ischaemic renal disease

Patrick G.J.F. Starremans Department of Paediatrics & Cell Physiology, University of Nijmegen, Nijmegen, The Netherlands
5.5 Hypokalaemic tubular disorders

Vladisav Stefanović Professor of Medicine, Institute of Nephrology and Haemodialysis, University School of Medicine, University of Niš, Niš, Yugoslavia
6.7 Balkan nephropathy

Coen A. Stegeman Associate Professor of Nephrology, Department of Nephrology, University Hospital Groningen, Groningen, The Netherlands
4.5.1 Pathogenesis of angiitis

Henk Stevens Consultant in Nuclear Medicine, Department of Nuclear Medicine, University Centre Utrecht, Utrecht, The Netherlands
1.6.1.vii Isotope scanning

Terry B. Strom Professor of Medicine, Harvard Medical School, Chief, Division of Immunology, BI-Deaconess Medical Center, Boston, Massachusetts, USA
13.2.1 The immunology of transplantation

Frank Strutz Universitätsklinikum/Innere Medizin, Abteilung für Nephrologie und Rheumatologie, Göttingen, Germany
6.1 Mechanisms of interstitial inflammation

Manikkam Suthanthiran Chief, Nephrology and Transplantation Medicine, Stanton Griffis Distinguished Professor of Medicine, Cornell University Medical College, New York, USA
13.2.1 The immunology of transplantation

Dante Tagliavini Cattedra di Nefrologia, Ospedale Maggiore, Parma, Italy
12.1 Dialysis strategies

Richard L. Tannen University of Pennsylvania School of Medicine, Philadelphia, Pennsylvania, USA
2.2 Hypo–hyperkalaemia

Antonio Tarantino Divisione Di Nefrologia, Ospedale Maggiore, IRCCS, Milan, Italy
4.6 The patient with mixed cryoglobulinaemia and hepatitis C infection

James Tattersall Department of Nephrology, St James's University Hospital, Leeds, UK
12.5 Adequacy of dialysis

C. Mark Taylor Department of Nephrology, Birmingham Children's Hospital, Birmingham, UK
10.6.3 Acute renal failure associated with microangiopathy (haemolytic–uraemic syndrome and thrombotic thrombocytopenic purpura)

Hans-Göran Tiselius Professor of Urology, Department of Urology, Huddinge University Hospital, Stockholm, Sweden
8.1 Aetiological factors in stone formation

Wai Y. Tse Department of Nephrology, Derriford Hospital, Plymouth, UK
6.3 Non-steroidal anti-inflammatory drugs and the kidney

A. Neil Turner Professor of Nephrology, University of Edinburgh, Renal & Autoimmunity Group, Royal Infirmary, Edinburgh, UK
3.2 Glomerular injury and glomerular response
3.11 Antiglomerular basement disease

William H. Turner Consultant Urologist, Addenbrooks NHS Trust, Cambridge, UK
18.4 Tumours of the bladder

Robert J. Unwin St Peter's Professor of Nephrology, Centre for Nephrology, Royal Free and University College Medical School, London, UK
5.1 The structure and function of tubules

Seppo Vainio Department of Biochemistry, University of Oulu, Linnanmaa, Finland
17.1 The development of the kidney and renal dysplasia

Bernard E. Van Beers Professor of Radiology, Universite Catholique de Louvain, Cliniques Universitaires Saint-Luc, Brussels, Belgium
1.6.1.v CT scanning and helical CT

Nele Van Den Noortgate Department of Internal Medicine, Division of Geriatric Medicine, Ghent University Hospital, Ghent, Belgium
10.7.4 The elderly

Charles van Ypersele Professor of Medicine, Universite Catholique de Louvain, Cliniques Universitaires Saint-Luc, Brussels, Belgium
6.8 Chinese herbs (and other rare causes of interstitial nephropathy)
10.6.6 Hantavirus infection
11.3.10 β2M Amyloidosis

William G. van't Hoff Consultant Paediatric Nephrologist, Great Ormond Street Hospital for Children, NHS Trust, London, UK
5.3 Fanconi syndrome
8.5 Renal and urinary tract stone disease in children

Raymond Camille Vanholder Nephrology Department, University Hospital Ghent, Ghent, Belgium
10.2 Acute renal failure: pathophysiology and prevention
10.7.4 The elderly
11.3.1 Uraemic toxicity

Patrick J.W. Venables Kennedy Institute of Rheumatology, Faculty of Medicine, The Charing Cross Hospital Campus, Arthritis Research Campaign Building, London, UK
4.10 The patient with Sjögren's syndrome and overlap syndromes

Christoph Wanner Department of Medicine, Division of Nephrology, University Hospital, Würzburg, Germany
11.3.4 Hypertension

Richard P. Wedeen Professor of Medicine, Professor of Preventive Medicine and Community Health, UMDNJ—New Jersey Medical School and Associate Chief of Staff for Research and Development, Department of Veterans Affairs New Jersey Health Care System, East Orange, New Jersey, USA
6.5 Nephrotoxic metals

Pieter M. Ter Wee Department of Nephrology, Vrije Universiteit Academic Medical Center, Amsterdam, The Netherlands
11.2 Assessment and initial management of the patient with failing renal function

Richard B. Weiner Clinical Assistant Professor of Psychiatry, SUNY Health Sciences Center at Brooklyn and Director, Children's Psychiatric Impatient Unit, Division of Child and Adolescent Psychiatry, Kings County Hospital Center, Brooklyn, New York, USA
12.7 Psychological aspects of treatment for renal failure

Ulrich Wenzel Department of Medicine, Division of Nephrology, Universitätsklinikum Hamburg-Eppendorf, Hamburg, Germany
9.4 The effects of hypertension on renal vasculature and structure

Jack F.M. Wetzels University Medical Center St Radboud, Division of Nephrology 545, Nijmegen, The Netherlands
1.8 Immunological investigation of the patient with renal disease

Peter Whelan Department of Urology, St James's University Hospital, Leeds, UK
18.3 Tumours of the renal pelvis and ureter

Hugh Whitfield Department of Urology, Battle Hospital, Reading, Berkshire, UK
8.3 The surgical management of renal stones

Alan H. Wilkinson Professor of Medicine, Director Kidney & Kidney/Pancreas Transplantation, David Geffen School of Medicine, University of California at Los Angeles, Los Angeles, California, USA
13.3.2 The early management of the recipient

Robert Wilkinson Department of Nephrology, The Freeman Hospital, High Heaton, Newcastle-upon-Tyne, UK
9.2 Clinical approach to hypertension

K. Martin Wissing Departement Medico-Chirurgical de Nephrologie, Dialyse et Transplantation, Hopital Erasme, Brussels, Belgium
13.2.2 Immunosuppression for renal transplantation

Oliver Wrong University College London, Department of Nephrology, Middlesex Hospital, London, UK
8.4 Nephrocalcinosis

Muhammad Magdi Yaqoob Professor and Lead Consultant in Nephrology, Department of Renal Medicine & Transplantation, The Royal London Hospital, Whitechapel, London, UK
17.3 The patient with urinary tract obstruction

Jerry Yee Division Head, Division of Nephrology and Hypertension, Department of Medicine, Henry Ford Hospital, Detroit, Michigan, USA
2.6 Clinical acid–base disorders

Michael Zellweger Nephrology Fellow, Research Center, Hôpital du Sacré-Coeur de Montréal, Montréal, Québec, Canada
5.6 Nephrogenic diabetes insipidus

Carla Zoja Mario Negri Institute for Pharmacological Research, Bergamo, Italy
11.3.12 Coagulation disorders

4

The kidney in systemic disease

4.1 The patient with diabetes mellitus

Ralf Dikow and Eberhard Ritz

Introduction

History

The development of proteinuria in patients with diabetes mellitus has been described in the eighteenth century by Cotugno and it was Richard Bright who postulated in 1836 that albuminuria reflects renal disease. Although renal lesions in diabetic patients have been well known in the nineteenth century, they were usually regarded as non-specific consequences of hypertension. It was only in 1936 that Kimmelstiel and Wilson recognized nodular homogenous glomerular lesions (nodular diabetic glomerulosclerosis) as a diabetes specific complication (Kimmelstiel and Wilson 1936). Lundbaek (1970) later documented that the renal lesion was part of the more general clinical syndrome of microangiopathy.

Keen *et al.* (1969) in the United Kingdom and Parving *et al.* (1976) in Denmark were the first to note that urinary albumin excretion rates are elevated in some patients with types 1 and 2 diabetes. There is now consensus that a lowish but supranormal albumin excretion rate in the urine ('microalbuminuria') is a powerful predictor of renal (and cardiovascular) events (Parving *et al.* 1982). Persistent albuminuria, that is, greater than 300 mg/24 h or 200 μg/min, is the clinical hallmark of the manifestation of diabetic nephropathy (DN). This clinical definition is valid in both types 1 and 2 diabetes.

It has long been thought that the renal prognosis is much more benign in type 2 than in type 1 diabetes (Farbre *et al.* 1982). In retrospect, this view is remarkably wrong, since today type 2 diabetes accounts for the majority of diabetic patients reaching endstage renal disease (ESRD) (Ritz and Stefanski 1996).

Dimension of the problem

In most Western countries, DN has become the leading cause of ESRD (Ritz *et al.* 1999). According to the United States Renal Data System (USRDS 2001), in 1999 DN was the primary diagnosis in 42.8 per cent (38,160 of 89,252) of incident patients (USRDS 2001), an increase by 238 per cent compared to 1990. In 2000, the proportion of diabetics amongst patients reaching ESRD varied considerably between different countries, for example, 14.6 per cent in the Netherlands, 22 per cent in Australia, 25 per cent in Sweden, and 36.1 per cent in Germany, but it was consistently on the increase in all countries (Table 1). The prevention and management of diabetes and its renal complications is thus an immense global challenge. Registry figures tend to underestimate the renal burden posed by diabetes because it is underrepresented as illustrated by our own observations (Schwenger *et al.* 2001). In 1998–2000, diabetes mellitus was found as a comorbid condition in no less than 48.9 per cent of patients admitted for renal replacement therapy in Heidelberg (Schwenger *et al.* 2001). Classical features of Kimmelstiel Wilson's disease were observed in only in 60 per cent, that is, large kidneys, massive proteinuria (>1 g/24 h) with or without retinopathy. Atypical presentation consistent with ischaemic nephropathy was seen in 13 per cent and known primary renal disease (e.g. polycystic kidney disease, analgesic nephropathy, glomerulonephritis) with superimposed diabetes in 27 per cent of cases. For the diabetic patient with ESRD, survival is similar irrespective of whether he or she suffers from DN or primary non-diabetic renal disease (Koch *et al.* 1993). Inadequate medical care for the diabetic with renal complications is illustrated by our finding that in 11 per cent of the patients the diagnosis of diabetes had not even been made at the time of admission to the renal unit. This may result from the fact that hyperglycaemia is often self-corrected when patients lose weight as a result of anorexia. This may also explain why several observers (Catalano *et al.* 1990; Ritz and Stefanski 1996) noted that at least 5 per cent of patients developed apparent *de novo* diabetes after they had been taken on dialysis. It has recently also been recognized that a substantial

Table 1 Incidence of patients with diabetes with ESRD: evolution during the last decade (after Ritz *et al.* 1999)

	1984	1994
Austria	7.3	18.0
Catalonia (Spain)	8.0	26.6
Denmark	6.5	16.9
Iceland	0.0	10.0
Lombardy (Italy)	6.5	13.0
The Netherlands	4.2	10.4
Norway	6.5	15.4
Sweden	15.3	23.4
Australia	4.0	14.0
New Zealand	6.0	28.0
Japan	23.4	66.0
Taiwan	—	59.0
United States	29.0	107.0

Note: Data expressed as patients per million population.

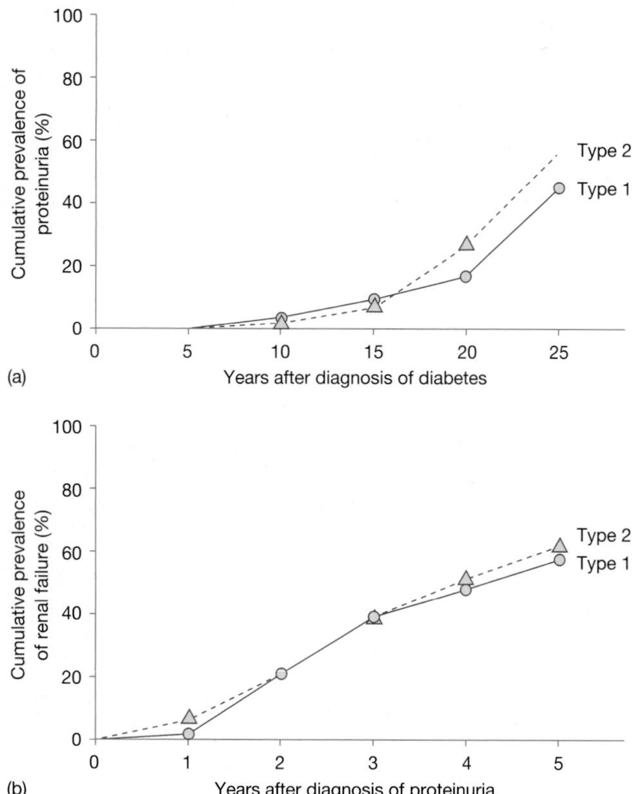

Fig. 1 Cumulative risks (a) to develop proteinuria and (b) to progress renal failure in patients with types 1 and 2 diabetes (after Hasslacher *et al.* 1989).

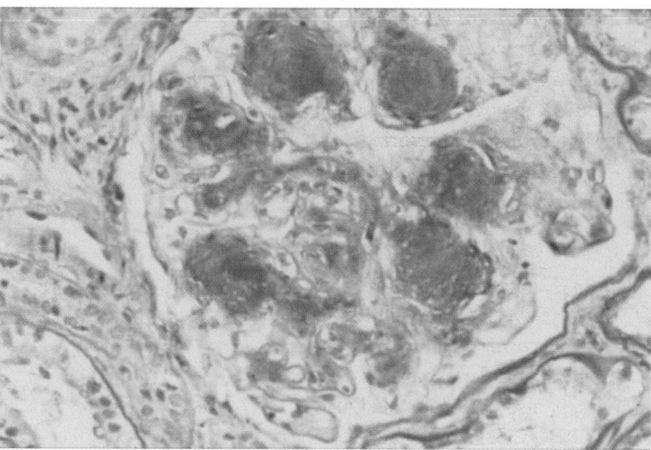

Fig. 2 Nodular diabetic glomerulosclerosis. PAS reaction. Magnification 100×. Courtesy of Prof R. Waldherr, Heidelberg, Germany.

proportion of transplanted patients develop diabetes mellitus, up to 21 per cent according to the Cleveland clinic (Cosio *et al.* 2001).

A great majority of patients entering ESRD with diabetes as a comorbid condition suffer from type 2 diabetes (Ritz *et al.* 1999); in our local experience (Schwenger *et al.* 2001) this is the case in 94 per cent. This finding thoroughly dispels the previous opinion that renal involvement and renal failure are rare in type 2 diabetes (Farbre *et al.* 1982). In the past, few patients with type 2 diabetes had a chance to live long enough to develop nephropathy. Today with better treatment of hypertension and of coronary heart disease, an increasing proportion survive and are exposed to the risk of developing nephropathy and ESRD (Lippert *et al.* 1995). The proportion of patients with types 1 and 2 diabetes who develop proteinuria and elevated serum creatinine is related to the duration of diabetes. As shown in Fig. 1, the cumulative risks to develop proteinuria and to progress in types 1 and 2 diabetes are practically superimposable (Hasslacher *et al.* 1989). Currently, the incidence, that is, the number of patients with diabetes requiring renal replacement therapy, is 98 per million population (pmp) per year in Germany (Schwenger *et al.* 2001) and 127 pmp in the United States (USRDS 2001). The risk is higher in Black patients and patients of Asian origin.

Pathomechanisms

Pathology

Macroscopic changes

Enlargement of the kidney is found in newly diagnosed patients with type 1 diabetes. Similarly, in experimental animals it is seen within 4 days of the onset of diabetes. It results from tubular hypertrophy and interstitial expansion (Bilous 1997). It is thought to be related to hyperfiltration and stimulated active reabsorption (Wolf and Ziyadeh 1997).

Light microscopic changes

The glomerulus

Glomerular enlargement is an early feature of both human and experimental diabetes and is the result of increases in capillary length and diameter.

Glomerular enlargement is also present in established nephropathy, mean glomerular volumes are 4–6 $\times 10^6$ μm^3 in patients with types 1 and 2 diabetes compared to normal values of 1–2.3 $\times 10^6$ μm^3 (White and Bilous 2000).

The reasons for enlargement are unclear—initially it may be because of altered glomerular haemodynamics and hyperfiltration, and later because of a compensatory response to capillary closure and global glomerulosclerosis.

The hallmark of diabetic glomerulopathy is diffuse mesangial expansion, associated with nodule formation in a minority of patients (Fig. 2). Most patients with long-standing diabetes show an increase in periodic acid–schiff (PAS)-positive matrix material, although these changes are much more prominent in those with clinical nephropathy. Initially, this material is central to the tuft but later it expands and effectively obliterates the capillaries eventually leading to global glomerulosclerosis (Bilous 1997).

Nodules are more or less pathognomonic for diabetes and were the first glomerular pathological abnormality described by Kimmelstiel and Wilson. They comprise acellular, eosinophilic, and lamellated structures, usually located at the periphery of the tuft. Their pathogenesis is unclear, but they may represent obliterated capillary microaneurysms, or result from focal mesangiolysis at the junction of the glomerular basement membrane (GBM) with the mesangium. This would lead to endothelial cell detachment and subsequent ballooning into the capillary, quickly followed by matrix deposition (Bilous 1997). These features are not universally found in patients with microalbuminuric type 2 diabetes patients (Fioretto *et al.* 1996). A proportion of these patients have an appearance which is more suggestive of glomerular ischaemia or tubulointerstitial disease. Patients with type 2 diabetes with clinical nephropathy or retinopathy have glomerular changes similar to type 1 diabetes (Olsen and Mogensen 1996).

Capsular drops of PAS-positive matrix material lying between the matrix membrane and parietal epithelium of Bowman's capsule are commonly seen, but their significance is unclear.

In ESRD, glomeruli appear as sclerosed hyalinized structures and a percentage is actually resorbed. This global sclerosis is due to a combination of mesangial expansion and ischaemia secondary to afferent arteriolar hyalinosis (Harris *et al.* 1991).

Tubulointerstitium

Armanni–Ebstein lesions, that is, glycogen-rich granules in proximal tubular cells, result from glucose overload and are preventable by reversing glycosuria.

Tubulointerstitial expansion contributes to whole kidney enlargement. It is also a feature of established nephropathy and is found even in a significant number of microalbuminuric type 2 diabetic patients. Its causes are almost certainly different in early diabetes and established nephropathy. Acute changes in the juxtaglomerular apparatus are seen within hours of development of diabetes in the rat. More subtle long-term abnormalities in this structure have also been described in patients with microalbuminuric type 1 diabetes and may reflect increased activity of the tubuloglomerular feedback mechanism and possibly an upregulation of the renin–angiotensin system (RAS) (Gulmann *et al.* 2001).

Afferent and efferent arteriolar hyalinosis is a characteristic feature of diabetic patients and is more prominent in those with microalbuminuria (Olsen 2000) or more advanced renal disease.

Immunofluorescence microscopy

Non-specific linear staining for immunoglobulin (IgG) (mainly IgG4) and albumin is found in the GBM, tubular basement membrane (TBM), and Bowman capsule. No direct correlation is found with the severity of glomerulopathy or nephropathy. Its pathophysiological significance is unclear (Bilous 1997).

Electronmicroscopy

Glomerulus

Its structure is normal at the onset of type 1 diabetes, but GBM thickening up to three times the normal range of 270–359 nm is an almost universal feature in patients with a duration of diabetes greater than 10 years. This thickening is more marked in patients with microalbuminuria and clinical nephropathy. There is an accumulation of type IV collagen with a net reduction in heparin sulfate proteoglycan. This combination disrupts both GBM structure and its electrostatic charge properties. It is thus thought to result in abnormal permselectivity and leakage of circulating proteins (Bilous 1997).

In normal man, the ratio of cellular to matrix components is about 1 : 1. The mean fractional volume of the mesangium is between 14–20 per cent of the glomerular tuft (Steffes *et al.* 1992). In contrast, in patients with DN, the mesangium can comprise over 40 per cent of the total tuft volume. This accumulation disrupts the microfibrillar structure of the mesangium, altering its porosity to proteins and weakening attachments to the endothelium and GBM, thus perhaps predisposing to nodule formation (Bilous 1997). Nodules comprise matrix of similar composition, but with a prominent accumulation of microfibrils.

In advanced nephropathy, thin irregular segments of GBM lined by an abnormal looking endothelium may be found, representing either new capillary growth or microaneurysms. This may lead to microscopic haematuria that is occasionally seen in diabetes as it is in thin basement membrane disease.

Tubulointerstitium

The structure of the TBM is largely similar to the GBM, but it is almost twice as wide. In diabetes, the TBM increases to about two to three times its normal width and often appears split (Ziyadeh and Goldfarb 1991), possibly permitting penetration of macromolecules into the interstitial space and thus favouring the development of fibrosis.

Early tubulointerstitial expansion results from an increase in cellular components (Lane *et al.* 1993) followed by collagen accumulation later.

Pathomechanisms of microvascular damage

The microvascular lesions of the kidney in diabetes mellitus had variably been ascribed to generation of advanced glycation endproducts (AGE), cumulation of sorbitol, activation of protein kinase C (PKC), and activation of the hexosamine pathway. A unifying concept has recently been proposed by Brownlee (2001). He provided evidence that in insulin-insensitive tissues hyperglycaemia increases the delivery of glucose-derived intermediates as the metabolic substrate for mitochondrial oxidation. Increased mitochondrial oxidation leads to the generation of reactive oxygen species (ROS). ROS are responsible for the following four metabolic abnormalities: (a) accumulation of methylglyoxal and other substrates leads to the generation of early Amadori products and late AGE respectively (see below), (b) furthermore activation of PKC by ROS, particularly the β-isoenzyme, (c) activation of the polyol pathway causing accumulation of sorbitol, and finally (d) also activation of the hexosamine pathway.

Major attention has recently been paid to the pathogenic role of AGE. As shown in Fig. 3, glucose (but more importantly also other compounds such as methylglyoxal) interact with the α and γ amino groups of amino acids to form Schiff bases that rearrange spontaneously to yield Amadori products. These are non-enzymatically transformed into highly reactive early Amadori products, for example, methylglyoxal, dideoxyglucosone, deoxyglucosone, etc. In the course of weeks, heterocyclic advanced fluorescent AGEs are generated, which cross-link proteins and interact with several receptors, the most important of which is receptor for AGE (RAGE).

Activation of the RAGE triggers ROS formation and promotes translocation of the transcription factor NF-κB, a central switch for inflammatory processes into the nucleus. The relevance of AGE for DN is illustrated by the fact that the course of DN is accelerated in animals, which are transgenic for RAGE (Sakurai *et al.* 2003).

Important secondary mediators for the development of renal damage are transforming growth factor β (TGFβ) (Sharma and Ziyadeh 1995), locally generated angiotensin II (Wolf and Ziyadeh 1997), endothelin, and several other cytokines.

Glucose		Aldimin		Ketoamin
H–C=O		H–C=N-Valyl		CH_2NH-Valyl
H–C–OH		H–C–OH		C=O
HO–C–H		HO–C–H	Amadori	HO–C–H
H–C–OH	+H_2N-Valyl →	H–C–OH	rearrangement →	H–C–OH
H–C–OH		H–C–OH		H–C–OH
CH_2OH		CH_2OH		CH_2OH

Fig. 3 Glucose (but more importantly also other compounds such as methylglyoxal) interact with the α and γ amino groups of amino acids to form Schiff bases, which rearrange spontaneously to yield Amadori products. These are non-enzymatically transformed into highly reactive early Amadori products, for example, methylglyoxal, dideoxyglucosone, or deoxyglucosone.

Renal pathophysiology

It has been known since decades that the glomerular filtration rate (GFR) is elevated in diabetes mellitus (Cambier 1934). This has now been well documented in type 1 diabetes (Mogensen 1971) and, although this has remained more controversial, equally in type 2 diabetes (Nowack *et al.* 1992).

The mechanisms underlying hyperfiltration have been clarified in animal experiments (Hostetter *et al.* 1981). In rats with diabetes, hyperfiltration as well as hyperperfusion and enhanced glomerular capillary hydraulic pressure have been well documented. This constellation is due to preferential afferent renal vasodilatation with the resulting impairment of renal autoregulation. This was also documented in patients with type 1 (Parving *et al.* 1984) and type 2 diabetes (Christensen *et al.* 1997). Dilatation of the preglomerular vessels will increase the vulnerability to hypertension (or conversely vulnerability to ischaemia from hypotension). A larger proportion of aortic blood pressure is transmitted into the glomerular capillary bed causing 'glomerular hypertension'. This fact also explains why even blood pressure (BP) values in the upper normal range are injurious to the vasodilated kidney of diabetic patients.

As shown in Fig. 4, glomerular hypertension resulting from afferent vasodilatation and efferent vasoconstriction, in conjunction with altered glomerular permeability causes proteinuria, activation of proximal tubular epithelial cells, renal fibrosis and ultimately nephron loss and renal failure. ACE inhibitors interfere with these processes as described in detail below.

Apart from elevated systemic and glomerular capillary pressure, proteinuria plays a major pathogenetic role. Remuzzi *et al.* (2002) had postulated that proteinuria is not only a marker of adverse renal prognosis, but actually a 'nephrotoxin'. This concept has been amply confirmed by studies showing that proximal tubular epithelial cells acquire an inflammatory phenotype and upregulate expression of

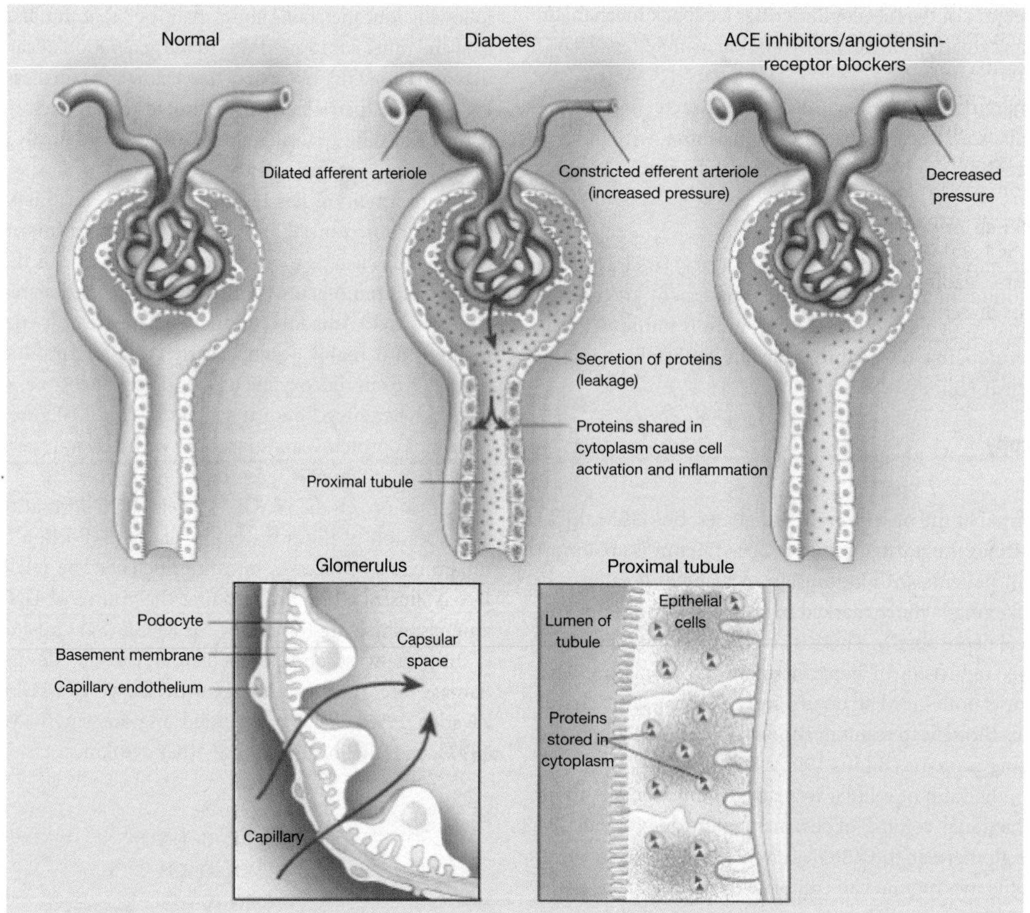

In diabetes glomerular capillary pressure is increased (glomerular hypertension) because of dilatation of the afferent artery and angiotensin II-dependent constriction of the efferent artery.

Glomerular hypertension and increased glomerular permeability cause high protein concentrations in the filtrate. Proteins are endocytosed by proximal tubular epithelial cells, which develop an inflammatory phenotype and stimulate interstitial fibrosis by secretion of agonists (angiotensin II, endothelin-1), cytokines, and chemokines.

ACE inhibitors reverse glomerular hypertension, improve glomerular permeability characteristics and are thus renoprotective.

Fig. 4 Schema of glomerular hypertension, injury from proteinuria, and the effect of ACE inhibitors.

angiotensinogen (Wolf and Ziyadeh 1997), endothelin (Zoja *et al.* 1999), and cytokines, when they have been confronted with a protein overload in the tubular fluid. Albumin was shown to be less injurious than complement factors, iron-containing proteins and oxidized lipids (Arici *et al.* 2003). Angiotensin II, endothelin, and cytokines are then secreted in an abluminal direction into the interstitium where they activate peritubular fibroblasts and lead to interstitial fibrosis. This sequence has also been shown *in vivo* by studies in the amphibian kidney (Gross *et al.* 2002).

In the past, it was felt to be a paradox that in diabetes the kidney responds so favourably to pharmacological blockade of the RAS, although the systemic RAS is suppressed. It has recently been documented, however, that hyperglycaemia upregulates the local synthesis of angiotensinogen (Wang *et al.* 1998) in proximal tubular epithelial cells, which possess all components of the RAS and are able to generate angiotensin II. In the tubular fluid and the interstitium, the concentration of angiotensin II is orders of magnitude greater than in the circulation (Nishiyama *et al.* 2002). Furthermore, the expression of the angiotensin II receptor subtype 1 is upregulated (Wagner *et al.* 1999). These facts may explain the finding that despite low plasma renin activity (PRA) in patients with diabetes, RAS blockade causes a pronounced increase in renal plasma flow (Price *et al.* 1999) under hyperglycaemic, but not under euglycaemic conditions (Miller 1999).

In diabetes, renal sodium (Na) handling is abnormal. This explains the frequent findings of Na retention and hypervolaemia. Proximal tubular reabsorption of Na is increased as a result of increased activity of the Na, glucose cotransporter (Skott 1993). As a result, distal Na delivery is diminished and GFR is increased via the tubuloglomerular feedback mechanism, leading to hyperfiltration (Woods *et al.* 1987). In addition, insulin directly increases distal tubular Na reabsorption (DeFronzo 1981). Furthermore, increased angiotensin II in tubular fluid was recently shown to also activate Na channels in the collecting duct (Nishiyama *et al.* 2002). Na retention is a prominent factor in the genesis of hypertension of the diabetic patient.

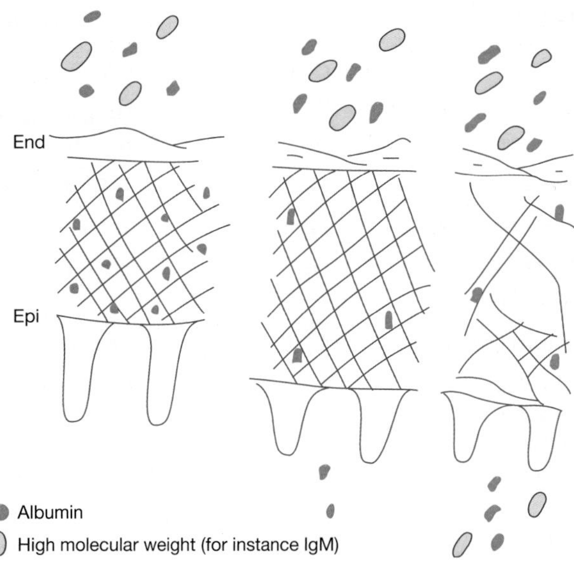

Fig. 5 Schema of the genesis of selective albuminuria and non-selective proteinuria.

Why do diabetic patients develop albuminuria and proteinuria?

In the past, it had been thought that negatively charged molecules of the GBM are reduced, particularly sialic acid and heparan sulfate, normally repel negatively charged anionic albumin. As a result glomerular permselectivity would be reduced so that albumin molecules can escape into the glomerular filtrate. Reduced negative charge density of the GBM has not been consistently confirmed (van den Born *et al.* 1995). It was also thought that in later stages of DN, disruption of the texture of the basal membrane creates gaps and holes (Fig. 5) and allows high molecular weight serum proteins to escape into the filtrate.

Recent insights into podocyte function and specifically identification of proteins of the slit membrane (Mundel and Shankland 2002) have led to the concept that the podocyte is a prime player in the genesis of proteinuria. Indeed, in experimental diabetes the expression of one permeability controlling protein, nephrin, is abnormally low and is restored by administration of angiotensin II receptor blockers (Bonnet *et al.* 2001; Mifsud *et al.* 2001). It is also of interest that in experimental diabetes, podocyte damage is the first sign of renal injury (Gross *et al.* 2003). Diminished podocyte numbers have been documented in animals and patients with diabetes (Steffes *et al.* 2001). Podocytes are postmitotic and can no longer proliferate. If glomeruli increase in size, each podocyte has to cover an ever larger domain, ultimately exceeding the capacity of the podocyte. This discrepancy causes loss of podocytes by desquamation, apoptosis or necrosis, denudation of the basement membrane, synechia formation, and ultimately glomerulosclerosis (Mundel and Shankland 2002).

When tubular epithelial cells are exposed to higher protein loads, they acquire an inflammatory phenotype and amplify renal damage as outlined above.

Pathophysiology of hypertension in diabetic nephropathy

There must be a relation between a genetic predisposition to hypertension (and cardiovascular disease) on the one hand and the propensity of diabetic patients to develop DN on the other hand. BP is higher in parents of patients with type 1 diabetes with nephropathy compared to parents of patients without DN (Fagerudd *et al.* 1998). As shown in Table 2, it is also higher in offspring of parents with type 2 diabetes as compared to offspring of parents without DN (Strojek *et al.* 1997). In addition, it has been noted that cardiovascular disease is more frequent in parents of patients with type 2 diabetes with nephropathy (Earle *et al.* 1992). In patients with type 2 diabetes, a history of hypertension and cardiovascular events in first degree relatives is a potent predictor of early onset of microalbuminuria (Keller *et al.* 1996). The hypothetical genes that code for hypertension, cardiovascular events, and nephropathy have not yet been identified.

As shown in Table 3 the relation between nephropathy and hypertension is somewhat different in types 1 and 2 diabetes.

Table 2 Blood pressure and urinary albumin excretion in offsprings of type 2 diabetics with nephropathy

	Controls (n = 30)	Offsprings of type 2 diabetic parents	
		Without nephropathy (n = 30)	With nephropathy (n = 30)
Age (years)	31.5 ± 5.4	33.0 ± 8.5	33.0 ± 6.5
Body mass index (kg/m^2)	25.5 ± 3.0	26.2 ± 5.1	26.6 ± 3.4
Systolic 24-h blood pressure (mmHg)	114 ± 8.5	117 ± 12.4	125 ± 16.9
Albuminuria (μg/min)	4.4 (0.16–18.4)	4.8 (0.36–17.5)	7.8 (1.04–19.5)
Increase of albuminuria after submaximal ergometry (*x*-fold)	4.8 (1.2–99)	6.3 (1.5–231)	16 (1.2–236)

Table 3 Hypertension in diabetes mellitus

Type 1	Renoparenchymal hypertension
Type 2	Primary hypertension (metabolic syndrome) + Superimposed renoparenchymal hypertension + High blood pressure amplitude (systolic hypertension)

Table 4 Blood pressure at the time of diagnosis of type 2 diabetes

Ambulatory 24-h blood pressure >130/80 mmHg	60%
<15% dipping of blood pressure at night-time	61%
Abnormal according to first or second criterion → only 21% normal blood pressure profile!	79%

If hypertension develops in a patient with type 1 diabetes it is almost always of renal parenchymal origin. In contrast, in patients with type 2 diabetes hypertension often precedes the onset of diabetes by years and decades. As shown in Table 4, at the time when type 2 diabetes is diagnosed (Keller *et al.* 1996) an abnormal BP and/or an abnormal circadian BP profile is found in 79 per cent of patients. If patients with type 2 diabetes develop nephropathy, the prevalence of hypertension increases and the degree of BP elevation is greater, but generally the relation between hypertension and nephropathy is less close than in type 1 diabetes.

In DN, it has been well documented that the nocturnal BP decrease is attenuated ('non-dipping') (Nielsen *et al.* 1995). Recently, it has also been found that non-dipping precedes the development of microalbuminuria in patients with type 1 diabetes (Lurbe *et al.* 2002). Even when the BP is normal under basal conditions, the BP response to exercise tends to be exaggerated (Karlefors 1966).

Is BP related to the onset or progression of DN?

Nelson *et al.* (1993) showed that prediabetic hypertension, that is, hypertension prior to the onset of type 2 diabetes, determines the risk to develop proteinuria 5 years after type 2 diabetes has been diagnosed (Table 5). The observation that non-dipping precedes the appearance of microalbuminuria (Lurbe *et al.* 2002) is also consistent with a causal role of BP in the genesis of DN.

Many observational studies in types 1 and 2 diabetes documented that elevated BP is correlated to the presence of DN (Parving *et al.* 1988; Gall *et al.* 1991) and is even predictive of its onset (Parving *et al.* 1981; Drury 1983). One example out of many is shown in Table 6. In patients with non-proteinuric type 2 diabetes, the prevalence of hypertension was much greater in those patients who subsequently developed overt nephropathy than in those who did not (Hasslacher *et al.* 1987).

Whilst such observational studies are strongly suggestive, a causal role could only be proven by interventional studies. Danish diabetologists were the first to provide the evidence that lowering of BP attenuates the rate of progression (Mogensen 1982; Parving *et al.* 1983). These observations have subsequently been amply confirmed by further studies (see below).

Table 5 Prediabetic hypertension and incidence of diabetic nephropathy in Pima Indians (after Nelson *et al.* 1993)

Blood pressure 1 year before onset of diabetes	Incidence of albuminuria 5 years after onset of diabetes (%)
Lower tertile	9
Mid tertile	16
Upper tertile	23

Which pathomechanisms lead to hypertension in DN? This is an important point because rational selection of antihypertensive agents requires understanding of the underlying pathophysiology. Previously, we have referred to the overriding role of Na retention and hypervolaemia and this explains why dietary Na restriction and diuretics are uniquely effective in DN.

We have also referred to activation of the local RAS in the kidney although PRA is suppressed at least early on in diabetics. In advanced stages, however, concentrations of angiotensin II in the circulation may also increase after the administration of diuretics (Bjorck 1990). The activation of the RAS, local or systemic, explains the unique efficacy of angiotensin-converting enzyme (ACE) inhibitors and angiotensin receptor blockers (Lewis *et al.* 1993, 2001; Brenner *et al.* 2001, see below).

The important role of the activation of the sympathetic nerve system in the genesis of renal hypertension has been appreciated only

Table 6 Hypertension predicts onset of proteinuria in non-proteinuric type 2 diabetic patients (after Hasslacher *et al.* 1987)

	Postprandial blood glucose (mg/dl)	Systolic blood pressure (mmHg)	Frequency of hypertension (%)[a]
Development of proteinuria (n = 63)	208 (139–295)	164 (105–215)	70
No development of proteinuria (n = 63)	199 (104–272)	149 (122–183)	43

[a] Blood pressure consistant or intermittent >160/95 mmHg.

recently (Adamczak *et al.* 2002). In renal disease, increased sympathetic nerve activity is demonstrable even when the GFR is still normal. This finding may explain, at least in part, why β-blockers are so effective in lowering BP in diabetic patients, with renal disease (Mogensen 1982; Parving *et al.* 1983). There is also recent experimental evidence that β-blockers cause BP-independent renoprotection (Amann *et al.* 2001).

Finally, endothelial cell dysfunction with impaired endothelial cell-dependent nitric oxide (NO)-mediated vasodilatation has been well documented in diabetes (Stehouwer *et al.* 1997), but this abnormality is currently not susceptible to specific intervention of proven clinical benefit.

Although diminished compliance of the central arteries in diabetes has been known for decades, the importance of the abnormalities of the pulsatile changes of BP, that is, increased peak systolic and decreased diastolic pressure causing an increased BP amplitude, have been appreciated only recently, particularly their relation to cardiovascular risk (London and Guerin 1999). Both pulse wave velocity and BP amplitude predict cardiovascular death (Blacher *et al.* 2003) and this has been documented in non-diabetic as well as in diabetic patients with ESRD. The greater BP amplitude resulting from increased aortic stiffness explains why isolated systolic hypertension is relatively common in patients with type 2 diabetes.

Extrarenal complications associated with diabetic nephropathy

The average diabetic patient seen by the nephrologist is much more severely ill than the average diabetic patient seen in the diabetes clinic. This is due to the fact that renal complications develop on average 15–20 years after the onset of diabetes at a time when the patient is at high risk of also developing microvascular and macrovascular complications. The most common ones are listed in Table 7.

Diabetic retinopathy is present in virtually all type 1 diabetic patients with nephropathy (Parving *et al.* 1988), but only 50–60 per cent of proteinuric patients with type 2 diabetes suffer from retinopathy (Gall *et al.* 1991), so that the absence of retinopathy does not preclude the diagnosis of Kimmelstiel Wilson glomerulosclerosis. Nevertheless absence of retinopathy is one argument, amongst others, favouring the indication for a renal biopsy (see below). The risk of blindness because of severe proliferative retinopathy or maculopathy is substantially greater in diabetic patients with nephropathy. Retinopathy tends also to progress more rapidly in patients with DN, so that more frequent ophthalmological examination is clearly indicated, that is, at yearly or half-yearly intervals.

Many patients with DN have polyneuropathy. Sensory polyneuropathy is an important aspect of the diabetic foot problem (see below).

Table 7 Major microvascular and macrovascular complications in patients with diabetic nephropathy

Microvascular complications
Retinopathy
Polyneuropathy including autonomic neuropathy
Gastroparesis, diarrhoea/obstipation, detrusor paresis, painless myocardial ischaemia, erectile impotence, and supine hypertension/orthostatic hypotension
Macrovascular complications
Coronary heart disease, left ventricular hypertrophy, and congestive heart failure
Cerebrovascular complications (stroke)
Peripheral artery occlusive disease
Mixed complications
Diabetic foot (neuropathic, vascular)

Motor and sensory neuropathy may cause areflexia, wasting, and sensory disturbances such as paraesthesia, anaesthesia, impaired perception of vibration, and pain, but the most vexing clinical problems are the result of autonomic polyneuropathy. It involves frequently the cardiocirculatory system (Standl and Schnell 2000) causing abnormally low pulse rate variability (RR interval) and unchanged heart rate in upright position, but more sophisticated techniques such as uptake of radioanalogues of norepinephrine by the heart show that subclinical abnormalities are practically always found. Further consequences of autonomic polyneuropathy are gastroparesis, that is, delayed emptying of gastric contents into the gut, and diarrhoea, or constipation (often alternating with each other). These problems are caused by impaired intestinal innervation, often complicated by intestinal bacterial overgrowth because of stasis. Finally, urogenital abnormalities are frequent such as erectile impotence or detrusor paresis with delayed and incomplete emptying of the bladder.

The major macroangiopathic complications are stroke, coronary heart disease, and peripheral vascular disease. These complications are again up to five fold more frequent in diabetic patients with and without DN.

The onset of DN is a turning point in the life of a patient with diabetes. The presence of DN greatly increases the mortality of a patient with types 1 and 2 diabetes. This had been documented by Borch-Johnsen *et al.* (1985), decades ago. They found that compared to the background population type 1 diabetic patients without proteinuria had only a slightly, that is, two- to threefold elevated, mortality. In contrast, mortality was increased by a factor of 20–200 in patients with proteinuria. The major increase in risk starts as soon as microalbuminuria has set in (Dinneen and Gerstein 1997), but a higher risk is found even in upper quartile of normal range albuminuria. The mechanistic link between microalbuminuria and cardiovascular death is not well understood. It is widely thought that the presence of microalbuminuria reflects generalized endothelial cell dysfunction and increased risk of atherogenesis. It is associated with many cardiovascular risk factors, such as elevated BP, dyslipoproteinaemia, increased platelet aggregation, increased C-reactive protein (CRP) concentration and others. An added risk factor is presumably the association of microalbuminuria with autonomic polyneuropathy (Standl and Schnell 2000), which predicts deaths from myocardial infarction or arrhythmia (sudden death). Further cardiac abnormalities associated with microalbuminuria are cardiac hypertrophy (Nielsen *et al.* 1997) and impaired left ventricular diastolic function.

The prognosis is even more grim in diabetic patients with proteinuria, that is, with clinically manifest DN (Borch-Johnsen *et al.* 1985). In the past, the estimated 10-year cumulative death rate was up to 70 per cent in type 1 (Andersen *et al.* 1983) as well as in patients with type 2 diabetes (Schmitz and Vaeth 1988). It has substantially decreased in recent years with better control of hypertension, better care of coronary heart disease, and improved management of patients by renal replacement therapy. For instance in the Heidelberg series, mortality decreased substantially in the decades between 1966 and 1985 (Hasslacher *et al.* 1990). There is an ongoing discussion whether the high death rate in DN is explained by established cardiovascular risk factors or whether uraemia amplifies the cardiovascular risk because of the presence of additional non-classical risk factors. In this context, it is of interest that experimentally even minor impairment of renal function, for example, uninephrectomy, causes drastic acceleration of atherogenesis (Buzello *et al.* 2003).

Diagnostic procedures

DN remains a clinical diagnosis based upon the detection of proteinuria, although many patients will also have hypertension and retinopathy. The diagnostic procedures to establish the diagnosis of DN and its complications comprise (a) determination of albuminuria or proteinuria, (b) blood pressure measurement, (c) estimation of GFR and in selected cases, and (d) renal biopsy.

Measurement of albuminuria/proteinuria

Microalbuminuria is defined as excretion of 30–300 mg albumin per 24 h in at least two out of three consecutive non-ketotic sterile urine samples. There is substantial intraindividual day to day variation (coefficient of variation 30–50 per cent). In this range of albumin concentrations, albumin is normally not detected using non-specific tests for protein (e.g. Biuret reaction). Albumin can be detected, however, using specific techniques such as dipstick, enzyme linked immunosorbent assay (ELISA), nephelometry or radioimmunoassay (RIA). If 24-h urine collections are not possible, the albumin concentration can be determined in spot urine or better morning urine samples. The normal range is 30–300 mg /l of albumin (Marshall 1991). The definition of the normal range of albumin excretion must be interpreted with caution because the risk of progression is definitely greater even in patients in the upper quartile of normal albumin excretion (see above).

The main advantage of determining microalbuminuria is that it predicts a high renal risk: 80 per cent of type 1 diabetic patients with microalbuminuria go on to develop clinical nephropathy. In patients with type 2 diabetes, the proportion is closer to 40 per cent. It also predicts a high cardiovascular risk. Annual screening of all patients is therefore recommended (American Diabetes Association 2002).

Although the correlation between renal histology and microalbuminuria is relatively loose, recent work shows that microalbuminuria is not only a marker of impending DN, but indicates presence of abnormal glomerular metabolic function. Increased mRNA for proteins involved in mesangial pathology such as collagen alpha 2 (IV) and connective tissue factor has been noted in biopsies of microalbuminuric as compared to non-microalbuminuric type 1 diabetic patients (Adler *et al.* 2001).

The measurement of microalbuminuria is only reliable if confounding factors have been excluded such as fever, physical exercise, urinary tract infection, non-diabetic renal disease, haematuria from other causes, heart failure, uncontrolled hypertension, or uncontrolled hyperglycaemia. A flow chart for the diagnosis of incipient and clinically overt nephropathy is given in Fig. 6.

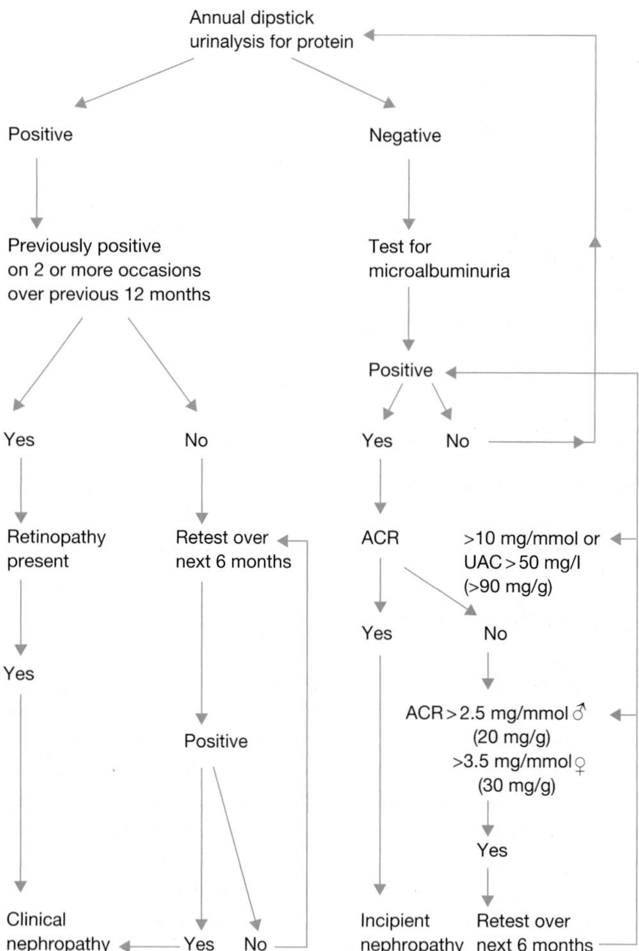

Fig. 6 Flow chart for diagnosis of incipient and advanced nephropathy.

By definition, clinically overt DN is present if the rate of albumin excretion exceeds 300 mg/day. At this point, usually urinary proteins other than albumin are excreted as well. The high sensitivity of urinary albumin to predict renal disease is due to the fact that under normal circumstances urinary protein excretion is no less than 150 mg/day, however, and albumin (and other serum proteins) comprises only a minute fraction so that its concentration is miniscule. The excreted proteins are mainly of tubular (e.g. Tamm–Horsfall glycoprotein) or postrenal origin (sexual glands). In patients with orthostatic proteinuria, however, serum proteins are excreted in the urine.

Measurement of blood pressure

When measuring the BP in a patient with diabetes one should be aware of several problems. In overweight patients with type 2 diabetes, the size of the cuff has to be adapted to the upper arm circumference. When this exceeds 32 cm, cuffs of 18 cm width are indicated. For unknown reasons, the prevalence of white coat hypertension is lower in diabetic patients with DN. Patients with severe autonomic polyneuropathy tend to develop orthostatic hypotension, that is, a decrease of systolic BP by more than 20 mmHg in the upright position. It is therefore advisable to measure BP in the upright position at regular intervals. In diabetic patients with sclerosis or calcification of the radial and brachial arteries pseudohypertension may occur, that is, spuriously elevated BP values despite normotension by intraarterial BP measurements. Suspicion of this condition should be raised if a discrepancy is found between modest target organ damage, for example, left ventricular hypertrophy and very high measured BP values. Such patients tend to develop marked hypotension even with relatively modest antihypertensive medication. The circadian BP profile tends to be abnormal in early stages (Lurbe *et al.* 2002) and even a paradoxical rise in the night-time BP is not rare. In the diabetic patient with nephropathy, it has been shown that a night-time increase in BP is independently associated with a 20-fold higher mortality and a higher risk of ESRD (Nakano *et al.* 1999). Occasional measurements of ambulatory BP are particularly useful to assess the efficacy of antihypertensive treatment.

Measurement/estimation of glomerular filtration rate

The gold standard for the measurement of the GFR is the inulin clearance or its equivalents such as radiochelate clearance or iothalamate clearance. In clinical practice, the serum creatinine concentration is most frequently used. The serum creatinine concentration may be grossly misleading if patients are wasted and have low muscle mass. This problem is particularly frequent in elderly female type 2 diabetic patients. The concentration of cystatin has the advantage that it is not affected by muscle mass (Fliser and Ritz 2001). The DOQI guidelines recommended to calculate an estimated GFR according to the Cockcroft Gault formula.

Renal biopsy

A final problem may be the issue whether renal dysfunction is the result of DN or the result of some non-diabetic renal disease. As shown in Table 8, renal biopsy is certainly not indicated when a type 1 diabetic patient has retinopathy and when the time course is consistent with DN. Renal biopsy should be considered, however, when proteinuria is present less than 10 years after the onset of type 1 diabetes. In type 2 diabetes, this argument is unreliable because the onset of type 2 diabetes is often not known. The presence of dysmorphic erythrocytes, erythrocyte casts, or cellular casts is not a feature of DN and should prompt investigations to exclude glomerulonephritis or vasculitis, if necessary by renal biopsy. Other indications are rapid deterioration of renal function or elevated serum creatinine without urine abnormalities. Finally, gross proteinuria is not infrequently associated with non-diabetic renal disease, for example, amyloid, focal–segmental glomerulosclerosis, etc. Needless to say that prior to renal biopsy renal ultrasonography is indicated which by itself may already yield a diagnosis.

Table 8 Potential indications for renal biopsy in patients with diabetes

Biopsy not indicated when
Typical evolution of renal disease
Concomitant retinopathy
Biopsy should be considered when
Renal manifestations are seen atypically (<10 years) early in type 1 diabetes
Dysmorphic erythrocytes/casts are found (nephritic sediment)
Rapid deterioration of renal function of unknown cause is noted
Elevated serum creatinine without urine abnormalities
Heavy proteinuria (>5–8 g/day) persists despite lowering of blood pressure

Natural history

Stages of diabetic nephropathy

There are few renal diseases where the course is as predictable as in DN. This has led to a scheme proposed by Mogensen (Table 9), which is valid in type 1 diabetes, but less consistently so in type 2 diabetes. An early stage of renal hyperfunction is followed by a stage of clinical latency which may last up to 20 years. It is subsequently followed in a very well-defined time course by the stages of microalbuminuria progressing to that of overt nephropathy and renal failure.

While this scheme emphasizes the early stages of DN, it does not provide a sensitive measure of renal dysfunction in later stages. For this reason, following the recommendations of the DOQI guidelines, the German Diabetes Association has proposed a modified scheme, which is given in Table 10.

Risk factors for development and progression of diabetic nephropathy

Stage of microalbuminuria

What is the frequency of microalbuminuria? The point prevalence of microalbuminuria in clinic populations of type 1 diabetics is approximately 20 per cent. Population-based studies, for example, a study from Norway using two-timed overnight urine collections and a cut-off of 15 μg/min found a prevalence of 12.5 per cent.

For patients with type 2 diabetes the range of reported values is much wider. Using a cut-off of 50–300 mg/l of albumin, the UKPDS study found a prevalence of 6.5 per cent (Adler *et al.* 2003). Using

Table 9 The stages of diabetic nephropathy

Stage	Glomerular filtration	Albuminuria	Blood pressure	Time interval[a]
Renal hyperfunction	Elevated	Absent	Normal	At diagnosis
Clinical latency	High normal	Absent		
Microalbuminuria	Within the normal range	20–200 μg/min (30–300 mg/day)	Rising within or above the normal range	5–15
Macroalbuminuria/ proteinuria (overt nephropathy)	Decreasing	200 μg/min (300 mg/day)	Increased	10–15
Renal failure	Diminished	Massive	Increased	15–30

[a] Time after diagnosis in patients with type 1 diabetes (not valid in type 2 diabetes because the diagnosis is often not made at the time of onset of diabetes).

Table 10 Classification of diabetic nephropathy (Guidelines of the German Diabetic Association)

Stage	Albuminuria (mg/l)	Creatinine clearance (ml/min)
Renal involvement with normal renal function		
Microalbuminuria	20–200	>90
Macroalbuminuria	>200	>90
Reduced renal function		
Mild	>200	60–89
Moderate	>200	30–59
Advanced	Decreased	15–29
Terminal	—	<15

albuminuria greater than 30 mg/day as the cut-off, a prevalence of 16 per cent was found in newly diagnosed patients with type 2 diabetes (Keller *et al.* 1996). Population-based studies showed point prevalence values ranging from 11 per cent in the United Kingdom to 42 per cent in Pacific islanders from Nauru, indicating that the prevalence depends heavily upon ethnicity.

It has been reported that in patients with type 1 diabetes, the incidence of *de novo* microalbuminuria is about 2 per cent per year. The annual increase of urinary albumin excretion is about 20 per cent both in type 1 (Borch-Johnsen *et al.* 1993) and patients with type 2 diabetes (Ravid *et al.* 1993).

Several relatively small studies showed that in type 1 diabetes microalbuminuria has approximately 70–85 per cent power to predict the development of DN (Parving *et al.* 1982; Viberti *et al.* 1982; Mogensen and Christensen 1984). The predictive value is less in type 2 diabetes. The relative risk of microalbuminuric type 2 diabetic patients to develop DN ranged from 4.4 to 21 in several series (Parving *et al.* 2002). In two large studies, Nelson *et al.* (1991) and Ravid *et al.* (1993) found that 34 and 42 per cent of microalbuminuric type 2 diabetics, respectively, developed DN. The variability is in part accounted for by the differences in observation periods and by different cut-off values for the diagnosis of albuminuria. The implications of microalbuminuria for cardiovascular risk and mortality have been dealt with above.

Which risk factors determine the risk to develop microalbuminuria in DN?

One can distinguish modifiable and non-modifiable risk factors. The higher frequency of DN in certain ethnic groups such as Indo-Asians, Africans, Hispanics, native Americans, Aboriginals in Australia, and Maori in New Zealand, suggests strong ethnic determination. There is also substantial familial clustering. Seaquist *et al.* (1989) showed that in a patient with type 1 diabetes who has a first degree relative with diabetes and nephropathy, the risk to develop DN is 83 per cent. The frequency is only 17 per cent if he or she has a first degree relative with diabetes but without nephropathy (Seaquist *et al.* 1989). In type 2 diabetes, familial clustering has been well documented in Pima Indians (Nelson *et al.* 1993) and a familial determinant is also suggested by the observation that albumin excretion rates are greater in offspring of type 2 diabetic patients with nephropathy (Strojek *et al.* 1997). The familial cumulation of DN has led to intense efforts to identify the genes that code for the development of DN. A recent study localized a susceptibility gene on chromosome 18q22.3–23 (Vardali *et al.* 2002). Several small studies yielded controversial results. Increased sodium–lithium countertransport, possibly a surrogate marker for Na^+/H^+ countertransport, has been identified as a potential intermediate phenotype in type 1 diabetes (Davies *et al.* 1992). The transport rate was also higher in skin fibroblasts cultured from type 1 diabetic patients with DN; this protocol excludes as a potential artefact that the high transport rate is the result of hyperglycaemia (Davies *et al.* 1992). There have been many conflicting studies concerning the D/I (deletion/insertion) polymorphism at intron 16 of the ACE gene. The polymorphism is associated with differenties in the activity of ACE in the circulation and in tissues. The D allele is associated with higher ACE activity and angiotensin II concentrations. There is very little evidence that this polymorphism predicts the risk to develop microalbuminuria, but it may be associated with more rapid progression of manifest DN (Marre *et al.* 1997; Solini *et al.* 2002). The association of DN with a family history of hypertension (Strojek *et al.* 1997; Fragerrudd *et al.* 1998) and of cardiovascular events (Keller *et al.* 1996) in relatives of patients with types 1 and 2 diabetes and DN suggests that the susceptibility genes for nephropathy also code for BP and cardiovascular risk factors, but details are unknown.

As an interesting hypothesis it has been proposed that the risk to develop DN can be traced back to the fetal period: severely growth retarded infants are thought to have fewer but bigger glomeruli, predisposing to the development of hypertension and renal disease later in life (Brenner *et al.* 1998). As far as the relation of fewer glomeruli to hypertension is concerned, this hypothesis has recently be confirmed (Keller *et al.* 2003), but whether this feature explains genetic predisposition to DN as well, is uncertain.

Further risk factors are:

(1) albumin excretion rates in the upper normal range (Microalbuminuria Collaborative Study Group UK 1993);

(2) gender (the risk being higher in males than in females, at least premenopause; Borch-Johnsen 1989; Gall *et al.* 1991);

(3) onset of type 1 diabetes before the age of 20 years (Krolewski *et al.* 1985); and

(4) elevated prorenin concentrations (Luetscher *et al.* 1985; Allen *et al.* 1996).

Of greater practical interest are modifiable risk factors which are susceptible to intervention (Table 11), such as hyperglycaemia, smoking, hypertension, and possibly high dietary protein intake and dyslipidaemia. In the following, we discuss the impact of the management of these factors on onset (primary prevention) and progression (secondary prevention) of DN.

Hyperglycaemia

Obviously there is no DN without hyperglycaemia. The role of hyperglycaemia in the development of DN is most convincingly demonstrated by transplantation studies. When normal kidneys are transplanted into diabetic recipients, they developed glomerulosclerosis in experimental or clinical observations (Mauer *et al.* 1976). More excitingly isolated pancreatic transplantation in patients with type 1 diabetes and nephropathy led gradually after several years to the regression of diabetic glomerulosclerosis (Fioretto *et al.* 1998). There exists a wealth of information on the association between hyperglycaemia or HbA1c concentrations and development of microalbuminuria (Prirart 1978; Feldt-Rasmussen and Deckert 1993; Krolewski *et al.* 1996; Rudberg and Dahlquist 1996).

The definite proof that the association is causal in nature has come from intervention trials, that is, the Diabetes Control and Complications Trial (DCCT) (The Diabetes Control and Complications Trial Research Group 1993) in type 1 diabetes and the Kumamoto trial (Shichiri *et al.* 1995) as well as the UKPDS study (UK Prospective Diabetes Study Group 1998) in type 2 diabetes (see below).

In the DCCT trial, patients in the intensively treated group had three or more insulin injections per day or used an infusion pump, performed four or more capillary glucose blood tests a day, and were seen monthly with regular telephone contact between visits. Despite the intensity of follow-up, less than 5 per cent achieved a consistently normal (<6.05 per cent) HbA1c throughout the study. After 9 years, the difference was approximately 7.1 versus 9.1 per cent for intensive versus conventional therapy. In the primary prevention cohort, the risk of developing microalbuminuria was reduced by 34 per cent, whereas in the secondary prevention cohort, the risk reduction was 43 per cent.

Table 11 Factors that increase the risk to develop diabetic nephropathy

Hyperglycaemia
Smoking
Hypertension
High protein intake?
Dyslipidaemia?

In an almost identical protocol, the Kumamoto study randomized Japanese patients with type 2 diabetes to intensive or conventional insulin treatment. Achieved HbA1c was 7.1 versus 9.4 per cent in the intensive versus conventional treatment groups achieving a 70 per cent risk reduction in developing nephropathy. These individuals were slim, relatively young, and normotensive. They differed therefore from typical European patients with type 2 diabetes. In the UKPDS trial, 3041 newly diagnosed, mostly Europid type 2 diabetic subjects were randomized to either conventional (target fasting plasma glucose <15 mmol/l) or intensive (fasting plasma glucose < 6 mmol/l) treatment with either insulin or oral therapy. Median follow-up was 10 years. Achieved HbA1c was 7 and 7.9 per cent for intensively and conventionally treated patients, respectively. At 9 years, 19.2 per cent had progressed in the intensively and 25.4 per cent in the conventionally treated group and the separation was sustained even after 15 years of follow-up. It had been claimed that a glycaemic threshold for the development of microalbuminuria exists at around 8.0 per cent HbA1c, but this has not been confirmed in subsequent studies. Unfortunately, efforts to intensify glycaemic control are associated with an increase in the frequency of severe hypoglycaemia: in the DCCT study, the frequency of severe hypoglycaemic episodes per 100 patient years was 88 at a HbA1c value of 6 per cent compared with 28 episodes at a HbA1c of 10 per cent. Consequently, the effort to obtain lower HbA1c values to benefit from a relatively small gain at lower HbA1c values must be balanced against the risk of hypoglycaemia, which may prove unacceptable for some patients.

Intensified glycaemic correction tends also to reduce the hyperfiltration of acute type 1 and newly presenting patient with type 2 diabetes, although the GFR values remain greater than the age- and sex-matched normal range in a significant proportion of patients. This has been found in several small studies, where as the impact on long-term renal outcome is unclear.

The effect of normoglycaemic control on renal structures is well investigated in experimental studies, where normoglycaemia was shown to prevent or reverse glomerulopathy in the diabetic rat. Human data on renal lesions in patients without clinically manifest nephropathy are lacking, but some studies showed a marginal effect on GBM thickening in microalbuminuric patients biopsied at baseline and 2–3 years later.

Smoking

Smoking is a potent predictor of a more frequent and premature onset of microalbuminuria in type 1 diabetes. A number of recent studies showed that microalbuminuria is also more frequent in patients with type 2 diabetes who smoke (Rossing *et al.* 2002). In microalbuminuric patients, the rate of progression to DN is accelerated. Furthermore, comparison of the rate of GFR loss in current smokers compared to non-smokers or ex-smokers documented that cessation of smoking was beneficial (Sawicki *et al.* 1994). Finally, Biesenbach *et al.* (1997) compared the rate of loss of measured creatinine clearance in smokers and non-smokers with types 1 and 2 diabetes and impaired renal function. He found that smokers had twice the rate of loss compared to non-smokers. The adverse effect of smoking was even demonstrable when patients with diabetes received ACE inhibitors and had well-controlled BP values, that is mean arterial pressure less than 100 mmHg (Chuahirun and Wesson 2002).

Hypertension

It is now recognized that systemic BP values are higher in those patients with type 1 diabetes who go on to develop microalbuminuria compared to those who have persistently normal albumin excretion rates. This is not surprising in view of the association of paternal hypertension and the risk of DN in the offspring (Strojek *et al.* 1997; Fragerudd *et al.* 1998). The association between prediabetic BP and onset of nephropathy after the onset of type 2 diabetes in Pima Indians is illustrated in Table 5. In view of such associations the question arises whether treatment with antihypertensive agents, particularly with ACE inhibitors, will reduce the risk to develop microalbuminuria and DN even in patients whose BP values are within the normal range. Unfortunately no conclusive information on this point is currently available, although the results of some studies are definitely intriguing (Chaturvedi *et al.* 1998).

In the EUCLID study, 440 initially normoalbuminuric type 1 diabetic patients with baseline BP less then 150/70–90 mmHg were randomized to receive lisinopril or placebo. A 30 per cent reduction in urinary albumin excretion was noted after 2 years, but the difference was not statistically significant.

The effect of BP on the risk to develop microalbuminuria in hypertensive patients is beyond doubt. As one example, in the UKPDS study, hypertensive patients with type 2 diabetes ($>$160/90 mmHg or antihypertensive treatment) were randomized to tight (target BP $<$ 150/85 mmHg) or less tight ($<$180/105 mmHg) BP control. A smaller number of patients developed microalbuminuria on tight as compared to less tight BP control, that is, 20.3 versus 28.5 per cent at 6 years. The frequency was similar in patients on atenolol or captopril.

Obesity

Obesity is increasingly prevalent in Western societies as exemplified in Fig. 7. There is undoubtedly a link between obesity and the development of type 2 diabetes, but there is also evidence that obese patients are more likely to have progressive renal disease (Praga 2002), although little specific information on DN is available. It is difficult to dissociate the effects of obesity *per se* from those of hypertension and hyperlipidaemia. An interesting hypothesis linking obesity and DN has recently been proposed by Wolf *et al.* (2002) based on the observation that leptin receptors are present in the glomerulus and that leptin has striking effects on renal function.

High protein intake

Animal models show a convincing association between dietary protein intake and progression of nephropathy in experimental diabetes. In type 1 diabetes, the EURODIAB cross-sectional survey found that a dietary protein intake accounting for greater than 20 per cent total energy was linked to the presence of microalbuminuria. Patients with less than 20 per cent dietary proteins were more likely to have an albumin excretion rate of less than 20 μg/min. This effect was more marked in those with hypertension (Toeller *et al.* 1997). The HOORN study (Bilous 1999) found an increased risk of microalbuminuria for every 0.1 g/kg body weight per day in dietary protein intake. In contrast to animal data, overall, the evidence for linking protein intake and DN in humans is not very strong, however. Dietary protein ingestion has effects on renal haemodynamics and this has been studied both in normal and patient with diabetes. Usually there is an increase in GFR and in renal plasma flow, possibly mediated by prostaglandins or glucagon. These effects are not seen when proteins from vegetable sources rather than animal sources are administered.

The American Diabetes Association Guidelines currently recommend an intake of 0.8 g/kg body weight per day.

Dyslipidaemia

A wealth of data from animal models suggest a role of circulating plasma lipoproteins in the genesis of progressive renal injury. Cultured mesangial cells possess low density lipoprotein (LDL) cholesterol receptors

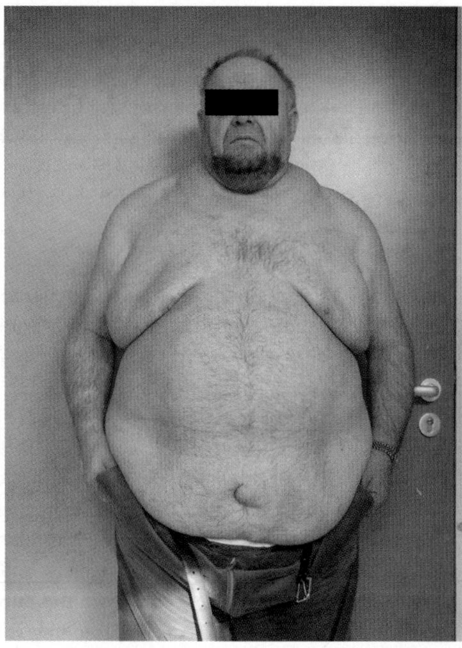

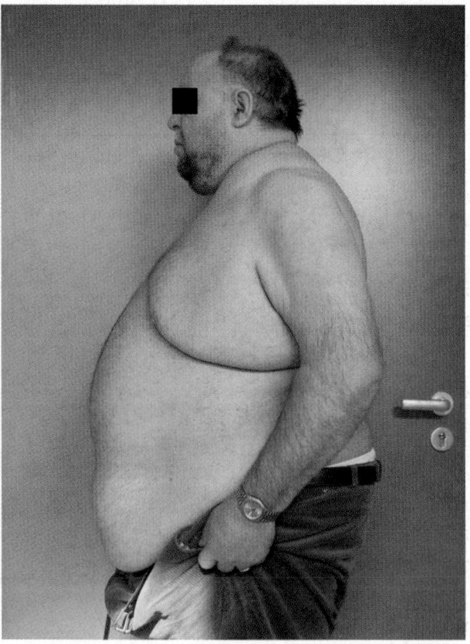

Fig. 7 A 64-year-old patient with type 2 diabetes and proteinuria of 5.1 g/day, body mass index 56.3, and blood pressure 164/103 mmHg.

(as well as scavenging receptors) and binding of LDL initiates a proliferative response. There is no definite proof, however, that dyslipidaemia is causally linked to the onset or progression of DN. Patients with established nephropathy have abnormally raised total and LDL cholesterol, apo-lipoprotein B, total and very low density lipoprotein (VLDL) triglycerides as well as reduced high density lipoprotein (HDL) (particularly HDL-2)-cholesterol. These abnormalities are present in microalbuminuric patients and almost certainly contribute to the observed increase in cardiovascular disease. Higher serum cholesterol concentrations were also associated with progressive loss of GFR in type 1 diabetic patients with nephropathy (Mulec *et al.* 1990). In patients, with type 2 diabetes plasma cholesterol greater than 5.25 mmol/l was associated with a more than 20-fold odds ratio for progression of microalbuminuria. Some association was also seen with HDL and LDL cholesterol (Smulders *et al.* 1997). Similar associations were found in Pima Indians, but they were only apparent after 10 years diabetes duration. High serum triglycerides were associated with an increase in the albumin excretion rate. The question whether the link between lipids and renal damage is causal, and whether lipid interventions are beneficial, is currently unresolved. Nevertheless, some preliminary observations in non-diabetic patients are encouraging: administration of statins lowered albumin excretion under conditions where confounding effects of BP changes can be excluded (Wierzbicki 2002).

Multifactorial management

It would be wrong to focus efforts in preventing onset or progression of nephropathy on one single factor only, for example, on hyperglycaemia. A recent study in high risk type 2 diabetic patients with microalbuminuria showed that target-driven long-term intensified intervention aimed at multiple risk factors caused dramatic reduction not only of the risk of cardiovascular, but also of renal events. Patients were randomly assigned either to management by general practitioners according to the guidelines of the Danish Diabetes Society or to intensified treatment in a diabetes clinic. In the latter, intervention included aggressive lowering of BP, administration of ACE inhibitors or angiotensin receptor blockers; administration of statins; dietary advise; and advise on life style modification. This strategy caused an impressive reduction of cardiovascular disease by 53 per cent and of nephropathy by 61 per cent. The authors had achieved striking differences in systolic BP, in fasting glucose, and in LDL cholesterol concentration. This was associated with decreased urinary albumin excretion in patients on intensified compared to an increase in patients on conventional treatment. The findings are more remarkable because only modest differences in HbA1c and no significant impact on cessation of smoking or resumption of physical exercise had been achieved (Gaede *et al.* 2003).

Interventions in overt diabetic nephropathy

It is didactically useful to separately discuss the most important factors that increase the risk of onset of microalbuminuria on the one hand and the most important factors that increase the risk of progression of DN ('progression promotors') on the other hand (Table 12).

In the normoalbuminuric diabetic patient, hyperglycaemia is the most potent predictor (Yokoyama *et al.* 1997). In contrast, in the patient with established DN, hypertension and proteinuria are the most potent progression promotors. Most studies dealing with the natural history of DN have demonstrated a relentless, often linear rate of decline in GFR which varies widely, however, between patients ranging from 2 to 20 ml/min/year. The mean value is 12 ml/min/year (Mogensen 1976; Parving *et al.* 1981; Viberti *et al.* 1983). Patients with type 2 diabetes suffering from nephropathy display the same degree of loss in filtration rate as do with type 1 diabetes patients (Gall *et al.* 1993; Nelson *et al.* 1996). Predictors of progression in patients with both types 1 and 2 diabetes are mesangial expansion in the glomeruli and tubulointerstitial lesions.

Table 12 Factors that increase the risk of progression of diabetic nephropathy to ESRD

Hypertension
Proteinuria
Smoking
Poor glycaemic control
Dyslipidaemia?
High dietary intake of protein?

Hypertension

A close correlation between BP and the rate of decline in GFR has been documented in patients with both types 1 and 2 diabetes (Krolewski *et al.* 1994; Taft *et al.* 1994; Breyer *et al.* 1996; Yokoyama *et al.* 1997; Rossing 1998; Hovind *et al.* 2001). The paradigms to explain the relation between BP and progressive renal injury have changed with time. In the past, it was felt that the effect of hypertension was mediated through vasoconstriction and nephrosclerosis (Jacobson 1991). Based on experimental studies, however, a new concept has been proposed, that is, that the kidney is vasodilated, loses autoregulation, and develops glomerular hypertension even when systemic BP values are still within the normotensive range (Imanishi *et al.* 1999). A number of studies on types 1 and 2 diabetes provided evidence that BP was a powerful predictor of GFR loss in DN (Mathiesen *et al.* 1995; Stephenson *et al.* 1995). The causal role of hypertension has been confirmed in numerous studies following the seminal observations of Mogensen (1982) and Parving *et al.* (1983). These authors had documented that lowering of BP attenuated the rate of loss of GFR. The beneficial effect of BP lowering *per se* is now beyond any doubt. The American Diabetes Association (2002) recommends a target BP of 125/75 mmHg for diabetic patients with proteinuria and this recommendation is also given by other societies (Kidney Disease Outcome Quality Initiative 2002). In experimental studies, it appeared that lowering of systemic BP alone without concomitant reduction in glomerular capillary pressure did not optimally protect against progression. This may explain, at least in part, the BP-independent renoprotective effects of ACE inhibitors (Lewis *et al.* 2001) and angiotensin receptor blockers (Brenner *et al.* 2001; Lewis *et al.* 2001) in types 1 and 2 diabetes, respectively, because the agents lower glomerular capillary pressure by dilating the efferent arteriole. Furthermore, angiotensin II, either circulating or generated locally by ACE-dependent or -independent pathways, has numerous adverse effects independent of haemodynamic actions, for example, activation of TGF β, upregulation of plasminogen activation inhibitor (PAI), activation of cytokines, injury to podocytes etc. This further explains why ACE inhibitors and angiotensin receptor blockers provide superior and in part BP-independent renoprotection compared to alternative antihypertensive agents.

More recently, it has also been shown that, in addition to hypertension, proteinuria *per se* accelerates the loss of GFR. This hypothesis originally proposed by Remuzzi and Bertani (1990) has been confirmed from observational studies showing a correlation between proteinuria and loss of GFR. More recently, however, intervention studies documented that the reduction in proteinuria is accompanied by more pronounced attenuation of GFR loss, even when corrections are made for the lowering of BP (IDNT) (Lewis *et al.* 2001).

A meta-analysis of 12 trials in 698 type 1 diabetic patients with microalbuminuria who were followed for at least 1 year has revealed that ACE inhibitors reduced the risk of progression to macroalbuminuria compared to that of the placebo group (odds ratio 0.38) (The ACE Inhibitors in Diabetic Nephropathy Trialist Group 2001). Regression to normoalbuminuria was three times more frequent than in patients receiving placebo. At 2 years the urinary albumin excretion rate was 50 per cent lower in patients taking ACE inhibitors than in those receiving placebo. This benefit persists over prolonged follow-up periods and is apparently associated with preservation of GFR (Mathiesen *et al.* 1999). It has even been shown that pharmacological blockade of the RAS has a beneficial impact on glomerular structural changes in types 1 and 2 diabetic patients with early diabetic glomerulopathy (Cordonnier *et al.* 1999; Rudberg *et al.* 1999; Osterby *et al.* 2000). Nevertheless controlled data suggest that long-acting dihydropyridine calcium antagonists were as effective as ACE inhibitors in delaying the occurrence of macroalbuminuria in normotensive patients with type 1 diabetes with persistent microalbuminuria (Crepaldi *et al.* 1998). In microalbuminuric type 2 diabetic patients ACE inhibitors were shown to prevent progression and development of nephropathy even in normotensive patients treated with enalapril or placebo (Ravid *et al.* 1993). Recently, there has been documentation of a BP-independent effect of angiotensin receptor blockers in patients with type 2 diabetes early in the course of DN, that is, hypertensive microalbuminuric patients (IRMA-2, Parving *et al.* 2001) and patients with advanced nephropathy (IDNT, Lewis *et al.* 2001; RENAAL, Brenner *et al.* 2001). In the IRMA-2 trial (Parving *et al.* 2001), hypertensive type 2 diabetic patients with microalbuminuria received either placebo (i.e. alternative antihypertensive agents) or Irbesartan at a dose of 150 or 300 mg daily. After 2 years of follow-up, 15.9 per cent of patients on placebo and only 5.2 per cent of patients on 300 mg Irbesartan had reached the primary endpoint of persistent albumin excretion greater 200 μg/min.

In advanced DN with heavy proteinuria (>900 mg/day) and elevated serum creatinine, both Losartan (RENAAL, Brenner *et al.* 2001) and Irbesartan (IDNT, Lewis *et al.* 2001) reduced the primary endpoint of progression, that is, doubling of serum creatinine significantly despite similar BP control, implying a BP-independent additional benefit from pharmacological blockade of the RAS. The effect on cardiovascular endpoints was not significant in either study, which were both underpowered to assess this issue.

Of interest with respect to the practical management of patients is that the benefit on the renal endpoint was greater, the lower the achieved BP. As a consequence, both a low target BP and pharmacological blockade of the RAS must be achieved. It is of note, however, that the median BP in both studies was still around 140/77 mmHg although the BP target was 135/85 mmHg in the Irbesartan group. It is quite difficult to lower BP sufficiently in these patients and on average administration of four to five classes of antihypertensive agents is necessary. A particularly neglected aspect is provision of a salt-restricted diet and administration of sufficient diuretics. In heavily proteinuric patients, the absolute free concentration of diuretics in the tubular lumen is reduced and higher doses are required than in normoproteinuric patients.

A new concept is that the treatment with ACE inhibitors or angiotensin receptor blockers should not be targeted to lowering BP alone, but also to reduction of proteinuria. The initial reduction of proteinuria, that is, 4 weeks after start of ACE inhibitor treatment, predicts the attenuation of the rate of loss of GFR in the subsequent observation period. It is therefore advisable to check the initial decrease of proteinuria. If this cannot be lowered to values less than 1 g/24 h, recent studies suggest that not infrequently an aldosterone escape has occurred, that is, a secondary increase of aldosterone concentration after an initial decrease (Epstein 2001). Administration of aldosterone receptor blockers has been shown to further reduce proteinuria despite no further lowering of BP, but whether this will affect the rate of loss of GFR in the long run has not been investigated.

It is currently unclear whether ACE inhibitors and angiotensin receptor blockers are equipotent in halting progression of diabetic nephropathy. Head-to-head comparisons of ACE inhibitors versus angiotensin receptor blockers suggest similar ability to reduce albuminuria and BP in proteinuric diabetic patients (Andersen *et al.* 2000; Lacourciere *et al.* 2000; Muirhead *et al.* 2002). The effect on the rate of loss of GFR in the long-term has not been explored.

More recently, it has been suggested that combination of ACE inhibitors and angiotensin receptor blockers is superior to the respective monotherapy. This has been proven with respect to reducing albuminuria (Mogensen *et al.* 2000; Viberti *et al.* 2002), but data on long-term effects on progression are not available in patients with diabetes. In non-diabetic patients, combination of the angiotensin receptor blocker Losartan and the ACE inhibitor Trandolapril, had been shown to reduce the proportion of patients doubling serum creatinine concentration compared to the respective monotherapies despite similar control of BP (Nakao *et al.* 2003). This study was performed with the doses of the respective drugs, which have been licensed for clinical use. Whether at higher doses an additive effect is still present, is currently unclear, but experimental studies in non-diabetic models suggest no further benefit (Ots *et al.* 1998; Peters *et al.* 1998).

When starting treatment with ACE inhibitors, as one would predict from reversing glomerular capillary hypertension, GFR decreases initially, causing an increase in serum creatinine concentration (Palmer 2002). This should not deter from continuation of treatment unless serum creatinine increases by more than 50 per cent, in which case clinical investigation to refute reversible causes, for example, volume depletion, coronary artery stenosis, etc. are indicated. It appears that the initial decline in GFR is largely, though not exclusively, a functional haemodynamic one associated with a subsequent slower decline of GFR (Hansen *et al.* 1997). A further potential complication of ACE inhibitor treatment is hyperkalaemia and aggravation of anaemia, which must be managed appropriately.

Glycaemia control

In the past, it has been felt that once clinically manifest DN was established, a 'point of no return' had been reached, where DN progressed autonomously independent of glycaemia and other interventions. This notion is in contrast with more recent findings, which show a definite impact of glycaemic control on progression (Nyberg *et al.* 1987; Mulec *et al.* 1995, 1998; Parving *et al.* 1995; Breyer *et al.* 1996; Alaveras *et al.* 1997; Yokoyama *et al.* 1997; Bangstad *et al.* 2002). Whilst this is true for type 1 diabetes, most, but not all, studies on proteinuric type 2 diabetic patients failed to show a benefit (Knowles 1974; Bjorn *et al.* 1995; Wu *et al.* 1997).

Dietary protein restriction

The rationale for dietary protein restriction is based on experimental studies which showed that this manoeuvre limits glomerular capillary pressures and flow rates in rats (Zatz *et al.* 1985; Zatz and Brenner 1986). Although short-term studies in normoalbuminuric, microalbuminuric, and macroalbuminuric type 1 diabetic patients showed that low protein diets reduce urinary albumin excretion and hyperfiltration, independently of glycaemic control and BP (Cohen *et al.* 1987; Hansen *et al.* 1999), the reported effects on progression are controversial (Walker *et al.* 1989; Parving 1990; Zeller *et al.* 1991).

It is therefore wise to stick to the recommendation of the American Diabetes Association to administer a diet with 0.8 g/kg/day and to avoid excess protein intake, but further lowering below recommended levels is beneficial. At any rate, the effect of dietary protein restriction is small in relation to what can be achieved by lowering of BP and administering ACE inhibitors.

This is also reflected by the fact that lowering of BP and of proteinuria are the most powerful interventions to reduce the rate of progression (Lewis *et al.* 1993, 2001; Brenner *et al.* 2001). In streptozotocin diabetic rats lowering of BP protected against development of proteinuria and glomerulosclerosis. Anderson *et al.* (1989) had documented years ago that ACE inhibitors afforded superior long-term protection compared to triple therapy with reserpin, hydralazine, and hydrochlorothiazide.

Pregnancy in women with diabetic nephropathy

Pregnancy outcomes in women with DN had improved over the last 20 years with reported fetal survival rates more than 95 per cent. The rates are not as good as in women with reduced GFR, as well as in women with manifest proteinuria. These women are more likely to be delivered earlier, around 31 weeks gestation in one series, and to have infants of low birth weight requiring neonatal intensive care.

The impact of pregnancy on renal function in women with nephropathy is variable. The early rise in GFR seen in normal pregnancy does not occur in around 50 per cent of women with nephropathy, but there is no firm evidence that pregnancy itself accelerates the rate of loss of GFR. A recent review of all reported series from 1981 to 1986 identified a total patient population of 315 pregnancies. Data were available on follow-up of 185 patients postpartum. Seventeen per cent of patients had developed ESRD after a mean surveillance of 35 months. Five per cent had died as a result of their renal disease.

Because they are contraindicated in pregnancy, ACE inhibitors and angiotensin II receptor blockers cannot be used and there is some concern that withdrawal of these drugs preconceptual and during pregnancy, may result in a loss of nephroprotection. One study from Israel suggested that vigorous treatment preconceptually with ACE inhibitors offered some protection throughout the pregnancy, although these results need verifying in a much larger series.

Proteinuria can increase to nephrotic levels, particularly by the third trimester. One study reported that 50 per cent of women will excrete more than 5 g/day by the time of delivery. In addition, the majority will have clinically significant hypertension (>140/90 mmHg) by the time of delivery. Proteinuria generally returns to preconceptual levels with 12 weeks postpartum.

Women with preconceptual microalbuminuria have been less well studied, but an increase in albuminuria by up to four times in the third trimester have been reported. Nephrotic range proteinuria occurred in four of 12 women with preconceptual microalbuminuria, but this phenomenon has also been noted in women who were normoalbuminuric prior to pregnancy. As with patients with clinical nephropathy, albuminuria returned to pregnancy levels in the majority by 12 weeks postpartum. GFR responses to pregnancy appear to be normal in women within this range of albuminuria.

Thus, women with well-preserved renal function and early or clinical nephropathy can expect a good outcome from pregnancy with little or no adverse effects on maternal kidney function. However, those with renal impairment have a more variable response and regular monitoring of GFR and proteinuria is required. These women need careful counselling prior to embarking upon a pregnancy and should be managed in specialized units by a multidisciplinary team of obstetricians, nephrologists, and diabetologists.

References

Adamczak, M., Zeier, M., Dikow, R., and Ritz, E. (2002). Kidney and hypertension. *Kidney International Supplement* **80**, 62–67.

Adler, A. I., Stevens, R. J., Manley, S. E., Bilous, R. W., Cull, C. A., and Holman, R. R. (2003). Development and progression of nephropathy in type 2 diabetes: The United Kingdom Prospective Diabetes Study (UKPDS 64). *Kidney International* **63**, 225–232.

Adler, S. G., Kang, S. W., Feld, S., Cha, D. R., Barba, L., Striker, L., Striker, G., Riser, B. L., LaPage, J., and Nast, C. C. (2001). Glomerular mRNAs in human type 1 diabetes: biochemical evidence for microalbuminuria as a manifestation of diabetic nephropathy. *Kidney International* **60** (6), 2330–2336.

Alavares, A., Thomas, S. M., Sagriotis, A., and Viberti, G. C. (1997). Promotors of progression of diabetic nephropathy: the relative roles of blood glucose and blood pressure control. *Nephrology, Dialysis, Transplantation* **12** (2), 71–74.

Allen, T. J., Cooper, M. E., Gilbert, R. E., Winikoff, J., Skinner, S. L., and Jerums, G. (1996). Serum total renin is increased before microalbuminuria in diabetes. *Kidney International* **50**, 902–907.

Amann, K., Koch, A., Hofstetter, J., Gross, M. L., Haas, C., Orth, S. R., Ehmke, H., Rump, L. C., and Ritz, E. (2001). Glomerulosclerosis and progression: effect of subantihypertensive doses of alpha and beta blockers. *Kidney International* **60** (4), 1309–1323.

American Diabetes Association (2002). Diabetic nephropathy. *Diabetes Care* **25**, S85–S89.

Andersen, A. R., Christiansen, J. S., Andersen, J. K., Kreiner, S., and Deckert, T. (1983). Diabetic nephropathy in type 1 (insulin-dependent) diabetes: an epidemiological study. *Diabetologia* **25**, 496–501.

Andersen, S., Tarnow, L., Rossing, P., Hansen, B. V., and Parving, H. H. (2000). Renoprotective effects of angiotensin II receptor blockade in type 1 diabetic patients with diabetic nephropathy. *Kidney International* **57**, 601–606.

Anderson, S., Rennke, H. G., Garcia, D. L., and Brenner, B. M. (1989). Short and long term effects of antihypertensive therapy in the diabetic rat. *Kidney International* **36**, 526–536.

Arici, M., Chana, R., Lewington, A., Brown, J., and Brunskill, N. J. (2003). Stimulation of proximal tubular cell apoptosis by albumin-bound fatty acids mediated by peroxisome proliferator activated receptor-gamma. *Journal of the American Society of Nephrology* **14**, 17–27.

Bangstad, H. J., Osterby, R., Rudberg, S., Hartmann, A., Braband, K., and Hanssen, K. F. (2002). Kidney function and glomerulopathy over 8 years in young patients with type I (insulin-dependent) diabetes mellitus and microalbuminuria. *Diabetologia* **45** (2), 253–261.

Biesenbach, G., Grafinger, P., Janko, O., and Zazgornik, J. (1997). Influence of cigarette-smoking on the progression of clinical diabetic nephropathy in type 2 diabetic patients. *Clinical Nephrology* **48**, 146–150.

Bilous, R. W. The pathology of diabetic nephropathy. In *International Textbook of Diabetes Mellitus* 2nd edn. (ed. K. G. M. M. Alberti, P. Zimmet, and R. A. de Fronzo), pp. 1349–1362. Chichester: John Wiley & Sons, 1997.

Bilous, R. W. Risk factors for the progression of renal disease in type 2 diabetes. In *Nephropathy in Type 2 Diabetes* (ed. E. Ritz and I. Rychlik), pp. 89–110. Oxford: Oxford University Press, 1999.

Bjorck, S. (1990). The renin angiotensin system in diabetes mellitus. A physiological and therapeutic study. *Scandinavian Journal of Urology and Nephrology Supplement* **126**, 1–51.

Bjorn, S. F., Bangstad, H. J., and Hanssen, K. F. (1995). Glomerular epithelial foot processes and filtration slits in IDDM diabetic patients. *Diabetologia* **38**, 1197–1204.

Blacher, J., Safar, M. E., Guerin, A. P., Pannier, B., Marchais, S. J., and London, G. M. (2003). Aortic pulse wave velocity index and mortality in end-stage renal disease. *Kidney International* **63**, 1852–1860.

Bonnet, F., Cooper, M. E., Kawachi, H., Allen, T. J., Boner, G., and Cao, Z. (2001). Irbesartan normalises the deficiency in glomerular nephrin expression in a model of diabetes and hypertension. *Diabetologia* **44**, 874–877.

Borch-Johnsen, K. (1989). The prognosis of insulin-dependent diabetes mellitus. An epidemiological approach. *Danish Medical Bulletin* **39**, 336–339.

Borch-Johnsen, K., Andersen, P. K., and Deckert, T. (1985). The effect of proteinuria on relative mortality in type 1 (insulin-dependent) diabetes mellitus. *Diabetologia* **28** (8), 590–596.

Borch-Johnsen, K., Wenzel, H., Viberti, G. C., and Mogensen, C. E. (1993). Is screening and intervention for microalbuminuria worthwhile in patients with insulin-dependent diabetes. *British Medical Journal* **306**, 1722–1725.

Brenner, B. M., Cooper, M. E., De Zeeuw, D., Keane, W. F., Mitch, W. E., Parving, H. H., Remuzzi, G., Snapinn, S. M., Zhang, Z., and Shahinfar, S. (2001). Effects of losartan on renal and cardiovascular outcomes in patients with type 2 diabetes and nephropathy. *New England Journal of Medicine* **345**, 861–869.

Brenner, B. M., Garcia, D. L., and Anderson, S. (1998). Glomeruli and blood pressure. Less of one, more the other? *American Journal of Hypertension* **1**, 335–347.

Breyer, J. A. *et al.* (1996). Predictors of the progression of renal insufficiency in patients with insulin-dependent diabetes and overt diabetic nephropathy. *Kidney International* **50**, 1651–1658.

Brownlee, M. (2001). Biochemistry and molecular cell biology of diabetic complications. *Nature* **414**, 813–820.

Buzello, M., Tornig, J., Faulhaber, J., Ehmke, H., Ritz, E., and Amann, K. (2003). The apolipoprotein e knockout mouse: a model documenting accelerated atherogenesis in uremia. *Journal of the American Society of Nephrology* **14**, 311–316.

Cambier, P. (1934). Application de la theorie de Rehberg a l'etude clinique des affections renales et du diabete. *Annals of Medicine* **35**, 273–299.

Catalano, C., Postorino, M., Kelly, P. J., Fabrizi, F., Enia, G, Goodship, T. H., Fulcher, G. R., and Maggiore, Q. (1990). Diabetes mellitus and renal replacement therapy in Italy: prevalence, main characteristics and complications. *Nephrology, Dialysis, Transplantation* **5**, 181–190.

Chaturvedi, N., Sjolie, A. K., Stephenson, J. M., Abrahamian, H., Keipes, M., Castellarin, A., Rogulja-Pepeonik, Z., and Fuller, J. H. (1998). Effect of lisinopril on progression of retinopathy in normotensive people with type 1 diabetes. The EUCLID Study Group. EURODIAB Controlled Trial of Lisinopril in Insulin-Dependent Diabetes Mellitus. *Lancet* **351**, 28–31.

Christensen, P. K., Hansen, H. P., and Parving, H. H. (1997). Impaired autoregulation of GFR in hypertensive non-insulin dependent diabetic patients. *Kidney International* **52**, 1369–1374.

Chuahirun, T. and Wesson, D. E. (2002). Cigarette smoking predicts faster progression of type 2 established diabetic nephropathy despite ACE inhibition. *American Journal of Kidney Diseases* **39**, 376–382.

Cohen, D., Dodds, R. A., and Viberti, G. C. (1987). Effect of protein restriction in insulin-dependent diabetics at risk of nephropathy. *British Medical Journal* **294**, 795–798.

Cordonnier, D. J. *et al.* (1999). Expansion of cortical interstitium is limited by converting enzyme inhibition in type 2 diabetic patients with glomerulosclerosis. *Journal of the American Society of Nephrology* **10**, 1253–1263.

Cosio, F. G., Pesavento, T. E., Osei, K., Henry, M. L., and Ferguson, R. M. (2001). Post-transplant diabetes mellitus: increased incidence in renal allograft recipients transplanted in recent years. *Kidney International* **59** (2), 732–737.

Crepaldi, G. *et al.* (1998). Effects of lisinopril and nifedipine on the progression of overt albuminuria in IDDM patients with incipient nephropathy and normal blood pressure. *Diabetes Care* **21** (1), 104–110.

Davies, J. E., Ng, L. L., Kofoed-Enevoldsen, A., Li, L. K., Earle, K. A., Trevisan, R., and Viberti, G. (1992). Intracellular pH and Na^+/H^+ antiport activity of cultured skin fibroblasts from diabetics. *Kidney International* **42**, 1184–1190.

DeFronzo, R. A. (1981). The effect of insulin on renal sodium metabolism. *Diabetologia* **21**, 165–171.

Dinneen, S. F. and Gerstein, H. C. (1997). The association of microalbuminuria and mortality in non-insulin-dependent diabetes mellitus. *Archives of Internal Medicine* **157**, 1413–1418.

Drury, P. L. (1983). Diabetes and arterial hypertension. *Diabetologia* **24**, 1–9.

Earle, K., Walker, J., Hill, C., and Viberti, G. C. (1992). Familial clustering of cardiovascular disease in patients with insulin-dependent diabetes and nephropathy. *New England Journal of Medicine* **326**, 673–677.

Epstein, M. (2001). Aldosterone as a mediator of progressive renal disease: pathogenic and clinical implications. *American Journal of Kidney Diseases* **37**, 677–688.

Fagerudd, J. A., Tarnow, L., Jacobsen, P., Stenman, S., Nielsen, F. S., Pettersson-Fernholm, K. J., Gronhagen-Riska, C., Parving, H. H., and Groop, P. H. (1998). Predisposition to essential hypertension and development of diabetic nephropathy in IDDM patients. *Diabetes* **47**, 439–444.

Farbre, J., Balant, L. P., Dayer, P. G., Fox, H. M., and Vernet, A. T. (1982). The kidney in maturity onset diabetes mellitus: a clinical studie of 510 patients. *Kidney International* **21**, 730–738.

Feldt-Rasmussen, B. and Deckert, T. (1993). Is metabolic control a determinant of renal disease progression in type I diabetic nephropathy. *Journal of Nephrology* **2**, 58–62.

Fioretto, P., Mauer, M., Brocco, E., Velussi, M., Frigato, F., Muollo, B., Sambataro, M., Abaterusso, C., Baggio, B., Crepaldi, G., and Nosadini, R. (1996). Patterns of renal injury in NIDDM patients with microalbuminuria. *Diabetologia* **39**, 1569–1576.

Fioretto, P., Steffes, M. W., Sutherland, D. E., Goetz, F. C., and Mauer, M. (1998). Reversal of lesions of diabetic nephropathy after pancreas transplantation. *New England Journal of Medicine* **339**, 69–75.

Fliser, D. and Ritz, E. (2001). Serum Cystatin C concentration as a marker of renal dysfunction in the elderly. *American Journal of Kidney Diseases* **37**, 79–83.

Gaede, P., Vedel, P., Larsen, N., Jensen, G. V., Parving, H. H., and Pedersen, O. (2003). Multifactorial intervention and cardiovascular disease in patients with type 2 diabetes. *New England Journal of Medicine* **348**, 383–393.

Gall, M. A. *et al.* (1991). Prevalence of micro- and macroalbuminuria, arterial hypertension, retinopathy and large vessel disease in European Type 2 (non-insulin-dependent) diabetic patients. *Diabetologia* **34**, 655–661.

Gall, M. A., Nielsen, F. S., Schmidt, U. M., and Parving, H. H. (1993). The course of kidney function in type 2 (non-insulin-dependent) diabetic patients with diabetic nephropathy. *Diabetologia* **36**, 1071–1078.

Gross, M. L., El-Shakmak, A., Szabo, A., Koch, A., Kuhlmann, A., Munter, K., Ritz, E., and Amann, K. (2003). ACE-inhibitors but not endothelin receptor blockers prevent podocyte loss in early diabetic nephropathy. *Diabetologia* **46**, 856–868.

Gross, M. L., Hanke, W., Koch, A., Ziebart, H., Amann, K., and Ritz, E. (2002). Intraperitoneal protein injection in the axolotl: the amphibia kidney as a novel model to study tubulointerstitial activation. *Kidney International* **62** (1), 51–59.

Gulmann, C., Osterby, R., Bangstad, H. J., and Rudberg, S. (2001). The juxtaglomerular apparatus in young type 1 diabetic patients with microalbuminuria. Effect of antihypertensive treatment. *Virchows Archive* **438**, 618–623.

Hansen, H. P., Christensen, P. K., Tauber-Lassen, E., Klausen, A., Jensen, B. R., and Parving, H. H. (1999). Low-protein diet and kidney function in insulin-dependent diabetic patients with diabetic nephropathy. *Kidney International* **55** (2), 621–628.

Hansen, H. P., Nielsen, F. S., Rossing, P., Jacobsen, P., Jensen, B. R., and Parving, H. H. (1997). Kidney function after withdrawal of long-term antihypertensive treatment in diabetic nephropathy. *Kidney International* **52** (63), S49–S53.

Harris, R. D., Steffes, M. W., Bilous, R. W., Sutherland, D. E. R., and Mauer, S. M. (1991). Global glomerular sclerosis and glomerular arteriolar hyalinosis in insulin dependent diabetes. *Kidney International* **40**, 107–114.

Hasslacher, C., Borgholte, G., Panradl, U., and Wahl, P. (1990). Improved prognosis of type 1 and type 2 diabetics with nephropathy. *Medizinische Klinik* **85**, 643–646.

Hasslacher, C., Ritz, E., Wahl, P., and Michael, C. (1989). Similar risks of nephropathy in patients with type I or type II diabetes mellitus. *Nephrology, Dialysis, Transplantation* **4** (10), 859–863.

Hasslacher, C., Wolfrum, M., Stech, G., Wahl, P., and Ritz, E. (1987). Diabetic nephropathy in type II diabetes: effect of metabolic control and blood pressure on its development and course. *Deutsche Medizinische Wochenschrift* **112** (38), 1445–1449.

Hostetter, T. H., Troy, J. L., and Brenner, B. M. (1981). Glomerular hemodynamics in experimental diabetes mellitus. *Kidney International* **19**, 410–415.

Hovind, P., Rossing, P., Tarnow, L., Schmidt, U. M., and Parving, H. H. (2001). Progression of diabetic nephropathy. *Kidney International* **59**, 702–709.

Imanishi, M. *et al.* (1999). Glomerular hypertension as one cause of albuminuria in type II diabetic patients. *Diabetologia* **42**, 999–1005.

Jacobson, H. R. (1991). Chronic renal failure: pathophysiology. *Lancet* **338**, 419–423.

Karlefors, T. (1966). Circulatory studies during exercise with particular reference to diabetics. *Acta Medica Scandinavica* **180**, S1–S87.

Keen, H., Chlouverakis, C., Fuller, J. H., and Jarrett, R. J. (1969). The concomitants of raised blood sugar: studies in newly-detected hyperglycaemics. II. Urinary albumin excretion, blood pressure and their relation to blood sugar levels. *Guy's Hospital Reports* **118**, 247–254.

Keller, C., Bergis, K. H., Fliser, D., and Ritz, E. (1996). Renal findings in patients with short term type 2 diabetes. *Journal of the American Society of Nephrology* **7**, 1636–1642.

Keller, G., Zimmer, G., Mall, G., Ritz, E., and Amann, K. (2003). Nephron number in patients with primary hypertension. *New England Journal of Medicine* **348**, 101–108.

Kidney Disease Outcome Quality Initiative (2002). K/DOQI clinical practice guidelines for chronic kidney disease: evaluation, classification, and stratification. *American Journal of Kidney Diseases* **39**, S1–S246.

Kimmelstiel, P. and Wilson, C. (1936). Intercapillary lesions in the glomeruli of the kidney. *American Journal of Pathology* **12**, 83–97.

Knowles, H. C. J. (1974). Magnitude of the renal failure problem in diabetic patients. *Kidney International* **6** (Suppl. 1), S2–S7.

Koch, M., Thomas, B., Tschöpe, W., and Ritz, E. (1993). Survival and predictors of death in dialysed diabetic patients. *Diabetologia* **36**, 1113–1117.

Krolewski, A. S., Warram, J. H., Christlieb, A. R., Busick, E. J., and Kahn, C. R. (1985). The changing natural history of nephropathy in type 1 diabetes. *American Journal of Medicine* **78**, 785–794.

Krolewski, A. S., Warram, J. H., and Christlieb, A. R. (1994). Hypercholesterolemia— a determinant of renal function loss and deaths in IDDM patients with nephropathy. *Kidney International* **45** (Suppl. 45), S125–S131.

Krolewski, M., Eggers, P. W., and Warram, J. H. (1996). Magnitude of end-stage renal disease in IDDM: a 35 year follow-up study. *Kidney International* **50**, 2041–2046.

Lacourciere, Y. *et al.* (2000). Long-term comparison of losartan and enalapril on kidney function in hypertensive type 2 diabetics with early nephropathy. *Kidney International* **58** (2), 762–769.

Lane, P. H., Steffes, M. W., Fioretto, P., and Mauer, S. M. (1993). Renal interstitial expansion in insulin-dependent diabetes mellitus. *Kidney International* **43**, 661–667.

Lewis, E. J., Hunsicker, L. G., Bain, R. P., and Rohde, R. D. (1993). The effect of angiotensin-converting-enzyme inhibition on diabetic nephropathy. *New England Journal of Medicine* **329**, 1456–1462.

Lewis, E. J., Hunsicker, L. G., Clarke, W. R., Berl, T., Pohl, M. A., Lewis, J. B., Ritz, E., Atkins, R. C., Rohde, R., and Raz, I. (2001). Renoprotective effect of the angiotensin-receptor antagonist irbesartan in patients with nephropathy due to type 2 diabetes. *New England Journal of Medicine* **345**, 851–860.

Lippert, J., Ritz, E., Schwarzbeck, A., and Schneider, P. (1995). The rising tide of endstage renal failure from diabetic nephropathy type II—an epidemiological analysis. *Nephrology, Dialysis, Transplantation* **10** (4), 462–467.

London, G. M. and Guerin, A. P. (1999). Influence of arterial pulse and reflected waves on blood pressure and cardiac function. *American Heart Journal* **138**, 220–224.

Luetscher, J. A., Kramer, F. B., Wilson, D. M., Schwartz, H. C., and Bryer-Ash, M. (1985). Increased plasma inactive renin in diabetes mellitus. A marker of microvascular complications. *New England Journal of Medicine* **312**, 1412–1417.

Lundbaek, K. (1970). Renal structure and function in early and diabetes long-term. *Revue Medical De La Suisse Romande* **90** (8), 603–614.

Lurbe, E., Redon, J., Kesani, A., Pascual, J. M., Tacons, J., Alvarez, V., and Batlle, D. (2002). Increase in nocturnal blood pressure and progression to microalbuminuria in type I diabetes. *New England Journal of Medicine* **347** (11), 797–805.

Marre, M. *et al.* (1997). Contribution of genetic polymorphism in the renin–angiotensin system to the development of renal complications in insulin-dependent diabetes. *Journal of Clinical Investigation* **99**, 1585–1595.

Mathiesen, E. R., Hommel, E., Hansen, H. P., Schmidt, U. M., and Parving, H. H. (1999). Randomised controlled trial of long term efficacy of captopril on preservation of kidney function in normotensive patients with insulin dependent diabetes and microalbuminuria. *British Medical Journal* **319**, 24–25.

Mathiesen, E. R., Ronn, B., Storm, B., Foght, H., and Deckert, T. (1995). The natural course of microalbuminuria in insulin dependent diabetes: a 10 year prospective study. *Diabetic Medicine* **12**, 482–487.

Mauer, S. M., Barbosa, J., Vernier, R. L., Kjellstrand, C. M., Buselmeier, T. J., Simmons, R. L., Najarian, J. S., and Goetz, F. C. (1976). Development of diabetic vascular lesions in normal kidneys transplanted into patients with diabetes mellitus. *New England Journal of Medicine* **295**, 916–920.

Microalbuminuria Collaborative Study Group UK (1993). Risk factors for development of microalbuminuria in insulin dependent diabetic patients: a cohort study. *British Medical Journal* **306**, 1235–1239.

Mifsud, S. A. *et al.* (2001). Podocyte foot process broadening in experimental diabetic nephropathy: amelioration with renin–angiotensin blockade. *Diabetologia* **44**, 878–882.

Miller, J. A. (1999). Impact of hyperglycemia on the renin angiotensin system in early human type 1 diabetes mellitus. *Journal of the American Society of Nephrology* **10**, 1778–1785.

Mogensen, C. E. (1971). Glomerular filtration rate and renal plasma flow in short-term and long-term juvenile diabetes mellitus. *Scandinavian Journal of Clinical and Laboratory Investigation* **28**, 91–100.

Mogensen, C. E. (1976). Progression of nephropathy in long-term diabetics with proteinuria and effect of initial antihypertensive treatment. *Scandinavian Journal of Clinical and Laboratory Investigation* **36**, 383–388.

Mogensen, C. E. (1982). Long-term antihypertensive treatment inhibiting progression of diabetic nephropathy. *British Medical Journal* **285**, 685–688.

Mogensen, C. E. and Christensen, C. K. (1984). Predicting diabetic nephropathy in insulin-dependent patients. *New England Journal of Medicine* **311**, 89–93.

Mogensen, C. E., Neldam, S., Tikkanen, I., Oren, S., Viskoper, R., Watts, R. W., and Cooper, M. E. (2000). Randomised controlled trial of dual blockade of renin–angiotensin system in patients with hypertension, microalbuminuria, and non-insulin dependent diabetes: the candesartan and lisinopril microalbuminuria (CALM) study. *British Medical Journal* **321**, 1440–1444.

Muirhead, N. *et al.* (2002). The effects of Valsartan and Captopril on reducing microalbuminuria in patients with type 2 diabetes mellitus: a placebo-controlled trial. *Current Therapeutic Research* **60** (12), 650 (Abstract).

Mulec, H., Blohme, G., Grande, B., and Bjorck, S. (1995). Progression of overt diabetic nephropathy (DN); role of metabolic control. *Journal of the American Society of Nephrology* **6**, 453.

Mulec, H., Blohme, G., Grande, B., and Bjorck, S. (1998). The effect of metabolic control on rate of decline in renal function in insulin-dependent diabetes mellitus with overt diabetic nephropathy. *Nephrology, Dialysis, Transplantation* **13**, 651–655.

Mulec, H., Johnson, S. A., and Björk, S. (1990). Relation between serum cholesterol and diabetic nephropathy. *Lancet* **335**, 1537–1538.

Mundel, P. and Shankland, S. J. (2002). Podocyte biology and response to injury. *Journal of the American Society of Nephrology* **13**, 3005–3015.

Nakao, N., Yoshimura, A., Morita, H., Takada, M., Kayano, T., and Ideura, T. (2003). Combination treatment of angiotensin-II receptor blocker and angiotensin-converting-enzyme inhibitor in non-diabetic renal disease (COOPERATION) randomised controlled trial. *Lancet* **361**, 117–124.

Nakano, S., Ogihara, M., Tamura, C., Kitazawa, M., Nishizawa, M., Kigoshi, T., and Uchida, K. (1999). Reversed circadian blood pressure rhythm independently predicts endstage renal failure in non-insulin-dependent diabetes mellitus subjects. *Diabetes Complications* **13**, 224–231.

Nelson, R. G., Knowler, W. C., Pettitt, D. J., Saad, M. F., Charles, M. A., and Bennett, P. H. (1991). Assessing risk of overt nephropathy in diabetic patients from albumin excretion in untimed urine specimens. *Archives of Internal Medicine* **151**, 1761–1765.

Nelson, R. G., Pettin, D. J., Baird, H. R., Charles, M. A., Liu, Q. Z., Bennett, P. H., and Knowler, W. C. (1993). Prediabetic blood pressure predicts urinary albumin secretion after the onset of type 2 (non-insulin dependent) diabetes mellitus in Pima Indians. *Diabetologia* **36**, 998–1001.

Nelson, R. G. *et al.* (1996). Development and progression of renal disease in Pima Indians with non-insulin-dependent diabetes mellitus. *New England Journal of Medicine* **335**, 1636–1642.

Nielsen, F. S. *et al.* (1995). On the mechanisms of blunted nocturnal decline in arterial blood pressure in NIDDM patients with diabetic nephropathy. *Diabetes* **44**, 783–789.

Nielsen, F. S. *et al.* (1997). Left ventricular hypertrophy in non-insulin diabetic patients with and without diabetic nephropathy. *Diabetic Medicine* **14**, 538–546.

Nishiyama, A., Seth, D. M., and Navar, L. G. (2002). Renal interstitial fluid angiotensin I and angiotensin II concentrations during local angiotensin-converting enzyme inhibition. *Journal of the American Society of Nephrology* **13**, 2207–2212.

Nowack, R., Raum, E., Blum, W., and Ritz, E. (1992). Renal hemodynamics in recent-onset type II diabetes. *American Journal of Kidney Diseases* **20** (4), 342–347.

Nyberg, G., Blohme, G., and Norden, G. (1987). Impact of metabolic control in progression of clinical diabetic nephropathy. *Diabetologia* **30**, 82–86.

Olsen, S. Light microscopy of diabetic glomerulopathy: the classic lesions. In *The Kidney and Hypertension in Diabetes Mellitus* 5th edn. (ed. C. E. Mogensen), pp. 201–210. Boston: Kluwer Academic Publishers, 2000.

Olsen, S. and Mogensen, C. E. (1996). How often is NIDDM complicated with non-diabetic renal disease? An analysis of renal biopsies and the literature. *Diabetologia* **39**, 1638–1645.

Osterby, R., Bangstad, H. J., and Rudberg, S. (2000). Follow-up study of glomerular dimensions and cortical interstitium in microalbuminuric type 1 diabetic patients with or without antihypertensive treatment. *Nephrology, Dialysis, Transplantation* **15** (10), 1609–1616.

Ots, M., Mackenzie, H. S., Troy, J. L., Rennke, H. G., and Brenner, B. M. (1998). Effects of combination therapy with enalapril and losartan on the rate of progression of renal injury in rats with 5/6 renal mass ablation. *Journal of the American Society of Nephrology* **9**, 224–230.

Palmer, B. F. (2002). Renal dysfunction complicating the treatment of hypertension. *New England Journal of Medicine* **347**, 1256–1261.

Parving, H. H. (1990). Low-protein diet and progression of renal disease in diabetic nephropathy (letter). *Lancet* **335**, 411.

Parving, H. H., Andersen, A. R., Smidt, U. M., and Svendsen, P. A. (1983). Early aggressive antihypertensive treatment reduces rate of decline in kidney function in diabetic nephropathy. *Lancet* **1**, 1175–1179.

Parving, H. H., Chaturvedi, N., Viberti, G., and Mogensen, C. E. (2002). Does microalbuminuria predict diabetic nephropathy? *Diabetes Care* **25**, 406–407.

Parving, H. H., Kastrup, J., Smidt, U. M., Andersen, A. R., Feldt-Rasmussen, B., and Christiansen, J. S. (1984). Impaired autoregulation of glomerular filtration rate in type 1 (insulin-dependent) diabetic patients with nephropathy. *Diabetologia* **27**, 547–552.

Parving, H. H., Lehnert, H., Bröchner-Mortensen, J., Gomis, R., Andersen, S., and Arner, P. (2001). The effect of irbesartan on the development of diabetic nephropathy in patients with type 2 diabetes. *New England Journal of Medicine* **345**, 870–878.

Parving, H. H., Oxenboll, B., Svendsen, P. A., Christiansen, J. S., and Andersen, A. R. (1982). Early detection of patients at risk of developing diabetic nephropathy. *Acta Endocrinologica* **100**, 550–555.

Parving, H. H., Rossing, P., Hommel, E., and Schmidt, U. M. (1995). Angiotensin converting enzyme inhibition in diabetic nephropathy: ten years experience. *American Journal of Kidney Diseases* **26**, 99–107.

Parving, H. H., Smidt, U. M., Friisberg, B., Bonnevie-Nielsen, V., and Andersen, A. R. (1981). A prospective study of glomerular filtration rate and arterial blood pressure in insulin-dependent diabetics with diabetic nephropathy. *Diabetologia* **20**, 457–461.

Parving, H. H. *et al.* (1976). The effect of metabolic regulation on microvascular permeability to small and large molecules in short-term juvenile diabetics. *Diabetologia* **12**, 161–166.

Parving, H. H. *et al.* (1988). Prevalence of microalbuminuria, arterial hypertension, retinopathy and neuropathy in patients with insulin-dependent diabetes. *British Medical Journal* **296**, 156–160.

Peters, H., Border, W. A., and Noble, N. A. (1998). Targeting TGF-beta overexpression in renal disease: maximising the antifibrotic action of angiotensin II blockade. *Kidney International* **54**, 1570–1580.

Praga, M. (2002). Obesity—a neglected culprit in renal disease. *Nephrology, Dialysis, Transplantation* **17** (7), 1157–1159.

Price, D. A., Porter, L. E., Gordon, M., Fisher, N. D., De'Oliveira, J. M., Laffel, L. M., Passan, D. R., Williams, G. H., and Hollenberg, N. K. (1999). The paradox of the low-renin-state in diabetic nephropathy. *Journal of the American Society of Nephrology* **10**, 2382–2391.

Prirart, J. (1978). Diabetes mellitus and its degenerative complications: a prospective study of 4400 patients observed between 1947 and 1973. *Diabetes Care* **1**, 168–188.

Ravid, M., Savin, H., Jutrin, I., Bental, T., Katz, B., and Lishner, M. (1993). Long-term stabilizing effect of angiotensin-converting enzyme inhibition on plasma creatinine and on proteinuria in normotensive type II diabetic patients. *Annals of Internal Medicine* **118**, 577–581.

Remuzzi, G. and Bertani, T. (1990). Is glomerulosclerosis a consequence of altered glomerular permeability to macromolecules? *Kidney International* **38**, 384–394.

Remuzzi, G., Schieppati, A., and Ruggenenti, P. (2002). Nephropathy in patients with type 2 diabetes. *New England Journal of Medicine* **346**, 1145–1151.

Ritz, E. and Stefanski, A. (1996). Diabetic nephropathy in type II diabetes. *American Journal of Kidney Diseases* **27**, 167–194.

Ritz, E., Rychlik, I., Locatelli, F., and Halimi, S. (1999). End-stage renal failure in type 2 diabetes: a medical catastrophe of worldwide dimensions. *American Journal of Kidney Diseases* **34**, 795–808.

Rossing, P. (1998). Promotion, prediction and prevention of progression in diabetic nephropathy. *Diabetic Medicine* **15** (11), 900–919.

Rossing, P., Hougaard, P., and Parving, H. H. (2002). Risk factors for development of incipient and overt diabetic nephropathy in type 1 diabetic patients: a 10-year prospective observational study. *Diabetes Care* **25**, 859–864.

Rudberg, S. and Dahlquist, G. (1996). Determinants of progression of microalbuminuria in adolescents with IDDM. *Diabetes Care* **19** (4), 369–371.

Rudberg, S., Osterby, R., Bangstad, H. J., Dahlquist, G., and Persson, B. (1999). Effect of angiotensin converting enzyme inhibitor or beta blocker on glomerular structural changes in young microalbuminuric patients with type I (insulin-dependent) diabetes mellitus. *Diabetologia* **42** (5), 589–595.

Sakurai, S., Yonekura, H., Yamamoto, Y., Watanabe, T., Tanaka, N., Li, H., Rahman, A. K., Myint, K. M., Kim, C. H., and Yamamoto, H. (2003). The AGE-RAGE system and diabetic nephropathy. *Journal of the American Society of Nephrology* **14** (Suppl. 3), S259–S263.

Sawicki, P. T., Didjurgeit, U., Muhlhauser, I., Bender, R., Heinemann, L., and Berger, M. (1994). Smoking is associated with progression of diabetic nephropathy. *Diabetes Care* **17**, 126–131.

Schmitz, A. and Vaeth, M. (1988). Microalbuminuria: a major risk factor in non-insulin-dependent diabetes. A 10-year follow-up study of 503 patients. *Diabetic Medicine* **5**, 126–134.

Schwenger, V., Mussig, C., Hergesell, O., Zeier, M., and Ritz, E. (2001). Incidence and clinical characteristics of renal insufficiency in diabetic patients. *Deutsche Medizinische Wochenschrift* **126**, 1322–1326.

Seaquist, E. R., Goetz, F. C., Rich, S., and Barbosa, J. (1989). Familial clustering of diabetic kidney disease. Evidence for genetic suspectibility to diabetic nephropathy. *New England Journal of Medicine* **320**, 1161–1165.

Sharma, K. and Ziyadeh, F. N. (1995). Hyperglycemia and diabetic kidney disease. The case for transforming growth factor-beta as a key mediator. *Diabetes* **44** (10), 1139–1146.

Shichiri, M., Kishikawa, H., Ohkubo, Y., and Wake, N. (2000). Long-term results of the Kumamoto Study on optimal diabetes control in type 2 diabetic patients. *Diabetes Care* **23**, S21–S29.

Skott, P. (1993). Lithium clearance in the evaluation of segmental renal tubular reabsorption of sodium and water in diabetes mellitus. *Danish Medical Bulletin* **41**, 23–37.

Smulders, Y. M., Rakic, M., Stehouwer, C. D., Weijers, R. N., Slaats, E. H., and Siberbusch, J. (1997). Determinants of progression of microalbuminuria in patients with NIDDM. A prospective study. *Diabetes Care* **20**, 999–1005.

Solini, A., Dalla, V. M., Saller, A., Nosadini, R., Crepaldi, G., and Fioretto, P. (2002). The angiotensin-converting enzyme DD genotype is associated with glomerulopathy lesions in type 2 diabetes. *Diabetes* **51**, 251–255.

Standl, E. and Schnell, O. (2000). A new look at the heart in diabetes mellitus: from ailing to failing. *Diabetologia* **43** (12), 1455–1469.

Steffes, M. W., Bilous, R. W., Sutherland, D. E. R., and Mauer, S. M. (1992). Cell and matrix components of the glomerular mesangium in type 1 diabetes. *Diabetes* **41**, 679–684.

Steffes, M. W., Schmidt, D., McCrery, R., and Basgen, J. M. (2001). Glomerular cell number in normal subjects and in type 1 diabetic patients. *Kidney International* **59**, 2104–2113.

Stehouwer, C. D. A., Lambert, J., Donker, A. J. M., and van Hinsbergh, V. W. M. (1997). Endothelial dysfunction and the pathogenesis of diabetic angiopathy. *Cardiovascular Research* **34**, 55–68.

Stephenson, J. M., Kenny, S., Stevens, L. K., Fuller, J. H., and Lee, E. (1995). Proteinuria and mortality in diabetes: the WHO multinational study of vascular disease in diabetes. *Diabetic Medicine* **12**, 149–155.

Strojek, K., Grzeszcak, W., Morawin, E., Adamski, M., Lacka, B., Rudzki, H., Schmidt, S., Keller, C., and Ritz, E. (1997). Nephropathy of type II diabetes: evidence for hereditary factors? *Kidney International* **51**, 1602–1607.

Taft, J. L., Nolan, C. J., Yeung, S. P., Hewitson, T. D., and Martin, F. I. R. (1994). Clinical and histological correlations of decline in renal function in diabetic patients with proteinuria. *Diabetes* **43**, 1046–1051.

The ACE Inhibitors in Diabetic Nephropathy Trialist Group (2001). Should all type 1 diabetic microalbuminuric patients receive ACE inhibitors? A meta-regression analysis. *Annals of Internal Medicine* **134**, 370–379.

The Diabetes Control and Complications Trial Research Group (1993). The effect of intensive treatment of diabetes on the development and progression of long-term complications in insulin-dependent diabetes mellitus. *New England Journal of Medicine* **329**, 977–986.

Toeller, M. *et al.* (1997). Protein intake and urinary albumin excretion in the EURODIAB IDDM Complications Study. *Diabetologia* **40**, 1219–1226.

UK Prospective Diabetes Study Group (1998). Tight blood pressure control and risk of macrovascular and microvascular complications in type 2 diabetes: UKPDS 38. *British Medical Journal* **317**, 703–713.

United States Renal Data System: (USRDS) (2001). National Institute of Diabetes and Digestive and Kidney Diseases. Annual Data Report, Bethesda. The National Institute of Health.

Van den Born, J., van Kraats, A. A., Bakker, M. A. H., Assmann, K. J. M., Dijkman, H. B. P. M., and Van der Laak, J. A. W. M. (1995). Reduction of heparan sulphate-associated anionic sites in the glomerular basement of rats with streptozotocin-induced diabetic nephropathy. *Diabetologia* **38**, 1169–1175.

Vardali, I., Baier, L. J., Hanson, R. L., Akkoyun, I., Fischer, C., Rohmeiss, P., Basci, A., Bartram, C. R., Van der Woude, F. J., and Janssen, B. (2002). Gene for susceptibility to diabetic nephropathy in type 2 diabetes maps to 18q22.3–23 **62**, 2176–2183.

Viberti, G., Wheeldon, N. M., and MicroAlbuminuria Reduction with VALsartan (MARVAL) Study Investigators (2002). Microalbuminuria reduction with valsartan in patients with type 2 diabetes mellitus: a blood pressure-independent effect. *Circulation* **106**, 671–678.

Viberti, G. C., Bilous, R. W., Mackintosh, D., and Keen, H. (1983). Monitoring glomerular function in diabetic nephropathy. *American Journal of Medicine* **74**, 256–264.

Viberti, G. C., Hill, R. D., Jarrett, R. J., Argyropoulos, A., Mahmud, U., and Keen, H. (1982). Microalbuminuria as a predictor of clinical nephropathy in insulin-dependent diabetes mellitus. *Lancet* **i**, 1430–1432.

Wagner, J., Gehlen, F., Ciechanowcz, A., and Ritz, E. (1999). Angiotensin II receptor type 1 gene expression in human glomerulonephritis and diabetes mellitus. *Journal of the American Society of Nephrology* **10**, 545–551.

Walker, J. D. *et al.* (1989). Restriction of dietary protein and progression of renal failure in diabetic nephropathy. *Lancet* **ii**, 1411–1415.

Wang, T. T., Wu, X. H., Zhang, S. L., and Chan, J. S. (1998). Effect of glucose on the expression of the angiotensinogen gene in opossum kidney cells. *Kidney International* **53**, 312–319.

White, K. E. and Bilous, R. W. (2000). Type 2 diabetic patients with nephropathy show structural–functional relationships that are similar to type 1 disease. *Journal of the American Society of Nephrology* **11**, 1667–1673.

Wierzbicki, A. S. (2002). Lipid lowering: another method of reducing blood pressure? *Journal of Human Hypertension* **16**, 753–760.

Wolf, G. and Ziyadeh, F. N. (1997). The role of angiotensin II in diabetic nephropathy: emphasised nonhemodynamic mechanisms. *American Journal of Kidney Diseases* **29** (1), 153–163.

Wolf, G., Chen, S., Han, D. C., and Ziyadeh, F. N. (2002). Leptin and renal disease. *American Journal of Kidney Diseases* **39** (1), 1–11.

Woods, L. L., Mizelle, H. L., and Hall, J. G. (1987). Control of renal hemodynamics in hyperglycemia. *American Journal of Physiology* **252**, F65–F73.

Wu, M. S. *et al.* (1997). Poor predialysis glycaemic control is a predictor of mortality in type II diabetic patients on maintenance haemodialysis. *Nephrology, Dialysis, Transplantation* **12**, 2105–2110.

Yokoyama, H. *et al.* (1997). Predictors of the progression of diabetic nephropathy and the beneficial effect of angiotensin-converting enzyme inhibitors in NIDDM patients. *Diabetologia* **40**, 405–411.

Zatz, R. and Brenner, B. M. (1986). Pathogenesis of diabetic microangiopathy. The hemodynamic view. *American Journal of Medicine* **80**, 443–453.

Zatz, R., Meyer, T. W., Rennike, H. G., and Brenner, B. M. (1985). Predominance of hemodynamic rather than metabolic factors in the pathogenesis of diabetic glomerulopathy. *Proceedings of the National Academy of Sciences USA* **82**, 5963–5967.

Zeller, K. R., Whittaker, E., Sullivan, L., Raskin, P., and Jacobson, H. R. (1991). Effect of restricting dietary protein on the progression of renal failure in patients with insulin-dependent diabetes mellitus. *New England Journal of Medicine* **324**, 78–84.

Ziyadeh, F. N. and Goldfarb, S. (1991). The renal tubulo-interstitium in diabetes mellitus. *Kidney International* **39**, 464–475.

Zoja, C., Benigni, A., and Remuzzi, G. (1999). Protein overload activates proximal tubular cells to release vasoactive and inflammatory mediators. *Experimental Nephrology* **7** (5–6), 420–428.

4.2 The patient with amyloid or immunotactoid glomerulopathy

4.2.1 Amyloidosis

Nicola Joss and Michael Boulton-Jones

Introduction

Rudolf Virchow is credited with describing and naming amyloid in 1854 while in Wurzburg, during a period of enforced political inactivity after his exertions in the revolution of 1848. Amyloid had probably been seen earlier and included in conditions of the liver covered by the adjectives *lardaceous* or *waxy*. Special stains were required to identify amyloid specifically, and it was the link between amyloid and the iodine–sulfuric acid reaction pattern which Virchow established. This, however, was not easy to use consistently and the next advance came with the introduction of the metachromatic stains derived from aniline dyes in 1875. These dyes had the property of changing colour when exposed to certain cellular structures. The ease with which they, and in particular dahlia or iodine-violet, identified amyloid quickly led to their widespread use and to recognition of some of the clinical syndromes with which amyloid was associated. The first report in which amyloid did not appear to be caused by an underlying infection is attributed to Wild in 1886, but it was not until 1929 that criteria were established to differentiate 'primary' and 'secondary' amyloidosis.

Congo red was discovered in 1883 and received its name after a conference held in Berlin in 1884–1885 to discuss the fate of the Congo in Africa. Although Congo red was used by histologists as soon as it was discovered, it was not until 1922 that its use in amyloid was recognized, first as a test of uptake following an intravenous injection, and then almost immediately as an histological stain. Six years later, the typical apple-green colour when viewed with polarized light was discovered, and this remains the hallmark of histological diagnosis.

Cohen first discovered the fibrillary nature of amyloid in 1959 shortly after electron microscopic (EM) techniques became available. The fibrils are 8–10 nm in diameter, of variable length, and do not branch. These characteristics comprise the second diagnostic criterion. Once methods had been developed for extracting and solubilizing the amyloid fibrils, it was possible to determine their structure and composition. In 1969, Cohen's group, using X-ray diffraction analysis, demonstrated that all types of amyloid shared a common structure in which the polypeptide backbone assumed a β-pleated sheet conformation and were orientated at right angles to the axis of the fibril. EM examination of tissue homogenates also led to the identification of a pentagonal structure about 9 nm in diameter derived from serum amyloid P protein.

It is striking that although amyloidogenic proteins are distinct with respect to their amino acid sequence, native folding, and function, the fibrils are structurally similar, and yet, each protein gives rise to a different syndrome. The reasons for their particular sites of deposition are largely unknown.

Definition

Amyloid is defined as an extracellular substance that stains apple-green with Congo red or Sirius red when viewed by birefringent light, and contains non-branching fibrils 8–10 nm in diameter when examined by EM. Either criterion is sufficient to make the diagnosis.

Classification

'Secondary amyloid' was the first form identified. This form occurred in patients with prolonged infections, such as osteomyelitis and tuberculosis. Some patients were identified who appeared to have no precipitating illness, and these were thought to have primary amyloid and the terms 'primary' and 'secondary' were used for 50 years. Patients with myeloma were known to have a syndrome identical to that associated with 'primary' amyloidosis and therefore this cause was said to lead to 'primary' amyloid, even though it was clearly 'secondary'. From the 1930s, the identification of families with amyloidosis causing different syndromes led to a separate group of inherited or familial amyloid syndromes, which were initially classified according to the clinical picture. Some forms of amyloid are localized to a single organ, but others are systemic.

The identification of the constituent proteins led to a new classification dependent on the protein involved (see Table 1 for details). Each is associated with a different clinical syndrome determined by the distribution of deposits. Twenty forms of amyloid have been recognized, some of which are rare, but others of which play a role in the pathogenesis of diseases affecting millions of patients.

Pathogenesis

Introduction

The mechanisms leading to amyloid deposition are under intense investigation. Certain clues are emerging and hypotheses being generated. All amyloid has a common conformation of the β-sheet when studied by X-ray diffraction. This conformation is made up of

Table 1 Classification of amyloidosis

Type	Protein	Organs affected	Clinical setting
Localized			
ACal	Calcitonin	Thyroid	Medullary carcinoma of the thyroid
AIAPP	Amylin (islet amyloid polypeptide)	Pancreas	Type 2 diabetes mellitus Insulinoma
AANF	Atrial natriuetic factor	Heart	Isolated atrial amyloid
Aβ	Aβ protein precursor	Brain	Alzheimer's disease Down syndrome
APro	Prolactin	Pituitary	Prolactinoma
APrP	Prion protein	Brain	Scrapie Creutzfeld Jacob Disease (CJD)
Senile			
ATTR	Transthyretin (wild type)	Heart	Senile cardiac amyloid
Systemic			
AA	Serum amyloid A	Kidneys, liver, spleen	Inflammatory disease, infection, and malignancy
AL	Light chain	Kidneys, heart, nerves	Multiple myeloma
AH	Heavy chain		Other plasma cell conditions
Aβ_2M	β_2 Microglobulin	Periarticular, ligaments	Long-term dialysis
Inherited			
AA	Serum amyloid A	Kidneys	FMF, Muckle–Wells, TRAPS
ATTR	Transthyretin (previously called prealbumin)	Nerves, heart	Familial amyloid polyneuropathy
ACys	Cystatin C	Cerebral arteries	Hereditary cerebral haemorrhage with amyloid (Icelandic)
AGel	Gelsolin	Eyes, cranial, and peripheral nerves	Finnish type familial amyloidosis
AFib	Fibrinogen Aα	Kidneys and liver	Hereditary non-neuropathic amyloidosis
AApoAI	Apolipoprotein AI	Kidneys and liver	Hereditary non-neuropathic and neuropathic amyloidosis
AApoAII	Apolipoprotein AII	Kidneys	Hereditary non-neuropathic amyloidosis
ALys	Lysozyme	Kidneys and liver	Hereditary non-neuropathic amyloidosis
Aβ	Aβ precursor protein	Cerebral arteries	Hereditary cerebral haemorrhage with amyloid (Dutch)

FMF, familial Mediterranean fever; TRAPS, tumour necrosis factor receptor antagonist periodic syndrome.

proteins bound parallel to each other by hydrogen bonds but with the *C*-terminal end of one protein next to the *N*-terminal end of its neighbours. The axis of these proteins is at right angles to the length of the fibril. It is this conformation which is responsible for the characteristic staining with Congo red. There is now some evidence about the circumstances in which proteins can be transformed in this way, but the mechanism varies from protein to protein.

1. *Proteolysis:* Some of the proteins recovered from amyloid fibrils are fragments of their parent protein. For example, AA protein is a proteolytic cleavage fragment from serum amyloid A (SAA). AL amyloid is made up of a fragment of light chains which includes the variable region. In other forms of amyloid, the deposited protein is identical to the circulating protein. A protein fragment may polymerize into the β-sheet conformation more readily because its secondary configuration is less stable than the complete molecule and more likely to refold in a way that leads to fibril formation.
2. *Increased availability:* Clinically significant amyloid is more likely to develop if its rate of formation is faster, which, in turn, is more likely to occur if the synthetic rate of the relevant protein is increased or, in the case of β_2 microglobulin, the excretion rate is reduced. A raised synthetic rate is not sufficient by itself since, for example, not all patients with inflammatory disease and raised SAA develop AA amyloidosis.
3. *Type of protein:* The properties of proteins capable of forming amyloid fibrils are unknown. It is interesting that 75 per cent of AL amyloid is derived from λ chains, whereas the amorphous deposits of light chain deposit disease (see Chapter 4.8) usually consist of κ chains. SAA1α appears more susceptible to amyloid transformation than the product of other alleles, at least in Caucasians.
4. *Mutation:* There are several examples of mutations causing a change in one amino acid that renders the protein amyloidogenic. These include all the familial forms of amyloidosis. In the

majority of these, the normal or wild form of the protein is not amyloidogenic.

Perhaps the most interesting example is that of *transthyretin*. The normal or wild form is associated with cardiac amyloidosis in a proportion of elderly subjects. Different point mutations in the molecule, of which more than 70 have been described, give rise to subtly different clinical syndromes. The exact mutation affects the principle site of deposits, the age of onset and the speed of progression of the disease. A mutation in the amino acid sequence on its own is not necessarily sufficient to result in amyloidosis as an identical mutation has been shown to be related to amyloid deposition in one kindred but not in another.

5. *Geographical factors:* It is difficult to separate genetic and environmental factors. AA amyloidosis is almost 10 times less common in patients with rheumatoid arthritis (RA) in the United States than in northern Europe. This has been attributed to a difference in treatment or to a different gene pool. However, the fact that AA amyloidosis associated with familial Mediterranean fever (FMF) is also less common in Armenians in the United States than in their kin in Eastern Europe makes either explanation less likely. It suggests that an environmental factor reduces the chances of a given individual developing this type of amyloid if he or she is raised in America. Another example is that the same genetic mutation of transthyretin occurs in several countries, but in the Swedish form the clinical onset is about 25 years later than the Portuguese or Japanese.

Assembly of fibrils

It has proved possible to make fibrils, which stain with Congo red and have the dimensions of amyloid on EM, from some of the parent proteins *in vitro*. The first success in this type of experiment came with light chains. In 1971, Glenner described how light chains exposed to trypsin yielded fragments which spontaneously formed fibrils with the properties of amyloid (Glenner *et al.* 1971). Twenty years later, tetrameric transthyretin was converted to a monomeric intermediary which spontaneously polymerized into a structure consistent with amyloid when the pH was reduced to 4 (Lai *et al.* 1996). There are several other examples. The major factors identified so far that contribute to fibril formation are the protein's amino acid sequence, oxidative stress (Hashimoto *et al.* 1999), pH (Ratnaswamy *et al.* 1999), ionic concentration (Mantyh *et al.* 1993), temperature, and the presence of associated proteins whose effect is described below.

The β-sheet configuration is unlikely to be the dominant conformation of most of the proteins that form amyloid, but it is a major component of the structure of the amyloid fibril. Therefore, the proteins comprising amyloid must undergo significant conformational change and/or partial degradation to form the fibril. Mutations or proteolysis produce forms which are more susceptible to this refolding and, in doing so, expose hydrophobic areas of the molecule which can coalesce together. In certain conditions, including super-saturation, these small polymers appear to form fibrils spontaneously. The process can be accelerated by seeding with small lengths of fibrils or by the poorly understood *amyloid enhancing factor* (Kisilevsky *et al.* 1992). Using techniques such as atomic force microscopy and X-ray diffraction, as well as EM, precursors to the fibrils have been demonstrated. Spherical aggregates are rearranged into beaded chains, which in turn form protofilaments and then the typical fibril. The transthyretin fibril, for example, consists of four protofilaments (Rochet and Lansbury 2000).

Other constituents

Amyloid deposits contain several other components, which may play a key role in fibril formation. These include collagen IV, laminin, and fibronectin, but the ones which have received most attention are serum amyloid P (SAP) (Hawkins *et al.* 1990), sulfated glycosaminoglycans (Kisilevsky and Fraser 1996) and apolipoprotein E.

Serum amyloid P is a normal serum glycoprotein produced in the liver and is a member of the pentraxin family. It was identified by extraction from amyloid material. Amyloid P (AP) component and SAP are identical and have a molecular weight of 25,000. Its functions are poorly understood. It is related to C-reactive protein (CRP) (Pepys *et al.* 1979), but is not an acute phase response protein in humans (as it is in mice). AP is a universal constituent of amyloid deposits and undergoes reversible calcium-dependent binding to all types of amyloid fibrils (Pepys and Dash 1977). AP has a tendency to form pentamers (MW 125,000), which appear like a pentagon on scanning EM, and comprises 15 per cent of the amyloid deposit.

AP may both enhance fibril formation and protect the formed fibrils from degradation. SAP has been shown to increase the amount of soluble, radiolabelled Aβ proteins precipitated *in vitro* in a calcium-dependent process and the amount precipitated varied with the dose of SAP added (Hamazaki 1995). This is consistent with the finding that AA amyloidosis formation in SAP knockout mice is slower than in normal animals (Botto *et al.* 1997). AP may protect amyloid fibrils from degradation *in vivo* by masking the abnormal fibrillar conformation that may otherwise trigger phagocytic clearance mechanisms (Emsley *et al.* 1994). This has been shown *in vitro*. Substances which can prevent or reverse the deposition of AP in amyloid deposits may offer a new approach to all forms of amyloidosis (Pepys *et al.* 2002).

Glycosaminoglycans are chains of repeating disaccharide units linked to a protein. That most commonly found in amyloid deposits is heparan sulfate proteoglycan (HSPG). It may interact with amyloid precursors and both enhance formation of and stabilize the formed β-pleated sheet. The dominant effect of HSPG is to influence proteins such as SAA and Aβ to undergo accelerated formation of β-pleated sheets (Kisilevsky and Fraser 1996), but it may also protect the fibril from proteolysis. It has been impossible to examine amyloidogenesis in heparan sulfate knockout mice because most animals die in gestation (Arikawa-Hirasawa *et al.* 1999).

Apolipoprotein E: ApoE4 was initially implicated in the development of Alzheimer's disease (Corder *et al.* 1993) where the protein was found in the senile plaques along with Aβ. Subsequently, apoE was found in all types of amyloid. Apo E knockout mice develop AA amyloidosis more slowly, again suggesting a role in pathogenesis (Bales *et al.* 1997).

Renal-specific factors

Renal amyloid is characterized by deposits found predominantly in the glomerular basement membrane, the subendothelial area and the extracellular mesangial system. This is the route of clearance of molecular debris deposited on the glomerular basement membrane. AA and AL amyloidosis are the most common forms causing renal disease and both are associated with protein overproduction. The precursor molecules have a molecular weight of 16 and 22 kDa respectively, and their molecular weight is such that they are filtered, but not quite freely. They will, therefore, be slowed in their passage through the glomerular capillary wall and have an opportunity to polymerize into fibrils. Once seeded, the process would accelerate.

Occasionally, tubular defects dominate the clinical picture. This presumably happens when filtered molecules are reabsorbed and extruded from the tubular cells in an amyloidogenic form. This may be the same mechanism that leads to dense deposits in κ chain nephropathy.

Diagnosis

Histological diagnosis

Amyloidosis can be diagnosed with certainty only by histological examination of tissue. Although the diagnosis is often suspected clinically, this is not always so, and all renal biopsies should be stained with Congo red or an equivalent stain. Any tissue biopsy may be used to confirm the diagnosis of amyloid. Kidney biopsies are positive for amyloid in over 90 per cent of cases of both AA and AL, whereas the diagnosis can be made by fat aspiration in 60–80 per cent, rectal biopsies in 50–70 per cent and skin biopsies in 50 per cent. Some advocate the use of fat aspiration or rectal biopsy as being less invasive and associated with fewer complications. However, if these less invasive tests are negative, a renal biopsy will still be required to determine the cause of proteinuria or renal failure. We, therefore, believe that renal biopsy is the investigation of choice in any patient suspected of amyloidosis who has renal abnormalities.

Renal biopsies acquired a reputation for being dangerous in patients with amyloidosis, supposedly as a result of stiff small blood vessels and subtle coagulation disorders (see below) which made postbiopsy haemorrhage more common and more severe. If this was ever true, most clinicians think the risk of complications is not increased with new techniques using direct ultrasound guidance and an automated Biopty© gun, rather than conventional Tru cut© or Beckton–Dickenson needles.

Adequate tissue specimens and skilled histological technique are necessary to maintain a high diagnostic sensitivity and specificity. However, a negative renal biopsy does not absolutely exclude the diagnosis of amyloidosis. Additional and alternative renal pathology may coexist in patients, particularly with AA amyloidosis. Mesangial proliferative and crescentic nephritis, often Henoch–Schönlein purpura, have been seen in FMF, while membranous and diabetic nephropathy can coexist with AA amyloidosis.

Light microscopy

The presence of amyloid is suggested by the appearance of amorphous, pink hyaline material in tissue sections which are stained with haematoxylin and eosin (Fig. 1a). The extracellular deposits are usually found in glomeruli and small arteries and arterioles of the kidney. The glomerular deposits are often mesangial, and can produce a lobulated appearance suggestive of mesangiocapillary glomerulonephritis or diabetic nephropathy. In contrast to these two conditions, however, the deposited material is negative on staining with silver methenamine. The amyloid is usually found also along the glomerular capillary

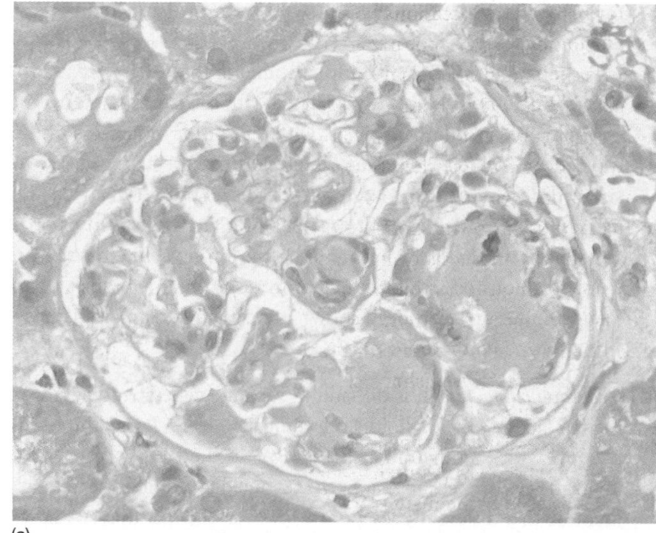

(a)

(b)

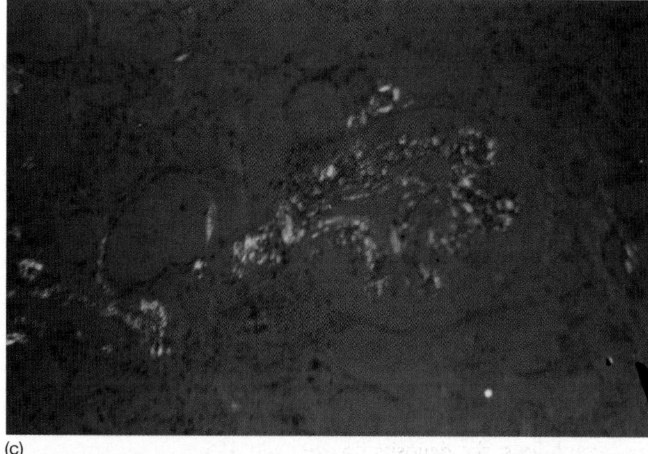

(c)

Fig. 1 (a) Haematoxylin and eosin (H&E) 250× in original magnification. Large eosinophilic deposits are present in the mesangium. The distribution of the deposits are asymmetrical. (b) Congo red staining of glomerulus viewed by normal light, 250×. The amyloid deposits are easily detected by uptake of Congo red, but this is not specific for amyloid. (c) Congo red staining of glomerulus viewed by birefringent light, 250×. The green colour is specific for amyloid.

walls, where it may occasionally evoke extracapillary spicular protrusions forming a 'brush' appearance, reminiscent on silver staining of the 'spikes' seen in membranous nephropathy, but longer and more irregular (Shiiki *et al.* 1989). Rarely, peritubular deposits are found, or even predominate. Small and medium-sized blood vessels within the kidney, may be infiltrated as elsewhere in the body, and again this site may rarely be predominant, with little glomerular involvement (Grcevska and Polenakovic 1993). After Congo red staining, the deposits appear red under normal conditions of light microscopy (Fig. 1b) and show the characteristic apple-green birefringence under polarized light (Fig. 1c). The best way to view the birefringence is to cut tissue sections of 6–8 μm rather than the usual 2–3 μm. Modifications of the Congo red method have been attempted to distinguish between AL and AA amyloid; these include pretreatment with potassium permanganate which causes the fibrils in AA, but not AL amyloidosis, to lose their affinity for Congo red. This test, however, is unreliable and has been made obsolete by the use of immunohistochemistry.

Immunohistochemistry

Immunohistochemistry is the most reliable way to distinguish between the various types of amyloid. Antisera to most fibril precursor proteins conjugated with fluorescein or peroxidase are commercially available. Immunohistochemistry gives reliable results in AA (Fig. 2a), transthyretin, and β2 microglobulin amyloidosis. It is less reliable in AL amyloidosis (Fig. 2b), since staining with λ and κ light chain antibodies gives positive results in only about 50 per cent of cases. This is because the fibrils are made up of the variable region of light chains, whereas the specificity of the antisera is usually directed at the constant regions. Therefore, the diagnosis of AL amyloidosis is often made by inference if the staining for AA amyloid is negative. This is a fair assumption, particularly if the patient has a monoclonal band on serum or urine electrophoresis. However, rare inherited causes of renal amyloidosis, which also result in negative AA staining, may be misdiagnosed. In one study, 10 per cent of 350 patients diagnosed as AL amyloidosis turned out to have an inherited form of amyloidosis, usually involving a mutation of fibrinogen A α-chain or transthyretin. Surprisingly, a low-grade monoclonal gammopathy was detected in nearly a quarter of these misdiagnosed patients, but none had light chains in the urine. None had a clear family history (Lachmann *et al.* 2002). If this experience were to be confirmed, the diagnostic criteria for AL amyloidosis may have to include genotyping in those with no light chain deposits in the glomeruli and no light chains in the urine.

Electron microscopy

By EM, amyloid deposits randomly orientated non-branching fibrils with a diameter of 8–10 nm (Fig. 3). In addition to the fibrils, EM also demonstrates the pentagonal amyloid P component of amyloid deposits. Fibrils are found in the glomeruli in other conditions. These include fibrillary/immunotactoid glomerulopathy (see Chapter 4.2.2), fibronectin glomerulopathy, and (rarely) diabetic nephropathy. In these conditions, the deposits do not stain with Congo red and the diameter of the fibrils is larger.

Problems with histological diagnosis

The unavoidable problem of sampling error means that biopsies may give false negative results. False positive results are rare if green staining with Congo red is identified using polarized light. Red staining with Congo or Sirius red is not as reliable because other tissues such as elastic fibres and collagen take up the stain. However, they do not stain green when viewed by polarized light.

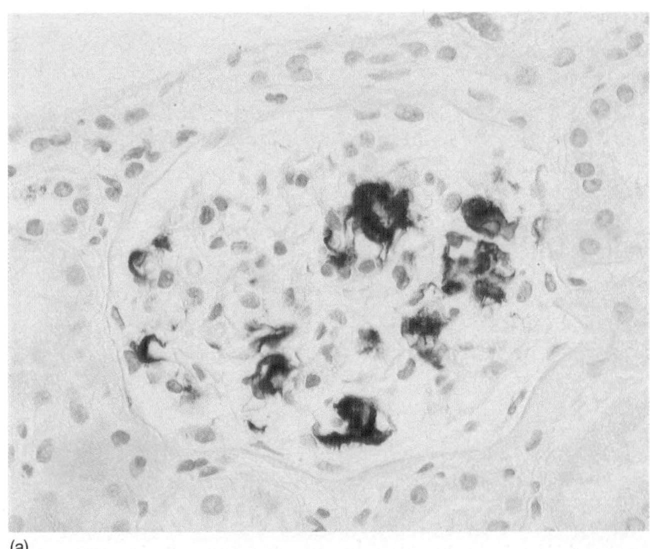

(a)

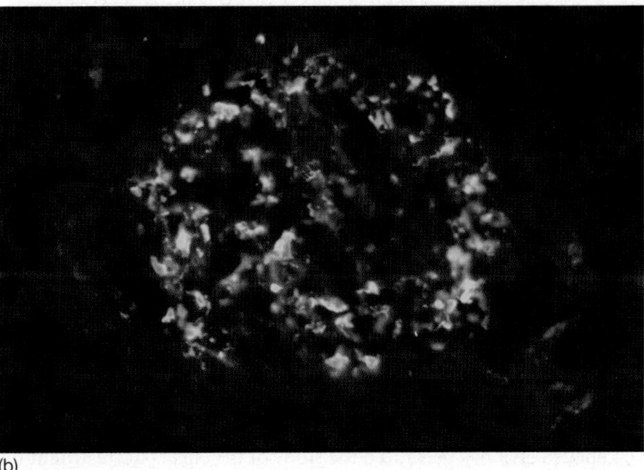

(b)

Fig. 2 (a) Immunohistochemical staining of glomerulus with antibody to amyloid A protein (original magnification 250×). The deposits of AA amyloid are in both the mesangium and the capillary walls. The antibody is tagged with alkaline phosphatase. (b) Staining of glomerulus with antibody to AL protein. This has been achieved on a frozen section using an antibody to λ light chain labelled with fluorescein.

Biopsies generally provide small samples of tissue and do not reveal the extent or distribution of amyloid. They are unsuitable for regular follow up of patients either to determine the natural history or to determine the response to treatment or transplantation.

Serum amyloid P scintigraphy

The finding that all amyloid deposits contain SAP led to the development of radiolabelled SAP as a tracer for targeting amyloid deposits *in vivo*. Radiolabelled ^{123}I-SAP is rapidly catabolized and excreted in patients without amyloidosis, but is taken up by the deposits in proportion to the amount of amyloid present (Fig. 4).

SAP scintigraphy is an exciting diagnostic tool. It has provided important observations in amyloidosis, including the demonstration

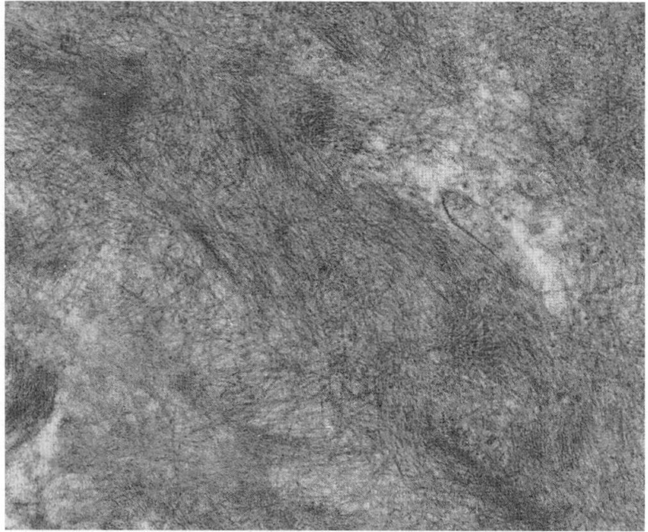

Fig. 3 EM view of amyloid fibrils in glomerular basement membrane and mesangium (30,000×). The fibrils are present throughout the GBM and are 8–10 nm in diameter and are arranged randomly.

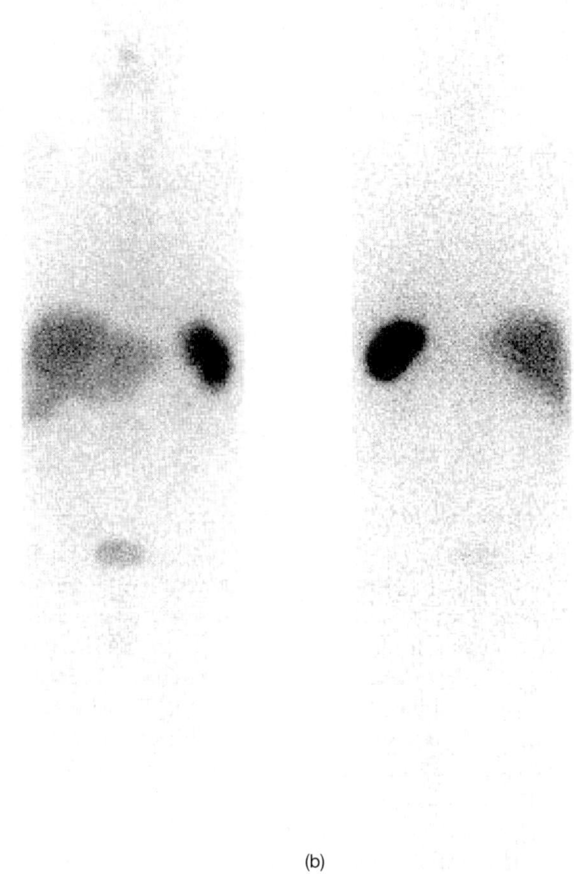

(a) (b)

Fig. 4 SAP scan of patient with AL amyloidosis showing uptake in spleen and liver. (a) Anterior and (b) posterior views.

of amyloid in sites not available for biopsy and that there is often a poor correlation between quantity of amyloid and the degree of organ dysfunction. SAP scintigraphy is both specific and sensitive for the evaluation of tissue distribution in AA amyloidosis. However, in a series of 100 patients with AL amyloidosis, positive scans were obtained in only 85 per cent of cases with histologically proven disease, and cardiac deposits were not consistently identified (Vigushin *et al.* 1994). SAP scintigraphy has also been used in dialysis-related amyloidosis, but shoulder deposits were not regularly identified (Nelson *et al.* 1991).

Labelled SAP has permitted the study of the effects of treatment on amyloid deposits. Until recently, it was thought that the deposition of amyloid was irreversible; SAP scintigraphy has now demonstrated regression of amyloid deposits following treatment in AL amyloidosis, AA amyloidosis (Gillmore *et al.* 2001a), dialysis-related amyloidosis (Tan *et al.* 1996), and transthyretin and apolipoprotein AI amyloidosis (Holmgren *et al.* 1993; Gillmore *et al.* 2000). This proves that the deposits are in a state of dynamic turnover.

Biopsy remains the gold standard of clinical practice, but has the disadvantage of requiring an invasive procedure with a variable false negative rate. SAP scintigraphy is not entirely specific and is available in only a few centres. They should be regarded as complementary diagnostic tools.

AA amyloidosis

Introduction

In modern times, AA amyloidosis (or 'secondary' amyloidosis as it was previously known), is a relatively rare disease in developed countries. A cause is usually found easily (Table 2), but may sometimes remain obstinately obscure. The most common chronic inflammatory conditions leading to AA amyloidosis in developed countries are juvenile chronic arthritis (JCA), RA, and ankylosing spondylitis. Amyloidosis is exceptionally rare in systemic lupus erythematosus, polymyalgia rheumatica, and ulcerative colitis, which probably reflects the modest rise in SAA associated with these conditions. Recently described associations include AA amyloidosis complicating cystic fibrosis and skin abscesses secondary to subcutaneous abuse of heroin. In the developing world, AA amyloidosis remains relatively common because chronic infections are still rife, in particular, tuberculosis, leprosy, and osteomyelitis.

The causes of AA amyloidosis have changed in developed countries over the last 40 years. Table 3 highlights the change from chronic infections to chronic rheumatological disorders which occurred around the 1960s. This change is a consequence of better treatment of chronic infections, and in particular, the elimination of tuberculosis as a cause of severe lung disease. The second finding is that AA amyloidosis appears to be much less common in America. Sixty-four patients were identified over a 33-year period in the Mayo clinic, while 75 patients were identified in a 12-year period in Bristol. A surprising finding was that there were no cases of tuberculosis in the Mayo series (Gertz and Kyle 1991).

Malignancies, particularly Hodgkin's disease and renal cell carcinoma, are much cited causes of AA amyloidosis. In practice, this association is rare: only five cases were reported in 219 cases (2 per cent) from 4 series (Triger and Joekes 1973; Browning *et al.* 1985; Gertz and Kyle 1991; Joss *et al.* 2000).

Epidemiology

It is difficult to obtain accurate figures for the incidence and prevalence of AA amyloidosis in the general population. Most information comes from autopsy data in which the prevalence varies between 0.53 and 0.86 per cent of unselected post mortems (Cohen 1968; Lofberg *et al.* 1987). Amyloid is found in about 2.5 per cent of renal biopsies, but this includes both AA and AL amyloidosis. The ratio of AA to AL amyloid is approximately 2 : 1 in our renal biopsy series and only slightly less in a German one (Bohle *et al.* 1993). AA amyloidosis was found in 0.76 per cent of renal biopsies in France (Chevrel *et al.* 2001). It is found more frequently in the elderly, in whom renal AL amyloid is one of the commoner causes of the nephrotic syndrome (see Chapter 1.5). None of these figures, however, gives any indication of the prevalence in the general population.

There is a startling difference in the frequency of AA amyloidosis worldwide among patients with chronic rheumatological disorders. In the United Kingdom, amyloidosis was found in 7.4 per cent of patients with JCA after 15 years (David *et al.* 1993), which is many times more than the 0.1 per cent recorded in equivalent patients in the United States. The highest prevalence (10.6 per cent) was reported in Polish patients (Filipowicz-Sosnowska *et al.* 1978).

Similar differences apply to AA amyloidosis complicating rheumatoid arthritis. Rates in post mortem series from the 1940s to 1960s ranged from 0 to 60 per cent (see Kennedy *et al.* 1974 for references). The highest prevalence was found in Finland, but there is more recent evidence of a substantial reduction from 60 to 5 per cent. (Myllykangas-Luosujarvi *et al.* 1999). This was corroborated by a fall in the percentage of positive biopsies in a hospital for rheumatic diseases from 10 to 5 per cent between 1987 and 1997 (Laiho *et al.* 1999) and by a reduction in the number of patients with amyloidosis taken onto dialysis in the last 12 years (see below). Other countries have failed to show such a dramatic reduction: for example, a recent study of Japanese patients with RA found no change in the frequency of AA amyloidosis between 1979–1988 and 1989–1996 (Nakano *et al.* 1998).

Thus, the causes of AA amyloidosis have altered from chronic infections to chronic rheumatological disorders in developed countries (Table 3). Interestingly, it appears to complicate similar diseases in Europe, Japan, and the United States, although with different levels of penetration. The incidence may be falling in Europe to the low levels found throughout the twentieth century in the United States. Chronic infection remains the major cause of AA amyloidosis in the developing world, principally tuberculosis, leprosy, and osteomyelitis.

Table 2 Conditions associated with AA amyloidosis

Chronic inflammatory diseases
Rheumatoid arthritis
Juvenile chronic arthritis
Ankylosing spondylitis
Psoriatic arthritis
Reiter's syndrome
Behçet's syndrome
Adult Still's disease
Crohn's disease
Chronic infections
Tuberculosis
Leprosy
Osteomyelitis
Bronchiectasis
Decubitus ulcers
Malignancies
Hodgkin's lymphoma
Castleman's disease
Renal cell carcinoma
Hairy cell leukaemia
Inherited
Familial Mediterranean fever
Muckle–Wells syndrome
TRAPS

Pathogenesis

AA protein was isolated from amyloid fibrils in 'reactive' systemic amyloidosis in 1971 (Benditt and Eriksen 1971). The AA protein is a proteolytic cleavage fragment of the circulating acute phase reactant SAA. Small variations in size and isoelectric points have been found in these fragments (Westermark 1982). SAA is mainly synthesized by

Table 3 Changes in causes of AA amyloidosis

Time period	Country	Number of patients	Chronic rheumatological disorders (%)	Chronic infections (%)
1949 (autopsy study)	America	30	7	63
1973 (1957–1970)	England	37	11	68
1974 (1963–1973)	Scotland	40	27	54
1985 (1973–1982)	England	75	73	17
1991 (1959–1989)	America	64	65	17
1994 (not given)	Holland	91	61	14
2000 (1985–1999)	Scotland	43	70	14

hepatocytes regulated by cytokines, in particular IL-1, IL-6, and tumour necrosis factor (TNF). The serum concentration can increase from less than 10 mg/l to over 1000 mg/l within 24–48 h of active inflammation. Other sites of synthesis include macrophages, atherosclerotic smooth muscle cells and synovium of rheumatoid joints.

SAA is an apolipoprotein, predominately associated with high-density lipoprotein particles. Its functions include upregulation of adhesion molecules (Preciado-Patt *et al.* 1996) and inhibition of platelet aggregation (Zimlichman *et al.* 1990). It is a chemotactic agent for inflammatory cells (Badolato *et al.* 1994) and activates neutrophils (Badolato *et al.* 2000). SAA also has cytokine like properties (Patel *et al.* 1998) and has been found to induce metalloproteinase production (Migita *et al.* 1998). Therefore, SAA may be actively involved in inflammatory disease processes.

There are four SAA genes located on chromosome 11. SAA1 and SAA2 are upregulated in the presence of inflammation, SAA3 is a pseudogene with no protein product and SAA4 is not up-regulated in response to inflammation. Three alleles of SAA1 ($\alpha\beta\gamma$) and two of SAA2 ($\alpha\beta$) have been described. SAA1 is the predominant isoform of SAA in AA amyloidosis. SAA1α and SAA1γ alleles differ at only one base and there is a difference in frequency of SAA1 alleles between races. All three alleles appear equally in the Japanese population, while the α allele is dominant in Caucasians. Certain polymorphisms in SAA1 have recently been found to be associated with an increased likelihood of developing AA amyloidosis. Homozygosity for the γ allele is a significant risk factor for AA amyloidosis in Japanese patients with RA (Moriguchi *et al.* 1999). In Caucasians with JCA and AA amyloidosis, there is a greater frequency of the SAA1α allele and in particular an increase in the homozygous SAA1α/SAA1α genotype. This is sufficiently marked for one group to recommend earlier and more intensive anti-inflammatory therapy in rheumatoid patients with the SAA1α genotype to reduce the probability of developing AA amyloid (Booth *et al.* 1998). The value of this advice remains unproven.

Long-standing inflammation and raised SAA concentrations are required for the development of AA amyloidosis, but they are not sufficient in isolation. The reason why only a small proportion of patients with a persistent acute phase response develop amyloidosis remains unclear. SAA concentrations are increased equally in rheumatoid patients with or without amyloidosis, but the type and size of the fragments of SAA may determine their amyloidogenic potential and site of deposition. Fragments of 4.5 and 6 kDa are found at higher concentrations in patients with RA and AA amyloidosis compared to patients with RA without amyloidosis despite similar SAA concentration. Fragments causing vascular deposits are of different size to fragments causing deposits in other sites (Westermark 1982).

Clinical findings and course

The natural history of untreated AA amyloidosisis is progressive, resulting in organ failure and death. The age at presentation depends on the nature of the underlying inflammatory disease. The latency between the onset of the inflammatory disease and clinical evidence of amyloidosis is usually about 15–18 years; however, it can be as short as 18 months or more than 30 years. AA amyloid deposition may be extensive without causing symptoms. Females are more often affected, reflecting the female bias in chronic rheumatological conditions. Clinical history and general examination of the patient rarely fails to reveal the cause, but elderly and Asian patients with AA amyloidosis may reveal evidence of prior tuberculosis only on radiography.

Renal findings

Renal involvement is the most common and most serious problem (Browning *et al.* 1985). The clinical manifestations vary with the site of the deposits in the kidney. The majority of patients have glomerular deposits resulting in proteinuria, which can vary from minimal asymptomatic proteinuria to an extreme nephrotic syndrome. The urine sediment is generally benign. Haematuria is present in about one-third of our patients on dipstick testing. Casts are rarely found. Extensive vascular deposits (Fig. 5) can result in chronic renal insufficiency with little proteinuria (Falck *et al.* 1983a). Tubular deposits are rare, but may cause any of the syndromes of tubular dysfunction. Massive glomerular amyloid infiltration is associated with little or no proteinuria in 5 per cent of cases, and nephrotic range proteinuria can occur even when amyloid is minimal on light microscopy (Fig. 6). Although it was originally believed that kidney size was increased in amyloidosis, it is usually normal and may decrease as renal failure progresses.

The rate of progression of renal failure from diagnosis was rapid at 1 ml/min/month in our series. It correlates with SAA concentration and the degree of albuminuria (Falck *et al.* 1983b; Joss *et al.* 2000). Occasionally, renal failure may be acute, as the Victorian physicians such as Dickinson knew with their huge experience of the condition. One patient presented with the nephrotic syndrome and a glomerular filtration rate (GFR) of 20 ml/min, only 6 weeks after the start of joint/bone sepsis from a neglected penetrating wound, which allowed accurate dating of onset. Treatment arrested, but did not reverse the condition (personal communication J.S. Cameron). Historically, renal failure was the predominant cause of death in patients with AA amyloidosis but this has changed with the wider availability of renal replacement therapy (see below).

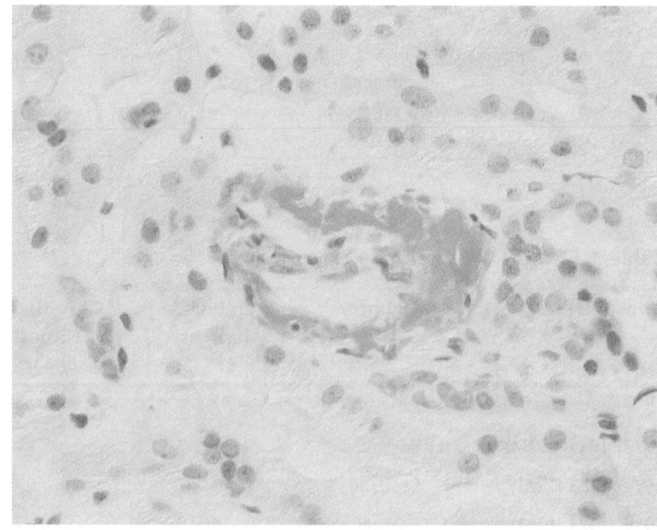

Fig. 5 Amyloid in renal arteriole (H&E 400×). Congo red stain showing a large deposit of amyloid (in this case AA amyloid) in an afferent glomerular arteriole.

Non-renal findings

Although the kidney is the organ that is most often affected and causes the most serious consequences, amyloid deposits in other sites can be important. The spleen is affected early and may lead to functional hyposplenism. The adrenal glands are infiltrated in approximately one-third of cases, and clinically significant adrenal suppression may occur and contribute to morbidity and mortality. Abnormal synacthen tests are found in 50 per cent. Amyloid is frequently deposited in the liver and hepatomegaly may be the presenting feature. Gastrointestinal disease may result from mucosal infiltration, neuromuscular infiltration or autonomic neuropathy. Mucosal lesions may cause gastrointestinal bleeding while chronic intestinal dysmotility may result in dysphagia, gastroparesis, malabsorption, and constipation. Amyloid deposition in the heart may occur in AA amyloid, but in sharp contrast to AL amyloid, generally does not cause clinical symptoms. The symptoms, on the rare occasions that they do occur, are related to restrictive cardiomyopathy and/or conduction defects. Glandular amyloid deposition can also occur, resulting in hypothyroidism and panhypopituitarism. Skin involvement, macroglossia, and peripheral neuropathy are seldom reported in AA amyloidosis.

The distribution of deposits is perhaps best demonstrated by SAP scintigraphy. AA amyloid was found in the spleen in all 80 patients, kidneys in 70 patients, adrenal glands in 46 patients, and the liver in 10 patients (Gillmore *et al.* 2001a). Autopsy studies in patients with AA amyloidosis have demonstrated amyloid deposits in kidneys and adrenal glands in all patients while gastrointestinal and hepatic deposits were an almost universal finding (Browning *et al.* 1985).

Table 4 highlights the main clinical findings in five major series. Note the higher cardiac and lower renal involvement in Japanese patients compared to American or Europeans.

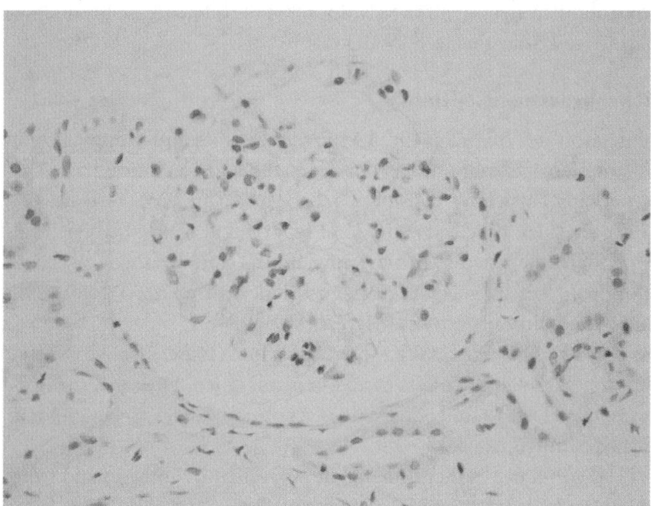

Fig. 6 Minimal amyloid deposits in a patient with AA amyloidosis secondary to rheumatoid arthritis who had severe nephrotic syndrome. Congo red, 250×.

Natural history

The long-term prognosis of untreated AA amyloidosis is usually poor. Prognosis is related to the degree of renal involvement and the diagnosis is often not made until substantial organ infiltration has occurred. Reports from renal units give a median survival between 24 and 31 months from the time of diagnosis, with one report quoting a median survival of only 18 months from when the serum creatinine reaches 150 μmol/l (Lindqvist *et al.* 1989). We found a median patient survival from time of diagnosis of 51 months (Joss *et al.* 2000) with a 5-year survival of 43 per cent. This compares to only 5 per cent in our previous series from 30 years ago (Kennedy *et al.* 1974). The improvement reflects in large part the increased availability of dialysis. In none of these series were details of treatment given, and most patients were probably given no specific treatment, apart from treatment of sepsis when required. Reports from rheumatological units do specify treatment and better survival was found in untreated patients with JCA who had a 5-year survival of 50 per cent, than in untreated RA patients, in whom the 5-year survival was only 27 per cent (Ahlmen *et al.* 1987; David *et al.* 1993).

In early studies, renal failure was the cause of death in 70 per cent of cases (David *et al.* 1993). Other common causes include infection, bowel perforation, gastrointestinal bleeding, and myocardial infarction (Janssen *et al.* 1986; Okuda *et al.* 1994). With the wider availability of renal replacement therapy, infection has replaced renal failure as the leading cause of death (48 per cent in our recent series). Amyloidosis as a cause of death in patients with JCA has fallen between 1969–1979 and 1980–1990; probably because of more intensive treatment of the later patients (Savolainen and Isomaki 1993).

Table 4 Clinical findings in AA amyloidosis (figures indicate percentage)

	America (Gertz and Kyle *et al.* 1991)	UK (Browning 1985)	Holland (Janssen *et al.* 1986)	Japan (Okuda *et al.* 1994)	UK (David *et al.* 1993)
Associated conditions	Mixed	Mixed	RA	RA	JCA
Renal involvement	91	75	85	56.9	100
Hepatomegaly	5	4	19	NK	21.5
GI disturbance	22	5	24	58.1	Diarrhoea 12.6
Cardiac	0	0	9	39.5	NK

RA, rheumatoid arthritis; JCA, juvenile chronic arthritis; NK, not known.

Factors which correlate with death or dialysis, have varied from study to study. A raised plasma creatinine, low serum albumin, high urinary protein, raised SAA, and CRP concentrations have been important in determining outcome in some studies (Joss *et al.* 2000; Gillmore *et al.* 2001a).

Treatment

The current treatment strategy in AA amyloidosis is to eliminate the supply of the precursor protein (SAA) by suppressing the acute phase response. This stops further amyloid deposition and may cause resorbtion of existing deposits.

There are several reports of dramatic responses following surgical resection of the underlying cause of amyloidosis. These include amputation of limbs affected by osteomyelitis, resection of Castelman's tumour, resection of bowel in Crohn's disease, and resection of renal cell carcinoma. Thus, removal of the cause may reverse proteinuria and renal failure to some extent. Unfortunately, these cases are exceptional today in the developed world, and medical treatment of the now more usual chronic inflammatory conditions is the standard approach.

Anti-inflammatory treatment

Alkylating agents are effective treatment for AA amyloidosis associated with chronic rheumatological conditions (Schnitzer and Ansell 1977; Falck *et al.* 1980; Ahlmen *et al.* 1987; Berglund *et al.* 1993; David *et al.* 1993; Chevrel *et al.* 2001). The trials which support this claim can be criticized for design flaws such as the use of historical controls and heterogeneity of the specific treatment used. Despite these criticisms, they are consistent in supporting the use of immunosuppressive agents. The response to treatment is generally defined in terms of organ function and patient survival rather than histological information of amyloid resorption, which is rarely available and difficult to interpret. Repeated SAP scanning has, however, confirmed that the amyloid load is reduced in some of these patients.

Chlorambucil has been used in patients with JCA since the early 1960s and considerable experience has been obtained with it (Schnitzer and Ansell 1977). Ten year survival increased to 80 per cent compared to 23.5 per cent for the untreated controls (David *et al.* 1993). The control patients were either from the prechlorambucil era or had refused treatment.

The use of chlorambucil or cyclophosphamide was examined in 14 patients with chronic rheumatological disorders (majority of patients had RA) in 22 treatment periods. Renal function improved, stabilized or deteriorated more slowly in 19/22 treatment periods. A 5-year survival figure of 93 per cent and a 10-year figure of 75 per cent was achieved (Berglund *et al.* 1993).

Oral daily cyclophosphamide and prednisolone (Falck *et al.* 1980) and pulsed intravenous cyclophosphamide (Chevrel *et al.* 2001) have proved remarkably effective in small trials. The median survival was 46 months in the untreated group and 165 months in the treated group (Chevrel *et al.* 2001).

There is only one randomized prospective trial that compared immunosuppressive treatment in 11 patients with AA amyloidosis complicating RA with 11 control patients. The treatment used was mainly podophylotoxin, a microtubule antagonist, but also included azathioprine, chlorambucil, and cyclophosphamide. Four patients received more than one treatment. Five-year survival was 89 per cent in the treated group and 27 per cent in the untreated group. Endstage renal disease occurred in two treated patients and in seven untreated patients (Ahlmen *et al.* 1987).

These studies are consistent in achieving a 5-year survival rate greater than 70 per cent with treatment compared to less than 30 per cent without (see Table 5). Although the use of immunosuppressive drugs causes infertility and increases the risk of malignancy in later life, they control inflammation effectively, suppress the acute phase production of SAA and delay the need for dialysis.

Other treatment options

The effect of *colchicine* in AA amyloidosis complicating chronic inflammatory conditions has not been studied in a clinical trial. This is perhaps surprising considering its efficacy in FMF (see below). However, there have been anecdotal reports that it may be beneficial, which include patients with AA amyloidosis complicating ankylosing spondylitis (Escalante *et al.* 1991), psoriatic arthropathy (Kagan *et al.* 1999), and ulcerative colitis (Meyers *et al.* 1988).

Dimethlysulfoxide (DMSO) has been shown to be effective in some reports, although the mode of action is unknown. However, the drug is associated with a foul odour and is very unpopular with patients and this has limited its use.

TNF-α plays a pathogenic role in inflammatory diseases and stimulates the production of SAA. The use of TNF-α antagonists may offer a new approach to the management of AA amyloidosis complicating inflammatory diseases (Camussi and Lupia 1998). Trials of anti-TNF-α in patients with RA have shown that the treatment is generally well tolerated with significant reductions in indices of disease activity

Table 5 Summary of treatment studies in AA amyloidosis

Authors	Cause	Number	Treatment	Control	Survival
David *et al.* (1993)	JCA	79	Chlorambucil ($n = 57$)	Nil ($n = 17$)	80 versus 23.5% at 10 years
Berglund *et al.* (1993)	Adult arthritis	14	Chlorambucil/ cyclophosphamide	No control group	75% at 10 years
Ahlmen *et al.* (1987)	RA	22	Various ($n = 11$)	Nil ($n = 11$)	89 versus 27% at 5 years
Chevrel *et al.* (2001)	RA	15	Pulsed cyclophosphamide ($n = 6$)	Nil ($n = 9$)	75 versus 22% at 5 years

RA, rheumatoid arthritis; JCA, juvenile chronic arthritis.

including IL-6, CRP, and SAA (Charles *et al.* 1999). However, long-term risks and benefits of these drugs are not yet known.

A new approach to treatment designed to strip out the AP component of amyloid deposits using *carboxy-pyrrolidin-hexanoyl-pyrrolidine-carboxylic acid* (CPHPC) has been described (Pepys *et al.* 2002).

In conclusion, the aim of treatment is to switch off the inflammatory process and keep SAA and CRP concentrations as close to normal as possible. However, supportive treatment is also important. Nephrotic syndrome can be treated by the usual non-specific measures (see Chapter 3.4). It is probable that angiotensin-converting enzyme (ACE) inhibitors have the same advantage in amyloid as in other causes of profuse proteinuria. Renal failure has been successfully treated with dialysis or transplantation (see below).

Monitoring

Prospective studies have shown the disease to be progressive in nearly all patients with a sustained acute phase response, although the rate varies both among individuals and among different organs in the same individual. If the acute phase response is controlled, SAP scintigraphy has demonstrated stabilization or regression of amyloid deposits (Gillmore *et al.* 2001a).

Measurement of serial SAA concentrations and serial SAP scintigraphy may provide a guide to the adequacy of treatment. SAA concentrations have been shown to be higher in patients whose amyloid deposits continued to accumulate. The 10 year survival of patients with SAA concentrations more than 10 mg/l was 40 per cent whereas it was 90 per cent in those whose SAA level was persistently less than 10 mg/l (Gillmore *et al.* 2001a). The closely related and more available CRP may be able to serve the same purpose.

Renal replacement therapy

Renal replacement programmes have improved the prognosis of patients with AA amyloidosis. The question of continuing immunosuppressive treatment for patients with no renal function is difficult. Renal failure is the most significant, but not the only clinical consequence of AA amyloidosis. Once on dialysis, there is no purpose in continuing treatment of which the major objective was renal protection, unless extra-renal amyloidosis becomes clinically significant without it. However, a major cause of death in patients with AA amyloidosis on dialysis is infection. Therefore, care must be taken when using immunosuppressive agents. Extra-renal amyloidosis is less likely to occur after renal transplantation as antirejection treatment may also control the chronic inflammatory condition. Recurrence of amyloid in the transplanted kidney can occur but is seldom clinically significant (see below).

Conclusion

The causes of AA amyloidosis are changing, particularly in developed countries. There is evidence that the incidence is falling in Finland, which had the highest rate. No good controlled trials have been conducted, but the evidence that immunosuppression improves prognosis is circumstantial but consistent. Serial measurements of SAA may be a good guide to the efficacy of treatment.

Inherited causes of AA amyloidosis

There are three causes of inherited AA amyloid, the most common of which is FMF. Some of the aspects of these three syndromes are summarized in Table 6.

Familial Mediterranean fever

Background

The creation of the state of Israel accelerated the understanding of FMF. Jews returned to Israel in large numbers after 1948 and thereby concentrated patients and effort.

FMF is transmitted by a recessive gene carried by one in seven of non-Ashkenazi Jews and Armenians. The Sephardi and Oriental Jews came from the Arab countries of the Near East and the southern Mediterranean. Ashkenazi Jews, who had settled in Russia, central Europe, and then the United States, are less often affected. Anatolian and Cypriot Turks, Arabs, Druze, and most other Mediterranean races carry the gene with variable frequency. The frequency with which amyloidosis complicates FMF also differs between the various races, from 3 per cent in Armenians to 60 per cent in Turks (Shohat *et al.* 1992 for review).

Table 6 Features of the three syndromes of periodic fevers associated with AA amyloidosis

	FMF	Muckle–Wells	TRAPS
Race	Jews, Armenians, Turks	North European	North European
Inheritance	Autosomal recessive	Autosomal dominant	Autosomal domininant
Chromosome	16	1	12
Gene/protein	MEFV/marenostrin	Cryopyrin	TNF receptor
Duration of fever	2–3 days		3 days to 3 weeks
Clinical features	Abdominal pain, athralgia, pleurisy, rash	Urticaria, arthralgia, progressive deafness	Rash, abdominal pain, arthralgia, conjunctivitis
Amyloid	Very variable	30%	25%
Treatment	Colchicine	None known	Prednisolone, etanercept

Inheritance

The MEditerranean FeVer (MEFV) gene is recessive and was found on the short arm of chromosome 16 by two groups working in France (The French FMF Consortium 1997) and the United States (The International FMF Consortium 1997). It codes for a protein named marenostrin (after Mare Nostrum, the Roman name for the Mediterranean) by the French and pyrin (after the pyrexia which is such a prominent part of the syndrome) by the Americans. Marenostrin/pyrin is expressed in neutrophils and has not been found in other cells. However, this finding has yet to lead to an improved understanding of the molecular basis of the disease. Sporadic reports of a dominant form of transmission have been claimed and recently corroborated through genetic studies of a small number of families (Booth *et al.* 2000).

Some 25 mutations have been described and most patients have two abnormal alleles. However, a substantial minority do not and some patients with two mutations do not have symptoms which meet the clinical criteria for a diagnosis of FMF (Grateau *et al.* 2000). Attempts have been made to relate particular mutations to clinical expression. M694V occurs in 20–67 per cent of cases and V726A in 7–35 per cent. The former is associated with the more severe phenotype (Drenth and van der Meer 2001). Homozygosity for M694V is also thought to increase the likelihood of developing amyloidosis (Cazeneuve *et al.* 1999; Livneh *et al.* 1999).

Therefore, the relationship between MEFV and FMF with or without amyloidosis is not simple. Other genes may be involved: for example, among Armenian patients with FMF, the risk of amyloid was increased in males and in those with the SAA1α/α genotype (Cazeneuve *et al.* 2000). If confirmed, this report, which is consistent with other studies of AA amyloidosis, establishes that amyloid is a polygenic complication of FMF.

Clinical features

The clinical presentation is often classical and easily diagnosed, provided that it is considered. Most patients experience their first attack before the age of 20 and 86 per cent of Jordanian children had developed symptoms before the age of 10 (Majeed *et al.* 1999). Males are affected slightly more frequently (ratio 1.7:1) (Shohat *et al.* 1992). The attacks usually start without warning in a previously fit individual. Various precipitating factors have been suggested including menstruation in women, stress, trauma, and exposure to cold. Pregnancy is often a period of relative calm. The attack evolves quickly with fever of about 40°C. Severe abdominal pains due to a sterile peritonitis develop in about 75–95 per cent. Fluid levels may be seen on abdominal X-rays. Laparotomy for suspected appendicitis is very common and some suggest that an elective appendicectomy should be carried out. Sometimes (about 3 per cent) adhesions form and obstruction may need surgical relief. Agonizing arthritis occurs in 50–75 per cent of patients and usually affects one of the larger joints in the legs. About one-third suffer pleurisy and radiologically there may be some blunting of the costophrenic angle. Less common manifestations are pericarditis, myalgia, scrotal inflammation, and an erysipiloid like erythema. About 25 per cent of attacks consist of fever alone. The attacks usually last 48–72 h and resolve spontaneously. During the attack, the white blood count, CRP, and other markers of inflammation are increased but return to normal between attacks. The frequency of attacks varies between weekly and 6-monthly.

Amyloidosis is the main life-threatening consequence of FMF. It is formed from a fragment of SAA and is laid down in many organs. The frequency with which it occurs varies from 0.4 per cent in Arabs to 90 per cent in Jews of North African origin (Pras *et al.* 1982; Majeed *et al.* 1999). Geographical or environmental influences are thought to account for the observation that Armenians living in America have less amyloidosis than those remaining in Armenia.

Renal involvement is the most serious manifestation and runs a similar course to that of acquired AA amyloidosis. Ninety per cent of patients with untreated amyloidosis are dead or on dialysis by the age of 40 (Zemer *et al.* 1993).

Intuitively, one would expect those with the most frequent and serious attacks to be most at risk, but that is not the case and some rare patients present with amyloidosis without previous events (so-called phenotype 2). The mechanism is unclear, since the indicators of inflammation revert to normal between attacks.

Treatment of FMF

Colchicine has revolutionized the outlook. In 1972, Goldfinger used it in a patient suffering from both gout and FMF. He noted an improvement in both syndromes and successfully extended this observation to other patients (Goldfinger 1972). His conclusion was supported by a controlled trial (Dinarello *et al.* 1974). Since then, colchicine 1–2 mg/day has proved to be a remarkably effective treatment. In a prospective study of 960 Israeli patients, 906 complied with treatment over 11 years and only 2 per cent developed amyloidosis. This compared with 49 per cent in the 54 patients who admitted poor compliance (Zemer *et al.* 1986). Compliance is more likely in patients who have symptoms that are relieved (phenotype 1) than in those who have few symptoms (phenotype 2). Treatment of renal disease, once established, is less successful, but may reduce proteinuria and delay renal failure. Dialysis and transplantation are successful in these patients particularly if they comply with colchicine treatment.

FMF—conclusion

The prognosis of this disease has been transformed by an accidental clinical observation of an acute observer. The identification of the gene has not yet led to a clear-cut diagnostic test, a new understanding of the pathogenetic process, or an explanation of the efficacy of colchicine. The relationship between MEFV genes and clinical picture is unusual although mutations are present most frequently in patients in whom the clinical diagnosis is most certain. The story remains incomplete.

Muckle–Wells syndrome

Muckle–Wells syndrome is another hereditary syndrome of periodic fever associated with AA amyloidosis. It is a rare autosomal dominant disease described first in a Derbyshire family in 1962 but subsequently over 100 cases have been reported in Northern Europe and North America and even in a family of Indian origin. The clinical characteristics are of attacks of urticaria, fever, and aches in the limbs usually starting in adolescence. These attacks are associated with a rise in acute phase proteins perhaps orchestrated by IL-6 (Gerbig *et al.* 1998). This is followed by the slow onset of sensorineural deafness. AA amyloidosis develops in about one-third of patients but different families seem to have different levels of susceptibility. Death from renal failure due to amyloidosis is common. Treatment with colchicine has been proposed.

The gene has been located on chromosome 1q44, and may be the same as the gene for *familial cold urticaria* which is very similar to the Muckle–Wells syndrome, including the development of AA amyloid, but without deafness (Hoffman *et al.* 2000). The protein for which this gene codes is a member of the pyrin family and has been named cryopyrin. It is found on the surfaces of leucocytes and may control apoptosis in the early stage of the inflammatory reaction.

Tumour necrosis factor receptor associated periodic syndrome or familial Hibernian fever

In 1982, a family of Scottish–Irish descent was described in Nottingham (Williamson *et al.* 1982). Affected members had episodes consisting of fever, lasting between a few days and some weeks, muscle pains, which may migrate during the attack, arthralgia of large joints, abdominal pains, and painful red eyes. Erythematous rashes on the limbs and migrating distally were common. Abdominal pain sometimes associated with vomiting and diarrhoea occured in over 90 per cent. These symptoms may be caused by a sterile peritonitis and lead to adhesions and obstruction. Pleurisy and pleural effusions are less common. Attacks may be precipitated by trauma and stress. A further 20 families have been described in Holland, France, Belgium, Finland, Australia, the United States, Puerto Rico, and in an Arab child in Israel.

CRP and erythrocyte sedimentation rate (ESR) are raised during the acute attack. Mild complement activation and a generalized rise in immunoglobulins, particularly IgA, occur. Levels of soluble TNF receptor are characteristically low.

Inheritance is by an autosomal dominant gene identified on the short arm of chromosome 12 coding for the receptor of type 1 TNF. Sixteen mutations have been identified and it is possible that they permit prolonged inflammation by preventing shedding of the extracellular part of the receptor which acts as an inhibitor of TNF-α.

The first association with AA amyloidosis was described in one of a Nottingham family who became nephrotic and developed progressive renal failure (McDermott *et al.* 1997). About 25 per cent of affected families have members who develop this complication (Drenth and van der Meer 2001).

Treatment has been unsatisfactory. Prednisolone in doses of more than 20 mg/day appears to reduce the severity and length of attacks if given early (McDermott *et al.* 1997). Etanercept, a fusion of TNF-α receptor and the Fc portion of IgG, has been reported to relieve symptoms (Drenth and van der Meer 2001) and reduce proteinuria and amyloid deposits in at least one patient with associated amyloidosis (Drewe *et al.* 2000). Future experience may show that etanercept offers specific and effective treatment for this rare disorder.

AL amyloidosis

AL amyloidosis is a rare disorder in which fragments of light chains, produced by monoclonal plasma cells, polymerize to form fibrils. About one-third of patients have overt myeloma, and conversely 10–15 per cent of patients with myeloma have AL amyloidosis (Kyle and Bayrd 1975; Buxbaum 1992). The overlap between those with and without myeloma is difficult to define, as most patients with AL amyloidosis have some evidence of a plasma cell dyscrasia. However, patients who present with 'primary' AL amyloidosis hardly ever develop overt myeloma, perhaps because of their poor prognosis. Some patients with other causes of monoclonal plasma cell proliferation, such as benign monoclonal gammopathy, may also develop AL amyloidosis.

Epidemiology

The epidemiology of AL amyloidosis has not been much studied. The incidence was found to be 8.9 per million per year in Olmstead County, United States (Kyle *et al.* 1992) and 4.5 per million per year in Boston (Simms *et al.* 1994). It appears to be less common in Europe and we estimate the incidence to be about 1–2 per million per year in the West of Scotland.

Pathogenesis

The protein recovered from amyloid deposits is the variable portion of a light chain (V_L) sometimes with the contiguous residues of the constant region. Overproduction of light chain is not the only factor in pathogenesis: its properties are also important. λ is three times as common as κ light chains in AL amyloid, but in normal subjects or those with myeloma, the ratio of κ to λ is about 3 : 2. Furthermore, among the subgroups of Vλ chains, Vλvi is most commonly involved (Comenzo *et al.* 1999). Certain changes in the protein appear to increase its amyloidogenicity. It is presumed that the loss of the constant moiety increases the potential for V_L to unfold. A similar effect may be achieved by key amino acid substitutions resulting from gene mutation which render parts of the molecule more hydrophobic and thus liable to aggregate. Amyloidogenic light chains have a lower pI and are more likely to be glycosylated than non-amyloidogenic ones, although it is not clear how these properties predispose to fibril formation (Dhodapkar *et al.* 1997). The properties of the protein rather than the host are crucial, as was shown by the ability of light chain from patients with AL amyloidosis to cause amyloid deposits when injected into mice and the failure of light chains from patients without amyloidosis to do so (Solomon *et al.* 1991).

Clinical features

AL amyloidosis is rare under the age of 40 and the median age at diagnosis is about 65. Males are affected slightly more frequently. Presenting symptoms can be non-specific and include tiredness, weight loss, oedema (which may conceal the weight loss), and breathlessness. These symptoms may develop insidiously leading to an average delay in diagnosis of 1–2 years (Kyle and Bayrd 1975; Gertz *et al.* 1999). Delays are less likely in those with nephrotic syndrome (median of 2.3 months) or cardiac failure (median of 3.6 months) (Kyle and Greipp 1983). There are four major clinical groupings, one of which usually dominates in an individual although most will have evidence of involvement of more than one system. These are renal, cardiac, neuropathic, and gastroenterological.

Renal group

This comprises about 40 per cent of patients with AL amyloidosis. Proteinuria is by far the commonest manifestation (about 70 per cent of all patients) and is of nephrotic proportions in about 30–40 per cent (Kyle and Bayrd 1975). Proteinuria ranged from 0.1–22.4 g/24 h in one series and was over 3 g/24 h in nearly 50 per cent (Kyle *et al.* 1997). Patients with λ light chains tend to have greater proteinuria. This is usually non-selective and the urinary sediment is unremarkable. The serum creatinine is raised in less than half at diagnosis. In an occasional patient, tubular defects predominate. Greater proteinuria is associated in general with a more rapid progression of renal failure, although no series has measured the rate of change of GFR. Interstitial fibrosis and cortical tubular loss are, as always, the best biopsy guides to renal prognosis, whereas the amount of amyloid deposited is not (Bohle *et al.* 1993). The median time from diagnosis to dialysis is 14 months (Gertz *et al.* 2002). Many patients who are not nephrotic at diagnosis become so subsequently, but patients who have no proteinuria at presentation, rarely develop it later. Hypertension is not as severe as in other glomerulopathies which may be because of autonomic neuropathy, or rarely, hypoadrenalism. Renal vein thrombosis, presenting with flank pain, haematuria, and loss of renal function, is a famous but fortunately rare event. Renal failure is the second most common cause of death, accounting for about 30 per cent (Cohen *et al.* 1987). The advent of dialysis offers an extension of life, but inevitably leaves the patient liable to other complications of the disease.

Cardiac group

About 25 per cent have a predominantly cardiological presentation, most of whom present with cardiac failure (Kyle and Bayrd 1975). The diagnosis should be considered in patients in cardiac failure without a history of ischaemic or valvular heart disease. ECHO may show a bright speckled pattern (Fig. 7). The other helpful ultrasonic feature is increased thickness of the atrial wall (Falk *et al.* 1987). Cardiac amyloid is the most common identifiable cause of a restrictive cardiomyopathy and this finding should raise the possibility. Arrhythmias are the second major cardiological complication. Palladini undertook 24 h ECG monitoring in 51 patients with AL amyloidosis affecting the heart (Palladini *et al.* 2001). Twenty-three percent had heart failure and 55 per cent had diagnostic changes on ECHO. Complex ventricular arrhythmias were present in 57 per cent of the recordings but the most dangerous finding was that couplets, found in 29 per cent, predicted earlier death. The median survival of this group was 23.4 months, which is surprisingly good, because cardiac involvement is the most serious prognostic event. Cardiac failure and sudden death, which may be the result of an arrhythmia, are the most common modes of death (about 40 per cent) (Cohen *et al.* 1987). In many studies, the median survival of those with cardiac involvement is only 6 months.

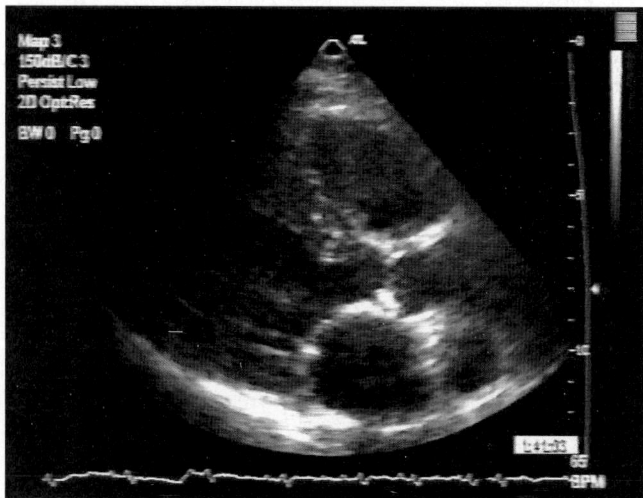

Fig. 7 Echocardiogram (transverse section) of a patient with AL amyloidosis. The speckled brightness of the ECHO pattern is due to cardiac amyloid infiltration and is relatively easily identified by an experienced operator.

Neuropathic group

Peripheral neuropathy, mainly sensory, and/or autonomic neuropathy are the main presentation in about 15 per cent of patients. Numbness of the extremities may be progressive and is sometimes painful. Postural hypotension can be so severe that patients have difficulty standing. Diarrhoea and vomiting may contribute to weight loss. Impotence is common in men.

Gastroenterological group

The most common finding is hard hepatomegaly which is present in 25 per cent and is often mistaken for malignant infiltration. It is associated with an increase in the serum alkaline phosphatase but minimal changes in bilirubin or hepatic enzymes. Splenomegaly is much less common and may be the site of haemorrhage (Fig. 8). Macroglossia occurs in about 10–15 per cent and may be striking with indentation of the teeth on the lateral surfaces (Fig. 9). Small bowel infiltration causes malabsorption in about 5 per cent. Sometimes, local accumulation of amyloid in the mucosa may mimic the effects of a tumour causing obstruction, ileus or haemorrhage (Koppelman *et al.* 2000; Gockel *et al.* 2001).

Other features

Purpura, particularly affecting the face and neck, may occur in response to straining or appear spontaneously. Localized amyloid deposits may appear in the skin and other tissues (Fig. 10). For example, carpal tunnel syndrome develops in as many as 25 per cent (Kyle and Greipp 1983). The shoulder-pad sign occurs as a result of infiltration of the periarticular tissues and is said to be pathognomic for AL amyloid (Liepnieks *et al.* 2001) but can also develop in dialysis related amyloid. Bone pain and even vertebral collapse due to amyloid infiltration have been reported. This may mimic osteolytic lesions due to myeloma and requires a biopsy to distinguish the cause. Amyloid infiltration of lachrymal or salivary glands leads to dry eyes or dry mouth.

Anaemia is common but rarely severe. A bleeding diathesis may be present. This may result from stiff, fragile small vessels or be due to a coagulation defect. Mumford studied 337 patients and found a history of bleeding, mostly affecting the skin, in 25 per cent of which it was the presenting symptom in 3 per cent. Half of all the patients had an abnormal clotting screen, which was more common in those with hepatic or renal infiltration (Mumford *et al.* 2000). Various clotting factors, particularly factor X are reduced, perhaps because of binding to amyloid fibrils.

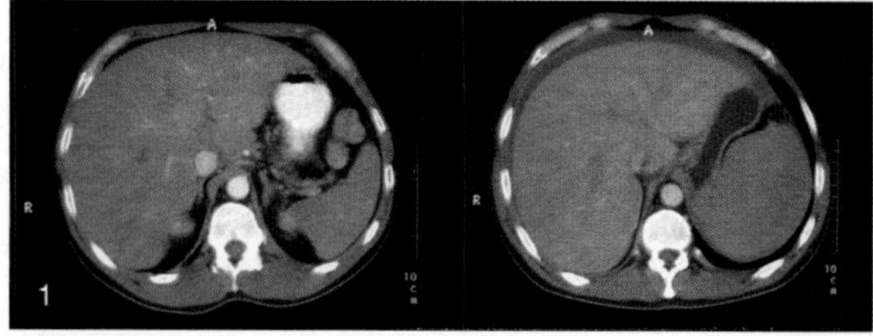

Fig. 8 CT scan of a 36-year-old man with AL amyloidosis before and after a splenic haemorrhage. These scans were taken 3 days apart. Note the increase in size of the spleen over that time. The patient underwent splenectomy.

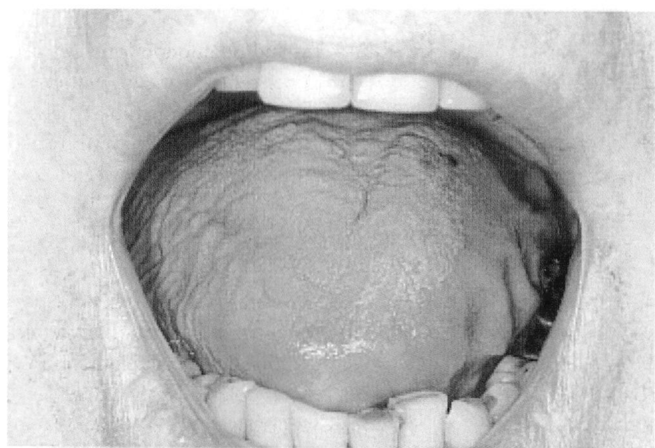

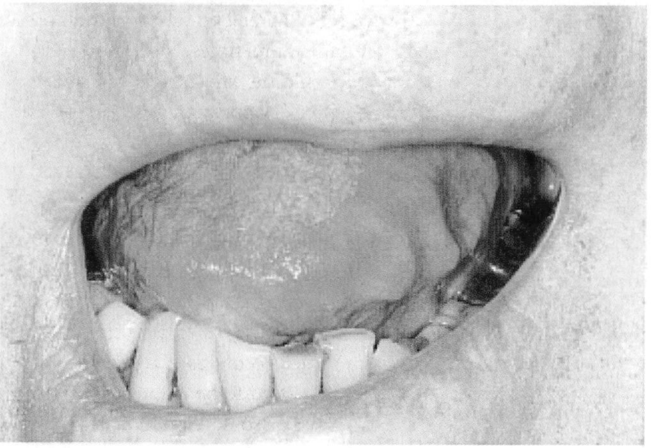

Fig. 9 Tongue of patient with AL amyloidosis showing macroglossia and imprints of teeth on the lateral surface.

Investigations

The diagnosis of amyloidosis has been discussed above. Clinical pointers suggesting AL amyloidosis may be present in a patient with proteinuria are greater age, and the presence of purpura or cardiac failure often together with hypotension and a low-voltage ECG. Renal biopsy is usually the biopsy of choice. EM is a more sensitive diagnostic test than conventional Congo red staining. The diagnosis of AL amyloid may be achieved by using specific immunohistochemical techniques (Fig. 2b), but false negative results are frequent—only 38 per cent of patients with AL amyloidosis had positive staining (Lachmann *et al.* 2002). In the remainder, it is necessary to show that the deposits are not due to other forms of amyloid, particularly AA. The absence of uptake of amyloid A antibody in a patient with a monoclonal band in blood or urine may be regarded as reasonable evidence of AL amyloidosis. However, patients with familial renal amyloidosis may be misdiagnosed using these criteria. This happened in 10 per cent of 350 patients diagnosed as AL amyloidosis, a minority of whom had a monoclonal band in their sera (Lachmann *et al.* 2002). However, since only 30 families with renal involvement due to hereditary amyloid (non-AA) syndromes have been identied (Lachmann *et al.* 2002), this report may exaggerate the problem. There is a major difference in the treatment of the different types of amyloid, so this problem needs resolving.

The identification of a monoclonal immunoglobulin or light chain in serum or urine is achieved in about 85 per cent of patients. Immunofixation is a more sensitive method than immunoelectrophoresis, and should be used because there may be only a small amount of protein. When found, a monoclonal band in either serum or urine provides good supporting evidence for AL amyloidosis. A monoclonal band was found in the serum of 71 per cent (IgG in 34 per cent and light chain in 23 per cent) and in the urine in 70 per cent (λ in 54 per cent and κ in 16 per cent of patients) (Kyle *et al.* 1997). The median size of the urinary monoclonal spike was 0.24 g/day and of the serum band was 5.3 g/l (Gertz *et al.* 1999).

The differentiation from frank myeloma is difficult. Five to ten per cent of plasma cells in the bone marrow is usual in AL amyloidosis, whilst over 20 per cent is present in myeloma, as are lytic lesions on X-ray and hypercalcaemia. The absence of all these features is diagnostic of 'primary' AL amyloidosis.

Treatment

Treatment is divided into measures aimed at reversing or arresting the disease process and measures to relieve or mitigate symptoms.

Curative treatment

The 'natural' history of AL amyloidosis is grim. The median survival in an early large series of those without myeloma was 14.7 months. However, there was a minority of patients, about 20 per cent, who survived 5 years. Some patients were treated, the effect of which is difficult to assess (Kyle and Bayrd 1975). The median survival in the only group of untreated patients was only 6 months. The principal causes of death were cardiac failure and sudden death (34 per cent), renal failure (31 per cent), and pulmonary involvement (14 per cent). The cause of death was unknown in 10 per cent (Cohen *et al.* 1987). The median survival of those whose AL amyloidosis was associated with myeloma was only 4 months (Kyle and Bayrd 1975).

Since AL amyloidosis is the result of a clonal proliferation of plasma cells with production of a monoclonal immunoglobulin or light chain, it is logical to consider treatment with regimens that ablate plasma cells. Rather oddly, the first efforts attempted to assess the efficacy of colchicine in AL amyloidosis, to see if its remarkable success in FMF could be transferred to another form of amyloid (Cohen *et al.* 1987). This trial used historical controls. Median survival for the control group was only 7 months compared to 18 months for the colchicine group. The differences were significant. There were no long-term survivors in the control group and only 5 per cent of the colchicine group survived 5 years. Therefore, all patients fared badly, but colchicine appeared to help.

This led to three randomized controlled trials that compared colchicine to treatment designed to reduce production of light chains. All trials were stratified for the major system involved at time of diagnosis (Kyle *et al.* 1985; Skinner *et al.* 1996; Kyle *et al.* 1997). All three trials showed that colchicine alone was inferior to the other arm of the study aimed at ablating plasma cell proliferation and the median survival was extended from about 6 months to 12–18 months (see Table 7).

These rather disappointing results were thought to be due to the limited effect of prednisolone and melphalan. Therefore, a trial comparing melphalan and prednisolone (M + P) with vincristine, carmustine, melphalan, cyclophosphamide, and prednisolone (VBMCP) was undertaken (Gertz *et al.* 1999). One hundred and one patients were randomly

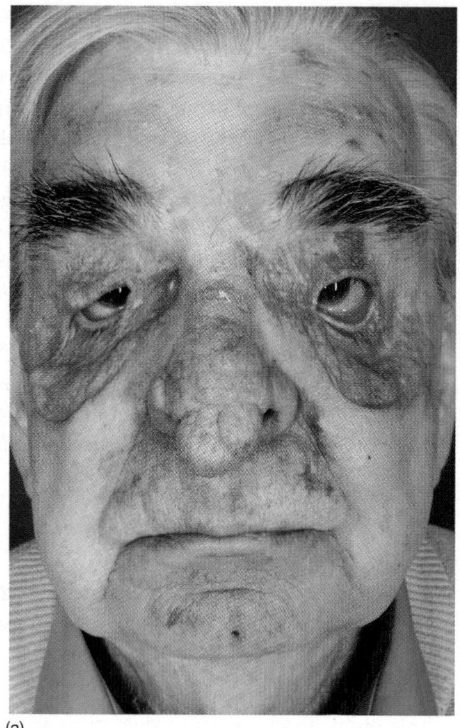
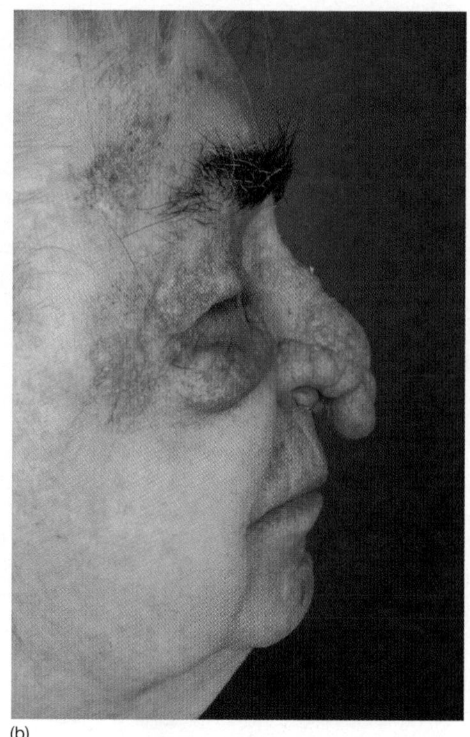

(a) (b)

Fig. 10 Face (a) and profile (b) of an elderly patient with AL amyloidosis showing both local subcutaneous deposits of amyloid and periorbital purpura.

Table 7 Median survival (months) achieved in studies of AL amyloidosis

Study	No treatment	Colchicine	M + P	MPC	VBMCP
Cohen *et al.* (1987)	7	18			
Kyle *et al.* (1985)		3	16		
Skinner *et al.* (1996)		6.7		12.2	
Kyle *et al.* (1997)		8.5	18	17	
Gertz *et al.* (1999)			29		29

M + P, melphalan + prednisolone; MPC, melphapan, prednisolone, and colchicine; VBMCP, vincrisitine, carmustine, melphalan, colchicine, and prednisolone.

allocated to the two groups after stratification according to disease severity. More severely ill patients were not enrolled. The median survival was 29 months in both groups. Various criteria of organ response were devised which included a renal response judged by a 50 per cent reduction in proteinuria. There were 10 renal responses in both groups.

The extension of the median survival to 29 months appears encouraging, but the patients enrolled did not have such advanced disease as in the earlier trials. For example, proteinuria and the size of the monoclonal spike in the urine were both less than in the previous studies. The apparent improvement in survival may have resulted from the exclusion of less fit patients or from earlier diagnosis.

It is possible that intensive chemotherapy with stem cell transplantation may be more effective. There have been no controlled trials of this treatment, but quite large series have been published which appear to offer promise (Moreau *et al.* 1998; Comenzo 2000; Dember *et al.* 2001; Sanchorawala *et al.* 2001). The Boston group has treated 205 patients, but the selection of patients excludes some of the frailer patients and those with cardiac involvement. Only 152 finished treatment, of whom 76 per cent survived 1 year and 60 per cent 4 years. Forty-seven per cent of survivors at 1 year were in complete haematological remission. The encouraging headline 4-year survival figures of 60 per cent cannot be compared directly with the results of the trials examined above. The procedure itself carries a mortality of about 20 per cent (Comenzo 2000). If the exclusion rate was 60 per cent (Dember *et al.* 2001) and 20 per cent die during the first 3 months from the start of treatment, then the 4-year survival rate of all patients was nearer 20 per cent which is very similar to the trials of M + P or MPC (Kyle *et al.* 1997). However, it is possible that the patients who do survive will survive longer because of a more complete haematological remission. Certainly, complete haematological response (defined by absence of M band in blood and urine and less than 5 per cent plasma cells in the bone marrow) was associated with renal remission (50 per cent reduction in proteinuria and stable renal function) in 79 per cent compared to 11 per cent of those with persistent haematological abnormalities. Complete remissions occurred in 36 per cent compared to 10 per cent of Skinner's trial (Skinner *et al.* 1996) and 18 per cent in Kyle's (Kyle *et al.* 1997). But once the exclusions discussed above are incorporated, the results are no better.

In summary, there have been several good studies during the last 15 years, but advances have been modest. The median survival of 14.7 months, much quoted since its publication in 1975, may have been unusually good for a largely untreated group. As shown in Table 7, the median survival in the untreated and colchicine groups was less than 10 months except in Cohen's 1987 study (Cohen *et al.* 1987). The M + P and MPC groups survived nearly twice as long with a median survival of about 18 months. The better figures achieved by Gertz and colleagues in their 1999 study and by stem cell transplantation may be largely due to selection. At present, M + P appears a reasonable treatment for both survival and renal response, but stem cell transplantation may prove its value once randomized controlled trials are undertaken.

Other treatments

High dose prednisolone with α-interferon

This has been used with some success in small numbers of patients (Dhodapkar *et al.* 1997).

Iodo-deoxydoxorubicin (I-DOX)

The substitution of an iodine atom for a hydroxyl group increases the hydrophobic and lipophilic properties of the parent molecule, doxorubicin. A small study showed some clinical effectiveness, for example, reduction of proteinuria in three out of four patients, without affecting the level of the paraprotein (Dhodapkar *et al.* 1997). It is thought that the drug binds avidly to all types of amyloid fibrils and may prevent or reduce further fibril formation (Palha *et al.* 2000).

Thalidomide

This has been used with some success in myeloma and its use is being explored in AL amyloid. Phase 2 trials are in progress. Early reports have been mixed with many suffering side effects. The median dose tolerated was 300 mg/day above which CNS side effects became intolerable. No haematological remissions have been reported but 25 per cent have a reduction in proteinuria (Seldin *et al.* 2003).

Carboxy-pyrrolidin-hexanoyl-pyrrolidone-carboxylic acid (CPHPC)

This molecule crosslinks with SAP forming compound molecules that are quickly cleared by the liver. It can be given orally, subcutaneously, or intravenously, and effectively depletes the animal or patient of SAP. AP contained in amyloid deposits is then mobilized and cleared. It appears to be effective in SAP knockout mice transgenic for human SAP given subcutaneous casein to induce AA amyloidosis (Pepys *et al.* 2002). CPHPC has also been assessed in human amyloidosis. Intravenous infusion led to a rapid and sustained fall in SAP. CPHPC has been given to 12 patients with AL amyloidosis and five with different types of inherited amyloidosis, over a period of up to 9 months. The patients all had advanced disease and had failed to respond to conventional treatments when available. The clinical condition appeared to stabilize over the period of treatment. The amyloid deposits at autopsy in one patient who died were found to contain about 15 per cent of the usual amount of AP (Pepys *et al.* 2002). These results are inconclusive, but potentially very interesting and applicable to all forms of amyloidosis.

None of these treatments has yet been shown to be effective in a formal trial.

Supportive treatment

Patients present with such a wide variety of symptoms and complications of AL amyloidosis that it is difficult to make general rules. The effect of treatment on the constitutional symptoms, often present at diagnosis, has not been well studied. They may be difficult to reverse, unless there is some haematological response.

Cardiac failure is relatively resistant to conventional treatment. Diuretics should be used cautiously in patients with a restrictive cardiomyopathy. Arrhythmias may be treated with the usual measures, but evidence of their effectiveness is lacking and ventricular arrhythmias resistant to treatment are a frequent fatal event.

The renal manifestations may be eased by conventional treatment of nephrotic syndrome. Fluid restriction, large doses of oral diuretics, and ACE inhibitors in the largest tolerated dose are standard, if unproven, measures. Intravenous frusemide with albumin may help patients with severe nephrotic syndrome.

Autonomic neuropathy varies in severity. Postural hypotension in its milder forms may be manageable with leg support stockings and asking the patient to rise slowly. Some recommend a small dose of fludrocortisone. When severe, it is almost impossible to manage satisfactorily. Diarrhoea and vomiting may be eased by the usual symptomatic measures. The pain of peripheral neuropathy may be helped by carbamazepine or amitriptyline.

Renal replacement therapy, usually with dialysis but sometimes with transplantation, has been used and remarkable successes have been achieved. One patient was still alive 21 years after diagnosis, treatment with chemotherapy, renal transplant, and dialysis (Goldsmith *et al.* 1996). Such patients are the exception: only 18 per cent of 221 patients survived long enough and were sufficiently well to be offered dialysis (Gertz *et al.* 1992). The median time of survival on dialysis is only 8 months and peritoneal dialysis is as effective as haemodialysis (Gertz *et al.* 1992). Transplantation should be reserved for patients who have survived two years in full haematological remission.

Monitoring

The importance of the haematological response and changes in proteinuria has already been emphasized. SAP scintigraphy has been used with some success. Serial studies were performed in 27 patients, 18 of whom underwent cytotoxic treatment. Regression of deposits was seen in one-third of treated patients (Hawkins *et al.* 1993).

Conclusion

AL amyloidosis is a rare and aggressive disease that frequently presents with proteinuria, the nephrotic syndrome, and progressive renal failure. Most have a monoclonal band of immunoglobulin or light chain in either blood or urine. Controlled trials have shown that a subset benefit from a combination of prednisolone and melphalan but it is difficult to identify these patients prospectively. There is no evidence that intensive chemotherapy with stem cell transplants is more effective in unselected patients but may be superior in those with a better prognosis who can survive the rigours of treatment.

Renal replacement therapy for amyloidosis

Amyloidosis as a cause of endstage renal disease

Renal failure was a major cause of death in patients with both AA and AL amyloidosis. The more widespread use of haemodialysis and transplantation has markedly improved prognosis, particularly in AA amyloidosis. Most information on renal replacement therapy does not distinguish between the types of amyloid; however experience is greater with AA amyloidosis.

Records from the ERA-EDTA surveying eight countries with adequate registries indicate that amyloidosis accounted for 1–3 per cent of patients accepted onto renal replacement programmes in the 1990s. However, there were marked differences between countries. Amyloidosis accounted for 11.6 per cent of patients starting renal replacement therapy in Finland in 1990 and this fell to 6.5 per cent in 1999. The incidence in Scotland has been constant during the decade at about 2 per cent. There appears to be a North–South divide in Europe, with amyloidosis accounting for only 0.2 per cent of patients starting RRT in Greece in 1999 (Data from ERA registry: personal communication). In the United States, between 1995 and 1999, amyloidosis accounted for only 0.3 per cent of patients starting renal replacement therapy (USRDS registry website). Northern Europe, and particularly Finland, therefore, appears to have an unusually high incidence.

Dialysis treatment

The median patient survival from time of starting dialysis varies between 8 and 52 months in different series (Port and Nissenson 1989; Martinez-Vea *et al.* 1990; Gertz and Kyle 1991; Moroni *et al.* 1992). None give details of patient selection for dialysis, so the results are difficult to interpret and variations may depend on the proportion of patients with AL amyloidosis.

In 1991, the EDTA reported a 5-year survival rate of 29 per cent in 2863 patients with amyloidosis on dialysis, three quarters of whom had AA amyloidosis (Fassbinder *et al.* 1991). The last ten years have seen no improvement with 1- and 5-year survival rates of 64 and 21 per cent, respectively. The median survival was 19 months (Fig. 11a).

Hospital haemodialysis is the most commonly used modality. Particular problems in these patients include persistent hypotension, gastrointestinal bleeding, and fistula failure (Martinez-Vea *et al.* 1990). There is much less experience with peritoneal dialyis, but the available information suggests that there is no difference in survival (Gertz and Kyle 1991; Moroni *et al.* 1992).

The poor survival rate of patients with amyloidosis on dialysis is largely due to cardiovascular diseases and infections. A rapid deterioration of renal function and short duration of disease predicts poor survival on dialysis in both AA and AL amyloidosis (Moroni *et al.* 1992). Cardiac amyloid is the most important predictor of poor survival in patients with AL amyloidosis undergoing dialysis (Gertz *et al.* 2002). Infection is the second major cause of death on dialysis accounting for between 15 and 65 per cent (Martinez-Vea *et al.* 1990; Joss *et al.* 2000). This is important because extra-renal amyloid deposition generally progresses when the patient is on renal replacement therapy unless the underlying cause of amyloidosis is treated. Gut and cardiac amyloid can become problematic even in patients with AA amyloidosis and some advocate intensive immunosuppression to prevent these complications. If infection is the major cause of death, this may not be justified.

Transplantation

Belzer in 1968 and Cohen in 1971 reported the first successful renal transplants in patients with amyloidosis. Most transplants have been performed in patients with AA amyloidosis, although it can be effective in AL amyloidosis too. Over the past 20 years, there have been substantial improvements in survival figures.

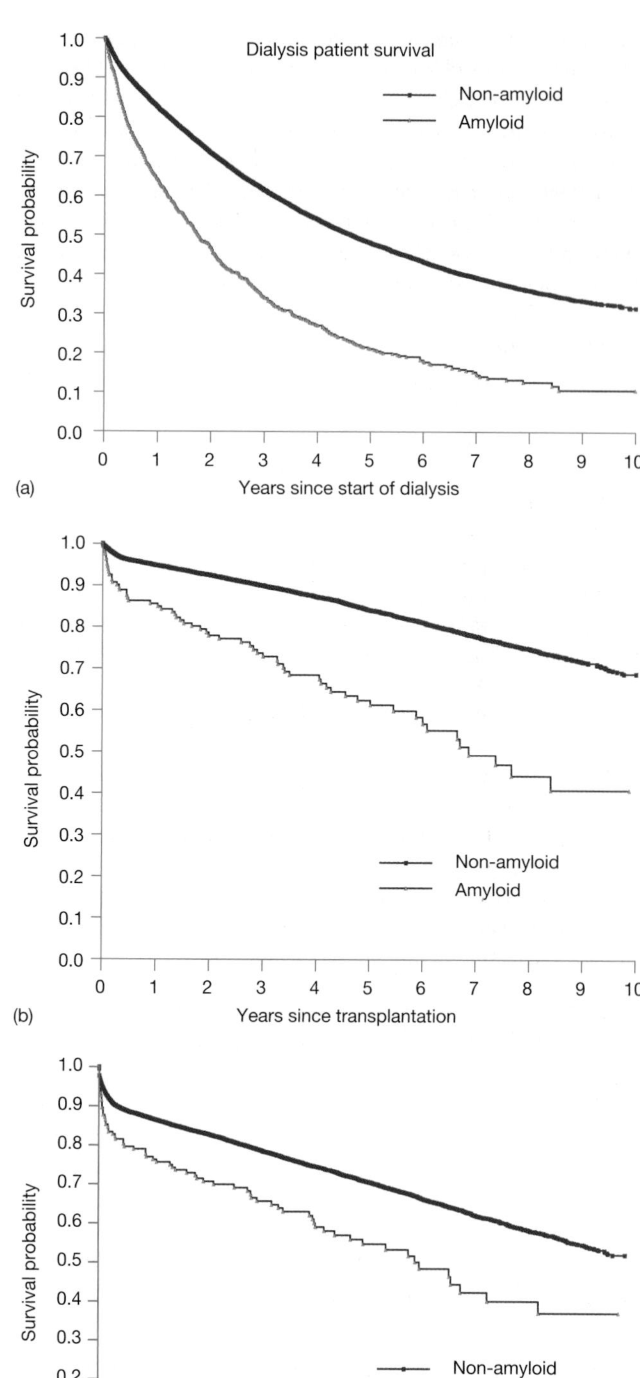

Fig. 11 (a) Patients with amyloidosis: survival on dialysis in Europe. This represents all patients taken onto dialysis in eight European countries between 1990 and 1999. (b) Patient survival after transplantation comparing those with amyloidosis to all other diagnoses. (c) Graft survival in patients with amyloidosis compared to graft survival in other diagnoses. (Data supplied by ERA-EDTA.)

In patients with amyloidosis who receive renal transplants, 5-year patient survival rates of between 39 and 65 per cent have been reported (Isoniemi *et al.* 1989; Hartmann *et al.* 1992). The early series found little difference between patient and graft survival rates, the majority of patients dying with a functioning graft. In one series, the three-year graft survival was 49 per cent compared to 53 per cent in patients without amyloidosis. However, patient survival was lower in those with amyloidosis, 50 versus 80 per cent. The major causes of death were again infection and cardiovascular disease (Pasternack *et al.* 1986).

More encouraging data have been reported in recent years. First, Heering *et al.* reviewed the Collaborative Transplant Study data ($n = 311$) and found that patient survival was 66 per cent and graft survival was 55 per cent at 5 years (Heering *et al.* 1998). Second, between 1990 and 1999, the ERA-EDTA found that 1.1 per cent ($n = 164$) of transplants performed were in patients with amyloidosis. Although the 5-year survival rate was lower than in patients without amyloidosis, the figure had improved to 61 per cent (cf. 84 per cent in non-amyloid patients) with a median survival of 67 months (Fig. 11b). This improvement may reflect better selection of patients and general improvements in transplant management. The mean age of patients with amyloidosis who were transplanted was 47 years compared to 60 years in those who were treated by dialysis alone. Graft survival rates are also less than in non-amyloid patients with 5-year survival of 55 per cent compared to 71 per cent (Fig. 11c).

Amyloid may recur in the transplanted kidney, but rarely causes graft failure (Hartmann *et al.* 1992). Progressive extrarenal amyloidosis appears to be much less common in transplanted patients compared to those who remain on dialysis, perhaps due to the antirejection regime. The long-term prognosis is determined by the presence of cardiac and adrenal amyloidosis.

Dialysis-related β-2 microglobulin amyloidosis

This subject is discussed in Chapter 13.3.2.

Hereditary amyloidosis

'Hereditary amyloidosis' is a collection of diseases, all of which result from mutations in genes encoding various proteins. They are inherited in an autosomal dominant fashion and can cause either localized or systemic disease. The major exception to this rule is FMF, which, together with other inherited febrile fevers leading to AA amyloidosis has been discussed above. The systemic forms of inherited amyloidosis are now classified by the protein involved, and not their clinical picture (Table 8).

Systemic inherited amyloidosis can be divided into the hereditary neuropathic and non-neuropathic subgroups. Hereditary neuropathic amyloidosis is usually caused by mutations in the gene encoding transthyretin. Ostertag first described the hereditary non-neuropathic amyloidoses in 1932 in patients who presented with nephrotic syndrome and hepatosplenomegaly (Ostertag 1932). It is now known that this is a heterogeneous group of diseases with amyloid fibrils composed of different proteins (Table 8).

Transthyretin

Mutations in the transthyretin gene are responsible for syndromes of hereditary neuropathic amyloidosis. First diagnosed in Portugal in 1952 (Andrade 1952), it was found subsequently in many parts of the world including Japan, Sweden (Sousa *et al.* 1993), and North West Ireland (Reilly *et al.* 1995).

Transthyretin, formerly known as prealbumin, is a tetrameric soluble protein. Over 90 per cent is produced in the liver and it has two known functions; it binds thyroxine, accounting for 20 per cent of plasma thyroxine binding in humans, and vitamin A. Wild transthyretin is associated with senile cardiac amyloid, while mutations in the gene increase the propensity of transthyretin to form amyloid. More than 70 mutations have been identified, the most common of which is the substitution of valine for methionine at position 30 (Val30Met).

Different mutations are responsible for variations in the age of onset, clinical picture, and rate of progression. In Portugal, the age of onset varies from 17 to 78 years in 1233 patients, with a median age

Table 8 Inherited amyloidosis excluding AA amyloid syndromes

Protein	First described clinically	Mutation identified	Clinical picture
Transthyretin	Andrade (1952)	Saraiva *et al.* (1985)	Peripheral and autonomic neuropathy + varying degrees of visceral involvement
Gelsolin	Meretoja (1969)	Maury (1991)	Cranial neuropathy Corneal lattice dystrophy Distal peripheral neuropathy
Apolipoprotein AI	Van Allen *et al.* (1969)	Nichols *et al.* (1988)	Renal Gastric ulcers Polyneuropathy
Apolipoprotein AII	Benson *et al.* (2001)	Benson *et al.* (2001)	Renal
Lysozyme	Zalin *et al.* (1991)	Pepys *et al.* (1993)	Renal
Fibrinogen Aα	Weiss and Page (1973)	Benson *et al.* (1993)	Renal and hepatomegaly

of 33 years (Sousa *et al.* 1995), while in Sweden the median age is 56.7 years (Sousa *et al.* 1993). This is interesting because the mutation is identical. In the United Kingdom, the median age of presentation is 67.5 years (Reilly *et al.* 1995). Predominant cardiac disease has been found to be associated with particular mutations (Jacobson *et al.* 1997).

The initial symptoms are the result of peripheral and autonomic neuropathy. The degrees of cardiac, gastrointestinal, and renal involvement are variable, but involvement of one of these systems is the usual cause of death. This form of inherited amyloidosis accounted for 13 of the 34 patients misdiagnosed with AL amyloidosis (Lachmann *et al.* 2002).

Until recently, the disease was invariably fatal after a period of 10–15 years. Orthotopic liver transplants are a logical treatment, since 95 per cent of the mutated protein is produced in the liver. The first operation was performed in Sweden in 1990 (Holmgren *et al.* 1991). Three out of four transplanted patients had marked symptomatic improvement, particularly of autonomic neuropathy (Holmgren *et al.* 1993) with reduction in the size of deposits as defined by serial SAP studies.

Apolipoprotein AI and AII

Van Allen *et al.* (1969) reported hereditary amyloidosis in settlers of British descent in Iowa. The clinical features were of lower limb neuropathy, gastric ulceration, and renal failure. The protein isolated from these amyloid deposits was identified as apolipoprotein AI (Nichols *et al.* 1988).

The clinical picture in this type of amyloidosis again varies with the mutation and can be either neuropathic or non-neuropathic. Patients generally develop extensive deposits affecting the liver, kidney, and spleen with variable involvement of the heart, nerves, and gastrointestinal tract. The progression of renal disease is often slow.

Eight apolipoprotein AI variants are associated with amyloidosis. The phenotypic expression of these mutations varies both between and within families (Soutar *et al.* 1992; Vigushin *et al.* 1994). Some mutations cause predominant cardiac disease (Arg173Pro and Leu74Ser) resulting in death from heart failure by the sixth decade (Hamidi *et al.* 1997; Obici *et al.* 1999). Others, for example, a unique deletion mutation, cause death from liver failure.

Apolipoprotein AI is part of the HDL complex and is encoded on chromosome 11. It has a role in reverse cholesterol transport. It is synthesized in approximately equal quantities by the liver and small intestine, but, perhaps surprisingly, a successful liver and kidney transplant has been performed in a patient with apolipoprotein AI amyloidosis. SAP studies failed to show re-accumulation of amyloid 24 months post transplant (Gillmore *et al.* 2001b).

A family with hereditary renal amyloidosis was discovered to have a mutation in the gene encoding apolipoprotein AII (Benson *et al.* 2001).

Lysozyme

An English family with renal amyloidosis and skin petechiae was described in 1991. It was originally thought that they had a defect in the apolipoprotein AI gene (Zalin *et al.* 1991). However, variant lysozyme was subsequently recovered from the amyloid fibril (Pepys *et al.* 1993). This family had a point mutation in the gene altering the amino acid 56 from isoleucine to threonine (Ile56Thr). A second English family was found to have variant lysozyme with a different point mutation, aspargine to histidine at position 67 (Asp67His) (Pepys *et al.* 1993). In this family, affected individuals presented between 23 and 50 years of age with renal involvement, but with wide variation in the rate of loss of renal function (Gillmore *et al.* 1999). Interestingly, another family with the identical mutation (Asp67His) presented with liver haemorrhage (Harrison *et al.* 1996). The clinical expression of hereditary lysozyme amyloidosis is variable, both within and between families. The prognosis varies; some patients survive for twenty years after diagnosis, while others die within one year.

Lysozyme is the major secreted product of macrophages and neutrophils discovered by Fleming in 1922. It is also produced by hepatocytes and gastrointestinal cells. Orthotopic liver transplantation is therefore impractical, and, at present, the only treatment is supportive management.

Fibrinogen Aα

The first reported mutation (Arg554Leu) in the fibrinogen Aα gene was identified in an individual of Peruvian descent (Benson *et al.* 1993). Subsequently, four further mutations have been reported (Gillmore *et al.* 2000) of which the Glu526Val is the most common in Britain. Nephropathy is the major clinical manifestation. It is the most common type of hereditary amyloidosis associated with nephropathy masquerading as AL amyloidosis (Lachamnn *et al.* 2002). In one case, a renal transplant was performed and amyloid deposits recurred within 2 years (Hamidi *et al.* 1997). However, in another kindred with the same mutation (Glu526Val), a hepatorenal transplant was successful with no re-accumulation of amyloid after 36 months (Gillmore *et al.* 2000).

Gelsolin

Hereditary amyloidosis of the Finnish type is the result of an autosomal dominant mutation, Asp187Asn, in the gelsolin protein (Maury 1991). This particular mutation has been found in all patients described from Finland, as well as occasional families from Japan and America. A different mutation at the same site (Asp187Try) results in a similar clinical disorder in Danish and Czech families (Maury *et al.* 2000). The clinical picture is one of corneal lattice dystrophy, cranial neuropathy, and peripheral neuropathy. There may be skin, renal, and cardiac involvement. The renal disease is particularly severe in homozygote patients and is usually mild, consisting of intermittent proteinuria in the heterozygote (Maury *et al.* 1992).

The gene for gelsolin is on chromosome 9 and gelsolin is a cytoplasmic actin modulating protein.

Cerebral amyloidosis

The brain is an important site of amyloid deposition but rarely coexists with renal involvement. The various syndromes are summarized in Table 9.

Localized non-inherited amyloid

There are several examples in this category, such as senile cardiac amyloid and medullary carcinoma of the thyroid. However, type 2 diabetes is of greater interest to nephrologists.

Table 9 The different forms of cerebral amyloidosis and the responsible protein

Syndrome	Precursor protein
Alzheimer's disease	
Sporadic	Aβ peptide
Familial	Aβ peptide
Associated with Down syndrome	Aβ peptide
Cerebral amyloid angiopathy	Aβ peptide
Hereditary cerebral haemorrhage with amyloidosis	
Dutch	Aβ peptide
Icelandic	Cystatin C
Cerebral amyloid with prion disease	
Gerstmann–Straussler–Scheinker disease	Prion peptide
Prion protein cerebral amyloid angiopathy	
Fatal familial insomnia	
Kuru	
Cruetzfeldt–Jacobs disease	

Amyloid of the islets of Langerhans

One of the commonest renal diseases in affluent countries is caused by type 2 diabetes. Amyloid is found in the pancreatic islets of about 90 per cent of patients and is more extensive in patients requiring insulin. Analysis of amyloid deposits has identified a product of the islet cells called islet amyloid polypeptide or amylin. The role of this form of amyloid in the aetiology of type 2 diabetes is controversial. It is unlikely to be the prime cause because it is not found in 10 per cent of patients. Insulin resistance, the primary defect of the condition, leads to increased secretion of insulin and amylin which are co-secreted. Increased production may be one of the factors leading to amyloid deposition because amino acid sequencing has shown the protein recovered from amyloid to be identical to secreted amylin. Its ability to refold into amyloid is enhanced by glycosylation. In monkeys, the deposition of amyloid accelerates the destruction of the islets and thereby loss of insulin production capacity, thus accelerating the evolution of the disease. Perlecan, a glycoprotein constituent of endothelial cell basement membranes accelerates fibril formation. No deposits of this type of amyloid have been found elsewhere in the body. If amylin amyloid formation could be prevented, the consequences of type 2 diabetes including nephropathy may be reduced or delayed (Hoppener *et al.* 2000).

References

Ahlmen, M., Ahlmen, J., Svalander, C., and Bucht, H. (1987). Cytotoxic drug treatment of reactive amyloidosis in rheumatoid arthritis with special reference to renal insufficiency. *Clinical Rheumatology* **6**, 27–38.

Andrade, C. (1952). A peculiar form of peripheral neuropathy: familial atypical generalised amyloidosis with special involvement of the peripheral nerves. *Brain* **75**, 408–427.

Arikawa-Hirasawa, E., Watanabe, H., Takami, H., Hassell, J. R., and Yamada, Y. (1999). Perlecan is essential for cartilage and cephalic development. *Nature Genetics* **23**, 354–358.

Badolato, R. *et al.* (1994). Serum amyloid A is a chemoattractant: induction of migration, adhesion, and tissue infiltration of monocytes and polymorphonuclear leukocytes. *Journal of Experimental Medicine* **180**, 203–209.

Badolato, R., Wang, J. M., Stornello, S. L., Ponzi, A. N., Duse, M., and Musso, T. (2000). Serum amyloid A is an activator of PMN antimicrobial functions: induction of degranulation, phagocytosis, and enhancement of anti-Candida activity. *Journal of Leukocyte Biology* **67**, 381–386.

Bales, K. R. *et al.* (1997). Lack of apolipoprotein E dramatically reduces amyloid beta-peptide deposition. *Nature Genetics* **17**, 263–264.

Benditt, E. P. and Eriksen, N. (1971). Chemical classes of amyloid substance. *American Journal of Pathology* **65**, 231–252.

Benson, M. D., Liepnieks, J., Uemichi, T., Wheeler, G., and Correa, R. (1993). Hereditary renal amyloidosis associated with a mutant fibrinogen alpha-chain. *Nature Genetics* **3**, 252–255.

Benson, M. D. *et al.* (2001). A new human hereditary amyloidosis: the result of a stop-codon mutation in the apolipoprotein AII gene. *Genomics* **72**, 272–277.

Berglund, K., Thysell, H., and Keller, C. (1993). Results, principles and pitfalls in the management of renal AA-amyloidosis; a 10–21 year followup of 16 patients with rheumatic disease treated with alkylating cytostatics. *Journal of Rheumatology* **20**, 2051–2057.

Bohle, A., Wehrmann, M., Eissele, R., von Gise, H., Mackensen-Haen, S., and Muller, C. (1993). The long-term prognosis of AA and AL renal amyloidosis and the pathogenesis of chronic renal failure in renal amyloidosis. *Pathology Research and Practice* **189**, 316–331.

Booth, D. R., Booth, S. E., Gillmore, J. D., Hawkins, P. N., and Pepys, M. B. (1998). SAA1 alleles as risk factors in reactive systemic AA amyloidosis. *Amyloid* **5**, 262–265.

Booth, D. R., Gillmore, J. D., Lachmann, H. J., Booth, S. E., Bybee, A., Soyturk, M., Akar, S., Pepys, M. B., Tunca, M., and Hawkins, P. N. (2000). The genetic basis of autosomal dominant familial Mediterranean fever. *Quarterly Journal of Medicine* **93**, 217–221.

Botto, M. *et al.* (1997). Amyloid deposition is delayed in mice with targeted deletion of the serum amyloid P component gene. *Nature Medicine* **3**, 855–859.

Browning, M. J. *et al.* (1985). Ten years' experience of an amyloid clinic—a clinicopathological survey. *Quarterly Journal of Medicine* **54**, 213–227.

Buxbaum, J. (1992). Mechanisms of disease: monoclonal immunoglobulin deposition. Amyloidosis, light and heavy chain deposition disease. *Haematology–Oncology Clinics of North America* **6**, 323–346.

Camussi, G. and Lupia, E. (1998). The future role of anti-tumour necrosis factor (TNF) products in the treatment of rheumatoid arthritis. *Drugs* **55**, 613–620.

Cazeneuve, C. *et al.* (1999). MEFV-gene analysis in Armenian patients with familial Mediterranean fever: diagnostic value and unfavorable renal prognosis of the M694V homozygous genotype—genetic and therapeutic implications. *American Journal of Human Genetics* **65**, 88–97.

Cazeneuve, C. *et al.* (2000). Identification of MEFV-independent modifying genetic factors for familial Mediterranean fever. *American Journal of Human Genetics* **67**, 1136–1143.

Charles, P. *et al.* (1999). Regulation of cytokines, cytokine inhibitors, and acute-phase proteins following anti-TNF-alpha therapy in rheumatoid arthritis. *Journal of Immunology* **163**, 1521–1528.

Chevrel, G., Jenvrin, C., McGregor, B., and Miossec, P. (2001). Renal type AA amyloidosis associated with rheumatoid arthritis: a cohort study showing improved survival on treatment with pulse cyclophosphamide. *Rheumatology (Oxford)* **40**, 821–825.

Cohen, A. S. (1968). Amyloidosis associated with rheumatoid arthritis. *Medical Clinics of North America* **52**, 643–653.

Cohen, A. S. *et al.* (1987). Survival of patients with primary (AL) amyloidosis. Colchicine-treated cases from 1976 to 1983 compared with cases seen in previous years (1961 to 1973). *American Journal of Medicine* **82**, 1182–1190.

Comenzo, R. L. (2000). Hematopoietic cell transplantation for primary systemic amyloidosis: what have we learned? *Leukaemia and Lymphoma* **37**, 245–258.

Comenzo, R. L. *et al.* (1999). Clonal immunoglobulin light chain variable region germline gene use in AL amyloidosis: association with dominant amyloid-related organ involvement and survival after stem cell transplantation. *British Journal of Haematology* **106**, 744–751.

Corder, E. H. *et al.* (1993). Gene dose of apolipoprotein E type 4 allele and the risk of Alzheimer's disease in late onset families. *Science* **261**, 921–923.

David, J., Vouyiouka, O., Ansell, B. M., Hall, A., and Woo, P. (1993). Amyloidosis in juvenile chronic arthritis: a morbidity and mortality study. *Clinical Experimental Rheumatology* **11**, 85–90.

Dember, L. M. *et al.* (2001). Effect of dose-intensive intravenous melphalan and autologous blood stem-cell transplantation on an amyloidosis-associated renal disease. *Annals of Internal Medicine* **134**, 746–753.

Dhodapkar, M. V., Merlini, G., and Solomon, A. (1997). Biology and therapy of immunoglobulin deposition diseases. *Hematology–Oncology Clinics of North America* **11**, 89–110.

Dinarello, C. A., Wolff, S. M., Goldfinger, S. E., Dale, D. C., and Alling, D. W. (1974). Colchicine therapy for familial Mediterranean fever. A double-blind trial. *New England Journal of Medicine* **291**, 934–937.

Drenth, J. P. and van der Meer, J. W. (2001). Hereditary periodic fever. *New England Journal of Medicine* **345**, 1748–1757.

Drewe, E., McDermott, E. M., and Powell, R. J. (2000). Treatment of the nephrotic syndrome with etanercept in patients with the tumor necrosis factor receptor-associated periodic syndrome. *New England Journal of Medicine* **343**, 1044–1045.

Emsley, J. *et al.* (1994). Structure of pentameric human serum amyloid P component. *Nature* **367**, 338–345.

Escalante, A., Ehresmann, G. R., and Quismorio, F. P., Jr. (1991). Regression of reactive systemic amyloidosis due to ankylosing spondylitis following the administration of colchicine. *Arthritis and Rheumatism* **34**, 920–922.

Falck, H. M., Skrifvars, B., and Wegelius, O. Treatment of amyloidosis secondary to rheumatoid arthritis with cyclophosphamide. In *Amyloid and Amyloidosis* (ed. G. Glenner, P. Costa, and F. de Freitas), pp. 592–594. Amsterdam: Excerpta Medica, 1980.

Falck, H. M., Tornroth, T., and Wegelius, O. (1983a). Predominantly vascular amyloid deposition in the kidney in patients with minimal or no proteinuria. *Clinical Nephrology* **19**, 137–142.

Falck, H. M., Maury, C. P., Teppo, A. M., and Wegelius, O. (1983b). Correlation of persistently high serum amyloid A protein and C-reactive protein concentrations with rapid progression of secondary amyloidosis. *British Medical Journal (Clinical Research Edition)* **286**, 1391–1393.

Falk, R. H. *et al.* (1987). Sensitivity and specificity of the echocardiographic features of cardiac amyloidosis. *American Journal of Cardiology* **59**, 418–422.

Fassbinder, W. *et al.* (1991). Combined report on regular dialysis and transplantation in Europe, XX, 1989. *Nephrology, Dialysis, Transplantation* **6** (Suppl. 1), 5–35.

Filipowicz-Sosnowska, A. M., Roztropowicz-Denisiewicz, K., Rosenthal, C. J., and Baum, J. (1978). The amyloidosis of juvenile rheumatoid arthritis—comparative studies in Polish and American children. I. Levels of serum SAA protein. *Arthritis and Rheumatism* **21**, 699–703.

Gerbig, A. W., Dahinden, C. A., Mullis, P., and Hunziker, T. (1998). Circadian elevation of IL-6 levels in Muckle–Wells syndrome: a disorder of the neuro-immune axis? *Quarterly Journal of Medicine* **91**, 489–492.

Gertz, M. A. and Kyle, R. A. (1991). Secondary systemic amyloidosis: response and survival in 64 patients. *Medicine (Baltimore)* **70**, 246–256.

Gertz, M. A., Kyle, R. A., and O'Fallon, W. M. (1992). Dialysis support of patients with primary systemic amyloidosis. A study of 211 patients. *Archives of Internal Medicine* **152**, 2245–2250.

Gertz, M. A., Lacy, M. Q., Lust, J. A., Greipp, P. R., Witzig, T. E., and Kyle, R. A. (1999). Prospective randomized trial of melphalan and prednisone versus vincristine, carmustine, melphalan, cyclophosphamide, and prednisone in the treatment of primary systemic amyloidosis. *Journal of Clinical Oncology* **17**, 262–267.

Gertz, M. A., Lacy, M. Q., and Dispenzieri, A. (2002). Immunoglobulin light chain amyloidosis and the kidney. *Kidney International* **61**, 1–9.

Gillmore, J. D., Booth, D. R., Madhoo, S., Pepys, M. B., and Hawkins, P. N. (1999). Hereditary renal amyloidosis associated with variant lysozyme in a large English family. *Nephrology, Dialysis, Transplantation* **14**, 2639–2644.

Gillmore, J. D. *et al.* (2000). Curative hepatorenal transplantation in systemic amyloidosis caused by the Glu526Val fibrinogen alpha-chain variant in an English family. *Quarterly Journal of Medicine* **93**, 269–275.

Gillmore, J. D., Lovat, L. B., Persey, M. R., Pepys, M. B., and Hawkins, P. N. (2001a). Amyloid load and clinical outcome in AA amyloidosis in relation to circulating concentration of serum amyloid A protein. *Lancet* **358**, 24–29.

Gillmore, J. D. *et al.* (2001b). Clinical and biochemical outcome of hepatorenal transplantation for hereditary systemic amyloidosis associated with apolipoprotein AI Gly26Arg. *Transplantation* **71**, 986–992.

Glenner, G. G., Ein, D., Eanes, E. D., Bladen, H. A., Terry, W., and Page, D. L. (1971). Creation of 'amyloid' fibrils from Bence Jones proteins *in vitro*. *Science* **174**, 712–714.

Gockel, I., Linke, R. P., Kupczyk-Joeris, D., and Peters, H. (2001). A lambda-amyloidosis of the gastrointestinal tract with recurrent incomplete ileus and gastrointestinal haemorrhage. *European Journal of Surgery* **167**, 463–466.

Goldfinger, S. E. (1972). Colchicine for familial Mediterranean fever. *New England Journal of Medicine* **287**, 1302.

Goldsmith, D. J., Sandooran, D., Short, C. D., Mallick, N. P., and Johnson, R. W. (1996). Twenty-one years survival with systemic AL-amyloidosis. *American Journal of Kidney Diseases* **28**, 278–282.

Grateau, G. *et al.* (2000). Clinical versus genetic diagnosis of familial Mediterranean fever. *Quarterly Journal of Medicine* **93**, 223–229.

Grcevska, L. and Polenakovic, M. (1993). Primary amyloidosis involving principally intrarenal blood vessels. *Nephrology, Dialysis, Transplantation* **8**, 296–300.

Hamazaki, H. (1995). Amyloid P component promotes aggregation of Alzheimer's beta-amyloid peptide. *Biochemical and Biophysical Research Communications* **211**, 349–353.

Hamidi, A. L. *et al.* (1997). Renal amyloidosis with a frame shift mutation in fibrinogen alpha-chain gene producing a novel amyloid protein. *Blood* **90**, 4799–4805.

Harrison, R. F., Hawkins, P. N., Roche, W. R., MacMahon, R. F., Hubscher, S. G., and Buckels, J. A. (1996). 'Fragile' liver and massive hepatic haemorrhage due to hereditary amyloidosis. *Gut* **38**, 151–152.

Hartmann, A. *et al.* (1992). Fifteen years' experience with renal transplantation in systemic amyloidosis. *Transplantation International* **5**, 15–18.

Hashimoto, M. *et al.* (1999). Oxidative stress induces amyloid-like aggregate formation of NACP/alpha-synuclein *in vitro*. *Neuroreport* **10**, 717–721.

Hawkins, P. N., Wootton, R., and Pepys, M. B. (1990). Metabolic studies of radioiodinated serum amyloid P component in normal subjects and patients with systemic amyloidosis. *Journal of Clinical Investigation* **86**, 1862–1869.

Hawkins, P. N. *et al.* (1993). Scintigraphic quantification and serial monitoring of human visceral amyloid deposits provide evidence for turnover and regression. *Quarterly Journal of Medicine* **86**, 365–374.

Heering, P., Hetzel, R., Grabensee, B., and Opelz, G. (1998). Renal transplantation in secondary systemic amyloidosis. *Clinical Transplantation* **12**, 159–164.

Hoffman, H. M., Wright, F. A., Broide, D. H., Wanderer, A. A., and Kolodner, R. D. (2000). Identification of a locus on chromosome 1q44 for familial cold urticaria. *American Journal of Human Genetics* **66**, 1693–1698.

Holmgren, G. *et al.* (1991). Biochemical effect of liver transplantation in two Swedish patients with familial amyloidotic polyneuropathy (FAP-met30). *Clinical Genetics* **40**, 242–246.

Holmgren, G. *et al.* (1993). Clinical improvement and amyloid regression after liver transplantation in hereditary transthyretin amyloidosis. *Lancet* **341**, 1113–1116.

Hoppener, J. W., Ahren, B., and Lips, C. J. (2000). Islet amyloid and type 2 diabetes mellitus. *New England Journal of Medicine* **343**, 411–419.

Isoniemi, H., Eklund, B., Hockerstedt, K., Salmela, K., and Ahonen, J. (1989). Renal transplantation in amyloidosis. *Transplantation Proceedings* **21**, 2039–2040.

Jacobson, D. R. *et al.* (1997). Variant-sequence transthyretin (isoleucine 122) in late-onset cardiac amyloidosis in black Americans. *New England Journal of Medicine* **336**, 466–473.

Janssen, S., Van Rijswijk, M. H., Meijer, S., Ruinen, L., and Van der Hem, G. K. (1986). Systemic amyloidosis: a clinical survey of 144 cases. *Netherlands Journal of Medicine* **29**, 376–385.

Joss, N., McLaughlin, K., Simpson, K., and Boulton-Jones, J. M. (2000). Presentation, survival and prognostic markers in AA amyloidosis. *Quarterly Journal of Medicine* **93**, 535–542.

Kagan, A., Husza'r, M., Frumkin, A., and Rapoport, J. (1999). Reversal of nephrotic syndrome due to AA amyloidosis in psoriatic patients on long-term colchicine treatment. Case report and review of the literature. *Nephron* **82**, 348–353.

Kennedy, A. C., Burton, J. A., and Allison, M. E. (1974). Tuberculosis as a continuing cause of renal amyloidosis. *British Medical Journal* **3**, 795–797.

Kisilevsky, R. and Fraser, P. (1996). Proteoglycans and amyloid fibrillogenesis. *Ciba Foundation Symposium* **199**, 58–67.

Kisilevsky, R., Lyon, A. W., and Young, I. D. (1992). A critical analysis of postulated pathogenetic mechanisms in amyloidogenesis. *Critical Reviews of Clinical and Laboratory Sciences* **29**, 59–82.

Koppelman, R. N., Stollman, N. H., Baigorri, F., and Rogers, A. I. (2000). Acute small bowel pseudo-obstruction due to AL amyloidosis: a case report and literature review. *American Journal of Gastroenterology* **95**, 294–296.

Kyle, R. A. and Bayrd, E. D. (1975). Amyloidosis: review of 236 cases. *Medicine (Baltimore)* **54**, 271–299.

Kyle, R. A. and Greipp, P. R. (1983). Amyloidosis (AL). Clinical and laboratory features in 229 cases. *Mayo Clinic Proceedings* **58**, 665–683.

Kyle, R. A., Greipp, P. R., Garton, J. P., and Gertz, M. A. (1985). Primary systemic amyloidosis. Comparison of melphalan/prednisone versus colchicine. *American Journal of Medicine* **79**, 708–716.

Kyle, R. A. *et al.* (1992). Incidence and natural history of primary systemic amyloidosis in Olmsted County, Minnesota, 1950 through 1989. *Blood* **79**, 1817–1822.

Kyle, R. A. *et al.* (1997). A trial of three regimens for primary amyloidosis: colchicine alone, melphalan and prednisone, and melphalan, prednisone, and colchicine. *New England Journal of Medicine* **336**, 1202–1207.

Lai, Z., Colon, W., and Kelly, J. W. (1996). The acid-mediated denaturation pathway of transthyretin yields a conformational intermediate that can self-assemble into amyloid. *Biochemistry* **35**, 6470–6482.

Lachmann, H. J. *et al.* (2002). Misdiagnosis of hereditary amyloidosis as AL (primary) amyloidosis. *New England Journal of Medicine* **346**, 1786–1789.

Laiho, K., Tiitinen, S., Kaarela, K., Helin, H., and Isomaki, H. (1999). Secondary amyloidosis has decreased in patients with inflammatory joint disease in Finland. *Clinical Rheumatology* **18**, 122–123.

Liepnieks, J. J., Burt, C., and Benson, M. D. (2001). Shoulder-pad sign of amyloidosis: structure of an Ig kappa III protein. *Scandinavian Journal of Immunology* **54**, 404–408.

Lindqvist, B., Andersen, S., Isacsson, B., and Lundberg, E. (1989). The course of renal amyloidosis with uraemia. *International Urology and Nephrology* **21**, 555–559.

Livneh, A. *et al.* (1999). MEFV mutation analysis in patients suffering from amyloidosis of familial Mediterranean fever. *Amyloid* **6**, 1–6.

Lofberg, H. *et al.* (1987). The prevalence of renal amyloidosis of the AA-type in a series of 1,158 consecutive autopsies. *Acta Pathologica, Microbiologica, et Immunologica Scandinavica[A]* **95**, 297–302.

Majeed, H. A., Rawashdeh, M., el Shanti, H., Qubain, H., Khuri-Bulos, N., and Shahin, H. M. (1999). Familial Mediterranean fever in children: the expanded clinical profile. *Quarterly Journal of Medicine* **92**, 309–318.

Mantyh, P. W. *et al.* (1993). Aluminum, iron, and zinc ions promote aggregation of physiological concentrations of beta-amyloid peptide. *Journal of Neurochemistry* **61**, 1171–1174.

Martinez-Vea, A., Garcia, C., Carreras, M., Revert, L., and Oliver, J. A. (1990). End-stage renal disease in systemic amyloidosis: clinical course and outcome on dialysis. *American Journal of Nephrology* **10**, 283–289.

Maury, C. P. (1991). Gelsolin-related amyloidosis. Identification of the amyloid protein in Finnish hereditary amyloidosis as a fragment of variant gelsolin. *Journal of Clinical Investigation* **87**, 1195–1199.

Maury, C. P., Kere, J., Tolvanen, R., and de la, C. A. (1992). Homozygosity for the Asn187 gelsolin mutation in Finnish-type familial amyloidosis is associated with severe renal disease. *Genomics* **13**, 902–903.

Maury, C. P., Liljestrom, M., Boysen, G., Tornroth, T., de la, C. A., and Nurmiaho-Lassila, E. L. (2000). Danish type gelsolin related amyloidosis: 654G-T mutation is associated with a disease pathogenetically and clinically similar to that caused by the 654G-A mutation (familial amyloidosis of the Finnish type). *Journal of Clinical Pathology* **53**, 95–99.

McDermott, E. M., Smillie, D. M., and Powell, R. J. (1997). Clinical spectrum of familial Hibernian fever: a 14-year follow-up study of the index case and extended family. *Mayo Clinic Proceedings* **72**, 806–817.

Meretoja, J. (1969). Familial systemic paramyloidosis with lattice dystrophy of the cornea, progressive cranial neuropathy, skin changes and various internal symptoms. A previously unrecognized heritable syndrome. *Annals of Clinical Research* **1**, 314–324.

Meyers, S. *et al.* (1988). Colchicine therapy of the renal amyloidosis of ulcerative colitis. *Gastroenterology* **94**, 1503–1507.

Migita, K., Kawabe, Y., Tominaga, M., Origuchi, T., Aoyagi, T., and Eguchi, K. (1998). Serum amyloid A protein induces production of matrix metalloproteinases by human synovial fibroblasts. *Laboratory Investigation* **78**, 535–539.

Moreau, P. *et al.* (1998). Prognostic factors for survival and response after high-dose therapy and autologous stem cell transplantation in systemic AL amyloidosis: a report on 21 patients. *British Journal of Haematology* **101**, 766–769.

Moriguchi, M. *et al.* (1999). Influence of genotypes at SAA1 and SAA2 loci on the development and the length of latent period of secondary AA-amyloidosis in patients with rheumatoid arthritis. *Human Genetics* **105**, 360–366.

Moroni, G. *et al.* (1992). Chronic dialysis in patients with systemic amyloidosis: the experience in northern Italy. *Clinical Nephrology* **38**, 81–85.

Mumford, A. D., O'Donnell, J., Gillmore, J. D., Manning, R. A., Hawkins, P. N., and Laffan, M. (2000). Bleeding symptoms and coagulation abnormalities in 337 patients with AL-amyloidosis. *British Journal of Haematology* **110**, 454–460.

Myllykangas-Luosujarvi, R., Aho, K., Kautiainen, H., and Hakala, M. (1999). Amyloidosis in a nationwide series of 1666 subjects with rheumatoid arthritis who died during 1989 in Finland. *Rheumatology (Oxford)* **38**, 499–503.

Nakano, M. *et al.* (1998). Analysis of renal pathology and drug history in 158 Japanese patients with rheumatoid arthritis. *Clinical Nephrology* **50**, 154–160.

Nelson, S. R. *et al.* (1991). Imaging of haemodialysis-associated amyloidosis with 123I-serum amyloid P component. *Lancet* **338**, 335–339.

Nichols, W. C., Dwulet, F. E., Liepnieks, J., and Benson, M. D. (1988). Variant apolipoprotein AI as a major constituent of a human hereditary amyloid. *Biochemical and Biophysical Research Communications* **156**, 762–768.

Obici, L. *et al.* (1999). The new apolipoprotein A-I variant leu(174) $\rightarrow$ Ser causes hereditary cardiac amyloidosis, and the amyloid fibrils are constituted by the 93-residue N-terminal polypeptide. *American Journal of Pathology* **155**, 695–702.

Okuda, Y., Takasugi, K., Oyama, T., Onuma, M., and Oyama, H. (1994). Amyloidosis in rheumatoid arthritis—clinical study of 124 histologically proven cases. *Ryumachi* **34**, 939–946.

Ostertag, B. (1932). Demonstration einer eigenartigen familiaren 'Paraamyloidose'. *Zentralblatt der Allgemeine Pathologie* **56**, 253–254.

Palha, J. A. *et al.* (2000). 4′-Iodo-4′-deoxydoxorubicin disrupts the fibrillar structure of transthyretin amyloid. *American Journal of Pathology* **156**, 1919–1925.

Palladini, G. *et al.* (2001). Holter monitoring in AL amyloidosis: prognostic implications. *Pacing Clinical Electrophysiology* **24**, 1228–1233.

Pasternack, A., Ahonen, J., and Kuhlback, B. (1986). Renal transplantation in 45 patients with amyloidosis. *Transplantation* **42**, 598–601.

Patel, H., Fellowes, R., Coade, S., and Woo, P. (1998). Human serum amyloid A has cytokine-like properties. *Scandinavian Journal of Immunology* **48**, 410–418.

Pepys, M. B. and Dash, A. C. (1977). Isolation of amyloid P component (protein AP) from normal serum as a calcium-dependent binding protein. *Lancet* **1**, 1029–1031.

Pepys, M. B., Baltz, M., Gomer, K., Davies, A. J., and Doenhoff, M. (1979). Serum amyloid P-component is an acute-phase reactant in the mouse. *Nature* **278**, 259–261.

Pepys, M. B. *et al.* (1993). Human lysozyme gene mutations cause hereditary systemic amyloidosis. *Nature* **362**, 553–557.

Pepys, M. B. *et al.* (2002). Targeted pharmological depletion of serum amyloid P component for treatment of human amyloidosis. *Nature* **417**, 254–259.

Port, F. K. and Nissenson, A. R. (1989). Outcome of end-stage renal disease in patients with rare causes of renal failure. II. Renal or systemic neoplasms. *Quarterly Journal of Medicine* **73**, 1161–1165.

Pras, M., Bronshpigel, N., Zemer, D., and Gafni, J. (1982). Variable incidence of amyloidosis in familial Mediterranean fever among different ethnic groups. *Johns Hopkins Medical Journal* **150**, 22–26.

Preciado-Patt, L., Hershkoviz, R., Fridkin, M., and Lider, O. (1996). Serum amyloid A binds specific extracellular matrix glycoproteins and induces the adhesion of resting CD4+ T cells. *Journal of Immunology* **156**, 1189–1195.

Ratnaswamy, G., Koepf, E., Bekele, H., Yin, H., and Kelly, J. W. (1999). The amyloidogenicity of gelsolin is controlled by proteolysis and pH. *Chemistry and Biology* **6**, 293–304.

Reilly, M. M., Staunton, H., and Harding, A. E. (1995). Familial amyloid polyneuropathy (TTR ala 60) in north west Ireland: a clinical, genetic, and epidemiological study. *Journal of Neurology, Neurosurgery and Psychiatry* **59**, 45–49.

Rochet, J. C. and Lansbury, P. T., Jr. (2000). Amyloid fibrillogenesis: themes and variations. *Current Opinion in Structural Biology* **10**, 60–68.

Sanchorawala, V. *et al.* (2001). An overview of the use of high-dose melphalan with autologous stem cell transplantation for the treatment of AL amyloidosis. *Bone Marrow Transplantation* **28**, 637–642.

Saraiva, M. J., Costa, P. P., and Goodman, D. S. (1985). Biochemical marker in familial amyloidotic polyneuropathy, Portuguese type. Family studies on the transthyretin (prealbumin)-methionine-30 variant. *Journal of Clinical Investigation* **76**, 2171–2177.

Savolainen, H. A. and Isomaki, H. A. (1993). Decrease in the number of deaths from secondary amyloidosis in patients with juvenile rheumatoid arthritis. *Journal of Rheumatology* **20**, 1201–1203.

Schnitzer, T. J. and Ansell, B. M. (1977). Amyloidosis in juvenile chronic polyarthritis. *Arthritis and Rheumatism* **20** (Suppl.) 245–252.

Seldin, D. C. *et al.* (2003). Tolerability and efficacy of thalidomide for the treatment of patients with light chain associated (AL) amyloidosis. *Clinical Lymphoma* **3**, 241–246.

Shohat, M., Danon, Y. L., and Rotter, J. I. (1992). Familial Mediterranean fever: analysis of inheritance and current linkage data. *American Journal of Medical Genetics* **44**, 183–188.

Shiiki, H., Shimokama, T., Yoshikawa, Y., Onoyama, K., Morimatsu, M., and Watanabe, T. (1989). Perimembranous-type renal amyloidosis: a peculiar form of AL amyloidosis. *Nephron* **53**, 27–32.

Simms, R. W., Prout, M. N., and Cohen, A. S. (1994). The epidemiology of AL and AA amyloidosis. *Bailliere's Clinical Rheumatology* **8**, 627–634.

Skinner, M. *et al.* (1996). Treatment of 100 patients with primary amyloidosis: a randomized trial of melphalan, prednisone, and colchicine versus colchicine only. *American Journal of Medicine* **100**, 290–298.

Solomon, A., Weiss, D. T., and Kattine, A. A. (1991). Nephrotoxic potential of Bence Jones proteins. *New England Journal of Medicine* **324**, 1845–1851.

Sousa, A., Andersson, R., Drugge, U., Holmgren, G., and Sandgren, O. (1993). Familial amyloidotic polyneuropathy in Sweden: geographical distribution, age of onset, and prevalence. *Human Heredity* **43**, 288–294.

Sousa, A., Coelho, T., Barros, J., and Sequeiros, J. (1995). Genetic epidemiology of familial amyloidotic polyneuropathy (FAP)-type I in Povoa do Varzim and Vila do Conde (north of Portugal). *American Journal of Medical Genetics* **60**, 512–521.

Soutar, A. K. *et al.* (1992). Apolipoprotein AI mutation Arg-60 causes autosomal dominant amyloidosis. *Proceedings of the National Academy of Sciences of the USA* **89**, 7389–7393.

Tan, S. Y. *et al.* (1996). Long term effect of renal transplantation on dialysis-related amyloid deposits and symptomatology. *Kidney International* **50**, 282–289.

The French FMF Consortium (1997). A candidate gene for familial Mediterranean fever. *Nature Genetics* **17**, 25–31.

The International FMF Consortium (1997). Ancient missense mutations in a new member of the RoRet gene family are likely to cause familial Mediterranean fever. *Cell* **90**, 797–807.

Triger, D. R. and Joekes, A. M. (1973). Renal amyloidosis—a fourteen-year follow-up. *Quarterly Journal of Medicine* **42**, 15–40.

Van Allen, M. W., Frohlich, J. A., and Davis, J. R. (1969). Inherited predisposition to generalized amyloidosis. Clinical and pathological study of a family with neuropathy, nephropathy, and peptic ulcer. *Neurology* **19**, 10–25.

Vigushin, D. M. *et al.* (1994). Familial nephropathic systemic amyloidosis caused by apolipoprotein AI variant Arg26. *Quarterly Journal of Medicine* **87**, 149–154.

Weiss, S. W. and Page, D. L. (1973). Amyloid nephropathy of Ostertag with special reference to renal glomerular giant cells. *American Journal of Pathology* **72**, 447–460.

Westermark, P. (1982). The heterogeneity of protein AA in secondary (reactive) systemic amyloidosis. *Biochimica et Biophysica Acta* **701**, 19–23.

Williamson, L. M., Hull, D., Mehta, R., Reeves, W. G., Robinson, B. H., and Toghill, P. J. (1982). Familial Hibernian fever. *Quarterly Journal of Medicine* **51**, 469–480.

Wisniewski, T. and Frangione, B. (1992). Apolipoprotein E: a pathological chaperone protein in patients with cerebral and systemic amyloid. *Neuroscience Letters* **135**, 235–238.

Zalin, A. M., Jones, S., Fitch, N. J., and Ramsden, D. B. (1991). Familial nephropathic non-neuropathic amyloidosis: clinical features, immunohistochemistry and chemistry. *Quarterly Journal of Medicine* **81**, 945–956.

Zemer, D., Pras, M., Sohar, E., Modan, M., Cabili, S., and Gafni, J. (1986). Colchicine in the prevention and treatment of the amyloidosis of familial Mediterranean fever. *New England Journal of Medicine* **314**, 1001–1005.

Zemer, D., Livneh, A., Pras, M., and Sohar, E. (1993). The kidney in familial Mediterranean fever. *Contributions to Nephrology* **102**, 187–197.

Zimlichman, S., Danon, A., Nathan, I., Mozes, G., and Shainkin-Kestenbaum, R. (1990). Serum amyloid A, an acute phase protein, inhibits platelet activation. *Journal of Laboratory and Clinical Medicine* **116**, 180–186.

4.2.2 Fibrillary and immunotactoid glomerulopathy

Stephen M. Korbet, Melvin M. Schwartz, and Edmund J. Lewis

Introduction

In 1977, Rosenmann and Eliakim (1977) reported an unusual glomerular lesion in a 45-year-old woman presenting with the nephrotic syndrome and renal insufficiency. Electron microscopy demonstrated electron-dense deposits with a high degree of organization in the form of fibrils which measured 10 nm in diameter. The deposits were associated with mesangial expansion and immune deposits of IgG, IgM, and C3 in a mesangial pattern. Congo-red stain of the deposits was negative and there was no clinical or serological evidence of a systemic disease. The deposits were interpreted to be 'amyloid-like' and it was speculated that they might represent a 'pre-amyloid' state. Shortly thereafter, Schwartz and Lewis (1980) reported a case of a 49-year-old man presenting with the nephrotic syndrome, with no evidence of systemic disease, who had a similar renal lesion: immune aggregates were associated with highly organized electron-dense deposits composed of microtubules. During 7 years of follow-up the patient progressed to renal failure but never demonstrated any clinical or serological evidence of a systemic disease. In order to distinguish this lesion from other disorders with renal lesions having glomerular immune deposits associated with highly organized microtubular or fibrillary structures such as amyloidosis, cryoglobulinaemia, paraproteinaemias, and systemic lupus erythematosus (SLE), the term 'immunotactoid glomerulopathy' (ITG) was introduced, reflecting the composition (immuno-) and polymeric morphology (tactoid) of the glomerular deposits.

Since these initial reports, more than 200 cases of ITG have been reported. Various synonyms have been used to refer to the lesion described in these reports, including fibrillary glomerulonephritis (FGN), non-amyloidotic fibrillary glomerulopathy, amyloid-like glomerulopathy, and amyloid-stain-negative microfibrillary glomerulopathy, but we believe they all represent the same or a similar disease process. The unifying feature in all the cases is the finding of highly organized ultrastructural deposits that appear to be composed of immunoglobulin and complement and are negative for amyloid by Congo-red stain.

Despite the increasing recognition of this lesion, ITG is an uncommon glomerulopathy which accounts for less than 4 per cent of renal biopsies done for the evaluation of nephrotic syndrome (Korbet *et al.* 1991, 1996; Iskander *et al.* 1992; Fogo *et al.* 1993; Pronovost *et al.* 1996; Brady 1998; Schwartz 1998). The clinical diagnosis of ITG is applied only after the exclusion of diseases known to be associated with organized glomerular immune deposits including amyloidosis, cryoglobulinaemia, paraproteinaemias, and SLE. Along with ITG, these disorders comprise the family of histopathological lesions referred to as the 'fibrillary glomerulopathies' (Table 1, Fig. 1). The disorders included in this classification are defined histochemically. In this schema, ITG represents one of the non-amyloid, immunoglobulin-mediated fibrillary glomerulopathies of which there is a differential diagnosis with diseases which must be excluded before the diagnosis of ITG is made. Many of the diseases associated with the fibrillary glomerulopathies have specific therapies and prognoses which differ significantly from that of ITG. As a result, it is critical that the clinician use a combined histological, clinical, and serological approach in reaching the correct diagnosis (Table 2, Fig. 1).

Table 1 Classification of the fibrillary glomerulopathies

Amyloid (Congo-red positive)
AL amyloid
Primary
Multiple myeloma
AA amyloid
Rheumatic diseases
Chronic suppurative and granulomatous inflammation
Tumours
Familial Mediterranean fever
Non-amyloid (Congo-red negative)
Immunoglobulin-derived fibrils
Cryoglobulinaemias
Mixed essential
Multiple myeloma
Chronic lymphocytic leukaemia
Monoclonal gammopathies
'Benign'
Multiple myeloma
Monoclonal immunoglobulin deposition disease
Chronic lymphocytic leukaemia
Systemic lupus erythematosus
Immunotactoid (fibrillary) glomerulopathy
Non-immunoglobulin-derived fibrils
Diabetes mellitus (diabetic fibrillosis)
Fibronectin nephropathy
Others

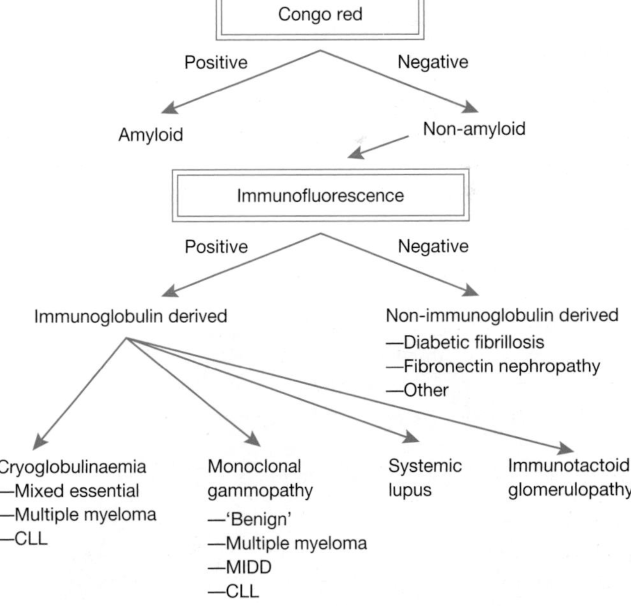

Fig. 1 Algorithm for the evaluation of a patient with fibrillary glomerulopathy. MIDD, monoclonal deposition disease; CLL, chronic lymphocytic leukaemia. Reproduced with permission (Korbet *et al.* 1994).

Pathology

The primary pathology of ITG is almost exclusively confined to the glomeruli, reflecting the location of the microfibrils in the mesangium and the glomerular capillary walls (Korbet *et al.* 1991; Schwartz 1998). By light microscopy mesangial expansion by periodic acid–Schiff (PAS) positive material with only a mild mesangial hypercellularity is almost always observed (Fig. 2). Glomerular capillary wall pathology may be focal or diffuse, and consists of thickening and complex staining patterns seen with methenamine silver-PAS (Jones) stain, including reticular patterns, spikes, and double contours (Fig. 3). Proliferative glomerulonephritis with cellular and fibrocellular crescents, and segmental necrotizing lesions have been described in a few patients

Table 2 Diagnostic features of fibrillary glomerulopathies

	Primary amyloid	MEC	LCDD	Systemic lupus	ITG
Systemic symptoms (%)	75	75	75	100	0
Cryoglobulins (%)	0	100	0	50	0
Paraproteins (%)	100	75	100	0	0
ANA (%)	0	0	0	100	20
C3/C4	NL	Low	NL	Low	NL
Microfibril diameter (nm)	8–10	6–62	10–15	8–25	10–49

MEC, mixed essential cryoglobulinaemia; LCDD, light chain deposition disease; ITG, immunotactoid glomerulopathy; NL, normal.

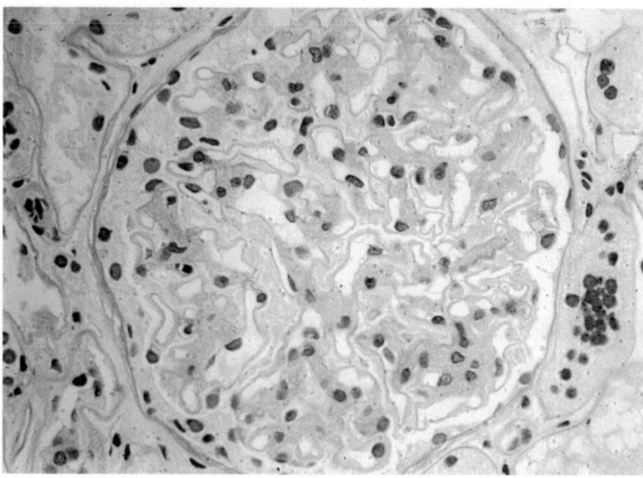

Fig. 2 Glomerulus with diffuse increase in mesangial matrix and normal capillary walls (PAS, 100×).

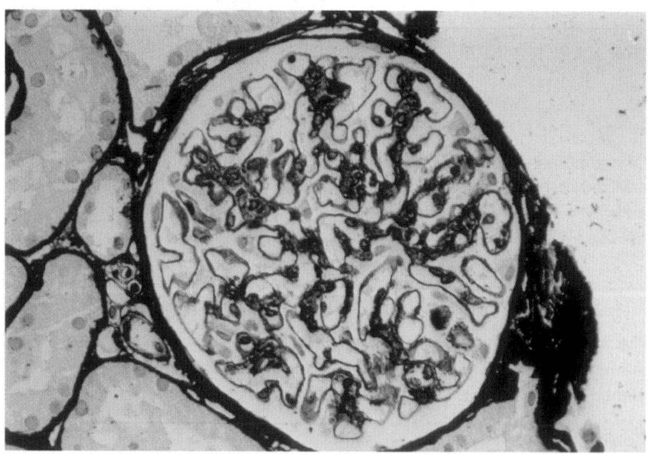

Fig. 3 The mesangium is diffusely expanded. The glomerular basement membrane has a complex appearance with diffuse thickening, focal spikes, and a reticular pattern (Jones, 100×).

(Duffy *et al.* 1983; Alpers *et al.* 1987; Iskander *et al.* 1992; Brady 1998). However, we have not seen these lesions in ITG when systemic diseases such as cryoglobulinaemia, paraproteinaemia, and SLE have been excluded. Most importantly, the glomeruli, tubulointerstitium, and vessels are negative for amyloid by Congo red and thioflavin-T stains. Evaluation of extraglomerular structures demonstrates no specific vascular or tubulointerstitial lesions in ITG.

The principal findings by fluorescence microscopy are the presence of immunoglobulins and complement in a pattern that precisely reflects the distribution of the fibrils by electron microscopy and glomerular mesangial and capillary wall pathology (Fig. 4) seen by light microscopy (Korbet *et al.* 1991; Schwartz 1998). The capillary wall deposits are either diffuse and coarsely granular or discontinuous and pseudolinear. Tubular basement membrane, interstitial and vascular deposits, determined by fluorescence microscopy, have not been observed. The immunoglobulin class is IgG in more than 90 per cent of cases, and the deposits usually contains both κ and λ light chains (Table 3). Despite the absence of a paraproteinaemia, monoclonal immunoglobulin deposits have been seen in approximately 20 per cent cases of ITG studied with light chain antisera, and κ light chain restriction was present in all cases, usually in combination with γ heavy chain (Korbet *et al.* 1991). A study of IgG subgroups found IgG4 as the dominant subclass with weak staining for IgG1 and absent IgG2

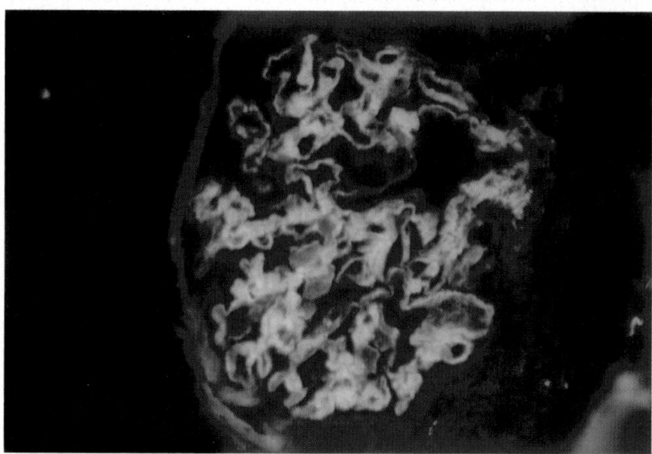

Fig. 4 Mesangial and peripheral capillary wall deposits of IgG. [Fluorescein isothiocynate conjugated rabbit anti-human immunoglobulin G (IgG), 100×.]

Table 3 Immunofluorescence features

Immune component	% positive
IgG	94
IgA	60
IgM	29
C3	96
κ only	23
κ and λ	77

Data from Korbet *et al.* (1991).

and IgG3 (Iskander *et al.* 1992) and monoclonal IgG3κ was reported in one case, not associated with a paraproteinaemia, with 35 nm microtubular deposits (Schwartz and Lewis 1980).

The ultrastructural appearance of ITG is characterized by the glomerular deposition of extracellular elongated, non-branching microfibrils/microtubules which have neither periodicity nor substructure. The microfibrils are seen in the same locations as the immune deposits seen by immunofluorescence microscopy suggesting that they are composed of immunoglobulin and complement. Thus, the microfibrils are seen in the mesangium, the primary site of deposition and often also seen in the glomerular capillary wall. The amount of tactoidal material present in the glomerular capillary wall seems to correlate with the extent of glomerular damage. Most commonly, they are present within a thickened basal lamina, but they are also present beneath the epithelial cell where they form large deposits that alternate with projections of basement membrane (spikes). Occasionally, the deposits are seen in the subendothelial space and within the capillary lumen. When fibrils are subepithelial or subendothelial, new layers of basement membrane form over them and incorporate the fibrils into a thickened, irregular capillary wall. Extraglomerular deposits involving the tubular basement membrane or interstitium have been demonstrated in only three cases of ITG (Duffy *et al.* 1983; Korbet *et al.* 1985; Alpers *et al.* 1987).

The size of the fibrils varies, but they are distinguished from amyloid by a larger diameter (Table 2). In most series the diameters have a mean value of 18–22 nm (Table 4, Fig. 5). However, the reported diameters have varied from slightly larger than amyloid (10–12 nm) to as large as 49 nm (Fig. 6). Even though there is variability of fibril size among cases, the fibrils in a given case are remarkably consistent in appearance wherever they appear in the glomerulus. The cross-sectional appearance varies from a solid dot to microtubules with either a thin or a thick wall. Examination of the fibrils at high magnification reveals a central core and a wall of varying thickness. Fibrils have a variable length and can appear long and straight or short and curved. They are usually present within a granular, electron-dense matrix suggesting that only part of the deposit is aggregated into fibrils. In most cases the microtubules are randomly arranged on cross-section with various elongated profiles seen in adjacent areas (Fig. 5). In other cases, the microtubules appear to be in tightly packed parallel bundles on cross-section, especially with larger fibrils, that have a paracrystalline appearance (Fig. 6).

It has been suggested that ITG should be separated into two categories based upon arbitrary ultrastructural criteria regarding fibril size and/or organization. The proponents of subdividing ITG suggest that the diagnosis of ITG be reserved for cases with larger (≤30 nm), parallel microtubules, and that FGN be applied to cases with smaller (<30 nm), randomly arranged fibrils (Alpers 1992; Iskander *et al.* 1992; Fogo *et al.* 1993). The rationale used for this subdivision is that the different morphological categories have significant clinical implications (D'Agati *et al.* 1991; Iskander *et al.* 1992; Alpers 1993; Fogo *et al.* 1993). Presently, there is no compelling reason to separately diagnose ITG and FGN on the basis of morphology alone as it has not been demonstrated that the ultrastructural features have significant pathogenetic or clinical implications (Pronovost *et al.* 1996; Brady 1998). Thus, we use the diagnosis of ITG to describe patients with both types of deposits, and reserve the term FGN to denote the broader category of diseases (Fig. 1) that are characterized morphologically by fibrils seen by electron microscopy without regard to their biochemical composition (Churg and Venkataseshan 1993; Korbet *et al.* 1994; Brady 1998).

Table 4 The range of microfibril diameter in ITG

Microfibril diameter (nm)	% of patients
<12	13
13–17	11
18–22	44
23–27	12
28–32	14
>32	6

Data from Korbet *et al.* (1994).

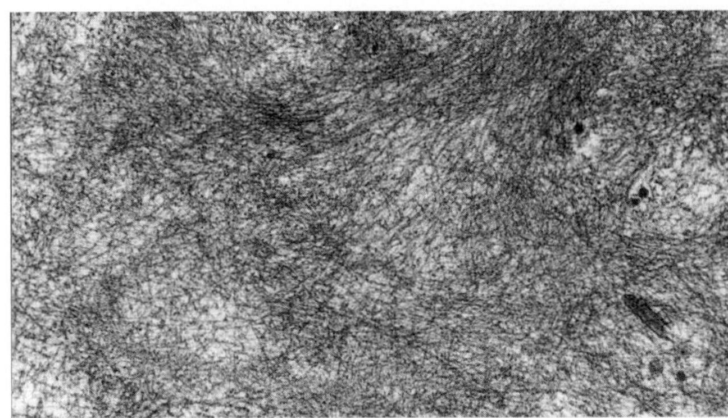

Fig. 5 Electron micrograph of glomerular fibrillar deposits showing a random arrangement and measuring 20 nm in diameter. (Uranyl acetate and lead citrate, 32,000×.)

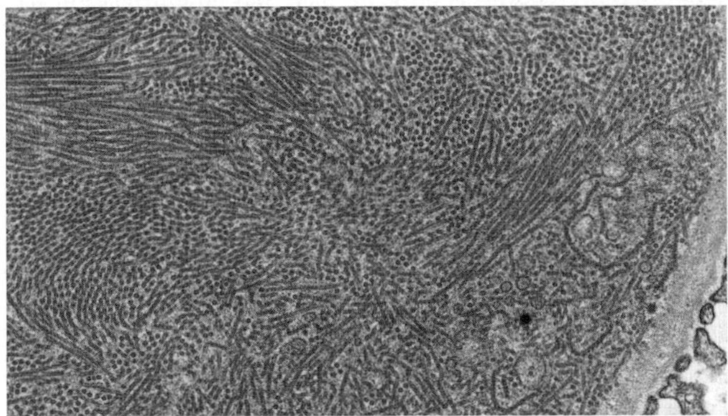

Fig. 6 Electron micrograph of glomerular microtubular deposits showing a parallel, packed arrangement and measuring 35 nm in diameter. (Uranyl acetate and lead citrate, 32,000×.)

Clinical and laboratory features

On clinical grounds there is nothing unique about the presentation or course of ITG that would allow one to distinguish this disorder from other primary glomerulopathies (Table 5). Patients with ITG range

Table 5 Presenting clinical features

	Korbet *et al.* (1991, 1996)	Pronovost *et al.* (1996)
n	62	186
Age range (mean)	10–80 (44 ± 15)	10–81
Male	61%	47%
White	92%	90%
Hypertension	66%	70%
Proteinuria	100%	100%
Nephrotic	61%	72%
Haematuria	78%	71%
Renal insufficiency	47%	53%

in age from 10 to 80 years but on average have been 44 years old at presentation (Korbet *et al.* 1991, 1994; Iskander *et al.* 1992; Pronovost *et al.* 1996; Brady 1998). Ninety per cent of the patients are White, and the distribution between men and women is approximately equal (Korbet *et al.* 1991, 1996; Iskander *et al.* 1992; Pronovost *et al.* 1996). The presenting feature in all patients is proteinuria, with over 60 per cent having the nephrotic syndrome. Hypertension and microscopic haematuria are common and present in more than 65 and more than 70 per cent of patients, respectively, and more than 45 per cent of patients have some degree of renal insufficiency at the time of diagnosis, indicating the chronic and progressive nature of ITG (Korbet *et al.* 1991; Iskander *et al.* 1992; Pronovost *et al.* 1996). In a review of 186 cases of ITG (Pronovost *et al.* 1996) there was no difference in the prevalence of hypertension, haematuria, nephrotic syndrome, or renal insufficiency at presentation when the diagnosis of ITG was subdivided based on differences in fibril size (>30 versus ≤30 nm) or arrangement (random versus parallel bundles).

The serological evaluation for cryoglobulins and paraproteins (by immunoelectrophoresis or immunofixation of serum and urine) is, by definition, negative in ITG and the serum complement levels are normal. However, up to 19 per cent of patients have a low titre antinuclear antibodies (ANA), often in a speckled pattern (Korbet *et al.* 1985; Iskander *et al.* 1992; Pronovost *et al.* 1996). Nonetheless, patients with ITG do not have clinical SLE and, in general, have no evidence of a systemic disease process.

ITG represents a primary glomerulopathy. Extrarenal involvement with organized immunoglobulin deposits has been described in only two cases (Korbet *et al.* 1990; Ozawa *et al.* 1991; Masson *et al.* 1992; Wallner *et al.* 1996). In both these cases, one involving the liver (Ozawa *et al.* 1991) and the other the lung (Masson *et al.* 1992), there were clinical evidences of disease. Unlike amyloidosis and other forms of monoclonal immunoglobulin deposition diseases, deposits have not been demonstrated in clinically uninvolved organs studied at autopsy (Korbet *et al.* 1990).

The overall prevalence of a lymphoproliferative malignancy in patients with ITG is low (<3 per cent). It has been suggested that these neoplasias are more frequently seen in patients whose deposits are composed of larger (>30 nm) microtubules. However, when patients with paraproteinaemia are excluded, there is no difference in the prevalence of lymphoproliferative disease based on differences in either fibril diameter or arrangement (Pronovost *et al.* 1996). Patients rarely develop clinical or serological evidence of a systemic disease or a dysproteinaemia (Korbet *et al.* 1991). Thus, the pathogenetic process in ITG primarily involves the glomeruli, which distinguishes the lesion from the other immunoglobulin-derived fibrillary glomerulopathies (Korbet *et al.* 1994) (Table 2).

Prognosis and treatment

The course of patients with ITG is one of progressive renal failure to the requirement of dialysis over 2–4 years in 50 per cent of patients (Korbet *et al.* 1991; Iskander *et al.* 1992; Pronovost *et al.* 1996). This is similar to other primary glomerulopathies but is distinct from that of the other fibrillary glomerulopathies which experience a more rapid decline to endstage renal disease (ESRD) (Korbet *et al.* 1994). Features at presentation, which appear to be associated with a poor renal prognosis, are hypertension, nephrotic syndrome, and the presence of decreased glomerular filtration rate at presentation (Korbet *et al.* 1985, 1991; Pronovost *et al.* 1996). Even though detailed analyses on the pathology of this lesion have been reported there has been little information regarding the prognostic significance of the various pathological features of ITG. Unsurprisingly, those patients with more extensive glomerular deposits have a poorer prognosis (Korbet *et al.* 1985).

Since ITG appears to be an immune-mediated lesion, immunosuppressive therapy has been attempted. While the reported experience is limited, therapeutic trials with steroids alone, steroids with cytotoxic agents, and steroids with plasmapheresis have rarely (<10 per cent) resulted in clinical remission of proteinuria (Schwartz and Lewis 1980; Alpers *et al.* 1987; Schifferli *et al.* 1987; D'Agati *et al.* 1991; Minami *et al.* 1997; Kurihara *et al.* 1998).

The overall survival of the patient with ITG is as one might expect with a primary glomerulopathy and no systemic disease. The survival at 1 year is 100 per cent with over 80 per cent of patients alive at 5 years (Korbet *et al.* 1985, 1991). As a result, renal transplantation should be a treatment consideration for ITG patients with ESRD. The outcome of renal transplantation has been reported in 15 ITG patients (Table 6) with 2–13 years of post-transplant follow-up (Alpers *et al.* 1987; Sturgil and Bolton 1989; Korbet *et al.* 1990; Fogo *et al.* 1993; Pronovost *et al.* 1996; Carles *et al.* 2000; Samaniego *et al.* 2001). Recurrence of ITG has been demonstrated in 46 per cent of these patients from 2 to 9 years after transplantation, and in three cases this resulted in the loss of the graft. In the remaining patients with recurrent disease, renal function continued to be adequate after 5–11 years of follow-up (Alpers *et al.* 1987; Korbet *et al.* 1990; Pronovost *et al.* 1996; Carles *et al.* 2000). The rate of deterioration in renal function in patients with recurrent disease has been shown to be slower than with their original disease. One possible explanation could be the effect of immunosuppression (Pronovost *et al.* 1996). In those patients with recurrent disease, the ultrastructural morphology in the transplants was similar to that originally seen in the native kidneys (Alpers *et al.* 1987; Korbet *et al.* 1990; Carles *et al.* 2000; Samaniego *et al.* 2001). Thus, while recurrent disease does occur in ITG, it usually occurs late post-transplantation and does not inevitably result in graft loss.

Table 6 Post-transplant course in ITG

Reference	Patients (*n*)	Follow-up (years)	Recurrence	ESRD
Alpers *et al.* (1987)	1	5	1 (5 years)	0
Sturgil *et al.* (1989)	1	2	0	0
Korbet *et al.* (1990)	2	5–6	1 (4.5 years)	1
Fogo *et al.* (1993)	2	??	0	0
Pronovost *et al.* (1996)	4	4–11	2 (? years)	1
Carles *et al.* (2000)	1	4	1 (1.5 years)	0
Samaniego *et al.* (2000)	4	3–13	2 (2 and 9 years)	1
Total	15	2–13	7	3

Pathogenesis and pathophysiology

The term immunotactoid was chosen to stress the organized orientation of the deposits and their immunoglobulin composition (Korbet *et al.* 1985). Using immunoelectron microscopy, it has been shown that the fibrils in patients with ITG contain immunoglobulins (both heavy and light chains) and complement as well as amyloid P component but do not contain other amyloid-associated, basement membrane-associated (type IV collagen and heparan-sulfate proteoglycans), or microfibril-associated (fibronectin and fibrillin) proteins (Casanova *et al.* 1992; Yang *et al.* 1992). The presence of amyloid P component raises the possibility that fibrillogenesis in ITG may be analogous to amyloidosis but without resulting in the critical β-pleated sheet formation.

In the usual physiological environment, intact normal ITG do not crystallize readily. In ITG, the propensity to form microtubular structures or tactoids suggests that the deposits are composed of a uniform substructure with strong intermolecular attraction. Therefore, one can speculate that the formation of immunotactoid deposits are the result of immune complexes having a uniform structure or an abnormal production of monoclonal immunoglobulins which perhaps have an unusual or abnormal structure. These may be produced in such small quantities that they escape detection with standard serological evaluation as patients with ITG, by definition, do not have evidence of a circulating cryoglobulin or a paraprotein. The deposition of the immunoglobulins within the glomerulus along the filtration surface of the glomerular capillary wall may be a consequence of the unique environment created by the ultrafiltration of plasma (Korbet *et al.* 1985). The increased concentration of protein occurring along the glomerular capillary as a consequence of ultrafiltration may account for the tendency of the deposits to form exclusively within the kidney.

Structural alterations along the filtration surface of the glomerulus may also be important and predispose to fibril formation. In mice, absence of CD2-associated protein (CD2AP), a protein which binds to nephrin and is important in the function of the podocyte slit diaphragm, results in congenital nephrotic syndrome and glomerular ultrastructural pathology similar to that seen in ITG in humans (Shih *et al.* 1999; Li *et al.* 2000; Shaw 2000). Thus, glomerular deposits in ITG may result from acquired defects in critical podocyte cellular functions involved in the clearance of filtered and retained immunoglobulin.

Although the cause of ITG is unknown, the heterogeneity of the immunopathology suggests that more than one aetiology is responsible for the production of fibrils with a common morphological appearance. In this respect, it may be similar to amyloid where it is well known that various disease states are capable of producing different proteins which have in common the capacity to form the highly organized β-pleated sheet structure. Since immunotactoids may be composed of either immune complexes or monoclonal proteins which are capable of forming tactoids or microtubules, the variability in the size and orientation of the tactoids from one patient to another may be a result of concentration or biochemical composition of the protein similar to that described in cryoglobulinaemia.

Alternatively, the variability in ultrastructural morphology among patients with ITG may be analogous to the morphological heterogeneity in haemoglobin S described in the haemoglobinopathy of sickle cell anaemia (Eaton and Hofrichter 1987). The morphology of deoxygenated haemoglobin S in sickle cell disease is dependent upon the concentration of haemoglobin S and the rate of tactoid formation. Under circumstances where they form slowly, the tactoids are aligned in parallel forming a paracrystalline structure. In contrast, the more rapidly the tactoids are formed the more random the orientation to one another (Eaton and Hofrichter 1987). Similarly, a patient with ITG has been described with biochemically identical fibrils in the glomeruli and in a serum precipitate that formed after 4 months in cold storage; however, the ultrastructural morphology differed significantly between the fibrils (Rostagno *et al.* 1996). The fibrils in the glomeruli were 15–20 nm in diameter while those in the serum precipitate were 90 nm. Thus, as in haemoglobin S, the variability in morphology observed in ITG may result from physiochemical factors involved in fibrillogenesis.

The pathogenesis of ITG may be immunochemically diverse with the unifying feature being the ultrastructural organization of the deposits. In the appropriate setting, immune complexes or immunoglobulins are capable of forming fibrils or microtubules (tactoids) in the glomerular capillary wall or mesangium. Unfortunately, the disease(s) responsible for the production of the immune material in the tactoids of ITG has not been determined in the patients who have been described to date.

References

Alpers, C. E. (1992). Immunotactoid (microtubular) glomerulopathy: an entity distinct from fibrillary glomerulonephritis? *American Journal of Kidney Diseases* **19**, 185–191.

Alpers, C. E. (1993). Fibrillary glomerulonephritis and immunotactoid glomerulopathy: two entities, not one. *American Journal of Kidney Diseases* **22**, 448–451.

Alpers, C. E., Rennke, H. G., Hopper, J., and Biava, C. G. (1987). Fibrillary glomerulonephritis: an entity with unusual immunofluorescence features. *Kidney International* **31**, 781–789.

Brady, H. R. (1998). Fibrillary glomerulopathy. *Kidney International* **53**, 1421–1429.

Carles, X., Rostaing, L., Modesto, A., Orfila, C., Cisterne, J. M., Delisle, M. B., and Durand, D. (2000). Successful treatment of recurrence of immunotactoid glomerulopathy in a kidney allograft recipient. *Nephrology, Dialysis, Transplantation* **15**, 897–900.

Casanova, S., Donini, U., Zucchelli, P., Mazzucco, G., Monga, G., and Linke, R. (1992). Immunohistochemical distinction between amyloidosis and fibrillary glomerulopathy. *American Journal of Clinical Pathology* **97**, 787–795.

Churg, J. and Venkataseshan, S. (1993). Fibrillary glomerulonephritis without immunoglobulin deposits in the kidney. *Kidney International* **44**, 837–842.

D'Agati, V., Sacchi, G., Truong, L., Venkataseshan, S., Kim, D., Kim, B., and Appel, G. (1991). Fibrillary glomerulopathy: defining the disease spectrum. *Journal of the American Society of Nephrology* **2**, 591 (abstract).

Duffy, J. L., Khurana, E., Susin, M., Gomez-Leon, G., and Churg, J. (1983). Fibrillary renal deposits and nephritis. *American Journal of Pathology* **113**, 279–290.

Eaton, W. and Hofrichter, J. (1987). Hemoglobin S gelation and sickle cell disease. *Blood* **70**, 1245–1266.

Fogo, A., Qureshi, N., and Horn, R. G. (1993). Morphologic and clinical features of fibrillary glomerulonephritis versus immunotactoid glomerulopathy. *American Journal of Kidney Diseases* **22**, 367–377.

Iskander, S. S., Falk, R. J., and Jennette, C. (1992). Clinical and pathological features of fibrillary glomerulonephritis. *Kidney International* **42**, 1401–1407.

Korbet, S. M., Genchi, R. M., Borok, R. Z., and Schwartz, M. M. (1996). The racial prevalence of glomerular lesions in nephrotic adults. *American Journal of Kidney Diseases* **27**, 647–651.

Korbet, S. M., Rosenberg, B. F., Schwartz, M. M., and Lewis, E. J. (1990). Course of renal transplantation in immunotactoid glomerulopathy. *American Journal of Medicine* **89**, 91–95.

Korbet, S. M., Schwartz, M. M., and Lewis, E. J. (1991). Immunotactoid glomerulopathy. *American Journal of Kidney Diseases* **17**, 247–257.

Korbet, S. M., Schwartz, M. M., and Lewis, E. J. (1994). The fibrillary glomerulopathies. *American Journal of Kidney Diseases* **23**, 751–765.

Korbet, S. M., Schwartz, M. M., Rosenberg, B. F., Sibley, R. K., and Lewis, E. J. (1985). Immunotactoid glomerulopathy. *Medicine* **64**, 228–243.

Kurihara, I., Saito, T., Sato, H., Chiba, J., Saito, J., Soma, J., and Ito, S. (1998). Successful treatment with steroid pulse therapy in a case of immunotactoid glomerulopathy with hypocomplementemia. *American Journal of Kidney Diseases* **32**, E4.

Li, C., Ruotsalainen, V., Tryggvason, K., Shaw, A. S., and Miner, J. H. (2000). CD2AP is expressed with nephrin in developing podocytes and is found widely in mature kidney and elsewhere. *American Journal of Physiology. Renal Physiology* **279**, F785–F792.

Masson, R. G., Rennke, H. G., and Gottlieb, M. N. (1992). Pulmonary hemorrhage in a patient with fibrillary glomerulonephritis. *New England Journal of Medicine* **326**, 36–39.

Minami, J., Ishimitsu, T., Inenaga, T., Ishibashi-Ueda, H., Kawano, Y., and Takishita, S. (1997). Immunotactoid glomerulopathy: report of a case. *American Journal of Kidney Diseases* **30**, 160–163.

Ozawa, K., Yamabe, H., Fukushi, K., Osawa, H., Chiba, N., Miyata, M., Seino, S., Inuma, H., Saki, T., Yoshikawa, S., and Onodera, K. (1991). Case report of amyloid-like glomerulopathy with hepatic involvement. *Nephron* **58**, 347–350.

Pronovost, P. H., Brady, H. R., Gunning, M. E., Espinoza, O., and Rennke, H. G. (1996). Clinical features, predictors of disease progression and results of renal transplantation in fibrillary/immunotactoid glomerulopathy. *Nephrology, Dialysis, Transplantation* **11**, 837–842.

Rosenmann, E. and Eliakim, M. (1977). Nephrotic syndrome associated with amyloid-like glomerular deposits. *Nephron* **18**, 301–308.

Rostagno, A., Vidal, R., Kumar, A., Chuba, J., Niederman, G., Gold, L., Frangione, B., Ghiso, J., and Gallo, G. R. (1996). Fibrillary glomerulonephritis related to serum fibrillar immunoglobulin-fibrinectin complexes. *American Journal of Kidney Diseases* **28**, 676–684.

Samaniego, M., Nadasdy, G. M., Laszik, Z., and Nadasdy, T. (2001). Outcome of renal transplantation in fibrillary glomerulonephritis. *Clinical Nephrology* **55**, 159–166.

Schifferli, J. A., Merot, Y., and Chatelanat, F. (1987). Immunotactoid glomerulopathy with leucocytoclastic skin vasculitis and hypocomplementemia: a case report. *Clinical Nephrology* **27**, 151–155.

Schwartz, M. M. Glomerular diseases with organized deposits. In *Heptinstall's Pathology of the Kidney* 5th edn. (ed. J. C. Jennette, J. Olson, M. M. Schwartz, and F. Silva), pp. 369–388. Philadelphia, PA: Lippincott-Raven, 1998.

Schwartz, M. M. and Lewis, E. J. (1980). The quarterly case: nephrotic syndrome in a middle-aged man. *Ultrastructural Pathology* **1**, 575–582.

Shaw, A. S. (2000). Congenital nephrotic syndrome in mice lacking CD2-associated protein. *Journal of the American Society of Nephrology* **11**, 19 (abstract).

Shih, N. Y., Li, J., Karpitskii, V., Nguyen, A., Dustin, M. L., Kanagawa, O., Miner, J. H., and Shaw, A. S. (1999). Congenital nephrotic syndrome in mice lacking CD2-associated protein. *Science* **286**, 312–315.

Sturgil, B. C. and Bolton, W. K. (1989). Non-amyloidotic fibrillary glomerulopathy. *Kidney International* **35**, 233 (abstract).

Wallner, M., Prischl, F. C., Hobling, W., Haidenthaler, A., Regele, H., Ulrich, W., and Kramar, R. (1996). Immunotactoid glomerulopathy with extrarenal deposits in the bone, and chronic cholestatic liver disease. *Nephrology, Dialysis, Transplantation* **11**, 1619–1624.

Yang, G. C. H., Nieto, R., Stachura, I., and Gallo, G. R. (1992). Ultrastructural immunohistochemical localization of polyclonal IgG, C3, and amyloid P component on the Congo red-negative amyloid-like fibrils of fibrillary glomerulopathy. *American Journal of Pathology* **141**, 409–419.

4.3 Kidney involvement in plasma cell dyscrasias

Pierre M. Ronco, Pierre Aucouturier, and Béatrice Mougenot

Introduction

Plasma cell dyscrasias are characterized by uncontrolled proliferation of a single clone of B cells at different maturation stages, with a more or less marked differentiation to immunoglobulin-secreting plasmocytes. They are thus usually associated with the production and secretion in blood of a monoclonal immunoglobulin or a fragment thereof. An ominous consequence of the secretion of monoclonal immunoglobulin products is their deposition in tissues. These proteinaceous deposits can take the form of casts (in myeloma cast nephropathy), crystals (in myeloma-associated Fanconi syndrome), fibrils (in light-chain and exceptional heavy-chain amyloidosis), or granular precipitates (in monoclonal immunoglobulin deposition disease). They may disrupt organ structure and function, inducing life-threatening complications. In a large proportion of patients with crystals, fibrils, or granular deposits of immunoglobulin products, major clinical manifestations and mortality are related to visceral immunoglobulin deposition rather than to expansion of the B-cell clone. Indeed, except for myeloma cast nephropathy which is generally associated with a malignancy with a large tumour mass, immunoglobulin precipitation or deposition diseases frequently occur in the course of a benign B-cell proliferation or of a low-grade myeloma.

The presence of abnormal urine components in a patient with severe bone pain and oedema was first recognized in the 1840s by Henry Bence Jones and William MacIntyre, who described unusual thermal solubility properties of urinary proteins, attributed much later to immunoglobulin light chains (Edelman and Gally 1962). Thus monoclonal light-chain proteinuria is often referred to as 'Bence Jones proteinuria'. However this term is not appropriate, because less than 50 per cent of light chains show thermal solubility. Renal damage characterized by large protein casts surrounded by multinucleated giant cells within distal tubules was identified in the early 1900s, and termed 'myeloma kidney'. However, this denomination must be abandoned also, because other patterns of renal injury were subsequently described in myeloma patients. The first of these was amyloidosis, in which tissue deposits are characterized by Congo red binding and fibrillar ultrastructure. Glenner *et al.* (1971) showed that the aminoacid sequence of amyloid fibrils extracted from tissue was identical to the variable region of a circulating immunoglobulin light chain, thus providing the first demonstration that an immunoglobulin component could be responsible for tissue deposition. The spectrum of renal diseases due to monoclonal immunoglobulin deposition has expanded dramatically with the advent of routine staining of renal biopsies with specific anti-κ- and anti-λ-light-chain antibodies, and of electron microscopy (Table 1). These morphological techniques, associated with more sensitive analyses of blood and urine monoclonal components, have led to the description of new entities, including non-amyloid monoclonal light-chain deposition disease (LCDD) (Antonovych *et al.* 1974; Randall *et al.* 1976), heavy-chain amyloidosis (Eulitz *et al.* 1990), non-amyloid heavy-chain deposition disease (HCDD) (Aucouturier *et al.* 1993b; Moulin *et al.* 1999), and chronic lymphocytic leukaemia-associated glomerulopathies with organized deposits (Touchard *et al.* 1989;

Table 1 Pathological classification of diseases featuring tissue deposition or precipitation of monoclonal immunoglobulin-related material

Organized			**Non-organized (granular)**	
Crystals	**Fibrillar**	**Microtubular**	**MIDD ('Randall type')**	**Other**
Myeloma cast nephropathy[a]	Amyloidosis (AL, AH)	Cryoglobulinaemia kidney	LCDD	Crescentic GN (IgA or IgM)
Fanconi syndrome	Non-amyloid	Immunotactoid (microtubular)	LHCDD	
Other (extrarenal)			HCDD	

[a] Crystals are predominantly localized within casts in the lumen of distal tubules and collecting ducts, but may also occasionally be found in the cytoplasm of proximal tubule epithelial cells.

AH, heavy-chain amyloidosis; AL, light-chain amyloidosis; GN, glomerulonephritis; HCDD, LCDD, LHCDD, MIDD, heavy, light, light and heavy chain, monoclonal immunoglobulin deposition disease, respectively.

Adapted from Preud'homme *et al.* (1994).

Moulin *et al.* 1992). These pathological entities principally involve the kidney, which thus appears as the main target for deposition of monoclonal immunoglobulin components. This is explained not only by the high renal plasma flow and glomerular filtration rate, but also by the prominent role of the renal tubule in light-chain handling and catabolism.

Polymorphism of renal lesions may be due to specific properties of immunoglobulin components influencing their precipitation, their interaction with renal tissue, or their processing after deposition. Alternatively, the type of renal lesions may be driven by the local response to immunoglobulin deposits, which may vary from one patient to another. That intrinsic properties of immunoglobulin components are responsible for the observed renal alterations was first suggested by *in vitro* biosynthesis of abnormal immunoglobulin by bone marrow cells from patients with lymphoplasmacytic disorders and visceral light-chain deposition (Preud'homme *et al.* 1980a) and by recurrence of nephropathy in renal grafts (Short *et al.* 2001). A further demonstration of the specificity of immunoglobulin component pathogenicity was provided by Solomon *et al.* (1991). They showed that the pattern of human renal lesions associated with the production of monoclonal light chains—myeloma cast nephropathy, LCDD, and AL amyloidosis—could be reproduced in mice injected intraperitoneally with large amounts of light chains isolated from patients with multiple myeloma or AL amyloidosis.

A normal immunoglobulin is composed of two light chains and two heavy chains covalently assembled by disulfide bonds. Light chains and heavy chains are themselves made up of the so-called constant (C) and variable (V) globular domains. While, a limited number of genes encode the constant region, multiple gene segments are rearranged to produce a variable domain unique to each chain. Diversity is further amplified by mutations and variations of the linking peptide segment. Light chains (and heavy chains) thus not only have many structural similarities, but also possess a unique sequence that may be responsible for physicochemical peculiarities, hence their deposition in tissue or interaction with tissue constituents. A number of structural and physicochemical abnormalities of immunoglobulin have already been described (reviewed by Cogné *et al.* 1992). They include deletions of C_H domains in HCDD (Aucouturier *et al.* 1993b; Moulin *et al.* 1999) and heavy-chain amyloidosis (Eulitz *et al.* 1990), shortened or lengthened light chains and abnormal light-chain glycosylation in LCDD (Preud'homme *et al.* 1980a; Cogné *et al.* 1991), and resistance to proteolysis of the V_L fragment in Fanconi syndrome (Aucouturier *et al.* 1993a; Leboulleux *et al.* 1995). Moreover, over-representation of certain V_L gene subgroups was also reported in amyloidosis (Solomon *et al.* 1982) and LCDD (Denoroy *et al.* 1994). However, some abnormal immunoglobulin chains produced in immunoproliferative disorders are not associated with any special clinical features. On the other hand, structural abnormalities of light chains are not a constant feature of diseases associated with light-chain deposition.

Because of the lack of specificity of clinical manifestations such as acute renal failure or the nephrotic syndrome, we have classified the various forms of renal involvement in plasma cell dyscrasias according to the lesions observed in renal biopsy. Elucidation of the pathophysiological mechanisms responsible for each type of lesion should result in the identification of patients at risk for this lesion and in the design of new therapeutic strategies. AL- and AH-amyloidosis and type I and type II cryoglobulinaemias that also belong to the family of plasma cell dyscrasias are described in other chapters.

Myeloma-associated tubulopathies

The overall prevalence of tubular lesions in myeloma patients is difficult to assess, because most patients do not undergo a renal biopsy, but it is most likely considerable. In Kapadia's (1980) autopsy series, 46 of 60 consecutive myeloma patients (77 per cent) had tubular atrophy and fibrosis, and 37 (62 per cent) had tubular hyaline casts, with a giant-cell reaction specific of myeloma cast nephropathy in 29 patients (48 per cent). Only three patients (5 per cent) had amyloidosis and seven patients (12 per cent) had apparently normal kidneys by light microscopic examination. In a more recent autopsy study including immunofluorescence (Ivanyi 1990), 18 of 57 patients (32 per cent) had cast nephropathy, while six (11 per cent) had renal amyloidosis and three (5 per cent) had κ-LCDD. The major prevalence of tubular alterations in patients with light-chain proteinuria is attested also by increased urinary concentrations of the low molecular weight proteins normally reabsorbed by the proximal tubule, increased urinary elimination of the tubular lysosomal enzyme β-acetyl-D-glucosaminidase (Cooper *et al.* 1984), and frequent abnormalities in renal tubular acidifying and concentrating ability (DeFronzo *et al.* 1978). However, myeloma-associated Fanconi syndrome remains exceptional: for example, it was not detected at all in the 42 myeloma patients whose tubular function was studied systematically by Coward *et al.* (1985).

Cast nephropathy is not only the most frequent lesion in myeloma patients, it is also the major cause of renal failure, as attested by its prevalence which is in the same range as that of renal insufficiency—22–50 per cent in more recent series of myeloma patients (Rayner *et al.* 1991; Knudsen *et al.* 1994; MacLennan *et al.* 1994; Blade *et al.* 1998; Knudsen *et al.* 2000). In nephrology departments, the prevalence of histologically assessed cast nephropathy varies from 60 to 87 per cent (Pozzi *et al.* 1987; Rota *et al.* 1987; Pasquali *et al.* 1990; Ganeval *et al.* 1992; Sakhuja *et al.* 2000) among azotaemic myeloma patients. It is most likely underestimated because patients with presumed cast nephropathy do not systematically undergo a renal biopsy, while those exhibiting significant albuminuria or *a fortiori* the nephrotic syndrome do, especially in the absence of amyloidotic deposits in non-renal biopsy specimens.

Myeloma cast nephropathy

Clinical presentation

Changing presentation of patients with myeloma-induced renal failure

When DeFronzo *et al.* reported the first series of 14 myeloma patients with acute renal failure in 1975, it was established that renal failure occurred at some time during the illness in approximately half of the patients, but that the mode of presentation was usually chronic with progression over a period of several months to years.

The mode of presentation of renal failure in myeloma has changed dramatically over the years. In their review of 141 patients treated in Nottingham between 1975 and 1988, Rayner *et al.* (1991) showed that the absence of severe renal impairment at presentation predicted a low probability of developing renal failure subsequently. In only five of 34 patients of our own renal series (Rota *et al.* 1987) did the diagnosis of myeloma antedated the discovery of renal failure by more than 1 month. In 64 per cent of the 53 cases collected in the Oxford series over the period 1989–1994 (Winearls 1995), renal failure was discovered within a month of the diagnosis of myeloma, and in more than half of the cases it antedated it. Such a change in epidemiology of renal failure may be interpreted in two ways. It is possible, although unlikely, that patients with established myeloma who subsequently develop renal failure are not referred for dialysis. Alternatively, more aggressive treatment of myeloma in the last two decades may have prevented light-chain precipitation within the tubule lumen, hence the development of cast nephropathy (Winearls 1995).

Demographic and haematological characteristics of patients with cast nephropathy-related renal failure

Table 2 summarizes the clinical and pathological data in four large series of myeloma patients with acute renal failure, in which a renal biopsy was performed in at least 40 per cent of the patients. A diagnosis of myeloma cast nephropathy was established histologically in 81 of 99 renal biopsies (82 per cent), and lesions compatible with this diagnosis were found in 10 further biopsy specimens (10 per cent). In comparison with the Mayo Clinic series of 869 unselected myeloma cases (Kyle 1975) in which the mean age was 62 years and the male to female ratio was 1.55, patients with acute renal failure did not show any particular features.

More than 72 per cent of patients in the renal series have a high tumour burden (Table 2). This is confirmed by Alexanian's series, which included 494 consecutive patients referred to an oncology centre (Alexanian *et al.* 1990). Only 3 per cent of patients with myeloma of low tumour mass had renal failure, while 40 per cent of those with high tumour burden had a serum creatinine greater than 180 μmol/l.

Another salient feature of myeloma associated with renal failure is the high prevalence of pure light-chain myelomas. While they represent only about 20 per cent of all myelomas referred to haematology or cancer centres, they are found in between 37 and 64 per cent of patients with renal failure of presumed or established tubulointerstitial origin. Development of cast nephropathy in the two studies in which this diagnosis was established histologically (Rota *et al.* 1987; Pasquali *et al.* 1990) was associated with urinary excretion of light chains exceeding 2 g/day in 53 and 72 per cent of the patients (Table 2). IgD myeloma has the greatest potential for causing renal disease (Blade *et al.* 1994). To give a balanced view on the prevalence of pure light-chain myeloma and on the output of urinary light chains in myeloma-associated renal failure, it is also necessary to analyse non-renal series (Alexanian *et al.* 1990). When specific disease features implicated in the pathogenesis of renal failure are examined, light-chain protein excretion emerges as a highly significant independent factor on multivariate analysis (Table 3). The risk of developing renal failure is twice as high in patients with pure light-chain myeloma, and five to six times greater in patients with light-chain proteinuria over 2.0 g/day compared to those with proteinuria below 0.05 g/day. This indicates that in patients producing complete immunoglobulin molecules, cast nephropathy essentially occurs in those synthesizing an excess of light chains. The frequency of renal failure is identical in patients excreting κ or λ light chains, as it is in most renal series.

The clinical and urinary syndrome of myeloma cast nephropathy

Cast nephropathy-induced renal failure is remarkably silent. Clinical accompanying signs are due to myeloma, including weakness, weight loss, bone pain, and infection. Because of their non-specificity and their frequency in older patients, they often do not lead patients to take medical advice or physicians to prescribe serum and urinary electrophoreses which are the key laboratory investigations for the diagnosis of myeloma. Peaks visible on serum or urine electrophoresis are then identified by immunoelectrophoresis.

The main urinary feature is the excretion of a monoclonal light chain which accounts for 70 per cent or more of total proteinuria in 80 per cent of patients (Rota *et al.* 1987). Light-chain proteinuria is not detected by urinary dipsticks, but only by techniques measuring total proteinuria. Certain light chains fail to react or react weakly in some widely used precipitation assays, such as the sulfosalicylic acid method, leading to falsely negative or underestimated results. The remaining

Table 2 Clinical and pathological characteristics of patients with myeloma-induced renal failure of presumed or established tubulointerstitial origin

Series	Number of patients	Age (years)	Male to Female ratio	Tumour mass (%)		Serum creatinine (μmol/l)	Urinary LC >2 g/day (%)	Renal lesions in biopsy specimen
				IIB[a]	IIIB[a]			
Rota *et al.* (1987)	34	66 (33–90)	0.88	15	73	975 (164–2000)	53	26 MCN 2 ATN 2 CIN
Pozzi *et al.* (1987)	50	63 (47–75)	1.38	12	82	798 (273–1518)	41[b]	16 'Myeloma kidney'[c] 8 Other
Pasquali *et al.* (1990)	25	60 (48–74)	2.12	24	72	891 (455–1391)	72	25 MCN
Winearls (1995)	42	66 (42–82)	2.0	'Majority' of patients		896 (302–2006)	NA	14 MCN 6 AIN[d]

[a] IIB, intermediate tumour mass; IIIB, high tumour mass.

[b] Total proteinuria, including LC.

[c] Presumably myeloma cast nephropathy.

[d] Compatible with myeloma.

AIN, acute interstitial nephritis; ATN, acute tubular necrosis; CIN, chronic interstitial nephritis; MCN, myeloma cast nephropathy; NA, not available; LC, light chain.

proteins are composed of albumin and low molecular weight globulins that have failed to be reabsorbed by proximal tubule cells. In the rare patients with albuminuria over 1 g/day, cast nephropathy is usually associated with glomerular lesions due to amyloidosis or monoclonal immunoglobulin deposition disease. There is no haematuria in pure cast nephropathy.

Precipitants of cast nephropathy

These are of paramount importance because of measures to prevent precipitation (Table 4). It is often difficult to identify a particular event responsible for precipitating renal failure, as these patients suffer many of the complications of the disease at once, a common thread of which seems to be an effect on renal perfusion.

Hypercalcaemia is an important precipitant found in 19–44 per cent of the renal series (Table 4), and in 57 per cent of the patients with renal failure in Alexanian's non-renal series (1990). In the latter series, hypercalcaemia was identified a major pathogenetic factor (Table 3). Presumably it acts by inducing dehydration as a result of emesis and a nephrogenic diabetes insipidus. It may also enhance light-chain toxicity (Smolens *et al.* 1987), and cause nephrocalcinosis. Calcium was shown to enhance the aggregation of light chains with Tamm–Horsfall protein (THP) (Huang and Sanders 1995).

Table 3 Features associated with renal failure in myeloma

	Number of patients[a]	Percentage with renal failure	*P*
All patients	494	18	
Urinary LC (g/day)			0.00001
>2.0	123	39	
0.05–2.00	149	17	
<0.05	222	7	
Myeloma protein type			0.0003
Only LC protein	93	31	
Other	401	15	
Serum calcium, mmol/l[b]			0.00001
>2.87	104	49	
≤2.87	390	10	

[a] This series included 494 consecutive, previously untreated patients with multiple myeloma.

[b] Corrected calcium (mmol/l).

LC, light chain.

From Alexanian *et al.* (1990).

Dehydration, with or without hypercalcaemia, and infection are other major risk factors for acute renal failure. Rota *et al.* (1987) found a high rate of urinary infections (10/34, 29 per cent) which were associated in three cases with an increased proportion of polymorphonuclear leucocytes in the renal biopsy, suggesting an aetiological link between infection and deterioration of renal function. Infection also operates by causing dehydration and prompting the use of nephrotoxic antibiotics.

Contrast media have hitherto been considered an important precipitant of acute renal failure. It was hypothesized that the contrast medium bound to intratubular proteins, especially the light-chain and THP, causing them to precipitate and obstruct tubular flow (Ronco *et al.* 1987). Contrast media also have vasoconstrictive effects, decreasing glomerular filtration rate and urinary output. McCarthy and Becker (1992) reviewed seven retrospective studies of myeloma patients receiving contrast media, involving 476 patients who had undergone a total of 568 examinations. The prevalence of acute renal failure (which was not defined) was 0.6–1.25 per cent, compared to 0.15 per cent in the general population. This is a low risk and contradicts the dogma that contrast media should not be used in myeloma patients. This change may reflect awareness of the risk and care taken to hydrate patients actively with alkaline solutes before and during the administration of contrast media. No clinical data currently support the preferential use of non-ionic agents in myeloma patients to decrease the risk of acute renal failure.

A number of drugs are noxious in myeloma patients. They include antibiotics, particularly aminoglycosides, and non-steroidal anti-inflammatory drugs (NSAIDs). Rota *et al.* (1987) first insisted on the harmful effects of NSAIDs, and suggested that the chance of recovery was diminished if NSAIDs were a precipitating factor. Angiotensin-converting enzyme (ACE) inhibitors can also precipitate renal failure in myeloma patients because they reduce glomerular filtration rate dramatically in dehydrated patients (Rabb *et al.* 1999). Their use as that of angiotensin type-1 receptor antagonists should be avoided in myeloma patients as long as a risk of decreased renal perfusion persists.

Renal pathology and the value of renal biopsy

A renal biopsy should not be systematically performed in patients with a presumed diagnosis of myeloma cast nephropathy. However, it is useful in two circumstances:

1. to analyse tubulointerstitial lesions and predict the reversibility of renal failure in patients with presumed cast nephropathy but multiple precipitating factors; and

Table 4 Precipitants of acute renal failure in myeloma

Series	Number of patients	Dehydration (%)	Infection (%)	Hypercalcaemia (%)	Contrast medium (%)	NSAIDs (%)	None (%)
Rota *et al.* (1987)	34[a]	65	44	44 (>2.60 mmol/l)	0	24	
Pozzi *et al.* (1987)	50[a]	24	10	34 (≥ 2.75 mmol/l)	4	0	44
Ganeval *et al.* (1992)	80[b]	10	9	30	11		35
Winearls (1995)	42[a]			19		10	71

[a] Renal lesions are described in Table 2.

[b] Includes 29 patients with renal biopsies: 19 with myeloma cast nephropathy, two with amyloidosis, and eight with LCDD.

Adapted from Rota *et al.* (1987) and Winearls (1995).

2. to identify glomerular lesions in patients with albuminuria over 1 g/day and no evidence of amyloid deposits in 'peripheral' biopsies (rectum, salivary glands, and abdominal fat).

Myeloma casts

Myeloma cast nephropathy (also inappropriately referred to as 'myeloma kidney'), is characterized by the presence of specific casts, associated with severe alterations of the tubule epithelium. Myeloma casts are large and usually numerous. Their prevailing localization is the distal tubule and the collecting duct, but they may also be found in the proximal tubule and even exceptionally in the glomerular urinary space. They often have a 'hard' and 'fractured' appearance, and show polychromatism upon staining with Masson's trichrome (Fig. 1a). Casts may also have a stratified or laminated appearance, and thus stain with Congo red, but only exceptionally do they show the typical yellow–green dichroism of amyloid under polarized light (see Chapter 4.2.1).

An important diagnostic feature of myeloma casts is the presence of *crystals*, which may be suspected by light microscopy (Pirani *et al.* 1987). Such casts are often angular or heterogeneous because they contain multiple rhomboid or needle-shaped crystals surrounded by amorphous material and cell debris.

Casts are frequently surrounded by mononuclear cells, exfoliated tubular cells, and more characteristically by multinucleated giant cells (Fig. 1a) whose macrophagic origin has been established by specific antibodies (Pirani 1988). These cells are often seen engulfing the casts and at times actually phagocytosing cast fragments. In some cases, the cellular reaction is made of polymorphonuclear leucocytes in the absence of urinary tract infection. Typical 'myeloma' casts with a giant, multinucleated cell reaction can be very occasionally detected in other haemopathies including μ-heavy chain disease (Preud'homme *et al.* 1997) and Waldenström's disease. In myeloma cast nephropathy, there is great variability in the percentages of typical myeloma casts and of non-specific hyaline casts. In some instances, most casts have

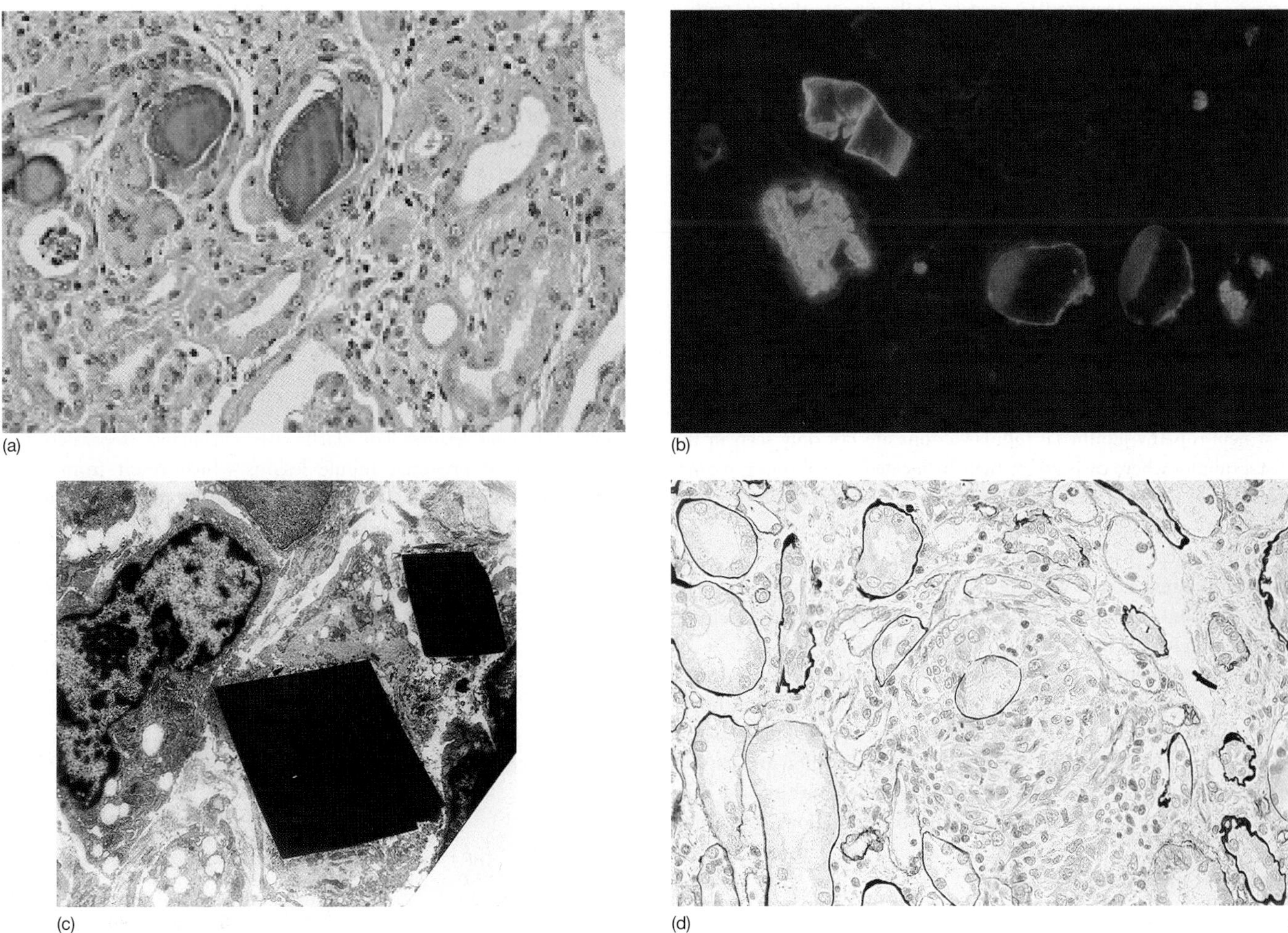

Fig. 1 Myeloma cast nephropathy. (a) Typical myeloma casts with fractured appearance are surrounded by multinucleated macrophagic cells in a patient with λ-light-chain myeloma (Masson's trichrome, 312×). (b) Several tubules contain large casts, one of which has an angular and fractured aspect. The stain with anti-κ antibody is more intense at the periphery of most casts (immunofluorescence 312×). (c) Rectangular crystals presumably composed of λ light chains in tubular cells (electron micrograph, uranyl acetate and lead citrate; original magnification 7000×). (d) Interstitial granulomatous-like formations with macrophages surrounding disrupted tubular basement membrane were numerous in this λ-light-chain cast nephropathy (silver stain, 312×).

non-specific characteristics by light microscopy even if by immunofluorescence the vast majority consists predominantly of one of the two light-chain types. The search for typical casts has to be conducted on all available sections if necessary (Pirani 1988).

By immunofluorescence, myeloma casts are essentially composed of the monoclonal light chains excreted by the patient, together with THP. In most cases, casts are stained exclusively or predominantly with either the anti-κ or the anti-λ antibody. However, in about 25 per cent of myeloma biopsies, casts stain for both antibodies because they contain polyclonal light chains, together with albumin and fibrinogen (Pirani *et al.* 1987). Staining of 'angular' casts is often irregular, and more intense at the periphery (Fig. 1b). In heterogeneous casts, the crystals themselves fail to stain while the matrix of the cast and the surrounding cellular debris and amorphous material often stain positively for one of the light chains.

Cast ultrastructure has been studied by electron microscopy in 24 biopsies of myeloma cast nephropathy by Pirani *et al.* (1987). Crystals were detected in 14 biopsies and suspected in another four. The authors have identified four major categories of casts, depending on their content and ultrastructural appearance. One category characterized by large rectangular crystals, or fragments thereof, with a pentagonal or hexagonal cross-section, is found only in myeloma cast nephropathy. It seems to be closely linked to the development of a giant-cell reaction around the cast. A second category also frequently contains crystals but these are small, electron-dense, and needle-shaped, and seemingly not associated with a cellular reaction. Similar large, rectangular and small, needle-shaped crystals can be found within plasma cells. They are also seen occasionally within the cytoplasm of either proximal or distal tubular cells (Fig. 1c), surrounded by a single smooth membrane, which suggests that they are located within lysosomes.

Tubules and interstitium

Considerable tubular damage is almost always present in myeloma cast nephropathy. Epithelial tubular lesions are not only seen in the distal tubules where casts are principally located, but also in proximal convoluted tubules, where the epithelium undergoes atrophy and degenerative changes. Frank tubular necrosis may also be seen, with or without typical myeloma cast nephropathy (Rota *et al.* 1987). By immunofluorescence, a variable number of tubule sections can be shown to contain numerous 'protein reabsorption droplets' staining for the monoclonal light chain (Cohen and Border 1980).

Interstitial lesions are often associated with the tubular damage. They may be mild and consist of inflammatory infiltrates and fibro-oedema, but fibrosis and its correlate, tubular atrophy, may also be fairly extensive. In severe cases with epithelial denudation and gaps in the continuity of the tubular basement membrane, often in close contact with myeloma casts, granulomatous-like formations containing macrophages and histiocytes develop around the ruptured tubules (Fig. 1d) (Cohen and Border 1980).

Glomeruli and vessels

The glomeruli are usually normal except for small clusters of globally sclerotic gomeruli and a mild thickening of the mesangial matrix. When mesangial thickening is more prominent, the possibility of an associated monoclonal immunoglobulin deposition disease (MIDD) should be considered (see below). Exceptionally, amorphous deposits reminiscent of myeloma casts can be seen in capillary loops or in the glomerular urinary space. In younger patients, severe chronic vascular lesions are sometimes observed, which may contribute to the progression of sclerosis.

Pathophysiology of myeloma cast nephropathy

Cast nephropathy occurs mainly in myeloma patients with a high light-chain secretion rate, which suggests that light chains play a key pathogenetic role. That light chains are the main culprits is supported also by the following clinical, pathological, and experimental data.

1. Renal lesions may recur on grafted kidneys (Short *et al.* 2001).
2. Similar crystals may occasionally be seen within casts, proximal tubule cells, and plasma cells (Pirani 1988). Their usual lack of staining with anti-light-chain antibody is most likely due to degradation or masking of the relevant epitopes.
3. Mice injected with light chains purified from patients with cast nephropathy developed extensive cast formation in the distal renal tubules (Koss *et al.* 1976; Solomon *et al.* 1991).

However, it is surprising that a number of patients produce large amounts of light chains and yet fail to present significant signs of renal involvement throughout the course of the disease. This may be related to the absence of the enhancing factors described above, but this also suggests that some light chains may be particularly likely to induce renal lesions, especially cast formation.

Because lesions observed in cast nephropathy associate cast formation with proximal tubule cell lesions, it is usually believed that light chains are directly toxic to epithelial cells, resulting in decreased proximal reabsorption of the light chains and increased delivery to the distal tubule in which they coprecipitate with THP. Tubular obstruction by large and numerous casts may also contribute to the development of tubular lesions. For clarity, we will analyse separately the pathogenesis of proximal tubule lesions which result from renal metabolism of light chains, the mechanisms of cast formation, and the respective role of tubular obstruction and tubular lesions in the genesis of renal failure (Fig. 2). This mode of presentation is also warranted by the observation that certain light chains damage the proximal

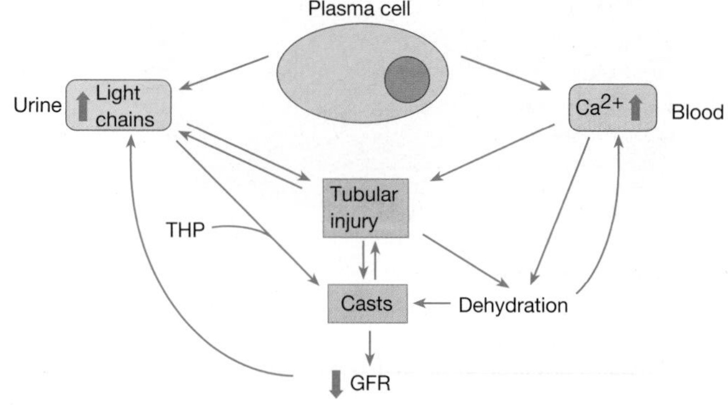

Fig. 2 Schematic representation of the pathogenesis of myeloma cast nephropathy (adapted from Winearls 1995).

tubule while others precipitate in the distal tubule, obstructing the nephron, when perfused in rat nephrons *in vivo* (Sanders *et al.* 1988a).

Renal metabolism of light chains and pathogenesis of proximal tubule lesions

An excess production of light chains over heavy chains appears to be required for efficient immunoglobulin synthesis, but it results in the release of free light chains, especially in myeloma. Light chains are normally filtered by the glomerulus, then reabsorbed by the proximal tubule (see Chapter 3.3). Lambda and to a lesser extent, κ light chains circulate mainly as covalently-linked dimers which have a mass-restricted glomerular filtration. In normal individuals, the small quantity of circulating free polyclonal light chains is filtered by glomeruli, and approximately 90 per cent of these are reabsorbed and catabolized by proximal tubular cells. Light chains bind to a single class of low-affinity, high-capacity non-cooperative binding sites described by Batuman *et al.* (1990) on both rat and human kidney brush-border membranes. These sites exhibit relative selectivity for light chains compared with albumin and β-lactoglobulin. They probably function as endocytotic receptors for light chains and possibly other low molecular weight proteins. It has been shown that light chains could bind to cubilin (Batuman *et al.* 1998), a multiligand receptor belonging to the large family of low-density lipoprotein receptors and located in the intermicrovillar areas of the brush border. After binding to the luminal domain of proximal tubular epithelial cells, light chains are incorporated in endosomes that fuse with primary lysosomes where proteases, mainly cathepsin B, degrade the proteins into amino acids, which are returned to the circulation by the basolateral route.

When the concentration of filtered light chains is increased, profound functional and morphological alterations of proximal tubule epithelial cells may occur. The functional disturbances include low molecular weight proteinuria (Cooper *et al.* 1984; Coward *et al.* 1985) and inhibition of sodium-dependent uptake of amino acids and glucose by brush-border preparations (Batuman *et al.* 1986). Morphologically, some of the light chains infused in mice (Koss *et al.* 1976) or rats (Smolens *et al.* 1986), or perfused in rat nephron *in vivo* (Sanders *et al.* 1987, 1988a), accumulate in endosomes and lysosomes of the proximal convoluted tubule and sometimes of the distal convoluted tubule. Similar observations were made in a rat model of multiple myeloma (Smolens *et al.* 1983). Crystalloid formations were frequently seen within phagolysosomes in proximal tubule cells, and lysosomes often appeared markedly enlarged and distorted (Smolens *et al.* 1983). Activation of the endosome/lysosome system was associated with mitochondrial alterations (Smolens *et al.* 1986), prominent cytoplasmic vacuolation, focal loss of the microvillous border, and epithelial cell exfoliation (Sanders *et al.* 1987).

These experiments establish that the proximal tubule epithelium is a main target of light-chain toxicity, but that not all light chains are toxic to this epithelium. However, they must be interpreted with caution. In most cases, large amounts of light chains were injected or microperfused. Moreover, clinical characteristics and renal lesions of the patients from whom light chains had been isolated were defined poorly or not at all. Because of the heterogeneity of myeloma-associated tubulopathies, it might well be that some of the light chains, especially those prone to form crystals, were produced by patients with Fanconi syndrome. On the other hand, these experiments suggested that the proximal tubule endocytotic and lysosomal system might be overwhelmed when large quantities of light chains were filtered, thereby allowing light chains to proceed to the distal nephron.

Pathogenesis of cast formation

Because myeloma casts are composed principally of the monoclonal light chains and THP, it has long been hypothesized that interaction of these two proteins was a key event in cast formation. THP is a highly glycosylated and acidic protein (isoelectric point, pI = 3.2), synthesized exclusively by the cells of the ascending limb of Henle's loop (Ronco *et al.* 1987). It is the major protein constituent of normal urine, and an almost universal component of casts. This 80 kDa protein is also remarkable because of its ability to form reversibly high molecular weight aggregates of about 7×10^6 Da at high but physiological concentrations of sodium and calcium, and at low urinary pH. The role of THP in cast formation has prompted a wealth of studies on its interactions with light chains. These studies were performed with the aim of defining a population of myeloma patients at risk of developing renal damage. The role of light-chain pI has long been suggested. As early as 1945, Oliver proposed that the occurrence of casts in the distal tubules was the result of coagulation of globulins with a low pI in an acid urine (Oliver 1945). Clyne *et al.* (1979) suggested that light chains with a high pI (>5.6) and THP could bear opposite charges in the normal urine pH range, and undergo polar interaction between charged groups and precipitation. Clyne's hypothesis was supported by Coward *et al.* (1984) who reported a significant negative correlation between pI and creatinine clearance. However, the nephritogenic potential of light chains with a high pI was not confirmed in further experimental and clinical studies (Smolens *et al.* 1983; Melcion *et al.* 1984; Johns *et al.* 1986; Rota *et al.* 1987).

In an elegant series of studies, Sanders and his coworkers implicated THP as a major pathogenetic factor in a rat model. Development of casts and injury to proximal tubule cells in renal tubules microperfused with human nephritogenic light chains were not correlated with light-chain pI, molecular form, or isotype (Sanders *et al.* 1988a). Intranephronal obstruction was aggravated by decreasing extracellular fluid volume or adding furosemide. In perfused loop segments, cast-forming light chains reduced chloride absorption directly, thus increasing tubule fluid [Cl^-] and promoting their own aggregation with THP (Sanders *et al.* 1990). Pretreatment of rats with colchicine, which prevents additon of sialic acid to the protein, completely prevented obstruction and cast formation in perfused nephrons (Sanders and Booker 1992) and THP from those rats did not aggregate with light chains *in vitro*, contrary to THP purified from control rats. *In vitro* studies suggest that THP can undergo both self (homotypic) aggregation and heterotypic aggregation with light chains (Huang and Sanders 1995). Homotypic aggregation is enhanced by calcium, furosemide, and low pH, and is dependent on the sialic acid content of THP. Heterotypic aggregation requires previous binding of light chain to the THP backbone (Huang *et al.* 1993). A 9-residue sequence of the THP was identified as the binding site of light chains, including a histidine at position 226 which explains, at least partially, the pH dependence of molecular interactions (Huang and Sanders 1997). Conversely, the binding site of immunoglobulin light chains for THP was mapped in the third complementarity-determining region (CDR3) (Ying and Sanders 2001). The sugar moiety is also essential for coaggregation of the light chain and THP, perhaps by facilitating homotypic aggregation of THP. THP from normal volunteers treated with colchicine had a lower sialic acid content and a decreased aggregation potential in the presence of pathogenic light chains (Huang and Sanders 1995).

These findings suggest that colchicine could be a useful treatment for preventing cast nephropathy, and that new therapeutic strategies aimed at reducing light chain—THP interactions can be envisioned. An increase in dietary salt and the loop diuretic, furosemide, may be harmful because they not only enhance THP homotypic aggregation, but also increase expression of this protein in the rat (Ying and Sanders 1998).

Cast formation may not rely only on interactions between light chains and THP. First, five of 12 light chains purified from the urine of patients with cast nephropathy failed to react with THP in the enzyme linked immunosorbent assay (ELISA) (Leboulleux *et al.* 1995). Second, myeloma casts occasionally do not stain for THP in human biopsies (Verroust *et al.* 1982), and casts induced in mice by light-chain injection do not seem to contain THP during the first 24 h (Koss *et al.* 1976), indicating that some light chains may undergo homotypic aggregation or precipitation in the absence of THP. This hypothesis is supported by size-exclusion chromatography studies showing that the deposition of certain light chains *in vivo* may be related to their capability to aggregate *in vitro* (Myatt *et al.* 1994). Other physicochemical properties of light chains may also play a pathogenetic role. Ten of the 12 light chains isolated from the urine of patients with cast nephropathy showed significant resistance to trypsin and/or pepsin, and cathepsin B, a lysosomal enzyme, yielded small amounts of the variable domain of the light chains in four cases (Leboulleux *et al.* 1995). Resistance of light chains to urinary and macrophage-released proteases may also participate in cast formation and persistence since cells surrounding casts seem incapable of degrading cast proteins.

Role of tubular obstruction by casts in the genesis of renal failure

The role of casts as plugs obstructing the tubules has been clearly shown in micropuncture studies (Weiss *et al.* 1981). In myeloma patients, the correlation between severity of renal insufficiency and the number of casts remains controversial. Hill *et al.* (1983) found a good correlation between the extent of cast formation and degree of renal failure, whereas others (Levi *et al.* 1968; DeFronzo *et al.* 1978; Rota *et al.* 1987) have failed to demonstrate this correlation. This may be explained partly by the prominent medullary localization of casts, whose count is therefore underestimated in superficial kidney cortex biopsy specimens. The first indication that antibodies to THP could serve as probes of tubular obstruction was provided by Cohen and Border (1980) who identified the protein in glomerular urinary spaces of two myeloma patients. This finding is indicative of intratubular urinary back-flow. THP was detected in glomerular urinary spaces in 16 of 18 biopsies of patients with myeloma cast nephropathy (Ronco *et al.* 1988) (Fig. 3). Forty-six per cent of the 119 glomeruli available for study stained for THP. In mice grafted with a light-chain-secreting murine plasmacytoma, which developed numerous lamellar casts and extensive tubular damage, glomerular deposits of THP were also found in 10 of 13 animals (Ronco *et al.* 1988). However, the proportion of affected tubules is too small to account by itself for renal failure. Renal failure induced by cast nephropathy is multifactorial, implicating also tubular epithelial cells and interstitial lesions. Tubule obstruction by casts may explain the slow recovery of renal function noted in many patients (Rota *et al.* 1987).

Interstitial deposits of THP were also found in eight of the 18 biopsies (44 per cent) examined with specific antibodies (Ronco *et al.* 1988). They probably result from a leakage of the protein through gaps in the tubular basement membrane. Clinical and experimental models have implicated

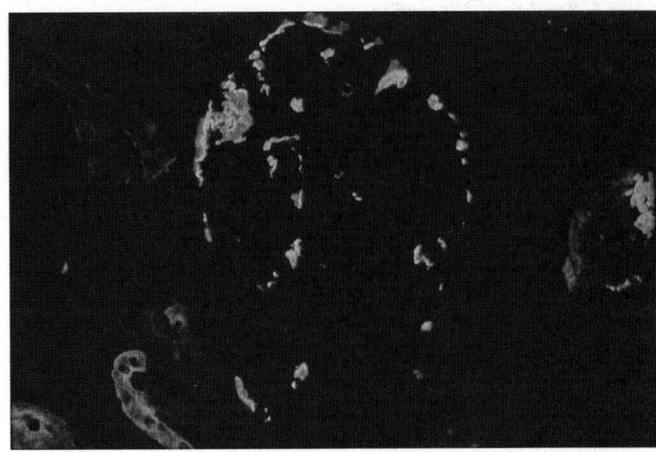

Fig. 3 Myeloma cast nephropathy. Immunofluorescence stain with anti-THP monoclonal antibody. Glomerular deposits in Bowman's space delineate the inner aspect of the Bowman's capsule and penetrate between lobules of the capillary tuft. Identification of THP in the urinary spaces of glomeruli supports the obstructive role of casts with reflux of tubular urine (312×).

the protein in the pathogenesis of tubulointerstitial nephritis. Thomas *et al.* (1993a,b) identified a single class of sialic-acid-specific cell surface receptors for THP on polymorphonuclear leucocytes, and further showed that *in vitro* activation of human mononuclear phagocytes by particulate THP led to the release of gelatinase and reactive oxygen metabolites, both probably contributing to tissue damage.

In conclusion, there is now considerable evidence that some light chains are intrinsically prone to induce tubular damage but the type of the predominant renal lesion, that is casts, crystals, or tubular epithelial cell alterations, varies from one light chain to another. In addition, extrinsic factors, including dehydration, hypercalcaemia, low urine pH, use of contrast medium or xenobiotics toxic to epithelial cells, most likely enhance light-chain toxicity. Tubular obstruction plays an important but not exclusive, role in the genesis of renal failure. Both tubular obstruction and acute tubular lesions are theoretically reversible.

Outcome and prognosis of myeloma cast nephropathy

Until the 1980s, myeloma-induced renal failure was associated with a very poor prognosis. In the first series reported by DeFronzo *et al.* (1975), only five of 14 patients survived the early period of acutely impaired renal function, and four of these died within only 2 months. Both renal prognosis and survival have significantly improved in the last 20 years, however.

Renal outcome and prognostic factors

About half of patients have complete or partial reversal of renal failure after weeks to months (see Table 5 for references), and some come off dialysis (Pichette *et al.* 1993). Ganeval *et al.* (1992) noticed that patients with improved renal function showed a phase of rapid decrease in serum creatinine within the first month, then a second phase of much slower improvement. The first phase of improvement is mostly independent of chemotherapy while the second phase is likely to be the

Table 5 Renal recovery, median survival, and prognostic indicators in patients with severe renal failure and myeloma

Series	Number of patients[a]	Renal recovery (%)	Median survival (months)	Pejorative renal predictors	Pejorative survival predictors
Rota *et al.* (1987)	34	47	19	Female gender Interstitial lesions, tubular atrophy	No renal recovery
Pozzi *et al.* (1987)	50	46	11	High serum creatinine Severity of renal lesions, number of casts	No renal recovery
Misiani *et al.* (1987)	23	83	9	NA	Poor response to chemotherapy
Pasquali *et al.* (1990)	37	43	17	NA	No renal recovery Hypercalcaemia, early infection Interstitial fibrosis, tubular atrophy No plasma exchange
Johnson *et al.* (1990)	21	57	22	Number of casts Response to chemotherapy	NA
Ganeval *et al.* (1992)[b]	78	62	20	High serum creatinine	Poor response to chemotherapy Disease stage Renal function after 1 month
Winearls (1995)	42	17	20	NA	NA
Blade *et al.* (1998)	94	26	10	Serum creatinine > 354 μmol/l Serum calcium < 2.88 mmol/l Proteinuria > 1 g/24 h	Poor response to chemotherapy Severity of renal failure No renal recovery
Knudsen *et al.* (2000)	225	58	—	High serum creatinine Normal calcaemia Low protein excretion	Stage III disease Hypercalcaemia High age Severity of renal failure No renal recovery

[a] Includes early deaths.

[b] Includes 29 patients with renal biopsies: 19 with myeloma cast nephropathy, 2 with amyloidosis, and 8 with LCDD.

NA: not available.

result of both chemotherapy (in responders) and continuation of measures undertaken to suppress the toxic renal effect of remnant light chains.

Elevated plasma creatinine concentration at presentation has been quoted as a marker of poor prognosis in four studies (Pozzi *et al.* 1987; Ganeval *et al.* 1992; Blade *et al.* 1998; Knudsen *et al.* 2000), implying that renal functional impairment of any degree should be treated as a medical emergency. In Rota *et al.*'s study (1987), main prognostic indicators were provided by renal histology. Return to normal renal function was seen only in patients with typical cast nephropathy and/or tubular necrosis in the absence of interstitial damage. Global tubular atrophy and interstitial fibrosis were associated with partially or totally irreversible renal failure, while the number of casts has a controversial predictive value (Pozzi *et al.* 1987; Rota *et al.* 1987; Johnson *et al.* 1990).

Survival and predictors

Myeloma patients with renal failure have a shorter survival than those with normal renal function. In the presence of renal failure mortality in the first three months is about 30 per cent (Pozzi *et al.* 1987; Ganeval *et al.* 1992; Blade *et al.* 1998), and median survival ranges from 9 to 22 months (Table 5). However, Rota *et al.* (1987) found that survival time was about 2 years in those patients whose serum creatinine returned to normal, compared to only 5 months in patients with irreversible renal failure. The effect of recovering renal function on survival was emphasized in other series (Pozzi *et al.* 1987; Pasquali *et al.* 1990; Ganeval *et al.* 1992; Blade *et al.* 1998; Knudsen *et al.* 2000) (Table 5). Response to chemotherapy is another important predictor (Table 5).

In Alexanian's series of 494 consecutive myeloma patients (Alexanian *et al.* 1990), a large tumour mass was the only significant variable adversely affecting survival ($p < 0.001$) on multivariate analysis. For comparable patients with high tumour mass, the frequency of response was less and the remission and survival times were shorter with more severe renal failure, but the differences were not significant. Reversal of renal failure did not confer a survival advantage, contrary to response to chemotherapy.

These data indicate that myeloma patients with renal failure should be treated with chemotherapy just as those without renal failure, and that any measures that could contribute to improved renal function should be taken from the day of diagnosis.

Treatment

The treatment of patients with cast-nephropathy-induced renal failure has two main objectives:

(1) to limit further cast precipitation by reducing the precipitability of the urinary light chains and light-chain production rate; and

(2) to avoid complications of uraemia by dialysis and sometimes by transplantation.

Even more importantly, preventive measures are essential to reduce the incidence of renal failure.

Decreasing precipitability of the urinary light chains by immediate symptomatic measures

Since coprecipitation in renal tubules of free light chains and THP is the main nephritogenic event, measures to reduce concentration and precipitability of both partners are essential and urgent. They include rehydration, correction of hypercalcaemia, stopping NSAID administration, and treatment of infections with non-nephrotoxic antibiotics. Despite controversy about the role of light-chain p*I* in cast formation, alkalinization of urine is still recommended because the solubility of THP is reduced at low pH. An acidic environment may also increase the interaction and aggregation of light chains with THP (Huang and Sanders 1995). Therefore, a daily urine output greater than 3 l and a urine pH above 7.0 should be reached in all patients whose cardiac and renal function can tolerate a deliberate expansion of the extracellular fluid volume. These measures alone are sufficient to improve renal function in the majority of patients with renal impairment at presentation (Alexanian *et al.* 1990). However, they must be completed by therapeutic means aimed at decreasing the amount of urinary light chains filtered by glomeruli.

Reducing the production rate (and concentration) of the monoclonal light chains

Most myeloma patients reported in renal series were treated with conventional chemotherapy—alkylating agents and high-dose corticosteroids. The response rate was 45 per cent (Ganeval *et al.* 1992), similar to that found in series with no or few patients with renal failure (Alexanian and Dimopoulos 1994). The drawbacks of this chemotherapy are slow antitumour action and necessity of reducing melphalan doses because the drug is eliminated through the kidneys, although pharmacokinetic data are controversial on this point. Regimens including vincristine and doxorubicin (VAD) induce earlier remission, which is an advantage in patients with hypercalcaemia and renal failure, and are safer in patients with renal failure since the cytotoxic drugs are metabolized in the liver. Although a higher proportion of patients achieve remission with this regimen, its long-term efficacy in term of median survival and duration of remission is not better than that of melphalan–prednisone. The VAD protocol is efficient in treatment of relapses (40 per cent remission) (Alexanian and Dimopoulos 1994) and of refractory myelomas (25 per cent remission). However, these therapeutic regimens have not radically changed the global prognosis of multiple myeloma.

In the past 10 years, the concept of high-dose chemotherapy regimens with haematopoietic stem cell support (to reduce the duration of the drug-induced myelosuppression with its high risks of morbidity and mortality) has modified the treatment of young patients with multiple myeloma (Munshi *et al.* 1999). Transplantation from an allogeneic donor may have the advantage over autotransplantation of a potential 'graft versus myeloma' effect, but the procedure still has a high level of related mortality. Many more patients are candidates for autologous transplantation that is now usually performed using peripheral blood stem cells. One can take advantage of $CD34^{+}$ cell selection to reduce the number of tumour cells in reinfused grafts. In 1996, a randomized controlled trial first demonstrated the benefits of high-dose therapy over conventional combination therapy in terms of complete remission rate, event-free survival and overall survival in myeloma patients with normal renal function (Attal *et al.* 1996). High-dose therapy with autotransplantation can lead to a median overall survival exceeding 5 years (Fermand *et al.* 1998).

However, until recently, high-dose therapy with stem cell transplantation had not been considered in patients with significant renal impairment. Small series now show that this procedure is feasible in renal patients, even in those on dialysis (Ballester *et al.* 1997; Badros *et al.* 2001). In the most recent series of 81 patients including 38 patients on dialysis (Badros *et al.* 2001), treatment-related mortality was 6 per cent and 13 per cent after the first and second autologous stem cell transplantation, respectively. Further studies are needed to define the risks and benefits in this patient population.

Plasmapheresis is logical but controversial (Winearls 1995) and clinical evidence conflicting. It has been advocated by many to reduce light-chain concentration rapidly, but its efficacy has not been established convincingly, except in patients with hyperviscosity syndrome. Two small randomized controlled trials have been published (Zucchelli *et al.* 1988; Johnson *et al.* 1990) but further trials enrolling larger numbers of patients are required.

Supportive therapy in the form of blood transfusion, analgesia, and biphosphonates are important adjuncts to treatment. The total dose of pamidronate does not need to be reduced in renal impairment but regular review of renal function is recommended.

Dialysis and renal transplantation

Dialysis is clearly indicated for the treatment of acute renal failure and endstage renal disease, except in patients with refractory myeloma (Sharland *et al.* 1997). It should be started early to avoid the added complications of uraemia and to compensate for the hypercatabolic state induced by the use of high doses of corticosteroids. If peritoneal dialysis is chosen, the early placement of a permanent indwelling dialysis catheter is recommended to avoid infectious peritonitis, the risk of which is increased by chemotherapy-induced leukopenia (Winearls 1995). Residual renal function must be carefully monitored because of possible improvement after several months of dialysis (Pichette *et al.* 1993). Two reports, from Great Britain (Iggo *et al.* 1989) and the United States (Port and Nissenson 1989) first suggested that chronic dialysis is a worthwhile treatment in patients with myeloma and renal failure. Survival at 1 year was 45 per cent in the British study (23 patients) and 54 per cent in the collected American series (731 patients). At 30 months, survival declined to 25 per cent compared with 66 per cent in non-diabetic endstage renal disease patients without myeloma (Port and Nissenson 1989). These data have been confirmed in a more recent series that showed a 1-year survival rate of 63 per cent and a median survival of 12–20 months in patients with myeloma undergoing haemodialysis (Clark *et al.* 1999). In another series (Sharland *et al.* 1997), there was no difference in outcome between patients with severe renal failure, those treated with dialysis, and those with milder impairment (median survival, 22 months in both groups). However, median survival was less in patients on haemodialysis with myeloma cast nephropathy (12 months) than in those with AL-amyloidosis (24 months) or with light chain deposition disease (48 months) (Montseny *et al.* 1998). Haemodialysis and chronic ambulatory peritoneal dialysis appear to be equally effective treatments, but most authors insist on the serious risk of infection in patients undergoing the latter treatment (Iggo *et al.* 1989). The experience with renal transplantation in myeloma is extremely limited.

Finally, if most cases of severe renal failure cannot be prevented because they occur simultaneously with the finding of myeloma, it is necessary to avoid or correct all precipitating factors of renal failure in patients with established myeloma. It is particularly important to reduce the use of NSAIDs as analgesic drugs, to detect and control hypercalcaemia as soon as possible, and to correct dehydration.

The Fanconi syndrome

The Fanconi syndrome (see Chapter 5.3) is characterized by renal glycosuria, generalized aminoaciduria, hypophosphataemia, and frequently chronic acidosis, hypouricaemia, and hypokalaemia. It often includes osteomalacia also, with pseudofractures. These manifestations result from functional impairment of the renal proximal tubule. Engle and Wallis (1957) identified crystal-like inclusions in both tumour cells and renal tubular epithelial cells, and suggested that a Fanconi syndrome and myeloma could be related. Costanza and Smoller (1963) described cytoplasmic inclusions as round or rod-like electron-opaque structures with longitudinally oriented fibrils. Lee *et al.* (1972) established clearly that myeloma was a cause of adult Fanconi syndrome. Maldonado *et al.* (1975) reported 17 cases of the Fanconi syndrome associated with plasma cell dyscrasias, and a recent study of 11 personal cases reviews also 57 published cases (Messiaen *et al.* 2000). Although fewer than 70 patients have been reported as yet the disease is most likely underdiagnosed. This rarity of a Fanconi syndrome in myeloma patients contrasts, however, with the high prevalence of morphological tubular alterations in myeloma autopsy series (Kapadia 1980) and after injection of light chains in animals. This suggests that unusual specific properties of light chains, mostly κ, are involved in the pathophysiology of the Fanconi syndrome.

Clinical presentation

The clinical features are summarized in Table 6 (Messiaen *et al.* 2000). Most patients are over 50 years of age with a slight female predominance. Most common initial manifestations are bone pain and weakness, principally due to osteomalacia. The major cause of this osteomalacia is hypophosphataemia, which results from increased urinary clearance of phosphate. Chronic acidosis and abnormal renal vitamin D metabolism further contribute to the development of bone lesions (see Chapter 5.1). Bone pain may also be the consequence of lytic lesions in patients with a high-mass myeloma. Other revealing signs are essentially due to the proximal tubule impairment or are related to hypokalaemia. Renal failure occurs more frequently than one would expect in a disease of the proximal tubule.

Criteria for the diagnosis of the Fanconi syndrome—'orthoglycaemic' glycosuria, increased phosphate and uric acid clearances, and generalized aminoaciduria—may not all be present together, especially in patients with renal failure. Generalized aminoaciduria is then a useful criterion in distinguishing the Fanconi syndrome from the non-specific proximal tubular transport abnormalities found in chronic renal failure (Lee *et al.* 1972).

The diagnosis of the Fanconi syndrome is usually missed, for a mean of 3 years, in patients presenting with proteinuria, bone pain, or renal failure. Typically, the diagnosis of the Fanconi syndrome precedes that of the plasma cell dyscrasia, most often a κ light-chain-excreting multiple myeloma, because the haematological disease has a low tumour burden and a slow progression. In 21 out of 66 published cases, even criteria for the diagnosis of myeloma are lacking, and patients were classified initially as having a benign monoclonal gammopathy. In some patients, the diagnosis of the plasma cell dyscrasia

Table 6 Clinical characteristics of patients with plasma cell dyscrasia-associated Fanconi syndrome[a]

Total number of patients	Age mean/extremes	Gender	Initial manifestations	Bone lesions	Renal Failure[b]	Plasma cell dyscrasia	Light chain isotype
68	57/22–81	30 males 38 females	Bone pain (25)[c] Weakness, fatigue (16) Weight loss (7) Polyuria-polydipsia (7) Hypokalaemia-related signs (4) Proteinuria (18) Renal failure (16) Renal glycosuria (13)	Osteomalacia (25) High-mass myeloma (12) Plasmacytoma (1)	54	Myeloma (36)[d] MGUS (21)[e] MGUS/myeloma (4)[f] Lymphoma/CLL (4)[g] 'Atypical' plasma cell dyscrasia (1)	49κ 7λ

[a] For references, see Messiaen *et al.* (2000).

[b] Serum creatinine > 130 μmol/l, or creatinine clearance < 80 ml/min.

[c] Related to osteomalacia.

[d] Including 12 patients with a high-mass myeloma.

[e] Monoclonal gammopathy of undetermined significance.

[f] Undetermined diagnosis, mostly due to cytoplasmic inclusions in plasma cells making interpretation of cytology difficult.

[g] Chronic lymphocytic leukaemia.

remains undetermined because it may be difficult to recognize the cytological characteristics of myeloma cells when their cytoplasm is stuffed with crystals.

Pathological data

Typically there are prominent crystals in enlarged proximal tubular cells and degenerative changes of proximal tubules (Messiaen *et al.* 2000). Proximal tubular cells are stuffed with microcrystals that stain red or green with Masson trichrome (Fig. 4) and are periodic acid-Schiff negative. In the most severely affected tubules, crystal-containing exfoliated cells are seen in the tubular lumen, while intracytoplasmic crystals are still present in atrophic tubules. In other cases, crystals can be only suspected by the presence of a finely granular material of glassy appearance in an enlarged proximal tubular epithelium. Their presence is more easily demonstrated by toluidine-blue staining of semi-thin sections and by haematoxylin–eosin staining of cryostat sections. In the same tubular section, all the cells are not equally affected: cells with a normal aspect coexist with those stuffed with crystals.

A universal feature is the additional presence of severe lesions of the proximal tubular epithelium devoid of crystals. Interstitial cellular infiltrate including plasma cells may contain analogous crystalline inclusion bodies. Patchy tubular atrophy and focal interstitial fibrosis together with a variable number of obsolescent glomeruli are commonly observed.

In several cases, attempts to characterize the crystal proteins with anti-immunoglobulin conjugates including anti-light-chain antibodies have failed. When immunohistochemical studies are positive, crystals stain only (or predominantly) for the monoclonal light chains, most often κ.

By electron microscopy, crystals of various size and shape surrounded by a single smooth membrane, are detected within the cytoplasm of proximal tubule cells [Fig. 5(3)] (Thorner *et al.* 1983; Pirani *et al.* 1987; Aucouturier *et al.* 1993a). In rare cases, crystals are also seen in distal tubule cells (Thorner *et al.* 1983; Orfila *et al.* 1991). In other cases, crystals are not seen by light microscopy, but electron microscopy shows enlarged vesicular bodies containing dense tubular and rod-like structures (Costanza and Smoller 1963; Lee *et al.* 1972; Maldonado *et al.* 1975; Uchida *et al.* 1990) or fibrils and needle-shaped deposits very close to crystalline structures (Orfila *et al.* 1991).

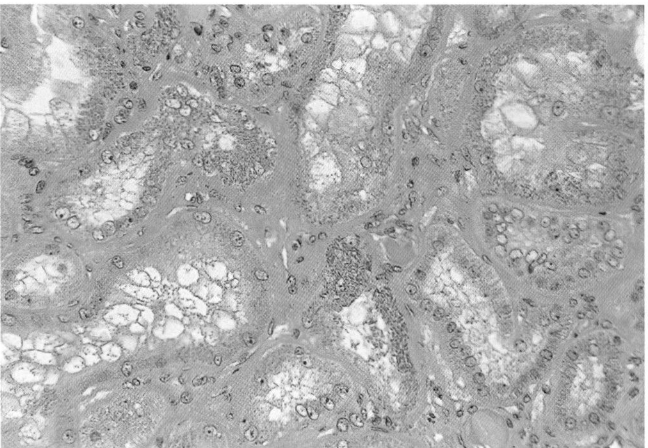

Fig. 4 Plasma cell dyscrasia-associated Fanconi syndrome. Small dense polychromatic crystals were abundant in the epithelium of most proximal tubules. Note also mild interstitial fibrosis (Masson's trichrome, 312×).

Crystal formation in plasma cell dyscrasia-associated Fanconi syndrome is not limited to renal tubule epithelium but also occurs in bone marrow and tissue infiltrating plasma cells, and in macrophages [Fig. 5(1 and 2)] (Engle and Wallis 1957; Costanza and Smoller 1963; Lee *et al.* 1972; Maldonado *et al.* 1975; Aucouturier *et al.* 1993a). The presence of crystals in macrophages close to the tumour plasma cells might result from endocytosis of either freshly secreted light chains or lysed plasma cells. In plasma cells, crystals are localized not only in lysosomes, but they are also frequently found inside the granular endoplasmic reticulum. These observations indicate that light chains accumulate in lysosomes and in endoplasmic reticulum. Crystal formation in these organelles therefore suggests incomplete proteolysis of light chains. The slow progression of myeloma disease in typical Fanconi syndrome associated with crystal formation may be explained by the deleterious effects on cell growth of the accumulation of crystalline inclusions in the tumour plasma cells.

Although crystals are a salient feature of the plasma cell dyscrasia-associated Fanconi syndrome, they are neither specific nor absolutely constant. They may also be found in proximal tubule epithelial cells of patients with cast nephropathy, but in low amounts (Pirani *et al.* 1987; Leboulleux *et al.* 1995), and occasionally in myeloma patients with isolated tubular lesions, that is, in the absence of distal nephron myeloma casts (Pasquali *et al.* 1987; Sanders *et al.* 1988b). In addition, recent pathological studies of 11 patients suggest that the Fanconi syndrome due to light chain nephropathy is more heterogeneous than expected (Messiaen *et al.* 2000).

Pathophysiology of plasma cell dyscrasia-associated Fanconi syndrome

The rare occurrence of Fanconi syndrome in multiple myeloma, the peculiar proneness of light chains to form crystals, and their unique

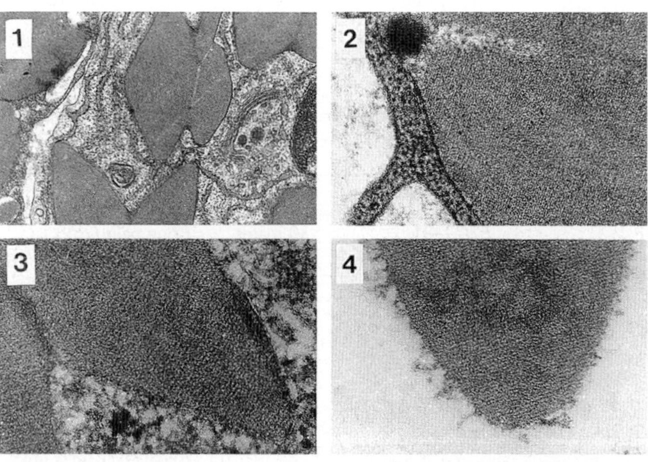

Fig. 5 Plasma cell dyscrasia-associated Fanconi syndrome. Electron microscopic study of intracellular (1, 2, and 3) and *in vitro*-formed (4) crystals in the same patient. (1) Bone marrow plasma cell (and a macrophage on the left) (original magnification, 8000×); (2) bone marrow macrophage (50,000×); (3) proximal convoluted tubular epithelial cell (50,000×); (4) crystal obtained *in vitro* from Sephadex G100 fraction from the patient's urine (by courtesy of the *Journal of Immunology*, Aucouturier *et al.* 1993a).

ability to alter proximal tubular transports, strongly suggest that light chains have unusual physicochemical properties. The peculiar propensity of certain light chains to form crystals *in vivo* is attested by experimental studies in mice (Solomon *et al.* 1991) and rats (Clyne *et al.* 1974; Sanders *et al.* 1987, 1988a). It is remarkable that the κ light chains that induced crystallization *in vivo*, also significantly reduced the glucose, chloride, and volume fluxes. The clinical characteristics of the patients from whom the light chains were isolated, especially the presence of Fanconi syndrome, were unfortunately not specified.

Crystal composition was analysed in a patient with myeloma-associated Fanconi syndrome and hexagonal crystals in kidney proximal tubular cells, bone marrow plasma cells, and phagocytes (Aucouturier *et al.* 1993a). *N*-terminal sequencing and mass spectrometry studies showed that a homogeneous, 107 amino acid fragment corresponding to the variable domain of the κ light chain (Vκ) was the essential component of crystals forming spontaneously from the patient's urine [Figs 5(4) and 6A]. Vκ was also crystallized alone using the hanging-drop technique (Fig. 6B). Crystals were hexagonal bipyramids and had the same 60 Å periodicity on electron micrographs as those found in the cells. In addition, *in vitro* trypsin and pepsin treatment of the native entire κ chain yielded a homogeneous V domain fragment (12 kDa) which, contrary to V domains of other monoclonal κ chains, was completely resistant to further proteolytic attack. The peculiar proneness of the V domain to resist proteolysis, to self-react, and to form crystals may explain its accumulation in phagolysosomes of plasma cells and proximal tubular cells. The resistance of light-chain V domains to proteolytic enzymes including cathepsin B (a lysosomal enzyme) was confirmed in further studies (Leboulleux *et al.* 1995; Messiaen *et al.* 2000) except in two patients with a high-mass myeloma and Fanconi syndrome. At variance with the observations made in patients with cast nephropathy (Huang *et al.* 1993; Leboulleux *et al.* 1995), light chains from patients with Fanconi syndrome did not bind THP except in one case where both syndromes were associated.

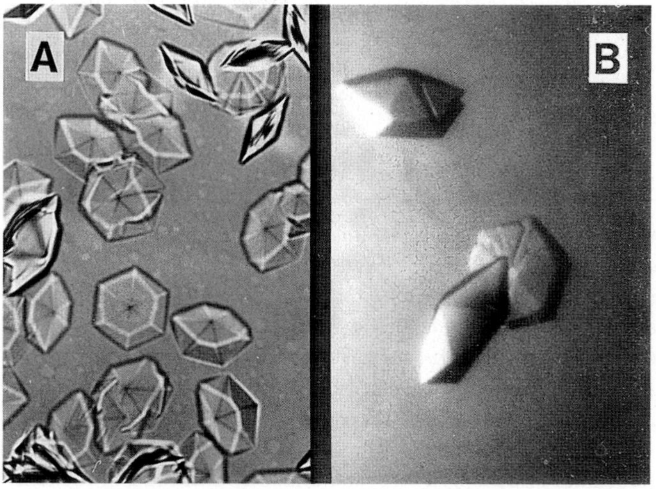

Fig. 6 Plasma cell dyscrasia-associated Fanconi syndrome. Same patient as in Fig. 5. Crystals spontaneously obtained *in vitro* from a Sephadex G100 fraction of the patient's urinary proteins (A) and by the hanging-drop technique from purified Vκ fragment (B). (A) Original magnification, 400× and (B) size of these crystals, 0.25 mm. (By courtesy of the *Journal of Immunology*, Aucouturier *et al.* 1993a.)

The unusual physicochemical behaviour of Fanconi syndrome κ chains was tentatively correlated with their structure in a number of cases (Deret *et al.* 1999). Sequence analyses showed that eight of nine (89 per cent) light chains belonged to the VκI variability subgroup while this subgroup only accounts for 56 per cent of all monoclonal κ light chains. The VκI appeared to originate from only two germline genes, *LCO2/O12* in five cases and *LCO8/O18* in three. Analyses of the DNA sequences suggested that all structure peculiarities arose from somatic mutations in the proliferating clone. In the eight available sequences, residues had never or rarely been reported among VκI subgroup light chains. The unusual presence of non-polar or hydrophobic amino acids in the CDR-L1 loop at position 30, together with a non-polar amino acid at position 50, seems to be specific for Fanconi syndrome light chains derived from gene *LCO2/O12*. These hydrophobic residues are exposed to the light-chain surface (Deret *et al.* 1999) and may be involved in the pathophysiology of Fanconi syndrome.

In summary, unusual properties of light chains associated with the Fanconi syndrome might explain crystal formation and/or accumulation in lysosomes. After endocytosis, light chains are processed in the endosomal and lysosomal compartment where 'normal' light chains are degraded. In Fanconi syndrome, accumulation of the protease-resistant V domain fragment generated by lysosomal enzymes may induce crystal formation. Clogging of the endolysosomal system may subsequently alter apical membrane recycling and/or ATP production (hence, Na^+,K^+-ATPase functioning) as suggested by mitochondrial injury (Lee *et al.* 1972), and lead to progressive impairment of sodium-dependent apical transports. However, we do not know why Fanconi syndrome does not occur in patients with apparently the same degree of distortion of the lysosomal compartment as can be seen in certain myeloma patients with or without cast nephropathy. The molecular mechanisms responsible for glycosuria, phosphaturia, generalized amino aciduria, and uric acid loss remain poorly understood.

Treatment

There has been little information about the response of the Fanconi syndrome to the treatment of multiple myeloma itself (Gailani *et al.* 1987; Uchida *et al.* 1990; Orfila *et al.* 1991; Messiaen *et al.* 2000). In patients with osteomalacia, considerable improvement can be obtained with vitamin D, calcium, and phosphorus supplementation. The effect of chemotherapy on the proximal tubule impairement is much more debated. Uchida *et al.* (1990) and Orfila *et al.* (1991) both reported that the treatment of underlying myeloma improves urinary signs and tubular transport abnormalities. On the other hand, it has been suggested (Levine and Bernstein 1985) that the presence of crystals within plasma cells should be added to the list of criteria defined by Kyle and Greipp (1980) against chemotherapy in myeloma.

Monoclonal immunoglobulin deposition disease

History and nomenclature

It was known from the late 1950s that non-amyloidotic forms of glomerular disease could occur in multiple myeloma. Kobernick and Whiteside (1957) and Sanchez and Domz (1960) first described glomerular nodules 'resembling the lesion of diabetic glomerulosclerosis', lacking the staining features and fibrillar organization of amyloid. The monoclonal light-chain content of these lesions was recognized in 1973 by Antonovych *et al.* (1974) and confirmed by Randall *et al.* (1976), who published the first description of the LCDD.

Monoclonal heavy chains were found together with light chains in the tissue deposits from certain patients (Preud'homme *et al.* 1980b), and the terms monoclonal immunoglobulin deposition disease (Ganeval *et al.* 1984) and light- and heavy-chain deposition disease (LHCDD) (Gallo *et al.* 1989; Buxbaum *et al.* 1990) were proposed. Deposits containing monoclonal heavy chains only, that is in the absence of detectable light chains, were first observed in 1993 in patients affected with otherwise typical Randall's disease (HCDD) (Aucouturier *et al.* 1993b), and two series of similar patients were published later (Moulin *et al.* 1999; Lin *et al.* 2001). More than 20 cases of HCDD have been reported so far, but this disease is most likely underdiagnosed. In two further cases, termed 'pseudo-γ HCDD', predominant γ_4 chain deposits were demonstrated with pathological aspects similar to MIDD; the authors suggested that misfolding or denaturation of the light chain was responsible for its non-reactivity with specific antibodies (Tubbs *et al.* 1992).

In clinical and pathological terms, LCDD, LHCDD, and HCDD are essentially similar and therefore will be described together. They differ from amyloidosis by the lack of affinity for Congo red and of fibrillar organization. The distinction also relates to different pathophysiology of amyloid which implicates one-dimensional elongation of a pseudocrystalline structure, and of MIDD which would rather involve a one-step precipitation of immunoglobulin chains.

Pathological features of monoclonal immunoglobulin deposition disease

Light microscopy

The morphological features of these disorders are well established, and in retrospect, cases of undiagnosed 'para-amyloid', or unidentified glomerulonephritis, or even 'diabetic' glomerulosclerosis in patients with normal glycaemic control were presumably MIDD. MIDD should not be considered a pure glomerular disease. In fact, tubular lesions may be more conspicuous than the glomerular damage.

Tubular lesions are characterized by the deposition of a refractile, eosinophilic, periodic acid-Schiff-positive, ribbon-like material along the outer part of the tubular basement membrane in virtually all patients with MIDD. The deposits predominate around the distal tubules, Henle's loops, and in some instances around the collecting ducts, whose epithelium is flattened and atrophied. Typical myeloma casts are only occasionally seen in pure forms of MIDD. In advanced stages, a marked interstitial fibrosis including refractile deposits is frequently associated with tubular lesions.

Glomerular lesions are much more heterogeneous (Ronco *et al.* 2001). Nodular glomerulosclerosis is the most characteristic (Fig. 7a) (Sanders *et al.* 1991), being found in 30–100 per cent of patients with LCDD (Lin *et al.* 2001; Ronco *et al.* 2001). Expansion of the mesangial matrix was observed in all cases of HCDD, with nodular glomerulosclerosis in almost all of them (Moulin *et al.* 1999; Lin *et al.* 2001). Mesangial nodules are composed of periodic-acid-Schiff-positive membrane-like material and are often accompanied by mild mesangial hypercellularity. The capillary loops stretch at the periphery of florid nodules and may undergo aneurysmal dilatation. The Bowman's capsule may contain a material identical to that present in the centre of the nodules. These lesions resemble nodular diabetic glomerulosclerosis, but some characteristics are distinctive: the distribution of the nodules is fairly regular in a given glomerulus; the nodules are often poorly argyrophilic; exudative lesions as 'fibrin caps' and extensive hyalinosis of the efferent arterioles are not observed. In occasional cases with prominent endocapillary cellularity and mesangial interposition, the glomerular features mimic a lobular glomerulonephritis.

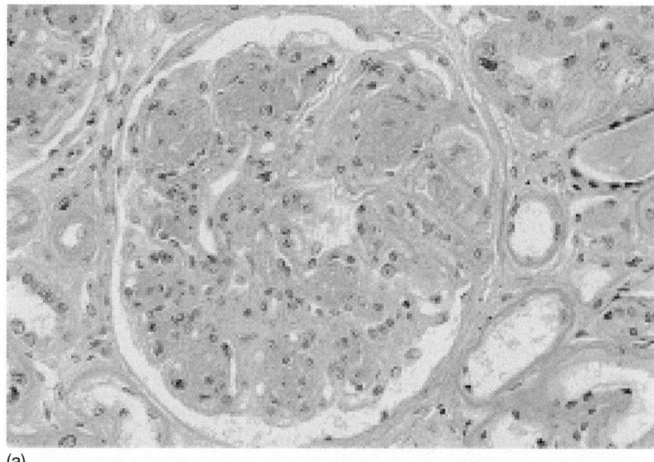

(a)

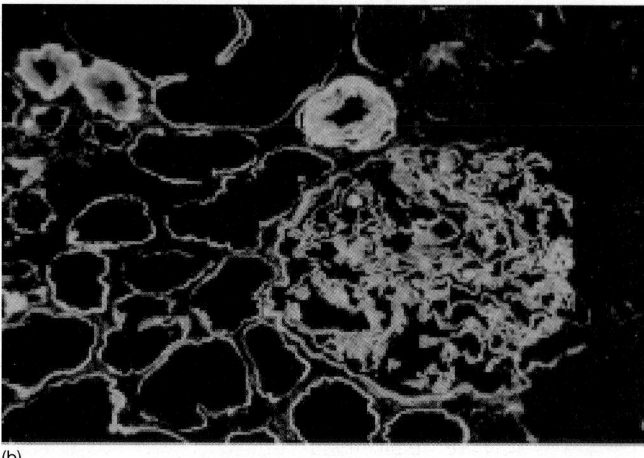

(b)

Fig. 7 Monoclonal immunoglobulin deposition disease. (a) Typical nodular glomerulosclerosis. Note membrane-like material in the centre of the nodules and nuclei at the periphery. Some glomerular capillaries show double contours. Note also thickening of the basement membrane of atrophic tubules. Light microscopy, Masson's trichrome, 312×. (b) Bright staining of tubular and glomerular basement membranes, and of mesangium and arteriolar wall with anti-κ antibody in a case of κ-light-chain deposition disease without nodular glomerular lesions. Immunofluorescence, 312×.

Milder forms simply show an increase in mesangial matrix and sometimes in mesangial cells, and a modest thickening of the basement membranes appearing abnormally bright and rigid. Glomerular lesions may not be detected by light microscopy, but require ultrastructural examination. These lesions may represent early stages of glomerular disease or be induced by light chains with a weak pathogenic potential. Their diagnosis would be unrecognized without the immunostaining results.

Arteries, arterioles, and peritubular capillaries may all contain deposits in close contact with their basement membranes.

Immunofluorescence

A key step in the diagnosis of the various forms of MIDD is immunofluorescence examination of the kidney. All biopsies show evidence of monotypic light- and/or heavy-chain fixation along tubular basement membranes (Fig. 7b). This criterion is required for the diagnosis of MIDD. In contrast with AL amyloidosis, the κ isotype is markedly predominant.

The tubular deposits stain strongly and predominate along the loops of Henle and the distal tubules, but they are also often detected along the proximal tubules. In contrast, the pattern of glomerular immunofluorescence displays marked heterogeneity. In patients with nodular glomerulosclerosis, deposits of monotypic immunoglobulin chains are usually found along the peripheral glomerular basement membranes and to a lesser extent in the nodules themselves. The staining in glomeruli is typically weaker than that observed along the tubular basement membranes. This may not be a function of the actual amount of deposited material, since several cases have been reported in which glomerular immunofluorescence was negative despite the presence of large amounts of granular glomerular deposits by electron microscopy (Pirani *et al.* 1987). Local modifications of deposited light chains might thus change their antigenicity (Ganeval *et al.* 1984). In patients without nodular lesions, glomerular staining occurs along the basement membrane, but it may involve the mesangium in some cases (Fig. 7b). Linear immunoglobulin chain staining is usually present along Bowman's capsule basement membrane. Deposits of immunoglobulin chains are constantly found in vascular walls (Fig. 7b).

In patients with HCDD, immunofluorescence with anti-light-chain antibodies is negative despite typical nodular glomerulosclerosis. Monotypic deposits of γ, α, or μ heavy chain may be identified. Any γ subclass may be observed. Analysis of the kidney biopsies with monoclonal antibodies directed to the various constant domains of the γ heavy chain showed that C_H1 domain determinants were undetectable in all tested cases (Moulin *et al.* 1999; Lin *et al.* 2001; Ronco *et al.* 2001) (Fig. 8). In addition, monoclonal antibodies to the $\gamma1$ C_H2 domain also failed to react with the renal deposits of one patient, due to a combined deletion of C_H1 and C_H2 domains (Aucouturier *et al.* 1993b). In most cases of HCDD, especially when a $\gamma1$ or $\gamma3$ chain is involved, complement components could be demonstrated in a granular or pseudolinear pattern. Complement deposits were often associated with signs of complement activation in serum (Moulin *et al.* 1999; Lin *et al.* 2001).

Electron microscopy

The most characteristic ultrastructural feature is the presence of finely to coarsely granular electron-dense deposits that delineate the outer aspect of the tubular basement membranes (Fig. 9a). They appear to be in contact with a well-preserved basal lamina. The deposits are usually quite large and may protrude into the adjacent part of the interstitium.

Ultrastructural glomerular lesions are characterized by the deposition of a non-fibrillar, electron-dense material in the mesangial nodules and along the glomerular basement membrane (Fig. 9b). The mesangial material is usually finely granular with a membranoid appearance, but in some cases it may contain strongly electron-dense granules identical to the peritubular deposits. The deposits along the glomerular basement membrane appear as a prominent but thin, continuous band delineating the endothelial aspect of the basement membrane. The limits between the deposits and the basement membrane may be difficult to distinguish. In rare cases the deposits invade the lamina densa. Glomerular endothelial cells are separated from this material by areas of electron-lucent fluffy material. Deposits can also be found in Bowman's capsules and in the wall of small arteries between the myocytes (Ronco *et al.* 2001).

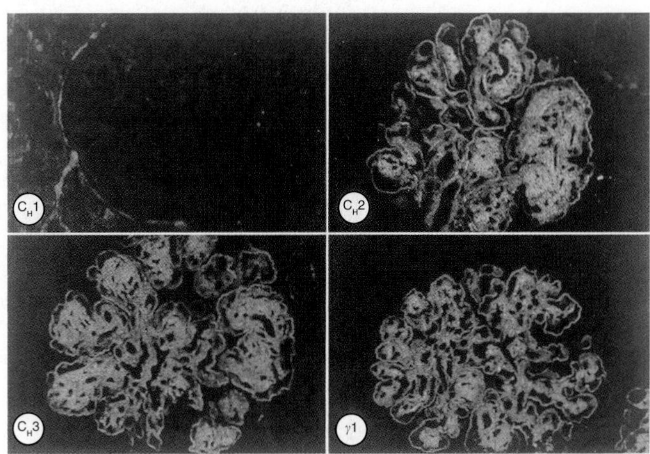

Fig. 8 Heavy-chain deposition disease. Nodular glomerulosclerosis. Mesangial and parietal deposits stain with a monoclonal antibody specific for the $\gamma1$ isotype in the absence of detectable light chain (bottom right). Immunofluorescence with a panel of monoclonal antibodies directed to the various constant domains of the γ heavy chain shows that the glomerular deposits are stained with anti-C_H2 and C_H3, but not with anti-C_H1 antibodies. Original magnification, 312×.

A common feature shared by most patients with MIDD is the dramatic accumulation of extracellular matrix. Nodules are made of normal constituents (Bruneval *et al.* 1985), and stain weakly for the small proteoglycans, decorin and biglycan (Stokes *et al.* 2000). In a series of 36 patients with light-chain-related renal diseases including AL amyloidosis, cast nephropathy, fibrillary glomerulopathy, and LCDD, transforming growth factor-β (TGF-β) was detected only in glomeruli of the three patients with LCDD and nodular glomerular lesions (Herrera *et al.* 1994). In the control series, it was essentially found in nodular diabetic glomerulosclerosis, which may suggest that distinct initial insults to the glomerular mesangium may trigger similar fibrogenetic pathways. A similar accumulation of matrix proteins was found in the perisinusoidal space of the liver of patients with LCDD (Bedossa *et al.* 1988).

Clinical presentation of monoclonal immunoglobulin deposition disease

Table 7 summarizes the main data from the five largest series (Ganeval *et al.* 1984; Confalonieri *et al.* 1988; Buxbaum *et al.* 1990; Heilman *et al.* 1992; Lin *et al.* 2001). They show an unexpectedly wide range of affected ages (31–79 years), with a slight male preponderance.

MIDD is a systemic disease with immunoglobulin chain deposition in a variety of organs leading to various clinical manifestations (Ronco *et al.* 2001), but visceral immunoglobulin chain deposits may be totally asymptomatic and found only at autopsy.

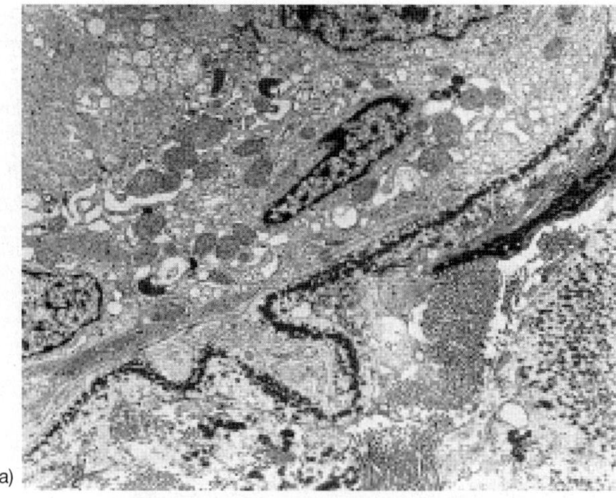

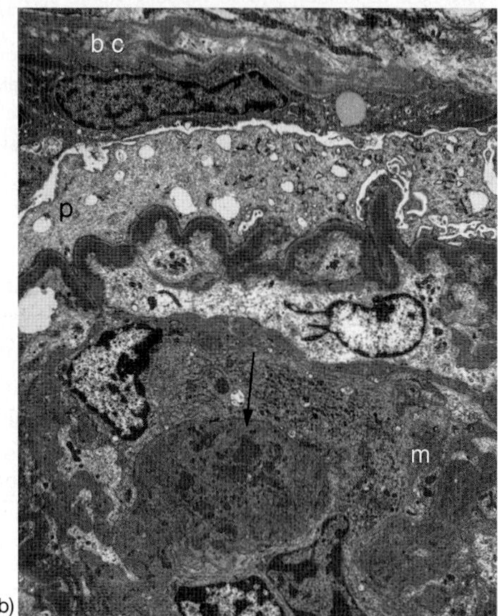

Fig. 9 Light-chain deposition disease. (a) Coarsely granular dense deposits lining the outer aspect of tubular basement membrane. Electron microscopy, uranyl acetate and lead citrate; original magnification, 6000× (by courtesy of Dr L. H. Noël). (b) Heavy granular deposits were identified along the glomerular basement membrane invading the lamina rara interna and the lamina densa. Foot process fusion was extensive. Some deposits were also seen in the mesangial nodule (arrow). Electron microscopy, uranyl acetate and lead citrate; original magnification 2500× (bc = Bowman's capsule; p = podocyte; m = mesangium).

Renal features

Renal involvement is a constant feature of MIDD, and renal symptoms, mostly proteinuria and renal failure, often dominate the clinical presentation (Table 7). In 23–67 per cent of the patients, albuminuria is associated with the nephrotic syndrome. However, in one quarter it is less than 1 g/24 h, and these patients exhibit mainly a tubulointerstitial syndrome. Albuminuria is not correlated with the existence of nodular glomerulosclerosis, at least initially, and may occur in the absence of significant glomerular lesions as detected by light microscopy. Haematuria is more frequent than one would expect for a nephropathy in which cell proliferation is usually modest, with a few exceptions.

Table 7 Clinical manifestations and renal lesions in patients with MIDD

Characteristics	Light- and light-plus heavy-chain (LCDD/LHCDD) deposition diseases	Heavy-chain (HCDD) deposition disease
Male–female ratio	1.4	0.8
Age (years)	55 (31–77)	57 (26–79)
Hypertension (%)	58	89
Renal failure (serum creatinine ≥ 130 μmol/l) (%)	90	85
Nephrotic syndrome (%)	38	32
Haematuria (%)	45	88
Nodular glomerulosclerosis (%)	31–100	100

The high prevalence, early appearance, and severity of renal failure are other salient features of MIDD (Randall *et al.* 1976; Tubbs *et al.* 1981; Lin *et al.* 2001; Ronco *et al.* 2001). In most cases, renal function declines rapidly, which is a main reason for referral. It occurs with comparable frequency in patients with either modest or heavy proteinuria, and thus presents in the form of a subacute tubulointerstitial nephritis or a rapidly progressive glomerulonephritis, respectively. The prevalence of hypertension is variable, but must be interpreted according to associated medical history.

Extrarenal manifestations

Liver and cardiac involvement are the most common features of LCDD and light- and heavy-chain deposition disease. Liver deposits were constant in patients whose liver was examined (Droz *et al.* 1984). They were either discrete, confined to sinusoids and basement membranes of biliary ductules without associated parenchymal lesions, or massive with marked dilatation and multiple ruptures of sinusoids resembling peliosis. Hepatomegaly with mild alterations of liver functional tests were the most usual symptoms, but several patients developed hepatic insufficiency and portal hypertension.

Cardiac involvement is also frequent and may be responsible for cardiomegaly and severe heart failure. As in the kidney and liver, in all autopsy cases immunofluorescence showed monotypic light-chain deposits in the vascular walls and perivascular areas of the heart (Ganeval *et al.* 1984).

Deposits may also occur along the nerve fibres and in the choroid plexus, as well as in the lymph nodes, bone marrow, spleen, pancreas, thyroid gland, submandibular glands, adrenal glands, gastrointestinal tract, abdominal vessels, lungs, and skin (Ronco *et al.* 2001).

Extrarenal deposits are less common in patients with HCDD. They have been reported in the heart, synovial tissue, skin, striated muscles, pancreas, around the thyroid follicles, and in Disse's spaces in the liver.

Haematological findings

Myeloma is diagnosed in about 40 per cent of the patients with LCDD and LHCDD, and in 25 per cent of those with HCDD.

MIDD was found at postmortem examination in 5 per cent of myeloma cases (Ivanyi 1990). MIDD, like AL-amyloidosis, is often the presenting disease leading to the discovery of myeloma at an early stage. In some patients who first presented with common myeloma and with normal-sized monoclonal immunoglobulin without kidney disease, LCDD occurred when the disease relapsed after chemotherapy, together with immunoglobulin structural abnormalities (Preud'homme *et al.* 1980b; Ganeval *et al.* 1984). Since melphalan can induce immunoglobulin gene mutations (Preud'homme *et al.* 1973), the disease in these patients might result from the emergence of a variant clone induced by the alkylating agent. Apart from myeloma, MIDD rarely complicates Waldenström's macroglobulinaemia, including its apparently non-secretory form (Preud'homme *et al.* 1980a). It often occurs in the absence of detectable malignant process even after prolonged (more than 10 years) follow-up. In such 'primary' forms, a monoclonal bone marrow plasma cell population is easily evidenced, whereas its detection requires a very careful analysis in primary amyloidosis (Preud'homme *et al.* 1988). This suggests that the plasma cell mass required for the clinical expression of the disease is larger in LCDD than in amyloidosis.

It is worth noting that in 15–30 per cent of patients with MIDD, there is no detectable monoclonal immunoglobulin in the serum and urine. Hence, some patients are affected with the so-called non-secretory myeloma or macroglobulinaemia. Non-secretory myeloma is unappropriately defined by the absence of detectable serum and urine monoclonal immunoglobulin. True non-secretion is probably very rare. In most cases, there is a secretion of abnormal immunoglobulin molecules which are either rapidly degraded postsynthetically or deposited in tissues (reviewed in Cogné *et al.* 1992).

Pathophysiology of monoclonal immunoglobulin deposition disease

The pathogenetic mechanisms leading to MIDD remain entirely hypothetical, because circulating or urinary monoclonal immunoglobulin chain precursors are frequently absent, or present at very low levels, making their purification and analysis particularly difficult, and data on the precise nature of the visceral deposits remains speculative. MIDD is due to monoclonal κ light chains in most cases, with a probable over-representation of the rare $V\kappa_{IV}$ variability subgroup (Denoroy *et al.* 1994); however, contrary to the $V\lambda_{VI}$ subgroup which was found exclusively on monoclonal light chains from AL amyloidosis patients (Ozaki *et al.* 1994), $V\kappa_{IV}$ light chains may be encountered in myeloma without renal involvement.

That immunoglobulin chain deposition involves unusual immunoglobulin chain properties is supported by the absence of detectable monoclonal component in the serum and urine in 15–30 per cent of patients with MIDD, the recurrence of the disease in the transplanted kidney, and the biosynthesis of abnormal light chains by bone marrow plasma cells (Preud'homme *et al.* 1980a,b; Buxbaum *et al.* 1990).

Abnormal glycosylation and structure of MIDD light chains

Structural abnormalities of immunoglobulins in MIDD have long been suggested by empirical studies of *in vitro* bone marrow cell biosynthesis products (Preud'homme *et al.* 1980a,b; Ganeval *et al.* 1984; Buxbaum *et al.* 1990). In a study of immunoglobulin biosynthesis by bone marrow plasma cells in eight consecutive patients (Ganeval *et al.* 1984), light chains were of normal size in two cases, and short or apparently large in the other six patients. These short or large light chains showed a striking ability to polymerize when secreted *in vitro*. Abnormal glycosylation may be responsible for an increase in apparent molecular weight of the corresponding light chain.

Undetectable circulating light chains were found to be *N*-glycosylated in all cases where they could be studied, either by *in vitro* inhibition of glycosylation with tunicamycin, analysis of the carbohydrate content of purified light chains (Ganeval *et al.* 1984), or by treatment with endoglycosidase-F (Denoroy *et al.* 1994). Thus, light-chain glycosylation might increase their propensity to precipitate in tissues and displace the equilibrium from soluble toward deposited forms so that they are no more detectable in the body fluids.

Sequence analysis

The first complete primary structure of a light chain in LCDD was determined by Cogné *et al.* in 1991. The 30 kDa κ chain found in the kidney was presumably identical to that secreted by the malignant plasma cells since they shared the same apparent molecular mass and 13 amino acid *N*-terminal sequence. It was encoded by a normal-sized κ mRNA and was *N*-glycosylated. The C region was entirely normal and the V region belonged to the $V\kappa_{IV}$ subgroup. Eight mutations were observed, including replacement of Pro95 (considered as essential for the conformation of the third hypervariable region). Replacement of Asp70 by Asn determined a *N*-glycosylation site.

The primary structures of a few further LCDD precursors were analysed at the complementary DNA (Khamlichi *et al.* 1992; Rocca *et al.* 1993) and protein levels (Bellotti *et al.* 1991). Most peculiarities are clustered in peptide loops corresponding to the CDRs, that is parts of the molecules normally implicated in antigen binding, suggesting that a first step of the pathogenesis could be a light-chain tropism for extracellular components behaving as antigen-like structures. The most remarkable observations were unusual hydrophobic residues at positions where they could either be exposed to the solvent or strongly modify the conformation, potentially leading to light-chain aggregation or interaction with other hydrophobic molecules.

However, as in AL-amyloidosis, extrinsic conditions may also contribute to aggregation of the light chain. The same light chain can form granular aggregates or amyloid fibrils depending on the environment, and different partially folded intermediates of this protein may be responsible for amorphous or fibrillar aggregation pathways (Khurana *et al.* 2001).

Heavy-chain deposition disease: a disease featured by heavy-chain deletions

A deletion of the first C domain C_H1 was found in the deposited or circulating heavy chain in the 11 patients with γ-HCDD where it was searched for (Lin *et al.* 2001; Ronco *et al.* 2001). A larger deletion also including the hinge and C_H2 domain was found in one case (Aucouturier *et al.* 1993b). In the blood, the deleted heavy chain was associated with light chains, mostly of the λ isotype, or circulated in small amounts as a free unassembled subunit (Moulin *et al.* 1999). It is likely that the C_H1 deletion facilitates the secretion of free heavy chains that are rapidly cleared from the circulation by organ deposition. Deletion of the C_H1 is also found in heavy-chain disease, a lymphoproliferative disorder with free heavy chain secretion without corresponding renal tissue deposition, and in AH-amyloidosis in which deposits have a fibrillar organization. In heavy-chain disease, however, the variable domain also is partially or completely deleted, which suggests that the V_H domain is required for tissue precipitation.

Sequence analysis of two HCDD proteins did show unusual amino acid substitutions in the V_H, which might change their physicochemical properties, including charge and hydrophobicity (Khamlichi *et al.* 1995).

Deposition does not mean pathogenicity

The finding by Solomon *et al.* (1991) of unexpectedly frequent (14 out of 40) deposition of human monoclonal light chains along basement membranes in a mouse experimental model, raises the question of the relationship between tissue precipitation and pathogenic effects. While approximately 80 per cent of MIDDs are caused by κ chains, human light chains which were found deposited along basement membranes in mice were predominantly of the λ type (nine out of 14). In addition, light-chain deposition, similar in aspect to LCDD by immunofluorescence but with only scanty granular electron-dense deposits in the tubular basement membrane, may occur in the absence of glomerular lesions and tubular basement membrane thickening (Gallo and Buxbaum 1988; Lin *et al.* 2001). In our opinion, the diagnosis of MIDD should be restricted to the patients with extracellular matrix accumulation.

Pathophysiology of extracellular matrix accumulation

A striking feature of MIDD is the dramatic associated accumulation of extracellular matrix. A role for TGF-β is supported by its strong expression in glomeruli of MIDD patients, and by *in vitro* experiments using cultured mesangial cells (Zhu *et al.* 1995). Incubation of mesangial cells with light chains from patients with MIDD induces cell changes, activation of PDGF-β and its receptor, production of monocyte chemoattractant protein-1 (MCP-1) as well as increased expression of Ki-67, a proliferation marker, whereas tubulopathic light chains chain have no effect (Russell *et al.* 2001). Because of the similarities between MIDD- and diabetes-induced nodular glomerulosclerosis, including the strong reactivity of lesions with the periodic-acid-Schiff reagent, it has been suggested that immunoglobulin chains might stimulate mesangial cells in a similar manner to advanced glycation-end products (AGEs).

Outcome and treatment of monoclonal immunoglobulin deposition disease

Survival from the onset of symptoms varies greatly from 1 month to 10 years, whereas by comparison, the prognosis of a related disease, AL amyloidosis, is much more homogeneous (see Chapter 4.2.1). In MIDD, Heilman *et al.* (1992) calculated that 5-year actuarial patient survival and survival free of endstage renal disease under chemotherapy were 70 and 37 per cent, respectively. The only predictor of renal and patient survival seems to be the initial serum creatinine at the time of biopsy, whereas the presence of myeloma did not seem to influence renal or patient survival (Lin *et al.* 2001). Outcomes in terms of renal and patient survival are significantly better in patients with pure MIDD, compared with those who present with LCDD and myeloma cast nephropathy (Lin *et al.* 2001).

As in AL amyloidosis, the therapeutic strategy should be aimed at reducing immunoglobulin production by chemotherapy, hence improving or stabilizing renal failure and preventing extrarenal deposition of light chains. Chemotherapy is logical in the patients with MIDD and myeloma, but is controversial in the absence of overt malignancy, given the uncertainties about the natural history of LCDD and the absence of reliable follow-up criteria, especially in patients without detectable monoclonal component. However, it has become general practice to treat patients with steroids plus melphalan or a cytotoxic agent, irrespective of the accompanying haematological disease (Ganeval 1988; Heilman *et al.* 1992; Lin *et al.* 2001).

It has been unclear, however, whether appropriate treatment can result in sustained remission in patients with LCDD. Barjon *et al.* (1992) first provided the demonstration of relatively rapid clearance of the deposits after syngeneic bone marrow transplantation to a patient with LCDD from his HLA-identical twin brother. Mariette *et al.* (1995) also observed a striking recovery from multiorgan failure and clearing of light-chain deposits in the heart and liver of a patient with LCDD after intensive chemotherapy. More recently, disappearance of nodular mesangial lesions and κ light-chain deposits was reported in a patient with LCDD after long-term chemotherapy (Komatsuda *et al.* 2000). These observations are of paramount importance. First, they demonstrate that fibrotic nodular glomerular lesions are reversible. Second, they argue for intensive chemotherapy with autologous blood stem cell transplantation, in patients with severe visceral involvement.

Kidney transplantation has been performed in a few patients with MIDD. Recurrence of the disease is usually observed (Spence *et al.* 1979; Scully 1981; Briefel *et al.* 1983; Gerlag *et al.* 1986). Therefore, because of shortage of kidney grafts, it would be logical to eradicate the light-chain secreting plasma-cell clone by intensive chemotherapy before kidney transplantation.

Combined glomerular and tubular lesions

Tubular lesions associated with glomerular and tubular light-chain deposits

The association of monoclonal light-chain deposits, mostly along renal tubular basement membranes, with typical myeloma cast nephropathy is more frequent than reported initially (Fig. 10). It was found in 11 of 34 (32 per cent) patients with MIDD (Lin *et al.* 2001). Nodular glomerulosclerosis is, however, infrequent (<10 per cent), and some ribbon-like tubular basement membranes are seen in fewer than half of the patients. In addition, one-third of the patients do not have granular-dense deposits by electron microscopy. The lack of matrix accumulation in most of these patients who present with acute renal failure in the setting of a true myeloma may relate to insufficient time for the development of fibrosis or to a weaker sclerogenic effect of the light chain, if any (Ronco *et al.* 2001). As discussed above, the presence of light-chain deposits along the tubular basement membrane is not sufficient to make a diagnosis of MIDD. Conversely, in patients with glomerular lesions associated with light chains, damage to proximal tubule epithelium frequently occurs and can become prominent in some patients (Sanders *et al.* 1988b) although typical myeloma casts are rare. In addition, the pattern of renal lesions may change with time under chemotherapy. In three patients with typical myeloma cast nephropathy on initial biopsy, casts were replaced by massive tissue deposits of light chains (κ chains in two, amyloid in one) (Hill *et al.* 1983), suggesting chemotherapy-induced mutation of the light chains

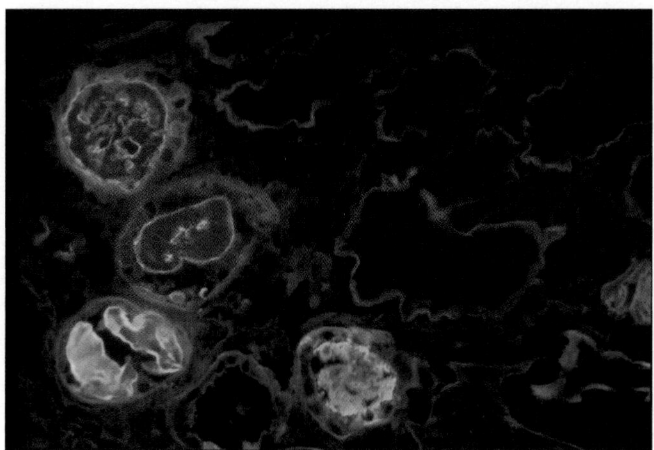

Fig. 10 Tubular light-chain deposits and myeloma cast nephropathy. Immunofluorescence for κ light chain revealed linear tubular basement membrane staining and strong staining of typical myelomatous casts. Original magnification 312×.

which might cause the light chains to be deposited in tissues rather than giving rise to myeloma casts (Preud'homme *et al.* 1973, 1980b).

More exceptional is the association of a Fanconi syndrome with AL amyloidosis. In three cases (Short and Smith 1959; Finkel *et al.* 1973; Maldonado *et al.* 1975), a Fanconi syndrome was not caused by amyloid infiltration of the kidney. Amyloid was diagnosed shortly before death or at autopsy. Finkel *et al.* (1973) noticed that nodular amyloid deposits were surrounded by atypical lymphoid cells containing numerous needle-shaped crystals, and first suggested that 'a product' from these cells 'may have been involved with both crystal formation and amyloid production'. Since the nucleation processes initiating amyloid and crystal formation may share similarities, it is tempting to speculate that the responsible light chain bore unusual physicochemical properties, inducing both pathological conditions.

Combined AL amyloidosis and monoclonal immunoglobulin deposition disease

Since the description of MIDD, it was expected that the two types of deposits might coexist at different sites in a single patient and this was reported by Jacquot *et al.* (1985). A review by Gallo *et al.* (1989) indicated that in approximately 7 per cent of 135 cases of LCDD, amyloid was found in one or more organs. Because amyloid deposits were focal, the true incidence of the association may be markedly underestimated. In patients with both types of deposits, amyloid P component was found in the fibrillar, but not the non-fibrillar light-chain deposits by immunohistochemical methods (Gallo *et al.* 1988). The pathophysiological significance of this association remains controversial. On the one hand, some light chains may possess intrinsic properties which make them prone to form both fibrillar and non-fibrillar deposits, depending on the tissue microenvironment (Khurana *et al.* 2001). On the other hand, in the absence of structural analysis of the deposited light chains, one cannot exclude that they are generated by different variant clones. In a patient with IgD myeloma, MIDD and amyloidosis were associated with cast nephropathy (Lam and Chan 1993).

Other dysproteinaemia-associated glomerular lesions

Glomerulonephritis with intracapillary thrombi of IgM

This glomerulonephritis is almost specific of Waldenström's macroglobulinaemia (Morel-Maroger *et al.* 1970). It is considered as the most common renal lesion with amyloidosis in this condition, but like amyloidosis, it has become a rare entity, probably because of the increased efficacy of chemotherapy. In the series of 16 autopsy and biopsy cases published by Morel-Maroger *et al.* (1970), this lesion was found in six cases, and was associated with a variable degree of proteinuria and normal or slightly altered renal function. It was characterized by periodic acid-Schiff-positive, non-congophilic endomembranous deposits in a variable number of capillary loops. Deposits were sometimes so voluminous as to occlude the capillary lumens partially or completely, thus forming thrombi. By immunofluorescence, thrombi and deposits stained with anti-IgM (three cases studied) and with anti-κ (one case studied). Two of the six patients had cryoglobulinaemia and slight glomerular cell proliferation. In the remaining four, the amount of circulating IgM was higher than in the other patients of the series with amyloidosis or no detectable renal lesion, which suggested that hyperviscosity could favour IgM deposition in glomerular capillaries where ultrafiltration further increases the protein concentration. This pathophysiological hypothesis is also supported by the case of Argani and Kipkie (1964) in which formation of diffuse intracapillary thrombi was probably precipitated by severe dehydration.

Since renal biopsy may be hazardous in patients with Waldenström's macroglobulinaemia who frequently have an increased bleeding time, it is wise to search for amyloid deposits first by a less invasive tissue biopsy. In these patients, amyloidosis is a major cause of morbidity, associated with a much shorter survival (Gertz *et al.* 1993).

Glomerulonephritis with non-amyloid organized monotypic deposits

These entities are characterized by fibrillar or microtubular deposits in mesangium and glomerular capillary loops which are readily distinguishable from amyloid by the larger thickness of fibrils and lack of Congo red staining and β-pleated sheet organization. They were termed 'fibrillary glomerulonephritis' by Alpers and associates (Alpers 1993) and 'immunotactoid glomerulopathy' by Korbet *et al.* (1985) (see also Chapter 4.2). However, the two denominations may cover partly different morphological entities, as defined by the size and aspect of organized structures. For Alpers the distinguishing morphological features of immunotactoid glomerulonephritis are organized deposits made of large, thick-walled microtubules, usually greater than 30 nm in diameter, at times arranged in parallel arrays. On the other hand, fibrillary glomerulonephritis is characterized by more amyloid-like deposits with smaller fibrils (12–20 nm).

Although these criteria remain controversial (Fogo *et al.* 1993), distinguishing immunotactoid from fibrillary glomerulonephritis may be of great clinical and pathophysiological interest, because the former seems to be more often associated with monotypic immunoglobulin deposits. In a recent study of 23 patients based on ultrastructural appearance of the deposits, deposits were monotypic in 13 of 14 patients with immunotactoid (microtubular) glomerulopathy (κ, seven cases; λ, six cases), and in only one of eight patients with fibrillary glomerulonephritis (Bridoux *et al.* 2002).

Patients with immunotactoid glomerulonephritis and monotypic immunoglobulin deposits have a mean age of 55–60 years (extremes: 19–76 years) with a male to female ratio of 2 (Moulin *et al.* 1992; Bridoux *et al.* 2002). They usually present with the nephrotic syndrome, microscopic haematuria and mild renal failure, mostly in the setting of chronic lymphocytic leukaemia or related lymphoma (seven of 14 patients in Bridoux's series, 2002). Renal biopsy showed either atypical membranous glomerulonephritis, often associated with segmental mesangial proliferation, or lobular membranoproliferative glomerulonephritis. A circulating monoclonal immunoglobulin of the same isotype as the deposited one was detected in only five of 14 patients by immunoelectrophoresis (Bridoux *et al.* 2002). Intracytoplasmic crystal-like immunoglobulin inclusions were found in three patients with chronic lymphocytic leukaemia and in the lymphoma patient (Bridoux *et al.* 2002). They showed the same microtubular organization and contained the same IgG subclass and light-chain type as renal deposits. Whether crystallization in lymphocytes and the glomerulus is due to unusual intrinsic physicochemical properties of the monoclonal immunoglobulin or to reactivity with a shared epitope remains to be established. These properties may also account for the rapid disappearance of the immunoglobulin from the blood and recurrence on renal graft noted in several patients (Pronovost *et al.* 1996). It is worth noting that corticosteroid and/or chemotherapy were associated with partial or complete remission of the nephrotic syndrome in most cases, with parallel improvement in haematological parameters.

A better understanding of these unusual glomerulopathies, which most likely make up a new form of monoclonal immunoglobulin-related deposition disease with microtubular organization of the deposits, will require

(1) detailed ultrastructural and immunomorphological characterization of the renal deposits;

(2) careful analysis of circulating immunoglobulin with sensitive techniques, including repeated search of cryoglobulins;

(3) studies on bone marrow and circulating lymphocytes (ultrastructure, *in vitro* immunoglobulin biosynthesis); as well as

(4) prolonged follow-up of patients to assess eventual occurrence of extrarenal manifestations and efficacy of treatment.

Immunotactoid (microtubular) glomerulopathies must now be added to the heterogeneous list of glomerulopathies caused by B-cell chronic lymphocytic leukaemia and related lymphomas, including AL amyloidosis and the larger cohort of cryoglobulinaemia-associated membranoproliferative glomerulonephritis (Table 8).

Other types of glomerulonephritis

Additional histological forms of glomerulonephritis have been described occasionally in B-cell proliferations, including crescentic and hypocomplementaemic membranoproliferative glomerulonephritis, apparently without cryoglobulinaemia, as reviewed by Meyrier *et al.* (1984). However, most of these observations are old. Careful immunomorphological, ultrastructural, and immunochemical studies should be performed before these histological forms are recognized as distinct entities.

Myeloma- and AL amyloidosis-induced renal failure account for less than 2 per cent of the patients admitted on a chronic dialysis programme each year. This is due in part to the relative rarity of these

Table 8 Renal lesions observed in B-cell proliferations

Renal lesions	Multiple myeloma	Waldenström's macroglobulinaemia	Chronic lymphocytic leukaemia and related lymphomas
Tubular lesions			
Cast nephropathy	+++	−	−
(Proximal) tubule lesions[a]	+	−	−
Fanconi syndrome	+ (smoldering)	−	−
Glomerular lesions[b]			
AL amyloidosis	++	+	+
MIDD (nodular, 'membranoproliferative', 'minimal change')	++	+	−
Non-amyloid organized deposits[c]	−	−	+
Type I and type II cryoglobulinaemia	+	++	++
IgM capillary thrombi	−	+	−
Other (crescentic, 'minimal change', etc.)	+	+	+
Interstitial lesions			
B-cell infiltrate	+[d]	++	++
Nephrocalcinosis	+	−	−
Pyelonephritis (infections)	+	−	−

[a] Without detectable myeloma casts, sometimes acute tubular necrosis.

[b] Glomerular involvement is usually but not always preponderant.

[c] Usually atypical membranous (or membranoproliferative) glomerulonephritis.

[d] Exceptionally, plasmacytoma.

− Not or exceptionally observed; + to ++, semiquantitative rating of the prevalence of renal lesions.

immunoproliferative diseases, but also to the deteriorated clinical condition of many patients at the time of endstage renal disease. A dramatic effort of prevention must therefore be undertaken, relying on a better understanding of the structural and physicochemical properties of immunoglobulin components leading to deposition or precipitation in tissues. Any progress in this field may also enlighten the pathogenesis of immunologically mediated renal diseases, especially glomerulonephritides, because properties of monoclonal immunoglobulin components favouring their deposition may also apply to polyclonal immunoglobulin involved in the formation of immune complexes. This is exemplified by type II mixed cryoglobulins that both contain a monoclonal immunoglobulin and form circulating immune complexes.

References

Alexanian, R. and Dimopoulos, M. (1994). The treatment of multiple myeloma. *New England Journal of Medicine* **330**, 484–489.

Alexanian, R., Barlogie, B., and Dixon, D. (1990). Renal failure in multiple myeloma: pathogenesis and prognostic implications. *Archives of Internal Medicine* **150**, 1693–1695.

Alpers, C. E. (1993). Fibrillary glomerulonephritis and immunotactoid glomerulopathy: two entities, not one. *American Journal of Kidney Diseases* **22**, 448–451.

Antonovych, T. T. *et al.* (1974). Light chain deposits in multiple myeloma (Abstract 3). 7th Annual Meeting, American Society of Nephrology, 1973. *Laboratory Investigation* **30**, 370A.

Argani, I. and Kipkie, G. F. (1964). Macroglobulinemic nephropathy. Acute renal failure in macroglobulinemia of Waldenström. *American Journal of Medicine* **36**, 151–157.

Attal, M. *et al.* (1996). A prospective, randomised trial of autologous bone marrow transplantation and chemotherapy in multiple myeloma. *New England Journal of Medicine* **35**, 91–97.

Aucouturier, P. *et al.* (1993a). Monoclonal Ig L chain and L chain V domain fragment crystallization in myeloma-associated Fanconi syndrome. *Journal of Immunology* **150**, 3561–3568.

Aucouturier, P. *et al.* (1993b). Brief report: heavy-chain deposition disease. *New England Journal of Medicine* **329**, 1389–1393.

Badros, A. *et al.* (2001). Results of autologous stem cell transplant in multiple myeloma patients with renal failure. *British Journal of Haematology* **114**, 822–829.

Ballester, O. F. *et al.* (1997). High dose chemotherapy and autologous peripheral blood stem cell transplantation in patients with multiple myeloma and renal insufficiency. *Bone Marrow Transplantation* **20**, 653–656.

Barjon, P. *et al.* (1992). Traitement de la maladie par dépôts de chaînes légères par greffe de moelle. *Néphrologie* **13**, 24.

Batuman, V., Sastrasinh, M., and Sastrasinh, S. (1986). Light chain effects on alanine and glucose uptake by renal brush border membranes. *Kidney International* **30**, 662–665.

Batuman, V., Dreisbach, A. W., and Cyran, J. (1990). Light-chain binding sites on renal brush-border membranes. *American Journal of Physiology* **258**, F1259–F1265.

Batuman, V. *et al.* (1998). Myeloma light chains are ligands for cubilin (gp 280). *American Journal of Physiology* **275**, F246–F254.

Bedossa, P. *et al.* (1988). Light chain deposition disease with liver dysfunction. *Human Pathology* **19**, 1008–1014.

Bellotti, V. *et al.* (1991). Amino acid sequence of κ Sci, the Bence Jones protein isolated from a patient with light chain deposition disease. *Biochimica et Biophysica Acta* **1097**, 177–182.

Blade, J., Lust, J. A., and Kyle, R. A. (1994). Immunoglobulin D multiple myeloma: presenting features, response to therapy and survival in a series of 53 cases. *Journal of Clinical Oncology* **12**, 2398–2404.

Blade, J. *et al.* (1998). Renal failure in multiple myeloma. *Archives of Internal Medicine* **158**, 1889–1893.

Bridoux, F. *et al.* (2002). Fibrillary glomerulonephritis and immunotactoid (microtubular) glomerulopathy are associated with distinct immunological features. *Kidney International* **62**, 1764–1775.

Briefel, G. R. *et al.* (1983). Renal transplantation in a patient with multiple myeloma and light chain nephropathy. *Surgery* **93**, 579–584.

Bruneval, P. *et al.* (1985). Glomerular matrix proteins in nodular glomerulosclerosis in association with light chain deposition disease and diabetes mellitus. *Human Pathology* **16**, 477–484.

Buxbaum, J. N. *et al.* (1990). Monoclonal immunoglobulin deposition disease: light chain and light and heavy chain deposition diseases and their relation to light chain amyloidosis. Clinical features, immunopathology, and molecular analysis. *Annals of Internal Medicine* **112**, 1990.

Clark, A. D., Shetty, A., and Soutar, R. (1999). Renal failure and multiple myeloma: pathogenesis and treatment of renal failure and management of underlying myeloma. *Blood Review* **13**, 79–90.

Clyne, D. H. *et al.* (1974). Renal effects of intraperitoneal kappa chain injection. Induction of crystals in renal tubular cells. *Laboratory Investigation* **31**, 131–142.

Clyne, D. H., Pesce, A. J., and Thompson, R. E. (1979). Nephrotoxicity of Bence Jones proteins in the rat: importance of protein isoelectric point. *Kidney International* **16**, 345–352.

Cogné, M. *et al.* (1991). Structure of a monoclonal kappa chain of the $V\kappa_{IV}$ subgroup in the kidney and plasma cells in light chain deposition disease. *Journal of Clinical Investigation* **87**, 2186–2190.

Cogné, M. *et al.* (1992). Structurally abnormal immunoglobulins in human immunoproliferative disorders. *Blood* **79**, 2181–2195.

Cohen, A. H. and Border, W. A. (1980). Myeloma kidney: an immunomorphogenetic study of renal biopsies. *Laboratory Investigation* **42**, 248–256.

Confalonieri, R. *et al.* (1988). Light chain nephropathy: histological and clinical aspects in 15 cases. *Nephrology, Dialysis, Transplantation* **2**, 150–156.

Cooper, E. H. *et al.* (1984). Proximal renal tubular function in myelomatosis: observations in the fourth Medical Research Council trial. *Journal of Clinical Pathology* **37**, 852–858.

Costanza, D. J. and Smoller, M. (1963). Multiple myeloma with the Fanconi Syndrome. Study of a case, with electron microscopy of the kidney. *American Journal of Medicine* **34**, 125–133.

Coward, R. A. *et al.* (1984). The importance of urinary immunoglobulin light chain isoelectric point (p*I*) in nephrotoxicity in multiple myeloma. *Clinical Science* **66**, 229–232.

Coward, R. A., Mallick, N. P., and Delamore, I. W. (1985). Tubular function in multiple myeloma. *Clinical Nephrology* **24**, 180–185.

DeFronzo, R. A. *et al.* (1975). Acute renal failure in multiple myeloma. *Medicine (Baltimore)* **54**, 209–223.

DeFronzo, R. A. *et al.* (1978). Renal function in patients with multiple myeloma. *Medicine (Baltimore)* **57**, 151–166.

Denoroy, L., Déret, S., and Aucouturier, P. (1994). Overrepresentation of the $V\kappa_{IV}$ subgroup in light chain deposition disease. *Immunology Letters* **42**, 63–66.

Deret, S. *et al.* (1999). Kappa light chain-associated Fanconi syndrome: molecular analysis of monoclonal immunoglobulin light chains from patients with and without intracellular crystals. *Protein Engineering* **12**, 363–369.

Droz, D. *et al.* (1984). Liver involvement in nonamyloid light chain deposits disease. *Laboratory Investigation* **50**, 683–689.

Edelman, G. M. and Gally, J. A. (1962). The nature of Bence Jones proteins: chemical similarities to polypeptide chains of myeloma globulins and normal γ-globulins. *Journal of Experimental Medicine* **116**, 207–227.

Engle, R. L. and Wallis, L. A. (1957). Multiple myeloma and the adult Fanconi syndrome. *American Journal of Medicine* **22**, 5–12.

Eulitz, M., Weiss, D. T., and Solomon, A. (1990). Immunoglobulin heavy-chain-associated amyloidosis. *Proceedings of the National Academy of Sciences of the United States of America* **87**, 6542–6546.

Fermand, J. P. *et al.* (1998). High dose therapy and autologous peripheral blood stem cell transplantation in multiple myeloma: up-front or rescue treatment? Results of a multicenter sequential randomized clinical trial. *Blood* **92**, 3131–3136.

Finkel, P. N. *et al.* (1973). Adult Fanconi syndrome, amyloidosis and marked kappa light chain proteinuria. *Nephron* **10**, 1–24.

Fogo, A., Qureshi, N., and Horn, R. G. (1993). Morphologic and clinical features of fibrillary glomerulonephritis versus immunotactoid glomerulopathy. *American Journal of Kidney Diseases* **22**, 367–377.

Gailani, S., Seon, B. K., and Henderson, E. S. (1987). κ-Light chain myeloma associated with adult Fanconi syndrome: response of the nephropathy to treatment of myeloma. *Medical and Pediatric Oncology* **4**, 141–147.

Gallo, G. and Buxbaum, J. Monoclonal immunoglobulin deposition disease: immunopathologic aspects of renal involvement. In *The Kidney in Plasma Cell Dyscrasias* (ed. L. Minetti, G. D'Amico, and C. Ponticelli), pp. 171–181. Dordrecht: Kluwer Academic Publishers, 1988.

Gallo, G. *et al.* (1988). Nonamyloidotic monoclonal immunoglobulin deposits lack amyloid P component. *Modern Pathology* **1**, 453–456.

Gallo, G. *et al.* (1989). The spectrum of monoclonal immunoglobulin deposition disease associated with immunocytic dyscrasias. *Seminars in Hematology* **26**, 234–245.

Ganeval, D. Kidney involvement in light chain deposition disease. In *The Kidney in Plasma Cell Dyscrasias* (ed. L. Minetti, G. D'Amico, and C. Ponticelli), pp. 221–228. Dordrecht: Kluwer Academic Publishers, 1988.

Ganeval, D. *et al.* (1984). Light-chain deposition disease: its relation with AL-type amyloidosis. *Kidney International* **26**, 1–9.

Ganeval, D. *et al.* (1992). Treatment of multiple myeloma with renal involvement. *Advances in Nephrology from Necker Hospital* **21**, 347–370.

Gerlag, P. G. G., Koene, R. A. P., and Berden, J. H. M. (1986). Renal transplantation in light chain nephropathy: case report and review of the literature. *Clinical Nephrology* **25**, 101–104.

Gertz, M. A., Kyle, R. A., and Noel, P. (1993). Primary systemic amyloidosis: a rare complication of immunoglobulin M monoclonal gammopathies and Waldenström's macroglobulinemia. *Journal of Clinical Oncology* **11**, 914–920.

Glenner, G. G. *et al.* (1971). Amyloid fibril proteins: proof of homology with immunoglobulin light chains by sequence analyses. *Science* **172**, 1150–1151.

Heilman, R. L. *et al.* (1992). Long-term follow-up and response to chemotherapy in patients with light-chain deposition disease. *American Journal of Kidney Diseases* **20**, 34–41.

Herrera, G. A. *et al.* (1994). Growth factors in monoclonal light-chain-related renal diseases. *Human Pathology* **25**, 883–892.

Hill, G. S. *et al.* (1983). Renal lesions in multiple myeloma: their relationship to associated protein abnormalities. *American Journal of Kidney Diseases* **2**, 423–438.

Huang, Z. Q. and Sanders, P. W. (1995). Biochemical interaction between Tamm–Horsfall glycoprotein and Ig light chains in the pathogenesis of cast nephropathy. *Laboratory Investigation* **73**, 810–817.

Huang, Z. Q. and Sanders, P. W. (1997). Localization of a single binding site for immunoglobulin light chains on human Tamm–Horsfall glycoprotein. *Journal of Clinical Investigation* **99**, 732–736.

Huang, Z. Q. *et al.* (1993). Bence Jones proteins bind to a common peptide segment of Tamm–Horsfall glycoprotein to promote heterotypic aggregation. *Journal of Clinical Investigation* **92**, 2975–2983.

Iggo, N. *et al.* (1989). Chronic dialysis in patients with multiple myeloma and renal failure: a worthwhile treatment. *Quarterly Journal of Medicine* **270**, 903–910.

Ivanyi, B. (1990). Frequency of light chain deposition nephropathy relative to renal amyloidosis and Bence Jones cast nephropathy in a necropsy study of patients with myeloma. *Archives of Pathology and Laboratory Medicine* **114**, 986–987.

Jacquot, C. *et al.* (1985). Association of systemic light-chain deposition disease and amyloidosis: a report of three patients with renal involvement. *Clinical Nephrology* **24**, 93–98.

Johns, E. A. *et al.* (1986). Isoelectric points of urinary light chains in myelomatosis: analysis in relation to nephrotoxicity. *Journal of Clinical Pathology* **39**, 833–837.

Johnson, W. J. *et al.* (1990). Treatment of renal failure associated with multiple myeloma. *Archives of Internal Medicine* **150**, 863–869.

Kapadia, S. B. (1980). Multiple myeloma: a clinicopathologic study of 62 consecutively autopsied cases. *Medicine* **59**, 380–392.

Khamlichi, A. A. *et al.* (1992). Primary structure of a monoclonal κ chain in myeloma with light chain deposition disease. *Clinical and Experimental Immunology* **87**, 122–126.

Khamlichi, A. A. *et al.* (1995). Structure of abnormal heavy chains in human heavy chain deposition disease. *European Journal of Biochemistry* **229**, 54–60.

Khurana, R. *et al.* (2001). Partially folded intermediates as critical precursors of light chain amyloid fibrils and amorphous aggregates. *Biochemistry* **40**, 3525–3535.

Knudsen, L. M. *et al.* (1994). Renal function in newly diagnosed multiple myeloma—a demographic study of 1353 patients. *European Journal of Haematology* **53**, 207–212.

Knudsen, L. M. *et al.* (2000). Renal failure in multiple myeloma: reversibility and impact on the prognosis. *European Journal of Haematology* **65**, 175–181.

Kobernick, S. D. and Whiteside, J. H. (1957). Renal glomeruli in multiple myeloma. *Laboratory Investigation* **6**, 478–485.

Komatsuda, A. *et al.* (2000). Disappearance of nodular mesangial lesions in a patient with light chain nephropathy after long-term chemotherapy. *American Journal of Kidney Diseases* **35**, E9.

Korbet, S. M. *et al.* (1985). Immunotactoid glomerulopathy. *Medicine (Baltimore)* **64**, 228–243.

Koss, M. N., Pirani, C. L., and Osserman, E. F. (1976). Experimental Bence Jones cast nephropathy. *Laboratory Investigation* **34**, 579–591.

Kyle, R. A. (1975). Multiple myeloma: review of 869 cases. *Mayo Clinic Proceedings* **50**, 29–40.

Kyle, R. A. and Greipp, P. R. (1980). Smoldering multiple myeloma. *New England Journal of Medicine* **302**, 1347–1349.

Lam, K. Y. and Chan, K. W. (1993). Unusual findings in a myeloma kidney: a light- and electron-microscopic study. *Nephron* **65**, 133–136.

Leboulleux, M. *et al.* (1995). Protease resistance and binding of Ig light chains in myeloma-associated tubulopathies. *Kidney International* **48**, 72–79.

Lee, D. B. N. *et al.* (1972). The adult Fanconi syndrome. Observations on etiology, morphology, renal function and mineral metabolism in three patients. *Medicine (Baltimore)* **51**, 107–138.

Levi, D. F., Williams, R. C. J., and Lindstrom, F. D. (1968). Immunofluorescent studies of the myeloma kidney with special reference to light chain disease. *American Journal of Medicine* **44**, 922–933.

Levine, S. B. and Bernstein, L. D. (1985). Crystalline inclusions in multiple myeloma. *Journal of the American Medical Association* **254**, 1985.

Lin, J. *et al.* (2001). Renal monoclonal immunoglobulin deposition disease: the disease spectrum. *Journal of the American Society of Nephrology* **12**, 1482–1492.

McCarthy, C. S. and Becker, J. A. (1992). Multiple myeloma and contrast media. *Radiology* **183**, 519–521.

MacLennan, I. C. M., Drayson, M., and Dunn, J. (1994). Multiple myeloma. *British Medical Journal* **308**, 1033–1036.

Maldonado, J. E. *et al.* (1975). Fanconi syndrome in adults. A manifestation of a latent form of myeloma. *American Journal of Medicine* **58**, 354–364.

Mariette, X., Clauvel, J. P., and Brouet, J. C. (1995). Intensive therapy in AL-amyloidosis and light-chain deposition disease. *Annals of Internal Medicine* **123**, 553.

Melcion, C. *et al.* (1984). Renal failure in myeloma: relationship with isoelectric point of immunoglobulin light chains. *Clinical Nephrology* **22**, 138–143.

Messiaen, T. *et al.* (2000). Adult Fanconi syndrome secondary to light chain gammopathy: clinicopathologic heterogeneity and unusual features in 11 patients. *Medicine (Baltimore)* **79**, 135–154.

Meyrier, A. *et al.* (1984). Rapidly progressive ('crescentic') glomerulonephritis and monoclonal gammapathies. *Nephron* **38**, 156–162.

Misiani, R. *et al.* (1987). Management of myeloma kidney: an anti-light-chain approach. *American Journal of Kidney Diseases* **10**, 28–33.

Montseny, J. J. *et al.* (1998). Long-term outcome according to renal histological lesions in 118 patients with monoclonal gammapathies. *Nephrology, Dialysis, Transplantation* **13**, 1438–1445.

Morel-Maroger, L. *et al.* (1970). Pathology of the kidney in Waldenström's macroglobulinemia. Study of sixteen cases. *New England Journal of Medicine* **283**, 123–129.

Moulin, B. *et al.* (1992). Glomerulonephritis in chronic lymphocytic leukemia and related B-cell lymphomas. *Kidney International* **42**, 127–135.

Moulin, B. *et al.* (1999). Nodular glomerulosclerosis with deposition of monoclonal immunoglobulin heavy chains lacking CH1. *Journal of the American Society of Nephrology* **10**, 519–528.

Munshi, N. C. *et al.* (1999). Novel approaches in myeloma therapy. *Seminars in Oncology* **26**, 28–34.

Myatt, E. A. *et al.* (1994). Pathogenic potential of human monoclonal immunoglobulin light chains: relationship of *in vitro* aggregation to *in vivo* organ deposition. *Proceedings of the National Academy of Sciences of the United States of America* **91**, 3034–3038.

Oliver, J. (1945). New directions in renal morphology: a method, its results and its future. *Harvey Lectures* **40**, 102–155.

Orfila, C. *et al.* (1991). Fanconi syndrome, kappa light-chain myeloma, non-amyloid fibrils and cytoplasmic crystals in renal tubular epithelium. *American Journal of Nephrology* **11**, 345–349.

Ozaki, S. *et al.* (1994). Preferential expression of human λ-light chain variable region subgroups in multiple myeloma, AL amyloidosis, and Waldenström's macroglobulinemia. *Clinical Immunology and Immunopathology* **71**, 183–189.

Pasquali, S. *et al.* (1987). Renal histological lesions and clinical syndromes in multiple myeloma. *Clinical Nephrology* **27**, 222–228.

Pasquali, S. *et al.* (1990). Long-term survival patients with acute and severe renal failure due to multiple myeloma. *Clinical Nephrology* **34**, 247–254.

Pichette, V. *et al.* (1993). Renal function recovery in end-stage renal disease. Biochemical characterization. *American Journal of Kidney Diseases* **22**, 398–402.

Pirani, C. L. Histological, histochemical and ultrastructural features of myeloma kidney. In *The Kidney in Plasma Cell Dyscrasias* (ed. L. Minetti, G. D'Amico, and C. Ponticelli), pp. 153–170. Dordrecht: Kluwer Academic Publishers, 1988.

Pirani, C. L. *et al.* (1987). Renal lesions in plasma cell dyscrasias: ultrastructural observations. *American Journal of Kidney Diseases* **10**, 208–221.

Port, F. K. and Nissenson, A. R. (1989). Outcome of end-stage renal disease in patients with rare causes of renal failure. II. Renal or systemic neoplasms. *Quarterly Journal of Medicine* **272**, 1161–1165.

Pozzi, C. *et al.* (1987). Prognostic factors and effectiveness of treatment in acute renal failure due to multiple myeloma: a review of 50 cases. Report of the Italian Renal Immunopathology Group. *Clinical Nephrology* **28**, 1–9.

Preud'homme, J. L., Buxbaum, J., and Scharff, M. D. (1973). Mutagenesis of mouse myeloma cells with Melphalan. *Nature* **245**, 320–322.

Preud'homme, J. L. *et al.* (1980a). Synthesis of abnormal immunoglobulins in lymphoplasmacytic disorders with visceral light chain deposition. *American Journal of Medicine* **69**, 703–710.

Preud'homme, J. L. *et al.* (1980b). Synthesis of abnormal heavy and light chains in multiple myeloma with visceral deposition of monoclonal immunoglobulin. *Clinical and Experimental Immunology* **42**, 545–553.

Preud'homme, J. L. *et al.* (1988). Immunoglobulin synthesis in primary and myeloma amyloidosis. *Clinical and Experimental Immunology* **73**, 389–394.

Preud'homme, J. L. *et al.* (1994). Monoclonal immunoglobulin deposition disease (Randall type). Relationship with structural abnormalities of immunoglobulin chains. *Kidney International* **46**, 965–972.

Preud'homme, J. L. *et al.* (1997). Cast nephropathy in μ heavy chain disease. *Clinical Nephrology* **48**, 118–121.

Pronovost, P. H. *et al.* (1996). Clinical features, predictors of disease progression and results of renal transplantation in fibrillary immunotactoid glomerulopathy. *Nephrology, Dialysis, Transplantation* **11**, 837–842.

Rabb, H. *et al.* (1999). Acute renal failure from multiple myeloma precipitated by ACE inhibitors. *American Journal of Kidney Diseases* **33**, E5.

Randall, R. E. *et al.* (1976). Manifestations of systemic light chain deposition. *American Journal of Medicine* **60**, 293–299.

Rayner, H. C. *et al.* (1991). Perspectives in multiple myeloma: survival, prognostic factors and disease complications in a single centre between 1975 and 1988. *Quarterly Journal of Medicine* **290**, 517–525.

Rocca, A. *et al.* (1993). Primary structure of a variable region of the $V\kappa_I$ subgroup (ISE) in light chain deposition disease. *Clinical and Experimental Immunology* **91**, 506–509.

Ronco, P. *et al.* (1987). Pathophysiologic aspects of Tamm–Horsfall protein: a phylogenetically conserved marker of the thick ascending limb of Henle's loop. *Advances in Nephrology from Necker Hospital* **16**, 231–250.

Ronco, P. *et al.* Pathophysiological aspects of myeloma cast nephropathy. In *The Kidney in Plasma Cell Dyscrasias* (ed. L. Minetti, G. D'Amico, and C. Ponticelli), pp. 93–104. Dordrecht: Kluwer Academic Publishers, 1988.

Ronco, P. *et al.* (2001). Light chain deposition disease: a model of glomerulosclerosis defined at the molecular level. *Journal of the American Society of Nephrology* **12**, 1558–1565.

Russell, W. *et al.* (2001). Monoclonal light chain-mesangial interactions: early signaling events and subsequent pathologic effects. *Laboratory Investigation* **81**, 689–703.

Rota, S. *et al.* (1987). Multiple myeloma and severe renal failure: a clinicopathologic study of outcome and prognosis in 34 patients. *Medicine (Baltimore)* **66**, 126–137.

Sakhuja, V. *et al.* (2000). Renal involvement in multiple myeloma: a 10-year study. *Renal Failure* **22**, 465–477.

Sanchez, L. M. and Domz, C. A. (1960). Renal patterns in myeloma. *Annals of Internal Medicine* **52**, 44–54.

Sanders, P. W. and Booker, B. B. (1992). Pathobiology of cast nephropathy from human Bence Jones proteins. *Journal of Clinical Investigation* **89**, 630–639.

Sanders, P. W., Herrera, G. A., and Galla, J. H. (1987). Human Bence Jones protein toxicity in rat proximal tubule epithelium *in vivo*. *Kidney International* **32**, 851–861.

Sanders, P. W. *et al.* (1988a). Differential nephrotoxicity of low molecular weight proteins including Bence Jones proteins in the perfused rat nephron *in vivo*. *Journal of Clinical Investigation* **82**, 2086–2096.

Sanders, P. W. *et al.* (1988b). Morphologic alterations of the proximal tubules in light-chain related renal disease. *Kidney International* **33**, 881–889.

Sanders, P. W. *et al.* (1990). Mechanisms of intranephronal proteinaceous cast formation by low molecular weight proteins. *Journal of Clinical Investigation* **85**, 570–576.

Sanders, P. W. *et al.* (1991). Spectrum of glomerular and tubulointerstitial renal lesions associated with monotypic immunoglobulin light chain deposition. *Laboratory Investigation* **64**, 527–537.

Scully, R. E. (1981). Case records of the Massachusetts General Hospital (case 1—1981). *New England Journal of Medicine* **304**, 33–43.

Sharland, A. *et al.* (1997). Hemodialysis: An appropriate therapy in myeloma-induced renal failure. *American Journal of Kidney Diseases* **30**, 786–792.

Short, I. A. and Smith, J. P. (1959). Myelomatosis associated with glycosuria and aminoaciduria. *Scottish Medical Journal* **4**, 89–93.

Short, A. K. *et al.* (2001). Recurrence of light chain nephropathy in a renal allograft. A case report and review of the literature. *American Journal of Nephrology* **21**, 237–240.

Smolens, P., Venkatachalam, M., and Stein, J. H. (1983). Myeloma kidney cast nephropathy in a rat model of multiple myeloma. *Kidney International* **24**, 192–204.

Smolens, P., Barnes, J. L., and Stein, J. H. (1986). Effect of chronic administration of different Bence Jones proteins on rat kidney. *Kidney International* **30**, 874–882.

Smolens, P., Barnes, J. L., and Kreisberg, R. (1987). Hypercalcemia can potentiate the nephrotoxicity of Bence Jones proteins. *Journal of Laboratory and Clinical Medicine* **110**, 460–465.

Solomon, A., Frangione, B., and Franklin, E. C. (1982). Bence Jones proteins and light chains of immunoglobulins: preferential association of the $V\lambda_{VI}$ subgroup of human light chains with amyloidosis AL (l). *Journal of Clinical Investigation* **70**, 453–460.

Solomon, A., Weiss, D. T., and Kattine A. A. (1991). Nephrotoxic potential of Bence Jones proteins. *New England Journal of Medicine* **324**, 1845–1851.

Spence, R. K. *et al.* (1979). Renal transplantation for end-stage myeloma kidney. Report of a patient with long-term survival. *Archives of Surgery* **114**, 950–952.

Stokes, M. B. *et al.* (2000). Expression of decorin, biglycan, and collagen type I in human renal fibrosing disease. *Kidney International* **57**, 487–498.

Thomas, D. B. L., Davies, M., and Williams, J. D. (1993a). Release of gelatinase and superoxide from human mononuclear phagocytes in response to particulate Tamm Horsfall protein. *American Journal of Pathology* **142**, 249–260.

Thomas, D. B. L. *et al.* (1993b). Tamm–Horsfall protein binds to a single class of carbohydrate specific receptors on human neutrophils. *Kidney International* **44**, 423–429.

Thorner, P. S., Bédard, Y. C., and Fernandes, B. J. (1983). λ-Light chain nephropathy with Fanconi syndrome. *Archives of Pathology and Laboratory Medicine* **107**, 654–657.

Touchard, G. *et al.* (1989). Nephrotic syndrome associated with chronic lymphocytic leukemia: an immunological and pathological study. *Clinical Nephrology* **31**, 107–116.

Tubbs, R. R. *et al.* (1981). Light chain nephropathy. *American Journal of Medicine* **71**, 263–269.

Tubbs, R. R. *et al.* (1992). Pseudo-γ heavy chain ($IgG_4\lambda$) deposition disease. *Modern Pathology* **5**, 185–190.

Uchida, S. *et al.* (1990). Adult Fanconi syndrome secondary to κ-light chain myeloma: improvement of tubular functions after treatment for myeloma. *Nephron* **55**, 332–335.

Verroust, P., Morel-Maroger, L., and Preud'homme, J. L. (1982). Renal lesions in dysproteinemias. *Springer Seminars in Immunopathology* **5**, 333–356.

Weiss, J. H. *et al.* (1981). Pathophysiology of acute Bence–Jones protein nephrotoxicity in the rat. *Kidney International* **20**, 198–210.

Winearls, C. G. (1995). Nephrology forum: acute myeloma kidney. *Kidney International* **48**, 1347–1361.

Ying, W. Z. and Sanders, P. W. (1998). Dietary salts regulate expression of Tamm-Horsfall glycoprotein in rats. *Kidney International* **54**, 1150–1156.

Ying, W. Z. and Sanders, P. W. (2001). Mapping the binding domain of immunoglobulin light chains for Tamm–Horsfall protein. *American Journal of Pathology* **158**, 1859–1866.

Zhu, L. *et al.* (1995). Pathogenesis of glomerulosclerosis in light chain deposition disease. Role of transforming growth factor-β. *American Journal of Pathology* **147**, 375–385.

Zucchelli, P. *et al.* (1988). Controlled plasma exchange trial in acute renal failure due to multiple myeloma. *Kidney International* **33**, 1175–1180.

4.4 The patient with sarcoidosis

Jean-Philippe Méry

Definition

Sarcoidosis is a chronic multisystem disorder characterized by the accumulation of non-caseating granulomas in multiple organs. It is more common in patients of African origin living in a Western environment, and usually presents under the age of 40 years. The sarcoid granuloma was first described by Schaumann (1933) and has since been studied extensively, particularly with regard to its structural and functional characteristics (Basset *et al.* 1988; Sheffield 1997; ATS/ERS/WASOG 1999). Typically, the florid granuloma is a rounded cellular collection composed of epithelioid and multinucleate giant cells surrounded by a rim of lymphocytes and macrophages in association with various degrees of fibrosis. Giant cells appear to result from the coalescence of epithelioid cells, both sharing the same ultrastructural characteristics, notably the presence of numerous cytoplasmic vesicles. Giant cells may contain inclusion bodies which are not specific. Lymphocytes are mainly T lymphocytes. While the central portion of the granuloma consists of predominantly $CD4^+$ lymphocytes, $CD8^+$ lymphocytes predominate in its peripheral rim. Unlike the situation in tuberculous granulomas, caseous necrosis is usually absent or restricted to small central areas of the granuloma. Despite advances made in understanding its pathogenesis, the cause of sarcoidosis remains unknown. The available evidence suggests a disordered cellular immune response to some yet unknown antigen(s). Recent studies have shed some light on the immunologic abnormalities found in patients with sarcoidosis (ATS/ERS/WASOG 1999; Agostini *et al.* 2000). The early sarcoid reaction is characterized by the accumulation of activated T-cells and macrophages at sites of ongoing inflammation. Activated T-helper lymphocytes release interleukin-2 and γ-interferon, and sarcoid macrophages release a great variety of cytokines and chemokines, most of them favouring granuloma formation (ATS/ERS/WASOG 1999).

Although any organ may be affected in sarcoidosis, pulmonary involvement being the most common, clinically important renal involvement is only an occasional problem in sarcoidosis (Newman *et al.* 1997). A spectrum of renal syndromes may be associated with sarcoidosis (Casella and Allon 1993; Göbel *et al.* 2001; Meyrier 2001) (Table 1). Renal involvement is most commonly due to disordered calcium metabolism. Granulomatous infiltration of the interstitium and, less frequently, a variety of glomerulopathies as well as granulomatous involvement of the renal vasculature and retroperitoneum may also be observed.

Table 1 A spectrum of renal syndromes associated with sarcoidosis

Consequences of abnormal calcium metabolism
Reduction in glomerular filtration rate
Impaired urinary concentration ability
Nephrocalcinosis
Nephrolithiasis
Granulomatous interstitial nephritis
Glomerulopathies
Membranous GN
Focal GN
IgA nephropathy
Diffuse endocapillary proliferative GN
Membranoproliferative GN
Crescentic GN
Miscellaneous
Amyloidosis
Retroperitoneal involvement
Granulomatous angiitis

GN, glomerulonephritis.

Renal consequences of abnormal calcium metabolism

Abnormal calcium metabolism resulting in hypercalcaemia and/or hypercalciuria is often present in sarcoidosis. Although the frequency of these calcium disorders cannot be assessed precisely, it is generally assumed that they account for renal impairment more frequently than does granulomatous interstitial nephritis. It is noteworthy that the two processes often coexist in the same patient. The reported incidence of *hypercalcaemia* in sarcoidosis varies from 10 to 63 per cent with an acceptable incidence of 11 per cent (Sharma 2000). The importance of hypercalciuria has been less thoroughly appreciated. Nevertheless, it seems three times more common than hypercalcaemia (Sharma 2000). The mechanism of hypercalcaemia in sarcoidosis is now well established. Early observations suggested that it was the consequence of an increase of calcium intestinal absorption. The occurrence in patients with sarcoidosis of low-dose vitamin D-induced episodes of hypercalcaemia or exacerbation of hypercalcaemia during the summer months suggested either an overproduction of or an hypersensitivity to vitamin D.

A major step in the understanding of the mechanisms of hypercalcaemia was taken when several groups demonstrated increased levels of serum $1{,}25(OH)_2D_3$ (calcitriol) in patients with active sarcoidosis

(Bell *et al.* 1979; Papapoulos *et al.* 1979; Zerwekh *et al.* 1980). While under normal physiological circumstances calcitriol is synthesized almost only by the kidney, Barbour *et al.* (1981) observed hypercalcaemia and increased serum calcitriol in an anephric patient with sarcoidosis, thus strongly arguing for an extrarenal source of the latter. A similar conclusion was reached by Maeseka *et al.* (1982) who found the same abnormalities in a patient with endstage renal disease. Adams *et al.* (1983) proved that the sarcoid granuloma was the site of the extrarenal calcitriol production. They demonstrated that alveolar macrophages of a patient with sarcoidosis were able to convert $25(OH)D_3$ to a calcitriol-like metabolite. The same was demonstrated by Mason *et al.* (1984) for a sarcoid lymph-node homogenate, whereas lymph nodes from normal controls failed to do so. Adams's group ultimately characterized this metabolite as calcitriol and demonstrated 1α-hydroxylation of vitamin D_3 by cultured alveolar macrophages from patients with sarcoidosis (Adams and Gacad 1985; Adams *et al.* 1985). Subcellular localization of macrophage 1α-hydroxylase is yet unknown; however, in an immortalized chick myelomonocytic cell line (HD-11) that constitutively expresses a $25(OH)D_3$–1α-hydroxylation, the enzyme activity has been shown to be localized in the mitochondrial fraction (Shany *et al.* 1993). Normally, the renal calcitriol synthesis (1α-hydroxylase activity) is regulated by changes of parathyroid hormone (PTH) and intracellular phosphate, as well as by the negative feedback of calcitriol on its own production. In contrast, extrarenal 1α-hydroxylase activity of sarcoid macrophages is not sensitive to changes in PTH and phosphate or calcitriol (Adams and Gacad 1985; Reichel *et al.* 1987; Adams *et al.* 1990a; Dusso *et al.* 1994). Nevertheless, Monkawa *et al.* (2000) showed that macrophage 1α-hydroxylase activity is mediated by the same enzyme as in the kidney. They also showed that γ-interferon increases macrophage 1α-hydroxylase levels by directly increasing gene expression of this enzyme. γ-Interferon seems also to play a role in the impairment of the calcitriol negative feedback (Dusso *et al.* 1997).

In active stages of the disease it seems likely that large amounts of calcitriol are released into the circulation with corresponding systemic consequences. It should be emphasized that macrophagic 1α-hydroxylase activity is not specific to sarcoid granulomas. Hypercalcaemia secondary to an extrarenal production of calcitriol has indeed been demonstrated in various other granulomatous diseases (Reichel *et al.* 1989). The mechanism of *hypercalciuria* in sarcoidosis appears to be threefold: (1) absorptive, associated with elevated serum calcitriol and abnormally high urinary calcium/creatinine ratio; (2) resorptive, associated with an extensive dissemination of sarcoidosis, including bones; and (3) associated with osteoclast activating factor (Meyrier *et al.* 1986; Sharma 2000).

The renal consequences of altered calcium metabolism comprise both functional and structural disorders. Reduction of the glomerular filtration rate, which often occurs in patients with sarcoidosis, is usually ascribed to the effects of hypercalcaemia on glomerular haemodynamics (see Chapter 2.3). Hypercalcaemia can also result in the impairment of urinary concentrating ability and in other tubular defects (see Chapter 2.3). It is uncertain whether hypercalciuria *per se* can induce tubular disorders; however, impaired urinary concentrating ability has been observed in some normocalcaemic hypercalciuric patients (Lebacq *et al.* 1970). Chronic hypercalcaemia and/or hypercalciuria may result in *nephrocalcinosis* and nephrolithiasis. Radiologically demonstrable nephrocalcinosis is rare in sarcoidosis, and is found in less than 5 per cent of cases (Freitag *et al.* 1997). Its true frequency is probably greater, particularly in patients with renal insufficiency (Coburn and Barbour 1984, p. 419). Calcium deposits in the glomeruli have been observed in three patients with sarcoidosis (Trillo *et al.* 1992). *Nephrolithiasis* occurs in about 10 per cent of sarcoid patients, and it may be responsible for obstructive nephropathy (Rodman and Mahler 2000). Occasionally, nephrolithiasis can be the presenting feature of sarcoidosis. In the prospective study made by Rizzato (2001) in 110 patients with histologically proven sarcoidosis, 3.6 per cent of cases presented with renal stones. Unlike the decrease of glomerular filtration rate and impairment of urinary concentrating ability, neither nephrocalcinosis nor nephrolithiasis regress after calcium metabolism returns to normal.

A low-calcium diet, adequate hydration, and minimization of exposure to ultraviolet light decrease the risk of hypercalcaemia. *Glucocorticoids* are the mainstay of therapy for hypercalcaemia when it occurs despite these preventive measures (ATS/ERS/WASOG 1999). Long before the pathogenesis of hypercalcaemia was clarified, their efficacy was taken as an argument supporting the hypothesis of increased intestinal calcium absorption. Glucocorticoids block extrarenal calcitriol synthesis by inhibiting macrophage 1α-hydroxylase activity and suppressing the immune activation of macrophages. They also diminish the effects of calcitriol on intestinal calcium absorption and bone resorption. Numerous studies using different glucocorticoids have been reported, all showing efficacy at relatively low doses. For example, Barbour *et al.* (1981) used prednisone at an initial daily dosage of 40 mg, which was tapered to 20 mg on alternate days 4 months later. Prednisone was also used successfully by Maesaka *et al.* (1982) at a lower dosage of 10 mg on alternate days. Nordal *et al.* (1985) used prednisolone at an initial daily dosage of 35 mg. The results of these studies suggest that glucocorticoids have a rapid effect, with a return to normal of both serum calcium and renal function within a few days. Following glucocorticoid therapy, serum calcium rapidly decreases, usually in parallel with a decrease of serum calcitriol whereas serum $25(OH)D_3$ remains normal; urinary calcium excretion decreases while faecal calcium excretion increases. However, increased urinary calcium may persist in some patients; this can be explained either by persistent bone resorption, on which glucocorticoids would be ineffective, or by secondary calcium mobilization from other body stores. The whole duration of treatment cannot be standardized; the decision for withdrawal of the drug is dependent upon the response of serum and urinary calcium levels following progressive tapering of dosage.

4-Aminoquinoline derivatives (chloroquine and hydroxychloroquine), and more recently ketoconazole, have been proposed as alternative treatments, particularly in cases of intolerance or contraindications to glucocorticoids. Hunt and Yendt (1963) had noticed that chloroquine successfully reduced both hypercalcaemia and disease activity in a patient with sarcoidosis. Long-term chloroquine therapy (500 mg/day) was followed by a return of blood and urinary calcium to normal, together with a decrease of calcitriol, in two patients with hypercalcaemia and hypercalciuria who were intolerant to glucocorticoids (O'Leary *et al.* 1986). Barré *et al.* (1987) described a patient with endstage renal failure who had experienced two renal transplant rejections. She had received haemodialysis for 4 years thereafter, when hypercalcaemia developed and sarcoidosis was diagnosed. Because of previous side-effects of glucocorticoid therapy, the patient was given hydroxychloroquine (500 mg/day). Serum calcium and calcitriol returned to normal within 24 weeks of treatment. Short-course chloroquine therapy also proved to be efficient. Three days of treatment was sufficient to decrease serum calcitriol in a patient described by Adams *et al.* (1989). The mechanism by which 4-aminoquinoline derivatives are effective in calcium disorders of sarcoidosis is unknown. The finding of a decrease of serum calcitriol while $25(OH)D_3$ remains normal, as in patients treated by glucocorticoids, similarly suggests an inhibition of the conversion of $25(OH)D_3$ to calcitriol. Indeed, Reichel *et al.* (1987) showed that chloroquine produces a dose-dependent inhibition of the $25(OH)D_3$ hydroxylation by cultured pulmonary alveolar macrophages from patients with sarcoidosis. The precise mechanism(s) by which chloroquine inhibits macrophage calcitriol synthesis is unknown. Barré *et al.* (1987) suggested that hydroxychloroquine inhibits the calcitriol-induced coalescence of mononuclear cells which results in the formation of multinucleate giant cells. This could impair granuloma formation and subsequently calcitriol-induced osteoclastic osteolysis. Thus, it could account for the successful result achieved by chloroquine in the patient described by Hunt and Yendt (1963) and in one of the patients described by O'Leary *et al.* (1986) in whom bone resorption was assumed to be responsible for persistent hypercalciuria.

The antifungal drug *ketoconazole*, a cytochrome P-450 inhibitor, has been shown to inhibit the production of several steroid hormones including calcitriol. Both renal and extrarenal production of calcitriol are inhibited. Inhibition of renal production of calcitriol has been demonstrated both *in vitro* (Henry 1985) and *in vivo* (Glass and Eil 1986, 1988). Ketoconazole has also been shown to lower serum calcitriol in hypercalcaemic patients with sarcoidosis (Adams *et al.* 1990b; Glass *et al.* 1990; Bia and Insogna 1991). It seems to act directly on 1α-hydroxylase, which is P-450 cytochrome-dependent, and not indirectly by reducing the serum calcium concentration. Indeed, in contrast with the sharp reduction in serum calcitriol concentration, the serum calcium concentration only decreases slightly or remains normal during ketoconazole administration in patients with sarcoidosis. However, the exact mechanism by which ketoconazole inhibits oxidative enzyme activity is not yet known. The rapid decrease in serum calcitriol appears to be dose-dependent. Oral ketoconazole (800 mg/day) decreased the serum calcitriol concentration by 73 per cent within 4 days in the patient described by Adams *et al.* (1990b). These authors have also shown that *in vitro* ketoconazole has a rapid-onset, concentration-dependent inhibitory effect on calcitriol synthesis by pulmonary alveolar macrophages from two hypercalcaemic patients with sarcoidosis. The two patients treated by Glass *et al.* (1990) and the single patient treated by Adams *et al.* (1990b) received ketoconazole for a short period (4, 6, and 9 days, respectively). The patient of Bia and Insogna (1991) is still the only reported patient who received ketoconazole for a prolonged period (800 mg/day for 2 years); the only side-effect was a slight decrease in serum testosterone accompanied by some decrease in libido. Although nephrotoxicity of ketoconazole has not been described, Glass *et al.* (1990) observed a deterioration of renal function during a short period of ketoconazole administration (4 and 6 days, respectively) in their two patients.

The efficacy of other modes of therapy is not conclusive. The use of various *calcium-binding agents* (inositol hexophosphate, cellulose phosphate, and orthophosphate) has led to conflicting results; moreover, it is frequently followed by serious intestinal side-effects.

In summary, glucocorticoids which offer constant and rapid efficacy remain the drugs of first choice. Chloroquine or hydroxychloroquine may be alternative choices in cases of intolerance or contraindications to glucocorticoids. They may be particularly efficient in those patients in whom abnormal calcium metabolism is presumed to be mostly the consequence of bone resorption. To date, too few patients have been treated with ketoconazole to allow any conclusions to be drawn on its indication in the treatment of sarcoid hypercalcaemia.

Granulomatous interstitial nephritis

The exact prevalence of granulomatous interstitial nephritis in sarcoidosis is ill defined; differing estimates have been reported from necropsy and biopsy series. It was found in 7 and 13 per cent of cases in the necropsy series of Longcope and Freiman (1952) and Branson and Park (1954), respectively. However, recent reviews of biopsy series from the literature showed a mean prevalence of 34 per cent (Romer 1980), with values ranging from 15 to 40 per cent (Muther *et al.* 1981). These discrepancies may reflect different attitudes among nephrologists to the requirement for renal biopsy in patients with sarcoidosis. Moreover, since granulomatous infiltration of the interstitium may be clinically silent and scarce granulomas absent in small biopsy specimens, the true frequency of granulomatous interstitial nephritis is likely to be underestimated.

Detailed descriptions of the pathology of sarcoid granulomatous interstitial nephritis have been made by Berger and Relman (1955) and MacDonald Cameron (1956). The extent of the granulomatous infiltration varies widely between cases. In some instances, granulomas are rare in the biopsy specimen while in others they are numerous and widespread throughout the interstitium both in the cortex and the medulla. They have the general appearance of sarcoid granulomas as described above (Fig. 1). Some granulomas may have small arteries at their centre (Bottcher 1959; Turner *et al.* 1977; Michielsen *et al.* 1985). Various degrees of fibrosis, which may result in tubular atrophy and degeneration, may be associated with cellular interstitial infiltration. Glomeruli appear normal or show only slight mesangial hypertrophy and thickening of the basement membrane. Electron microscopy has occasionally shown fusion of epithelial foot processes (Falls *et al.* 1972; Farge *et al.* 1986). No significant immune deposits in either glomeruli or tubules have been shown by immunofluorescence microscopy, except for the case described by Cuppage *et al.* (1988) in which IgA and IgG were found within the cytoplasm of some interstitial cells. Cells infiltrating the interstitium in two patients with sarcoidosis were characterized with monoclonal antibodies by Cheng *et al.* (1989). They comprised a significant number of B-cells, plasma cells, and T-cells,

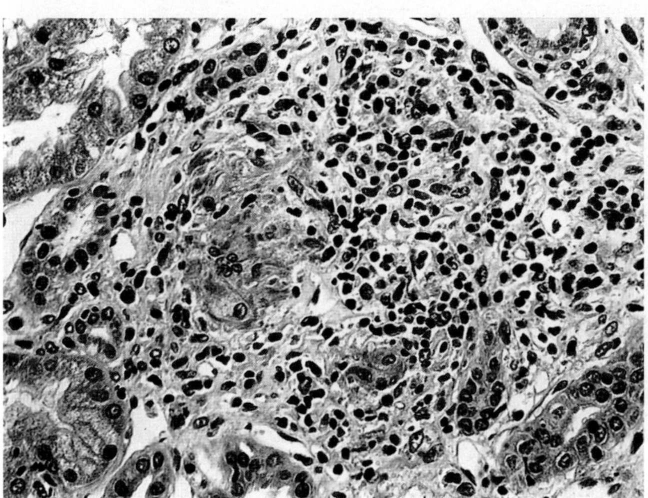

Fig. 1 Renal biopsy. Interstitial granuloma. Note the presence of lymphocytes, histiocytes, a few polymorphonuclear leucocytes, and foci of epithelioid cells. (Masson's trichrome; magnification, 900×.) (Courtesy of Dr Béatrice Mougenot.) (Reproduced with permission from Méry and Kenouch 1988.)

with a predominance of T-helper lymphocytes. Eosinophils were also seen. These workers also found an increased tubular display of HLA DR compared with controls, and suggested that this could result in the activation of T-helper lymphocytes and propagation of the immune local reaction. Immunofluorescence with an anti-angiotensin-converting enzyme (anti-ACE) serum has been performed in two renal biopsies (Méry and Kenouch 1988, p. 71; Ito *et al.* 1994). In both cases ACE was localized in granulomas in addition to the normal staining of the brush border of the proximal tubules (Fig. 2). Pertschuk *et al.* (1981), using an anti-ACE serum to study sarcoid and non-sarcoid granulomas of tissues other than the kidney, found that positive staining was obtained only in sarcoid granulomas. However, Grönhagen-Riska *et al.* (1988) found positive staining with anti-ACE serum in other diseases: both histiocytes of a pleural rheumatoid nodule and macrophages of a renal transplant (during an acute rejection reaction) stained positively.

Sarcoid infiltration of the kidney presents as renal failure in most cases. Indeed, in a review of 59 cases in the literature, Méry and Kenouch (1988, p. 73) found only three patients whose renal function was normal; among the others, serum creatinine was greater than 800 μmol/l in 12 (20 per cent). Since, as discussed above, hypercalcaemia results from an increased production of calcitriol by granulomas, it is frequently observed in association with granulomatous interstitial nephritis and may contribute to the renal insufficiency. Decline of renal function usually progresses slowly over weeks or months and can reach endstage renal disease in some patients (Coutant *et al.* 1999; Tsiouris *et al.* 1999). Occasionally, some patients may present with acute renal failure (Korzets *et al.* 1985; Michielsen *et al.* 1985; Tanneau *et al.* 1987; Cuppage *et al.* 1988; Warren *et al.* 1988; Berner *et al.* 1999; O'Riordan *et al.* 2001). Proteinuria is either absent or mild, with a tubular pattern on electrophoresis. Leucocytes and granular casts are often present in the urine. Mills *et al.* (1994) described a patient in whom sarcoid interstitial nephritis presented as a frank haematuria which lasted several weeks. Tubular abnormalities are found in about 50 per cent of cases investigated (Muther *et al.* 1981; Méry and Kenouch 1988, p. 74). Orthoglycaemic glycosuria, urinary wasting of potassium or sodium, Fanconi syndrome, decreased urinary concentrating ability or overt nephrogenic diabetes insipidus, and proximal or distal tubular acidosis have all been described. It is uncertain whether the presence of interstitial lesions is the only factor responsible for the tubular abnormalities, and both hypercalcaemia and hypergammaglobulinaemia may also play a pathogenetic role. Hypertension, which is usually absent early in the course of the nephropathy, often occurs later, secondary to progressive sclerosis of the parenchyma and may be related to long-term corticotherapy.

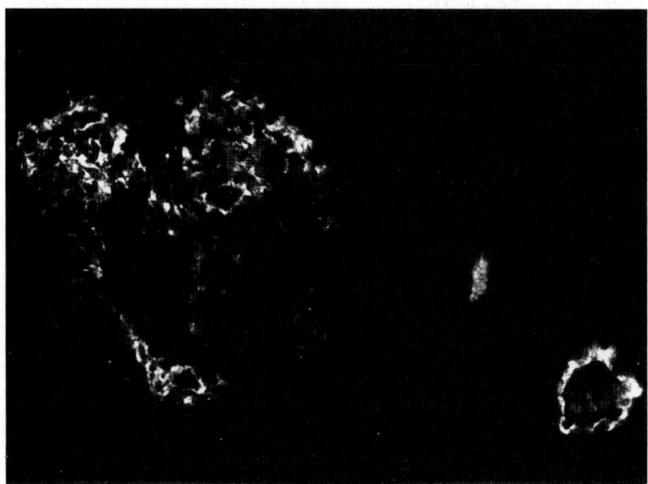

Fig. 2 Renal biopsy. Immunofluorescence with anti-ACE serum. Top left: bright staining of epithelioid cells of an interstitial granuloma. Bottom right: normal staining of epithelial cells of proximal convoluted tubule. (Masson's trichrome; magnification, 900×.) (Courtesy of Dr Béatrice Mougenot; the antiserum was kindly provided by Dr François Alhenc-Gélas.) (Reproduced with permission from Méry and Kenouch 1988.)

Granulomatous infiltration of the kidney often results in enlarged kidneys which may even mimic polycystic kidney disease (Coburn *et al.* 1967; Guédon *et al.* 1967) or renal carcinoma (Leng-Lévy *et al.* 1965; Amouroux *et al.* 1967; Rohatgi *et al.* 1990; Schillinger *et al.* 1999). In such cases, abdominal sonogram and computed tomographic study have demonstrated bilateral masses which were either hyper- or hypoechoic in comparison to the adjacent renal parenchyma and of low density on computed tomography (Herman *et al.* 1997; Alkilic-Genauzeau *et al.* 1999). A ^{67}Ga citrate scan may show an uptake of the tracer by the kidneys but it can also be negative in active granulomatous interstitial nephritis (Méry and Kenouch 1988, p. 73). Moreover, it appears of little value in the assessment of evolution under treatment (Pagniez *et al.* 1987). The same reservations apply to serum ACE concentration; indeed, it has been found to be normal in cases of active granulomatous interstitial nephritis with severe renal failure (Farge *et al.* 1986; Singer and Evans 1986; Pagniez *et al.* 1987; Hannedouche *et al.* 1990).

In most cases, the association of granulomatous interstitial nephritis with extrarenal manifestations and/or hypercalcaemia makes the diagnosis of sarcoidosis easy. In some patients, however, renal involvement is isolated, preceding other localizations of the disease for several months or years (Guédon *et al.* 1967; Ford *et al.* 1978; Nédelec *et al.* 1986; Utas *et al.* 1999; Göbel *et al.* 2001). It is possible that some cases published as isolated granulomatous interstitial nephritis are in fact localized forms of sarcoidosis (Bolton *et al.* 1976; Barbiano di Belgioioso 1980; Caruana *et al.* 1982). In such circumstances, it is important to rule out drug-induced interstitial nephritis which are more frequent than interstitial nephritis due to sarcoidosis. The relation between sarcoidosis and the 'TINU' syndrome described by Dobrin *et al.* (1975) must be remembered; it is characterized by an association of acute interstitial nephritis, anterior uveitis, and epithelioid granulomas in bone marrow and lymph nodes. The renal lesion consists of an interstitial infiltrate mainly composed of mononuclear cells with a few eosinophils. Although no 'mature' interstitial granulomas are found in Dobrin syndrome, the cellular composition of the interstitial infiltrate does not differ from that observed in sarcoidosis and in some cases the cellular arrangement almost outlines a granuloma. Therefore, it is possible that some cases described as Dobrin syndrome could in fact be atypical forms of sarcoidosis (Kenouch *et al.* 1989).

It is generally agreed that sarcoid granulomatous interstitial nephritis should be treated with *glucocorticoids*. To be effective, initial treatment usually requires a daily dosage of prednisone or prednisolone of 1–1.5 mg/kg body weight. Following initiation of corticosteroid therapy, renal function can improve dramatically. For example, it was possible to discontinue peritoneal dialysis after 15 days of prednisolone therapy in the patient described by Singer and Evans (1986) who had initially a severe renal failure. Renal tubular disorders regress concurrently with improvement of renal function. It is most important to recognize the necessity for prolonged glucocorticoid treatment. Indeed, treatment of less than 6 months duration is frequently followed by a relapse of the nephropathy (Guénel and Chevet 1988). In our opinion, the initial dose should be progressively tapered after 2 months and then switched to an alternate-day regimen. Treatment should be maintained for at least 1 year. Serial renal biopsies usually show regression of granulomas in parallel with the improvement of renal function (Farge *et al.* 1986; Méry and Kenouch 1988, p. 75). However, such a parallel course is not always seen (Guénel and Chevet 1988). Interstitial fibrosis often develops in association with focal glomerulosclerosis and vascular lesions; the latter, which are ascribed to long-term corticotherapy, may be responsible for the delayed occurrence of hypertension which in turn may contribute to the progression of renal failure. Successful *renal transplantation* has been carried out in patients with sarcoidosis (Padilla *et al.* 1997). Recurrence of sarcoid granulomatous nephritis in the transplant has been reported (Shen *et al.* 1986; Brown *et al.* 1992). Motte *et al.* (2001) reported on a case of granulomatous interstitial nephritis occurring 4 years after a lung transplantation for endstage pulmonary sarcoidosis. At the time of transplantation, there was no extrarenal localization of sarcoidosis.

Glomerular involvement

Glomerular involvement is not common in sarcoidosis although about 50 cases of glomerular lesions associated with pulmonary sarcoidosis have been reported. Various types of glomerulonephritis have been observed: membranous (Jones and Fowler 1989; Oliver Rotellar *et al.* 1990; Khan *et al.* 1994; Dimitriades *et al.* 1999; Göbel *et al.* 2001), focal and segmental (Hakaim *et al.* 1992; Peces *et al.* 1993; Veronese *et al.* 1998), IgA nephropathy (Vanhille *et al.* 1986; Murray *et al.* 1987; Chung-Park *et al.* 1990; Anwar and Gokal 1993; Taylor and Ansell 1996; Nishiki *et al.* 1999), diffuse endocapillary proliferative (Michaels *et al.* 2000), membranoproliferative (Molle *et al.* 1986), and crescentic glomerulonephritis (Shintaku *et al.* 1989; Auinger *et al.* 1997; Van Umm *et al.* 1997). The mechanism by which glomerular injury occurs in sarcoidosis is not known, nor is a causal relationship to sarcoidosis proved and some cases may be coincidental. However, it is likely that abnormalities of both the humoral and the cellular immune system present in patients with sarcoidosis predispose to the development of immune complex-type glomerulonephritis.

Membranous glomerulonephritis seems particularly frequent. Among the 39 cases of glomerular lesions reviewed by Vanhille *et al.* (1986), there were 13 cases of membranous glomerulonephritis, which in most cases occurred late in the course of an overt sarcoidosis. Beneficial effects of high-dose prednisone therapy have been reported in a few patients (Jones and Fowler 1989; Oliver Rotellar *et al.* 1990; Khan *et al.* 1994). A recent experimental study sheds light on a possible mechanism of membranous glomerulonephritis associated with sarcoidosis. Maruyama *et al.* (1999) induced subepithelial deposits in pigs injected with heterologous antibody to ACE. Confocal microscopy clearly identified colocalization of granular deposits of ACE and anti-ACE goat IgG on the outer aspect of the glomerular basement membrane. It is possible that a similar autoimmune process may operate in membranous glomerulonephritis associated with sarcoidosis.

The nephrotic syndrome associated with *minimal-change disease* has been reported in two patients, one by Mündlein *et al.* (1996) and the other by Parry and Falk (1997). We have observed a 31-year-old Black woman with sarcoidosis of 6 years duration who developed massive proteinuria (6 g/day) together with a relapse of the disease. While she was undergoing evaluation, proteinuria disappeared. A renal biopsy showed normal glomeruli by both light and immunofluorescence microscopy; electron microscopy was not performed. Two weeks later, she had a transient recurrence of massive proteinuria (10 g/day), which again spontaneously disappeared after a few days. Corticosteroid therapy was started because of pulmonary involvement. Four months later, at her latest evaluation, proteinuria had not recurred. Such a case could be explained by a functional and transient increase of glomerular permeability to proteins secondary to the release of some lymphokines by activated immune cells.

Miscellaneous

A few cases of renal amyloidosis associated with sarcoidosis have been reported (Rainfray *et al.* 1988; Tchénio *et al.* 1996). It was proved to be AA amyloidosis in the only case of Tchénio *et al.* A few cases of obstructive uropathy secondary to retroperitoneal involvement with resolution of ureteral compression with corticosteroid therapy have been reported (Castrignano *et al.* 1988; Tamella *et al.* 1989; Miyazaki *et al.* 1996). Godin *et al.* (1980) described a patient with sarcoidosis in whom hypertension developed. Aortography showed extensive stenosis of the right renal artery. Surgical exploration disclosed extensive periaortic and perirenal fibrosis which caused extrinsic compression of the right renal artery. In addition, pathological examination disclosed an epithelioid infiltration in the adventitia of the renal artery, suggestive of sarcoid angiitis. Widespread giant cell vasculitis affecting renal arteries, arterioles, and veins was found in association with interstitial sarcoid granulomas in the patient described by Marcussen and Lund (1989). A case of granulomatous inflammation involving small renal vessels was reported by Shintaku *et al.* (1989), and association of microscopic polyangiitis and sarcoidosis was reported in two patients (Kwong *et al.* 1994; Watson *et al.* 1996).

References

Adams, J. S. and Gacad, M. A. (1985). Characterization of 1α-hydroxylation of vitamin D_3 sterols by cultured alveolar macrophages from patients with sarcoidosis. *Journal of Experimental Medicine* **161**, 755–765.

Adams, J. S. *et al.* (1983). Metabolism of 25-hydroxyvitamin D_3 by cultured pulmonary alveolar macrophages in sarcoidosis. *Journal of Clinical Investigation* **72**, 1856–1860.

Adams, J. S. *et al.* (1985). Isolation and structural identification of 1,25-dihydroxyvitamin D_3 produced by cultured alveolar macrophages in sarcoidosis. *Journal of Clinical Endocrinology and Metabolism* **60**, 960–966.

Adams, J. S., Diz, M. M., and Sharma, O. P. (1989). Effective reduction in the serum 1,25-dihydroxyvitamin D and calcium concentration in sarcoidosis-associated hypercalcemia with short-course chloroquine therapy. *Annals of Internal Medicine* **111**, 437–438.

Adams, J. S. *et al.* (1990a). A role for endogenous arachidonate metabolites in the regulated expression of the 25-hydroxyvitamin D-1-hydroxylation reaction in cultured alveolar macrophages from patients with sarcoidosis. *Journal of Clinical Endocrinology and Metabolism* **70**, 595–600.

Adams, J. S. *et al.* (1990b). Ketoconazole decreases the serum 1,25-dihydroxyvitamin D and calcium concentration in sarcoidosis-associated hypercalcemia. *Journal of Clinical Endocrinology and Metabolism* **70**, 1090–1095.

Agostini, C., Adami, F., and Semenzato, G. (2000). New pathogenetics insights into the sarcoid granuloma. *Current Opinion in Rheumatology* **12**, 71–76.

Alkilic-Genauzeau, I. *et al.* (1999). Radiological diagnosis of renal sarcoidosis. *Journal of Radiology* **80**, 1672–1675.

Amouroux, J. *et al.* (1967). Sarcoïdose pseudo-tumorale du rein. *Archives d'Anatomie Pathologique* **15**, A301–A303.

Anwar, N. and Gokal, R. (1993). Simultaneous occurrence of IgA nephropathy and sarcoidosis in the context of pre-existent minimal change nephrotic syndrome. *Nephron* **65**, 310–312.

ATS/ERS/WASOG (1999). Statement on sarcoidosis. *Sarcoidosis, Vasculitis and Diffuse Lung Diseases* **16**, 149–173.

Auinger, M. *et al.* (1997). Normocalcaemic hepatorenal sarcoidosis with crescentic glomerulonephritis. *Nephrology, Dialysis, Transplantation* **12**, 1474–1477.

Barbiano di Belgioioso, G. Granulomatous interstitial nephritis as a possible isolated manifestation of sarcoidosis: report of a case. In *Abstracts of the 17th Congress of European Dialysis and Transplantation Association*, p. 27, 1980.

Barbour, G. L. *et al.* (1981). Hypercalcemia in an anephric patient with sarcoidosis: evidence for extra-renal generation of 1,25-dihydroxyvitamin D. *New England Journal of Medicine* **305**, 440–443.

Barré, P. E. *et al.* (1987). Hydroxychloroquine treatment of hypercalcemia in a patient with sarcoidosis undergoing hemodialysis. *American Journal of Medicine* **82**, 1259–1262.

Basset, F., Soler, P., and Hance, A. J. Sarcoidosis—from granuloma formation to fibrosis. In *Sarcoidosis and Other Granulomatous Disorders* (ed. C. Grassi, G. Rizzato, and E. Pozzi), pp. 235–246. Amsterdam: Elsevier, 1988.

Bell, N. H. *et al.* (1979). Evidence that increased circulating 1α,25-dihydroxyvitamin D is the probable cause for abnormal calcium metabolism in sarcoidosis. *Journal of Clinical Investigation* **64**, 218–225.

Berger, K. W. and Relman, A. S. (1955). Renal impairment due to sarcoid infiltration of the kidney. Report of a case proved by renal biopsies before and after treatment with cortisone. *New England Journal of Medicine* **252**, 44–49.

Berner, B. *et al.* (1999). Rasch-progrediente Niereninsuffizienz als Primärmanifestation einer systematischen Sarkoidose. *Medizinische Klinik* **94**, 690–694.

Bia, M. J. and Insogna, K. (1991). Treatment of sarcoidosis-associated hypercalcemia with ketoconazole. *American Journal of Kidney Diseases* **18**, 702–705.

Bolton, W. K. *et al.* (1976). Reversible renal failure from isolated granulomatous renal sarcoidosis. *Clinical Nephrology* **5**, 88–92.

Bottcher, E. (1959). Disseminated sarcoidosis with a marked granulomatous arteritis. *Archives of Pathology* **68**, 419–423.

Branson, J. H. and Park, J. H. (1954). Sarcoidosis hepatic involvement: presentation of case with fatal liver involvement, including autopsy findings and review of evidence for sarcoid involvement of liver as found in literature. *Annals of Internal Medicine* **40**, 111–114.

Brown, J. H. *et al.* (1992). Sarcoid-like granulomata in a renal transplant. *Nephrology, Dialysis, Transplantation* **7**, 173.

Caruana, R. J., Carr, A. A., and Rao, R. N. (1982). Idiopathic granulomatous nephritis in a patient with hypertension and an atrophic kidney. *Nephron* **32**, 83–86.

Casella, F. J. and Allon, M. (1993). The kidney in sarcoidosis. *Journal of the American Society of Nephrology* **3**, 1555–1562.

Castrignano, L. *et al.* Retroperitoneal involvement in sarcoidosis. In *Sarcoidosis and Other Granulomatous Disorders* (ed. C. Grassi, G. Rizzato, and E. Pozzi), pp. 383–384. Amsterdam: Elsevier, 1988.

Cheng, H. F. *et al.* (1989). HLA DR display by renal tubular epithelium and phenotype of infiltrate in interstitial nephritis. *Nephrology, Dialysis, Transplantation* **4**, 205–215.

Chung-Park, M., Lam, M., and Yazdy, A. M. (1990). IgA nephropathy associated with sarcoidosis. *American Journal of Kidney Diseases* **15**, 601–602.

Coburn, J. W. and Barbour, G. L. Vitamin D intoxication and sarcoidosis. In *Hypercalciuric States. Pathogenesis, Consequences and Treatment* (ed. F. L. Coe), pp. 379–433. Orlando: Grune and Stratton, 1984.

Coburn, J. W. *et al.* (1967). Granulomatous sarcoid nephritis. *American Journal of Medicine* **42**, 273–283.

Coutant, R. *et al.* (1999). Renal granulomatous sarcoidosis in childhood: a report of 11 cases and a review of the literature. *European Journal of Pediatrics* **158**, 154–159.

Cuppage, F. E., Emmott, D. F., and Duncan, K. A. (1988). Renal failure secondary to sarcoidosis. *American Journal of Kidney Diseases* **11**, 519–520.

Dimitriades, C. *et al.* (1999). Membranous nephropathy associated with childhood sarcoidosis. *Pediatric Nephrology* **13**, 444–447.

Dobrin, R. S., Vernier, R. L., and Fish, A. J. (1975). Acute eosinophilic interstitial nephritis and renal failure with bone marrow-lymph node granulomas and anterior uveitis. A new syndrome. *American Journal of Medicine* **59**, 325–333.

Dusso, A., Brown, A., and Slatopolsky, E. (1994). Extrarenal production of calcitriol. *Seminars in Nephrology* **14**, 144–155.

Dusso, A. S. *et al.* (1997). γ-Interferon-induced resistance to 1,25-$(OH)_2D_3$ in human monocytes and macrophages: a mechanism for the hypercalcemia of various granulomatoses. *Journal of Clinical Endocrinology and Metabolism* **82**, 2222–2232.

Falls, W. F. *et al.* (1972). Nonhypercalcemic sarcoid nephropathy. *Archives of Internal Medicine* **130**, 285–291.

Farge, D. *et al.* (1986). Granulomatous nephritis and chronic renal failure in sarcoidosis. Long-term follow-up studies in two patients. *American Journal of Nephrology* **6**, 22–27.

Ford, M. J., Anderton, J. L., and MacLean, N. (1978). Granulomatous sarcoid nephropathy. *Postgraduate Medical Journal* **54**, 416–417.

Freitag, J. *et al.* (1997). Consider sarcoidosis in patients with nephrocalcinosis, even if the chest roentgenogram is normal. *Nephrology, Dialysis, Transplantation* **12**, 2151–2155.

Glass, A. R. and Eil, C. (1986). Ketoconazole-induced reduction in serum 1,25-dihydroxyvitamin D. *Journal of Clinical Endocrinology and Metabolism* **63**, 766–769.

Glass, A. R. and Eil, C. (1988). Ketoconazole-induced reduction in serum 1,25-dihydroxyvitamin D and total serum calcium in hypercalcemic patients. *Journal of Clinical Endocrinology and Metabolism* **66**, 934–938.

Glass, A. R. *et al.* (1990). Ketoconazole reduces elevated serum levels of 1,25-dihydroxyvitamin D in hypercalcemic sarcoidosis. *Journal of Endocrinological Investigation* **13**, 407–413.

Göbel, U. *et al.* (2001). The protean face of renal sarcoidosis. *Journal of the American Society of Nephrology* **12**, 616–623.

Godin, M. *et al.* (1980). Sarcoidosis. Retroperitoneal fibrosis, renal arterial involvement, and unilateral focal glomerulosclerosis. *Archives of Internal Medicine* **140**, 1240–1242.

Grönhagen-Riska, C. *et al.* ACE in physiologic and pathologic conditions. In *Sarcoidosis and Other Granulomatous Disorders* (ed. C. Grassi, G. Rizzato, and E. Pozzi), pp. 203–211. Amsterdam: Elsevier, 1988.

Guédon, J. *et al.* (1967). Sarcoïdose rénale à forme pseudo-tumorale révélatrice de l'affection. *Presse Médicale* **75**, 265–268.

Guénel, J. and Chevet, D. (1988). Néphropathies interstitielles de la sarcoïdose. Effet de la corticothérapie et évolution à long terme. Etude rétrospective de 22 observations. *Néphrologie* **9**, 253–257.

Hakaim, A. G. *et al.* (1992). Successful renal transplantation in a patient with systemic sarcoidosis and renal failure due to focal glomerulosclerosis. *American Journal of Kidney Diseases* **19**, 493–495.

Hannedouche, T. *et al.* (1990). Renal granulomatous sarcoidosis: report of six cases. *Nephrology, Dialysis, Transplantation* **5**, 18–24.

Henry, H. L. (1985). Effect of ketoconazole and miconazole on 25-hydroxyvitamin D3 metabolism by cultured chick kidney cells. *Journal of Steroid Biochemistry* **23**, 991–994.

Herman, T. E., Shackelford, G. D., and McAlister, W. H. (1997). Pseudotumoral sarcoid granulomatous nephritis in a child: case presentation with sonographic and CT findings. *Pediatric Radiology* **27**, 752–754.

Hunt, B. J. and Yendt, E. R. (1963). The response of hypercalcemia in sarcoidosis to chloroquine. *Annals of Internal Medicine* **59**, 554–565.

Ito, Y. *et al.* (1994). A case of renal sarcoidosis showing central necrosis and abnormal expression of angiotensin converting enzyme in the granuloma. *Clinical Nephrology* **42**, 331–336.

Jones, B. and Fowler, J. (1989). Membranous nephropathy associated with sarcoidosis. Response to prednisone. *Nephron* **52**, 101–102.

Kenouch, S. *et al.* (1989). Un nouveau syndrome: les néphropathies interstitielles aiguës avec uvéite. *Annales de Médecine Interne* **140**, 169–172.

Khan, I. H. *et al.* (1994). Membranous nephropathy and granulomatous interstitial nephritis in sarcoidosis. *Nephron* **66**, 459–461.

Korzets, Z. *et al.* (1985). Acute renal failure due to sarcoid granulomatous infiltration of the renal parenchyma. *American Journal of Kidney Diseases* **6**, 250–253.

Kwong, T. *et al.* (1994). Systemic necrotizing vasculitis associated with childhood sarcoidosis. *Seminars in Arthritis and Rheumatism* **23**, 388–395.

Lebacq, E., Desmet, V., and Venhaegen, H. (1970). Renal involvement in sarcoidosis. *Postgraduate Medical Journal* **46**, 526–529.

Leng-Lévy, J. *et al.* (1965). Maladie de Besnier–Boeck–Schaumann à localisation rénale. *Bulletins et Mémoires de la Société Médicale des Hôpitaux de Paris* **116**, 907–911.

Longcope, W. T. and Freiman, D. G. (1952). A study of sarcoidosis based on combined investigation of 160 cases including 30 autopsies from Johns Hopkins Hospital and Massachusetts General Hospital. *Medicine* **31**, 132–140.

MacDonald Cameron, H. (1956). Renal sarcoidosis. *Journal of Clinical Pathology* **9**, 136–141.

Maesaka, J. K. *et al.* (1982). Elevated 1,25-dihydroxyvitamin D levels in a patient with sarcoidosis and end-stage renal disease. *Archives of Internal Medicine* **142**, 1206–1207.

Marcussen, N. and Lund, C. (1989). Combined sarcoidosis and disseminated visceral giant cell vasculitis. *Pathology Research and Practice* **184**, 325–330.

Maruyama, S. *et al.* (1999). Membranous glomerulonephritis induced in the pig by antibody to angiotensin-converting enzyme: considerations on its relevance to the pathogenesis of human idiopathic membranous glomerulonephritis. *Journal of the American Society of Nephrology* **10**, 2102–2108.

Mason, R. S. *et al.* (1984). Vitamin D conversion by sarcoid lymph node homogenate. *Annals of Internal Medicine* **100**, 59–61.

Méry, J. Ph. and Kenouch, S. Les atteintes de l'interstitium rénal au cours des maladies systémiques. In *Séminaires d'uro-néphrologie Pitié-Salpêtrière* (ed. C. Chatelain and C. Jacobs), pp. 57–89. Paris: Masson, 1988.

Meyrier, A. (2001). Sarcoidosis: the nephrologist's view. *Annales de Médecine Interne* **152**, 45–50.

Meyrier, A. *et al.* (1986). Different mechanisms of hypercalciuria in sarcoidosis. *Annals of the New York Academy of Sciences* **465**, 575–586.

Michaels, S. *et al.* (2000). Renal sarcoidosis with superimposed postinfectious glomerulonephritis presenting as acute renal failure. *American Journal of Kidney Diseases* **36**, E4.

Michielsen, P. *et al.* (1985). Insuffisance rénale aiguë: première manifestation d'une sarcoïdose familiale. *Néphrologie* **6**, 151–152.

Mills, P. R. *et al.* (1994). Granulomatous sarcoid nephritis presenting as frank hematuria. *Nephrology, Dialysis, Transplantation* **9**, 1649–1651.

Miyazaki, E. *et al.* (1996). Sarcoidosis presenting as bilateral hydronephrosis. *Internal Medicine* **35**, 579–582.

Molle, D. *et al.* (1986). Membranoproliferative glomerulonephritis associated with pulmonary sarcoidosis. *American Journal of Nephrology* **6**, 386–387.

Monkawa, T. *et al.* (2000). Identification of 25-hydroxyvitamin D_3 1α-hydroxylase gene expression in macrophages. *Kidney International* **58**, 559–568.

Motte, G. *et al.* (2001). Renal involvement after lung transplantation for sarcoidosis. *Clinical Nephrology* **56**, 411–412.

Mündlein, E., Greten, T., and Ritz, E. (1996). Graves' disease and sarcoidosis in a patient with minimal-change nephropathy. *Nephrology, Dialysis, Transplantation* **11**, 860–862.

Murray, F. E. *et al.* (1987). Simultaneous presentation of IgA nephropathy and sarcoidosis. *Sarcoidosis* **4**, 134–136.

Muther, R. S., McCarron, D. A., and Bennett, W. M. (1981). Renal manifestations of sarcoidosis. *Archives of Internal Medicine* **141**, 643–645.

Nédelec, G. *et al.* (1986). Néphropathie interstitielle et insuffisance rénale dans la sarcoïdose. *Presse Médicale* **15**, 623.

Newman, L. S., Rose, C. S., and Maier, L. A. (1997). Sarcoidosis. *New England Journal of Medicine* **336**, 1224–1234.

Nishiki, M. *et al.* (1999). Steroid-sensitive nephrotic syndrome, sarcoidosis and thyroiditis—a new syndrome? *Nephrology, Dialysis, Transplantation* **14**, 2008–2010.

Nordal, K. P. *et al.* (1985). Rapid effect of prednisolone on serum 1,25-dihydroxycholecalciferol levels in hypercalcemic sarcoidosis. *Acta Medica Scandinavica* **218**, 519–523.

O'Leary, T. J. *et al.* (1986). The effects of chloroquine on serum 1,25-dihydroxyvitamin D and calcium metabolism in sarcoidosis. *New England Journal of Medicine* **315**, 727–730.

O'Riordan, E. *et al.* (2001). Isolated sarcoid granulomatous interstitial nephritis: review of five cases at one center. *Clinical Nephrology* **55**, 297–302.

Oliver Rotellar, J. A., Garcia Ruiz, C., and Martinez Vea, A. (1990). Response to prednisone in membranous nephropathy associated with sarcoidosis. *Nephron* **54**, 195.

Padilla, M. L., Schilero, G. J., and Teirstein A. S. (1997). Sarcoidosis and transplantation. *Sarcoidosis, Vasculitis and Diffuse Lung Diseases* **14**, 16–22.

Pagniez, D. C. *et al.* (1987). Gallium scan in the follow-up of sarcoid granulomatous nephritis. *American Journal of Nephrology* **7**, 326–327.

Papapoulos, S. E. *et al.* (1979). 1,25-Dihydroxycholecalciferol in the pathogenesis of the hypercalcaemia of sarcoidosis. *Lancet* **i**, 627–630.

Parry, R. G. and Falk, M. C. (1997). Minimal-change disease in association with sarcoidosis. *Nephrology, Dialysis, Transplantation* **12**, 2159–2160.

Peces, R. *et al.* (1993). Focal segmental glomerulosclerosis associated with pulmonary sarcoidosis. *Nephron* **65**, 656–657.

Pertschuk, L. P., Silverstein, E., and Friedland, J. (1981). Immunohistologic diagnosis of sarcoidosis. Detection of angiotensin-converting enzyme in sarcoid granulomas. *American Journal of Clinical Pathology* **75**, 350–354.

Rainfray, M. *et al.* (1988). Renal amyloidosis complicating sarcoidosis. *Thorax* **43**, 422–423.

Reichel, H. *et al.* (1987). Regulation of 1,25-dihydroxyvitamin D_3 production by cultured alveolar macrophages from normal human donors and from patients with pulmonary sarcoidosis. *Journal of Clinical Endocrinology and Metabolism* **65**, 1201–1209.

Reichel, H., Koeffler, H. P., and Norman, A. W. (1989). The role of the vitamin D endocrine system in health and disease. *New England Journal of Medicine* **320**, 980–991.

Rizzato, G. (2001). Extrapulmonary presentation of sarcoidosis. *Current Opinion in Pulmonary Medicine* **7**, 295–297.

Rohatgi, P. K., Liao, T. E., and Borts, F. T. (1990). Pseudotumor of left kidney due to sarcoidosis. *Urology* **35**, 271–275.

Rodman, J. S. and Mahler, R. J. (2000). Kidney stones as a manifestation of hypercalcemic disorders. *Urologic Clinics of North America* **27**, 275–285.

Romer, F. K. (1980). Renal manifestations and abnormal calcium metabolism in sarcoidosis. *Quarterly Journal of Medicine* **49**, 233–247.

Schaumann, J. (1933). Etude anatomo-pathologique et histologique sur les localisations viscérales de la lymphogranulomatose bénigne. *Bulletin de la Société Francaise de Dermatologie et de Syphiligraphie* **40**, 1167–1178.

Schillinger, F. *et al.* (1999). Sarcoïdose rénale avec localisation pyélique pseudotumorale. *Presse Médicale* **28**, 683–685.

Shany, S. *et al.* (1993). Subcellular localization and partial purification of the 25-hydroxyvitamin D_3 1-hydroxylation reaction in the chick myelomonocytic cell line HD-11. *Journal of Bone and Mineral Research* **8**, 269–276.

Sharma, O. P. (2000). Hypercalcemia in granulomatous disorders: a clinical review. *Current Opinion in Pulmonary Medicine* **6**, 442–447.

Sheffield, E. A. (1997). Pathology of sarcoidosis. *Clinics in Chest Medicine* **18**, 741–754.

Shen, S. Y. *et al.* (1986). Recurrent sarcoid granulomatous nephritis and reactive tuberculin skin test in a renal transplant recipient. *American Journal of Medicine* **80**, 699–702.

Shintaku, M. *et al.* (1989). Generalized sarcoidlike granulomas with systemic angiitis, crescentic glomerulonephritis, and pulmonary hemorrhage. *Archives of Pathology and Laboratory Medicine* **113**, 1295–1298.

Singer, D. R. J. and Evans, D. J. (1986). Renal impairment in sarcoidosis: granulomatous nephritis as an isolated cause (two case reports and review of the literature). *Clinical Nephrology* **26**, 250–256.

Tamella, T. *et al.* (1989). Sarcoidosis of the bladder: a case report and review of the literature. *Journal of Urology* **141**, 608–609.

Tanneau, R. *et al.* (1987). Insuffisance rénale aiguë anurique par infiltration interstitielle granulomateuse révélatrice d'une sarcoïdose. *Annales de Médecine Interne* **138**, 147.

Taylor, J. E. and Ansell, I. D. (1996). Steroid-sensitive nephrotic syndrome and renal impairment in a patient with sarcoidosis and IgA nephropathy. *Nephrology, Dialysis, Transplantation* **11**, 355–356.

Tchénio, X. *et al.* (1996). Amylose rénale AA au cours d'une sarcoïdose. *Revue des Maladies Respiratoires* **13**, 601–602.

Trillo, A., Orozco, R., and Jindal, K. (1992). Glomerular calcinosis in sarcoidosis. *Archives of Pathology and Laboratory Medicine* **116**, 1221–1225.

Tsiouris, N. *et al.* (1999). End-stage renal disease in sarcoidosis of the kidney. *American Journal of Kidney Diseases* **34**, E21.

Turner, M. C., Shin, M. L., and Ruley, E. J. (1977). Renal failure as a presenting sign of diffuse sarcoidosis in an adolescent girl. *American Journal of Diseases of Children* **131**, 997–1000.

Utas, C. *et al.* (1999). Granulomatous interstitial nephritis in extrapulmonary sarcoidosis. *Clinical Nephrology* **51**, 252–254.

Vanhille, Ph. *et al.* (1986). Glomérulonéphrite rapidement progressive à dépôts mésangiaux d'IgA au cours d'une sarcoïdose. *Néphrologie* **5**, 207–209.

Van Umm, S. H. M. *et al.* (1997). A 58-year-old man with sarcoidosis complicated by focal crescentic glomerulonephritis. *Nephrology, Dialysis, Transplantation* **12**, 2703–2707.

Veronese, F. J. V. *et al.* (1998). Pulmonary sarcoidosis and focal segmental glomerulonephritis. *Nephrology, Dialysis, Transplantation* **13**, 493–495.

Warren, G. V., Sprague, S. M., and Corwin, H. L. (1988). Sarcoidosis presenting as acute renal failure during pregnancy. *American Journal of Kidney Diseases* **12**, 161–163.

Watson, I. *et al.* (1996). Sarcoidosis and primary systemic vasculitis. *Nephrology, Dialysis, Transplantation* **11**, 1631–1633.

Zerwekh, J. E., Pak, C. Y. C., and Kaplan, R. A. (1980). Pathogenetic role of 1-alpha, 25-dihydroxyvitamin D in sarcoidosis and absorptive hypercalciuria: different response to prednisone therapy. *Journal of Clinical Endocrinology and Metabolism* **51**, 381–386.

4.5 The patient with vasculitis

4.5.1 Pathogenesis of angiitis

Coen A. Stegeman and
Cees G.M. Kallenberg

Introduction

Angiitis, or vasculitis, is a clinicopathological process defined by inflammation and damage to blood vessels. Inflammatory cell infiltration in some or all tissue layers of blood vessels cause swelling, necrosis, and disruption of vessel wall structures such as the internal elastic lamina and endothelium, compromising antithrombotic activity, vessel patency, and integrity. In addition, the inflammatory response can lead to remodelling and proliferation of vascular structures causing fibrosis and thickening of media and intima compromising the vessel lumen. Vessel wall inflammation may even extend into the tissues adjacent to the vessels causing perivascular or angiocentric inflammation. The inflammatory changes and loss of vascular functions lead to diverse sequelae such as aneurysmatic vessel dilatation, tissue ischaemia, and organ dysfunction, necrosis, and bleeding.

The clinical syndromes caused by vasculitic diseases are broad and heterogeneous, as most forms are not—or only partially—restricted to single organs, certain vessel types, or sizes. Therefore, vasculitis usually is a systemic, multiorgan disease, although its presentation may be dominated by a single or limited number of clinical organ manifestations. In clinical practice, the most common forms of vasculitis affect the smaller blood vessels, primarily arterioles, capillaries, and postcapillary venules. Given the extensive presence of small vascular structures in the kidney, it is not surprising that renal involvement is a frequent finding in systemic vasculitic syndromes.

In the approach to the patient with suspected vasculitis, it is important to realize that vasculitis may be the primary manifestation of a disease, or, alternatively, be a secondary manifestation of another underlying disease. The distinction between primary and secondary forms of vasculitis is important as their pathophysiologies may be completely different, which has prognostic and therapeutic consequences. From a pathophysiological point of view, many of the secondary forms of vasculitis are associated with immune complex formation and deposition, or direct infiltration of the vascular tissue by infectious agents. For most of the primary vasculitic syndromes, the pathogenesis is less clear. Classification of human vasculitic syndromes partly reflects this distinction, but syndromes are mainly categorized by the vessel size primarily involved, and the histopathological characteristics of the lesions (Table 1) (Jennette *et al.* 1994; Jennette and Falk 1997). This chapter will discuss the pathogenesis of human vasculitis with respect to general pathogenetic patterns and more specific pathogenetic pathways related to primary and secondary syndromes.

Table 1 Categories of primary and secondary vasculitic syndromes according to the predominant vessel size involved (Jennette *et al.* 1994; Jennette and Falk 1997)

Large vessel vasculitis (aorta and major arterial branches)
Giant cell arteritis
Takayasu's arteritis
Medium-sized vessel vasculitis (larger muscularized arteries)
Polyarteritis nodosa
Kawasaki's disease
Primary granulomatous vasculitis of the central nervous system
Small vessel vasculitis (small arteries, arterioles, capillaries, venules)
ANCA-associated vasculitis
Microscopic polyangiitis
Wegener's granulomatosis
Churg–Strauss syndrome
Drug-induced ANCA-associated vasculitis
Immune-complex small vessel vasculitis
Henoch–Schönlein purpura
Cryoglobulinaemic vasculitis
Connective tissue disease associated vasculitis, e.g. systemic lupus erythematosus, Sjögren's syndrome, rheumatoid arthritis
Hypocomplementaemic urticarial vasculitis
Behçet's disease
Goodpasture syndrome
Serum sickness
Drug-induced immune complex vasculitis
Infection induced immune complex vasculitis
Paraneoplastic small vessel vasculitis

Immunopathological aspects of the vasculitic inflammation

The pathogenesis of vasculitis is complex, and involves different mechanisms that may operate simultaneously or sequentially. It was long thought that antigen–antibody complex formation at the site of the vessel wall was the primary pathological process in all forms of vasculitis. The clinical association of infections or drugs with the development of vasculitis, in which immune depositions in the lesions could be demonstrated, substantiated this concept. From earlier work on experimental serum sickness and other models, Fauci proposed a multiple-step hypothesis for the development of necrotizing vasculitis in which antigen exposure and subsequent antibody formation would lead to circulating antigen–antibody complexes which, under specific circumstances, would be deposited in blood vessel walls causing complement activation, recruitment and, activation of leucocytes, vessel wall damage, and necrosis (Fauci *et al.* 1978). Although operative in many secondary forms of vasculitis, the uniformity of the concept is challenged by the absence of demonstrable immune complexes in early lesions of most forms of vasculitis. In addition, in certain vasculitides the vessel wall is infiltrated by activated T-lymphocytes and macrophages in the absence of both neutrophils and immune deposits.

Immune complex-mediated vasculitis

The role of immune complexes in the pathogenesis of vasculitis

The role of antigen–antibody complex formation in the development of vasculitis has been demonstrated in animal models of serum sickness and the Arthus reaction. In the acute serum sickness model in rabbits following a single intravenous dose of heterologous serum albumin necrotizing arteritis, glomerulonephritis and arthritis develop after 10–14 days (Dixon *et al.* 1958). The lesions develop at the moment when complexes of serum albumin, antibody, and complement can be demonstrated in the circulation and in the vessel wall of arteries and glomeruli. As heterologous antigen cannot be demonstrated in the vessel wall prior to the formation of circulating and deposited immune complexes, *in situ* complex formation is not involved (Dixon *et al.* 1958). Chronic serum sickness with daily administration of heterologous protein results in a variety of sequelae, ranging from absence or resolution of the vasculitic process due to tolerance or rapid clearance of the antigen to chronic immune complex glomerulonephritis and leucocytoclastic small vessel vasculitis (Brentjens *et al.* 1975; Christian and Sergent 1976). A likely explanation for the differences observed between acute and chronic serum sickness and the inconsistent features of vasculitis in animal and human immune complex disease is that physical and immunological characteristics of complexes vary greatly. These differences in characteristics are caused by quantitative and qualitative differences both in the immune response and the antigen load, leading to different composition and size of the antigen–antibody complexes, depending on the relative amounts of antigen and antibody present. In addition, non-specific binding characteristics and size of the antigen, affinity and isotype of the antibody, and binding of complement determine the fate of these complexes (Cochrane and Hawkins 1968; Fauci *et al.* 1978). Antibodies present in immune complexes are frequently of the IgG isotype, but IgM and IgA have also been demonstrated in circulating and deposited immune complexes. The mere presence of circulating immune complexes is, however, not sufficient to produce vasculitis (Fig. 1). Experimental data have shown that vasoactive amines

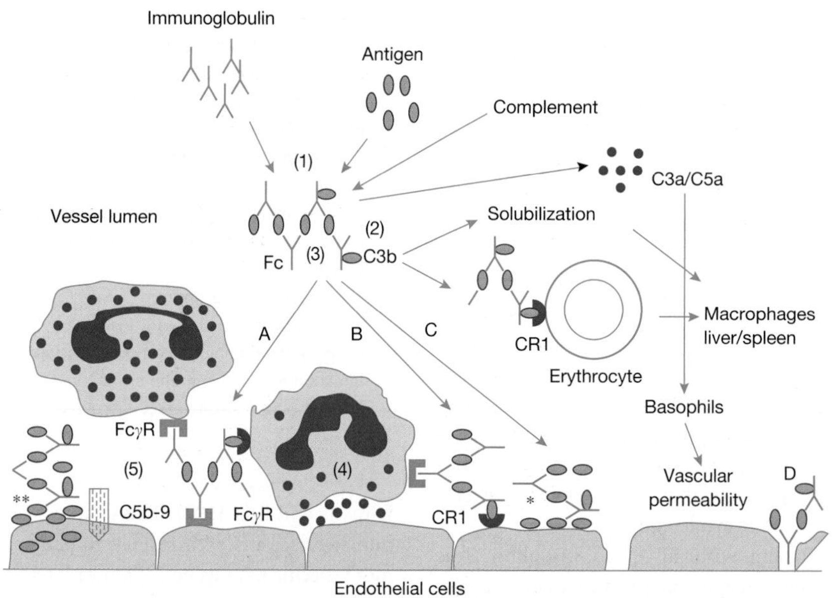

Fig. 1 Schematic representation of the processes involved in immune complex formation in the vessel lumen or at the endothelial cells, immune complex deposition, and initial inflammatory events in immune complex mediated vasculitis. (1) Immune complexes are formed between circulating or endothelial bound (*) or produced antigen(s) (**) and immunoglobulins. (2) Complement will be activated by the complexes through the classical or alternate pathway resulting in release of complement fragments C3a and C5a, which will attract neutrophils and stimulate basophils to release vasoactive amines. C3b will bind to the immunoglobulin of the complexes and facilitate solubilization of the complex and binding to complement 1 receptors on macrophages or erythrocytes. (3) Circulating complexes not eliminated by binding to erythrocytes or macrophages can be deposited on the endothelial cells by: (A) binding of the Fc part of the complexed immunoglobulin to the Fcγ-receptors (FcγR) or (B) binding of complex bound C3b to complement receptor 1 (CR1) expressed on capillaries and postcapillary venules; (C) binding of antigen to endothelial cell membranes by charge interaction; (D) trapping of complexes with binding to subendothelial matrix due to increased vascular permeability caused by vasoactive amines. (4) Neutrophils attracted by chemotactic factors complement C3a, C5a, and locally produced cytokines (not depicted) will bind to the complexes with Fcγ-receptors (FcγR) and complement receptor 1 (CR1). Neutrophil activation and degranulation will occur with subsequent lytic and oxidative damage to the endothelial cells. In addition, bound complexes will lead to full complement activation with formation and membrane insertion of the membrane attack complex (C5b-9).

increasing vascular permeability derived form platelets, mast cells, and basophils are necessary for tissue deposition of immune complexes and that treatment with antihistamines prevents or attenuates vasculitis (Henson and Cochrane 1971; McCluskey and Fienberg 1983). The fact that deposited immune complexes and vascular lesions are preferentially found at vessel branching sites, heart valves, sites of tissue trauma, and dependent body areas point to the necessity of certain microcirculatory circumstances for deposition and inflammation to occur (Ball and Bridges 2002). In addition to low-flow velocities, capillaries and postcapillary venules can express receptors for the Fc fragment of immunoglobulins and for complement C3b facilitating binding of complexes (Claudy 1998) (Fig. 1). This explains, in part, the predilection for these vessels in immune complex-mediated vasculitis.

Inflammatory reactions following immune complex deposition

Following the deposition of immune complexes in vessel walls, the inflammatory reaction is driven by complement activation which will lead to the formation of chemotactic factors C3a and C5a causing recruitment, infiltration, and activation of leucocytes (Gower *et al.* 1977) (Fig. 1). The acute phase is characterized by necrosis of endothelium and disruption of the basement membrane of capillaries and postcapillary venules due to the formation of complement C5b-9 complexes and the release of lytic enzymes and oxygen radials from activated polymorph mononuclear cells. In larger vessels, this process leads to infiltration of the adventitia and media and disruption of the elastic lamina. Concomitantly, the physical integrity and antithrombotic capacity of the endothelium is lost, causing deposition in the vessel wall of plasma proteins and fibrin. In the model of acute serum sickness, rabbits that have been depleted of circulating complement by treatment with cobra venom do not develop vasculitis: deposited immune complexes can be demonstrated, but no complement is found and neutrophil infiltration with necrosis of vessel wall structures is absent (Henson and Cochrane 1971). Likewise, induced neutropenia or absence of Fcγ-receptors will prevent the development of inflammation and vasculitis, pointing to the essential role of complement activation, neutrophil recruitment, and Fcγ-receptor engagement with immune complexes in the early stages of the process (Sylvestre and Ravetch 1994).

The endothelial cells are, however, by no means injured, innocent bystanders of the attack. Early expression of P-selectin on endothelial cells activated by histamine, thrombin, and complement components (C5b-9) and of endothelial E-selectin by activation with tumour necrosis factor-α (TNF-α) and interleukin-1β (IL-1β) are essential for leucocyte rolling and adherence through binding to sialyl Lewis-X and L-selectin expressed on neutrophils. The endothelial selectin expression peaks within hours and disappears by 24 h, but is taken over and superseded by endothelial expression of intercellular adhesion molecule-1 (ICAM-1) and vascular cell adhesion molecule-1 (VCAM-1). These adhesion molecules form ligands for CD11/CD18 integrins expressed on leucocytes and expression will result in strong and irreversible binding and subsequent transendothelial migration of the leucocytes (Sais *et al.* 1997; Claudy 1998). Activated neutrophils and monocytes will produce IL-8, which will further stimulate neutrophil migration and activation. The activated and transmigrated neutrophils will rapidly degrade the immune complexes, which will no longer be detectable after 24–48 h (Grunwald *et al.* 1997). The temporal pattern of expression of endothelial adhesion molecules in combination with secreted chemokines such as monocyte chemoattractant protein-1 (MCP-1) and regulated upon activation of normal T-cell expressed and secreted (RANTES) will change the infiltrate from predominantly neutrophilic to mono- and lymphocytic.

Immune complexes in human vasculitis

Detection of immunoglobulin and complement in human leucocytoclastic vasculitis, which is the histopathological prototype of human immune complex vasculitis, provides circumstantial evidence for a role of immune complexes in the pathogenesis. These immune complexes, either deposited from the circulation or formed *in situ*, are found in Henoch–Schönlein purpura, vasculitis associated with cryoglobulinaemia, hepatitis B-associated polyarteritis nodosa, and many cases of the secondary vasculitides. The complexes involved are supposedly composed of antibodies bound to microbial antigens in case of underlying infectious diseases, autoantigens in the connective tissue diseases, and non-microbial exogenous antigens in the hypersensitivity disorders (Table 2). The immune complex-associated vasculitides (Table 1) are all associated with the presence of circulating immune complexes and vascular deposits composed of combinations of IgM, IgG, IgA, and complement C3, suggesting a role of these complexes in their pathogenesis. Definite support for a pathogenetic role of immune complexes requires the simultaneous detection of a relevant antigen and specific antibody in the circulation and the vasculitic lesions. With the exception of the small- and medium-sized vessel vasculitis associated with chronic hepatitis B infection, in which hepatitis B surface antigen–antibody complexes have been demonstrated in the circulation and in lesions of muscular arteries, dermal vessels, and glomeruli (Trepo *et al.* 1974; Michalak 1978), the specificities of the antigens and their corresponding antibodies have not been identified in most of the cases. Although

Table 2 Secondary vasculitides: antigens and antigen sources presumably involved in immune complex formation

Exogenous antigens
Microbial antigens
Bacterial
Streptococci
Staphylococci
Mycobacterium leprae
Treponema pallidum
Others
Viral
Hepatitis B/C virus
Human immunodeficiency virus
Cytomegalovirus
Epstein–Barr virus
Others
Protozoal
Plasmodia
Non-microbial antigens
Heterologous proteins (therapeutic monoclonal or polyclonal antibodies)
Allergens
Drugs
Tumour antigens (?)
Autologous antigens
Nuclear antigens (antinuclear antibodies)
Immunoglobulin G (rheumatoid factor, cryoglobulins)
Others

circulating immune complexes can be demonstrated in many patients with vasculitis, this finding is very aspecific as many patients with chronic hepatitis B or other infections, connective tissue diseases, or tumours have circulating immune complexes, of which only a very small fraction will develop vasculitis and glomerulonephritis (McDougal and MacDuffie 1985; McMahon *et al.* 1989).

Factors leading to immune complex formation and disease in humans

The fact that immune complex formation occurs frequently under pathological and probably also under physiological conditions, while vasculitis or other sequelae secondary to these complexes are rare, suggests that specific conditions have to be met for immune complexes to lead to immune complex vasculitis (Table 3). Normally, immune complexes form only transiently and are rapidly cleared from the circulation. Persistent or recurrent exposure to antigens in the circulation in combination with the presence of specific antibodies may lead to circulating complexes. Chronic infections such as hepatitis B and C or endocarditis, increased permeability for gastrointestinal antigens in Henoch–Schönlein purpura, and release of endogenous antigens in systemic lupus erythematosus or rheumatoid arthritis are all thought to provide these antigens and, in the presence of binding antibodies, to result in persistent or recurrent immune complex formation. On the other hand, the efficiency with which immune complexes are cleared from the circulation may be an important determinant. Activation of the classical and alternative complement pathways by the immune complexes will lead to adherence of C3b and C4b. C3b binding facilitates solubilization of immune complexes and uptake of the complex by interaction with the complement receptor type 1 (CR1) on cells of the reticuloendothelial system, especially the Kupffer cells in the sinoids of the liver. In addition, CR1 is abundantly present on the surface of erythrocytes (Fig. 1). Binding of immune complexes to these receptors on erythrocytes inhibits their precipitation and allows their transport to liver and spleen macrophages (Schifferli *et al.* 1986). In patients with

Table 3 Factors possibly influencing the *in situ* formation or deposition of circulating immune complexes and development of vasculitis

Immune complex characteristics
Concentration of circulating immune complexes
Size and composition of the immune complexes
  Ratio of antigens and antibodies
  Immunoglobulin class(es) and subclass(es)
Properties of the antigen
  Charge of the antigen
  Site of production of the antigen
Complement activating capacity

Patient characteristics
Capacity to efficiently remove circulating immune complexes
  Expression and affinity of complement and Fcγ-receptors on reticuloendothelial and other cells
  Intact complement system
Haemodynamic conditions or factors influencing vascular permeability facilitating antigen trapping or immune complex deposition
Propensity to chronic or intermittent antigen exposure due to chronic or recurrent infection(s) or increased gastrointestinal permeability for antigens

systemic lupus erythematosus, a decreased density of CR1 receptors on erythrocytes has been found, resulting in decreased binding of immune complexes to erythrocytes (Miyakawa *et al.* 1981; Lobatto *et al.* 1988). The association of genetic deficiencies of complement components and immune complex diseases suggests that complement-mediated clearance *in vivo* is important in preventing immune complex deposition. Immune complex uptake is also mediated by the interaction of the Fc part of complexed immunoglobulins and Fcγ-receptors on mononuclear phagocytic cells. Functional polymorphisms in the human Fcγ-receptors II and III have been described that lead to differences in affinity for different IgG subclasses. Associations between these functional polymorphisms and reduced clearance of immune complexes and risk for immune complex-mediated diseases such as systemic lupus erythematosus have been described (van der Pol and van de Winkel 1998; Dijstelbloem *et al.* 2000).

Amounts of circulating immune complexes are often higher in patients with vasculitic disease activity compared to those without the activity, in diseases such as rheumatoid arthritis associated with vasculitis, and in Henoch–Schönlein purpura. Also, in individual patients, circulating immune complex levels can fluctuate in relation with disease activity. The relation between levels of circulating immune complexes and vasculitis is, however, by no means absolute. Size and composition of the immune complexes are important: in experimental models only complexes with certain sedimentation characteristics are deposited in vessel walls (Cochrane and Hawkins 1968). In patients with drug-induced and Henoch–Schönlein purpura, the development of leucocytoclastic vasculitis coincides with the presence of large IgA and C3-containing complexes in the circulation which disappear when the patient recovers (Kauffmann *et al.* 1980). The size of the immune complex determines its fate as circulating and deposited IgA–immune complexes are found in both patients with IgA nephropathy and Henoch–Schönlein purpura, but these complexes are smaller in IgA nephropathy than in Henoch–Schönlein purpura (Davin and Weening 2001).

Specific characteristics of the immunoglobulin component or the antigen present in the complex may determine its propensity to be formed or deposited at certain vascular sites. IgA1 present in immune complexes in Henoch–Schönlein purpura has been found to be abnormally glycosylated, especially when nephritis is present (Allen *et al.* 1998) (see Chapter 3.6). Likewise, in hepatitis C virus-associated mixed cryoglobulinaemia, which is present in 50 per cent of patients with chronic hepatitis C, the small minority who develop cryoglobulinaemic vasculitis have more often IgG3 subclass in their complexes (Dammacco *et al.* 2001) (see Chapter 4.9). Binding of endogenous antigens such as nuclear histones or bacterial antigens such as Staphylococcal neutral phosphatase to (glomerular) basement membranes or endothelial cells due to charge interactions may result in deposition or *in situ* formation of immune complexes. Finally, endothelial cells may be infected by microbial agents such as cytomegalo- or other herpes viruses, Parvo B19 virus, hepatitis C virus, or intracellular growing bacteria, which, in addition to direct endothelial cell damage, may result in local release of antigen and thereby formation of immune complexes with subsequent inflammatory response (Somer and Finegold 1995; Kallenberg and Heeringa 1998).

'Pauci-immune' systemic vasculitis

In contrast to secondary vasculitides, primary vasculitides are, with the exception of Henoch–Schönlein purpura and vasculitis associated with essential cryoglobulinaemia, characterized by a paucity of immune deposits in the lesions. The pathogenesis of most of the primary vasculitic syndromes is unclear, but autoantibodies and T-cell mediated cellular immune reactions may be involved and will be discussed. The primary vasculitic syndromes are classified based on the size of the vessels involved, the histopathology of the lesions, and the presence of characteristic clinical symptoms. A classification scheme as well as definitions for the various vasculitic syndromes have been proposed by an International Consensus Group in 1993 (Table 4). Potential pathogenetic pathways play only a very limited role in this classification, although the association of certain small- vessel vasculitic syndromes with the presence of circulating antineutrophil cytoplasmic antibodies (ANCA) is recognized.

Autoantibodies in primary vasculitis

As for the large vessel vasculitides, no disease-specific autoantibodies have been described until now. Also in medium-sized vessel vasculitis, specific autoantibodies are lacking. In contrast, some forms of primary small vessel vasculitis are strongly associated with the presence of circulating ANCA directed against proteinase 3 (PR3) and myeloperoxidase (MPO), which are cytoplasmic constituents of neutrophils and monocytes. Furthermore, antiendothelial cell antibodies (AECA) have been described in patients with primary vasculitis. The potential role of both groups of antibodies in the pathogenesis of vasculitis will be discussed.

Pathogenic potential of antineutrophil cytoplasmic antibodies in systemic vasculitis

Following the preliminary reports on the associations of antineutrophil autoantibodies with idiopathic necrotizing glomerulonephritis and vasculitis (Davies *et al.* 1982; Hall *et al.* 1984), van der Woude described in 1985 the presence of autoantibodies producing a characteristic cytoplasmic immunofluorescence pattern on ethanol-fixed neutrophils in sera of a large series of patients with active Wegener's granulomatosis (van der Woude *et al.* 1985). Since then the close association between antibodies directed against either proteinase 3 or myeloperoxidase and Wegener's granulomatosis, microscopic polyangiitis, renal limited vasculitis (isolated pauci-immune necrotizing glomerulonephritis), and,

Table 4 Names, definitions, and description of usual features of vasculitides adopted by the Chapel Hill Consensus Conference on the nomenclature of systemic vasculitis (Jennette *et al.* 1994)

Large vessel vasculitis

Giant cell (temporal) arteritis

Granulomatous arteritis of the aorta and its major branches, with a predilection for the extracranial branches of the carotid artery

Features: Often involves temporal artery. Usually in patients older than 50 years and is often associated with polymyalgia rheumatica

Takayasu's arteritis

Granulomatous inflammation of the aorta and its major branches

Features: Usually occurs in patients younger than 50 years

Medium-sized vessel vasculitis

Polyarteritis nodosa

Necrotizing inflammation of medium-sized and small arteries without glomerulonephritis or vasculitis in arterioles, capillaries, or venules

Kawasaki's disease

Arteritis involving large, medium-sized, and small arteries and associated with mucocutaneous lymph node syndrome

Features: Coronary arteries often involved. Aorta and veins may be involved. Usually occurs in children

Small-vessel vasculitis

Wegener's granulomatosis

Granulomatous inflammation involving the respiratory tract and necrotizing vasculitis affecting small- to medium-sized vessels (e.g. capillaries, venules, arterioles, and arteries)

Features: Necrotizing glomerulonephritis is common. Strongly associated with the presence of antineutrophil cytoplasmic antibodies

Churg–Strauss syndrome

Eosinophil-rich and granulomatous inflammation involving the respiratory tract and necrotizing vasculitis affecting small- to medium-sized vessels and associated with asthma and eosinophilia

Features: Associated with the presence of antineutrophil cytoplasmic antibodies

Microscopic polyangiitis

Necrotizing vasculitis with few or no immune deposits affecting small vessels (capillaries, venules, or arterioles)

Features: Necrotizing arteritis involving small- and medium-sized arteries may be present. Necrotizing glomerulonephritis is very common. Pulmonary capillaritis often occurs. Strongly associated with the presence of antineutrophil cytoplasmic antibodies

Henoch–Schönlein purpura

Vasculitis with IgA-dominant immune deposits affecting small vessels (capillaries, venules, or arterioles)

Features: Typically involves skin, gut, and glomeruli and is associated with arthralgias or arthritis

Essential cryoglobulinaemic vasculitis

Vasculitis with cryoglobulin immune deposits affecting small vessels (capillaries, venules, or arterioles) and associated with cryoglobulins in serum

Features: Skin and glomeruli are often involved

Cutaneous leucocytoclastic angiitis

Isolated cutaneous leucocytoclastic angiitis without systemic vasculitis or glomerulonephritis to a lesser extent, Churg–Strauss syndrome has been extensively described (Falk and Jennette 1988; Cohen Tervaert *et al.* 1991; Kallenberg *et al.* 1994; Hagen *et al.* 1998; Savige *et al.* 2000). Based on a relation, albeit not absolute, between the level of these autoantibodies and disease activity of the associated vasculitic syndromes, the autoantibodies were suggested to be involved in the pathogenesis of the associated diseases (Cohen Tervaert *et al.* 1990; Kallenberg *et al.* 1995; Boomsma *et al.* 2000; Harper and Savage 2000). This hypothesis also more firmly positions these diseases within the spectrum of autoimmune disorders.

In humans, direct evidence for a pathogenic role of ANCA is not available. Associations between the mere presence or increases in ANCA directed against PR3 and, to a lesser extent, MPO and risk for vasculitic disease activation have been described and debated. Indeed, episodes of disease activity at diagnosis or during relapse of Wegener's granulomatosis, microscopic polyangiitis, and renal limited vasculitis are nearly always accompanied by the concomitant presence of ANCA. However, many patients who have been treated for one of the latter diseases and are in complete remission remain ANCA positive. Clearly, the mere presence of ANCA directed against PR3 or MPO is not sufficient for vasculitic disease activity to occur, while on the other hand ANCA is, if not directly involved in the pathogenesis, an important marker for disease activity. Certain *in vitro* data and results of a limited number of experimental animal models suggest that ANCA may have effects that play a role in small vessel vasculitic disease activity (Fig. 2).

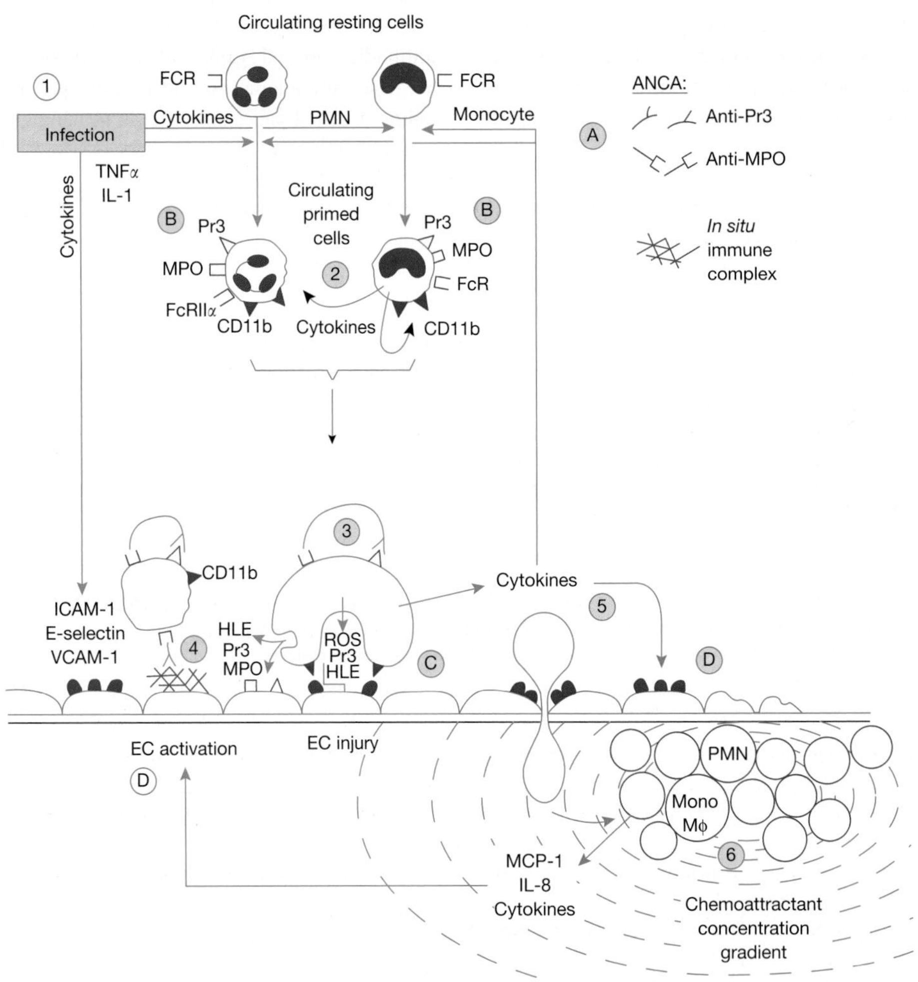

Fig. 2 Schematic representation of the immune mechanisms supposedly involved in the pathophysiology of ANCA-associated vasculitides.
(1) Cytokines released due to (local) infection cause upregulation of adhesion molecules on the endothelium and priming of neutrophils and/or monocytes.
(2) Circulating primed neutrophils and/or monocytes express the ANCA antigens on the cell surface. (3) Adherence of primed neutrophils and/or monocytes to the endothelium, followed by activation of these cells by ANCA. Activated neutrophils and/or monocytes release reactive oxygen species (ROS) and lysosomal enzymes, which leads to endothelial cell injury and eventually to necrotizing inflammation. (4) Degranulation of proteinase 3 and myeloperoxidase by these ANCA-activated neutrophils and/or monocytes results in endothelial cell activation, endothelial cell injury, or even endothelial cell apoptosis. Furthermore, bound Pr3 and MPO serve as planted antigens, resulting in *in situ* immune complexes, which in turn attract other neutrophils.
(5) ANCA-induced monocyte activation leads to production of monocyte chemoattractant protein-1 (MCP-1) and interleukin-8 (IL-8) production by these cells. The release of these chemoattractants by these cells amplifies monocytes and neutrophil recruitment possibly leading to granuloma formation
(6). (A)–(D) represent the four prerequisites for endothelial cell damage by ANCA: (A) the presence of ANCA; (B) expression of the target antigens for ANCA on primed neutrophils and monocytes; (C) the necessity of an interaction between primed neutrophils and endothelium via β_2-integrins; and finally (D) activation of endothelial cells. (Reprinted with permission from Muller Kobold *et al.* 1999.)

Experimental and laboratory data on pathophysiological effects of ANCA (Fig. 2)

In vitro, ANCA are able to activate neutrophils to produce reactive oxygen species and to degranulate with the release of lytic enzymes such as elastase and PR3 (Falk *et al.* 1990). In order to get activated by ANCA, *in vitro*, neutrophils must be in a state of preactivation ('primed'). Priming occurs in the presence of low amounts of proinflammatory cytokines such as TNF-α, IL-1, and IL-8. Although low levels of PR3 may be constitutively expressed on neutrophils, priming results in enhanced expression of the target antigens of ANCA, that is, PR3 and MPO, at the cell surface, makes these antigens accessible for interaction with ANCA (Muller Kobold *et al.* 1998a; Harper *et al.* 2001). *In vivo* priming may be induced by infections or colonization of the upper airways by *Staphylococcus aureus*, a potent neutrophil activator, as this was found to be associated with increased risk for relapse of ANCA-associated vasculitis (Stegeman *et al.* 1994). More recently, it was found that the level of constitutional expression of PR3 on neutrophils was highly variable between different individuals but stable within one person. A high level of constitutional PR3 expression was found to be a risk factor for PR3–ANCA-related vasculitis in one study (Witko-Sarsat *et al.* 1999), and a risk factor for relapse in another study (Rarok *et al.* 2002).

ANCA-induced neutrophil activation requires not only binding of the antibodies via their F(ab′)$_2$-fragments to surface expressed PR3 or MPO, but also interaction of their Fc-fragments with Fc-receptors on neutrophils, particularly with the Fcγ RIIa- and Fcγ RIIIb-receptor (Mulder *et al.* 1994; Porges *et al.* 1994; Kocher *et al.* 1998). Additional studies have shown that especially ANCA of the IgG3 subclass interact efficiently with the Fcγ RIIa-receptor, and the *in vitro* capacity of sera to activate primed neutrophils was found to be closely related to the IgG3–ANCA titre than to the total IgG–ANCA titre (Mulder *et al.* 1995). Also, IgG isolated from sera from patients who were still PR3–ANCA positive during remission of the disease were shown to have lower amounts of IgG3–PR3–ANCA and a lesser *in vitro* neutrophil stimulating capacity than sera collected at the moment of active vasculitis. Finally, studies on Fcγ IIa- and IIIb-receptor polymorphisms in humans with ANCA-associated vasculitis have shown that certain phenotypes with a high affinity for IgG3 subclass antibodies may be associated with more severe disease and disease relapse (Edberg *et al.* 1997; Dijstelbloem *et al.* 1999; Tse *et al.* 2000). However, a large prospective study showed that assessment of levels of IgG3–PR3–ANCA was not better in predicting relapse of vasculitic disease activity than that of total IgG–PR3–ANCA (Boomsma *et al.* 2000).

Binding of membrane expressed antigen and Fcγ-receptor interaction by ANCA results in activation of neutrophils through intracellular pathways involving tyrosine phosphorylation, protein-kinase C translocation, and phosphatidyl-inositol 3-kinase activation leading to activation of neutrophil respiratory burst with release of reactive oxygen products, degranulation of azurophilic granules, and secretion of leukotrienes and inflammatory cytokines (Falk *et al.* 1990; Brooks *et al.* 1996; Grimminger *et al.* 1996; Savage 2001). ANCA-induced neutrophil activation occurs efficiently when neutrophils are adherent to an endothelial surface, a process in which β2-integrins are involved (Reumaux *et al.* 1995; Radford *et al.* 2000). *In vitro* studies have demonstrated that ANCA are able to induce stable adherence of rolling neutrophils to endothelial cell monolayers expressing adhesion molecules and that endothelial cells can be lysed by neutrophils in the presence of ANCA (Ewert *et al.* 1992; Savage *et al.* 1992; Radford *et al.* 2001). *In vivo*, this process is assumed to occur at the endothelial surface of small vessels. Indeed, activated neutrophils adherent to the endothelium are observed in renal biopsies from patients with ANCA-associated necrotizing crescentic glomerulonephritis (Brouwer *et al.* 1994a). In addition, activated neutrophils are found within the circulation of patients with active vasculitis, and their degree of activation correlates with disease activity (Muller Kobold *et al.* 1998b). The presence of circulating activated neutrophils may lead to trapping within dense capillary systems such as pulmonary alveoli and the glomerulus, with subsequent damage to endothelial cells (Harper and Savage 2000). This latter concept is in agreement with the description of early vasculitic lesions found in Wegener's granulomatosis with local small vessel thrombosis and necrosis with lysed neutrophils (Donald *et al.* 1976; Brouwer *et al.* 1994a).

Neutrophils are not the only cells expressing the ANCA target antigens PR3 and MPO. Monocytes are known to contain and express PR3 and MPO, and can interact with ANCA. *In vitro*, activation of monocytes by ANCA has been shown with release of IL-8 and MCP-1 (Casselman *et al.* 1995; Ralston *et al.* 1997). Priming with TNF-α is not a prerequisite for monocyte activation by ANCA, but does lead to stronger activation. Infiltration by activated monocytes in crescentic glomerulonephritis associated with ANCA-related vasculitis has been shown. It is mediated by chemotaxis induced by fibrin and MCP-1 produced within the glomeruli and VCAM-1 expression on glomerular endothelium (Pall *et al.* 1996; Rastaldi *et al.* 1996). Whether endothelial cells themselves express ANCA-antigens, such as PR3, has been a subject of controversy. Some data suggest that endothelial cells express PR3, particularly when activated, and that, subsequently, ANCA can bind to surface-expressed PR3 resulting in upregulation of adhesion molecules and further activation of those cells or complement-dependent damage (Mayet *et al.* 1993). Others, however, have not been able to confirm PR3 expression by endothelial cells (Pendergraft *et al.* 2000), but demonstrated that both PR3 and MPO bind to endothelial cells and can be targetted by ANCA leading to complement-dependent damage (Savage *et al.* 1992; Taekema-Roelvink *et al.* 2000). PR3 may also have direct effects on endothelial cells by promoting apoptosis and enhancing vascular permeability, endothelial cell detachment, and expression of adhesion molecules, thereby increasing local inflammation and damage (Ballieux *et al.* 1994; Taekema-Roelvink *et al.* 1998, 2001). Likewise, there is controversy whether glomerular epithelial cells express PR3 and whether or not local glomerular epithelial expression of PR3 is involved in the pathogenesis of PR3–ANCA-associated glomerulonephritis (King *et al.* 1995; Schwarting *et al.* 2000).

ANCA directed against PR3 may reversibly bind to PR3 and interfere with the binding of PR3 with its main inhibitor α1-antitrypsin. This may lead to diminished clearance of PR3. *In vitro* this inhibition of PR3–α1-antitrypsin complexation can be demonstrated and was found to correlate with disease activity (Dolman *et al.* 1993). Also, congenital α1-antitrypsin deficiency with an over-representation of PiZ and PiZZ alleles is associated with PR3–ANCA-related vasculitis, or to a more severe outcome of the disease. This suggests that interference with the regulation of the enzymatic activity of PR3 may be involved in the pathogenesis of PR3–ANCA-related vasculitis (Harper and Savage 2000). Likewise, binding to MPO of MPO–ANCA may interfere with the physiological inhibition of MPO by ceruloplasmin binding.

Animal models of antineutrophil cytoplasmic antibody-associated vasculitis

More definite evidence for a pathophysiological role of ANCA may come from animal models. Until recently, fully satisfactory models for

ANCA-associated glomerulonephritis were not available (reviewed by Heeringa *et al.* 1998). Passive transfer of ANCA in primates or inducing an autoimmune response to MPO in rats did not result in renal lesions (Brouwer *et al.* 1993). When, however, the products of activated neutrophils such as MPO, and its substrate H_2O_2, are perfused into the renal artery in rats immunized with MPO, severe pauci-immune NCGN develops. Interestingly, very early in this model immune complexes, probably consisting of MPO and anti-MPO antibodies, can be demonstrated. These results suggest that cationic proteins such as MPO from activated neutrophils can also adhere to the glomerular capillary wall *in vivo* and are bound by their cognate antibodies. The immune complexes formed *in situ* activate the complement system, resulting, amongst other events, in attraction of neutrophils. These neutrophils are subsequently activated by ANCA, and degrade the immune complexes that were initially present. The potential of ANCA to augment an inflammatory reaction *in vivo* has been demonstrated also in an animal model of antiglomerular basement membrane (anti-GBM) disease (Heeringa *et al.* 1996). Injection of a subclinical dose of heterologous anti-GBM antibodies in rats, which resulted in deposition of immunoglobulins along the GBM but not in severe glomerulonephritis, resulted in severe necrotizing and crescentic glomerulonephritis when rats were immunized with human MPO, which led to the development of anti-MPO antibodies cross-reacting with their own MPO. These experiments show the phlogistic potential of ANCA.

Other models in which vasculitis and/or crescentic glomerulonephritis develops spontaneously in conjunction with autoantibodies to MPO have been described. The autoantibody response to MPO in these models is, however, part of a more polyclonal autoantibody response, which does not allow the analysis of the specific contribution of anti-MPO to the development of vasculitis. Recently, however, more definite proof of the role of antibodies directed to MPO in the pathophysiology of necrotizing glomerulonephritis and vasculitis was obtained. Transfer of splenocytes from MPO-deficient mice immunized with MPO to Rag2$^{-/-}$ knock-out mice, which lack functional B- and T-lymphocytes but not neutrophils and monocytes, led to the development of severe necrotizing and crescentic glomerulonephritis, while splenocytes from animals immunized with bovine serum albumin did not (Xiao *et al.* 2002). The fact that also direct administration of anti-MPO antibodies raised in MPO-deficient mice to wild-type or Rag2$^{-/-}$ mice resulted in glomerulonephritis provides strong evidence for the pathophysiological role of these antibodies. With respect to PR3–ANCA, there are currently no models available with the exception of the anti-anti-idiotypic model, which awaits confirmation as well as further analysis of the lesions (Blank *et al.* 1995).

Antiendothelial cell antibodies in primary systemic vasculitis

Nearly three decades ago, antibodies which specifically stained the vascular endothelium on mouse kidney sections as a substrate were reported for the first time (Lindquist and Osterland 1971). Later, these AECA have been described not only in the primary vasculitides but also in secondary vasculitides, connective tissue diseases, and a variety of other (inflammatory) disorders (Belizna and Cohen Tervaert 1997). AECA represent a heterogeneous group of antibodies and their target antigens are, generally, poorly characterized. AECA are generally detected by enzyme-linked immunosorbent assays using as a substrate cultured human umbilical vein endothelial cells. AECA react with different endothelial antigens ranging in molecular weight from 25 to 200 kDa. However, most of the antigens recognized by AECA are not specific for endothelial cells as these antibodies also react with fibroblasts or peripheral blood mononuclear cells (Belizna and Cohen Tervaert 1997). Whether the antigens recognized by AECA on endothelial cells are expressed constitutively or upon activation of endothelial cells or are so-called 'planted' antigens that adhere to endothelial cells by charge interaction is unclear. Potential candidate antigens that indeed can adhere to endothelial cells and to which antibodies can be detected in AECA assays are β_2-glycoprotein and deoxyribonucleic acid (Kallenberg and Cohen Tervaert 2002). On the other hand, AECA from a patient with Takayasu's arteritis proved to react specifically with large vessel endothelial cells (Blank *et al.* 1999).

AECA have been reported in extremely varying frequencies in patients with all forms of primary systemic vasculitis, but are clinically of little value due to lack of disease specificity. Possibly, full characterization of the target antigens will improve their diagnostic significance. However, serial levels of AECA have been reported to correlate with disease activity in primary small vessel vasculitis and Kawasaki disease, which may point to a pathogenetic role, although the possibility that AECA are a result and not a cause of endothelial cell injury clearly exists (Leung *et al.* 1986; Chan *et al.* 1993).

In vitro, AECA have been shown to mediate complement and cellular-dependent cytotoxicity against cultured endothelial cell monolayers (Savage *et al.* 1991; Del Papa *et al.* 1992). Binding of AECA to endothelial cells also results in endothelial cell activation with expression of IL-1, -6, and -8, monocyte MCP-1, ICAM-1, and VCAM-1 (Del Papa *et al.* 1996; Carvalho *et al.* 1999). Other *in vitro* effects of AECA on endothelial cells that have been reported are promotion of thrombotic events with increased production of tissue factor and von Willebrand factor, shedding of heparin sulfate, and inhibition of prostacyclin production (Frampton *et al.* 1990; Savage *et al.* 1991; Lindsey *et al.* 1994; Ihrcke *et al.* 1996). Finally, it has recently been shown that AECA from patients with systemic vasculitis may induce apoptosis of endothelial cells (Bordron *et al.* 1998).

A definite animal model supporting a pathophysiological role for AECA in the development of vasculitis has not yet been discovered. However, injection of antibodies to known endothelial antigens such as angiotensin-converting enzyme or factor VIII von Willebrand complex induces lung vasculitis and glomerulonephritis in rabbits and rats (Belzina and Cohen Tervaert 1997). Together, all these findings suggest that AECA may have a direct role in the induction of endothelial damage but a definite role in the pathogenesis of vasculitis is unproven.

T-cell activity in primary vasculitis

The role of T-lymphocytes in different forms of primary vasculitis is suggested to be important, but remains far from fully characterized. Human biopsy material and animal models suggest that in small vessel vasculitis the vasculitic lesions develop over time from a predominantly polymorph neutrophil lesion into a lesion in which activated mononuclear cells, that is, monocytes/macrophages and T-lymphocytes, predominate. Experimental evidence exists that vasculitis in mice strongly resembling some forms of human vasculitis can be induced by T-lymphocytes that have been sensitized to microvascular smooth muscle cells *in vitro* (Hart *et al.* 1985). In addition, lymphocytes isolated from autoimmune mice that spontaneously develop arteritis react to and destroy cultured syngenic vascular smooth muscle cells *in vitro* (Moyer and Reinisch 1984). Activated T-lymphocytes can be clearly demonstrated in lesions of human necrotizing small vessel vasculitis in renal, lung, and nasal biopsies. In addition, the occurrence of granulomas in Wegener's granulomatosis and Churg–Strauss syndrome indicate the activation of these cell types. The activated T-cells in these types of vasculitides are predominantly $CD4^+$ with a Th1-dominant profile characterized by high interferon-γ (INF-γ) and low IL-4 and -5 production (Gephardt *et al.* 1983; Csernok *et al.* 1999; Cunningham *et al.* 1999). Patients with the ANCA-associated vasculitides also show activated T-lymphocytes in their peripheral blood, a pattern that persists even when the disease is in remission (Ludviksson *et al.* 1998; Popa *et al.* 1999). This pattern of activated T-cells is also reflected by increased serum levels of soluble T-cell acivation markers (Stegeman *et al.* 1993). Finally, antigen-specific T cells recognizing the ANCA antigens PR3 and MPO have been identified in the peripheral blood of patients with ANCA-associated vasculitis (Brouwer *et al.* 1994b; Griffith *et al.* 1996; King *et al.* 1998; van der Geld *et al.* 2000). However, neither a clear association between these findings and disease activity has been found, nor have these antigen specific cells been isolated from vasculitic lesions. As the predominant type of T-cells is $CD4^+$, it is possible that these cells mainly are responsible for antigen specific B-cell help, a concept entirely compatible with the IgG-class high affinity type of autoantibodies that ANCA are.

A role for T-cell-mediated immunity is more firmly established, albeit by circumstantial evidence, in the large vessel vasculitides. The most common form is giant cell arteritis, its name derived from the presence of many Langhans' giant cells in the lesions. The vasculitis, involving large muscular arteries with a predilection for the temporal artery, is characterized by a granulomatous inflammatory reaction within the medial vessel wall with accumulation of $CD4^+$ T-cells, macrophages, multinucleated giant cells, and disruption of the internal elastic lamina (Weyand and Goronzy 1999). The predilection of the disease for white people from northern European countries and northern areas in the United States suggests that besides environmental factors, genetic factors are also involved. HLA-typing has shown an association with class II HLA–DR4 and with HLA–DRB1 alleles, particularly with DRB*0401, *0404, and *0408, which points to the involvement of antigen-specific T-lymphocytes in the pathogenesis and is in line with the predominance of $CD4^+$ T-cell involvement seen in this disease. Clonally expanded T-cells, as detected by T-cell receptor β chain analysis in biopsies from involved temporal arteries, have been found at different sites in the biopsy but not in the peripheral blood. *In vitro* some of these T-cell clonotypes showed proliferation when incubated with monocytes pulsed with temporal artery extracts from patients but not with extracts from control temporal arteries (Brack *et al.* 1997).

These data point to an (auto)antigen-specific T-cell response in which a modified antigen present in diseased arteries may be involved. Actinically degenerated elastic tissue has been suggested as the relevant autoantigen, although characterization of the precise antigenic structures and their modification(s) has not been accomplished. Viral or bacterial infections have also been implicated in triggering the disease as temporal associations of giant cell arteritis with parvovirus B19 infection, parainfluenza type I infection, influenza vaccination, and *Chlamydia pneumoniae* infection have been described and parvovirus B19 and *Chlamydia pneumoniae* DNA have been found in diseased arteries (Levine and Hellmann 2002). Analysis of cytokine patterns in biopsies from patients with GCA shows mRNA expression of IL-2 and IFN-γ as well as IL-1β but not of IL-10 (Weyand *et al.* 1997). In contrast to giant cell arteritis, the infiltrate in Takayasu's arteritis predominantly consists of $CD8^+$ and natural killer (NK) T cells, which is in line with the finding that the disease is associated with HLA class I antigens of the B-locus and not with class II antigens. Moreover, the T-cell receptor α- and β-chains of these infiltrating cells show a restricted use of variable genes, which is similar within the lesions (Seko 2002). These data suggest that the infiltrating cells are directed against a specific antigen.

As some have found an association with responses to *Mycobacterium tuberculosis*, especially heat-shock protein (HSP)-65, the hypothesis that contact with microbacteria may elicit the disease in susceptible individuals has been put forward. Further evidence for a cytotoxic T-cell response in the pathogenesis of Takayasu's arteritis is found in an animal model in pigs in which granulomatous large vessel vasculitis strongly resembling Takayasu's arteritis is induced by a cytotoxic T-cell response following gene transfer of a foreign HLA class I antigen to the vessel (Nabel *et al.* 1990).

Thus, T-cell based autoimmunity seems to underlie giant cell arteritis and Takayasu's arteritis, although the relevant autoantigen(s) and epitopes, whether or not constitutive or modified proteins, are not identified. The disruption of vascular structures and expression of growth factors like platelet-derived growth factors A and B, and tumour growth factor β by the inflammatory infiltrate will lead to aneurysmatic dilatation and migration and proliferation of myofibroblasts in the intima and media with subsequent fibrosis and stenosis.

In other forms of primary vasculitis, T-cells may be involved, but how and to what extent is unclear. In Kawasaki's disease, the infiltrate in small- and medium-sized vessels is predominantly mononuclear. Some have suggested an association of this disease with certain HLA class II antigens, but this could not be confirmed by others. Likewise, data compatible with massive, antigen unrestricted, T-cell stimulation by superantigens from *Staphylococcus* spp. and *Streptococcus* spp. have been reported in this disease, but others failed to confirm this association. In polyarteritis nodosa, the inflammatory vascular infiltrate predominantly consists of $CD8^+$ T-cells and macrophages suggesting cell-mediated immune mechanism in the pathogenesis of this disease (Panegyres *et al.* 1990). The precise role of these cells and the antigen or antigens against which these cells are directed are not known.

General discussion

Despite clear advances made in the last decades in the understanding of mechanisms involved, the pathogenesis of angiitis is not fully understood. General patterns of involvement of both the innate and adaptive immune system have been found and allows categorizing of the inflammatory response of the vasculitic syndromes into primarily immune complex mediated, autoantibody mediated, or T-cell mediated (Table 5). From the pathophysiology of the different syndromes discussed above, it is clear that this pathophysiological distinction into three groups is a gross oversimplification, and that in many forms of vasculitis different forms of immune responses are concurrently or sequentially operative. The proof that autoreactive immunoglobulin response or autoreactive T-cells are definitely the cause of vasculitis is for most vasculitic diseases absent. Furthermore, the antigens to which the autoreactive B- or T-cell response is directed are either not characterized or are tissue non-specific structures that are ubiquitously

Table 5 Immune response pathways presumed to be involved in the pathogenesis of primary systemic vasculitis

Vasculitic syndrome	Immune complexes	Autoantibodies	(Auto-)Reactive T-cells	Known autoantigens	Complement
Giant cell arteritis	−	−	+	−	−
Takayasu's arteritis	−	±	+	−	−
Polyarteritis nodosa	+[a]	−	±	−	−
Kawasaki's syndrome	−	±	±	−	−
Microscopic polyangiitis	−	++	±	+	−
Wegener's granulomatosis	−	++	±	+	−
Churg–Strauss syndrome	−	+	−	−	−
Henoch–Schönlein purpura	++	−	−	−	±
Essential cryoglobulinaemic vasculitis	++	−	−	−	+
Cutaneous leucocyclastic angiitis	++	−	−	−	+

−, not involved in pathogenesis; +, likely to be involved; ±, potentially involved, but maybe only in effector phase; ++, involved in pathogenesis.

[a] In hepatitis B-associated cases.

present. As vasculitic diseases are infrequent, it is clear that very specific circumstances have to be met with respect to the antigens, modified or not, and the response to these antigens. Likewise, the seemingly more elucidated pathogenesis of immune complex vasculitis is not understood, as far as factors resulting in excessive immune complex formation and especially the fact that only a minority of these complex result in vasculitis are concerned. How this occurs in a given patient at a given time is currently unclear. Models using inbred or genetically manipulated animals have provided proof of concept for some pathophysiological hypotheses like the role of cytotoxic T-cells in granulomatous large vessel vasculitis, immune complex mediated vasculitis, and ANCA-related vasculitis.

References

Allen, A. C. *et al.* (1998). Abnormal IgA glycosylation in Henoch–Schönlein purpura restricted to patients with clinical nephritis. *Nephrology, Dialysis, Transplantation* **13**, 930–934.

Ball, G. V. and Bridges, S. L., Jr. (2002). Pathogenesis of vasculitis. In *Vasculitis* (ed. G. V. Ball and S. L. Bridges, Jr.), pp. 34–52. Oxford: Oxford University Press.

Ballieux, B. E. P. B. *et al.* (1994). Detachment and cytolysis of human endothelial cells by proteinase 3. *European Journal of Immunology* **24**, 3211–3215.

Belizna, C. and Cohen Tervaert, J. W. (1997). Specificity, pathogenicity, and clinical value of anti endothelial cell antibodies. *Seminars in Arthritis and Rheumatism* **27**, 98–109.

Blank, M. *et al.* (1995). Immunization with anti-neutrophil cytoplasmic antibody (ANCA) induces the production of mouse ANCA and perivascular lymphocyte infiltration. *Clinical and Experimental Immunology* **102**, 120–130.

Blank, M. *et al.* (1999). Monoclonal anti-endothelial cell antibodies from a patient with Takayasu arteritis activate endothelial cells from large vessels. *Arthritis and Rheumatism* **42**, 1421–1432.

Boomsma, M. M. *et al.* (2000). Prediction of relapses in Wegener's granulomatosis by measurement of antineutrophil cytoplasmic antibody levels: a prospective study. *Arthritis and Rheumatism* **43**, 2025–2033.

Bordron, A. *et al.* (1998). The binding of some human antiendothelial cell antibodies induces endothelial cell apoptosis. *Journal of Clinical Investigation* **101**, 2029–2035.

Brack, A. *et al.* (1997). Giant cell arteritis is a T-cell dependent disease. *Molecular Medicine* **3**, 530–543.

Brentjens, J. R. *et al.* (1975). Experimental chronic serum sickness in rabbits that received daily multiple and high doses of antigen: a systemic disease. *Annals of the New York Academy of Sciences* **254**, 603–613.

Brooks, C. J. *et al.* (1996). IL-1β production by human polymorphonuclear leukocytes stimulated by anti-neutrophil cytoplasmic autoantibodies: relevance to systemic vasculitis. *Clinical and Experimental Immunology* **106**, 273–279.

Brouwer, E. *et al.* (1993). Anti-myeloperoxidase associated proliferative glomerulonephritis: an animal model. *Journal of Experimental Medicine* **177**, 905–914.

Brouwer, E. *et al.* (1994a). Neutrophil activation *in vitro* and *in vivo* in Wegener's granulomatosis. *Kidney International* **45**, 1120–1131.

Brouwer, E. *et al.* (1994b). T cell reactivity to proteinase 3 and myeloperoxidase in patients with Wegener's granulomatosis (WG). *Clinical and Experimental Immunology* **98**, 448–453.

Carvalho, D. *et al.* (1999). IgG anti-endothelial cell autoantibodies from patients with systemic lupus erythematosis or systemic vasculitis stimulate release of two endothelial cell-derived mediators, which enhance adhesion molecule expression and leukocyte adhesion in an autocrine manner. *Arthritis and Rheumatism* **42**, 631–640.

Casselman, B. *et al.* (1995). Antibodies to neutrophil cytoplasmic antigens induce monocyte chemoattractant protein-1 secretion from human monocytes. *Journal of Laboratory and Clinical Medicine* **126**, 495–502.

Chan, T. M. *et al.* (1993). Clinical significance of anti-endothelial cell antibodies in systemic vasculitis: a longitudinal study comparing anti-endothelial cell antibodies and anti-neutrophil cytoplasm antibodies. *American Journal of Kidney Diseases* **22**, 387–392.

Christian, C. L. and Sergent, J. S. (1976). Vasculitis syndromes: clinical and experimental models. *American Journal of Medicine* **61**, 385–392.

Claudy, A. (1998). Pathogenesis of leukocytoclastic vasculitis. *European Journal of Dermatology* **8**, 75–79.

Cochrane, C. G. and Hawkins, D. (1968). Studies on circulating immune complexes. III. Factors governing the ability of circulating complexes to localize in blood vessels. *Journal of Experimental Medicine* **127**, 137–154.

Cohen Tervaert, J. W. *et al.* (1990). Prevention of relapses in Wegener's granulomatosis by treatment based on antineutrophil cytoplasmic antibody titre. *Lancet* **336**, 709–711.

Cohen Tervaert, J. W. *et al.* (1991). Detection of autoantibodies against myeloid lysosomal enzymes: a useful adjunct to classification of patients with biopsy-proven necrotizing arteritis. *American Journal of Medicine* **91**, 59–66.

Csernok, E. *et al.* (1999). Cytokine profiles in Wegener's granulomatosis: predominance of type 1 (Th1) in granulomatous inflammation. *Arthritis and Rheumatism* **42**, 742–750.

Cunningham, M. *et al.* (1999). Predominance of cell-mediated immunity effectors in pauci-immune glomerulonephritis. *Journal of the American Society of Nephrology* **10**, 499–506.

Dammacco, F. *et al.* (2001). The cryoglobulins: an overview. *European Journal of Clinical Investigation* **31**, 628–638.

Davies, D. J. *et al.* (1982). Segmental necrotising glomerulonephritis with antineutrophil antibody: possible arbovirus aetiology? *British Medical Journal* **285**, 606.

Davin, J.-C. and Weening, J. J. (2001). Henoch–Schönlein purpura nephritis: an update. *European Journal of Pediatrics* **160**, 689–695.

Del Papa, N. *et al.* (1992). Antibodies to endothelial cells in primary vasculitides mediate *in vitro* endothelial cytotoxicity in the presence of normal peripheral blood mononuclear cells. *Clinical Immunology and Immunopathology* **63**, 267–274.

Del Papa, N. *et al.* (1996). Anti-endothelial cell IgG antibodies from patients with Wegener's granulomatosis bind to human endothelial cells *in vitro* and induce adhesion molecule expression and cytokine excretion. *Arthritis and Rheumatism* **39**, 758–766.

Dijstelbloem, H. M. *et al.* (1999). Fcγ receptor polymorphisms in Wegener's granulomatosis: risk factors for disease relapse. *Arthritis and Rheumatism* **42**, 1823–1827.

Dijstelbloem, H. M. *et al.* (2000). Fcγ receptor polymorphisms in systemic lupus erythematosus: association with disease and in vivo clearance of immune complexes. *Arthritis and Rheumatism* **43**, 2793–2800.

Dixon, F. J. *et al.* (1958). Pathogenesis of serum sickness. *Archives of Pathology* **65**, 18–28.

Dolman, K. M. *et al.* (1993). Relevance of classic anti-neutrophil cytoplasmic autoantibody (C-ANCA)-mediated inhibition of proteinase-α 1-antitrypsin complexation to disease activity in Wegener's granulomatosis. *Clinical and Experimental Immunology* **93**, 405–410.

Donald, K. J., Edwards, R. L., and McEvoy, J. D. S. (1976). An ultrastructural study of the pathogenesis of tissue injury in limited Wegener's granulomatosis. *Pathology* **8**, 161–169.

Edberg, J. C. *et al.* (1997). Analysis of FcγRII gene polymorphisms in Wegener's granulomatosis. *Experimental and Clinical Immunogenetics* **14**, 183–195.

Ewert, B. H., Jennette, J. C., and Falk, R. J. (1992). Anti-myeloperoxidase antibodies stimulate neutrophils to damage human endothelial cells. *Kidney International* **41**, 375–383.

Falk, R. J. and Jennette, J. C. (1988). Anti-neutrophil cytoplasmic autoantibodies with specificity for myeloperoxidase in patients with systemic vasculitis and idiopathic necrotizing glomerulonephritis. *New England Journal of Medicine* **318**, 1651–1657.

Falk, R. J. *et al.* (1990). Anti-neutrophil cytoplasmic autoantibodies induce neutrophils to degranulate and produce oxygen radicals in vitro. *Proceedings of the National Academy of Sciences of the United States of America* **87**, 4115–4119.

Fauci, A. S., Haynes B. F., and Katz, P. (1978). The spectrum of vasculitis. Clinical, pathologic, immunologic, and therapeutic considerations. *Annals of Internal Medicine* **89**, 660–676.

Frampton, G. *et al.* (1990). Autoantibodies to endothelial cells and neutrophil cytoplasmic antigens in systemic vasculitis. *Clinical and Experimental Immunology* **82**, 227–232.

van der Geld, Y. M. *et al.* (2000). In vitro T lymphocyte responses to proteinase 3 (PR3) and linear peptides of PR3 in patients with Wegener's granulomatosis (WG). *Clinical and Experimental Immunology* **122**, 504–513.

Gephardt, G. N., Ahmad, M., and Tubbs, R. R. (1983). Pulmonary vasculitis (Wegener's granulomatosis). Immunohistochemical study of T and B cell markers. *American Journal of Medicine* **74**, 700–704.

Gower, R. G. *et al.* (1977). Leukocytoclastic vasculitis: sequential appearance of immunoreactants and cellular changes in serial biopsies. *Journal of Investigative Dermatology* **69**, 477–484.

Griffith, M. E., Coulthart, A., and Pusey, C. D. (1996). T cell responses to myeloperoxidase (MPO) and proteinase 3 (PR3) in patients with systemic vasculitis. *Clinical and Experimental Immunology* **103**, 253–258.

Grimminger, F. *et al.* (1996). Neutrophil activation by anti-proteinase 3 antibodies in Wegener's granulomatosis: role of exogenous arachidonic acid and leukotriene B4 generation. *Journal of Experimental Medicine* **184**, 1567–1572.

Grunwald, M. H. *et al.* (1997). Leukocytoclastic vasculitis—correlation between different histological stages and direct immunofluorescence results. *International Journal of Dermatology* **36**, 349–352.

Hagen, E. C. *et al.* (1998). Diagnostic value of standardised assays for anti-neutrophil cytoplasmic antibodies in idiopathic systemic vasculitis: EC/BCR Project for ANCA assay standardization. *Kidney International* **53**, 743–753.

Hall, J. B. *et al.* (1984). Vasculitis and glomerulonephritis: a subgroup with an antineutrophil cytoplasmic antibody. *Australian and New Zealand Journal of Medicine* **14**, 277–278.

Harper, L. and Savage, C. O. S. (2000). Pathogenesis of ANCA-associated systemic vasculitis. *Journal of Pathology* **190**, 349–359.

Harper, L. *et al.* (2001). Neutrophil priming and apoptosis in ANCA-associated vasculitis. *Kidney International* **59**, 1729–1738.

Hart, M. N. *et al.* (1985). Autoimmune vasculitis resulting from in vitro immunization of lymphocytes to smooth muscle. *American Journal of Pathology* **119**, 448–455.

Heeringa, P. *et al.* (1996). Autoantibodies to myeloperoxidase aggravate mild anti-glomerular-basement-membrane-mediated glomerular injury in the rat. *American Journal of Pathology* **149**, 1695–1706.

Heeringa, P. *et al.* (1998). Animal models of anti-neutrophil cytoplasmic antibody associated vasculitis. *Kidney International* **53**, 253–263.

Henson, P. M. and Cochrane, C. G. (1971). Acute immune complex disease in rabbits. The role of complement and of a leukocyte-dependent release of vasoactive amines from platelets. *Journal of Experimental Medicine* **133**, 554–571.

Ihrcke, N. S. and Platt, J. L. (1996). Shedding of heparin sulphate proteoglycan by stimulated endothelial cells: evidence for proteolysis of cell-surface molecules. *Journal of Cellular Physiology* **168**, 625–637.

Jennette, J. C. *et al.* (1994). Nomenclature of systemic vasculitides. Proposal of an International Consensus Conference. *Arthritis and Rheumatism* **37**, 187–192.

Jennette, J. C. and Falk, R. J. (1997). Small-vessel vasculitis. *New England Journal of Medicine* **337**, 1512–1523.

Kallenberg, C. G. M. and Heeringa, P. (1998). Pathogenesis of vasculitis. *Lupus* **7**, 280–284.

Kallenberg, C. G. M. and Cohen Tervaert, J. W. (2002). Autoantibodies in vasculitis. In *Inflammatory Diseases of Blood Vessels* (ed. G. S. Hoffman and C. M. Weyand), pp. 37–56. New York: Marcel Dekker, Inc.

Kallenberg, C. G. M. *et al.* (1994). Anti-neutrophil cytoplasmic antibodies: current diagnostic and pathophysiologic potential. *Kidney International* **46**, 1–15.

Kallenberg, C. G. *et al.* (1995). ANCA-pathophysiology revisited. *Clinical and Experimental Immunology* **100**, 1–3.

Kauffmann, R. H. *et al.* (1980). Circulating and tissue-bound immune complexes in allergic vasculitis: relationship between immunoglobulin class and clinical features. *Clinical and Experimental Immunology* **41**, 459–470.

King, W. J. *et al.* (1995). Endothelial cells and renal epithelial cells do not express the Wegener's autoantigen, proteinase 3. *Clinical and Experimental Immunology* **102**, 98–105.

King, W. J. *et al.* (1998). T lymphocyte responses to anti-neutrophil cytoplasmic autoantibody (ANCA) antigens are present in patients with ANCA-associated systemic vasculitis and persist during disease remission. *Clinical and Experimental Immunology* **112**, 539–546.

Kocher, M. *et al.* (1998). Antineutrophil cytoplasmic antibodies preferentially engage FcγRIIIb on human neutrophils. *Journal of Immunology* **161**, 6909–6914.

Leung, D. Y. M. *et al.* (1986). Two monokines, IL-1 and TNF, render cultured vascular EC susceptible to lysis by antibodies circulating during Kawasaki syndrome. *Journal of Experimental Medicine* **164**, 1958–1972.

Levine, S. M. and Hellmann, D. B. (2002). Giant cell arteritis. *Current Opinion in Rheumatology* **14**, 3–10.

Lindquist, K. J. and Osterland, C. K. (1971). Human antibodies to vascular endothelium. *Clinical and Experimental Immunology* **9**, 753–762.

Lindsey, N. J. *et al.* (1994). Inhibition of prostacyclin release by endothelial binding anticardiolipin antibodies in thrombosis-prone patients with SLE and the anti-phospholipid syndrome. *British Journal of Rheumatology* **33**, 20–26.

Lobatto, S. *et al.* (1988). Abnormal clearance of soluble aggregates of human immunoglobulin G in patients with systemic lupus erythematosus. *Clinical and Experimental Immunology* **72**, 55–59.

Ludviksson, B. *et al.* (1998). Active Wegener's granulomatosis is associated with HLA-DR+ CD4+ T cells exhibiting an unbalanced Th1-type T cell cytokine pattern: reversal by IL-10. *Journal of Immunology* **160**, 3602–3609.

McCluskey, R. T. and Fienberg, R. (1983). Vasculitis in primary vasculitides, granulomatoses, and connective tissue diseases. *Human Pathology* **14**, 302–315.

McDougal, J. S. and MacDuffie, F. C. (1985). Immune complexes in man: detection and clinical significance. *Advances in Clinical Chemistry* **28**, 1–60.

McMahon, B. J. *et al.* (1989). Hepatitis B-associated polyarteritis nodosa in Alaskan Eskimos: clinical and epidemiologic features and long-term follow up. *Hepatology* **9**, 97–101.

Mayet, W. J. *et al.* (1993). Human endothelial cells express proteinase 3, the target antigen of anti-cytoplasmic antibodies in Wegener's granulomatosis. *Blood* **82**, 1221–1229.

Michalak, T. (1978). Immune complexes of hepatitis B surface antigen in the pathogenesis of periarteritis nodosa. A study of seven necropsy cases. *American Journal of Pathology* **90**, 619–632.

Miyakawa, Y. *et al.* (1981). Defective immune-adherence (C3b) receptor on erythrocytes from patients with systemic lupus erythematosus. *Lancet* **2**, 493–497.

Moyer, F. and Reinisch, C. L. (1984). The role of vascular smooth muscle cells in experimental autoimmune vasculitis. I. The initiation of delayed type hypersensitivity angiitis. *American Journal of Pathology* **117**, 380–390.

Mulder, A. H. L. *et al.* (1994). Activation of granulocytes by anti-neutrophil cytoplasmic antibodies (ANCA); a FcγRII-dependent process. *Clinical and Experimental Immunology* **78**, 270–278.

Mulder, A. H., Stegeman, C. A., and Kallenberg, C. G. (1995). Activation of granulocytes by anti-neutrophil cytoplasmic antibodies (ANCA) in Wegener's granulomatosis: a predominant role for the IgG3 subclass of ANCA. *Clinical and Experimental Immunology* **101**, 227–232.

Muller Kobold, A. C. *et al.* (1998a). Are circulating neutrophils intravascularly activated in patients with anti-neutrophil cytoplasmic antibody (ANCA)-associated vasculitides? *Clinical and Experimental Immunology* **114**, 491–498.

Muller Kobold, A. C., Kallenberg, C. G. M., and Cohen Tervaert, J. W. (1998b). Leukocyte membrane expression of proteinase 3 correlates with disease activity in patients with Wegener's granulomatosis. *British Journal of Rheumatology* **37**, 901–907.

Muller Kobold, A. C. *et al.* (1999). Pathophysiology of ANCA-associated glomerulonephritis. *Nephrology, Dialysis, Transplantation* **14**, 1366–1375.

Nabel, E. G., Plautz, G., and Nabel, G. J. (1990). Transduction of a foreign histocompatibility gene into the arterial wall induces vasculitis. *Proceedings of the National Academy of Sciences of the United States of America* **89**, 5157–5161.

Pall, A. A. *et al.* (1996). Glomerular vascular cell adhesion molecule-1 expression in renal vasculitis. *Journal of Clinical Pathology* **49**, 238–242.

Panegyres, P. *et al.* (1990). Vasculitis of peripheral nerve and skeletal muscle: clinicopathological corrleation and immunopathic mechanisms. *Journal of Neurological Science* **100**, 193–202.

Pendergraft, W. F. *et al.* (2000). ANCA antigens, proteinase 3 and myeloperoxidase, are not expressed in endothelial cells. *Kidney International* **57**, 1981–1990.

Pol, W. L. van der and Winkel, J. G. J. van de (1998). IgG receptor polymorphisms: risk factor for disease. *Immunogenetics* **48**, 222–232.

Popa, E. R. *et al.* (1999). Differential B- and T-cell activation in Wegener's granulomatosis. *Journal of Allergy and Clinical Immunology* **103**, 885–894.

Porges, A. J. *et al.* (1994). Anti-neutrophil cytoplasmic antibodies engage and activate human neutrophils via Fc gamma RIIa. *Journal of Immunology* **153**, 1271–1278.

Radford, D. J., Savage, C. O. S., and Nash, G. B. (2000). Activation of neutrophil β2-integrin and induction of firm adhesion by anti-neutrophil cytoplasm autoantibodies (ANCA). *Arthritis and Rheumatism* **43**, 1337–1345.

Radford, D. J. *et al.* (2001). Antineutrophil cytoplasmic antibodies stabilize adhesion and promote migration of flowing neutrophils on endothelial cells. *Arthritis and Rheumatism* **44**, 2851–2861.

Ralston, D. *et al.* (1997). Antineutrophil cytoplasmic antibodies induce monocyte IL-8 release. Role of surface proteinase-3, alpha1-antitrypsin, and Fcγ receptors. *Journal of Clinical Investigation* **100**, 1416–1424.

Rarok, A. A. *et al.* (2002). Membrane expression of neutrophil proteinase 3 (PR3) is related to relapse in PR3–ANCA associated vasculitis. *Journal of the American Society of Nephrology* **13**, 2232–2238.

Rastaldi, M. *et al.* (1996). Intraglomerular and interstitial leukocyte infiltration, adhesion molecules, and interleukin-1 alpha expression in 15 cases of antineutrophil cytoplasmic autoantibody-associated renal vasculitis. *American Journal of Kidney Diseases* **27**, 48–57.

Reumaux, D. *et al.* (1995). Effect of tumor necrosis factor-induced integrin activation on Fc gamma receptor II-mediated signal transduction: relevance for activation of neutrophils by anti-proteinase 3 or anti-myeloperoxidase antibodies. *Blood* **86**, 3189–3195.

Sais, G. *et al.* (1997). Adhesion molecule expression and endothelial cell activation in cutaneous leukocytoclastic vasculitis. *Archives of Dermatology* **133**, 443–450.

Savage, C. O. S. (2001). ANCA-associated renal vasculitis. *Kidney International* **60**, 1614–1627.

Savage, C. O. S. *et al.* (1991). Vascular damage in Wegener's granulomatosis and microscopic polyarteritis: presence of anti-endothelial antibodies and their relation to anti-neutrophil cytoplasmic antibodies. *Clinical and Experimental Immunology* **85**, 14–19.

Savage, C. O. S. *et al.* (1992). Autoantibodies developing to myeloperoxidase and proteinase 3 in systemic vasculitis stimulate neutrophil cytotoxicity toward cultured endothelial cells. *American Journal of Pathology* **141**, 335–342.

Savige, J. *et al.* (2000). Antineutrophil cytoplasmic antibodies and associated diseases: a review of the clinical and laboratory features. *Kidney International* **57**, 846–862.

Schifferli, J. A., Ng, Y. C., and Peters, D. K. (1986). The role of complement and its receptor in the elimination of immune complexes. *New England Journal of Medicine* **315**, 488–495.

Schwarting, A. *et al.* (2000). Proteinase-3 mRNA expressed by glomerular epithelial cells correlates with crescent formation in Wegener's granulomatosis. *Kidney International* **57**, 2412–2422.

Seko, Y. Takayasu's arteritis: pathogenesis. In *Inflammatory Diseases of Blood Vessels* (ed. G. S. Hoffman and C. M. Weyand), pp. 443–453. New York: Marcel Dekker, Inc, 2002.

Somer, T. and Finegold, S. M. (1995). Vasculitides associated with infections, immunization and antimicrobial drugs. *Clinics of Infectious Diseases* **20**, 1010–1036.

Stegeman, C. A. *et al.* (1993). Serum markers of T cell activation in relapses of Wegener's granulomatosis. *Clinical and Experimental Immunology* **91**, 415–420.

Stegeman, C. A. *et al.* (1994). Association of chronic nasal carriage of *Staphylococcus aureus* and higher relapse rates in Wegener granulomatosis. *Annals of Internal Medicine* **120**, 12–17.

Sylvestre, D. L. and Ravetch, J. V. (1994). Fc receptors initiate the Arthus reaction: redefining the inflammatory cascade. *Science* **265**, 1095–1098.

Taekema-Roelvink, M. E. *et al.* (1998). Effect of anti-neutrophil cytoplasmic antibodies on proteinase 3-induced apoptosis of human endothelial cells. *Scandinavian Journal of Immunology* **48**, 37–43.

Taekema-Roelvink, M. E. *et al.* (2000). Proteinase 3 interacts with a 111-kD membrane molecule of human umbilical vein endothelial cells. *Journal of the American Society of Nephrology* **11**, 640–648.

Taekema-Roelvink, M. E. *et al.* (2001). Proteinase 3 enhances endothelial monocyte chemoattractant protein-1 production and induces increased adhesion of neutrophils to endothelial cells by upregulating intercellular cell adhesion molecule-1. *Journal of the American Society of Nephrology* **12**, 932–940.

Trepo, C. G. *et al.* (1974). The role of circulating hepatitis B antigen/antibody immune complexes in the pathogenesis of vascular and hepatic manifestations in polyarteritis nodosa. *Journal of Clinical Pathology* **27**, 863–868.

Tse, W. Y. *et al.* (2000). Neutrophil FcgammaRIIIb allelic polymorphism in anti-neutrophil cytoplasmic antibody (ANCA)-positive systemic vasculitis. *Clinical and Experimental Immunology* **119**, 574–577.

Van der Woude, F. J. *et al.* (1985). Autoantibodies to neutrophils and monocytes: a new tool for diagnosis and a marker of disease activity in Wegener's Granulomatosis. *Lancet* **ii**, 425–429.

Weyand, C. M. *et al.* (1997). Disease patterns and tissue cytokine profiles in giant cell arteritis. *Arthritis and Rheumatism* **40**, 19–26.

Weyand, C. M. and Goronzy, J. J. (1999). Arterial wall injury in giant cell arteritis. *Arthritis and Rheumatism* **42**, 844–853.

Witko-Sarsat, V. *et al.* (1999). A large subset of neutrophils expressing membrane proteinase 3 is a risk factor for vasculitis and rheumatoid arthritis. *Journal of the American Society of Nephrology* **10**, 1224–1233.

Xiao, H. *et al.* (2002). Antineutrophil cytoplasmic autoantibodies specific for myeloperoxidase cause glomerulonephritis and vasculitis in mice. *Journal of Clinical Investigation* **110**, 955–963.

4.5.2 The nephritis of Henoch–Schönlein purpura

Rosanna Coppo and Alessandro Amore

Definition and diagnostic criteria

The association of 'petechial haemorrhages on lower limbs, joint and abdominal pains, bloody stools, and urine tinged with blood' was first reported by Heberden at the beginning of the nineteenth century (Heberden 1801). A few decades later, Schönlein named the association of purpura and joint pain 'peliosis (purpura) rheumatica' (Schönlein 1832), and his pupil Henoch reported the frequent presence of gastrointestinal symptoms and kidney involvement (Henoch 1868). Henoch–Schönlein purpura (HSP) is the most common definition of a vasculitis of the small blood vessels with clinical presentation of a multiorgan involvement syndrome with variable expression in skin, gastro-intestinal tract, joints, and kidneys (Meadow *et al.* 1972; Mills *et al.* 1990). The combination of various systemic and renal symptoms leads to apparently different clinical entities and often overlaps the features of autoimmune diseases. The difficulty of correctly interpreting the frequently associated cutaneous allergic reactions to drugs and the role played by infectious agents led to the past ambiguous definitions of hypersensitivity angiitis, anaphylactoid purpura, or streptococcal rheumatic peliosis.

In 1990, the American College of Rheumatology considered that for the diagnosis of HSP the presence of two of the four criteria—palpable purpura, age less than 20 years at disease onset, bowel angina, and cutaneous biopsy showing granulocytes in the walls of small arterioles or venules (leucocytoclastic vasculitis)—yields a sensitivity of 87 per cent and a specificity of 88 per cent (Mills *et al.* 1990). The diagnostic power of the IgA vascular deposits was stressed by the 1994 Consensus Conference on Nomenclature of Systemic Vasculitides which defined HSP as a small vessel vasculitis (involving capillaries, arterioles, venules) with IgA-dominant immune deposits, typically involving skin, gut, and glomeruli and associated with arthralgias or arthritis (Jennette *et al.* 1994).

Clinical and laboratory features

Epidemiology and enhancing factors

In children, HSP is the most frequent vasculitis (Meadow *et al.* 1972) and accounts for about 14/100,000 cases/year (Nielsen 1988). The median age at onset is about 4 years and rarely affects children under 2 years of age (Cameron 1984). HSP is more frequent in males, with a 1.5–2 : 1 preponderance (Habib and Cameron 1982). HSP is a relatively uncommon disease in adults, though it can occasionally affect old people. In part, the lower frequency is consequent upon difficulties in the differential diagnosis, sometimes overlapping other forms of more frequent systemic vasculitides in adults. However, it is evident that children are far more commonly affected than adults, for unknown reasons. Renal involvement also is most frequent in the first and second decades of life (Lévy *et al.* 1976; Rieu and Noel 1999). The geographical distribution is somehow similar to primary IgA nephropathy (IgAN), HSP being more common in Europe, particularly in France, Italy, Spain, the United Kingdom (Meadow *et al.* 1972), and Finland, and in Asia, including Japan (Yoshikawa *et al.* 1987), Singapore, and China, while it is less common in North America and Africa. Racial differences may play a role as Blacks and Indians are rarely affected (Emancipator 1998).

Aetiology

The aetiology of HSP is unknown. Triggering factors are reported in about two-thirds of the cases (Lévy *et al.* 1976), mostly infections and particularly in children. Streptococcus β, Yersina, Mycoplasma, Toxoplasma, varicella, measles, rubella, adenovirus, HIV, and several other agents have been sporadically recorded among the enhancing factors, but without evidence of causality (Davin *et al.* 2001). There is a peak incidence in winter in North Europe and in June in Italy (Coppo *et al.* 1999). A coincident role of allergic reactions to vaccination against smallpox or influenza (Patel *et al.* 1988), drugs (including ciprofloxacin, angiotensin converting enzyme inhibitors and angiotensin II receptor antagonists, vancomycin, minocycline, carbazepine, caridopa/levodopa, and others), or other allergens has also been strongly suspected in some cases (Davin *et al.* 2001).

Cancer, monoclonal IgA gammopathy, chronic alcoholic liver disease, trauma, and a number of other miscellaneous factors have been reported to be associated to HSP (Rostoker 2001).

Some familial cases and restricted epidemic clusters of HSP have been observed (Farley *et al.* 1989).

Systemic manifestations

Children, more frequently than adults, present with systemic extrarenal clinical picture of multiorgan involvement and of particular severity (Lévy *et al.* 1976; Coppo *et al.* 1997a, 1999).

Skin

The skin lesions are characteristic and consist of slightly raised 'palpable' purpuric macules that do not disappear on pressure and are not related to thrombocytopenia. Typically, the skin lesions begin with erythematous macules, some of which develop into slightly raised urticarial papules, which soon become purpuric and eventually take a fawn colour as they fade. The purpuric rash is symmetrically distributed over the extensor surfaces of the lower limbs and forearms and over the sides of buttocks (Fig. 1) and may be confluent in large patches.

The purpura is mostly present in the ankle area and in the milder cases it presents only there. It is also common in pressure areas such as occurs with belts and pants. The purpuric lesions occasionally affect earlobes, nose, and genitalia. Fever and general malaise may accompany the rash. At the beginning the picture is hardly distinguishable from infectious purpuras or allergic reactions.

At microscopic examination, the lesions consist of leucocytoclastic vasculitis of dermal vessels with IgA deposits in the vascular walls (Fig. 2).

The purpura lasts for a few days, often relapses in new crops of lesions when the first eruption ceases. It recurs in almost one-third of cases, up to 10 times during the follow-up (Coppo *et al.* 1997a), sometimes in association with the other symptoms, but this is generally unrelated to the severity of renal lesions.

Gastrointestinal tract

The abdominal manifestations include diffuse abdominal pain, increasing after meals, referred to as 'bowel angina', often accompanied by vomiting, haematemesis, and melena (Mills *et al.* 1990). In some cases, the pain is so severe that it mimics an acute surgical emergency, although intussusception, intestinal infarction, bowel perforation are very rare events. In these cases laparotomy is often necessary; however, a spontaneous reduction may be induced by relieving bowel-wall oedema using antihistamine and steroid therapy.

The gastrointestinal symptoms are reported in 50–70 per cent of all cases (Meadow *et al.* 1972), more frequently in children (62 per cent) than adults (47 per cent) (Coppo *et al.* 1999), and incidence rises to 90 per cent in patients with renal involvement when mucosal purpura is checked by gastroscopy or colonoscopy.

Joints

Transient arthralgias due to oligoarticular synovitis, mostly involving lower limb articulations, ankles, and knees, are reported in 50–70 per cent of all cases (Meadow *et al.* 1972). A periarticular oedema may be present. These lesions do not evolve into joint erosions or deformities.

Other extrarenal manifestations

Convulsions, encephalopathy, chorea, or blindness occasionally occur due to cerebral vasculitis (Yoshikawa 1997). Other rare manifestations include pulmonary–renal syndrome, cardiopulmonary syndrome,

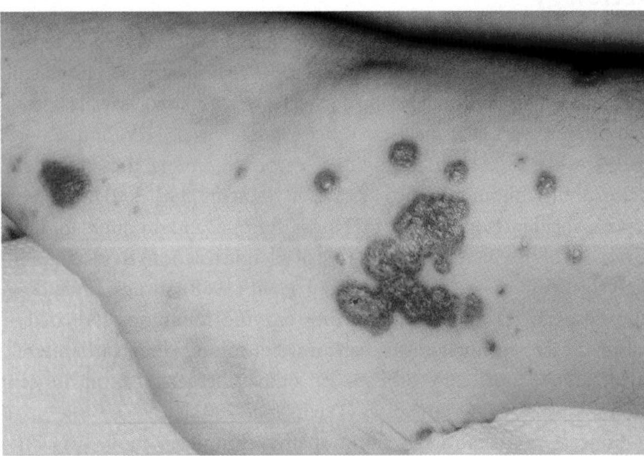

Fig. 1 Purpuric rash of Henoch–Schönlein purpura.

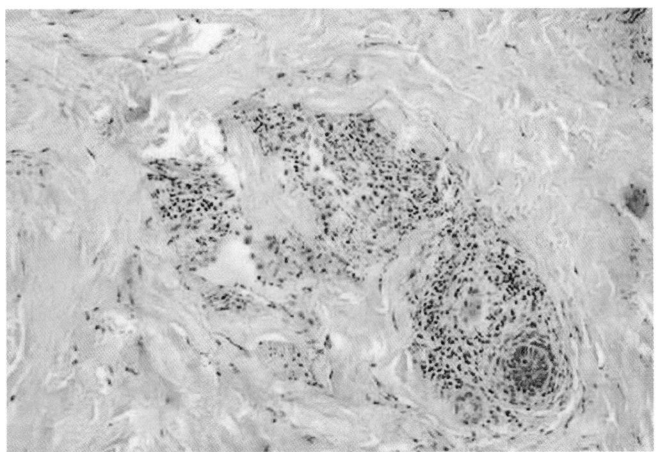

(a)

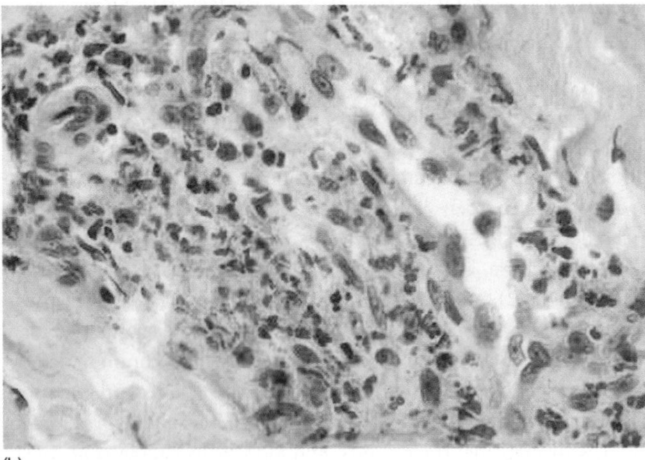

(b)

Fig. 2 Skin biopsy of HSP lesion. Leucocytoclastic vasculitis in the wall of a small dermal vessel: (a) haematoxylin and eosin stain 100×; (b) haematoxylin and eosin stain 400×.

pancreatitis, adrenal bleeding, or testicular, rather than ovarian involvement mimicking torsion (Davin *et al.* 2001).

Haemorrhagic ureteritis is a clinical feature sometimes occurring in children, usually below the age of 5 years (Kher *et al.* 1983). The clinical presentation is haematuria, associated with loin pain and renal colic. The necrotizing vasculitis and ureteritis may lead to ureteral obstruction, occasionally bilateral (Bruce *et al.* 1997; Garcia-Nieto and Claverie-Martini 1998). Ureteric lesions, when healed by, may progress to ureteral stenosis often requiring surgical correction.

Kidney

The proportion of childhood patients with renal involvement has been reported to range from 20 to 100 per cent (Yoshikawa 1997) according to the preselection of the cohorts investigated (Meadow *et al.* 1972; Lévy *et al.* 1976; Habib and Cameron 1982; Yoshikawa *et al.* 1987; Nielsen 1988). The frequencies vary according to the inclusion of serial urinalyses in the routine laboratory tests performed. Moreover, renal lesions may occur without clinical signs, or be evident only after some careful follow-up. Indeed, the percentage of renal involvement increases progressively to 35 per cent after 1 year and continues to increase thereafter (Kaku *et al.* 1998). Hence, late renal involvement can be missed in mild cases not sequentially investigated.

In unselected cohorts of children, the prevalence of the renal involvement during the course of HSP is a mean of 33 per cent, whereas in adults it is much more frequent (mean 63 per cent) (Rieu and Noel 1999) (Fig. 3).

A 50 per cent renal involvement with urinary abnormalities was detected in adults diagnosed by means of the very specific criteria of presence of leucocytoclastic skin vasculitis with IgA vascular deposits (Tancrede-Bohin *et al.* 1997). Even if it cannot be excluded that mildest cases of renal involvement among children could be underdiagnosed, and that some adult patients could be misdiagnosed as primitive vasculitis, the more frequent development of renal disease in older patients remains unquestionable and unexplained.

In cohorts of patients selected for a kidney disease severe enough to warrant renal biopsy, the prevalence of the glomerulonephritis secondary to HSP of all renal diseases is higher in children: 11.6 versus 3.5 per cent in the whole cohort in the Italian register of renal biopsies (Coppo *et al.* 1998), data comparable to French series (10–15 per cent of glomerulonephritis in children versus 2 per cent in adults) (Rieu and Noel 1999).

General paediatricians often report a systemic disease with modest and transient urinary abnormalities (Farine *et al.* 1986), whereas paediatric nephrologists and nephrologists describe much more severe and often chronic renal involvement both in children (Lévy *et al.* 1976; Yoshikawa *et al.* 1981; Goldstein *et al.* 1992) and in adults (Fogazzi *et al.* 1989; Rieu and Noel 1999). The HSP manifestations range from isolated microscopic haematuria, gross haematuria, proteinuria, to nephrotic syndrome (Rieu and Noel 1999). When the analysis is made on HSP patients with a renal disease severe enough to warrant renal biopsy, the severity of the clinical presentation is similar in adults and children except for a higher frequency of nephrotic syndrome in children (Coppo *et al.* 1997a; Coppo and Amore 2001).

Isolated microscopic haematuria is the more frequent clinical presentation of HSP nephritis in non-selected cohorts, particularly the paediatric ones (Farine *et al.* 1986; Blanco *et al.* 1997). Haematuria is detected within 4 weeks of onset of illness in 80 per cent of cases. It is often transient, detectable only by routine urinalysis during the acute illness, and followed by a complete and lasting remission. Instead, when haematuria persists, the nephritis become chronic, and proteinuria often develops. In non-selected series of children, nephrotic syndrome is detected less frequently than in adults. Renal function is often normal at the beginning, particularly in children, but sometimes there is

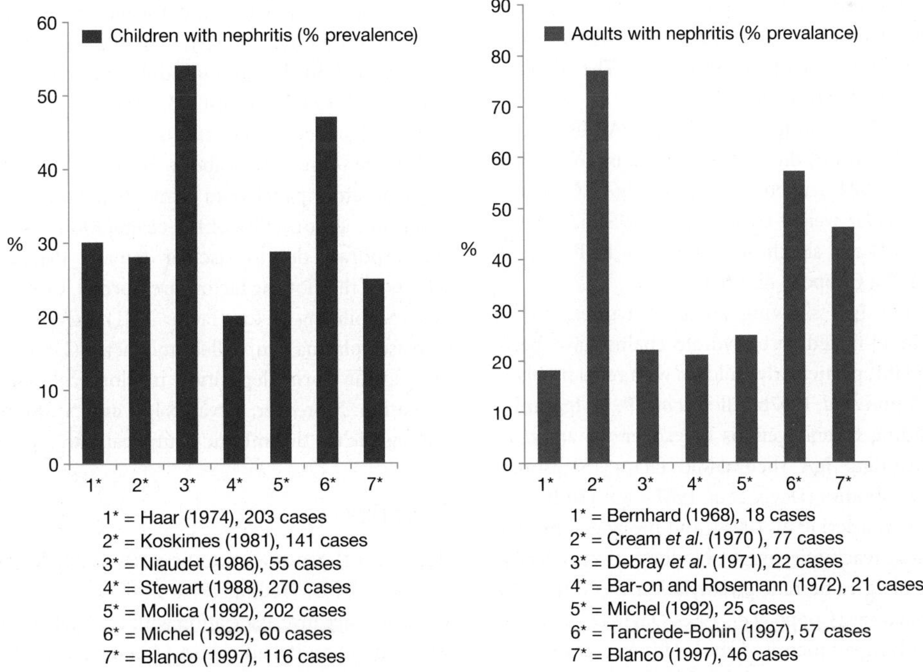

Fig. 3 Renal involvement detected by urinalysis in unselected cohorts of patients with Henoch–Schönlein purpura.

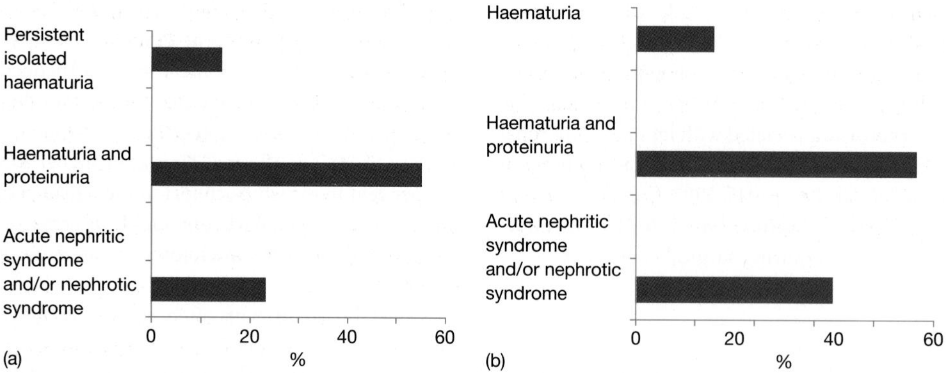

Fig. 4 Renal clinical features in patients with nephritis of Henoch–Schönlein purpura. (a) Cumulative series of children with renal involvement (666) patients (Koskimies 1981; Niaudet *et al.* 1986; Stewart 1988; Michel 1992; Mollica 1992; Blanco 1997). (b) Cumulative series of adults with renal involvement (184 patients) (Bernhard 1968; Cream *et al.* 1970; Debray *et al.* 1971; Bar-on and Rosemann 1972; Blanco 1997).

a functional impairment at onset. Acute nephritic syndrome, often with hypertension is observed in about half of the cases. In rare cases, the disease rapidly progress to renal insufficiency (Rieu and Noel 1999) (Fig. 4).

Palpable purpura often precedes or is coincident with the onset of nephritis, nevertheless in 10 per cent of the cases purpura follows renal symptoms by weeks or months, leading to initial diagnosis of idiopathic IgAN (Coppo *et al.* 1997a). These observations confirm the weak distinction between idiopathic IgAN and HSP nephritis discussed later. However, it is interesting that macroscopic haematuria coincident with upper respiratory tract infections, so common in IgAN patients, was reported in only 7 per cent of patients needing renal biopsy (4 per cent of adults and 19 per cent of children) (Coppo and Amore 2001).

Serum abnormalities

Mean serum IgA concentrations are increased, as in the idiopathic IgAN, but the increase is often limited to the acute illness, and serum IgA returns within normal values as the disease heals. The increase mainly involves polymeric IgA1 (Davin *et al.* 2001).

IgA immune complexes (IC), and IgA1/IgA1IC or IgA/fibronectin aggregates have been detected mostly during the acute phases or during relapses (Coppo *et al.* 1982, 1984; Jennette *et al.* 1991), IgA1IC, mixed IgA/IgGIC, and high molecular weight complexes (>19S) have been reported to be more frequent and significantly higher in HSP than in IgAN (Kauffmann *et al.* 1980; Coppo *et al.* 1984).

Aberrantly glycosylated IgA showing signs of truncation of GalNAC-Gal sequence in *O*-linked carbohydrate chains have been detected in patients with HSP, particularly children with renal involvement (Saulsbury 1997; Coppo *et al.* 1997b; Allen *et al.* 1998). IgA antibodies with specific binding to endogenous or exogenous antigens have been reported, including IgA rheumatoid factor (Saulsbury 1986), anti-α-galactosyl antibodies (Davin *et al.* 1987), IgA binding to mesangial cell antigens (Fornasieri *et al.* 1995), and mesangial matrix (Coppo *et al.* 1993). These reactivities might be due to lectin–lectin interactions consequent to IgA aberrant glycosylation more than to true antigen–antibody reactions (Coppo *et al.* 1993; Davin *et al.* 2001).

In HSP with renal involvement increased levels of IgA reacting with sonicated neutrophil extracts (antineutrophil cytoplasm antibodies of the IgA isotype, IgA–ANCA) and with purified cytoplasmatic antigens (myeloperoxidase) have been detected (Ronda *et al.* 1994; Coppo *et al.* 1997b). The presence and the meaning of IgA–ANCA is still debated, and lectin-like interactions are likely to play a role in this reactivity as discussed above.

IgA-producing T-cells are increased in circulation during the acute phase of the disease and abnormalities of T-suppressor activity are limited to the acute phase (Casanueva *et al.* 1990). Transforming growth factor (TGF) β-secreting T-cells have been detected in circulation during the phases of clinical activity of HSP, while resolved during recovery (Davin *et al.* 2001). In patients with HSP nephritis a reduction in Fcγ, C3b, and Fn receptor function of mononuclear phagocytes has been reported (Davin *et al.* 1985). These abnormalities were transient, probably secondary to saturation of receptors more than a primary event. Plasma IgE levels are increased in HSP, and significantly higher than in IgAN (Davin *et al.* 1994). Serum eosinophil cationic protein is elevated in HSP (Namgoong *et al.* 1997). Serum C3 and C4 values are within the normal ranges, even though CH50 and properdin are often reduced. These data, together with the frequent increase in C3d detected in adults and children (Coppo *et al.* 1982; Smith *et al.* 1997), suggest C3 activation, possibly via the alternative pathway, balanced by enhanced factor synthesis.

If there is any doubt about the aetiology of the purpura, the clotting laboratory panel gives elements for the differential diagnosis. No significant abnormality of the coagulation cascade is detectable, since the purpura is due to vascular damage. Platelet count as well as the activity of the clotting factors are normal. Conversely, abnormalities in fibrin-stabilizing factor (factor XIII) have been reported along with increased plasma von Willebrand factor (De Mattia *et al.* 1995), which may favour fibrin deposition in glomerular structures and crescent formation. Moreover, elevated IgA anticardiolipin antibodies may be responsible for thrombotic complications.

Genetics

HLA Class II genes seem to be a risk factor for HSP. A positive association with DRB1*01 and DRB1*11 (64 versus 48 per cent in the controls) as well as a negative association with HLA DRB1*07 was first reported by our group in an Italian cohort (Amoroso *et al.* 1997) and confirmed in an Hispanic cohort (Amoli *et al.* 2001b). In Japanese patients, there is an increase in DQA1*0301 (Jin *et al.* 1996). Genetic studies on Class III region have shown an increased frequency of homozygous C4A or C4B null phenotype in Caucasians (Mc Lean *et al.* 1984) and in Japanese patients (Jin *et al.* 1996). We, as well as others, failed to detect any association with manifestations or progression of HSP nephritis and the ACE–gene polymorphism (Amoroso *et al.* 1998). It has been recently reported that the polymorphism of the intracellular adhesion molecule 1 (ICAM-1) decreases the risk of developing severe gastrointestinal complications and may reduce the risk of renal sequelae (Amoli *et al.* 2001a).

Histopathology

Light microscopy

HSP nephritis is characterized by mesangial damage with different degrees of hypercellularity (Fig. 5), ranging from focal–segmental endocapillary proliferation to crescent formations.

These lesions are extremely variable among patients and during the course of the disease in the single case (Lévy *et al.* 1976). The classification of renal damage considered the severity of the proliferative intra- and extracapillary lesions (Meadow *et al.* 1972; Emancipator 1998).

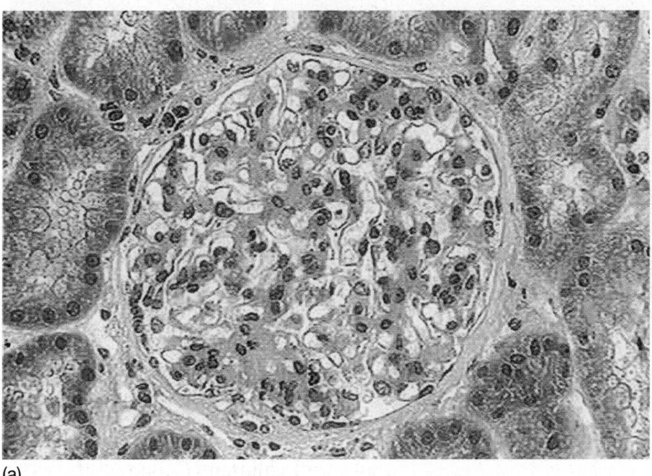

(a)

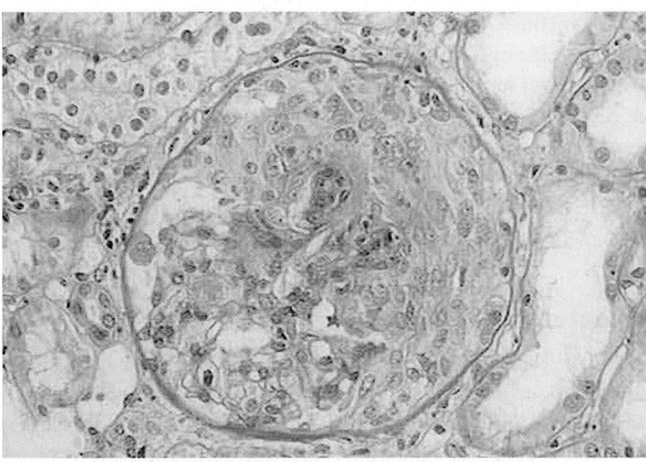

(b)

Fig. 5 Renal biopsy specimen from a patient with nephritis of Henoch–Schönlein purpura showing (a) expansion of the mesangial matrix and mild increase in mesangial cellularity (Trichrome 250×); (b) a circumferential cellular crescent (PAS 250×).

Six histological classes are distinguished according to presence/absence and extension of extracapillary proliferation, with subclasses defining the characteristics of the endocapillary lesions (Table 1).

The segmental proliferative lesions frequently show adhesions of the tuft to parietal epithelium in coincidence of which are sometimes found splitting and duplication of basal membranes. Only in rare cases, is there a severe mesangial proliferation associated with mesangial interposition in which cells and matrix migrate into the capillary walls, between the basement membrane and endothelial cytoplasm, mimicking a membranoproliferative glomerulonephritis. When proliferation is severe, polymorphonuclear cells may infiltrate the glomerular tufts, sometimes as severely as in acute poststreptococcal glomerulonephritis. Lobules with extensive intracapillary and extracapillary proliferation may undergo necrosis, or rarely mesangiolysis, with aneurismal capillary dilation. Focal fibrinoid necrosis is often present at onset, which corresponds, at a later time, to disorganized sclerosis. Intracapillary glomerular thrombi can be observed.

Crescents involve from a few lobules to the entire capsular circumference. At onset crescents are cellular, then evolve into fibrous crescents, generating segmental scars or global sclerosis. Adhesions between visceral and parietal epithelium may occur, leading to obliteration of the urinary space. The most common histological feature is a predominance of small crescents, with some large ones and only rarely repair without fibrosis, the latter indicates more severe cases and the fibrous evolution is common.

In patients, either adults or children having a disease so severe to warrant renal biopsy, extracapillary proliferation is detected in half or more of the cases (Yoshikawa *et al.* 1987; Coppo *et al.* 1997a). When present, proliferative extracapillary lesions often involve less than 50 per cent of glomeruli (class III) and are associated with polymorphonuclear

Table 1 Classification of Henoch–Schönlein nephritis lesions according to Emancipator (1998)

Class I	Minimal glomerular lesions and absence of crescents
Class II	No crescents IIa: pure mesangial proliferation IIb: focal–segmental endocapillary proliferation IIc: diffuse endocapillary proliferation
Class III	Presence of extracapillary cellular proliferation in <50% of glomeruli IIIa: in association with focal and segmental endocapillary proliferation IIIb: with diffuse endocapillary proliferation
Class IV	Florid extracapillary proliferation in 50–75% of glomeruli IVa: in association with focal and segmental endocapillary proliferation IVb: with diffuse endocapillary proliferation
Class V	extracapillary proliferation in >75% of glomeruli Va: in association with focal and segmental endocapillary proliferation Vb: with diffuse endocapillary proliferation
Class VI	Pseudo-membranoproliferative glomerulonephritis

glomerular infiltration. In some biopsies (2 per cent of adults and 15 per cent of children), periglomerular inflammatory infiltrates, mostly associated with crescents, can be observed (Coppo *et al.* 1997a).

Blood vessels may show medial hypertrophy and intimal fibroelastosis. Hyalin change and/or accumulation of fibrinoid material, or necrosis with inflammatory infiltration and clear findings of vasculitis can be present. In the past, these lesions were considered of diagnostic value; nevertheless, the presence of capillary necrosis even in idiopathic IgAN invalidates this putative criterion.

Necrosis of the capillary tuft has been reported in 10 per cent of adults and 8 per cent of children, coincident with extracapillary proliferation. In 30 per cent of the biopsies (both adult and paediatric cases), atherosclerotic lesions and arteriolar hyalinosis lesions have been reported (Coppo *et al.* 1997a).

Degenerative tubular alterations with flattening, vacuolization, desquamation, and loss of the brush-border microvilli are often detected, focally, in the cortical tubuli and they are more frequent than in the idiopathic IgAN (Emancipator 1998). Tubular cylinders and blood casts are detected in 30 per cent of patients. Tubular focal atrophy is common. A severe lymphomonocytic interstitial infiltration characterizes the progressive cases.

Immunohistochemistry

The characteristic feature is granular mesangial IgA deposition which, in contrast with the frequent focal and segmental proliferative changes, is always diffuse as in primary IgAN (Fig. 6).

IgA1 is the dominant subclass with equal distribution of light chains. The J-chain is generally present indicating deposits of dimeric IgA, whereas the secretory tract is absent. Extensive subendothelial deposits are associated with the most severe histological forms with endocapillary proliferation and/or crescent formation.

As for idiopathic IgAN, C3 is codeposited in 75–85 per cent of the cases. The membrane attack complex C5–C9 and the alternative complement pathway components are regularly detected (Evans *et al.* 1973). Early classical pathway complement components C1q and C4 are present only rarely and stain with low intensity (Emancipator 1998). IgG and IgM codeposits are present in 40 per cent of the cases. Fibrin/fibrinogen deposits are found in 60–70 per cent of patients, both in mesangial and in parietal areas, often coincident with mesangial proliferation suggesting a role of the clotting cascade activation. Glomerular fibrin-related deposits are much more frequently present in HSP nephritis than in IgAN (Habib and Cameron 1982), and are often related to active disease with extracapillary proliferation. In cases with severe glomerular changes, deposits of IgA and C3 can be found in arterioles and/or cortical peritubular capillaries.

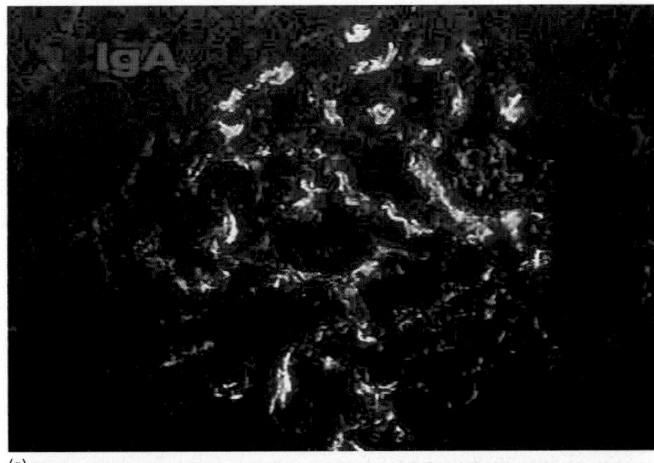

(a)

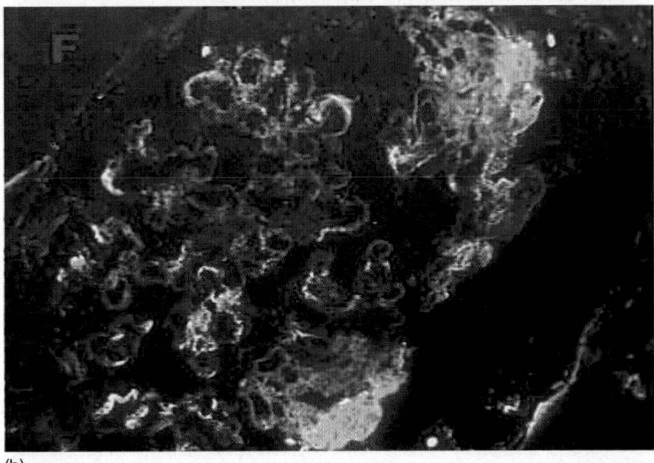

(b)

Fig. 6 Immunopathology of Henoch–Schönlein nephritis: (a) mesangial deposits of IgA (anti-IgA 250×); (b) segmental positivity of fibrinogen in the area of necrotizing extracapillary proliferation (anti-fibrinogen 250×).

Electron microscopy

Mesangial matrix expansion and variable degree of cellular hyperplasia are evident together with electron-dense deposits (Emancipator 1998). These deposits are initially paramesangial and small sized (100–120 nm), then they become larger (up to 800 nm) of non-uniform density, in strict connection with the mesangial matrix. Mostly the deposits have a mesangial site with parietal extensions (60 per cent), whilst only in 30 per cent of the cases are they purely mesangial. The parietal, paramesangial electron-dense material is generally subendothelial, more rarely subepithelial, and it is smaller sized. Sometimes, electron-dense deposits that are 'humps'-like with 'garland' shape or fluffy aspect are detectable, along with other with a 'woolly' aspect in the external rara lamina, placed in the periphery of the capillary loops and delimited by a thick layer of new basement membrane. The presence of parietal deposits modifies the capillary basal membrane profile because of the widening of the rara internal and external lamina, with neoformed layers, as a possible consequence of the membrane reactivity to immune deposits.

Repeated renal biopsy

Studies of serial biopsies in children with HSP (Niaudet *et al.* 1984) showed a good correlation between the histological changes, clinical data, and outcome. When patients undergo clinical resolution, mesangial proliferation disappears, small crescents regress while others leave place to floccular adhesion synechiae. IgA deposits substantially decrease and a complete disappearance has been seldom reported. Conversely, when repeat biopsies were performed in patients with persistently active or progressing nephritis, proliferation pursued and evolution into fibrotic lesions was common. This study reports a good correlation between clinical and histological data, stressing the importance of careful clinical monitoring during the follow-up.

Extrarenal lesions

The typical leucocytoclastic vasculitis—with fragmented nuclei of leucocytes in and around arterioles, capillaries, and venules, surrounded by infiltrating neutrophils and monocyte cells in the presence of nuclear residues (nuclear dust) in the wall of arterioles (Fig. 1)—is detectable in the kidneys and in other areas, particularly in the skin and gut. Fibrinoid accumulations and arteriolar and venular necrosis can be found.

Deposits of IgA and C3 are present in the capillary derma in purpuric lesions and uninvolved skin and are considered a valid diagnostic criteria, with 100 per cent specificity in combination with leucocytoclastic vasculitis. Co-deposits of IgG and IgM can be present in about 20 per cent of the cases, while C1q and C4 are absent. Similar deposits have been reported in superficial derma capillaries of IgAN patients. In dermatitis herpetiformis IgA deposits are found as well, but they are located on the top of the derma papilla. In SLE the dermal–epidermal junction is mostly positive for IgG, C1q, and C4.

Differential diagnosis

In children, the purpuric lesions are typical in aspect and distribution and usually the diagnosis is easy. The diagnosis is more difficult in the infrequent cases in which skin eruption entirely consists of urticaria without purpura. Hypersensitivity vasculitis is sometimes overlapping but the IgA vascular deposits are specific for dermal HSP lesions.

In adults, the presence of glomerular disease associated with joint pain and cutaneous lesions renders mandatory the differential diagnosis with SLE, polyarteritis nodosa (Cream *et al.* 1970), as well as microscopic polyangiitis (see Chapters 4.5.1 and 4.5.3). The light microscopy findings of systemic lupus erythematosus nephritis and those of nephritis of HSP may be undistinguishable. At immunofluorescence, glomerular IgA deposits are prevalent on the other immunoglobulin classes in HSP, while IgG deposits are usually prevalent in lupus nephritis. Similarly, the differential diagnosis between HSP nephritis and microscopic polyarteritis is based on the presence of mesangial IgA deposits when tuft necrosis, shared by either pathology, is present.

Clinicopathological correlations at onset

In the Italian series of 219 renal biopsies (Coppo *et al.* 1997a, 1999), patients with minimal proteinuria had higher prevalence of lesions of classes I and II, without crescents. In patients with significant proteinuria more severe renal lesions were frequently found, nevertheless with low predictive value for the single case. In children particularly, cases with non-nephrotic proteinuria had often extracapillary proliferation. Gross haematuria at presentation was associated with crescent formations in 22 per cent of the cases, independent of the patient's age. Renal functional impairment at onset had a predictive value of severe histological lesions. Similar figures have been reported in other cohorts of either children or adults (Droz 1955; Cream *et al.* 1970).

Clinical course and prognosis

The proportion of HSP nephritis in comparison of other renal diseases as a cause of endstage renal failures (ESRF) is minimal—0.05 per cent—in adults, while it is up to 5.1 per cent in children (Meadow *et al.* 1972; Lévy *et al.* 1976).

The long-term outcome in chronic renal failure varies according to the cohorts examined, being, in general, worse in adults than in children, particularly in unselected cases. When patients who have had renal biopsy are compared, the difference is less evident (Fig. 7).

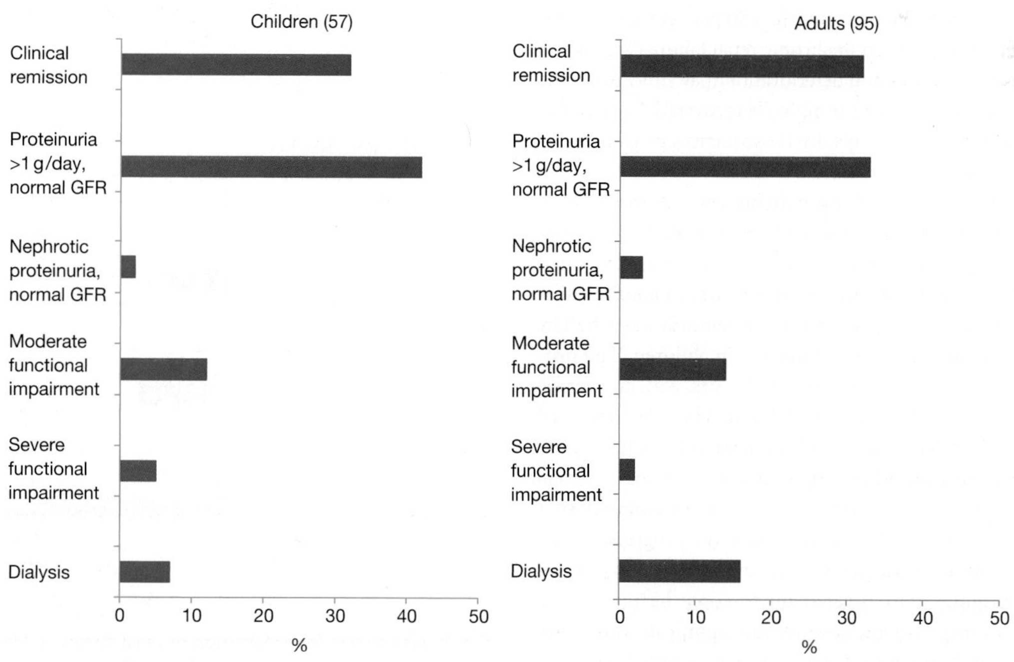

Fig. 7 Long-term renal outcome (mean 5 years) of patients with Henoch–Schönlein nephritis severe enough to warrant renal biopsy (Italian Group of Renal Immunopathology. Coppo *et al.* 1997a).

In unselected settings HSP is a mild disease, with renal involvement in a minority of cases, mostly presenting isolated haematuria and/or minimal proteinuria and long-term morbidity has been reported to involve no more than 1 per cent of patients (Lévy *et al.* 1976; Koskimies *et al.* 1981).

When considering hospital series (Koskimies *et al.* 1981; Farine *et al.* 1986; Stewart *et al.* 1988) of non-selected children admitted into General Paediatric Hospitals, the reports indicate that 20–28 per cent had urinary sediment that was abnormal for more than 1 month. After a decade of follow-up about 2–3 per cent of the children with initial signs of renal involvement progressed to ESRF (Hotta *et al.* 1996).

Tertiary Reference Centres report remission rates below 50 per cent and a poor outcome in 10–25 per cent of children (Lévy *et al.* 1976; Goldstein *et al.* 1992). The outcome of patients selected on the need for renal biopsy is much more severe and long-term analyses show that 15–30 per cent of patients progress to renal failure with wide variability depending on the initial selection criteria and follow-up duration (Rieu and Noel 1999).

In a long-term follow-up study over about 25 years late progression was observed in 25 per cent of children admitted to a Paediatric Nephrology Reference Centre, even after initial clinical improvement (Goldstein *et al.* 1992). It reported that 15 per cent of patients with a nephritic onset or persistent heavy proteinuria, 40 per cent of those with a nephritic presentation and 50 per cent of those with mixed nephritic–nephrotic syndrome at onset have ongoing urinary abnormalities and that many of these patients end in chronic renal failure. This progression can occur more than a decade after the initial presentation. The disease is more severe in adults, where the progression to renal failure is reported in 8–68 per cent of the cases (Fogazzi *et al.* 1989; Rieu and Noel 1999).

An important factor for individual prognosis is the presence and extent of extracapillary proliferation. The relationship is particularly strict for Classes IV and V, showing extensive glomerular involvement by crescents. In a Japanese series, 33 per cent of Class IV and 83 per cent of Class V, displaying, respectively, greater than 50 per cent and greater than 75 per cent of crescents ended in chronic renal failure (Yoshikawa *et al.* 1987). However, renal function deterioration may show up in the follow-up even in cases that seemed completely recovered 2 years after onset (Goldstein *et al.* 1992), perhaps due to sequences of glomerular hypertension.

In the Italian multicentre study on patients with a renal disease severe enough to warrant kidney biopsy (Coppo *et al.* 1997a), after 1–20 (mean 5) years one-third of the cases were in remission, often complete and without significant urinary anomalies. In another one-third of patients, only minimal or moderate proteinuria was left. The outcome was substantially similar in adults and in children. The progression to dialysis varied from a few days to 20 years, with an average of 3 years in the adults and 10 years in children. The actuarial renal survival of HSP nephritis in patients with indication for renal biopsy resulted in similar results for adults and children, with loss of renal function in 26 per cent of adults and in 27 per cent of children after 10 years (Coppo *et al.* 1997a). The comparison of the progression rate in HSP and IgAN is difficult due to the different indications to renal biopsy in IgAN, ranging from isolated microscopic haematuria to severe renal function impairment; however, no significant difference in progression rate can be envisaged, since IgAN is reported to have a 10-year progression rate of 15–25 per cent according to the biopsy criteria adopted (Yoshikawa 1997).

Risk factors for progression

As reported above, in non-selected series of HSP nephritis greater age is associated with a higher risk of progression, but in biopsied patients this correlation is not evident. A good correlation between the clinical presentation and the long-term outcome is reported in a paediatric series (Blanco *et al.* 1997). In some reports, nephrotic syndrome and/or renal insufficiency at onset were risk factors (44 per cent) for renal failure after two decades of follow-up (Goldstein *et al.* 1992) (Fig. 8).

In the cohorts of children and adults having had renal biopsy (Coppo *et al.* 1997a) the most unfavourable prognostic factor was renal function impairment at presentation: 45 per cent of adults with severe renal failure and 18 per cent of those with moderate functional impairment eventually required chronic dialysis, versus only 2 per cent of adults with normal renal function at onset. This association was not found in children, who experienced progression to renal failure even in cases with normal renal function at onset.

Hypertension was a negative prognostic factor particularly in adults, in whom it was more constant and associated with renal function impairment.

The predictive value of proteinuria produced different results in adults and children: in both cohorts absent or mild proteinuria or, on the contrary, nephrotic-range levels, were, respectively, associated with high frequency of remission or functional deterioration. However, adult patients who were moderately proteinuric only seldom showed extracapillary proliferation, while children with mild proteinuria frequently displayed severe histological lesions, with extracapillary proliferation. Among adults, a proteinuria greater than 1.5 g/day resulted in unfavourable outcome (Coppo *et al.* 1997a). On the contrary, nephrotic and non-nephrotic children had similar outcomes.

Extent and activity of extracapillary proliferation are important risk factors (Yoshikawa *et al.* 1981). The predictive value of mild extracapillary proliferation was low when crescents involved less than 50 per cent of glomeruli (Class III) (renal failure in 39 per cent of

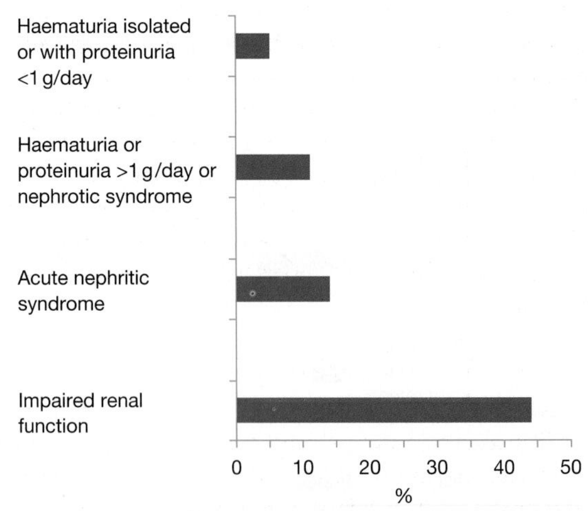

Fig. 8 Risk factors for progression of renal disease in Henoch–Schönlein purpura nephritis (Goldstein *et al.* 1992). Cumulative series of 77 patients with renal involvement. Data from: Koskimie (1981); Yoshikawa (1981, 1987); Stewart (1988); Goldstein *et al.* (1992); Niaudet (1993).

adults and in 18 per cent of children with crescents), since cases without crescents also experienced an unfavourable outcome (19 per cent of adults and 23 per cent of children).

HSP nephritis and renal transplantation

In patients transplanted after ERSF from HSP nephritis, extrarenal systemic recurrence is rare, or very mild, while IgA mesangial deposits may recur in allografts. The actuarial risk for histological/immunofluorescent renal recurrence is 35 per cent at 5 years, with loss of the graft in 11 per cent (Meulders *et al.* 1994; Kessler *et al.* 1996). In most patients, no clinical manifestations or minimal haematuria accompanies histological recurrence in grafted kidneys (Cameron 1993). Recurrence was more frequent in rapidly progressive cases, occurred even after a delay of 1 year between systemic signs and transplantation, and was not prevented by triple therapy, including cyclosporin (Meulders *et al.* 1994). The recurrence rate appears to be increased in recipients of living-related grafts, suggesting a role for genetic factors and arguing against the use of living donors for renal transplantation in HSP, even though this association is still controversial (Ramos 1991; Muller *et al.* 1998).

Therapy

Non-renal cases

No treatment is required for mild cases, provided an efficient urine monitoring is ensured to detect modifications in the clinical follow-up, mostly during the first 2–3 months after the purpuric rash.

Corticosteroids are generally considered to be effective in controlling the extrarenal signs, particularly abdominal pain and arthritis, hastening resolution. Severe recurrent necrotizing purpura as well as abdominal pain have been successfully treated by immunoglobulin intravenous infusions (Heldrich *et al.* 1993).

An important issue is whether medium doses of prednisone (1–2.5 mg/kg/day for 1–3 weeks) in children with normal urinalysis are able to prevent the development of nephropathy. This preventive effect has been debated using retrospective data analysis, which compared treated versus untreated patients. However, a selection bias may have influenced the treatment choice, often reserved to the more active cases (Buchanec 1988; Saulsbury 1993). A prospective study (albeit not strictly randomized) has contradicted the previous negative conclusions, suggesting a protective effect of small doses of prednisone for 2 weeks (Mollica *et al.* 1992). However, very small amounts of microscopic haematuria are not likely to be a risk for progression to renal failure. Thus, the prevention of mild nephropathy may not affect the risk of progression of HSP nephritis.

Treatment of HSP nephritis of moderate severity

For long steroids have been thought to be ineffective for treating established HSP nephritis, based on observations dating back to a few decades. Indeed, in a retrospective analysis no benefit of prednisone was demonstrated in the attempt to treat children with HSP nephritis (Counahan *et al.* 1977). However, the severity of the disease was a major determinant in the decision to treat, leading a selection bias favouring treatment of more severe cases. More recently, positive results were reported by treating patients with moderately severe renal involvement for almost 1 year by means of oral prednisone and azathioprine (Foster *et al.* 2000), when compared with historical untreated cases (Lévy *et al.* 1976). Since it is likely that the historical group included more severe cases, no recommendation for treatment of moderately severe HSP nephritis is presently made (Wyatt and Hogg 2001).

Finally, also reports on tonsillectomy do not support the recommendation of this intervention in the treatment of mild forms of this nephropathy (Sanai and Kudoh 1996).

Treatment of severe HSP nephritis with extensive crescents

Great interest is focused on the possibility of reducing or stopping the progression to renal failure of HSP nephritis with severe endocapillary and extracapillary proliferation, clinical presentation of nephritic or nephritic syndrome with impaired renal function, which present with an evolutive course. A favourable clinical outcome was reported in 11/12 children with 60–90 per cent glomeruli with crescent formations by using a triple therapy (Oner *et al.* 1955) of 30 mg/kg intravenous pulses for 3 days followed by 6 months of prednisone, dipyridamole, and cyclophosphamide for 3 months. More than 60 per cent of these patients experienced a complete remission.

Larger series (Niaudet and Habib 1998) confirmed that a similar prednisone regimen, in some cases associated with a 2-month course of oral cyclophosphamide, induced a clinical recovery in 71 per cent of children with nephritic syndrome and/or crescentic involvement of 50 per cent of the glomeruli, versus 40 per cent in untreated children. The most significant results have been obtained in paediatric patients with epithelial crescents involving more than 50 per cent of glomeruli or with nephrotic syndrome. It is of interest to notice that in the same cohort, no effect of treatment was found when crescents involved less than 50 per cent of glomeruli.

In children having HSP nephritis with greater than 50 per cent glomeruli involved in crescent formations, good results were reported by using oral prednisone treatment pursued for 4 months in association with 2 months of cyclophosphamide and 4 months of heparin or warfarin (Iijima *et al.* 1998). Positive results were obtained with a combination of prednisone, azathioprine, or cyclophosphamide (Bergstein *et al.* 1998; Flynn *et al.* 2001).

Our group (Coppo *et al.* 1985) and, more recently, others (Hattori *et al.* 1999) successfully treated patients with rapidly progressive HSP nephritis with plasma exchange, corticosteroids, and cytotoxic drugs. In the follow-up of our cases, even though some patients experienced a complete remission, most had subsequent renal relapses, and, in spite of a new cycle of plasma exchange, the renal function could not be improved again and patients had a final outcome in ESRF. The estimated progression was delayed by 1–4 years. In the Japanese experience after 10 years 60 per cent of the treated patients had a complete remission of renal disease. A German series (Scharer *et al.* 1999) similarly showed that aggressive treatment including PE may delay the rate of progression, but not prevent chronic ESRF in the majority of severe crescentic HSP nephritis.

To summarize, uncontrolled studies of combined treatment with steroids (either intravenous pulses or oral therapy) and immunosuppressive drugs (cyclophosphamide or azathioprine), sometimes in association with anticoagulants (warfarin or dipyridamole), in patients with nephrotic-range proteinuria and/or important extracapillary proliferation on biopsy can retard and sometimes halt renal function deterioration, if the therapy is initiated early enough, before a non-return stage characterized by the establishment of fibrous crescents and glomerular or interstitial changes.

Intravenous immunoglobulin therapy

In addition to steroid and cytotoxic therapy, favourable results with decrease in proteinuria and improvement of histological index of renal activity have been reported in potentially progressive patients with heavy proteinuria, using immunoglobulin intravenous infusions (Rostoker *et al.* 1994; Kasuda *et al.* 1999). However, a rebound was noticed shortly after the therapeutic cycles, which somehow negated the positive results obtained (Rostoker *et al.* 1994).

Pathogenesis

The histological feature distinguishing HSP nephritis from other systemic vasculitides or collagen diseases with similar multiorgan involvement is mesangial IgA deposition. Hence, as for primary IgAN, interest has been focused on this class of immunoglobulins.

IgA is found in serum and mostly in external secretions, where it plays a major role in mucosal immunity. IgA exists as two distinct subclasses, IgA1 and IgA2, differing as an insertion of 19 aminoacids, peculiar to IgA1 and deleted in IgA2 subclass (Kerr 1990). Either subclass is synthesized by plasma cells as a 155-kDa protein consisting of two α-chains and two light chains, or as dimers or polymers of the basic four-chain immunoglobulin structure, with molecular weights in multiples of 155 kDa. Dimers are joined by a J-chain and can be transported from the basolateral to the luminal surface of the secretory epithelium via a specialized glycoprotein receptor (secretory component). In humans, serum IgA is predominantly monomeric, of the IgA1 subclass, and it is derived from plasmocytes within the marrow and spleen. Mucosal-derived plasmocytes produce predominantly dimeric IgA containing J-chain (Mestecky and McGhee 1987). Glomerular deposits in HSP as well as in primary IgAN are made of polymeric IgA1, leaving open the possibility of either bone-marrow or mucosal origin, by a somehow disturbed synthetic pathway (Emancipator 1992).

Since IgA is the major immunoglobulin in mucosal secretions working as a defence against viral and bacterial agents, and since HSP can be enhanced by mucosal infections, an extensive search for peculiar antigens was performed. Alimentary antigens or infectious organisms have been advocated (Ackroyd 1953; Miescher *et al.* 1956). However, the search for an eliciting antigen remained elusive (Coppo *et al.* 1988, 1992; Emancipator 1990).

HSP has been assumed to be an antigen-dependent process, on the basis of the cross-reactivity between eluted mesangial IgA with the mesangial area of other biopsy samples from different HSP patients (Tomino *et al.* 1983). The concept of HSP as an antigen-dependent process was further emphasized by an experimental observation that most closely reproduces HSP: systemic vasculitis and nephritis was obtained by injecting animals with a complement activating carbohydrate antigen (Rifai *et al.* 1987; Montinaro *et al.* 1991).

HSP nephritis has been ascribed to the accumulation of IgAIC within glomeruli, as for idiopathic IgAN. Many studies revealed high levels of IgAIC during clinically active phases of HSP nephritis (Kauffman *et al.* 1980; Coppo *et al.* 1982, 1984; Davin *et al.* 1987), often coincidentally with the development of clinical signs of nephritis and in correlation with urinary activity. However, the correlation with renal involvement was not completely satisfying and the search of eliciting antigens in humans remained elusive (Emancipator 1992), reducing the support to the hypothesis of circulating IgAIC as the unique pathogenetic mechanism.

Several studies accumulated evidence of a large spectrum of abnormal reactivities of circulating IgA in HSP patients, particularly those with nephritis, including anti-α-galactosyl antibodies (Davin *et al.* 1987), IgA binding to fibronectin (Jennette *et al.* 1991), lectin-like molecules mostly gluten-derived (Coppo *et al.* 1991) or mesangial matrix glycoproteins (Coppo *et al.* 1993), IgA binding to endothelial cells (Fornasieri *et al.* 1995). Hence, we and others postulated that these reactions were not due to true antigen–antibody reactions but to some kind of affinity of circulating IgA to various molecules.

Attention has been focused on the carbohydrate moieties of IgA. Human IgA1, the predominant subclass deposited in both primary IgAN and HSP nephritis, is highly glycosylated (Kerr 1990). In addition to the *N*-linked oligosaccharides typically present in the carboxyl terminal portion of all classes of the immunoglobulin heavy chain, IgA1 contains five short *O*-linked oligosaccharide chains composed of *N*-acetylgalactosamine, galactose, and sialic acid. These oligosaccharides are coupled to serine and/or threonine residues which lie in the hinge region connecting the CH1 and CH2 domains, at the junction between the Fab and the Fc portions of the IgA molecule (Kerr 1990).

Several studies support the hypothesis of defective immunoregulation leading to aberrant IgA glycosylation not only in patients with primary IgAN but also in HSP patients (Saulsbury 1997; Coppo *et al.* 1997b; Allen *et al.* 1998) (see Chapter 3.6).

A genetic defect with inadequate activity of β1–3 galactosyltransferase in B-cells has been hypothesized as for primary IgAN (Allen *et al.* 1997). An imbalance in lymphocyte function, with a prevalence of Th2 over Th1 T-cell subsets, can lead to altered IgA glycosylation in mice (Chintalacharuvu and Emancipator 1997), similar abnormalities could derive from genetic conditioning (but the search is till now inconclusive) or from *de novo* somatic mutations. Such aberrantly glycosylated IgA can circulate in monomeric form or participate in the formation of self-aggregates or true IC. *In vitro*, desialylated or degalactosylated IgA shows a high tendency to self-aggregate, forming macromolecules with a molecular weight similar to IgAIC (Kokubo *et al.* 1998).

Whether bound in IC or in self-aggregates, such aberrantly glycosylated IgA likely escapes clearance by hepatic receptors (ASGPR) for asialoglycoproteins (Roccatello *et al.* 1993) because of the lack of galactose and possibly because the size of the aggregates excludes them from the space of Disse.

In addition, by virtue of enhanced lectin-like reactivity with the fibronectin, laminin, and collagen within the mesangial matrix (Coppo *et al.* 1993), abnormally glycosylated IgA deposits in glomeruli more readily than does normal IgA. Finally, mesangial catabolism of aberrantly glycosylated IgA may be diminished. In combination, these factors can lead to increased accumulation and/or prolonged persistence of IgA deposits within the mesangium.

However, there is enhanced interaction with Fcα receptors on mesangial cells, resulting in cellular activation and phlogistic mediator synthesis. Our group has demonstrated that mesangial cells increase expression of integrin adhesion molecules (Peruzzi *et al.* 2000), and of the inducible form of nitric oxide synthase (Amore *et al.* 2001) in response to coincubation with aggregated forms of desialylated or desialylated/degalactosylated IgA. The resultant increase in the production of intraglomerular nitric oxide may lead to peroxidative damage, apoptosis, and sclerosis. The effect can be further enhanced by the concomitant depressed expression of vascular endothelial growth factor induced by aberrantly glycosylated IgA on mesangial cells, leading to an impaired repair process (Amore *et al.* 2000).

Aggregates of IgA also stimulate the synthesis of a variety of cytokines (IL-6, PDGF, IL-1, TNF-α, TGF-β), vasoactive factors (prostaglandins, thromboxane, leukotrienes, endothelin, PAF, NO), or chemokines (MCP-1, IL-8, MIP-1, RANTES) by mesangial cells (Gesualdo *et al.* 1994; Grandaliano *et al.* 1996).

In the pathogenesis of HSP nephritis, a particular role could be played by complement activation, which shows some signs in circulation. It is of interest that aberrantly glycosylated IgA can activate complement more efficiently than normal IgA (Nikolova *et al.* 1994).

IgA–ANCA have been reported in adults with active HSP (Vander Wall Bake *et al.* 1987; Ronda *et al.* 1994) but other reports were negative (Sinico *et al.* 1994). We demonstrated that IgA molecules from children and adults with HSP nephritis are provided by reactivities due to abnormal glycosylation and increased binding to sonicated neutrophil extracts, and due to purified myeloperoxidase (MPO) (Coppo *et al.* 1997b). No increased binding was found to serine protease 3. It is interesting to note that, this reactivity was never observed in sera of patients with primary IgAN, even though they have aberrantly glycosylated IgA. This binding was affected by electrical charge and carbohydrate interactions. The glycoprotein Fibronectin and the lectin Jacalin, which can bind IgA and the carbohydrate moieties of other glycoproteins, enhanced the binding of IgA to MPO. These data were consistent with a lectin-like binding of IgA to neutrophil cytoplasmic antigens.

We speculate that aberrantly glycosylated IgA in HSP patients—having among other reactivities also high affinity for antineutrophil cytoplasm antibodies (ANCA) antigens—may form circulating aggregates, which, in presence of increased levels of eosinophilic cationic proteins (Namgoong *et al.* 1997) as well as other phlogistic mediators (Ranieri *et al.* 1996; Smith *et al.* 1997), may favour the vascular deposition of IgA. The presence of IgA instead of IgG ANCA may avoid the precipitous and disastrous reactions that characterize IgG ANCA vasculitides.

Relationship between HSP and primary IgAN

The relationship between HSP nephritis and primary IgAN is complex, since the elements in common, like the immunopathological findings, are so strong that they support the identity of the two nephropathies, while the peculiar clinical features, like the recovery capacity of HSP (even at histological level) versus the persistence and progression of renal damage in primary IgAN, argue in favour of two different disease entities.

Paediatric nephrologists are so frequently facing an acute, benign illness, provided with a strong recovery potential, that they are more prone to conceive the two diseases as different entities, with different needs and clinical evolution. Besides the acute, mild, and reversible forms of HSP nephritis affecting children, which are typical of HSP only, the two entities become very similar when the disease is chronic and severe enough to warrant renal biopsy. The histological lesions and the clinical outcome of this peculiar subset of HSP patients are identical to primary IgAN, supporting the hypothesis of only an nephrological entity. For these reasons, most nephrologists working with adult patients consider primary IgAN as HSP nephritis without purpura.

Several reports support a common origin for the two diseases, such as the recurrence of IgAN in transplanted kidneys of patients on dialysis for HSP nephritis, or the development of HSP in primary IgAN patients. In several families, the two diseases coexist in different members of the same family (Huges *et al.* 1988). In a French national survey on 40 families with two or more members affected by primary IgAN, five had members presenting with complete HSP syndrome, confirming a possible genetic link between the two diseases (Lévy 2001); in HSP as well as in primary IgAN an increased frequency of HLA BW35 has been reported (Davin *et al.* 2001).

From an immunological point of view the two diseases seem to share similar disturbances in the IgA system. High levels of serum IgA are detectable in both HSP and primary IgAN, along with high levels of circulating IgAIC, IgA1 IC, and IgA/fibronectin aggregates, as discussed above, but at higher levels in HSP (Coppo *et al.* 1984; Jennette *et al.* 1991).

Aberrantly glycosylated IgA have been detected in children with HSP nephritis, more frequently than in subjects with extrarenal vasculitis only (Saulsbury 1997; Coppo *et al.* 1997b; Allen *et al.* 1998).

The reason why some patients with IgAN develop a systemic vasculitis and present with the full expression of HSP is the clue of the problem of different pathogenesis in these two entities.

A greater complement activation by aberrantly glycosylated IgA might represent the distinct pathogenetic mechanism inducing the vasculitic lesions that differentiate patients with HSP from those with primary IgAN (Coppo *et al.* 1982; Smith *et al.* 1997).

IgA–ANCA have been reported in active HSP only (Ronda *et al.* 1994; Coppo *et al.* 1997b), while they were never found in primary IgAN. Since this reaction is an indirect expression of altered glycosylation of the IgA molecule, it is tempting to speculate that the clue to the problem of the difference between HSP and IgAN is the quality and extent of aberrant glycosylation of IgA, which favours different reactivities and capacities of activating complement as well as other flogistic mediators. The involvement of a particular mediator pathway is suggested by the increase in IgE (Davin *et al.* 1994) and eosinophilic cationic proteins (Namgoong *et al.* 1997). This inflammatory potential in HSP is more time-limited than in primary IgAN, where it lasts lifelong. In HSP, there may be a clue to the role of a switch-on enhancing factor leading to an acute illness, often self-limiting and allowing a repair process. Genetic as well as acquired mechanisms might be responsible for this fine tuning.

Acknowledgements

The authors are grateful to Dr Franco Ferrario, Renal Immunopathology Center, San Carlo Borromeo Hospital, Milan, for the pathology illustrations.

References

Ackroyd, J. F. (1953). Allergic purpura, including purpura due to food, drugs and infections. *American Journal of Medicine* **14**, 605–614.

Allen, A. C. *et al.* (1997). Leucocyte beta 1,3 galactosyltransferase activity in IgA nephropathy. *Nephrology, Dialysis, Transplantation* **12**, 701–706.

Allen, A. C. *et al.* (1998). Abnormal IgA glycosylation in Henoch–Schönlein purpura restricted to patients with clinical nephritis. *Nephrology, Dialysis, Transplantation* **13**, 930–934.

Amoli, M. M. *et al.* (2001a). Polymorphism at codon 469 of the intercellular adhesion molecule-1 locus is associated with protection against severe gastrointestinal complications in Henoch–Schönlein purpura. *Journal of Rheumatology* **28**, 1014–1018.

Amoli, M. M. *et al.* (2001b). HLA-DRB1*01 association with Henoch–Schönlein purpura in patients from Northwest Spain. *Journal of Rheumatology* **28**, 1266–1270.

Amore, A. *et al.* (2000). Aberrantly glycosylated IgA molecules downregulate the synthesis and secretion of vascular endothelial growth factor in human mesangial cells. *American Journal of Kidney Diseases* **36**, 1242–1252.

Amore, A. *et al.* (2001). Glycosylation of circulating IgA in patients with IgA nephropathy modulates proliferation and apoptosis of mesangial cells. *Journal of the American Society of Nephrology* **12**, 1862–1871.

Amoroso, A. *et al.* (1997). Immunogenetics of Henoch–Schönlein disease. *European Journal of Immunogenetics* **2**, 323–333.

Amoroso, A. *et al.* (1998). Polymorphism in angiotensin-converting enzyme gene and severity of renal disease in Henoch–Schönlein patients. *Nephrology, Dialysis, Transplantation* **13**, 3184–3188.

Bar-on, H. and Rosemann, E. (1972). Schönlein–Henoch syndrome in adults. *Israel Journal of Medical Science* **8**, 1702–1715.

Bergstein, J. *et al.* (1998). Response of crescentic Henoch–Schönlein purpura nephritis to corticosteroid and azathioprine therapy. *Clinical Nephrology* **49**, 9–14.

Bernhart, J. P. (1968). La néphropathie du syndrome de Schönlein–Henoch chez l'adulte. *Seminaires des Hopitaux de Paris* **57**, 70–88.

Blanco, R. *et al.* (1997). Henoch–Schönlein purpura in adulthood and childhood: two different expressions of the same syndrome. *Arthritis and Rheumatism* **40**, 859–864.

Bruce R. G. *et al.* (1997). Bilateral ureteral obstruction associated with Henoch–Schönlein purpura. *Pediatric Nephrology* **11**, 347–349.

Buchanec, J. *et al.* (1988). Incidence of renal complications in Schönlein–Henoch purpura syndrome in dependence on an early administration of steroids. *International Journal of Urology and Nephrology* **20**, 409–412.

Cameron, J. S. (1984). Henoch–Schönlein purpura: clinical presentation. *Contributions to Nephrology* **40**, 246–256.

Cameron, J. S. (1993). Recurrent diseases in renal allografts. *Kidney International* **43** (Suppl.), S91–S94.

Casanueva, B. *et al.* (1990). Autologous mixed lymphocyte reaction and T-cell suppressor activity in patients with Henoch–Schönlein purpura and IgA nephritis. *Nephron* **54**, 224–228.

Chintalacharuvu, S. R. and Emancipator, S. N. (1997). The glycosylation of IgA produced by murine B cells is altered by Th2 cytokines. *Journal of Immunology* **159**, 2327–2333.

Coppo, R. and Amore, A. Vasculitis (ANCA negative): Henoch–Schönlein purpura. In *Rheumatology and the Kidney* (ed. D. Adu, P. Emery, and M. Madaio), pp. 246–257. New York: Oxford University Press, 2001.

Coppo, R. *et al.* (1982). Circulating immune complexes containing IgA, IgG and IgM in patients with primary IgA nephropathy and with Henoch–Schönlein nephritis. Correlation with clinical and histologic signs of activity. *Clinical Nephrology* **18**, 230–239.

Coppo, R. *et al.* (1984). IgA1 and IgA2 immune complexes in primary IgA nephropathy and Henoch–Schönlein nephritis. *Clinical and Experimental Immunology* **57**, 583–590.

Coppo, R. *et al.* (1985). Plasma exchange in primary IgA nephropathy and Henoch–Schönlein syndrome nephritis. *Plasma Therapy and Transfusion Technology* **6**, 705–723.

Coppo, R. *et al.* (1988). The pathogenetical potential of environmental antigens in IgA nephropathy. *American Journal of Kidney Diseases* **5**, 420–424.

Coppo, R. *et al.* (1991). IgA antibodies to dietary antigens and lectin-binding IgA in sera from Italian, Australian and Japanese IgA nephropathy patients. *American Journal of Kidney Diseases* **17**, 480–487.

Coppo, R., Amore, A., and Roccatello, D. (1992). Dietary antigens and primary immunoglobulin A nephropathy. *Journal of the American Society of Nephrology* **2**, S173–S180.

Coppo, R. *et al.* (1993). Serum IgA and macromolecular IgA reacting with mesangial matrix components. *Contributions to Nephrology* **104**, 162–171.

Coppo, R. *et al.* for the Italian Group of Renal Immunopathology (1997a). Long-term prognosis of Henoch–Schönlein nephritis in adults and in children. *Nephrology, Dialysis, Transplantation* **12**, 2277–2283.

Coppo, R. *et al.* (1997b). Properties of circulating IgA molecules in Henoch–Schönlein purpura nephritis with focus on neutrophil cytoplasmic antigen IgA binding (IgA-ANCA): new insight into a debated issue. *Nephrology, Dialysis, Transplantation* **12**, 2269–2276.

Coppo, R. *et al.* (1998). Frequency of renal diseases and clinical indications for renal biopsy in children (report of the Italian National Registry of Renal Biopsies in Children). *Nephrology, Dialysis, Transplantation* **13**, 293–297.

Coppo, R. *et al.* (1999). Clinical features of Henoch–Schönlein purpura. *Annales Medicine Interne* **150**, 143–150.

Counahan, R. *et al.* (1977). Prognosis of Henoch–Schönlein purpura nephritis in children. *British Medical Journal* **2**, 11–14.

Cream, J. I., Gumpel, J. M., and Peachey, R. D. (1970). Schönlein–Henoch purpura in the adult. *Quarterly Journal of Medicine* **39**, 461–484.

Davin, J. C. *et al.* (1985). Sequential measurements of the reticulo-endothelial system function in Henoch–Schönlein disease in childhood. Correlation with various immunological parameters. *Acta Pediatrica Scandinavica* **74**, 201–206.

Davin, J. C. *et al.* (1987). Anti-alpha-galactosyl antibodies and immune complexes in children with Henoch–Schönlein purpura or IgA nephropathy. *Kidney International* **31** (5), 1132–1139.

Davin, J. C. *et al.* (1994). Possible pathogenetic role of IgE in Henoch–Schönlein purpura. *Pediatric Nephrology* **8**, 169–171.

Davin, J. C., Berge, I. J., and Weening, J. J. (2001). What is the difference between IgA nephropathy and Henoch–Schönlein purpura nephritis? *Kidney International* **59**, 823–834.

Debray, J., Krulik, M., and Giorgi, H. L. (1971). Le purpura rhumatoide (syndrome de Schönlein–Henoch). *Seminaires Hopitaux de Paris* **47**, 1805–1819.

DeMattia, D. *et al.* (1995). Von Willebrand factor XIII in children with Henoch–Schönlein purpura. *Pediatric Nephrology* **9**, 603–605.

Droz, D. La biopsie rénale dans les glomérulopathies à dépots mésangiaux d'IgA. In *Maladie de Berger et purpura rheumatoide. Biopsie rénale.* (ed. D. Droz and B. Lantz), pp. 151–166. Paris INSERM, 1955.

Emancipator, S. N. (1990). Immunoregulatory factors in the pathogenesis of IgA nephropathy. *Kidney International* **38**, 1216–1229.

Emancipator, S. N. IgA nephropathy and Henoch–Schönlein purpura. In *Heptinstall's Pathology of the Kidney* (ed. J. C. Jennette, J. L. Olson, M. M. Schwartz, and F. G. Silva), pp. 556–572. Philadelphia: Lippincott-Raven, 1998.

Evans, D. J. *et al.* (1973). Glomerular deposition of properdin in Henoch–Schönlein syndrome and idiopathic focal nephritis. *British Medical Journal* **3**, 326–328.

Farine, M. *et al.* (1986). Prognostic significance of urinary findings and renal biopsies in children with Henoch–Schönlein nephritis. *Clinical Paediatrics* **25**, 257–259.

Farley, T. A. *et al.* (1989). Epidemiology of a cluster of Henoch–Schönlein purpura. *American Journal of Diseases in Children* **143**, 798–803.

Flynn, J. T. *et al.* (2001). Treatment of Henoch–Schönlein purpura glomerulonephritis in children with high-dose corticosteroids plus oral cyclophosphamide. *American Journal of Nephrology* **21**, 128–133.

Fogazzi, G. B. *et al.* (1989). Long-term outcome of Schönlein–Henoch nephritis in the adult. *Clinical Nephrology* **83**, 60–66.

Fornasieri, A. *et al.* (1995). Anti-mesangial and anti-endothelial cell antibodies in IgA mesangial nephropathy. *Clinical Nephrology* **44**, 71–79.

Foster, B. J. *et al.* (2000). Effective therapy for Henoch–Schönlein purpura nephritis with prednisone and azathioprine: a clinical and histopathologic study. *Journal of Paediatrics* **136**, 370–375.

Garcia-Nieto, V. and Claverie-Martin, F. (1998). Additional cases of ureteral obstruction associated with Henoch–Schönlein purpura. *Pediatric Nephrology* **12**, 168–169.

Gesualdo, L. *et al.* (1994). Expression of platelet-derived growth factor receptors in normal and diseased human kidneys. An immunochemistry and *in situ* hybridization study. *Journal of Clinical Investigation* **94**, 50–58.

Goldstein, A. R. *et al.* (1992). Long-term follow-up of childhood Henoch–Schönlein nephritis. *Lancet* **339**, 280–282.

Grandaliano, G. *et al.* (1996). Monocyte chemoattractant peptide-1 expression in acute and chronic human nephritides: a pathogenetical role in interstitial monocyte recruitment. *Journal of the American Society of Nephrology* **7**, 906–913.

Habib, R. and Cameron, J. S. Schönlein–Henoch purpura. In *The Kidney Rheumatic Disease* (ed. P. A. Bacon and M. N. Hadler), pp. 232–253. London: Butterworth Scientific, 1982.

Hattori, M. *et al.* (1999). Plasmapheresis as the sole therapy for rapidly progressive Henoch–Schönlein purpura nephritis in children. *American Journal of Kidney Diseases* **33**, 427–433.

Heberden, W. *Commentaria di morboriana: historia and curatione*. London: Payne, 1801.

Heldrich, F. J., Minkin, S., and Gatdula, C. L. (1993). Intravenous immunoglobulin in Henoch–Schönlein purpura: a case study. *Medical Journal* **42**, 577–579.

Henoch, E. H. (1868). Verhandlungen arztlicher Gesellschaffen. *Berlier Klinische Wochenschrift* **5**, 517–530.

Hotta, O. *et al.* (1996). Long-term effects of intensive therapy combined with tonsillectomy in patients with IgA nephropathy. *Acta Otolaryngologica (Stockh) Supplement* **523**, 165–168.

Huges, F. J., Wolfish, N. M., and McLaine, P. N. (1988). Henoch–Schönlein syndrome and IgA nephropathy: a case report suggesting a common pathogenesis. *Pediatric Nephrology* **2**, 389–392.

Iijima, K. *et al.* (1998). Multiple combined therapy for severe Henoch–Schönlein nephritis in children. *Pediatric Nephrology* **12**, 244–248.

Jennette, J. C. *et al.* (1991). Serum IgA-fibronectin aggregates in patients with IgA nephropathy and Henoch–Schönlein purpura: diagnostic value and pathogenic implications. The Glomerular Disease Collaborative Network. *American Journal of Kidney Diseases* **18**, 466–471.

Jennette, J. C. *et al.* (1994). Nomenclature of systemic vasculitides. Proposal of an International Consensus Conference. *Arthritis and Rheumatism* **2**, 187–192.

Jin, D. K. *et al.* (1996). Complement 4 locus II gene deletion and DQA1*0301 gene: genetic risk factors for IgA nephropathy and Henoch–Schönlein nephritis. *Nephron* **73**, 390–395.

Kaku, Y., Nohara, K., and Honda, S. (1998). Renal involvement in Henoch–Schönlein purpura: a multivariate analysis of prognostic factors. *Kidney International* **53**, 1755–1759.

Kasuda, A. *et al.* (1999). Successful treatment of adult-onset Henoch–Schönlein purpura nephritis with high-dose immunoglobulins. *Internal Medicine* **38**, 376–379.

Kauffman, R. H. *et al.* (1980). Circulating immune complexes in Henoch–Schönlein purpura. A longitudinal study of their relationship to disease activity and vascular deposition of IgA. *American Journal of Medicine* **69**, 859–866.

Kessler, M. *et al.* (1996). Recurrence of immunoglobulin A nephropathy after renal transplantation in the cyclosporine era. *American Journal of Kidney Diseases* **28**, 99–104.

Kerr, M. A. (1990). The structure and function of human IgA. *Biochemistry Journal* **271**, 285–296.

Kher, K. K., Sheth, K. J., and Makker, S. P. (1983). Stenosing ureteritis in Henoch–Schönlein purpura. *Journal of Urology* **129**, 1040–1041.

Kokubo, T. *et al.* (1998). Protective role of IgA1 glycans against IgA1 self-aggregation and adhesion to extracellular matrix proteins. *Journal of the American Society of Nephrology* **9**, 2048–2054.

Koskimies, O. *et al.* (1981). Henoch–Schöenlein nephritis: long-term prognosis of unselected patients. *Archives of Disease in Childhood* **56**, 482–484.

Lévy, M. (2001). Familial cases of Berger's disease and anaphylactoid purpura. *Kidney International* **60**, 1611–1612.

Lévy, M. *et al.* Anaphylactoid purpura nephritis in childhood natural history and immunopathology. In *Advances in Nephrology Necker Hospital* (ed. J. Hamburger, J. Crosnier, and M. H. Maxwell), pp. 183–228. Chicago: Year Book Medical, 1976.

Meadow, S. R., Glasgow, E. F., and White, R. H. R. (1972). Schönlein–Henoch nephritis. *Quarterly Journal of Medicine* **41**, 241–258.

Mestecky, J. and McGhee, J. R. (1987). Immunoglobulin A (IgA): molecular and cellular interactions involved in IgA biosynthesis and immune response. *Advances in Immunology* **40**, 153–168.

Meulder, Q. *et al.* (1994). Course of Henoch–Schönlein nephritis after renal transplantation: report on ten patients and review of the literature. *Transplantation* **58**, 1179–1186.

Mc Lean, R. H., Wyatt, R. J., and Julian, B. A. (1984). Complement phenotypes in glomerulonephritides: increased frequency of homozygous null C4 phenotypes in IgA nephropathy and Henoch–Schönlein purpura. *Kidney International* **26**, 855–860.

Michel, B. A. *et al.* (1992). Hypersensibility vasculitis and Henoch–Schönlein purpura: a comparison between the two disorders. *Journal of Rheumatology* **19**, 721–728.

Miescher, P. A., Reymond, A., and Ritter, O. (1956). Le role de l'allergie bactérienne dans la pathogénèse de certaines vasculites. *Schwed Medizinische Wochenschrift* **86**, 799–808.

Mills, J. A. *et al.* (1990). The American College of Rheumatology 1990 criteria for the classification of Henoch–Schönlein purpura. *Arthritis and Rheumatism* **33**, 1114–1121.

Mollica, F. *et al.* (1992). Effectiveness of early prednisone treatment in preventing the development of nephropathy in anaphylactoid purpura. *European Journal of Paediatrics* **151**, 140–144.

Montinaro, V. *et al.* (1991). Antigen as mediator of glomerular injury in experimental IgA nephropathy. *Laboratory Investigation* **64**, 508–519.

Muller, T. *et al.* (1998). Recurrence of renal disease after kidney transplantation in children: 24 years of experience in a single center. *Clinical Nephrology* **49**, 272–274.

Namgoong, M. K., Lim, B. K., and Kim, J. S. (1997). Eosinophil cationic protein in Henoch–Schönlein purpura and in IgA nephropathy. *Pediatric Nephrology* **11**, 703–706.

Niaudet, P. and Habib, R. (1998). Methylprednisone pulse therapy in the treatment of severe forms of Schönlein–Henoch purpura nephritis. *Pediatric Nephrology* **12**, 238–243.

Niaudet, P. *et al.* (1984). Clinicopathologic correlations in severe forms of Henoch–Schönlein purpura nephritis based on repeat biopsies. *Contributions to Nephrology* **40**, 250–254.

Niaudet, P., Lenoir, G. D., and Habib, R. (1986). La néphropathie du purpura rhumatoide chez l'enfant. *Journées Parisiennes de Pédiatrie*, 145–150.

Nielsen, H. E. (1988). Epidemiology of Schönlein–Henoch purpura. *Acta Paediatrica Scandinavica* **77**, 125–131.

Nikolova, E. B., Tomana, M., and Russell, M. W. (1994). The role of the carbohydrate chains in complement (C3) fixation by solid-phase-bound human IgA. *Immunology* **82**, 321–327.

Oner, A., Tinaztepe, K., and Erdogan, O. (1955). The effect of triple therapy on rapidly progressive type of Henoch–Schönlein purpura nephritis. *Pediatric Nephrology* **9**, 6–10.

Patel, U. *et al.* (1988). Henoch–Schönlein purpura after influenza vaccination. *British Medical Journal of Clinical and Medical Research Education* **298**, 1800.

Peruzzi, L. *et al.* (2000). Integrin expression and IgA nephropathy: *in vitro* modulation by IgA with altered glycosylation and macromolecular IgA. *Kidney International* **58**, 2331–2340.

Ramos, E. L. (1991). Recurrent diseases in the renal allograft. *Journal of the American Society of Nephrology* **2**, 109–121.

Ranieri, E. *et al.* (1996). Urinary IL6/EGF ratio: a useful prognostic marker for the progression of renal damage in IgA nephropathy. *Kidney International* **50**, 1990–2001.

Rieu, P. and Noel, L. H. (1999). Henoch–Schönlein nephritis in children and adults. *Annales de Medicine Interne* **150**, 151–158.

Rifai, A., Chen, A., and Imai, H. (1987). Complement activation in experimental IgA nephropathy: an antigen-mediated process. *Kidney International* **32**, 838–844.

Roccatello, D. *et al.* (1993). Removal systems of immunoglobulin A and immunoglobulin A containing complexes in IgA nephropathy and cirrhosis patients. The role of asialoglycoprotein receptors. *Laboratory Investigation* **69**, 714–723.

Ronda, N. *et al.* (1994). Antineutrophil cytoplasm antibodies (ANCA) of IgA isotype in adult Henoch–Schönlein purpura. *Clinical and Experimental Immunology* **95**, 49–55.

Rostoker, G. (2001). Schöenlein–Henoch purpura in children and adults: diagnosis, pathophysiology and management. *BioDrugs* **15**, 99–138.

Rostoker, G. *et al.* (1994). High dose immunoglobulin therapy for severe IgA nephropathy and Henoch–Schönlein purpura. *Annals of Internal Medicine* **120**, 476–484.

Sanai, A. and Kudoh, F. (1996). Effects of tonsillectomy in children with IgA nephropathy, purpura nephritis, or other chronic glomerulonephritides. *Acta Otolaryngologica (Stockh) Supplement* **523**, 172–174.

Saulsbury, F. T. (1986). IgA rheumatoid factor in Henoch–Schönlein purpura. *Journal of Pediatrics* **108**, 71–76.

Saulsbury, F. T. (1993). Corticosteroid therapy does not prevent nephritis in Henoch–Schönlein purpura. *Pediatric Nephrology* **7**, 69–71.

Saulsbury, F. T. (1997). Alteration in the *O*-linked glycosylation of IgA1 in children with Henoch–Schönlein purpura. *Journal of Rheumatology* **24**, 2246–2249.

Scharer, K. *et al.* (1999). Clinical outcome of Schönlein–Henoch purpura nephritis in children. *Pediatric Nephrology* **13**, 816–823.

Schonlein, J. L. *Allgemeine und Specielle Pathologie und Therapie.* Wurtzberg: Etlinger, 1832.

Sinico, R. A. *et al.* (1994). Lack of IgA antineutrophil cytoplasmic antibodies in Henoch–Schönlein purpura and IgA nephropathy. *Clinical Immunology and Immunopathology* **73**, 19–26.

Smith, G. C. *et al.* (1997). Complement activation in Henoch–Schönlein purpura. *Pediatric Nephrology* **11**, 477–480.

Stewart, M., Savage, J. M., and McCord, B. (1988). Long-term renal prognosis of Henoch–Schönlein purpura in an unselected childhood population. *European Journal of Pediatrics* **147**, 113–115.

Tancrede-Bohin, E. *et al.* (1997). Schönlein–Henoch purpura in adult patients: predictive factors for IgA glomerulonephritis in a retrospective study of 57 cases. *Archives of Dermatology* **133**, 438–518.

Tomino, Y. *et al.* (1983). Cross-reactivity of eluted antibodies from renal tissues of patients with Henoch–Schönlein nephritis and IgA nephropathy. *American Journal of Nephrology* **3**, 218–223.

Van der Wall Bake, A. W. L. *et al.* (1987). IgA antibodies directed against cytoplasmic antigens of polymorphonuclear leukocytes in patients with Henoch–Schönlein purpura. *Advances in Experimental Medical Biology* **216B**, 1593–1598.

Wyatt, R. J. and Hogg, R. J. (2001). Evidence-based assessment of treatment options for children with IgA nephropathies. *Pediatric Nephrology* **16**, 156–167.

Yoshikawa, N. Henoch–Schönlein purpura. In *Immunologic Renal Diseases* (ed. E. G. Neilson and W. G. Couser), pp. 1119–1131. Philadelphia: Lippincott-Raven Publishers, 1997.

Yoshikawa, N. *et al.* (1981). Prognostic significance of the glomerular changes in Henoch–Schönlein nephritis. *Clinical Nephrology* **5**, 223–229.

Yoshikawa, N. *et al.* (1987). Henoch–Schönlein nephritis in children: comparison of clinical course. *Clinical Nephrology* **27**, 233–237.

4.5.3 Systemic vasculitis

Gillian Gaskin

The term 'systemic vasculitis' encompasses a variety of conditions that may affect the kidney by damaging its vasculature. Virtually any size or type of vessel may be involved; involvement of glomerular capillaries leads to focal necrotizing glomerulonephritis, while disease affecting larger arteries causes renal infarction and ischaemia.

Historical aspects

Disease characterized by vascular inflammation was first reported by Kussmaul and Maier (1866). They described a clinical picture of fever, muscle, gastrointestinal, and renal disease, with nodular swellings along the course of medium-sized arteries and histological evidence of inflammatory change in the vessel wall and named the condition 'periarteritis nodosa'. When it was later appreciated that the pathological process arose from within rather than around the arterial wall, the term 'polyarteritis' came into general use. In the early part of the twentieth century, the term was applied to a heterogeneous group of vasculitic illnesses, within which distinctive clinical and histological patterns gradually emerged, leading to the classifications that we use today.

Differentiation of primary vasculitic syndromes

Wegener's granulomatosis

The first description of the clinical syndrome now known as Wegener's granulomatosis came from Klinger (1931), who described a patient with nephritis and uraemia, together with destructive sinusitis, systemic arteritis, and splenic granulomas. Friedrich Wegener, a German pathologist, reported clinical and pathological findings in three patients with the same pattern of disease (Wegener 1936) and he went on to describe this illness in detail (Wegener 1939). As further reports appeared during the 1940s, the disease took his name. Fahey *et al.* (1954) published a series of seven further cases, and the pathological findings were analysed and reviewed by Godman and Churg (1954). They defined the illness by the presence of necrotizing granulomatous lesions in the respiratory tract, a generalized vasculitis involving both arteries and veins, and a focal necrotizing glomerulonephritis with evolution of a granulomatous pattern. Pathological confirmation of all three features was required to make a firm diagnosis. It was later realized that Wegener's granulomatosis is not invariably a severe and generalized illness: in some cases with typical histology, the disease appears to be localized to one or two organ systems. Carrington and Liebow (1966) designated this 'limited' disease.

Microscopic polyarteritis

A microscopic form of polyarteritis was first identified at postmortem by Davson *et al.* (1948), in a subgroup of patients diagnosed in life with polyarteritis nodosa. They exhibited a febrile illness with respiratory, abdominal, and rheumatic symptoms; four of the nine died in uraemia with normal blood pressure. All but one showed patchy fibrinoid necrosis of glomerular tufts and there were varying degrees of crescent formation. The pathological findings in a further six patients were reported by Wainwright and Davson (1950). The name 'microscopic polyarteritis' was not universally accepted, with some authors using the term 'hypersensitivity vasculitis' and others reporting 'necrotizing glomerulonephritis with vasculitis'.

Churg–Strauss syndrome

Churg and Strauss (1951) described the pathological features of another variant of polyarteritis nodosa, which previously had been recognized clinically by Rackemann and Greene (1939) and Harkavy (1941). They studied 13 cases with asthma, fever, hypereosinophilia, cardiac failure, peripheral neuropathy, and gastrointestinal and renal disease. There were nodular swellings in the small arteries of many organs, characterized microscopically by segmental fibrinoid necrosis of the vessel wall, aneurysm formation, and an inflammatory response containing many eosinophils in and around the vessel. Inflammatory extravascular lesions were noted, eosinophils being the predominant early cell type. Giant cells were prominent in older lesions and granulomatous nodules were identified, with necrosis and eosinophils at the core. Renal findings commonly included vasculitis in arcuate arteries, afferent arterioles, and glomerular capillaries, often with intense eosinophil infiltration. Focal segmental glomerular lesions were present in most cases but rarely involved the majority of glomeruli. Interstitial nephritis with a heavy eosinophilic infiltrate was also described. They concluded that this represented a discrete syndrome, and named it 'allergic granulomatosis and angiitis'. This condition is now referred to as the Churg–Strauss syndrome.

Polyarteritis nodosa

Rose and Spencer (1957) studied a group of 111 patients given a diagnosis of polyarteritis nodosa at nine British teaching hospitals. The patients with lung disease and a tendency to form granulomas could be classified as having either the allergic granulomatosis and angiitis of Churg and Strauss, or as having Wegener's granulomatosis. The term polyarteritis nodosa could then be reserved for the cases without granulomas, characterized by a necrotizing vasculitis involving medium-sized muscular arteries and leading to aneurysm formation.

Discovery of the association with antineutrophil cytoplasmic antibodies

A major breakthrough came with the discovery of antibodies against neutrophil cytoplasmic antigens (ANCA). They were first described in illnesses compatible with systemic vasculitis, thought to be associated with viral infection, by Davies *et al.* (1982). van der Woude *et al.* (1985) were the first to appreciate an association with Wegener's granulomatosis, detecting ANCA by indirect immunofluorescence on normal human neutrophils in 25 of 27 patients with active disease. Soon afterwards, other workers confirmed a close association of these antibodies with generalized Wegener's granulomatosis and described a correlation with disease activity. They appeared to occur less frequently in patients with more limited disease.

Much subsequent work focused on defining the spectrum of diseases associated with ANCA and the nature of their antigens (reviewed by van der Woude *et al.* 1989). It is now clear that they are not unique to Wegener's granulomatosis; they are also closely associated with microscopic polyangiitis and renal-limited vasculitis (i.e. isolated focal necrotizing glomerulonephritis) and Churg–Strauss syndrome (Hagen *et al.* 1998). An indirect immunofluorescence assay on ethanol-fixed neutrophils differentiates two main patterns of staining by vasculitis sera (Fig. 1). The first, termed 'cytoplasmic' or 'c-ANCA', is a diffuse granular staining throughout the neutrophil cytoplasm. It usually corresponds to specificity for the primary granule enzyme proteinase 3 and is particularly associated with Wegener's granulomatosis, The second pattern, termed 'perinuclear' or 'p-ANCA', is a concentration of fluorescence around the nucleus. This pattern is usually associated with antibodies directed against the neutrophil granule enzyme myeloperoxidase and is commonly seen in patients with microscopic polyangiitis, renal-limited vasculitis and Churg–Strauss syndrome. Patients with polyarteritis nodosa generally do not have ANCA. Other neutrophil proteins reported as occasional targets for ANCA in vasculitis include elastase, α-enolase; lactoferrin, bactericidal/permeability increasing protein, and h-lamp-2 though these are not important in clinical practice.

ANCA have also been detected in other conditions outside the spectrum of primary systemic vasculitis, including inflammatory bowel disease and primary sclerosing cholangitis (reviewed by Roozendaal and Kallenberg 1999) and rheumatoid disease (Schnabel *et al.* 1996). Indeed, nuclear staining of neutrophils by rheumatoid sera (granulocyte-specific antinuclear antibodies) was first reported by Wiik *et al.* (1974). ANCA in these disorders tend to recognize neutrophil constituents other than proteinase 3 and myeloperoxidase, including lactoferrin and cathepsin G. A number of 'false positive ANCA' have been reported in other diseases including certain infections, and in general, perinuclear ANCA without antimyeloperoxidase activity has a low specificity for vasculitis. An apparently high rate of false positives appears when using immunofluorescence screening assays alone in populations with a low pretest probability of vasculitis. In contrast, when the combination of immunofluorescence and well-validated solid-phase essays are applied in suspected vasculitis and its mimics, a high specificity for vasculitis can be demonstrated (Hagen *et al.* 1998). Numerous recommendations for the optimal use of ANCA testing have been published (Savige *et al.* 1999; Wiik 2001).

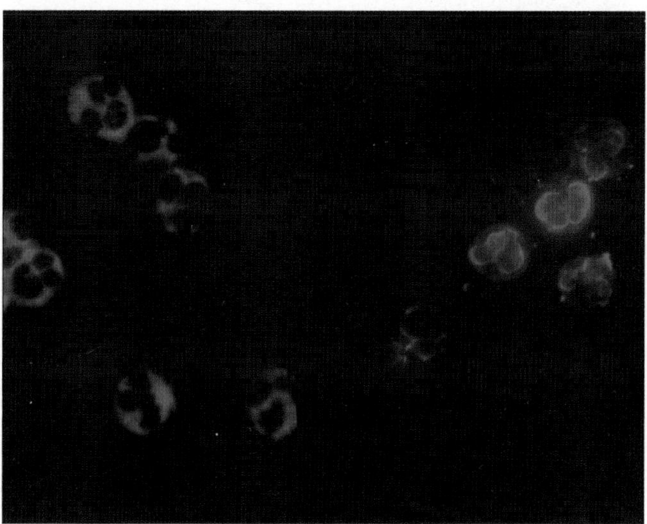

Fig. 1 Detection of ANCA using indirect immunofluorescence on ethanol-fixed neutrophils, illustrating patterns of c-ANCA (on left) and p-ANCA (on right).

Classification

A move from anatomical to clinical criteria

The strict pathological criteria for diagnosing Wegener's granulomatosis devised by Godman and Churg (1954) were only usable because most cases came to autopsy. Fauci *et al.* (1983) adopted a more flexible definition that allowed living patients to be classified. A definite diagnosis required a patient to have clinical evidence of disease in at least two of: the upper airways, the lungs (both in the form of a granulomatous vasculitis), and the kidneys (in the form of a glomerulonephritis). Histological confirmation was required from at least one, and preferably two, of these sites. This definition has been widely used, but in practice, it can be difficult to demonstrate granulomas. Our own approach has been to diagnose Wegener's granulomatosis in patients with a multisystem vasculitis affecting small vessels, with prominent involvement of the upper and lower respiratory tracts and kidneys. Our usual source of histological confirmation is a renal biopsy showing focal necrotizing glomerulonephritis.

Diagnostic criteria for Churg–Strauss syndrome have evolved similarly. Churg and Strauss devised diagnostic criteria from post-mortem studies, requiring demonstration of necrotizing vasculitis, eosinophilic tissue infiltration, and extravascular granulomas. Lanham *et al.* (1984) offered a clinical definition: this demanded the coexistence of systemic vasculitis involving two or more extra-pulmonary organs with asthma and peripheral blood eosinophilia (in excess of 1.5×10^9 per litre), and did not require the demonstration of granulomas.

Current approaches to the nomenclature of vasculitis

ACR 1990 criteria for the classification of vasculitis

The American College of Rheumatologists (ACR) (Hunder *et al.* 1990) created classification criteria, based on the clinical features most commonly and most specifically associated with certain diagnostic labels within the spectrum of vasculitis. They were intended to identify groups of similar patients for research studies and were not intended as diagnostic criteria for individual patients. Unfortunately for the nephrologist, they did not distinguish patients with small-vessel vasculitis, reflected in focal necrotizing glomerulonephritis, from those with classical polyarteritis nodosa.

Chapel Hill consensus criteria for the nomenclature of vasculitis

Debate about the ACR criteria stimulated an alternative approach: the Chapel Hill consensus nomenclature (Jennette *et al.* 1994), which will be used throughout this chapter. According to this system, the distinction between syndromes depends principally on the size of vessel affected (see Fig. 2), with recognition of characteristic features in some. Its salient features are illustrated in Table 1. Not all of the conditions listed are covered in this chapter, which will concentrate on the small- and medium-sized vessel vasculitides which regularly affect the kidney. Henoch–Schönlein purpura (Chapter 4.5.2) and mixed essential cryoglobulinaemia (Chapter 4.6) are described in detail elsewhere. Systemic lupus erythematosus (Chapter 4.7.2) and rheumatoid disease (Chapter 4.9) were not discussed at Chapel Hill, but may cause the combination of vasculitis and glomerulonephritis, and are covered separately.

Three aspects of the nomenclature require comment. First, a syndrome is classified by the smallest vessel affected, rather than the largest. Thus, while a diagnostic label of Wegener's granulomatosis (typically a small-vessel vasculitis) may be given to a patient who also has involvement of muscular arteries, a diagnosis of polyarteritis nodosa may not be given to a patient with necrotizing glomerulonephritis. This means (i) that a diagnosis of polyarteritis nodosa is made only rarely, and (ii) that patients with a syndrome previously considered to be an 'overlap' in view of the heterogeneity of vessel size involved are now readily classified.

Second, the term 'microscopic polyangiitis' replaces 'microscopic polyarteritis' since capillaries and veins may be affected, as well as arterioles and arteries. This term would be applied to a small-vessel vasculitis affecting the respiratory tract without granulomatous inflammation, typically taking the form of an alveolar capillaritis.

Finally, the classification does not deal specifically with 'idiopathic rapidly progressive glomerulonephritis'—focal necrotizing and crescentic glomerulonephritis without antiglomerular basement membrane (anti-GBM) antibodies. Even before the widespread availability of ANCA testing, many authors considered this to a renal-limited form

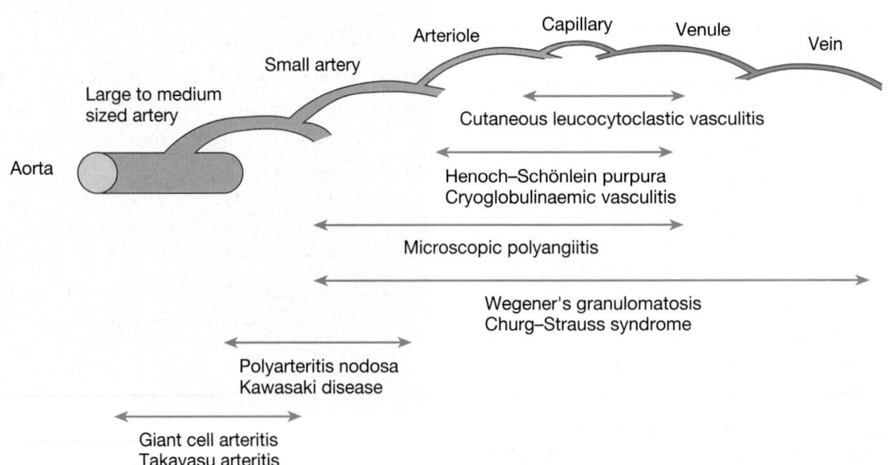

Fig. 2 Diagrammatic representation of Chapel Hill consensus nomenclature of vasculitis [modified from Jennette *et al.* (1994), with permission].

Table 1 Nomenclature of systemic vasculitis—the Chapel Hill consensus

*Small-vessel vasculitis**	
Wegener's granulomatosis	Granulomatous inflammation involving the respiratory tract and necrotizing vasculitis affecting small- to medium-sized vessels
Churg–Strauss syndrome	Eosinophil-rich and granulomatous inflammation involving the respiratory tract, and necrotizing vasculitis affecting small- and medium-sized vessels, associated with asthma and eosinophilia
Microscopic polyangiitis	Necrotizing vasculitis, with few or no immune deposits, affecting small vessels
Henoch–Schönlein purpura	Vasculitis, with IgA-dominant immune deposits, affecting small vessels
Essential cryoglobulinaemic vasculitis	Vasculitis, with cryoglobulin immune deposits, affecting small vessels, and associated with cryoglobulins in serum
Cutaneous leucocytoclastic angiitis	Isolated cutaneous leucocytoclastic angiitis without systemic vasculitis or glomerulonephritis
Medium-sized vessel vasculitis	
Polyarteritis nodosa	Necrotizing inflammation of medium-sized or small arteries without glomerulonephritis or vasculitis in arterioles, capillaries or venules
Kawasaki disease	Arteritis involving large, medium-sized, and small arteries, and associated with mucocutaneous lymph node syndrome
Large-vessel vasculitis	
Giant cell (temporal) arteritis	Granulomatous arteritis of the aorta and its major branches, with a predilection for the extracranial branches of the carotid artery
Takayasu arteritis	Granulomatous inflammation of the aorta and its major branches

* Small vessels are capillaries, venules, and arterioles.

of vasculitis. Their conclusions were based on clinical features in common (age at presentation, non-specific constitutional symptoms, laboratory findings), identical histological changes on renal biopsy, and a similar response to steroids and immunosuppressive therapy. Furthermore, some patients presenting with isolated rapidly progressive glomerulonephritis subsequently developed extrarenal vasculitis. The detection of ANCA in both conditions (Falk and Jennette 1988; Bindi *et al.* 1993; Angangco *et al.* 1994; Hagen *et al.* 1998) provides confirmatory evidence that they represent different parts of the spectrum of primary systemic vasculitis, and in the remainder of this chapter the term renal-limited vasculitis will be used.

ANCA and classification of vasculitis

Many recent publications have not distinguished between the clinical syndromes of Wegener's granulomatosis, microscopic polyangiitis, and renal-limited vasculitis, but have simply combined them as 'ANCA-associated vasculitis and glomerulonephritis'. However, since the full clinical implications of a given ANCA specificity have not been determined, this chapter will subdivide patients as far as possible according to clinical characteristics rather than their autoantibodies. Within those syndromes, data on the relevance of ANCA will be discussed.

Epidemiology of vasculitis

Incidence and demography

In 1982, Scott *et al.* estimated an incidence of 4.6 new cases per year of systemic vasculitis of the polyarteritis type per million of population, based on experience in a district hospital over a period of 8 years (Scott *et al.* 1982). The number of diagnosed cases has risen over the last decade, but it is unclear whether this reflects a genuine increase in incidence, improved diagnosis, or increased consideration of elderly patients for treatment. Data from Norfolk in 1993–1997 indicated an incidence of ANCA-associated vasculitis of 22.4/million/year (Watts *et al.* 2000) and in the United States in 1986–1990, the prevalence of Wegener's granulomatosis was estimated at 26/million.

It is unclear whether Wegener's granulomatosis and microscopic polyangiitis differ in true incidence, since there is variation between centres relating to referral bias and the use of different nomenclatures. There is an impression that microscopic polyangiitis is more common in southern Europe, and Wegener's granulomatosis more prevalent in northern Europe. However, a German vasculitis register has not demonstrated any difference between the North and South of the country (Reinhold-Keller *et al.* 2002). Both Wegener's granulomatosis and microscopic polyangiitis appear to be more common than Churg–Strauss syndrome.

In the 1980s, small-vessel vasculitis was reported most commonly in middle-age, with a slight male predominance, but the peak incidence is now in the 65–74 age-group, at 60.1/million/year in the Norfolk population (Watts *et al.* 2000). Older patients may also present with more organ damage. Mean age at entry to a European vasculitis trial for patients with creatinine greater than 500 μmol/l was 65, significantly higher than in trials for patients with lesser degrees of renal impairment (Gaskin *et al.* 2002). This is likely to have a significant impact on future treatment policies and outcomes, as both age and renal failure are associated with an increased mortality. Small-vessel vasculitis can also present in childhood, although clinical features and course in children may be atypical (Rottem *et al.* 1993).

Most reported cases of small-vessel vasculitis are in European Caucasoids; 97 per cent of the 158 patients with Wegener's granulomatosis reported from the National Institutes of Health were of this racial group (Hoffman *et al.* 1992a). Nonetheless, there are series reported from the Indian subcontinent and a number of reports from Japan.

Aetiological factors

Genetic factors

The influence of genetic factors in the development of vasculitis has recently been reviewed by Kallenberg *et al.* (2002). Familial vasculitis is rare, but there are accounts of siblings with Wegener's granulomatosis, siblings with polyarteritis nodosa, cases of both Wegener's granulomatosis and polyarteritis nodosa in the same family, and siblings with lung haemorrhage, glomerulonephritis, and myeloperoxidase-specific p-ANCA associated with low levels of the C4 component of complement. The latter abnormality is not usually detected in sporadic cases.

A number of systematic studies have investigated immunoregulatory genes (reviewed by Griffith and Pusey 1997). Comparisons of MHC types in vasculitis patients with control populations have yielded conflicting results and it seems very unlikely that there are strong HLA associations. Two studies linked susceptibility with complement components: Müller *et al.* (1984) demonstrated an association of the properdin factor B phenotype, BfF, with idiopathic rapidly progressive glomerulonephritis, while Finn *et al.* (1994), reported a relative risk of developing vasculitis of 2.6 in heterozygotes and 5.1 in homozygotes for the C3F allele. Investigations of immunoglobulin FcγRIIa and IIIb receptor polymorphisms have failed to demonstrate a significant difference between patients and control populations, although an association of certain alleles (FcγRIIa R131 and FcγRIIIa F158) with increased risk of relapse in Wegener's granulomatosis has been suggested (see Chapter 4.5.1 for a more detailed discussion). Recent studies have suggested an association of Wegener's granulomatosis with IL-10 polymorphisms: (i) with a single nucleotide polymorphism of the IL-10 promoter which leads to lower IL-10 production (Murakozy *et al.* 2001), and (ii) with a microsatellite polymorphism linked to greater antibody production (Zhou *et al.* 2002). These findings remain to be confirmed. A single study suggests an association with a CTLA4 polymorphism (Huang *et al.* 2000). Significant associations with polymorphisms in tumour necrosis factor TNF-α (Huang *et al.* 2000) or TGF-β (Murakozy *et al.* 2001) have not been demonstrated.

Interest has also focused on polymorphisms of α1-antitrypsin, which is the major physiological inhibitor of the c-ANCA antigen, proteinase 3. The frequency of deficient 'Z' alleles appears to be increased in vasculitis patients with ANCA directed against proteinase 3 (see, e.g. Esnault *et al.* 1993) and in one report was greater in those with severe lung haemorrhage (O'Donoghue *et al.* 1993). Furthermore, there appears to be an increase in frequency of the 'S' allele in vasculitis patients with myeloperoxidase-specific ANCA (Griffith *et al.* 1996). The pathogenetic significance of these findings is unknown.

Environmental factors

Certain drugs are associated with the development of an ANCA-associated illness (Merkel 1998), most notably D-penicillamine, propylthiouracil and hydralazine. D-penicillamine treatment may be associated with a rapidly progressive glomerulonephritis, with or without lung haemorrhage (numerous accounts reviewed by Devogelaer *et al.* 1987) and associated with myeloperoxidase-specific ANCA (Gaskin *et al.* 1995). The link with the antithyroid drug Propylthiouracil, first reported by Dolman *et al.* (1993), is most commonly, but not exclusively, with antimyeloperoxidase antibody-associated disease. The extent of organ damage is variable, but can be life-threatening. A significant proportion of patients on long-term treatment with the drug develop antibodies, even without overt vasculitis.

The recently introduced leukotriene antagonists, montelukast, zafirlukast, and pranlukast, used in troublesome asthma, have been linked to an increase in cases of Churg–Strauss syndrome (Wechsler *et al.* 1999). It is hypothesized that by allowing a reduction in steroid therapy, these drugs unmask Churg–Strauss syndrome, but a direct effect of the drugs has not been excluded (reviewed by Noth *et al.* 2003).

Silica exposure has been postulated as a risk factor for the development of vasculitis (reviewed by Tervaert *et al.* 1998). Patients with silicosis have an increased incidence of ANCA and risk of renal damage, and case–control studies have suggested an increased frequency of silica exposure in patients with ANCA-associated crescentic glomerulonephritis and Wegener's granulomatosis. An increase in the incidence of antimyeloperoxidase antibody-associated vasculitis, with prominent respiratory involvement, following the Kobe earthquake prompted further speculation on the role of environmental dust exposure (Yashiro *et al.* 2000).

Various reports suggest a possible link between vasculitis and infection, though there are different associations in small- and medium-vessel disease. Davies *et al.* (1982) reported a vasculitis-like illness, associated with ANCA, in patients with serological evidence of infection with an arbovirus, Ross River virus; while Falk *et al.* (1990) and Geffriaud-Ricouard *et al.* (1993) noted a seasonal variation in presentation of ANCA-associated disease. There is a single report associating Wegener's granulomatosis with parvovirus B19 infection (Finkel *et al.* 1994) and there are also reports of chronic parvovirus B19 infection in three patients with polyarteritis nodosa (Corman and Dolson 1992; Finkel *et al.* 1994). However, there was no evidence of infection with this virus when 38 French patients with polyarteritis nodosa were tested (Leruez-Ville *et al.* 1994). An association of hepatitis B infection with polyarteritis nodosa was first recognized over 30 years ago (Gocke *et al.* 1970), but it has not been reproduced in series concentrating on microscopic polyangiitis. There have also been reports of necrotizing vasculitis associated with infection by the human immunodeficiency virus (HIV) (Calabrese *et al.* 1989). Arteritis has long been recognized as a possible complication of streptococcal infection, with or without a typical postinfectious glomerulonephritis (Fordham *et al.* 1964; David *et al.* 1993).

There are numerous reports of active vasculitis presenting shortly after vaccination against influenza virus (see, e.g. Mader *et al.* 1993 and Yanai-Berar *et al.* 2002). There are also reports of vasculitis developing after vaccinations against pneumococcus, hepatitis A, and hepatitis B, and after administration of tetanus toxoid.

Finally, it is worth remembering that vasculitis may occur in association with both solid organ tumours and haematological malignancy, and this possibility should always be considered in the presence of atypical features.

Wegener's granulomatosis and microscopic polyangiitis

Clinical and pathological features

Spectrum and severity of disease

According to the Chapel Hill consensus criteria (Jennette *et al.* 1994), Wegener's granulomatosis is characterized by granulomatous inflammation involving the respiratory tract, together with necrotizing vasculitis affecting small- to medium-sized vessels. Microscopic polyangiitis is a necrotizing vasculitis, with few or no immune deposits, affecting small vessels, but without granulomatous inflammation. Since small-vessel vasculitis is present in both syndromes, they share many clinical features. Indeed any or all of the features of microscopic polyangiitis may occur in Wegener's granulomatosis, but the converse is not true. The overall clinical picture varies considerably from patient to patient and may also change in any one patient as the illness progresses.

Features specific to Wegener's granulomatosis

Upper respiratory tract

Upper airways disease occurs in over 90 per cent of patients (Fauci *et al.* 1983; Hoffman *et al.* 1992a) and is characterized histologically by necrotizing, loosely formed granulomas and vasculitis, although the full constellation of features is detected in only a minority of head and neck biopsies (Devaney *et al.* 1990). Nasal involvement may present with epistaxis, rhinorrhoea, and nasal discomfort, or with symptoms resulting from obstruction of drainage of the paranasal sinuses or nasolacrimal duct. Destruction of cartilage may follow soft-tissue necrosis and lead to the characteristic saddle-nose deformity, shown in Fig. 3. Gross destruction of bone or of the overlying skin is unusual and should raise suspicions of lethal midline granuloma or other underlying neoplasm. Cocaine abuse has in recent years become an additional differential diagnosis for destructive lesions.

Disease within the sinuses causes facial pain and symptoms of purulent sinusitis and may be confirmed by plain radiography or computed tomography (CT) scanning, but it should be remembered that sinusitis and soft-tissue thickening on radiographs are common in the 'healthy' population. Otitis media and conductive hearing loss are frequently observed and may result from middle ear involvement or granulomatous tissue in the nasopharynx. Mastoid and tympanic granulomas have also been recognized.

Inflammation may also involve the larynx, trachea, and large airways (Hoffman *et al.* 1992a). While this can lead to haemoptysis or hoarseness, it may sometimes only become apparent when the airways are visualized at bronchoscopy, or may reveal itself later when critical subglottic stenosis occurs. Pulmonary function tests, with analysis of the inspiratory limb of a flow-volume loop, are useful in the detection of extrathoracic airway narrowing.

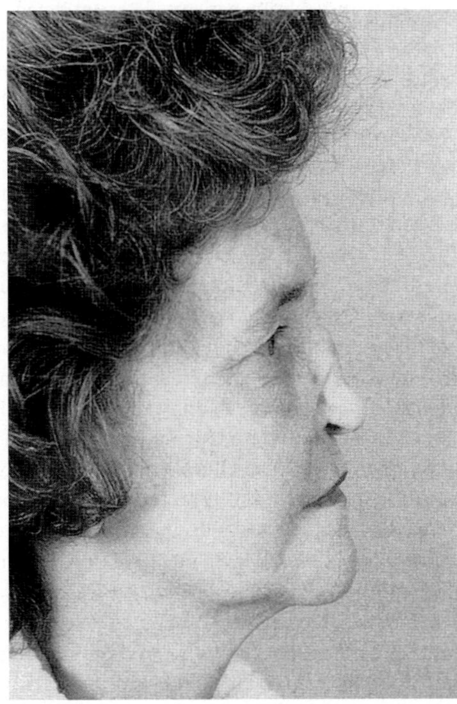

Fig. 3 Typical appearances of nasal collapse in Wegener's granulomatosis.

Pulmonary disease

Manifestations of lung involvement are apparent at presentation in around 90 per cent of patients. Symptoms are not specific and include cough, dyspnoea, haemoptysis, and chest pain, with or without pleuritic characteristics. Lesions may occur in the lung parenchyma, typically in the form of granulomas seen as rounded, and frequently cavitating, lesions on radiography (Fig. 4); histology may be required to distinguish these from neoplasms if diagnostic features in other organs are absent. Microscopically these lesions contain areas of necrosis with granuloma formation.

Granulomas in the bronchi may contribute to haemoptysis, or may be revealed by bronchoscopy. Cicatricial bronchial stenosis, with a tendency to distal infection, may result. One particularly ominous, though not specific, manifestation of disease in the lungs is alveolar haemorrhage (Haworth *et al.* 1985). This is discussed in detail below, as a manifestation of small-vessel vasculitis. Many patients simply have

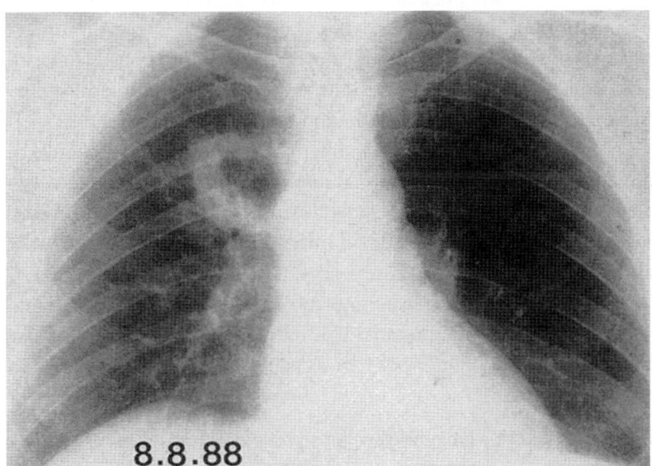

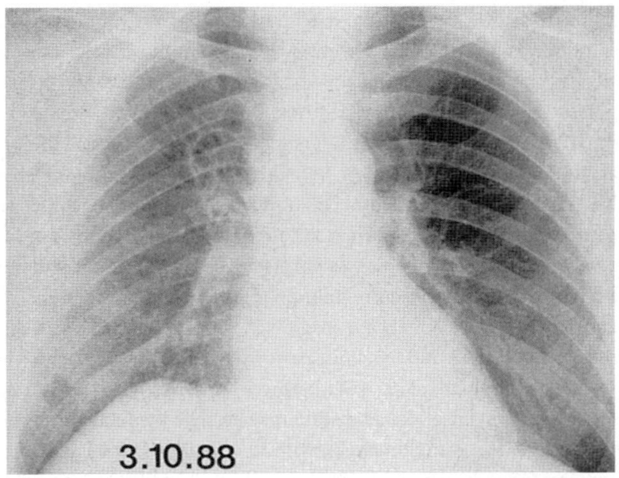

Fig. 4 Chest radiographs from a patient with Wegener's granulomatosis, demonstrating resolution of a cavitating granuloma with immunosuppressive therapy.

ill-defined infiltrates apparent on chest radiography and some have pleural effusions.

Histological studies have revealed a variety of patterns in Wegener's granulomatosis. In a report of 87 open-lung biopsies (Travis *et al.* 1991), the three major findings were parenchymal necrosis (neutrophilic microabscesses and larger areas of geographical necrosis), vasculitis (of arteries, veins, and capillaries), and poorly formed granulomas, accompanied by a mixed inflammatory infiltrate. Minor findings were interstitial fibrosis, alveolar haemorrhage, tissue eosinophilia, and bronchial and bronchiolar lesions.

Granulomatous inflammation outside the respiratory tract

Granulomatous inflammation can affect many parts of the body, including the kidney. Interstitial granulomas can be demonstrated unequivocally in only a minority of renal biopsies (Ronco *et al.* 1983; Bajema *et al.* 1997). A granulomatous reaction may occur around glomeruli severely damaged by necrosis (Yoshikawa and Watanabe 1984) or where there is crescent formation associated with exudation of immunoglobulins and complement components into Bowman's space (Bhathena *et al.* 1987); this may not be specific to Wegener's granulomatosis.

Cerebral complications may result from locally arising granulomas or occasionally from spread of disease from the nasopharynx (Drachman 1962). Anterior and posterior pituitary disease with diabetes insipidus have both been reported by Haynes and Fauci (1978) and in numerous reports subsequently. Overall, however, granulomatous lesions are less common than vasculitic lesions as a cause of neurological symptoms and signs in Wegener's granulomatosis (Nishino *et al.* 1993).

Localized or infiltrative inflammatory masses are also recognized, and have been reported in unusual sites (Lie 1997), including the salivary glands, urogenital tract retroperitoneum, mediastinum, and breast, in addition to well-recognized sites such as the orbit (Bullen *et al.* 1983) and gingiva, causing 'strawberry gums'. Granulomatous inflammation in the skin may be found in a minority of biopsies taken from patients with Wegener's granulomatosis. This frequently presents as a nodular lesion, usually on the upper limbs or trunk, and sometimes ulcerates (Barksdale *et al.* 1995).

Generalized versus limited Wegener's granulomatosis

Not all series describe the same spectrum or severity of disease. The early reports of Wegener (1936) and Fahey *et al.* (1954) were of disseminated disease progressing relentlessly to death from renal and respiratory failure; lack of effective treatment presumably allowed study of the full natural history. Carrington and Liebow (1966) reported patients with a more restricted pattern of disease that they termed 'limited Wegener's granulomatosis'. Their patients had abnormal chest radiographs and 14 of 16 had constitutional symptoms, but other extrapulmonary disease was limited; none had unequivocal evidence of a glomerulonephritis, although five had granulomas in the kidney at autopsy. The disease was not always benign, since five patients died as a direct result of severe pulmonary lesions. Limited Wegener's granulomatosis does not always progress inexorably to generalized disease: some patients avoid renal disease for very many years, even without therapy (Luqmani *et al.* 1994a); others appear to have generalized disease from the outset. Renal disease may even be the first manifestation of Wegener's granulomatosis, with lung lesions following several years later (Woodworth *et al.* 1987). The ELK classification, popularized by DeRemee, and the disease extent index (de Groot *et al.* 2001b) recognize that different combinations of organ may be involved; for example, 'LK' disease involves only the lung and kidney.

Clinical features of generalized vasculitis

Non-specific features

Constitutional symptoms are common in both Wegener's granulomatosis (Pinching *et al.* 1983) and microscopic polyangiitis (Savage *et al.* 1985), with many patients reporting malaise and weight loss or fever and flu-like symptoms at presentation.

Renal disease

This is common but rarely leads to symptoms. Renal involvement should be suspected in patients with microscopic haematuria, proteinuria, and granular and red cell casts, even when excretory function is within normal limits. Renal dysfunction can progress over days or weeks to oliguria and dialysis-dependent renal failure. Heavy proteinuria and macroscopic haematuria occur in a minority of patients (Bindi *et al.* 1993; Geffriaud-Ricouard *et al.* 1993). Hypertension may be seen at presentation in fewer than half (Savage *et al.* 1985; Coward *et al.* 1986; Adu *et al.* 1987; Bindi *et al.* 1993; Geffriaud-Ricouard *et al.* 1993) but fluid overload and the presence of long-standing renal disease may be important contributory factors.

Renal biopsy generally shows focal segmental necrotizing glomerulonephritis, which may become diffuse in advanced disease. Extracapillary proliferation and crescent formation are seen in cases with a clinically rapidly progressive nephritis. Glomerular lesions of varying ages may coexist (Fig. 5); there may be a mixture of normal glomeruli, glomeruli showing active necrosis or crescent formation, and glomeruli which are segmentally or globally sclerosed. Evidence of chronic damage tends to be more marked at presentation in patients with microscopic polyangiitis and in those with ANCA specific for myeloperoxidase; there is more glomerulosclerosis, more interstitial fibrosis, more tubular atrophy, and there are fewer normal glomeruli (Franssen *et al.* 1995; Hauer *et al.* 2002c). It is unclear whether this reflects later presentation or differences in pathogenesis.

Brouwer *et al.* (1994) identified activated neutrophils within the glomerulus in biopsies from patients with untreated Wegener's granulomatosis, and their number correlated with the severity of renal impairment. Müller *et al.* (1988) demonstrated CD8-positive lymphocytes within the glomeruli and monocyte/macrophages in Bowman's space. Macrophages are also present in active glomerular lesions, and display activation markers (Rastaldi *et al.* 2000). Studies of MHC expression are contradictory; das Neves *et al.* (1991) demonstrated intense HLA DR expression in the glomerular tuft and crescents, while Müller *et al.* (1988) reported a reduction in glomerular expression, commensurate with the degree of glomerular damage, but an increase in expression by tubular cells. Studies of the expression of leucocyte–endothelial adhesion molecules have not demonstrated a unique pattern of abnormality, although intercellular adhesion molecule-1 (ICAM-1) expression may be increased in affected glomeruli (Fuiano *et al.* 1991), and in cellular crescents (Moon *et al.* 2002) while vascular cell adhesion molecule-1 (VCAM-1) expression is increased on renal tubular epithelial cells (Seron *et al.* 1991). The cellular composition of glomerular crescents and the cellular markers seen in crescentic glomerulonephritis are discussed in further detail in Chapter 3.10 and the role of leucocyte–endothelial adhesion in vasculitic injury is discussed in greater detail in Chapter 4.5.1.

The necrotizing glomerulonephritis is commonly accompanied by an interstitial infiltrate, containing T lymphocytes, predominantly of the CD4 phenotype, in both Wegener's granulomatosis (ten Berge *et al.* 1985) and microscopic polyangiitis (Müller *et al.* 1988). CD8 lymphocytes may also be present in abundance (das Neves *et al.* 1991). In certain patients, interstitial nephritis may be the predominant finding (Cameron 1991). Vasculitis may be found within the kidney, typically affecting interlobular arteries and arterioles (Novak *et al.* 1982; Bindi *et al.* 1993), but it is not detected in the majority of biopsies (Savage *et al.* 1985; Hoffman *et al.* 1992a).

Glomerulonephritis in this condition is usually considered to be 'pauci-immune', though sparse deposits of immunoglobulin and complement are often seen, particularly in necrotic or sclerotic lesions. Electron microscopy only rarely shows immune deposits (Ronco *et al.* 1983; Jennette *et al.* 1989; Bindi *et al.* 1993). The histology of the renal lesion appears similar whether or not immune deposits are detected.

Muscle and joint symptoms

Arthralgia and myalgia are common; arthritis occurs less commonly (Savage *et al.* 1985; Noritake *et al.* 1987), and there may rarely be erosive changes (Jacobs *et al.* 1987).

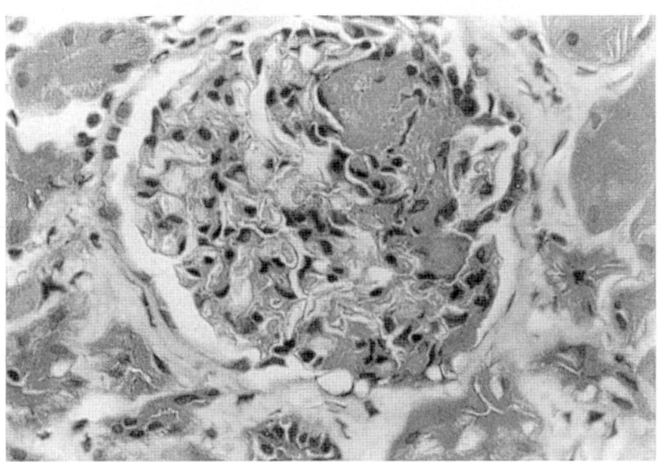

(a)

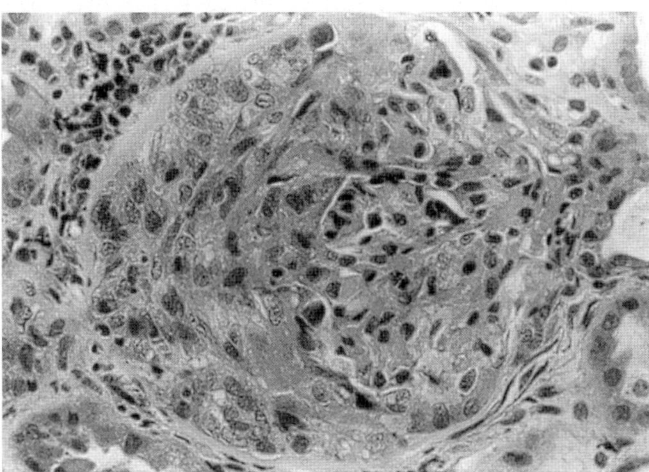

(b)

Fig. 5 Light microscopy of a renal biopsy from a patient with Wegener's granulomatosis, demonstrating (a) segmental necrosis and (b) cellular crescent formation with compression of glomerular tuft.

Eye involvement

The spectrum of eye disease is greatest in Wegener's granulomatosis and includes conjunctivitis, episcleritis, corneal ulceration, uveitis, retinal vasculitis, and optic neuropathy, as well as orbital involvement and obstruction of the nasolacrimal duct due to granulomatous masses. Eye involvement occurs in up to 50 per cent of patients (Fauci *et al.* 1983) and carries significant ocular morbidity. Bullen *et al.* (1983) reported the need for enucleation of three eyes in a series of 40 patients with ophthalmic disease. Episcleritis also occurs in microscopic polyangiitis, affecting 24 per cent of patients in one series (Savage *et al.* 1985).

Nervous system involvement

Necrotizing vasculitis may affect the brain, cranial, or peripheral nerves (Moore and Fauci 1981; and reviewed by Tervaert and Kallenberg 1993). Cerebral vasculitis may lead to major neurological deficits due to the involvement of large arteries (Satoh *et al.* 1988), or more subtle physical signs due to small-vessel vasculitis. Subclinical abnormalities of cognitive function have recently been identified, in association with subcortical abnormalities on magnetic resonance imaging (MRI) scanning (Mattioli *et al.* 2002). Seizures may occur, although metabolic abnormalities may also contribute in patients in renal failure. Cerebrospinal fluid analysis may reveal pleocytosis or a raised protein, and CT or MRI of the brain may be helpful, although there are no changes which are pathognomonic of small-vessel vasculitis. Isolated cranial nerve lesions are also well recognized. Peripheral nerve lesions are more common than central abnormalities, typically causing an asymmetrical mononeuritis multiplex, or occasionally a distal sensory neuropathy.

Cutaneous involvement

Cutaneous manifestations have been described in detail by Jennette *et al.* (1989), Daoud *et al.* (1994), and Barksdale *et al.* (1995). Palpable purpura (Fig. 6), isolated necrotic lesions, nailbed infarcts and splinter haemorrhages occur frequently. Soft-tissue infarction of the extremities, although more often associated with large-vessel vasculitides, has also been observed. Necrotizing leucocytoclastic vasculitis is the most common histological finding, and may affect small arteries, veins, or capillaries. The paucity of immune deposits excludes the diagnosis of

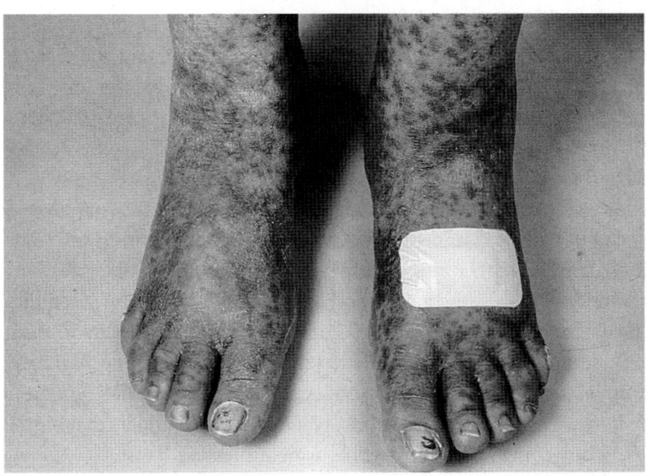

Fig. 6 Vasculitic rash in a patient with microscopic polyangiitis. A plaster covers the site of skin biopsy.

cryoglobulinaemic vasculitis or Henoch–Schönlein purpura, although the clinical presentation may be similar. Panniculitis may result from the involvement of deeper vessels and pyoderma gangrenosum-like ulceration is also reported.

Gastrointestinal tract vasculitis

Gastrointestinal disease may present with abdominal pain, diarrhoea, or gastrointestinal bleeding (Camilleri *et al.* 1983). Inspection of the intestinal mucosa, either at endoscopy or surgery, reveals scattered purpuric lesions with ulceration. Serious complications of major bleeding or bowel perforation may occur. Severe ulceration of the oral mucosa occurs in a number of patients. Gut vasculitis occurs in both Wegener's granulomatosis and microscopic polyangiitis, although perhaps more frequently in the latter, affecting up to 30 per cent of patients (Savage *et al.* 1985).

Alveolar haemorrhage

Systemic vasculitis is (confusingly!) the most common cause of 'Goodpasture's syndrome', the combination of rapidly progressive glomerulonephritis and alveolar haemorrhage. The alveolar haemorrhage results from a pauci-immune alveolar capillaritis (Bosch *et al.* 1994) and usually presents with haemoptysis and dyspnoea, together with anaemia, hypoxia, and diffuse alveolar shadowing on radiography (Fig. 7); increased transfer factor for carbon monoxide provides diagnostic confirmation. As a non-granulomatous form of vasculitis, it is not exclusive to Wegener's granulomatosis (Haworth *et al.* 1985) and microscopic polyangiitis is the most common single cause of alveolar haemorrhage. There is no association with cigarette smoking (unlike the lung haemorrhage of anti-GBM antibody-mediated disease), but clinical experience suggests that intercurrent infection and fluid overload may lead to exacerbations.

Cardiac involvement

Cardiac involvement is relatively unusual in Wegener's granulomatosis and microscopic polyangiitis. Dysrhythmias and cardiac failure have been reported, together with rarer clinical findings such as dilated cardiomyopathy (Fauci *et al.* 1983), pericarditis clearly attributable to vasculitis (Hoffman *et al.* 1992a), and valvular lesions. In Wegener's granulomatosis mimicking infective endocarditis (Gerbracht *et al.* 1987).

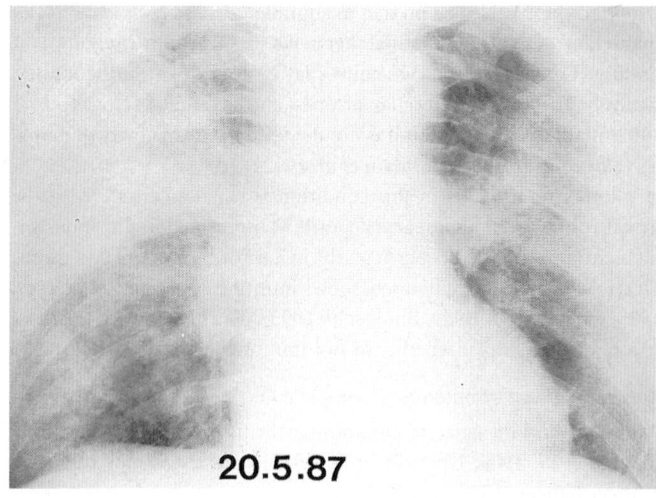

(a)

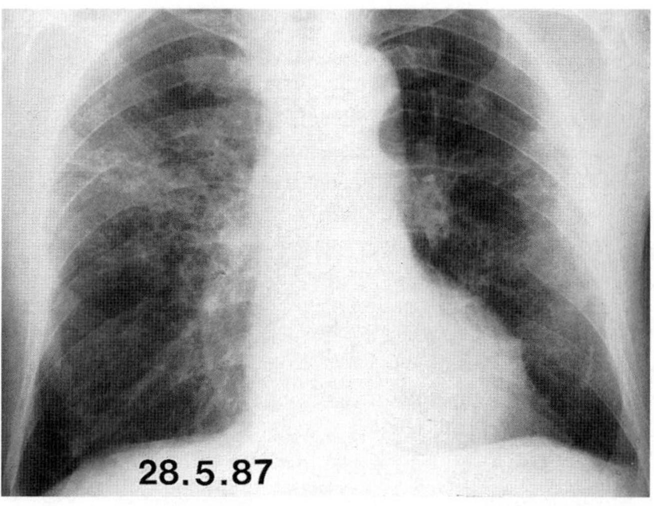

(b)

Fig. 7 Chest radiograph from a patient with microscopic polyangiitis, demonstrating the appearances of diffuse alveolar haemorrhage, with rapid resolution following immunosuppressive therapy including plasma exchange.

Relationship of clinical features to ANCA

Features of the presenting illness segregate to some extent with the main ANCA specificities. c-ANCA with specificity for proteinase 3 are particularly associated with sinus disease and granulomatous lung vasculitis (Jennette *et al.* 1989; Cohen Tervaert *et al.* 1990a), and therefore with a diagnosis of Wegener's granulomatosis (Hagen *et al.* 1998). p-ANCA with specificity for myeloperoxidase are associated with renal-limited vasculitis (Falk and Jennette 1988), microscopic polyangiitis (Geffriaud-Ricouard *et al.* 1993) and Churg–Strauss syndrome (Cohen Tervaert *et al.* 1991). The distinction is not absolute, as exemplified by the studies of Geffriaud-Ricouard *et al.* (1993) and Hagen *et al.* (1998), and there are undoubtedly differences between series because different diagnostic criteria are used. Patients with myeloperoxidase-specific ANCA appear to have a greater degree of chronic renal damage on initial renal biopsies, when compared with patients with proteinase 3-specific ANCA, though the extent to which this results from later diagnosis in the absence of specific extrarenal symptoms is unclear. A minority of patients with small-vessel vasculitis have ANCA of specificities other than proteinase 3 and myeloperoxidase, including bactericidal/permeability-increasing protein and elastase, but there are no clear associations with particular clinical characteristics.

The tendency to relapse also appears to segregate with ANCA specificity. Our data suggest that proteinase 3-specific ANCA are associated with a relapse rate up to fourfold higher than that associated with myeloperoxidase-specific ANCA when patients are treated with the same protocol (Gaskin and Pusey 1995). A difference in relapse rate has also been demonstrated by others (Geffriaud-Ricouard *et al.* 1993; Booth *et al.* 2003).

Vasculitis in children

Hall *et al.* (1985b) reported four children with Wegener's granulomatosis, whose initial features, including cutaneous vasculitis and nephritis in four and gastrointestinal symptoms in two, mimicked Henoch–Schönlein purpura, and in whom institution of appropriate therapy was delayed. Typical respiratory manifestations emerged during follow-up.

Rottem *et al.* (1993) compared the features of Wegener's granulomatosis in 23 children and 135 adults treated at the National Institutes of Health. The mean age at onset in the children was 15.4 years, with a range of 9.3–19.4 years, and the clinical spectrum of disease varied from anatomically limited and indolent, to generalized and life-threatening vasculitis. In comparison with adults, childhood-onset patients were more often female and were five times more likely to have subglottic stenosis and twice as likely to have nasal deformities.

Diagnosis

Confirmation of diagnosis depends on establishing the presence of small-vessel vasculitis, together with granulomatous inflammation in the respiratory tract in Wegener's granulomatosis. Ultimately, this requires proof by histology, but many other investigations, including assays for ANCA, can yield supporting evidence. When combined with a typical clinical appearance, these investigations are usually sufficient to justify the commencement of therapy.

Haematology and biochemistry

Routine blood count frequently demonstrates anaemia, typically with a normocytic normochromic pattern but occasionally with iron deficiency due to lung or gastrointestinal haemorrhage. A neutrophil leucocytosis is common (Savage *et al.* 1985; Hoffman *et al.* 1992a), but low levels of eosinophilia have also been reported (Ronco *et al.* 1983). Thrombocythaemia is frequently seen and the mean platelet count in one series (Pinching *et al.* 1983) was 612×10^9 per litre. Erythrocyte sedimentation rate (ESR) will invariably be elevated (Fauci *et al.* 1983) as will C-reactive protein, and the latter is more specific in renal failure. As part of the same acute-phase response, albumin may be low and alkaline phosphatase elevated. There may be hyperglobulinaemia, especially affecting IgA in some cases (see, e.g. ten Berge *et al.* 1985), but mainly IgG in others.

Serum urea and creatinine may be increased, commensurate with the degree of renal damage, but values in the normal range do not exclude significant renal inflammation. Proteinuria indicates the presence of glomerular disease, but is only rarely in the nephrotic range. The urine sediment will usually show red cells and granular and red cell casts, but in some cases shows less abnormality than expected from the histological severity of nephritis. These and other non-specific findings are summarized in Table 2.

Immunology

Antineutrophil cytoplasmic antibodies

Assays for ANCA have become integral to the assessment of patients with suspected vasculitis. The most widely used assay is the internationally validated indirect immunofluorescence assay (Wiik 1989) using ethanol-fixed neutrophils and able to differentiate c-ANCA and p-ANCA. This should be used in conjunction with solid-phase assays using purified proteinase 3 and myeloperoxidase (Hagen *et al.* 1998; Savige *et al.* 1999; Wiik 2001).

A positive ANCA in the clinical setting of suspected vasculitis, particularly if specific for proteinase 3 or myeloperoxidase, is highly suggestive that the diagnosis is correct (Niles *et al.* 1991; Hagen *et al.* 1998), although the majority of clinicians would still seek biopsy confirmation. c-ANCA is more specific for vasculitis than p-ANCA determined by immunofluorescence only, since perinuclear staining is not only produced by antimyeloperoxidase antibodies, but also by antinuclear antibodies and antibodies to a variety of neutrophil components which are not strongly associated with vasculitis. A negative ANCA in the setting of limited Wegener's granulomatosis is common, and negative ANCA has been reported in a minority of cases with generalized small-vessel vasculitis (Bindi *et al.* 1993; Adu *et al.* 1995) even when well-validated assays are used (Hagen *et al.* 1998).

The majority of assays detect circulating ANCA of IgG specificity; subclasses IgG1 and IgG4 predominate. It has been suggested that significant levels of IgG3 ANCA may be found in addition when renal involvement is present (Brouwer *et al.* 1991), when the disease is active (Jayne *et al.* 1991), and when ANCA are specific for proteinase 3 (Segelmark and Wieslander 1993). An early report suggested an association of ANCA of IgM class only with pulmonary haemorrhage (Jayne *et al.* 1989), although a later study detected coexisting IgG and IgM ANCA in such patients (Esnault *et al.* 1992), and other studies have not confirmed an association of IgM antimyeloperoxidase ANCA with any particular syndrome (Kokolina *et al.* 1994).

ANCA coexisting with circulating and deposited anti-GBM antibodies have been described (Jayne *et al.* 1990). Data using purified antigen assays suggest that ANCA may be detected in 10–20 per cent of patients with anti-GBM disease, while anti-GBM antibodies specific for the 'Goodpasture antigen', the α-3 chain of type 4 collagen, may be found in 2–3 per cent of patients with ANCA (Short *et al.* 1993). The usual sequence of the two immune reponses is uncertain: Wahls *et al.* (1987) reported anti-GBM disease as a secondary event, while O'Donoghue *et al.* (1989) reported the development of systemic vasculitis following the diagnostic features of anti-GBM disease. Patients with both antibodies are more likely to have myeloperoxidase-specific ANCA (Bosch *et al.* 1991; Niles *et al.* 1991), may have evidence of renal vasculitis (Weber *et al.* 1992), frequently have evidence of systemic disease outside the kidneys and lungs (Jayne *et al.* 1990), and respond to immunotherapy in a way more typical of vasculitis than of typical anti-GBM disease, particularly if the ANCA titre is high (Bosch *et al.* 1991). Furthermore, like vasculitis patients, they are at significant risk of relapse (Jayne *et al.* 1990). These data have management implications;

Table 2 Non-specific laboratory findings in vasculitis

Haematology
Anaemia
Leucocytosis
Thrombocytosis
Elevated ESR
Biochemistry
Evidence of renal impairment
Elevated alkaline phosphatase
Hypoalbuminaemia
Elevated C-reactive protein
Urine findings
Proteinuria
Microscopic haematuria
Granular and red cell casts
Immunology
Hyperglobulinaemia
Immune complexes
Rheumatoid factors

aggressive treatment is justified for dialysis-dependent patients and long-term therapy should be modelled on regimens for vasculitis. It would seem appropriate to use plasma exchange in the acute phase, to remove circulating anti-GBM antibodies, although the proof that this is obligatory is lacking.

Other immunological abnormalities

No other investigations offer the same predictive value as assays for ANCA. The concentrations of complement components are usually normal or increased, and this may help to distinguish small-vessel vasculitis from systemic lupus erythematosus, cryoglobulinaemic vasculitis, and infective endocarditis with glomerulonephritis. Rheumatoid factors and immune complexes are common, but not specific for vasculitis (Pinching *et al.* 1983; Ronco *et al.* 1983). Antibodies binding to cultured endothelial cells have been identified in the sera of patients with systemic vasculitis, including Wegener's granulomatosis, but they are not invariably present and they have also been detected in other rheumatological disorders. This topic is discussed in greater detail in Chapter 4.5.1.

Radiology

Pulmonary imaging

In Wegener's granulomatosis, the most specific findings are rounded opacities corresponding to granulomas (Fig. 5), which may cavitate. CT may confirm the presence of lesions poorly visualized on plain radiography (Cordier *et al.* 1990; Lee *et al.* 2003), and may be valuable in follow-up (Reuter *et al.* 1998). Bronchial lesions may now be assessed non-invasively using CT virtual bronchoscopy with a sensitivity of around 80 per cent (Summers *et al.* 2002).

A diffuse alveolar shadowing pattern may indicate alveolar haemorrhage, although the differential diagnoses of pulmonary oedema and severe infection must always be considered. A typical pattern is illustrated in Fig. 7, which shows the appearance before treatment and a week afterwards. There is usually a rapid resolution with immunosuppressive therapy. Patchy infiltration is a less specific finding, and pleural effusions may be seen in both vasculitic syndromes.

Upper respiratory tract imaging

In Wegener's granulomatosis, radiological sinus abnormalities, including fluid levels and soft-tissue thickening, are very common. The combination of bone destruction and new bone formation on CT, in the absence of previous surgery is highly suggestive of Wegener's granulomatosis (Lloyd *et al.* 2002). Tracheal disease may be assessed using spiral CT (Screaton *et al.* 1998). MRI may demonstrate abnormalities, especially of the paranasal sinuses, in up to 90 per cent of patients with Wegener's granulomatosis (Muhle *et al.* 1997) and offers an alternative method for imaging the laryngeal region (Hoffman *et al.* 1992a). MR is also an excellent modality for imaging the orbits (Courcoutsakis *et al.* 1997) and avoids the radiation exposure associated with repeated CT scanning.

Renal imaging

This is usually unremarkable, although renal echogenicity may be increased in the presence of glomerulonephritis. The principal reason for imaging is to exclude other causes of renal dysfunction, and to guide renal biopsy.

Angiography

According to the Chapel Hill consensus approach to the classification of vasculitis (Jennette *et al.* 1994), involvement of medium-sized arteries is compatible with a diagnosis of microscopic polyangiitis or Wegener's granulomatosis, although it is neither diagnostic nor common. Coeliac or renal angiography is not, therefore, part of routine investigation when these diagnoses are suspected, although it may be warranted in the light of certain clinical symptoms and may demonstrate the presence of aneurysms or, less specifically, irregularities of calibre and arterial occlusions. It may also be used therapeutically, to occlude bleeding vessels in patients with gastrointestinal involvement.

Radiolabelled leucocyte scanning

Indium-labelled leucocyte scanning may be used to identify neutrophil migration into areas affected by vasculitis, including the gut (Reuter *et al.* 1993). Early images may also identify increased margination of neutrophils into the lungs in vasculitis (Jonker *et al.* 1992), although this does not currently have diagnostic significance.

Histopathology

Pathological confirmation of Wegener's granulomatosis requires demonstration of the presence of necrotizing granulomas. Upper airways biopsies are easy to take but only rarely show a full house of vasculitis, necrosis, and granulomatous infiltration. Distinction from other important conditions may, therefore, be difficult (Devaney *et al.* 1990). Taking multiple biopsies improves the diagnostic yield (Anderson *et al.* 1992). Lung histology obtained at open-lung biopsy is more reliable (Travis *et al.* 1991), but this is invasive. Imaging-guided biopsies may give sufficient information to distinguish between important differential diagnoses (active disease or infection) during follow-up (Carruthers *et al.* 2000). Transbronchial biopsy has been advocated, but the specimens are often too small and fragmented to be of value. By comparison, renal biopsy is more likely to give an adequate amount of tissue, and will usually show a focal necrotizing glomerulonephritis; granulomas and vascular lesions are much less commonly seen.

Definitive diagnosis of microscopic polyangiitis similarly requires histological confirmation, almost invariably from renal biopsy showing a pauci-immune focal necrotizing glomerulonephritis with crescent formation. Biopsy from other organs, such as skin or intestine, may confirm the presence of a vasculitis.

Investigations and differential diagnosis

Other investigations will often be needed to exclude other possible diagnoses. The combination of arthralgia and clinical evidence of nephritis is compatible with both systemic lupus erythematosus (Chapter 4.7.2) and primary systemic vasculitis. While the age, gender, and racial background of the patient might favour one syndrome rather than the other, the final distinction must be made by assay for ANCA, antinuclear and anti-double-stranded DNA antibodies, estimation of serum complement, and renal biopsy, with immunohistology.

Lung haemorrhage and rapidly progressive nephritis should provoke a search for anti-GBM antibodies (Chapter 3.12), although a clinical picture of widespread systemic disease favours small-vessel vasculitis. As already discussed, infrequently there is evidence of both diseases simultaneously.

Mixed essential cryoglobulinaemia (Chapter 4.6) and Henoch–Schönlein purpura (Chapter 4.5.2) also enter the differential diagnosis of small-vessel vasculitis with glomerulonephritis, but may be distinguished by the nature and extent of immune deposits; detectable cryoglobulins and hypocomplementaemia point to a diagnosis of mixed essential cryoglobulinaemia.

Differentiation of Wegener's granulomatosis from Churg–Strauss syndrome can occasionally be difficult, though the distinction may not actually influence treatment. Cases are reported in which marked tissue eosinophilia was seen in the absence of peripheral blood eosinophilia or asthma. Symptoms resulting from nasal polyps in Churg–Strauss syndrome may also cause initial confusion.

There are reports of detectable ANCA in patients with endocarditis and glomerulonephritis (Wagner *et al.* 1991; Soto *et al.* 1994) and clinically the features may be very similar to those of systemic vasculitis. Current experience suggests that further investigations, including repeated blood cultures, trans-oesophageal echocardiography, serum complement estimation, purified antigen ANCA assays, and renal biopsy with immunofluorescence microscopy staining are advisable. Disseminated cholesterol emboli may occasionally cause similar confusion (Peat and Mathieson 1996).

Assessment of disease activity

Long-term management entails balancing the risks of treatment toxicity against the risk of disease recurrence or progression. The ability to diagnose active disease, and to identify patients at risk from relapse is critically important. Assessment of disease activity depends chiefly on a clinical assessment and clinical scoring systems are presently the mainstay of clinical trial evaluations (Luqmani *et al.* 1994b; Stone *et al.* 2001a). Abnormalities of routine investigations such as haemoglobin, leucocyte and platelet counts, renal function, urinary sediment, and the chest radiograph often accompany relapse. The ESR is slow to reflect changes in disease activity, and estimations of C-reactive protein are more reliable (Hind *et al.* 1984; Jayne *et al.* 1995). Nonetheless, these markers are not specific, and sometimes reflect infection rather than active vasculitis. Furthermore, abnormalities tend to coincide with relapse, and are of little help in predicting imminent disease activity.

Initial optimism that ANCA changes correlate tightly enough with disease activity to dictate therapy (Cohen Tervaert *et al.* 1990b) has not been sustained, and subclass assays do not improve the predictive value (Boomsma *et al.* 2000; Ara *et al.* 1999). Nonetheless, relapses occur more frequently in patients with persisting ANCA or rising - concentrations (see, e.g. Gaskin *et al.* 1991; Jayne *et al.* 1995; Kyndt *et al.* 1999; Boomsma *et al.* 2000), which should act as a warning signal. This is true for both anti-proteinase 3 and antimyeloperoxidase ANCA.

Other potential markers of active vasculitis have been examined in research studies, although they have no place in current clinical practice. They include circulating soluble leucocyte–endothelial adhesion molecules: levels of soluble ICAM-1 and VCAM-1 are higher in vasculitis patients than in healthy controls (Ara *et al.* 2001; Takizawa *et al.* 2001), though some authors attribute the elevation to the presence of renal failure. Concentrations of soluble IL-2 receptor are also raised (see, e.g. Lai and Lockwood 1993; Schmitt *et al.* 1998), but a close relationship with disease activity following treatment is doubtful, and levels may also rise in the presence of intercurrent infection (Arranz *et al.* 2000; Christensson *et al.* 2000). Circulating levels of soluble CD14 are raised in patients with ANCA-associated vasculitis but remain elevated after the induction of clinical remission (Nowack *et al.* 2001). The proportion of neutrophils with membrane proteinase 3 expression is higher in patients with Wegener's granulomatosis than in healthy controls, and patients who relapse have a higher level of surface expression than those who do not (Rarok *et al.* 2002).

Treatment and outcome

Historical aspects

Evidence for steroids and cyclophosphamide

Historically, the outcome of untreated Wegener's granulomatosis was poor, with a mean survival of 5 months (Walton 1958). Eighty per cent of patients died within 1 year; survival to 4 years was exceptional. The presence of progressive renal failure was particularly ominous before dialysis was generally available, although death from respiratory failure was also common. Corticosteroids were the first agents to make an impact: an early report by Fahey *et al.* (1954) described the benefit of cortisone and adrenocorticotrophic hormone treatment in one patient and commented on 'good evidence that these drugs controlled the intensity of the inflammatory process'. Walton (1958) later described temporary remissions in two patients and by 1967, 26 steroid-treated patients had been reported in the literature and mean survival was 12.5 months (Hollander and Manning 1967). Unfortunately, despite the use of high doses of prednisone (a mean of 44 mg daily), the disease eventually became refractory. Thus, while corticosteroids represented the first step in development of therapy, their use alone was inadequate.

Fahey *et al.* (1954) had used intravenous nitrogen mustard in a patient with Wegener's granulomatosis who became resistant to steroid therapy, and reported a temporary improvement in symptoms. Use of the alkylating agents chlorambucil (Hollander and Manning 1967) and cyclophosphamide (Novack and Pearson 1971) followed. Fauci *et al.* (1971) treated nine patients, seven of whom had generalized disease, with oral cyclophosphamide alone at an initial dose of 100–125 mg daily; all showed clinical improvement within 3 weeks of commencing therapy. A consistent regimen of cyclophosphamide and corticosteroids was subsequently developed, and by 1983, Fauci *et al.* (1983) were able to report use of these drugs in 85 patients with follow-up of up to 21 years.

The earliest attempts to treat microscopic polyangiitis and classical polyarteritis used oral corticosteroids alone, with an improvement in survival from 13 per cent at 5 years in untreated patients to around 50 per cent (Frohnert and Sheps 1967; Sack *et al.* 1975). Fauci and co-workers added cyclophosphamide in steroid-resistant disease (Fauci *et al.* 1979), using a dose of 2 mg/kg daily. Leib *et al.* (1979), treating 64 patients with polyarteritis, preferred azathioprine as the additional agent in the majority. It is not clear how many had predominantly small-vessel disease and only 22 had abnormal renal function, but the response to therapy was dramatic. Five-year survival was 12 per cent in untreated patients, 53 per cent in patients treated with steroids alone, and 80 per cent in those treated with a combination of steroids and cytotoxic agents. A retrospective study of a similar group of patients by Cohen *et al.* (1980) found less convincing benefit from combined therapy, but it seems likely that the patients selected to receive additional treatment were those with the most severe disease at the outset. In subsequent reports of patients with microscopic polyangiitis and focal segmental necrotizing glomerulonephritis (see, e.g. Serra *et al.* 1984; Savage *et al.* 1985), a combination of steroids and cytotoxic agents was generally used.

These early studies did not resolve whether cyclophosphamide should be preferred to azathioprine in microscopic polyangiitis and polyarteritis nodosa, and it is possible that the two conditions may require different approaches. We treat microscopic polyangiitis with the same cyclophosphamide-based regimen that we use for Wegener's granulomatosis, and the approach of the European Vasculitis Study group has been similar (Jayne 2001). Cyclophosphamide may be less crucial in some cases of polyarteritis nodosa. Guillevin *et al.* (2003) developed a five-factor score, based on renal function, proteinuria, cardiac, gastrointestinal, and neurological involvement to distinguish between good and bad prognosis patients with Churg–Strauss syndrome and polyarteritis nodosa. His group, analysing pooled data from a variety of trials, suggests that addition of cyclophosphamide to corticosteroids prolongs survival only in poor-prognosis patients (Gayraud *et al.* 2001).

The NIH steroid and cyclophosphamide regimen

Fauci *et al.* (1983) reported from the United States National Institutes of Health (NIH) the treatment of 85 patients with Wegener's granulomatosis. The treatment regimen is summarized in Table 3. The daily steroids were continued for 1–2 weeks, and then converted to an alternate day regimen. A dose of 20 mg on alternate days was usually achieved by 6–12 months. The drug was then tailed off, leaving the patient on cyclophosphamide alone, provided there was no evidence of disease activity. The cyclophosphamide was continued at the starting dose, toxicity permitting, until the patient had been in complete clinical remission for at least 1 year, and then reduced by 25 mg every 2–3 months and either stopped completely or maintained at a dose above that at which the patient had evidence of disease activity. To minimize the risk of infection, the total white cell was not allowed to fall to less than 3000–3500 per mm^3. Fauci's treatment rapidly became the 'gold standard' with which to compare other treatment strategies, and was also used to treat paediatric patients at the NIH (Rottem *et al.* 1993).

Although this regimen was vastly superior to any previous approach, long-term follow-up revealed a high level of morbidity from both the disease and its treatment (Hoffman *et al.* 1992a). Adverse effects of treatment ranged from the cosmetic to the life-threatening. Mild to moderate hair loss affected 17 per cent and cushingoid features developed transiently in all patients. Diabetes was induced in 8 per cent, cataracts in 21 per cent, bony fractures in 11 per cent and aseptic bone necrosis in 3 per cent. Significant infections occurred during follow-up in 46 per cent of the patients; half of the serious bacterial, pneumocystis, and fungal infections occurred during the period of daily steroid therapy. Cohen *et al.* (1982), in a separate study, had identified the dose of steroids as the most important factor predisposing to infection in patients treated for immune-mediated renal diseases.

Table 3 NIH treatment regimen

Induction
Prednisolone
1 mg/kg daily
Cyclophosphamide
2 mg/kg daily
Fulminant disease
Prednisolone
2 mg/kg daily
Cyclophosphamide
4–5 mg/kg daily
Maintenance
Prednisolone
tapering alternate day dose
Cyclophosphamide
starting dose maintained until remission >1 year

Urothelial toxicity of cyclophosphamide was an important problem. Haemorrhagic cystitis, which is mediated by a cyclophosphamide metabolite, acrolein, occurred in 43 per cent of the patients reported by Hoffman *et al.* (1992a), and 15 per cent of a similar group of patients reported by Stilwell *et al.* (1988). Bladder cancer developed in approximately 2.5 per cent of the patients in each series, representing a 33-fold increase in risk, and the incidence had risen to 5 per cent in a further follow-up study on the NIH cohort (Talar-Williams *et al.* 1996) after a median follow-up of 8.5 years. Bladder toxicity is dose-dependent: Stillwell *et al.* (1988) reported a higher cumulative dose of cyclophosphamide in those developing haemorrhagic cystitis, and in six of the seven patients developing cancer in Talar-Williams' series (1996), the total cumulative cyclophosphamide dose exceeded 100 g, and the cumulative duration of cyclophosphamide therapy exceeded 2.7 years.

The gonadal toxicity of cyclophosphamide in both males and females is well-recognized from its use in malignant disease, though the quantitative impact at the doses used in vasculitis is less certain. Hoffman *et al.* (1992a) noted that after 1 year of the drug, 57 per cent of women between 18 and 35 years of age were amenorrhoeic, unable to conceive, or had evidence of ovarian failure. Haubitz *et al.* (1998a) reported higher FSH levels, implying worse gonadal injury, in men treated with oral cyclophosphamide than those treated with a pulse regimen that delivered a lower total dose.

Long-term haematological abnormalities attributed to cyclophosphamide include persistent hypogammaglobulinaemia and myelodysplastic syndromes and the development of haematological malignancies, including lymphomas and myeloid leukaemias. Hoffman *et al.* (1992a) calculated that the risk of lymphoma was increased 11-fold.

Rottem *et al.* (1993) examined the side-effects of the standard NIH regimen when used to treat children with Wegener's granulomatosis. The spectrum of complications were similar to those reported in adults, with the exception of malignancies, which were not detected in any of the children during the period of follow-up (up to 18 years; mean 8.7 years).

Since the risks of cyclophosphamide are associated with the duration and total dose of treatment, refinement of treatment in recent years has concentrated on induction regimens employing lower doses, and maintenance regimens avoiding the use of cyclophosphamide completely.

Current approaches to initial therapy

Early conversion to azathioprine maintenance therapy

For over 20 years, our practice in ANCA-associated vasculitis has been to commence treament with oral cyclophosphamide and steroids, but to substitute azathioprine maintenance therapy for cyclophosphamide after approximately 3 months. Many other European groups have used a similar approach. A comparison of this approach with the use of 1 year's cyclophosphamide has recently been made in a European randomized controlled trial, which demonstrated equal efficacy in the first 18 months of treatment. (Jayne *et al.* 1999). Azathioprine maintenance therapy is not completely free of risk; data from a Swedish cancer registry demonstrated a significant increase in skin cancer risk associated with its use in vasculitis patients (Westman *et al.* 1998).

Alternatives to oral cyclophosphamide

Pulsed intravenous cyclophosphamide Pulsed cyclophosphamide offers two potential advantages over continuous oral cyclophosphamide.

The first of these is a reduction in the total dose administered; the second is that it facilitates the concomitant use of mesna to prevent bladder toxicity. The success of pulsed intravenous cyclophosphamide in the treatment of lupus nephritis has led to a number of systematic studies in systemic vasculitis.

Pulsed cyclophosphamide has been tested in groups of patients with Wegener's granulomatosis, patients with ANCA-associated glomerulonephritis and vasculitis, and patients with a mixture of primary vasculitic disorders. Regimens have varied in dose size, frequency, and route of administration. De Groot *et al.* (2001a) pooled data from 11 non-randomized studies; the key outcomes are shown in Table 4. Use of a higher individual dose (Hoffman *et al.* 1990) increased adverse effects but not efficacy. Pulsed therapy appeared to be less successful in patients with relapsed disease (Hoffman *et al.* 1990), perhaps because these patients have already declared their disease harder to control, and in predominantly non-renal Wegener's granulomatosis (Reinhold Keller *et al.* 1994).

There have also been three randomized controlled trials (Adu *et al.* 1997; Guillevin *et al.* 1997b; Haubitz *et al.* 1998c) in which pulses were usually, but not invariably, given intravenously. Adu and coworkers, from Birmingham, administered both cyclophosphamide and corticosteroids as oral pulses after the first month (Adu *et al.* 1997); their complex regimen is described in detail in the study of relapse by Gordon *et al.* (1993). The three studies varied in the dose adjustments made for renal failure, age, and leucopenia, and in the details of concurrent therapy and, strictly speaking, Adu's trial (1997) was a comparison of two different treatment regimens rather than a direct comparison of two types of cyclophosphamide administration. Notwithstanding these differences, the data from the three studies have been combined in a meta-analysis by de Groot and colleagues (2001a). The odds ratios are shown in Table 5. They concluded that pulsed therapy was more likely to induce remission and was associated with less infection, though this did not reduce overall mortality. It is worth noting that the oral regimens tested in these controlled studies were lengthy, and permitted significant leucopenia, and so significant toxicity is unsurprising. An apparently higher rate of relapse in pulse-treated patients did not reach statistical significance. The question of whether cyclophosphamide should be given continuously or in pulses has still not been resolved, but further data will be available soon from another European study. Nor has the optimum dose and interval for pulse therapy been defined.

Table 4 Summary of non-randomized studies of pulsed cyclophosphamide (taken from de Groot *et al.* 2001a)

Regimen	
Dose	375–1000 mg/m^2
Interval	Weekly to monthly
Outcome	
Complete remission	In 112/191 evaluable patients
Partial remission	In 23/191 evaluable patients
Relapse	In 68/135 patients

This includes treatment of initial disease and treatment of relapse.

Table 5 Results of a meta-analysis of 143 patients with Wegener's granulomatosis and microscopic polyangiitis in three randomized controlled trials of pulsed cyclophosphamide (de Groot *et al.* 2001a)

	Odds ratio pulsed : continuous cyclophosphamide
Failure to induce remission	0.29 (95% CI 0.12–0.73)
Infection	0.45 (95% CI 0.23–0.89)
Leucopenia	0.36 (95% CI 0.17–0.78)
Relapse	1.79 (95% CI 0.85–3.75)

Methotrexate Weekly methotrexate, widely used in rheumatoid arthritis, has been tested in patients with Wegener's granulomatosis as a possible alternative to cyclophosphamide. Twenty-nine patients with active Wegener's granulomatosis were studied initially (Hoffman *et al.* 1992b); two had relapsed off therapy and the remainder had been partially treated. None had life-threatening disease, although more than half had previous or active glomerulonephritis; six had renal impairment at entry, although a creatinine greater than 221 μmol/l was generally considered a contraindication. Methotrexate was commenced at 0.3 mg/kg/week, administered orally, and a mean stable weekly dose of 20 mg was reached; oral corticosteroids were also given. Twenty-two of the 29 patients responded to the treatment. A follow-up report extended the experience to 42 patients (Sneller *et al.* 1995), with a similar response rate (remission in 30/41, at a median of 4.2 months). Patients were treated for 1 year after remission was achieved; seven patients relapsed on treatment and four relapsed after its discontinuation. Drug toxicity described in both reports included abnormal liver enzymes necessitating a dose reduction (in 24 per cent) and methotrexate-induced pneumonitis which reversed on discontinuation of the drug (in 7 per cent). Two patients died from *Pneumocystis carinii* infection when taking methotrexate and high-dose oral steroids; the overall incidence of opportunist infections was 9.5 per cent. Methotrexate has recently been tested in a European randomized controlled trial (NORAM) against cyclophosphamide in patients with early disease with minimal evidence of nephritis (de Groot *et al.* 2002). Preliminary data suggest that initial control of disease was comparable in the two trial limbs, but relapse rates were unacceptably high in both limbs when immunosuppressive therapy was stopped at 1 year.

Mycophenolate mofetil Many renal transplant centres now use mycophenolate mofetil in place of azathioprine as part of maintenance antirejection therapy. Unsurprisingly, it has now been tested, and in some centres routinely adopted, as a maintenance agent in vasculitis. To date, the supporting literature is small and there are no published randomized trials. The largest series was reported by Nowack *et al.* (1999), who used the drug at a dose of 2 g per day in conjunction with oral steroids. The combination was able to maintain remission after cyclophosphamide-based induction therapy in 10 of the 11 patients studied. One patient in this series and another reported separately (Woywodt *et al.* 2000) developed cytomegalovirus colitis while on the drug. Haubitz and de Groot (2002) suggested that toxicity may be more pronounced in vasculitis patients with end-stage renal failure, and that dose reduction may be appropriate.

Antitumour necrosis factor therapy An anti-TNF strategy is a logical approach, since TNF has been implicated as a priming factor for neutrophil-mediated endothelial injury in vasculitis, and anti-TNF treatment has significant potential to turn off inflammation rapidly, and so reduce long-term organ damage. In an animal model of crescentic glomerulonephritis, anti-TNF treatment reduced renal injury, even when administered after the onset of nephritis (Karkar *et al.* 2001). Anti-TNF therapy is firmly established in the treatment of rheumatoid arthritis and Crohn's disease, and may take one of two forms: a chimeric monoclonal neutralising antibody directed against TNF (Infliximab) or a soluble TNF receptor fusion protein (etanercept). Stone *et al.* (2001b) have conducted an open-label study of etanercept added to conventional therapies in 20 patients with active, but not life-threatening, Wegener's granulomatosis. Adverse effects were few, and a randomized trial (WGET) is now underway to test efficacy. Lamprecht *et al.* (2002) used Infliximab to treat four patients successfully for refractory Wegener's granulomatosis, and this agent is also being used in clinical trials.

Cyclosporin Cyclosporin A is not a first-line agent for the treatment of ANCA-associated vasculitis but may have a role in selected patients. For example, Haubitz *et al.* (1998b) reported benefit of adding cyclosporin in seven patients with relapsing disease.

Intravenous immunoglobulin Another immunomodulatory treatment which has been used with some success in vasculitis is intravenous immunoglobulin (IVIg). Following successes in individual patients using 'Sandoglobulin' 0.4 g/kg/day for 5 days, Jayne *et al.* (2000) conducted a placebo-controlled trial in previously treated vasculitis patients with active disease; other medication was not altered. Treatment responses, defined by clinical and laboratory parameters, were found in 14/17 of the IVIg group and 6/17 of the placebo group; the effect was short-lived. Seventeen adverse effects occurred after IVIg and six after placebo: they were mostly mild, although reversible rises in serum creatinine occurred. Nephrotoxicity is a recognized complication of IVIg, affecting 6.7 per cent of patients in one series and may not always be reversible (Levy and Pusey 2000). It does not appear to be related to the sucrose content of the preparation used, although this had previously been implicated. Other small studies of IVIg in vasculitis have yielded mixed results.

Treatment of limited disease

In limited disease, and specifically in non-renal Wegener's granulomatosis, when there are no immediately life-threatening features, the risks of drug toxicity must be carefully balanced against the benefits of treatment. Regimens for limited disease designed to be less toxic than the NIH regimen include methotrexate, as described above, pulsed intravenous cyclophosphamide (D'Cruz *et al.* 1989), and a combination of azathioprine and corticosteroids (Harrison 1989).

Cotrimoxazole Cotrimoxazole has long been proposed for the treatment of Wegener's granulomatosis, although its usefulness has been hotly debated (DeRemee 1988; Leavitt *et al.* 1988). Reinhold-Keller *et al.* (1993) used it as induction therapy for limited Wegener's granulomatosis and saw improvement in 11 of 17 patients, but progression of disease six. They also tested it as maintenance therapy for generalized Wegener's granulomatosis; remission was maintained in only 14 of 32 patients, after a mean of 36.5 months' treatment. Stegeman *et al.* (1996) tested cotrimoxazole as an adjunctive agent to maintain remission in Wegener's granulomatosis, in a placebo-controlled prospective study. Although 19 per cent of the patients discontinued cotrimoxazole due to adverse effects, a significant reduction in relapses was achieved in the treated group.

Taken together, these data suggest a possible role for cotrimoxazole in Wegener's granulomatosis: as an induction agent for limited disease and as an adjunctive agent to maintain remission. They do not support its use as a first-line agent in severely ill patients, or as a single agent for maintenance therapy of generalized disease. There are no data on its use in microscopic polyangiitis.

Why should cotrimoxazole modify the course of Wegener's granulomatosis? It may reduce the frequency of infection, which appears to provoke relapse in some patients (Pinching *et al.* 1980). In support of this hypothesis, it has been shown that patients with Wegener's granulomatosis who carry *Staphylococcus aureus* in the nose have an increased incidence of relapse (Stegeman *et al.* 1994), although it is also possible that abnormalities of the nasal mucosa due to low-grade disease activity (preceding overt relapse) predispose to colonization.

Renal-limited vasculitis

Many reports of outcome in patients treated for focal necrotizing glomerulonephritis include both patients with systemic vasculitis and those with isolated, or 'idiopathic', rapidly progressive glomerulonephritis. Since there is reason to believe that this is a renal-limited form of small-vessel vasculitis, we adopt the same treatment regimen and use a combination of steroids and cytotoxic agents. The treatment of crescentic and necrotizing glomerulonephritis in general is discussed further in Chapter 3.10.

Treatment of severe disease

Additional strategies are needed for the treatment of fulminant disease. Two therapies, used as adjuncts to conventional drugs, have gained considerable acceptance. They are plasma exchange and pulsed intravenous methylprednisolone.

Plasma exchange The use of plasma exchange to treat crescentic nephritis due to Wegener's granulomatosis was introduced in the 1970s, with the rationale that humoral factors involved in pathogenesis might be removed (Lockwood *et al.* 1977) and a number of other uncontrolled series followed; its contribution in these patients is difficult to assess. Randomized controlled trials of plasma exchange in patients with vasculitis and crescentic glomerulonephritis have been undertaken and are summarized in Table 6. Adjunctive plasma exchange does not appear to confer benefit in the majority of patients. However, it appears to improve the renal recovery rate in the subgroup that are dialysis-requiring. In the controlled trial by Pusey *et al.* (1991), 10 of 11 dialysis-dependent patients who were randomized to plasma exchange discontinued dialysis; only 3/8 patients in the control group did so. The number of dialysis-requiring patients in the other studies is too small to draw conclusions. Our experience suggests that plasma exchange may also be useful for severe non-renal vasculitis, including pulmonary haemorrhage and neurological involvement, but this has not been tested in a randomized study.

Protein A immunoadsorption is a modification of plasma exchange, removing IgG, but not other components, from separated plasma, and it avoids the need for replacement solutions. It is compelling to speculate that the removal of IgG ANCA is the reason for the benefit of plasma exchange, and that this could be reproduced by immunoadsorption. Palmer *et al.* (1991) added protein A immunoadsorption to a regimen of pulsed methylprednisolone, oral prednisolone, and cyclophosphamide in seven patients with ANCA-associated rapidly progressive glomerulonephritis; six were able to discontinue dialysis, although most were left with significant renal impairment. Three patients had significant infections during follow-up. The contribution of the immunoadsorption to the improvement is unclear. A recent Scandinavian study (Stegmayr *et al.* 1999) suggested that immunoadsorption could be substituted for

Table 6 Randomized controlled trials of plasma exchange

Trial	Number of patients	Drugs	Plasma exchange	Benefit?
Glockner *et al.* (1998) GN with >70% crescents various aetiologies CrCL <50 ml/min	26	P, Cyc then Aza	50 ml/kg 2–3 per week × 4 weeks	No
Pusey *et al.* (1991) pauci-immune necrotizing GN All levels of renal function	48	P, Cyc ± Aza	4 l at least 5 in first week	If dialysis-requiring
Cole *et al.* (1992) idiopathic RPGN >50% crescents	32	MeP, P Aza	One plasma volume at least 10 in first 16 days	No
Guillevin *et al.* (1997a) Microscopic polyangiitis Churg–Strauss syndrome Only 32 had GN	140	P ± Cyc	60 ml/kg 12 in first 2 months	No

GN, glomerulonephritis; MP, microscopic polyangiitis; CSS, Churg–Strauss syndrome; P, prednisolone; Cyc, cyclophosphamide; Aza, azathioprine; MeP, methylprednisolone.

plasma exchange in rapidly progressive glomerulonephritis with no significant difference in outcome.

Pulsed intravenous methylprednisolone Bolus doses of intravenous methylprednisolone have also been used as an adjunct to conventional immunosuppression in groups of patients with oliguric crescentic nephritis (Bolton and Couser 1979; Stevens *et al.* 1982; Bolton and Sturgill 1989), ANCA-associated renal disease (Falk 1990), fulminant systemic vasculitis (Fuiano *et al.* 1988), or a mixture of these (Levy and Winearls 1994). There have been no controlled trials. The doses, concurrent therapy, and outcomes reported vary. Bolton and Sturgill (1989), used three pulses of 30 mg/kg in addition to oral prednisolone and reported discontinuation of dialysis in 16/23 patients, in contrast to 0/9 patients given only oral medication. Falk *et al.* (1990) used lower doses (7 mg/kg) added to varying regimens of prednisolone and cyclophosphamide and reported that 6/12 patients were able to discontinue dialysis. Andrassy *et al.* (1991) used even lower doses in patients with Wegener's granulomatosis: 250 mg pulses were administered on days 1–3, with excellent renal outcomes. Other series report selected use of methylprednisolone, typically at doses of 1 g daily, with sustained benefit. Like plasma exchange, pulsed intravenous methylprednisolone has been used, together with oral steroids and cytotoxic agents, for severe extrarenal vasculitis.

Which adjunctive therapy is superior? Both treatments have disadvantages; plasma exchange needs vascular access, is costly, mainly due to the need for albumin replacement solutions, and carries the risks of allergic reactions, transfer of infection, bleeding due to anticoagulation, and depletion of clotting factors. Methylprednisolone is cheaper, but not without risk: administration may induce arrhythmias in hypokalaemic or volume-depleted patients, and other short-term toxicity includes risk of infection, hypertension, and diabetes. Serious long-term effects may occur, particularly when high-dose oral steroids are continued, including cataracts (in up to 25 per cent) and avascular necrosis of bone. Risk of infection seems likely to be a greater problem with methylprednisolone than with plasma exchange: steroid dose has been particularly associated with infection in previous studies of vasculitis treatment (Cohen *et al.* 1982), while suggestions from early studies that plasma exchange is associated with increased infection risk have not been confirmed (Pohl *et al.* 1991). In general, plasma exchange is well tolerated (Sutton *et al.* 1989).

A controlled comparison of plasma exchange and methylprednisolone has not been made until recently. Overall, the best results reported with each type of adjunctive therapy are similar, although probably best of all in the trial reported by Pusey *et al.* (1991). McLelland *et al.* (1989), Bruns *et al.* (1989), and Levy and Winearls (1994) found plasma exchange and intravenous methylprednisolone to be equally effective in uncontrolled series. The European Vasculitis Study Group has conducted a randomized controlled trial (MEPEX) comparing the two modalities. Patients with ANCA-associated vasculitis, active necrotizing glomerulonephritis, and creatinine greater than 500 μmol/l, were randomized to receive either three pulses of methylprednisolone (each of 15/mg/kg to a maximum of 1 g) or seven plasma exchanges in the first 2 weeks (each of 60 ml/kg to a maximum of 4 l). Preliminary analysis indicates that plasma exchange is superior in securing renal recovery, with 80 per cent of survivors dialysis-independent at 3 months, compared with 59 per cent in the methylprednisolone group (Gaskin *et al.* 2002).

Might the combination of conventional drugs with both pulsed methylprednisolone and plasma exchange offer even greater benefits? Levy and Winearls (1994) combined the treatments successfully, while others (Adu *et al.* 1987; Rondeau *et al.* 1989) have drawn attention to the risk of sepsis in patients in whom multiple immunosuppressive strategies are combined. In the MEPEX study, the overall mortality was significant, although not different in the two treatment limbs, nor surprising in the light of published data. It emphasized the toxicity of combined immunosuppressive strategies in predominantly elderly patients with advanced renal failure and suggests that the quest should be for a safer approach, rather than one which seeks to produce more renal recoveries.

Treatment of refractory disease

A minority of patients show relentless progression of disease on conventional therapy, or continue to show disease activity for such prolonged periods that toxicity of conventional treatment becomes limiting. In this 'refractory' group, 15-deoxyspergualin has shown promise in an open-label study (Birck *et al.* 2003), but the main developments have been within the biological therapies able to deplete lymphocytes or interfere with leucocyte adhesion. Following success with a single patient (Mathieson *et al.* 1990), Lockwood *et al.* (1993) went on to treat three more patients with a combination of two humanized anti-T lymphocyte monoclonal antibodies, CAMPATH 1H, directed against CDw52, and an anti-CD4 antibody. The treatment achieved remission in all four patients, which was sustained in three and responded to retreatment in the fourth. Despite the production of marked lymphopenia, no opportunist infections were seen. Polyclonal anti-T cell antibodies, in the form of rabbit antithymocyte globulin, were used by Hagen *et al.* (1995) to treat five patients with Wegener's granulomatosis; four showed a favourable response. Infliximab, an anti-TNF antibody has also been used in refractory disease, as outlined above, and recently the anti-CD20 (anti-B lymphocyte) chimeric monoclonal antibody Rituximab has been used with sustained benefit in conjunction with high-dose steroids (Specks *et al.* 2001). Lockwood *et al.* (1999) used an anti-CD18 antibody in five patients with severe vasculitic tissue injury with apparent benefit in four.

Maintenance therapy

While there is broad agreement that a regimen including corticosteroids and cyclophosphamide is appropriate for the initial therapy of small-vessel vasculitis, there is little agreement about how to maintain remission thereafter. Long-term data from the NIH (Hoffman *et al.* 1992a) indicate that simply continuing the same drugs carries excessive risk, and alternative approaches include early cessation of therapy and conversion to safer agents. A survey of 15 specialist units in Europe participating in the ECSYSVASTRIAL studies showed wide variations in policy (Rasmussen *et al.* 1995). Eight different drug combinations were used for maintenance therapy in the first year, and there was even greater variability in the second. Patients in four centres discontinued therapy completely during the first year; a further four typically used only a single agent in the second year.

Is maintenance therapy necessary? Our unit believes so. In the 1970s, our policy was to discontinue therapy in most patients during the first year; 25 per cent of patients relapsed during the first year. Following the introduction of maintenance therapy continuing to and beyond 12 months, the proportion of patients relapsing was reduced to 11 per cent. Similarly, as our treatment progressively lengthened, the relapse rate fell from 53 per cent at 5 years to 22 per cent (Gaskin and Pusey 1995). The majority of our patients are now still taking a cytotoxic agent, which is usually azathioprine, in the third year. Data from other groups reinforce the view that relapse is a major problem during follow-up (Gordon *et al.* 1993), and that early discontinuation of therapy is associated with recurrence of disease (Coward *et al.* 1986). This is underlined by the NORAM study (de Groot *et al.* 2002).

Our practice is progressively to reduce prednisolone to a maintenance dose of around 5 mg daily and to substitute azathioprine for cyclophosphamide, dose-for-dose, once remission has been achieved. The dose is then tapered to a maintenance level not higher than 1 mg/kg. Azathioprine is usually well tolerated, although a small minority of patients display an allergy to it, and it maintains remission in most patients. Some patients relapse and require reversion to cyclophosphamide; however, such relapse is rarely severe and permanent renal damage is unusual if diagnosed promptly. We consider that the probable small increase in frequency of relapse on azathioprine, compared with cyclophosphamide, is compensated for by the preservation of reproductive capacity and reduced risk of haematological and urothelial malignancy. Other strategies being used for maintenance therapy include combinations of the newer agents employed in induction therapy—intravenous immunoglobulin, methotrexate, and pulsed intravenous cyclophosphamide, but none of these has been formally compared with a combination of low-dose steroids and azathioprine.

The optimal duration of therapy is unknown. It is increasingly apparent that relapse can occur years after initial presentation; our record is a first relapse at 27 years! It can also have devastating consequences. However, it is likely that the risk of toxicity of treatment will outweigh the benefits if it is indiscriminately continued in every patient. The hope is that identification of markers of impending relapse will in the future allow targeting of therapy to those at greatest risk. Our current impression is that patients with persisting ANCA, irrespective of specificity, and patients whose disease was initially associated with proteinase 3-specific ANCA are at greatest risk of relapse.

Outcome with current therapy

Induction of remission

Complete control of disease activity can be achieved with first-line therapy in 70–90 per cent of patients, with cyclophosphamide or methotrexate-based treatment (Fauci *et al.* 1983; Hoffman *et al.* 1992a, Sneller *et al.* 1995; de Groot *et al.* 2001a). Median time to complete remission varies in published series from 3 to 12 months.

Renal function

We have analysed outcome in 80 patients with an initial creatinine greater than 500 μmol/l who were treated with a combination of oral steroids, cyclophosphamide, and five or more plasma exchanges; 73 per cent were alive with improved renal function 2 months after presentation. Table 7 summarizes data from several other studies of patients with small-vessel vasculitis and severe renal dysfunction. It is important to note from these data that recovery from dialysis dependence is common, even when the biopsy shows a high percentage of crescents (Andrassy *et al.* 1991) and immunosuppressive therapy should not be withheld due to pessimism about renal outcome. In this respect, the rapidly progressive nephritis of small-vessel vasculitis differs from that of anti-GBM disease (see Chapter 3.12). Sometimes renal recovery is delayed; Coward *et al.* (1986) described renal recovery as late as 4 months after presentation. In the majority of patients in the European MEPEX study, renal outcome at 3 months was representative of renal outcome at 1 year.

A proportion of the patients with independent renal function after induction therapy later progress to end-stage renal failure, as illustrated by the Kaplan–Meier analysis of renal survival depicted in Fig. 8. Many of these patients present with a long history of untreated or partially treated disease, make an incomplete recovery with initial treatment, and lose renal function progressively, presumably due to scarring. Their initial biopsy usually reveals extensive glomerular sclerosis and interstitial damage (Andrassy *et al.* 1991; Bindi *et al.* 1993). A second group of patients who progress to dialysis comprises those who sustain further renal damage during relapse. In our experience, patients who make a good response to initial therapy, and who remain in remission, usually maintain stable and independent renal function during long-term follow-up. This experience is shared by other groups (Coward *et al.* 1986; Adu *et al.* 1987; Andrassy *et al.* 1991; Grotz *et al.* 1991). Repeat

Table 7 Renal response to therapy in severe vasculitis-associated glomerulonephritis

Author (no. of patients)	Type of patients	Treatment	Initial response: per cent alive with independent renal function
Fuiano *et al.* (1988) (n = 5)	WG, MP Creat >600	Mix of MP, P, Cyc, A, PE	60
Bindi *et al.* (1993) (n = 17)	ANCA + GN Creat >600	P and/or MP, Cyc, PE in 6	47
Hammersmith data (n = 80)	WG, MP, RLV Creat >500	P, Cyc, PE	73
Coward *et al.* (1986) (n = 18)	WG, MP Dial-dept	Mix of MP, P, Cyc, A, PE	50
Falk *et al.* (1990) (n = 12)	ANCA + GN Dial-dept	Mix of MP, P, i.v., or oral Cyc	50
Andrassy *et al.* (1991) (n = 14)	WG Dial-dept	P, i.v. Cyc, MP PE in 2	93
Garrett *et al.* (1992) (n = 19)	ANCA + GN Dial-dept	Mix of P, Cyc, A MP, PE	41
Cole *et al.* (1992) (n = 11)	RLV Dial-dept	MP, P, A MP, P, A, PE	29 75
Levy and Winearls (1994) (n = 20)	WG, MP, RLV Dial-dept	P, Cyc, PE and/or MP	70
Haubitz *et al.* (1998) (n = 20)	WG, MP Dial-dept	MP, P, oral Cyc MP, P, i.v. Cyc	50 20

Patients: ANCA+ GN, ANCA-associated glomerulonephritis; WG, Wegener's granulomatosis; MP, microscopic polyangiitis; RLV, renal-limited vasculitis.
Treatment: P, oral prednisolone; MP, pulsed methylprednisolone; Cyc, cyclophosphamide, administered orally unless stated; A, azathioprine; P, plasma exchange.

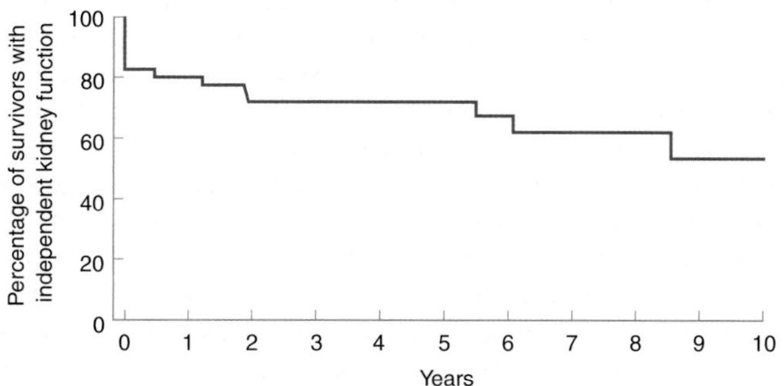

Fig. 8 Renal survival after severe glomerulonephritis due to small-vessel vasculitis; patients with creatinine greater than 500 μmol/l treated with prednisolone, cyclophosphamide, and plasma exchange.

renal biopsies suggest that no new glomeruli are recruited into the inflammatory process, and there may even be a degree of healing (Hauer *et al.* 2002a).

Andrassy *et al.* (1992) have reported patients with Wegener's granulomatosis with a pauci-immune focal necrotizing glomerulonephritis at presentation, who developed mesangial IgA deposits on follow-up biopsy, performed to investigate declining renal function and an abnormal urinary sediment. The prognostic and therapeutic significance of this development is not clear.

Deaths due to infection

Serious infections account for half to two-thirds of early deaths. Infection is a common complication of treatment (Hoffman *et al.* 1992a), and even when it is not life-threatening, it has significant resource implications: Aasarod and colleagues (2000) reported that 32 per cent of patients treated in Norway for Wegener's granulomatosis with renal involvement needed hospitalization for infection during a median follow-up period of 41.5 months.

Pneumocystis carinii (PCP) is the most commonly reported opportunist pathogen, affecting 6–20 per cent of patients in series reported prior to the use of cotrimoxazole prophylaxis. PCP in patients treated for Wegener's granulomatosis tended to occur 2–4 months from commencement of therapy (Jarrousse *et al.* 1993; Ognibene *et al.* 1995). The highest incidence (6/23 patients) was reported by Jarrousse *et al.* (1993) in recruits to a randomized controlled trial; the final incidence of PCP in the trial was 20 per cent (Guillevin *et al.* 1997b). Godeau *et al.* (2000) examined risk factors for the development of PCP. The lymphocyte count fell in all patients during induction immunosuppression, but lymphopenia was more marked in those developing PCP, in terms of mean lymphocyte count (1060 versus 1426 per mm^3), lowest absolute lymphocyte count (244 versus 738 per mm^3) and number of patients with lymphocytes less than 600 per mm^3 in the first 3 months (10/12 versus 11/32), and a multivariate analysis demonstrated that the infected group had a lower count prior to immunosuppressive treatment. Since the appreciation of PCP as an important opportunist pathogen in patients treated for ANCA-associated vasculitis, it has become common practice to use low-dose cotrimoxazole prophylaxis. It seems particularly prudent to use it in patients with a marked fall in lymphocyte count.

Tuberculosis is reported (Bindi *et al.* 1993) and isoniazid prophylaxis should be considered in patients with a previous history of exposure, to prevent reactivation. Cytomegalovirus, *Nocardia, Aspergillus,* and other fungal infections are well recognized. Herpes zoster is common (Hoffman *et al.* 1992a) and may occasionally be fatal (Bindi *et al.* 1993). Bacterial infections, with a variety of organisms and at a variety of sites, may also lead to death. The use of granulocyte colony-stimulating factor (G-CSF) can limit the risk of overwhelming sepsis due to neutropenia, although there are anecdotal reports that its use precipitates relapse; in other contexts it has been associated with the development of vasculitis.

Overall survival

One-year patient survival in patients with vasculitis-associated and isolated pauci-immune rapidly progressive glomerulonephritis is 60–80 per cent (see, e.g. Coward *et al.* 1986; Adu *et al.* 1987; Booth *et al.* 2003).

Late deaths include a small number due to relapse, which is often unexpected when it occurs many years after initial presentation, and a proportion due to adverse effects of therapy, including haematological malignancies in patients with prolonged exposure to cyclophosphamide. The remainder are attributable to unrelated causes in a predominantly elderly population. Prognosis improved during the 1980s, with early recognition of disease activity and the more judicious use of immunosuppression. Data from Guy's Hospital indicate a marked improvement in actuarial survival at 5 years, from 38 per cent (Serra *et al.* 1984) to 77 per cent (Fuiano *et al.* 1988). Indeed, 5-year survivals of 55–75 per cent are the norm, even when many of the patients present with advanced renal impairment.

Risk factors for poor prognosis

Based on the consistent themes which emerge from published series, it is possible to predict which groups of patients will do well and which will fare badly. It is harder to predict prognosis in individual patients.

Presence and severity of renal involvement Mortality in Wegener's granulomatosis is higher in patients with renal disease than those without. For example, Luqmani *et al.* (1994a) reported three early deaths and three late deaths in 28 patients with renal involvement, but no deaths in 22 patients without it. Similarly, Anderson *et al.* (1992) calculated a median survival of 7.1 years in 154 patients with renal involvement, compared with a median survival in excess of 11 years in 92 patients without.

Furthermore, the severity of renal impairment is highly relevant. A recent multivariate analysis of patients treated in London over a 5-year period confirmed an association between risk of death and creatinine less than 200 μmol/l (Booth *et al.* 2003). Indeed, oliguria and advanced renal failure at presentation have been confirmed as risk factors for high mortality in many recent series.

Age Older patients have been demonstrated to be at greater risk in many series (see, e.g. Rondeau *et al.* 1989; Garrett *et al.* 1992; Booth *et al.* 2003). Excess deaths are usually due to infective complications. Our experience is that these can be reduced by modification of immunosuppressive regimens, and satisfactory outcomes achieved (Gaskin and Pusey 1993). Age is an increasingly important risk factor, as the age of the presenting population increases (Watts *et al.* 2000).

Extrarenal vasculitis Whether the presence of systemic disease associated with renal vasculitis alters the prognosis is open to debate. Weiss and Crissman (1985) found no difference in outcome, while Croker *et al.* (1987) found a higher morbidity in patients without systemic disease. They attributed the difference to later presentation with more advanced renal damage in cases where medical help was not sought for systemic symptoms. This is consistent with our experience; in an analysis of 22 patients without extrarenal vasculitis, 15 required dialysis at presentation.

Outcome differences may also be explained by differences in the intensity of treament. In general, cytotoxic drugs have been used less frequently in isolated rapidly progressive glomerulonephritis than in systemic vasculitis. Bindi *et al.* (1993) found that a smaller number of extrarenal organs involved was associated with a better prognosis when differences in treatment were excluded.

Alveolar haemorrhage One systemic manifestation clearly associated with a high early mortality is the presence of lung haemorrhage (Jennette *et al.* 1989; Bindi *et al.* 1993) and its importance as a manifestation of small-vessel vasculitis is increasingly recognized (Haworth *et al.* 1985; Travis *et al.* 1990; Bosch *et al.* 1994; Lauque *et al.* 2000). We analysed 50 patients treated in our unit for varying degrees of alveolar haemorrhage; 19 patients required assisted ventilation shortly after admission, of whom 10 died without discontinuing ventilation. Gallagher *et al.* (2002) recently emphasized the potentially poor outcome in this group of patients.

ANCA and specific diagnosis Neither ANCA specificity, nor differentiation into Wegener's granulomatosis or microscopic polyangiitis, seems to influence the initial response to therapy and survival (Falk 1990; Geffriaud-Ricouard *et al.* 1993).

Factors influencing renal prognosis Oliguria (Serra *et al.* 1984), severe renal impairment (Heilman *et al.* 1987), and an initial requirement for dialysis (Andrassy *et al.* 1991) have been highlighted as risk factors for permanent renal failure. In a study from North Carolina (Hogan *et al.* 1996), advanced renal failure at presentation was associated with a very low probability of dialysis-independence 5 years later. In biopsy studies, renal prognosis is most closely associated with the presence of normal glomeruli and with chronic damage (Bajema *et al.* 1999; Haroun *et al.* 2002; Hauer *et al.* 2002b). The extent of active lesions correlates with the change in GFR with treatment (Hauer *et al.* 2002b). An equation incorporating the initial GFR, influenced by the degree of chronic damage, and biopsy parameters of activity gave the best prediction of outcome in one recent study (Hauer *et al.* 2002b).

Further prognostic information is yielded by the response to initial therapy. Grotz *et al.* (1991) found creatinine at 2 weeks to be predictive of long-term renal outcome. In general, patients who make a good response to initial therapy, and who remain in remission, maintain stable renal function.

Morbidity

Patients responding to initial therapy do not invariably remain in good health, even if in remission, due to the combination of irreversible organ damage from past vasculitis and the adverse effects of treatment. Hoffman *et al.* (1992b) calculated that these problems affected 86 per cent and 42 per cent respectively, of patients under long-term follow-up for Wegener's granulomatosis. This may translate into poor perception of health and impaired ability to carry out activities of daily living, and there may be significant socioeconomic impact (Cotch 2000).

In the series of Hoffman *et al.* (1992b), morbidity in Wegener's granulomatosis included unilateral or bilateral hearing loss (35 per cent), cosmetic and functional nasal deformities (28 per cent), tracheal stenosis (13 per cent), and visual loss, usually due to retro-orbital granuloma (8 per cent). Previous vasculitis was felt to contribute, together with treatment, to chronic sinus disease and pulmonary insufficiency.

Pulmonary dysfunction due to diffuse pulmonary fibrosis may also occur in patients with microscopic polyangiitis, using p-ANCA with antimyeloperoxidase specificity. In our experience, this is an ominous complication, with a high proportion of the patients dying due to respiratory failure. The association between pulmonary fibrosis and vasculitis seems too common to be due to chance: three cases were reported by Nada *et al.* (1990), lung fibrosis is listed as a clinical feature in a small number of patients in published vasculitis series, and a number of cases have been reported more recently from Japan. We believe that fibrosis may develop as a consequence of alveolar capillaritis, and this is supported by the sequence of changes in pathological studies (Jennette *et al.* 1989).

Other residual organ damage due to non-granulomatous manifestations of vasculitis includes neurological abnormalities. Recovery from severe mononeuritis is usually slow and often incomplete. Patients with vasculitis affecting the cerebral circulation may also be left with irreversible deficits.

Relapse

Between one-third and one-half of patients with small-vessel vasculitis relapse during follow-up (Hoffman *et al.* 1992a; Gordon *et al.* 1993). Proteinase 3-specific ANCA seems to confer increased risk of relapse when compared with myeloperoxidase-specific ANCA, irrespective of the clinical diagnosis (Geffriaud-Ricouard *et al.* 1993; Booth *et al.* 2003), and overall, relapse appears to be more frequent in Wegener's granulomatosis than in microcopic polyangiitis (Gordon *et al.* 1993).

When do patients relapse? Hoffman *et al.* (1992a) reported relapses occurring from 3 months to 16 years after induction of complete remission, and we have documented first relapses between 4 months and 27 years from presentation. Relapse may occur during reduction of immunosuppressive therapy or following discontinuation (Fauci *et al.* 1983; Coward *et al.* 1986; Geffriaud-Ricouard *et al.* 1993), suggesting that withdrawal of treatment should be gradual, only performed when there is no evidence of disease activity and accompanied by close monitoring for early signs of recurrence. Assays for ANCA may assist the identification of patients at particular risk of relapse, as discussed earlier in this chapter. Pinching *et al.* (1980) reported that relapse was provoked by infection in some patients. Unfortunately, a minority of patients relapse despite continuing therapy at comparable doses to those who remain in remission (Gordon *et al.* 1993), and with no other apparent explanation. Early reporting of new symptoms, coupled with regular follow-up to detect asymptomatic changes in urine sediment and renal function, remain invaluable to detect relapse before significant organ damage accrues.

Recurrent disease may also be seen in patients on long-term dialysis and after transplantation, and may affect the transplanted kidney (Nachman *et al.* 1999). Relapse appears to be less common in patients on antirejection drugs than in those on dialysis (Allen *et al.* 1998) and transplant outcomes are rarely prejudiced by recurrent disease (Allen *et al.* 1998; Nachman *et al.* 1999). The lower frequency of relapse in endstage renal failure patients means that diagnosis may be delayed or attributed to a complication of renal replacement therapy. The examples we have seen are pulmonary haemorrhage misdiagnosed as fluid overload and intestinal vasculitis with perforation treated as peritonitis associated with peritoneal dialysis; the true diagnoses were revealed at autopsy.

The characteristics of relapse are not necessarily those of the original presentation (Gordon *et al.* 1993). We have treated one patient who presented with isolated necrotizing glomerulonephritis but developed extrarenal vasculitis during relapse, and have also treated a patient with features of microscopic polyangiitis at presentation, who developed necrotizing pulmonary granulomas during a third relapse 12 years later.

The consequences of relapse can be severe. Gordon *et al.* (1993) reported that of 42 relapses, two led to death and two to chronic dialysis. Our own experience with a larger group of patients is similar: four of 139 relapses led to death and 10 of 139 to chronic dialysis; the most severe relapses occurred in patients no longer taking immunosuppressive therapy (Gaskin and Pusey 1995).

Outcome on renal replacement therapy

Dialysis Prognosis on renal replacement therapy is satisfactory, with no major problems related to either haemodialysis or chronic ambulatory peritoneal dialysis (Coward *et al.* 1986), although Andrews *et al.* (1996) suggested an increased risk of peritoneal infection in patients who had previously received steroid treatment. A review of outcome of end-stage renal disease due to rare causes by Nissenson and Port (1990) showed a survival in the polyarteritis group of illnesses comparable with that in control populations: 62 per cent at 3 years. This is confirmed in published data from our own group (Allen *et al.* 1998).

Transplantation Patients in several series, including our own (Allen *et al.* 1998), have undergone successful kidney transplants. There are no firm data to guide the optimal timing: a successful outcome has been achieved when the patient is in remission (Hoffman *et al.* 1992a), but the minimum duration of remission required is unclear. A positive ANCA at the time of transplantation is not a contraindication, and there are no clear requirements for particular antirejection drugs. Transplantation in vasculitis has been reviewed recently by Schmitt and van der Woude (2003).

Pregnancy in vasculitis patients

There are numerous reports of successful outcome, when conception occurs during disease remission (reviewed by Langford and Kerr 2002), but relapses during pregnancy have also been reported, and the overall evidence is limited. Close monitoring is advised.

Polyarteritis nodosa

Definition

Polyarteritis nodosa, as first described by Kussmaul and Maier (1866), is characterized clinically by fever, muscular, gastrointestinal, and renal disease, and pathologically by nodular swellings along the course of medium-sized arteries with histological evidence of inflammation in the outer part of the vessel wall. Thus, it is a necrotizing vasculitis involving medium-sized muscular arteries and leading to aneurysm formation.

Clinical features

Polyarteritis nodosa is typically a disease of men in middle life, with a male : female ratio of 2 : 1 and presentation in the fifth or sixth decades (Frohnert and Sheps 1967; Sack *et al.* 1975; Guillevin *et al.* 1988). The reported association with hepatitis B virus infection appears to be more common in France, occurring in up to 36 per cent of cases (Ronco *et al.* 1983; Guillevin *et al.* 1988), than in the United Kingdom (Scott *et al.* 1982). A similar clinical picture has been described in intravenous drug users (Citron *et al.* 1970) and in those with HIV infection (Calabrese *et al.* 1989).

The clinical features are those of tissue infarction, haemorrhage, and organ dysfunction, typically affecting the gastrointestinal tract, nervous system, muscles, and soft tissues. Constitutional features are common. The reported frequency of hypertension varies from 25 (Sack *et al.* 1975) to 71 per cent (Travers *et al.* 1979); systemic features of accelerated phase hypertension are sometimes seen (Guillevin *et al.* 1988). The typical subcutaneous nodules overlying arteries are not invariably seen in life (Sack *et al.* 1975; Travers *et al.* 1979). Renal involvement may present with loin pain and haematuria due to renal infarction, or renal impairment due to ischaemia. Glomerulonephritis has been reported, presumably due to coexisting microvascular disease, but this would now exclude a diagnosis of polyarteritis nodosa according to the Chapel Hill consensus criteria (Jennette *et al.* 1994). Indeed, the strict application of these criteria makes polyarteritis nodosa a much rarer disease, since the coexistence of small- and medium-vessel vasculitis leads to a diagnosis of microscopic polyangiitis instead.

Diagnosis

Non-specific indices of inflammation are usually seen (Table 2). While both c-ANCA and p-ANCA have been occasionally been reported, the majority of patients with true polyarteritis nodosa, without small- vessel involvement, are ANCA-negative (Hagen *et al.* 1998). The use of differing diagnostic criteria in many of the reported studies has made it difficult to address the question of ANCA in polyarteritis nodosa satisfactorily, and it is sometimes hard to exclude covert small-vessel involvement. ANCA have been detected in hepatitis B-associated disease, typically with a perinuclear immunofluorescence pattern (Hauschild *et al.* 1994).

Confirmation of diagnosis requires the demonstration of medium-sized artery involvement. Typically, this leads to formation of multiple aneurysms with vessel narrowing and irregularity, which may be seen on arteriography. These findings may often be demonstrable in the renal circulation, although studies of the hepatic circulation are said to give the best diagnostic yield (Travers *et al.* 1979).

The diagnosis may be confirmed morphologically, and muscle biopsy has been widely used. Renal biopsy is logical in the presence of clinical evidence of renal involvement and is an effective means of diagnosis (Ronco *et al.* 1983), but carries a greater than usual risk of bleeding or formation of an arteriovenous fistula (Curran *et al.* 1967). The histological picture is one of fibrinoid necrosis of arcuate or occasionally of interlobular arteries, with a marked inflammatory response within and surrounding the vessel. Destruction of the internal elastic lamina may be seen, even in healed or healing lesions, and aneurysms may be observed. Hypertensive changes may be seen in smaller arteries and arterioles, but are clearly not specific. There may be evidence of ischaemic damage, with tubular atrophy and periglomerular fibrosis, and occasionally areas of infarction.

Treatment

Treatment conventionally involves corticosteroids, but many authors would advocate using an additional cytotoxic agent (Fauci *et al.* 1979; Leib *et al.* 1979). We use the same protocol as for small-vessel vasculitis. Guillevin *et al.* (1988) previously used a combination of steroids and plasma exchange with or without cyclophosphamide, but more recently suggested that plasma exchange did not confer additional benefit (Guillevin *et al.* 1992). Patients with a low 'five factor' prognostic score may not even need a cytotoxic agent (Guillevin *et al.* 1996). Cases associated with hepatitis B require special consideration; Guillevin *et al.* (1994) used a combination of plasma exchange and α-interferon.

Outcome

The prognosis has improved steadily over the last two decades, as outlined above. Most recently, Guillevin *et al.* (1988, 1992) have reported 5-year survivals of 60–80 per cent in different treatment groups. In general, disease-related deaths are most likely to be due to extrarenal vasculitis: life-threatening features include severe intestinal vasculitis, cerebral vessel involvement, and massive bleeding from aneurysmal vessels, which may now be treated by angiographic placement of intra-arterial coils (Hachulla *et al.* 1993). As in small-vessel vasculitis, older patients have a poorer outcome (Sack *et al.* 1975).

Churg–Strauss syndrome

Clinical features

Extrarenal disease

Lanham *et al.* (1984) documented the clinical features in 16 patients and reviewed the literature for details in a further 138 cases. Respiratory disease is characterized by asthma, usually of relatively late onset. Infiltrates on the chest radiograph are common, although often transient, and pleural effusions, which may contain large numbers of eosinophils, are described. Disease of the upper respiratory tract is common in the form of allergic rhinitis and nasal polyps. The symptoms of respiratory involvement often antedate the appearance of vasculitis by several years. Eosinophilia exceeding 1.5×10^9 per litre occurred in all Lanham's patients, with a mean peak eosinophil count of 8.4×10^9 per litre. This is considerably higher than the small elevations in eosinophil count sometimes seen in polyarteritis nodosa and Wegener's granulomatosis. Eosinophilic tissue infiltrates may occur in the absence of peripheral blood eosinophilia. Treated patients may not show the characteristic eosinophilia, since this is rapidly suppressed by corticosteroids. Vasculitic manifestations of the disease affect particularly the heart, skin, bowel, and the musculoskeletal and nervous systems. Mononeuritis multiplex is described in two-thirds of cases (Lanham *et al.* 1984; Sehgal *et al.* 1995). Serious ocular complications, including optic neuropathy and retinal artery occlusion are increasingly recognized. Cardiac involvement includes coronary vasculitis and myocardial infiltration causing ventricular dysfunction and arrhythmias (Kozak *et al.* 1995). As in other forms of small-vessel vasculitis, life-threatening alveolar haemorrhage may occur (Clutterbuck and Pusey 1987) although this is rare. Involvement of medium-sized arteries can be confirmed at arteriography. The clinical and laboratory features have recently been reviewed by Noth *et al.* (2003).

Renal disease

Renal disease is not a major feature although histological changes in the kidney were clearly described by Churg and Strauss. In an unselected series of 30 patients reported by Chumbley *et al.* (1977), only one patient had 'renal failure', six had microscopic haematuria, and three had slight elevations of urea and creatinine. The Hammersmith experience differs, but referral bias may have led to an over-representation of severe vasculitis and renal disease. In Lanham's (1984) series, most of the patients had some degree of renal involvement, and Clutterbuck *et al.* (1990) described renal disease in 16 of 19 patients; nephrotic syndrome occurred in three and serum creatinine concentration was greater than 500 μmol/l in four patients. The urine sediment was abnormal in all but one patient with renal disease, generally with microscopic haematuria and granular casts, and proteinuria was detected in 12 of the 16. The dominant histological pattern was a focal segmental glomerulonephritis. In general, vascular lesions and eosinophilic infiltration were less common, although in one biopsy an intense interstitial infiltrate was seen.

Antineutrophil cytoplasmic antibodies in Churg–Strauss syndrome

ANCA are detectable in around 60 per cent of patients with Churg–Strauss syndrome (Cohen Tervaert *et al.* 1991; Hagen *et al.* 1998), and typically show specificity for myeloperoxidase. The presence of ANCA in Churg–Strauss syndrome illustrates the immunological relationship with other forms of systemic vasculitis.

Treatment

Corticosteroids have been the mainstay of therapy in most reported series (Chumbley *et al.* 1977; Lanham *et al.* 1984). Most patients responded well, but doses were sometimes high and side-effects troublesome, and cytotoxic agents were added in a minority of cases. In Clutterbuck's (1990) series, which had a greater proportion of renal disease, additional immunosuppression was used in 11 of 19, with plasma exchange in five. Guillevin *et al.* (1992) suggested that steroids alone may be adequate in 80 per cent of patients and can be used with confidence in those whose clinical features suggest a good prognosis (Gayraud *et al.* 1997). We add cyclophosphamide in patients with significant renal involvement or other 'organ-threatening' disease.

The vasculitic illness is usually of limited duration, and gradual reduction or withdrawal of treatment is, therefore, possible. Occasionally, disease activity continues or recurs and maintenance therapy with a combination of prednisolone and azathioprine is suggested (Lanham *et al.* 1984). Interferon-alpha has been used successfully in small numbers of patients for particularly difficult disease (Tatsis *et al.* 1998); clinical improvement was associated with a suppression of eosinophilia.

Outcome

The prognosis of Churg–Strauss syndrome is generally good (Guillevin *et al.* 1999, and reviewed by Noth *et al.* 2003). Initial therapy is effective in most patients and long-term survival is usual. The same is true even in cases with more severe renal disease; 10 of 19 patients in Clutterbuck's (1990) series had a normal serum creatinine at 2–10 years after diagnosis. However, abnormal renal function and proteinuria, together with gastrointestinal, central nervous system and cardiac disease, mark out a worse prognosis overall (Guillevin *et al.* 1996). Cardiac disease is the single most common cause of death, and a patient treated by cardiac transplantation has been reported; unfortunately, the disease recurred in the transplanted heart (Henderson *et al.* 1993). Late relapse may sometimes occur, but is less frequent than in Wegener's granulomatosis.

Renal disease in other vasculitic illnesses

Giant cell arteritis

Giant cell arteritis is predominantly a disease of the elderly, usually characterized clinically by temporal arteritis or polymyalgia rheumatica. The major complications are ophthalmic, and overt renal disease is rare, although microscopic haematuria and low levels of proteinuria with normal renal function may occur at presentation (Sonnenblick *et al.* 1989). More noteworthy are occasional reports of widely disseminated visceral giant cell arteritis, affecting both large arteries in various organs and smaller vessels within the kidney (Lie 1978). Elling and Kristensen (1980) reported a patient with polymyalgia rheumatica who developed fatal renal failure associated with florid intrarenal vasculitis affecting all the intrarenal arteries and arterioles. Others (see, e.g. O'Neill *et al.* 1976 and Canton *et al.* 1992) have reported the coexistence of typical giant cell arteritis affecting the temporal arteries and focal necrotizing glomerulonephritis, leading to marked renal impairment. One case of temporal arteritis with membranous nephropathy has been described (Truong *et al.* 1985), and there are numerous reports of the development of renal amyloidosis.

The distinction between giant cell arteritis and other vasculitides more frequently associated with renal disease is not always clear-cut. There are reports of temporal artery involvement in other syndromes, including Wegener's granulomatosis, Churg–Strauss syndrome, and polyarteritis nodosa.

Takayasu's arteritis

Takayasu's arteritis is typically a disease of young women which causes inflammation in large arteries, particularly the aorta and its main branches. Stenoses and occlusions, and also dilatations and aneurysms result. The main renal arteries are frequently involved (Hall *et al.* 1985a) but glomerular disease is rare. Minor mesangial proliferative changes have been reported by Takagi *et al.* (1984) and others, and membranoproliferative nephritis has also been reported. Focal segmental necrotizing glomerulonephritis with crescent formation has been described in one case, which responded to treatment with pulse methylprednisolone (Hellman *et al.* 1987).

Behçet's syndrome

This disease is characterized clinically by ocular inflammation, oral and genital ulceration, and variable thrombotic, neurological, pulmonary, and rheumatic features, and pathologically by a leucocytoclastic vasculitis chiefly involving veins, venules, and capillaries. Renal dysfunction in Behçet's syndrome may be a side-effect of therapy rather than a reflection of intrinsic renal disease. Both cyclosporin A and FK506 have been used, with frequent reports of nephrotoxicity.

There are numerous reports of necrotizing or crescentic glomerulonephritis attributed to the disease process, although it is sometimes difficult to be certain from the clinical features described that the diagnosis was Behçet's syndrome, rather than microscopic polyangiitis or Wegener's granulomatosis (see, e.g. Landwehr *et al.* 1980 and Donnelly *et al.* 1989). Yang *et al.* (1993) reported a patient with oral and vaginal ulceration, uveitis, and arthralgias, thus meeting criteria for the diagnosis of Behçet's syndrome, who also had cutaneous vasculitis, and renal failure associated with globally and segmentally sclerosed glomeruli, and c-ANCA by immunofluorescence. Other reported patterns of renal pathology include IgA nephropathy, minimal change nephrotic syndrome complicated by renal vein thrombosis and amyloidosis, reported in long-standing Behçet's syndrome. The range of glomerular lesions have been reviewed by Akpolat *et al.* (2002) and Altiparmak *et al.* (2002); they rarely cause significant renal impairment.

Relapsing polychondritis

This is another rare inflammatory condition in which glomerulonephritis has been recognized. It is characterized by episodic inflammation and destruction of cartilaginous structures, with diverse clinical manifestations including features of systemic vasculitis in some patients. ANCA have occasionally been detected (Geffriaud-Ricouard *et al.* 1993).

Chang-Miller *et al.* (1987) summarized a variety of case reports showing renal involvement, typically in the form of a segmental necrotizing glomerulonephritis, with a rapidly progressive course and crescent formation in some. They also reviewed 129 patients with relapsing polychondritis seen at the Mayo Clinic over a period of 40 years, and estimated an incidence of renal involvement of 22 per cent. Renal biopsies were performed in 11 cases; mesangial proliferation was seen in all, and segmental necrotizing glomerulonephritis in eight. Renal disease was diagnosed more commonly in older patients, and evidence of systemic vasculitis was more likely in those patients with renal disease. Actuarial survival was significantly worse in the presence of renal involvement, and cytotoxic therapy in addition to corticosteroids was advocated for most patients with glomerular disease.

Kawasaki's disease

Kawasaki's disease, or mucocutaneous lymph node syndrome, is a febrile illness of childhood characterized by a multisystem disease with systemic vasculitis, often with life-threatening coronary involvement. Lytic antiendothelial antibodies have been identified in this condition (see Chapter 4.5.1) and antineutrophil cytoplasmic antibodies may also be detected (Savage *et al.* 1989). Renal disease is not usually a feature. Renal histology was reported in one case with microscopic haematuria and proteinuria to show mesangial hypercellularity and interstitial infiltrates, without renal vasculitis (Salcedo *et al.* 1988). Interstitial nephritis leading to acute renal failure has also been reported (Veiga *et al.* 1992; Bonany *et al.* 2002).

References

Aasarod, K. *et al.* (2000). Wegener's granulomatosis: clinical course in 108 patients with renal involvement. *Nephrology, Dialysis, Transplantation* **15**, 611–618.

Adu, D. *et al.* (1987). Polyarteritis and the kidney. *Quarterly Journal of Medicine* **62**, 221–237.

Adu, D. *et al.* (1995). ANCA positive and ANCA negative microscopic polyarteritis. *Clinical and Experimental Immunology* **101** (Suppl. 1), 62.

Adu, D. *et al.* (1997). Controlled trial of pulse versus continuous prednisolone and cyclophosphamide in the treatment of systemic vasculitis. *Quarterly Journal of Medicine* **90**, 401–409.

Akpolat, T. *et al.* (2002). Renal Behçet's disease: a cumulative analysis. *Seminars in Arthritis and Rheumatism* **31**, 317–337.

Allen, A. R., Pusey, C. D., and Gaskin, G. (1998). Outcome of renal replacement therapy in ANCA-associated systemic vasculitis. *Journal of the American Society of Nephrology* **9**, 1258–1263.

Altiparmak, M. R. *et al.* (2002). Glomerulonephritis in Behçet's disease: report of seven cases and review of the literature. *Clinical Rheumatology* **21**, 14–18.

Anderson, G. *et al.* (1992). Wegener's granuloma. A series of 265 British cases seen between 1975 and 1985. A report by a sub-committee of the British Thoracic Society Research Committee. *Quarterly Journal of the Medicine* **83**, 427–438.

Andrassy, K. *et al.* (1991). Wegener's granulomatosis with renal involvement: patient survival and correlations between initial renal function, renal histology, therapy and renal outcome. *Clinical Nephrology* **35**, 139–147.

Andrassy, K., Waldherr, R., Erb, A., and Ritz, E. (1992). *De novo* glomerulonephritis in patients during remission from Wegener's granulomatosis. *Clinical Nephrology* **38**, 295–298.

Andrews, P. A., Warr, K. J., Hicks, J. A., and Cameron, J. S. (1996). Impaired outcome of continuous ambulatory peritoneal dialysis in immunocompromised patients. *Nephrology, Dialysis, Transplantation* **11**, 1104–1108.

Angangco, R. *et al.* (1994). Does truly 'idiopathic' crescentic glomerulonephritis exist? *Nephrology, Dialysis, Transplantation* **9**, 630–636.

Ara, J. *et al.* (1999). Relationship between ANCA and disease activity in small vessel vasculitis patients with anti-MPO ANCA. *Nephrology, Dialysis, Transplantation* **14**, 1667–1672.

Ara, J. *et al.* (2001). Circulating soluble adhesion molecules in ANCA-associated vasculitis. *Nephrology, Dialysis, Transplantation* **16**, 276–285.

Arranz, O. *et al.* (2000). Serum levels of soluble interleukin-2 receptor in patients with ANCA-associated vasculitis. *Journal of Nephrology* **13**, 59–64.

Bajema, I. M. *et al.* (1997). Renal granulomas in systemic vasculitis. EC/BCR project for ANCA-assay standardization. *Clinical Nephrology* **48**, 16–21.

Bajema, I. M. *et al.* (1999). Kidney biopsy as a predictor for renal outcome in ANCA-associated necrotizing glomerulonephritis. *Kidney International* **56**, 1751–1758.

Barksdale, S. K. *et al.* (1995). Cutaneous pathology in Wegener's granulomatosis. A clinicopathologic study of 75 biopsies in 46 patients. *American Journal of Surgical Pathology* **19**, 161–172.

Bhathena, D. B. *et al.* (1987). Morphologic and immunohistochemical observations in granulomatous glomerulonephritis. *American Journal of Pathology* **126**, 581–591.

Bindi, P. *et al.* (1993). Necrotizing crescentic glomerulonephritis without significant immune deposits: a clinical and serological study. *Quarterly Journal of Medicine* **86**, 55–68.

Birck, R. *et al.* (2003). 15-Deoxyspergualin in patients with refractory ANCA-associated systemic vasculitis: a six-month open-label trial to evaluate safety and efficacy. *Journal of the American Society of Nephrology* **14**, 440–447.

Bolton, W. K. and Couser, W. G. (1979). Intravenous pulse methylprednisolone therapy of acute crescentic rapidly progressive glomerulonephritis. *American Journal of Medicine* **66**, 495–502.

Bolton, W. K. and Sturgill, B. C. (1989). Methylprednisolone therapy for acute crescentic rapidly progressive glomerulonephritis. *American Journal of Nephrology* **9**, 368–375.

Bonany, P. J. *et al.* (2002). Acute renal failure in typical Kawasaki disease. *Pediatric Nephrology* **17**, 329–331.

Boomsma, M. M. *et al.* (2000). Prediction of relapses in Wegener's granulomatosis by measurement of antineutrophil cytoplasmic antibody levels: a prospective study. *Arthritis and Rheumatism* **43**, 2025–2033.

Booth, A. D. *et al.* (2003). Outcome of ANCA-associated renal vasculitis: a 5 year retrospective study. *American Journal of Kidney Disease* **41**, 776–784.

Bosch, X. *et al.* (1994). Antineutrophil cytoplasmic autoantibody-associated alveolar capillaritis in patients presenting with pulmonary haemorrhage. *Archives of Pathology and Laboratory Medicine* **118**, 517–522.

Bosch, X. *et al.* (1991). Prognostic implication of anti-neutrophil cytoplasmic autoantibodies with myeloperoxidase specificity in anti-glomerular basement membrane disease. *Clinical Nephrology* **36**, 107–113.

Brouwer, E. *et al.* (1991). Predominance of IgG1 and IgG4 subclasses of anti-neutrophil cytoplasmic autoantibodies (ANCA) in patients with Wegener's granulomatosis and clinically related disorders. *Clinical and Experimental Immunology* **83**, 379–386.

Brouwer, E. *et al.* (1994). Neutrophil activation *in vitro* and *in vivo* in Wegener's granulomatosis. *Kidney International* **45**, 1120–1131.

Bruns, F. J., Adler, S., Fraley, D. S., and Segel, D. P. (1989). Long-term follow-up of aggressively treated idiopathic rapidly progressive glomerulonephritis. *American Journal of Medicine* **86**, 400–406.

Bullen, C. L., Liesegang, T. J., McDonald, T. J., and DeRemee, R. A. (1983). Ocular complications of Wegener's granulomatosis. *Ophthalmology* **90**, 279–290.

Calabrese, L. H. *et al.* (1989). Systemic vasculitis in association with human immunodeficiency virus infection. *Arthritis and Rheumatism* **32**, 569–576.

Cameron, J. S. Renal vasculitis: microscopic polyarteritis and Wegener's granuloma. In *Renal Involvement in Systemic Vasculitis* (ed. A. Sessa, M. Meroni, and G. Battini), pp. 38–46. Basel: Karger, 1991.

Camilleri, M., Pusey, C. D., Chadwick, V. S., and Rees, A. J. (1983). Gastrointestinal manifestations of systemic vasculitis. *Quarterly Journal of Medicine* **52**, 141–149.

Canton, C. G. *et al.* (1992). Renal failure in temporal arteritis. *American Journal of Nephrology* **12**, 380–383.

Carrington, C. B. and Liebow, A. (1966). Limited forms of angiitis and granulomatosis of Wegener's type. *American Journal of Medicine* **41**, 497–527.

Carruthers, D. M. *et al.* (2000). Percutaneous image-guided biopsy of lung nodules in the assessment of disease activity in Wegener's granulomatosis. *Rheumatology (Oxford)* **39**, 776–782.

Chang-Miller, A. *et al.* (1987). Renal involvement in relapsing polychondritis. *Medicine* **66**, 202–217.

Christensson, M., Pettersson, E., Sundqvist, K. G., and Christensson, B. (2000). T cell activation in patients with ANCA-associated vasculitis: inefficient immune suppression by therapy. *Clinical Nephrology* **54**, 435–442.

Chumbley, L. C., Harrison, E. G., and DeRemee, R. A. (1977). Allergic granulomatosis and angiitis (Churg–Strauss syndrome). Report and analysis of 30 cases. *Mayo Clinic Proceedings* **52**, 477–484.

Churg, J. and Strauss, L. (1951). Allergic granulomatosis, allergic angiitis and periarteritis nodosa. *American Journal of Pathology* **27**, 277–301.

Citron, B. P. *et al.* (1970). Necrotizing angiitis associated with drug abuse. *New England Journal of Medicine* **283**, 1003–1011.

Clutterbuck, E. J., Evans, D. J., and Pusey, C. D. (1990). Renal involvement in Churg–Strauss syndrome. *Nephrology, Dialysis, Transplantation* **5**, 161–167.

Clutterbuck, E. J. and Pusey, C. D. (1987). Severe alveolar haemorrhage in Churg–Strauss syndrome. *European Journal of Respiratory Diseases* **71**, 158–163.

Cohen, J., Pinching, A. J., Rees, A. J., and Peters, D. K. (1982). Infection and immunosuppression. A study of the infective complications of 75 patients with immunologically-mediated renal disease. *Quarterly Journal of Medicine* **51**, 1–15.

Cohen, R. D., Conn, D. L., and Illstrup, D. M. (1980). Clinical features, prognosis and response to treatment in polyarteritis. *Mayo Clinic Proceedings* **55**, 140–155.

Cohen Tervaert, J. W. *et al.* (1990a). Autoantibodies against myeloid lysosomal enzymes in crescentic glomerulonephritis. *Kidney International* **37**, 799–806.

Cohen Tervaert, J. W. *et al.* (1990b). Prevention of relapses in Wegener's granulomatosis by treatment based on antineutrophil cytoplasmic antibody titre. *Lancet* **336**, 709–711.

Cohen Tervaert, J. W. *et al.* (1991). Antimyeloperoxidase antibodies in Churg–Strauss syndrome. *Thorax* **46**, 70–71.

Cole, E. *et al.* (1992). A prospective randomized trial of plasma exchange as additive therapy in idiopathic crescentic glomerulonephritis. *American Journal of Kidney Diseases* **20**, 261–269.

Cordier, J. F. *et al.* (1990). Pulmonary Wegener's granulomatosis. A clinical and imaging study of 77 cases. *Chest* **97**, 900–912.

Corman, L. C. and Dolson, D. J. (1992). Polyarteritis nodosa and parvovirus B19 infection. *Lancet* **339**, 491.

Cotch, M. F. (2000). The socioeconomic impact of vasculitis. *Current Opinion in Rheumatology* **12**, 20–23.

Cotch, M. F. *et al.* (1996). The epidemiology of Wegener's granulomatosis. Estimates of the five-year period prevalence, annual mortality, and geographic disease distribution from population-based data sources. *Arthritis and Rheumatism* **39**, 87–92.

Courcoutsakis, N. A. *et al.* (1997). Orbital involvement in Wegener granulomatosis: MR findings in 12 patients. *Journal of Computer Assisted Tomography* **21**, 452–458.

Coward, R. A., Hamdy, N. A. T., Shortland, J. S., and Brown, C. B. (1986). Renal micropolyarteritis: a treatable condition. *Nephrology, Dialysis, Transplantation* **1**, 31–37.

Croker, P. B., Lee, T., and Gunnells, J. C. (1987). Clinical and pathological features of polyarteritis nodosa and its renal-limited variant: primary crescentic and necrotizing glomerulonephritis. *Human Pathology* **18**, 38–44.

Curran, R. E., Steinberg, I., and Hagstrom, J. W. C. (1967). Arteriovenous malformation complicating percutaneous renal biopsy in polyarteritis nodosa. *American Journal of Medicine* **43**, 465–470.

D'Cruz, D. P., Baguley, E., Asherson, R. A., and Hughes, G. R. V. (1989). Ear, nose and throat symptoms in subacute Wegener's granulomatosis. *British Medical Journal* **299**, 419–422.

Daoud, M. S. *et al.* (1994). Cutaneous Wegener's granulomatosis: clinical, histopathologic, and immunopathologic features of thirty patients. *Journal of the American Academy of Dermatology* **31**, 605–612.

das Neves, F. C. *et al.* Cell activation and the role of cell-mediated immunity in vasculitis. In *Renal Involvement in Systemic Vasculitis* (ed. A. Sessa, M. Meroni, and G. Battini), pp. 13–21. Basel: Karger, 1991.

David, J., Ansell, B. M., and Woo, P. (1993). Polyarteritis nodosa associated with streptococcus. *Archives of Diseases in Childhood* **69**, 685–688.

Davies, D. J., Moran, J. E., Niall, J. F., and Ryan, G. B. (1982). Segmental necrotizing glomerulonephritis with antineutrophil antibody: possible arbovirus aetiology? *British Medical Journal* **285**, 606.

Davson, J., Ball, J., and Platt, R. (1948). The kidney in periarteritis nodosa. *Quarterly Journal of Medicine* **17**, 175–202.

de Groot, K., Adu, D., and Savage, C. O. S. (2001a). The value of pulse cyclophosphamide in ANCA-associated vasculitis: meta-analysis and critical review. *Nephrology, Dialysis, Transplantation* **16**, 2018–2027.

de Groot, K., Gross, W. L., Herlyn, K., and Reinhold-Keller, E. (2001b). Development and validation of a disease extent index for Wegener's granulomatosis. *Clinical Nephrology* **55**, 31–38.

de Groot, K., Rasmussen, N., Cohen Tervaert, J. W., and Jayne, D. (2002). Randomized trial of cyclophosphamide versus methotrexate for induction of remission in non-renal ANCA-associated vasculitis. *Journal of the American Society of Nephrology* **13**, 2A.

DeRemee, R. A. (1988). The treatment of Wegener's granulomatosis with trimethoprim/sulfamethoxazole: illusion or vision? *Arthritis and Rheumatism* **31**, 1068–1072.

Devaney, K. O. *et al.* (1990). Interpretation of head and neck biopsies in Wegener's granulomatosis: a pathologic study of 126 biopsies in 70 patients. *American Journal of Surgical Pathology* **14**, 555–564.

Devogelaer, J.-P. *et al.* (1987). D-Penicillamine induced crescentic glomerulonephritis: report and review of the literature. *Journal of Rheumatology* **14**, 1036–1041.

Dolman, K. M. *et al.* (1993). Vasculitis and antineutrophil cytoplasmic autoantibodies associated with propylthiouracil therapy. *Lancet* **342**, 651–652.

Donnelly, S., Jothy, S., and Barre, P. (1989). Crescentic glomerulonephritis in Behçet's syndrome—results of therapy and review of the literature. *Clinical Nephrology* **31**, 213–218.

Drachman, D. A. (1962). Neurological complications of Wegener's granulomatosis. *Archives of Neurology* **8**, 45–55.

Elling, H. and Kristensen, I. B. (1980). Fatal renal failure in polymyalgia rheumatica caused by disseminated giant cell arteritis. *Scandinavian Journal of Rheumatology* **9**, 200–208.

Esnault, V. L. M. *et al.* (1992). Association of IgM with IgG ANCA in patients presenting with pulmonary haemorrhage. *Kidney International* **41**, 1304–1310.

Esnault, V. L. M. *et al.* (1993). Alpha 1-antitrypsin genetic polymorphism in ANCA-positive systemic vasculitis. *Kidney International* **43**, 1329–1332.

Fahey, J. L., Leonard, E., Churg, J., and Godman, G. (1954). Wegener's granulomatosis. *American Journal of Medicine* **17**, 168–179.

Falk, R. J. (1990). ANCA-associated renal disease. *Kidney International* **38**, 998–1010.

Falk, R. J. and Jennette, J. C. (1988). Anti-neutrophil cytoplasmic autoantibodies with specificity for myeloperoxidase in patients with systemic vasculitis and idiopathic necrotizing and crescentic glomerulonephritis. *New England Journal of Medicine* **318**, 1651–1657.

Falk, R. J., Hogan, S., Carey, T. S., and Jennette, J. C. (1990). Clinical course of anti-neutrophil cytoplasmic autoantibody-associated glomerulonephritis and systemic vasculitis. *Annals of Internal Medicine* **113**, 656–663.

Fauci, A. S., Wolff, S., and Johnson, J. S. (1971). Effect of cyclophosphamide upon the immune response in Wegener's granulomatosis. *New England Journal of Medicine* **285**, 1493–1496.

Fauci, A. S., Katz, P., Haynes, B. F., and Wolff, S. M. (1979). Cyclophosphamide therapy of severe necrotising vasculitis. *New England Journal of Medicine* **301**, 235–238.

Fauci, A. S., Haynes, B. F., Katz, P., and Wolff, S. (1983). Wegener's granulomatosis: prospective clinical and therapeutic experience with 85 patients over 21 years. *Annals of Internal Medicine* **98**, 76–85.

Finkel, T. H. *et al.* (1994). Chronic parvovirus B19 infection and systemic necrotising vasculitis: opportunistic infection or aetiological agent? *Lancet* **343**, 1255–1258.

Finn, J. E. *et al.* (1994). Molecular analysis of C3 allotypes in patients with systemic vasculitis. *Nephrology, Dialysis, Transplantation* **9**, 1564–1567.

Fordham, C. C. I., Epstein, F. H., Hiffines, W. D., and Harrington, J. T. (1964). Polyarteritis and acute post-streptococcal glomerulonephritis. *Annals of Internal Medicine* **61**, 89–97.

Franssen, C. F. *et al.* (1995). Differences between anti-myeloperoxidase and anti-proteinase 3-associated renal disease. *Kidney International* **47**, 193–199.

Frohnert, P. P. and Sheps, S. G. (1967). Long-term follow-up study of periarteritis nodosa. *American Journal of Medicine* **43**, 8–14.

Fuiano, G. *et al.* (1988). Improved prognosis of renal microscopic polyarteritis in recent years. *Nephrology, Dialysis, Transplantation* **3**, 383–391.

Fuiano, G. *et al.* Expression of intercellular adhesion molecule in idiopathic crescentic glomerulonephritis. In *Renal Involvement in Systemic Vasculitis* (ed. A. Sessa, M. Meroni, and G. Battini), pp. 81–88. Basel: Karger, 1991.

Gallagher, H., Kwan, J. T., and Jayne, D. R. (2002). Pulmonary renal syndrome: a 4-year, single-center experience. *American Journal of Kidney Diseases* **39**, 42–47.

Garrett, P. J. *et al.* (1992). Renal disease associated with circulating antineutrophil cytoplasm activity. *Quarterly Journal of Medicine* **85**, 731–749.

Gaskin, G. and Pusey, C. D. (1993). ANCA-associated renal disease. *Quarterly Journal of Medicine* **86**, 138–139.

Gaskin, G. and Pusey, C. D. (1995). Prevention of relapse in systemic vasculitis, *Journal of the American Society of Nephrology* **6**, 921.

Gaskin, G. *et al.* (1991). Anti-neutrophil cytoplasmic antibodies and disease activity during long-term follow-up of 70 patients with systemic vasculitis. *Nephrology, Dialysis, Transplantation* **6**, 689–694.

Gaskin, G., Thompson, E. M., and Pusey, C. D. (1995). Goodpasture-like syndrome associated with anti-myeloperoxidase antibodies following penicillamine treatment. *Nephrology, Dialysis, Transplantation* **10**, 1925–1928.

Gaskin, G., Jayne, D., and European Vasculitis Study Group (2002). Adjunctive plasma exchange is superior to Methylprednisolone in acute renal failure due to ANCA-associated glomerulonephritis. *Journal of the American Society of Nephrology* **13**, 2A.

Gayraud, M. *et al.* (1997). Treatment of good-prognosis polyarteritis nodosa and Churg–Strauss syndrome: comparison of steroids and oral or pulse cyclophosphamide in 25 patients. French Cooperative Study Group for Vasculitides. *British Journal of Rheumatology* **36**, 1290–1297.

Gayraud, M. *et al.* (2001). Long-term follow-up of polyarteritis nodosa, microscopic polyangiitis, and Churg–Strauss syndrome: analysis of four prospective trials including 278 patients. *Arthritis and Rheumatism* **44**, 666–675.

Geffriaud-Ricouard, C. *et al.* (1993). Clinical spectrum associated with ANCA of defined antigen specificities in 98 selected patients. *Clinical Nephrology* **39**, 125–136.

Gerbracht, D. D., Savage, R. W., and Scharff, N. (1987). Reversible valvulitis in Wegener's granulomatosis. *Chest* **92**, 182–183.

Glockner, W. *et al.* (1988). Plasma exchange and immunosuppression in rapidly progressive glomerulonephritis: a controlled multi-centre study. *Clinical Nephrology* **29**, 1–88.

Gocke, D. J. *et al.* (1970). Association between polyarteritis and Australia antigen. *Lancet* **ii**, 7684–1153.

Godeau, B. *et al.* (2000). Factors associated with *Pneumocystis carinii* pneumonia in Wegener's granulomatosis. *Annals of the Rheumatic Diseases* **54**, 991–994.

Godman, G. C. and Churg, J. (1954). Wegener's granulomatosis: pathology and review of the literature. *Archives of Pathology* **58**, 533–553.

Gordon, M. *et al.* (1993). Relapses in patients with a systemic vasculitis. *Quarterly Journal of Medicine* **86**, 779–789.

Griffith, M. E. and Pusey, C. D. (1997). HLA genes in ANCA-associated vasculitides. *Experimental and Clinical Immunogenetics* **14**, 196–205.

Griffith, M. E. *et al.* (1996). C-antineutrophil cytoplasmic antibody positivity in vasculitis is associated with Z allele of alpha-1-antitrypsin and P-antineutrophil cytoplasmic antibody positivity with the S allele. *Nephrology, Dialysis, Transplantation* **11**, 438–443.

Grotz, W. *et al.* (1991). Crescentic glomerulonephritis in Wegener's granulomatosis: morphology, therapy, outcome. *Clinical Nephrology* **35**, 243–251.

Guillevin, L. *et al.* (1988). Clinical findings and prognosis of polyarteritis nodosa and Churg Strauss angiitis: a study in 165 patients. *British Journal of Rheumatology* **27**, 258–264.

Guillevin, L. *et al.* (1992). Lack of superiority of steroids plus plasma exchange to steroids alone in the treatment of polyarteritis nodosa and Churg–Strauss syndrome. A prospective randomised trial in 78 patients. *Arthritis and Rheumatism* **35**, 208–215.

Guillevin, L. *et al.* (1994). Treatment of polyarteritis nodosa related to hepatitis B virus with interferon-alpha and plasma exchanges. *Annals of Rheumatic Diseases* **53**, 334–337.

Guillevin, L. *et al.* (1996). Prognostic factors in polyarteritis nodosa and Churg–Strauss syndrome. A prospective study in 342 patients. *Medicine (Baltimore)* **75**, 17–28.

Guillevin, L. *et al.* (1997a). Treatment of glomerulonephritis in microscopic polyangiitis and Churg–Strauss syndrome. Indications of plasma exchanges: meta-analysis of 2 randomized studies on 140 patients, 32 with glomerulonephritis. *Annales de Medicine Interne, Paris* **148**, 198–204.

Guillevin, L. *et al.* (1997b). A prospective, multicenter, randomized trial comparing steroids and pulse cyclophosphamide versus steroids and oral cyclophosphamide in the treatment of generalized Wegener's granulomatosis. *Arthritis and Rheumatism* **40**, 2187–2198.

Guillevin, L. *et al.* (1999). Churg–Strauss syndrome. Clinical study and long-term follow-up of 96 patients. *Medicine (Baltimore)* **78**, 26–37.

Guillevin, L. *et al.* (2003). Treatment of polyarteritis nodosa and microscopic polyangiitis with poor prognosis factors: a prospective trial comparing glucocorticoids and six or twelve cyclophosphamide pulses in sixty-five patients. *Arthritis and Rheumatism* **49**, 93–100.

Hachulla, E. *et al.* (1993). Embolization of two bleeding aneurysms with platinum coils in a patient with polyarteritis nodosa. *Journal of Rheumatology* **20**, 158–161.

Hagen, E. C. *et al.* (1995). Compassionate treatment of Wegener's granulomatosis with rabbit anti-thymocyte globulin. *Clinical Nephrology* **43**, 351–359.

Hagen, E. C. *et al.* (1998). Diagnostic value of standardized assays for anti-neutrophil cytoplasmic antibodies in idiopathic systemic vasculitis. EC/BCR project for ANCA assay standardization. *Kidney International* **53**, 743–753.

Hall, S. *et al.* (1985a). Takayasu arteritis: a study of 32 North American patients. *Medicine* **64**, 89–99.

Hall, S. J. *et al.* (1985b). Wegener granulomatosis in pediatric patients. *Journal of Pediatrics* **106**, 739–744.

Harkavy, J. (1941). Vascular allergy. Pathogenesis of bronchial asthma with recurrent pulmonary infiltrations and eosinophilic polyserositis. *Archives of Internal Medicine* **67**, 709.

Haroun, M. K., Stone, J. H., Nair, R., Racusen, L., Hellmann, D. B., and Eustace, J. A. (2002). Correlation of percentage of normal glomeruli with renal outcome in Wegener's granulomatosis. *American Journal of Nephrology* **22**, 497–503.

Harrison, D. F. N. (1989). Ear, nose and throat symptoms in subacute Wegener's granulomatosis. *British Medical Journal* **299**, 791.

Haubitz, M. and de Groot, K. (2002). Tolerance of mycophenolate mofetil in end-stage renal disease patients with ANCA-associated vasculitis. *Clinical Nephrology* **57**, 421–424.

Haubitz, M. *et al.* (1998a). Reduced gonadal toxicity after i.v. cyclophosphamide administration in patients with nonmalignant diseases. *Clinical Nephrology* **49**, 19–23.

Haubitz, M., Koch, K. M., and Brunkhorst, R. (1998b). Cyclosporin for the prevention of disease reactivation in relapsing ANCA-associated vasculitis. *Nephrology, Dialysis, Transplantation* **13**, 2074–2076.

Haubitz, M. *et al.* (1998c). Intravenous pulse administration of cyclophosphamide versus daily oral treatment in patients with anti-neutrophil cytoplasmic antibody-associated vasculitis and renal involvement: a prospective, randomized study. *Arthritis and Rheumatism* **41**, 1835–1844.

Hauer, H. A. *et al.* (2002a). Long-term renal injury in ANCA-associated vasculitis: an analysis of 31 patients with follow-up biopsies. *Nephrology, Dialysis, Transplantation* **17**, 587–596.

Hauer, H. A. *et al.* (2002b). Determinants of outcome in ANCA-associated glomerulonephritis: a prospective clinico-histopathological analysis of 96 patients. *Kidney International* **62**, 1732–1742.

Hauer, H. A. *et al.* (2002c). Renal histology in ANCA-associated vasculitis: differences between diagnostic and serologic subgroups. *Kidney International* **61**, 80–89.

Hauschild, S., Csernok, E., Schmitt, W. H., and Gross, W. L. (1994). Antineutrophil cytoplasmic antibodies in systemic polyarteritis nodosa with and without hepatitis B virus infection and Churg–Strauss syndrome—62 patients. *Journal of Rheumatology* **21**, 1173–1174.

Haworth, S. J. *et al.* (1985). Pulmonary haemorrhage complicating Wegener's granulomatosis and microscopic polyarteritis. *British Medical Journal* **290**, 1775–1778.

Haynes, B. F. and Fauci, A. S. (1978). Diabetes insipidus associated with Wegener's granulomatosis successfully treated with cyclophosphamide. *New England Journal of Medicine* **299**, 764.

Heilman, R. L., Offord, K. P., Holley, K. E., and Velosa, J. A. (1987). Analysis of risk factors for patient and renal survival in crescentic glomerulonephritis. *American Journal of Kidney Diseases* **9**, 98–107.

Hellman, D. B., Hardy, K., Lindenfield, S., and Ring, E. (1987). Takayasu's arteritis associated with crescentic glomerulonephritis. *Arthritis and Rheumatism* **30**, 451–454.

Henderson, R. A., Hasleton, P., and Hamid, B. N. (1993). Recurrence of Churg Strauss vasculitis in a transplanted heart. *British Heart Journal* **70**, 553.

Hind, C. R. K. *et al.* (1984). Objective monitoring of activity in Wegener's granulomatosis by measurement of serum C-reactive protein concentration. *Clinical Nephrology* **21**, 341–345.

Hoffman, G. S. *et al.* (1990). Treatment of Wegener's granulomatosis with intermittent high dose intravenous cyclophosphamide. *American Journal of Medicine* **89**, 403–410.

Hoffman, G. S. *et al.* (1992a). Wegener granulomatosis: an analysis of 158 patients. *Annals of Internal Medicine* **116**, 488–498.

Hoffman, G. S., Leavitt, R. Y., Kerr, G. S., and Fauci, A. S. (1992b). The treatment of Wegener's granulomatosis with glucocorticoids and methotrexate. *Arthritis and Rheumatism* **35**, 1322–1329.

Hogan, S. L. *et al.* (1996). Prognostic markers in patients with anti-neutrophil cytoplasmic autoantibody-associated microscopic polyangiitis and glomerulonephritis. *Journal of the American Society of Nephrology* **7**, 23–32.

Hollander, D. and Manning, R. T. (1967). The use of alkylating agents in the treatment of Wegener's granulomatosis. *Annals of Internal Medicine* **67**, 393–398.

Huang, D., Giscombe, R., Zhou, Y., and Lefvert, A. K. (2000). Polymorphisms in CTLA-4 but not tumor necrosis factor-alpha or interleukin 1beta genes are associated with Wegener's granulomatosis. *Journal of Rheumatology* **27**, 397–401.

Hunder, G. G. *et al.* (1990). The American College of Rheumatology 1990 criteria for the classification of vasculitis. *Arthritis and Rheumatism* **33**, 1065–1145.

Jacobs, R. P., Moore, M., and Brower, A. (1987). Wegener's granulomatosis presenting with erosive arthritis. *Arthritis and Rheumatism* **30**, 943–946.

Jarrousse, B. *et al.* (1993). Increased risk of *Pneumocystis carinii* pneumonia in patients with Wegener's granulomatosis. *Clinical and Experimental Rheumatology* **11**, 615–621.

Jayne, D. (2001). Update on the European Vasculitis Study Group trials. *Current Opinion in Rheumatology* **13**, 48–55.

Jayne, D. R. W. *et al.* (1989). Severe pulmonary haemorrhage and systemic vasculitis in association with circulating anti-neutrophil cytoplasm antibodies of IgM class only. *Clinical Nephrology* **32**, 101–106.

Jayne, D. R. W., Marshall, P. D., Jones, S. J., and Lockwood, C. M. (1990). Autoantibodies to GBM and neutrophil cytoplasm in rapidly progressive glomerulonephritis. *Kidney International* **37**, 965–970.

Jayne, D. R. W., Weetman, A. P., and Lockwood, C. M. (1991). IgG subclass distribution of autoantibodies to neutrophil cytoplasmic antigens in systemic vasculitis. *Clinical and Experimental Immunology* **84**, 476–481.

Jayne, D. R. W., Gaskin, G., Pusey, C. D., and Lockwood, C. M. (1995). ANCA and prediction of relapse in systemic vasculitis. *Quarterly Journal of Medicine* **88**, 127–133.

Jennette, J. C., Wilkman, A. S., and Falk, R. J. (1989). Anti-neutrophil cytoplasmic autoantibody-associated glomerulonephritis and vasculitis. *American Journal of Pathology* **135**, 921–930.

Jayne D., Gaskin, G., and European Vasculitis Study Group (1999). Randomised trial of cyclophosphamide versus azathioprine during remission in ANCA-associated vasculitis (CYCAZAREM). *Journal of the American Society of Nephrology* **10**, 101A.

Jayne, D. R. *et al.* (2000). Intravenous immunoglobulin for ANCA-associated systemic vasculitis with persistent disease activity. *Quarterly Journal of Medicine* **93**, 433–439.

Jennette, J. C. *et al.* (1994). Nomenclature of systemic vasculitides. Proposal of an international consensus conference. *Arthritis and Rheumatism* **37**, 187–192.

Jonker, N. D. *et al.* (1992). A retrospective study of radiolabelled granulocyte kinetics in patients with systemic vasculitis. *Journal of Nuclear Medicine* **33**, 491–497.

Kallenberg, C. G., Rarok, A., and Stegeman, C. A. (2002). Genetics of ANCA-associated vasculitides. *Cleveland Clinic Journal of Medicine* **69** (Suppl. 2), SII61–SII63.

Karkar, A. M., Smith, J., and Pusey, C. D. (2001). Prevention and treatment of experimental crescentic glomerulonephritis by blocking tumour necrosis factor-alpha. *Nephrology, Dialysis, Transplantation* **16**, 518–524.

Klinger, H. (1931). Grenzformen der Periarteritis nodosa. *Frankfurter Zeitschrift für Pathologie* **42**, 455–480.

Kokolina, E. *et al.* (1994). Isotype and affinity of anti-myeloperoxidase autoantibodies in systemic vasculitis. *Kidney International* **46**, 177–184.

Kozak, M., Gill, E. A., and Green, L. S. (1995). The Churg–Strauss syndrome. A case report with angiographically documented coronary artery involvement and a review of the literature. *Chest* **107**, 578–580.

Kussmaul, A. and Maier, R. (1866). Uber eine bischer nicht beschriebere eigenthumliche Arterienerkrankung (Periarteritis Nodosa), die mit Morbus Brightii und rapid fortschreitender allemeiner Muskellahmung einhergeht. *Deutsche Archiv für Klinische Medizin* **1**, 484–516.

Kyndt, X. *et al.* (1999). Serial measurements of antineutrophil cytoplasmic autoantibodies in patients with systemic vasculitis. *American Journal of Medicine* **106**, 527–533.

Lai, K. N. and Lockwood, C. M. (1993). Serum soluble interleukin 2 receptor levels in anti-neutrophil cytoplasmic autoantibodies—positive systemic vasculitis. *Postgraduate Medical Journal* **69**, 708–711.

Lamprecht, P. *et al.* (2002). Effectiveness of TNF-alpha blockade with infliximab in refractory Wegener's granulomatosis. *Rheumatology (Oxford)* **41**, 1303–1307.

Landwehr, D. M., Cooke, C. L., and Rodriguez, G. E. (1980). Rapidly progressive glomerulonephritis in Behçet's syndrome. *Journal of American Medical Association* **244**, 1709–1711.

Langford, C. A. and Kerr, G. S. (2002). Pregnancy in vasculitis. *Current Opinion in Rheumatology* **14**, 36–41.

Lanham, J. G., Elkon, K. B., Pusey, C. D., and Hughes, G. R. (1984). Systemic vasculitis with asthma and eosinophilia: a clinical approach to the Churg–Strauss syndrome. *Medicine* **63**, 65–81.

Lauque, D. *et al.* (2000). Microscopic polyangiitis with alveolar hemorrhage. A study of 29 cases and review of the literature. Groupe d'Etudes et de Recherche sur les Maladies Orphelines Pulmonaires (GERMOP). *Medicine (Baltimore)* **79**, 222–233.

Leavitt, R. Y., Hoffman, G. S., and Fauci, A. S. (1988). Response: the role of trimethoprim/sulphamethoxazole in the treatment of Wegener's granulomatosis. *Arthritis and Rheumatism* **31**, 1073–1074.

Lee, K. S. *et al.* (2003). Thoracic manifestation of Wegener's granulomatosis: CT findings in 30 patients. *European Radiology* **13**, 43–51.

Leib, E. S., Restivo, C., and Paulus, H. E. (1979). Immunosuppressive and corticosteroid therapy of polyarteritis nodosa. *American Journal of Medicine* **67**, 941–945.

Leruez-Ville, M. *et al.* (1994). Polyarteritis nodosa and parvovirus B19. *Lancet* **344**, 263–264.

Levy, J. B. and Pusey, C. D. (2000). Nephrotoxicity of intravenous immunoglobulin. *Quarterly Journal of Medicine* **93**, 751–755.

Levy, J. B. and Winearls, C. G. (1994). Rapidly progressive glomerulonephritis: what should be first-line therapy? *Nephron* **67**, 402–407.

Lie, J. T. (1978). Disseminated giant cell arteritis. Histopathological description and differentiation from other granulomatous vasculitides. *American Journal of Clinical Pathology* **69**, 299–305.

Lie, J. T. (1997). Wegener's granulomatosis: histological documentation of common and uncommon manifestations in 216 patients. *Vasa* **26**, 261–270.

Lloyd, G., Lund, V. J., Beale, T., and Howard, D. (2002). Rhinologic changes in Wegener's granulomatosis. *Journal of Laryngology and Otology* **116**, 565–569.

Lockwood, C. M. *et al.* (1977). Plasma-exchange and immunosuppression in the treatment of fulminant immune-complex crescentic nephritis. *Lancet* **i**, 63–67.

Lockwood, C. M. *et al.* (1993). Long-term remission of intractable systemic vasculitis with monoclonal antibody therapy. *Lancet* **341**, 1620–1622.

Lockwood, C. M. *et al.* (1999). Anti-adhesion molecule therapy as an interventional strategy for autoimmune inflammation. *Clinical Immunology* **93**, 93–106.

Luqmani, R. A. *et al.* (1994a). Classical versus non-renal Wegener's granulomatosis. *Quarterly Journal of Medicine* **87**, 161–167.

Luqmani, R. A. *et al.* (1994b). Birmingham Vasculitis Activity Score in systemic necrotizing vasculitis. *Quarterly Journal of Medicine* **87**, 671–678.

Mader, R. *et al.* (1993). Systemic vasculitis following influenza vaccination—report of 3 cases and literature review. *Journal of Rheumatology* **20**, 1429–1431.

Mathieson, P. W. *et al.* (1990). Monoclonal antibody therapy in systemic vasculitis. *New England Journal of Medicine* **323**, 250–254.

Mattioli, F. *et al.* (2002). Frequency and patterns of subclinical cognitive impairment in patients with ANCA-associated small vessel vasculitides. *Journal of the Neurological Sciences* **195**, 161–166.

McLelland, P., Williams, P. S., Stevens, M. E., and Bone, J. M. (1989). *Nephrology, Dialysis, Transplantation* **4**, 917 (letter).

Merkel, P. A. (1998). Drugs associated with vasculitis. *Current Opinion in Rheumatology* **10**, 45–50.

Moon, K. C. *et al.* (2002). Expression of intercellular adhesion molecule-1 and vascular cell adhesion molecule-1 in human crescentic glomerulonephritis. *Histopathology* **41**, 158–165.

Moore, P. M. and Fauci, A. S. (1981), Neurologic manifestations of systemic vasculitis. A retrospective and prospective study of the clinicopathologic features and responses to therapy in 25 patients. *American Journal of Medicine* **71**, 517–524.

Muhle, C. *et al.* (1997). MRI of the nasal cavity, the paranasal sinuses and orbits in Wegener's granulomatosis. *European Radiology* **7**, 566–570.

Müller, G. A. *et al.* (1984). Association between rapidly progressive glomerulonephritis and the properdin factor BfF and different HLA-D region products. *Kidney International* **25**, 115–118.

Müller, G. A. *et al.* (1988). Renal major histocompatibility complex antigens and cellular components in rapidly progressive glomerulonephritis identified by monoclonal antibodies. *Nephron* **49**, 132–139.

Murakozy, G. *et al.* (2001). Gene polymorphisms of immunoregulatory cytokines and angiotensin-converting enzyme in Wegener's granulomatosis. *Journal of Molecular Medicine* **79**, 665–670.

Nachman, P. *et al.* (1999). Recurrent ANCA-associated small vessel vasculitis after transplantation: a pooled analysis. *Kidney International* **56**, 1544–1550.

Nada, A. K. *et al.* (1990). Pulmonary fibrosis as an unusual clinical manifestation of a pulmonary-renal vasculitis in elderly patients. *Mayo Clinic Proceedings* **65**, 847–856.

Niles, J. L. *et al.* (1991). Antigen-specific radioimmunoassays for anti-neutrophil cytoplasmic antibodies in the diagnosis of rapidly progressive glomerulonephritis. *Journal of the American Society of Nephrology* **2**, 27–36.

Nishino, H. *et al.* (1993). Neurological involvement in Wegener's granulomatosis: an analysis of 324 consecutive patients at the Mayo Clinic. *Annals of Neurology* **33**, 4–9.

Nissensen, A. R. and Port, F. K. (1990). Outcome of end-stage renal disease in patients with rare causes of renal failure. III: systemic/vascular disorders. *Quarterly Journal of Medicine* **74**, 65–74.

Noritake, D. T. *et al.* (1987). Rheumatic manifestations of Wegener's granulomatosis. *Journal of Rheumatology* **14**, 949–951.

Noth, I., Strek, M. E., and Leff, A. R. (2003). Churg–Strauss syndrome. *Lancet* **361**, 587–594.

Novack, S. and Pearson, C. M. (1971). Cyclophosphamide therapy in Wegener's granulomatosis. *New England Journal of Medicine* **284**, 938–941.

Novak, R. F., Christiansen, R. G., and Sorensen, E. T. (1982). The acute vasculitis of Wegener's granulomatosis in renal biopsies. *American Journal of Clinical Pathology* **78**, 367–371.

Nowack, R. *et al.* (1999). Mycophenolate mofetil for maintenance therapy of Wegener's granulomatosis and microscopic polyangiitis: a pilot study in 11 patients with renal involvement. *Journal of the American Society of Nephrology* **10**, 1965–1971.

Nowack, R. *et al.* (2001). ANCA titres, even of IgG subclasses, and soluble CD14 fail to predict relapses in patients with ANCA-associated vasculitis. *Nephrology, Dialysis, Transplantation* **16**, 1631–1637.

O'Donaghue, D. J. *et al.* (1989). Sequential development of systemic vasculitis with anti-neutrophil cytoplasmic antibodies complicating anti-glomerular basement membrane disease. *Clinical Nephrology* **32**, 251–255.

O'Donoghue, D. J., Guickian, M., Blundell, G., and Winney, R. J. Alpha-1-proteinase inhibitor and pulmonary haemorrhage in systemic vasculitis. In *ANCA-Associated Vasculitides: Immunological and Clinical Aspects* (ed. W. L. Gross), pp. 331–335. New York: Plenum Press, 1993.

O'Neill, W. M. J., Hammar, S. P., and Bloomer, A. (1976). Giant cell arteritis with visceral angiitis. *Archives of Internal Medicine* **136**, 1157–1160.

Ognibene, F. P. *et al.* (1995). *Pneumocystis carinii* pneumonia: a major complication of immunosuppressive therapy in patients with Wegener's granulomatosis. *American Journal of Respiratory and Critical Care Medicine* **151**, 795–799.

Palmer, A. *et al.* (1991). Treatment of rapidly progressive glomerulonephritis by extracorporeal immunoadsorption, prednisolone and cyclophosphamide. *Nephrology, Dialysis, Transplantation* **6**, 536–542.

Peat, D. S. and Mathieson, P. W. (1996). Cholesterol emboli may mimic systemic vasculitis. *British Medical Journal* **313**, 546–547.

Pinching, A. J. *et al.* (1980). Relapses in Wegener's granulomatosis: the role of infection. *British Medical Journal* **281**, 836–838.

Pinching, A. J. *et al.* (1983). Wegener's granulomatosis: observations on 18 patients with severe renal disease. *Quarterly Journal of Medicine* **52**, 435–460.

Pohl, M., Lan, S., Berl, T., and The Lupus Nephritis collaborative study group (1991). Plasmapheresis does not increase the risk for infection in immunosuppressed patients with severe lupus nephritis. *Annals of Internal Medicine* **114**, 924–929.

Pusey, C. D. *et al.* (1991). Plasma exchange in focal necrotizing glomerulonephritis without anti-GBM antibodies. *Kidney International* **40**, 757–763.

Rackemann, F. M. and Greene, J. E. (1939). Periarteritis nodosa and asthma. *Transactions of the Association of American Physicians* **54**, 112–118.

Rarok, A. A., Stegeman, C. A., Limburg, P. C., and Kallenberg, C. G. (2002). Neutrophil membrane expression of proteinase 3 (PR3) is related to relapse in PR3-ANCA-associated vasculitis. *Journal of the American Society of Nephrology* **13**, 2232–2238.

Rasmussen, N. *et al.* (1995). European therapeutic trials in ANCA-associated systemic vasculitis: disease scoring, consensus regimens and proposed clinical trials. *Clinical and Experimental Immunology* **101** (Suppl. 1), 29–34.

Rastaldi, M. P. *et al.* (2000). Glomerular monocyte–macrophage features in ANCA-positive renal vasculitis and cryoglobulinemic nephritis. *Journal of the American Society of Nephrology* **11**, 2036–2043.

Reinhold-Keller, E. *et al.* (1993). Trimethoprim–sulphamethoxazole (T/S) in the long-term treatment of Wegener's granulomatosis. *Clinical and Experimental Immunology* **93** (Suppl. 1), 38.

Reinhold Keller, E. *et al.* (1994). Influence of disease manifestation and antineutrophil cytoplasmic antibody titer on the response to pulse cyclophosphamide therapy in patients with Wegener's granulomatosis. *Arthritis and Rheumatism* **37**, 919–924.

Reinhold-Keller, E. *et al.* (2002). No difference in the incidences of vasculitides between north and south Germany: first results of the German vasculitis register. *Rheumatology (Oxford)* **41**, 540–549.

Reuter, H., Qasim, F. J., Wraight, P., and Lockwood, C. M. (1993). The clinical significance of 111-Indium leucocyte imaging in systemic vasculitis. *Clinical and Experimental Immunology* **93** (Suppl. 1), 36.

Reuter, M. *et al.* (1998). Pulmonary Wegener's granulomatosis: correlation between high-resolution CT findings and clinical scoring of disease activity. *Chest* **114**, 500–506.

Ronco, P. *et al.* (1983). Immunopathological studies of polyarteritis nodosa and Wegener's granulomatosis: a report of 43 patients with 51 renal biopsies. *Quarterly Journal of Medicine* **52**, 212–223.

Rondeau, E. *et al.* (1989). Plasma exchange and immunosuppression for rapidly progressive glomerulonephritis: prognosis and complications. *Nephrology, Dialysis, Transplantation* **4**, 196–200.

Roozendaal, C. and Kallenberg, C. G. (1999). Are anti-neutrophil cytoplasmic antibodies (ANCA) clinically useful in inflammatory bowel disease (IBD)? *Clinical and Experimental Immunology* **116**, 206–213.

Rose, G. A. and Spencer, H. (1957). Polyarteritis nodosa. *Quarterly Journal of Medicine* **26**, 43–81.

Rottem, M. *et al.* (1993). Wegener granulomatosis in children and adolescents: clinical presentation and outcome. *Journal of Pediatrics* **122**, 26–31.

Sack, M., Cassidy, J. T., and Bole, G. G. (1975). Prognostic factors in polyarteritis. *Journal of Rheumatology* **2**, 411–420.

Salcedo, J. R., Greenberg, L., and Kapur, S. (1988). Renal histology of mucocutaneous lymph node syndrome (Kawasaki disease). *Clinical Nephrology* **29**, 47–51.

Satoh, J. *et al.* (1988). Extensive cerebral infarction due to involvement of both anterior cerebral arteries by Wegener's granulomatosis. *Annals of the Rheumatic Diseases* **47**, 606–611.

Savage, C. O. S. *et al.* (1985). Microscopic polyarteritis: presentation, pathology and prognosis. *Quarterly Journal of Medicine* **56**, 467–483.

Savage, C. O. S. *et al.* (1989). Anti-neutrophil cytoplasm antibodies in Kawasaki syndrome. *Archives of Disease in Childhood* **64**, 462.

Savige, J. A. *et al.* (1995). α1-Antitrypsin deficiency and anti-proteinase 3 antibodies in anti-neutrophil cytoplasmic antibody (ANCA)-associated systemic vasculitis. *Clinical and Experimental Immunology* **100**, 194–197.

Savige, J. *et al.* (1999). International Consensus Statement on testing and reporting of antineutrophil cytoplasmic antibodies (ANCA). *American Journal of Clinical Pathology* **111**, 507–513.

Schmitt, W. H. and van der Woude, F. J. (2003). Organ transplantation in the vasculitides. *Current Opinion in Rheumatology* **15**, 22–28.

Schmitt, W. H. *et al.* (1998). Churg–Strauss syndrome: serum markers of lymphocyte activation and endothelial damage. *Arthritis and Rheumatism* **41**, 445–452.

Schnabel, A., Hauschild, S., and Gross, W. L. (1996). Anti-neutrophil cytoplasmic antibodies in generalized autoimmune diseases. *International Archives of Allergy and Immunology* **109**, 201–206.

Scott, D. G. I. *et al.* (1982). Systemic vasculitis in a district general hospital 1972–1980: clinical and laboratory features, classification and prognosis of 80 cases. *Quarterly Journal of Medicine* **51**, 292–311.

Screaton, N. J., Sivasothy, P., Flower, C. D., and Lockwood, C. M. (1998). Tracheal involvement in Wegener's granulomatosis: evaluation using spiral CT. *Clinical Radiology* **53**, 809–815.

Segelmark, M. and Wieslander, J. (1993). IgG subclasses of antineutrophil cytoplasm autoantibodies (ANCA). *Nephrology, Dialysis, Transplantation* **8**, 696–702.

Sehgal, M., Swanson, J. W., DeRemee, R. A., and Colby, T. V. (1995). Neurologic manifestations of Churg–Strauss syndrome. *Mayo Clinic Proceedings* **70**, 337–341.

Seron, D., Cameron, J. S., and Haskard, D. O. (1991). Expression of VCAM-1 in the normal and diseased kidney. *Nephrology, Dialysis, Transplantation* **6**, 917–922.

Serra, A. *et al.* (1984). Vasculitis affecting the kidney: presentation, histopathology and long-term outcome. *Quarterly Journal of Medicine* **53**, 181–207.

Short, A. K., Esnault, V. L. M., and Lockwood, C. M. ANCA and anti-GBM antibodies in RPGN. In *ANCA-Associated Vasculitides: Immunological and Clinical Aspects* (ed. W. L. Gross), pp. 441–444. New York: Plenum Press, 1993.

Sneller, M. C. *et al.* (1995). An analysis of forty-two Wegener's granulomatosis patients treated with methotrexate and prednisone. *Arthritis and Rheumatism* **38**, 608–613.

Sonnenblick, M., Nesher, G., and Rosin, A. (1989). Nonclassical organ involvement in temporal arteritis. *Seminars in Arthritis and Rheumatism* **19**, 183–190.

Soto, A. *et al.* (1994). Endocarditis associated with ANCA. *Clinical and Experimental Rheumatology* **12**, 203–204.

Specks, U., Fervenza, F. C., McDonald, T. J., and Hogan, M. C. (2001). Response of Wegener's granulomatosis to anti-CD20 chimeric monoclonal antibody therapy. *Arthritis and Rheumatism* **44**, 2836–2840.

Stegeman, C. A. *et al.* (1994). Association of chronic nasal carriage of *Staphylococcus aureus* and higher relapse rates in Wegener granulomatosis. *Annals of Internal Medicine* **120**, 12–17.

Stegeman, C. A., Cohen Tervaert, J. W., de Jong, P. E., and Kallenberg, C. G. M. (1996). Trimethoprim–sulphamethoxazole (Co-trimoxazole) for the prevention of relapses of Wegener's granulomatosis. Dutch Co-Trimoxazole Wegener study group. *New England Journal of Medicine* **335**, 16–20.

Stegmayr, B. G. *et al.* (1999). Plasma exchange or immunoadsorption in patients with rapidly progressive crescentic glomerulonephritis. A Swedish multi-center study. *International Journal of Artificial Organs* **22**, 81–87.

Stevens, M. E., McConnell, M., and Bone, J. M. (1982). Aggressive treatment with pulse methylprednisolone or plasma exchange is justified in rapidly progressive glomerulonephritis. *Proceedings of the European Dialysis and Transplant Association* **19**, 724–731.

Stillwell, T. J. *et al.* (1988). Cyclophosphamide-induced bladder toxicity in Wegener's granulomatosis. *Arthritis and Rheumatism* **31**, 465–470.

Stone, J. H. *et al.* (2001a). A disease-specific activity index for Wegener's granulomatosis: modification of the Birmingham Vasculitis Activity Score. International Network for the Study of the Systemic Vasculitides (INSSYS). *Arthritis and Rheumatism* **44**, 912–920.

Stone, J. H. *et al.* (2001b). Etanercept combined with conventional treatment in Wegener's granulomatosis: a six-month open-label trial to evaluate safety. *Arthritis and Rheumatism* **44**, 1149–1154.

Summers, R. M. *et al.* (2002). CT virtual bronchoscopy of the central airways in patients with Wegener's granulomatosis. *Chest* **121**, 242–250.

Sutton, D. M., Nair, R. C., and Rock, G. (1989). Complications of plasma exchange. *Transfusion* **29**, 124–127.

Takagi, M. *et al.* (1984). Renal histological studies in patients with Takayasu's arteritis. Report of 3 cases. *Nephron* **36**, 68–73.

Takizawa, M. *et al.* (2001). Correlation between the levels of circulating adhesion molecules and PR3-ANCA in Wegener's granulomatosis. *Auris, Nasus, Larynx* **28** (Suppl.), S59–S62.

Talar-Williams, C. *et al.* (1996). Cyclophosphamide-induced cystitis and bladder cancer in patients with Wegener granulomatosis. *Annals of Internal Medicine* **124**, 477–484.

Tatsis, E., Schnabel, A., and Gross, W. L. (1998). Interferon-alpha treatment of four patients with the Churg-Strauss syndrome. *Annals of Internal Medicine* **129**, 370–374.

ten Berge, I. J. M. *et al.* (1985). Clinical and immunological follow-up of patients with severe renal disease in Wegener's granulomatosis. *American Journal of Nephrology* **5**, 21–29.

Tervaert, J. W. and Kallenberg, C. (1993). Neurologic manifestations of systemic vasculitides. *Rheumatic Disease Clinics of North America* **19**, 913–940.

Tervaert, J. W., Stegeman, C. A., and Kallenberg, C. G. (1998). Silicon exposure and vasculitis. *Current Opinion in Rheumatology* **10**, 12–17.

Travers, R. L., Allison, D. J., Brettle, R. P., and Hughes, G. R. V. (1979). Polyarteritis nodosa: a clinical and angiographic analysis of 17 cases. *Seminars in Arthritis and Rheumatism* **8**, 184–199.

Travis, W. D., Colby, T. V., Lombard, C., and Carpenter, H. A. (1990). A clinicopathologic study of 34 cases of diffuse pulmonary haemorrhage with lung biopsy confirmation. *American Journal of Surgical Pathology* **14**, 1112–1125.

Travis, W. D. *et al.* (1991). Surgical pathology of the lung in Wegener's granulomatosis: review of 87 open lung biopsies from 67 patients. *American Journal of Surgical Pathology* **15**, 315–333.

Truong, L., Kopelman, R. G., Williams, G. S., and Pirani, C. L. (1985). Temporal arteritis and renal disease. Case report and review of the literature. *American Journal of Medicine* **78**, 171–175.

van der Woude, F. J. *et al.* (1985). Autoantibodies against neutrophils and monocytes: tool for diagnosis and marker of disease activity in Wegener's granulomatosis, *Lancet* **i**, 425–429.

van der Woude, F. J., Daha, M. R., and van Es, L. A. (1989). The current status of neutrophil cytoplasmic antibodies. *Clinical and Experimental Immunology* **78**, 143–148.

Veiga, P. A., Pieroni, D., Baier, W., and Feld, L. G. (1992). Association of Kawasaki disease and interstitial nephritis. *Pediatric Nephrology* **6**, 421–423.

Wagner, J., Andrassy, K., and Ritz, E. (1991). Is vasculitis in subacute bacterial endocarditis associated with ANCA? *Lancet* **337**, 799–800.

Wahls, T. L., Bonsib, S. M., and Schuster, V. L. (1987). Coexistent Wegener's granulomatosis and anti-glomerular basement membrane disease. *Human Pathology* **18**, 202–205.

Wainwright, J. and Davson, J. (1950). The renal appearances in the microscopic form of periarteritis nodosa. *Journal of Pathology and Bacteriology* **62**, 189–196.

Walton, E. W. (1958). Giant-cell granuloma of the respiratory tract (Wegener's granulomatosis). *British Medical Journal* **2**, 265–270.

Watts, R. A., Lane, S. E., Bentham, G., and Scott, D. G. I. (2000). Epidemiology of systemic vasculitis. *Arthritis and Rheumatism* **43**, 414–419.

Weber, M. F. *et al.* (1992). Antineutrophil-cytoplasmic antibodies and antiglomerular basement membrane antibodies in Goodpasture's syndrome and in Wegener's granulomatosis. *Journal of the American Society of Nephrology* **2**, 1227–1234.

Wechsler, M. E., Pauwels, R., and Drazen, J. M. (1999). Leukotriene modifiers and Churg–Strauss syndrome: adverse effect or response to corticosteroid withdrawal? *Drug Safety: An International Journal of Medical Toxicology and Drug Experience* **21**, 241–251.

Wegener, F. (1936). Uber generalisierte, septische Gefasserkrankungen. *Verhandlungen der Deutschen Pathologischen Gesellschaft* **29**, 202–210.

Wegener, F. (1939). Uber eine eigenartige rhinogene Granulomatose mit besonderer Beteiligung des Arteriensystems und der Nieren. *Beitrage der Pathologische Anatomie* **102**, 30–68.

Weiss, M. A. and Crissman, J. D. (1985). Segmental necrotizing glomerulonephritis: diagnostic, prognostic and therapeutic significance. *American Journal of Kidney Diseases* **6**, 199–211.

Westman, K. W. *et al.* (1998). Relapse rate, renal survival, and cancer morbidity in patients with Wegener's granulomatosis or microscopic polyangiitis with renal involvement. *Journal of the American Society of Nephrology* **9**, 842–852.

Wiik, A. (1989). Delineation of a standard procedure for indirect immunofluorescence detection of anti-neutrophil cytoplasmic antibodies (ANCA). *Acta Pathologica, Microbiologica, et Immunologica Scandanavica* **97** (Suppl. 6), 12–13.

Wiik, A. (2001). Methods for the detection of anti-neutrophil cytoplasmic antibodies. Recommendations for clinical use of ANCA serology and laboratory efforts to optimize the informative value of ANCA test results. *Springer Seminars in Immunopathology* **23**, 217–229.

Wiik, A., Jensen, E., and Friis, J. (1974). Granulocyte-specific antinuclear factors in synovial fluids and sera from patients with rheumatoid arthritis. *Annals of Rheumatic Diseases* **33**, 515–522.

Woodworth, T. G., Abuelo, J. G., Austin, H. A., and Esparza, A. (1987). Severe glomerulonephritis with late emergence of classic Wegener's granulomatosis: report of 4 cases and review of the literature. *Medicine* **66**, 181–191.

Woywodt, A. *et al.* (2000). Cytomegalovirus colitis during mycophenolate mofetil therapy for Wegener's granulomatosis. *American Journal of Nephrology* **20**, 468–472.

Yanai-Berar, N., Ben-Itzhak, O., Gree, J., and Nakhoul, F. (2002). Influenza vaccination induced leukocytoclastic vasculitis and pauci-immune crescentic glomerulonephritis. *Clinical Nephrology* **58**, 220–223.

Yang, C. W. *et al.* (1993). Antineutrophil cytoplasmic autoantibody associated vasculitis and renal failure in Behçet disease. *Nephrology, Dialysis, Transplantation* **8**, 871–873.

Yashiro, M. *et al.* (2000). Significantly high regional morbidity of MPO–ANCA-related angiitis and/or nephritis with respiratory tract involvement after the 1995 great earthquake in Kobe (Japan). *American Journal of Kidney Diseases* **35**, 889–895.

Yoshikawa, Y. and Watanabe, T. (1984). Granulomatous glomerulonephritis in Wegener's granulomatosis. *Virchows Archiv. A. Pathological Anatomy and Histopathology* **402**, 361–372.

Zhou, Y., Giscombe, R., Huang, D., and Lefvert, A. K. (2002). Novel genetic association of Wegener's granulomatosis with the interleukin 10 gene. *Journal of Rheumatology* **29**, 317–320.

4.6 The patient with mixed cryoglobulinaemia and hepatitis C infection

Antonio Tarantino

Definition of mixed cryoglobulinaemia

The term 'cryoproteins' was first introduced in 1933 by Wintrobe and Buell to designate a group of proteins that precipitate or form gel in the cold. In 1947, Lerner and Watson provided evidence that cold-insoluble proteins are immunoglobulins. Purification and immunochemical analysis of cryoprecipitable immunoglobulins has permitted classification of these proteins (Brouet *et al.* 1974). Type I cryoglobulin is a single monoclonal immunoglobulin and is associated with multiple myeloma, Waldenström's macroglobulinaemia, or idiopathic monoclonal gammopathy. Type II cryoglobulins are mixed cryoglobulins, consisting of a monoclonal antiglobulin (usually IgM and more rarely IgA or IgG) plus polyclonal IgGs. Type III cryoglobulins are mixed polyclonal immunoglobulins. Type I and II cryoglobulins are usually present in large amounts in serum (often >5 mg/ml), while type III cryoglobulins are present in relatively low concentration (<1 mg/ml). In about 60–75 per cent of cases, circulating cryoglobulins are found in patients with connective tissue diseases, infections, lymphoproliferative disorders, hepatobiliary diseases, or immunologically mediated glomerular diseases. These cases are generally considered as 'secondary mixed cryoglobulinaemias'. The so-called 'essential mixed cryoglobulinaemias', not related to any of the aforementioned diseases, first described by Meltzer *et al.* (1966), are clinically characterized by purpura, weakness, arthralgias, and in some patients, by renal involvement.

Mechanisms of cryoprecipitation

Two main mechanisms have been identified: intrinsic physicochemical properties of immunoglobulins or factors dependent on antigen–antibody interaction. Intrinsic physicochemical properties, such as particular heavy chain class, IgG subclass, heavy and light chain subgroups, structural modification in the variable regions of heavy and light chains have been described for type I cryoproteins. All these structural changes make the immunoglobulin hydrophobic and thus enhance its insolubility. The isolated components from mixed cryoglobulins cannot precipitate by themselves, both immunoglobulins are required for precipitation. An enrichment in the IgG3 subclass has been found in the cryoprecipitates. They have a peculiar cryogenic property stemming from their ability to assemble themselves through spontaneous Fc–Fc interactions (Musset *et al.* 1992). IgM rheumatoid factors (IgM RFs) with the specificity of anti-IgG3 activity are more potent for the generation of cryoglobulins than those lacking anti-IgG3 activity. Fibronectin, an adhesive glycoprotein of 440 kDa, coprecipitates with all types and classes of cryoglobulins. In addition, IgM k RFs, isolated by cryoglobulins, have a great affinity for immobilized cellular fibronectin present in some glomerular cells (monocytes, endothelial, epithelial, and mesangial cells) (Fornasieri *et al.* 1996).

Aetiology

Viruses and mixed cryoglobulinaemia

The aetiological role of the hepatitis B virus (HBV) was initially overemphasized (Levo *et al.* 1977). Since the development in 1989 of a test for the detection of antibodies to hepatitis C virus (HCV), it has been established that almost all cases of mixed cryoglobulinaemia (MC) previously called 'essential' are in fact related to chronic HCV infection (Pascual *et al.* 1990). The incidence of HCV infection in MC ranges from 40 to 100 per cent in the reported case series and in different geographical areas. In the Mediterranean area, almost all cases of MC are HCV positive (Dammacco and Sansonno 1997). The aetiological role of HCV in MC is based on the following facts: (a) the concentration of HCV-RNA in the cryoprecipitate is from 10- to 1000-fold greater than in supernatants; (b) most of the known viral antigens (core, E1, E2, NS3, NS4, NS5) and their corresponding antibodies are detected in both cryoprecipitates and vascular lesions in tissue sections (Munoz-Fernandes *et al.* 1994; Sansonno *et al.* 1995); (c) the presence of HCV-RNA sequence in bone marrow cells and peripheral blood mononuclear cells (Gabrielli *et al.* 1994).

The strong association between MC and HCV infection suggests that the term 'essential' cryoglobulinaemia should be changed in 'HCV-related cryoglobulinaemia'.

Pathogenesis of tissue damage

The mechanisms by which HCV elicits the formation of cryoglobulins only in some patients, are not well defined. It is thought that the cryoglobulinaemic syndrome may be the consequence of interaction between exogenous agents and a host characterized by a particular genetic background, but HLA expression has been investigated in MC patients with controversial results (Nightingale *et al.* 1981; Amoroso *et al.* 1998; Lenzi *et al.* 1998).

The strong association of HCV infection with MC and the presence of viral antigens, antibodies against viral antigenes, and RFs mostly mounting WA idiotype in the cryoglobulins are compelling evidence that the virus is directly involved in production of the monoclonal RFs and in the pathophysiology of MC. Recent identification of intrahepatic clonal B cells capable of RF production, of selective infection of B cells over T cells and of an HCV receptor on B lymphocytes strongly supports a central role for these cells in the immune response to HCV infection. In particular, CD5+ B cells which are capable of producing natural antibodies with autoreactive specifities are likely to be important in the development of HCV-associated autoimmunity and lymphoproliferation. In cutaneous vasculitis, which is the most prevalent clinical feature of the disease, the HCV virion is found in association with IgM and IgG. HCV alone is detected in some vessel walls and in skin and ductal epithelium and in vascular endothelium in inflamed, but not normal skin. Moreover, the extent of cutaneous lesions correlated with levels of viraemia (Agnello and Abel 1997). Upregulation of LDL receptors on keratinocytes is detected in inflamed, but not normal skin. These data show that HCV is present in the cutaneous vasculitic lesions most likely in complexes with IgG and IgM formed *in situ*. The presence of HCV in keratinocytes, ductal epithelial and vascular endothelial cells may be considered as indirect evidence that *in vivo* endocytosis of HCV is provided by LDL receptors.

A second point concerns the mechanisms by which RFs are produced (Fig. 1). HCV–VLDL complexes that contain apo E2 are poorly endocytosed by LDL receptors, which is the major route of entry of the virus to the cell. It has been proposed that HCV complexed to VLDL is the superantigen that directly stimulates the proliferation of the primordial type B cells bearing the CD5 marker and the synthesis of RFs. On the other hand, monoclonal RFs may prevent the spread of infection to hepatocytes and other permissive and non-permissive cells by blocking endocytosis of HCV–VLDL complexes by LDLR (Ramos-Casals *et al.* 2000).

In contrast to cutaneous vasculitis, HCV-RNA has not been prominently detected in immune complexes in renal lesions and has not been detected at all in the peripheral neuropathy lesions. These preliminary observations suggest that different pathophysiologic processes may be involved in these lesions and in cutaneous vasculitis (Agnello 1997). These conclusions are supported by the recent identification of CD81 as a HCV receptor on B lymphocytes that provides another mechanism by which B cells are infected with or activated by HCV. Binding of HCV to CD81, which complexes with CD21 and CD19, may lower the activation threshold of B cells and result in the production of RFs of IgM molecule capable of immune complex formation (Pileri *et al.* 1998). On the other hand, in evaluating the clonality and antibody specificity of 20 cryoprecipitates, Mondelli *et al.* (1998) found a marked preponderance of IgG3 (12/14), whereas specificity studies revealed that polyclonal IgGs1 were reactive with HCV structural proteins but IgG3 subclass was apparently not involved in HCV nucleoprotein binding. These findings do not support a direct link between monoclonal cryoglobulins and immune response to HCV. Therefore, other cooperative mechanisms will be responsible for the formation of cryoprecipitable RFs, their continuous production, and the expansion of monoclonal B cells.

Looking at experimental models of MC nephritis (Spertini *et al.* 1989; Fornasieri *et al.* 1993; Taneda *et al.* 2001), none of them fits the spontaneous disease in humans, mostly because of the lack of long-lasting viral infection. Only the spontaneous Aleutian disease of mink might be identified as the animal counterpart of MC in humans. These animals have a chronic viral infection, develop hypergammaglobulinaemia, and a progressive glomerulopathy, which is the cause of death. The glomerular lesions are characterized by proliferative changes, monocyte/macrophage infiltration of glomeruli, subendothelial deposition of electron-dense granular material with crystalloid structure resembling that observed in human pathology (Fig. 2), and accumulation of similar-appearing material in the cytoplasms of mesangial and inflammatory cells (Henson *et al.* 1967). Fluorescence for IgG and complement appears in capillary wall and in eosinophilic thrombi, a lesser degree of fluorescence is commonly seen in mesangial areas while fibrin and albumin are not detectable (Pan *et al.* 1970). A restudy of Aleutian disease could be fruitful in delineating morphologic and

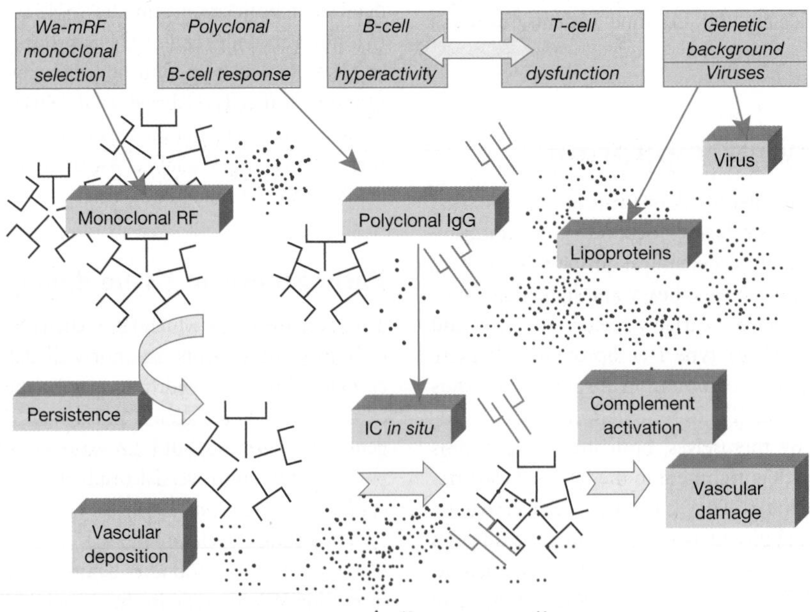

Fig. 1 Pathogenesis of tissue damage in 'mixed cryoglobulinaemia' modified from Ramos-Casals *et al.* 2000.

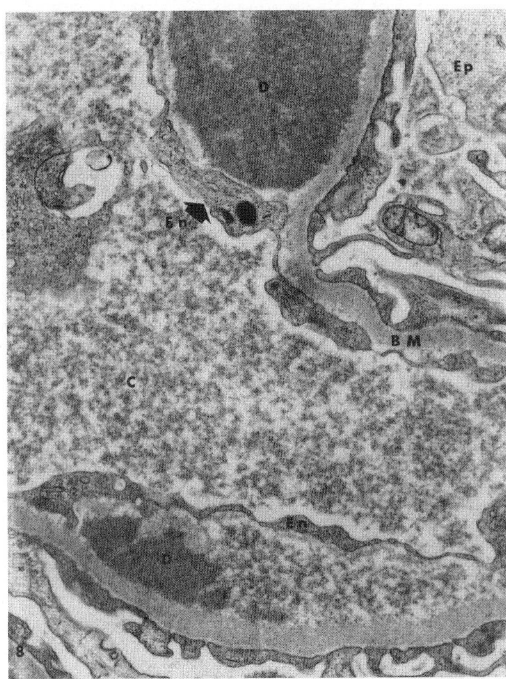

Fig. 2 Aleutian nephropathy: subendothelial electron-dense deposits (D) in the capillary loop (C) show a crystalloid appearance. Reproduced from: *Laboratory Investigation* **17**, 131 (1967). EM 22,750×.

pathogenetic mechanisms of all the events responsible for these two diseases.

Composition of circulating immune complexes

The interaction between cryoprecipitable IgM RF and polyclonal IgG has been generally considered as the binding of $F(ab)_2$ fragments of the RF to the Fc component of the corresponding autoantigenic IgG. In 1980, Geltner *et al.* for the first time, demonstrated that IgM cryoglobulins, isolated from 11 MC patients, endowed with a double reactivity: the classical RF reactivity against the Fc fragment of IgG and an anti-idiotypic reactivity against the $F(ab)_2$ fragment of both autologous and isologous IgG (Geltner *et al.* 1980). In addition, they showed that four out of five tested IgGs had anti-HBsAg reactivity which was inhibited by the addition of the putative HBV antigen(s), thus suggesting that the antigen combining site of IgG was implicated in the reactivity with IgM antiglobulins and therefore that the last had to be considered as an anti-idiotype. These result further researches about the nature of the binding characteristics of the cryoprecipitable IgM RF–IgG complexes. It has been reported that IgM fractions of cryoglobulins preferentially bound to the autologous cryoglobulins IgG, whereas a weak binding of IgM RF to the autologous F(ab) papain digestion fractions of IgG was found (Renversez *et al.* 1984). Therefore, the immune complex should be composed by an IgM RF reacting with the Fc portion of the IgG and an anti-idiotypic IgG reacting with the $F(ab)_2$ portion of IgM. This double reactivity could explain the increased binding affinity of the complex and its reduced solubility in the cold. In this view, a chronic viral infection would elicit an antibody production against the responsible viruses, with subsequent induction of RF and/or autoanti-idiotypic antibodies, via the idiotypic network (either of the IgG or IgM isotype). The absence of antigen-related proteins at sites of immune complex deposition could afford the possibility that, once the nominal antigen is long lost from the circulation, only RFs and/or the autoanti-idiotypic reaction between the cryoprecipitable Igs remain operative in tissue deposition of circulating immune complexes. The possible involvement of idiotype–anti-idiotype interaction in the generation of these cryoglobulins was challenged by Stone *et al.* (1988), who using rabbit antibodies to human pepsin agglutinator site, which recognizes epitopes on $F(ab)_2$ exposed by pepsin digestion, were unable to detect idiotype interaction between cryoprecipitable IgM and the $F(ab)_2$ fragment of IgGs from 10 MC patients. On the other hand, after the discovery of the association between HCV infection and MC, one cannot exclude that all these complex interactions are targeted to eliminate HCV viruses throughout the immune precipitation and the cellular phagocytosis. Therefore, the physicochemical characteristics of MC macromolecular aggregates are different from those identified in experimental glomerulonephritides in which the deposition of circulating immune complexes is regulated by solubility, antigen excess, and low-affinity and -avidity between antigen and antibodies.

Microheterogeneity of cryoglobulins

The classification of cryoglobulins into three types on the basis of their immunochemical properties offers a good correlation with associated diseases and clinical manifestations. There are, however, unusual cryoglobulins whose immunochemical structure cannot be fitted into these classes. Mixed cryoglobulins formed by oligoclonal IgM and traces of polyclonal IgG have been described (Musset *et al.* 1992). This IgM heterogeneity might provide indirect evidence of a possible transition from type III to type II. The transformation from polyclonal (type III) to oligoclonal (type III–II) and finally to monoclonal RF (type II) may somehow be induced by the duration of B-cell stimulation caused by infectious or other exogenous agents.

HCV, MC, and lymphoproliferative malignancy

The quasispecies nature of HCV allows it to escape the immune surveillance and favours the persistence of infection in the host, mainly in lymphoid cells. Evidence for a correlation between chronic HCV infection, cryoglobulinaemia, and non-Hodgkin's lymphoma is based on clinical and epidemiological observations and on several biological considerations: (a) mono- or polyclonal B-lymphocyte expansion is present in MC and is responsible for cryoglobulin production (Perl *et al.* 1989; Shorki *et al.* 1991); (b) in about 5–8 per cent of cases, MC may evolve into a B-cell malignancy (Gorevic and Frangione 1991); (c) reduction or disappearance of signs of lymphoproliferation after eradication of the HCV (Mazzaro *et al.* 1996); (d) an increased prevalence of B-cell lymphoma in hepatopathic patients (Satoh *et al.* 1997; De Vita *et al.* 1998); (e) the frequent observation of monoclonal gammopathies in HCV positive patients with liver diseases (Andreone *et al.* 1998); (f) the presence of genome sequences and viral proteins in the neoplastic and reactive lymphadenopathies of patients with chronic HCV infection (Sansonno *et al.* 1996). In HCV patients, lymphoproliferation and its evolution from a benign disorder such as MC to a malignant neoplasia such as lymphoma is probably a multifactorial and multistep process in which infectious agents and genetic environmental factors may be involved.

Clinical features of HCV-related mixed cryoglobulinaemia

The first clinical manifestations of type II MC usually appear in the fourth to fifth decades of life. Women outnumber men, its incidence varies in different geographical areas, the majority of cases reported being from Mediterranean countries, Italy, Spain, France, and Israel. After the initial description of symptoms associated with cryoglobulinaemia, purpura, arthralgias, and weakness, it became apparent that its clinical picture is very heterogenous and protean (Table 1). Purpura is the main clinical sign of MC. The frequency of the other systemic symptoms is extremely variable and most of them play only a minor part in the clinical characterization of MC because their relevance in the clinical picture of MC is limited only to a few occasional cases. Thus, only purpura, liver, and renal disease will be described in detail.

Purpura

The most frequent manifestations of MC are recurrent purpuric episodes accompanied by torpid leg ulcers (Fig. 3). Lesions primarily appear on the lower limbs, less frequently on the buttocks and trunk, and very rarely on the face. Purpura varies greatly in frequency, is not triggered by a particular cause, and is usually preceded by paresthaesias or local pricking sensations. Ulcers appear above the malleoli spontaneously regressing and leaving discoloured skin patches formed by haemosiderin deposits. Purpuric eruptions, in a few patients, however, are never seen even after a longer follow-up. A leucocytoclastic small-vessel vasculitis is the usual finding at skin biopsy. Sometimes, an urticaria-like rash characterizes skin lesions as an eruption of transient erythematosus, oedematous swelling of the dermis, or subcutaneous tissues mostly due to venulitis. More rarely, skin lesions present as deep necrotizing cutaneous vasculitis (Fig. 4) or as severe digital gangrene that requires digital amputation.

Liver disease

Although hepatomegaly and splenomegaly are frequent findings on physical examination of MC patients, abnormal liver function tests are found in a small number of patients. Levo *et al.* (1977) reported clinical or biochemical evidence of liver dysfunction in 84 per cent. In spite of persistently abnormal biochemical test findings, hepatomegaly, and pathologic chronic changes in the liver, only two had clinically overt liver disease at the time of diagnosis, and only two others developed clinically significant liver disease during the course of their illness. Liver failure was the cause of death in only one patient. Other reports found a relatively low incidence of liver disease (about 25 per cent) and of death from liver failure in these patients (Tarantino 1981; Cordonnier *et al.* 1987; Frankel *et al.* 1992). These conflicting results are antecedent to the discovery of HCV and its striking association with MC. Recently, it has been reported that HCV-positive patients

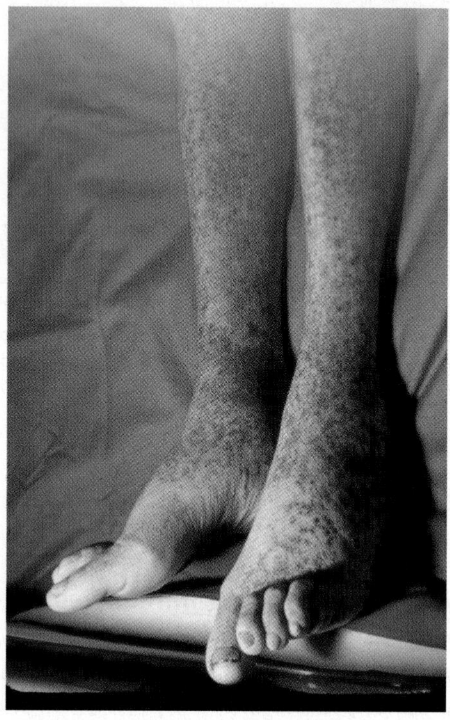

Fig. 3 Purpuric eruptions involving lower legs. Skin brownish pigmentation resulting from chronic haemosiderin deposits.

Table 1 Frequency of clinical manifestations in 'mixed cryoglobulinaemias'

	Gorevic et al. (1980)	**Monti et al. (1995)**	**Tarantino et al. (1995)**	**Dammacco et al. (2001)**
Patients	40	654	105	>200
Signs and/or symptoms (%)				
Purpura	100	80.7	94	90
Hepatomegaly	70	—	91	70
Arthralgia	72.5	10.1[a]	81	60
Asthenia	—	—	—	60
Splenomegaly	52.5	—	57	50
Raynaud's phenomenon	25	21.3	—	40
Polyneuropathy	—	22.2	38	36
Leg ulcers	39	—	—	35
Abdominal pain	20	—	27	1
Liver disease	70	44	—	~66
Renal disease	55	22	100	~25

[a] Evaluated at the time of diagnosis.

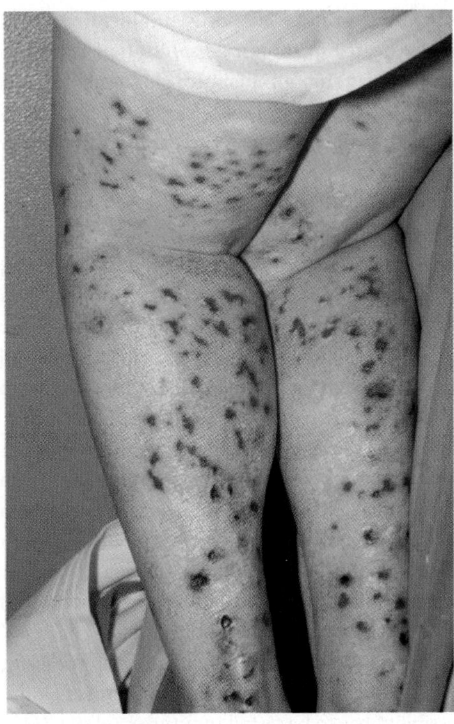

Fig. 4 Widespread necrotizing skin lesions involving lower legs.

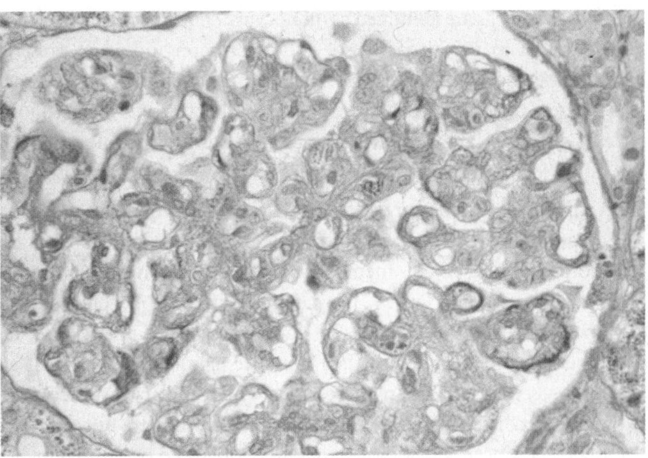

Fig. 5 Diffuse mesangial enlargement with moderate increase of cellularity, the capillary walls are diffusely thickened and show in some loops a 'double contour' appearance, in some others, protein deposits in subendothelial location are present (AFOG 400×).

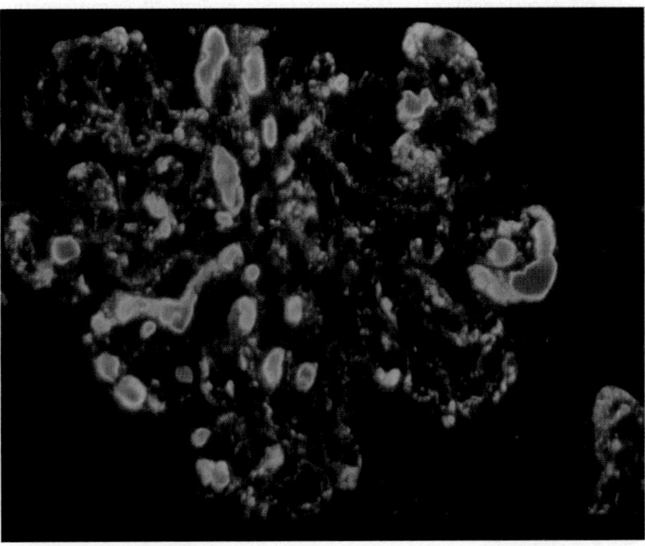

Fig. 6 On immunofluorescence, fine and coarse granular deposits of IgM are present in mesangial and parietal distribution with intracapillary pseudo-thrombi (IgM antiserum 250×).

with active infection have expansion of CD5+ B lymphocytes, which is associated with the production of RFs and protection against development of progressive liver disease (Curry *et al.* 2000).

Renal disease

The incidence of renal disease in MC varies from 8 to 58 per cent of patients. Generally, systemic symptoms antedate renal involvement, but renal and extrarenal manifestations appear concomitantly in some patients. In very few patients, the renal disease can be the first and unique presenting manifestation which makes diagnosis of MC possible. More than a half have proteinuria and/or haematuria only. A nephrotic syndrome is diagnosed in about 20 per cent of cases and an acute nephritic syndrome, defined by haematuria, proteinuria, hypertension, and a sudden rise in serum creatinine, develops in a similar proportion. Often both nephritic and nephrotic syndromes are simultaneously present. In 10 per cent of patients, acute oliguric renal failure is the first indicator of renal disease. Arterial hypertension is a frequent symptom, affecting more than 50 per cent of patients at the time of diagnosis. This complication is often severe and requires vigorous therapy. In some patients, a malignant hypertension is associated with rapidly progressive nephritis, while in others refractory hypertension is independent of the severity of kidney disease.

Morphological features of MC nephritis

Glomerular histological changes are seen only in patients with clinical or laboratory evidence of renal disease. Apart from a few cases in which glomerular lesions are characterized by the thickening of the glomerular basement membranes without cell proliferation, all biopsy specimens of kidneys from patients with MC nephritis show various degrees of endocapillary proliferation. In two-thirds of cases, the proliferative changes together with the thickening of glomerular basement membrane or its reduplication assume the picture of membranoproliferative glomerulonephritis (Fig. 5). Extracapillary proliferation with focal and segmental distribution is less frequent. On immunofluorescence, deposition of immunoglobulins and complement component are invariably present. More diffuse and intense is the fixation of anti-IgM serum along the capillary loops (Fig. 6), whereas C3 and early complement components deposits are less frequently observed and generally with low intensity.

Tubular and interstitial compartments show non-specific changes. A periglomerular or perivascular mononuclear cell infiltrate may be present. These cells are identified as monocytes, dendritic cells, or T lymphocytes. A scarring of renal tissue is not common and when present can be observed in patients with long-lasting renal involvement and some degree of chronic renal insufficiency. Some features make it possible to distinguish this glomerulonephritis from idiopathic or other secondary forms of type I membranoproliferative glomerulonephritis:

1. Under light microscopy, the most striking finding is the presence of numerous, 'hyaline thrombi' lying on the endothelial side of glomerular basement membrane and/or occluding the lumina of capillary loops (Fig. 7). They are present in 72 per cent of cases and their extent is variable. In some cases they are very rare, in others abundant. Usually, their presence parallels the acute onset of the renal disease. In these cases, endocapillary proliferation may be reduced or even absent. Hyaline thrombi are not amyloid deposits, since they do not stain with Congo red or thioflavine T. Electron microscopy has revealed the exact characteristics of these deposits. In addition to classical immune complex-like deposits, one can observe a peculiar fibrillar or crystalloid material, which in a cross-sectional view appears to be made up of tubular units, while longitudinal sections reveal parallel fibrils (Fig. 8). Deposits with such a structure may be seen in subendothelial, mesangial and occasionally in extramembranous regions. It is noteworthy that the serum cryoprecipitate is structurally similar to the deposits in the glomeruli and that the structure of deposits varies according to the relative amounts of IgG and IgM as well as to the heavy-chain classes present in both cryoprecipitate and glomerular deposits (Cordonnier *et al.* 1975; Feiner and Gallo 1977). On cross-section these deposits appear as annular bodies, having a light centre, a dense ring and a lighter peripheral coat. The total diameter measures 62–63 nm, thus making it possible to distinguish cryoglobulins from other fibrillary structures such as in amyloidosis 10 nm, fibrillary glomerulonephritis 20 nm, and immunotactoid glomerulopathy 30 nm (Iskandar *et al.* 1992).
2. Leucocytes and especially monocytes massively infiltrate glomerular structures. Four times more cells per glomerulus can be counted in this disease than in severe diffuse proliferative lupus nephritis, whereas the degree of monocyte infiltration is almost inexistent in idiopathic membranoproliferative glomerulonephritis (Ferrario *et al.* 1985; Mazzucco *et al.* 1986). Moreover, markers of monocyte activation and proliferation (27E10) are mostly negative in sharp contrast with the findings observed in monocytes infiltrating glomerular structure in ANCA-positive renal vasculitis (Rastaldi *et al.* 2000). These results can be interpreted as proof that monocytes, in MC nephritis, are involved in the deposit degradation as suggested by the close contact of monocytes to immune deposits and by the presence of protein droplets of different osmophilia in the cytoplasm of monocytes. These intracellular protein droplets do not show a crystalloid structure, indicating that the cryoglobulin lose their structure during phagocytosis (Mihatsch and Banfi 1986). Alternatively, monocyte/macrophage infiltration of glomerular capillary loops has been mainly observed in glomerular injury secondary to infectious agents as in acute post-streptococcal glomerulonephritis and in membranoproliferative glomerulonephritis associated with ventriculoatrial shunt infection. These observations could support the hypothesis that monocyte might assure the supply of viral or bacterial antigens throughout their function as antigen presenting cells, thus enhancing the *in situ* formation of immune complexes at glomerular level. This possibility has to be tested in future studies.
3. Vascular lesions characterized by fibrinoid necrosis of vessel walls and infiltration by inflammatory cells affecting small- and medium-sized arteries is found in 5–30 per cent of biopsy specimens (Fig. 9). They can also be found in the absence of obvious glomerular damage. IgG and IgM deposits may be localized in vessel walls without evidence of crystalloid structure.

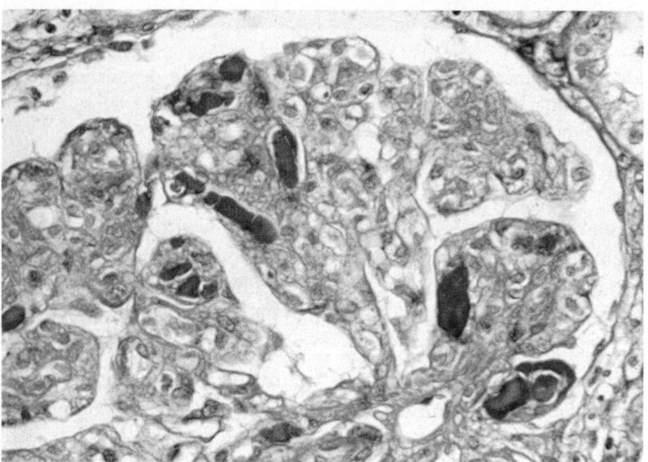

Fig. 7 Numerous capillary loops contain intraluminal proteinaceous pseudo-thrombi; in one of them (upper left) concomitant large subendothelial deposits are present (AFOG 400×).

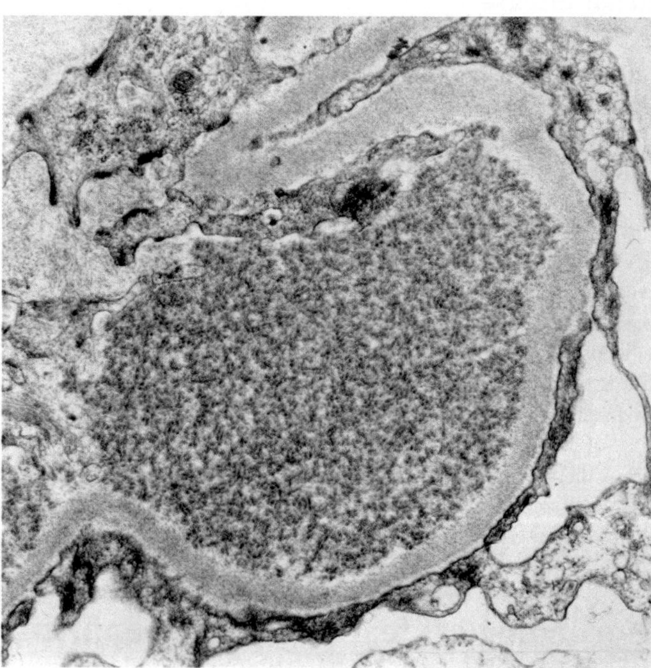

Fig. 8 Electron microscopy shows a massive electron-dense deposit with crystalloid structure occluding a glomerular capillary lumen (EM 7081×).

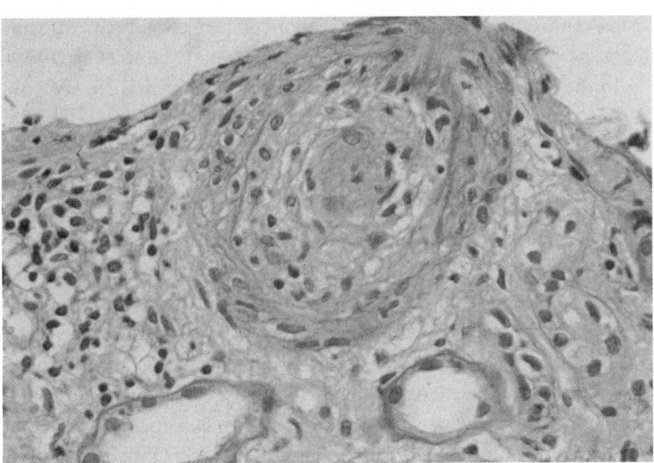

Fig. 9 A medium-sized arteriole shows proliferative endoarteritis occluding the lumen (PAS 480×).

Clinical course and prognosis

Patients with only systemic signs of MC may have an indolent outcome for years, with alternating periods of exacerbations and periods of spontaneous quiescence. As already mentioned, only rarely in individual patients does one of these manifestations become severe enough to cause a life-threatening complication. Renal damage has been considered as the consequence of long-lasting injury caused by cryoprecipitating immune complexes or in early severe kidney impairment as a feature of the most aggressive forms of MC. In both cases the prognosis of MC patients is worsened by renal disease. In a series of Gorevic *et al.* (1980), 14 out of 20 patients with renal disease died compared to four out of 13 without renal involvement after an average follow-up of 7.4 years. Invernizzi *et al.* (1983) followed up 35 MC patients for 8–17 years, 15 of them developed a glomerulonephritis that led to endstage renal failure in 13, four developed liver cirrhosis, three Waldenström macroglobulinaemia, non-Hodgkin-lymphoma or chronic lymphoid leukaemia, 12 had only arthralgias and purpura. In another series of 18 type II MC with nephropathy, three had been lost for follow-up, 10 died, four of acute respiratory failure or of unexplained myocardiopathy, two patients died at home between dialysis sessions. Of the remaining five, one had to be submitted to regular dialysis. The interval between diagnosis and death was more than 10 years in two cases, 2–4 years in four patients, and less than 1 year in the other four cases (Cordonnier *et al.* 1987).

Reviewing the literature of 11 patients with nephritic syndrome and renal function impairment who received supportive treatment alone, four died or showed progressive renal failure, in two patients, renal insufficiency remained stable while spontaneous improvement occured in the other five patients. This retrospective experience demonstrates that a spontaneous remission of renal manifestations may occur and that the role of immunosuppression in influencing the outcome of acute nephritic episodes is questionable (Ponticelli *et al.* 1986). In the large series of MC patients, all with nephritis, studied in Milan, the outcome of membranoproliferative glomerulonephritis was variable; 30 per cent had persistent but mild abnormalities of renal function, 50 per cent had a relapsing/remitting but generally benign course, whereas 15 of 105 patients required regular dialysis after a mean follow-up of 131 months. However, 42 patients died of extrarenal complications: cardiovascular disease in 12 patients, infections in nine, liver failure in eight, and haematological malignancies in four. The 10-year probability of survival without dialysis was 49 per cent. Significant clinical and/or laboratory covariates associated with patient's death or dialysis were age more than 50 years, recurrent purpura, splenomegaly, cryocrit level more than 10 per cent, C3 plasma levels less than 54 mg/dl, and plasma creatinine not less than 1.5 mg/dl at the time of kidney biopsy. There was a trend towards a worse prognosis in severely hypertensive patients although it did not reach statistical significance (Tarantino *et al.* 1995). These results show that MC patients had a bad prognosis. Even if the number of patients who developed chronic renal failure is relatively small, indicating that nephritis '*per se*' has not an ominous prognosis, death is mainly related to cardiovascular disease. It is likely that hypertension and generalized vasculitis contributed to the high death rate in these patients. Indeed, widespread vasculitis, involving small- and medium-sized vessels in the heart, gastrointestinal tract, nervous system, muscles, skin, lung and adrenals, in various combinations, is usually found in postmortem autopsies.

Laboratory findings

The concentration of circulating cryoglobulins expressed as a percentage of a given volume of serum or as protein concentration (mg/ml) has a large interpatient and intrapatient variability (from 1 to 70 per cent). There is, however, no correlation between the amount of cryoglobulins and systemic or renal symptoms. However, high cryoglobulin concentration correlated with a bad prognosis at least in patients with overt renal disease (Tarantino *et al.* 1986).

The serum complement profile is highly suggestive of MC with early component (C1q, C4, C2) markedly depressed and C3 slightly reduced, while late component (C5–C9) tend to be greater than in normal controls. This complement pattern changes little with disease activity, since early components are persistently low even in the period of quiescence. This prevalent consumption of the early complement components, with sparing of C3, has been attributed to a regulatory mechanism of the classical pathway C3 convertase mediated by two normal serum protein: the C4 binding protein and the C3b inactivator (Haydey *et al.* 1980). Supportive evidence for such a mechanism derives from the observation that complement anaphylatoxin C5a was not detectable in plasma from 21 patients with MC (Miadonna *et al.* 1985).

Therapy

A few years ago, we reviewed the available therapy and compared the results of supportive therapy with that of prolonged treatment with oral corticosteroids given alone or in association with cytotoxic drugs (Ponticelli *et al.* 1986). The risk of renal failure, the probability of reversal of renal function and the probability of maintaining a plasma creatinine were similar between the two groups (36 versus 37 per cent; 45 versus 48 per cent; 18 versus 15 per cent, respectively). Based on the above results, prolonged immunosuppression does not appear to be justified in patients with MC. Moreover, both systemic and renal manifestations of MC are characterized by an alternance of quiescence and exacerbations. Spontaneous remission of acute exacerbations are not uncommon. Thus, it is useful to consider separately the therapy of acute flares from maintenance or chronic treatment.

Therapy of acute flares

Acute nephritic and/or severe vasculitic flare-ups may be treated with high dose intravenous steroid pulses followed by a short-term course of oral prednisone and cytotoxic drugs. Among 27 episodes of renal exacerbations treated with this immunosuppressive regimen, plasma creatinine tended to decrease within one week in 86 per cent of cases, while proteinuria and cryocrit levels decreased more slowly. Although the observation is not controlled and it cannot be excluded that some patients improved spontaneously, the fact that in most patients plasma creatinine improved within 1 week seems to be a strong argument in favour of the effectiveness of this treatment. In addition, extrarenal manifestations (fever, arthralgias, abdominal pain, and leg ulcers) promptly improved after steroid administration. During acute flares, life-threatening refractory symptoms may be considered as an indication for plasmapheresis or cryofiltration apheresis. In combination with steroids and cytotoxic agents, these procedures were successful in reversing severe symptoms including demyelinating neuropathy (Kiyomoto *et al.* 1997; Suzuki *et al.* 2000). Long-term treatment with these agents should be avoided as it does not protect against renal and extrarenal flares, while exposing the patient to the risk of infections, hypertension, cardiovascular disease and neoplasia. Lastly, a prolonged immunosuppressive therapy may enhance viral replication and worsen clinical manifestations of MC.

The proved association between MC and HCV infection has changed the rationale for the treatment of systemic symptoms and its renal complication by the use of antiviral drugs.

Results of interferon therapy

The introduction of interferon in the management of MC dates from prior to the demonstration of its close relationship with HCV. In 1987, Bonomo *et al.* obtained a therapeutic response in 77 per cent of patients treated with 3 million U/day of interferon for 3 months (Bonomo *et al.* 1987). In five prospective randomized trials, the success rate of interferon was evaluated by disappearance of HCV-RNA, improvement in cutaneous vasculitis, and reduction in the amount of cryocrit, plasma creatinine, and RF titre.

The virological and clinical response rate was similar in these studies, between 42 and 73 per cent of cases. However, the long-term response was disappointingly low (0–22 per cent) in all studies indicating that relapse is very common after treatment withdrawal (Casato *et al.* 1991; Ferri *et al.* 1993; Dammacco *et al.* 1994; Misiani *et al.* 1994; Adinolfi *et al.* 1997).

Combination therapy with interferon and ribavirin

Ribavirin may inhibit viral replication through an imbalance between proinflammatory (Th 1-like) and anti-inflammatory (Th 2-like) cytokines rather than eradicating the virus or by anti-inflammatory properties. In patients with HCV and chronic hepatitis, when ribavirin is added to natural or pegilated interferon (which can only be administered once weekly) the sustained virological response is 54 versus 47 per cent in patients given interferon alone. Among patients with HCV genotype 1, the corresponding sustained virological responses are 42 and 33 per cent respectively, whereas it is about 80 per cent for patients with genotypes 2 and 3 irrespective of treatment group (Manns *et al.* 2001).

To the best of my knowledge at the time of writing there are only 11 MC patients being treated with combined antiviral therapy (Zuckerman *et al.* 2000; Garini *et al.* 2001). Five out of 11 have renal involvement (two renal insufficiency, two nephrotic syndrome). Response to combination therapy is reported in Table 2.

In summary, the benefit of interferon, administered as a single therapy is transient and is confined to only a few patients with mild and/or quiescent renal disease. It remains unproven whether interferon has a favourable effect on patients with flares of renal activity or with stabilized renal insufficiency. Of note, interferon may even be contraindicated in patients with active disease, as its immunostimulating effect might worsen renal disease and vasculitic lesions (Bojic *et al.* 1994; Roitthinger *et al.* 1995; Cid *et al.* 1999; Ohta *et al.* 1999). Lastly, interferon therapy is poorly tolerated by many patients. In addition to flu-like syndrome, psychic depression and ischaemic heart disease are possible severe complications of interferon therapy.

Combined therapy (peginterferon and ribavirin) seems to be the best option for HCV-positive MC patients, but its efficacy should be evaluated by a prospective, randomized, controlled trial. Patients should be stratified for the presence or absence of renal disease and for HCV genotype. In acute severe flares of renal or systemic signs, MP pulses followed by oral, low-dose corticosteroids, cyclophosphamide with or without plasmapheresis remain the best therapeutic approach.

Clinical aspects of cryoglobulinaemia during renal replacement therapy or organ transplantation

There are only a few reports concerning the outcome of patients with MC treated with chronic dialysis or organ allotransplantation. Tarantino *et al.* (1994) described 17 of 133 patients with MC nephritis who had to be submitted to regular dialysis because of endstage renal disease. The life expectancy for MC patients was similar to that of patients dialysed because of other primary diseases. The 5-year survival rate reached 85 per cent when four patients who died soon after starting dialysis because of devastating vasculitis were excluded. It can be concluded that patients who were submitted to dialysis with very active disease have a bad prognosis because of complications caused by MC and/or side-effects of an aggressive immunosuppresive therapy. The majority of patients who started dialysis after a slowly progressive renal disease showed a good survival rate and a reduction of the disease activity under dialysis. In HCV-positive patients without MC, a reduction of viral load after haemodialysis procedure has been detected. This reduction was partially attributed to the absorption of HCV by the dialysis membranes, and by the passage of HCV virions or HCV-RNA fragments into the dialysate or ultrafiltrate compartments. An alternative explanation is the release of interferon-like substances favoured by the the contact with dialysis membrane. *In vivo* and *in vitro* experiments resulted in an increase of interferon levels at the end of haemodialysis. This increase was due to the blood-membrane interactions (Fabrizi *et al.* 2000).

Seven patients with endstage renal disease due to MC nephritis were given renal allografts (Andrejak *et al.* 1978; Hiesse *et al.* 1989; Tarantino *et al.* 1994). HCV status either before or after transplantation

Table 2 Virological and clinical response to ribavirin and interferon therapy

Patient	Cryoglobulin response	Clinical response	Biochemical response (ALT)	Virological response	Duration of post-treatment follow-up (months)	Outcome during follow-up
1	CR	CR	—	No	9	Relapse of MC symptoms
2	CR	CR	NR	No	6	Relapse of MC symptoms
3	CR	CR	CR	No	8	Sustained remission of MC symptoms
4	CR	CR	CR	Yes	7	Sustained virological and clinical response
5	CR	CR	NR	No	7	Sustained remission of MC symptoms
6	PR	PR	NR	No	6	Relapse of MC symtoms
7	CR	CR	CR	Yes	6	Sustained virological and clinical response
8	PR	PR	NR	No	7	Relapse of MC symptoms
9	CR	CR	NR	No	6	Sustained improvement in MC symptoms
10	CR	CR	—	Yes	12	Sustained virological and clinical response
11	PR	PR	CR	Yes	12	Sustained improvement in MC symptoms

CR, complete remission; NR, no response; PR, partial response; MC, mixed cryoglobulinaemia.

is not reported. Five of them had an early recurrence after transplantation. There was a short observation period so that it is difficult to assess whether the recurrence of MC nephritis may interfere with the evolution of the transplanted kidney. In some patients the recurrence of MC nephritis does not preclude a favourable course even in the long term.

Some authors have observed that HCV infection predisposes patients to acute glomerular lesions in the allograft. Cosio *et al.* (1996) reported a high incidence (around 50 per cent) of acute transplant glomerulopathy in HCV-positive transplant recipients. In addition, *de novo* glomerular diseases with or without MC are the most consistent renal lesions associated with HCV chronic infection in renal allograft (Roth *et al.* 1995; Cruzado *et al.* 1996; Morales *et al.* 1997; Cruzado *et al.* 2001). HCV infection is the most common reason for liver transplantation in the majority of transplant units throughout the world. Both circulating cryoglobulins and glomerular lesions were detected either before or after liver transplantation (Gournay *et al.* 1996; Cantarell *et al.* 1999).

Acknowledgements

The author wishes to thank Mr Andrea Centa for his technical assistance. I also thank Dr G. Banfi (Ospedale Maggiore-IRCCS, Divisione di Nefrologia e Dialisi, Milano, Italy) and M.J. Mihatsch (Kantonsspital Basel, Universitätskliniken, Institut für Pathologie, Basel, Switzerland) for providing the histological and ultrastructural illustrations.

References

Adinolfi, L. E. *et al.* (1997). Effects of long-term course of alpha interferon in patients with chronic hepatitis C associated to mixed cryoglobulinemia. *European Journal of Gastroenterology and Hepatology* **11**, 1067–1072.

Agnello, V. (1997). The etiology and pathophysiology of mixed cryoglobulinemia secondary to hepatitis C virus infection. *Springer Seminars in Immunopathology* **19**, 111–129.

Agnello, V. and Abel, G. (1997). Localization of hepatitis C virus in cutaneous vasculitis lesions in patients with type II cryoglobulinemia. *Arthritis and Rheumatism* **40**, 2007–2015.

Amoroso, A. *et al.* (1998). Are HLA class II and immunoglobulin constant region genes involved in the pathogenesis of mixed cryoglobulinemia type II after hepatitis C virus infection? *Journal of Hepatology* **29**, 36–44.

Andrejak, M. *et al.* (1978). Cryoglobulinaemia in renal transplant recipients. *Transplantation* **26**, 446–447.

Andreone, P. *et al.* (1998). Prevalence of monoclonal gammopathies in patients with hepatitis C virus infection. *Annals of Internal Medicine* **129**, 294–298.

Bojic, I., Lilic, D., Radojcic, C., and Mijuskovic, P. (1994). Deterioration of mixed cryoglobulinemia during treatment with interferon alpha-2a. *Journal of Gastroenterology* **29**, 369–371.

Bonomo, L., Casato, M., Afeltra, A., and Caccavo, D. (1987). Treatment of idiopathic mixed cryoglobulinemia with alpha interferon. *American Journal of Medicine* **83**, 726–730.

Brouet, J. P. *et al.* (1974). Biologic and clinical significance of cryoglobulins. A report of 86 cases. *American Journal of Medicine* **57**, 775–788.

Cantarell, M. C. *et al.* (1999). Outcome of hepatitis C virus-associated membranoproliferative glomerulonephritis after liver transplantation. *Transplantation* **68**, 1131–1134.

Casato, S. *et al.* (1991). Long-term results of therapy with interferon-alpha for type II essential mixed cryoglobulinemia. *Blood* **78**, 3142–3147.

Cid, C. M. *et al.* (1999). Interferon-α may exacerbate cryoglobulinemia-related ischemic manifestations. *Arthritis and Rheumatism* **42**, 1051–1055.

Cordonnier, D. *et al.* (1975). Mixed IgG-IgM cryoglobulinemia with glomerulonephritis. Immunochemical, fluorescent and ultrastructural study of kidney and *in vitro* cryoprecipitate. *American Journal of Medicine* **59**, 867–872.

Cordonnier, J. D., Renversez, J. C., Vialtel, P., and Dechelette, E. (1987). The kidney in mixed cryoglobulinemias. *Springer Seminars in Immunopathology* **9**, 395–415.

Cosio, F. G. *et al.* (1996). The high prevalence of severe early posttransplant renal allograft pathology in hepatitis C positive recipients. *Transplantation* **62**, 1054–1059.

Cruzado, M. J. *et al.* (1996). Hepatitis C virus-associated membranoproliferative glomerulonephritis in renal allografts. *Journal of the American Society of Nephrology* **7**, 2469–2475.

Cruzado, M. J., Carrera, T. S., and Grinyó, M. J. (2001). Hepatitis C virus infection and *de novo* glomerular lesions in renal allografts. *American Journal of Transplantation* **1**, 171–178.

Curry, M. P. *et al.* (2000). Expansion of peripheral blood CD5+ B cells is associated with mild disease in chronic hepatitis C virus infection. *Journal of Hepatology* **32**, 121–125.

Dammacco, F. and Sansonno, D. (1997). Mixed cryoglobulinemia as a model of systemic vasculitis. *Clinical Reviews in Allergy & Immunology* **15**, 99–119.

Dammacco, F. *et al.* (1994). Natural interferon-α versus its combination with 6-methyl-prednisolone in the therapy of type II mixed cryoglobulinemia: a long-term, randomized, controlled study. *Blood* **84**, 3336–3343.

Dammacco, F. *et al.* (2001). The cryoglobulins: an overview. *European Journal of Clinical Investigation* **31**, 628–638.

De Vita, S. *et al.* (1998). Hepatitis C virus, non-Hodgkin's lymphomas and hepatocellular carcinoma. *British Journal of Cancer* **77**, 2032–2035.

Fabrizi, F., Martin, P., Luvighi, G., and Locatelli, F. (2000). Membrane compatibility, flux and HCV infection in dialysis patients: newer evidence. *International Journal of Artificial Organs* **23**, 296–304.

Feiner, H. and Gallo, G. (1977). Ultrastructure in glomerulonephritis associated with cryoglobulinemia. *American Journal of Pathology* **88**, 145–155.

Ferrario, F. *et al.* (1985). The detection of monocytes in human glomerulonephritis. *Kidney International* **28**, 513–519.

Ferri, C. *et al.* (1993). Interferon-alpha in mixed cryoglobulinemia patients: a randomized crossover-controlled trial. *Blood* **81**, 1132–1136.

Fornasieri, A. *et al.* (1993). Glomerulonephritis induced by human IgMk–IgG cryoglobulins in mice. *Laboratory Investigation* **69**, 531–540.

Fornasieri, A. *et al.* (1996). High binding of immunoglobulin Mk rheumatoid factor from type II cryoglobulins to cellular fibronectin: a mechanism for induction of *in situ* immune complex glomerulonephritis? *American Journal of Kidney Diseases* **27**, 476–483.

Frankel, A. H. *et al.* (1992). Type II essential mixed cryoglobulinaemia: presentation, treatment and outcome in 13 patients. *Quarterly Journal of Medicine* **82**, 101–124.

Gabrielli, A. *et al.* (1994). Active hepatitis C virus infection in bone marrow and peripheral blood mononuclear cells from patients with mixed cryoglobulinemia. *Clinical and Experimental Immunology* **97**, 87–93.

Garini, G. *et al.* (2001). Interferon-α in combination with ribavirin as initial treatment for hepatitis C virus-associated cryoglobulinemic membranoproliferative glomerulonephritis. *American Journal of Kidney Diseases* **38**, E35.

Geltner, D., Franklin E. C., and Frangione B. (1980). Antidiotypic activity in the IgM fractions of mixed cryoglobulins. *Journal of Immunology* **125**, 1530–1534.

Gorevic, P. D. and Frangione, B. (1991). Mixed cryoglobulinemia cross-reactive idiotypes: implications for the relationship of MC to rheumatic and lymphoproliferative diseases. *Seminars in Hematology* **28**, 79–94.

Gorevic, P. D. *et al.* (1980). Mixed cryoglobulinemia: clinical aspects and long-term follow-up of 40 patients. *American Journal of Medicine* **69**, 287–308.

Gournay, J. *et al.* (1997). Renal disease in hepatitis C-positive liver transplant recipients. *Transplantation* **63**, 1287–1293.

Haydey, R. P., Patarroyo de Royas, M., and Gigli, I. A. (1980). A newly described control mechanism of complement activation in patients with mixed cryoglobulinemia (cryoglobulins and complement). *Journal of Investigative Dermatology* **74**, 328–333.

Henson, J. B., Gorham, J. R., and Tanaka, Y. (1967). Renal glomerular ultrastructure in mink affected by Aleutian disease. *Laboratory Investigation* **17**, 123–139.

Hiesse, C. *et al.* (1989). Recurrent essential mixed cryoglobulinemia in renal allografts. Report of two cases and review of the literature. *American Journal of Nephrology* **9**, 150–154.

Invernizzi, F. *et al.* (1983). Secondary and essential cryoglobulinemias. Frequency, nosological classification and long-term follow-up. *Acta Haematologica (Basel)* **70**, 73–82.

Iskandar, S. S., Falk, J. R., and Jennette, C. J. (1992). Clinical and pathologic features of fibrillary glomerulonephritis. *Kidney International* **42**, 1401–1407.

Kiyomoto, H. *et al.* (1997). The effect of combination therapy with interferon and cryofiltration on mesangial proliferative glomerulonephritis originating from mixed cryoglobulinemia in chronic hepatitis C virus infection. *Therapeutic Apheresis* **3**, 329–333.

Lenzi, M. *et al.* (1998). Haplotype HLA-B8-DDR confers susceptibility to hepatitis C virus-related cryoglobulinemia. *Blood* **91**, 2062–2066.

Lerner, A. B. and Watson, C. J. (1947). Studies of cryoglobulins. I. Unusual purpura associated with the presence of high concentration of cryoglobulin (cold precipitable serum globulin). *American Journal of Medical Science* **214**, 410–415.

Levo, Y. *et al.* (1977). Association between hepatitis B virus and essential mixed cryoglobulinemia type II. *New England Journal of Medicine* **297**, 946–948.

Manns, P. M. *et al.* (2001). Peginterferon alpha-2b plus ribavirin compared with interferon alpha-2b plus ribavirin for initial treatment of chronic hepatitis C: a randomized trial. *Lancet* **358**, 958–965.

Mazzaro, C. *et al.* (1996). Regression of monoclonal B-cell expansion in patients affected by mixed cryoglobulinemia responsive to α-interferon therapy. *Cancer* **77**, 2604–2613.

Mazzucco, G., Monga, G., Casanova, S., and Cagnoli, L. (1986). Cell interposition in glomerular capillary walls in cryoglobulinemic glomerulonephritis. Ultrastructural investigation of 23 cases. *Ultrastructural Pathology* **10**, 355–361.

Meltzer, M. *et al.* (1966). Cryoglobulinemia—a clinical and laboratory study. II. Cryoglobulins with rheumatoid factor activity. *American Journal of Medicine* **40**, 837–856.

Miadonna, A. *et al.* (1985). Complement anaphylatoxins in idiopathic mixed cryoglobulinemia. *International Archives of Allergy and Applied Immunology* **76**, 120–125.

Mihatsch, J. M. and Banfi, G. Ultrastructural features in glomerulonephritis in essential mixed cryoglobulinemia. In *Antiglobulins, Cryoglobulins and Glomerulonephritis* (ed. C. Ponticelli, L. Minetti, and G. D'Amico), pp. 211–218. Dordrecht: Martinus Nijhoff, 1986.

Misiani, R. *et al.* (1994). Interferon alpha-2a therapy in cryoglobulinemia associated with hepatitis C virus. *New England Journal of Medicine* **330**, 751–756.

Mondelli, M. U. *et al.* (1998). Clonality and specificity of cryoglobulins associated with HCV: pathophysiological implications. *Journal of Hepatology* **29**, 879–886.

Monti, G. *et al.* (1995). Cryoglobulinaemias: a multi-centre study of the early clinical and laboratory manifestations of primary and secondary disease. *Quarterly Journal of Medicine* **88**, 115–126.

Morales, J. M. *et al.* (1997). Membranous glomerulonephritis associated with hepatitis C virus infection in renal transplant recipients. *Transplantation* **63**, 1634–1639.

Munoz-Fernandes, S. *et al.* (1994). Evidence of hepatitis C virus antibodies in the cryoprecipitate of patients with mixed cryoglobulinemia. *Journal of Rheumatology* **21**, 229–233.

Musset, L. *et al.* (1992). Characterization of cryoglobulins by immunoblotting. *Clinical Chemistry* **38**, 798–802.

Nightingale, S. D. *et al.* (1981). Inheritance of mixed cryoglobulinemia. *American Journal of Human Genetics* **33**, 735–744.

Ohta, S. *et al.* (1999). Exacerbation of glomerulonephritis in subjects with chronic hepatitis C virus infection after interferon therapy. *American Journal of Kidney Diseases* **33**, 1040–1048.

Pan, I. C., Tsai, K. S., and Karstad, L. (1970). Glomerulonephritis in Aleutian disease of mink: histological and immunofluorescence studies. *Journal of Pathology* **101**, 119–127.

Pascual, M., Perrin, L., Giostra, E., and Schifferli, J. A. (1990). Hepatitis C virus in patients with cryoglobulinemia type II. *Journal of Infective Diseases* **169**, 569–570.

Perl, A. *et al.* (1989). Clonal B cell expansion in patients with essential mixed cryoglobulinemia. *Clinical and Experimental Immunology* **76**, 54–560.

Pileri, P. *et al.* (1998). Binding of hepatitis C virus to CD81. *Science* **282**, 938–940.

Ponticelli, C. *et al.* Treatment of renal disease in essential mixed cryoglobulinemia. In *Antiglobulins, Cryoglobulins and Glomerulonephritis* (ed. C. Ponticelli, L. Minetti, and G. D'Amico), pp. 265–271. Dordrecht: Martinus Nijhoff, 1986.

Ramos-Casals, M. *et al.* (2000). Mixed cryoglobulinemia: new concepts. *Lupus* **9**, 83–91.

Rastaldi, M. P. *et al.* (2000). Glomerular monocyte-macrophage features in ANCA-positive renal vasculitis and cryoglobulinemic nephritis. *Journal of American Society of Nephrology* **11**, 2036–2043.

Renversez J. C. *et al.* (1984). Idiotypic interactions in type II mixed cryoglobulins. *Revue Franciase de Transfusion et Immuno-Hematologie* **27**, 737–755.

Roitthinger, F. X. *et al.* (1995). A lethal course of chronic hepatitis C, glomerulonephritis, and pulmonary vasculitis unresponsive to interferon treatment. *American Journal of Gastroenterology* **90**, 1006–1008.

Roth, D. *et al.* (1995). *De novo* membranoproliferative glomerulonephritis in hepatitis C virus-infected renal allograft recipients. *Transplantation* **59**, 1676–1682.

Sansonno, D. *et al.* (1995). Localization of hepatitis C virus antigens in liver and skin tissues of chronic hepatitis C virus-infected patients with mixed cryoglobulinemia. *Hepatology* **21**, 305–312.

Sansonno, D. *et al.* (1996). Detection and distribution of hepatitis C virus-related proteins in lymph nodes of patients with type II mixed cryoglobulinemia and neoplastic or non-neoplastic lymphoproliferation. *Blood* **88**, 4638–4645.

Satoh, T. *et al.* (1997). The relationship between primary splenic malignant lymphoma and chronic liver disease associated with hepatitis C virus infection. *Cancer* **80**, 1981–1988.

Shorki, F. *et al.* (1991). Quantification of cross-reactive idiotype-positive rheumatoid factors produced in autoimmune rheumatic diseases. An indicator of clonality and B cell proliferative mechanisms. *Clinical and Experimental Immunology* **85**, 20–27.

Spertini, F. *et al.* (1989). Prevention of murine cryoglobulinemia and associated pathology by monoclonal anti-idiotypic antibody. *Journal of Immunology* **143**, 2508–2513.

Stone, G. L., Nardella, F. A., Oppliger, I. R., and Mannick, M. (1988). Absence of anti-idiotypic activity between the IgM and IgG fractions of human mixed cryoglobulins. *Journal of Immunology* **140**, 3114–3119.

Suzuki, H., Takai, T., Tsujic, H., and Nishikawa, T. (2000). Membranoproliferative glomerulonephritis and demyelinating neuropathy caused by type II cryoglobulinemia associated with HCV infection. *Internal Medicine* **39**, 397–400.

Taneda, S. *et al.* (2001). Cryoglobulinemic glomerulonephritis in thymic stromal lymphopoietin transgenic mice. *American Journal of Pathology* **159**, 2355–2369.

Tarantino, A. *et al.* (1981). Renal disease in essential mixed cryoglobulinemia. Long-term follow-up of 44 patients. *Quarterly Journal of Medicine* **197**, 1–30.

Tarantino, A. *et al.* Prognostic factors in essential mixed cryoglobulinemia nephropathy. In *Antiglobulins, Cryoglobulins and Glomerulonephritis* (ed. C. Ponticelli, L. Minetti, and G. D'Amico), pp. 219–225. Dordrecht: Martinus Nijhoff, 1986.

Tarantino, A. *et al.* (1994). Renal replacement therapy in cryoglobulinemic nephritis. *Nephrology, Dialysis, Transplantation* **9**, 1426–1430.

Tarantino, A. *et al.* (1995). Long-term predictors of survival in essential mixed cryoglobulinemic nephropathy. *Kidney International* **47**, 618–623.

Wintrobe, M. M. and Buell, M. W. (1933). Hyperproteinemia associated with multiple myeloma. With report of a case in which an extraordinary hyperproteinemia was associated with thrombosis of the retinal veins and symptoms suggesting Raynaud's disease. *Bullettin of Johns Hopkins Hospital* **52**, 156–165.

Zuckerman, E. *et al.* (2000). Treatment of refractory, symptomatic, hepatitis C virus related mixed cryoglobulinemia with ribavirin and interferon-γ. *Journal of Rheumatology* **27**, 2172–2178.

4.7 The patient with systemic lupus erythematosus

4.7.1 The pathogenesis of systemic lupus erythematosus

L.J. Mason and David A. Isenberg

Introduction

Systemic lupus erythematosus (SLE) is an autoimmune rheumatic disease. Classification of the disease is based on a set of criteria published by the American College of Rheumatology (Tan *et al.* 1982) updated by Hochberg (1997). This is a multisystem disease, exhibiting a wide diversity of clinical expression, the muscoskeletal and dermatological manifestations are most frequent but there is often involvement of kidney, heart, lungs, and central nervous system (CNS). Despite the wide ranging nature of SLE, all presentations of the disease are usually characterized by the presence of circulating autoantibodies against a multiplicity of cellular antigens. The pathogenesis of SLE is an immunological jigsaw puzzle, some pieces of which are missing or have not yet fallen into place. The initial stimulus for the disease is likely to be one or more environmental factors which interact with susceptibility genes in predisposed individuals. Once the critical threshold is breached, there is a failure of the immune system to down regulate the ensuing abnormal immune response. Key questions include what are the disease mechanisms which allow the availability of autoantigens and the breakdown of tolerance to give rise to pathogenic autoantibodies and what are the roles played by elements such as cytokines, adhesion molecules, complement, and apoptosis in this process? This chapter discusses current knowledge of the pathogenesis of SLE in general, but will focus on the pathogenic factors in the evolution of lupus nephritis.

Glomerulonephritis in SLE

Renal involvement, whilst no longer as life-threatening as it once was, remains a major cause of morbidity in patients with SLE. The World Health Organization (WHO) has divided renal lupus into six categories based upon histological analysis of kidney biopsies. The groups are broadly defined as minimal or mesangial change; mild or focal proliferative; severe or diffuse proliferative, membranous, and end-stage sclerosing nephritis. There are also two distinct manifestations of glomerulonephritis not included within the WHO score—tubulointerstitial disease and renal vascular thrombosis. The remainder of this chapter will deal in detail with the immunological pathogenesis of SLE, but since it is important to consider that these different patterns of inflammation may have varying pathogenic mechanisms (Couser 1998), we will briefly summarize them here.

Proliferative glomerulonephritis

Proliferative glomerulonephritis can be subdivided with increasing severity into mesangial, focal, or diffuse proliferative disease with crescent formation. The main pathological agents in this form of glomerulonephritis are autoantibodies and complement components. The major features of proliferative nephritis are hypercellularity and often crescent formation due to the large infiltration of mononuclear cells, which are also the primary source of cytokines and complement proteins. Tissue injury is caused by toxic oxidants released by neutrophils, which localize in the glomeruli by interaction with adhesion molecules, and by macrophages which also produce proteases and a tissue factor which facilitates fibrin deposition. The glomerular cells themselves are not innocent bystanders, with endothelial, epithelial, and mesangial cells all producing proinflammatory mediators including complement, cytokines, oxidants, and proteases.

Membranous nephritis

Membranous nephritis is characterized histologically by immunoglobulin and complement deposition in the subepithelium and the relative lack of an inflammatory cell infiltrate. The major clinical feature is a high degree of proteinuria but the mechanisms involved are not yet fully understood. In the animal model (Heymann nephritis), glomerular immune deposit formation is facilitated by binding to a cell surface glycoprotein and the C5b-9 membrane attack complex of complement mediates renal injury. In membranous nephritis in humans, the cell surface antigen has not been confirmed but there is interest in heparan sulfate and laminin.

Tubulointerstitial nephritis

The pathogenesis of tubulointerstitial disease is not yet well understood. Tubular epithelial cells undergo a series of structural and functional changes and produce mediators, which trigger interstitial inflammation, cellular crescents, and fibrosis. It appears that these events are triggered by mediators arising systemically, in the tubular lumen or from other renal cells (Harris 2001). MRL-*lpr/lpr* mice and patients with interstitial nephritis, have infiltrates of activated T cells in the interstitium, these are thought to cause direct tissue damage by release of cytokines and cytolysis (Shlomchik *et al.* 2001).

Renal thrombosis

Patients with renal vascular thrombosis normally have impaired renal function due to multiple small thrombi, but have minimal proteinuria. Intraglomerular thrombosis can occur either due to the presence of antiphospholipid antibodies or commonly in patients with focal and diffuse proliferative glomerulonephritis, it is associated with the deposition of complement and immune complexes in the absence of antiphospholipid antibodies.

Autoantibodies

Spectrum of autoantibodies

A major serological feature of SLE is the presence of circulating autoantibodies against a multiplicity of nuclear, cytoplasmic, and membrane antigens. Intriguingly, although there are at least 2000 potential intracellular targets, the autoimmune response is confined to 30–40 of these. These antibodies are predominantly targeted at intracellular nucleoprotein particles, with 98 per cent of patients having antinuclear antibodies (ANA). These include the 70 per cent (approximately) of patients who have antibodies against double-stranded DNA (dsDNA), high titres of which are virtually confined to SLE, and have been eluted from affected kidney and skin samples. Antibodies to both native/dsDNA and denatured/single-stranded (ssDNA) can be present in SLE patients, but the former are more strongly associated with the renal pathology. Although attention has focused on anti-DNA antibodies in renal disease, many other autoantibodies have been implicated in the pathogenesis of SLE, some linked to particular clinical subsets of the disease (Table 1).

Origin of autoantibodies

The origin of anti-DNA antibodies remains one of the greatest enigmas of SLE (reviewed by Kalsi *et al.* 1999). The question, whether the antibodies to dsDNA present in patients with SLE, are antigen-driven autoantibodies or derive from a pool of germline gene-encoded natural autoantibodies, is still a matter of debate. Murine models of SLE have a background of random polyclonal B cell activation. However, due to their relatively restricted nature, the autoantibodies found in human SLE patients are thought likely to arise due to an antigen-driven T helper cell-dependent response, possibly in combination with a limited and educated polyclonal activation. The anti-DNA antibody response in SLE has been shown to be heterogeneous, with anti-DNA antibodies recognizing multiple epitopes on diverse molecules (Stollar 1986). This finding together with the fact that mammalian DNA is non-immunogenic, suggest that naked DNA itself is unlikely to be the original immunogen for what we observe as anti-DNA antibodies. So what is the source of the antigen which promotes T cell help?

Bacterial DNA has been shown to be much more antigenic than mammalian DNA, which would support the idea of an antigen-driven origin for the autoantibodies, however, research exploring the role of bacteria as the inciting stimulus to dsDNA antibody production in humans is unconvincing (Gilkeson *et al.* 1993). Polyomavirus transcription factor T antigen can induce anti-DNA antibodies in mice and antibodies to dsDNA were found in patients with frequent polyomavirus reactivations (Rekvig *et al.* 1997). The possible role of viruses, such as retroviruses and Epstein–Barr virus (EBV), as causative agents is discussed later.

DNA linked to histones, as found abundantly in apoptotically released nucleosomes, is prime suspect to be the stimulating antigen (reviewed by Berden 1997). As discussed later, it is believed that defective removal of apoptosing cells in patients with lupus, may lead to the availability of autoantigens, which can drive the immune

Table 1 Autoantibodies associated with clinical subsets of SLE

Location	Antibody	Antigen/epitope	Prevalence (%)	Clinical association
Intracellular	DNA	dsDNA	40–90	Renal and cardiovascular/pulmonary disease
	Histones	H1, 2A, 2B, H3 & H4	30–80	Drug induced lupus (>95% positive)
	Sm	B/B′ & D	50–70 (Afro-Carribeans) 10–20 (Caucasians)	SLE specific (Afro-Carribeans associated with DR2 and nephritis)
	U1 RNP	68 kDa RNP	20–30	Mild disease (associated with DR4 and reduced risk of nephritis)
	Ro	60 and 52 kDa protein	25–40	Sjögren's syndrome, photosensitivity, and neonatal lupus syndrome
	La	47 kDa protein	10–15	Sjögren's syndrome and neonatal lupus syndrome
	Heatshock proteins	Hsp 90 (Hsp 70)	50 (40 mainly IgM)	Cardiovascular/pulmonary disease
	Ribosome P proteins	P0, P1, and P2	15–35	Link to lupus psychosis is controversial
Cell membrane	Cardiolipin	Phospholipids and DNA	20–40	Recurrent abortion and thrombosis
	Neuronal	Neuronal antigen	70–90 (+CNS) 10 (−CNS)	In serum and central nervous system
	Lymphocyte	HLA/CD4/CD8 markers	~74 (IgM) ~47 (IgG)	80% are cytotoxic (T cells affected more than B cells)
	Red cells and platelets	Non-Rhesus related	<10	Haemolytic anaemia and ITP, respectively
Extracellular	Complement	C1q	~56	Rising titres indicative of proliferative glomerular nephritis
	Rheumatoid factor	Fc region of IgG	~25	Usually IgM (may be linked to erosive disease)

dsDNA, double-stranded DNA; RNP, ribonucleoprotein; ITP, idiopathic thrombocytopenic purpura.

response. In mouse models of SLE, autoantibodies were found, at disease onset, which recognized conformational epitopes of nucleosome particles, before those antibodies which recognised dsDNA or histones. Recent work has revealed a dominant pathogenic autoepitope, the histone peptide $H1'_{22-42}$ was processed and presented on major histocompatibility complex (MHC) class II molecules, by antigen presenting cells (APCs) which had been fed crude chromatin (Kaliyaperumal *et al.* 2002). It has also been suggested that activated phagocytic cells can release highly reactive oxygen species, which can penetrate cell membranes and alter nuclear DNA causing it to become antigenic (Berden 1997).

Epitope spreading is a hypothetical mechanism by which autoantibodies could develop to a wide variety of specificities, as found in SLE, possibly through molecular mimicry and antibody crossreactivity. This hypothesis suggests that if a single epitope on a self protein is targeted, the immune response can spread to other epitopes on the same molecule and subsequently to epitopes on other closely related molecules. An octapeptide (PPPGMRPP), derived from SmB/B′, is potentially one of the early targets of the autoimmune response in SLE. NZW rabbits immunized with this peptide not only produced antibodies specific for the immunizing peptide but developed autoantibodies to related spliceosomal antigens, dsDNA, and exhibited clinical features, suggestive of lupus, such as proteinuria and seizures (James *et al.* 1995). However, other workers have been unable to reproduce this model of epitope spreading (Mason *et al.* 1999; Vlachoyiannopoulos *et al.* 2000). Several papers have suggested that idiopeptides derived from anti-DNA antibodies themselves trigger reciprocal T-B determinant (epitope) spreading resulting in expansion of cells producing autoantibodies. This has been extensively shown in mouse models (reviewed in Singh and Hahn 1998), but experimental evidence that this mechanism applies to human lupus is still limited. Whatever the initiating mechanism, the consensus appears to be that antibody production in SLE is antigen driven. This observation emphasizes that impaired tolerance must be the central defect in SLE and once triggered abnormal immunoregulation leads to persistence of the immune response.

Pathogenic role of autoantibodies

Autoantibodies which bind dsDNA are of paramount importance in SLE and especially in lupus nephritis. The pathogenic role of these antibodies is indicated by correlation between disease activity and levels of anti-dsDNA antibodies in many patients, elution of antibodies from kidneys of patients and the fact that these antibodies are hardly ever found in relatives of patients with SLE (reviewed Kalsi *et al.* 1999). However, it has been shown in both patients and murine models that only a subset of circulating anti-DNA antibodies deposit in the kidney and are pathogenic, indeed only 30–50 per cent of SLE patients with such antibodies develop lupus nephritis (ter Borg *et al.* 1990). It is not clear at present, which features distinguish pathogenic and non-pathogenic dsDNA antibodies. High-affinity anti-dsDNA antibodies of the IgG isotype, which have narrow crossreactivity for antigens other than naked DNA, are believed to be the major culprits in the pathogenesis of lupus nephritis. DNA binding is often enhanced by the presence of cationic amino acids, probably arising by somatic mutation, in the complementarity determining regions. Anti-DNA antibodies which can also bind nucleosomes appear to be particularly pathogenic, this polyreactivity of anti-DNA antibodies may be due to multiple variable binding sites or to shared epitopes on different antigens.

Assessing pathogenicity of anti-DNA antibodies

Murine monoclonal anti-DNA antibodies have been extensively produced and studied. Over 20 murine monoclonal anti-DNA antibodies produced from MRL-*lpr/lpr*, SNF1 or NZW lupus-prone mice were administered to normal mice, the pattern of immune deposit formation and resulting nephritis varied, presumably depending on specific properties of the individual antibodies (Vlahakos *et al.* 1992). Transgenic mice have been produced which contain genes encoding the heavy- and light-chains of a pathogenic murine IgG antibody to dsDNA, facilitating a longer term study of the role of this particular antibody (Tsao *et al.* 1992). A human anti-dsDNA IgG light chain transgenic mouse has recently been described, however, this does not appear to be associated with any significant pathology (Ravirajan *et al.* 2001).

Human anti-DNA monoclonal antibodies, especially high-affinity antibodies of the IgG isotype, have been much harder to produce than their murine counterparts, with most published work describing low-affinity IgM antibodies. However, some groups have produced high-affinity, IgG-secreting human hybridomas from patients with active lupus, including a total of 13 published IgG clones from the laboratories of Kalden and Isenberg (Winkler *et al.* 1991; Ehrenstein *et al.* 1993; Ravirajan *et al.* 1998). Interestingly, high-affinity IgG-secreting hybridomas appear to be more likely when the peripheral blood lymphocytes are derived from a patient with active renal disease. Fusion with cells from patients with inactive disease usually results in IgM anti-DNA hybridomas, this switch possibly reflects the increased proportion of IgG antibodies during active disease.

As with the murine monoclonal antibodies, not all human anti-dsDNA monoclonal antibodies bind to the kidney when implanted into SCID mice and individual antibodies exhibit different localization of binding and varying degrees of pathogenicity. Investigation of the 13 human IgG anti-DNA monoclonals from these two laboratories showed varying ability of these antibodies to also bind histones, nucleosomes, heparan sulfate, and laminin. When implanted in SCID mice, two of these clones bound to the kidney glomeruli and another two penetrated cell nuclei of the kidney and other organs (Ehrenstein *et al.* 1995). These four antibodies also resulted in proteinuria production in these mice, but only one antibody RH14, caused pathological changes resembling those in patients with lupus nephritis, as a result of deposition in the kidney (Ravirajan *et al.* 1998).

Influence of sequence and structure on the binding of anti-dsDNA antibodies

The amino acid sequences of monoclonal anti-DNA antibodies, have been determined in an attempt to identify structural features, which might confer greater pathogenic potential to particular antibodies (reviewed Kalsi *et al.* 1999). It is striking that monoclonal antibodies derived from different mouse models often use the same V_H and/or V_L genes, V_H genes of the J558 family are commonly used, the sequences of over 300 murine monoclonal anti-DNA antibodies have been reviewed (Radic and Weigert 1994).

The picture is less clear-cut for human anti-DNA antibodies, although at least 50 human monoclonal anti-DNA antibody sequences are known, most of these are polyreactive IgM antibodies, which bind DNA with low affinity. Only a few human IgG anti-DNA antibodies have been sequenced, most of these use genes of the V_H3 or V_H4 families, but the significance of this finding is uncertain since most functional human V_H genes are members of V_H1, V_H3, or V_H4 families.

As yet, there is no data to show preferential use of a particular human V_H or V_L gene family in human anti-DNA antibodies. Fetally expressed genes, V3-23, V3-30, and V6-1, are commonly used. It may be that these genes include complementarity-determining region (CDR) sequences, which lend themselves to the formation of a DNA binding site (Rahman *et al.* 1998).

Evidence suggests that somatic mutations lead to an increase in the number of positively charged amino acid residues such as arginine and lysine, in anti-DNA antibodies, especially within the CDR3 region. It has been postulated that the presence of these positively charged residues might enhance binding to the DNA molecule, which carries an array of negative charges. Accumulated replacement mutations have been described in the CDRs of monoclonal anti-DNA antibodies derived from mouse models of lupus and these monoclonal antibodies showed a high frequency of positively charged arginine residues in the CDR3 of the heavy chain (Radic and Weigert 1994). As in mouse models, positively charged residues in CDRs are a recurring feature of human monoclonal anti-DNA antibodies (Winkler *et al.* 1992; Rahman *et al.* 1998). However, charge and affinity for dsDNA may not be adequate predictors of anti-DNA antibody pathogenicity, which may be more related to their fine specificities or the precise location of the arginine/lysine residues in the CDRs (Putterman *et al.* 1996; Cabral and Alarcon-Segovia 1997).

In order to study some of the monoclonal anti-DNA antibodies and the hypotheses about their binding properties, it has been necessary to develop expression systems to produce mutated antibodies or antibody fragments. The majority of this work has been performed using mouse antibodies expressed either in heavy chain loss variants (HCLV) or bacterial systems and is reviewed in detail elsewhere (Kalsi *et al.* 1999). Overall, these experiments using HCLV and bacterial expression systems underline the importance of V_H CDR3 and arginine residues, but show that mutations in other areas of the sequence, including some framework regions, can be involved in the fine-binding specificity of anti-DNA antibodies.

One exciting use of expression systems is their potential to produce a large enough quantity of antibody to allow X-ray crystallographic analysis of human anti-DNA antibodies. This has been done for murine antibodies (reviewed Kalsi *et al.* 1999) but not as yet with human anti-DNA antibodies, and no crystal structure yet exists of a human anti-dsDNA antibody complexed with its antigen. To predict antibody–DNA interaction, sequence data can be employed in computer modelling of the three-dimensional structure of anti-DNA antibodies. The modeller can then hypothesize which amino acid groups may enhance or reduce binding to DNA. This technique has been used to model several human anti-dsDNA monoclonal antibodies, including one designated B3. Modelling of B3 revealed that the binding groove contained three arginines, one each in the CDR1 and CDR2 of the light chain and in the CDR2 of the heavy chain, which might stabilize the binding of B3 to dsDNA (Kalsi *et al.* 1996).

Kidney localization of pathogenic autoantibodies

In lupus nephritis, the pathogenic antibodies appear to deposit preferentially in the kidney. Three hypothetical mechanisms may account for this localization, the circulating immune complex hypothesis, the crossreactive antibody hypothesis, and the planted antigen hypothesis (Davis *et al.* 1996; Lefkowith and Gilkeson 1996; van Bruggen *et al.* 1996). It was originally thought that circulating immune complexes of DNA–anti-DNA antibodies became passively trapped in the glomerulus, but the presence of such complexes in human lupus sera is controversial. It has been shown that injected complexes bind poorly to glomerular basement membrane (GBM) and that such complexes would be rapidly cleared by the liver. The premise of the crossreactive antigen hypothesis is that anti-DNA antibodies are broadly reactive, binding a wide array of molecules such as GBM components. This theory is a variant on the molecular mimicry theme, but it is thought that the polyreactivity of antibodies is less likely to occur than binding to their cognate antigen. Recent evidence supports the 'planted antigen' mechanism, which suggests that circulating, non-complexed cationic anti-DNA antibodies bind to collagen type IV and the heparan sulfate glycosaminoglycan component of the GBM, via a complex of histones and DNA, in the form of nucleosomes.

Nucleosomes are chromatin complexes generated during apoptosis which contain 180–200 bp pieces of DNA around histone proteins. It has been shown *in vitro* that autoreactive T cells from lupus patients recognize nucleosomes preferentially to DNA or histones alone. The formation of nucleosome-specific antibodies may precede the development of both anti-dsDNA and antihistone antibodies. Also it has been demonstrated that antinucleosome IgG antibodies are a more sensitive diagnostic marker of SLE than anti-DNA antibodies, these antibodies, therefore, play a central role in the antinuclear response in lupus (reviewed Amoura *et al.* 2000). The possibility of other glomerular antigens as targets for anti-DNA antibody binding, notably alpha-actinin found on kidney podocyte cells, was suggested by the binding of pathogenic but not non-pathogenic murine anti-DNA monoclonal antibodies (Mostoslavsky *et al.* 2001).

There are a number of *in vivo* studies suggesting that anti-DNA, anti-U1 RNP, and antiribosomal P antibodies can penetrate living cells and potentially induce renal disease by intracellular effects, such as inducing loss of tolerance to self by modification of apoptotic events (Cabral and Alarcon-Segovia 1997). It has been proposed that a subset of anti-DNA antibodies can bind to myosin 1 on the cell surface, become internalized and cause glomerular hypercellularity and proteinuria (Yanase *et al.* 1997). Other researchers suggest that antibody penetration depends on a membrane determinant resembling DNA (Zack *et al.* 1996). Recent *in vitro* work has demonstrated monoclonal anti-dsDNA antibodies from MRL/*lpr*/*lpr* mice penetrate live renal tubular cells. Human anti-DNA monoclonal antibody B3, has been shown to penetrate glomerular cells when implanted in SCID mice (Ehrenstein *et al.* 1995). It thus appears that a subset of anti-DNA antibodies, might exert their pathogenic effect by cellular penetration and nuclear localization (reviewed by Madaio and Yanase 1998).

Cellular involvement in the evolution of systemic autoimmunity

Loss of B- and T-cell tolerance

As discussed earlier, SLE appears to result from a series of interactions in the immune system that ultimately lead to the loss of self-tolerance to nuclear autoantigens. A model has been proposed, which emphasizes that autoimmunity is initiated by a loss of peripheral rather than central tolerance (Shlomchik *et al.* 2001). The presence of self-reactive lymphocytes is a prerequisite for autoimmunity, but the hypothesis of this model is that intact central tolerance eliminates high-affinity anti-self lymphocytes but peripheral tolerance breaks down allowing expansion of lower-affinity self-reactive T and B cells. Somatic hypermutation and selection can then result in the generation of high-affinity B cells, producing the high-affinity autoantibodies seen in SLE patients, from low-affinity precursors, provided that T cell help is available.

In summary, the model proposed by both Shlomchik *et al.* (2001) and Mamula (1998) assumes initial presentation, of either foreign crossreactive antigens or cryptic self-determinants, by professional APCs [dendritic cells (DCs) or macrophages] which activates T cells. Costimulation is required for this first step, aberrations in these processes in lupus are described later. Normal T cells when exposed to self-antigen in the periphery would become tolerized but either this is circumvented by molecular mimicry or lupus T cells have a lowered threshold of T cell activation in SLE, which might allow normally cryptic self-peptides to initiate autoimmunity (reviewed Lehmann *et al.* 1998). The activated T cells provide help to autoreactive B cells, allowing expansion of these B cell clones. In the second stage, these autoreactive B cells, which have surface immunoglobulin receptors, can bind and process any available multideterminant autoantigens and present novel self-peptides to further T cells; this whole process resulting in a positive feedback cycle of activation and expansion of the autoimmune response. The resulting tissue damage provides further self-antigenic material to fuel the whole cascade. Activated T cells can also directly cause pathology by migrating to the target organ and mediating cytotoxicity and releasing cytokines.

Cellular abnormalities

SLE is characterized by multiple functional defects among cells of the immune system including T and B lymphocytes, DCs, natural killer (NK) cells, and accessory cells (APCs). Numbers of circulating lymphocytes may be altered profoundly, hyperactive B cells are increased in number with coexistent T lymphocytopenia (T cell death).

B lymphocytes

The most marked defect in SLE is the increase in numbers of activated B lymphocytes, which contributes to the hypergammaglobulinaemia associated with reactivity to self-antigens. However, secretion of autoantibody is not the only role played by B cells in SLE, as already mentioned B cells are extremely efficient APCs for antigens taken up specifically through the B cell receptor (Ig receptor). B cells thus play an important role activating T cells, as shown by experiments using a strain of autoimmune prone mice that have B cells which cannot secrete antibodies, these mice still develop interstitial nephritis, vasculitis, and glomerulonephritis (Chan *et al.* 1999). In addition, elimination of B cells in lupus prone mice results in a complete abrogation of pathology including T cell interstitial infiltration (Chan *et al.* 1999). In a preliminary study, eight patients who had failed conventional therapy, steroids, and azathioprine and/or cyclophosphamide, were given B cell depleting anti-CD20 and cyclophosphamide with encouraging clinical and serological benefit (Leandro *et al.* 2002).

Altering the expression of molecules that control B cell activation often results in lupus-like disease in gene-targeted mouse models, the elucidation of whether these molecules are altered in lupus patients is an active area of research. One particular population of B cells which has attracted interest, are the CD1 positive marginal zone B cells which are expanded at an early stage in NZB/W mice (Zeng *et al.* 2000). The CD1 family of MHC class 1-like proteins present lipid antigens to T cells. Double-negative T cells lack the CD4 and CD8 markers and are increased in lupus patients, these cells provide help for CD1c+ B cells for IgG production and are restricted by CD1c (Sieling *et al.* 2000). IgG helper activity for CD1c+ B cells was weaker or undetectable among the double-negative T cells from healthy donors. Double-negative T cell help for IgG production was mediated through CD1c, IL-4, and CD40.

T lymphocytes

The increase in B cells is accompanied by T lymphocytopenia, especially of cells bearing the CD4+/CD45R+ phenotype. This population of cells 'helps' to induce suppression by providing a signal to the CD8+ population. The reduction in this subset may contribute to the failure of the T cells to suppress the hyperactive B cells. Anti-T-cell antibodies may be responsible for the depletion of this cellular subset. CD45 autoantibodies mediate neutralization of activated T cells from lupus patients through anergy or apoptosis (Mamoune *et al.* 2000). A study has reported that the titre of anti-T cell antibodies is directly proportional to the ratio of CD4/CD8 killing and that flares of disease are associated with an increase in CD4/CD8 killing and disease remission is accompanied by a corresponding decrease in the ratio. Parallel changes in anti-T cell titres reflect the disease activity (Yamada *et al.* 1993). CD8+ cells and NK cells may behave aberrantly by providing help, rather than suppression, to B cells and hence stimulating production of autoantibodies. Increased mutations have been found in the DNA of T cells in patients with lupus, which may result in T cell death by necrosis and the release of non-degraded DNA contributing to anti-DNA antibody production.

T cells from lupus patients have been cloned *in vitro*; only 15 per cent of these T cells provided help for B cells to make pathogenic anti-DNA antibodies. Of these, the majority (83 per cent) of cells were CD4+ with the classical $\alpha\beta$ T cell receptor (TCR) and were class II restricted, the remaining 17 per cent were double-negative and not class II restricted. The presence of double-negative T cells is a feature of SLE and of murine lupus models. As double-negatives these T cells probably escape thymic deletion. Only 30 per cent of double-negative T cells have the classical $\alpha\beta$ TCR chains, 70 per cent express the alternative $\gamma\delta$ TCR. Subsequent sequencing of the TCRs has revealed Vδ and Vγ gene usage not found in normal adults but resembling that of fetal thymocytes (Rajagopalan *et al.* 1992).

The appearance of class II molecules, usually HLA-DR, on T cells is taken as a marker of activation. Peripheral T cells with increased expression of HLA-DP at the cell surface and as mRNA transcripts have been found in lupus patients. The frequency of HLA-DP expression exceeded that of HLA-DR and correlated well with disease activity. HLA-DR restricted T cells have been cloned from a lupus patient and shown to induce IgG anti-DNA antibodies *in vitro* from high-density (activated) B cells from DR-matched patients with lupus, and IgM anti-DNA antibodies from B cells from DR-matched normal individuals (Murakami *et al.* 1992).

There is very little published data linking TCR gene usage to lupus in humans or in lupus-prone mice strains. Sequencing of the TCRα and β chain genes derived from 42 CD4+ lines from five lupus patients revealed recurrent motifs of highly charged residues in their CDR3 loops. Four of the five patients displayed the Vα8 gene family (Desai-Mehta *et al.* 1995). Indiscriminate sequencing of γ and δ chains of the TCR from peripheral blood of patients with lupus showed oligoclonal expansion of $\gamma\delta$ T cells in lupus (Alarcon-Segovia and Cabral 1996). The p70 (Ku) autoantigen has been described as a non-histone nuclear protein recognized by antibodies from lupus patients. It has been shown that the p70 antigen is a DNA-binding protein and specifically binds to the TCRβ-chain gene enhancer thus playing a role in regulation of TCRβ gene expression (Messier *et al.* 1993). Antigen-specific T cells have now been cloned from patients with SLE. Nucleosome-specific T cells have attracted much interest and peptide autoepitopes in core histones of nucleosomes, are recurrently recognized by the autoimmune T cells derived from lupus patients (Lu *et al.* 1999).

Accessory cells

A number of studies have shown that SLE patients exhibit deficient APC function for allogeneic T cells, deficient APC function for the presentation of exogenous antigen, and reduced stimulation of autologous T cell proliferation in the autologous mixed lymphocyte reaction (MLR). The frequencies of DCs in peripheral blood are consistently reduced in SLE patients as compared with healthy controls (Scheinecker *et al.* 2001). This reduction results mainly from diminished proportions of CD11c+ (germinal centre or myeloid related) DCs. These observations may explain the reduction in CD4+ T cells, since mature CD4+ T cells need peripheral class II MHC expression, such as that found on DCs for survival. These DCs also exhibit reduced expression of costimulatory molecules, B7-2 and CD40, although B7-1 was not significantly different from controls.

Monocytes are the precursors of DCs, monocytes from SLE patients but not normal monocytes, are potent activators of naive T cells *in vitro*. Furthermore, when stimulated with SLE serum, normal monocytes develop DC-like morphology, phenotype and function, including the ability to engulf apoptotic cells and present the associated antigens to $CD4^+$ T cells. These results indicate that in SLE, there might be mass differentiation of monocytes into DCs. The exodus of activated DCs into tissues could account for their reduced numbers in SLE blood. Increased levels of interferon α (IFNα) are found in SLE patients and this cytokine is a potent activator of DCs. Consistent with a role for IFNα, the DC-stimulating capacity of SLE serum was found to correlate with the levels of this cytokine (Blanco *et al.* 2001).

Macrophage and NK cell cytotoxicity is impaired in patients with SLE, as is the clearance of immune complexes by the mononuclear phagocytic system. NK cells are large granular cells expressing CD16 and CD56, and constitute 15 per cent of peripheral blood mononuclear cells (PBMCs) in normal individuals. The numbers of NK cells are significantly reduced in active SLE and particularly in patients with renal involvement. A recent study confirms that non-MHC-restricted cytotoxicity, shared by NK, NK-like (T cells positive for CD3, CD16, and CD56) and γ/δ T cells may be down-regulated in SLE patients (Riccieri *et al.* 2000). In addition to the numbers of NK cells being reduced in SLE patients, those present are probably skewed towards B-cell help rather than suppression.

As mentioned, another dysfunction of the mononuclear phagocyte system in SLE, is in immune-complex clearing. This is partly attributed to abnormalities of the surface receptors for the Fc of IgG (FcγR). Many cellular abnormalities are due to genetic defects, an example being the FcγRIIA-H131 allele. The FcγRIIA receptor, on phagocytes, recognizes and aids clearance of pathogenic IgG2 antibodies/complexes and the lack of this allele is associated with lupus nephritis in blacks (Salmon *et al.* 1996). FcγRIIIA alleles with reduced affinity for IgG1 and IgG3 have also been shown to be associated with increased severity of SLE, with a significantly increased frequency of the low-affinity allele in SLE patients from diverse ethnic groups (Wu *et al.* 1997). Increased numbers of apoptotic neutrophils, and impaired monocyte/macrophage clearance of apoptotic cells have been demonstrated in SLE. CD44 is implicated in the clearance of apoptotic neutrophils and it has been shown that CD44 expression is reduced on monocytes and neutrophils in SLE, which may contribute to their impaired recognition and clearance (Cairns *et al.* 2001).

Macrophage accumulation is a prominent feature of most types of human glomerulonephritis. In particular, tubulointerstitial macrophage accumulation correlates with renal dysfunction and is predictive of disease progression. Tubular epithelial cells are a major source of chemokines and adhesion molecules which promote macrophage infiltration and activation. Depletion studies have shown that macrophages can induce glomerular injury in experimental models and inhibiting macrophage accumulation, by targeting chemokines and adhesion molecules, suppresses progressive renal injury in these models. Macrophages can release many inflammatory mediators but the precise mechanisms of renal damage are yet to be determined (reviewed by Nikolic-Paterson and Atkins 2001).

Cell signalling

It may be that patients with lupus have a primary T-cell signalling disorder, whereby T-cell dysfunction is a by-product of abnormal biochemical pathways, which result in altered regulation of effector function (reviewed by Tsokos *et al.* 2000). Whether a lymphocyte is activated, anergic, or undergoes apoptosis, depends on the summation of the signals which it receives after binding of antigen to its cell surface receptors. Signals are either delivered by cytokines or engagement of costimulatory molecules with T-cell surface receptor molecules. Such antigen-receptor signalling events are abnormal in lupus lymphocytes, manifested by increased calcium responses and hyperphosphorylation of several cytosolic protein substrates.

T cells from SLE patients showed impaired protein kinase A (PKA)-catalyzed protein phosphorylation, due to a deficiency in PKA-1 isozyme (reviewed Dayal and Kammer 1996). PKA is responsible for phosphorylation and activation of cAMP's second messenger role. Alterations in the cellular protein phosphorylation pattern may alter homeostasis and disturb the immune function of the cell. Impaired protein phosphorylation could affect gene transcription resulting in an imbalance of protein synthesis within cells, for example, altering the pattern of cytokine production. There is also a CD3-mediated increase in free intracytoplasmic calcium, which occurs specifically in T cells from patients with lupus.

This increased calcium may account for alterations in PKA function, altered apoptosis, or decreased IL-2 production. In comparison with T cells from normal individuals, those from patients with lupus show markedly abnormal 'capping' of the cell surface proteins, CD4 and CD8. This process is controlled by the cAMP pathway, and in patients with lupus there is decreased cAMP production, resulting in an inability to switch phenotype and express suppressor activity. Furthermore, potential molecular defects may involve gene methylation. Inhibition of T-cell gene methylation has been associated with autoreactivity due to overexpression of lymphocyte function associated antigen 1, leading to increased T cell homing to target tissues.

Following activation, T lymphocytes from lupus patients demonstrate increased downstream signalling, at the gene transcription level, and also have reduced TCR ζ chain, a critical signalling molecule. This may be partly explained by the increased expression of FcϵRIγ chain, that functions as an alternate ζ chain, in a large proportion of SLE T cells (Enyedy *et al.* 2001). Another defect that has been well described in T cells is the deficient synthesis of IL-2 when T cells are stimulated by mitogens, this defect also extending to NK cells. This defect may be explained by the finding that freshly isolated SLE T cells demonstrate a TCR-mediated defect in the activation of NF-κB (Wong *et al.* 1999). This is mediated by decreased p65-Rel A protein, which is responsible for the inducible NF-κB activity.

Costimulation

Activation of antigen-specific T cells requires at least two distinct signals. The first is antigen-specific via the TCR–CD3 complex and the second is a costimulatory signal. The most prominent costimulatory pathway involves the B7 family of molecules, B7-1(CD80) and B7-2(CD86), expressed on the APC and CD28 on mature T cells. The expression of CTLA-4 (CD152), also found on T cells, is dependent on CD28/B7 engagement. CTLA-4 negatively regulates T cell function, subsequently providing self-regulation of the immune response and is involved in the maintenance of tolerance. The complexities of these pathways in autoimmunity have recently been reviewed (Salomon and Bluestone 2001).

The role of CD28/B7 costimulation has been analysed in the murine lupus models. Treatment with CTLA-4Ig, to block the CD28/B7 interaction, prevented disease in the NZB/NZW F1 model, as did a combination of antibodies against both B7-1 and B7-2. MRL-*lpr/lpr* mice that were injected with both anti-B7-1 and anti-B7-2 expressed significantly lower anti-snRNP and anti-dsDNA autoantibodies than untreated mice. Interestingly, anti-B7-2 alone only inhibited anti-dsDNA expression, not anti-snRNP and treatment with anti-B7-1 alone did not change the levels of either antibody. MRL-*lpr/lpr* mice deficient in B7-1 exhibited a more severe glomerulonephritis whilst B7-2 deficient MRL-*lpr/lpr* mice had mild or absent kidney pathology compared to wild-type mice (Liang *et al.* 1999). These findings underline the importance of both costimulation pathways, although indicating that CD28/B7-2 may play the major role in murine lupus. It also seems apparent from these experiments that in the absence of either B7 molecule an alternative or compensatory pathway exists.

The production of pathogenic antibodies also requires cognate interaction between CD40 ligand (CD40L or CD154) on T cells and CD40 on B cells. Recent data from SLE patients and murine lupus models have demonstrated prolonged expression of CD40L on lupus T cells and its capacity to mediate excessive B cell activation (reviewed by Crow and Kirou 2001).

A study of the expression of costimulatory molecules on the peripheral blood lymphocytes of SLE patients, during active and inactive disease, has recently been reported (Bijl *et al.* 2001). Almost all CD4+ cells expressed CD28 both in patients and controls. B7-1 expression on CD19+ B cells was low in both patients and controls and did not correlate with disease activity. In contrast, the percentage of CD19+ B cells expressing B7-2 was increased in patients with SLE, even when disease was inactive. However, the highest expression of B7-2 was in active disease and levels correlated with the SLEDAI score of disease activity and with levels of anti-dsDNA antibodies. No changes were found in the levels of CD40 or CD40L. Defective responses to recall antigens have been recognized for lupus immune cells and the upregulation of B7-1 on lupus APCs has been found to be defective.

Cell adhesion molecules

Adhesion molecules are classified into selectin, integrin, and immunoglobulin supergene family groups. Leucocyte adhesion is regulated by changes in adhesion molecule expression and avidity, dependent on the extent of cellular activation. During the inflammatory or autoimmune response, adhesion molecules mediate the interactions between lymphocytes and vascular endothelial cells during extravasation and homing as well as allowing local retention of cells in the extracellular matrix. Adhesion molecules also play an important role in the interaction between APCs and T cells, ensuring effective T cell help or cytotoxic T cell function. In SLE E-selectin, lymphocyte function-associated antigen-1 (LFA-1)/intercellular adhesion molecule-1 (ICAM-1) and very late antigen-4 (VLA-4)/vascular cell adhesion molecule-1 (VCAM-1) appear to provide the predominant adhesive interactions at inflammatory sites (reviewed by McMurray 1996).

Skin biopsies from lupus patients show upregulation of surface expression of E-selectin, VCAM-1, and ICAM-1 on dermal vessel endothelial cells. Levels of adhesion molecules directly correlated with disease activity and in several cases decreased with clinical improvement. Patients with active lupus have also been shown to have elevated levels of the soluble adhesion molecules, soluble E-selectin, sICAM-1 and sVCAM-1 in their sera, as compared with normal controls, levels of which in some studies correlated with disease activity. A recent study showed that the levels of soluble markers CD14, ICAM-1, and E-selectin were elevated in active lupus and that the levels of these soluble adhesion molecules in lupus were similar to patients with sepsis (Egerer *et al.* 2000).

Increased glomerular expression of ICAM-1, and also VLA-3, has been found in patients with SLE who had rapidly progressive glomerulonephritis. These patients also express elevated levels of E-selectin on glomerular and tubular epithelium, and VCAM-1 is upregulated on the endothelium of interstitial vessels. Peripheral blood lymphocytes from patients with SLE show increased expression of LFA-1 as compared to controls and LFA-1 and VLA-4 are increased in SLE patients with vasculitis. ICAM-1 expression has been shown to be increased by ultraviolet (UV) irradiation of keratinocytes *in vitro*, modulated by cytokine release which *in vivo* could culminate in photosensitive lupus. Agents such as procainamide or hydralazine which can cause drug-induced lupus, have been shown *in vitro*, to induce LFA-1 overexpression and subsequent autoreactivity due to their ability to inhibit T cell DNA methylation.

These findings fit with observations in murine lupus, where upregulation of both ICAM-1 and VCAM-1 have been found in nephritic kidneys from MRL-*lpr/lpr* mice. Kidney sections from these mice show increased adhesion of T cell and macrophage cell lines. *In vitro* studies have shown that IL-1, TNFα, and IFNγ stimulate upregulation of adhesion molecule expression on glomerular mesangial cells. The expression of ICAM-1 and VCAM-1 have been shown to be induced by TNFα and IL-1 in MRL-*lpr/lpr* mice (McHale *et al.* 1999). T-cell clones derived from kidney-infiltrating lymphocytes of MRL-*lpr/lpr* mice induced ICAM-1 expression *in vitro*, which was blocked by an anti-IFNγ monoclonal antibody. Mrl/mpj-fas(lpr), a lupus mouse strain that is deficient in ICAM-1, have reduced tissue inflammation and prolonged survival (Bullard *et al.* 1997). The effect of anti-adhesion molecule therapy in patients with SLE is not yet known. Targeting lymphocyte adhesion molecules or their ligands is likely to be used to induce tolerance in patients.

Cytokines

The aberrant cellular effector mechanisms seen in SLE are closely connected to the interaction of cells with their extracellular environment, which critically involves cellular messengers, the cytokines. T-helper cells are characterized into different subsets dependent on their cytokine profile. In general, Th1 cells support cell-mediated immunity and produce proinflammatory cytokines, such as IFNγ, TNFα, and IL-12 whereas Th2 cells provide B-cell help and suppress cell-mediated immunity via cytokines including IL-4, IL-5, and IL-10.

Cytokine paradigm

Several autoimmune diseases may now be classified according to the predominance of a particular T-helper cell subset. With the caveat that a rigid distinction between Th1 and Th2 diseases is probably incorrect, one might predict, therefore, that SLE would be a predominantly Th2 cell-mediated disease, resulting in excess help for B cells, polyclonal B cell activation and production of pathogenic autoantibodies. In support of this concept, increased IL-10 has been found in lupus patients and this cytokine suppresses Th1 cells and thus impairs cell mediated immunity, a characteristic feature of SLE. In mice, continuous administration of anti-IL-10 delays the onset of disease. The shift from a predominantly Th0 population of T cells, producing both Th1 and Th2 cytokines towards a Th2 predominance, might arise as a result of altered regulation or expression of genes, due to a biochemical or signalling defect. A further subset of CD4+ T cells has recently been characterized, Th3 cells produce transforming growth factor β (TGFβ), IL-4, and IL-10. Th3 cells play a regulatory role, down regulating APCs, and are important in induction of immune tolerance. The Th1/Th2/Th3 paradigm is limited because not all cytokines are produced by T cells, in fact, IL-6 and IL-10 are mainly synthesized by monocytes.

Role of cytokines in SLE

An inflammatory reaction such as the one occurring in lupus can thus be understood in terms of an imbalance of these opposing cytokines, or their inhibitory receptors. The balance of cytokines may determine disease activity in general and the particular organ involvement. There is an increase in proinflammatory cytokines such as IL-6 in lupus nephritis. TGFβ has been implicated in preventing renal disease and decreased levels have been found in renal tissue. A recent paper suggests that differential expression of cytokines within the kidney itself, may dictate the clinical manifestation of nephritis. The intrarenal gene expression of various cytokines were measured by reverse-transcriptase-polymerase chain reaction (RT-PCR) in biopsies from 54 patients with proliferative glomerulonephritis and 42 with non-proliferative glomerulonephritis. Th1, proinflammatory cytokines were more abundant in proliferative glomerulonephritis and correlated with unfavourable disease parameters (Kim *et al.* 2001). Serum levels of cytokines are difficult to interpret as they may be affected by soluble cytokine receptors which are shed from cells, IL-1, IL-2, IL-6, TNFα, and IFNγ, all have such soluble receptors. Serum levels may not reflect the local levels of cytokines produced in the tissues where they are acting. When looking at *in vitro* cytokine production by immune cells, it is important to differentiate between spontaneous and stimulated cytokine production. It is also important to note that experiments and potential treatments which simply target a particular cytokine in isolation may not provide meaningful data since the cytokine network is so interrelated and cytokines may compensate for each other. All of these factors have led to many contradictory reports in this field. We present a simplified summary of the major findings in this area (see Dean *et al.* 2000 for a full review). A synthesis of the function of the cytokines in SLE is summarized in Table 2.

TNFα

The genes for both tumour necrosis factors, TNFα and TNFβ, are closely linked and located within the MHC. *In vitro* TNFα production by mitogen-activated peripheral blood lymphocytes varies according to the HLA Class II haplotype of the donor with some haplotypes associated with predisposition for lupus nephritis as shown in Table 2 (Jacob *et al.* 1990). It seems that genetic predisposition towards a strong TNFα response is protective against developing lupus nephritis.

TNFα and IL-6 are increased in patients with active SLE but the ratio of TNFα to its soluble receptor is significantly lower in SLE when compared to patients with rheumatoid arthritis. This suggests that there is a relative deficiency of active TNFα in patients with SLE. High levels of TNFα are frequently associated with rheumatoid arthritis and therapeutic benefit has been reported using monoclonal antibodies to TNFα. Two of 20 RA patients treated with anti-TNFα antibody developed anti-dsDNA antibodies and other serological abnormalities characteristic of lupus although neither developed clinical symptoms of SLE. All antibodies disappeared when therapy was stopped (Charles *et al.* 2000). The proinflammatory cytokines IL-6, IL-1, and TNFα, are thought to induce the release from the liver of acute phase proteins, C reactive protein (CRP), and serum amyloid P (SAP), which bind to apoptotic fragments, so promoting clearance of potential autoantigens. Data correlating levels of these cytokines with levels of CRP and circulating autoantibodies are, however, inconclusive.

IL-6

Patients with lupus nephritis have increased plasma concentrations of IL-6 and soluble IL-6 receptor (sIL-6R) as compared with normal controls. The ratio of IL-6/sIL-6R is increased in lupus nephritis, suggesting an increased effective level of IL-6 in these patients. IL-6 protein and mRNA have been found in kidney biopsies from patients with lupus nephritis, indicating local production of IL-6. High levels of IL-6 are also found in the urine of these patients. It has been suggested that IL-6 is involved in maintaining B cell hyperactivity via an autocrine route, IL-6 receptors are constitutively expressed on B cells from patients with SLE, unlike healthy controls. MRL-*lpr/lpr* mice given anti-IL-6 antibody showed a decrease in renal damage and in levels of anti-dsDNA antibodies.

IL-10

Apart from IL-6, IL-10 is another potent stimulator of B cell proliferation and differentiation (see Table 2 for summary), IL-10 increases *in vitro* IgG production by PBMCs, from patients with SLE (reviewed

Table 2 Role of cytokines in SLE

Cytokine	Clinical and experimental observations
IL-1	↓ Production in lupus patients. T cells unresponsive, possibly defective IL-1R
IL-2	Normal or ↓ production by CD4 and CD8, ↓ T cell maturation and ↓ CD8 suppressor function. Functional activity may reflect ↑ soluble IL-2R and CD4 cells have low-affinity IL-2 receptors
IL-4	↑ Secretion by antigen-primed T cells
IL-6	↑ Levels in sera and cerebral spinal fluid of lupus patients. Localized in nephritic kidneys and detectable in urine of these patients. ↑ mRNA in PBMCs from patients B cells have ↑ IL-6R and spontaneously produce IL-6 (autocrine) and ↑ Ab production
IL-10	↑ In sera of patients with SLE, suppresses Th1 cells and impairs cell mediated immunity ↑ Production by macrophages and B cells → defective B7-1 expression → ↓ APC function ↑ B cell function and ↑ production of pathogenic autoantibodies, by autocrine pathway Anti IL-10 blocks anti-DNA Ab production by PBMCs from lupus patients in SCID mice IL-10 accelerated disease and anti IL-10 delayed disease onset in the NZB/W murine model Disease severity correlates with increased ratio of IL-10:IFNγ secretion in lupus PBMCs
IL-12	↓ In patients (in most reports) especially in glomerulonephritis patients
IL-16	↑ In patients, correlates with disease activity
IL-17	↑ In patients
IL-18	↑ In patients, lymphocytes hyper-responsive to IL-18
IFNα	May activate immature dendritic cells, ↑ APC function may drive B/T cell autoimmunity
IFNγ	Normal production in patients, but macrophage and NK cell-mediated cytotoxicity impaired. Recombinant IFNγ exacerbated disease in patients and lupus prone mice
TNFα	Protective role in lupus. Produced by Th1 cells, B cells, NK cells, and mononuclear phagocytes MHC linked production: ↑ TNFα seen in haplotypes, DR3 and DR4 ↓ incidence of lupus nephritis ↓ TNFα seen in haplotypes, DR2 and DqW1, associated with lupus nephritis
TGFβ	↓ In lupus, low level may contribute to renal pathology since TGFβ suppresses IgG production
BlyS	↑ Serum level in patients. Inhibition of BlyS improves survival in murine lupus models

IL, interleukin; R, receptor; Ab, antibody; PBMC, peripheral blood mononuclear cell; APC, antigen presenting cell; IFN, interferon; NK, natural killer cell; SCID, severe combined immunodeficient mice; MHC, major histocompatibility complex; ssDNA, single-stranded DNA; dsDNA, double-stranded DNA; BlyS, B cell stimulator; NZB/W, New Zealand Black/New Zealand White F1.

by Lauwerys and Houssiau 1998). Serum titres of IL-10 are positively correlated with anti-dsDNA antibody titre and disease activity. Twin and family studies suggest that genetic regulation of IL-10 is important in most patients with SLE and this is effected at the transcriptional level. An association between distinct polymorphisms at the human IL-10 promoter locus and SLE have been described. A recent paper measured cytokine production by PBMCs and serum cytokine in 52 SLE patients and 29 healthy controls. They confirmed earlier reports that SLE patients have both increased production and serum levels of the Th2 cytokines IL-6 and IL-10. Although the serum levels of IL-10 correlated with anti-dsDNA titres, they report no correlation between IL-6 and IL-10 with disease activity score or clinical profiles, suggesting that the increased cytokine production is constitutive (Grondal *et al.* 2000).

IL-1

Accessory cells in lupus seem to produce insufficient amounts of IL-1 to provide the necessary activation signal for T cells. This effect cannot be overcome *in vitro* by the addition of exogenous IL-1 suggesting that a defect may exist at the level of the IL-1 receptor on T cells. Alternatively, the defect could exist at a distal point in a biochemical pathway.

IL-2

Aberrations of IL-2 production and IL-2 receptor expression in lupus are summarized in Table 2. The complex role of IL-2 in SLE is reviewed by Crispin and Alcocer-Varela (1998).

Apoptosis

Apoptosis is the term used to describe programmed cell death, the process which is initiated by ligand–receptor interaction, as compared with cell necrosis caused by toxic insults. The strict regulation of cell death is of vital importance in ensuring a competent but not autoreactive lymphocyte repertoire. Apoptosis appears to have a dual role in lupus pathogenesis. First, this process is an important mechanism for deletion of autoreactive lymphocytes and second, apoptosis results in the availability of autoantigens which can be presented to the immune system. It is the latter that has generated most interest in recent years. The process of apoptosis involves complex biochemical pathways, whose final stages probably involve a DNase and a protease. The activation of DNase causes cleavage of internucleosomal DNA-releasing nucleosomes. Circulating nucleosomes have been detected in patients with lupus whose disease is active, as already discussed, these may be an important immunogen for the production of autoantibodies to DNA. Normally, apoptotic cells are rapidly cleared by macrophages but recent evidence had demonstrated that there is a profound defect in this clearance pathway in lupus patients (Herrmann *et al.* 1998). When macrophages from a subgroup of SLE patients were differentiated *in vitro*, they displayed markedly impaired phagocytosis of apoptotic cells, leading to the accumulation of secondary necrotic cells. This subject has been recently reviewed (Lorenz *et al.* 2000).

Evidence from a number of animal models supports the idea that defective clearance of apoptotic cells lies at the heart of the pathogenesis of lupus (Walport 2000). Thus, a lupus type phenotype occurs in mice lacking C1q, which, together with other complement proteins, helps to clear immune complexes and apoptotic cells. Deletion of the gene encoding SAP, which binds chromatin and may mask it from the immune system, results in antinuclear autoimmunity and glomerulonephritis. A similar phenotype is observed in mice lacking secreted IgM, implicated in clearing effete cells. Mice that lack DNase1 develop lupus autoimmunity, the ability of DNAase to digest DNA prevents an immune response. The importance of removing apoptotic cells is explained by the appearance of a variety of nuclear autoantigens which are sequestered in blebs on the surface of apoptotic cells, and may become accessible for DCs (Andrade *et al.* 2000). DCs, but not macrophages, efficiently present antigen derived from apoptotic cells to class I restricted autologous cytotoxic T cells (Albert *et al.* 1998). In individuals with a defective clearance, sun exposure may result in accumulation of non-ingested apoptotic cells and nuclear autoantigens in the skin, which is a highly immune-competent tissue. This fact presumably explains the disease and flare-inducing capabilities of exposure to UV light.

Evidence from experimental models of lupus has suggested that murine lupus can arise from failure to delete autoreactive lymphocytes. The *Fas* protein has been intimately linked with apoptosis and is normally expressed on the cell surface (CD95). MRL-*lpr/lpr* mice have an endogenous retroviral DNA sequence integrated into the *Fas* gene, which results in incorrect membrane expression of the *Fas* protein and loss of apoptosis. This abnormality would result in failure of self-reactive T cells to undergo apoptosis in the thymus and may account for the accumulation of double negative T cells (CD4–CD8), which infiltrate many tissues in these mice. Although defects in the apoptotic gene Fas lead to autoimmunity in mice, there is little evidence to suggest that such defects are involved in the development of human lupus. A recent study demonstrated increased levels of *in vitro* apoptosis in SLE in a patient population with inactive disease and without use of immunosuppressive medication, factors which might have influenced results from previous studies (Bijl *et al.* 2001).

Bcl-2 is a proto-oncogene, located at the inner membrane of mitochondria, the endoplasmic reticulum, and the nuclear membrane. *Bcl-2* exerts a regulatory function during development and maintenance of adult tissue, by preventing apoptosis in specific cell types. It is involved in T cell development and thymic selection and is found in long-lived B lymphocytes within the follicular mantle zone. Over-expression of *bcl-2* in mice leads to increased B cell longevity and an increased response to foreign antigens, and, in some genetic backgrounds autoimmunity. It is peripheral rather than central tolerance that is defective in these mice. Elevated Bcl-2 levels have been found in lymphocytes derived from a proportion of lupus patients and a number of cytokines (IL-2, IL-4, IL-7, and IL-15) can increase this expression, and prevent cellular apoptosis, preferentially in lupus patients (Graninger *et al.* 2000). CD28 costimulation induces increased expression of the antiapoptotic protein Bcl-X_L that promotes cell survival (Salomon and Bluestone 2001).

However, current dogma is that there is little wrong with apoptosis *per se* in patients with lupus, but the major defect lies in the removal of apoptotic cells. Recent work supports this hypothesis showing impaired uptake of early apoptotic cells into tingible body macrophages (TBM) in the germinal centres of patients with SLE (Baumann *et al.* 2002). Apoptosis is, therefore, allowed to continue into secondary necrosis with released autoantigens, bound by complement components, being retained on the surface of follicular DCs. This could lead to the undue persistence of potential autoantigens and circumvent B cell tolerance mechanisms.

Complement

The complement system consists of approximately 20 plasma proteins, which mediate inflammatory responses to immune complexes and are crucial for phagocytosis of infectious microbes. Inherited complement deficiencies are rare but occur with increased frequency in SLE, the frequency of a lupus-like disease developing is greater than 50 per cent, in patients with homozygous deficiencies of the early classical complement pathway components C1, C4, and C2 (reviewed by Carroll 1998). In contrast, SLE is very seldom associated with late complement component deficiencies. The strength of the association is inversely correlated with the position of these complement components in the classical activation pathway. Thus, deficiency in C1q leads to a lupus-like disease in 95 per cent of cases, C4 57 per cent, and C2 10 per cent. C3 deficiency leads to a somewhat different clinical picture of recurrent pyogenic infections, membranoproliferative glomerulonephritis, and rashes. A recent clinical evaluation of 53 patients, revealed that although decreases in complement levels were not consistently associated with SLE flares, decreasing complement was associated with a concurrent increase in renal and haematologic SLE activity (Ho *et al.* 2001).

Complement deficiencies are genetically determined, since two alleles are inherited for each component complement, deficiencies may be partial (heterozygous) or complete (homozygous). Homozygous C1q deficiency is a very rare disorder and patients suffer from a particularly severe form of SLE with glomerulonephritis and skin manifestations. Gene-targeted C1q-deficient mice have also been shown to develop a syndrome reminiscent of SLE with antinuclear autoantibodies and proliferative glomerulonephritis. A recent paper demonstrates that the effect of C1q deficiency in this mouse model is strongly influenced by the genetic background, only accelerating disease in lupus-prone mouse models when imposed on the MRL/Mp+/+ background (Mitchell *et al.* 2002). Congenital defects in C2 and C4 are often found in patients with MHC haplotypes DR3 and DR2. Complete C2 or C4 deficiencies are rare and can be associated with a mild form of lupus, limited to skin and joint involvement. The C4 proteins, C4A and C4B, bind immune complexes preventing their immunoprecipitation. Mice deficient in C4 spontaneously develop autoantibodies against nuclear antigens and this is independent of C3 (Einav *et al.* 2002). Homozygous C4A deficiency occurs in 10–15 per cent of Caucasian lupus patients despite being rare in the healthy population. Partial C4A deficiency occurs in 50–80 per cent of SLE patients but only 10–20 per cent of controls. A C4A null allele is transmitted as part of the extended HLA-A7, B8, DR3 haplotype which is associated with SLE in Caucasians. Mannose-binding protein (MBP) is an acute phase protein that activates both the classical and alternative complement pathways. A defective allele, incapable of activating complement, has been associated with SLE in several ethnic populations.

The mechanism that links these deficiencies in the early components of complement to pathogenesis of SLE are not entirely clear. Perhaps the most favoured explanation is that complement proteins play a vital role in the processing and clearing of immune complexes and also in the clearance of apoptotic cells, which as discussed earlier is thought to be defective in SLE. C1q has been shown to bind directly to apoptotic blebs and mice deficient in C1q or C4 have defects in the clearance of injected apoptotic thymocytes, also apoptotic bodies are found in the glomeruli of the C1q-deficient mice. A second model proposes that the innate immune system including complement is protective against SLE by enhancing negative selection of self-reactive B cells. It is hypothesized that innate proteins such as SAP, DNase I, natural IgM, C1q, or C4 ensure efficient localization and presentation of self antigens such as dsDNA within the primary lymphoid compartment, thus resulting in the elimination of potential self-reactive B cells. Therefore, deficiency in these innate proteins including complement components could lead to an escape from negative selection and potential activation of self-reactive B cells in the periphery, given the presence of cognate T cell help and available antigens (Carroll 2001).

The levels of complement receptors, CR1 and CR2 are also altered in SLE. CR1 binds activated complement components C3b and C4b and their associated immune complexes. The receptor is present on peripheral B lymphocytes, erythrocytes, monocytes, and tissue macrophages and binds, internalizes, processes, and transports immune complexes which have activated complement. Low expression of CR1 on erythrocytes and peripheral blood leucocytes was described in SLE patients and their healthy family members (Walport and Lachmann 1988). This was originally interpreted as an inherited defect which could predispose to SLE. More recently, this defect is thought to be acquired since normal erythrocytes infused into SLE patients also showed a decrease in CR1 receptors. Levels of CR1 deficiency in SLE patients correlate with disease activity. Controversy still abounds in this area as to the precise nature of this defect and is confounded further by the possibility of a functional defect of CR1 receptors on polymorphonuclear neutrophils.

Complement receptor 2, CR2 (CD21) is found on 10–40 per cent of peripheral blood T cells, B cells, and follicular DCs and binds C3d, C3g, and EBV. In patients with active lupus, CR2 expression is significantly reduced on B cells, which may reflect the highly activated state of these cells. CR2 may be lost as the activated B cells differentiate into immunoglobulin-secreting plasma cells or the levels may be modulated by high levels of circulating immune complexes. CR2 expression is increased on T cells from patients with active lupus but is normal on those with inactive disease. CR2 is important in signalling and increased expression of this receptor may play a role in cell adhesion or cytotoxicity (Levy *et al.* 1992).

Genetic factors

Genetic predisposition plays a crucial role in susceptibility to SLE, both in patients and animal models. Evidence stems from the higher rate of concordance for this disease in monozygotic twins (25 per cent) compared to dizygotic twins (3 per cent), the increased frequency of lupus and immunological abnormalities in relatives of lupus patients compared to healthy controls and the fact that lupus occurs more frequently in certain ethnic groups. In addition to those genetic predisposing factors for SLE already described in the context of complement deficiencies, T and B cell receptor gene usage and altered expression of phagocyte Fcγ receptor alleles, the genes which determine gender, race, and tissue type (human leucocyte antigen, HLA) are believed to influence pathogenicity.

Candidate genes

Recent workers have made great progress in murine systems and human linkage studies and the list of candidate genes is expanding fast (reviewed by Wakeland *et al.* 2001). The emerging picture clearly indicates that multiple genes contribute to SLE and that susceptibility is inherited in a fashion similar to other complex genetic diseases. Several genome scans have been published for SLE, their results varying substantially presumably because of heterogeneity of sample populations and differing methods of analysis. These studies have identified several chromosomal regions indicating possible linkages with SLE. In some cases, chromosomal regions containing genes already known to be associated were identified, such as FcγRIIA on 1q23. In other cases, the same region has been identified in humans and mice, for example Sle1, Lbw7, and Nba2 on chromosome1, map to a region syntenic to human chromosome 1q21–1q23 (Tsao 2000). A region on chromosome 1q41–q42 has been linked to human SLE by nearly all the mapping studies reported to date, this is also syntenic to a murine susceptibility region. It is interesting to note that none of the chromosome 1 regions were identified in the Icelandic patients. Other regions have been identified as a cluster of autoimmune loci, including 19q, which has linkage to MS and IDDM and contains candidate genes such as CD22, a negative regulator of B cell activation, and TGFβ which plays numerous roles in controlling immune reactions.

Major histocompatibility complex

The HLA region is a gene rich and transcriptionally active segment which encodes many immunologically important genes, including those encoding MHC classes I and II. There is evidence that HLA haplotypes spanning the MHC class II region are genetic risk factors in several ethnic populations. The DR-B1 alleles, D2 and D3, have shown associations with SLE in European-Caucasians. HLA associations in many non-Caucasian populations are not so convincing, although in American Blacks DRw52b is positively associated with renal disease and negatively associated with antinuclear RNP antibodies. Interestingly, DR/DQ alleles show stronger association with the autoantibody profiles observed in SLE than with the disease expression itself. DR3 (DRw17) and DQw2 are highly associated with the ability to produce anti-Ro/anti-La antibodies. DR4 is associated with the ability to make anti-RNP and with a reduced risk for lupus nephritis. In contrast to the protection conferred by DR4, DR2 confers susceptibility to nephritis. Compared to the normal ethnic population,

Afro-Caribbean patients with antibodies to Sm have an increased frequency of DR2 and a reduced frequency of DR3, regardless of anti-DNA antibody status.

Ethnic background

SLE shows an ethnic bias with more Afro-Caribbeans (1/250) being affected than Orientals (1/1000), who in turn, are more affected than Caucasians (1/4300). Black race is an independent risk factor for developing SLE. African-Americans and Afro-Caribbeans, living in the United Kingdom/United States, are at greatest risk of developing SLE, develop the disease earlier in life, and have an increased frequency and severity of renal pathology. Also of note and not satisfactorily explained, SLE is rare in native Africans. A study in Birmingham demonstrated major differences in the incidence and prevalence rates of SLE in the United Kingdom depending on ethnic group, the observed prevalence in females was 206/100,000 among Afro-Caribbeans, 91/100,000 among Asians, and 36/100,000 among Caucasians. These results were irrespective of place of birth (Johnson *et al.* 1995).

Sex hormones

SLE occurs nine times more often in females, than in males (9 : 1 ratio) and sex hormones are known to influence disease in both mice and humans with autoimmune disease (reviewed by McMurray 2001). Prior to puberty, the ratio of females : males is lower at approximately 3 : 1 and after menopause, the ratio also falls. In humans where pregnancy occurs during active disease, exacerbations often occur as oestrogen levels rise. On a basic level, androgens are immunosuppressive and oestrogens are immunoenhancing. The spontaneous antibody production in mixed strains of mice (NZB × CBA and NZB × C3H) is reduced by androgens and enhanced by oestrogens. In MRL-*pr/lpr* mice testosterone treatment reduces lupus-like symptoms without affecting lympho-proliferation. Abnormal oestrogen metabolism has been described in women with SLE, which results in an excess of 16-α-hydroxyestrone and estrol metabolites, with chronic hyperestrogenism. The anterior pituitary hormone, prolactin has been found to be immunostimulatory in SLE and has been reported to be elevated in several studies of both male and female patients. Recent research has suggested that there is an interdependence of the neuroendocrine and immune systems, involving many different hormones. Although these data may be interpreted as indicating the possible role of sex hormones in the aetiopathology of lupus, they do not prove it. Much remains to be done before our understanding of why women in particular get lupus is truly clarified.

Environmental factors

Infectious agents

A common but still to be proven hypothesis is that SLE, and other autoimmune diseases, are triggered by infectious agents including viruses (reviewed by James *et al.* 2001). Coimmunization with virus-self complexes has been shown to be a possible mechanism capable of breaking tolerance and generating autoimmunity. As described earlier, a role for BK polyoma viruses in the development of anti-dsDNA autoantibodies has been supported by animal experiments (Rekvig *et al.* 1997), but their role in human SLE is still unknown. Using the technique of epitope mapping, antigenic epitopes of Sm and nRNP autoantigens have been identified and researchers have found a striking similarity between these regions and antigenic peptides derived from EBV nuclear antigen, EBNA-1, suggesting a possible role for these agents in the aetiology of lupus. A significant increase in the prevalence of EBV infection was found in paediatric patients with lupus compared to controls (reviewed by James and Harley 1998). SLE patients produce high titre antibodies to various retroviral proteins, including Gag, Env, and Nef of human immunodeficiency virus (HIV) and human T-cell leukaemia virus (HTLV), in the absence of overt retroviral infection. A recent article reviews the role of human endogenous retroviruses (HERVs) in SLE and proposes that molecular mimicry between HTLV-1-related endogenous sequence (HRES-1) and the snRNP complex initiates autoantibody formation (Adelman and Marchalonis 2002). The role of viruses in the pathogenesis of SLE continues to be a controversial issue, which is frequently revisited.

Other environmental triggers

UV radiation has been shown to trigger and exacerbate the photosensitive lupus rash, but there is also evidence that UV light may actually be capable of altering the structure of DNA leading to the genesis of autoantibodies. UV light has also been shown to induce apoptosis in human keratinocytes resulting in blebs of nuclear and cytoplasmic autoantigens on the cell surface. This provides a mechanism whereby nuclear antigens, which are frequent autoantibody targets, can reach the cell surface. Antihypertensive drugs among others have been shown to give rise to drug-induced lupus, however, this disease is associated with antibodies to ssDNA and histones rather than dsDNA. Although skin and joint disease are common, renal or CNS pathology is virtually unknown and the disease is reversed on curtailment of the drug involved.

Animal models

Throughout this chapter, we have referred to several of the spontaneous lupus-prone mouse models which include the F1 progeny of New Zealand black × New Zealand white mice (NZB × NZW)F1 or (BWF1), (NZB), MRL-+/+, MRL-*lpr/lpr*, BXSB, Moth-eaten, and (SWR × NZB)F1. Most of these exhibit varying degrees of glomerulonephritis, especially the females and are valuable tools for studying renal presentations of lupus although it is important to remember the contrasts between experimental models and human lupus. These models are extensively reviewed elsewhere (Peutz-Kootstra *et al.* 2001).

Recently, the number of mouse models has rapidly increased with the introduction of many gene-targeted mice such as single gene knock-outs, as well as gene overexpression and transgenic (knock-in) models. We have referred to several of these such as C1q knock-outs during the course of this chapter. These gene-targeted models enable researchers to dissect the role of an immunological component in the pathogenesis of lupus. Table 3 summarizes current mouse models of lupus, which have resulted from gene-targeting experiments.

Table 3 Mouse models of lupus arising from gene targeting experiments

Gene targeted	Background	Glomerular nephritis	Postulated mechanism
Autoimmunity through lack of clearance of apoptotic cells			
SAP (KO)	129 × C57BL/6	Immune complex GN	Binds apoptotic cells/nuclear debris—aiding their clearance
DNAse-1 (KO)	C57BL/6	Immune complex GN IgG and C3 deposits	Removes DNA from antigenic nucleoprotein complexes
C1q (KO)	129 × C57BL/6	Proliferative GN, C3 and apoptotic body deposits	Promotes clearance of apoptotic cells
Serum IgM (KO)	129 × C57BL/6	Immune complex GN IgG and C3 deposits	Alters antigen clearance, binds nuclear debris
Negative regulators of B-cell activation			
FcγRIIB (KO)	129 × C57BL/6	Glomerular sclerosis IgG deposits	Inhibitory receptor gating of BCR, induces B cell apoptosis
CD22 (KO)	129 × C57BL/6	Immune complex GN	Negative regulator of BCR
Lyn (KO)	E14 × C57BL/6	FSGS, crescentic GN IgG deposits	Negative signal transduction in BCR pathway, eliminates autoreactive B cells
Dysregulated B- and T-cell proliferation			
Eμ-bcl-2-22 (transgene)	C57BL/6 × SJL	Immune complex GN IgM, IgG, C3 deposits	Expansion of B-cell population ↑ Autoreactive B-cell precursors
BAFF (Blys/THANK/ zTNF4/TALL-1) (transgene)	C57BL/6J × DBA	Immune complex GN C3 and IgG deposits	Proliferation of activated autoreactive B cells, suppression of protective effect of dendritic cells against autoreactive T cells
CD45 (point mutation inhibitory wedge)	129 × C57BL/6	Diffuse membranous proliferative GN	Inappropriate lymphocyte activation Polyclonal T- and B-cell activation
P21 (KO)	C57BL/6 × 129/5V	Immune complex GN IgG deposits	Sustained CD4+ and CD8+ T-cell proliferation. Exposure to antinuclear antigens from excess apoptotic bodies
Cbl-b (KO)	C57BL/6	Interstitial nephritis Leucocyte infiltration	Negative molecular adaptor on lymphocyte activation pathway
Enzymes affecting TCR recruitment			
Mgat5 (KO)	129	Glomerular nephritis	Enhanced TCR recruitment Sustained T-cell activation
M11(KO)	C57BL/6	Immune complex GN	Enhanced TCR recruitment Sustained T-cell activation
Lack of apoptosis of activated B and T cells			
Pten +/−	129 × C57BL/6	Immune complex GN Segmental sclerosis	Negatively regulates Akt survival signals and thus promotes Fas-mediated cell death

SAP, serum amyloid P; KO, knock-out; GN, glomerular nephritis; BCR, B-cell receptor; FSGS, focal segmental glomerular sclerosis; TCR, T-cell receptor.

Conclusion

Our understanding of the pathogenesis of SLE is advancing more rapidly than ever before, with major contributions being made on many fronts utilizing the increasingly sophisticated research tools available. With this increased knowledge of how the disease is initiated and perpetuates, we can attempt to develop carefully targeted therapies for patients with SLE.

References

Adelman, M. K. and Marchalonis, J. J. (2002). Endogenous retroviruses in systemic lupus erythematosus: candidate lupus viruses. *Clinical Immunology* **102**, 107–116.

Alarcon-Segovia, D. and Cabral, A. R. (1996). Autoantibodies in systemic lupus erythematosus. *Current Opinion in Rheumatology* **8**, 403–407.

Albert, M. L., Sauter, B., and Bhardwaj, N. (1998). Dendritic cells acquire antigen from apoptotic cells and induce class I-restricted CTLs. *Nature* **392**, 86–89.

Amoura, Z., Koutouzov, S., and Piette, J. C. (2000). The role of nucleosomes in lupus. *Current Opinion in Rheumatology* **12**, 369–373.

Andrade, F., Casciola-Rosen, L., and Rosen, A. (2000). Apoptosis in systemic lupus erythematosus. Clinical implications. *Rheumatic Diseases Clinics of North America* **26**, 215–227.

Baumann, I. *et al.* (2002). Impaired uptake of apoptotic cells into tingible body macrophages in germinal centers of patients with systemic lupus erythematosus. *Arthritis and Rheumatism* **46**, 191–201.

Berden, J. H. (1997). Lupus nephritis. *Kidney International* **52**, 538–558.

Bijl, M. *et al.* (2001). Expression of costimulatory molecules on peripheral blood lymphocytes of patients with systemic lupus erythematosus. *Annals of the Rheumatic Diseases* **60**, 523–526.

Blanco, P. *et al.* (2001). Induction of dendritic cell differentiation by IFN-alpha in systemic lupus erythematosus. *Science* **294**, 1540–1543.

Bullard, D. C. *et al.* (1997). Intercellular adhesion molecule-1 deficiency protects MRL/MpJ-Fas(lpr) mice from early lethality. *Journal of Immunology* **159**, 2058–2067.

Cabral, A. R. and Alarcon-Segovia, D. (1997). Autoantibodies in systemic lupus erythematosus. *Current Opinion in Rheumatology* **9**, 387–392.

Cairns, A. P. *et al.* (2001). Reduced expression of CD44 on monocytes and neutrophils in systemic lupus erythematosus: relations with apoptotic neutrophils and disease activity. *Annals of the Rheumatic Diseases* **60**, 950–955.

Carroll, M. (2001). Innate immunity in the etiopathology of autoimmunity. *Nature Immunology* **2**, 1089–1090.

Carroll, M. C. (1998). The role of complement and complement receptors in induction and regulation of immunity. *Annual Review of Immunology* **16**, 545–568.

Chan, O. T., Madaio, M. P., and Shlomchik, M. J. (1999). B cells are required for lupus nephritis in the polygenic, Fas-intact MRL model of systemic autoimmunity. *Journal of Immunology* **163**, 3592–3596.

Chan, O. T. *et al.* (1999). A novel mouse with B cells but lacking serum antibody reveals an antibody-independent role for B cells in murine lupus. *Journal of Experimental Medicine* **189**, 1639–1648.

Charles, P. J. *et al.* (2000). Assessment of antibodies to double-stranded DNA induced in rheumatoid arthritis patients following treatment with infliximab, a monoclonal antibody to tumor necrosis factor alpha: findings in open-label and randomized placebo-controlled trials. *Arthritis and Rheumatism* **43**, 2383–2390.

Couser, W. G. (1998). Pathogenesis of glomerular damage in glomerulonephritis. *Nephrology, Dialysis, Transplantation* **13**, 10–15.

Crispin, J. C. and Alcocer-Varela, J. (1998). Interleukin-2 and systemic lupus erythematosus—fifteen years later. *Lupus* **7**, 214–222.

Crow, M. K. and Kirou, K. A. (2001). Regulation of CD40 ligand expression in systemic lupus erythematosus. *Current Opinion in Rheumatology* **13**, 361–369.

Davis, J. C., Tassiulas, I. O., and Boumpas, D. T. (1996). Lupus nephritis. *Current Opinion in Rheumatology* **8**, 415–423.

Dayal, A. K. and Kammer, G. M. (1996). The T cell enigma in lupus. *Arthritis and Rheumatism* **39**, 23–33.

Dean, G. S. *et al.* (2000). Cytokines and systemic lupus erythematosus. *Annals of the Rheumatic Diseases* **59**, 243–251.

Desai-Mehta, A. *et al.* (1995). Structure and specificity of T cell receptors expressed by potentially pathogenic anti-DNA autoantibody-inducing T cells in human lupus. *Journal of Clinical Investigation* **95**, 531–541.

Egerer, K. *et al.* (2000). Increased serum soluble CD14, ICAM-1 and E-selectin correlate with disease activity and prognosis in systemic lupus erythematosus. *Lupus* **9**, 614–621.

Ehrenstein, M., Longhurst, C., and Isenberg, D. A. (1993). Production and analysis of IgG monoclonal anti-DNA antibodies from systemic lupus erythematosus (SLE) patients. *Clinical and Experimental Immunology* **92**, 39–45.

Ehrenstein, M. R. *et al.* (1995). Human IgG anti-DNA antibodies deposit in kidneys and induce proteinuria in SCID mice. *Kidney International* **48**, 705–711.

Einav, S. *et al.* (2002). Complement C4 is protective for lupus disease independent of C3. *Journal of Immunology* **168**, 1036–1041.

Enyedy, E. J. *et al.* (2001). Fc epsilon receptor type I gamma chain replaces the deficient T cell receptor zeta chain in T cells of patients with systemic lupus erythematosus. *Arthritis and Rheumatism* **44**, 1114–1121.

Gilkeson, G. S. *et al.* (1993). Molecular characterization of anti-DNA antibodies induced in normal mice by immunization with bacterial DNA. Differences from spontaneous anti-DNA in the content and location of VH CDR3 arginines. *Journal of Immunology* **151**, 1353–1364.

Graninger, W. B. *et al.* (2000). Cytokine regulation of apoptosis and Bcl-2 expression in lymphocytes of patients with systemic lupus erythematosus. *Cell Death and Differentiation* **7**, 966–972.

Grondal, G. *et al.* (2000). Cytokine production, serum levels and disease activity in systemic lupus erythematosus. *Clinical and Experimental Rheumatology* **18**, 565–570.

Harris, D. C. (2001). Tubulointerstitial renal disease. *Current Opinion in Nephrology and Hypertension* **10**, 303–313.

Herrmann, M. *et al.* (1998). Impaired phagocytosis of apoptotic cell material by monocyte-derived macrophages from patients with systemic lupus erythematosus. *Arthritis and Rheumatism* **41**, 1241–1250.

Ho, A. *et al.* (2001). A decrease in complement is associated with increased renal and hematologic activity in patients with systemic lupus erythematosus. *Arthritis and Rheumatism* **44**, 2350–2357.

Hochberg, M. C. (1997). Updating the American College of Rheumatology revised criteria for the classification of systemic lupus erythematosus. *Arthritis and Rheumatism* **40**, 1725.

Jacob, C. O. *et al.* (1990). Heritable major histocompatibility complex class II-associated differences in production of tumor necrosis factor alpha: relevance to genetic predisposition to systemic lupus erythematosus. *Proceedings of the National Academy of Sciences USA* **87**, 1233–1237.

James, J. A. *et al.* (1995). Immunoglobulin epitope spreading and autoimmune disease after peptide immunization: Sm B/B′-derived PPPGMRPP and PPPGIRGP induce spliceosome autoimmunity. *Journal of Experimental Medicine* **181**, 453–461.

James, J. A. and Harley, J. B. (1998). B-cell epitope spreading in autoimmunity. *Immunological Reviews* **164**, 185–200.

James, J. A., Harley, J. B., and Scofield, R. H. (2001). Role of viruses in systemic lupus erythematosus and Sjögren syndrome. *Current Opinion in Rheumatology* **13**, 370–376.

Johnson, A. E. *et al.* (1995). The prevalence and incidence of systemic lupus erythematosus in Birmingham, England. Relationship to ethnicity and country of birth. *Arthritis and Rheumatism* **38**, 551–558.

Kaliyaperumal, A., Michaels, M. A., and Datta, S. K. (2002). Naturally processed chromatin peptides reveal a major autoepitope that primes pathogenic T and B cells of lupus. *Journal of Immunology* **168**, 2530–2537.

Kalsi, J. K. *et al.* (1996). Functional and modelling studies of the binding of human monoclonal anti-DNA antibodies to DNA. *Molecular Immunology* **33**, 471–483.

Kalsi, J. K. *et al.* Structure–function analysis and the molecular origins of anti-DNA antibodies in systemic lupus erythematosus. In *Expert Reviews in Molecular Medicine*. Cambridge: Cambridge University Press, 1999 (http://www-ermm.cbcu.cam.ac.uk/99000423h.htm).

Kim, Y. S. *et al.* (2001). Differential expression of various cytokine and chemokine genes between proliferative and non-proliferative glomerulonephritides. *Clinical Nephrology* **56**, 199–206.

Lauwerys, B. R. and Houssiau, F. A. (1998). Cytokines: clues to the pathogenesis of SLE. *Lupus* **7**, 211–213.

Leandro, M. J. *et al.* (2002). An open study of B lymphocyte depletion in systemic lupus erythematosus. *Arthritis and Rheumatism* **46**, 2673–2677.

Lefkowith, J. B. and Gilkeson, G. S. (1996). Nephritogenic autoantibodies in lupus: current concepts and continuing controversies. *Arthritis and Rheumatism* **39**, 894–903.

Lehmann, P. V., Targoni, O. S., and Forsthuber, T. G. (1998). Shifting T-cell activation thresholds in autoimmunity and determinant spreading. *Immunological Reviews* **164**, 53–61.

Levy, E. *et al.* (1992). T lymphocyte expression of complement receptor 2 (CR2/CD21): a role in adhesive cell–cell interactions and dysregulation in a patient with systemic lupus erythematosus (SLE). *Clinical and Experimental Immunology* **90**, 235–244.

Liang, B. *et al.* (1999). B7 costimulation in the development of lupus: autoimmunity arises either in the absence of B7.1/B7.2 or in the presence of anti-b7.1/B7.2 blocking antibodies. *Journal of Immunology* **163**, 2322–2329.

Lorenz, H. M. *et al.* (2000). Role of apoptosis in autoimmunity. *Apoptosis* **5**, 443–449.

Lu, L. *et al.* (1999). Major peptide autoepitopes for nucleosome-specific T cells of human lupus. *Journal of Clinical Investigation* **104**, 345–355.

Madaio, M. P. and Yanase, K. (1998). Cellular penetration and nuclear localization of anti-DNA antibodies: mechanisms, consequences, implications and applications. *Journal of Autoimmunity* **11**, 535–538.

Mamoune, A. *et al.* (2000). CD45 autoantibodies mediate neutralization of activated T cells from lupus patients through anergy or apoptosis. *Lupus* **9**, 622–631.

Mamula, M. J. (1998). Epitope spreading: the role of self peptides and autoantigen processing by B lymphocytes. *Immunological Reviews* **164**, 231–239.

Mason, L. J. *et al.* (1999). Immunization with a peptide of Sm B/B′ results in limited epitope spreading but not autoimmune disease. *Journal of Immunology* **162**, 5099–5105.

McHale, J. F. *et al.* (1999). TNF-alpha and IL-1 sequentially induce endothelial ICAM-1 and VCAM-1 expression in MRL/lpr lupus-prone mice. *Journal of Immunology* **163**, 3993–4000.

McMurray, R. W. (1996). Adhesion molecules in autoimmune disease. *Seminars in Arthritis and Rheumatism* **25**, 215–233.

McMurray, R. W. (2001). Sex hormones in the pathogenesis of systemic lupus erythematosus. *Frontiers in Bioscience* **6**, E193–E206.

Messier, H. *et al.* (1993). p70 lupus autoantigen binds the enhancer of the T-cell receptor beta-chain gene. *Proceedings of the National Academy of Sciences USA* **90**, 2685–2689.

Mitchell, D. A. *et al.* (2002). C1q deficiency and autoimmunity: the effects of genetic background on disease expression. *Journal of Immunology* **168**, 2538–2543.

Mostoslavsky, G. *et al.* (2001). Lupus anti-DNA autoantibodies cross-react with a glomerular structural protein: a case for tissue injury by molecular mimicry. *European Journal of Immunology* **31**, 1221–1227.

Murakami, M. *et al.* (1992). *In vitro* induction of IgG anti-DNA antibody from high density B cells of systemic lupus erythematosus patients by an HLA DR-restricted T cell clone. *Clinical and Experimental Immunology* **90**, 245–250.

Nikolic-Paterson, D. J. and Atkins, R. C. (2001). The role of macrophages in glomerulonephritis. *Nephrology, Dialysis, Transplantation* **16** (Suppl. 5), 3–7.

Peutz-Kootstra, C. J. *et al.* (2001). Lupus nephritis: lessons from experimental animal models. *Journal of Laboratory and Clinical Medicine* **137**, 244–260.

Putterman, C. *et al.* (1996). The double edged sword of the immune response: mutational analysis of a murine anti-pneumococcal, anti-DNA antibody. *Journal of Clinical Investigation* **97**, 2251–2259.

Radic, M. Z. and Weigert, M. (1994). Genetic and structural evidence for antigen selection of anti-DNA antibodies. *Annual Review of Immunology* **12**, 487–520.

Rahman, M. A. *et al.* (1998). Properties of whole human IgG molecules produced by the expression of cloned anti-DNA antibody cDNA in mammalian cells. *Journal of Autoimmunity* **11**, 661–669.

Rajagopalan, S., Mao, C., and Datta, S. K. (1992). Pathogenic autoantibody-inducing gamma/delta T helper cells from patients with lupus nephritis express unusual T cell receptors. *Clinical Immunology and Immunopathology* **62**, 344–350.

Ravirajan, C. T. *et al.* (1998). Genetic, structural and functional properties of an IgG DNA-binding monoclonal antibody from a lupus patient with nephritis. *European Journal of Immunology* **28**, 339–350.

Ravirajan, C. T. *et al.* (2001). Human pathogenic anti-DNA light chain failed to induce nephritis without an appropriate heavy chain: demonstration using human light chain only transgenic animals. *Arthritis and Rheumatism* **44** (Abstracts Suppl.), S76.

Rekvig, O. P. *et al.* (1997). Experimental expression in mice and spontaneous expression in human SLE of polyomavirus T-antigen. A molecular basis for induction of antibodies to DNA and eukaryotic transcription factors. *Journal of Clinical Investigation* **99**, 2045–2054.

Riccieri, V. *et al.* (2000). Down-regulation of natural killer cells and of gamma/delta T cells in systemic lupus erythematosus. Does it correlate to autoimmunity and to laboratory indices of disease activity? *Lupus* **9**, 333–337.

Salmon, J. E. *et al.* (1996). Fc gamma RIIA alleles are heritable risk factors for lupus nephritis in African Americans. *Journal of Clinical Investigation* **97**, 1348–1354.

Salomon, B. and Bluestone, J. A. (2001). Complexities of CD28/B7: CTLA-4 costimulatory pathways in autoimmunity and transplantation. *Annual Review of Immunology* **19**, 225–252.

Scheinecker, C. *et al.* (2001). Alterations of dendritic cells in systemic lupus erythematosus: phenotypic and functional deficiencies. *Arthritis and Rheumatism* **44**, 856–865.

Shlomchik, M. J., Craft, J. E., and Mamula, M. J. (2001). From T to B and back again: positive feedback in systemic autoimmune disease. *Nature Reviews. Immunology* **1**, 147–153.

Sieling, P. A. *et al.* (2000). Human double-negative T cells in systemic lupus erythematosus provide help for IgG and are restricted by CD1c. *Journal of Immunology* **165**, 5338–5344.

Singh, R. R. and Hahn, B. H. (1998). Reciprocal T-B determinant spreading develops spontaneously in murine lupus: implications for pathogenesis. *Immunological Reviews* **164**, 201–208.

Stollar, B. D. (1986). Antibodies to DNA. *CRC Critical Reviews in Biochemistry* **20**, 1–36.

Tan, E. M. *et al.* (1982). The 1982 revised criteria for the classification of systemic lupus erythematosus. *Arthritis and Rheumatism* **25**, 1271–1277.

ter Borg, E. J. *et al.* (1990). Measurement of increases in anti-double-stranded DNA antibody levels as a predictor of disease exacerbation in systemic lupus erythematosus. A long-term, prospective study. *Arthritis and Rheumatism* **33**, 634–643.

Tsao, B. P. (2000). Lupus susceptibility genes on human chromosome 1. *International Reviews of Immunology* **19**, 319–334.

Tsao, B. P. *et al.* (1992). Failed self-tolerance and autoimmunity in IgG anti-DNA transgenic mice. *Journal of Immunology* **149**, 350–358.

Tsokos, G. C. *et al.* (2000). Immune cell signaling in lupus. *Current Opinion in Rheumatology* **12**, 355–363.

van Bruggen, M. C., Kramers, C., and Berden, J. H. (1996). Autoimmunity against nucleosomes and lupus nephritis. *Annales de Medecine Interne (Paris)* **147**, 485–489.

Vlachoyiannopoulos, P. G. *et al.* (2000). No evidence of epitope spreading after immunization with the major Sm epitope P-P-G-M-R-P-P anchored to sequential oligopeptide carriers (SOCs). *Journal of Autoimmunity* **14**, 53–61.

Vlahakos, D. V. *et al.* (1992). Anti-DNA antibodies form immune deposits at distinct glomerular and vascular sites. *Kidney International* **41**, 1690–1700.

Wakeland, E. K. *et al.* (2001). Delineating the genetic basis of systemic lupus erythematosus. *Immunity* **15**, 397–408.

Walport, M. J. (2000). Lupus, DNase and defective disposal of cellular debris. *Nature Genetics* **25**, 135–136.

Walport, M. J. and Lachmann, P. J. (1988). Erythrocyte complement receptor type 1, immune complexes, and the rheumatic diseases. *Arthritis and Rheumatism* **31**, 153–158.

Winkler, T. H., Fehr, H., and Kalden, J. R. (1992). Analysis of immunoglobulin variable region genes from human IgG anti-DNA hybridomas. *European Journal of Immunology* **22**, 1719–1728.

Winkler, T. H., Jahn, S., and Kalden, J. R. (1991). IgG human monoclonal anti-DNA autoantibodies from patients with systemic lupus erythematosus. *Clinical and Experimental Immunology* **85**, 379–385.

Wong, H. K. *et al.* (1999). Abnormal NF-kappa B activity in T lymphocytes from patients with systemic lupus erythematosus is associated with decreased p65-RelA protein expression. *Journal of Immunology* **163**, 1682–1689.

Wu, J. *et al.* (1997). A novel polymorphism of FcgammaRIIIa (CD16) alters receptor function and predisposes to autoimmune disease. *Journal of Clinical Investigation* **100**, 1059–1070.

Yamada, A. *et al.* (1993). Changes in subset specificity of anti-T cell autoantibodies in systemic lupus erythematosus. *Autoimmunity* **14**, 269–273.

Yanase, K. *et al.* (1997). Receptor-mediated cellular entry of nuclear localizing anti-DNA antibodies via myosin 1. *Journal of Clinical Investigation* **100**, 25–31.

Zack, D. J. *et al.* (1996). Mechanisms of cellular penetration and nuclear localization of an anti-double strand DNA autoantibody. *Journal of Immunology* **157**, 2082–2088.

Zeng, D. *et al.* (2000). Cutting edge: a role for CD1 in the pathogenesis of lupus in NZB/NZW mice. *Journal of Immunology* **164**, 5000–5004.

4.7.2 Systemic lupus erythematosus (clinical)

Claudio Ponticelli, Giovanni Banfi, and Gabriella Moroni

Epidemiology

Systemic lupus erythematosus (SLE) is predominantly a disease of women. In general, the female to male ratio is about 7 : 1 with an 11 : 1 female to male ratio during childbearing years (Manzi 2001). Over 80 per cent of cases occur in women during their childbearing years, but SLE spares neither the neonatal nor advanced age. Its prevalence ranges between 14.6 and 50.8 per 100,000 general Caucasian population (Hochberg 1997a). Surveys based on patients admitted to hospital reported a considerably greater incidence in black (McCarthy *et al.* 1995) and Asian people (Johnson *et al.* 1995), living in Western countries. However, the actual difference in racial prevalence remains difficult to estimate as long as studies do not include both in- and outpatients. The incidence of SLE has increased approximately three-fold over the past two decades (Voss *et al.* 1998; Uramoto *et al.* 1999). At least in part, these data reflect an easier detection of the SLE, thanks to the continuous improvement of diagnostic tools.

Clinical features

At presentation, SLE may be multisystemic, or may involve only one organ system with additional manifestations later. In some patients, the clinical diagnosis is preceded for months or years by insidious symptoms, in others the presentation is dramatic, with severe or even life-threatening manifestations.

General manifestations

Systemic symptoms are usually prominent and include fatigue, malaise, weakness, fever, lymphadenopathy, anorexia, nausea, vomiting, and unintentional weight loss. These symptoms may be mild or severe, fleeting or persistent.

Mucocutaneous lesions

The skin and mucous membranes are symptomatically involved in 60–80 per cent of patients. Their frequency may be altered by the concurrent treatment of the systemic disease. Mucocutaneous lesions may accompany or precede other signs or symptoms of SLE.

The specific cutaneous lesions may be classified as acute, subacute, and chronic. The acute lesions generally present as malar rash or butterfly dermatitis. These lesions are photosensitive and are often associated with systemic manifestations. They are characterized by confluent, symmetric erythema and oedema centred over the malar eminence. The subacute lesions consist of nonscarring papulosquamous or annular lesions which are exquisitely photosensitive. They initially present as erythematous macules or papules which evolve into scaly papulosquamous or annular, polycyclic plaques. Chronic lesions are mostly represented by discoid lupus with flat, erythematous, demarcated macules or papulae evolving into coin-shaped, demarcated plaques. Merging of several discoid plaques may cause disfiguration. Hyperkeratosis, verrucous dermatitis, or panniculitis are rare forms of chronic lesions. The sun-exposed areas of the skin are the common sites of cutaneous lesions caused by lupus erythematosus (Sontheimer and Provost 1997).

Gastrointestinal manifestations

Gastrointestinal symptoms are common in patients with SLE and can be due to primary gastrointestinal disorders, complications of therapy, or SLE itself. A number of patients complain of oesophageal disturbances with dysphagia, often without radiographic abnormalities. Mesenteric vasculitis may cause an acute abdomen (Buck *et al.* 2001). Acute pancreatitis may be caused by vasculitis or by the use of steroids. Liver involvement is unusual. The association of liver abnormalities with positive antinuclear antibodies (lupoid hepatitis) is more consistent with chronic active hepatitis.

Musculoskeletal symptoms

Arthralgia and arthritis are reported by almost all patients with SLE. Symptoms are often asymmetrical and migratory. All major and minor joints may be affected. Fingers, hands wrists, knees, ankles, elbows, and shoulders are the most affected joints. Pain is often out of proportion to physical findings. Deformities and erosions may occur (Boumpas *et al.* 1992). Myalgias occur in 40–80 per cent of patients and are most marked in proximal muscles. Tendonitis and inflammatory myositis may also be present. As a consequence of musculoskeletal symptoms, up to 80 per cent of patients with SLE are treated with anti-inflammatory drugs (Ostensen and Villiger 2001) and may develop side-effects related to these agents.

Neuropsychiatric manifestations

Anxiety and depression are not uncommon in patients with lupus and may be worsened by corticosteroid therapy. Frank psychosis may develop. Phobias and obsessive behaviour may even precede the diagnosis of lupus (Khan *et al.* 2000). Headache is frequent and several patients suffer from migraine.

About 28 per cent of patients with SLE may have definite central nervous system disease, which is associated with antiphospholipid antibodies in half of these cases (Toubi *et al.* 1995). Any region of the brain can be involved. Neurological events may be isolated or multiple, but usually occur in the presence of active disease. Mild mental dysfunction is the most frequent manifestation. Seizures are frequent. Other neurological disorders include delirium, confusional state, aseptic meningitis, mononeuritis multiplex, ascending or transverse myelitis, peripheral or cranial neuropathy, chorea, cerebellar ataxia, headache, pseudotumour cerebri, migraine, and acute psychosis (Wallace and Metzger 1997). Intravenous cyclophosphamide appears to be an effective treatment for some patients with severe neuropsychiatric SLE (Neuwelt *et al.* 1995). The differential diagnosis between organic brain disease and psychological reaction may be difficult. Psychological tests, magnetic resonance, evoked potentials, and cerebrospinal fluid analysis can help in discriminating functional from organic disturbances.

Cardiovascular manifestations

Cardiac disease is common in patients with lupus. Pericardial effusion, usually clinically silent, may occur in up to half of patients (Moder *et al.* 1999). Myocardial dysfunction can cause arrhythmias and cardiac failure. Verrucous endocarditis, secondary either to infections or to antiphospholipid antibodies, is often underdiagnosed, but can be responsible for valvular defects (Moroni *et al.* 1995). Mitral valve prolapse is frequent and valvular disease may occur in one-fourth of patients. Transoesophageal echocardiography has been recommended to detect cardiac abnormalities, which may be oligosymptomatic, but may lead in the long-term to stroke, heart failure, or endocarditis (Roldan *et al.* 1996). Coronary artery disease and myocardial infarction are frequent complications. These complications are favoured by the use of corticosteroids and by changes in serum cholesterol, and blood pressure, but accelerated atherosclerosis can also be independent of traditional risk factors, suggesting a role for disease-related factors in atherogenesis (Roman *et al.* 2003).

Recurrent deep vein and/or arterial thrombosis are more frequent in patients with antiphospholipid antibodies (Levine *et al.* 2002).

Pulmonary manifestations

Pleurisy and pleural effusions are common. Lupus pneumonitis is characterized by recurrent pulmonary infiltrates with fever, dyspnoea, and cough. Radiography shows acinar infiltrates, especially in the lower lobes. Subsequently, diffuse interstitial infiltrates, fibrosis, and progressive pulmonary dysfunction develop. Pulmonary hypertension may rarely complicate SLE. Treatment with corticosteroids and cyclophosphamide may be effective if administered in the early stage (Tanaka *et al.* 2002).

Ophthalmological disorders

Keratoconjunctivitis sicca is the most common ocular disorder (Gilboe *et al.* 2001). Retinal vasculitis with cotton wool exudates is rare. Episcleritis and scleritis are also rare. Cases of transient amaurosis may occur in patients with antiphospholipid antibodies (Donders *et al.* 1998).

Vascular manifestations

Raynaud's phenomenon and livedo reticularis may occur in patients with SLE. Recurrent thromboembolism and phlebitis are probably caused by antiphospholipid antibodies that can initiate clotting (Levine *et al.* 2002). Vasculitis may be responsible for mucocutaneous purpura or ulcers particularly in the legs. Rarely, vasculitis can cause major abdominal crises. Blindness can develop as a consequence of retinal vasculitis with infarct.

Haematological disorders

Anaemia occurs in most patients with active SLE. Haemolytic anaemia with an elevated reticulocyte count, reduced haptoglobin concentrations, and a positive direct Coombs' test has been noted in 10–40 per cent of patients. Tzioufas *et al.* (1997) detected autoantibodies to erythropoietin in 15 per cent of SLE patients. The prevalence of autoantibodies was higher in anaemic patients. Patients with antibodies had higher disease activity scores than patients without antibodies. Leucopenia is common. It may result from antineutrophil antibodies, immune complexes, or medications. Mild thrombocytopenia is common. Severe thrombocytopenia with haemorrhage and purpura occurs in less than 5 per cent of cases. It should be remembered that most patients with Evans' syndrome, that is, haemolytic anaemia and idiopathic thrombocytopenic purpura, have also SLE.

Kidney involvement

Renal involvement is frequent: overt clinical evidence of renal disease varies from 35–75 per cent of patients with well-documented systemic lupus (Nossent *et al.* 1989; Wallace *et al.* 1997). Lupus nephritis usually develops within 3 years after diagnosis of SLE. However, clinical data probably underestimate the prevalence of lupus nephritis. Studies with renal biopsies show that SLE involves the kidney in almost all cases in which enough tissue is available for analysis. Even in the absence of proteinuria or abnormal urinary sediment, the renal biopsy is rarely free of detectable abnormalities, especially if evaluated by immunofluorescence or electron microscopy (Cavallo *et al.* 1977; Mahajan *et al.* 1977; Font *et al.* 1987).

The clinical features of lupus nephritis will be detailed later in this chapter.

Diagnosis

Clinical criteria

In 1971 a subcommittee of the American Rheumatism Association proposed a classification of SLE that was mainly based upon clinical criteria (Cohen *et al.* 1971). These criteria were revised by Tan *et al.* (1982) and more recently by Hochberg (1997b). The new classification takes into account 11 criteria, including some serological tests widely used in clinical practice (Table 1). According to this classification a diagnosis of SLE should be made if any four or more of the 11 criteria are present serially or simultaneously during any interval of observation. The purpose of the classification was to operationalize the definition of lupus and to allow comparison among data from different sources. However, the diagnosis of lupus in the individual patient could be made without regard to the above mentioned criteria.

Serological and immunological tests

Antibodies (see also Chapter 4.7.1)

More than 95 per cent of patients with SLE have antinuclear antibodies which may be present many years before the diagnosis of SLE

Table 1 Revised criteria for classification of SLE (Hochberg 1997b)

Malar rash
Discoid rash
Photosensitivity
Oral ulcers
Arthritis (two or more joints)
Pleurisy-pericarditis
Renal abnormalities (persistent proteinuria >0.5 g daily, cellular casts)
Neurological disorders (seizures, psychosis)
Haematological disorders (haemolytic anaemia, leucopenia, lymphocytopenia, thrombocytopenia)
Immunological disorders (anti-DNA, anti-Sm antibodies, abnormal serum level of IgG or IgM anticardiolipin antibodies, a positive lupus anticoagulant, false positive serologic test for syphilis)
Antinuclear antibody

(Arbuckle *et al.* 2003). However, antinuclear antibodies are not specific as they can be present in other rheumatic diseases, chronic infections, chronic liver diseases, neoplastic syndromes, as well as in the elderly. The method of choice for the detection of antinuclear antibodies is the indirect immunofluorescence, usually on acetone-fixed epithelial cells. Antibodies to DNA can be divided into two categories corresponding to the two macromolecular forms of DNA (Hahn 1998). These are native (double-stranded or ds) and denatured (single-stranded or ss) DNA. Anti-nDNA antibodies display a 95 per cent specificity for the diagnosis of SLE, although they can be negative in few patients with inactive lupus. Anti-ssDNA antibodies can also be found in patients with other connective tissue diseases or infectious diseases. The methods for the detection of anti-DNA antibodies are: the Farr assay, the Crithidia luciliae indirect immunofluorescent test, and solid-phase ELISA. The Crithidia test is the more accurate test for diagnostic screening, the Farr test is more predictive of flares, and the ELISA method is the simplest test for monitoring the SLE activity although it may give false positive results. The nucleosome is the basic structure of chromatin. It consists of pairs of the four core histones forming the histone-octamer around which 145 basis pair of DNA are wound twice. Nucleosomes are probably the major autoantigens that drive the autoimmune response in lupus. The presence of antibodies that react exclusively with the nucleosome, but not with its constituents, DNA or histones, has been reported in as many as 80 per cent of patients with lupus (Berden 1997).

Patients with SLE also develop antibodies to non-DNA-containing, soluble antigens, such as histones, Sm, ribonucleoprotein, Ro, and La. Anti-SM antibodies have been found only in SLE. All the other antibodies can be present also in other rheumatic diseases. Autoantibodies to C1q were reported to be present in lupus (Uwatoko *et al.* 1984) and lupus nephritis. Autoantibodies to endothelial cells are also frequently found in patients with SLE (D'Cruz *et al.* 1991; Perri *et al.* 1993).

Another group of antibodies is directed against negatively charged phospholipids. This group includes antibodies detectable by the anticardiolipin solid-phase assay, and/or by the prolongation of the phospholipid-dependent coagulation assays, the so-called lupus 'anti-coagulant'. Less frequently, antiphospholipid antibodies can be responsible for the false positivity of serological tests for syphilis (Cuadradao and Hughes 2001). Antiphospholipid antibodies have been shown to be directed against phospholipid-binding proteins, rather than to phospholipid themselves. Two major phospholipid-binding proteins have been identified: beta2 glycoprotein1 and prothrombin (Roubey 2000). Beta2 glycoprotein1 has been suggested to be the major target in the solid phase assay and beta2 glycoprotein1-dependent antiphospholipid antibodies assays are currently required as diagnostic tools for antiphospholipid antibodies (Roubey 2000). Antiphospholipid antibodies are found in 44–53 per cent of patients with SLE being more frequent in those with active disease (Love and Santoro 1990). However, these antibodies are not specific: they have been observed in Sjögren's syndrome, rheumatoid arthritis, systemic sclerosis, malignancy, and infectious disease, as well as in the so-called primitive antiphospholipid syndrome. Antiphospholipid antibodies may be associated with widespread arterial and venous thrombosis, neurological disorders, recurrent abortion, thrombocytopenia, haemolytic anaemia, leg ulcers, and endocardial valve disease (Levine *et al.* 2002). An association between antiphospholipid antibodies and the presence of arteriolar and glomerular capillary thrombosis at renal biopsy has also been reported (Glueck *et al.* 1985; Frampton *et al.* 1991; Farrugia *et al.* 1992).

Hypocomplementaemia

In SLE, there is an activation of the classic complement cascade with consumption of the early components C1q, C4, and C3. Serum C4 generally decreases earlier and to a greater extent than C3 in the disease exacerbations. The alternate pathway of complement can also be activated in SLE; this may account for the low C3 found in patients with congenital deficiency of C2, Clr, or Cls, which are essential components of the classical pathway. Some patients with null C4 alleles have C4 about 50 per cent all the time. The specificity of hypocomplementaemia for the diagnosis of SLE is not agreed upon. However, the presence of both low C3 and increased anti-DNA antibody titres is 100 per cent correct in predicting the diagnosis of SLE when applied to a population of patients in which that diagnosis is considered (Weinstein *et al.* 1983). Serum C3 is usually lower in patients with nephritis than in those without renal involvement. Patients with milder renal disease have higher serum C3 concentrations (Houissau *et al.* 1991).

Clinical features of lupus nephritis

Renal syndromes at presentation

Only 25–50 per cent of patients who develop lupus nephritis present with renal disease as the first manifestation (Cameron 1999). In several cases, renal involvement develops 5 or more years after the diagnosis of lupus. Arthritis and/or facial rash usually precede nephritis. The involvement of the kidneys in SLE may manifest itself clinically with virtually any possible form of presentation of renal disease.

Some patients with lupus nephritis initially show only mild urinary abnormalities such as microhaematuria, red-cell casts, or asymptomatic proteinuria. These abnormalities may be intermittent. This should be kept in mind by the physician as urine can appear 'normal' when examined sporadically. Other patients show, at onset, a frank nephrotic syndrome, or a nephritic syndrome and various degrees of renal functional impairment. More rarely, patients present with a rapidly progressive renal failure or an established chronic renal failure. These renal disorders are often associated with some other signs or symptoms of SLE and with the typical serological abnormalities. In few cases, however, glomerulonephritis is the only initial manifestation of SLE.

Acute renal failure can exceptionally represent the first manifestation of the disease. There are several possible patterns. In some patients, often with high titres of antiphospholipid antibodies, heavy glomerular involvement with widespread capillary thrombi can be found. More rarely, extensive crescents are seen at renal biopsy in anuric patients. An isolated acute interstitial nephritis may be responsible of acute renal failure in few other cases. Finally, renal vessel thrombosis can precipitate an acute renal failure both in patients with or without antiphospholipid antibodies (Cameron 2001).

Sometimes the first renal symptoms are related to an incomplete or complete renal tubular acidosis, which has been ascribed to mononuclear cell infiltration, deposition of tubular antigen–antibody complexes, or the formation of antibodies directed against the tubular basement membranes.

The clinical course of lupus nephritis

The clinical outcome of lupus nephritis is highly variable. Moreover, most patients with SLE and renal involvement are given corticosteroid and/or cytotoxic agents, which can modify the course of the disease. It is therefore difficult to assess the natural history for these patients. Bearing in mind that there are many exceptions and that transitions between groups can occur, it is possible to attempt to categorize the clinical course of lupus nephritis into the following groups.

Some patients maintain asymptomatic proteinuria and microhaematuria over a long period. In these patients, the final outcome is predominantly determined by the severity of the disease in other systems rather than by the renal disease. However, patients with clinically mild or silent renal disease may eventually develop severe kidney involvement.

In other patients, the renal involvement manifests itself with a picture of nephrotic syndrome accompanied by microhaematuria and 'telescoped' urinary sediment, with or without hypertension. The natural clinical course may be slowly progressive, with about 50 per cent of patients developing hypertension and uraemia within 10 years. The extrarenal and serological activities of SLE are usually mild to moderate in these patients.

In a third group of patients, nephrotic syndrome, haematuria, hypertension, and renal insufficiency, generally accompanied by other signs and symptoms of SLE activity, may be present from the onset or can develop early after the diagnosis of nephritis. The nephrotic syndrome and renal insufficiency can remit if adequate therapy is instituted. The disease course may be punctuated by renal and/or extrarenal flares alternating with periods of quiescence. When untreated or undertreated, most patients with such clinical features progress to endstage renal failure or die from other complications of SLE within 2 years from clinical onset (Pollak *et al.* 1964). Several parameters have been claimed to be predictive of renal relapses, including changes of antibodies to C1q (Coremans *et al.* 1995; Moroni *et al.* 2001), the appearance of urinary red blood cell/white blood cell casts (Hebert *et al.* 1995), or an increase in the antibodies against double-stranded DNA (Bootsma *et al.* 1995).

A few patients can manifest a tumultuous, progressive course with death or irreversible renal failure in spite of therapy. They show marked hypertension, papilloedema, heart failure, encephalopathy, and subacute renal failure. This clinical picture strongly suggests a severe underlying vascular involvement. Patients with SLE may also develop acute anuric renal failure, either related to an exacerbation of the disease or to the use of non-steroidal anti-inflammatory drugs. A syndrome resembling thrombotic thrombocytopenic purpura with thrombocytopenia, microangiopathic haemolytic anaemia, seizures, and renal dysfunction may also complicate the course of systemic lupus in exceptional cases. Although this syndrome more often occurs in pregnant women with lupus anticoagulant (Kincaid-Smith *et al.* 1988), it has also been observed outside pregnancy either in patients with clinically and serologically quiescent SLE or during a flare-up of the disease (Gelfand *et al.* 1985).

Pathological features of lupus nephritis

Basic lesions

Hypercellularity of the glomerular tuft is frequent. It can be segmental or global, focal or diffuse, but characteristically is almost never uniform and may vary widely from one glomerulus to another. Hypercellularity may be due to proliferation of mesangial, endothelial, and epithelial cells, and to some extent to monocytes and polymorphonuclear cell exudation. There are often areas of necrosis of the tuft, usually confined to a lobule. They are composed of granular and ill-defined material, weakly eosinophilic or staining for fibrin ('fibrinoid necrosis'). Nuclear fragments and polymorphs intermingle with this material. Proliferating epithelial cells may encircle the necrotic area and adhere to the Bowman capsule-forming crescent. In fewer than 10 per cent of cases, haematoxylin bodies can be found in the areas of necrosis or inflammation, at times in the capillary lumen. Haematoxylin bodies, the only pathognomonic lesion in the nephritis of SLE, are mainly observed in florid cases and rarely, if ever, in doubtful ones, where they might be of use. They appear on haematoxylin–eosin staining as round or oval, violet–pink, amorphous structures without a limiting membrane (Fig. 1). On ultrastructural examination they are electron-dense nuclear masses with light areas in the centre, sometimes surrounded by degenerated cytoplasm.

The presence of immune deposits in the glomeruli is the hallmark of lupus nephritis. The amount and location of deposits are closely related to the severity and pattern of glomerular changes (Dujovne *et al.* 1972). Mesangial deposits are usually present, even in patients without overt renal disease. Subepithelial and/or subendothelial deposits may be associated with these in the mesangial region. They are often irregularly distributed, and when massive, give the rigid and refractile appearance of the classic 'wire loops' to the thickened capillary wall (Fig. 1). Subepithelial deposits are usually uneven in size and distribution, in contrast to idiopathic membranous nephritis. The amount of subepithelial deposits is often inversely correlated with that of subendothelial deposits. Subendothelial deposits may be so prominent as to bulge out into the lumen forming the so-called hyaline thrombi (Fig. 1). True fibrin thrombi, although rare, may be observed at the same time as severe glomerular lesions.

Immunofluorescence invariably reveals the presence, in glomerular deposits, of strong staining for IgG, followed in intensity by IgM and IgA, although sometimes IgA may be dominant. All complement components may be found, the most usual being C3, C1q, and C4. A 'full house' of these immunoreactants is found in some 25 per cent of patients and is highly characteristic of lupus nephritis (Cameron 1989).

On electron microscopy, electron-dense deposits may appear more granular than those in other types of glomerulonephritis. In about 6 per cent of cases, a substructure with a fingerprint-like pattern can be seen (Fig. 2a). This finding, although not specific has been regarded as a sensitive marker of concomitant or subsequent development of overt lupus nephritis (Alpers *et al.* 1984). Other findings that are frequent in lupus while exceptional in other diseases are tubuloreticular inclusions resembling myxoviruses (Fig. 2b). They are mostly located within the cytoplasm of endothelial cell of glomeruli, interstitial capillary, and arterioles. Originally thought to represent viral material, they seem more probably derived from degenerative cellular changes.

Fig. 1 Diffuse proliferative lupus glomerulonephritis. Diffuse wiry appearance of the thickened capillary walls. Some loops are stuffed with inflammatory cells, while others are plugged by so-called hyaline thrombi (arrow) (Masson, 480×). Insert: haematoxylin body (arrow) (H&E, 1200×).

Classification of glomerular lesions (the WHO classification)

The World Health Organization classification remains the most commonly adopted in clinical nephrology because it is easy to learn, ready to use, and reproducible (McCluskey 1975) (Fig. 3). Over the years the original classification has been the object of different revised versions (Churg and Sobin 1982; Churg *et al.* 1995), until the 2003 classification of the International Society of Nephrology/Renal Pathology Society (Weening *et al.* 2004) (Tables 2 and 3).

Class I: normal kidney

Completely normal glomeruli not only at light microscopy but also on immunofluorescence and electron microscopy may be seen in patients with SLE (Cavallo *et al.* 1977; Mahajan *et al.* 1977; Lee *et al.* 1984; Font *et al.* 1987). This condition is almost exceptional in patients with renal manifestations. In some cases with inconstant and mild urinary abnormalities, biopsy may show normal glomeruli at light microscopy, but very scanty mesangial deposits on immunofluorescence (subgroup IB). In the recently revised classification (Weening *et al.* 2004), class I is used for mesangial accumulation of immune deposits without hypercellularity and class II for mesangial immune deposits with hypercellularity.

Class II: mesangial glomerulonephritis

This is observed in 10–30 per cent of patients depending on the criteria used as indications for renal biopsy. The changes are characterized by the presence of IgG, C3, and sometimes IgM and IgA deposits confined

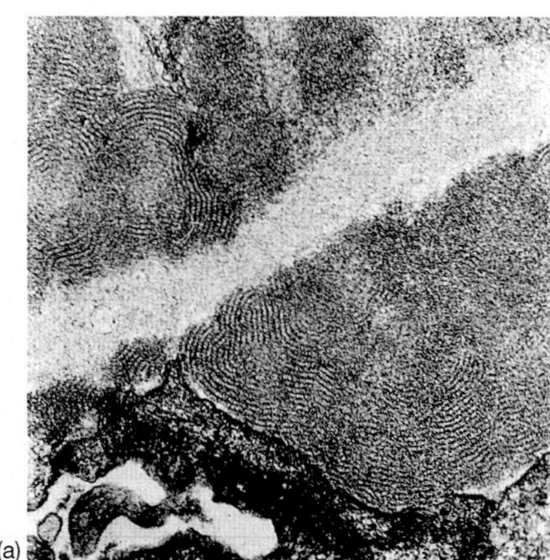
(a)

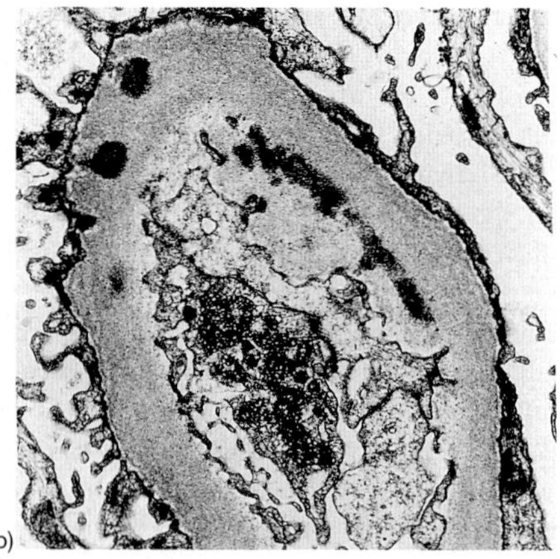
(b)

Fig. 2 (a) Fingerprint-like appearance of electron-dense subendothelial and subepithelial deposits (85,000×). (b) 'Virus-like' particles in the cytoplasm of an endothelial cell (20,000×).

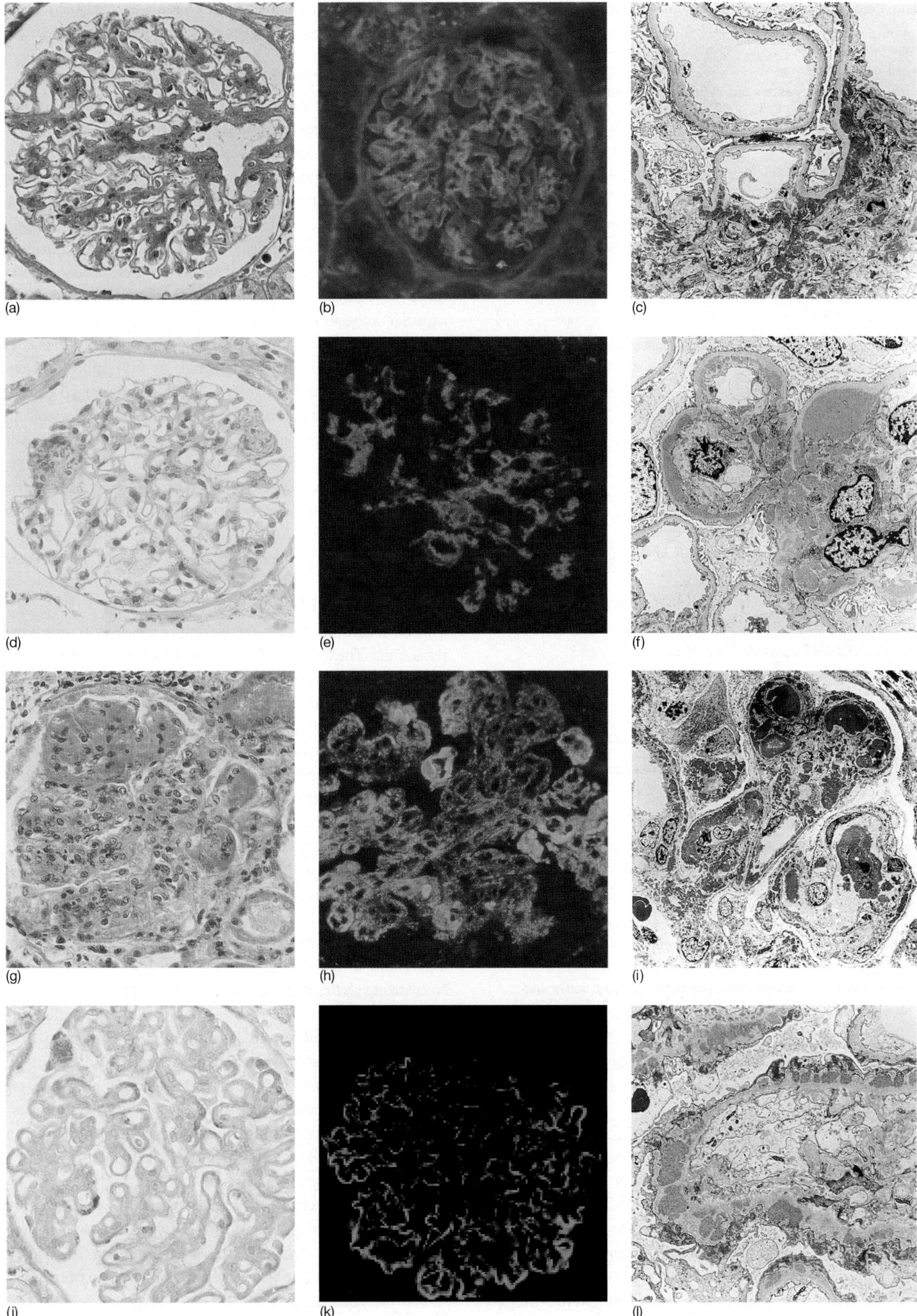

Fig. 3 Main histological patterns of the WHO classes of lupus nephritis.

Table 2 The 1995 WHO classification of lupus nephritis

I	Normal glomeruli (A) Normal by all techniques (B) Normal on light microscopy but deposits on immunohistology and/or electron microscopy
II	Pure mesangial alterations (A) Mesangial widening and or mild hypercellularity (B) Mesangial cell prolfieration
III	Focal segmental glomerulonephritis (associated with mild/moderate mesangial alterations, and/or segmental epimembranous deposits) (A) Active necrotizing lesions (B) Active and sclerosing lesions (C) Sclerosing lesions
IV	Diffuse glomerulonephritis (severe mesangial/mesangiocapillary with extensive subendothelial deposits. Mesangial deposits always present, and frequently subepithelial deposits) (A) With segmental lesions (B) With active necrotizing lesions (C) With active and sclerosing lesions (D) With sclerosing lesions
V	Diffuse membranous glomerulonephritis (A) Pure membranous glomerulonephritis (B) Associated with lesions of category II (A or B)
VI	Advanced sclerosing glomerulonephritis

Table 3 The 2003 ISN/RPS classification of lupus nephritis

I	Minimal mesangial lupus nephritis Normal glomeruli but mesangial immune deposits by immunofluorescence
II	Mesangial proliferative lupus nephritis Mesangial hypercellularity with mesangial immune deposits
III	Focal lupus nephritis Active or inactive focal, segmental, or global endo- or extracapillary glomerulonephritis involving $<50\%$ of all glomeruli. Active lesions (A), active and chronic lesions (A/C), chronic lesions (C)
IV	Diffuse lupus nephritis Active or inactive diffuse, segmental, or global endo- or extracapillary glomerulonephritis involving $\geqslant 50\%$ of all glomeruli. IV-S when $\geqslant 50\%$ of the involved glomeruli have segmental lesions. IV-G when $\geqslant 50\%$ of involved glomeruli have global lesions. Active lesions (A), active and chronic lesions (A/C), chronic lesions (C)
V	Membranous lupus nephritis Global or segmental subepithelial deposits with or without mesangial alterations. Class V may occur in combination with class III or IV or may show advanced sclerosis
VI	Advanced sclerosis lupus nephritis $\geqslant 90\%$ of glomeruli globally sclerosed

to the mesangium. This class has been subdivided into two subgroups: IIA, characterized by pure mesangial deposits on immunofluorescence without glomerular changes, and IIB in which some degree of mesangial hypercellularity is also present. Most class IIA patients do not have detectable urinary abnormalities. Conversely, the majority of class IIB patients have some abnormalities of the urinary sediment, and mild to moderate proteinuria. Nephrotic syndrome is exceptional. In these cases, diffuse glomerular podoyte changes compatible with the picture of 'minimal change disease' have been noted (Dube *et al.* 2002).

Class III: focal proliferative glomerulonephritis

Some 10–25 per cent of patients present with this form of nephritis. Glomerular changes involving not only the mesangium but also the periphery of the tuft are limited to 50 per cent or fewer of the glomeruli. At light microscopy, they are characterized by sharply delineated areas of segmental proliferation. In these areas, subendothelial immune deposits are irregularly distributed along the capillary walls. Neutrophil and mononuclear cell infiltration, foci of fibrinoid necrosis with karyorrhexis and crescent formation may be associated with proliferative lesions. Other glomeruli may show healing stages with scars, capsular adhesions, and/or global sclerosis. Mild, diffuse mesangial enlargement may accompany segmental lesions, but the capillary walls of uninvolved segments are normal. At immunofluorescence all the glomeruli appear to be involved. There are mesangial deposits of IgG, C3, and frequently also of IgM, IgA, and Clq. On electron microscopy there are subendothelial and more rarely subepithelial deposits, mainly confined to segmental proliferative lesions.

These patients generally have proteinuria and erythrocyturia. Nephrotic syndrome is present in about one-third of patients. Renal insufficiency is rare. Anti-DNA antibodies are elevated in almost all patients and in 50 per cent of the cases C3 and C4 are lowered.

Class IV: diffuse proliferative glomerulonephritis

This form accounts for 20–60 per cent of the cases in series coming from renal units. The lesions are quite similar to those of class III but differ in extension and severity. The proliferative lesions involve more than 50 per cent of glomeruli. They may have a sharp segmental distribution which forms the basis to subclassification in the 2003 classification: class IV-segmental, or may extend to most of the tuft, in a more membranoproliferative pattern, classified as class IV-global. The capillary walls are generally thickened, with a 'wire-loop' appearance caused by extensive subendothelial deposits. Segmental necrosis with leucocyte infiltration is frequent. Crescent formation may also occur. This finding is usually associated with severe renal disease. Haematoxylin bodies may occasionally be observed in these areas. A variant of class IV is the membranoproliferative form in which circumferential subendothelial extension of mesangial cells is a prominent feature, giving rise to the lobular aspect and to the double-contour appearance of the capillary loops. Necrotizing changes and crescent formation are less frequent.

Immunofluorescence studies show diffuse mesangial, subendothelial, and endomembranous staining in class IV disease. Subepithelial deposits are less abundant and are irregularly distributed. IgG and C3 are constantly found, while IgM and IgA are often present but fainter. Clq is almost universally present, brighter at times than C3. Ultrastructural study confirms the presence of numerous and often confluent mesangial and parietal deposits, which in severe cases permeate the capillary wall from side to side.

Patients with class IV disease usually have heavy proteinuria, haematuria, and 'telescoped' sediment. Many of them are hypertensive and have variable degrees of renal insufficiency. Most patients have positive anti-DNA antibodies and hypocomplementaemia.

Class V: membranous glomerulonephritis

The membranous form is observed in 10–20 per cent of patients with lupus nephritis. It shares the main histological features and staging criteria of the idiopathic form. A characteristic feature is the rather uniform thickening of capillary walls due to the presence of numerous subepithelial and intramembranous immune deposits. Immunofluorescent microscopy shows diffuse granular staining with IgG, IgM, C3, and Clq. The subclass IgG3 is prevalent in lupus, whereas IgG4 is more frequent in non-lupus membranous glomerulonephritis (Haas 1994). The presence of C4 and Clq distinguish sharply lupus from idiopathic membranous nephritis. Subepithelial deposits are usually more irregular in shape and in size than in the idiopathic form. In some patients, a diffuse mesangial expansion and proliferation, of slight or moderate entity, is present together with mesangial deposits which are usually absent in the idiopathic form. These features, together with the occasional finding of 'fingerprint' deposits, should raise the suspicion of lupus.

Moderate to severe proteinuria is the dominant urine abnormality. About two-thirds of the patients become nephrotic. Haematuria is found in about 50 per cent of the patients, while moderate renal insufficiency and hypertension are noted in some 25 per cent of cases at presentation. DNA binding is moderately elevated, whereas antinuclear antibodies may be negative.

Serum complement and C4 may be normal or slightly reduced. In some patients, membranous nephritis may occur months or even years before systemic manifestations and clear-cut immunological features of SLE develop.

Unusual lesions of lupus nephritis

Necrotizing pauci-immune lupus nephritis

Rarely a necrotizing form of glomerulonephritis with segmental cellular proliferation, but without demonstrable immune deposits, is observed in patients with lupus (Schwartz *et al.* 1983; Akhtar *et al.* 1994). Usually, serological markers of disease activity is either normal or slightly abnormal in these patients. When searched for, antineutrophil cytoplasmic antibodies were absent. Clinical information on the few cases since now reported are very limited and the long-term prognosis of these patients remain unknown.

Crescentic glomerulonephritis

Crescents are frequently noted in classes III and IV, where they are usually segmental and focal in distribution. In rare cases, epithelial proliferation is so prominent and diffuse as to give rise to the picture of severe crescentic nephritis with a rapid downhill course.

Other unusual forms of glomerulonephritis

In a few patients with lupus, mild mesangial hypercellularity with almost exclusively deposits of IgA and C3 in the mesangium have been found at biopsy (Mac-Moune Lai *et al.* 1995). As for many patients with idiopathic IgA nephropathy, renal disease may run a favourable indolent course. An unusual form of non-proliferative lupus nephritis, characterized by predominant large, ribbon-like, subendothelial IgA deposits associated with sparse subepithelial deposits of IgG and C3, has been recently reported in a patient with nephritic syndrome and a very poor renal outcome despite immunosuppressive therapy (Florquin *et al.* 2001).

Interstitial nephritis

About 60–70 per cent of patients with lupus nephritis show some degree of interstitial inflammation, tubular damage, and interstitial fibrosis. Together with inflammatory lesions, some 30–50 per cent of cases show immune deposits (mostly IgG and C3) along tubular basement membranes, into the interstitium, and along peritubular capillary and arteriolar walls (Brentjens *et al.* 1975; Park *et al.* 1986). Usually, the degree of interstitial lesions correlates with the severity of glomerular changes. On rare occasions, however, severe and predominant interstitial nephritis without glomerular involvement may cause clinical manifestations of renal disease such as tubular acidosis, salt-losing nephritis, Fanconi syndrome (Caruana *et al.* 1985), and sometimes acute renal failure (Cameron 2001). Most patients have a benign steroid-responsive course, but in some cases a progressive decline of renal function is observed (Singh *et al.* 1996).

Lupus renal vasculopathies

Lupus vasculitis

True inflammatory lesions of the arteries as observed in systemic vasculitis are exceptional in SLE; the reported incidence varies from 0 to 5 per cent.

Non-inflammatory necrotizing vasculopathy

A non-inflammatory renal microangiopathy can be observed in about 10 per cent of patients, mostly in those with diffuse proliferative nephritis (Banfi *et al.* 1991; Descombes *et al.* 1997). Although similar to the microangiopathic lesions seen in malignant hypertension or in thrombotic thrombocytopenic purpura, this vasculopathy has some distinctive features. Lesions involve arterioles and interlobular arteries. They are characterized by destruction of the endothelial layer and massive precipitation in the intima mainly of IgG, C3, but also of IgM, IgA and, in some cases, fibrin deposits; sometimes the elastic membrane is disrupted and deposits spread into the media with necrosis of the adjacent myocytes. Occlusion of the lumen with the same immunoglobulin components or sometimes with fibrin, frequently accompanies mural lesions (Fig. 4). The prominence of immunoreactants in the arteriolar and the association with glomerular hyaline thrombi precipitates indicate that the first step of these lesions is represented by the deposition of these components, which trigger thrombosis as secondary phenomenon (Bhathena *et al.* 1981; Appel *et al.* 1994). A link between this form of vasculopathy and antophospholipid antibodies, suggested in the past, has not been confirmed in more recent studies (Descombes *et al.* 1997). Surprisingly, the long-term outcome of these patients is not worse than that of those with diffuse lupus nephritis class IV (Descombes *et al.* 1997).

Thrombotic microangiopathy

The incidence of thrombotic microangiopathy varies from less than 1–8 per cent of patients with lupus nephritis (Banfi *et al.* 1991; Descombes *et al.* 1997; Huong *et al.* 1999). It may be associated with any class of lupus nephritis, and may develop independently of the activity of the systemic disease. The sudden onset of malignant hypertension may herald the occurrence of the microangiopathy. The renal prognosis is poor.

Glomerular thrombosis

Intraglomerular thrombotic lesions (Kant *et al.* 1981) isolated or associated to thrombotic microangiopathic lesions, seem to be fairly unusual and in most cases associated with the presence of antiphospholipid antibodies. In some patients these lesions may precede the onset of SLE by several years.

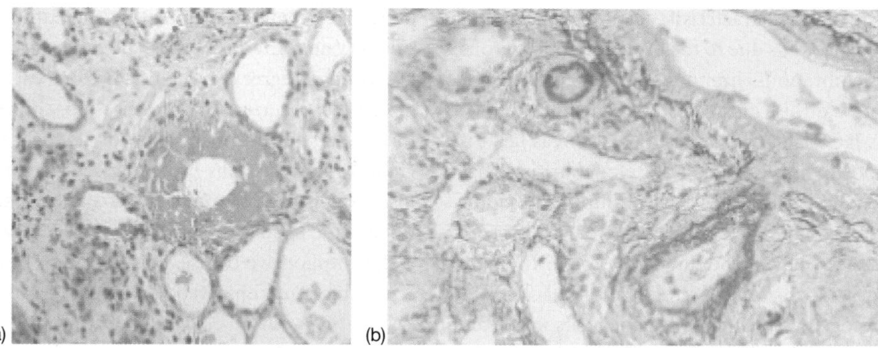

Fig. 4 Different aspects of lupus vasculitis. Left: an interlobular artery shows circumferential lumpy and massive proteinaceous deposits permeating the intima and partially extending to the media. Note the absence of cellular inflammatory reaction. Right: a small arteriole (upper left) is occluded by fibrinoid material that extends to the intima; another segment of interlobular artery (lower right) shows massive infiltration of the intima with fibrinoid material focally invading the muscular layer. Fluffy material also accumulates beneath the swollen endothelial cells (Masson, 250×).

Transformations

Transformations among forms can occur either spontaneously or as a result of treatment. The exact rate of transformation is difficult to assess because of the different criteria used for classification, the changing therapeutic attitude in the last years, and mostly the small number of patients undergoing second biopsies. Transformation from mild to severe forms has been reported more frequently than the converse. Class II may transform into class III or IV in some 15–20 per cent of cases. Baldwin (1982) regarded this event as the real occurrence of renal disease rather than as a transformation. Class III seems the most unstable form with a rate of transformation (mainly to class IV) of between 20 and 40 per cent. Transition from class V to either class III or class IV is rather unusual, being reported in some 7 per cent of cases. Classes II and IV appear to transform to class V at an even lower rate (2.5 per cent). The rarity of transformation between membranous and proliferative glomerulonephritis could suggest the existence of different pathological mechanisms in these types of nephritis.

Clinicopathological correlations

The histological form of nephritis at initial renal biopsy may help to predict the outcome. Although some patients may show a late transformation into severe forms and may eventually progress to uraemia, most patients of class II usually have an excellent prognosis even in the long term.

Much controversy exists on the validity of distinction between classes III and IV. Today, most investigators agree that involvement of under 50 per cent of glomeruli (class III) identifies patients with distinctly better kidney survival than those with more extensive lesions (class IV). The prognosis is more severe for segmental glomerulonephritis extended to more than 50 per cent of glomeruli, now classified as class IV-segmental (Weening *et al.* 2004). In the long term, these patients may have a survival rate similar (Appel *et al.* 1987) or even worse (Najafi *et al.* 2001) than that of those in class IV. This observation is in disagreement with the opinion that histopathological and clinical features of lupus nephritis follow a continuum with the prognosis being correlated simply to the proportion of injured glomeruli. Diffuse proliferative nephritis (class IV) has been considered to have an ominous prognosis, and in many series still has the worst outcome when compared to other forms. Nevertheless, some recent papers have reported a long-term survival rate of over 80 per cent in diffuse proliferative lupus nephritis, with many patients maintaining prolonged stabilization of renal function (Austin *et al.* 1986; Ponticelli 1997; Cameron 1999).

Membranous lupus nephritis may have a relatively indolent course for some years. However the few studies reporting the long-term outcome reported that some 40–50 per cent of patients either die or enter endstage renal failure within 10 years from diagnosis (Donadio 1992; Bono *et al.* 1999). The prognosis is more severe for patients with membranous nephropathy associated with proliferative or necrotic lesions in half or more glomeruli (Najafi *et al.* 2001). There is the impression, however, that adequate treatment can allow excellent renal survival even in these patients (Pasquali *et al.* 1993; Moroni *et al.* 1998).

Although there is a trend for distinctive clinical features and long-term outcome in the different histological categories, they do not represent absolute and distinct clinicopathological entities. In individual patients, the characteristic and the distribution of inflammatory lesions may have different prognostic weight in the same category of nephritis. For this reason, it is recommended that renal pathologists, through an accurate morphological description, identify the original categorization for segmental glomerulonephritis, diffuse glomerulonephritis, and mixed membranous and proliferative glomerulonephritis (Lewis *et al.* 2001). This would have practical consequences, as patients with segmental lesions involving more than 50 per cent of glomeruli, as well as patients with mixed membranous and proliferative lesions are at risk of developing renal failure and require more aggressive and prolonged therapies than usually adopted.

Though in the majority of early untreated cases the renal lesions in individual patients fall into one of the major patterns, in about 10–20 per cent mixed forms are present that cannot easily be classified. Cases that develop transformation are not rare and frequently present mixed patterns with active and sclerosing lesions. For these reasons, a modified version of the WHO classification, proposed in 1982, included subclasses with a mixed pattern (Churg and Sobin 1982). As the outcome of the class Vc (association of V and III) and Vd (association of V and IV) is comparable to that of class IV, in the 1995 WHO classification (Churg *et al.* 1995) they were included in class IV, with the disappointment of some authors (Lewis *et al.* 2001). In the most recent classification the subclassification into V a, b, c, and d has been changed into mentioning both classes when two types of involvement are diagnosed, for example class III and V or IV-S and class V (Weening *et al.* 2004).

The 'activity' and 'chronicity' indices

As first emphasized by Pollak and Pirani (1969), the predictive power of renal biopsy may be improved by a semiquantitative evaluation of findings indicating either florid or irreversible lesions. The Bethesda group has proposed the so-called chronicity and activity indices, obtained by summing the scores attributed to certain histological features. For activity index, they scored from 0 to 3 cellular proliferation, hyaline thrombi and wire loops, leucocyte infiltration, and tubulointerstitial mononuclear infiltration, while fibrinoid necrosis and cellular creascents were weighted by a factor of 2. For the chronicity index they scored from 0 to 3 glomerular sclerosis, fibrous crescents, interstitial fibrosis, and tubular atrophy. These investigators found that both indices are useful in assessing the renal prognosis in patients with diffuse lupus nephritis (Carette *et al.* 1983; Austin *et al.* 1986). The reliability of the chronicity index would be particularly important. In their experience, patients with a high chronicity index had much poorer preservation of renal function at 5 years than those with a low index. The association of a high chronicity index with a poor renal prognosis was confirmed by several studies (Parichatikanond *et al.* 1986; Rush *et al.* 1986; Appel *et al.* 1987; Esdaile *et al.* 1991; Moroni *et al.* 1999), but other investigators could not find any correlation between chronicity index and renal outcome (Magil *et al.* 1988; Schwartz *et al.* 1989). While chronicity index indicates the degree of irreversible lesions, the activity index shows the degree of florid potentially reversible lesions and is particularly useful in deciding whether a treatment should be aggressive or not.

A new morphological, index has been found to correlate better than activity and chronicity index with clinical and outcome parameters (Hill *et al.* 2000). This biopsy index comprised four elements: (a) a glomerular activity index with the addition of glomerular monocytes and elimination of interstitial inflammation, (b) a tubulointerstitial activity index which includes interstitial inflammation and excludes tubular atrophy, (c) chronic lesion index which adds glomerular scars to the standard chronicity index, and (d) immunofluorescence index, a semiquantitative index for six standard antisera, for glomerular capillary, mesangial, tubulointerstitial, and vascular elements. A better correlation with renal outcome was found when this index was evaluated in protocol biopsy performed after treatment, while it was weak at the time of biopsy performed at presentation.

Prognosis

Patient survival

A progressive improvement in the survival rate of patients with lupus nephritis has been noted in recent years. By reviewing the published literature, Cameron (1999) found that the life expectancy at 5 years increased from 44 per cent in the period 1953–1969 to 82 per cent in the period 1980–1995. Recent papers reported a 10-year survival rate of 90 per cent (Huong *et al.* 1999), the long-term prognosis being exceptionally good for those patients who had had treatment-free remission for at least one year (Drenkard *et al.* 1996). Earlier diagnosis and therapy as well as advances in specific and symptomatic treatment probably account for this better survival.

Several factors may influence the survival of patients with SLE. Epidemiological studies identified black race (Reveille *et al.* 1990), male gender (Iseki *et al.* 1994), and poor socioeconomic status (Studenski *et al.* 1987) as variables predictive of a worse outcome. There is more uncertainty about age. Some have reported a bad prognosis for children (Lévy *et al.* 1994; Berden 1997), but others did not (Cameron 1994). A benign course has been predicted for older patients (Baker *et al.* 1979), but other studies showed a negative prognostic impact of age (Reveille *et al.* 1990). The severity of underlying renal disease may also influence survival.

Lupus activity, infection, and thromboses are the most frequent causes of death in the first few years after diagnosis (Cervera *et al.* 1999). In the long term, active SLE may persist or reappear in the course of the disease, accounting for some deaths. However, late mortality is mainly due to cardiovascular disease. With improvement of survival, coronary disease leading to angina, myocardial infarction or congestive heart failure are becoming an increasing problem. Corticosteroid therapy, hypertension, nephrotic syndrome, hyperlipidaemia, and renal failure may all contribute to the development of an accelerated atherosclerosis. Circulating antiphospholipid antibodies (Font *et al.* 2001), which are frequently found in patients with SLE, can expose them to an increased risk of intracoronary thrombosis. Some 15 per cent of patients with lupus have hyperhomocysteinaemia. In these patients, there is a significant association between elevated plasma homocysteine and stroke or arterial thrombosis (Petri *et al.* 1996). On the other hand, in the long-term many patients suffer the consequences of valvular defects, which are probably caused by an often underdiagnosed verrucous endocarditis in the active stages of SLE (Moroni *et al.* 1995; Moder *et al.* 1999).

Malignancy is a less frequent cause of late mortality. Some studies reported no change in the overall cancer rate in patients with lupus but an increase in non-Hodgkin's lymphoma (Abu-Sharka *et al.* 1996; Nived *et al.* 2001) while other studies found an elevation in the overall cancer rate (Mellemkjaer *et al.* 1997; Cibere *et al.* 2001).

Kidney survival

While in the past most patients with kidney involvement died or developed endstage renal failure within a few years (Pollak *et al.* 1964), more recent series reported that more than 80 per cent of patients still retained adequate renal function 10 years after diagnosis (Iseki *et al.* 1994; Bono *et al.* 1999; Cameron 1999).

Predictors of renal failure include elevated plasma creatinine, nephrotic proteinuria, male gender, young age, Black race, and low socioeconomic status (Austin *et al.* 1994; Dooley *et al.* 1996; Berden 1997). The prognostic significance of histological lesions has already been discussed. Flares of active nephritis are associated with an increased risk of progressive renal disease (Korbet *et al.* 2000). In a study, the occurrence of a nephritic flare increased the risk of doubling the plasma creatinine of 6.8 times. The risk increased to 27 times when flares were associated with an acute elevation of plasma creatinine (Moroni *et al.* 1996). A strong association between antiphospholipid antibodies and development of chronic renal insufficiency has also been showed (Moroni *et al.* 2004).

Therapy

The main goals of therapy in lupus nephritis are (a) to control the activity of a disease which may affect many systems, (b) to prevent the progression of renal lesions, and (c) to minimize the side-effects of a treatment, which should be prolonged and often aggressive.

Unfortunately, lupus may have Protean clinical manifestations, a capricious and unpredictable course, and a different response to therapy. Moreover, all the drugs which proved to be effective in lupus have a low therapeutic index. For these reasons, treatment of lupus nephritis is one of the most difficult tasks in clinical medicine and it is not surprising that a number of different therapeutical approaches have been proposed. On the other hand, if still there is no agreement about the optimal therapeutic strategy, there is little doubt that the refinement of therapy allowed a tremendous improvement in the prognosis of the disease.

Bearing in mind that lupus is a 'systemic' disease, we will focus, in this chapter, on the treatment of renal disease. For the sake of clarity we will review the possible treatments of different clinical–pathological groups of lupus nephritis.

Mild renal lesions

Patients with minor renal abnormalities (proteinuria < 1 g/day, inactive urine sediment, normal renal function and blood pressure) and with minimal or mesangial lesions at kidney biopsy do not require specific therapy. However, their periodic clinical surveillance is mandatory to allow early diagnosis and treatment of possible transformations. While renal disease remains clinically silent, therapeutic measures should be aimed at controlling the extrarenal activity of systemic lupus. Exposure to ultraviolet light should be avoided to prevent skin lesions and reactivation of the disease. Arthralgias, arthritis, myalgias, and fever may respond to rest and salicylates in about 50 per cent of cases. Patients with SLE are, however, at risk of hepatitis and diminished renal function from salicylates, which therefore need to be used with caution. Chloroquine (250–500 mg daily) or hydroxychloroquine (200–400 mg daily) have been used successfully for the same symptoms as well as for control of cutaneous manifestations. These agents may produce dermatitis, nausea, or leucopenia in 5–10 per cent of patients. A rare but severe side-effect is retinopathy, initially characterized by small, paracentral, relative scotomas, which can progress to a bilateral, permanent abnormality of the visual field. Periodic ophthalmic evaluation is therefore needed in patients taking these drugs (Jones 1999). Non-steroidal anti-inflammatory drugs can be helpful in controlling arthralgias, myalgias, and fever. However, these agents should be handled with caution, as they may produce a deterioration in renal function through their interference with vasodilating prostaglandin production. When these measures are insufficient or contraindicated, small doses of prednisone (0.2–0.5 mg/kg body weight per day) may be used. Whenever possible corticosteroids should be given in a single dose, between 7 and 9 a.m., in order to reduce their side-effects. Large doses of corticosteroids should be reserved for severe extrarenal manifestations, namely cerebritis, carditis, pleuritis, haemolytic anaemia, leucopenia, and thrombocytopenia. The treatment of antiphospholipid syndrome is still debated. Low-dose aspirin (75 mg daily) is the first-line choice for the prevention of thrombotic complications, but patients with high levels of antiphospholipid antibodies and previous episodes of major thrombosis can require long-term, and even lifelong, warfarin or coumarin treatment. A target international ratio of 2.5 is a reasonable aim in to prevent recurrence (Greaves 1999). Recurrence of thrombosis has been reported after the withdrawal of anticoagulation (Schulman *et al.* 1998).

Focal proliferative glomerulonephritis

Whether to treat patients with focal lesions affecting only a minority of glomeruli is still controversial. If there are neither clinical nor severe histological features of disease activity, we prefer to spare powerful but toxic drugs and go on with symptomatic treatment alone. Others suggest the use of small doses of corticosteroid and/or cytotoxic agents to inhibit the immunological activity and to prevent potential transformation into more severe forms of lupus nephritis (Lee *et al.* 1984). Patients with diffuse segmental lesions, important proteinuria, elevated serum creatinine, and nephritic sediment should be treated similarly to those with diffuse proliferative lupus glomerulonephritis.

Membranous glomerulonephritis

Patients with membranous lupus nephritis, symptomless proteinuria, and stable renal function should be given only symptomatic treatment in order to control extrarenal disease. The management of patients with nephrotic syndrome is still controversial. However, it seems that prolonged treatment may reduce the risk of renal failure. Pasquali *et al.* (1993) reported the outcome for 42 patients; 26 had pure membranous nephropathy and 16 had mixed membranous and proliferative lesions. All were treated with corticosteroids and 28 were also given cytotoxic drugs. There were seven complete remissions in the pure form and only one in the mixed disease. The 10-year kidney survival rate was 100 per cent in the pure form and 83 per cent in the patients with proliferative lesions. In a retrospective study, Moroni *et al.* (1998) treated eight patients with corticosteroids alone and 11 with methylprednisolone alternated with chlorambucil for 6 months, a schedule often adopted in idiopathic membranous nephropathy (Ponticelli *et al.* 1989). The demographic characteristics of the two groups were similar. After a mean follow-up of 8 years, three patients given steroids alone and one given steroids and chlorambucil entered end stage renal failure. There were four partial remissions in the steroid group and seven complete remissions plus three partial remissions in the group given steroids and chlorambucil.

Radhakrishnan *et al.* (1994) treated 10 nephrotic patients with cyclosporin (4–6 mg/kg per day) for up to 43 months. In six patients, the proteinuria declined to less than 1 g daily; in two others it decreased to 1–2 g daily. Serum creatinine did not change during the follow-up. Control renal biopsy showed a decrease in SLE activity, but an increase in the chronicity index.

On the basis of these data, in patients with nephrotic syndrome we suggest to give corticosteroids alternated with a cytotoxic drug every other month for 6 months. This treatment may offer stable remission in responders and protection of renal function in the long-term. For patients who do not respond or have contraindications to steroids or cytotoxic drugs, administration of cyclosporin may be useful to reduce proteinuria and related complication. However, most patients show an increase of proteinuria when cyclosporin is stopped.

Diffuse proliferative and severe focal proliferative glomerulonephritis

These are the most serious forms of renal disease in SLE. Vigorous therapy is recommended when nephritic sediment, renal insufficiency, and/or nephrotic syndrome are present. There is more uncertainty about the cases of clinically silent or mild lupus nephritis; whether to treat these patients is still controversial. Probably low-dose corticosteroid and/or cytotoxic therapy is sufficient to prevent possible impairment of renal function without exposing an asymptomatic patient to the iatrogenic risks of a vigorous treatment. Aggressive approaches should be reserved for treating severe extrarenal flares or clinically active renal disease.

Several different therapeutic agents and schedules have been suggested for the management of severe lupus nephritis.

Corticosteroids

Corticosteroids are the cornerstone of the treatment of SLE, but how to give these agents in severe lupus nephritis is a matter of debate. In the early 1960s, Pollak *et al.* (1964) reported that low-dose prednisone was unable to interfere with the downhill course of diffuse proliferative lupus glomerulonephritis, while high-dose prednisone could improve the outcome, at least in some patients. Since then, many clinicians have started treatment with prednisone at doses of 1–2 mg/kg body weight per day, whenever a diagnosis of diffuse lupus nephritis is made. The doses are tapered only when renal disease and serological measures improve. This may happen only after several months in some patients, and others may continue to manifest active and progressive renal disease, which is often refractory to an increased dosage of prednisone. As a consequence, many patients treated with high-dose prednisone suffer from invalidating and even life-threatening complications. Because of the poor results in the long-term, even Pollak *et al.* (1991) suggested to limit the use of high-dose prednisone to the acute phases of lupus nephritis. In patients with less severe disease, the initial dosage of prednisone should not exceed 1 mg/kg body weight per day and should be tapered after 4–8 weeks. Patients with a good clinical response should be allocated to low-dose maintenance therapy and switched to an alternate-day regimen when possible. For patients resistant to this schedule, alternative approaches can be tried.

Today, a number of units treat diffuse lupus nephritis and renal flares with high-dose steroid 'pulses'. Intravenous pulse methylprednisolone in doses of 0.5–1 g/day is given for three or more consecutive days, followed by oral prednisone in decreasing doses. Pulse therapy may obtain rapid resolution of clinical extrarenal symptoms and a slower improvement in serological activity. Serum creatinine may rapidly decrease, particularly in patients who had rapid deterioration of their renal function, but in other cases renal function tends to improve slowly. Reduction of urinary protein excretion is also variable but usually occurs more slowly than the improvement in renal function, often after several weeks or some months (Ponticelli *et al.* 1987). There is a general impression that once remission has been achieved with methylprednisolone pulse therapy it can be maintained by low-dose prednisone, preventing most steroid-related side-effects.

In summary, in view of the need for protracted corticotherapy in most patients with SLE, schedules that maximize the therapeutic index of steroids should be preferred. These could be based upon short courses of intravenous, high-dose methylprednisolone whenever renal and extrarenal flares occur followed by moderate doses of oral prednisone. The maintenance treatment with oral prednisone should be given in a single morning dose and kept at the lowest possible dosage: it is worth pointing out that many patients with lupus nephritis can maintain stable remission with 0.2–0.5 mg/kg body weight per day oral prednisone. An alternate-day regimen may further protect from steroid toxicity. On the other hand, in patients with persisting activity of SLE, combination with a cytotoxic agent and/or further course of steroid pulse therapy may be considered.

Immunosuppressive agents

In order to reduce the doses of prednisone and to reinforce the efficacy of treatment, many investigators combined small doses of corticosteroids with immunosuppressive agents, namely cyclophosphamide and/or azathioprine. When the data of the available trials were controlled in a pooled analysis, it clearly appeared that the risk of renal death was significantly lower for patients assigned to receive immunosuppressive agents than for those given steroids alone (Felson and Anderson 1984). In 1986, Austin *et al.* (1986) reported the long-term results of a controlled trial in which patients with lupus nephritis were randomized to be given high-dose prednisone alone or moderate doses of prednisone in association with oral cyclophosphamide or with azathioprine or with azathioprine plus oral cyclophosphamide or with monthly intravenous pulses of high-dose cyclophosphamide. While there was no difference between the five groups until the fifth year, the kidney survival was significantly worse at 10 years in patients who were given corticosteroids alone than in those given intravenous cyclophosphamide. There was a trend to a better outcome for the group assigned to intravenous cyclophosphamide than for those given various types and combinations of oral immunosuppressive drugs, but this difference was marginal and not statistically significant.

The same group of the National Institutes of Health in Bethesda performed a further controlled trial. Eighty-two patients with proliferative lupus nephritis were randomly assigned to receive one of the three regimens: (a) intravenous methylprednisolone 1 g/m^2 every month for at least 12 months and up to 36 months, (b) intravenous cyclophosphamide 1 g/m^2 every month for 6 months and then once every 3 months for at least 24 months, or (c) the combination of the previous two regimens. All patients were also given moderate doses of oral prednisone (Boumpas *et al.* 1992; Gourley *et al.* 1996). After a median follow-up of 11 years, the rate of treatment failure (defined as need for supplemental immunosuppression or doubling of serum creatinine or death) was significantly lower in the cyclophosphamide and combined groups. The proportion of patients who doubled their serum creatinine was significantly lower in the combination group than in the cyclophosphamide group (Illei *et al.* 2001). There was no difference between cyclophosphamide and combined regimen in side-effects. About 31 per cent of patients developed avascular necrosis, 19 per cent osteoporosis, 48 per cent became amenorrheic, 16 per cent developed infections, another 22 per cent had herpes zooster; and five of 27 patients in the cyclophosphamide group, five of 28 in the combined group, and one of 27 in methylprednisolone group died. According to the authors, the combination therapy should be considered the treatment of choice for patients with severe disease, being more effective and equally tolerated than intravenous cyclosphosphamide.

The efficacy of intravenous cyclophosphamide has been confirmed by a number of studies and today this therapy is adopted by many physicians for treating lupus nephritis, although there is no clear evidence that this regimen is superior to schedules based on oral cyclophosphamide (Korbet *et al.* 2000). Two important advantages of intravenous over oral treatment are rarer malignancy and better compliance of the patient. On the other hand, intravenous cyclophosphamide may have some drawbacks, (a) the patient has to spend many hours at hospital to receive adequate hydration in order to prevent bladder toxicity, (b) nausea and vomiting are relatively frequent, (c) alopecia and irreversible ovarian failure are common, and (d) the use of a fixed schedule may expose some patients with milder forms of lupus nephritis to the risk of overimmunosuppression.

Individualizing therapy according to activity of the disease

Lupus is a heterogenous disease with profound inter- and intraindividual variations. There may be large differences in activity and severity among patients with diffuse proliferative nephritis; even in the same patient alternance of activity and quiescence of renal disease may be frequent. Finally, it is possible that lesions leading to chronic renal failure are the results of incompletely reversed acute injury rather than the consequence of a chronic ongoing immunological aggression (Pollak *et al.* 1991; Balow *et al.* 1996). For these reasons it might be tempting to adapt therapy to the clinical and biological conditions of the patient rather than using fixed protocols. Accordingly, the active phase of lupus nephritis should be treated aggressively while low-dose maintenance therapy should be given in the quiescent periods.

There are two main problems with such an approach. The first is to decide when an exacerbation of renal activity should be treated aggressively. As there is evidence that renal flares strongly influence the prognosis of lupus nephritis (Moroni *et al.* 1996), we give treatment whenever one of the two types of renal flare-up occur: (a) nephritic flare, defined as an increase in plasma creatinine of at least 30 per cent over the basal, associated with a nephritic sediment and generally increased proteinuria; and (b) proteinuric flare defined by a strong increase in proteinuria (>2 g per day, or doubling if proteinuria was already in a nephrotic range). A second problem is the choice of treatment. Aggressive treatments are necessary to control the renal and extrarenal activity of lupus. On the other hand, as iatrogenic side-effects may be responsible of severe morbidity and mortality, every effort should be made to improve the therapeutic index of 'induction' treatments while trying to reduce to the minimum the maintenance therapy.

The severe lupus nephritis and the flares can be treated with three intravenous methylprednisolone pulses (0.5–1 g each). After steroid pulses, oral prednisone is started in a single morning administration, at doses ranging between 0.5 and 1 mg per kg body-weight, according to the severity of the disease. Prednisone may be continued at the initial dose for 1–2 months, then may be gradually reduced to a maintenance of 10 mg per day or 20 mg every other day.

Immunosuppressive agents should be added from the beginning in case of fibrinoid necrosis or cellular crescents at renal biopsy, increase in plasma creatinine or full-blown nephrotic syndrome. Cyclophosphamide (1.5–2 mg/kg) is the preferred agent. When possible it should be given for no longer than twelve weeks because of bladder, gonadal, or oncogenic risk. Afterwards the patient may be given azathioprine (1.5–2 mg/kg), which seems to be less effective than cyclophosphamide, but better tolerated in the long-term (Ponticelli 1997; Cameron 1999).

The results with such a fexible strategy have been excellent in our experience. We followed 66 patients with diffuse proliferative nephritis for a mean period of 10 ± 6.7 years. The patient survival rate was 97 per cent at 10 years and 83 per cent at 20 years. Three patients died of cerebral haemorrhage, one of lung cancer, and one of car accident. Kidney survival, including death, was 93 per cent at 10 years and 72 per cent at 20 years (Moroni and Ponticelli 2001).

Plasma exchange

Controlled trials failed to show any favourable effect of plasma exchange in patients with diffuse lupus nephritis (Derksen *et al.* 1988; Lewis *et al.* 1992; Wallace *et al.* 1998). Although plasma exchange might be useful in controlling severe cerebritis or devastating cutaneous manifestations of SLE, its indications in lupus nephritis should be reappraised. However, this therapy might have some role in the rare cases of haemolytic–uraemic syndrome complicating SLE (Gelfand *et al.* 1985; Kincaid-Smith *et al.* 1988).

Cyclosporin

A number of small non-comparative trials with cyclosporin have been carried out in patients with lupus. Usually, there was a good response to treatment with improvement of proteinuria and a reduction in steroid use. However, proteinuria often relapsed when cyclosporin was stopped (Miescher *et al.* 1944; Noble and Wagstaff 1997). In an open prospective study (Tam *et al.* 1998) 14 patients with type IV lupus nephritis were treated with cyclosporin and prednisolone up to 4 years. A significant improvement of proteinuria and serum albumin was noted after one month. Improvement was maintained in all but three patients who showed relapse of the nephrotic syndrome under treatment. There was no modification of serum creatinine, while repeat renal biopsy at 12 months showed histological improvement with transformation to type II and reduction in activity index. Corticosteroid-sparing effects were noted. In a paediatric study, 40 children with lupus nephritis were randomized to receive cyclosporin or cyclophosphamide, plus prednisone, for 1 year. Proteinuria significantly decreased in both groups. However, children given cyclosporin had a higher mean growth rate (8.2 versus 2.7 cm/year). No change in creatinine clearance was observed (Fu *et al.* 1998).

In summary, low-dose cyclosporin could be an alternative to other immunosuppressive agents as a maintenance treatment. In most patients cyclosporin may also allow reduction of the doses of corticosteroids and of related side-effects. The initial doses should not exceed 4 mg/kg per day with the new microemulsion (Neoral), renal function and blood pressure should be monitored under treatment. Patients with impaired renal function, severe hypertension and/or diffuse interstitial fibrosis at initial biopsy are bad candidates for cyclosporin treatment.

Mycophenolate mofetil

Mycophenolate mofetil is an inhibitor of purine synthesis which is largely used in organ transplantation for the prevention and treatment of rejection. Non-controlled studies with few patients and short follow-ups, reported promising results with this agent as an alternative to cyclophosphamide (Dooley *et al.* 1999; Gaubitz *et al.* 1999). In a randomized controlled trial, Chan *et al.* (2000) assigned 42 Chinese patients with diffuse lupus nephritis to a regimen with prednisolone and mycophenolate mofetil for 12 months or to prednisolone and oral cyclophosphamide for 6 months followed by prednisolone and azathioprine for other 6 months. After one year, the improvement in proteinuria, serum albumin, and serum creatinine were similar in the two groups. Also side-effects were not significantly different. There was a non-significant trend to a greater number of complete remission in the mycophenolate group. In another prospective trial 59 patients with lupus nephritis were assigned to long-term therapy with intravenous cyclophosphamide or to short-term therapy with intravenous cyclophosphamide followed by maintenance therapy with mycophenolate mofetil or azathioprine. The 72-month renal survival including death was 85 per cent for the group given mycophenolate mofetil, 74 per cent for azathioprine group, and 43 per cent for the group treated with intravenous cyclophosphamide (Contreras *et al.* 2004).

Clearly, further studies with larger number of patients and longer follow-up are required to better assess the role of mycophenolate mofetil in lupus nephritis, but even today this drug may represent a promising alternative option to the available drugs.

Intravenous immunoglobulins

Anedoctal cases of improvement of lupus nephritis with high-dose intravenous immunoglobulins have been reported. In a pilot study, the administration of intravenous immunoglobulins to five patients for 18 months was found to be a promising alternative to intravenous cyclophosphamide (Boletis *et al.* 1999).

Ablative therapy with stem cell reconstitution

Ablative chemotherapy with high-dose intravenous cyclophosphamide, methylprednisolone, and antithymocyte globulins may provide a window of time free of memory-T cell influence, so that the maturation of new lymphocyte progenitors would occur without recruitment to anti-self reactivity. The infusion of peripheral stem cells (either autologous or haploidentical) may reconstitute the recipient bone marrow. Autologous haematopoietic stem cell infusion after intense immunosuppression could maintain seven patients with severe disease free from active lupus with no immunosuppression or small doses of prednisone after a mean follow-up of 25 months (Traynor *et al.* 2000). However, another group reported one case of relapse of lupus out of three patients who received high-dose chemotherapy and haematopoietic stem-cell transplantation (Rosen *et al.* 2001).

Synopsis

Several options are available today for the treatment of patients with diffuse proliferative lupus nephritis. In choosing the therapeutic strategy, the clinician should remember that aggressive treatment is needed in patients with high clinical or histological activity in order to prevent irreversible deterioration of renal function, and that in most patients therapy should be continued for years or even decades in order to control the activity of SLE. Some physicians face these problems by following fixed therapeutic regimens drawn from protocols originally studied for controlled trials. This choice has the advantage of using an extensively investigated therapy, of which the benefits and the side-effects are well recognized. The potential disadvantage of fixed schedules is unnecessary overtreatment in patients with milder disease. Others prefer a more flexible strategy based on short courses of vigorous therapy during flares of the disease and on low-dose treatment during quiescent phases. This choice may be biased by the subjectivity of the clinician but can allow better modulation of therapy accordingly to the activity of SLE.

Among the fixed schedules, that of monthly intravenous pulse cyclophosphamide, combined with intravenous methylprednisolone in the more severe cases, seems to be safer and more effective than others. Monthly cyclophosphamide (and methylprednisone when necessary) pulses should be continued for 6 months. Then pulses should be given every 3 months until a remission of lupus nephritis has been sustained for 1 year. Patients should also receive moderate doses of oral prednisone every day or every other day (Balow *et al.* 1996). The long-term risks of such prolonged treatment have been already described.

The flexible strategies are usually based on a course of three intravenous pulses of methylprednisolone of 0.5–1 g each at the diagnosis of diffuse lupus nephritis. The course is repeated whenever severe renal or extrarenal exacerbations occur. After pulse therapy, oral prednisone is given in a single morning dose of 0.5–1 mg/kg per day and progressively tapered to the lowest dose possible. Oral cyclophosphamide, 1–2 mg/kg per day, for 2–3 months, followed by azathioprine, 1.5–2 mg/kg per day, if prolonged treatment is foreseen, are added in patients with more active disease. As an alternative treatment, it is possible to replace azathioprine with cyclosporin which can exert an important antiproteinuric effect and may allow a further reduction of steroid doses. Another alternative may be represented by mycophenolate mofetil which may replace cyclophosphamide, so preventing the toxicity related to excessive cumulative doses. In patients showing a long-lasting remission under low-dose treatment, a careful attempt of completely stopping any specific therapy may be done. Although ablative therapy with stem cell reconstitution is a promising approach, it should be limited to few selected cases, due to the risks of morbidity and mortality.

Is it possible to stop treatment in diffuse lupus nephritis?

Since protracted therapy with corticosteroids or cytotoxic agents may expose the patient to the risk of disabling or even life-threatening complications, it is important to know whether and when therapy can eventually be stopped in patients with diffuse proliferative lupus nephritis. In our experience, we stopped treatment in 27 patients with previous diffuse proliferative lupus nephritis. Most of them were in complete renal remission when treatment was stopped. After treatment was withdrawn, 12 patients did not show any sign of relapse after a mean follow-up of 142 months. The other 15 patients had a flare-up of activity which needed to restart therapy. At the last visit, 10 of the 15 patients were in complete remission and five had proteinuria lower than 1 g per day. The only difference between the two groups was the mean period of therapy between beginning and stopping treatment. It was 67 months in patients who did not relapse and 27 months in those who relapsed (Ponticelli and Moroni 2000).

Thus, in patients with stable renal function and minimal or absent proteinuria, a cautious trial of stopping treatment may be done. We suggest to try to stop treatment only in patients showing an inactive disease for at least 3 years, to taper off therapy very slowly, and to monitor carefully the clinical and the renal status of the patient. Obviously, in case of a flare of renal or extrarenal activity treatment should be started as soon as possible.

Endstage renal disease

Dialysis

Even during dialysis treatment, patients with SLE maintain the characteristics of a variable and erratic disease. Many patients, usually those who had slowly progressive renal dysfunction and inactive disease before dialysis, are easy to manage, show decreased clinical and serological activity, and have a life expectancy similar to that of dialysis patients with disorders other than SLE (Nossent *et al.* 1990; Mojcik and Klippel 1996). Another subset of patients, more often those who reached dialysis after a rapidly progressive course, maintain clinical and serological activity. Many of them die shortly after starting dialysis, but 10–28 per cent may recover renal function and discontinue dialysis (Cheigh and Stenzel 1993) either spontaneously or after methylprednisolone therapy. The choice of therapy in these instances is critical. Aggressive treatment might favour a recovery of renal function in a consistent proportion of patients and might prevent deaths from active lupus. On the other hand, uraemia increases the risks of iatrogenic complications, particularly infection and bone marrow suppression. There are no rules that may substitute for clinical practice in these difficult instances.

After the first few months, patients generally do well whether they are treated with haemodialysis or peritoneal dialysis. Clinical and serological manifestations of SLE improve, probably as a result of the reduction in immune responsiveness induced by uraemia and corticosteroid as well as cytotoxic agents, can be completely stopped. Rehabilitation is excellent, and many patients return to normal physical activity. However, some patients may manifest clinical flares, including fever, rash, myalgias, serositis, cerebritis, and haematological abnormalities, usually associated with serological activity. These patients require maintenance prednisone therapy, which exposes them to increased risks of infection and atherogenesis. Exceptionally the clinical activity is particularly severe and refractory to corticosteroids.

No specific dialysis-related problems have been reported in patients with SLE. Since *in vitro* studies suggested that recombinant erythropoietin might augment immune response (Grimm *et al.* 1990; Kimata *et al.* 1991), one might have some concern that the drug can reactivate SLE. However, a clinical study found no evidence that recombinant erythropoietin increases autoimmunity in patients with SLE (Hebert *et al.* 1994). There is some increased risk of fistula thrombosis in patients with high-titre anticardiolipin antibodies. More frequent peritonitis may also be expected in heavily immunosuppressed patients on peritoneal dialysis (Huang *et al.* 2001).

Renal transplantation

Some studies reported that patient and graft survival rates of patients with lupus nephritis are similar to those of patients with other primary renal diseases (Clark and Jevnikar 1999; Alarcon-Segovia 2000; Ward 2000), while others found a lower graft survival rate in lupus patients (Stone 1998). The variations in the outcome of allografts may depend on differences in criteria of acceptance for transplantation, type of immunosuppression, and composition of the control group. Lupus nephritis may recur in 3–9 per cent (Mojcik and Klippel 1996; Stone 1998) although a report found recurrence in 30 per cent of cases (Goral *et al.* 2003). The histological picture usually is not severe. It can include mesangial, focal proliferative and only exceptionally diffuse proliferative glomerulonephritis (Moroni *et al.* 2003). However, the major post-transplant problems are not caused by recurrence but by extrarenal complications related either to disease itself or to previous steroid or immunosuppressive therapy. As a matter of fact, even before transplant, many patients with lupus are affected by complications such as hyperlipidaemia, hypoalbuminaemia, arterial hypertension, and hyperhomocysteinaemia, which can expose to severe cardiovascular disease after transplantation. Most patients received long-term corticosteroid therapy which not only exposes to cardiovascular complications, but may also cause diabetes, osteoporosis, infection, myopathy, and cataracts. The prolonged use of immunosuppressive drugs before transplantation may expose to an increased risk of infections and malignancy, which is further increased by the continuous post-transplant immunosuppression.

Thus, it may be advisable, to postpone transplantation by at least 1 year after entry to dialysis to allow a 'wash-out' of previous corticosteroid and cytotoxic therapy in a patient who has been, and will be, immunosuppressed for years. This strategy may also allow to see whether a patient may have a late reversal of renal failure, which is a rare but possible event.

Lupus remains inactive in the majority of renal transplant recipients (Nossent *et al.* 1992). Serological parameters appear to be unreliable markers of outcome or recurrence. The rate of graft loss and the number of rejection episodes are similar in patients with and without anticardiolipin antibodies. However, antiphospholipid antibody-positive patients are particularly exposed to thrombotic complications and may require prophylactic anticoagulation (McIntyre *et al.* 2001).

A completely different issue concerns the possibility of transplanting the kidneys of a donor affected by lupus nephritis. Lipkowitz *et al.* (2000) reported the outcomes for two patients who received the kidneys fom a cadaveric donor with a histological class II–V lupus nephritis. Complete resolution of electron dense and immunofluorescent deposits was seen at repeat biopsies in the recipients. At 3 years after transplantation, both the recipients showed normal renal function and urinalysis.

References

Abu-Sharka, M., Gladmann, D. D., and Urowitz, M. B. (1996). Malignancy in systemic lupus erythematosus. *Arthritis and Rheumatism* **6**, 1050–1054.

Akhtar, M., Al Dalaan, A., and El Ramahi, K. M. (1994). Pauci-immune necrotizing lupus nephritis: report of two cases. *American Journal of Kidney Diseases* **23**, 320–325.

Alarcon-Segovia, D. (2000). Kidney transplantation is a safe therapeutic tool in systemic lupus erythematosus. *Clinical Experimental Rheumatology* **18**, 185–186.

Alpers, C. E., Hopper, J., Jr., Bernstein, M. J., and Biava, C. G. (1984). Late development of systemic lupus erythematosus in patients with glomerular 'finger-print' deposits. *Annals of Internal Medicine* **100**, 66–68.

Appel, G. B. *et al.* (1987). Long-term follow-up of patients with lupus nephritis. *American Journal of Medicine* **83**, 877–885.

Appel, G. B., Pirani, C. L., and D'Agati, V. (1994). Renal vascular complications of systemic lupus erythematosus. *Journal of the American Society of Nephrology* **4**, 1499–1515.

Arbuckle, M. R. *et al.* (2003). Development of autoantibodies before the clinical onset of systemic lupus erythematosus. *New England Journal of Medicine* **349**, 1526–1533.

Austin, H. A., III *et al.* (1986). Therapy of lupus nephritis: controlled trial of prednisone and cytotoxic drugs. *New England Journal of Medicine* **314**, 614–619.

Austin, H. A., III, Boumpas, D. T., Vaughan, E. M., and Balow, J. E. (1994). Predicting renal outcomes in severe lupus nephritis: contributions of clinical and histologic data. *Kidney International* **45**, 544–550.

Baker, S. B., Rovira, J. R., Campion, E. W., and Mills, J. A. (1979). Late onset of systemic lupus erythematosus. *American Journal of Medicine* **66**, 727–732.

Baldwin, D. S. (1982). Clinical useful of the morphology classification of lupus nephropathy. *American Journal of Kidney Diseases* **2**, 142–149.

Balow, J. E., Boumpas, D. T., Fessler, B. J., and Austin, H. A. (1996). Management of lupus nephritis. *Kidney International* **49** (Suppl. 53), 88–92.

Banfi, G. *et al.* (1991). Renal vascular lesions as a marker of poor prognosis in patients with lupus nephritis. *American Journal of Kidney Diseases* **18**, 240–248.

Berden, J. H. M. (1997). Lupus nephritis. *Kidney International* **52**, 538–558.

Bhathena, D. B., Sobel, B. J., and Migdal, S. D. (1981). Noninflammatory renal microangiopathy of systemic lupus erythematosus (lupus vasculitis). *American Journal of Nephrology* **1**, 144–159.

Boletis, J. N., Ioannidis, J. P. A., Boki, K. A., and Moutsopoulos, H. M. (1999). Intravenous immunoglobulin compared with cyclophosphamide for proliferative lupus nephritis. *Lancet* **ii**, 569–570.

Bono, I., Cameron, J. S., and Hicks, J. A. (1999). The very long-term prognosis and complications of lupus nephritis and its treatment. *Quarterly Journal of Medicine* **92**, 211–218.

Bootsma, H. *et al.* (1995). Prevention of relapses in systemic lupus erythematosus. *Lancet* **345**, 1595–1599.

Boumpas, D. T. *et al.* (1992). Controlled trial of pulse methylprednisolone with two regimens of pulse cyclophosphamide in severe lupus nephritis. *Lancet* **ii**, 41–45.

Brentjens, J. R. *et al.* (1975). Interstitial immune complex nephritis in patients with systemic lupus erythematosus. *Kidney International* **7**, 342–350.

Buck, A. C., Serebro, L. H., and Quinet, R. J. (2001). Subacute abdominal pain requiring hospitalization in a systemic lupus erythematosus patient: a retrospective analysis and review of the literature. *Lupus* **10**, 491–495.

Cameron, J. S. (1989). The treatment of lupus nephritis. *Pediatric Nephrology* **3**, 350–362.

Cameron, J. S. (1994). Lupus nephritis in childhood and adolescence. *Pediatric Nephrology* **8**, 230–249.

Cameron, J. S. (1999). Lupus nephritis. *Journal of American Society of Nephrology* **10**, 413–424.

Cameron, J. S. Clinical manifestations of lupus nephritis. In *Rheumatology and the Kidney* (ed. D. Adu, P. Emery, and M. Madaio), pp. 16–32. Oxford: Oxford University Press, 2001.

Carette, S. *et al.* (1983). Controlled studies of oral immunosuppressive drugs in lupus nephritis. *Annals of Internal Medicine* **99**, 1–8.

Caruana, R. J., Barish, C. F., and Buckalew, V. M. (1985). Complete distal renal tubular acidosis in systemic lupus: clinical and laboratory findings. *American Journal of Kidney Diseases* **6**, 59–63.

Cavallo, T., Cameron, W. R., and Lapenas, D. (1977). Immunopathology of early and clinically silent lupus nephropathy. *American Journal of Pathology* **87**, 1–15.

Cervera, R. *et al.* (1999). Morbidity and mortality in systemic lupus erythematosus during a 5-year period. *Medicine* **78**, 167–175.

Chan, T. M. *et al.* (2000). Efficacy of mycophenolate mofetil in patients with diffuse proliferative lupus nephritis. *New England Journal of Medicine* **343**, 1156–1162.

Cheigh, J. S. and Stenzel, K. H. (1993). End-stage renal disease in systemic lupus erythematosus. *American Journal of Kidney Diseases* **21**, 2–8.

Churg, J. and Sobin, L. H. Lupus nephritis. In *Renal Disease* (ed. J. Churg and L. H. Sobin), pp. 127–131. Tokyo: Igaku-Shoin, 1982.

Churg, J., Dernstein, J., and Glassock, R. J. *Classification and Atlas of Glomerular Diseases* 2nd edn., pp. 151–156. Tokyo, New York: Igakou-Shoin, 1995.

Cibere, J., Sibley, J., and Haga, M. (2001). Systemic lupus erythematosus and the risk of malignancy. *Lupus* **10**, 394–400.

Clark, W. F. and Jevnikar, A. M. (1999). Renal transplantation for end stage renal disease caused by systemic lupus erythematosus. *Seminars of Nephrology* **19**, 77–85.

Cohen, A. S. *et al.* (1971). Preliminary criteria for the classification of systemic lupus erythematosus. *Bulletin of Rheumatic Diseases* **21**, 643–648.

Contreras, G. *et al.* (2004). Sequential therapies for proliferative lupus nephritis. *New England Journal of Medicine* **350**, 971–980.

Coremans, I. E. M. *et al.* (1995). Changes in antibodies to C1q predict renal relapses in systemic lupus erythematosus. *American Journal of Kidney Diseases* **26**, 595–601.

Cuadradao, M. J. and Hughes, G. R. V. (2001). Hughes (antiphospholipid) syndrome: clinical features. *Rheumatological Diseases Clinics of North America* **27**, 507–524.

D'Cruz, D. P. *et al.* (1991). Antibodies to endothelial cells in systemic lupus erythematosus: a potential marker for nephritis and vasculitis. *Clinical and Experimental Immunology* **85**, 254–261.

Derksen, R. H. *et al.* (1988). Prospective multicentre trial on the short-term effects of plasma exchange versus cytotoxic drugs in steroid-resistant lupus nephritis. *Netherlands Journal of Medicine* **33**, 168–177.

Descombes, E. *et al.* (1997). Renal vascular lesions in lupus nephritis. *Medicine* **76**, 355–368.

Donadio, J. V. (1992). Treatment of membranous nephropathy in systemic lupus erythematosus. *Nephrology, Dialysis, Transplantation* **7** (Suppl. 1), 97–104.

Donders, R. C. *et al.* (1998). Transient monocular blindness and antiphospholipid antibodies in systemic lupus erythematosus. *Neurology* **51**, 535–540.

Dooley, M. A., Hogan, S., Jennette, C., and Falk, R. for the Glomerular Disease Collaborative Network (1996). Cyclophosphamide therapy for lupus nephritis. *Kidney International* **51**, 1188–1195.

Dooley, M. A. *et al.* (1999). Mycophenolate mofetil therapy in lupus nephritis: clinical observations. *Journal of American Society of Nephrology* **10**, 833–839.

Drenkard, C. *et al.* (1996). Remission of systemic lupus erythematosus. *Medicine* **75**, 88–98.

Dube, K. C. *et al.* (2002). Minimal change disease and systemic lupus erythematosus. *Clinical Nephrology* **190**, 104–109.

Dujovne, I., Pollak, V. E., Pirani, C. L., and Dillan, M. C. (1972). The distribution and character of glomerular deposits in systemic lupus erythematosus. *Kidney International* **2**, 33–50.

Esdaile, J. M. *et al.* (1991). Predictors of one year outcome in lupus nephritis: the importance of renal biopsy. *Quarterly Journal of Medicine* **81**, 907–918.

Farrugia, E. *et al.* (1992). Lupus anticoagulant in systemic lupus erythematosus: a clinical and renal pathological study. *American Journal of Kidney Diseases* **20**, 463–471.

Felson, D. T. and Anderson, J. (1984). Evidence for the superiority of immunosuppressive drugs and prednisone over prednisone alone in lupus nephritis. *New England Journal of Medicine* **311**, 1528–1533.

Florquin, S. *et al.* (2001). Severe non-proliferative lupus nephritis with predominant sub-endothelial IgA deposits. *Nephrology, Dialysis, Transplantation* **16**, 1479–1482.

Font, J., Torras, A., Cervera, R., Darnell, A., Revert, L., and Ingelmo, M. (1987). Silent renal disease in systemic lupus erythematosus. *Clinical Nephrology* **27**, 79–84.

Font, J. *et al.* (2001). Cardiovascular risk factors and the long-term outcome of lupus nephritis. *Quarterly Journal of Medicine* **94**, 19–26.

Frampton, G., Hicks, J., and Cameron, J. S. (1991). Significance of antiphospholipid antibodies in patients with lupus nephritis. *Kidney International* **39**, 1225–1231.

Fu, L. W., Yang, L. Y., Chen, W. P., and Lin, C. Y. (1998). Clinical efficacy of cyclosporin A Neoral in the treatment of paediatric lupus nephritis with heavy proteinuria. *British Journal of Rheumatology* **37**, 217–221.

Gaubitz, M. *et al.* (1999). Mycophenolate mofetil for the treatment of systemic lupus erythematosus: an open pilot trial. *Lupus* **8**, 731–736.

Gelfand, J. *et al.* (1985). Thrombotic thrombocytopenic purpura syndrome in systemic lupus erythematosus: treatment with plasma infusion. *American Journal of Kidney Diseases* **6**, 154–160.

Gilboe, I. M., Kvien, T. K., Uhlig, T., Husby, G. (2001). Sicca syndrome and secondary Sjoegren's syndrome in systemic lupus erythematosus: comparison with rheumatoid arthritis and correlation with disease variables. *Annals of Rheumatic Diseases* **12**, 1103–1109.

Glueck, H. I. *et al.* (1985). Thrombosis in systemic lupus erythematosus: relationship with the presence of circulating anticoagulants. *Archives of Internal Medicine* **1450**, 1389–1395.

Goral, S. *et al.* (2003). Recurrent lupus nephritis in renal transplant recipients revisited: it is not rare. *Transplantation* **75**, 651–656.

Gourley, M. F. *et al.* (1996). Methylprednisolone and cyclophosphamide alone or in combination in patients with lupus nephritis. A randomized controlled trial. *Annals of Internal Medicine* **125**, 549–557.

Greaves, M. (1999). Antiphospholipid antibodies and thrombosis. *Lancet* **353**, 1348–1353.

Grimm, P. C. *et al.* (1990). Effects of recombinant human erythropoietin on HLA sensitization and cell mediated immunity. *Kidney International* **38**, 12–18.

Haas, M. (1994). IgG subclass deposits in glomeruli of lupus and non-lupus membranous nephropathies. *American Journal of Kidney Diseases* **23**, 358–364.

Hahn, B. H. (1998). Antibodies to DNA. *New England Journal of Medicine* **338**, 1359–1368.

Hebert, L. A. *et al.* (1994). Effect of recombinant erythropoietin therapy on autoimmunity in systemic lupus erythematosus. *American Journal of Kidney Diseases* **24**, 25–32.

Hebert, L. A. *et al.* (1995). Relationship between appearances of urinary red blood cell/white blood cell casts and the onset of renal relapse in systemic lupus erythematosus. *American Journal of Kidney Diseases* **26**, 432–438.

Hill, G. *et al.* (2000). A new morphologic index for the evaluation of renal biopsies in lupus nephritis. *Kidney International* **58**, 1160–1173.

Hochberg, M. C. (1997a). The epidemiology of systemic lupus erythematosus. In *Dubois' Lupus Erythematosus* 5th edn. (ed. D. J. Wallace and B. H. Hahn), pp. 49–68. Baltimore: Williams and Wilkins, 1997a.

Hochberg, M. C. (1997b). Updating the American College of Rheumatology Revised Criteria for the classification of systemic lupus erythematosus. *Arthritis and Rheumatism* **40**, 1725.

Houissau, F. A., D'Cruz, D., Vianna, J., and Hughes, G. R. (1991). Lupus nephritis: the significance of serological tests at the time of biopsy. *Clinical and Experimental Rheumatology* **9**, 345–349.

Huang, J. W. *et al.* (2001). Systemic lupus erythematosus and peritoneal dialysis. Outcomes and infections complications. *Peritoneal Dialysis International* **21**, 143–148.

Huong, D. L. T. *et al.* (1999). Renal involvement in systemic lupus erythematosus. *Medicine* **78**, 148–166.

Illei, G. G. *et al.* (2001). Combination therapy with pulse cyclophosphamide plus pulse methylprednisolone improves long-term renal outcome without adding toxicity in patients with lupus nephritis. *Annals of Internal Medicine* **135**, 248–257.

Iseki, K. *et al.* (1994). An epidemiologic analysis of end-stage lupus nephritis. *American Journal of Kidney Diseases* **23**, 547–554.

Jones, S. K. (1999). Ocular toxicity and hydroxychloroquine: guidelines for screening. *British Journal of Dermatology* **140**, 3–7.

Johnson, A. E., Gordon, C., Palmer, R. G., and Bacon, P. A. (1995). The prevalence and incidence of systemic lupus erythematosus in Birmingham, England: relationship to ethnicity and country of birth. *Arthritis and Rheumatism* **38**, 551–558.

Kant, K. S., Pollak, V. E., Weiss, M. A., Glueck, H. I., Miller, M. A., and Hess, E. V. (1981). Glomerular thrombosis in systemic lupus erythematosus: prevalence and significance. *Medicine* **60**, 71–86.

Khan, S., Haddad, P., Montague, L., and Summerton, C. (2000). Systemic lupus erythematosus presenting as mania. *Acta Psychiatrica Scandinavica* **101**, 406–408.

Kimata, H., Yoshida, A., Ishioka, C., and Mikawa, H. (1991). Erythropoietin enhances immunoglobulin production and proliferation by human plasma cells in a serum-free medium. *Clinical Immunology and Immunopathology* **59**, 495–501.

Kincaid-Smith, P., Fairley, K. F., and Kloss, M. (1988). Lupus anticoagulant associated with renal thrombotic microangiopathy and pregnancy-related renal failure. *Quarterly Journal of Medicine* **69**, 795–815.

Korbet, S. M. *et al.* (2000). Factors predictive of outcome in severe lupus nephritis. Lupus Nephritis Collaborative Group. *American Journal of Kidney Diseases* **35**, 904–914.

Lee, H. S. *et al.* (1984). Course of renal pathology in patients with systemic lupus erythematosus. *American Journal of Medicine* **77**, 612–622.

Leehey, D. J. *et al.* (1982). Silent diffuse lupus nephritis: long-term follow-up. *American Journal of Kidney Diseases* **2** (Suppl.), 188–196.

Levine, J. S., Branch, D. W., and Rauch, J. (2002). The antiphospholipid syndrome. *The New England Journal of Medicine* **346**, 752–763.

Lévy, M., Montes de Oca, M., and Claude-Babron, M. (1994). Unfavourable outcomes (end-stage renal failure/death) in childhood onset systemic lupus erythematosus: a multicenter study in Paris and its environs. *Clinical Experimental Rheumatology* **12** (Suppl. 10), S63–S68.

Lewis, E. J., Hunsicker, L. G., Lan, S. P., Rhode, R. D., and Lachin, J. M. (1992). A controlled trial of plasmapheresis therapy in severe lupus nephritis. *New England Journal of Medicine* **326**, 1373–1379.

Lewis, E. J., Schwartz, M. M., and Korbet, S. M. (2001). Severe lupus nephritis: importance of re-evaluating the histologic classification and the approach to patient care. *Journal of Nephrology* **14**, 223–227.

Lipkowitz, G. S. *et al.* (2000). Transplantation and 2-year follow-up of kidneys procured from a cadaver donor with a history of lupus nephritis. *Transplantation* **69**, 1221–1224.

Love, P. E. and Santoro, S. A. (1990). Antiphospholipid antibodies: anticardiolipin and the lupus anticoagulant in systemic lupus erythematosus (SLE) and in non SLE disorders. *Annals of Internal Medicine* **112**, 682–698.

Mac-Moune Lai, F. *et al.* (1995). IgA nephropathy: a rare lesion in systemic lupus erythematosus. *Modern Pathology* **8**, 5–10.

Magil, A. B. *et al.* (1988). Prognostic factors in diffuse proliferative lupus glomerulonephritis. *Kidney International* **34**, 511–517.

Mahajan, S. K. *et al.* (1977). Lupus nephropathy without clinical renal involvement. *Medicine* **54**, 493–501.

Manzi, S. (2001). Epidemiology of systemic lupus erythematosus. *American Journal of Management and Care* **7** (Suppl. 16), S474–S479.

McCarthy, D. J. *et al.* (1995). Incidence of systemic lupus erythematosus: race and gender differences. *Arthritis and Rheumatism* **38**, 1260–1270.

McCluskey, R. T. Lupus nephritis I. In *Kidney Pathology Decennial 1966–1975* (ed. S. C. Sommers), pp. 435–460. New York: Appleton Century Crofts, 1975.

McIntyre, J. A. *et al.* (2001). Antiophospholipid antibodies: risk assessments for solid organ, bone marrow and tissue transplantation. *Rheumatic Disease Clinical of North America* **27**, 611–632.

Mellemkjaer, L. *et al.* (1997). Non-Hodgkin's lymphoma and other camcers among a cohort of patients with systemic lupus erythematosus. *Arthritis and Rheumatism* **40**, 761–768.

Miescher, P. A., Fauvre, H., Lemoine, R., and Huang, Y. P. (1994). Drug combination therapy of systemic lupus erythematosus. *Springer Seminars of Immunopathology* **16**, 295–304.

Moder, K. G. *et al.* (1999). Cardiac involvement in systemic lupus erythematosus. *Mayo Clinic Proceedings* **74**, 275–284.

Mojcik, C. F. and Klippel, J. H. (1996). End-stage renal disease and systemic lupus erythematosus. *American Journal of Medicine* **101**, 100–107.

Moroni, G. and Ponticelli, C. Lupus nephritis: treatment with continuous therapies. In *Rheumatology and the Kidney* (ed. D. Adu, P. Emery, and M. P. Madaio), pp. 93–107. Oxford: Oxford University Press, 2001.

Moroni, G. *et al.* (1995). Cardiologic abnormalities in patients with long-term lupus nephritis. *Clinical Nephrology* **43**, 20–28.

Moroni, G. *et al.* (1996). Nephritis flares, are predictors of bad long-term outcome in lupus nephritis. *Kidney International* **50**, 2047–2053.

Moroni, G. *et al.* (1998). Treatment of membranous lupus nephritis. *American Journal of Kidney Diseases* **31**, 681–686.

Moroni, G. *et al.* (1999). Clinical and prognostic value of serial renal biopsies in lupus nephritis. *American Journal of Kidney Diseases* **34**, 530–539.

Moroni, G. *et al.* (2001). Anti-C1q antibodies may help in diagnosing a renal flare in lupus nephritis. *American Journal of Kidney Diseases* **37**, 490–498.

Moroni, G., Tantardini, F., and Ponticelli, C. (2003). Renal replacement therapy in lupus nephritis. *Journal of Nephrology* **16**, 787–791.

Moroni, G. *et al.* (2004). Antiphospholipid antibodies are associated with an increased risk for chronic renal insufficiency in patients with lupus nephritis. *American Journal of Kidney Diseases* **43**, 28–36.

Najafi, C. C. *et al.* (2001). Significance of histologic patterns of glomerular injury upon long-term prognosis in severe lupus glomerulonephritis. *Kidney International* **59**, 2156–2163.

Neuwelt, C. M. *et al.* (1995). Role of intravenous cyclophosphamide in the treatment of severe neuropsychiatric systemic lupus erythematosus. *American Journal of Medicine* **98**, 32–41.

Nived, O. *et al.* (2001). Malignancies during follow-up in an epidemiologically defined systemic lupus erythematosus inception cohort in southern. *Sweden-Lupus* **10**, 500–504.

Noble, S. and Wagstaff, A. J. (1997). Cyclosporin—a review of its pharmacology and clinical potential in the treatment of systemic lupus erythematosus. *BioDrugs* **7**, 483–501.

Nossent, H. C., Bronsveld, W., and Swaak, A. J. (1989). Systemic lupus erythematosus. III. Observations on clinical renal involvement and follow up of renal function: duct experience with 110 patients studied prospectively. *Annals of Rheumatic Diseases*, **48**, 810–816.

Nossent, J. C., Swaak, A. J. G., Berden, J. H. M. (1990). Systemic lupus erythematosus. Analysis of disease activity in 55 patients with end stage renal failure treated with hemodialysis or continuous peritoneal dialysis. *American Journal of Medicine* **89**, 169–174.

Nossent, J. C., Swaak, T. J., and Berden, J. H. (1992). Systemic lupus erythematosus after renal transplantation: patient and graft survival and disease activity. *Annals of Internal Medicine* **114**, 183–188.

Ostensen, M. and Villiger, P. M. (2001). Nonsteroidal anti-inflammatory drugs in systemic lupus erythematosus. *Lupus* **10**, 135–139.

Parichatinond, P. *et al.* (1986). Lupus nephritis: clinic pathological studies in 162 cases in Thailand. *Journal of Clinical Pathology* **39**, 160–166.

Park, M. H., D'Agati, V., Appel, G. B., and Pirani, C. L. (1986). Tubulointerstitial disease in lupus nephritis: relationship to immune deposits, interstitial inflammation, glomerular changes, renal function and prognosis. *Nephron* **44**, 309–319.

Pasquali, S. *et al.* (1993). Lupus membranous nephropathy: long-term outcome. *Clinical Nephrology* **39**, 175–182.

Perri, G. J. *et al.* (1993). Antiendothelial cell antibodies in lupus: correlations with renal injury and circulating markers of endothelial damage. *Quarterly Journal of Medicine* **86**, 727–734.

Petri, M. *et al.* (1996). Plasma homocysteine as a risk factor for atherothrombotic events in systemic lupus erythematosus. *Lancet* **ii**, 1120–1124.

Pollak, V. E. and Pirani, C. L. (1969). Renal histologic findings in systemic lupus erythematosus. *Mayo Clinic Proceedings* **44**, 630–644.

Pollak, V. E., Pirani, C. L., and Schwartz, F. D. (1964). The natural history of the renal manifestations of systemic lupus erythematosus. *Journal of Laboratory and Clinical Medicine* **63**, 537–550.

Pollak, V. E., Kant, K. S., and Hariharan, S. (1991). Diffuse and focal proliferative lupus nephritis: treatment approaches and results. *Nephron* **59**, 177–193.

Ponticelli, C. (1997). Treatment of lupus nephritis—the advantages of a flexible approach. *Nephrology, Dialysis, Transplantation* **12**, 2057–2059.

Ponticelli, C. and Moroni, G. (2000). Lupus nephritis. *Journal of Nephrology* **13**, 385–399.

Ponticelli, C., Zucchelli, P., Moroni, G., Cagnoli, L., Banfi, G., and Pasquali, S. (1987). Long-term prognosis of diffuse lupus nephritis. *Clinical Nephrology* **28**, 263–271.

Ponticelli, C. *et al.* (1989). A randomized trial of methylprednisolone and chlorambucil in idiopathic membranous nephropathy. *New England Journal of Medicine* **320**, 8–13.

Radhakrishnan, J., Kunis, C. L., D'Agati, V., and Appel, G. B. (1994). Cyclosporine treatment of lupus membranous nephropathy. *Clinical Nephrology* **42**, 147–154.

Rahman, P., Gladman, D. D., and Urowitz, M. B. (1998). Clinical predictors of fetal outcome in systemic lupus erythematosus. *Journal of Rheumatology* **25**, 1526–1530.

Reveille, J. D., Bartolucci, A., and Alarcon, G. S. (1990). Prognosis in systemic lupus erythematosus. Negative impact of increasing age at onset. Black race and thrombocytopenia as well as causes of death. *Arthritis and Rheumatism* **33**, 37–48.

Roldan, C. A., Shively, B. K., and Crawford, M. H. (1996). An echocardiographic study of valvular heart disease associated with systemic lupus erythematosus. *New England Journal of Medicine* **335**, 1424–1430.

Roman, M. J. *et al.* (2003). Prevalence and correlates of accelerated atherosclerosis in systemic lupus erythematosus. *New England Journal of Medicine* **25**, 2399–2406.

Rosen, O. *et al.* (2001). Relapse of systemic lupus erythematosus. *Lancet* **i**, 807–808.

Roubey, R. A. (2000). Antiphospholipid syndrome: antibodies and antigens. *Current Opinion in Hematology* **7**, 316–320.

Rush, P. J., Banmal, R., Shore, A., Balfe, J. W., and Schreiber, M. (1986). Correlation of renal histology with outcome in children with lupus nephritis. *Kidney International* **29**, 1060–1071.

Schulman, S., Svenungsson, E., and Granavist, S. (1998). Anticardiolipin antibodies predict early recurrence of thromboembolism and death among patients with venous thrombolism following anticoagulant therapy. *American Journal of Medicine* **104**, 332–333.

Schwartz, M. M., Roberts, J. L., and Lewis, E. J. (1983). Necrotizing glomerulitis of systemic lupus erythematosus. *Human Pathology* **14**, 158–167.

Schwartz, M. M. *et al.* (1989). Predictive value of renal pathology in diffuse proliferative lupus glomerulonephritis. *Kidney International* **36**, 831–896.

Singh, I. A. K., Ucci, A., and Madias, N. E. (1996). Predominant tubulointerstitial lupus nephritis. *American journal of Kidney Diseases* **27**, 273–278.

Sontheimer, R. D. and Provost, T. T. Cutaneous manifestation of lupus erythematosus. In *Dubois' Lupus Erythematosus* 5th edn. (ed. D. J. Wallace and B. H. Hahn), pp. 569–623. Baltimore: Williams and Wilkins, 1997.

Stone, J. H. (1998). End-stage renal disease in lupus: disease activity, dialysis and the outcome of transplantation. *Lupus* **7**, 654–659.

Studenski, S. *et al.* (1987). Survival in systemic lupus erythematosus. *Arthritis and Rheumatism* **30**, 1326–1332.

Tam, L. S. *et al.* (1998). Long-term treatment of lupus nephritis with cyclosporin A. *Quarterly Journal of Medicine* **91**, 573–580.

Tan, E. M. *et al.* (1982). The 1982 revised criteria for the classification of systemic lupus erythematosus. *Arthritis and Rheumatism* **25**, 1271–1277.

Tanaka, E. *et al.* (2002). Pulmonary hypertension in systemic lupus erythematosus: evaluation of clinical characteristics and response to immunosuppressive therapy. *Journal of Rheumatology* **29**, 282–287.

Ter Borg, E. J. *et al.* (1990). Measurement of increases in anti-double stranded DNA antibody levels as a predictor of disease exacerbation in systemic lupus erythematosus. *Arthritis and Rheumatism* **33**, 634–643.

Toubi, E., Khamashata, M. A., Panarra, A., and Hughes, G. R. V. (1995). Association of antiphospholipid antibodies with central nervous system disease in systemic lupus erythematosus. *American Journal of Medicine* **99**, 397–401.

Traynor, A. E. *et al.* (2000). Treatment of severe systemic lupus erythematosus with high-dose chemotherapy and haemopoietic stem-cell transplantation: a phase I study. *Lancet* **ii**, 701–707.

Tzioufas, A. G., Kokon, S. I., Petrovas, C. I., and Moutsopoulos, H. M. (1997). Autoantibodies to human recombinant erythropoietin in patients with systemic lupus erythematosus. *Arthritis and Rheumatism* **40**, 2212–2216.

Uramoto, K. M. *et al.* (1999). Trends in the incidence and mortality of systemic lupus erythematosus 1950–1992. *Arthritis and Rheumatism* **42**, 46–50.

Uwatoko, S. *et al.* (1984). Characterization of C1q-binding IgG complexes in systemic lupus erythematosus. *Clinical Immunology Immunopathology* **30**, 104–116.

Voss, A., Green, A., and Junker, P. (1998). Systemic lupus erythematosus in Denmark: clinical and epidemiological characterization of a county-based cohort. *Scandinavian Journal of Rheumatology* **27**, 98–105.

Wallace, D. J. and Metzger, A. L. Systemiclupus erythematosus and the nervous system. In *Dubois' Lupus Erythematosus* 5th edn. (ed. D. J. Wallace and B. H. Hahn), pp. 723–754. Baltimore: Williams and Wilkins, 1997.

Wallace, D. J., Hahn, B. H., and Klippel, J. H. Lupus nephritis. In *Dubois' Lupus Erythematosus* 5th edn. (ed. D. J. Wallace and B. H. Hahn), pp. 1053–1065. Baltimore: Williams and Wilkins, 1997.

Wallace, D. J. *et al.* (1998). Randomized controlled trila of pulse/synchonization cyclophosphamide/apheresis for proliferative lupus nephritis. *Journal of Clinical Apheresis* **13**, 163–166.

Ward, M. M. (2000). Outcomes of renal transplantation among patients with end-stage renal disease caused by lupus nephritis. *Kidney International* **57**, 2136–2143.

Weening, J. J. *et al.* (2004). The classification of glomerulonephritis in systemic lupus erythematosus revisited. *Journal of the American Society of Nephrology* **15**, 241–250.

Weinstein, A. *et al.* (1983). Antibodies to native DNA and serum complement (C3) levels. *American Journal of Medicine* **74**, 206–216.

Yanase, K. *et al.* (1997). Receptor-mediated cellular entry of nuclear localizing anti-DNA antibodies via myosin 1. *Journal of Clinical Investigation* **100**, 25–31.

Zack, D. J. *et al.* (1996). Mechanisms of cellular penetration and nuclear localization of an anti-double strand DNA autoantibody. *Journal of Immunology* **157**, 2082–2088.

Zeng, D. *et al.* (2000). Cutting edge: a role for CD1 in the pathogenesis of lupus in NZB/NZW mice. *Journal of Immunology* **164**, 5000–5004.

4.8 The patient with scleroderma—systemic sclerosis

Carol M. Black and Christopher P. Denton

Background

Systemic sclerosis (SSc) is an autoimmune rheumatic disease characterized by organ-based fibrosis. A number of different renal pathologies occur in SSc and these are considered in this chapter, although the major emphasis will be on the clinical features, management, and pathology of the typical scleroderma renal crisis (SRC). Although complicating a minority (around 5–10 per cent overall) of cases, this remains one of the most important and immediately life-threatening of complications of SSc. It is however, also a treatable complication, and one for which management might be further improved by better physician and patient education and earlier diagnosis.

Recent figures of prevalence of clinically significant renal disease attributable to SSc from our own unit are given in Table 1. It is likely, however, that less extensive or severe involvement is much more frequent. This is evident from early autopsy series, as well as from imaging and functional assessments of renal function and perfusion in unselected SSc patients. The renal manifestations of SSc emphasize the vascular pathology of the disease although there is also clear evidence that inflammatory and fibrotic processes occur and contribute. Interestingly, another vascular complication that is now recognized in up to 15 per cent of SSc cases is pulmonary arterial hypertension. The histological features of these two manifestations are remarkably similar, although in the pulmonary circulation the changes appear to occur over a longer time than in renal crisis and effects on the haemodynamics are likely to be more direct with obliteration of pulmonary vasculature, in contrast to SRC, in which systemic hypertension probably reflects secondary systemic changes in vascular tone in part due to renal haemodynamic changes.

Table 1 Prevalence of scleroderma renal disease

Subset	Number of cases	Renal SSc (%)
LcSSc	497	1.6
DcSSc	256	12.4
Overall	753	5.3

Patients attending Royal Free Rheumatology Unit, 1990–2000, fulfilling ACR preliminary criteria for SSc.

Diagnosis

Systemic sclerosis is clinical diagnosis for which serological and other investigations are confirmatory. Thorough systematic investigation of new cases is appropriate to determine the pattern and extent of internal organ involvement. This should include renal assessment by urinalysis (see Chapter 1.2), serum biochemistry, and an estimation of glomerular filtration rate (see Chapter 1.4). Important causes for renal involvement in SSc are summarized in Table 2.

In early diffuse scleroderma clinical features may be non-specific, and a high level of suspicion in the early oedematous phase of the disease is vital, bearing in mind that clinical differentiation between rheumatoid arthritis, dermatomyositis, scleroderma, or an overlap syndrome with features of more than one of these diagnoses can be extremely difficult. The subsequent development of firm, taut, hide-bound skin proximal to the metacarpophalangeal joints permits a definite diagnosis of SSc in over 90 per cent of patients (Masi *et al.* 1980).

Classification of scleroderma subsets

Clinical descriptions over the past 100 years have identified a spectrum of sclerodermatous disease that varies widely in severity and extent from single patches of hard skin (morphoea) of no more than cosmetic importance, to life-threatening systemic illness (LeRoy 1985). In its localized form, although the skin shows a marked inflammatory and fibrotic reaction in general, there are no systemic features (Jablonska and Lovell 1988). The most widely used classification of scleroderma-spectrum disorders is shown in Table 3. The two-subset model divides the disease into limited cutaneous systemic sclerosis (lcSSc) and diffuse cutaneous systemic sclerosis (dcSSc) (LeRoy *et al.* 1988; Table 4). Over 60 per cent of SSc patients fall into the subset lcSSc, where visceral involvement is a late event and tends to occur 10–30 years after the onset of Raynaud's phenomenom. The term lcSSc is preferable to CREST because cutaneous manifestations often extend beyond sclerodactyly and calcinosis may be present only late or radiologically. dcSSc has a much more rapid onset, with organ failure often present within 5 years of the first symptoms. In the diffuse form of the disease skin involvement extends widely over the limbs and trunk, whereas in lcSSc involvement is generally confined to the extremities, face, and neck. Other clinical manifestations also vary between these different forms of disease, for example, vascular abnormalities such as telangiectasia and Raynaud's phenomenon are often more prominent in lcSSc, whereas severe renal involvement or pulmonary fibrosis are typically seen in the dcSSc. Some of the features of the two major subsets of SSc

Table 2 Renal pathology in systemic sclerosis

Manifestation	Comments
Scleroderma renal crisis	Accelerated phase hypertension, otherwise unexplained progressive renal impairment, microangiopathic anaemia, end-organ damage including encephalopathy and flash pulmonary oedema. See main text for detailed description
Chronic scleroderma nephropathy	Interstitial renal fibrosis. Possible microvasculopathy. Clinically manifests as reduced glomerular filtration rate with out active urinary sediment or other underlying pathology. Prevalence unknown
Overlap glomerulonephritis	Primarily glomerular process with proliferative and/or membranous changes. Clinically may present with haematuria, proteinuria, renal impairment, or hypertension. Associated with serological evidence of vasculitis (ANCA—often atypical and rarely anti-PR3 specific) or lupus (anti-U1RNP, anti-Ro, anti-dsDNA). Biopsy series suggests that up to 20% of SSc patients developing acute progressive renal failure may fall into this category, emphasizing the importance of renal biopsy in management of these cases
Drug toxicity	Nephrotoxic agents including cyclosporin and NSAIDs may cause renal impairment. Some evidence that drugs may precipitate SRC (high-dose corticosteroids or cyclosporin). D-Penicillamine now rarely used in SSc but renal toxicity well recognized
Renovascular disease	Macrovascular disease reported to have increased prevalence in SSc. Incidental renovascular disease may contribute to hypertension and ACEI treatment can be hazardous. Ultrasound assessment of renal size essential if clinical suspicion and nuclear renal perfusion scan or arteriography may be necessary

Table 3 Spectrum of scleroderma and scleroderma-like syndromes

Raynaud's phenomenon	Primary Raynaud's Secondary Raynaud's
Scleroderma—localized	Morphoea (plaque, guttate, generalized) Linear *En coup de sabre*
Scleroderma—systemic	Limited cutaneous systemic sclerosis Diffuse cutaneous systemic sclerosis Scleroderma sine scleroderma
Chemically induced	Environmental/occupational
Scleroderma-like diseases	Metabolic Immunological/inflammatory Localized systemic sclerosis and visceral diseases

Table 4 Subsets of scleroderma (systemic sclerosis)

'Prescleroderma'
Raynaud's phenomenon plus nailfold capillary changes, disease-specific circulating antinuclear autoantibodies [antitopoisomerase-1, anticentromere (ACA), or nucleolar], and digital ischaemic changes
Diffuse cutaneous SSc (dcSSc)
Onset of skin changes within 1 year of onset of Raynaud's phenomenon
Truncal and acral skin involvement
Presence of tendon friction rubs
Early and significant incidence of interstitial lung disease, oliguric renal failure, diffuse gastrointestinal disease, and myocardial involvement
Nailfold capillary dilatation and drop out
Antitopoisomerase-1 (Scl-70) antibodies (30% of patients)
Limited cutaneous SSc (lcSSc)
Raynaud's phenomenon for years (occasionally decades)
Skin involvement limited to hands, face, feet, and forearms (acral)
A significant (10–15%) late incidence of pulmonary hypertension, with or without interstitial lung disease, skin calcification, telangiectasiae, and gastrointestinal involvement
A high incidence of ACA (70–80%)
Dilated nailfold capillary loops, usually without capillary dropout
Scleroderma sine scleroderma
Raynaud's phenomenon +/−
No skin involvement
Presentation with pulmonary fibrosis, scleroderma renal crisis, cardiac or gastrointestinal disease
Antinuclear antibodies may be present (Scl70, ACA, nucleolar)

are shown in Fig. 1(a–c). Also, the clinical course of lcSSc is generally more protracted than dcSSc, often with Raynaud's symptoms preceding skin disease by many years, although pathological hallmarks of tissue fibrosis, immunological abnormalities, and endothelial cell activation and damage are common to both subsets (Fleischmajer 1977). Some of the autoantibodies occurring in SSc are specific for different disease subsets (see Table 5), for example, antitopoisomerase-1 (scl-70) and anti-RNA polymerase (anti-RNAP) antibodies are typically associated with dcSSc. In contrast, anticentromere antibody occurs in lcSSc (Bona and Rothfield 1994).

A suggestion has been put forward recently that the classification of SSc should be broadened to include patients who have Raynaud's phenomenon and a hallmark antibody abnormality of SSc such as antitopoisomerase-1, anti-RNAPI or -III, or anticentromere antibody. This implies that such individuals progress to SSc. Others suggest classification as SSc only if additional clinical features are present. Thus, the terms 'prescleroderma' and 'limited systemic sclerosis' have been proposed. It seems appropriate that some patients with mild limited disease be included, and these patients are missed if the American College of Rheumatology (ACR) preliminary classification criteria are rigidly applied. Many of the experts originally involved in this classification would now favour broader inclusivity. In addition, these criteria do not take account of hallmark SSc antibodies and modern investigative techniques such as high resolution CT scanning of the chest to ascertain interstitial lung involvement. Nevertheless, the term

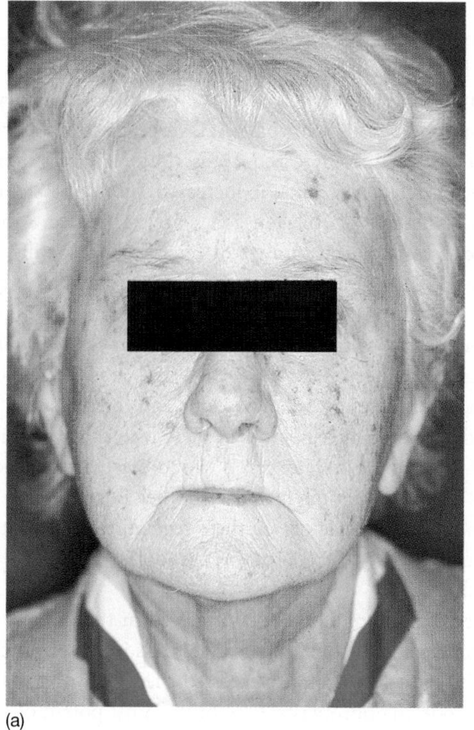

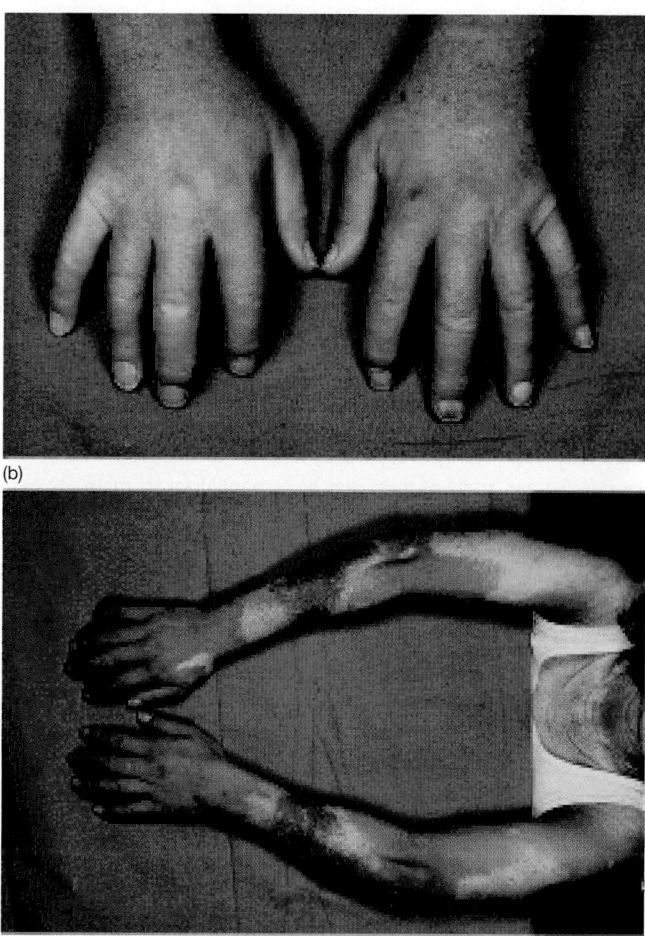

(a) (b) (c)

Fig. 1 Cutaneous features of scleroderma. The typical facial (a) and hand (b) changes associated with the limited form of scleroderma are shown. Telangiectasia are widespread but skin sclerosis is confined to the fingers and face. In contrast, the changes in skin texture are much more widespread in diffuse scleroderma and are often accompanied in dark skin by altered pigmentation (c).

Table 5 Autoantibodies in systemic sclerosis with clinical associations

Autoantibody specificity	Frequency (%)	Disease subset
ANA	70	Diffuse, speckled pattern. Non-specific
ACA	30	Associated with limited cutaneous subset of SSc (CREST variant)
Antitopoisomerase-1	20	Associated with diffuse cutaneous subset, and with increased frequency of lung fibrosis in both dcSSc and lcSSc
Anti-RNA polymerase	15	Associated with poor prognosis dcSSc, for RNAP I and III mutually exclusive from antitopoisomerase-1. High incidence of renal involvement
Anti-PM-Scl	4	Associated with systemic sclerosis–polymyositis overlap
Antifibrillarin	5	Poor outcome in the context of dcSSc. Renal, cardiac, and pulmonary vascular disease. Myositis
Anti-snU1-RNP	5–10%	Overlap features of lupus, arthritis, or myositis
Anti-Th/To	<5%	Not mutually exclusive. Identifies a poor prognosis subgroup of lcSSc

'autoimmune Raynaud's phenomenon' is probably valid and appropriate for patients with isolated Raynaud's phenomenon and an antinuclear autoantibody. Around 10 per cent of such cases appear to progress to a defined connective tissue disease, which suggests that a substantial number do not, making the terms 'prescleroderma' and 'limited systemic sclerosis' unsatisfactory.

Epidemiology of systemic sclerosis

Scleroderma is an uncommon disorder and virtually all of the descriptive epidemiology is derived from retrospective or prospective reviews of patients attending hospitals or institutions serving a defined denominator population: there is only one true population-based study (Maricq *et al.* 1989). Although there are apparently different disease frequencies between populations, some of these may be accounted for by methodological factors. Interestingly, although the prevalence in the United Kingdom was previously estimated in a large West Midlands population as several-fold lower than in Maricq's study, other reports observe a higher frequency, in line with that in North America and Australia. Currently, the best estimate for UK prevalence overall is approximately 120 per million of the population. Its relative rarity suggests that the genetic and/or environmental exposures necessary for disease susceptibility occur infrequently in the population. Scleroderma has a female excess (4F : 1M overall, and in the child-bearing years 15F : 1M). A number of geographical clusters have been reported. Clustering has been described close to international airports in the United Kingdom (Silman 1995), with a variety of autoimmune rheumatic diseases in the Republic of Georgia (Freni-Titulaer *et al.* 1989), and a clearer cluster of SSc in a region of Italy close to Rome (Valesini *et al.* 1993). In North America, a high prevalence has been observed in one population of Choctaw native Americans in Oklahoma. There is growing evidence for a genetic basis for this high prevalence and on-going studies are defining this in detail.

Aetiology and pathogenesis of systemic sclerosis

The pathogenesis of SSc is likely to be complex and multifactorial, since the heterogeneous nature of SSc implies variability in pathogenic mechanisms. The relative contribution of genetic and environmental factors is unclear. Three inter-related processes are involved: immunological activation, vascular damage, and fibrosis.

Fibrosis

Excess deposition of collagen and extracellular matrix protein in the skin and internal organs of patients with SSc was first demonstrated histopathologically many years ago, and this was confirmed by physical and biochemical means. Subsequently, techniques for culturing fibroblasts have provided valuable insight into the mechanisms involved in the synthesis of extracellular matrix components. The observation that skin fibroblasts from SSc synthesize increased quantities of fibronectin, proteoglycan core proteins, and particularly collagens types I and III and to a lesser degree IV and VI was inferred from *ex vivo* studies of skin biopsies, but the intriguing finding that this phenotype of matrix overproduction persists in tissue culture and could be passed on at cell division has provided a paradigm for the mechanisms underlying the development of fibrosis secondary to vascular and immunological perturbation. Overproduction of type I collagen is a reflection of increased transcriptional activation of the two pro(I)collagen genes and of increased transcript stability. Transcriptional regulation of collagen genes has itself been a major area of biological study and a number of important cis-acting regulatory regions and factors interacting with these regions have been identified. More recent studies have implicated several ubiquitous transcription factors in collagen gene activation in SSc fibroblasts including the heterotrimeric factor CBF, the GC-sequence binding protein Sp1, and most recently Smad proteins and their coactivators. It seems likely that upstream regulators of these factors are disturbed in SSc and that this leads to greater levels or more active phosphorylated forms of the transcription factors. Another possibility is that genetic differences in these factors or their regulation contribute to severity or susceptibility to scleroderma, as part of the polygenic background to this disease.

Profibrotic cytokines are likely to be involved in the initiation of fibrosis in scleroderma and constitutive alterations in the production of some growth factors or responsiveness to their actions has been observed in scleroderma fibroblasts. One of the most potent of these is connective tissue growth factor, and a body of evidence now suggests that this could be an important autocrine factor in the maintenance of the scleroderma fibroblast phenotype. Modern molecular genetic methods are now being applied to understanding scleroderma, as for other diseases. This includes approaches such as high-density genetic marker maps being used in pedigree and association studies to identify disease-associated loci, and especially the application of methods for parallel assessment of protein and gene expression. Different studies have identified various genes, including established candidates already suggested by linkage studies and novel factors such as protease nexin-1 and CTGF.

Vascular lesions

The most prevalent clinical manifestation of vascular abnormality is Raynaud's phenomenon, which is present in over 95 per cent of SSc patients. The pathological features of vascular damage, immune cell activation, and fibrosis are closely linked in scleroderma. In both localized and generalized disease many histological features are often shared, but the remainder of this discussion will focus on SSc. Detailed studies suggest that in both the skin and internal organs one of the earliest features is endothelial cell injury, initially at the ultrastructural level, and that this is temporally and spatially associated with activation of perivascular fibroblasts and subsequent deposition of increased amounts of structurally normal extracellular matrix components.

Many factors may be important in the vascular damage but it is the endothelial cell that is thought to have a pivotal role. The endothelium is now known to produce numerous molecules and to regulate many aspects of vascular stability including control of vascular tone, permeability, thrombotic potential, and leucocyte trafficking (Pearson 1990; Kahaleh and Mattuci-Cerinic 1995). Markers of endothelial cell activation have consistently been found to be elevated in SSc, especially in association with renal involvement (Denton *et al.* 1995;

Stratton *et al.* 1998). There is considerable evidence that endothelial cell activation and damage are early events in lesional and prelesional tissues, but their importance in initiating or sustaining abnormalities in other cell types remains uncertain.

Immunolopathology

Immunogenetics

There are several lines of evidence indicating familial or genetic predisposition to SSc. Although rare, there are familial clusters of SSc and related diseases, particularly Raynaud's phenomenon. As one of the primary roles of MHC class II molecules is the presentation of processed antigen to the T-cell receptor on helper T-lymphocytes resulting in an antigen-specific immune response, autoantibody subsets in scleroderma might be expected to show correlations with class II MHC polymorphism and indeed they do, although again, they appear to be complex. Anticentromere antibody was initially reported to be associated with HLA-DR5 (-DR11), -DR4 (-D13 subtypes), -DR1, and -DR8. These findings appear to reflect linkage disequilibrium of *HLA-DR5* (*-DR11*) and many *HLA-DR4* (*-D13* subtypes) with *HLA-DQ7*, and *-DR1* with *-DQ5*. These HLA-DR specificities share no unique amino acid sequences, which raised the possibility that another linked gene might be more highly correlated with this antibody response. In a study, oligotyping showed that the anticentromere antibody response was most closely associated with *HLA-DQB1* alleles in linkage disequilibrium with *HLA-DR1, -DR4, -DR5* (*-DR11*), and *-DR8*. These *HLA-DQB1* alleles had in common a polar tyrosine or a glycine at position 26 of the outermost domain of the HLA-DQB molecule, as opposed to a hydrophobic leucine residue. In a British study (Briggs *et al.* 1993), implication of the *HLA-DQB1* locus was inferred, as virtually all of the anticentromere antibody-positive patients had either HLA-DR1 or -DR4. However, McHugh *et al.* (1994) have indicated that, although at least one *HLA-DQB1* allele not coding at position 26 of the first domain appears necessary, it may not be sufficient for the generation of anticentromere antibody. Reveille and colleagues have also extended the known associations of antitopoisomerase antibodies with HLA-DR5, -DR2, and -DR52a to include four *HLA-DQB1* alleles. Japanese workers have found a similar allele association (Kuwana *et al.* 1994). Recently, in a mixed UK population, association with topoisomerase-1 has been linked to HLA-DPB1*1301 (Gilchrist *et al.* 2001).

Important racial and ethnic differences in the frequencies of these autoantibodies have been described, with Western Europeans and North American Whites having a significantly higher frequency of anticentromere autoantibodies and a lower frequency of antitopoisomerase-1 than American Blacks, Choctaw native Americans, Thai, and Italians. Particular forms of the disease may not be so strongly influenced by gender. For example, certain chemically induced SSc-like disorders tend to be associated with males, partly due to an occupational bias. There are some MHC associations with the environmentally induced cases, for example, toxic oil syndrome is characterized by a raised incidence of HLA-DR4, while vinyl chloride-induced disease is primarily associated with HLA-DR5, HLA-DR3 being a marker of severity. Although there has been much speculation about a possible association of silicone-containing cosmetic prostheses and the development of connective tissue disease, several well-conducted studies and reviews have failed to show any statistically significant association between these and SSc. Hochberg (1994) has carefully reviewed the epidemiological aspects of the literature and has reasonably concluded that none of the available studies has demonstrated a statistical association between augmentation mammoplasty with silicone gel-filled prostheses and scleroderma or other autoimmune rheumatic disorders.

Immune dysfunction and autoantibodies

There is considerable evidence for T-cell activation in SSc, including an increased ratio of circulating CD4+ : CD8+ cells, reflecting an increased number of CD4+ and/or a reduced number of CD8+ lymphocytes. A particular role for $\gamma\delta$ T-cells has been suggested and others have reported increased numbers of lymphokine-activated killer and natural killer cells in blood samples from patients with SSc. Furthermore, several studies have found increased soluble interleukin-2 receptor in scleroderma, sometimes appearing to correlate with disease activity (Kahaleh 1991). Support for the possibility that activated T-cells are important in pathogenesis is provided by the presence of infiltrates of CD3+, CD4+, CD450+, interleukin-2-producing, HLA-DR-positive+, leucocyte function-associated antigen-1-positive+, a/β T-cells in lesional tissues (Prescott *et al.* 1992).

More than 95 per cent of SSc patients have detectable antinuclear antibodies when HEp-2 cell lines are used as the detection tissue (Table 5). Characteristic staining patterns for antinuclear antibodies within the nuclear and subnuclear structures are relatively specific and can be confirmed by more sophisticated tests. A diffusely grainy pattern of staining is associated with the presence of antibodies to topoisomerase-1 (Scl-70), the major DNA uncoiling enzyme. An anticentromere staining pattern occurs in up to 80 per cent of patients with the limited form of SSc. Antigens recognized by positive sera have been identified as CENP-A, CENP-B, and CENP-C, with molecular weights of 19, 80, and 140 kDa, respectively. A correlation has been shown between anticentromere antibodies and aneuploidy in patients with SSc. Anti-RNAP antibodies occur mainly in patients with diffuse disease (Bunn *et al.* 1998), and antibodies against RNAPI, -II, and -III have been described (Bona and Rothfield 1994). The RNAPs are multiprotein complexes and are components of the transcription complex. Each RNAP is composed of collections of smaller proteins shared by other RNAPs and two large distinct proteins. RNAPI synthesizes ribosomal RNA precursors in the nucleoli, whereas RNAPII and -III are found in the nuclei. RNAPII synthesizes most of the small nuclear RNAs found in ribonucleoprotein particles that mediate pre-mRNA splicing and synthesize precursors of mRNA, and RNAPIII synthesizes small RNAs including single-strand ribosomal RNA and transfer RNA. Antifibrillarin (U3-RNP) is another SSc hallmark antibody that is associated with a poor outcome due to increased frequency of internal organ complications (Tormey *et al.* 2001). Other autoantibodies have also been detected in SSc as well as localized scleroderma, such as those reacting against the microfibrillar protein fibrillin-1 and antibodies against a number of different cytokines. These reactivities appear more likely to be related to abnormal protein expression or processing for these antigens, and may provide insight into the biochemical processes which are perturbed in scleroderma spectrum disorders although it seems unlikely that they are directly involved in disease pathogenesis. It would appear that certain of these antibodies are closely related to particular *HLA* alleles, for example, it has recently been shown that class II MHC haplotype is an important factor determining *in vitro* responsiveness to topoisomerase antigen, both in patients with SSc and in healthy control individuals (Kuwana *et al.* 1993). It is important to consider that there may be racial differences in HLA associations for the various autoantibodies.

Initiating events

The initiating stimulus in idiopathic scleroderma is unknown, although the identification of chemical precipitants for environmentally induced SSc as discussed above (e.g. vinyl chloride and epoxy resin) may provide some clues to the processes involved, particularly in view of the similar immunogenetic associations for both idiopathic and chemically induced disease (Black *et al.* 1983). The most obvious major targets for the immune response in SSc are endothelial cells and the fibroblasts. Stimulation of collagen synthesis could involve an increasing number of cytokines known to modulate the properties of fibroblasts. It is possible that cascades of such cytokines or autocrine/paracrine loops stimulate or maintain the disease process. It is now appreciated that the repertoire of mediators and cytokines produced by immune cells, fibroblasts, and endothelial cells is large. It is possible that the aberrant properties of connective tissue cells (e.g. excess synthesis of collagen, fibronectin, and glycosaminoglycans) and the endothelial-cell damage and vasculopathy are consequences of the immunological events in SSc.

Oxidant stress in scleroderma pathogenesis

There is considerable evidence that oxidant stress may play a role in pathogenesis of SSc. It is potentially involved in the fragmentation of autoantigens to expose cryptic epitopes and facilitate the development of antibodies. This has been shown for RNAP and topoisomerase-1 and may be catalyzed by heavy metal ions. There are some data to support an additional association between heavy metal exposure and the development of autoantibodies. The combination of an appropriate HLA haplotype and exposure to appropriate immunogenic epitopes offers a unifying hypothesis to link different hallmark events in scleroderma. Since tissue hypoxia may occur secondary to Raynaud's phenomenon and the vasculopathy of scleroderma, perhaps in concert with the relative tissue hypoxia of the established lesional tissue it is possible that oxidant stress may promote disease development. Moreover, there is additional evidence that oxidative modification of proteins may facilitate development of scleroderma. Antioxidant strategies for therapy offer an exciting possibility for treatment and are being pursued.

Microchimerism in scleroderma pathogenesis

The observation that fetal cells and even naked fetal DNA may persist in the maternal circulation after pregnancy has fuelled the hypothesis that some of these fetal cells may become reactivated and that scleroderma could represent a graft-versus-host disease. Indeed, it has even been suggested that maternal cells passed to the fetus may persist, allowing an allo-reactive process to be implicated in male patients with scleroderma. Although the concept is attractive, there is only weak evidence to support it and recent data suggest that differences between scleroderma and control levels of foreign DNA are at most quantitative rather than absolute.

Treatment of systemic sclerosis

There have been major advances in treating many of the organ-specific complications of SSc. Thus, critical ischaemia and severe Raynaud's phenomenon are improved by parenteral prostacyclin analogues; the management and outcome of SRC has been transformed by use of angiotensin-converting enzyme (ACE) inhibitor agents, and the morbidity from oesophagitis has been drastically cut by use of proton pump inhibitors. Added to this are the exciting developments in treating pulmonary hypertension and several encouraging retrospective studies suggesting that immunosuppression using cyclophosphamide may be effective in slowing the progression of SSc-associated fibrosing alveolitis. Added to these developments is a much clearer understanding of the heterogeneity and natural history of the major subsets of SSc and an appreciation that risk stratification, the use of serological markers, and proactive regular screening of patients for early signs of complications. Together these factors make SSc a much more manageable disease than ever (Denton and Black 2000), although such positive developments must be tempered by the assertion that so far no agent has been proven to be an effective disease-modifying therapy.

The choice and evaluation of any treatment regimen are not easy because the disease is complex and the pathogenesis poorly understood; the disorder is heterogeneous and its extent, severity, and rate of progression are highly variable—therapy must therefore be closely tailored to the individual patient systems involved; there is a tendency towards spontaneous stabilization and/or regression after a few years, particularly within the more benign and numerically larger subset of lcSSc; and there is a paucity of both clinical and laboratory features for ascertaining improvement (or deterioration) in the disease, especially with respect to visceral change (Denton and Black 2000).

Efforts over the last several years in trying to develop effective disease-modifying treatments for SSc have ensured that there is now a robust infrastructure for conducting prospective clinical trials in SSc and much more insight than previously into the nature of the endpoints that are likely to yield interpretable data during a clinical trial and appreciation of the likely requirements of licensing bodies in demonstrating that agents are beneficial in SSc. Ultimately, it is hoped that a better understanding of the pathogenesis of SSc, especially in its aggressive diffuse form, will identify key factors, pathways, or processes that can be targeted therapeutically. It is possible that targets will be stage or subset specific. There are already examples of pilot studies of anticytokine therapies using neutralizing antibodies or soluble receptors. Ultimately, small molecules that inhibit key pathways are likely to be the most successful form of treatment but these are presently a long way off.

Renal manifestations of systemic sclerosis

Renal disease

This remains one of the most important complications of SSc and is amenable to treatment, although the prognosis is much better if appropriate management is instituted early. As with pulmonary hypertension, renal scleroderma is mainly a vascular disease. Both post- and antemortem studies suggest that epithelial and endothelial renal lesions occur before there is clinical evidence of renal disease in SSc (Kovalchik *et al.* 1978), and certainly precede any histological evidence of fibrosis. This supports the view that epithelial, and particularly endothelial, damage are important early events in the pathogenesis of scleroderma (Prescott *et al.* 1992).

Management of renal SSc requires a high index of suspicion to enable early diagnosis and treatment of the renal crisis. Creatinine clearance or isotope glomerular filtration rate should be checked twice yearly in dcSSc for the first 5 years, and annually thereafter. In lcSSc there is much less risk, and a less frequent measurement of the glomerular filtration rate is sufficient. Blood pressure should be well controlled (often antihypertensive treatments also help Raynaud's symptoms) and in dcSSc the use of ACE inhibitors is particularly appropriate since there is some anecdotal evidence that they protect from hypertensive crisis (Steen *et al.* 1990). High-dose corticosteroids have now been formally demonstrated in a case–control study to increase the risk of renal crisis in dcSSc, and doses above 20 mg prednisolone equivalent daily should be avoided (Steen and Medsger 1998).

Table 6 Renal involvement in systemic sclerosis

Renal vascular pathologic features	60–80%
Decreased renal blood flow or GFR	50%
Clinical 'markers' of renal disease	45%
Proteinuria (1+ or greater)	36%
Hypertension (BP > 140/90)	24%
Uraemia (BUN > 25 mg/dl)	19%
Rapidly progressive acute renal failure associated with accelerated hypertension (scleroderma renal crisis)	10–15%

Historical perspective of renal scleroderma

The earliest reports did not suggest a direct relationship between skin disease and the kidney. In describing the first reported case, Auspitz (1863) concluded that 'there is no evidence to support the causal relationship between the kidney disease and skin disease as such'. Eighty years later clear descriptions of the histological changes emerged. Masugi and Ya-Shu (1938) and Talbott *et al.* (1939) described intimal hyperplasia and fibrinoid degeneration in the interlobular renal arteries, and Goetz (1945) described the widespread pathological changes in the small blood vessels. However, it was not until the early 1950s that the direct relationship between SSc and acute renal failure was accepted, after Moore and Sheehan (1952) described the clinical and histological abnormalities in the kidneys of three patients with scleroderma who were dying of uraemia.

The overall significance of renal disease in SSc before the introduction of ACE inhibitors in the mid-1970s is clearly illustrated in the survival figures reported by Medsger *et al.* (1971). In their initial study, all 16 patients who developed renal scleroderma were dead within 1 year. In a later study, all 17 patients with kidney involvement died within 10 months of onset, and the overall cumulative survival rate was 35 per cent after 7 years of follow-up (Medsger and Masi 1973). The factors indicating a worse prognosis included older age, male sex, and Black race. Renal disease was more often observed in the context of extensive diffuse skin disease. The reported frequency and type of renal involvement in SSc varies, depending on the clinical and pathological criteria used, and how they were defined. Features of renal involvement in SSc, compiled by Shapiro and Medsger (1988), are shown in Table 6. A glomerular filtration rate of less than 60 ml/min, protein excretion of more than 500 mg/24 h, or sustained hypertension should prompt treatment as suggested in Fig. 2.

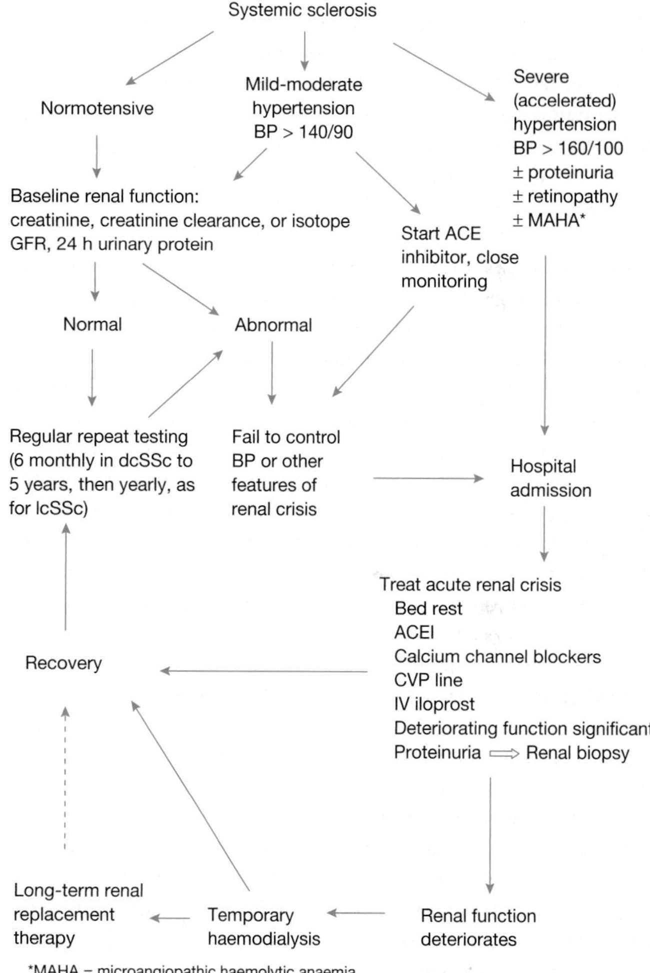

Fig. 2 Algorithm for the management of scleroderma renal disease.

Spectrum of renal disease

Scleroderma renal crisis

The best characterized pattern of SSc renal involvement is an acute or subacute renal hypertensive crisis (SRC). This generally occurs in patients with diffuse SSc within 5 years of disease onset. Patients usually present with the clinical features of severe hypertension including headaches, visual disturbances, hypertensive encephalopathy (especially seizures), and pulmonary oedema. The overall incidence of SRC is uncertain, with differences in the reported frequency even in series from the same unit. This variation probably reflects differences in incidence in the various SSc subsets. In high-risk patients the incidence may be as great as 20 per cent, but overall is probably less than 10 per cent (Steen *et al.* 1984, 1994). Traub (1983) proposed the following criteria to diagnose SRC abrupt onset of arterial hypertension greater than 160/90 mmHg; hypertensive retinopathy of at least grade III severity; rapid deterioration of renal function and elevated plasma renin activity (PRA). Other typical features include the presence of a microangiopathic haemolytic anaemia (MAHA) and hypertensive encephalopathy, often complicated by generalized convulsions. It is generally considered to be important to perform a renal biopsy once hypertension has been adequately controlled, especially if renal replacement therapy is being contemplated. This allows histological confirmation of the diagnosis and exclusion of other causes for abrupt onset renal failure such as glomerulonephritis, perhaps as part of an overlap syndrome, or the haemolytic–uraemic syndrome. Histologically, SSc renal crisis typically shows fibrinoid necrosis, mucoid or fibromucoid proliferative intimal lesions (when extensive, termed onion-skinning) in renal arteries, particularly the arcuate and interlobular vessels, glomerular thrombi, and ultimately glomerulosclerosis. The extent of the glomerular lesion can be useful in predicting the degree of functional recovery which can ultimately occur. Occasionally, a similar pattern of renal dysfunction occurs without hypertension (normotensive renal crisis), suggesting that the pathological features are not simply the end-organ consequences of raised arterial pressure (Helfrich *et al.* 1989).

Symptoms of the crisis usually present abruptly. The pulse rate is increased and patients develop headaches, visual phenomena, and convulsions due to accelerated hypertension. Features of left ventricular failure may follow rapidly. The glomerular filtration rate and renal blood flow are decreased, and serum creatinine increases. Oliguria and anuria may follow and death from renal failure can occur within a short time in untreated patients. Proteinuria is almost universal; although it may present long before the renal crisis develops, it often increases with the crisis, though not to nephrotic levels. Microscopic haematuria and granular casts may be present, as in other forms of accelerated hypertension; this situation may be complicated by MAHA. Although SRC usually occurs in patients with established SSc it can occasionally be the presenting feature of the disease. For this reason, the hands and face of any patient presenting with unexplained severe or accelerated hypertension should be examined for an underlying connective tissue disorder such as SSc, with appropriate investigations including autoimmune serology and nailfold capillaroscopy.

The rapid development of renal failure is the other hallmark of renal crisis and is alone sufficient to make the diagnosis, especially as there are several reports of normotensive renal failure in SSc (Moore and Sheehan 1952; Dichoso 1976; Helfrich *et al.* 1989). This suggests that a large change in blood pressure may not be required to precipitate vascular damage. Additional mechanisms which may be operative in SRC in some patients include hyper-reactivity of blood vessels or blood pressure to a number of mediators such as catecholamines—these mechanisms may be enhanced by a drop in temperature (Rodnan *et al.* 1964; Winkelman *et al.* 1977). Reperfusion injury, particularly with the formation of free radical species, is another potentially important mechanism for renal damage. Once diagnosed, an acute renal crisis in SSc must be treated as a medical emergency. The patient should be admitted immediately and reasonable control of the blood pressure is a priority. Although some specialists advocate quite rapid and aggressive control of blood pressure (Steen and Medsger 2000a,b), our practice is to use relative caution to avoid a precipitous or excessive drop in arterial pressure and also to prevent relative or actual hypovolaemia associated with vasodilatation of constricted vascular beds, both of which can further diminish renal perfusion and compound the renal lesion of SSc. It is likely that the severity and duration of SRC prior to treatment is relevant and that milder or earlier disease may be. For this reason, powerful parenteral antihypertensives (e.g. intravenous nitroprusside or labetolol) should be avoided; an internal jugular or subclavian venous cannula should be inserted to monitor central venous filling pressure, and an indwelling arterial cannula for monitoring of pressure should be considered.

Hypertension should be treated with ACE inhibitors (captopril up to maximum dose is often used initially as its short duration of action allows therapy to be titrated according to blood pressure response) and calcium-channel blockers (starting with long-acting nifedipine initially), aiming to reduce both diastolic and systolic pressure by 20 mmHg in the first 48 h and ultimately maintaining diastolic pressure at 80–90 mmHg. Intravenous prostacyclin, which is believed to help the microvascular lesion without precipitating hypotension, is often administered from diagnosis. Refractory hypertension may require addition of doxazosin. The effectiveness or rationale of combining angiotensin receptor blockers (e.g. losartan) with ACE inhibitors remains uncertain. Fish-oil capsules are sometimes prescribed in view of their unproven but theoretically beneficial properties. Renal function should be closely monitored by twice-weekly creatinine clearance and daily serum creatinine estimations. Regular full blood counts, clotting screening, and estimations of fibrin degradation product are important to monitor the degree of MAHA, which often reflects the activity of the disease process. Short-term haemodialysis should be given if necessary, and peritoneal dialysis often works well if long-term renal replacement therapy is needed (Steen and Medsger 2000a,b).

Interestingly, it has been observed that after a renal crisis, skin sclerosis and other features of SSc improve (Denton *et al.* 1994), particularly if a patient is undergoing maintenance dialysis. The reason for this is unknown; it may result from the removal or inactivation of circulating mediators or simply reflect the natural history of the disease. It should be remembered that there is also often considerable recovery in renal function after an acute crisis, sometimes allowing dialysis to be discontinued, and improvement can continue for up to 2 years (Abbott *et al.* 2002). Therefore, any decisions regarding renal transplantation should not be made before this time.

The renin–angiotensin system in scleroderma renal crisis

Plasma renin activity increases markedly with the onset of renal injury and may rise acutely to extreme levels, but there is no convincing evidence that a rise precedes the onset of SRC. Traub (1983) reported 13 cases in which PRA was coincidentally measured from 1 week to 1 year prior to the development of the renal crisis: none of the patients had significantly increased levels. Similar results have been reported by others (Fleischmajer and Gould 1975; Fiocco *et al.* 1978). A functional Raynaud's-like renal vasoconstriction may be superimposed on more chronic structural changes; this hypothesis is consistent with the data provided by Kovalchik *et al.* (1978) who performed renal biopsies on nine patients with scleroderma and normal renal function. Xenon clearance studies provide additional support for the importance of functional vascular narrowing (Urai *et al.* 1958; Cannon *et al.* 1974). In these studies, renal cortical perfusion was found to be decreased in SSc patients, and much more so at times of renal crisis.

Other abnormalities of renal function

Although the most prominent renal event in SSc is the acute hypertensive SRC, it is likely that more subtle abnormalities in renal physiology occur in the disease. A study by Clements *et al.* (1994) outlined some of these. Renal plasma flow (assessed by PAH clearance) was diminished in many SSc patients and PRA increased. Stress tests to determine the responsiveness of the renin–angiotensin system were performed and confirmed elevated levels in many patients. Although no factors were identified which were associated with an increased frequency of SRC, the authors did observe that stimulated PRA levels correlated with survival. Thus, the absence of an exaggerated PRA response to sodium depletion (single dose frusemide) was associated with reduced survival. It is suggested that this might reflect the failure of a homeostatic mechanism for maintenance of intravascular volume, for example, reflecting a non-reactive vascular bed. Overall, however, elevated levels of PRA, or reduced PAH did not correlate with either increased incidence of renal crises or worse survival. The widespread elevation of PRA in scleroderma is further evidence that the renin–angiotensin system is active in the disease and perhaps explains why ACE inhibitors are helpful in this condition. Moreover, the specific angiotensin antagonist saralasin has been shown to reduce blood pressure in the context of SRC (Clements *et al.* 1994). Clearly, the regulation of renal blood flow is complex in SSc; endothelin levels, when measured, have been found to be elevated in SRC, but whether this represents a primary or secondary phenomenon is unclear (Vancheeswaran *et al.* 1994).

Elevated levels of endothelin might simply reflect endothelial damage associated with SRC. Some support for this comes from reports of correlation between circulating soluble forms of the endothelial adhesion molecule VCAM-1 and renal dysfunction in SSc, with particularly high levels associated with SRC (Denton *et al.* 1995). There is evidence of differential EC activation in SSc renal and pulmonary hypertensive disease (Stratton *et al.* 1998). It has been suggested that intravenous prostacyclin may have a specific beneficial effect in treating SRC. There is evidence that renal blood flow improved in SSc patients with evidence of increased renal vascular resistance. In addition, iloprost downregulates CTGF expression in the skin and may do so in other organs in SSc and reduces expression of markers of endothelial cell activation (Della Bella *et al.* 2001).

A syndrome of renal and pulmonary hypertension has been suggested, based upon a small case series (Gunduz *et al.* 2001). This is intriguing considering the similarity between the histological features of these complications. It must be remembered that the chronology of the two processes is typically distinct. Assessment of pulmonary arterial hypertension can be difficult in the context of acute systemic hypertension.

Genetic studies have implicated the renin–angiotensin axis as well as other vasoactive regulatory pathways including endothelin and eNOS. Data so far are conflicting. This may reflect the complexity of these interacting pathways or the small numbers of samples studied and the importance of matching for known associated cardiovascular disease.

Histopathology of renal scleroderma

Arterial lesions

Microscopically, there are two types of arterial lesion in the acute renal disease of scleroderma. The first, affecting small interlobular and arcuate arteries, is characteristic of scleroderma. The second, involving the small arteries and arterioles supplying the glomeruli and glomerular capillaries, is indistinguishable from changes seen in malignant hypertension. Larger arteries (outer diameters $> 500\ \mu m$) are normal or show atherosclerotic changes.

The earliest change in acute renal disease is oedema, followed by marked proliferation of intimal cells and accumulation of mucoid ground substance composed of glycoproteins and mucopolysaccharides. This proliferation may damage the internal elastic lamina allowing smooth muscle-like cells, capable of synthesizing collagen and elastin, to migrate into the intima from the media, which is often stretched and thinned. Fibrous thickening in the adventitia and periadventitial tissue is another feature of SSc, seldom found in other causes of malignant hypertension (Fig. 3). Gross narrowing of the blood vessels results in vascular insufficiency with atrophy of perused tissue; thrombosis can also lead to necrosis and infarction of glomeruli and tubules.

Subintimal or intramural fibrinoid necrosis of the small arteries and arterioles supplying glomeruli and glomerular capillaries is the second typical lesion of scleroderma (Fig. 4). These changes are indistinguishable from those found in malignant hypertension and can occur in patients with SSc but without previously elevated blood pressure or clinical renal disease (D'Angelo *et al.* 1969). Glomerular changes which have been reported include focal or diffuse basement membrane thickening, with progressive glomerulosclerosis. There may also be non-specific hyperplasia of the juxtaglomerular apparatus. The tubules appear to be secondarily affected by the vascular insufficiency and the most prominent changes are flattening of the epithelial cells with hyaline droplet degeneration. The interstitial stroma may show a marked increase in fibrous tissue and small collections of lymphocytes and/or plasma cells. Immunohistological studies are inconclusive and non-specific. Deposits of immunoglobulins, most notably IgM, complement components (including Clq, C3, and C4), and fibrinogen have occasionally been reported (Lapernas *et al.* 1978). However, C3 deposition has also been reported in patients without clinical renal disease (Kovalchik *et al.* 1978). In a few cases, antinuclear antibodies have been eluted from the kidney, raising the possibility that immune complexes are involved in the pathogenesis. However, electron-dense material has not been found on electron microscopy. The identification of factor VIII in vessel walls may be due

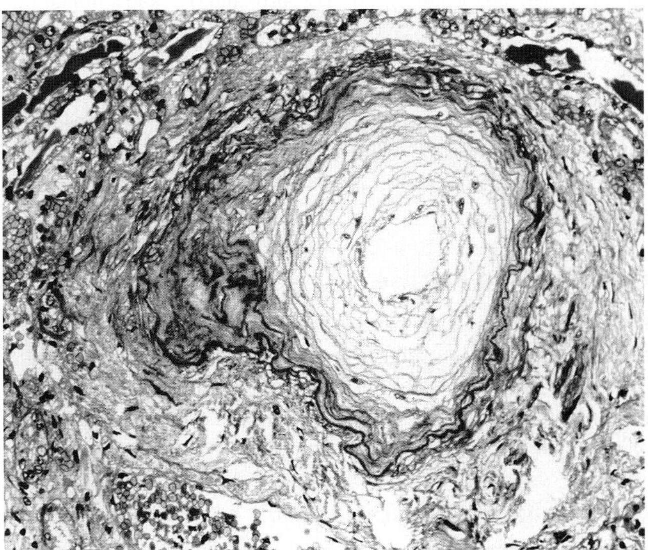

Fig. 3 Interlobular artery, showing intimal thickening and accumulation of mucin (haematoxylin and eosin, ×250).

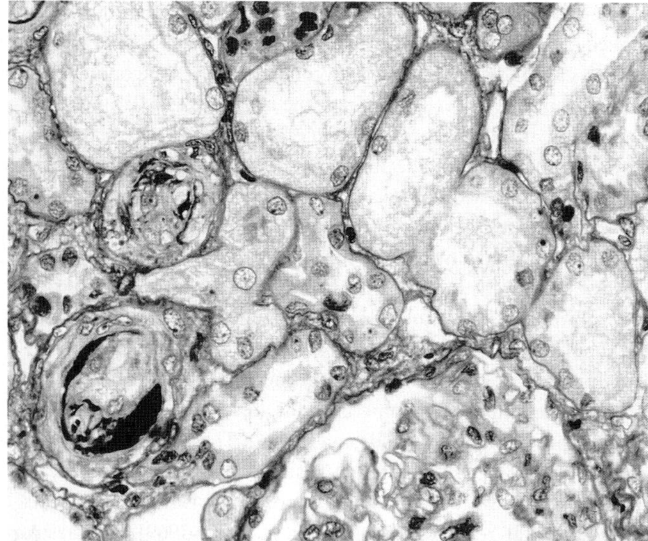

Fig. 4 Renal cortex with two arterioles showing fibrinoid necrosis and thrombus formation (haematoxylin and eosin, ×500).

to activation of the coagulation cascade (Kahaleh *et al.* 1981) or may merely reflect vascular injury; this observation has been extended by the recent report of an inverse correlation between glomerular filtration rate and circulating factor VIII levels in scleroderma patients (Scheja *et al.* 1994).

Fibrotic change

There are histological changes in the renal blood vessels and the interstitium as well as changes in the amount of basement membrane and other matrix collagens. The distribution of the collagens I, III, IV, and V in normal kidneys has been described by Roll *et al.* (1980) and Black *et al.* (1983) [Fig. 5(a–d)]. Immunofluorescent studies with type-specific anticollagen antibodies have revealed a marked increase in Type III collagen around large blood vessels and throughout the kidney, but particularly in the interstitium [Fig. 5(b) and (f)], and a similar but less obvious increase in Type I collagen [Fig. 5(a) and (e)]. The tubular and glomerular basement membranes also appear thickened and show an increased intensity of staining with antibody to Type IV collagen [Fig. 5(c) and (g)]. There is increased Type V collagen in the glomerular mesangial matrix as well as the interstitium [Fig. 5(d) and (h)]. These changes are found even in patients without clinical evidence of renal disease.

Chronic renal disease

Patients who survive SRC may develop similar but less florid proliferative changes in the interlobular and arcuate arteries. Even those who have never had a renal crisis may show reduplication of elastic fibres, sclerosed glomeruli tubular atrophy, and interstitial fibrosis, presumably reflecting the chronic changes of scleroderma.

Other renal manifestations of systemic sclerosis

A more insidious pattern of SSc renal involvement is also reported in which there is a slow reduction in glomerular filtration rate accompanied by proteinuria. This is believed to reflect a more benign

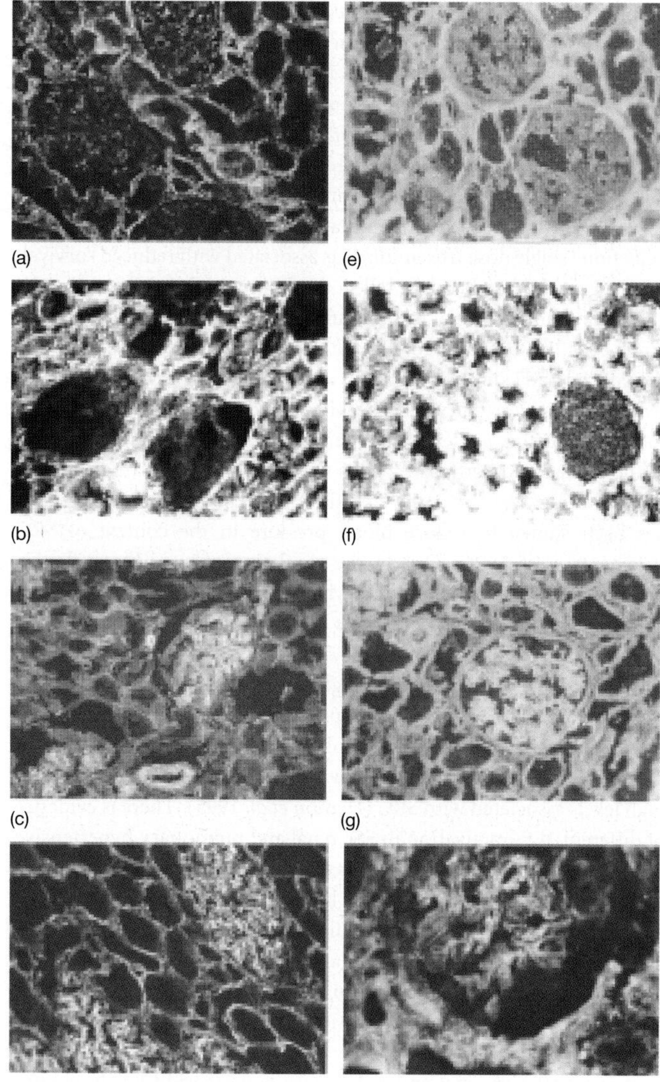

Fig. 5 Immunofluorescent staining of normal (a–d) and scleroderma kidney (e–h) stained with antibodies to type I (a–e), type III (b and f), type IV (c and g), and type V (d and h) collagen, ×100. An increase in staining is evident for all types of collagen, but is particularly marked for type III.

vascular and fibrotic process than SRC. There are well-recognized co-occurrences of other acute renal pathologies in scleroderma. This is especially seen in scleroderma overlap syndromes with lupus nephritis. There may be serological clues that a patient is evolving within the connective tissue disease spectrum that anticipates clinical changes, such as the development or a rise in titre of an associated anti-dsDNA antibody. It has been suggested that antineutrophil cytoplasmic antibody (ANCA) reactivity may predict unusual renal complications of SSc. There are cases of anti-MPO reactivity associated with glomerulonephritis or with renal vasculitis, and some additional reports of anti-PR3 or uncharacterized ANCA reactivities (Locke *et al.* 1997). Some of these changes are in patients who have received D-penicillamine therapy (Hillis *et al.* 1997). This agent is not used in most centres, but has been associated with antibody generation including ANCA.

Renal transplantion in scleroderma

It should be remembered that there is also often considerable recovery in renal function after an acute hypertensive renal crisis, sometimes allowing dialysis to be discontinued, and improvement can continue for up to 2 years. Therefore, any decisions regarding renal transplantation should not be made before this time. A recent comprehensive analysis of US renal transplantation experience suggested graft survival in SSc was comparable to that seen in other autoimmune rheumatic diseases including SLE (Chang and Spiera 1999). It is possible that immunosuppressive regimens post-transplant may have beneficial effects on underlying disease that diminish involvement in the grafted kidney. Nevertheless, there are clear examples of recurrent scleroderma renal disease in grafted organs, including a grafted kidney from an HLA identical twin.

Pregnancy in scleroderma

The predilection for scleroderma to affect women in the child-bearing years is well recognized, and it is not surprising therefore that the issue of pregnancy in this disease is frequently raised. The effect of pregnancy on the SSc disease process must be considered, as well as the potential increase in fetal and maternal complications which might occur during pregancy in a SSc sufferer (Black 1990). It has been noted that SSc onset or exacerbation is often temporally related to the puerperium. This provides indirect evidence for the important hormonal factors in disease pathogenesis, although the mechanisms for this are uncertain. The most feared complication in pregnancy is renal disease, which usually presents with hypertension especially in the third trimester, and is thus difficult to distinguish from toxaemia. Renal scleroderma should be considered in all but the most typical cases of pre-eclamptic toxaemia (PET). In contrast to PET, patients with SSc can be vulnerable in the postpartum period, and must be watched very carefully.

Advice to patients with SSc at pregnancy is difficult, since studies are limited and retrospective. It is our policy to recommend that patients who have active diffuse SSc avoid pregancy, especially if significant visceral disease has been confirmed. If such patients become pregnant, especially if lung, renal, or cardiac involvement is present, then they should be offered therapeutic abortion. Patients with limited disease should be told of the possible development of complications, and the variable and unpredictable outcome; the patients may then request abortion. Very close monitoring of any patient with SSc is then necessary throughout pregnancy.

Conclusions

Renal scleroderma was the first complication of this disorder which has been amenable to effective treatment. Some of the advances reflect overall progress in management of renal failure but there have also been more specific improvements in the diagnosis and management of SSc renal crisis. In particular, ACE inhibitors are especially effective in treating the hypertension in SSc and may have a renoprotective effect. Also, it has been shown that some therapies for SSc appear to increase the incidence of acute renal crisis, such as high-dose corticosteroids or cyclosporin-A and this will hopefully lead to changes in clinical practice (Steen and Medsger 1998).

However, treatment to modify the underlying disease processes in SSc has proven extremely difficult. No agent has emerged which, when tested in a controlled manner, can halt either the excessive fibrosis or vascular damage in the skin or internal organs (Steen and Medsger 2000a,b). Current therapy is, therefore, directed towards reducing the clinical effects of the disease (Denton and Black 2000) and providing a general understanding of the process which helps both the patient and family cope with the various problems associated with a chronic disease. Other potential advances in the management of renal disease in scleroderma may come as changes in circulating vascular markers, such as endothelin or soluble adhesion molecules, are elucidated. Finally, drawing analogy from work on scleroderma lung disease, serological and immunogenetic markers may soon be identified which can be used to stratify the risk to individual patients of renal involvement, thereby allowing management to become more proactive.

References

Abbott, K. C., Trespalacios, F. C., Welch, P. G., and Agodoa, L. Y. (2002). Scleroderma at end stage renal disease in the United States: patient characteristics and survival. *Journal of Nephrology* **15**, 236–240.

Auspitz, H. (1863). Ein Beitrag zur Lehre vom Haut-Sklerem der Erwachsenen. *Wiener Medizinische Wochenschrift* **13**, 739 (see also p. 755, 772, 788).

Black, C. M. (1990). Systemic sclerosis and pregnancy. *Baillière's Clinical Rheumatology* **4**, 105–124.

Black, C. M. *et al.* (1983). An investigation of the biochemical and histological changes in the collagen of the kidney and skeletal muscle in systemic sclerosis. *Collagen Related Research* **3**, 231–244.

Bona, C. and Rothfield, N. (1994). Autoantibodies in scleroderma and tight-skin mice. *Current Opinions in Immunology* **6**, 931–937.

Briggs, D. *et al.* (1993). A molecular and serologic analysis of the major histocomatibility complex and complement component C4 in systemic sclerosis. *Arthritis and Rheumatism* **36**, 943–954.

Bunn, C. C., Denton, C. P., Shi-Wen, X., Knight, C., and Black, C. M. (1998). Anti-RNA polymerases and other autoantibody specificities in systemic sclerosis. *British Journal of Rheumatology* **37**, 15–20.

Cannon, P. J. *et al.* (1974). The relationship of hypertension and renal failure in scleroderma (progressive systemic sclerosis) to structural and functional abnormalities of the renal cortical circulation. *Medicine* **53**, 1–46.

Chang, Y. J. and Spiera, H. (1999). Renal transplantation in scleroderma. *Medicine (Baltimore)* **78**, 382–385.

Clements, P. J. *et al.* (1994). Abnormalities of renal physiology in systemic sclerosis. A prospective study with 10-year followup. *Arthritis and Rheumatism* **37**, 67–74.

D'Angelo, W. A. *et al.* (1969). Pathologic observations in systemic sclerosis (scleroderma). A study of 58 autopsy cases and 58 matched controls. *American Journal of Medicine* **46**, 428–440.

Della Bella, S., Molteni, M., Mocellin, C., Fumagalli, S., Bonara, P., and Scorza, R. (2001). Novel mode of action of iloprost: *in vitro* down-regulation of endothelial cell adhesion molecules. *Prostaglandins* **65**, 73–83.

Denton, C. P. and Black, C. M. (2000). Scleroderma and related disorders: therapeutic aspects. *Baillière's Best Practice and Research Clinical Rheumatology* **14**, 17–35.

Denton, C. P. *et al.* (1994). Acute renal failure occurring in scleroderma treated with cyclosporin A—a report of three cases. *British Joural of Rheumatology* **33**, 90–92.

Denton, C. P. *et al.* (1995). Serial circulating adhesion molecule levels reflect disease severity in systemic sclerosis. *British Journal of Rheumatology* **34**, 1048–1054.

Dichoso, C. C. The kidney in progressive systemic sclerosis (scleroderma). In *The Kidney in Systemic Disease—Perspectives in Nephrology and Hypertension* Vol. 3 (ed. W. N. Suki and G. Eknoyan), pp. 57–74. New York: Wiley, 1976.

Fiocco, U. *et al.* (1978). Plasma renin activity in progressive systemic sclerosis. *Bollettino della Societa Italiana di Biologia Sperimentale* **54**, 2507–2510.

Fleischmajer, R. (1977). The pathophysiology of scleroderma. *International Journal of Dermatology* **16**, 310.

Fleischmajer, R. and Gould, A. P. (1975). Serum renin and renin substrate levels in scleroderma. *Proceedings of the Society for Experimental Biology and Medicine* **150**, 374–379.

Freni-Titulaer, L. J. W. *et al.* (1989). Connective tissue disease in South Eastern Georgia: a case–control study. *American Journal of Epidemiology* **130**, 404–409.

Gilchrist, F. C. *et al.* (2001). Class II HLA associations with autoantibodies in scleroderma: a highly significant role for HLA DP. *Genes and Immunity* **2**, 76–81.

Goetz, R. H. (1945). The pathology of progressive systemic sclerosis (generalised scleroderma) with special reference to changes in viscera. *Clinical Proceedings* **4**, 337–392.

Gunduz, O. H., Fertig, N., Lucas, M., and Medsger, T. A., Jr. (2001). Systemic sclerosis with renal crisis and pulmonary hypertension: a report of eleven cases. *Arthritis and Rheumatism* **44**, 1663–1666.

Helfrich, D. J. *et al.* (1989). Renal failure in normotensive patients with systemic sclerosis. *Arthritis and Rheumatism* **32**, 1128–1134.

Hillis, G. S., Khan, I. H., Simpson, J. G., and Rees, A. J. (1997). Scleroderma, D-penicillamine treatment, and progressive renal failure associated with positive antimyeloperoxidase antineutrophil cytoplasmic antibodies. *American Journal of Kidney Diseases* **30**, 279–281.

Hochberg, M. C. (1994). Silicone breast implants and rheumatic disease. *British Journal of Rheumatology* **33**, 601–602.

Jablonska, S. and Lovell, C. R. Localized scleroderma. In *Systemic Sclerosis—Scleroderma* (ed. M. I. V. Jayson and C. M. Black), pp. 303–318. Chichester: Wiley, 1988.

Kahaleh, M. B. (1991). Endothelin, an endothelial-dependent vasoconstrictor in scleroderma. *Arthritis and Rheumatism* **34**, 978–983.

Kahaleh, M. B. and Mattuci-Cerinic, M. (1995). Raynaud's phenomenon and scleroderma: dysregulated neuroendothelial control of vascular tone. *Arthritis and Rheumatism* **38**, 1–4.

Kahaleh, M. B., Osborn, I., and LeRoy, E. C. (1981). Increased factor VIII/von Willebrand factor antigen and von Willebrand factor activity in scleroderma and in Raynaud's phenomenon. *Annals of Internal Medicine* **94**, 482–484.

Kovalchik, M. T. *et al.* (1978). The kidney in progressive systemic sclerosis. A prospective study. *Annals of Internal Medicine* **89**, 881–887.

Kuwana, M. *et al.* (1993). The HLA DR and DQ genes control the autoimmune response to DNA topoisomerase 1 in systemic sclerosis (scleroderma). *Journal of Clinical Investigation* **92**, 1296–1301.

Kuwana, M. *et al.* (1994). Clinical and prognostic associations based on serum antinuclear antibodies in Japanese patients with systemic sclerosis. *Arthritis and Rheumatism* **37**, 75–83.

Lapernas, D. *et al.* (1978). Immunopathology of the renal vascular lesion of progressive systemic sclerosis (scleroderma). *American Journal of Pathology* **91**, 243–256.

LeRoy, E. C. Scleroderma (systemic sclerosis). In *Textbook of Rheumatology* 2nd edn. (ed. W. N. Kelly, E. D. Harris, Jr., S. Ruddy, and C. B. Sledge), pp. 1183–1205. Philadelphia: Saunders, 1985.

LeRoy, E. C. *et al.* (1988). Scleroderma (systemic sclerosis): classification, subsets, and pathogenesis. *Journal of Rheumatology* **15**, 202–205.

Locke, I. C., Worrall, J. G., Leaker, B., Black, C. M., and Cambridge, G. (1997). Autoantibodies to myeloperoxidase in systemic sclerosis. *Journal of Rheumatology* **24**, 86–89.

Maricq, H. R. *et al.* (1989). Prevalence of scleroderma spectrum disorders in the general population of South Carolina. *Arthritis and Rheumatism* **32**, 998–1006.

Masi, A. T. *et al.* (1980). Preliminary criteria for the classification of systemic sclerosis (scleroderma). *Arthritis and Rheumatism* **23**, 581–590.

Masugi, M. and Ya-Shu (1938). Die diffuse Sklerodermia und ihre Geffasveränderung. *Virchows Archiv [Pathologie und Anatomie]* **302**, 39–62.

McHugh, N. J. *et al.* (1994). Anti-centromere antibodies (ACA) in systemic sclerosis patients and their relatives: a serological and HLA study. *Clinical and Experimental Immunology* **96**, 267–274.

Medsger, T. A., Jr. and Masi, A. T. (1973). Survival with scleroderma-II. A life-table analysis of clinical and demographic factors in 358 US veteran patients. *Journal of Chronic Diseases* **26**, 647–660.

Medsger, T. A., Jr. *et al.* (1971). Survival with systemic sclerosis (scleroderma). *Annals of Internal Medicine* **75**, 369–376.

Moore, H. C. and Sheehan, H. L. (1952). The kidney of scleroderma. *Lancet* **i**, 68–70.

Pearson, J. D. (1990). The endothelium: its role in systemic sclerosis. *Annals of the Rheumatic Diseases* **50**, 866–871.

Prescott, R. J. *et al.* (1992). Sequential dermal microvascular and perivascular changes in the development of scleroderma. *Journal of Pathology* **166**, 255–263.

Rodnan, G. P., Shapiro, A. P., and Krifcher, E. (1964). The occurrence of malignant hypertension and renal insufficiency in progressive systemic sclerosis (diffuse scleroderma) (abstract). *Annals of Internal Medicine* **60**, 737.

Roll, F. J., Madri, J. A., Albert, J., and Furthmayr, H. (1980). Codistribution of collagen types IV and AB2 in basement membranes and mesangium of the kidney. *Journal of Cell Biology* **85**, 597–616.

Scheja, A. *et al.* (1994). Inverse relation between plasma concentration of von Willebrand factor and CrEDTA clearance in systemic sclerosis. *Journal of Rheumatology* **21**, 639–642.

Shapiro, A. P. and Medsger, T. A., Jr. Renal involvement in systemic sclerosis. In *Diseases of Kidney* 4th edn. (ed. R. Schreiner and C. Gottschalk), pp. 2272–2283. Boston: Little Brown & Co, 1988.

Silman, A. J. (1995). Scleroderma and survival: a review. *Annals of the Rheumatic Diseases* **50**, 267–269.

Steen, V. D. and Medsger, T. A., Jr. (1998). Case–control study of corticosteroids and other drugs that either precipitate or protect from the development of scleroderma renal crisis. *Arthritis and Rheumatism* **41**, 1613–1619.

Steen, V. D., and Medsger, T. A., Jr. (2000a). Long-term outcomes of scleroderma renal crisis. *Annals of Internal Medicine* **133**, 600–603.

Steen, V. D. and Medsger, T. A., Jr. (2000b). Severe organ involvement in systemic sclerosis with diffuse scleroderma. *Arthritis and Rheumatism* **43**, 2437–2444.

Steen, V. D. *et al.* (1984). Factors predicting the development of renal involvement in progressive systemic sclerosis. *American Journal of Medicine* **76**, 779–786.

Steen, V. D. *et al.* (1990). Outcome of renal crisis in systemic sclerosis: relation to the availibility of converting enzyme inhibitors (ACE). *Annals of Internal Medicine* **113**, 352–357.

Stratton, R. J. *et al.* (1998). Different patterns of endothelial cell activation in renal and pulmonary vascular disease in scleroderma. *Quarterly Journal of Medicine* **91**, 561–566.

Talbott, J. H. *et al.* (1939). Dermatomyositis with scleroderma, calcinosis and renal endarteritis associated with focal cortical necrosis. *Archives of Internal Medicine* **63**, 476–496.

Tormey, V. J., Bunn, C. C., Denton, C. P., and Black, C. M. (2001). Anti-fibrillarin antibodies in systemic sclerosis. *Rheumatology (Oxford)* **40**, 1157–1162.

Traub, X. M. (1983). Hypertension and renal failure (scleroderma renal crisis) in progressive systemic sderosis. Review of a 25 year experience with 68 cases. *Medicine* **62**, 335–352.

Urai, L., Nagy, Z., Szinay, G., and Waltner, W. (1958). Renal function in scleroderma. *British Medical Journal* **2**, 1264–1266.

Valesini, G. *et al.* (1993). Geographical clustering of scleroderma in a rural area in the province of Rome. *Clinical and Experimental Rheumatology* **11**, 41–47.

Vancheeswaran, R. *et al.* (1994). Circulating ET-1 levels in systemic sclerosis—a marker of fibrosis or vascular dysfunction. *Journal of Rheumatology* **21**, 1838–1844.

Winkelman, R. K. *et al.* (1977). Influence of cold on catecholamine response of vascular smooth muscle strips from resistance vessels of scleroderma skin. *Angiology* **28**, 33–39.

4.9 The patient with rheumatoid arthritis, mixed connective tissue disease, or polymyositis

Paul Emery and Dwomoa Adu

Introduction

Renal disease is a well-recognized cause of ill health and death in patients with rheumatoid arthritis. Three broad categories of renal disease occur in such patients. The first—and by far the most common—arises from the *nephrotoxicity* of the drugs used in treatment of the arthritis. Gold and penicillamine may lead to proteinuria and a glomerulonephritis in between 10 and 30 per cent of patients (see Chapter 19.1), and this is often severe enough to cause a nephrotic syndrome. Non-steroidal anti-inflammatory drugs (NSAIDs) are widely used for pain relief, and all are associated with the development of a variety of renal syndromes, ranging from a reversible reduction in glomerular filtration rate (GFR) to acute renal failure, in turn due either to an acute tubular necrosis or to an acute interstitial nephritis. The latter may be complicated by nephrotic-range proteinuria (see Chapter 6.3). Finally, cyclosporin has been extensively used in the treatment of patients with rheumatoid arthritis and is associated with significant nephrotoxicity and hypertension (see Chapter 13.2.2).

A second major but diminishing cause of renal disease in rheumatoid arthritis is *amyloidosis* (see Chapter 4.2.1). The clinical presentation is with proteinuria, a nephrotic syndrome, or renal impairment; progression to renal failure is inevitable. There is now good evidence that rheumatoid arthritis may be associated with the development of a *glomerulonephritis* (Adu *et al.* 1993). The main types described are a mesangial proliferative glomerulonephritis with or without IgA deposits, a membranous nephropathy, and a focal segmental necrotizing glomerulonephritis of the vasculitic type.

Prevalence and patterns of renal disease in rheumatoid arthritis

The prevalence of renal disease in rheumatoid arthritis has been examined using two types of study, based either on death certificates or on autopsy. Each has its limitations, and there is still no agreement on the incidence of renal disease in patients with rheumatoid arthritis.

Death certificates

Studies of mortality in patients with rheumatoid arthritis based on death certificates show that there is an excess of deaths from renal failure accounting for between 3 and 12 per cent of fatalities. Renal amyloid was reported as the cause of death in 1.5–9 per cent of cases (Table 1) (Cobb *et al.* 1953; Rasker and Cosh 1981; Prior *et al.* 1984; Laakso *et al.* 1986). Interpretation of these studies is complicated by differences in the definitions of rheumatoid arthritis, the duration of disease at death, the treatment received, the accuracy of death certification, and the method of statistical analysis.

Table 1 Incidence of renal disease in rheumatoid arthritis: death certificate studies

Study	Country	Number of patients	Renal amyloid (%)	Renal failure (%)
Cobb *et al.* (1953)	USA	130	3.1	10
Rasker and Cosh (1981)	UK	43	7	11.6
Prior et *al.* (1984)	UK	199	1.5	3.0
Laasko *et al.* (1986)	Finland	356	8.7	11.8

Autopsy studies (Table 2)

In autopsy studies the proportion of patients with renal failure ranged from 9 to 27 per cent, and of renal amyloid from 8 to 17 per cent (Missen and Taylor 1956; Mutru *et al.* 1976; Ramirez *et al.* 1981; Boers *et al.* 1987; Suzuki *et al.* 1994). In the study of Mutru *et al.* (1976), 27 per cent of patients with rheumatoid arthritis died from renal failure compared with 3 per cent of age- and sex-matched controls. In the patients with rheumatoid arthritis, 17 per cent had renal amyloidosis compared with 1 per cent of controls. This high prevalence of renal failure in the autopsy studies is at variance with clinical experience.

Autopsy renal pathology

In addition to renal amyloid, autopsy studies in the 1940s showed a proliferative glomerulonephritis in between 13 per cent (Fingerman and Andrus 1943) and 63 per cent (Baggenstoss and Rosenberg 1943) of cases. However, many of these patients had infections, and it is probable that these caused their glomerulonephritis (see Chapter 3.12). Subsequently, autopsy studies have differed in the pattern of renal disease seen (Table 2). It is likely that some of these differences are due to selection bias and referral patterns. Thus, some studies have shown a high incidence of glomerulonephritis and renal vasculitis (Ramirez *et al.* 1981; Boers *et al.* 1987) with little in the way of renal papillary necrosis. In contrast in the study of Nanra and Kincaid-Smith (1975), 30 per cent of patients had a renal papillary necrosis, and no mention was made of either glomerulonephritis or amyloid.

Table 2 Autopsy studies in rheumatoid arthritis

Study	Country	Number of patients	Renal amyloid (%)	Renal failure (%)
Missen and Taylor (1956)	UK	47	17	
Mutru *et al.* (1976)	Finland	41	17	27
Ramirez *et al.* (1981)	USA	76	8	9
Boers *et al.* (1987)	Holland	132	11	23
Suzuki *et al.* (1994)	Japan	81	21	9.9

Renal biopsy studies in rheumatoid arthritis

Clinical studies in patients with rheumatoid arthritis have not provided evidence of a consistent pattern of renal disease in this disorder. The first renal biopsy studies in such patients were done to ascertain whether or not there was a specific 'rheumatoid glomerulonephritis'. Most patients biopsied had minimal or minor urinary abnormalities, and these studies were characterized by a high proportion of normal biopsies and the almost complete absence of glomerulonephritis (Pollak *et al.* 1962; Brun *et al.* 1965). These careful studies laid the foundation for the belief that patients with rheumatoid arthritis did not develop a glomerulonephritis other than as a consequence of treatment with gold or penicillamine.

Later studies investigated patients with rheumatoid arthritis and significant renal disease; these have provided good evidence of glomerulonephritis in patients who had never been treated with gold or penicillamine (Salomon *et al.* 1974; Ørjavik *et al.* 1981; Sellars *et al.* 1983; Hordon *et al.* 1984; Helin *et al.* 1986; Korpela *et al.* 1990; Adu *et al.* 1993; Nakano *et al.* 1998). None of these studies (Table 3) has compared the prevalence of glomerulonephritis in patients with rheumatoid arthritis with that in healthy controls. Ideally, such a study should be done to establish beyond all argument that glomerulonephritis may develop as a consequence of rheumatoid arthritis. This seems likely and is important for two reasons: first, the development of proteinuria and renal impairment in a patient with rheumatoid arthritis does not always indicate renal amyloid, with its inexorable progression to renal failure, and second because some types of renal disease, such as vasculitis, are amenable to treatment with steroids and cyclophosphamide (see below).

With more aggressive treatment of rheumatoid arthritis with disease modifying drugs, there does seem to be a lessening of the incidence and severity of renal disease associated with this disorder. Two recent studies reported that renal failure was not now an important cause of death in rheumatoid arthritis (Wolfe *et al.* 1994; Kroot *et al.* 2000), which contrasts with findings in studies reported during the 1980s and earlier.

Amyloidosis (see Chapter 4.2.1)

Amyloidosis is the extracellular deposition of the fibrillary protein amyloid at one or more sites in the body. Generalized, non-hereditary forms occur in association with monoclonal gammopathy (AL amyloid) or chronic inflammatory disease (AA amyloid). The other major type of amyloid protein is Aβ_2M found in dialysis amyloidosis. A full discussion of the various forms of amyloidosis, including the hereditary forms and their biochemical structures, are given in Chapters 4.2.1 and 11.3.11.

There are two aspects of relevance to rheumatic diseases. The first is the clinical situation where amyloidosis mimics arthritis, and the second is the much greater problem of secondary amyloidosis occurring in patients with rheumatoid arthritis.

Rheumatic symptoms in amyloidosis

Rheumatic symptoms occur in the following contexts:

1. Haemodialysis arthropathy, in which an increased plasma β_2-microglobulin concentration in plasma results in deposition of fibrils, producing the characteristic clinical picture of an entrapment neuropathy (especially carpal tunnel syndrome), bone cysts, and destructive arthropathy with a predilection for the shoulder and wrist.
2. Amyloidosis that involves articular structures and mimics other rheumatic complaints.

Only in the amyloidosis associated with a monoclonal gammopathy do joint symptoms occur frequently. Here, a clinical picture of symmetrical small-joint involvement with subcutaneous nodules can lead to the erroneous diagnosis of rheumatoid arthritis. Neuropathy (10 per cent) and carpal tunnel syndrome (20 per cent) also occur. Purpura is common and when accompanied by factor X deficiency (due to the increased affinity of AL for factor X), severe haemorrhage may occur. Helpful distinguishing features are that in myeloma stiffness is short-lived, the joints are rarely very tender, erosions are uncommon, and there is often excessive soft tissue swelling for the degree of inflammation: in the shoulder this produces a characteristic 'shoulder pad' appearance. However, the best discriminator is the fact that, despite the presence of nodules, the serum does not contain IgM rheumatoid factor. The most severe manifestations of myeloma and haemodialysis-associated amyloid are seen in the heart and kidneys (Chapter 4.2.1).

Secondary (AA) amyloidosis (Chapter 4.2.1; Lachmann and Hawkins 2001)

Frequency

Rheumatoid arthritis and juvenile chronic arthritis are the most common causes of AA amyloidosis in developed countries, accounting for between 60 and 70 per cent of all cases (Browning *et al.* 1985; Gertz and Kyle 1991; Toyoshima *et al.* 1993; Joss *et al.* 2000). There are no precise figures on the prevalence of the disorder and wide geographical variations occur. Rheumatoid arthritis-associated AA amyloid is more common in Europe than in the United States, and appears to be particularly common in Japan. Autopsy studies in Europe in the 1970s showed a prevalence rate of AA amyloid of 8–17 per cent (Mutru *et al.* 1976) and renal biopsy studies showed a prevalence rate of 5–10 per cent (Tribe 1966). More recent studies in Europe show a prevalence of approximately 3 per cent in clinical series (Fonseca *et al.* 2001) and 5 per cent in autopsy series (Myllykangas-Luosujarvi *et al.* 1999), whilst in Japan it exceeds 20 per cent in autopsy series (Toyoshima *et al.* 1993; Suzuki *et al.* 1994). There is thus evidence for a decline in prevalence of amyloid in

Table 3 Renal biopsy studies in rheumatoid arthritis

Study	Number of patients	Clinical Status	Normal	Mesangial proliferative glomerulonephritis	Membranous glomerulonephritis	Amyloid	Tubulointerstitial nephritis	Other
Pollak *et al.* (1962)	41	Normal, proteinuria	21	0	0	4	0	16
Brun *et al.* (1965)	32	Normal, proteinuria, renal impairment	11	0	1	4	9	7
Salomon *et al.* (1974)	18	Normal, proteinuria, microscopic haematuria	11	7	0	0	0	0
Orjavik *et al.* (1981)	14	Proteinuria, nephrotic syndrome	0	5	0	7	0	2
Sellars *et al.* (1983)	30	Proteinuria, microscopic haematuria, nephrotic syndrome	0	13	9	1	4	3
Horden *et al.* (1984)	21	Microscopic haematuria	1	15	1	0	1	3
Helin *et al.* (1986)	39	Proteinuria, nephrotic syndrome, renal impairment	3	11	9	16	0	0
Adu *et al.* (1993)	90	Proteinuria, nephrotic syndrome, renal impairment	0	10	18	13	14	35
Korpela *et al.* (1990)	74	Not given	7	23	13	20	3	8
Nakano *et al.* (1998)	158	Proteinuria, nephrotic syndrome haematuria, renal impairment	20	54	49	30		

Western Europe over the last 20 years, and in the last 5 years this fall has been dramatic. The reason is likely to be a greater awareness of the harmful effect of the acute-phase response, and the use of serum amyloid A and C-reactive protein as a measure of this. The current approach has led to much more aggressive therapy, with fewer patients being left with a persistently elevated acute-phase response; certainly the severity of arthritis is a known risk factor for the development of amyloid.

Clinical presentation

Renal problems are the chief clinical manifestation of AA amyloidosis and a major cause of death. In one study, only 3 per cent of patients with rheumatoid arthritis and amyloidosis did not have pathological changes in the kidney (Wegelius *et al.* 1980). Proteinuria, often with a nephrotic syndrome, is the most common clinical presentation; others include acute or chronic renal failure. Occasionally, there may be gastric bleeding or malabsorption, or heart failure from cardiac amyloid—although these are much less common than in AL amyloidosis.

Pathology

The diagnosis of amyloid is based on histological examination of either a rectal biopsy or abdominal fat aspiration. In patients with renal abnormalities a renal biopsy is indicated (Fig. 1a). Congo red

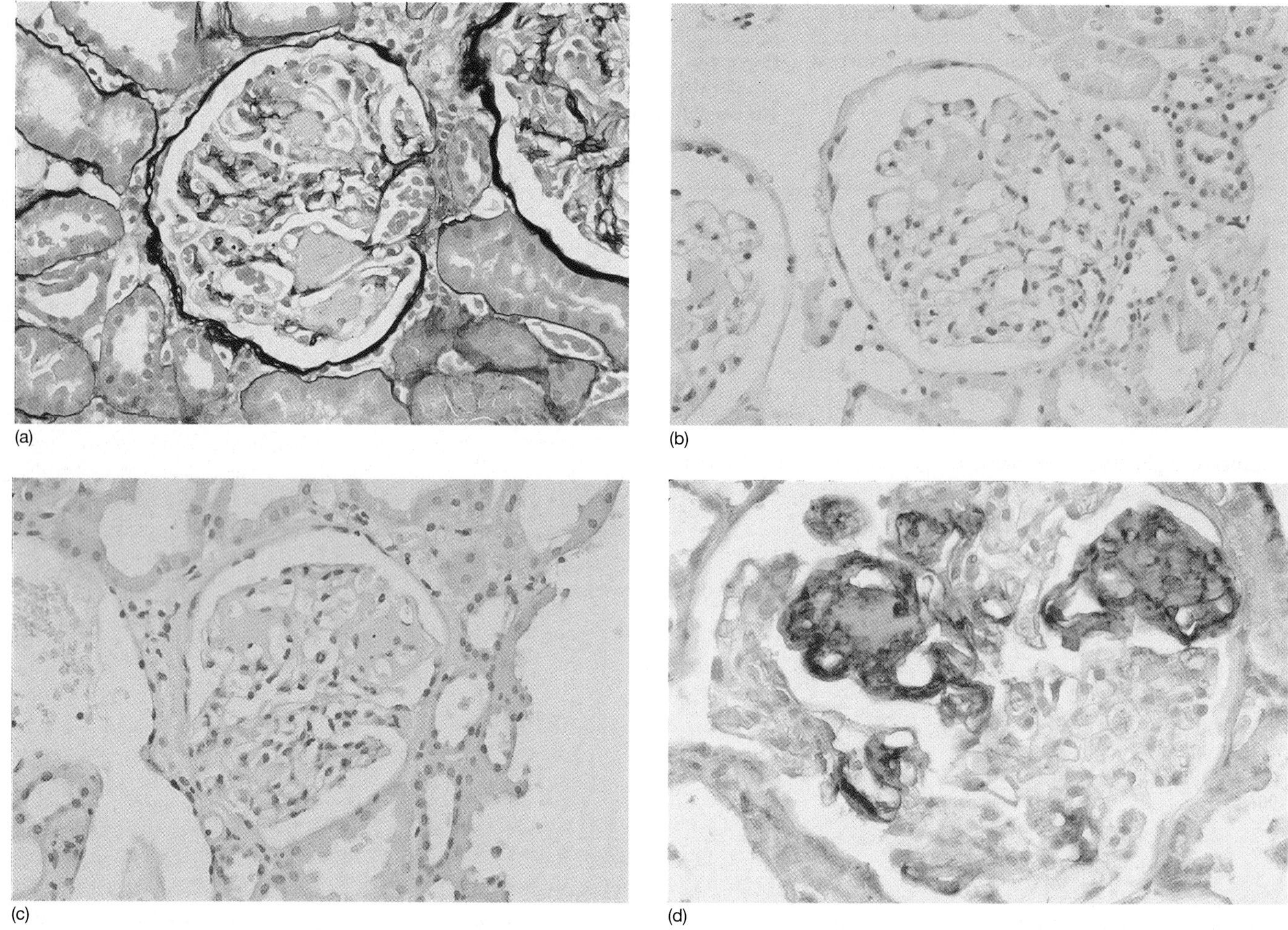

Fig. 1 (a) Photomicrograph of a renal biopsy showing glomerular deposits of amyloid. Periodic acid–methenamine silver, original magnification 100×. (b) Photomicrograph of a renal biopsy showing staining of amyloid deposits by Congo red. Original magnification 100×. (c) Photomicrograph of a renal biopsy. Congo red staining abolished by potassium permanganate. Original magnification 100×. (d) Photomicrograph of a renal biopsy showing staining of amyloid deposits by a monoclonal antibody to amyloid-A protein. Immunoperoxidase staining, original magnification 160×. (All photomicrographs by courtesy of Dr A.H. Howie.)

staining that is birefringent under polarized light is characteristic of amyloid in histological preparations (Fig. 1b). This staining is abolished by potassium permanganate in reactive AA amyloidosis (Fig. 1c) but not in primary AL amyloidosis. Monoclonal and polyclonal antibodies that specifically bind AA are now available, and these are of use for histological diagnosis (Fig. 1d) (see Chapter 4.2.1). Immunohistology using antibodies to κ- and λ-light chains may also confirm AL amyloid but this is not very reliable. In one study only 38 per cent of AL fibrils were identified by immunohistochemical staining (Lachmann *et al.* 2002).

Prognosis of untreated amyloidosis

After diagnosis of amyloid, mean survival in untreated patients with AA amyloidosis is poor, at about 24–48 months (Browning *et al.* 1985; Myllykangas-Luosujarvi *et al.* 1999; Chevrel *et al.* 2001) and this is worse in patients with renal impairment at diagnosis (Lindqvist *et al.* 1989).

Treatment of amyloidosis (see Chapter 4.2.1)

There is no specific therapy for AA amyloid, the general principle being that sustained suppression of the acute phase response can lead to regression of amyloid deposits. Because of the poor prognosis of untreated AA amyloid, alkylating agents have been used in treatment. Long-term treatment with chlorambucil was reported in uncontrolled studies to be effective in treating amyloidosis in children with juvenile chronic arthritis (Schnitzer and Ansell 1977). Evidence from uncontrolled studies also suggests that aggressive treatment of rheumatoid arthritis may be effective in delaying the deterioration of renal function in patients with renal amyloid. In a randomized controlled trial comparing treatment with a variety of cytotoxic drugs against no treatment, Ahlmen *et al.* (1987) reported a 5-year patient survival of 89 per cent in treated patients as compared to 29 per cent in untreated patients. Renal function was also better preserved in the treated patients. Several other uncontrolled studies have shown benefit in terms of survival and of renal function in patients treated with chlorambucil or cyclophosphamide (Hajzok *et al.* 1976; Falck *et al.* 1979a; Berglund *et al.* 1987, 1993; Mody and Meyers 1988; Maezawa *et al.* 1994; Shapiro and Spiera 1995).

Treatment of endstage renal failure from AA amyloid is by dialysis and renal transplantation. The median survival on dialysis ranges between 25 and 52 months (Martnez-Vea *et al.* 1990; Moroni *et al.* 1992; Joss *et al.* 2000).

Glomerulonephritis in rheumatoid arthritis

Proliferative glomerulonephritis

A proliferative glomerulonephritis is rare in rheumatoid arthritis. In the autopsy study of Boers *et al.* (1987), 5 of 132 cases had a proliferative glomerulonephritis (diffuse in one and focal in four). However, recent biopsy studies in patients with rheumatoid arthritis have reported little in the way of proliferative glomerulonephritis.

Mesangial proliferative glomerulonephritis

Recently, several studies in patients with rheumatoid arthritis and microscopic haematuria have reported a mild mesangial proliferative glomerulonephritis. Sellars *et al.* (1983) described a mesangial proliferative glomerulonephritis in 13 of 30 patients. The biopsies of nine were examined by immunofluorescence microscopy, and showed mesangial IgA deposits in two. Helin *et al.* (1986) reported a mild mesangial glomerulonephritis in 11 of 19 patients with rheumatoid arthritis and haematuria or proteinuria; 3 of the 11 had glomerular mesangial IgA deposits and a further seven had deposits of IgM, IgG, and C3. Details of these and other studies (Salomon *et al.* 1974; Ørjavik *et al.* 1981; Hordon *et al.* 1984) are summarized in Table 3. The majority of these patients were taking, or had recently been taking, gold or penicillamine, suggesting that their mild mesangial proliferative glomerulonephritis was drug related.

Mesangial IgA glomerulonephritis

In the studies of Sellars *et al.* (1983), Helin *et al.* (1986), and Korpela *et al.* (1990), several patients were described with a mesangial proliferative glomerulonephritis and mesangial IgA deposits. In most patients, mesangial IgA nephropathy is idiopathic (Berger and Hinglais 1968), but it has also been reported in patients with cirrhosis of the liver, dermatitis herpetiformis, mycosis fungoides, arthritis after yersinia infection, and seronegative spondyloarthritis (see Table 13, Chapter 3.9). We reported four patients with rheumatoid arthritis, microscopic haematuria, and proteinuria in whom renal biopsy showed a mesangial IgA glomerulonephritis; we also reviewed the literature on this association (Beaman *et al.* 1987). Three of these patients had never received gold or penicillamine, and in the one patient who had received gold this had been discontinued at least 10 years before presentation. These data provide circumstantial evidence of an association between rheumatoid arthritis and mesangial IgA nephropathy. As in idiopathic mesangial IgA nephropathy, the pathogenetic mechanisms of this disorder in patients with rheumatoid arthritis are unclear. It may be relevant that increased serum IgA, and also IgA rheumatoid factors, are found in some patients with rheumatoid arthritis. There are no long-term studies of renal function in patients with rheumatoid arthritis and mesangial IgA glomerulonephritis.

Membranous nephropathy

The most common cause of membranous nephropathy in patients with rheumatoid arthritis is gold or penicillamine therapy. However, there are now many reports of such patients who had never been on gold or penicillamine, and who have a membranous nephropathy unrelated to drug treatment. The numbers of reported cases make it unlikely that this association is coincidental. Honkanen *et al.* (1987) reported on four patients with rheumatoid arthritis and membranous nephropathy, and reviewed the literature. Only one of their four patients had received gold and that was 16 years before the renal biopsy. We also observed six patients with rheumatoid arthritis and a membranous nephropathy (Adu *et al.* 1993), none of whom had been treated with penicillamine, although two had received gold that was discontinued 17 and 13 years before renal biopsy. None of the patients in our study or in the previous reports (reviewed by Honkanen *et al.* 1987) had clinical or serological evidence of systemic lupus erythematosus (SLE), which may show membranous nephropathy (see Chapter 4.7.1).

Renal vasculitis (see also Chapters 4.5.1 and 4.5.3)

Introduction

The clinical spectrum of rheumatoid arthritis includes a systemic vasculitis, with involvement of blood vessels ranging in size from capillaries to small- and medium-sized arteries. The clinical presentation includes nailfold infarcts, a leucocytoclastic vasculitis, a peripheral neuropathy, pericarditis, gastrointestinal infarcts, and renal vasculitis (Scott *et al.* 1981). Data from one health district in the United Kingdom (Norwich Health Authority) suggests an overall annual incidence of systemic rheumatoid vasculitis of 12.5 per million population (Watts *et al.* 1994). Although renal abnormalities are found in about 25 per cent of patients with rheumatoid vasculitis (Scott *et al.* 1981) there are few reports of the renal histology in these patients.

Pathogenesis

The pathogenesis of vasculitic glomerulonephritis in rheumatoid arthritis is unknown. The majority of renal biopsies in the patients with this lesion show no significant immune deposits (Kuznetsky *et al.* 1986; Harper *et al.* 1997; Messiaen *et al.* 1998). This 'pauci-immune' vasculitic glomerulonephritis is similar to that seen in microscopic polyangiitis and Wegener's granulomatosis (see Chapters 4.5.1 and 4.5.2). Several patients with rheumatoid arthritis and a vasculitic glomerulonephritis have had antineutrophil cytoplasmic antibodies (ANCA) (Harper *et al.* 1997) and in some studies these were directed against myeloperoxidase (Messiaen *et al.* 1998; Yorioka *et al.* 1999). It is, however, difficult to establish a pathogenic role for ANCA in rheumatoid vasculitis. Approximately 20– 40 per cent of patients with rheumatoid arthritis have a positive ANCA (Savige *et al.* 1991;

Coremans *et al.* 1992; Mulder *et al.* 1993). The major antibody specificity is against lactoferrin, but between 4 and 12 per cent of patients have antimyeloperoxidase antibodies (Savige *et al.* 1991; Coremans *et al.* 1993; Cambridge *et al.* 1994).

Pathology

An autopsy study by Boers *et al.* (1987) of 132 patients with rheumatoid disease found a large vessel renal vasculitis in 8 of 18 cases with systemic vasculitis, and in four patients there was an extracapillary proliferative glomerulonephritis. There are now several case reports and small series of necrotizing and crescentic glomerulonephritis in patients with rheumatoid arthritis (Breedveld *et al.* 1985; Kuznetsky *et al.* 1986; Harper *et al.* 1997; Messiaen *et al.* 1998; Yorioka *et al.* 1999; Qarni and Kohan 2000). The renal pathology is of a vasculitic glomerulonephritis with focal and segmental necrosis of glomerular capillaries, breaks in the capillary walls, and extracapillary proliferation with a crescentic glomerulonephritis (Kuznetsky *et al.* 1986; Harper *et al.* 1997; Messiaen *et al.* 1998) (Fig. 2). Only 23 per cent of renal biopsies show significant glomerular immune deposits. An extraglomerular renal vasculitis is found in only 12 per cent of cases. Occasional patients may have other glomerular lesions such as a membranous nephropathy (Kuznetsky *et al.* 1986; Harper *et al.* 1997) or amyloidosis (Kiyama *et al.* 1991; Harper *et al.* 1997). Similar glomerular lesions have also been reported in patients with rheumatoid arthritis and other disorders who were treated with penicillamine.

Clinical presentation

The median age at onset from the published studies was 62 years with a range of 22–76 years and the median duration of rheumatoid arthritis of 13 years (range 1–40 years). Both genders are equally affected. Eighty-five per cent of patients are seropositive and 50 per cent of patients have extrarenal vasculitis. The clinical presentation is with microscopic haematuria and proteinuria in 90 per cent of cases and all patients have renal impairment or renal failure, which may be severe enough to require dialysis.

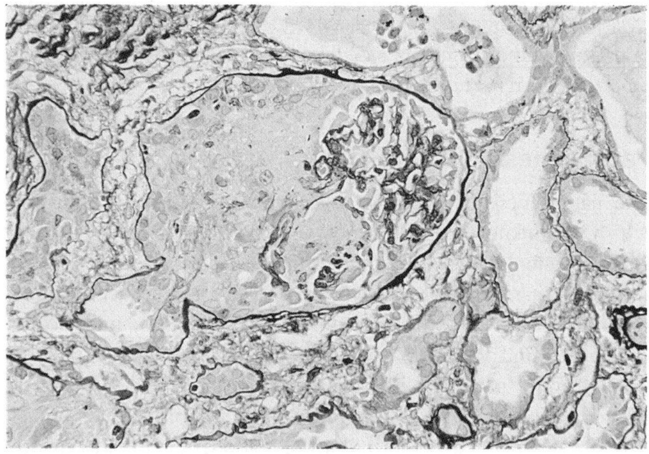

Fig. 2 Photomicrograph of a renal biopsy showing a segmental necrotizing glomerulonephritis with thrombosis and disruption of glomerular capillary loops and overlying extracapillary proliferation (crescents). Periodic acid–methenamine silver, original magnification 200×. (By courtesy of Dr A.H. Howie.)

Treatment and outcome

Treatment is with prednisolone and cyclophosphamide in the doses used to treat microscopic polyangiitis (see Chapter 4.5.3). The prognosis is reasonable with 95 per cent of patients surviving the acute illness. However, renal failure may be irreversible and require long-term dialysis. These studies show that, in addition to a renal arteritis, patients with rheumatoid arthritis may develop a vasculitic glomerulonephritis that by light microscopy appears similar to that seen in microscopic polyarteritis and Wegener's granulomatosis.

Renal disease in juvenile chronic arthritis

Renal failure accounts for 38 per cent of deaths in patients with juvenile chronic arthritis. The clinical spectrum of renal involvement in juvenile chronic arthritis has been reviewed by Anttila (1972). Proteinuria is found in between 3 and 12 per cent, and microscopic haematuria in 3–8 per cent of these patients. Nephrotic-range proteinuria is commonly due to renal amyloid, found in between 1.2 and 6.7 per cent of patients with juvenile chronic arthritis, whilst haematuria and proteinuria may be due to amyloid or gold treatment.

In one study, 47 of 638 patients (7.4 per cent) with juvenile chronic arthritis had renal disease (Anttila and Laaksonen 1969). In a study of renal histology (57 renal biopsy, three autopsy) in a relatively unselected group of patients with juvenile chronic arthritis renal amyloid was detected in two (3.3 per cent) and interstitial nephritis in eight patients (13.3 per cent) (Anttila 1972). There are unexplained geographical variations in the prevalence of amyloidosis in patients with juvenile chronic arthritis. In the United Kingdom the prevalence 7.4 per cent (Schnitzer and Ansell 1977), in America 1.8 per cent, and in Poland 10.6 per cent (Filipowicz-Sosnowska *et al.* 1978).

Renal amyloidosis with endstage renal failure accounted for between 33 and 50 per cent of deaths in juvenile chronic arthritis (Schnitzer and Ansell 1977). In the 1960s, Ansell introduced the use of chlorambucil for the treatment of children with juvenile rheumatoid arthritis and amyloidosis, and showed this to be of benefit in improving survival using historical controls (Ansell *et al.* 1971). Subsequent uncontrolled studies have confirmed the benefits of chlorambucil in these children (Schnitzer and Ansell 1977; Deschenes *et al.* 1990; David *et al.* 1993). In the study of David *et al.*, 80 per cent of patients treated with chlorambucil were alive at 10 years as compared with 25 per cent of untreated patients. Chlorambucil is an alkylating agent, and in addition to marrow suppression leads to gonadal failure and is oncogenic (Woo 1994). Clearly there is a need for studies into safer alternative therapies.

Tubulointerstitial nephritis in association with arthritis

Renal biopsy studies in patients with rheumatoid arthritis and juvenile chronic arthritis have reported that up to 28 per cent of patients with renal abnormalities have a tubulointerstitial nephritis (Brun *et al.* 1965; Anttila 1972; Sellars *et al.* 1983). This is often attributed to the renal toxicity of analgesic agents, including NSAIDs. It is, however, probable that these disorders may, in themselves, be associated with the development of tubulointerstitial nephritis.

Renal disease in ankylosing spondylitis

Amyloidosis with renal involvement develops in approximately 5 per cent of patients with ankylosing spondylitis (Gratacos *et al.* 1997). In addition, there are several reports of an association between ankylosing spondylitis and IgA nephropathy (Kanterewicz *et al.* 1987; Chen *et al.* 1988). Finally, patients with ankylosing spondylitis may develop NSAID-induced nephrotoxicity.

Gold and D-penicillamine-associated nephropathy

There is no cure for patients with rheumatoid arthritis. The aim of disease-modifying antirheumatic drugs, therefore, is to suppress disease activity. Gold and D-penicillamine are the prototypes of this group of drugs, and despite the introduction of alternatives these remain frequently prescribed. Despite intense investigation, the mode of action of neither of these drugs is known, although the immunological consequences of an improvement in disease activity are well documented. They have the greatest prevalence of side-effects produced by any drugs outside those used in malignancy. The incidence of toxicity is up to 70 per cent, and withdrawal of the drugs as a result of these adverse reactions occurs in around 40 per cent of patients (Huskisson *et al.* 1974). Therefore, the avoidance or reduction of toxicity would greatly improve patient care.

Clinical features of drug-induced disease

In general, gold and D-penicillamine produce very similar problems (Huskisson *et al.* 1974), and where not specifically mentioned, the following discussion applies to both drugs. The side-effects of these drugs can be divided temporally into two groups. The first group consists of those side-effects occurring early in therapy. These are believed to be due to a direct toxic effect of the drug, and include anorexia and rashes. The second group consists of those reactions that occur after 3 months and maximally around 6 months. These are believed to have an immunological basis and renal toxicity comes within this category.

The immunological reactions most frequently observed are glomerulonephritis and thrombocytopenia. Drug-induced autoimmune disorders such as SLE (D-penicillamine) occur less frequently (Emery and Panayi 1989). The prevalence of side-effects increases with the dose of D-penicillamine (Williams *et al.* 1983). This has not been shown for gold, probably because it is given intermittently according to a fixed regimen.

The most frequent presenting feature is proteinuria; haematuria is relatively rare (and seen more frequently with penicillamine). Proteinuria occurs in approximately 10 per cent of patients receiving gold and up to 30 per cent of patients taking penicillamine. This progresses to the nephrotic syndrome in 30 and 16 per cent, respectively. Haematuria occurring in the context of therapy with these drugs still requires the exclusion of other causes.

Renal function

In general, these drugs do not produce a significant reduction in GFR, although a wide range of renal function has been documented. A reduction in GFR may occur secondarily to hypovolaemia, and renal damage in severe cases of the nephrotic syndrome. Furthermore, there is no significant deterioration in renal function with time, provided the drug is stopped.

Histopathology

Membranous glomerulonephritis

About 80 per cent of patients who present with D-penicillamine- or gold-induced proteinuria will have a membranous glomerulonephritis. Epimembranous 'spikes' and a mild increase in mesangial cells are usually seen, and the diagnosis can be confirmed with immunofluorescence/immunoperoxidase microscopy, which shows granular subepithelial deposits of predominantly IgG. On electron microscopy, electron-dense deposits are seen (see Chapter 3.7).

Mesangial glomerulonephritis

Mesangial glomerulonephritis is found in patients with rheumatoid arthritis irrespective of therapy. The prevalence is probably increased after treatment with disease-modifying antirheumatic drugs, and for gold at least there is an increased association between this histological appearance and haematuria.

Immunofluorescence may reveal either granular deposits of immunoglobulin (predominantly IgG) and complement, or may be negative, particularly in the case of D-penicillamine-induced disease.

Minimal-change nephropathy

This can occur in association with the use of disease-modifying antirheumatic drugs (Lee 1965). Electron microscopy shows fusion of epithelial-cell foot processes (see Chapter 3.5).

Tubulointerstitial disease

This is found in up to 10 per cent of patients in association with mild, low-molecular-weight proteinuria and enzymuria. The outlook is good, with rapid resolution on withdrawal of the drug (see Chapter 19.2).

Crescentic glomerulonephritis

Penicillamine may lead to the development of a rapidly progressive glomerulonephritis (Williams *et al.* 1986; Almirall *et al.* 1993), the clinical picture of Goodpasture's syndrome (Sternlieb *et al.* 1975; Gibson *et al.* 1976) (Chapter 3.11) and also a renal vasculitis (Falck *et al.* 1979b; Banfi *et al.* 1983) (see Chapter 4.5.1).

Autoantibody production

D-Penicillamine therapy has been associated with a wide range of autoantibodies. Antibodies against DNA may lead to a drug-induced syndrome of SLE. Whilst most drug-induced lupus syndromes have antibodies directed against histones, occasionally patients with D-penicillamine-induced disease may have antibodies against double-stranded DNA and may develop significant renal disease (Chalmers *et al.* 1982) (see Chapter 4.7.1).

Management

An increasing experience of patients with renal toxicity to D-penicillamine and gold has revealed a benign long-term outcome following withdrawal of the drug (Collins 1987; Hall *et al.* 1987, 1988). The management of renal toxicity occurring *de novo* on therapy is now determined by practical issues. These include the response of the patient, the amount of proteinuria, and the presence of any deterioration in renal function. In general, a declining albumin, proteinuria greater than 2 g/24 h, or a, reduced GFR are considered indications for stopping treatment. No specific immunosuppression is required for the drug-induced disorder, although supportive measures are given as indicated.

In those patients without renal abnormalities before treatment, renal biopsy should be confined to those who have deteriorating renal function, or who fail to improve after withdrawal of the drug. In practice, therefore, patients who develop proteinuria are often managed empirically by a reduction in either the frequency or the size of the dose of the drug, with withdrawal of the drug only if any of the adverse factors are present. Regular monitoring of proteinuria and GFR are mandatory. Haematuria, unless it resolves when the drug is stopped, requires investigation in the usual manner.

Long-term outcome

After cessation of the drug, proteinuria peaks at around a month then gradually disappears; the majority of patients will have clear urine by 1 year and almost all will achieve this by 2 years (Fig. 3) (Hall *et al.* 1987, 1988). Renal function does not deteriorate in uncomplicated cases. If membranous nephropathy is present, the renal histology reverts towards normal although iterative renal biopsies are rarely needed. Given the genetic basis (the same for both drugs, see below) of most renal toxicities, it is not surprising that re-challenge with the same drug at the same dose usually leads to a recurrence of the renal problem, although a lower dose may be tolerated. The dilemma of whether to restart the drug is now less of a problem because of the increasing number of alternative therapies.

Predicting toxicity

HLA and drug toxicity

Soon after the demonstration of an increased prevalence of the class II major histocompatibility complex antigen HLA-DR4 in patients with rheumatoid arthritis, it was shown that the risk of developing certain immunological adverse reactions to gold was increased in patients

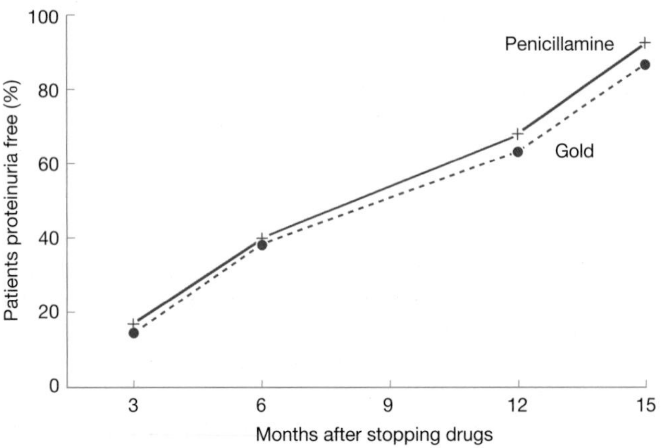

Fig. 3 Percentage of patients free of proteinuria after discontinuing gold or penicillamine (Hall *et al.* 1987, 1988).

with HLA-DR3 (Panayi *et al.* 1978; Wooley *et al.* 1980). Several studies have now confirmed this observation and it has been extended to D-penicillamine. Seventy-five per cent of patients with idiopathic membranous glomerulonephritis are HLA-DR3 positive (see Chapter 3.8) and HLA-DR3 confers a relative risk of 14.0–32.0 for gold-induced nephropathy and 3.2–10.0 for D-penicillamine-induced nephropathy (Klouda *et al.* 1979).

Metabolic factors that determine disease-modifying drug-induced toxicity

It is known that polymorphisms exist for certain enzymes which are largely genetically determined, and can be investigated using probe drugs. Adverse reactions to drugs metabolized by these pathways occur only, or much more severely, in the individuals who metabolize poorly. The sulfoxidation ability was originally assessed in patients with toxicity due to D-penicillamine because of the similarity between the structure of the drug and the probe-drug carbocysteine. The relative risk of toxicity was found to be 7.5 in those patients with low sulfoxidation activity. HLA-DR3 status was also assessed, and although the two risk factors were not additive, the possession of either DR3 or poor sulfoxidation produced a relative risk of 25.0 (Emery *et al.* 1984). Subsequently, poor sulfoxidation ability has been examined in patients treated with gold and has been shown to be a significant risk factor for gold toxicity also (Madhok *et al.* 1987). The mechanism for the association between sulfoxidation status and toxicity is unknown. As the only common structural similarity between gold and penicillamine is a thiol group (gold is usually given as aurothiomalate), the metabolism of this may be the critical determinant of toxicity. However, it is known that poor sulfoxidation is part of a number of other genetically determined 'linked' enzyme systems (e.g. glucuronidation and *S*-methylation) and it is possible that one of these is important in inducing the immunological abnormalities.

Cyclosporin nephrotoxicity (see Chapter 13.2.2)

Cyclosporin is licensed for the treatment of rheumatoid arthritis. Despite its less dramatic effect on the acute-phase response, studies have shown it to be better than placebo and equal to most other second-line drugs (Yocum *et al.* 1988). Furthermore, it has been shown to reduce the rate of occurrence of radiological erosions. The renal toxicity of cyclosporin in rheumatoid arthritis is well-documented (Boers *et al.* 1990; Cohen and Appel 1992). In these patients, cyclosporin should be started at a dose of 2.5 mg/kg per day and not exceed 5 mg/kg per day, with a reduction of cyclosporin dosage if creatinine increases to 130 per cent of baseline (Group 1989). Indeed, so sensitive is the increase in creatinine in patients with rheumatoid arthritis that other measures of renal function are used only to confirm changes. This arises from an (initially reversible) afferent arteriolar vasoconstriction (Chapter 13.2.2). Cyclosporin has been successfully combined with other agents, including methotrexate, the concern here being that the reduction in GFR affects renal excretion of methotrexate (Tugwell *et al.* 1995). The nephrotoxicity of cyclosporin is increased by NSAIDs (Berg *et al.* 1989).

Measurement of the blood concentration of cyclosporin is rarely required in rheumatoid arthritis, the limitation nearly always being renal toxicity and hypertension. Cyclosporin can lead also to chronic, irreversible renal failure with interstitial fibrosis, which is more common with doses in excess of 5 mg/kg, in patients with pre-existing renal impairment, in elderly patients, and in patients treated for longer than 6 months. Renal function should be carefully monitored in patients on cyclosporin therapy.

Analgesic nephropathy (see Chapter 6.2)

Patients with rheumatoid arthritis often take analgesics over many years. Until the 1960s, analgesia was obtained with aspirin or less commonly with compound analgesic drugs. More recently, NSAIDs have been used, such as the COX-1/COX-2 inhibitors, of which the prototype is indomethacin (although itself little used today because of gastrointestinal toxicity), and more recently the COX-2-selective NSAIDs, such as rofecoxib and celecoxib.

Renal papillary necrosis and chronic tubulointerstitial nephritis leading to renal failure was a well-recognized complication of compound analgesics, in particular of those that contained phenacetin (Cove-Smith and Knapp 1978). These renal complications also occurred in patients with rheumatoid arthritis (Cove-Smith and Knapp 1978). Most patients with rheumatoid arthritis were, however, treated with aspirin as the sole analgesic agent, and the occasional observation at autopsy of renal papillary necrosis in these patients led to suggestions that aspirin on its own was nephrotoxic (Lawson and Maclean 1966; Nanra and Kincaid-Smith 1975). The New Zealand Rheumatism Association (1974) study of 763 patients with rheumatoid arthritis and 145 patients with osteoarthritis, however, found no association between aspirin intake and renal dysfunction, and concluded that the risk of nephrotoxicity from this drug was of a very low order (Study 1974).

Phenacetin was withdrawn by the 1970s, and at this time aspirin was supplanted by the newer NSAIDs and paracetamol. NSAIDs are potentially nephrotoxic (Dunn 1984) and their renal side-effects are described in Chapter 6.3. In patients with rheumatoid arthritis, these drugs may lead to a reversible reduction in GFR, acute tubular necrosis, an acute interstitial nephritis, often with heavy proteinuria, renal papillary necrosis, and chronic tubulointerstitial nephritis (Adams *et al.* 1986). Recent data show that the COX-2-selective inhibitors have renal side-effects comparable to those seen with the non-selective COX-1 NSAIDs (see Chapter 6.3). Both rofecoxib (Rocha and Fernandez-Alonso 1946) and celecoxib (Henao *et al.* 2002) have been reported to cause an interstitial nephritis.

Paracetamol is also widely used and there are suggestions that it also may be nephrotoxic (Sandler 1989; Perneger *et al.* 1994).

Methotrexate

Methotrexate is widely used as a disease-modifying drug in rheumatoid arthritis. The major metabolite of methotrexate, 7-hydroxy methotrexate, is renally excreted and accumulates in renal impairment, which may lead to toxicity (Ellman and Ginsberg 1990; Kraus and Alarcon-Segovia 1991). The concurrent administration of NSAIDs and methotrexate is widespread, and is apparently safe. However, the potential nephrotoxicity of NSAIDs means that renal function should be monitored in patients on this combination of drugs.

Mixed connective tissue disease

Some patients with a connective tissue disorder do not fit easily into the accepted definitions of a single disease. Sharp *et al.* (1972) reported on 25 patients in whom there was an overlap of the clinical features of SLE, systemic sclerosis, and polymyositis. Sera from all of these patients contained antibodies to an RNAase-sensitive, extractable nuclear antigen subsequently shown to be ribonucleoprotein (RNP). These patients lacked antibody to Sm antigen, had infrequent and low titres of antibody to double-stranded DNA, and normal or increased serum complement. They termed this disorder *mixed connective tissue disease* (MCTD). The antibody specificity was later shown to be directed at the 70 kDa polypeptide of the uridine rich (U1) small nuclear RNP (U1 sn RNP) or against U1 RNA (Burdt *et al.* 1999). Subsequent studies have included patients with features at onset similar to rheumatoid arthritis and have emphasized the asynchronous development of overlapping clinical features of different connective tissues in this syndrome (Bennett and O'Connell 1980). There is still debate on whether MCTD is a distinctive autoimmune disorder.

In the original report of Sharp *et al.* (1972), of 25 patients with MCTD, only one patient developed evidence of renal disease. A follow-up study 4–5 years later showed that renal disease remained an infrequent complication of MCTD (Nimelstein *et al.* 1980). Subsequent studies in patients with MCTD have, however, shown that the prevalence of renal involvement was high, ranging from 10 to 40 per cent in adults (reviewed by Kitridou *et al.* 1986; Burdt *et al.* 1999) and up to 47 per cent in children (Singsen 1980).

Clinical presentation

Most patients (90 per cent) are female and the clinical presentation is with Raynaud's phenomenon and swollen hands. There may be features of SLE such as polyarthritis, lymphadenopathy, facial erythema, pericarditis or pleurisy, leucocytosis, and thrombocytopenia. The patients may also have systemic sclerosis-like features such as sclerodactyly, pulmonary fibrosis, and oesophageal hypomotility. Finally, patients may have features of polymyositis with muscle weakness and a raised creatinine kinase (Burdt *et al.* 1999). Other studies have included patients with features at onset similar to rheumatoid arthritis, and have emphasized the development of overlapping clinical features of different connective tissues in this syndrome (Bennett and O'Connell 1980).

The clinical presentation of renal disease in patients with MCTD usually takes the form of asymptomatic proteinuria or haematuria, often with mild renal impairment. In the study of Kitridou *et al.* (1986), 75 per cent of patients with renal disease developed a nephrotic syndrome, 42 per cent hypertension, and 17 per cent progressed to chronic renal failure.

Histological changes

Kitridou *et al.* (1986) reported on the renal histological changes in 12 patients with MCTD and reviewed previous reports in 64 patients. Membranous nephropathy and a mesangial proliferative glomerulonephritis were the most common histological changes, found in 34 and 30 per cent of cases, respectively. A focal or diffuse proliferative glomerulonephritis was found in 17 per cent, a mixed lesion with membranous nephropathy in 5 per cent, and in 7 per cent renal histology was normal. Seventeen per cent of patients had evidence of vascular sclerosis, a feature also emphasized in the autopsy study of Sawai *et al.* (1994). Immunofluorescence microscopy of glomeruli in patients with MCTD has shown immunoglobulin and complement deposits; on electron microscopy, dense deposits are found consistent with an immune complex-mediated glomerulonephritis (Bennett and Spargo 1977; Kitridou *et al.* 1986). Similar glomerular findings have been reported in children, but in addition widespread intimal proliferation was seen (Singsen *et al.* 1980).

Treatment

Treatment of renal failure in MCTD is with steroids initially in high doses, subsequently tapering to a maintenance at low dose over weeks (Glassock *et al.* 1982; Kitridou *et al.* 1986). In the study of Kitridou *et al.* (1986), treatment with high-dose steroids of patients with a nephrotic syndrome was associated with a significant reduction of proteinuria in 62 per cent of episodes. Whether patients with renal disease resistant to steroids would benefit from the addition of immunosuppressant drugs is not known. Some 14 per cent of patients with MCTD and renal involvement reviewed by Kitridou *et al.* (1986) developed chronic renal failure. The long-term overall mortality of MCTD has varied from 7 per cent over a mean follow-up of 7 years (Sharp *et al.* 1972) to 20–30 per cent over a period of 3–25 years after onset of disease (Nimelstein *et al.* 1980; Burdt *et al.* 1999).

Polymyositis

Inflammatory diseases of skeletal muscle may be idiopathic or secondary to a wide variety of disorders (Targoff 1993). Primary adult idiopathic polymyositis usually presents with insidious, proximal muscle weakness and muscle pain, often without previous illness, although some patients have a preceding febrile illness, Raynaud's phenomenon, or arthralgia. Rarely, severe muscle weakness develops abruptly and this may be associated with myoglobinuria and diagnosed by raised serum creatinine kinase.

Acute renal failure has been reported infrequently in patients with polymyositis, and this has been attributed to rhabdomyolysis and myoglobinuria (Sloan *et al.* 1978; Swainson *et al.* 1984). The clinical evolution of the acute renal failure is similar to that seen with other causes of non-traumatic rhabdomyolysis. There are occasional reports of a mesangial proliferative glomerulonephritis with mesangial deposits of immunoglobulin and complement in patients with polymyositis (Dyck *et al.* 1979; Valenzuela *et al.* 2001). Treatment with high-dose steroids and methotrexate or azathioprine is of benefit in patients with polymyositis (Mastaglia 2000).

Rheumatological complications of renal disease and dialysis (Karim et al. 2001)

Pseudogout (pyrophosphate arthropathy)

Calcium pyrophosphate deposition (CPPD) can lead to acute synovitis. This is less common in patients with renal disease than urate or basic CPPD disease, and is rare in dialysis patients. There is an association with Bartter's syndrome. The disease can present as acute, monoarticular, or pauciarticular arthritis (known as pseudogout), or as a chronic arthritis resembling degenerative joint disease (Ferrari 1996). It is important to remember that pseudogout can coexist with other disorders and can exacerbate existing joint conditions.

The pathology is a consequence of deposition of crystals in the articular cartilage. The natural history of attacks is more variable than gout, and prolonged symptoms may occur partly due to the common association between CPPD disease and osteoarthritis. Predisposing factors/associations include hyperparathyroidism, age, trauma, meniscectomy, hypomagnesaemia, hypothyroidism, hypophosphataemia, and haemochromatosis.

The treatment of coexisting conditions may have a variable impact on the arthritis. It is important to remember that infection also can coexist with the presence of CPPD in the synovial fluid. The therapy of this condition is limited; oral colchicine may be effective as a prophylaxis, but is not commonly used in patients with renal failure. Local intra-articular corticosteroids are the most effective and commonly used treatment, and have been shown to shorten acute attacks when compared to treatment with NSAIDs alone (O'Duffy 1976).

Septic arthritis

Septic arthritis should always be considered whenever a joint becomes swollen in a patient with renal disease. Infectious complications are common in transplant recipients, and opportunistic organisms such as *mycobacteria* and fungi as well as common pathogens should be considered. Impaired host defences secondary to underlying renal disease or immunosuppression, and pre-existing joint damage are all contributors to the risk of septic arthritis post-transplant (Vincenti *et al.* 1982). A particular problem occurs in those patients requiring joint replacement post-transplantation (Tannenbaum *et al.* 1997). Sepsis usually occurs in a single joint and most commonly within 18 months of transplant. Gram-negative joint infections have been associated with concurrent urinary tract infection. It is important to remember that crystal arthritis and infection may coexist and a thorough assessment of the synovial fluid is required to distinguish these conditions (Sinnott and Holt 1989).

Haemarthroses

Haemarthroses can occur in two major groups, first, those patients with bleeding diatheses and second, patients with degenerative joint disease. Furthermore, blood can appear in the synovial fluid as a consequence of a traumatic joint aspiration. Whatever the aetiology of the haemarthrosis, blood within the joint is known to be harmful and the correct therapy is aspiration as speedily as possible. Although lacking in objective evidence, clinical experience suggests that rapid aspiration of the blood with injection of corticosteroid produces the most beneficial result.

Joint effusions

Joint effusions can be either acute or chronic. Acute joint effusions should be aspirated to establish the cause and to prevent distension of the capsule and subsequent laxity and instability, which will contribute to degeneration. Acute benign joint effusions may occur in transplant recipients, in association with episodes of acute rejection. Chronic effusions are more difficult to treat and are often a consequence of mechanical factors. Intra-articular corticosteroid injection of the acute rather than chronic joint effusion is more likely to produce benefit.

β2-Microglobulin arthropathy (see Chapter 11.3.11)

Dialysis-related amyloidosis is a severe arthropathy that is seen with increasing frequency with age and time spent on dialysis (Chazot *et al.* 1993) and is the result of deposition of retained circulating β_2-microglobulin. Dialysis arthropathy frequently presents with pain and stiffness, usually in the shoulder joints and often bilateral and also with a carpal tunnel syndrome and hip and knee pain (Sethi *et al.* 1990). The pain may be worse at night and exacerbated by haemodialysis. Effusions may develop with a destructive spondyloarthropathy particularly of the cervical spine. Radiology may be helpful in diagnosis with bone cysts away from the synovial lining being seen and the joint often remaining normal.

Soft tissue calcification

Basic calcium phosphate can deposit at a periarticular site and cause acute inflammatory episodes such as rotator cuff tendinitis. When deposits occur within the joint this can produce non-inflammatory degeneration and destruction.

Transplant-related bone and joint disease

Osteoporosis

Osteoporosis has a high prevalence in renal transplant recipients, and arises from a variety of factors, including high-dose corticosteroid therapy. By the time of transplantation, bone density is almost always already less than normal, and this may be due to prior corticosteroid therapy and long-standing metabolic acidosis (Ferrari 1996). Following transplantation loss of bone mineral density (BMD) is more rapid than that seen in other patient groups, and the prevalence of significant osteoporosis is considerably greater in this population. The greatest bone loss occurs within the first 6–12 months after transplantation (Epstein *et al.* 1995; Grotz *et al.* 1995a,b) and predominantly affects cancellous (trabecular) bone, consistent with a dominant corticosteroid effect. In the first year, bone loss continues with a reduction in bone density of between 6 and 15 per cent (Epstein *et al.* 1995; Arlen and Adachi 1999), subsequent years see a loss of 1–2 per cent (Grotz *et al.* 1995b). The pathogenesis of rapid bone loss is multifactorial. Possible factors contributing to this include hyperparathyroidism, which reduces cortical bone, uraemia, aluminium accumulation, and osteomalacia. Genetic factors may also be implicated, with vitamin D receptor polymorphisms playing a role in bone loss. Other factors relating to the risk of bone loss include prednisolone dosage, whereas vitamin D therapy and physical activity counterbalance loss. Decrease in BMD is minimized if the prednisolone dose is maintained at less than 7.5 mg per day.

The mechanisms by which corticosteroids increase bone loss are exacerbated by chronic renal failure, which acts by inhibiting the formation and accelerating the resorption of bone. Corticosteroids inhibit calcium absorption from the gastrointestinal tract, and induce calcium loss; these effects lead to secondary hyperparathyroidism with further loss of skeletal calcium. It is recommended that patients be assessed with Dual energy X-ray absorptiometry scanning prior to transplantation. Therapy to reduce bone loss should be instituted during the waiting period, with all patients receiving calcium and vitamin D therapy as appropriate. Post-transplantation patients should receive the recommended daily allowance of calcium and vitamin D. Some studies have recommended pharmacological doses of vitamin D but this can lead to hypercalcaemia.

There are no large randomized trials of the effects of biphosphonates on post-transplant steroid-induced osteoporosis. These patients have pretransplant metabolic bone disease that is heterogeneous in its pathogenesis. In the absence of firm evidence it is difficult to give clear guidelines on the use of biphosphonates. One approach would be to identify patients with low bone density in the pretransplant period and to treat such individuals with biphosphonates. Current studies are evaluating the efficacy of biphosphonates in preventing post-transplant osteoporosis. They appear to be effective but require long-term use. The impact of newer, much higher potency biphosphonates is awaited.

Avascular necrosis of bone

The presence of avascular necrosis (osteonecrosis) in transplant recipients was reported in the past to affect up to 40 per cent of patients (Ferrari 1996) but more recent data suggest a prevalence of about 5 per cent (Le Parc *et al.* 1996). The femoral head is most commonly involved, but avascular necrosis has also been described in the humeral head and distal femur. Risk factors for this complication include high-dose corticosteroids (Lausten *et al.* 1998) and pretransplant hyperparathyroidism. Patients may describe pain when weight-bearing and also at rest. Later, they may develop a reduced range of movement. In the early stages radiographs are usually unhelpful, and bone scintigraphy and magnetic resonance imaging (MRI) are needed for diagnosis. MRI may detect lesions prior to symptoms. Therapy remains controversial and the options include conservative management (Kyd 1979) or decompression (Grevitt and Spencer 1995). Ultimately, joint replacement is often required.

Acute bone pain

This syndrome occurs in renal transplant recipients receiving cyclosporin (Lucas *et al.* 1991; Gauthier and Barbosa 1994; Stevens *et al.* 1995) and has a prevalence of 19 per cent (Barbosa *et al.* 1995). Symptoms develop up to 2 years post-transplant and usually disappear within 2–6 weeks of stopping the usage of cyclosporin (Lucas *et al.* 1990). The pain is usually bilateral and acute in onset, but may be episodic with a deep aching sensation that can last for several hours at a time. The pain characteristically affects the lower limb but can affect the upper limb, the shoulders, and the thighs. The pain is worse at night and when lying flat. There may be an association with increased cyclosporin levels, and reduction in dose may improve symptoms (Lucas *et al.* 1990). Examination and investigations are unrevealing and the ideal therapy is withdrawal of cyclosporin and conversion to tacrolimus. More specifically, nifedipine has been shown to be effective in one group of patients (Barbosa *et al.* 1995). The response to calcium channel blockade suggests a vascular aetiology.

Reflex sympathetic dystrophy

Reflex sympathetic dystrophy (RSD) can occur usually within 2–3 months postrenal transplant with an incidence of around 2–2.5 per cent (Munoz-Gomez *et al.* 1991). The pain is symmetrical, usually in the lower limbs and affecting the ankles and knees. Physical findings include periarticular soft tissue swelling and vasomotor changes, investigations show patchy osteoporosis on radiographs and increased epiphyseal uptake of 99m-Technetium with a periarticular distribution. Patients tend to be on cyclosporin therapy with blood levels greater than 200 ng/ml, and symptoms improve when the dose of cyclosporin is reduced and blood levels fall. Treatment with calcitonin and calcium channel blockers has been reported to be effective (Grandtnerova *et al.* 1998) as has been treatment with corticosteriods (Munoz-Gomez *et al.* 1991). It is possible that steroids may protect against the development of a full RSD pattern. Given the similar features between RSD and acute bone pain syndrome, it is possible that acute bone pain syndrome is part of the spectrum of RSD and that the signs are masked by concurrent corticosteroid use.

References

Adams, D. H. *et al.* (1986). Non-steroidal anti-inflammatory drugs and renal failure. *Lancet* **i**, 57–60.

Adu, D. *et al.* (1993). Glomerulonephritis in Rheumatoid Arthritis. *British Journal of Rheumatology* **32**, 1008–1011.

Ahlmen, M. *et al.* (1987). Cytotoxic drug treatment of reactive amyloidosis in rheumatoid arthritis with special reference to renal insufficiency. *Clinical Rheumatology* **6**, 27–38.

Almirall, J. *et al.* (1993). Penicillamine-induced rapidly progressive glomerulonephritis in a patient with rheumatoid arthritis. *American Journal of Nephrology* **13**, 286–288.

Ansell, B. M., Eghtedari, A., and Bywaters, E. G. (1971). Chlorambucil in the management of juvenile chronic polyarthritis complicated by amyloidosis. *Annals of the Rheumatic Diseases* **30**, 331.

Anttila, R. (1972). Renal involvement in juvenile rheumatoid arthritis. A clinical and histopathological study. *Acta Paediatrica Scandinavica* **227**, 1–73.

Anttila, R. and Laaksonen, A. L. (1969). Renal disease in juvenile rheumatoid arthritis. *Acta Rheumatologica Scandinavica* **15**, 99–111.

Arlen, D. J. and Adachi, J. D. (1999). Are bisphosphonates useful in the management of corticosteroid induced osteoporosis in transplant patients? *Journal of Nephrology* **12**, 5–8.

Baggenstoss, A. H. and Rosenberg, E. F. (1943). Visceral lesions associated with chronic infectious (rheumatoid) arthritis. *Archives of Pathology & Laboratory Medicine* **35**, 503–516.

Banfi, G. *et al.* (1983). Extracapillary glomerulonephritis with necrotizing vasculitis in D-penicillamine-treated rheumatoid arthritis. *Nephron* **33**, 56–60.

Barbosa, L. M., Gauthier, V. J., and Davis, C. L. (1995). Bone pain that responds to calcium channel blockers. A retrospective and prospective study of transplant recipients. *Transplantation* **59**, 541–544.

Beaman, M. *et al.* (1987). Rheumatoid arthritis and IgA nephropathy. *British Journal of Rheumatology* **26**, 299–302.

Bennett, R. M. and Spargo, B. H. (1977). Immune complex nephropathy in mixed connective tissue disease. *American Journal of Medicine* **63**, 534–541.

Bennett, R. M. and O'Connell, D. J. (1980). Mixed connective tisssue disease: a clinicopathologic study of 20 cases. *Seminars in Arthritis and Rheumatism* **10**, 25–51.

Berg, K. J. *et al.* (1989). Renal side effects of high and low cyclosporin A doses in patients with rheumatoid arthritis. *Clinical Nephrology* **31**, 232–238.

Berger, J. and Hinglais, N. (1968). [Intercapillary deposits of IgA-IgG]. *Journal of Urology and Nephrology (Paris)* **74**, 694–695.

Berglund, K., Keller, C., and Thysell, H. (1987). Alkylating cytostatic treatment in renal amyloidosis secondary to rheumatic disease. *Annals of the Rheumatic Diseases* **46**, 757–762.

Berglund, K., Thysell, H., and Keller, C. (1993). Results, principles and pitfalls in the management of renal AA-amyloidosis; a 10–21 year followup of 16 patients with rheumatic disease treated with alkylating cytostatics. *Journal of Rheumatology* **20**, 2051–2057.

Boers, M. *et al.* (1987). Renal findings in rheumatoid arthritis: clinical aspects of 132 necropsies. *Annals of the Rheumatic Diseases* **46**, 658–663.

Boers, M. *et al.* (1990). Reversible nephrotoxicity of cyclosporine in rheumatoid arthritis. *Journal of Rheumatology* **17**, 38–42.

Breedveld, F. C. *et al.* (1985). Rapidly progressive glomerulonephritis with glomerular crescent formation in rheumatoid arthritis. *Clinical Rheumatology* **4**, 353–359.

Browning, M. J. *et al.* (1985). Ten years' experience of an amyloid clinic—a clinicopathological survey. *Quarterly Journal of Medicine* **54**, 213–227.

Brun, C. *et al.* (1965). Renal biopsy in rheumatoid arthritis. *Nephron* **2**, 65–81.

Burdt, M. A. *et al.* (1999). Long-term outcome in mixed connective tissue disease: longitudinal clinical and serologic findings. *Arthritis and Rheumatism* **42**, 899–909.

Cambridge, G. *et al.* (1994). Anti-myeloperoxidase antibodies in patients with rheumatoid arthritis: prevalence, clinical correlates, and IgG subclass. *Annals of the Rheumatic Diseases* **53**, 24–29.

Chalmers, A. *et al.* (1982). Systemic lupus erythematosus during penicillamine therapy for rheumatoid arthritis. *Annals of Internal Medicine* **97**, 659–663.

Chazot, C. *et al.* (1993). Functional study of hands among patients dialysed for more than 10 years. *Nephrology, Dialysis, Transplantation* **8**, 347–351.

Chen, A. *et al.* (1988). Immunoglobulin A nephropathy and ankylosing spondylitis. Report of two patients in Taiwan and review of the literature. *Nephron* **49**, 313–318.

Chevrel, G. *et al.* (2001). Renal type AA amyloidosis associated with rheumatoid arthritis: a cohort study showing improved survival on treatment with pulse cyclophosphamide. *Rheumatology* **40**, 821–825.

Cobb, S., Andersen, F., and Baur, W. (1953). Length of life and cause of death in rheumatoid arthritis. *New England Journal of Medicine* **249**, 553–556.

Cohen, D. J. and Appel, G. B. (1992). Cyclosporine: nephrotoxic effects and guidelines for safe use in patients with rheumatoid arthritis. *Seminars in Arthritis and Rheumatism* **21**, 43–48.

Collins, A. J. (1987). Gold treatment for rheumatoid arthritis: reassurance on proteinuria. *British Medical Journal (Clinical Research Edition)* **295**, 739–740.

Coremans, I. E. *et al.* (1992). Antilactoferrin antibodies in patients with rheumatoid arthritis are associated with vasculitis. *Arthritis and Rheumatism* **35**, 1466–1475.

Coremans, I. E. *et al.* (1993). Anti-lactoferrin antibodies in patients with rheumatoid arthritis with vasculitis. *Advances in Experimental Medicine and Biology* **336**, 357–362.

Cove-Smith, J. R. and Knapp, M. S. (1978). Analgesic nephropathy: an important cause of chronic renal failure. *Quarterly Journal of Medicine* **295**, 49–69.

David, J. *et al.* (1993). Amyloidosis in juvenile chronic arthritis: a morbidity and mortality study. *Clinical & Experimental Rheumatology* **11**, 85–90.

Deschenes, G. *et al.* (1990). Renal amyloidosis in juvenile chronic arthritis: evolution after chlorambucil treatment. *Pediatric Nephrology* **4**, 463–469.

Dunn, M. J. (1984). Non-steroidal anti-inflammatory drugs and renal function. *Annual Review of Medicine* **35**, 411–428.

Dyck, R. F. *et al.* (1979). Glomerulonephritis associated with polymyositis. *Journal of Rheumatology* **6**, 336–344.

Ellman, M. H. and Ginsberg, D. (1990). Low-dose methotrexate and severe neutropenia in patients undergoing renal dialysis. *Arthritis and Rheumatism* **33**, 1060–1061.

Emery, P. and Panayi, G. In *Autoimmunity and Toxicology Autoimmune Reactions to* D*-Penicillamine* (ed. M. E. Kanmuller, N. Bloksma, and W. Seinan), pp. 167–182. Amsterdam: Elsevier, 1989.

Emery, P. *et al.* (1984). D-Penicillamine induced toxicity in rheumatoid arthritis: the role of sulphoxidation status and HLA-DR3. *Journal of Rheumatology* **11**, 626–632.

Epstein, S., Shane, E., and Bilezikian, J. P. (1995). Organ transplantation and osteoporosis. *Current Opinion in Rheumatology* **7**, 255–261.

Falck, H. *et al.* (1979a). Resolution of renal amyloidosis secondary to rheumatoid arthritis. *Acta Medica Scandinavica* **205**, 651–656.

Falck, H. M. *et al.* (1979b). Fatal renal vasculitis and minimal change glomerulonephritis complicating treatment with penicillamine. Report on two cases. *Acta Medica Scandinavica* **205**, 133–138.

Ferrari, R. (1996). Rheumatologic manifestations of renal disease. *Current Opinion in Rheumatology* **8**, 71–76.

Filipowicz-Sosnowska, A. M. *et al.* (1978). The amyloidosis of juvenile rheumatoid arthritis—comparative studies in Polish and American children. I. Levels of serum SAA protein. *Arthritis and Rheumatism* **21**, 699–703.

Fingerman, D. L. and Andrus, F. C. (1943). Visceral lesions associated with rheumatoid arthritis. *Annals of the Rheumatic Diseases* **3**, 168–181.

Fonseca, J. E. *et al.* (2001). Amyloidosis in a series of 964 Portuguese rheumatoid arthritis patients: comment on the article by Myllykangas-Luosujarvi *et al. Rheumatology* **40**, 944–945.

Gauthier, V. J. and Barbosa, L. M. (1994). Bone pain in transplant recipients responsive to calcium channel blockers. *Annals of Internal Medicine* **121**, 863–865.

Gertz, M. A. and Kyle, R. A. (1991). Secondary systemic amyloidosis: response and survival in 64 patients. *Medicine* **70**, 246–256.

Gibson, T., Burry, H. C., and Ogg, C. (1976). Goodpasture's syndrome and D-penicillamine. *Annals of Internal Medicine* **84**, 100–101.

Glassock, R. J. *et al.* (1982). Recurrent acute renal failure in a patient with mixed connective tissue disease. *American Journal of Nephrology* **2**, 282–290.

Grandtnerova, B. *et al.* (1998). Reflex sympathetic dystrophy of the lower limbs after kidney transplantation. *Transplant International* **11**, S331–S333.

Gratacos, J. *et al.* (1997). Secondary amyloidosis in ankylosing spondylitis. A systematic survey of 137 patients using abdominal fat aspiration. *Journal of Rheumatology* **24**, 912–915.

Grevitt, M. P. and Spencer, J. D. (1995). Avascular necrosis of the hip treated by hemiarthroplasty. Results in renal transplant recipients. *Journal of Arthroplasty* **10**, 205–211.

Grotz, W. H. *et al.* (1995a). Bone mineral density after kidney transplantation. A cross-sectional study in 190 graft recipients up to 20 years after transplantation. *Transplantation* **59**, 982–986.

Grotz, W. H. *et al.* (1995b). Bone loss after kidney transplantation: a longitudinal study in 115 graft recipients. *Nephrology, Dialysis, Transplantation* **10**, 2096–2100.

Group, C. C. E. R. (1989). Randomized trial of low dose cyclosporin A in severe RA. *Arthritis and Rheumatism* **97** (Suppl.), 517.

Hajzok, O., Tomik, F., and Hajzokova, M. (1976). Amyloidosis in rheumatoid arthritis. A study of 48 histologically confirmed cases. *Zeitschrift fur Rheumatologie* **35**, 356–362.

Hall, C. L. *et al.* (1987). The natural course of gold nephropathy: long term study of 21 patients. *British Medical Journal (Clinical Research Edition)* **295**, 745–748.

Hall, C. L. *et al.* (1988). Natural course of penicillamine nephropathy: a long term study of 33 patients. *British Medical Journal* **296**, 1083–1086.

Harper, L. *et al.* (1997). Focal segmental necrotizing glomerulonephritis in rheumatoid arthritis. *Quarterly Journal of Medicine* **90**, 125–132.

Helin, H. *et al.* (1986). Mild mesangial glomerulopathy—a frequent finding in rheumatoid arthritis patients with hematuria or proteinuria. *Nephron* **42**, 224–230.

Henao, J. *et al.* (2002). Celecoxib-induced acute interstitial nephritis. *American Journal of Kidney Diseases* **39**, 1313–1317.

Honkanen, E. *et al.* (1987). Membranous glomerulonephritis in rheumatoid arthritis not related to gold or D-penicillamine therapy: a report of four cases and review of the literature. *Clinical Nephrology* **27**, 87–93.

Hordon, L. D. *et al.* (1984). Haematuria in rheumatoid arthritis: an association with mesangial glomerulonephritis. *Annals of the Rheumatic Diseases* **43**, 440–443.

Huskisson, E. C. *et al.* (1974). Trial comparing D-penicillamine and gold in rheumatoid arthritis. Preliminary report. *Annals of the Rheumatic Diseases* **33**, 532–535.

Joss, N. *et al.* (2000). Presentation, survival and prognostic markers in AA amyloidosis. *Quarterly Journal of Medicine* **93**, 535–542.

Kanterewicz, E. *et al.* (1987). IgA nephropathy in a young female with ankylosing spondylitis. *British Journal of Rheumatology* **26**, 396–397.

Karim, Z., Lawson, C., and Emery, P. Rheumatological complications of renal disease and transplantation. In *Rheumatology and the Kidney* (ed. D. Adu, P. Emery, and M. Madaio), pp. 519–534. Oxford: Oxford University Press, 2001.

Kitridou, R. C. *et al.* (1986). Renal involvement in mixed connective tissue disease: a longitudinal clinicopathologic study. *Seminars in Arthritis and Rheumatism* **16**, 135–145.

Kiyama, S. *et al.* (1991). Crescentic glomerulonephritis associated with renal amyloidosis. *Japanese Journal of Medicine* **30**, 238–242.

Klouda, P. T. *et al.* (1979). Strong association between idiopathic membranous nephropathy and HLA-DRW3. *Lancet* **2**, 770–771.

Korpela, M. *et al.* (1990). Immunological comparison of patients with rheumatoid arthritis with and without nephropathy. *Annals of the Rheumatic Diseases* **49**, 214–218.

Kraus, A. and Alarcon-Segovia, D. (1991). Low dose MTX and NSAID induced 'mild' renal impairment and severe neutropenia. *Journal of Rheumatology* **18**, 1274.

Kroot, E. J. *et al.* (2000). No increased mortality in patients with rheumatoid arthritis: up to 10 years of follow up from disease onset. *Annals of the Rheumatic Diseases* **59**, 954–958.

Kuznetsky, K. A. *et al.* (1986). Necrotizing glomerulonephritis in rheumatoid arthritis. *Clinical Nephrology* **26**, 257–264.

Kyd, R. J. (1979). Bone and joint complications of maintenance haemodialysis and renal transplantation. *New Zealand Medical Journal* **89**, 4–7.

Laakso, M. *et al.* (1986). Mortality from amyloidosis and renal diseases in patients with rheumatoid arthritis. *Annals of the Rheumatic Diseases* **45**, 663–667.

Lachmann, H. J. *et al.* (2002). Misdiagnosis of hereditary amyloidosis as AL (primary) amyloidosis. *New England Journal of Medicine* **346**, 1786–1791.

Lausten, G. S. *et al.* (1998). Necrosis of the femoral head after kidney transplantation. *Clinical Transplantation* **12**, 572–574.

Lawson, A. A. and Maclean, N. (1966). Renal disease and drug therapy in rheumatoid arthritis. *Annals of the Rheumatic Diseases* **25**, 441–449.

Le Parc, J. M. *et al.* (1996). Osteonecrosis of the hip in renal transplant recipients. Changes in functional status and magnetic resonance imaging findings over three years in three hundred five patients. *Revue du Rhumatisme, English Edition* **63**, 413–420.

Lee, J. C. *et al.* (1965). Renal lesions associated with gold therapy: light and electron microscopic studies. *Arthritis and Rheumatism* **8**, 1–13.

Lindqvist, B. *et al.* (1989). The course of renal amyloidosis with uraemia. *International Urology and Nephrology* **21**, 555–559.

Lucas, V. *et al.* (1990). Epiphyseal bone pain caused by cyclosporin A in 28 patients with renal transplantation. *Revue du Rhumatisme et des Maladies Osteo-Articulaires* **57**, 79–84.

Lucas, V. P. *et al.* (1991). Musculoskeletal pain in renal-transplant recipients. *New England Journal of Medicine* **325**, 1449–1450.

Madhok, R., Capell, H. A., and Waring, R. (1987). Does sulphoxidation state predict gold toxicity in rheumatoid arthritis? *British Medical Journal (Clinical Research Edition)* **294**, 483.

Maezawa, A. *et al.* (1994). Combined treatment with cyclophosphamide and prednisolone can induce remission of nephrotic syndrome in a patient with renal amyloidosis, associated with rheumatoid arthritis. *Clinical Nephrology* **42**, 30–32.

Martnez-Vea, A. *et al.* (1990). End stage renal disease in systemic amyloidosis: clinical course and outcome on dialysis. *American Journal of Nephrology* **10**, 283–289.

Mastaglia, F. L. (2000). Treatment of autoimmune inflammatory myopathies. *Current Opinion in Neurology* **13**, 507–509.

Messiaen, T. *et al.* (1998). MPO–ANCA necrotizing glomerulonephritis related to rheumatoid arthritis. *American Journal of Kidney Diseases* **32**, E6.

Missen, G. A. K. and Taylor, J. D. (1956). Amyloidosis in rheumatoid arthritis. *Journal of Pathology and Bacteriology* **71**, 179–192.

Mody, G. M. and Meyers, O. L. (1988). Clinical regression of amyloid nephropathy in a patient with rheumatoid arthritis. A case report. *South African Medical Journal* **73**, 55–56.

Moroni, G. *et al.* (1992). Chronic dialysis in patients with systemic amyloidosis: the experience in northern Italy. *Clinical Nephrology* **38**, 81–85.

Mulder, A. H. *et al.* (1993). Antineutrophil cytoplasmic antibodies in rheumatoid arthritis. Characterization and clinical correlations. *Arthritis and Rheumatism* **36**, 1054–1060.

Munoz-Gomez, J. *et al.* (1991). Reflex sympathetic dystrophy syndrome of the lower limbs in renal transplant patients treated with cyclosporin A. *Arthritis and Rheumatism* **34**, 625–630.

Mutru, O., Koota, K., and Isomaki, H. (1976). Causes of death in autopsied RA patients. *Scandinavian Journal of Rheumatology* **5**, 239–240.

Myllykangas-Luosujarvi, R. *et al.* (1999). Amyloidosis in a nationwide series of 1666 subjects with rheumatoid arthritis who died during 1989 in Finland. *Rheumatology* **38**, 499–503.

Nakano, M. *et al.* (1998). Analysis of renal pathology and drug history in 158 Japanese patients with rheumatoid arthritis. *Clinical Nephrology* **50**, 154–160.

Nanra, R. S. and Kincaid-Smith, P. (1975). Renal papillary necrosis in rheumatoid arthritis. *Medical Journal of Australia* **1**, 239–240.

Nimelstein, S. H. *et al.* (1980). Mixed connective tissue disease: a subsequent evaluation of the original 25 patients. *Medicine* **59**, 239–248.

O'Duffy, J. D. (1976). Clinical studies of acute pseudogout attacks: comments on prevalence, predispositions, and treatment. *Arthritis and Rheumatism* **19**, 349–352.

Ørjavik, O. *et al.* (1981). A renal biopsy study with light and immunofluorescent microscopy in rheumatoid arthritis. *Acta Medica Scandinavica* **645** (Suppl.), 9–14.

Panayi, G. S., Wooley, P., and Batchelor, J. R. (1978). Genetic basis of rheumatoid disease: HLA antigens, disease manifestations, and toxic reactions to drugs. *British Medical Journal* **2**, 1326–1328.

Perneger, T. V., Whelton, P. K., and Klag, M. J. (1994). Risk of kidney failure associated with the use of acetaminophen, aspirin, and nonsteroidal anti-inflammatory drugs. *New England Journal of Medicine* **331**, 1675–1679.

Pollak, V. E. *et al.* (1962). The kidney in rheumatoid arthritis: studies by renal biopsy. *Arthritis and Rheumatism* **5**, 1–9.

Prior, P. *et al.* (1984). Causes of death in rheumatoid arthritis. *British Journal of Rheumatology* **23**, 92–99.

Qarni, M. U. and Kohan, D. E. (2000). Pauci-immune necrotizing glomerulonephritis complicating rheumatoid arthritis. *Clinical Nephrology* **54**, 54–58.

Ramirez, G., Lambert, R., and Bloomer, H. A. (1981). Renal pathology in patients with rheumatoid arthritis. *Nephron* **29**, 124–126.

Rasker, J. J. and Cosh, J. A. (1981). Cause and age at death in a prospective study of 100 patients with rheumatoid arthritis. *Annals of the Rheumatic Diseases* **40**, 115–120.

Rocha, J. L. and Fernandez-Alonso, J. (1946). Acute tubulointerstitial nephritis associated with the selective COX-2 enzyme inhibitor, rofecoxib. *Lancet* **357**, 1946–1947.

Salomon, M. I. *et al.* (1974). The kidney in rheumatoid arthritis: a study based on renal biopsies. *Nephron* **12**, 297–310.

Sandler, D. P. (1989). Analgesic use and chronic renal disease. *New England Journal of Medicine* **320**, 1238–1243.

Savige, J. A. *et al.* (1991). Anti-neutrophil cytoplasm antibodies in rheumatoid arthritis. *Clinical and Experimental Immunology* **86**, 92–98.

Sawai, T., Murakami, K., and Kurasono, Y. (1994). Morphometric analysis of the kidney lesions in mixed connective tissue disease (MCTD). *Tohoku Journal of Experimental Medicine* **174**, 141–154.

Schnitzer, T. J. and Ansell, B. M. (1977). Amyloidosis in juvenile chronic polyarthritis. *Arthritis and Rheumatism* **20**, 245–252.

Scott, D. G., Bacon, P. A., and Tribe, C. R. (1981). Systemic rheumatoid vasculitis: a clinical and laboratory study of 50 cases. *Medicine* **60**, 288–297.

Sellars, L. *et al.* (1983). Renal biopsy appearances in rheumatoid disease. *Clinical Nephrology* **20**, 114–120.

Sethi, D. *et al.* (1990). Dialysis arthropathy: a clinical, biochemical, radiological and histological study of 36 patients. *Quarterly Journal of Medicine* **77**, 1061–1082.

Shapiro, D. L. and Spiera, H. (1995). Regression of the nephrotic syndrome in rheumatoid arthritis and amyloidosis treated with azathioprine. A case report. *Arthritis and Rheumatism* **38**, 1851–1854.

Sharp, G. C. *et al.* (1972). Mixed connective tissue disease—an apparently distinct rheumatic disease syndrome associated with a specific antibody to an extractable nuclear antigen (ENA). *American Journal of Medicine* **52**, 148–159.

Singsen, B. H. *et al.* (1980). A histologic evaluation of mixed connective tissue disease in childhood. *American Journal of Medicine* **68**, 710–717.

Sinnott, J. T. and Holt, D. A. (1989). Cryptococcal pyoarthrosis complicating gouty arthritis. *Southern Medical Journal* **82**, 1555–1556.

Sloan, M. F. *et al.* (1978). Acute renal failure due to polymyositis. *British Medical Journal* **1**, 1457.

Sternlieb, I., Bennett, B., and Scheinberg, I. H. (1975). D-Penicillamine induced Goodpasture's syndrome in Wilson's disease. *Annals of Internal Medicine* **82**, 673–676.

Stevens, J. M., Hilson, A. J., and Sweny, P. (1995). Post-renal transplant distal limb bone pain. An under-recognized complication of transplantation distinct from avascular necrosis of bone? *Transplantation* **60**, 305–307.

Study, N. Z. R. A. (1974). Aspirin and the kidney. *British Medical Journal* **1**, 595–596.

Suzuki, A. *et al.* (1994). Cause of death in 81 autopsied patients with rheumatoid arthritis. *Journal of Rheumatology* **21**, 33–36.

Swainson, C. P., Lynn, K. L., and Bailey, R. R. (1984). Acute renal failure and polymyositis: case report. *New Zealand Medical Journal* **97**, 288–289.

Tannenbaum, D. A., Matthews, L. S., and Grady-Benson, J. C. (1997). Infection around joint replacements in patients who have a renal or liver transplantation. *Journal of Bone and Joint Surgery—American Volume* **79**, 36–43.

Targoff, I. N. (1993). Humoral immunity in polymyositis/dermatomyositis. *Journal of Investigative Dermatology* **100**, 116S–123S.

Toyoshima, H., Kusaba, T., and Yamaguchi, M. (1993). Cause of death in autopsied RA patients. *Ryumachi* **33**, 209–214.

Tribe, C. R. Amyloidosis in rheumatoid arthritis. In *Modern Trends in Rheumatology* (ed. H. A. G. S. Hill), pp. 121–138. London: Butterworth, 1996.

Tugwell, P. *et al.* (1995). Combination therapy with cyclosporine and methotrexate in severe rheumatoid arthritis. The Methotrexate–Cyclosporine Combination Study Group. *New England Journal of Medicine* **333**, 137–141.

Valenzuela, O. F., Reiser, I. W., and Porush, J. G. (2001). Idiopathic polymyositis and glomerulonephritis. *Journal of Nephrology* **14**, 120–124.

Vincenti, F. *et al.* (1982). Septic arthritis following renal transplantation. *Nephron* **30**, 253–256.

Watts, R. A. *et al.* (1994). The incidence of rheumatoid vasculitis in the Norwich Health Authority. *British Journal of Rheumatology* **33**, 832–833.

Wegelius, O. *et al.* Follow up of amyloidosis secondary to rheumatic disease. In *Amyloid and Amyloidosis* (ed. G. G. Glenner, P. P. de Costa, and A. F. de Freitas), pp. 337–342. Amsterdam: Excerpta Medica, 1980.

Williams, H. J. *et al.* (1983). Low-dose D-penicillamine therapy in rheumatoid arthritis. A controlled, double-blind clinical trial. *Arthritis and Rheumatism* **26**, 581–592.

Williams, A. J. *et al.* (1986). Progressive proliferative glomerulonephritis in a patient with rheumatoid arthritis treated with D-penicillamine. *Annals of the Rheumatic Diseases* **45**, 82–84.

Wolfe, F. *et al.* (1994). The mortality of rheumatoid arthritis. *Arthritis and Rheumatism* **37**, 481–494.

Woo, P. (1994). Amyloidosis in children. *Baillieres Clinical Rheumatology* **8**, 691–697.

Wooley, P. H. *et al.* (1980). HLA-DR antigens and toxic reaction to sodium aurothiomalate and D-penicillamine in patients with rheumatoid arthritis. *New England Journal of Medicine* **303**, 300–302.

Yocum, D. E. *et al.* (1988). Cyclosporin A in severe, treatment-refractory rheumatoid arthritis. A randomized study. *Annals of Internal Medicine* **109**, 863–869.

Yorioka, N. *et al.* (1999). Chronic rheumatoid arthritis complicated by myeloperoxidase antineutrophil cytoplasmic antibody-associated nephritis. *American Journal of Nephrology* **19**, 527–529.

4.10 The patient with Sjögren's syndrome and overlap syndromes

Patrick J.W. Venables

Sjögren's syndrome and the overlap syndromes, including mixed connective tissue disease (see also Chapter 4.9), represent a substantial part of the clinical load of the rheumatologist. In these conditions, overt renal disease is rare, occurring in about 10 per cent of patients. The most common route of presentation to a nephrologist is therefore by a rheumatological referral. Occasionally the patients present with renal disease, in which case the underlying connective tissue disease is usually obvious. However, Sjögren's syndrome may not be recognized, as the dominant symptoms and signs of the disease, xerostomia, and xerophthalmia are easily missed.

Sjögren's syndrome

Classification

Sjögren's syndrome represents a group of diseases characterized by a common pathological feature: namely, inflammation and destruction of exocrine glands. The salivary and lachrymal glands are principally involved, giving rise to dry eyes and mouth. Other exocrine glands, including those of the pancreas, sweat glands, and mucus-secreting glands of the bowel, bronchial tree, and vagina may be affected. It was originally described as the triad of dry eyes, dry mouth, and rheumatoid arthritis (Sjögren 1933). It is now classified as:

(1) primary Sjögren's syndrome where the disease exists on its own, and

(2) secondary Sjögren's syndrome, where it is associated with other autoimmune rheumatic diseases.

Primary Sjögren's syndrome

Primary Sjögren's syndrome occurs when the disease predominantly affects exocrine glands. Most of the patients have systemic or extraglandular features, which, by definition, are not numerous enough to fulfil criteria for other connective tissue diseases.

Secondary Sjögren's syndrome

Secondary Sjögren's syndrome occurs when sicca symptoms are associated with another connective tissue diseases, particularly rheumatoid arthritis, which accounts for approximately one-third of patients. The ocular and oral symptoms of Sjögren's syndrome with rheumatoid arthritis are similar to those of primary Sjögren's syndrome, although they usually occur after the onset of the arthritis and are relatively mild. Secondary Sjögren's syndrome also occurs in the autoimmune connective diseases, systemic lupus erythematosus, scleroderma, polymyositis, and primary biliary cirrhosis.

Clinical features

Exocrinopathy

Sjögren's syndrome is the second most common autoimmune rheumatic disease (Shearn 1977). The exact prevalence is not known as there are thought to be many sufferers whose symptoms are so mild that they do not seek medical advice. It is nine times more common in women than men and its onset is any age from 15 to 65 years. The patients rarely complain of dry eyes, but rather a gritty sensation, soreness, photosensitivity, or intolerance of contact lenses. In early disease, patients occasionally complain of excessive watering or deposits of dried mucus in the corner of the eye and recurrent attacks of conjunctivitis. The dry mouth is often manifest as the 'cream cracker' sign, inability to swallow dry food without fluid, or the need to wake up in the night to take sips of water. About half of the patients complain of recurrent parotid swelling, sometimes misdiagnosed as recurrent mumps. When the swelling is excessively painful it is often due to secondary bacterial infection.

On examination, xerostomia can be detected as a diminished salivary pool, a dried fissured tongue, often complicated by angular stomatitis and chronic oral candidiasis. The eyes may be reddened and roughened due to shallow erosions in the conjunctiva. Occasionally, the front of the eye is eroded to reveal strands of underlying collagen leading to the appearance of filamentary keratitis.

Exocrine glands other than salivary and lachrymal may be affected. Dry skin and dry hair are symptoms frequently elicited on direct questioning. About 30 per cent of patients have diminished vaginal secretions and may present with dyspareunia. Involvement of the gastrointestinal tract leads to reflux oesophagitis or gastritis due to lack of protective mucus secretion, and some patients complain of constipation which may be attributed to defective mucus in the colon and rectum. Pancreatic failure leading to malabsorption syndromes occurs rarely.

Extraglandular features

Sjögren's syndrome is a systemic disease. Almost all patients complain of fatigue and depression. Occasionally, weight loss and fever, mimicking an occult malignancy, may be the presenting symptoms. Other features are those attributable to circulating immune complexes, particularly in those patients with antibodies to Ro (SS-A) and La (SS-B). Prominent amongst these are non-erosive arthritis, Raynaud's phenomenon, and a purpuric vasculitis on the lower legs associated with ankle oedema. A high incidence of pulmonary function abnormalities has been described, although these are rarely clinically significant. Patients may present with a syndrome indistinguishable from polymyalgia rheumatica and it is well recognized that polymyositis may be associated with Sjögren's syndrome. Alexander *et al.* (1986) have noted a wide range of neurological diseases, including central nervous system disorders resembling multiple sclerosis (MS) in up to 30 per cent of patients. However, some selection bias may account for the unusually high frequency of such complications in their patients. More recent reports suggest that the MS-like syndromes, predominantly a transverse myelitis, occur in about 1 per cent of patients (Vincent *et al.* 2003).

Sjögren's lymphoma

About 5 per cent of patients with Sjögren's syndrome eventually develop lymphomas. These may present as progressive (as opposed to intermittent) massive enlargement of the salivary glands, with diffuse lymphadenopathy or with skin deposits. This malignant change, which is thought to arise as a result of chronic B-cell stimulation, may be much more common than previously thought, since a substantial proportion of patients with extraglandular disease show evidence of oligoclonal B-cell hyperactivity.

Interstitial cystitis

Chronic cystitis, in the absence of bacterial infection, has long been known to complicate what used to be called 'collagen vascular disease'. More recent studies have suggested that many of these patients have primary Sjögren's syndrome (Van de Merwe *et al.* 1993). The symptoms are very similar to those of bacterial infection, though cultures are repeatedly negative. The diagnosis is confirmed by cystoscopy and biopsy. Although more in the province of the urologist rather than the nephrologist, it is important to recognize this syndrome, because patients referred with mild proteinuria or haematuria may well be suffering from bladder inflammation rather than renal disease.

Diagnostic tests

Tests for keratoconjunctivitis sicca and xerostomia

Keratoconjunctivitis sicca can be detected by Schirmer's test, tear break-up time and Rose Bengal staining (Kincaid 1987), and xerostomia by a reduced salivary flow rate and by reduced uptake and clearance on isotope scans (Daniels 1987). It is important to remember that salivary and lachrymal function decline with age and may be impaired in conditions other than Sjögren's syndrome. One cause of diagnostic confusion arises from treatment with drugs with anticholinergic side-effects, the most frequent being the tricyclic antidepressants. It is also now recognized that dry eyes and dry mouth can occur in patients with variants of chronic fatigue syndrome or fibromyalgia. We have termed this syndrome dry eyes and mouth syndrome (DEMS) (Price and Venables 2002). It is distinguishable from primary Sjögren's syndrome by the patient's tendency to report symptoms out of proportion to physical signs, by the absence of systemic manifestations beyond arthralgia and by normal salivary gland biopsies.

Labial gland biopsies

Biopsy and histology of the labial glands from behind the lower lip provide the most definitive diagnostic test. The area is anaesthetized with lignocaine containing adrenaline, and an incision 1.5 cm long allows access to 5–10 glands of diameter 2–4 mm, which are removed by simple blunt dissection. A diagnosis of Sjögren's syndrome depends on finding foci of periductular infiltrates of at least 50 lymphocytes and/or plasma cells at a density of more than one focus/4 mm^2 (Fig. 1).

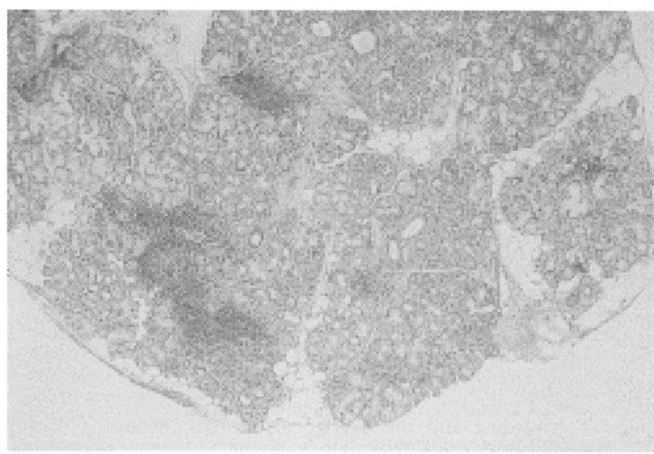

Fig. 1 Biopsy of minor salivary gland from a patient with Sjögren's syndrome. There is a dense inflammatory infiltrate surrounding the ducts, with the acini being relatively spared.

Haematology and chemical pathology

The majority of patients with Sjögren's syndrome have an increased erythrocyte sedimentation rate (ESR) and a mild normocytic anaemia. Leucopenia and thrombocytopenia occur in about 50 per cent of patients, and a referral from the haematology department with leucothrombocytopenia is an increasingly common route of presentation. One of the most remarkable features of primary Sjögren's syndrome is a polyclonal hypergammaglobulinaemia which can result in concentrations of IgG of up to 50 g/l. Complement is usually normal, even in the presence of immune complex disease, although C4 can sometimes be reduced, because of the link between Sjögren's syndrome and the C4A null gene.

Anti-Ro (SS-A) and La (SS-B)

Antibodies to the ribonucleoprotein antigens Ro (SS-A) and La (SS-B) are found in about 65 per cent and 50 per cent, respectively, of patients with primary Sjögren's syndrome (Alspaugh *et al.* 1976; Venables *et al.* 1989). Anti-La (SS-B) is virtually restricted to patients with primary Sjögren's syndrome or Sjögren's syndrome/systemic lupus erythematosus, whereas anti-Ro (SS-A) occurs with other diseases, particularly systemic lupus erythematosus, and occasionally polymyositis, rheumatoid arthritis, and in apparently healthy subjects.

Other autoantibodies

Rheumatoid factors, as measured by routine assays, occur in all forms of Sjögren's syndrome. They do not distinguish Sjögren's syndrome/rheumatoid arthritis from other forms of Sjögren's syndrome, and their detection in primary Sjögren's syndrome is a common reason for misdiagnosing such patients as having rheumatoid arthritis. Similarly, antinuclear antibodies detected by immunofluorescence, often in the absence of anti-Ro (SS-A) or anti-La (SS-B), can occur. Both rheumatoid factors and antinuclear antibodies, although not diagnostically specific, can help in distinguishing Sjögren's syndrome from non-autoimmune causes of sicca symptoms (Fox *et al.* 1986). Antisalivary gland antibodies have been reported in patients with Sjögren's syndrome and rheumatoid arthritis, though the assay has not been established as a useful diagnostic test. More recently, fodrin (a protein involved in apoptosis) and the muscurinic acetylcholine receptor (Haneji *et al.* 1997; Waterman *et al.* 2000) have been reported as Sjögren's syndrome autoantigens. Although attractive as potential antigens in pathogenesis, the specificity of their respective antibodies to Sjögren's syndrome has yet to be confirmed in independent studies.

Immunogenetics

Primary Sjögren's syndrome is strongly associated with HLA-DR3, the linked genes B8 and DQ2, and C4A null gene (Harley *et al.* 1986). Within the primary Sjögren's syndrome group, those with anti-La represent a subset which show an even more striking association with HLA-DR3: 90–100 per cent of patients with this antibody being HLA-DR3 positive. This suggests that the anti-La positive patients with Sjögren's syndrome may be the most homogeneous subgroup both clinically and immunogenetically. Anti-Ro is associated with DR2 and the linked DQ1 gene, as well as DR3, and this may reflect the wider diagnostic associations of this antibody. Rheumatoid arthritis with secondary Sjögren's syndrome is associated with DR4, not DR3 (Price and Venables 1995). There are no clear tissue types related to scleroderma with Sjögren's syndrome.

Diagnostic criteria

The application of diagnostic criteria, although not important in clinical practice, is essential for the standardization of any research involving patient groups, particularly with a disease, or group of diseases, as heterogeneous as Sjögren's syndrome. Currently used criteria include the so-called 'Copenhagen criteria' (Manthorpe *et al.* 1981), the 'Californian criteria' (Fox *et al.* 1986), and the 'European criteria' (Vitali *et al.* 1993). Those of Vitali *et al.* are based on the results of a multicentre European study and are probably the most thoroughly evaluated and simplest to apply. They are based on a short questionnaire of ocular and oral symptoms. Other essential criteria are: ocular signs (by Schirmer's test or Rose Bengal staining), lymphocytic infiltrates on lip biopsy; salivary gland involvement (scintigraphy, sialography, or decreased salivary flow rate), demonstration of serum autoantibodies (rheumatoid factors, antinuclear antibodies, and/or Ro or La antibodies).

Aetiopathogenesis of Sjögren's syndrome

Aetiology

Obvious aetiogical candidates for triggering autoimmunity in Sjögren's syndrome are viruses which infect the salivary gland. Sialotropic viruses such as Epstein–Barr virus and cytomegalovirus have been examined, with conflicting reports of abnormal responses to infection (reviewed in Price and Venables 1995). Epstein–Barr virus DNA has been detected in salivary and lachrymal glands although the evidence to date suggests that the virus is simply using the glands as a site of persistence rather than causing the inflammation in Sjögren's syndrome. Nevertheless, Epstein–Barr virus is still considered a candidate for involvement in the pathogenesis of this syndrome.

Retroviruses have been implicated in Sjögren's syndrome, as they are known to infect cells of the immune system and can cause abnormalities of immune regulation. A subgroup of patients with human immunodeficiency virus (HIV) infection develop diffuse infiltrative lymphocytosis of salivary glands and other organs, including the kidneys, with predominantly CD8+ T cells (Itescu and Winchester 1992). Clinical presentation can be very similar to Sjögren's syndrome. Interestingly, those with renal involvement develop renal tubular acidosis (as with idiopathic primary Sjögren's syndrome). More recent large-scale studies have suggested that patients with diffuse infiltrative lymphocytosis comprise between 3–8 per cent of HIV infections (Kordossis *et al.* 1998). A similar syndrome has also been described in association with the other major human retroviral pathogen, human T leukaemia retrovirus-I (HTLV-I). Although rare in the United Kingdom, HTLV-I is though to underlie up to 20 per cent of patients presenting with Sjögren's syndrome in endemic areas such as Japan (Terada *et al.* 1994). Conversely, sicca symptoms are found in about 3 per cent of patients infected with HTLV-I.

Given that diseases resembling Sjögren's syndrome occur in a proportion of infections with the two known major retroviruses in humans, the search has been on for novel retroviruses in idiopathic disease. The earliest positive finding was the demonstration of retroviral A-type particles were identified in lymphoblastoid cells co-cultured with homogenates of salivary glands from patients with Sjögren's syndrome (Garry *et al.* 1990). Our own group subsequently identified a novel retroviral sequence from a patient with Sjögren's syndrome, though we were unable to link it to the disease (Rigby *et al.* 1997). Animal models provide support for the role of retroviruses in Sjögren's syndrome. Mice with murine acquired immune deficiency, caused by the murine leukaemia virus, develop lymphocytic infiltrates of their salivary glands and other organs. Although the histology of the gland is very similar to that seen in Sjögren's syndrome, it could be argued that this model has a closer resemblance to the HIV infected patients with diffuse infiltrative lymphocytosis. The HTLV-I *tax* transgenic mouse described by Green *et al.* (1989) develops a sialadenitis characterized by focal proliferation of ductal epithelial cells within the major and minor salivary glands, followed by lymphocytic infiltration. This model is of interest because it demonstrates how a single viral gene product can generate inflammation (reviewed in Hollsberg 1999) and also explores how HTLV-I (and potentially other viruses) can cause the chronic inflammation of Sjögren's syndrome.

Thus, a number of studies provide quite compelling indirect evidence for the involvement of retroviruses in Sjögren's syndrome, though careful and systematic searches for a single agent have yet to be successful.

Pathogenesis

The most remarkable finding in inflamed salivary glands is dense epithelial class II (and to a lesser extent class I) antigen expression (Fox *et al.* 1985; Lindahl *et al.* 1985) on ducts and acini. The majority of the lymphocytes infiltrating the salivary gland are of the CD4 helper/inducer phenotype, with a relative paucity of CD8 (suppressor/cytotoxic) cells. Some restriction of T-cell receptor gene usage to Vβ 6.7b and Vβ13.2, and a profile of cytokine production consistent with Th1-type cells has been observed in affected tissues (reviewed by Price and Venables 1995). About 10 per cent of the lymphocytes are B cells. There are also plentiful plasma cells, which appear to be producing autoantibody and rheumatoid factors within the gland (Horsfall *et al.* 1989). Recently, dysregulation of apoptosis has attracted interest as a mechanism for autoimmunity. In Sjögren's syndrome it is now agreed that the rate of apoptosis is increased in glandular epithelium but decreased in the infiltrating lymphocytes. There is concordant over expression of proapoptotic markers such as Fas and Bax in the epithelium and anti-apoptotic markers such as Bcl-2 in the lymphocytes (reviewed by Patel and McHugh 2000).

These findings have led to the hypothesis that the hub of the disease is activation and apoptosis of exocrine tubular epithelial cells. It is not known what initiates this activation, but the elusive virus, or viruses, could be candidates. It is known, however, that certain autoantigens, including Ro and La, play an active part in this process and are expressed on the membrane of apoptotic cells. Co-expression of HLA class II and other adhesion molecules on epithelial cells leads to activation of infiltrating lymphocytes which results in a chronic immune attack on salivary epithelium. The production of autoantibodies result in the formation of immune complexes, which in turn leads to the extraglandular features of the disease.

Renal disease in Sjögren's syndrome

Clinically significant renal disease is rare in Sjögren's syndrome, and most descriptions in the literature are based on accumulated single-case reports. In a study of 89 patients with Sjögren's syndrome in our unit (Pease *et al.* 1989), clinically significant renal disease, manifest as proteinuria, hyperchloraemia, or acidosis, was detected in four patients. Three of 42 patients with primary Sjögren's syndrome had renal tubular acidosis, and one patient with Sjögren's syndrome/systemic lupus erythematosus overlap had glomerulonephritis. Subsequent studies have revealed a similar frequency of clinically significant renal disease, around 5 per cent, including a large recent study (Goules *et al.* 2000), which documented disease, confirmed by biopsy, in 4.2 per cent of 471 patients. Several smaller studies, for example, Bossini *et al.* (2001), suggest that if more sensitive tests of tubular or glomerular function are performed, such as water deprivation or acid load tests, the frequency of subclinical renal disease rises to around 30 per cent. These studies also agree that the prevalence of clinically significant disease is around 5 per cent.

The two major immunopathological lesions of Sjögren's syndrome, the exocrinopathy and the circulating immune complex disease, reflect the major types of lesions seen in the kidney. The first of these is the interstitial nephritis, in which plasma cells and lymphocytes surround the tubules; a pathological change which is strikingly reminiscent of the changes around the ducts in the inflamed salivary gland. The second is immune complex glomerulonephritis, often present in the Sjögren's syndrome/systemic lupus erythematosus overlap group.

Interstitial nephritis

Interstitial glomerulonephritis in Sjögren's syndrome results predominantly in tubular dysfunction. This was initially reported as nephrogenic diabetes insipidus in 10 out of 62 patients by Bloch *et al.* (1965). Kassan and Talal (1987) suggested that this lesion may have been secondary to hypokalaemia associated with renal tubular acidosis, rather than a direct effect of the inflammation itself. However, in a more recent study (Shiozawa *et al.* 1987), defective urinary concentration ability, as measured by the Fishberg test, was detected in nine of 11 patients with primary Sjögren's syndrome, and there was no relationship between this defect and renal tubular acidosis. This provided evidence that the failure to concentrate urine was not secondary to renal tubular acidosis, and may have been a direct result, or even a very sensitive indicator, of subclinical interstitial nephritis.

The classical lesion of Sjögren's syndrome is type I renal tubular acidosis (affecting the distal convoluted tubule) (see Chapter 5.4) which results in defective hydrogen ion excretion, leading to hyperchloraemic acidosis with secondary hypokalaemia. The mechanism for this is thought to be an increased leak of bicarbonate ions through the distal tubules due to increased permeability caused by inflammation (Zawadzki 1998) or by the absence of H(+)-ATPase in the intercalated cells (Joo *et al.* 1998). Type II renal tubular acidosis, involving the proximal tubule and leading to impaired bicarbonate reabsorption, is less frequent (Kassan and Talal 1987), although it has been described in association with Fanconi's syndrome (Shearn and Tu 1965). In these patients, severe pathological changes, such as tubular atrophy and extensive fibrosis, were present. More subtle changes in proximal tubular function, detected as reduced phosphate reabsorption in association with normal parathormone, were found in six of 17 patients with subclinical renal disease (Shiozawa *et al.* 1987). In one study (Cohen *et al.* 1992), it was suggested that the failure of acidification of urine was due to the absence of H^+-ATPase in cortical collecting tubules.

At least half the patients presenting with renal tubular acidosis have Sjögren's syndrome (Talal 1971). In patients with severe renal tubular acidosis complicated by nephrolithiasis, the frequency is nearly 90 per cent (Eriksson *et al.* 1996). Conversely, clinically important renal tubular acidosis occurs in about 5 per cent of patients with Sjögren's syndrome. Latent disease, detected only by means of of an acid load test in patients with normal plasma bicarbonate or chloride concentrations, occurs in about one-third of patients with primary Sjögren's syndrome or with Sjögren's syndrome/systemic lupus erythematosus overlap (Shearn and Tu 1965; Shiozawa *et al.* 1987; Siamopoulos *et al.* 1994) and rarely in Sjögren's syndrome/rheumatoid arthritis. The study by Shiozawa *et al.* (1987) suggested that the frequency of mild interstitial nephritis may be even greater than this. Among seven renal biopsies from patients with Sjögren's syndrome, five showed interstitial inflammation, although only two of the patients had evidence of renal tubular acidosis.

Presenting features

Renal tubular acidosis usually presents as a biochemical defect rather than with any clinical symptoms or signs. In one study reporting clinical features, Shioji *et al.* (1970) described muscle weakness in three of four patients with Sjögren's syndrome and renal tubular acidosis. The weakness was reversed by treatment with alkalis in all three cases, suggesting it was due to the renal tubular acidosis rather than the Sjögren's syndrome. There have been isolated reports of life-threatening paralysis due to hypokalaemia amounting to a total of 12 in 1993 with up to four cases per year reported since. Osteomalacia and/or nephrocalcinosis may also be rare presenting features of renal tubular acidosis (Moutsopoulos *et al.* 1991; Aerts *et al.* 1994). The most common biochemical abnormalitites indicating subclinical renal tubular acidosis are hypokalaemia and hyperchloraemia (Shearn and Tu 1965; Shiozawa *et al.* 1987; Siamopoulos *et al.* 1994), but the plasma bicarbonate concentration is an insensitive screening test. In some patients with minor biochemical abnormalities, a history of muscle cramps may be elicited on direct questioning (Venables, unpublished observations). Under these circumstances, a trial of treatment with alkalis may be worthwhile. Urinary findings are generally unimpressive (Kassan and Talal 1987; Shiozawa *et al.* 1987), with mild proteinuria and occasional hyaline casts or white cells.

Histology

As in the salivary gland, the target cells for the inflammatory response in the kidney appear to be the tubular epithelial cells. These are surrounded by lymphocytes and plasma cells (Fig. 2). In three reported cases where both renal and salivary gland biopsies were available in the same patients, the density of inflammation was much less in the kidney than in the salivary gland (Shioji *et al.* 1970). In the salivary gland, aggregates amounting to ectopic lymphoid follicles were seen, whereas in the corresponding renal tissue the infiltrates were much more scattered. Supporting Talal's prediction that similar pathological processes were occurring in the two tissues (Talal 1971) is the finding that, as in the salivary gland, most of the infiltrating T cells in the kidney are CD4 positive (Takaya *et al.* 1985; Rosenberg *et al.* 1988). In the majority of cases, the tubular epithelium appears normal (Shioji *et al.* 1970). In severe disease, there may be tubular atrophy or even necrosis of renal tubules, which can lead rarely to glomerular hyalinization and renal failure (Gerhardt *et al.* 1978). Interstitial fibrosis is a common finding which appears to occur roughly in proportion to disease duration.

Immunopathogenesis

In early studies, the pathogenesis of the lesion was thought to be related to the hypergammaglobulinaemia characteristic of Sjögren's syndrome (McCurdy *et al.* 1967). Two possible mechanisms have been proposed: the first, that filtered immunoglobulin damages the renal tubules; and the second, that hypergammaglobulinaemia leads to increased plasma viscosity, which, in turn, causes disturbances in the tubular microcirculation. In favour of such a link has been the known association between renal tubular acidosis and hyperglobulinaemia, both in idiopathic renal tubular acidosis and other diseases in which renal tubular acidosis is found, such as systemic lupus erythematosus, primary biliary cirrhosis, and other connective tissue diseases, all of which may be characterized by very high IgG concentrations in the serum. On the other hand, Shioji *et al.* (1970) found no difference between the serum IgG in patients with Sjögren's syndrome, with or without renal tubular acidosis. They also described a patient with severe interstitial nephritis in whom immunoglobulins were normal. In the same study, a careful search revealed no significant vascular abnormalities in renal biopsies from four patients with renal tubular acidosis.

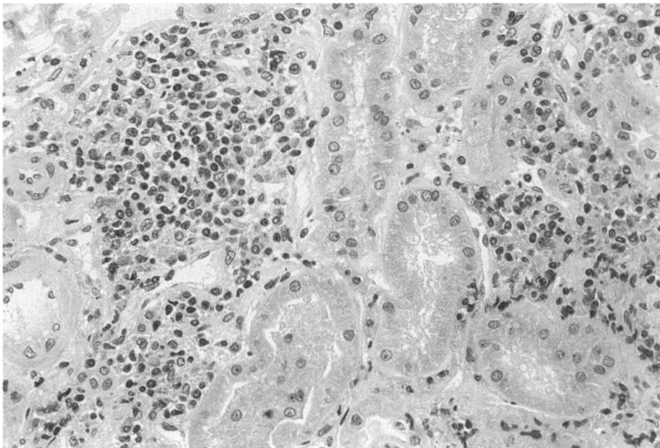

Fig. 2 Renal biopsy from a patient with renal tubular acidosis. There is an infiltrate of lymphocytes and plasma cells around the tubules, with complete sparing of the glomeruli.

It is now generally thought that Sjögren's syndrome itself, rather than the associated hypergammaglobulinaemia, is causally linked with interstitial nephritis. Kassan and Talal (1987) argued that most of the connective tissue diseases associated with hypergammaglobulinaemia and renal tubular acidosis are also associated with Sjögren's syndrome. Evidence in support of this was provided by Graninger *et al.* (1991), who described two of 109 patients with systemic lupus erythematosus who had renal tubular acidosis with interstitial nephritis. On further examination, both had features of Sjögren's syndrome. It has also been suggested that many patients with apparently idiopathic renal tubular acidosis have Sjögren's syndrome if it is looked for (Kassan and Talal 1987). Talal (1971), noting the analogy between the peritubular infiltrates in the kidney with the periductular lesion within the salivary gland, speculated that viruses within epithelial glands could be responsible for the local accumulation of inflammatory cells. It is tempting to speculate that the high frequency of occult inflammatory liver disease (Trevino *et al.* 1987) in primary Sjögren's syndrome may be due to similar mechanisms involving biliary ducts.

Diagnosis and treatment

Renal tubular acidosis requires treatment only if there are overt clinical or biochemical abnormalities such as hyperchloraemia, hypokalaemia, or evidence of acidosis, or there are complications such as osteomalacia or nephrocalcinosis. The investigations require nothing more than routine examination of the blood electrolytes, including chloride and bicarbonate, and the urine. An acid load test may be performed to confirm the diagnosis. A renal biopsy is rather academic unless glomerulonephritis needs to be excluded. Rather less invasive and often more informative is a labial biopsy for the diagnosis of the associated Sjögren's syndrome. The biopsy is more reliable than Schirmer's test, which may miss early disease (Shioji *et al.* 1970; Venables *et al.* 1989). Antibodies to Ro and La are useful serological markers.

Renal tubular acidosis is best treated with sodium bicarbonate in a sufficient dose to return plasma bicarbonate and chloride to normal. Secondary features such as hypokalaemia and osteomalacia will be corrected, and even mild azotaemia and proteinuria disappear (Kassan and Talal 1987). Renal tubular acidosis in itself is not usually an indication for treatment of the underlying Sjögren's syndrome, although there is good evidence that it responds to either steroids or cyclophosphamide (100 mg/day) (Talal and Moutsopoulos 1987) if they are used for other, more serious, manifestations of the disease. Recently, hydroxychloroquine (400 mg/day) has become routine immunomodulatory treatment for primary Sjögren's syndrome in many units. Although there have been no large scale controlled trials, a number of small open label studies have shown that the drug lowers the ESR, total immunoglobulin levels and has a modest benefit on symptoms such as fatigue and arthralgia. This may be mediated by its inhibitory effect on B cell cytokines such as IL-6 (Tishler *et al.* 1999). There are no studies of its effects on renal tubular function, but its may well be worth examining as a non-toxic disease modifying drug in the future.

Immune complex glomerulonephritis

Prevalence

Glomerulonephritis is very rare in Sjögren's syndrome. Even in patients with Sjögren's syndrome and fully developed systemic lupus erythematosus the frequency of nephritis is only 10 per cent, considerably less than the frequency in systemic lupus erythematosus without Sjögren's syndrome (Venables 1986; Pease *et al.* 1989). The observation by Wasicek and Reichlin (1982) that patients with systemic lupus erythematosus and anti-La (SS-B) had a relatively low frequency of renal disease would suggest that the immunopathology of Sjögren's syndrome may, in some way, be protective against nephritis.

Immunohistology

Membranous nephritis is the most common reported glomerular lesion in Sjögren's syndrome. Moutsopoulos *et al.* (1978) described three cases, two with some proliferative features. All three had primary Sjögren's syndrome, although extraglandular features were prominent, suggesting that they were tending towards the Sjögren's syndrome/systemic lupus erythematosus overlap part of the spectrum. More recently, two of 36 patients with Sjögren's syndrome in Greece were described with membranous or membranoproliferative lesions (Siamopoulos *et al.* 1994). In the largest series reported to date, Goules *et al.* (2000) described eight biopsy proven cases of membranous nephritis in over 400 cases (around 2 per cent). Occasional cases of proliferative nephritis have also been described. These are associated with cryoglobulinaemia, hypocomplementaemia, and evidence of widespread immune complex disease (Kassan and Talal 1987).

Overlap syndromes

The literature is full of case reports of various patterns of renal disease occurring in almost every conceivable type of overlap syndrome. As one might predict, the pattern of renal disease tends to reflect the dominant component of the overlap. In this chapter, two overlap syndromes which are thought to have their own distinct identity are reviewed: mixed connective tissue disease and the Jo-1 syndrome.

Mixed connective tissue disease (see also Chapter 4.9)

Definition

Mixed connective tissue disease is an overlap syndrome combining features of systemic lupus erythematosus, scleroderma, and polymyositis. It was originally defined by the finding of an antibody to an RNAse-sensitive component of a tissue extract called extractable nuclear antigen (Sharp *et al.* 1972). The major antigenic component of this mixture subsequently turned out to be the polypeptides of a nuclear ribonucleoprotein termed U1 RNP (Venables 1998). The clinical features included a high frequency of Raynaud's phenomenon, arthritis, polymyositis, and fibrosing alveolitis, and a low frequency of renal disease. The importance of the recognition of this syndrome was based on the claim that it had a good prognosis and response to steroid therapy.

Mixed connective tissue disease as a distinct entity

The association between antinuclear ribonucleoprotein and the clinical features described by Sharp *et al.* (1972) have been confirmed by a number of workers. Whether this constitutes a distinct entity or not has been the subject of continuous, and often fruitless, arguments over the past 15 years. Our own studies of patients presenting with polymyositis (Venables 1986) or fibrosing alveolitis (Chapman *et al.* 1984) suggested that patients with antinuclear ribonucleoprotein seemed to merge into the spectrum of autoimmune rheumatic diseases rather than appearing particularly distinctive.

Prognosis and response to treatment

The original claims that patients with the disease had a good prognosis or had a particularly good response to steroids have not stood the test of time (Venables 1998). Adult patients with mixed connective tissue disease have subsequently developed typical scleroderma, and children with features of the disease have evolved into typical patients with systemic lupus erythematosus. The mortality of mixed connective tissue disease (about 5 per cent in 5 years) is similar to that of systemic lupus erythematosus. There is no evidence that differentiating mixed connective tissue disease significantly alters treatment. Patients with mixed connective tissue disease require the same treatment for their dominant clinical problem, whether or not they have anti-U1RNP antibody.

Membranous nephritis

When originally described, mixed connective tissue disease was associated with a low frequency of renal disease (Sharp *et al.* 1972). Subsequent studies would suggest a frequency of about 10 per cent, though it is even more common (up to 47 per cent) in children with MCTD (Michels 1997). These considerations are of limited significance to renal physicians, as many of these patients would be diagnosed as having systemic lupus erythematosus and treated as such. Such treatment would be entirely appropriate, since over 60 per cent of patients with mixed connective tissue disease also fulfil criteria for systemic lupus erythematosus (Venables 1986). A diagnosis of mixed connective tissue disease or systemic lupus erythematosus represents an arbitrary choice of nomenclature. The link between anti-U1 RNP and membranous nephritis may reflect the high frequency of antibodies to ribonucleoproteins in membranous nephritis in systemic lupus erythematosus (Venables *et al.* 1983; Field *et al.* 1988). As in systemic lupus erythematosus, membranous nephritis in mixed connective tissue disease is rather slow to evolve and responds relatively poorly to steroids (Venables 1998).

Other systemic lupus erythematosus-like renal lesions

Because mixed connective tissue disease is closely related to systemic lupus erythematosus, any lupus-associated renal lesion can be found. This is particularly important in children, as mixed connective tissue disease can differentiate rapidly into full-blown lupus with severe proliferative glomerulonephritis.

Scleroderma kidney

A few cases of vascular intimal hyperplasia affecting renal vessels, indistinguishable from scleroderma kidney, have also been described in association with mixed connective tissue disease (reviewed in Satoh *et al.* 1994). Such patients have developed accelerated hypertension and renal failure, as in idiopathic scleroderma. Treatment is with angiotensin-converting enzyme inhibitors and analogues of prostaglandin E1.

The Jo-1 (tRNA synthetase) syndrome

When originally described, anti-Jo-1 (named after the prototype patient) was thought to be a 'marker' antibody for polymyositis. It is now appreciated that the antibody is associated with more widespread systemic manifestations with overlapping features of polymyositis, scleroderma, and lupus (reviewed in Venables 1998). When it was found that the antigen was histidyl tRNA synthetase, the syndrome has been given the alternative, if somewhat cumbersome, title of a 'tRNA synthetase' syndrome. Renal disease is rare in the Jo-1 syndrome and when it occurs it tends to be a mild mesangial glomerulonephritis (Frost *et al.* 1993). The importance of recognizing the syndrome is not so much for the renal disease, but for the potentially lethal complications of polymyositis or fibrosing alveolitis which occur in more than 50 per cent of the patients.

Sjögren's syndrome and overlap syndromes: conclusion

Both Sjögren's syndrome and mixed connective tissue disease overlap with systemic lupus erythematosus and thus, many of the renal manifestations are familiar to nephrologists who see lupus patients. The tubular disease associated with Sjögren's syndrome is also easily recognized but the underlying diagnosis may be missed. At present, this may not be of importance, but as more specific treatments of Sjögren's syndrome evolve, diagnosis of this rather neglected syndrome may be central to novel disease-specific therapies.

References

Aerts, J., Vigouroux, C., Fournier, P., Cariou, D., and Pasquier, P. (1994). Osteomalacia of renal origin disclosing Gougerot–Sjögren syndrome. *Revue de Medecine Interne (Paris)* **15**, 43–47.

Alexander, E. L., Malinow, K., Lijewski, J. E., Jerdan, M. S., Provost, T. T., and Alexander, G. E. (1986). Primary Sjögren's syndrome with central nervous system dysfunction mimicking multiple sclerosis. *Annals of Internal Medicine* **104**, 323–330.

Alspaugh, M. A., Talal, N., and Tan, E. M. (1976). Differentiation and characterization of autoantibodies and their antigens in Sjögren's syndrome. *Arthritis and Rheumatism* **19**, 216–222.

Bloch, K. J., Buchanan, W. W., Wohl, M. J., and Bunim, J. J. (1965). Sjögren's syndrome: a clinical, pathological and serological study of sixty-two cases. *Medicine (Baltimore)* **44**, 187–231.

Bossini, N. *et al.* (2001). Clinical and morphological features of kidney involvement in primary Sjögren's syndrome. *Nephrology, Dialysis, Transplantation* **16**, 2328–2336.

Chapman, J. R. *et al.* (1984). Definition and clinical relevance of antibodies to nuclear ribonucleoprotein and other nuclear antigens in patients with cryptogenic fibrosing alveolitis. *American Review of Respiratory Disease* **130**, 439–443.

Cohen, E. P., Bastani, B., Cohen, M. R., Kolner, S., Hemken, P., and Gluck, S. L. (1992). Absence of H(+)-ATPase in cortical collecting tubules of a patient with Sjögren's syndrome and distal tubular acidosis. *Journal of the American Society of Nephrology* **3**, 264–271.

Daniels, T. E. Oral manifestations of Sjögren's syndrome. In *Sjögren's Syndrome: Clinical and Immunological Aspects* (ed. N. Talal, H. M. Moutsopoulos, and S. S. Kassan), pp. 15–24. Berlin: Springer-Verlag, 1987.

Eriksson, P., Denneberg, T., Enestrom, S., Johansson, B., Lindstrom, F., and Skogh, T. (1996). Urolithiasis and distal renal tubular acidosis preceding primary Sjögren's syndrome: a retrospective study 5–53 years after the presentation of urolithiasis. *Journal of Internal Medicine* **239**, 483–488.

Field, M., Williams, D. G., Charles, P., and Maini, R. N. (1988). Specificity of anti-Sm antibodies by ELISA for systemic lupus erythematosus: increased sensitivity for detection using purified peptide antigens. *Annals of the Rheumatic Diseases* **47**, 820–825.

Fox, R. I., Bumol, T., Fantozzi, R., Bone, R., and Schreiber, R. (1985). Expression of histocompatibility antigen HLA DR by salivary epithelial cells in Sjögren's syndrome. *Arthritis and Rheumatism* **29**, 1105–1111.

Fox, R. I., Robinson, C., Kozin, F., and Howell, F. V. (1986). Sjögren's syndrome: proposed criteria for classification. *Arthritis and Rheumatism* **29**, 577–585.

Frost, N. A., Morand, E. F., Hall, C. L., Maddison, P. J., and Bhalla, A. K. (1993). Idiopathic polymyositis complicated by arthritis and mesangial proliferative glomerulonephritis: case report and review of the literature. *British Journal of Rheumatology* **32**, 929–931 (review).

Garry, R. F., Fermin, C. D., Hart, D. J., Alexander, S. S., Donehower, L. A., and Hong, L. Z. (1990). Detection of a human intracisternal A-type retroviral particle antigenically related to HIV. *Science* **250**, 1127–1129.

Gerhardt, R. E., Loebl, D. H., and Rao, R. N. (1978). Interstitial immunofluoresence in nephritis of Sjögren's syndrome. *Clinical Nephrology* **10**, 201–207.

Goules, A., Masouridi, S., Tzioufas, A. G., Ioannidis, J. P., Skopouli, F. N., and Moutsopoulos, H. M. (2000). Clinically significant and biopsy-documented renal involvement in primary Sjögren syndrome. *Medicine (Baltimore)*, **79**, 241–249.

Graninger, W. B., Steinberg, A. D., Meron, G., and Smolen, J. S. (1991). Interstitial nephritis in patients with systemic lupus erythematosus: a manifestation of concomitant Sjögren's syndrome? *Clinical and Experimental Rheumatology* **9**, 41–45.

Green, J. E., Hinrichs, S. H., Vogel, J., and Jay, G. (1989). Exocrinopathy resembling Sjögren's syndrome in HTLV-1 tax transgenic mice. *Nature* **341**, 72–74.

Haneji, N. *et al.* (1997). Identification of alpha-fodrin as a candidate autoantigen in primary Sjögren's syndrome. *Science* **276**, 604–607.

Harley, J. B., Reichlin, M., Arnett, F. C., Alexander, E. L., Bias, W. B., and Provost, T. T. (1986). Gene interaction at HLA-DQ enhances autoantibody production in primary Sjögren's syndrome. *Science* **232**, 1145–1147.

Hollsberg, P. (1999). Mechanisms of T-cell activation by human T-cell lymphotropic virus type I. *Microbiology and Molecular Biology Reviews* **63**, 308–333.

Horsfall, A. C., Venables, P. J. W., Allard, S. A., and Maini, R. N. (1989). Coexistent anti-La antibodies and rheumatoid factors bear distinct idiotypic markers. *Scandinavian Journal of Rheumatology* **75** (Suppl.), 84–88.

Itescu, S. and Winchester, R. (1992). Diffuse infiltrative lymphocytosis syndrome: A disorder occurring in human immunodeficiency virus-1 infection that may present as a sicca syndrome. *Rheumatic Diseases Clinics of North America* **18**, 683–697.

Joo, K. W. *et al.* (1998). Absence of H(+)-ATPase in the intercalated cells of renal tissues in classic distal renal tubular acidosis. *Clinical Nephrology* **49**, 226–231.

Kassan, S. S. and Talal, N. Renal disease in Sjögren's syndrome. In *Sjögren's Syndrome: Clinical and Immunological Aspects* (ed. N. Talal, H. M. Moutsopoulos, and S. S. Kassan), pp. 96–101. Berlin: Springer-Verlag, 1987.

Kincaid, M. C. The eye in Sjögren's syndrome. In *Sjögren's Syndrome: Clinical and Immunological Aspects* (ed. N. Talal, H. M. Moutsopoulos, and S. S. Kassan), pp. 25–33. Berlin: Springer-Verlag, 1987.

Kordossis, T. *et al.* (1998). Prevalence of Sjögren's-like syndrome in a cohort of HIV-1-positive patients: descriptive pathology and immunopathology. *British Journal of Rheumatology* **37**, 691–695.

Lindahl, G., Hedfors, E., Klareskog, L., and Forsum, U. (1985). Epithelial HLA-DR expression and T lymphocyte subsets in salivary glands in Sjögren's syndrome. *Clinical and Experimental Immunology* **61**, 475–482.

Manthorpe, R., Frost-Larsen, K., Isager, H., and Prause, J. U. (1981). Sjögren's syndrome: a review with emphasis on immunological features. *Allergy* **36**, 139–153.

McCurdy, D. K., Cornwell, G. G., and DePratti, V. J. (1967). Hyperglobulinaemic renal tubular acidosis. Report of two cases. *Annals of Internal Medicine* **67**, 110–117.

Michels, H. (1997). Course of mixed connective tissue disease in children. *Annals of Medicine* **29**, 359–364.

Moutsopoulos, H. M., Balow, J. E., Cawley, J. T., Stahl, N. I., Autonovych, T. T., and Chused, T. M. (1978). Immune complex glomerulonephritis in sicca syndrome. *American Journal of Medicine* **64**, 955–960.

Moutsopoulos, H. M., Cledes, J., Skopouli, F. N., Elisaf, M., and Youinou, P. (1991). Nephrocalcinosis in Sjögren's syndrome: a late sequelae of renal tubular acidosis. *Journal of Internal Medicine* **203**, 187–191.

Patel, Y. I., and McHugh, N. J. (2000). Apoptosis—new clues to the pathogenesis of Sjögren's syndrome? *Rheumatology* **39**, 119–121.

Pease, C. T., Shattles, W., Charles, P. J., Venables, P. J. W., and Maini, R. N. (1989). Clinical, serological and HLA phenotypes subsets in Sjögren's syndrome. *Clinical and Experimental Rheumatology* **17**, 185–190.

Price, E. J. and Venables, P. J. W. (1995). The aetiopathogenesis of Sjögren's syndome. *Seminars in Arthritis and Rheumatism* **25**, 117–133.

Price, E. J. and Venables, P. J. (2002). Dry eyes and mouth syndrome—a subgroup of patients presenting with sicca symptoms. *Rheumatology (Oxford)* **41**, 416–422.

Rigby, S. P., Griffiths, D. J., Weiss, R. A., and Venables, P. J. (1997). Human retrovirus-5 proviral DNA is rarely detected in salivary gland biopsy tissues from patients with Sjögren's syndrome. *Arthritis and Rheumatism* **11**, 2016–2021.

Rosenberg, M. E., Schendel, P. B., McCurdy, F. A., and Platt, J. L. (1988). Characterisation of immune cells in kidneys from patients with Sjögren's syndrome. *American Journal of Kidney Diseases* **11**, 20–22.

Satoh, K., Imai, H., Yasuda, T., Wakui, H., Miura, A. B., and Nakamoto, Y. (1994). Sclerodermatous renal crisis in a patient with mixed connective tissue disease. *American Journal of Kidney Diseases* **24**, 215–218.

Sharp, G. C., Irwin, W. S., Tan, E. M., Gould, R. G., and Holman, H. R. (1972). Mixed connective tissue disease—an apparently distinct rheumatic disease syndrome associated with antibody to extractable nuclear antigen. *American Journal of Medicine* **52**, 148–159.

Shearn, M. A. (1977). Sjögren's syndrome. *Medical Clinics of North America* **61**, 271–282.

Shearn, M. A. and Tu, W. H. (1965). Nephrogenic diabetes insipidus and other defects of renal tubular dysfunction in Sjögren's syndrome. *American Journal of Medicine* **39**, 312–318.

Shioji, R., Furuyama, T., Onodera, S., Saito, H., Ito, H., and Sasaki, Y. (1970). Sjögren's syndrome and renal tubular acidosis. *American Journal of Medicine* **48**, 456–463.

Shiozawa, S., Shiozawa, K., Shimizu, S., Nakada, M., Isobe, T., and Fugita, T. (1987). Clinical studies of renal disease in Sjögren's syndrome. *Annals of the Rheumatic Diseases* **46**, 768–772.

Siamopoulos, K. C., Elisaf, M., and Moutsopoulos, H. M. (1994). Hypokalaemic paralysis as the presenting manifestation of primary Sjögren's syndrome. *Nephrology, Dialysis, Transplantation* **9**, 1176–1178.

Sjögren, H. (1933). Zur Kenntnis der keratoconjunctivitis sicca (keratitis filiformis bei hypofunktion der tranendrusen). *Acta Ophthalmologica* **11**, 1–15.

Takaya, M. *et al.* (1985). T lymphocyte subsets of the infiltrating cells in the salivary gland and kidney of a patient with Sjögren's syndrome associated with nephritis. *Clinical and Experimental Rheumatology* **3**, 259–263.

Talal, N. (1971). Sjögren's syndrome, lymphoproliferation and renal tubular acidosis. *Annals of Internal Medicine* **74**, 633–634.

Talal, N. and Moutsopoulos, H. M. Treatment of Sjögren's syndrome. In *Sjögren's Syndrome: Clinical and Immunological Aspects* (ed. N. Talal, H. M. Moutsopoulos, S. S. Kassan), pp. 291–295. Berlin: Springer-Verlag, 1987.

Terada, K. *et al.* (1994). Prevalence of serum and salivary antibodies to HTLV-1 in Sjögren's syndrome. *Lancet* **344**, 1116–1119.

Tishler, M. (1999). Hydroxychloroquine treatment for primary Sjögren's syndrome: its effect on salivary and serum inflammatory markers. *Annals of the Rheumatic Disease* **58**, 253–236.

Trevino, H., Tsianos, E. B., and Schenker, S. Gastrointestinal and hepatobiliary features in Sjögren's syndrome. In *Sjögren's Syndrome: Clinical and Immunological Aspects* (ed. N. Talal, H. M. Moutsopoulos, S. S. Kassan), pp. 96–101. Berlin: Springer-Verlag, 1987.

Van de Merwe, J., Kamerling, R., Arendsen, E., Mulder, D., and Hooijkaas, H. (1993). Sjögren's syndrome in patients with interstitial cystitis. *Journal of Rheumatology* **20**, 962–966.

Venables, P. J. W. (1986). Antibodies to nucleic acid binding proteins: their clinical and aetiological significance. MD Thesis, University of Cambridge.

Venables, P. J. W. Overlap syndromes. In *Rheumatology* (ed. J. H. Klippel and P. A. Dieppe), pp. 7.33.1–7.33.8. Mosby-Year Book, 1998.

Venables, P. J. W., Shattles, W., Pease, C. T., Ellis, J. E., Charles, P. J., and Maini, R. N. (1989). Anti-La (SS-B): a diagnostic criterion for Sjögren's syndrome. *Clinical and Experimental Rheumatology* **7**, 181–185.

Venables, P. J. W, Tung, Y., Woodrow, D. F., Moss, J., and Maini, R. N. (1983). Relationship of antibodies to soluble cellular antigens with histological manifestations of renal disease in SLE. *Annals of the Rheumatic Diseases* **42**, 17–22.

Vincent, T. L., Richardson, M. P., Mackworth-Young, C. G., Hawke, S. H., and Venables, P. J. (2003). Sjogren's syndrome-associated myelopathy: response to immunosuppressive treatment. *American Journal of Medicine* **114**, 145–148.

Vitali, C. *et al.* (1993). Preliminary criteria for the classification of Sjögren's syndrome: results of a prospective concerted action supported by the European Community. *Arthritis and Rheumatism* **36**, 340–348.

Waterman, S. A., Gordon, T. P., and Rischmueller, M. (2000). Inhibitory effects of muscarinic receptor autoantibodies on parasympathetic neuro-transmission in Sjögren's syndrome. *Arthritis and Rheumatism* **43**, 1647–1654.

Wasicek, C. A. and Reichlin, M. (1982). Clinical and serological differences between systemic lupus erythematosus patients with antibodies to Ro versus patients with antibodies to Ro and La. *Journal of Clinical Investigation* **69**, 835–843.

Zawadzki, J. (1998). Permeability defect with bicarbonate leak as a mechanism of immune-related distal renal tubular acidosis. *American Journal of Kidney Diseases* **31**, 527–532.

4.11 The patient with sickle-cell disease

Ralph Caruana

Sickle-cell disease

Introduction

Sickle-cell disease is a worldwide health problem predominantly affecting members of the Black race. 'Sickle-cell disease' is said to be present in individuals heterozygous or homozygous for the haemoglobin S (HbS) gene. 'Sickle-cell anaemia' is said to be present in patients who are homozygous for HbS.

Sickle-cell anaemia—a worldwide health problem

History

James Herrick provided the first description of the clinical findings and red blood cell morphology (Fig. 1) of the entity now called sickle-cell anaemia (Herrick 1910). The index case was a young Black dental student from Grenada who was living in Chicago at the time. Herrick noted unusual poikilocytosis on the patient's peripheral blood smear while evaluating him for anaemia. The patient later had a painful crisis, which Herrick suggested might be due to his abnormal red cells. The patient graduated and returned to Grenada where he died of pneumonia at age 32. When knowledge of West African sources was later evaluated, it became clear that Herrick did not really 'discover' sickle-cell disease, since local oral and written sources clearly document a knowledge, dating back centuries, of an intermittently painful condition which ran in families.

Although Herrick mentioned abnormalities of the urinary sediment and low urine specific gravity in his patient, Sydenstricker *et al.* (1923) at the Medical College of Georgia were the first to report autopsy evidence of gross and microscopic renal alterations. These investigators described light microscopic findings of enlarged glomeruli distended with sickled red blood cells, as well as stainable iron in renal tubular cells.

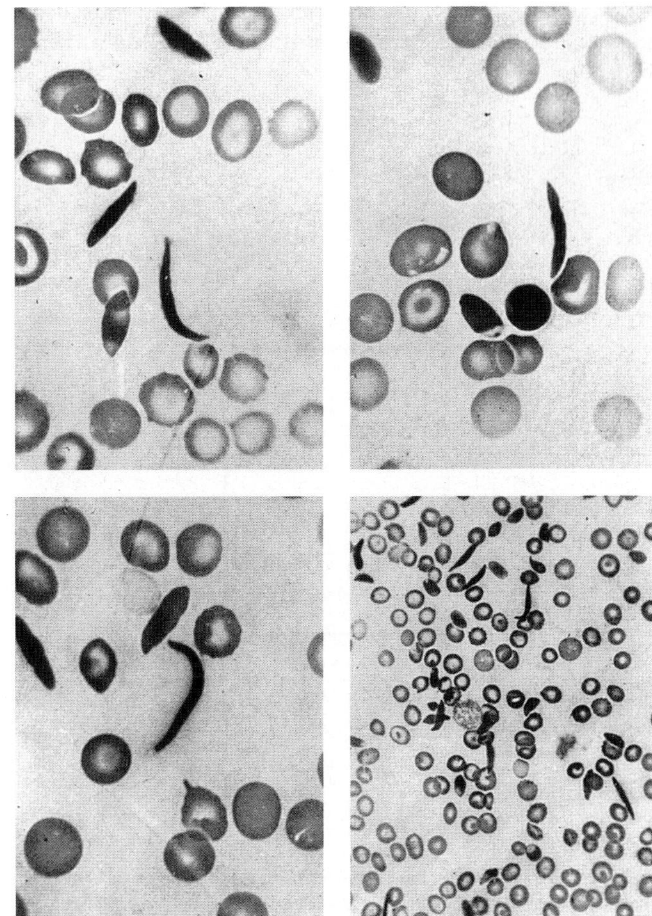

Fig. 1 Photomicrographs of red blood cell morphology in sickle-cell anaemia from Herrick's original case published in 1910 (Herrick 1910, with permission).

Ranney (1994) summarized the subsequent developments in the study of sickle-cell disease. The first breakthrough occurred in 1949 when a group led by Linus Pauling demonstrated that sickle-cell anaemia was the result of an abnormality in the haemoglobin molecule, thus ushering in the era of 'molecular diseases'. Pauling's group found that haemoglobin from patients with sickle-cell anaemia differed electrophoretically from normal haemoglobin, and later demonstrated that relatively asymptomatic patients who were presumed to be heterozygous for the condition had, in fact, a mixture of normal and sickle haemoglobin. Soon after these discoveries, Harris found that deoxygenated HbS had a propensity for gellation, while Perutz and his group demonstrated that crystals of HbS were birefringent and less soluble than normal haemoglobin. In 1953, Singer and Singer showed that polymerization of deoxyHbS was inhibited by fetal haemoglobin (HbF). This provided a plausible explanation for why newborns who later developed full-blown sickle-cell anaemia were spared from clinical manifestations immediately after birth, a time when HbF concentrations are at their highest. In 1956, Ingram reported results obtained from electrophoretic and chromatographic studies which showed that the β-chain of the sickle-cell globin molecule differed from the β-chain of normal globin by a single substitution of valine for glutamic acid at the sixth residue. This substitution of the uncharged, poorly water-soluble valine for the charged, highly soluble glutamic acid alters the three-dimensional spatial configuration of the haemoglobin molecule. Adherence of haemoglobin molecules to each other is enhanced by this substitution, permitting the formation of elongated haemoglobin polymers that give sickle cells their characteristic sickle shape. Later, the discovery of other haemoglobin variants revealed the existence of hybrid sickling disorders, such as haemoglobin SC (HbSC) and sickle cell–thalassaemia variants with characteristic red cell morphology and clinical characteristics (Fig. 2).

Epidemiology

The current state of knowledge about the origins and dispersion of the sickle gene has recently been summarized by Nagel (1994). Since homozygotes for the βS gene develop full-blown sickle-cell anaemia, a condition which has a marked survival disadvantage, the high frequency of the heterozygous state must indicate balanced polymorphism; that is, the disadvantages of the homozygous state must in some way be balanced by the advantages of the heterozygous state. The survival of the sickle-cell gene in the world gene pool has long been attributed to the observed attenuation of clinical symptoms of malaria in heterozygotes. Eaton (1994) has provided a lucid description of the relationship between malaria and the sickle-cell gene. The precise protective function of small amounts of HbS against the malarial parasite has not been totally explained, but increased removal of parasitized HbAS cells by the spleen, persistence of haemoglobin F, and vascular adherence properties of parasitized HbAS cells have all been implicated. Clearly, worldwide distribution of the HbS genotype and the reservoirs of falciparum malaria infection show striking congruence. The rise of malaria as an endemic disease and the resulting preservation of the sickle-cell gene may have been triggered by the beginnings of slash and burn agriculture in the previously dense West African rainforest, an ecological change which provided sun-drenched, treeless areas with standing water, a hospitable milieu for breeding of the *Anopheles* mosquito, the most effective insect vector for *Plasmodium falciparum*. Restriction enzyme techniques have allowed identification of five major βS haplotypes, Benin, Bantu (formerly Central African Republic or CAR), Senegal, Cameroon, and Arab–Indian (Fig. 3), all of which are thought to have arisen independently of each other (Nagel 1994). The predominant Benin type spread from West Africa to North Africa, western Arabia and the Mediterranean basin, including the Levant, Greece, and Italy. The Senegal and Cameroon haplotypes are still confined mainly to West Africa, but the Bantu haplotype spread across the continent, reaching the eastern coast. The Arab–Indian haplotype probably arose in the Indus Valley. It is the most common haplotype of the tribal peoples of India, central Asia, and the eastern province of Saudi Arabia. The West African slave trade, commencing in the seventeenth century, transported individuals with the HbS gene to the Caribbean islands and continental North and South America.

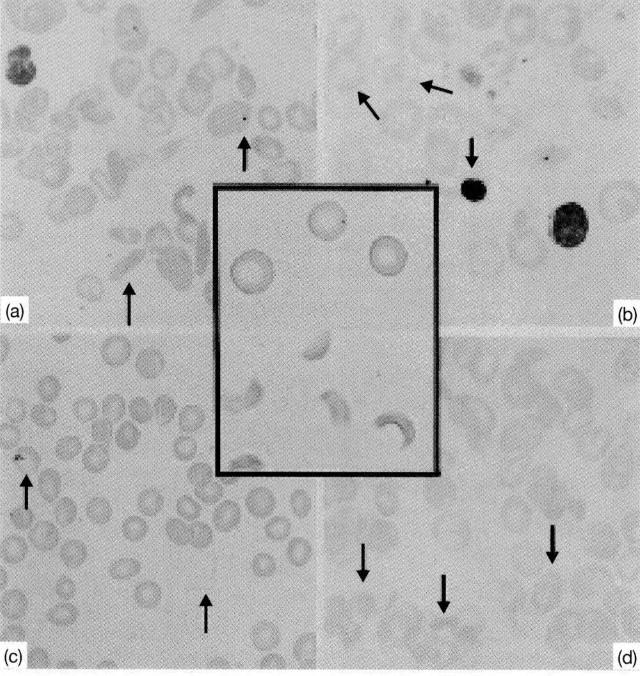

Fig. 2 The peripheral blood in sickle-cell disease. (a) Sickle-cell anaemia. The hallmark of the blood film in sickle-cell anaemia is the irreversibly sickled cell, a dense, pointed, elongated cell (lower arrow), scattered throughout the film. Also typical are Howell–Jolly bodies (upper arrow) which are nuclear remnants. (b) HbS–β°-thalassaemia. In addition to the rare sickle cell there is microcytosis, target cells, hypochromia (left arrow), basophilic stippling (uppermost arrow), and a nucleated erythrocyte (lower arrow). (c) HbS–β^{+}-thalassaemia. Microcytosis and hypochromia are characteristic of this condition and sickled cells are rarely seen when high levels of non-S haemoglobins are present. (d) HbSC disease. A dense spherocytic cell (left arrow), HbC crystal (middle arrow), folded cell (right arrow), target cells, and irregularly contracted erythrocytes are seen. Inset: a sodium metabisulfite sickling preparation in an individual with sickle-cell trait. The upper panel shows normal-appearing cells prior to the addition of sodium metabisulfite. The lower panel shows sickled forms following the addition of this agent. Tests of this sort were often used to diagnose sickle-cell disease, but have been supplanted by haemoglobin electrophoresis, other protein-based tests, and DNA-based means (from Ranney 1994, with permission).

Up to one-fourth of newborn babies in the West African endemic area carry the gene, compared to 8 per cent of Afro-Americans. The lower gene frequency in North America may reflect reduced heterozygote advantage in an area in which malaria has been eradicated, but even today, with one in 600 Afro-Americans being homozygous for HbS, sickle-cell anaemia is a major public health problem in the United States. Clinical manifestations in African homozygotes are more severe than those in Asian or New World populations. In all areas of the world, the Bantu haplotype is that most associated with severe organ failure syndromes, including chronic renal failure (Powars *et al.* 1990).

Pathophysiology

When present in sufficient amounts, HbS can undergo a spatial molecular rearrangement leading to an orderly alignment of haemoglobin molecules into chain-like formations. This process changes the shape of the normally biconcave red blood cells and increases their rigidity (Mohandas and Ballas 1994). Although sickled cells can revert to normal if the stimulus for sickling abates, some cells become irreversibly sickled and are referred to as dense cells (Fig. 4). The severity of haemolytic anaemia at any given time will be proportional to the number of these mechanically fragile and poorly deformable erythrocytes.

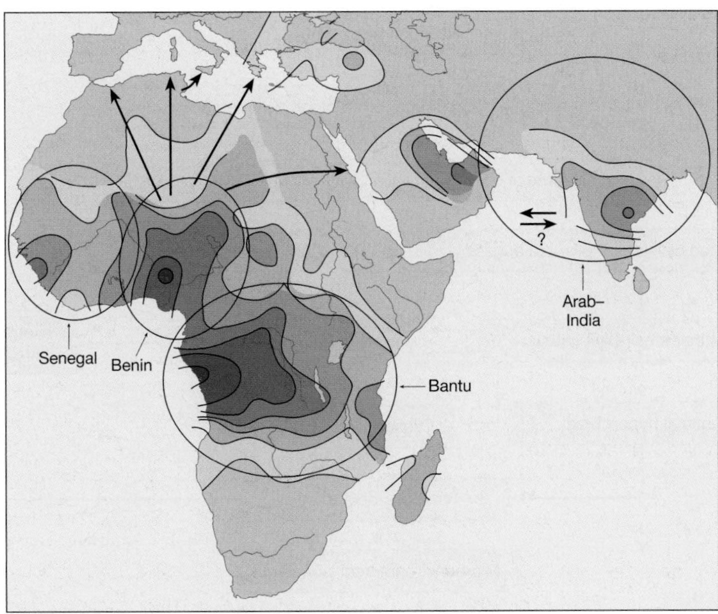

Fig. 3 Shaded areas in this map represent progressively increased frequencies (in direct proportion to darker intensity) of the βS gene. Circles define geographical areas in which the Senegal, Benin, Bantu, and Arab–Indian haplotypes are found at extreme high frequency (over 94%) linked to the βS gene and involving major populations (from Nagel 1994, with permission).

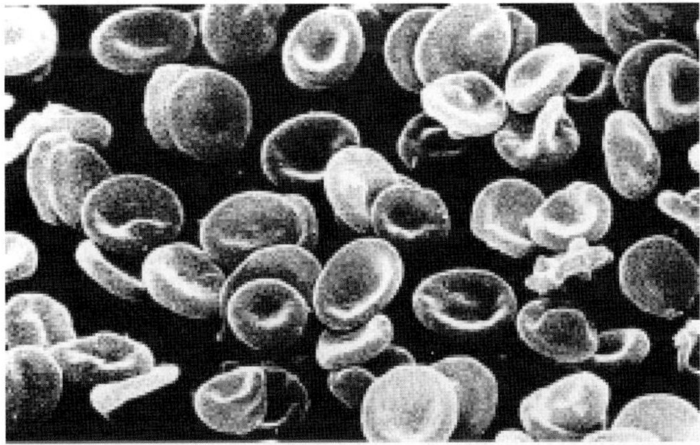

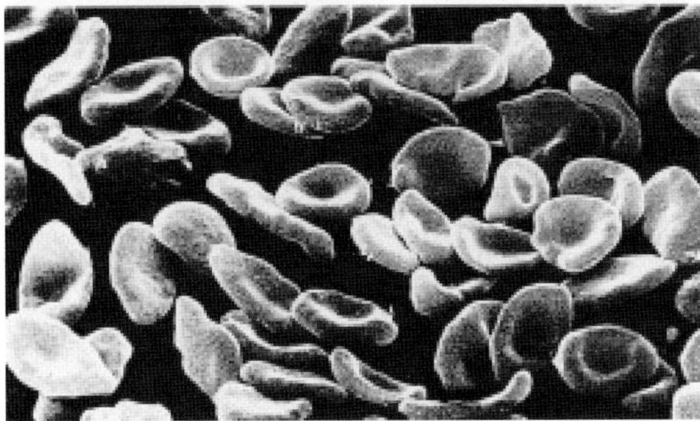

Fig. 4 Scanning electron micrographs of low-density (top) and high-density (bottom) oxygenated sickle cells. Discoid morphology is the dominant feature of the low-density cells, while irreversibly sickled red cells are enriched in the high-density fraction (from Mohandas and Ballas 1994, with permission).

The permanently sickled cells tend to have the least concentration of haemoglobin F and contain reduced amounts of 2,3-diphosphoglycerate. When present in large numbers these deformed, rigid red blood cells with low oxygen carrying capacity reduce tissue oxygenation and increase blood viscosity, leading to microvascular sludging which prevents the less affected red blood cells from delivering oxygen to tissues. The results of this cascade are small vessel thrombosis and infarction, which are responsible for the acute and chronic multiorgan manifestations of sickle-cell anaemia (Fig. 5). Vaso-occlusion is most probably multifactorial in pathogenesis, being influenced by the amount of HbS polymer, the fraction of dense sickle cells, blood viscosity, the coagulation cascade, platelet activation, vascular tone, vascular diameter, and adherence of sickled cells to vascular endothelium (Fig. 6). Thus, the existence of multiple activating pathways allows a variety of pathophysiological triggering mechanisms, including infection, hypoxaemia, volume depletion, acidosis, hypothermia, and hyperosmolality to initiate a vaso-occlusive crisis (Francis and Hebbel 1994).

Natural history of sickle-cell anaemia

Childhood and adolescence

Haematological complications

Baseline profile From early childhood, severe anaemia is the rule in homozygotes (SS genotype) who generally have baseline haemoglobin between 50 and 100 g/l. Growth and sexual development may be delayed but better attention to nutrition and aggressive treatment of infections have made the 'classic' extreme ectomorphic body habitus rare in industrialized countries. There is mounting evidence that patients with sickle-cell disease have chronic, covert inflammatory responses that result in cytokine release and can contribute to

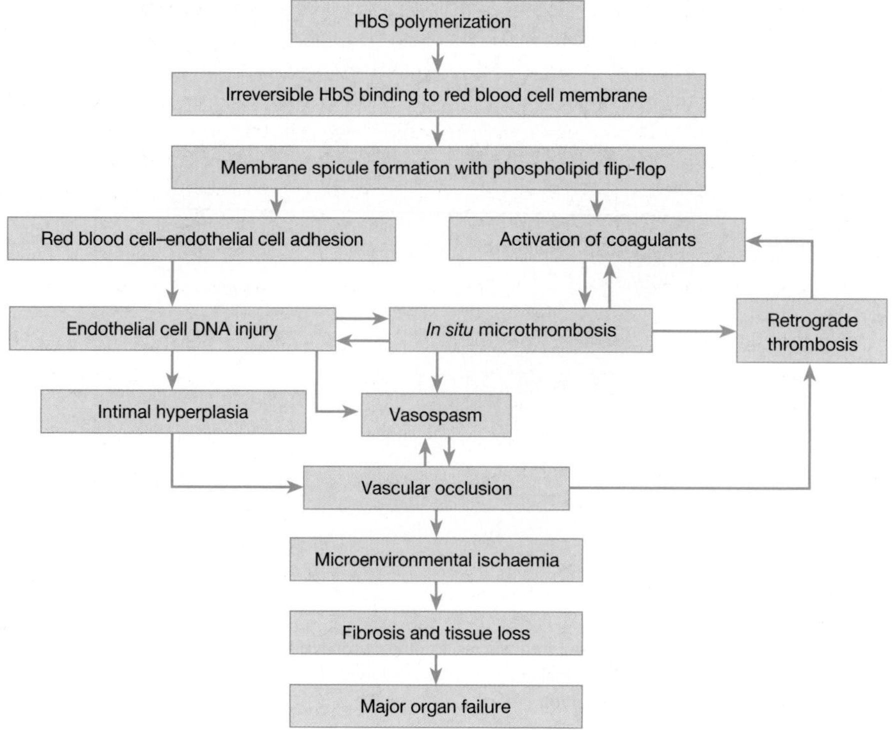

Fig. 5 Schematic representation depicting potential pathophysiological mechanisms by which the sickle cell induces vascular damage and irreversible major organ failure (reprinted from Powars 1994, by courtesy of Marcel Dekker, Inc.).

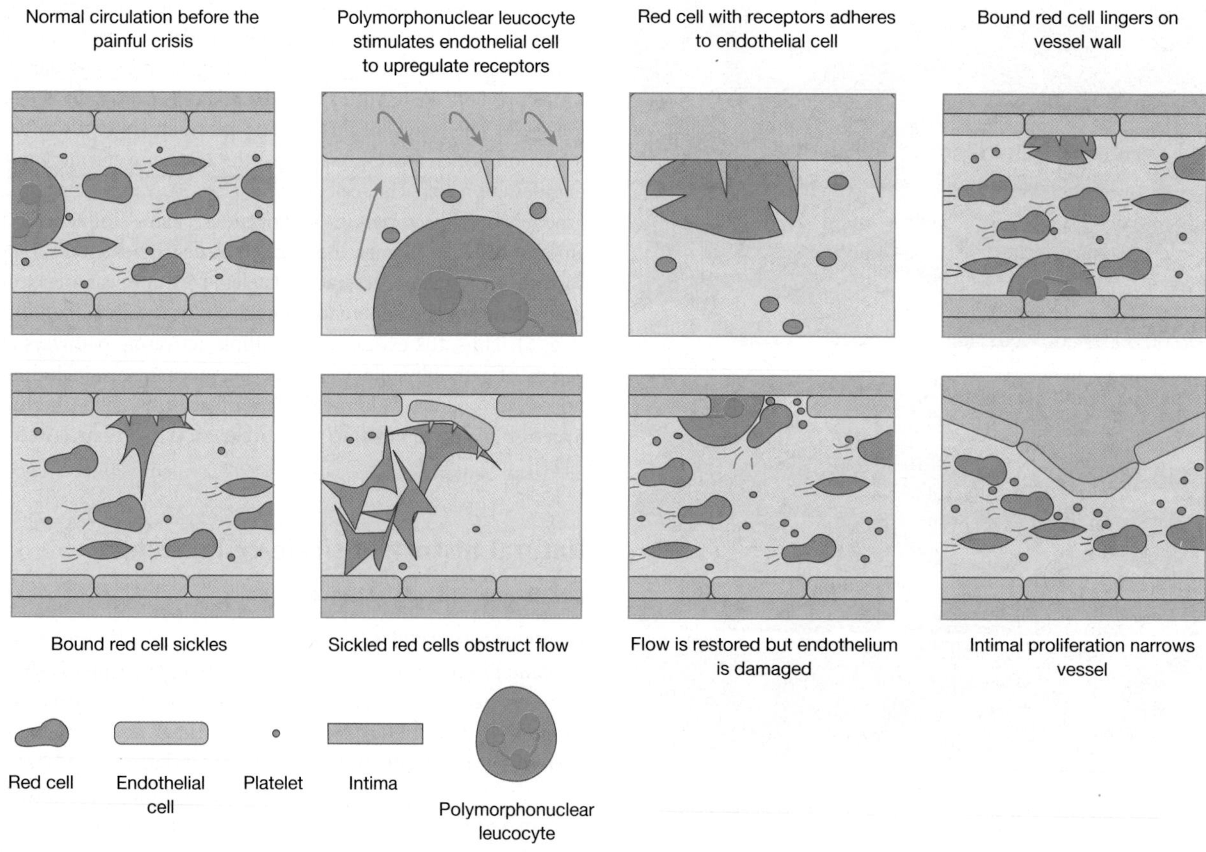

Fig. 6 Possible pathophysiological mechanisms of damage to vessels in sickle-cell disease (reprinted by permission of *The New England Journal of Medicine*, Platt 1994).

a chronic catabolic state with growth retardation in some settings (Singhal *et al.* 1993). Patients with sickle-cell anaemia may have 80 per cent or more of their haemoglobin as HbS, with most of the remainder being HbF. Patients who carry the gene for persistence of HbF have even greater amounts of HbF and, perhaps more importantly, a more uniform distribution of HbF throughout their red cells. Such individuals may have a normal red blood cell count and no clinical manifestations of sickle-cell anaemia since significant amounts of HbF, as mentioned above, can inhibit polymerization and sickling of HbS.

Sickle-cell anaemia patients usually have normocytic red blood cell indices. In their steady state these individuals have chronic, low-grade haemolysis with a reticulocytosis of up to 20 per cent and an average red blood cell survivals of about 30 days (25 per cent of normal). This level of haemolysis is accompanied by elevations of serum bilirubin and lactate dehydrogenase. Chronically elevated bilirubin predisposes to formation of calcium bilirubinate gallstones in children as young as 2 years. By the age of 18, 50 per cent of sickle-cell anaemia patients may have gallstones, the removal by surgery of which is indicated only when frank episodes of biliary colic or cholecystitis occur (Pearson 1989). An excellent review of the laboratory manifestations of sickle-cell anaemia has recently been provided by Steinberg and Mohandas (1994).

Haemolytic, aplastic, and sequestration crises In acute haemolytic crisis, which may be triggered by infection or other physiological stress, accelerated haemolysis outstrips the baseline replacement rate (Shapiro and Ballas 1994). Careful examination of the peripheral blood smear may show obvious evolution of red blood cell morphology as the crisis builds, peaks, and remits (Fig. 7). Generalized weakness and increasing jaundice may be the most prominent symptoms. Aplastic crisis occurs when reticulocyte production lags, often as the result of infection with parvovirus B19. A sequestration crisis occurs when large-scale splenic trapping of red blood cells sequesters a large percentage of the total red cell mass. This can result in acute, painful enlargement of the spleen and circulatory collapse. Less commonly, bone marrow necrosis contributes to worsening of anaemia when microinfarction of the marrow complicates a painful crisis. A rare but potentially lethal complication of haemolytic crisis is thrombotic thrombocytopenic purpura (Bolanos-Meade *et al.* 1999).

Immune defects Recurrent painful or clinically silent splenic infarction commonly produces functional asplenia early in life and predisposes patients to severe pneumococcal infection and sepsis (Pearson 1989). This is the first manifestation of a lifelong opsonic defect resulting in an inability of serum to support neutrophil phagocytosis of *Streptococcus pneumoniae* and other bacteria (Table 1). Other abnormalities in immune function noted in patients with sickle-cell anaemia include low circulating levels of IgM, chronic activation of the complement system, and a deficiency of tuftsin, a splenic derived cytokine which

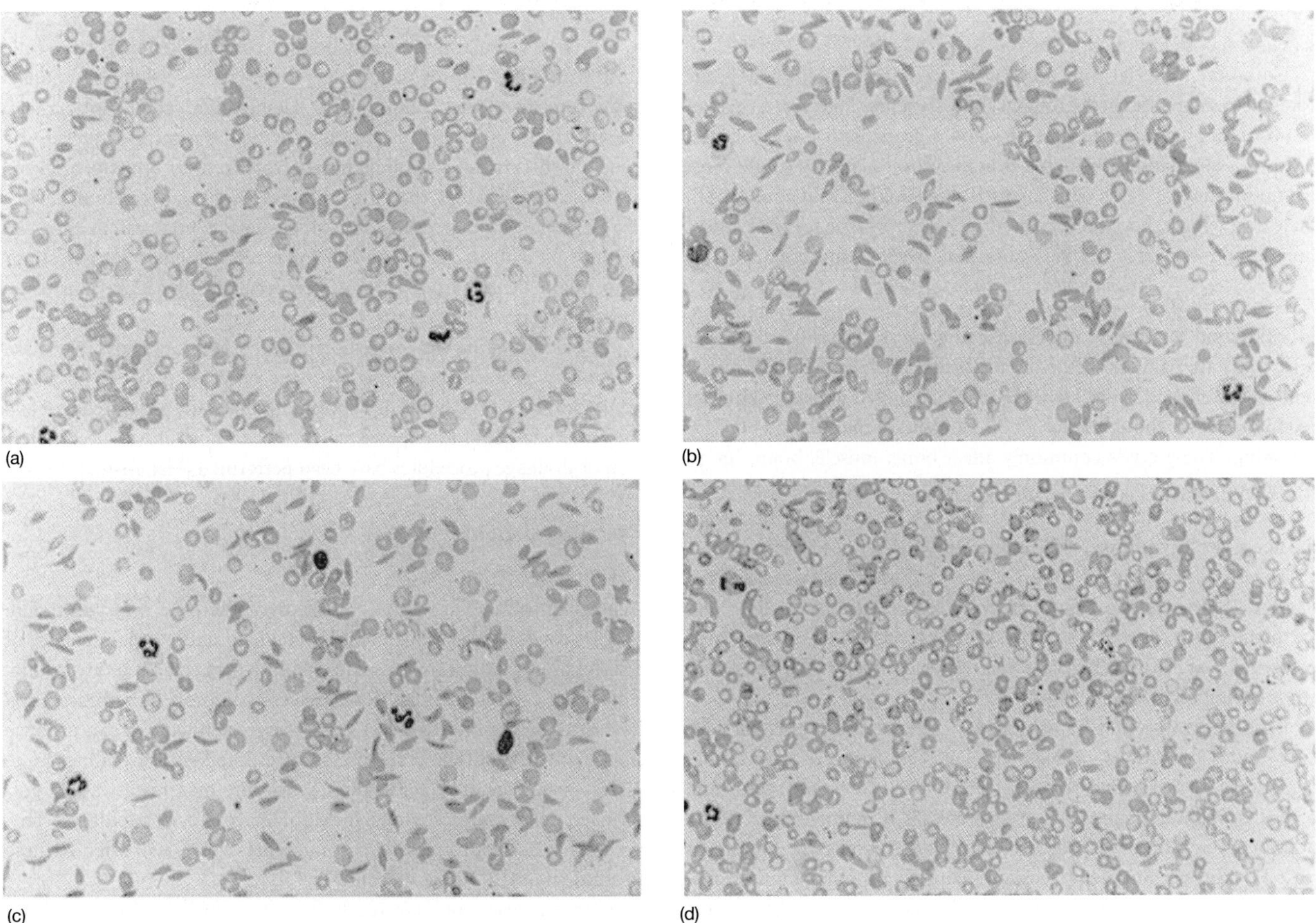

Fig. 7 Typical changes in the peripheral smear during the evolution of the painful sickle-cell crisis. Erythrocyte morphology (a) in the steady state; (b) on day 5 of crisis; (c) on day 6; and (d) on day 11 (from Shapiro and Ballas 1994, with permission).

Table 1 Bacteria and viruses that most frequently cause serious infection in patients with sickle-cell disease (from Buchanan 1994, with permission)

Micro-organism	Type of infection	Comments
Streptococcus pneumoniae	Septicaemia	Common despite prophylactic penicillin and pneumococcal vaccine
	Meningitis	Less frequent than in years past
	Pneumonia	Rarely documented except in infants and young children
	Septic arthritis	Uncommon
Haemophilus influenzae, type *b*	Septicaemia, meningitis, pneumonia	Much less common in recent years because of immunization with conjugate vaccine
Salmonella species	Osteomyelitis, septicaemia	Most common cause of bone and joint infection
Escherichia coli and other Gram-negative enteric pathogens	Septicaemia, urinary tract infection, osteomyelitis	Focus sometimes inapparent
Staphylococcus aureus	Osteomyelitis	Uncommon
Mycoplasma pneumoniae	Pneumonia	Pleural effusions; multilobe involvement
Chlamydia pneumoniae	Pneumonia	
Parvovirus B19	Bone marrow suppression (aplastic crisis)	High fever common; rash and other organ involvement infrequent
Hepatitis viruses (A, B, and C)	Hepatitis	Marked hyperbilirubinaemia

activates granulocytes, monocytes, and tissue macrophages. The relative contribution of these defects to clinical infection in this patient group remains to be determined.

Common bacterial infections with even intermittent low-grade bacteraemias are life threatening in these patients. The greatest risk of death occurs between the ages of 1 and 3 years, with pneumococcal sepsis, a potentially preventable complication, being the single most common cause of death (Buchanan 1994). Children and adults, both male and female, have an increased incidence of urinary tract infections (Zarkowsky *et al.* 1998; Pastore *et al.* 1999; Bruno *et al.* 2001).

Vaso-occlusive complications

In childhood and early adolescence the most clinically important symptoms are pain and acute organ dysfunction secondary to recurrent vaso-occlusive crises (Powars 1994). As noted above, sickling of red blood cells is thought to be an essential factor in initiation of vaso-occlusion. These crises commonly affect bone, muscle, brain, lungs, spleen, kidneys, and bone marrow. Common sequelae include aseptic necrosis of bone, rhabdomyolysis, stroke, splenic and renal infarction, the acute chest syndrome, and priapism.

The first clinical manifestation of vaso-occlusive bone damage is the hand–foot syndrome, a painful osteitis accompanied by swelling and erythema which can occur as early as the first year. Later, osteonecrosis involving the heads of the femur and humerus may produce pain and chronic disability (Powars 1994).

Rhabdomyolysis may be provoked by strenuous exercise, particularly under conditions of high ambient temperature and volume depletion (Devereux and Knowles 1985). The acute chest syndrome results from pulmonary vaso-occlusion and is defined as an acute pulmonary infiltrate with hypoxaemia severe enough to require at least 3 l of O_2 per minute by mask to maintain a haemoglobin saturation of 90 per cent (van Agtmael *et al.* 1994). Acute renal cortical infarction (Granfortuna *et al.* 1986) is fortunately a rare manifestation of vaso-occlusive crisis but may be accompanied by acute multiorgan failure, particularly if fat embolism or sepsis supervenes (Hassell *et al.* 1994).

Cerebral vascular disease may become clinically manifest before the third year of life. Approximately 6 per cent of sickle-cell disease patients suffer cerebrovascular complications. Hemiparetic strokes, intracranial haemorrhage, and cerebral atrophy can be devastating sequelae of a generalized cerebral vasculopathy characterized by both thromboses and vascular stenoses that involve large and small cerebral vessels. Transcranial Doppler evaluation of the intracranial vasculature can identify patients at increased risk for cerebrovascular complications who might benefit from chronic, recurrent prophylactic transfusion therapy (Adams 1994, 2000).

Vascular sludging and congestion in the corpora cavernosa may make priapism a problem beginning with the onset of puberty. As young adulthood is reached bouts of priapism may become more frequent and may ultimately lead to impotence, whether or not surgical decompression or drainage procedures have been performed (Hakim *et al.* 1994).

The adult patient

Sickle-cell anaemia

Acute painful and haemolytic crises may continue into adulthood. Problems with social adjustment, opiate habituation, maintenance of employment, and family relationships may reach a crescendo. Thrombotic cerebral infarctions are less common but intracerebral haemorrhages are more likely. Progressive osteonecrosis can produce significant disability and require surgical intervention (Milner *et al.* 1994). Recurrences of acute chest syndrome may result in cor pulmonale. Renal manifestations, including haematuria, papillary necrosis, nephrotic syndrome, and chronic renal failure, will often become prominent at this time (see below).

Liver involvement may result from transfusional iron overload, viral hepatitis, hepatic infarction, hepatic sequestration, or gallstone-associated cholangitis. Acute gouty arthritis, chronic skin ulcers, most

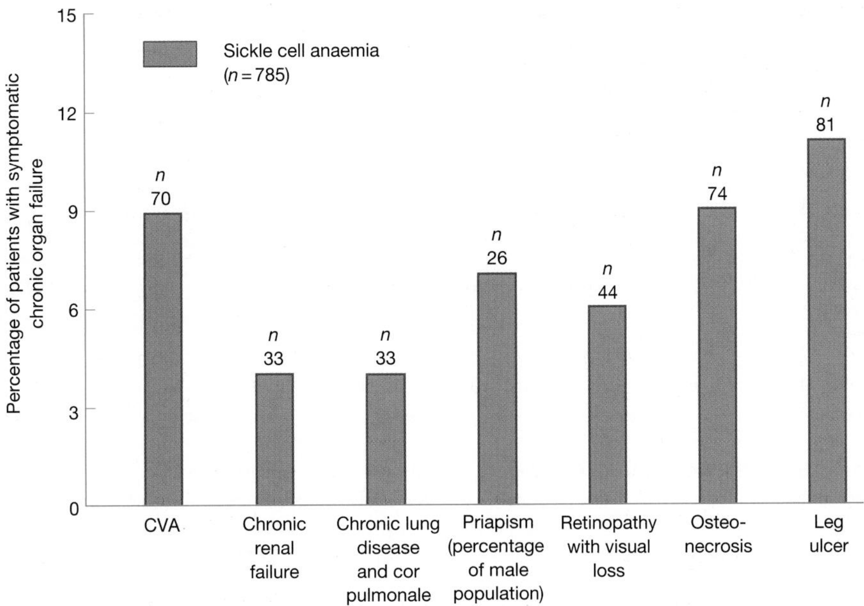

Fig. 8 The frequency of major organ failure in sickle-cell anaemia patients (reprinted from Powars 1994, by courtesy of Marcel Dekker, Inc.).

Table 2 Age of onset of clinically evident organ damage (reprinted from Powars 1994, by courtesy of Marcel Dekker, Inc.)

Clinical event	n	%	Median	Range
CVA	69	8.8	13.1	0.6–47.1
Priapism[a]	26	6.7	22.3	6.2–47.9
Osteonecrosis	74	9.4	23.1	1.3–60.9
SCLD	33	4.2	24.2	6.0–43.3
Leg ulcer	80	10.2	24.5	4.0–52.5
SRF	32	4.1	25.1	12.8–62.9
Retinopathy	44	5.6	25.8	8.9–65.3

[a] Percentage of male patients.

CVA, cerebrovascular accident; SCLD, sickle-cell lung disease; SRF, sickle renal failure.

characteristically over the malleolar areas, cardiomyopathy, and retinal neovascularization with haemorrhage may add to functional disability (Charache 1994a). Figure 8 and Table 2 show the prevalence and median age of onset of major organ syndromes in sickle-cell anaemia.

Survival and causes of death

Platt *et al.* (1994) have provided the most comprehensive analysis of life expectancy and risk factors for early death in sickle-cell anaemia in their analysis of data from the Cooperative Study of Sickle Cell Disease, a multicentre study conducted at 23 sites. The database included 2542 patients with sickle-cell anaemia, 844 with HbSC, and 388 with sickle cell-β-thalassaemia variants. This study reviewed the data on 3764 patients who were enrolled at ages ranging from birth to 66 years of age. The median age of death was 42 years for males and 48 years for females in patients with sickle-cell anaemia (Fig. 9). By comparison, the median age of death for patients with HbSC was 60 years for males and 68 years for females. In sickle-cell anaemia, 33 per cent of deaths occurred during an acute sickle crisis (78 per cent with painful crisis, the acute chest syndrome, or both; 22 per cent with stroke). Eighteen per cent of deaths were ascribed to chronic end-organ involvement, predominantly renal. Increased risk for early death correlated significantly with the presence of renal failure, seizures, acute chest syndrome, and a low level of HbF. The risk analysis incorporated data from 209 patients with sickle-cell anaemia who were 20 years of age or older when they died. Forty-five patients died during a crisis with 25/45 having concomitant acute chest syndrome. Nine patients died with acute chest syndrome without crisis. Fifteen deaths were due to stroke, with documented haemorrhage in 11. Although 13 patients died of infection there was no dominant pathogen. The decrease in life expectancy for adults with sickle-cell anaemia is thus 25–30 years as compared to the entire Afro-American population. Leikin *et al.* (1989), reporting data on 2824 patients less than 20 years of age, found that the most important cause of death between the ages of 1 and 3 years was infection, but after the age of 10 years stroke and trauma became the most important causes. In the period from 1968 to 1992 mortality rates of Black children with sickle-cell disease fell 41–53 per cent in all age groups (Davis *et al.* 1997).

Sickle-cell trait

Patients with sickle-cell trait (AS genotype) have 30–45 per cent of their haemoglobin as HbS and are not usually anaemic. Under conditions of severe stress, exhaustion, or hypoxaemia they may develop rhabdomyolysis (see below), haemolytic anaemia and, rarely, sickle-cell crises. In general, patients with sickle-cell trait do not have excess mortality compared to individuals without the trait. Splenic infarction at high altitudes is rare unless individuals with sickle-cell trait are exposed to altitudes of 3000 m or more in unpressurized aeroplane cabins (Sears 1978).

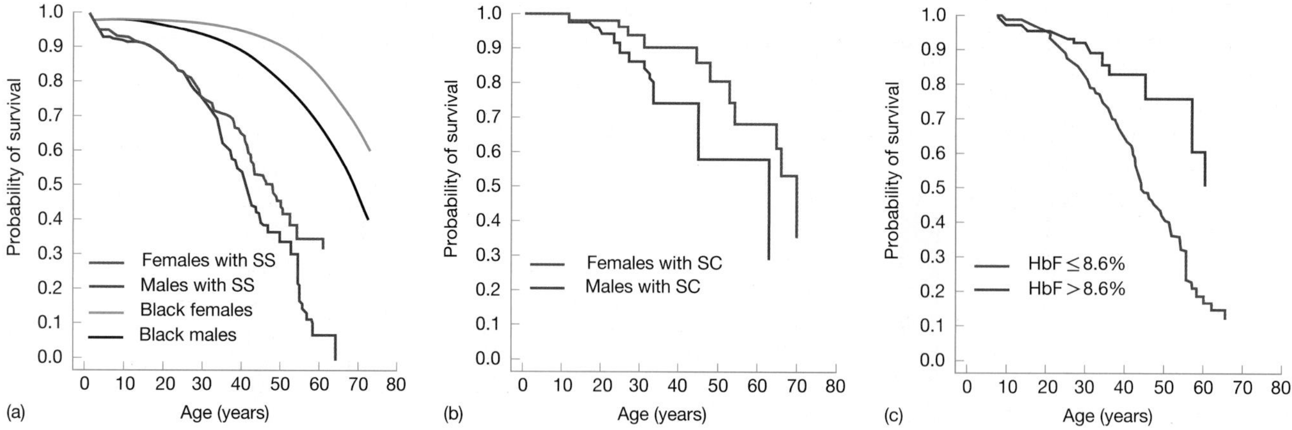

Fig. 9 Survival of patients in the Cooperative Study of Sickle Cell Disease. (a) Male and female patients with sickle-cell anaemia (SS) compared with Black males and females in the general population (data are from the National Center for Health Statistics 1988). (b) Male and female patients with sickle cell–haemoglobin C disease (SC). (c) Patients over 5 years of age with sickle-cell anaemia who had fetal haemoglobin (HbF) levels at or below the 75th percentile (8.6%) (reprinted by permission of *The New England Journal of Medicine*, Platt *et al.* 1994).

Treatment

General care

Exposure to altitudes over 2500 m should be avoided unless pressurized aircraft cabins or supplementary oxygen are available. Strenuous exercise can be accompanied by volume depletion, hypoxaemia, and lactic acidosis, and should be avoided in sickle-cell anaemia patients because of the danger of precipitating a crisis. Transfusions should be given during sepsis, blood loss, and before surgery. Prophylactic penicillin is efficacious in preventing infection but inhibits development of natural immunity by suppressing nasopharyngeal colonization and has the potential to select for development of resistant strains of *S. pneumoniae* and *H. influenzae*. Immunization against *S. pneumoniae*, *H. influenzae*, and *Neisseria meningitidis* is recommended but is not always successful. Supplementation with folic acid is usually required because of high red blood cell turnover. Fluids should never be restricted and daily intakes in the range of 2 l are recommended. Iron overload may have to be treated with chelation therapy, particularly in young patients who have received over 100 units of transfused red cells.

Treatment of a painful crisis has traditionally focused on replacement of fluid deficits, correction of acidosis, analgesia with frequent opiate injections at fixed intervals or patient-controlled analgesia, and antibiotics when bacterial infection is diagnosed or suspected. Patient-controlled analgesia with infusion pumps for opiate administration has become the standard approach to pain control. Perlin *et al.* (1994) and others have found that administration of ketorolac tromethamine for pain can reduce total opioid dose and length of hospital stay without adverse renal effects. Griffin *et al.* (1994), in a randomized placebo-controlled study of 56 pain episodes, found that high-dose intravenous methylprednisolone (15 mg/kg) given on two consecutive days aborted painful crises in an average of 41 h, compared to 71 h for standard therapy. Duration and total doses of narcotic agents were reduced, although rebound crises were more commonly observed in the methylprednisolone group.

Transfusion therapy

Although red cell transfusions may be required for acute situations such as acute blood loss or splenic sequestration crisis and to prepare patients for elective or emergency surgery (Scott-Conner and Brunson 1994), the goal of chronic intermittent transfusion therapy in sickle-cell anaemia is the prevention of vaso-occlusive phenomena by the dilution and replacement of sickle cells with normal red blood cells. Such therapy is most often used in an attempt to prevent further progression of pre-existing chronic complications of sickle-cell anaemia such as cerebrovascular disease, pulmonary vascular disease, priapism, and skin ulcers. Frequent transfusion is required if HbS is to be kept less than the target value of 30 per cent. If racially unmatched blood is transfused, the risks of alloimmunization and delayed transfusion reactions have been reported to be as high as 30 per cent and 11 per cent, respectively (Vichinsky *et al.* 1990). Other risks of transfusion in this population are not trivial and include acute hyperviscosity syndrome, precipitation of painful crises, pulmonary oedema, iron overload, viral hepatitis, and transmission of HIV infection.

Pharmacological therapy

Steinberg (1999) recently reviewed the principles of pharmacological therapy in patients with sickle-cell anaemia. Early interest in urea and cyanate as antisickling agents faded when pilot studies showed little clinical effect. A practical problem with any putative antisickling compound is the high dosing requirements and high blood concentrations required to stabilize a clinically significant percentage of a patient's β globin molecules. The major agents currently under investigation which are likely to help sickle-cell anaemia patients in the near future, therefore, are drugs capable of increasing endogenous synthesis of haemoglobin F (Charache 1994b).

On a biophysical basis, high levels of HbF would be expected to ameliorate the sickling phenomena by two mechanisms. By its simple presence HbF reduces the concentration of HbS within the erythrocyte and thus attenuates HbS polymerization. Secondly, HbF tetramers will not undergo polymerization with any HbS polymers being formed. Recent interest has focused on combination therapy employing hydroxyurea and recombinant erythropoietin (Rodgers *et al.* 1993a). When combined with adequate iron supplementation, this regimen is quite effective in increasing HbF and can be used as a form of salvage therapy for patients with severe disease. It should be noted that the recombinant erythropoietin doses required are very high, up to 3000 units/kg/week. Although the high amounts of HbF present in newborn babies and in patients with the various forms of hereditary persistence of HbF appear to ameliorate the severity of clinical manifestations, a direct relationship between HbF and attenuation of disease expression does not seem to exist.

A recent study sponsored by the National Heart, Lung, and Blood Institute (Charache *et al.* 1995) was terminated early when it became obvious that hydroxyurea therapy clearly reduced the incidence and severity of painful crises in patients with sickle-cell anaemia. This was a double-blind placebo-controlled study started in 1991, the goal of which was to determine whether daily administration of hydroxyurea would reduce the frequency of painful episodes by 50 per cent. The study was conducted by 21 clinical centres and enrolled 299 adult patients who had experienced at least three painful crises over the previous year. The study was terminated when it became clear that the treatment group would clearly demonstrate a significant reduction in painful episodes, hospital admissions, and episodes of acute chest syndrome. Caution must be exercised when hydroxyurea, which is eliminated by both renal and non-renal mechanisms, is used in patients with renal insufficiency, since these individuals may accumulate sufficient drug to experience life-threatening myelosuppression (Gwilt and Tracewell 1998).

Newer experimental therapies include agents targeted to increase HbF (short chain fatty acids, e.g. butyrate), membrane active drugs (clotrimazole, magnesium salts), surfactant compounds, nitric oxide and agents with primarily rheological effects (Gwilt and Tracewell 1998; Orringer *et al.* 2001).

Bone marrow transplantation

Bone marrow transplantation to correct the basic defect in sickle-cell anaemia has been employed in only a small number of patients worldwide. Therapeutic success has been obtained in about 90 per cent of cases with only 4 per cent perioperative mortality (Johnson *et al.* 1994). In a recent review, Hoppe and Walters (2001), reviewed the current status of bone marrow transplantation for sickle-cell anaemia. At that time fewer than 200 children worldwide had received matched sibling donor bone marrow transplantation for sickle-cell disease. The authors emphasized that with current, myeloablative conditioning regimens, serious postoperative problems of graft versus host disease, neurological events and gonadal dysfunction diminish the applicability of bone marrow transplantation as a mainstream treatment modality for sickle-cell anaemia.

Clearly, the youngest patients with the least irreversible organ damage might be in a position to benefit the most from bone marrow transplantation. However, this is the group in which the risk of perioperative mortality, although relatively low, might be judged unacceptable, particularly since accurate estimation of future risk of death or debilitating complications in young patients is problematic.

Waiting for the most severe cases to declare themselves makes the risks more acceptable, but allows development of severe end-organ damage which is unlikely to be reversed by successful marrow transplantation. The cost of marrow transplantation is high but may not exceed the cost of health care and disability experienced by many patients. Finally, the living related donor pool is relatively small since fully HLA-matched sibling donors without sickle-cell disease will not be available for more than 20–30 per cent of patients (Mentzer *et al.* 1994). Wider application of this mode of therapy awaits larger scale studies focusing on patient selection, risk–benefit and cost–benefit ratios, and strategies for increasing the potential donor pool.

The kidney in sickle-cell disease

Introduction

Renal manifestations of sickle-cell anaemia are multiple and diverse. They include abnormalities of tubular function and transport, haematuria and papillary necrosis, blood pressure and erythropoietin modulation, proteinuria, and renal failure of both acute and chronic types. In the next section of this chapter current knowledge in these areas is reviewed.

Glomerular filtration and renal blood flow

Several well-designed studies have shown that in young patients with sickle-cell anaemia renal blood flow, renal plasma flow, and glomerular filtration rates (GFRs) are increased by as much as 50 per cent (Etteldorf *et al.* 1952; Hatch *et al.* 1970; Sklar *et al.* 1990a). The filtration fraction is usually decreased, indicating that increases in GFR are not proportional to increases in renal blood and plasma flow. Anaemia *per se* probably has some influence on these abnormalities since similar findings were observed by Bruck (1953) in children with β-thalassaemia. However, other factors must be involved, since transfusion-associated increases in haematocrit do not cause the renal haemodynamic parameters to revert to normal (Statius van Eps *et al.* 1967). Hyperfiltration in sickle-cell anaemia does not usually persist into adulthood, but some adults may sustain this physiological pattern well into middle age (Morgan and Serjeant 1981; Sklar *et al.* 1990a). These renal haemodynamic changes may have important influences on renal tubular function, blood pressure regulation, and development of a hyperfiltration-induced chronic nephropathy with nephrosis similar to diabetic kidney disease. These issues are discussed in depth in subsequent sections of this chapter.

Two well-designed studies have focused on abnormal prostaglandin metabolism as an explanation for these haemodynamic alterations (de Jong *et al.* 1980; Allon *et al.* 1988). Neither study found increased basal excretion of vasodilator prostaglandin metabolites in patients with sickle-cell anaemia but de Jong's group reported decreased excretion of vasoconstrictor prostaglandin metabolites in these patients. This finding suggested that an abnormal ratio of vasodilator to vasoconstrictor prostaglandins, rather than a simple excess of vasodilator prostaglandins, was responsible for the observed haemodynamic parameters in sickle-cell anaemia. In both studies, indomethacin reduced elevated GFRs by 10–20 per cent. It is attractive to postulate that renal ischaemia in sickle-cell anaemia, which has been shown to stimulate the renin–angiotensin system (Hatch *et al.* 1970), triggers a shift to vasodilator prostaglandin predominance which modulates renal blood flow and GFR. In a similar manner, Bank *et al.* (1994) recently studied the mechanism of hyperfiltration in a transgenic sickle-cell mouse model in which hyperfiltration can be studied without the confounding variable of anaemia. These investigators concluded that renal synthesis of nitric oxide by the L-arginine pathway was increased in the transgenic mice and correlated positively with GFR. Whether this mechanism of hyperfiltration could be operative in humans, remains to be shown.

Renal pathological findings in young patients with sickle-cell anaemia include glomerular enlargement, with glomerular diameters

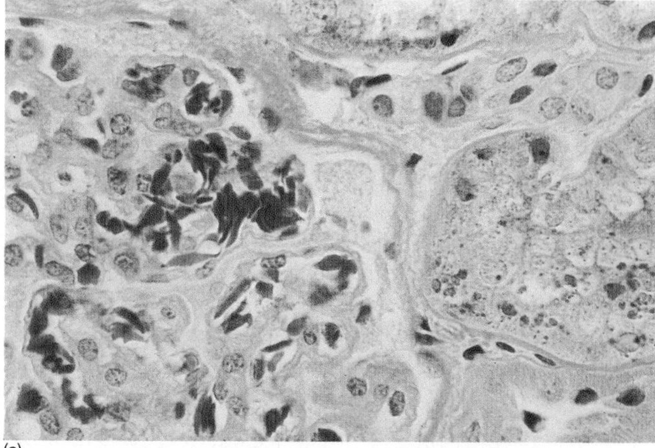

(a)

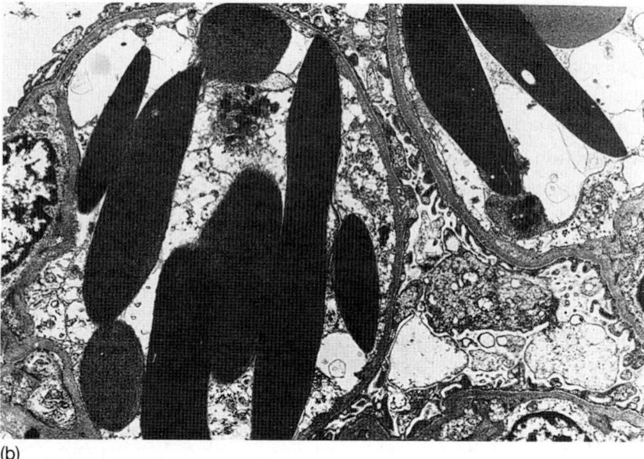

(b)

Fig. 10 (a) Sickle-cell anaemia. Sickled erythrocytes in capillary loops. Haemosiderin deposits in tubular cells. Masson trichrome (by courtesy of J. Charles Jennette). (b) Ultrastructural features of a large, congested glomerulus. The capillary lumina are distended by numerous sickled erythrocytes. Uranyl acetate and lead citrate; magnification 6380× (from Weidner and Buckalew 1994, with permission).

50 per cent greater than normal and glomerular areas almost twice normal, as well as an increased number of capillary lumens and epithelial, endothelial, and mesangial cells (Tejani *et al.* 1985; Bhathena and Sondheimer 1991; Falk *et al.* 1992). Other findings may include congestion of capillary loops with sickled erythrocytes and haemosiderin deposition in tubular cells (Fig. 10). Falk *et al.* (1992) have pointed out the similarity of these changes to those observed with cyanotic heart disease and morbid obesity with sleep apnoea, other conditions in which the kidney is subjected to conditions of increased blood viscosity and local hypoxaemia.

Tubular function

Proximal tubular abnormalities

The increased GFR present early in life are accompanied by evidence of enhanced proximal tubular function. Tubular creatinine secretion is elevated to such a degree that measured creatinine clearance will overestimate GFR determined by inulin or iodothalamate clearance by 25 per cent or more in younger patients (de Jong *et al.* 1980). In the older patient creatinine secretion seems to decline since creatinine clearance underestimates GFR in this age group (Aparicio *et al.* 1990). Similarly, uric acid clearance is elevated early in life to such a degree that hyperuricaemia does not occur despite elevated uric acid production resulting from haemolysis. Hyperuricaemia only develops later in life, usually when GFR has been reduced by development of a chronic nephropathy (Ball and Sorenson 1970; Diamond *et al.* 1975). Proximal tubular reabsorption of sodium and phosphate is also elevated in younger patients (de Jong *et al.* 1978; Smith *et al.* 1981) and may represent a manifestation of glomerular–tubular feedback, which is appropriate when GFR is supranormal.

Distal tubular abnormalities

Impaired concentrating ability

Hatch *et al.* (1967) demonstrated convincingly that impaired concentrating ability could occur in patients with sickle-cell anaemia. This impairment of concentrating ability is evident in childhood and has been observed in SS, SA, and SC genotypes. By the time adolescence is reached these patients may be unable to reach a urine osmolality of 500 mOsmol/kg, a value less than half of the expected normal maximum (Statius van Eps *et al.* 1970a).

In young children, but not in adults, transfusions of normal blood may completely restore concentrating ability (Statius van Eps *et al.* 1967). The usual explanation for this is that, in childhood, sickling in the vasa recta, promoted by contact with the relatively hypertonic inner medulla, disrupts normal function of the countercurrent multiplier system, making maximal concentrating impossible. The fact that this defect improves with indomethacin suggests that a prostaglandin-dependent reduction in sodium absorption in the medullary thick ascending limb prevents generation of adequate hypertonicity in this region (Allon *et al.* 1988). Since transfusion of normal blood decreases the fraction of sickle cells passing through the vasa recta, less sludging occurs and a more normal microvascular flow pattern through the inner medulla can be maintained. The reversibility of the defect by transfusion in young individuals, and the similarity of the defect to that seen in papillectomized rats, led to the suggestion that young patients with sickle-cell anaemia display a state of functional papillectomy (Buckalew 1970).

The failure of transfusion to correct the abnormality in concentrating ability in older subjects suggests that by adulthood irreversible anatomical changes have occurred. In fact, microradioangiographic studies have shown that with age the vasa recta become totally obliterated, resulting in a loss of the juxtamedullary nephrons with long loops of Henle which are required for maximal water conservation (Statius van Eps *et al.* 1970b). The outer medullary and cortical nephrons have capillary beds less susceptible to damage from sickling and the relative sparing of these nephrons gives sickle cell patients intact diluting capacity. This renal concentrating defect is usually asymptomatic although it may contribute to enuresis in childhood (Readett *et al.* 1990) and inability to defend total body water under conditions of extreme heat, fluid deprivation, or gastrointestinal fluid losses from vomiting or diarrhoea.

Impaired urinary acidification and potassium excretion

Many individuals with sickle-cell disease may evidence a form of incomplete distal renal tubular acidosis. In 1968, Ho Ping Kong and

Alleyne reported eight Jamaican patients with sickle-cell disease who had an abnormal urinary pH response to a standard ammonium chloride loading protocol (Ho Ping Kong and Alleyne 1968). Oster *et al.* (1976a) found a similar defect in lowering urinary pH in 6/20 SS patients studied in Miami. In another study, Oster *et al.* (1976b) found normal urine acidification in nine patients with sickle-cell trait studied at the same centre. In contrast to classical, hereditary, type I renal tubular acidosis, acidaemia is rare in sickle-cell anaemia unless the GFR is reduced to less than one-half of normal. Other differentiating points from classical renal tubular acidosis type I include the absence of hypokalaemia, hypercalciuria, nephrocalcinosis, and nephrolithiasis.

In 1979, DeFronzo and coworkers reported data showing impaired excretion of an intravenous potassium load in patients with sickle-cell anaemia who had normal GFRs but impaired acidification according to the acid loading protocol (DeFronzo *et al.* 1979). These patients had normal function of the renin–angiotensin–aldosterone axis. A subsequent study Batlle *et al.* (1982) described their evaluation of six patients with sickle haemoglobinopathies who had both hyperkalaemia and hyperchloraemic metabolic acidosis. Five of these patients had clearly diminished renal excretory function with serum creatinine of 1.5–5.1 mg/dl. Patients were categorized as having either hyperkalaemic distal renal tubular acidosis (inability to maximally lower urinary pH) or selective aldosterone deficiency (maximal urinary pH lowering normal, ammonium excretion reduced, aldosterone inappropriately low). According to this classification one patient had both defects, four patients had hyperkalaemic distal renal tubular acidosis, and one had selective aldosterone deficiency. The failure of either hydrogen ion secretion or potassium ion secretion to increase with sodium sulfate infusion confirmed the hypothesis of Buckalew (1970) that a state of functional papillectomy was present in sickle-cell anaemia.

Finally, DeFronzo *et al.* (1979) pointed out that if the hydrogen and potassium secretory defects were maintained because of a defect in sodium reclamation in the distal nephron, volume depletion could precipitate dangerous degrees of acidosis and hyperkalaemia, both by further reducing GFR and by reducing the supply of sodium available for cation exchange in the already functionally impaired distal nephron. We have, in fact, seen this sequence of events occur on several occasions in patients with sickle-cell anaemia.

Management of tubular abnormalities

The concentrating defect is usually subclinical and requires no specific treatment. Allopurinol and/or colchicine prophylaxis may be required if hyperuricaemia results in attacks of gout. Early in the course of chronic renal failure, alkali therapy for acidosis should be administered and dietary potassium and phosphorus restriction begun. Potassium-binding resins and phosphate binders may be needed as chronic renal failure progresses. In some cases, thiazide or loop diuretics may be used to increase potassium excretion by the kidney.

Drugs capable of causing hyperkalaemia, particularly angiotensin-converting enzyme inhibitors (ACE-I), non-steroidal anti-inflammatory drugs, β-blockers, and heparin should be used with caution in sickle-cell anaemia, particularly if renal insufficiency is already present. There is probably no situation in which a potassium-sparing diuretic would be considered indicated or safe. Similarly, the clinician should be aware of the recently recognized ability of trimethoprim and pentamidine to display an amiloride-like effect on distal potassium secretion, particularly when used in high doses in HIV patients with pneumocystis pneumonia.

Haematuria

Haematuria is a common manifestation of sickle-cell anaemia, sickle-cell trait, and the hybrid sickling disorders (Chapman *et al.* 1955; Mostofi *et al.* 1957). Microscopic haematuria may be a chronic finding which is punctuated by intermittent episodes of gross haematuria. Haematuria is the result of microthrombotic infarction and extravasation of blood in the inner medulla and renal papillae, areas whose hypertonic and relatively hypoxic milieu favour sickling in the adjacent vasa recta. Since the vasa recta and the capillaries of the renal pelvic mucosa both arise from the efferent arterioles of the juxtamedullary nephrons, obliteration of the vasa recta may lead to shunting of blood to the pelvic capillaries with subsequent extravasation into the collecting system (Weidner and Buckalew 1994). Gross haematuria is more common in males than in females, commonly occurs more often from the left kidney, but may be bilateral in origin. Blood loss during episodes of gross haematuria may be severe enough to require blood transfusion, and clots passed into the urinary collecting system may be large enough to cause renal colic and urinary tract obstruction. Since pyuria may accompany haematuria in this setting an inappropriate diagnosis of acute pyelonephritis may be made. Bleeding usually remits spontaneously but may in some cases persist for weeks or months. Haemorrhage into the subcapsular or perinephric spaces is an uncommon complication.

Treatment measures employed have included intravenous distilled water, sodium bicarbonate, diuretics, hyperbaric oxygen, ε-aminocaproic acid, irrigation of the pelvocalyceal system with silver nitrate, nephrectomy, and autotransplantation. Early enthusiasm for ε-aminocaproic acid was based on the work of Black *et al.* (1976) who reported treating 22 patients with complete resolution in all without any complications. However, most clinicians have found that supportive care with analgesics, fluid and blood replacement, and bladder catheterization for clot removal are effective in most cases. In our experience, ε-aminocaproic acid often results in the formation of larger, obstructing clots which are more difficult for the patient to pass.

Papillary necrosis

Harrow *et al.* (1963) were the first to emphasize the association between sickle-cell anaemia and renal papillary necrosis. This complication may be seen in sickle-cell disease, sickle-cell trait, and the hybrid sickle disorders. Papillary necrosis is most frequently found as an incidental finding during renal imaging procedures, formerly intravenous pyelography (Fig. 11a–d), but now more commonly ultrasound, computed axial tomography (CAT) scan or magnetic resonance imaging (MRI). The most detailed analysis of reported series (Vaamonde 1984) found 131 cases of papillary necrosis in 334 patients with sickle-cell anaemia (39 per cent), with the incidence ranging from 23 to 67 per cent in the individual series (Table 3).

Since many cases will be asymptomatic or have only microscopic haematuria which is not evaluated by imaging procedures, the true incidence of this complication is probably higher. The mean age of discovery was 21 ± 1 years with a range of 4–68 years. Painless gross haematuria is the most common presentation, but some patients may have fulminant presentations with colic and obstruction due to sloughed papillae, infection, and septicaemia, or even acute renal failure. In some cases, the pyuria and haematuria combined with flank

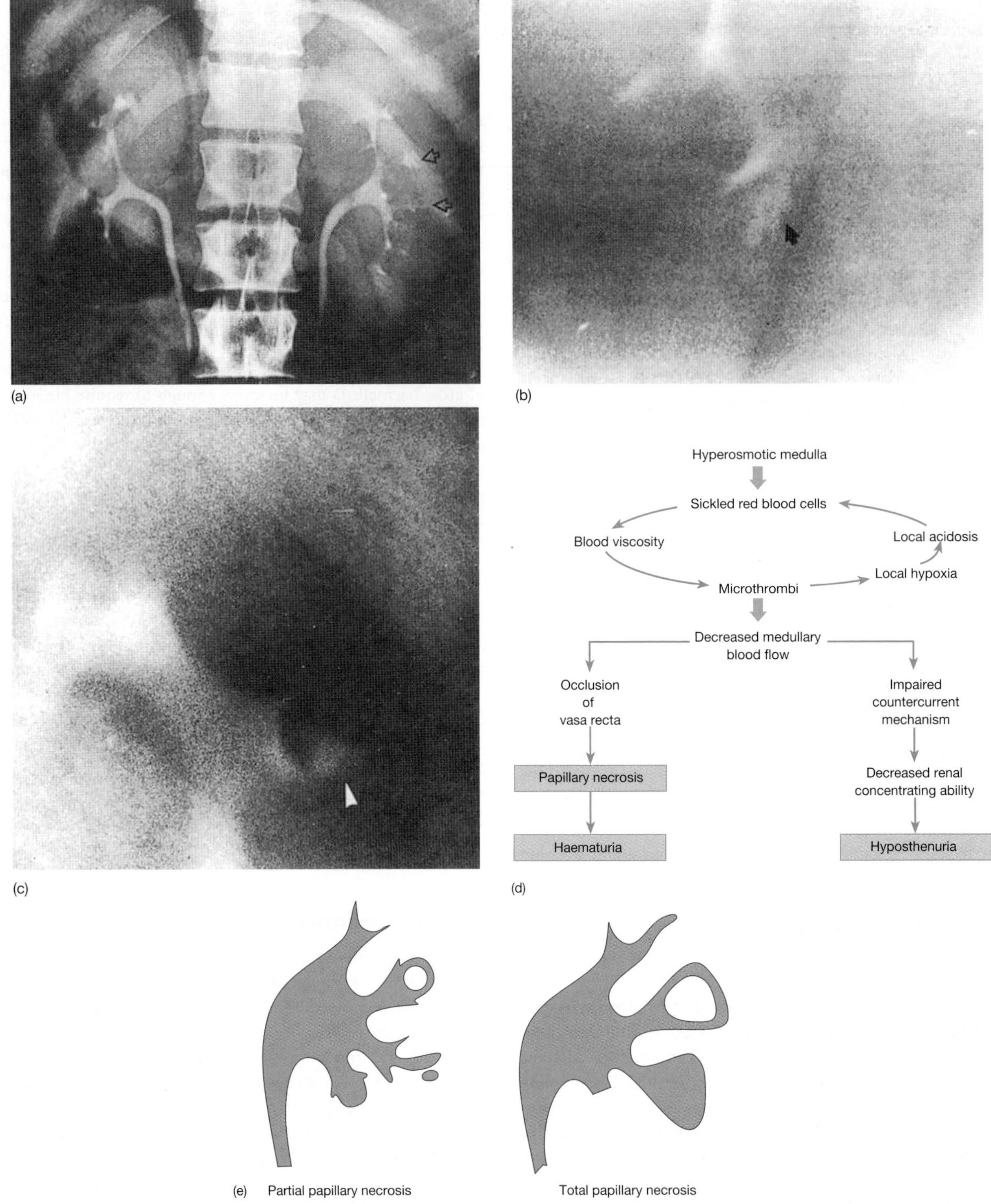

Fig. 11 (a–e) *Papillary necrosis and its genesis.* (a–c) Renal papillary necrosis with various forms of cavitation in a 33-year-old man with SC haemoglobinopathy and haematuria. Kidneys are normal sized and smooth in contour. (a) Central cavitation is present in many papillae, particularly in right interpolar areas (arrows). Right lower and upper poles are magnified in B and C. (b) Ill-defined smudge (arrow) represents early cavitation. Lucent oblique line is psoas margin, not medial border of kidney. (c) Eccentric, irregular cavity near forniceal angle (arrow) (from Davidson and Hartman 1994, with permission). (d) Schematic diagram of the radiographic patterns of renal papillary necrosis observed in patients with sickle-cell haemoglobinopathies. Left: partial papillary necrosis (medullary type). The top calyx is normal. Other calyces show intact fornices with a medullary ring, a sinus, and a small cavity, respectively. Right: total papillary necrosis (papillary type). Early destruction of fornices in the top calyx. Other calyces show ring shadows due to the presence of sequestered papilla, caliectasis ('clubbed calyx'), and an amputated calyx, respectively. The patterns of partial papillary necrosis predominate in patients with sickle-cell disorders (from Vaamonde 1984, with permission). (e) Mechanism of renal papillary necrosis in sickle-cell disorders (from Vaamonde 1984, with permission).

Table 3 Incidence of renal necrosis (RPN) in 334 patients with sickle-cell haemoglobinopathies (HbS). Evlauated by intravenous pyelography (IVP) (from Vaamonde 1984, *Seminars in Nephrology* **1** (49), with permission)

Ref.	No. of patients with HbS	No. of patients with RPN (%)	HbS type				Characteristics of study
			AS	SS	SC	S–Thal	
Eckert *et al.* (1974)	16	9 (56)	8/14	1/2	—	—	Retrospective review of IVP in 33 Black patients with known Hb type. Seventeen patients with HbAA had normal IVP
Eckert *et al.* (1974)	17	8 (47)	8/15	—	0/2	—	Prospective IVP study of 200 Black patients with known Hb type referred to radiology department for any clinical indication: six patients with HbAC had normal IVP, 177 patients with HbAA had normal IVP
Pandya *et al.* (1976)	35	23 (65)	11/18	9/10	3/5	0/2	Retrospective review of 35 patients with HbS attending haemoglobin clinic with urological symptoms
Pandya *et al.* (1976)	37	25 (67)	1/3	16/22	3/4	5/8	Prospective study of 37 patients with HbS from haemoglobin clinic without history of laboratory evidence of urinary tract disease
McCall *et al.* (1978)	189	44 (23)	—	44/189	—	—	Prospective IVP study of 189 patients with HbSS attending a sickle-cell clinic without acute symptoms at time of evaluation
Ballas *et al.* (1982)	40	22 (55)	—	11/25	11/15	—	Retrospective study of 40 patients with HbSS or HbSC attending a sickle-cell centre
Total percentage	334	131 (39)	28/50 56	81/248 33	17/26 65	5/10 50	

pain suggest a diagnosis of acute pyelonephritis, and only careful examination of the urinary sediment and urine cultures may lead to a definitive diagnosis.

Sickling of red blood cells in the vasa recta can result in medullary infarction and extravasation of red blood cells (Fig. 12). In the renal medulla, and especially the papilla, sickling of red blood cells is promoted by the ambient hypertonicity, hypoxia, and low pH in this area (Fig. 11e). The kidney has an exceptionally high rate of oxygen consumption which is second only to that of the myocardium. Consequently, the kidneys are very susceptible to injury induced by decrements in oxygen delivery caused by sickling and sludging of red blood cells in the renal microvasculature. It is not surprising that renal dysfunction and anatomical injury occurs in a setting in which a relentless cycle of sickling and hypoxaemia can develop. On rare occasions, papillary necrosis may progress to overt cortical infarction with or without development of perirenal haematoma.

Vaamonde (1984) has categorized papillary necrosis according to severity (Fig. 11d). The less severe variety is referred to as the medullary or partial papillary form and is usually confined to the tip of the papilla. Initially, involvement is patchy but may eventually extend to involve multiple papillae. Early on, before sequestration of necrotic papillae has occurred, diagnosis by intravenous pyelogram may be impossible. When more advanced, the forniceal architecture is preserved but types of involvement may include the ring sign (indicative of a necrotic papilla which has not been sloughed), sinus tract formation, and cavity formation involving loss of part or all of the papilla. Further progression to the total papillary stage includes sinus tract formation at the fornices, ever larger ring shadows indicative of larger sequestered papillae, caliectasis, and amputated calyces. At any stage calcification may occur within sequestered papillae. Totally sloughed papillae may be seen as filling defects in the pelves, ureters, or bladder. Cortical scars may occur and represent atrophy, scarring, and retraction rather than cortical necrosis.

On gross examination at autopsy or nephrectomy necrotic areas have sharp borders and appear yellowish or greyish red. On microscopic examination the perinecrotic areas may be rimmed by belts of polymorphonuclear leucocytes. Changes in the medulla and papillae include vascular congestion, oedema, infarcts, necrosis in the papillary region, and changes of chronic interstitial nephritis, including fibrosis and tubular atrophy. Mononuclear infiltrates may be present in the fibrotic areas. Thickness of the cortex may be reduced and cortical scars or abscesses present, but frank cortical necrosis is rare. Despite

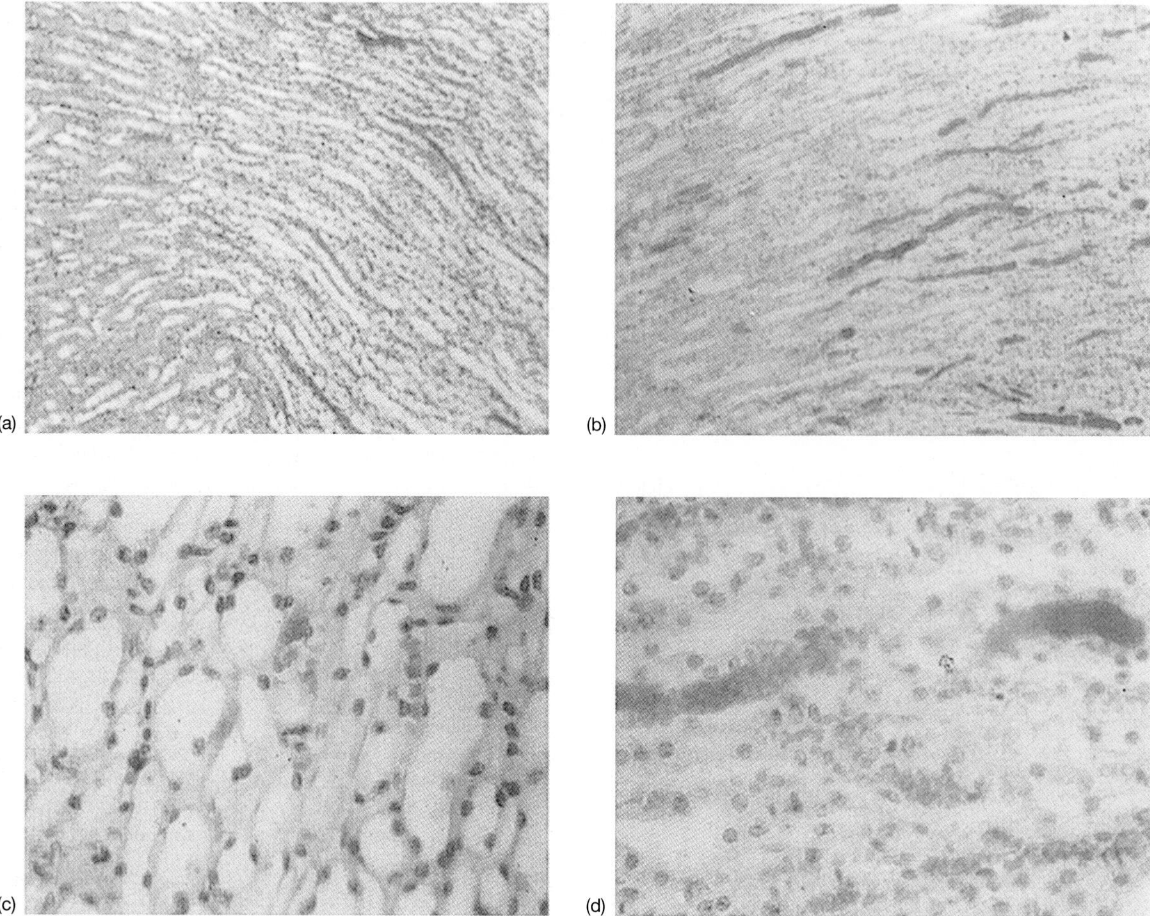

Fig. 12 Photomicrographs of renal papillae from transgenic mice under ambient (a, b) and hypoxic conditions (c). Note that in the transgenic animal under ambient conditions some vessels are congested but are not distended. Under hypoxic conditions, more capillaries show congestion and the capillaries are distended (from Fabry 1994, with permission).

the prominence of these lesions, progressive interstitial nephritis leading to uraemia is decidedly rare, perhaps because involvement is patchier and infection rates lower than in papillary necrosis due to conditions such as analgesic nephropathy.

Blood pressure regulation

Afro-Americans have a prevalence of hypertension approaching 30 per cent, but in gender- and age-matched sickle-cell anaemia patients the prevalence of hypertension is much lower. At all age levels and in both genders systolic and diastolic blood pressures are lower in sickle-cell anaemia patients than in normal individuals (Grell *et al.* 1981; Johnson and Giorgio 1981; de Jong *et al.* 1982). Johnson and Giorgio (1981) determined that the expected prevalence of hypertension in their Los Angeles population would have been 30 per cent, but their study of 187 patients found a prevalence of only 3.2 per cent. Overall, mean blood pressure in the sickle cell group was 116/70 mmHg. Even adjusting for age and gender did not obliterate the large differences in blood pressure (10–20 mmHg for both systolic and diastolic blood pressure in all age groups) between sickle-cell patients and normal individuals (Fig. 13). Furthermore, age-related blood pressure increases were not observed in the sickle cell group. Grell *et al.* (1981), reporting on Jamaican patients, found similar differences. De Jong *et al.* (1982) found the same trend in Curacao, although the magnitude of the difference was smaller. In our experience (Sklar *et al.* 1990a) hypertension only develops in sickle-cell anaemia patients when advanced renal failure develops.

A recent study of over 3000 patients with sickle-cell disease (Pegelow *et al.* 1997) conclusively demonstrated that blood pressure was significantly lower in patients with sickle-cell disease than in normal age-, race-, and gender-matched populations. Blood pressure in the sickle cell group correlated with body mass index, haemoglobin, age, and measures of renal function. Higher blood pressures predicted increased risk of stroke and all-cause mortality in this patient group. The possible risks of 'relative hypertension', that is, blood pressure higher than the sickle cohort but lower than the usual 140/90 mmHg cutoff, are unclear at this time. This situation is analogous to that seen in young insulin dependent diabetics. Interestingly, the prevalence of hypertension in patients with HgbS-C disease approximates the incidence in age, size, and gender matched Afro-Americans without haemoglobinopathy (Koduri *et al.* 2001).

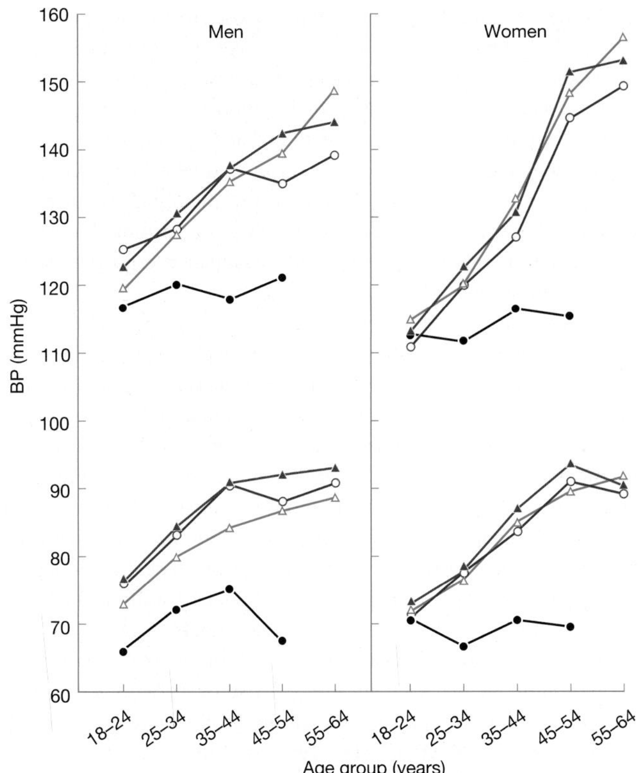

Fig. 13 Mean systolic and diastolic blood pressures (BPs) in sickle-cell disease and Afro-Americans by age and gender (Public Health Service 1976, 1977). Closed circles represent patients with sickle-cell disease; open circles, persons residing in large metropolitan areas, abstracted from the data of the Health and Nutrition Examination Survey (HANES); closed triangles, persons included in the HANES; and open triangles, persons included in the Health Examination Survey (from Johnson and Giorgio 1981, with permission).

The blood pressures of patients with sickle-cell anaemia, while lower than those of the general population, are greater than those of patients with β-thalassaemia and similar degrees of anaemia (Rodgers *et al.* 1993b). Whether this 'relative' hypertension is a cause or an effect of the renal abnormalities in sickle-cell anaemia is not clear. What is obvious, however, is that 'essential hypertension', as commonly defined in an Afro-American population, is rarely observed in sickle-cell anaemia, and is an unlikely contributor to chronic renal failure in this patient group. The precise reasons for this relative hypotension are not well defined. Peripheral resistance may be reduced in anaemias because of endogenous vasodilatory substances recruited to enhance tissue oxygenation. As noted above, evidence exists to suggest that a relative excess of vasodilator prostaglandins and nitric oxide may be present. Some degree of salt wasting has been described, and the increased renal blood flow described above, combined with possible natriuretic effects of prostaglandins, may be involved. Hatch *et al.* (1989) described elevated renin and decreased responsiveness to the vasoconstrictor effects of angiotensin in these patients. These features are reminiscent of Bartter's syndrome, another condition in which normotension and elevated renin levels occur in the context of relative excess of vasodilator prostaglandins.

Women with sickle-cell trait, however, are at increased risk for hypertensive disorders of pregnancy including pre-eclampsia (Larrabee and Monga 1997). In a study of 1584 women, which included 162 women with sickle-cell trait, these authors found that the incidence of pre-eclampsia in the sickle-cell trait positive women was more than double that of the other patients (24.7 versus 10.3 per cent). The women with sickle-cell trait had a significantly lower gestational age at delivery and a lower birth weight.

Erythropoietin physiology

Endogenous serum erythropoietin is elevated in sickle-cell anaemia but not to the degree observed in other disorders characterized by severe anaemia (Sherwood *et al.* 1986). This finding may be explained by the lower oxygen affinity of HbS, which may attenuate tissue hypoxia at steady state haemoglobin concentrations. Alternatively, the synthetic functions of the tubular cells responsible for erythropoietin synthesis may be disturbed by intrarenal factors related to sickling. Finally, the low serum creatinines seen in patients with sickle-cell anaemia and reduced muscle mass may obscure renal insufficiency as a cause of inadequate erythropoietin response, particularly in older patients. Clearly, anaemia tends to worsen as overt renal failure develops in these patients. Significant haematological responses to pharmacological doses of recombinant erythropoietin have not been reported in dialysis or predialysis patients, but successful renal transplantation tends to restore the haematocrit to its preuraemic values. Although Steinberg (1991) has reported that very high doses of recombinant erythropoietin may return sickle-cell dialysis patients to their baseline haematocrit, our experience has been that recombinant erythropoietin therapy in dialysis patients with sickle-cell anaemia, sickle cell–β-thalassaemia, or sickle-cell disease, even at doses of 450 units/kg three time per week, has little effect on transfusion requirements, haemoglobin, or haematocrit.

Acute renal failure

Given the multiple renal abnormalities described above, the propensity of these patients to develop severe infections, their predisposition to volume depletion, and the large number of potentially nephrotoxic agents to which they are exposed, it is surprising that the literature on sickle-cell anaemia so rarely describes acute renal failure. The first carefully described entity was acute renal failure secondary to rhabdomyolysis. Exertional rhabdomyolysis occurring in the setting of training of military recruits with sickle-cell trait was first reported by Jones *et al.* (1970). Other small series were reported over the next two decades, but the work of Kark *et al.* (1987) definitively demonstrated a 28-fold increased risk for sudden unexplained death in black military recruits with sickle-cell trait, with deaths clearly attributed to rhabdomyolysis, heat stroke, cardiac arrest, and arrhythmias.

Devereux and Knowles (1985) were the first to report non-traumatic rhabdomyolysis during sickle-cell crisis. Subsequent reports have verified the occurrence of non-traumatic rhabdomyolysis in many cases of severe painful crisis (Kelly and Singer 1986; Sklar *et al.* 1990b; Hassell *et al.* 1994). The latter investigators further demonstrated that severe rhabdomyolysis during painful crises was a common finding in many patients experiencing acute multiorgan failure comprising the acute chest syndrome, acute renal failure, and liver dysfunction.

Sklar *et al.* (1990a) tried to assess the incidence of acute renal failure in those patients in hospital with sickle-cell disease. By case–control methods, 12 out of 116 patients (10.3 per cent) had at least a doubling of their serum creatinine. Patients with acute renal failure were more likely to have been admitted with infection and had lower mean haemoglobin. Volume depletion was the most common identifiable cause for acute renal failure. Two of three patients with severe acute renal failure required dialytic support. Ten of the 12 acute renal failure patients survived and subsequently recovered renal function.

Sickle-cell nephropathy

Over the past 20 years, the most intensively studied aspect of renal dysfunction in sickle-cell disease has been the entity now referred to as sickle cell nephropathy. This term has come to refer to a condition usually commencing in adulthood which is characterized by the development of proteinuria, progressing to nephrotic-range proteinuria, renal insufficiency, and terminating in endstage renal disease (ESRD). Several excellent reviews on this condition have been published recently (Wong *et al.* 1996; Saborio and Scheinman 1999; Ataga and Orringer 2000; Phuong-Thu *et al.* 2000).

Proteinuria

In many sickle-cell anaemia clinical reports, proteinuria has been reported using semiquantitative methods such as urine dipstick values and graded from 0 to 4+. The first report dealing with the prevalence of proteinuria in sickle-cell anaemia was that of Henderson (1950) who reported 31 per cent prevalence in 54 patients. In a later study, McCall *et al.* (1978) reported a prevalence of 15 per cent. One of the first analyses of any size was that of Sklar *et al.* (1990a) who found dipstick proteinuria of 1+ or greater in 78 out of 368 patients (20.6 per cent). Falk *et al.* (1992) found proteinuria of at least 1+ in 101 out of 381 patients (26 per cent) and Wigfall *et al.* (1994) reported proteinuria of 2+ or greater in 21 out of 211 patients (10 per cent). In a more detailed study the same authors found proteinuria in 6.2 per cent of 442 paediatric sickle-cell patients with a higher rate of 12 per cent in older teenagers (Wigfall *et al.* 2000). In all studies the incidence of proteinuria increased with age, and the presence of proteinuria was associated with increased serum creatinine.

Case reports and small series of patients with nephrotic syndrome associated with sickle-cell anaemia began to appear in the medical literature more than 20 years ago (McCoy 1969; Walker *et al.* 1971; Elfenbein *et al.* 1974; Pardo *et al.* 1975; Strauss *et al.* 1975; Roy *et al.* 1976). Pathological findings reported at that time included poststreptococcal glomerulonephritis, membranous glomerulonephritis, membranoproliferative glomerulonephritis, and focal segmental glomerulosclerosis. Although poststreptococcal glomerulonephritis was one of the first glomerular lesions described, subsequent studies have not indicated an increased incidence of poststreptococcal glomerulonephritis in sickle-cell anaemia patients. Immune complexes containing renal tubular antigens (Ozawa *et al.* 1976) have been localized in the capillary loops, and iron–protein complexes have been described in a mesangial pattern (McCoy 1969). As described below, larger studies have not verified that immune complex glomerulonephritis is a common cause of proteinuria, nephrotic syndrome, or chronic renal failure in sickle-cell anaemia. Renal vein thrombosis was rarely reported in these early studies and limited data from this era did not suggest responsiveness of proteinuria to corticosteroids or cyclophosphamide.

The report of Tejani *et al.* (1985), which described 13 children with proteinuria or nephrotic syndrome, was one of the first to point out the frequency of focal segmental glomerulosclerosis (Fig. 14a–d) in sickle-cell anaemia. In 1987, Bakir and coworkers reported 12 adult cases of nephrotic syndrome in sickle-cell anaemia and reviewed the literature on 37 additional cases. Nine of the authors' 12 cases, 19 out of 37 previously reported adult cases, and 10 out of 31 paediatric cases were described as having mesangial expansion and reduplication of the basement membranes compatible with a form of membranoproliferative glomerulonephritis. Lobular architecture was not a prominent feature but basement membrane splitting with mesangial interposition was a frequent finding (Fig. 14e–h).

Haemosiderin was prominent in tubules and interstitium but not in glomeruli. There were variable degrees of focal, global, periglomerular, and interstitial fibrosis. These authors concluded that membranoproliferative glomerulonephritis and focal segmental glomerulosclerosis accounted for most cases of nephrotic syndrome in sickle-cell disease, with membranoproliferative glomerulonephritis being the more common lesion in adults. The membranoproliferative lesions described differ from idiopathic membranoproliferative glomerulonephritis by having ill-defined or absent immune complex or dense deposit deposition. Systematic biopsy analysis of two subsequent studies (Bhathena and Sondheimer 1991; Falk *et al.* 1992), describing 16 cases of nephrotic syndrome, indicated that focal segmental glomerulosclerosis was the more common lesion, even in adults. In some patients parvovirus infection appears to be capable of causing proliferative or sclerosing glomerular lesions (Wierenga *et al.* 1995; Tolaymat *et al.* 1999).

We view the focal and incompletely elaborated mesangial interposition in most sickle cell 'membranoproliferative glomerulonephritis' cases and the general absence of immunoglobulin and electron-dense deposits as arguments against a close relationship between sickle cell nephropathy and idiopathic membranoproliferative glomerulonephritis.

Hostetter *et al.* (1981) have shown that in a rat remnant kidney model, single nephron glomerular capillary plasma flow and transcapillary pressures are increased and, over time, glomerulomegaly, expansion of the mesangial matrix, mesangial proliferation, and glomerulosclerosis ensue. Anderson *et al.* (1985) demonstrated that in this rat model reduction of intraglomerular pressures could attenuate renal injury. This model is considered by many to be an analogue of hyperfiltration-induced renal injury in diabetes mellitus. As in diabetic kidney disease, in early life the kidneys of SSD patients with sickle-cell disease are commonly enlarged (Walker *et al.* 1996), and renal blood flow and GFR are higher than normal.

Since ACE-I are thought to reduce intraglomerular pressures in diabetic kidney disease, Falk and Jennette (1992) studied the effect of enalapril on sickle-cell nephropathy patients with proteinuria. They found that 2 weeks of enalapril therapy at doses of 5–10 mg/day (which did not alter systemic blood pressure) reduced proteinuria in all patients (mean decrement 57 per cent; range 23–79 per cent). In subsequent uncontrolled (Aoki and Soad 1995) and controlled (Foucan *et al.* 1998) studies, chronic ACE-I therapy dramatically reduced proteinuria in sickle-cell patients for a period of 6 months. In these two studies, ACE-I significantly reduced blood pressure, however, so that specific antiproteinuric effects of the drugs could not be fully separated from a non-specific antiproteinuric effect of blood pressure reduction. Further studies will be required to determine whether this mode of therapy will slow progression of renal insufficiency in patients with sickle-cell nephropathy.

The characteristics of the proteinuria in sickle cell patients have been intensely studied over the last decade. It appears that early in the

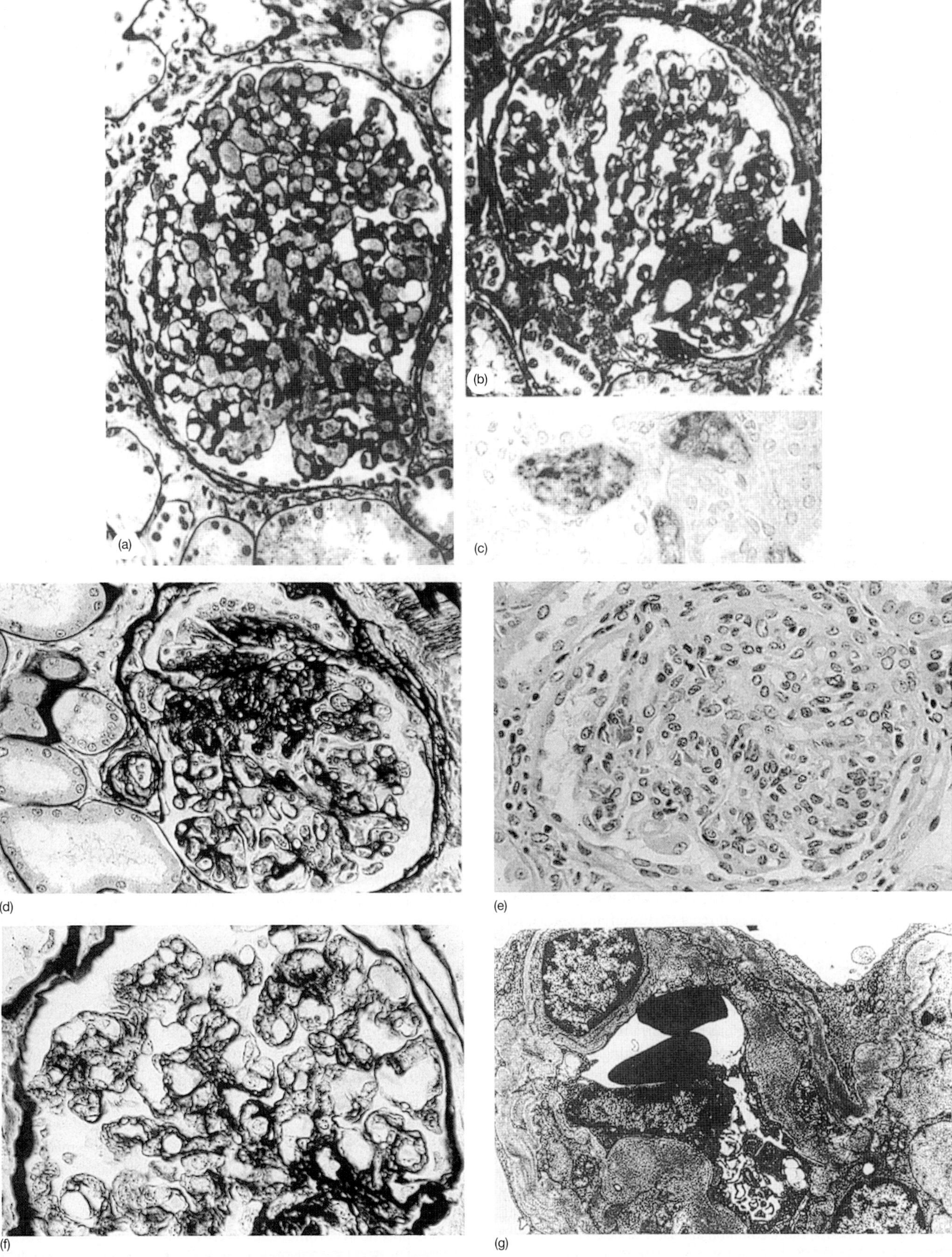

Fig. 14 Continued.

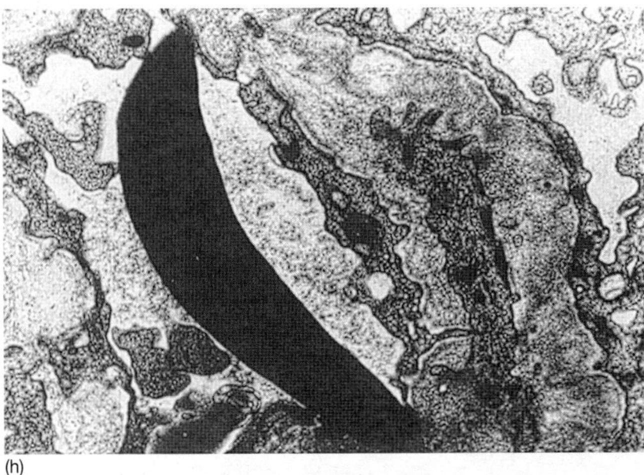
(h)

Fig. 14 (a) Large glomerulus in a patient with sickle-cell anaemia showing distended, congested capillary loops (silver methenamine; magnification 465×). (b) Glomerulus from the same patient exhibiting a segmental sclerosing lesion (arrowheads) (silver methenamine; original magnification 385×). (c) Proximal convoluted tubules from the same patient containing abundant haemosiderin pigment (Prussian blue; magnification 205×) (from Weidner and Buckalew 1994, with permission). (d) Sickle-cell anaemia. Focal segmental glomerulosclerosis (Jones silver stain with haematoxylin and eosin counterstain) (by courtesy of J. Charles Jennette). (e) Sickle-cell anaemia. Membranoproliferative lesion (haematoxylin and eosin) (by courtesy of J. Charles Jennette). (f) Sickle-cell anaemia. Reduplication of glomerular basement membranes (Jones silver stain) (by courtesy of J. Charles Jennette). (g) Electron micrograph from the same patient as in (f), showing a peripheral capillary loop containing marked peripheral mesangial interposition producing reduplication (arrow) of the basement membrane (uranyl acetate and lead citrate; magnification 380×) (from Weidner and Buckalew 1994, with permission). (h) More highly magnified field from the same patient as in (f) and (g) (second biopsy specimen) showing peripheral mesangial extension producing reduplication of the glomerular basement membrane. Adjacent capillary lumen contains a sickled erythrocyte (uranyl acetate and lead citrate; magnification 10, 440×) (from Weidner and Buckalew 1994, with permission).

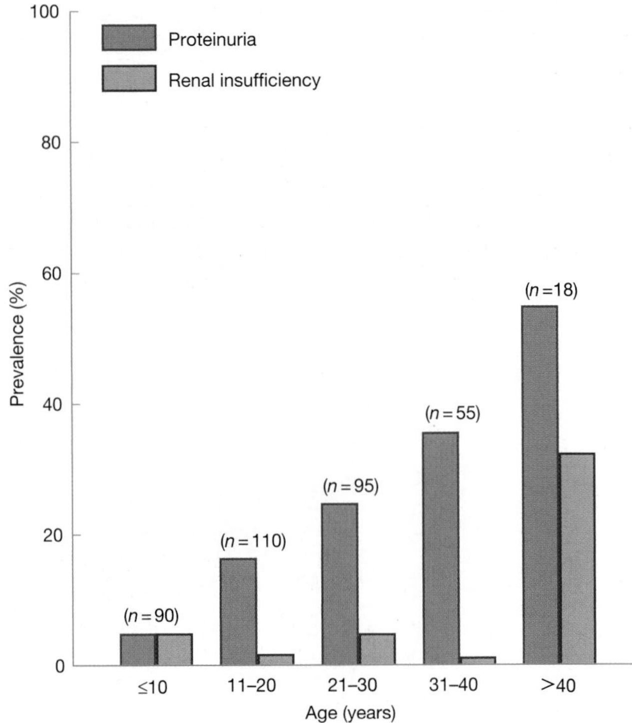

Fig. 15 Prevalence rates of proteinuria and renal insufficiency per decade of life (from Sklar 1990a, with permission).

course of sickle-cell nephropathy glomerular ultrafiltration coefficient is increased (Schmitt *et al.* 1998), possibly as a result of podocyte stretch lesions induced by increased renal perfusion and subsequent glomerular hypertrophy. This suggests that hyperfiltration in early sickle-cell nephropathy is the result of both glomerular hyperperfusion and increased glomerular permeability. Observations by Guasch *et al.* (1996) however, had shown that in older adults, presumably with further advanced nephropathy, the glomerular ultrafiltration coefficient was reduced and permselectivity impaired indicating a reduction in the number of membrane pores with an increase in average pore radius.

Chronic renal failure

The prevalence and natural history of chronic renal failure in this patient population became evident as survival of sickle-cell anaemia patients into middle age became more common and large-scale epidemiological studies were reported. Morgan and Serjeant (1981) quantitated renal function of 25 Jamaican sickle-cell anaemia patients aged between 40 and 64 years. Six of 25 patients had creatinine clearances less than the fifth percentile for age and gender. These investigators noted the association of proteinuria with low creatinine clearance but reported no patients with heavy or nephrotic-range proteinuria. In the absence of biopsy material they proposed that these individuals had a form of chronic interstitial nephritis.

Thomas *et al.* (1982) were the first to point out the contribution of renal disease to mortality in older sickle-cell anaemia patients. They found that renal failure contributed to death in 17 out of 95 (18 per cent) of patients over the age of 20. Significant blood pressure elevations, rare in sickle-cell anaemia, were common in the renal failure group. At autopsy the renal failure patients had shrunken, endstage kidneys. Sklar *et al.* (1990a) in a study of 368 patients found a 4.6 per cent prevalence of chronic renal insufficiency. In this study, the increasing prevalence of proteinuria and renal insufficiency with age was obvious (Fig. 15).

Powars *et al.* (1991) reported data on chronic renal failure from a prospective 25-year longitudinal study of 725 patients with sickle-cell anaemia and 209 patients with HbSC. Renal failure was diagnosed in 4.2 per cent of the sickle-cell anaemia patients and 2.4 per cent of the HbSC patients. The diagnosis of renal failure was made significantly earlier in the sickle-cell anaemia patients (23.1 versus 49.9 years). Relative risk for mortality in the group of sickle-cell anaemia patients with renal failure was 1.42 (Fig. 16). Case–control analysis of the renal failure group (n = 36) revealed several preazotaemic indicators of future renal disease, including proteinuria, haematuria, hypertension, nephrotic syndrome, and severity of anaemia. Without further elaboration the authors said that autopsy data on the 18 patients dying of renal failure showed glomerulosclerosis as the major lesion. Platt *et al.* (1994) reported data from Cooperative Study of Sickle Cell Disease, a multicentre database including 3764 patients of all ages. Eighteen per cent of deaths in adults were associated with some form of chronic organ failure associated with sickle-cell disease and 22 of these 38 deaths occurred in patients with chronic renal failure.

These investigators also found that in a subgroup of patients with severe renal failure 9 out of 10 had the Bantu (CAR) βS haplotype (Table 4). Guasch *et al.* (1999), however, found no association between the occurrence of albuminuria and β-globin haplotype in a study of 76 adult sickle-cell patients. Instead, these investigators found that microdeletions at the α-globin gene locus appeared to reduce the likelihood of nephropathy in this patient group.

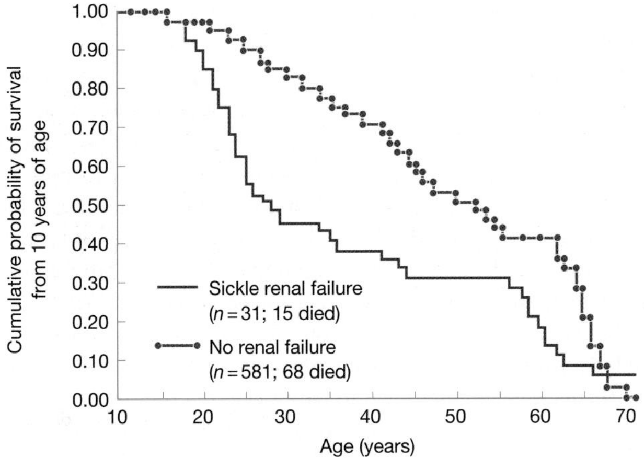

Fig. 16 Cumulative probability of survival (beginning at age 10 years) of patients with sickle-cell anaemia. Patients with sickle renal failure were compared with a cohort comprising the Los Angeles population that had not developed renal failure. After 10 years of age, endstage renal disease is a significant cause of death during young adult life (log-rank test, $P = 0.02$) (from Powars *et al.* 1991, with permission).

Management of endstage renal disease

Dialysis

It has been 20 years since the first reports of successful treatment and long-term survival of sickle-cell patients treated with dialysis appeared in the medical literature (Friedman *et al.* 1974; Gold 1974; Cruz *et al.* 1982). Both haemodialysis and peritoneal dialysis have been used in the treatment of sickle-cell disease patients with ESRD, although the total number of patients treated appears to be quite small. Nissenson and Port (1989) reviewed data from the Forum of Endstage Renal Disease Networks, which represented the best available data in the era before the United States Renal Data System (USRDS) was organized. In a 3-year period covering 1983–1985 there were 77 incident cases of ESRD ascribed to sickle-cell disease. Ninety-six per cent of patients were Black and 60 per cent were male. Fifty-seven per cent were between 20 and 39 years of age at the time of diagnosis, and 31 per cent were aged between 40 and 59. Eighty-two per cent were initially treated with haemodialysis, 17 per cent with peritoneal dialysis, and 1 per cent with cadaveric transplantation. The 30-month survival of these patients was 59 per cent. From 1992 to 1997 the USRDS received data from dialysis centres documenting 345 new cases of ESRD attributed to sickle-cell nephropathy (USRDS 1998). Based on these limited data, dialytic treatment of sickle-cell disease patients can be expected to produce clinical outcomes similar to those achieved in other chronic multisystem diseases. Clinical data from dialysis centres caring for patients with sickle-cell anaemia have not reported problems with increased frequency of crises attributable to the dialysis procedure itself. This is somewhat surprising since the hypoxaemia, hypotension, and cytokine activation occurring during haemodialysis might have been expected to promote sickle-cell crises.

Table 4 Genetic characteristics of patients with sickle-cell disease who developed sickle-cell failure (from Powars *et al.* 1991, with permission)

Patient	Sex	Haemoglobin	Fetal haemoglobin saturation (%)	α-Gene status	β-Gene cluster haplotype	Age at diagnosis of sickle renal failure (years)	Survival time (years)	Terminating renal event
1	F	SS	6	α–/αα	CAR/Benin	14	8.3	Dialysis
2	F	SS	4	αα/αα	CAR/CAR	19	1.5	Dialysis (death 2.1 years later)
3	M	SS	3	αα/αα	CAR/Camaroon	40	3.8	Dialysis
4	M	SS	3	αα/αα	CAR/CAR minor II	26	2.8	Dialysis
5	M	SS	1	αα/αα	CAR/C	15	2.8	Dialysis
6	F	SS	7	αα/αα	Benin/Camaroon	46	1.8	Dialysis (death 0.8 years later)
7	M	SS	6	αα/αα	CAR/Benin	30	2.4	Dialysis (death 3.0 years later)
8	F	SS	10	αα/αα	CAR/Benin	44	2.1	Alive (creatinine, 282 μmol/l)
9	M	SC	3	αα/αα	CAR/C	31	5.6	Death
10	M	SC	1	α–/αα	CAR/C	65	4.8	Dialysis

Survival time is the time in years from diagnosis to dialysis, renal transplantation, or death. SS, sickle-cell anaemia; SC, sickle-cell disease; CAR, Central African Republic (Bantu).

Transplantation

Early experiences at single centres reported high rates of graft loss due to sickling crisis and rejection (Barber *et al.* 1987) but subsequent larger studies have refuted this impression.

Chatterjee (1987) has reported on the natural history of renal allografts in sickle-cell disease and trait in the United States. Seventy-nine per cent of centres in the United States responded to a questionnaire and reported a total of 45 transplants in 40 patients. Eleven were from living related donors and 34 from cadaveric donors. Thirteen recipients had sickle-cell disease and 27 had sickle-cell trait. Patient survival at 1 year was 88 per cent. Graft survival at 1 year was 82 per cent in living donor recipients and 62 per cent in cadaveric recipients.

Recent studies of renal transplantation in both children and adults have confirmed the work of Chatterjee (Warady and Sullivan 1998; Ojo *et al.* 1999). These two studies verified that 1-year graft survival rates in sickle-cell nephropathy patients are not significantly different from patients with ESRD of other causes. Despite the fact that long-term graft survival is significantly shorter than that observed in other patient groups, life expectancy in the transplanted group is higher than that of other sickle-cell nephropathy patients on waiting lists who are maintained with dialysis.

Painful crises occurred in 12 out of 40 patients reported by Chatterjee (1987) in the first year after transplantation. Several studies have similarly documented painful crises after successful transplantation, but it is by no means clear whether crises became more frequent after successful transplantation (Spector *et al.* 1978; Barber *et al.* 1987; Montgomery *et al.* 1994). Increases in haematocrit occurring after transplantation and standard three-drug maintenance therapy (prednisone, azathioprine, and cyclosporin), therefore, have not been shown conclusively to increase the frequency of painful crises. Montgomery *et al.* (1994) found that crises were temporally related to monoclonal antibody therapy in two patients. These investigators suggested that antilymphocyte preparations that can induce a cytokine-release syndrome should be avoided in patients with sickle-cell nephropathy, but confirmation of this recommendation awaits further studies. Similarly, the single report of recurrent sickle-cell nephropathy in an allograft (Miner *et al.* 1987) does not provide a basis for assessing the risk of this complication.

Renal medullary carcinoma

Over the last 7 years, there have been numerous descriptions of a hitherto unreported association of sickle-cell trait and clinically aggressive, renal medullary carcinoma (Davidson *et al.* 1995; Davis *et al.* 1995; Khan *et al.* 2000).

As of 2002 there have been over 60 cases reported in the literature. The report of Davis *et al.* (1995) clearly defined an important clinical entity. Reviewing a 22-year experience, these authors collected 33 examples of a highly aggressive neoplasm which they and their colleagues at the Armed Forces Institute of Pathology had previously classified as variants of renal pelvic carcinoma. Closer review of pathological and clinical features of these patients led these investigators to conclude that these 34 cases represented, in fact, a distinct pathological and clinical entity.

The location of these tumours, many of which seemed to be centred near the renal pyramids, and their unusual histological features had previously led the investigators to uncertainty as to whether the tumours represented variants of renal pelvic tumours or metastatic lesions. The authors described the composite description of these tumours as 'a lobulated neoplasm' occupying chiefly the renal medulla, firm or rubbery, tan to gray, with variable haemorrhage and necrosis. The gross appearance and appearance on CT scan are demonstrated in Fig. 17.

The clinical features were, upon close review, similarly distinct (Table 5). All 25 of the 33 patients whose race was known were Black. All patients were either known to have sickle-cell trait or to have had sickled erythrocytes demonstrated in pathological specimens. The patients ranged in age from 11 to 39 years with 22 being males and 11 being female. The most common presenting symptoms were gross haematuria, abdominal pain, or flank pain. At the time of diagnosis, all tumours demonstrated lymphatic, vascular, or perinephric invasion. Fourteen patients had liver or lung metastases at the time of diagnosis. Mean survival from the time of surgery was 15 weeks.

The subsequent reports from other centres closely resemble the profile of the AFIP study. No patient reported to date has survived more than 15 months after diagnosis. Tumour or metastatic lesion growth after diagnosis has in several cases been characterized as 'explosive'. Neither surgery nor chemotherapy appear to significantly prolong survival. All studies comment on the difficulty of diagnosis in

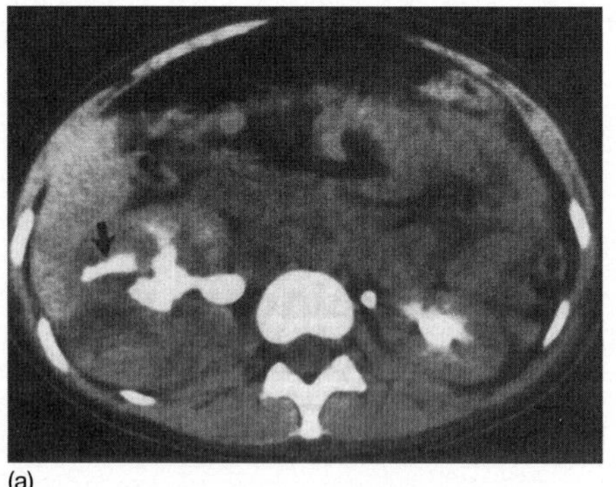
(a)

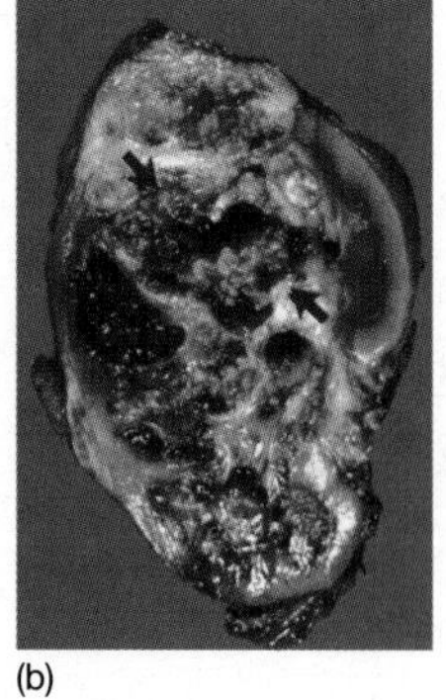
(b)

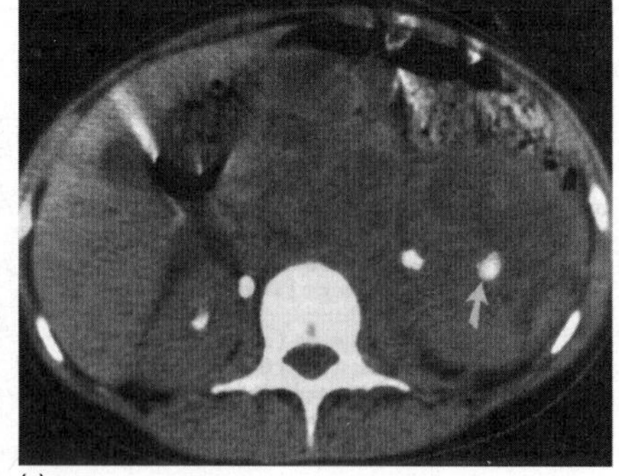
(c)

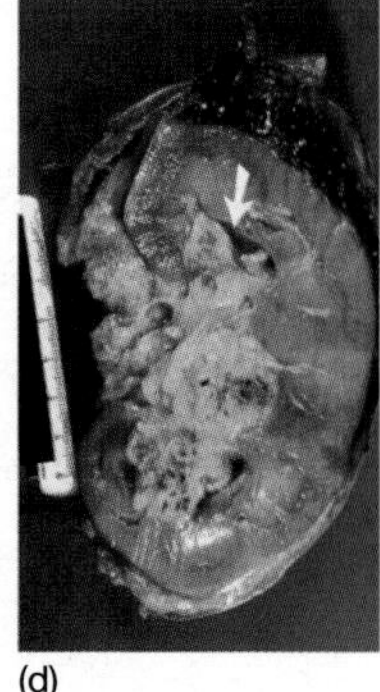
(d)

Fig. 17 Left panel (a) contrast enhanced CT scan of a 21-year-old Black female with sickle-cell trait. An extensive, centrally located mass is demonstrated in the right kidney. Arrow indicates a necrotic cavity communicating with the collecting system. Right panel (b) gross specimen of the medullary carcinoma shows preservation of reniform shape, diffuse infiltration, and a necrotic cavity (arrow) (from Davidson *et al.* 1995, with permission). Left panel (c) contrast-enhanced CT scan in a 23-year-old Black female with sickle-cell trait. The left kidney demonstrates infiltrative growth of a large central mass. Right panel (d) gross specimen of the medullary carcinoma demonstrates a large tumour around the renal sinus and central kidney with an isolated, dilated calyx (arrow) (from Davidson *et al.* 1995, with permission).

Table 5 Clinicopathological features of renal medullary carcinoma (from Davis *et al.* 1995, with permission)

Age and sex	Presenting symptoms	Duration of symptoms	Extent of tumour at diagnosis	Survival after diagnosis
20 M	Pain, fever, wt loss	6 weeks	Perinephric[a] and rt pleural effusion	3 weeks
16 M	Haematuria	3 months	Nodes[b], RV	?
20 F	Haematuria, pain	?	Nodes	?
11 M	Haematuria	3 months	Nodes, adrenal	4 months
17 M	?	?	Nodes	4 weeks
27 M	Fever, wt loss	4 weeks	Cervical node	4 months
15 M	Haematuria, pain	?	Lung METS 1 week postop	?
16 M	Palpable mass	?	Nodes, liver	4 months
21 M	?	?	Perinephric disease	?
22 F	?	?	Nodes	~12 months
20 M	?	?	Nodes, peritoneum	?
19 M	Haematuria	?	Nodes, massive retroperitoneal disease	4 months
21 M	Haematuria, wt loss, pain	5 months	Liver, extensive perinephric disease	8 months
12 M	Haematuria, pain	5 weeks	Nodes, liver, adrenal	2 months (lung METS)
27 M	Haematuria	?	Nodes	4 months (lung METS)
19 M	Haematuria	1 week	Nodes, adrenal	5 months
32 M	?	?	Perinephric disease	6 weeks (lung and peritoneal METS)
35 M	?	?	Nodes	9 weeks, extensive retroperitoneum
21 M	Nausea, vomiting, pain	?	Nodes, liver, lungs	?
14 M	Wt loss, pain	3 months	Pericaval, lungs	10 weeks
21 F	Massive haematuria, pain	?	Nodes, RV, mesentery	8 weeks (general METS: lungs, liver, thyroid, others)
33 M	Haematuria	?	Perinephric disease	3 months
23 F	?	?	Nodes, lung	?
16 F	Wt loss, fever	2 months	Nodes, adrenal, lungs	?
23 M	Pain	2 months	Nodes, liver	3 months
29 F	Haematuria, mass	?	Nodes, adrenal	7 weeks (lung, liver METS)
27 M	Weight loss	4 months	Nodes, adrenal, lungs	3 months
11 M	Pain	2 months	Nodes, RV, lungs, liver	?
28 F	Pain, mass	2 months	Nodes, RV, adrenal	?
39 F	?	?	Nodes	?
34 F	Haematuria, pain, acute retention	'Few weeks'	Extensive retroperitoneal disease	?
32 F	Haematuria	?	Nodes	?
27 F	Haematuria	?	Nodes, adrenal, lungs	?

Wt, weight; RV, renal vein; METS, metastasis.

[a] Perinephric refers to soft tissue peripheral to the kidney or renal pelvis.

[b] Nodes refers to those in or near renal hilum and adjacent retroperitoneum.

a patient group in which gross haematuria and flank pain, the major presenting symptoms of this tumour, are common manifestations of sickle-cell trait itself.

References

Adams, R. J. Neurologic complications. In *Sickle Cell Disease: Basic Principles and Clinical Practice* (ed. S. H. Embury *et al.*), pp. 599–622. New York: Raven Press, 1994.

Adams, R. J. (2000). Lessons from the Stroke Prevention Trial in Sickle Cell Anemia (STOP) Study. *Journal of Child Neurology* **15**, 344–349.

Allon, M. *et al.* (1988). Effects of nonsteroidal anti-inflammatory drugs on renal function in sickle cell anaemia. *Kidney International* **34**, 500–506.

Anderson, S. *et al.* (1985). Control of glomerular hypertension limits glomerular injury in rats with reduced renal mass. *Journal of Clinical Investigation* **76**, 612–619.

Aoki, R. Y. and Saad, T. O. (1995). Enalapril reduces the albuminuria of patients with sickle cell disease. *American Journal of Medicine* **98**, 432–434.

Aparicio, S. A. J. R. *et al.* (1990). Measurement of glomerular filtration rate in homozygous sickle cell disease: a comparison of ^{51}Cr-EDTA clearance, creatinine clearance, serum creatinine and beta 2 microglobulin. *Journal of Clinical Pathology* **43**, 370–372.

Ataga, K. I. and Orringer, E. P. (2000). Renal abnormalities in sickle cell disease. *American Journal of Hematology* **63**, 205–211.

Bakir, A. A. *et al.* (1987). Prognosis of the nephrotic syndrome in sickle glomerulopathy. *American Journal of Nephrology* **7**, 110–115.

Ball, G. V. and Sorenson, L. B. (1970). The pathogenesis of hyperuricemia and gout in sickle cell anaemia. *Arthritis and Rheumatism* **13**, 846–848.

Ballas, S. K. *et al.* (1982). Clinical, hematological, and biochemical features of HbSc disease. *American Journal of Hematology* **13**, 37–51.

Bank, N. *et al.* (1994). Increased abundance of nitric oxide synthases in kidneys of transgenic sickle cell mice. *Journal of the American Society of Nephrology* **5**, 573.

Barber, W. H. *et al.* (1987). Renal transplantation in sickle cell anaemia and sickle cell disease. *Clinical Transplantation* **1**, 169–175.

Batlle, D. C. *et al.* (1982). Hyperkalemic hyperchloremic metabolic acidosis in sickle cell haemoglobinopathies. *American Journal of Medicine* **72**, 188–192.

Bhathena, D. B. and Sondheimer, J. H. (1991). The glomerulopathy of homozygous sickle haemoglobin (SS) disease: morphology and pathogenesis. *Journal of the American Society of Nephrology* **1**, 1241–1252.

Black, W. D., Hatch, F. E., and Acchiardo, S. (1976). Epsilon amino caproic acid in prolonged hematuria of patients with sickle cell anaemia. *Archives of Internal Medicine* **136**, 678–681.

Bolanos-Meade, J. *et al.* (1999). Thrombotic thrombocytopenic purpura in a patient with sickle cell crisis. *Annals of Hematology* **78**, 558–559.

Bruck, E. (1953). Renal function in anaemia. *American Journal of Diseases of Children* **86**, 511–512.

Bruno, D. *et al.* (2001). Genitourinary complications of sickle cell disease. *Journal of Urology* **166**, 803–811.

Buchanan, G. R. Infection. In *Sickle Cell Disease: Basic Principles and Clinical Practice* (ed. S. H. Embury *et al.*), pp. 567–587. New York: Raven Press, 1994.

Buckalew, V. M., Jr. (1970). Sickle cell nephropathy. *Annals of Internal Medicine* **73**, 488.

Chapman, Z. A. *et al.* (1955). Gross hematuria in sickle cell trait and sickle cell haemoglobin C disease. *American Journal of Medicine* **19**, 773–782.

Charache, S. Natural history of disease: adults. In *Sickle Cell Disease: Basic Principles and Clinical Practice* (ed. S. H. Embury *et al.*), pp. 413–421. New York: Raven Press, 1994a.

Charache, S. (1994b). Experimental therapy of sickle cell disease. Use of hydroxyurea. *American Journal of Pediatric Hematology and Oncology* **16**, 62–66.

Charache, S. *et al.* (1995). Effect of hydroxyurea on the frequency of painful crises in sickle cell anemia. *New England Journal of Medicine* **332**, 1317–1323.

Chatterjee, S. N. (1987). National study of natural history of renal allografts in sickle cell disease or trait: a second report. *Transplantation Proceedings* **19**, 33–35.

Cruz, I. A. *et al.* (1982). Advanced renal failure in patients with sickle cell anaemia: clinical course and prognosis. *Journal of the National Medical Association* **74**, 1103–1109.

Davidson, A. J. and Hartman, D. S. *Radiology of the Kidney and Urinary Tract* 2nd edn. Philadelphia: W.B. Saunders, 1994.

Davidson, A. J. *et al.* (1995). Renal medullary carcinoma associated with sickle cell trait: radiologic findings. *Radiology* **195**, 83–85.

Davis, C. J., Jr., Mostofi, F. K., and Sesterhenn, I. A. (1995). Renal medullary carcinoma. The seventh sickle cell nephropathy. *American Journal of Surgical Pathology* **19**, 1–11.

Davis, H. *et al.* (1997). National trends in the mortality of children with sickle cell disease, 1968–1992. *American Journal of Public Health* **87**, 1317–1322.

DeFronzo, R. A. *et al.* (1979). Impaired renal tubular potassium secretion in sickle cell disease. *Annals of Internal Medicine* **90**, 310–316.

de Jong, P. E., de Jong-van de Berg, L. T. W., and van Eps Statius, L. W. (1978). The tubular reabsorption of phosphate in sickle cell nephropathy. *Clinical Science and Molecular Medicine* **55**, 429–434.

de Jong, P. E., Landman, H., and van Eps Statius, L. W. (1982). Blood pressure in sickle cell disease. *Archives of Internal Medicine* **142**, 1239–1240.

de Jong, P. E. *et al.* (1980). The influence of indomethacin on renal hemodynamics in sickle cell anaemia. *Clinical Science* **59**, 245–250.

Devereux, S. and Knowles, S. M. (1985). Rhabdomyolysis and acute renal failure in sickle cell anaemia. *British Medical Journal* **290**, 1707–1709.

Diamond, H. S. *et al.* (1975). Hyperuricosuria and increased tubular secretion of urate in sickle cell anaemia. *American Journal of Medicine* **59**, 796–802.

Eaton, J. W. Malaria and the selection of the sickle cell gene. In *Sickle Cell Disease: Basic Principles and Clinical Practice* (ed. S. H. Embury *et al.*), pp. 13–18. New York: Raven Press, 1994.

Eckert, D. E. *et al.* (1974). The incidence and manifestations of urographic papillary abnormalities in patients with S haemoglobinopathies. *Radiology* **113**, 59–63.

Elfenbein, J. B. *et al.* (1974). Pathology of the glomerulus in sickle cell anaemia with and without nephrotic syndrome. *American Journal of Pathology* **77**, 357–376.

Etteldorf, J. N., Tuttle, A. H., and Clayton, G. W. (1952). Renal function studies in pediatrics: I. Renal hemodynamics in children with sickle cell anaemia. *American Journal of Diseases of Children* **83**, 185–191.

Fabry, M. Transgenic animal models. In *Sickle Cell Disease: Basic Principles and Clinical Practice* (ed. S. H. Embury *et al.*), pp. 105–120. New York: Raven Press, 1994.

Falk, R. J. and Jennette, J. C. (1992). Sickle cell nephropathy. *Advances in Nephrology from the Neckar Hospital* **23**, 133–147.

Falk, R. J. *et al.* (1992). Prevalence and pathologic features of sickle cell nephropathy and response to inhibition of angiotensin-converting enzyme. *New England Journal of Medicine* **326**, 910–915.

Foucan, L. *et al.* (1998). A randomized trial of captopril for microalbuminuria in normotensive adults with sickle cell anemia. *American Journal of Medicine* **104**, 339–342.

Francis, R. B. and Hebbel, R. P. Hemostasis. In *Sickle Cell Disease: Basic Principles and Clinical Practice* (ed. S. H. Embury *et al.*), pp. 299–310. New York: Raven Press, 1994.

Friedman, E. A. *et al.* (1974). Uremia in sickle cell anaemia treated by maintenance hemodialysis. *New England Journal of Medicine* **291**, 431–435.

Gold, D. D. (1974). Hemodialysis and transfusions for uremic patients with sickle cell disease. *New England Journal of Medicine* **291**, 1361–1364.

Granfortuna, J., Zamkoff, K., and Urrutia, E. (1986). Acute renal infarction in sickle cell disease. *American Journal of Hematology* **23**, 59–64.

Grell, G. A. C., Alleyne, G. A. O., and Serjeant, G. R. (1981). Blood pressure with homozygous sickle cell disease. *Lancet* **2**, 1166.

Griffin, T. C., McIntire, D., and Buchanan, G. R. (1994). High-dose intravenous methylprednisolone therapy for pain in children and adolescents with sickle cell disease. *New England Journal of Medicine* **330**, 733–737.

Guasch, A., Cua, M., and Mitch, W. E. (1996). Early detection and the course of glomerular injury in patients with sickle cell anemia. *Kidney International* **49**, 786–791.

Guasch, A. *et al.* (1999). Evidence that microdeletion in the alpha globin gene protect against the development of sickle cell glomerulonephropathy in humans. *Journal of the American Society of Nephrology* **10**, 1014–1019.

Gwilt, P. R. and Tracewell, W. G. (1998). Pharmacokinetics and pharmacodynamics of hydroxyurea. *Clinical Pharmacokinetics* **34**, 347–358.

Hakim, L. S. *et al.* Priapism. In *Sickle Cell Disease: Basic Principles and Clinical Practice* (ed. S. H. Embury *et al.*), pp. 633–644. New York: Raven Press, 1994.

Harrow, B. R., Sloane, J. A., and Liebman, N. (1963). Roentgenologic demonstration of renal papillary necrosis in sickle-cell trait. *New England Journal of Medicine* **268**, 969–976.

Hassell, K. L., Eckman, J. R., and Lane, P. A. (1994). Acute multiorgan failure syndrome: a potentially catastrophic complication of severe sickle cell pain episodes. *American Journal of Medicine* **96**, 155–162.

Hatch, F. E., Culbertson, J. W., and Diggs, L. W. (1967). Nature of the renal concentrating defect in sickle cell disease. *Journal of Clinical Investigation* **46**, 336–345.

Hatch, F. E. *et al.* (1970). Renal circulatory studies in young adults with sickle cell anaemia. *Journal of Laboratory and Clinical Medicine* **76**, 632–640.

Hatch, F. E. *et al.* (1989). Altered vascular reactivity in sickle haemoglobinopathy: a possible protective factor from hypertension. *American Journal of Hypertension* **2**, 2–8.

Henderson, A. B. (1950). Sickle cell anaemia. Clinical study of fifty-four cases. *American Journal of Medicine* **9**, 757–765.

Herrick, J. B. (1910). Peculiar elongated and sickle shaped red blood corpuscles in a case of severe anaemia. *Archives of Internal Medicine* **6**, 517–520.

Ho Ping Kong, H. and Alleyne, G. A. O. (1968). Defect in urinary acidification in adults with sickle-cell anaemia. *Lancet* **1**, 954–955.

Hoppe, C. C. and Walters, M. C. (2001). Bone marrow transplantation in sickle cell anemia. *Transplantation* **13**, 85–90.

Hostetter, T. H. *et al.* (1981). Hyperfiltration in remnant nephrons: a potentially adverse response to renal ablation. *American Journal of Physiology* **241**, F85–F93.

Johnson, C. S. and Giorgio, A. J. (1981). Arterial blood pressure in adults with sickle cell disease. *Archives of Internal Medicine* **141**, 891–893.

Johnson, F. L. *et al.* (1994). Bone marrow transplantation for sickle cell disease. *American Journal of Pediatric Hematology & Oncology* **16**, 22–26.

Jones, S. R., Binder, R. A., and Donowho, E. M. (1970). Sudden death in sickle cell trait. *New England Journal of Medicine* **282**, 323–325.

Kark, J. A. *et al.* (1987). Sickle cell trait as a risk factor for sudden death in physical training. *New England Journal of Medicine* **317**, 781–788.

Kelly, C. J. and Singer, I. (1986). Acute renal failure in sickle-cell disease. *American Journal of Kidney Diseases* **8**, 146–150.

Khan, A. *et al.* (2000). Renal medullary carcinoma: sonographic, computed tomography magnetic resonance and angiographic findings. *European Journal of Radiology* **35**, 1–7.

Koduri, P. R., Agbemadzo, B., and Nathan, S. (2001). Hemoglobin S-C disease revisited: a clinical study of 106 adults. *American Journal of Hematology* **68**, 298–300.

Larrabee, K. D. and Monga, M. (1997). Women with sickle cell trait are at increased risk for preeclampsia. *American Journal of Obstetrics and Gynecology* **177**, 425–428.

Leikin, S. L. *et al.* (1989). Mortality in children and adolescents with sickle cell disease. *Pediatrics* **84**, 500–508.

McCall, I. A. *et al.* (1978). Urographic findings in homozygous sickle cell disease. *Radiology* **126**, 99–104.

McCoy, R. C. (1969). Ultrastructural alterations in the kidney with sickle cell disease and the nephrotic syndrome. *Laboratory Investigation* **21**, 85–95.

Mentzer, W. C. *et al.* (1994). Availability of related donors for bone marrow transplantation in sickle cell anaemia. *American Journal of Pediatric Hematology and Oncology* **16**, 27–29.

Milner, P. F. *et al.* Bone and joint disease. In *Sickle Cell Disease: Basic Principles and Clinical Practice* (ed. S. H. Embury *et al.*), pp. 645–662. New York: Raven Press, 1994.

Miner, D. J. *et al.* (1987). Recurrent sickle cell nephropathy in a transplanted kidney. *American Journal of Kidney Diseases* **10**, 306–313.

Mohandas, N. and Ballas, S. K. Erythrocyte density and heterogeneity. *In Sickle Cell Disease: Basic Principles and Clinical Practice* (ed. S. H. Embury *et al.*), pp. 195–203. New York: Raven Press, 1994.

Montgomery, R. *et al.* (1994). Renal transplantation in patients with sickle cell nephropathy. *Transplantation* **58**, 618–620.

Morgan, A. G. and Serjeant, G. R. (1981). Renal function in patients over 40 with sickle-cell disease. *West Indian Medical Journal* **36**, 241–250.

Mostofi, F. K., Vorger Bruegge, C. F., and Diggs, L. W. (1957). Lesions in kidneys removed for unilateral hematuria in sickle cell disease. *Archives of Pathology (Chicago)* **63**, 336–351.

Nagel, R. L. Origins and dispersion of the sickle cell gene. In *Sickle Cell Disease: Basic Principles and Clinical Practice* (ed. S. H. Embury *et al.*), pp. 353–380. New York: Raven Press, 1994.

National Center for Health Statistics. *Vital Statistics of the United States, 1985*. Vol. II. *Mortality*. Part A. Section 6, *Life tables*. DHHS publication no. (PHS) 88–1101. Washington, DC: Government Printing Office, 1988.

National Heart, Lung, and Blood Institute. Multicenter study of hydroxyurea in sickle cell anaemia. Clinical Alert U.S.D.H.H.S. U.S.P.H.S. January 30, Bethesda, MD, 1995.

Nissenson, A. R. and Port, F. K. (1989). Outcome of end-stage renal disease in patients with rare causes of renal failure. I. Inherited and metabolic disorders. *Quarterly Journal of Medicine* **73**, 1055–1062.

Ojo, A. O. *et al.* (1999). Renal transplantation in end-stage sickle cell nephropathy. *Transplantation* **67**, 291–295.

Orringer, E. P. *et al.* (2001). Purified Poloxamer 188 for treatment of acute vaso-occlusive crisis of sickle cell disease. A randomized controlled trial. *Journal of American Medical Association* **286**, 2099–2106.

Oster, J. R. *et al.* (1976a). Renal acidification in sickle-cell disease. *Journal of Laboratory and Clinical Medicine* **88**, 389–401.

Oster, J. R. *et al.* (1976b). Renal acidification in sickle cell trait. *Archives of Internal Medicine* **136**, 30–35.

Ozawa, T. *et al.* (1976). Autologous immune complex nephritis associated with sickle cell trait: diagnosis of the haemoglobinopathy after renal structural and immunological studies. *British Medical Journal* **1**, 369–371.

Pandya, K. K. *et al.* (1976). Renal papillary necrosis in sickle cell haemoglobinopathies. *Journal of Urology* **115**, 497–501.

Pardo, V. *et al.* (1975). Nephropathy associated with sickle cell anaemia: an autologous immune complex nephritis. II. Clinicopathologic study of seven patients. *American Journal of Medicine* **59**, 650–659.

Pastore, L. M., Savitz, D. A., and Thorp, J. M., Jr. (1999). Predictors of urinary tract infections at the first prenatal visit. *Epidemiology* **10**, 282–287.

Pearson, H. A. (1989). The kidney, hepatobiliary system, and spleen in sickle cell anaemia. *Annals of the New York Academy of Sciences* **565**, 120–125.

Pegelow, C. H. *et al.* (1997). Natural history of blood pressure in sickle cell disease: risks for stroke and death associated with relative hypertension in sickle cell anemia. *American Journal of Medicine* **102**, 171–177.

Perlin, E. *et al.* (1994). Enhancement of pain control with ketorolac tromethamine in patients with sickle cell vaso-occlusive crisis. *American Journal of Hematology* **46**, 43–47.

Phuong-Thu, T. *et al.* (2000). Renal abnormalities in sickle cell disease. *Kidney International* **57**, 1–8.

Platt, O. S. (1994). Easing the suffering caused by sickle cell disease. *New England Journal of Medicine* **330**, 783–784 (editorial).

Platt, O. S. *et al.* (1994). Mortality in sickle cell disease. Life expectancy and risk factors for early death. *New England Journal of Medicine* **330**, 1639–1644.

Powars, D. R. Natural history of sickle cell disease: the first two decades. In *Sickle Cell Disease: Basic Principles and Clinical Practice* (ed. S. H. Embury *et al.*), pp. 395–412. New York: Raven Press, 1994.

Powars, D. R. *et al.* (1990). The variable expression of sickle cell disease is genetically determined. *Seminars in Hematology* **27**, 360–376.

Powars, D. R. *et al.* (1991). Chronic renal failure in sickle cell disease: risk factors, clinical course, and mortality. *Annals of Internal Medicine* **115**, 614–620.

Public Health Service (1964). Blood pressure of adults by race and area, United States, 1960–1962, National Health Survey, Vital and Health Statistics Series II, No. 5. Washington DC: US Department of Health, Education and Welfare.

Public Health Service. Blood pressure levels of persons 6–74 years, United States (1971–1974), National Health Survey, Vital and Health Statistics Series II, No. 203. Washington DC: US Department of Health, Education, and Welfare, 1977.

Ranney, H. M. Historical milestones. In *Sickle Cell Disease: Basic Principles and Clinical Practice* (ed. S. H. Embury *et al.*), pp. 1–5. New York: Raven Press, 1994.

Readett, D. J. R., Morris, J., and Serjeant, G. R. (1990). Determinants of nocturnal enuresis in homozygous sickle cell disease. *Archives of Diseases in Childhood* **65**, 615–618.

Rodgers, G. P. *et al.* (1993a). Augmentation by erythropoietin of the fetal-haemoglobin response to hydroxyurea in sickle cell disease. *New England Journal of Medicine* **328**, 73–80.

Rodgers, G. P., Walker, E. C., and Podgor, M. J. (1993b). Is 'relative' hypertension a risk factor for vaso-occlusive complications in sickle cell disease? *American Journal of Medical Science* **305**, 150–156.

Roy, S. *et al.* (1976). Sickle-cell disease and poststreptococcal acute glomerulonephritis. *American Journal of Clinical Pathology* **66**, 986–990.

Saborio, P. and Scheinman, J. I. (1999). Sickle cell nephropathy. *Journal of the American Society of Nephrology* **10**, 187–192.

Scott-Conner, C. E. and Brunson, C. D. (1994). The pathophysiology of the sickle cell haemoglobinopathies and implications for perioperative management. *American Journal of Surgery* **168**, 268–274.

Schmitt, F. *et al.* (1998). Early glomerular dysfunction in patients with sickle cell anemia. *American Journal of Kidney Diseases* **32**, 208–214.

Sears, D. A. (1978). The morbidity of sickle cell trait. A review of the literature. *American Journal of Medicine* **64**, 1021–1036.

Shapiro, B. S. and Ballas, S. K. The acute painful episode. In *Sickle Cell Disease: Basic Principles and Clinical Practice* (ed. S. H. Embury *et al.*), pp. 531–543. New York: Raven Press, 1994.

Sherwood, J. B. *et al.* (1986). Sickle cell anaemia patients have low erythropoietin levels for their degree of anaemia. *Blood* **67**, 46–49.

Singhal, A. *et al.* (1993). Is there an acute-phase response in steady-state sickle cell disease? *Lancet* **341**, 651–653.

Sklar, A. H. *et al.* (1990a). A population study of renal function in sickle cell anaemia. *International Journal of Artificial Organs* **13**, 231–236.

Sklar, A. H. *et al.* (1990b). Acute renal failure in sickle cell anaemia. *International Journal of Artificial Organs* **13**, 347–351.

Smith, E. C. *et al.* (1981). Serum phosphate abnormalities in sickle cell anaemia. *Proceedings of the Society for Experimental Biology and Medicine* **168**, 254–258.

Spector, D. *et al.* (1978). Painful crises following renal transplantation in sickle cell anaemia. *American Journal of Medicine* **64**, 835–838.

Statius van Eps, L. W. *et al.* (1967). The influence of red blood cell transfusion on the hyposthenuria and renal hemodynamics of sickle cell anaemia. *Clinica Chimica Acta* **17**, 449–461.

Statius van Eps, L. W. *et al.* (1970a). The relation between age and renal concentrating capacity in sickle cell disease and haemoglobin C disease. *Clinica Chemica Acta* **27**, 501–511.

Statius van Eps, L. W. *et al.* (1970b). Nature of concentrating defect in sickle cell nephropathy, microradioangiographic studies. *Lancet* **1**, 450–452.

Steinberg, M. H. (1991). Erythropoietin for anaemia of renal failure in sickle cell disease. *New England Journal of Medicine* **324**, 1369–1370.

Steinberg, M. H. (1999). Drug therapy: management of sickle cell disease. *New England Journal of Medicine* **340**, 1021–1030.

Steinberg, M. H. and Mohandas, N. Laboratory values. In *Sickle Cell Disease: Basic Principles and Clinical Practice* (ed. S. H. Embury *et al.*), pp. 469–483. New York: Raven Press, 1994.

Strauss, J. *et al.* (1975). Nephropathy associated with sickle cell anaemia: an autologous immune complex nephritis. I. Studies on the nature of glomerular bound antibody and antigen identification in a patient with sickle cell disease and immune deposit glomerulonephritis. *American Journal of Medicine* **58**, 382–387.

Sydenstricker, V. P., Mulherin, W. A., and Houseal, R. W. (1923). Peculiar elongated and sickle-shaped red blood corpuscles in a case of severe anaemia. *American Journal of Diseases of Children* **26**, 132–154.

Tejani, A. *et al.* (1985). Renal lesions in sickle cell nephropathy in children. *Nephron* **39**, 352–356.

Thomas, A. N., Pattison, C., and Serjeant, G. R. (1982). Causes of death in sickle-cell disease in Jamaica. *British Medical Journal* **285**, 633–635.

Tolaymat, A. *et al.* (1999). Parvovirus glomerulonephritis in a patient with sickle cell disease. *Pediatric Nephrology* **13**, 340–342.

USRDS (1998). Annual data report: incidence and prevalence of ESRD. *American Journal of Kidney Diseases* **32** (Suppl.), 38–49.

Vaamonde, C. A. (1984). Renal papillary necrosis in sickle cell haemoglobinopathies. *Seminars in Nephrology* **1**, 48–64.

van Agtmael, M. A., Cheng, J. D., and Nossent, H. C. (1994). Acute chest syndrome in adult Afro–Caribbean patients with sickle cell disease. Analysis of 81 episodes among 53 patients. *Archives of Internal Medicine* **154**, 557–561.

Vichinsky, E. P. *et al.* (1990). Alloimmunozation in sickle cell anaemia and transfusion of racially unmatched blood. *New England Journal of Medicine* **322**, 1617–1621.

Walker, B. R. *et al.* (1971). Glomerular lesions in sickle cell nephropathy. *Journal of the American Medical Association* **215**, 437–440.

Walker, T. M. *et al.* (1996). Renal length in sickle cell disease: observations from a cohort study. *Clinical Nephrology* **46**, 384–388.

Warady, B. A. and Sullivan, E. K. (1998). Renal transplantation in children with sickle cell disease: a report of the North American Pediatric Renal Transplant Cooperative Study (NAPRTCS). *Pediatric Transplantation* **2**, 130–133.

Weidner, N. and Buckalew, V. M., Jr. Sickle cell anaemia, sickle cell trait, and polycythemic states. In *Renal Pathology with Clinical and Functional Correlations* (ed. C. C. Tisher and B. M. Brenner), pp. 1491–1510. Philadelphia: J.B. Lippincott, 1994.

Wierenga, K. J. *et al.* (1995). Glomerulonephritis after human parvovirus infection in homozygous sickle-cell disease. *Lancet* **346**, 475–476.

Wigfall, D. R. *et al.* (1994). Predictors of glomerular disease in children and adults with sickle cell anaemia. *Journal of the American Society of Nephrology* **5**, 344.

Wigfall, D. R. *et al.* (2000). Prevalence and correlates of glomerulopathy in children with sickle cell disease. *Journal of Pediatrics* **136**, 749–753.

Wong, W. Y., Elliott-Mills, D., and Powars, D. (1996). Renal failure in sickle cell anemia. *Hematology-Oncology Clinics of North America* **10**, 1321–1331.

Zarkowsky, H. S. *et al.* (1998). Bacteremia in sickle hemoglobinopathies. *Journal of Pediatrics* **109**, 579–585.

4.12 The patient exposed to substance misuse, organic solvents, and smoking

4.12.1 Substance misuse, organic solvents, and kidney disease

Gordon M. Bell and Matthew L.P. Howse

Introduction

Man has used drugs for recreational purposes as long as history itself. Arabic traders smoked heroin in the third century BC and the Aztecs enjoyed the effects of hallucinogenic mushrooms at a similar time. In the United Kingdom, the arrival of the '*club scene*' in the late 1980s increased the misuse of drugs, particularly stimulants. A recent estimate suggested that one-third of British adults have used illicit drugs at sometime, rising to half in the 16–24-year-old age group (Drug Scope 2000).

In the next section, we review the association of misused substances and renal pathology. While some substances are directly nephrotoxic, a number of other mechanisms are also involved in the development of kidney disease.

Renal effects of abuse of drugs and chemical agents

Ecstasy and other amphetamines

Ecstasy (3,4-methylenedioxymethamphetamine, MDMA), originally patented in 1914 as an appetite suppressant, is now a commonly used recreation drug in the UK club scene. MDMA is rapidly absorbed from the gastrointestinal tract, reaching plasma peak concentrations in approximately 2 h. Subsequently, it is metabolized by the liver and the metabolites are excreted by the kidney. Since 1977, it has been listed as a class A drug in the United Kingdom under the Misuse of Drugs Act, 1971 (Crowe *et al.* 2000).

In Europe, MDMA and amphetamines are generally taken by mouth during prolonged group dancing while attending 'rave' parties or clubs. The increased physical activity, overheated environments, and dehydration can result in hyperthermia. In experimental animals, MDMA has been shown to cause fever even in the absence of strenuous exercise. Unwanted effects may be minor—loss of appetite, nausea, vomiting, headaches, trismus, and cramps; or serious—convulsions, hyperpyrexia, hepatic dysfunction, rhabdomyolysis, disseminated intravascular coagulation (Henry *et al.* 1992), and acute renal failure (Fahal *et al.* 1992), The patient with rhabdomyolysis typically presents with muscle pain and tenderness, and is found to be in acute renal failure with hyperkalaemia, hyperphosphataemia, and raised creatine kinase (see Chapters 10.2 and 10.3). Myoglobin and granular casts are found in the urine. Following vigorous rehydration and cooling measures the treatment of these patients is supportive. The muscle relaxant, dantrolene, has been advocated by some but there is no consensus, or trials of its efficacy, in the treatment of MDMA-induced hyperpyrexia.

Following extensive press coverage, drug abusers are becoming aware of the risk of dehydration and often drink large quantities of water after taking ecstasy to try to prevent this. As a consequence, hyponatraemia, catatonic states, and cerebral oedema have occurred (Maxwell *et al.* 1993). The dilutional hyponatraemia, due to excessive fluid ingestion, may also involve inappropriate antidiuretic hormone secretion. 'Chill out' rooms are now provided in an attempt to prevent hyperthermia. In the United States, ecstasy has not been taken as a dance drug and consequently the spectrum of unwanted effects is different with cardiac arrhythmias being more common (Crowe *et al.* 2000).

As ecstasy has marked sympathomimetic effects, it is not surprising that cases of accelerated hypertension with associated acute renal failure have been described. Similarly, urinary retention due to bladder neck closure has been associated with its use (Crowe *et al.* 2000).

Two case reports have reported a further association with ingestion of MDMA or methamphetamine and the development of severe acute renal failure with, on renal histology, fibrinoid necrosis of the renal arterioles and consequent glomerular ischaemia and infarction (Woodrow *et al.* 1995; Bingham *et al.* 1998). Both the patients were hypertensive and failed to recover renal function in the medium term. In one case following a dialysis-dependent period of 5 months there was progressive improvement (but not normalization) of kidney function (Woodrow and Turney 1999). Cerebral vasculitis has been reported more frequently than renal vasculitis in association with the abuse of various substances, including amphetamines. In both situations the pathogenetic mechanisms remain unknown.

Cocaine

Cocaine is an alkaloid extracted from a shrub (*Erythroxylon coca*) that grows in the Andes mountains and can be absorbed through any mucous membrane, smoked, or injected intravenously or intramuscularly. It has an estimated half-life of 30–90 min: 80–90 per cent of cocaine is metabolized, while the remainder is excreted unchanged in the urine, in which its metabolites can be detected for 36–48 h (Crowe *et al.* 2000). The euphoria of cocaine is caused by the blocking of the reuptake of dopamine in the central nervous system, while the hypertensive effects are caused by inhibition of reuptake of noradrenaline throughout the vascular tree. It is also a vasoconstrictor through calcium influx in vascular smooth muscle cells, release of endothelin 1, and decreased production of nitric oxide, which is a potent vasodilator (Lange and Hillis 2001).

A wide spectrum of renal complications can occur with both acute and chronic use of cocaine (Crowe *et al.* 2000; Nzerue *et al.* 2000). Acute renal failure can occur as a result of rhabdomyolysis (see Chapters 10.2 and 10.3). In one series, 24 per cent of patients seen in an emergency department with cocaine-associated complaints presented with concentrations of creatine kinase of more than 1000 U/l (Welch *et al.* 1991) and up to one-third of such patients develop acute renal failure (Roth *et al.* 1988). Muscle ischaemia caused through prolonged vasoconstriction of intramuscular arteries, generalized seizures, coma with secondary muscle compression, or direct myofibrillar damage are different mechanisms of cocaine-induced rhabdomyolysis. Cocaine may be contaminated with arsenic, strychnine, amphetamine, and phencyclidine, which may also cause seizures and rhabdomyolysis.

There are a number of reports of acute renal failure secondary to accelerated hypertension in cocaine users. This has been associated with thrombotic microangiopathy (Roth *et al.* 1988) and less frequently with a renal scleroderma-like syndrome with fibrinoid necrosis involving the small interlobular arterioles. (Lam and Ballou 1992). To date, several other cases of scleroderma associated with cocaine use have been reported, with scleroderma renal crisis occurring in two cases (Nzerue *et al.* 2000). In pregnancy, acute renal failure secondary to abruptio placentae or pre-elampsia has been linked to cocaine use.

Cocaine-induced premature coronary artery disease is a well-described clinical entity, but less well known is that cocaine can cause renal atherosclerosis and infarction. Anecdotal reports linking cocaine with cases of Goodpasture's syndrome, interstitial nephritis, and Henoch–Schönlein vasculitis with nephritis require corroboration by larger studies (Nzerue *et al.* 2000).

The relationship between recurrent cocaine use and chronic hypertension is more complex with conflicting data. In a study of 301 cocaine users admitted to hospital for treatment of their addiction, there was no significant difference in blood pressure or microalbuminuria when compared to a demographically matched non-abusing control group (Brecklin *et al.* 1998). The authors concluded that cocaine use was more likely to be associated with acute but not chronic hypertension. However, two studies of urban dialysis populations suggest that chronic cocaine use may accelerate both hypertensive and intrinsic renal disease especially in black males (Dunea *et al.* 1995; Norris *et al.* 2001). Proving a direct cause and effect relationship is difficult because of confounding factors; for example, patients who smoke cocaine often abuse other drugs such as tobacco and heroin. Unpredictability and compliance issues would make prospective studies challenging in such a population.

While the clinical data suggest that cocaine may exacerbate pre-existing renal disease rather than cause *de novo* disease, animal models suggest that it may cause mesangial proliferation by increasing the release of interleukin-6 by macrophages.

Opiates

Heroin (diacetylmorphine, diamorphine) is the most commonly abused drug in this group. It can be sniffed ('snorting'), eaten, smoked ('chasing the dragon'), injected subcutaneously ('skin popping'), or injected intravenously ('mainlining'). It is often injected in combination with cocaine ('speed-balling'). Heroin has a half-life of 3 min and is rapidly metabolized to morphine, which is mainly responsible for the pharmacological actions of heroin. Heroin is excreted in the urine as free and unconjugated morphine. There are several renal complications from its abuse (Sreepada Rao *et al.* 1977; Crowe *et al.* 2000). Coma from overdose or underestimated drug potency leads to pressure-induced muscle damage and rhabdomyolysis during unconsciousness. Hypotension, hypoxia, acidosis, and dehydration may aggravate this state. Others have demonstrated rhabdomyolysis in the absence of coma or evidence of muscle compression, and suggest that this could be due to a direct toxic effect or an allergic response to heroin or the components in adulterated heroin (Grossman *et al.* 1974).

There is a high rate of viral, bacterial, and fungal contamination associated with intravenous drug misuse, including heroin, and consequently users are at risk of a variety of infections. Glomerulonephritis (GN) may be associated with these chronic infections. Local pyogenic abscesses, secondary to skin contamination with *Staphylococcus aureus*, have been associated with GN, thought to be due to deposition of immune complexes formed in response to the organism. Other bacterial and fungal endocarditis can also cause immune-complex-mediated GN. Hepatitis B has also been associated with GN, usually of membranous type, and with polyarteritis nodosa. Hepatitis C causes mesangiocapillary GN with associated cryoglobulinaemia (Crowe *et al.* 2000) (see Chapter 4.6).

Secondary (AA) amyloidosis (see Chapter 4.2.1) has increased in frequency as a cause of renal disease in chronic parenteral drug users, particularly among those who inject drugs subcutaneously ('skin poppers') and are subject to chronic infection. With continued abuse, the majority of such patients progress to endstage renal failure. Various drug treatments have been tried, but drug abstinence appears to be the most important factor in treatment and complete resolution following abstinence from subcutaneous drug abuse has been reported. (Crowe *et al.* 2000).

During the 1970s and 1980s, *heroin-associated nephropathy* (HAN) was described, presenting as nephrotic syndrome and progressing rapidly to endstage renal failure. Occasionally, the process reversed with abstinence from further heroin use (Sreepada Rao *et al.* 1977) and renal biopsy usually showed a focal segmental glomerulosclerosis (Cunningham *et al.* 1980). The pathogenesis of this syndrome is unclear; earlier studies suggested that heroin, or one of its adulterants, acted as an antigen leading to renal deposition of immune complexes in the kidney. More recent animal studies have shown that morphine may have a direct effect on the glomerulus, causing proliferation of fibroblasts and a decrease in degradation of type IV collagen. In North America (where it was particularly common), a decrease in the incidence of HAN among intravenous heroin addicts has been observed (Friedman and Tao 1995) (Fig. 1). 'Street' heroin has become increasingly pure, and it may be that addicts are now exposed to lower doses of possibly nephrotoxic adulterants with which street heroin was (and is) often mixed to extend its value through an increase in weight or bulk.

In parallel with the declining incidence of HAN, human immunodeficiency virus-associated nephropathy (HIVAN) is being diagnosed more frequently among heroin addicts with HIV infection (see Chapter 3.12). HIVAN also presents with nephrotic syndrome and rapidly progressing renal failure, and in some inner-city communities of the United States, it can cause up to 38 per cent of endstage renal failure. Renal biopsy usually reveals characteristic collapsing glomerular tuft with epithelial cell prominence. Localized segmental sclerosis of the tuft can also occur. A recent report of a case of clinical and histological

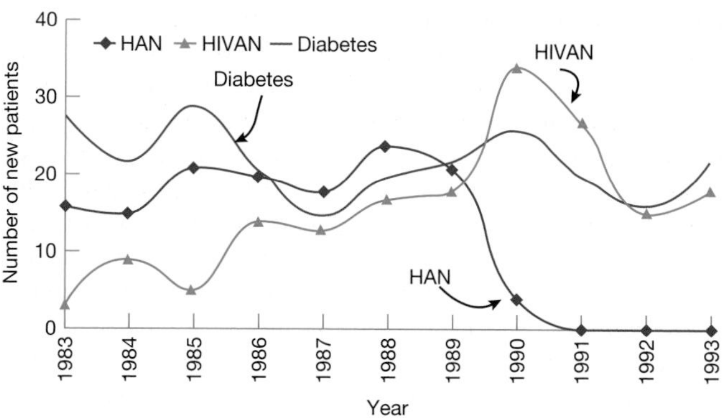

Fig. 1 Incidence of endstage renal disease by renal diagnosis at King's County Hospital, New York City. Note that heroin-associated nephropathy (HAN) decreased sharply in 1990 and was absent from 1991 to 1993. New cases of HIV-associated nephropathy (HIVAN) decreased from 1990, but still amounted to 15–23 cases per year. (Reproduced from Friedman and Jao, 1995, with permission.)

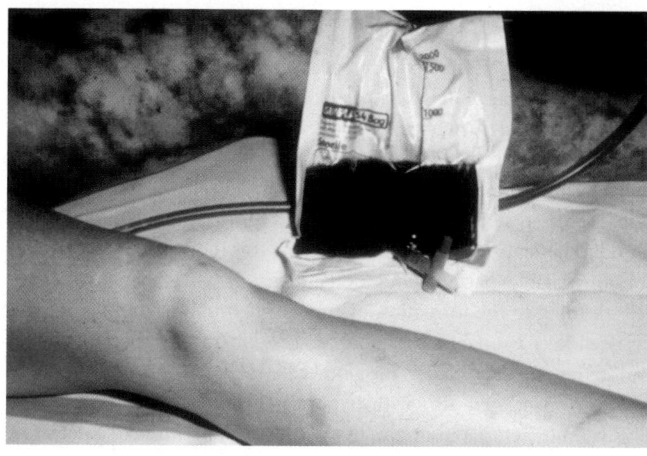

Fig. 2 The characteristic ischaemic mottling of the left leg as a consequence of inadvertent femoral intra-arterial injection of temazepam. The urine is dark with myoglobinuria.

resolution of HIVAN following treatment with triple antiretroviral therapy and reduction in viral load supports the hypothesis that the virus has a direct cytopathic effect on the kidney (Crowe *et al.* 2000).

A postmortem study from the Institute of Forensic Medicine, University of Bonn, reviewed 179 renal specimens from autopsies of Caucasian individuals known to be intravenous drug addicts (Dettmeyer *et al.* 1998). One hundred and five specimens (61.7 per cent) showed a monolymphocytic membranoproliferative GN and 48 specimens (45.7 per cent) deposits of IgM. No cases with focal segmental glomerulosclerosis, as reported in male African-American intravenous drug addicts, were found.

Benzodiazepines

Abused temazepam and diazepam usually originate from legal prescriptions or thefts from pharmacies. Temazepam is now a controlled drug and may be taken alone or as part of a 'cocktail' of drugs. Approximately 70 per cent of injecting drug users have used temazepam at some time (Crowe *et al.* 2000). Acute renal failure has been described following inadvertent intra-arterial temazepam injection. This provokes limb ischaemia as a result of particulate embolization and subsequent rhabdomyolysis and myoglobinuria (Fig. 2). Severe but temporary dialysis-dependent renal failure was present in several patients in one series (Deighan *et al.* 2000).

The liquid contents of the original gelatin capsule were reformulated to a hard gel to make temazepam more resistant to misuse. Despite this, misusers were still able to inject the gel by prewarming it in a microwave oven. Temazepam is now only available in tablet form, so some of the worse complications of its injection can now be prevented.

Mushrooms

The mushroom species *Panaeolus muscaria* and *Psilocybe* (including *Psilocybe semilanceata*—'liberty cap', 'magic mushrooms') are hallucinogenic when ingested (Crowe *et al.* 2000). In the United Kingdom, it is legal to pick and eat these mushrooms but not to prepare them in any way. They are not themselves nephrotoxic; however, correct mushroom identification is difficult and inadvertent ingestion of poisonous species is not uncommon. *Cortinarius* mushrooms which contain the nephrotoxic substance orellanine (see Chapter 10.2) can also masquerade as 'magic mushrooms' (Crowe *et al.* 2000). Oliguric renal failure may develop over 5–12 days after ingestion of *Cortinarius*. In some patients the renal failure is transient but in others it may be irreversible.

Cannabis and tobacco smoking

Renal complications are rare following cannabis abuse, but one case of renal infarction has been reported in a heavy cannabis smoker perhaps due to peripheral vasodilatation from tetrahydrocannobinol (Crowe *et al.* 2000). The renal complications of tobacco smoking are discussed in Chapter 4.12.2.

Solvents

The deliberate inhalation of volatile solvents ('glue sniffing') first emerged as a form of substance abuse in the early 1960s with the inhalation of glues used most frequently in the construction of model aeroplanes. The practice has diversified to include the use of adhesive cements, aerosol paints, lacquer thinners, typewriter correction fluids, and fuels (Ramsay *et al.* 1989). These products contain a number of volatile substances including toluene, *n*-hexane, methyl ketones, chlorohydrocarbons, and benzene. The 'high' from solvent inhalation is similar to alcohol intoxication. In addition, solvents can rapidly cause hallucinations of short duration (15–30 min). Serious cardiac, pulmonary, hepatic, neurological, and renal complications may develop, as well as sudden death (Crowe *et al.* 2000).

The nephrotoxic insult of volatile glues appears to be principally due to toluene. Various renal lesions have been associated with its abuse: microhaematuria, pyuria and proteinuria, distal renal tubular acidosis and Fanconi's syndrome, urinary calculi, GN, Goodpasture's syndrome, acute tubular necrosis, hepatorenal syndrome, and acute and chronic interstitial nephritis (Crowe *et al.* 2000). Toluene is thought to cause renal tubular acidosis by inducing permeability changes in the nephron allowing retrograde diffusion of the secreted acid. Chronic acid retention causes titration of alkaline bone salts leading to calcium mobilization, hypercalcuria, and hence urinary calculi (Crowe *et al.* 2000).

Alcohol

In postmortem studies 50–100 per cent of patients with hepatic cirrhosis due to alcohol have an associated glomerulopathy, histologically identical to IgA nephropathy (Newell 1987). In life, the disease is characterized by microhaematuria and proteinuria, but tends to remain clinically silent. Macrohaematuria and renal insufficiency are rare. Increased serum polymeric IgA and IgA immune complexes are found in patients with alcoholic cirrhosis. It is thought that portacaval shunting enables bacterial and food antigens to bypass hepatic Kupffer cells, leading to the formation of circulating immune complexes. The diseased liver is unable to catabolize these or transfer them into bile, and so they are deposited in the glomeruli. Heavy alcohol consumption has been associated also with hypomagnesaemia (see Chapter 2.5). This is multifactorial in origin, but is at least in part due to a defect in renal tubular function.

Summary

The abuse of substances both causes, and exacerbates, a wide spectrum of kidney disease. This spectrum will hopefully change as users modify their behaviour as a result of fashion and health consciousness in the face of health promotion messages. Increasingly, and unfortunately, drug abuse now must be considered in the differential diagnosis of any patient with unexplained renal pathology.

Exposure to organic solvents and renal disease

Although the nitro-, amino-, or chloro-derivatives of benzene have a known association with uroepithelial tumours (Andrews and Snyder 1991) (see Chapter 18.3); there is now a considerable body of evidence suggesting a role for organic solvent exposure, usually at the worksite, in the development of non-neoplastic renal diseases (Bell and Mason 2000). The term 'organic solvents' refers to hydrocarbons such as aliphatic, alicyclic, aromatic, halogenated hydrocarbons (carbon tetrachloride, trichloroethylene), and the commonly abused solvents toluene and xylene. Hydrocarbons are often used as solvents in industrial manufacturing practices because of their lipid solubility. Solvents are absorbed through the lungs, skin, and gastrointestinal tract (Andrews and Snyder 1991) and are metabolized usually by cytochrome P450-dependent enzymes present in the liver, kidneys, lungs, and other tissues. Solvents are known to be neurotoxicants affecting both the peripheral and central nervous systems. Occupational exposure to hydrocarbons with resulting nephrotoxicity may be a factor in the preponderance of male patients in dialysis programmes for endstage renal failure (Finn and Harmer 1979). In this section, we review the evidence linking organic solvents from occupational or environmental exposure and the development of renal disease.

Case reports and experimental studies

Case reports describe an association between organic-solvent exposure and the development of acute tubular necrosis (Landry and Langlois 1998; Li *et al.* 1999), chronic tubulointerstitial damage (Navarte *et al.* 1989), and different types of GN and Goodpasture's syndrome (Klavis and Drommer 1970; Beirne and Brennan 1972; Cagnoli *et al.* 1980; Daniell *et al.* 1988). In parallel with these clinical observations, experimental studies in animals have identified organic-solvent exposure as a factor in the development of both tubular and glomerular lesions (Bell and Mason 2000). Thus, glomerular lesions similar to those found in Goodpasture's disease have been induced in rats exposed to petroleum vapours (Klavis and Drommer 1970) and the nephrotic syndrome with severe GN and renal impairment, which is not dependent on either deposition of fibrin or coagulative mechanisms, has been induced in rats fed *N,N'*diacetylbenzidine (*N,N'*-DAB) (Harman 1970). Similarly, mesangial proliferative GN and tubulointerstitial disease, which again did not appear to be mediated by glomerular deposits of antigen–antibody complexes, has been described in rats after the administration of carbon tetrachloride (Zimmerman *et al.* 1983). For a more detailed review of this area the reader is referred to Ravnskov (2000).

Case–control studies

The majority of case–control studies from different research groups have reported a significantly greater exposure to organic solvents in patients with GN compared with control groups (Bell and Mason 2000) and have demonstrated substantial evidence in favour of a role for chronic solvent exposure in the development of various types of GN such as proliferative GN, IgA nephropathy, membranous GN, post-streptococcal GN, or rapidly progressive GN. Among the 16 studies in which estimated relative risks were either reported or calculated, there was a 1.7–10.5-fold increase in risk for the development of GN with renal impairment among solvent-exposed individuals (Ravnskov 2000).

The evidence presented in approximately one-third of these studies may be criticized on one of the following grounds: (i) the unsatisfactory nature of the control group; (ii) the possible bias of the unblinded interviewers; (iii) the failure to consider recall bias; (iv) failure to define a credible measure of solvent exposure; and (v) the diversity of glomerular disease patterns.

The most recent studies have addressed these criticisms. In one study (Yaqoob *et al.* 1992), exposure to solvents was assessed blindly by telephone interview and questionnaire in patients with endstage renal disease due to biopsy-proven primary GN and in whom there was no evidence of systemic disease. Their solvent exposure was compared with that of closely matched control groups of normal subjects and patients with other forms of kidney disease. Solvent-exposure scores derived from the results of the blind questionnaires were significantly higher in the patients with primary GN than the normal subjects and the internal control group. Moreover, more detailed assessment of the type of solvent exposure in patients with GN compared with normal controls showed significantly greater exposure scores in the patients to petroleum products, greasing/degreasing agents, and paints/glue and a resulting estimated relative risk of developing GN with each type of solvent exposure, respectively, of 15.5, 5.3, and 2.0 times greater than normal. Furthermore, in patients with primary GN the solvent-exposure score was related to their serum creatinine concentration at the time of presentation suggesting a dose–effect relationship (Fig. 3). There was no significant difference in tobacco and alcohol consumption among subjects in the different groups, and it was concluded that occupational exposure to organic solvents may play an important role in the development of primary GN with renal impairment.

A further possible link between renal impairment at presentation in patients with different forms of GN and solvent exposure was identified

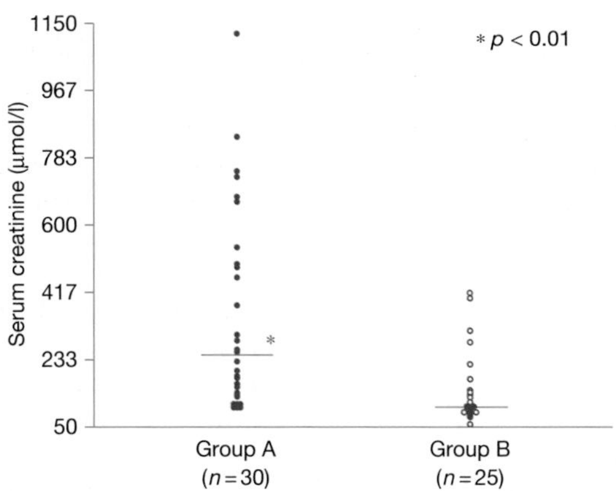

Fig. 3 Plasma creatinine (μmol/l) in patients with primary GN with heavy (group A) and moderate to low (group B) hydrocarbon exposure at the time of their presentation. Bar indicates mean and * indicates the level of significance. (Reproduced from Yaqoob *et al.* 1992, with permission of Oxford University Press.)

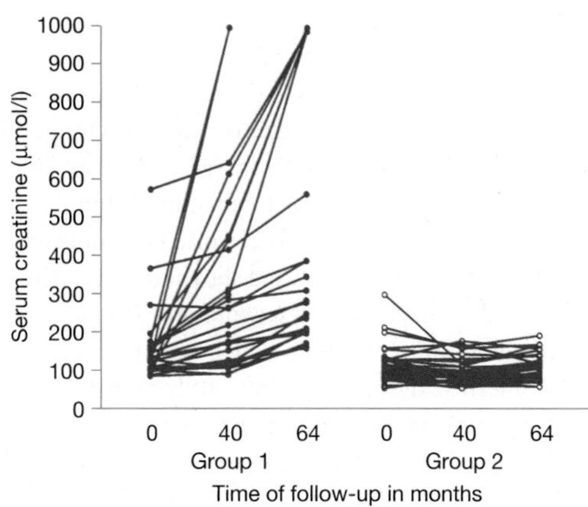

Fig. 4 Plasma creatinine concentration in group 1 GN patients with progressive renal impairment associated with high occupational organic-solvent exposure compared to group 2 GN patients without progressive renal impairment and associated with low occupational organic-solvent exposure. (Reproduced from Yaqoob *et al.* 1993a,b, with permission of Oxford University Press.)

by Stengel *et al.* (1995). This large study identified, in patients with different forms of GN, that the likelihood of previous organic-solvent exposure was greatest in those patients presenting with renal failure. A recent meta-analysis of 16 patient groups from 14 case–control studies (Ravnskov 2000) investigated this association in more detail by calculating the relative risk of development of GN in solvent-exposed individuals according to the stage of disease at presentation. The likelihood of previous solvent exposure was found to increase according to the level of renal impairment at presentation from 0.95 in patients with early or acute GN to 3.1 in chronic renal failure increasing to 5.9 in patients with endstage renal failure secondary to GN. This meta-analysis further strengthens the association between hydrocarbon exposure and progressive renal impairment in patients with diverse histological forms of GN.

This association is not confined to only patients with progressive GN. In a carefully designed study, the role of solvent exposure was investigated in the development of diabetic nephropathy (Yaqoob *et al.* 1994b). Exposure scores to solvents were significantly greater in patients with incipient (microalbuminuria) and overt (macroalbuminuria) diabetic nephropathy than those with no clinical evidence of nephropathy ($r = 0.4$, $p < 0.01$) suggestive of a dose–effect relationship also in patients with diabetic nephropathy. One conclusion of this study suggested that solvent exposure may play a role in the progression of diabetic nephropathy in patients with insulin-dependent diabetes mellitus (IDDM).

Solvent exposure and progression of renal failure

Further studies have demonstrated that both the histological severity of proliferative GN (Bell *et al.* 1985a) and the level of renal impairment at presentation (Yaqoob *et al.* 1992) are associated with the intensity and duration of antecedent solvent exposure. Likewise, accelerated progression of renal failure in patients with GN and continued heavy solvent exposure has been reported (Bell *et al.* 1985b; Ravnskov 1986). More recently, a cohort study specifically investigated the role of solvent exposure in the progression of renal failure in patients with primary GN (Yaqoob *et al.* 1993a,b). The results of this study suggested that such patients with progressive renal failure had greater solvent exposure and worse renal impairment at presentation than those with stable or improving renal function. Moreover, the patients with declining renal function were more likely to have had continued occupational solvent exposure following the diagnosis of GN (Fig. 4). They were also more likely to have persistent heavy proteinuria and to develop hypertension than those without progressive renal failure. Tubular damage, as suggested by biochemical parameters of increased tubular enzymuria and low molecular weight proteinuria, was also significantly worse in the patients with progressive renal failure, which indicates that this defect also played a part in the progression of their renal disease. This study highlights an additional important role for continued solvent exposure in the progression of renal failure in patients with primary GN.

Histological evidence of tubulointerstitial damage in primary glomerular disorders appears to correlate with severity of renal impairment and can predict the future outcome of renal disease (Cameron 1992). The relationship between solvent exposure and morphological parameters of tubulointerstitial damage was carefully examined in 59 patients with biopsy proven primary GN (Yaqoob *et al.* 1994a). Solvent exposure correlated significantly with both relative interstitial volume, an index of tubulointerstitial damage, and serum creatinine. Furthermore, solvent-exposure scores were significantly greater in patients with progressive renal failure compared with those with stable or improving renal function, suggesting a close and possibly causal relationship between occupational organic-solvent exposure, tubulopathy, and progressive renal failure in patients with GN.

Cross-sectional studies

The rarity of GN in the general population makes a prospective cohort analytic study of solvents in exposed populations logistically impossible. Cross-sectional studies comparing parameters of renal dysfunction in solvent-exposed and matched non-exposed workers is feasible and the few such studies performed suggest an association between solvent exposure and renal damage (Pai *et al.* 1998; Bell and Mason 2000). Thus, in one study, workers exposed to moderate amounts of styrene, toluene, and a mixture of mainly aromatic compounds were found to have slightly but significantly increased urinary excretions of erythrocytes, white/tubular epithelial cells, and albumin compared with a non-exposed group. Likewise, workers mainly exposed to aliphatic and acyclic hydrocarbons were shown to have increased proteinuria and tubular enzymuria (lysozyme and β-glucuronidase) in the absence of albuminuria, findings which were indicative of tubular rather than glomerular dysfunction. In a study of 20,000 workers the prevalence of proteinuria was found to be higher in those exposed to hydrocarbons than in those who were not. A significant shift of the cumulative frequency distribution of the urinary albumin concentration towards higher values has also been shown in workers exposed to styrene.

Two other studies have used more sensitive markers of kidney damage. In one, male oil refinery workers with exposures to hydrocarbons below the current US threshold limit values were found to have significantly higher urinary excretions of albumin and brush-border renal tubular antigen and a higher prevalence of circulating antilaminin antibodies than a non-exposed group. In the other, the study population was classified into heavy, moderate, and low hydrocarbon-exposure groups (based on retrospective lifelong hydrocarbon-exposure scores using a method similar to that used in a recent study by Yaqoob *et al.* 1992) and the findings were compared with those of a control group. The control group was unsatisfactory because 50 per cent of the controls had a past history of heavy metal exposure. Despite introducing this bias, the workers exposed to hydrocarbons were found to have an increase in the urinary excretion of glycosaminoglycans (a marker of glomerular basement-membrane damage) and fractional albumin clearance. The latter effect may have been secondary to an interaction between hypertension and hydrocarbon exposure. Further studies have suggested that this interaction was significantly associated with abnormal proteinuria, an increased serum laminin concentration, albumin excretion rate, and NAG activity. Furthermore, exposure to hydrocarbons seemed to accelerate the age-dependent decline in kidney function (Bell and Mason 2000).

Similarly, two recent studies yielded contrasting conclusions about renal function in subjects occupationally exposed to perchloroethylene. In one (Solet and Robins 1991), no association could be found between exposure and renal outcome in workers exposed to perchloroethylene in dry cleaning shops. In the other, the findings were consistent with both glomerular and tubular dysfunction in workers exposed to low levels of perchloroethylene in dry cleaning (Fig. 5) and indicated that solvent-exposed workers, especially dry cleaners, may need to be monitored for the possible development of chronic renal disease (Mutti *et al.* 1992).

In view of the ongoing controversy in this area of nephrology we undertook one further such cross-sectional study in car manufacturing plant workers exposed to various solvents at their worksite (Yaqoob *et al.* 1993a,b). The paint sprayers exposed to paint-based solvents had a significantly higher prevalence of renal impairment than the other groups (Fig. 6) and a higher prevalence of abnormal total proteinuria and enzymuria than controls. Workers exposed to petroleum-based paints had a significantly higher prevalence of abnormal proteinuria, transferrinuria, tubular proteinuria, and enzymuria but albuminuria was similar in all groups. These results suggested that chronic solvent exposure may be associated with both clinical and subclinical renal dysfunction.

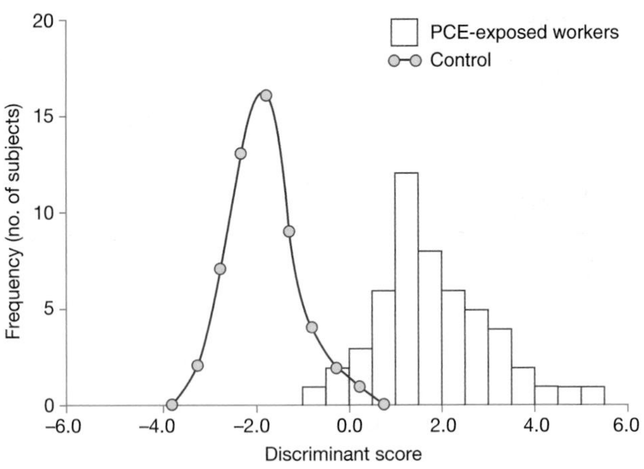

Fig. 5 Distribution of workers exposed to perchloroethylene (PCE) and matched controls classified on the basis of 13 selected early markers of renal damage. According to discriminant function 87 per cent of subjects were correctly classified ($\chi^2 = 69.9$, 13 df, $p < 0.001$). [Reproduced from Mutti *et al.*, 1992, with permission of Elsevier Science (*The Lancet*, 1992, 340, 189–193).]

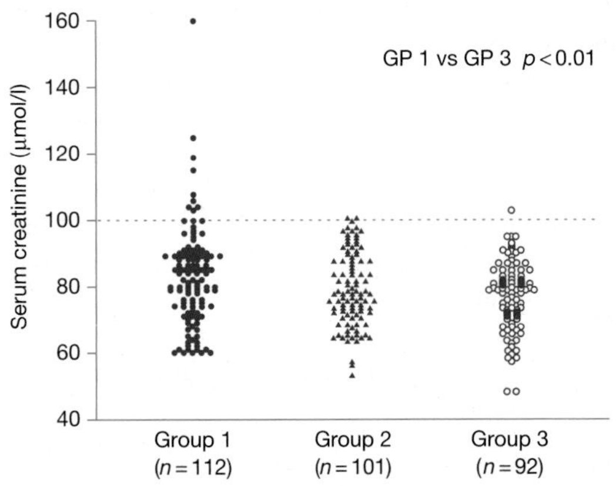

Fig. 6 Plasma creatinine concentrations in three groups of workers in a car plant. Group 1 (paint sprayers) had a significantly different distribution from group 2 (transmission shop workers) and group 3 (body shop workers). Evidence of renal improvement was present in 11 per cent of group 1. The dotted line represents the upper reference limit derived from external controls. (Reproduced from Yaqoob *et al.* 1993a,b, with permission of Oxford University Press.)

Recently, we have found evidence of endothelial activation and early basement-membrane disturbance resulting in autoantibody production as suggested by depressed serum laminin (marker of basement-membrane turnover) and elevated autoantibodies to laminin and Goodpasture's antigen in individuals occupationally exposed to paint- and petroleum-based solvents (Fig. 7). Unfortunately, there are no follow-up data on the renal outcome of these subjects. However, a recent study (Pai *et al.* 1998) of a matched cohort of paint sprayers from a

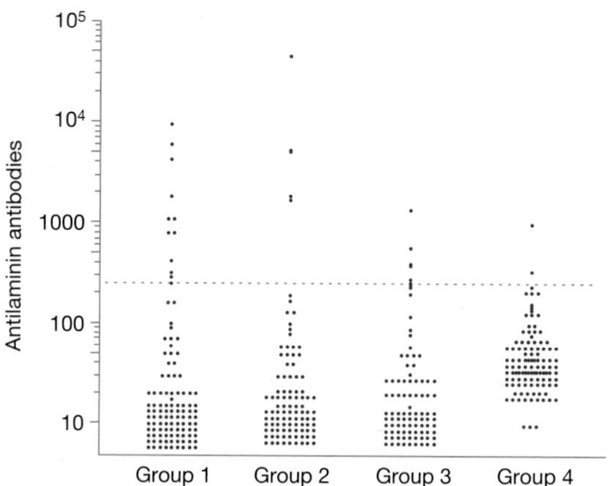

Fig. 7 Distribution of levels of serum antilaminin antibodies in three groups of workers in a car plant (group 1, paint sprayers; group 2, transmission workers; group 3, body shop workers; and group 4, normal external controls). In group 1 there was approximately a sixfold increase in the proportion of subjects with antilaminin antibody results compared with controls. (Reproduced from Stevenson *et al.* 1995, with permission of Oxford University Press.)

different car plant suggested that proximal tubular damage and renal dysfunction may be reduced by improved respiratory and skin protection at the work site.

Cohort studies

A cohort study involves a sample of a population exposed to solvents who are compared with an age- and sex-matched cohort of unexposed individuals who are then followed for an outcome assessment such as mortality due to renal failure. Such studies may offer valuable information in the investigation of the association between solvent exposure and renal diseases. However, the diagnostic categories of 'nephritis and nephrosis' or 'genitourinary diseases' are likely to be invalid representations of renal mortality. Thus, in four large cohort studies of solvent-exposed workers the risk of death (standardized mortality ratios) from renal causes was lower than otherwise expected in occupationally exposed cohorts (Bell and Mason 2000). The basic assumption for mortality studies is that the toxic effects are lethal. Such studies cast little light upon possible slight-to-moderate effects of exposure. Furthermore, the outcomes of 'register studies' are always difficult to interpret; diagnostic criteria may vary between and even within studies and the exposures are often vaguely or too generally defined. This may partly be explained by the influence of the well-documented 'healthy worker effect' on non-cancer mortality frequently observed in occupational cohorts. Moreover, mortality studies do not take into consideration those workers who take early retirement on health grounds (e.g. patients with endstage renal failure requiring dialysis treatment), although the medical condition may eventually account for the individual's death (Bell and Mason 2000).

Mechanisms of solvent-induced nephrotoxicity

The mechanism underlying solvent-induced nephropathy remains speculative and controversial despite solvents being well-recognized tubulotoxins in both clinical and experimental settings (Stevenson *et al.* 1995). GN appears to be mainly an immune-mediated disease and there is experimental and clinical evidence of an immunosuppressive potential of various solvents (Bekesi *et al.* 1978; Ravnskov 1985). Experimentally, solvent exposures have induced glomerular lesions in the presence of concomitant tubulointerstitial injury (Bell and Mason 2000). It is therefore possible to speculate that in susceptible individuals low-grade tubular damage from chronic exposure to solvents may provoke local autoimmunity by releasing either sequestered or altered tubular and basement-membrane antigens (antibodies to proximal tubular antigens, laminin, Goodpasture's antigens) with activation or damage of the overlying endothelium (Stevenson *et al.* 1995), which results in the development of GN (Nishikawa *et al.* 1993). Autoimmunity may be favoured by the immunosuppressive effects of solvent exposure (Bekesi *et al.* 1978; Ravnskov 1985). Furthermore, carbon tetrachloride nephrotoxicity can be inhibited by whole body irradiation exposed at each injection (Ogawa *et al.* 1992), favouring the role of primary tubular damage and local autoimmunity in the pathogenesis of solvent-induced nephropathy.

An alternative hypothesis is that potentially glomerulotoxic immune factors arise independently of solvent exposure and that solvents merely facilitate the deposition of these mediators of immune damage in renal tissue (Bell and Mason 2000). However, occupational exposure to solvents is widespread and GN and tubular interstitial disease are infrequently seen, which could suggest the operation of possible genetic or idiosyncratic factors in this association.

However, a recent report of a significant difference in the prevalence of polymorphisms of phase II solvent-metabolizing enzymes, GSTmu and NAT, in patients with membranous nephropathy (Pai *et al.* 1997) were not confirmed in a larger study (Gradden *et al.* 2001). Nonetheless, with improved worksite protection and monitoring of exposed subjects the potential risks of nephrotoxicity from solvent exposure should gradually reduce. Should genetic associations be identified, however, ethical issues regarding workforce screening and genetic suitability for employment in solvent-related industries may prove more difficult issues.

Acknowledgements

The section on organic solvents is an abbreviated, amended, and updated version of a chapter: Organic solvents and renal disease, by M. Yaqoob and G.M. Bell. In *Horizons in Medicine No. 6*. Royal Collage of Physicians, published by Blackwell Science Ltd in 1995, and appears with permission of the publisher.

The section on substance misuse is an abbreviated, amended and updated version of an article by A. Crowe, M. Howse, G.M. Bell, and J. Henry. In *Quarterly Journal of Medicine*, 2000, **93**, 147–152 and appears with permission of Oxford University Press.

References

Andrews, L. S. and Snyder, R. Toxic effects of solvents and vapors. In *Casarett and Doull's Toxicology; The Basic Science of Poisons* (ed. M. O. Amdur, J. Doull, and C. D. Klaussen), pp. 681–721. New York: Pergamon Press, 1991.

Beirne, G. J. and Brennan, J. T. (1972). Glomerulonephritis associated with hydrocarbon solvents. *Archives of Environmental Health* **25**, 365–369.

Bekesi, J. G. *et al.* (1978). Lymphocyte function of Michigan dairy farmers exposed to polybrominated diphenyls. *Science* **199**, 1207–1209.

Bell, G. M. *et al.* (1985a). Proliferative GN and exposure to organic solvents. *Nephron* **40**, 161–165.

Bell, G. M. *et al.* (1985b). End-stage renal disease associated with occupational exposure to organic solvents. *Proceedings EDTA-ERA* **22**, 725–729.

Bell, G. M. and Mason, H. Nephrotoxic effects of workplace exposures. In *Hunter's Disease of Occupations* 9th edn. (ed. P. J. Baxter, P. H. Adams, T. Aw, A. Cockroft, and J. M. Harrington), pp. 854–866. London: Arnold, 2000.

Bingham, C., Beaman, M., Nicholls, A. J., and Anthony, P. P. (1998). Necrotising renal vasculopathy resulting in chronic renal failure after ingestion of methamphetamine and 3,4-methylenedioxymethamphetamine. *Nephrology, Dialysis, Transplantation* **13**, 2654–2655.

Brecklin, C. S. *et al.* (1998). Prevalence of hypertension in chronic cocaine users. *American Journal of Hypertension* **11**, 1279–1283.

Cagnoli, L. *et al.* (1980). Relationship between hydrocarbon exposure and the nephrotic syndrome. *British Medical Journal* **280**, 1068–1069.

Cameron, J. S. (1992). Tubular and interstitial factors in the progression of GN. *Paediatric Nephrology* **6**, 292–303.

Crowe, A. V. *et al.* (2000). Substance abuse and the kidney. *Quarterly Journal of Medicine* **93**, 147–152.

Cunningham, E. E. *et al.* (1980). Heroin nephropathy. A clinicopathologic and epidemiologic study. *American Journal of Medicine* **68**, 47–53.

Daniell, W. E., Couser, W. G., and Rosenstock, L. (1988). Occupational solvent exposure and GN. *Journal of the American Medical Association* **259**, 2280–2283.

Deighan, C. J., Wong, K. M., McLaughlin, K. J., and Harden, P. (2000). Rhabdomyolysis and acute renal failure resulting from alcohol and drug abuse. *Quarterly Journal of Medicine* **93**, 29–33.

Dettmeyer, R., Wessling, B., and Madea, B. (1998). Heroin associated nephropathy—a post-mortem study. *Forensic Science International* **95**, 109–116.

Drugscope. *The UK Drug Situation 2000.* The UK report to the European Monitoring Centre for Drugs and Drug Addiction (EMCDDA). London, 2000.

Dunea, G. *et al.* (1995). Role of cocaine in end-stage renal disease in some hypertensive African-Americans. *American Journal of Nephrology* **15**, 5–9.

Fahal, I. H., Sallomi, D. F., Yaqoob, M., and Bell, G. M. (1992). Acute renal failure after ecstasy. *British Medical Journal* **307**, 1399.

Finn, R. and Harmer, D. (1979). Aetiological implications of sex ratio in GN. *Lancet* **1**, 1194.

Friedman, E. A. and Tao, T. K. (1995). Disappearance of uraemia due to heroin-associated nephropathy. *American Journal of Kidney Diseases* **25**, 689–693.

Gradden, C. W. *et al.* (2001). Membranous nephropathy, hydrocarbon exposure and genetic variants of hydrocarbon detoxification. *Quarterly Journal of Medicine* **94**, 79–87.

Grossman, R. A. *et al.* (1974). Non-traumatic rhabdomyolysis and acute renal failure. *New England Journal of Medicine* **291**, 807–811.

Harman, J. W. (1970). Chronic GN and nephrotic syndrome induced in rats with *N, N'*-diacetyl benzidine. *Journal of Pathology* **104**, 119–128.

Henry, J. A. *et al.* (1992). Toxicity and deaths from 3,4-methylenedioxymethamphetamine ('ecstasy'). *Lancet* **340**, 384–387.

Klavis, G. and Drommer, W. (1970). Goodpasture's syndrome and the effects of benzene. *Archives of Toxicology* **26**, 40–55.

Lam, S., and Ballou, S. P. (1992). Reversible scleroderma renal crisis after cocaine use. *New England Journal of Medicine* **326**, 1435.

Landry, J. and Langlois, S. (1998). Acute exposure to aliphatic hydrocarbons: an unusual case of acute tubular necrosis. *Archives of Internal Medicine* **158**, 1821–1823.

Lange, R. A. and Hillis, L. D. (2001). Cardiovascular complications of cocaine use. *New England Journal of Medicine* **345**, 351–358.

Li, F. K. *et al.* (1999). Acute renal failure and immersion in sea water polluted by diesel oil. *American Journal of Kidney Diseases* **34**, 1–5.

Maxwell, D. L., Polkey, M. I., and Henry, J. A. (1993). Hyponatraemia and catatonic stupor after taking 'ecstasy'. *British Medical Journal* **307**, 1399.

Mutti, A. *et al.* (1992). Nephropathies and exposure to perchloroethylene in dry cleaners. Lancet **340**, 189–193.

Navarte, J., Saba, S. R., and Ramirez, G. (1989). Occupational exposure to organic solvents causing chronic tubulo-interstitial nephritis. *Archives of Internal Medicine* **149**, 154–159.

Newell, C. G. (1987). Cirrhotic GN: incidence, morphology, clinical features, and pathogenesis. *American Journal of Kidney Diseases* **9**, 183–190.

Nishikawa, K. *et al.* (1993). Antibodies to intercellular adhesion molecule 1/lymphocyte function associated antigen 1 prevent crescent formation in rat auto-immune GN. *Journal of Experimental Medicine* **177**, 667–677.

Norris, K. C. *et al.* (2001). Cocaine use, hypertension and end-stage renal disease. *American Journal of Kidney Diseases* **38**, 523–528.

Nzerue, C. M., Hewan-Lowe, K., and Riley, L. J., Jr. (2000). Cocaine and the kidney: a synthesis of pathophysiologic and clinical perspectives. *American Journal of Kidney Diseases* **35**, 783–795.

Ogawa, M. *et al.* (1992). Studies on chronic renal injuries induced by carbon tetrachloride; selective inhibition of the nephrotoxicity by irradiation. *Nephron* **60**, 68–73.

Pai, P. *et al.* (1997). Genetic variants of microsomal metobolism and susceptibility to hydrocarbon-associated GN. *Quarterly Journal of Medicine* **90**, 693–698.

Pai, P., Stevenson, A., Mason, H., and Bell, G. M. (1998). Occupational hydrocarbon exposure and nephrotoxicity; a cohort study and literature review. *Postgraduate Medical Journal* **741**, 225–228.

Ramsay, J. D., Anderson, H. R., Bloor, K., and Flanagan, R. J. (1989). An introduction to the practice, prevalence, and chemical toxicology of volatile substance abuse. *Human Toxicology* **8**, 261–269.

Ravnskov, U. (1985). Possible mechanisms of hydrocarbon associated glomerulo-nephritis. *Clinical Nephrology* **23**, 294–298.

Ravnskov, U. (1986). Influence of hydrocarbon exposure on the course of glomerulo-nephritis. *Nephron* **42**, 156–160.

Ravnskov, U. (2000). Hydrocarbons may worsen renal function in glomerulonephritis a meta-analysis of the case–control studies. *American Journal of Industrial Medicine* **37**, 599–606.

Roth, D. *et al.* (1988). Acute rhabdomyolysis associated with cocaine intoxication. *New England Journal of Medicine* **319**, 673–677.

Solet, D. and Robins, T. G. (1991). Renal function in dry cleaning workers exposed to perchloroethylene. *American Journal of Industrial Medicine* **20**, 601–614.

Sreepada Rao, T. K. S., Nicastri, A. D., and Friedman, E. A. (1977). Renal consequences of narcotic abuse. *Advances in Nephrology* **7**, 261–290.

Stengel, B. *et al.* (1995). Organic solvent exposure may increase the risk of glomerular nephropathies with chronic renal failure. *International Journal of Epidemiology* **24**, 427–434.

Stevenson, A. *et al.* (1995). Biochemical markers of basement membrane disturbances and occupational exposure to hydrocarbons and mixed solvents. *Quarterly Journal of Medicine* **88**, 23–28.

Welch, R. D., Todd, K., and Krause, G. S. (1991). Incidence of cocaine-associated rhabdomyolysis. *Annals of Emergency Medicine* **20**, 154–157.

Woodrow, G. and Turney, J. H. (1999). Ecstasy-induced renal vasculitis. *Nephrology, Dialysis, Transplantation* **14**, 798.

Woodrow, G., Harnden, P., and Turney, J. H. (1995). Acute renal failure due to accelerated hypertension following ingestion of ecstasy. *Nephrology, Dialysis, Transplantation* **10**, 399–400.

Yaqoob, M., Bell, G. M., Percy, D., and Finn, R. (1992). Primary GN and hydrocarbon exposure: a case–control study and literature review. *Quarterly Journal of Medicine* **301**, 409–418.

Yaqoob, M. *et al.* (1993a). Renal impairment due to hydrocarbon exposure. *Quarterly Journal of Medicine* **86**, 165–174.

Yaqoob, M., Stevenson, A., Mason H., and Bell, G. M. (1993b). Hydrocarbon exposure and tubular damage: additional factors in the progression of renal failure in primary GN. *Quarterly Journal of Medicine* **86**, 661–667.

Yaqoob, M. *et al.* (1994a). Relationship between hydrocarbon exposure and nephropathology in primary GN. *Nephrology, Dialysis, Transplantation* **9**, 1575–1579.

Yaqoob, M. *et al.* (1994b). High hydrocarbon exposure in diabetic nephropathy. *Diabetic Medicine* **11**, 789–793.

Zimmerman, S. W., Norbach, D. P., and Powers, K. (1983). Carbon tetrachloride nephrotoxicity in rats with reduced renal mass. *Archives of Pathology and Laboratory Medicine* **17**, 264–269.

4.12.2 Smoking and the kidney

Stephan R. Orth

> I saw several Spaniards on the island of Hispaniola who were reproached because of their bad habits. They answered that it was impossible for them to stop these habits. I cannot understand what kind of pleasure and which advantages they derive from smoking
>
> Bartholome de las Casas (*Historia de las Indias, 1527*)

> Smoking cessation is still the best medicine
>
> J. Taylor Hays *et al.* (*Postgraduate Medicine, 1998*)

Introduction

In his manual '*Tobacco and the Organism*' Lickint (1939) reviewed the association between smoking and renal damage. In more recent times Christiansen (1978) noted that smoking confers an increased risk for the development of diabetic nephropathy in patients with type 1 diabetes mellitus. Although these early findings had been confirmed by others, including patients with type 2 diabetes, it was not until 1997 that the nephrological community became aware of smoking as a 'new' renal risk factor (Orth *et al.* 1997). Since then, interest in the topic and knowledge about the adverse renal effects of smoking has increased continuously.

Although large prospective studies are lacking, there is convincing epidemiological evidence that smoking must be considered as one of the most important renal risk factors, particularly for patients with pre-existing renal disease (Table 1). Recent evidence suggests that smoking may impair renal function in patients with apparently normal kidneys. Once in endstage renal failure (ESRF), continued smoking adversely affects the prognosis of patients both on renal replacement therapy and following transplantation, mainly by increasing the risk of cardiovascular complications. Finally, discontinuation of smoking has been shown to be the single most effective measure of prolonging life (Hays *et al.* 1998). This is particularly true in patients with a high cardiovascular risk and there is good evidence that smoking cessation is probably the single most effective measure to retard progression of renal failure (Orth 2002).

Table 1 Epidemiological evidence for smoking-induced impairment of renal function

Subjects with apparently normal kidneys
Dose-dependent increase of urinary albumin excretion rate/proteinuria in cigarette smokers
Dose-dependent increase of the risk of ESRF in male cigarette smokers of the general population
Independent predictor of (micro)albuminuria in patients with primary hypertension
Most powerful predictor of renal functional decline in patients with primary hypertension
Patients with primary or secondary renal disease
Increased risk for progression of renal failure in patients with primary renal disease
In types 1 and 2 diabetes mellitus: independent risk factor for the onset of microalbuminuria, for progression of microalbuminuria to manifest proteinuria (i.e. diabetic nephropathy) and for acceleration of the rate of progression of diabetic nephropathy to ESRF
Patients with a renal transplant
Increased risk for renal allograft loss

Evidence for adverse renal effects of smoking in the general population

Effect of smoking on urinary albumin/protein excretion

The nephrotoxic effect of smoking in the general population is documented by a cross-sectional study in non-diabetic subjects (Pinto-Sietsma *et al.* 2000) which reports that urinary albumin excretion rate correlated to daily cigarette consumption. After adjustment for several potential confounding factors, subjects who smoked less than 20 or greater than 20 cigarettes/day showed a dose-dependent association between smoking and high normal albuminuria relative risk, (RR: 1.33 and 1.98, respectively) and microalbuminuria (RR: 1.92 and 2.15, respectively). In another large study, smoking was associated with increased urinary albumin concentrations far below the microalbuminuric range (Janssen *et al.* 2000). Analysis of a well defined non-diabetic and non-hypertensive subgroup in this latter study revealed that smoking was independently associated with microalbuminuria (Hillege *et al.* 2001). Halimi *et al.* (2000) documented a marked risk of irreversible proteinuria despite moderate smoking. These European results have been confirmed in a large cross-sectional sample of adults in the United States (Hogan *et al.* 2001a).

Effect of smoking on renal function

The question arises as to whether the increase in albuminuria/proteinuria attributable to smoking is paralleled by an increased risk for renal functional deterioration. Halimi *et al.* (2000) found that smokers did not exhibit lower creatinine clearances than those who had never smoked but was even slightly higher in current smokers, even when normotensive and hypertensive subjects were analysed separately. The difference was, however small, particularly in women. The effect of current smoking on creatinine clearance was reversible on stopping smoking. In contrast, data from the prospective Multiple Risk Factor Intervention Trial (MRFIT) indicate that smoking increases the renal risk in the general male population (Klag *et al.* 1996): a dose-dependent increase of the relative risk for ESRF was found in smokers as compared to non-smokers (RR up to 1.69 for heavy smokers) (Whelton *et al.* 1995). The increase in risk was independent of age, ethnicity, income, blood pressure (BP), diabetes mellitus, prior history of myocardial infarction, or serum cholesterol. Unfortunately, this data have only ever been published in abstract form. Information is available only from a retrospective case–control study of 4142 non-diabetic participants in the Cardiovascular Health Study Cohort, all greater than or equal to 65 years of age, who had two measurements of serum creatinine performed at least 3 years apart (Bleyer *et al.* 2000). In this elderly population, the number of cigarettes smoked was highly associated with an increase in serum creatinine (>27 μmol/l). The definition of renal functional deterioration in this study is undoubtedly weak, but smoking may be one of the factors explaining why an impairment of renal function is observed in some but not all elderly subjects. This assumption is in line with data from Minnesota (Goetz *et al.* 1997), in that the decrease in creatinine clearance was greater in ex-smokers and current smokers than in non-smokers.

Thus, we can conclude that (a) smoking definitely increases the risk of albuminuria/proteinuria and (b) there is some evidence indicating that smoking increases the risk of renal functional impairment in the general population, particularly elderly men. However, a large prospective study investigating hard end-points, for example, time to doubling of serum creatinine, is needed for a definite answer.

Adverse renal effects of smoking in patients with primary hypertension

Effect on urinary albumin/protein excretion

Proteinuria is found in 4–18 per cent and albuminuria in 10–25 per cent of patients with primary hypertension. Albuminuria (and even more strongly proteinuria) is an independent predictor of cardiovascular mortality in such patients (Ruilope *et al.* 2001).

The results of earlier studies indicating that smoking confers an increased risk for the presence of micro/macroalbuminuria in patients with primary hypertension have recently been confirmed. The Heart Outcomes Prevention Evaluation (HOPE) Study (Gerstein *et al.* 2000) documented that smoking was an independent determinant of microalbuminuria in all participants (approximately 50 per cent being hypertensive), that is, non-diabetic and diabetic patients with a high cardiovascular risk profile. Furthermore, a recent study (Wachtell *et al.* 2002) found that patients with hypertension and left ventricular hypertrophy smoking greater than 20 cigarettes/day had a 1.6-fold greater prevalence of microalbuminuria and a 3.7-fold higher prevalence of macroalbuminuria than those who have never smoked.

Effect on renal function

Important new information has become available concerning the negative impact of smoking on renal functional deterioration in hypertensive patients. A prospective study of 51 patients with primary hypertension had a mean follow-up of 35.5 months after which, despite reduction of mean arterial BP, plasma creatinine had increased (Regaldo *et al.* 2000). Factors that independently predicted a decline in renal function were smoking, greater initial plasma creatinine, and Black ethnicity, of which smoking was by far the strongest and the only remediable factor. However, the mean rate of increase in plasma creatinine in this small study was more than expected for a representative sample of patients with primary hypertension. Indeed another large prospective study (Perry *et al.* 1995) including Black and non-Black hypertensive male subjects did not find a relation between smoking and the risk of ESRF during prolonged follow-up (minimum of 13.9 years).

Thus, the issue whether or not smoking increases the rate of progression in patients with primary hypertension remains controversial. Considering the proven effects of smoking on albuminuria/proteinuria it is, however, cautious to conclude that smoking has to be considered as a renal risk factor in hypertensive patients.

Adverse renal effects of smoking in patients with renal disease

The effect of smoking in patients with renal disease is of major interest, because it can be anticipated that this population is particularly susceptible to smoking-induced renal damage.

Diabetic nephropathy

The first well-documented reports of an increased risk in smokers were mostly retrospective studies in patients with type 1 diabetes, in whom an increased risk of developing diabetic nephropathy was noted amongst smokers (Christiansen 1978; Telmer *et al.* 1984). In the latter study, the prevalence of diabetic nephropathy was significantly greater among subjects smoking less than 10 or greater than 10 cigarettes/day for more than 1 year (19.2 versus 12.1 per cent) and an increasing frequency of nephropathy was found with increasing cigarette consumption: 13 per cent in patients smoking less than 10 cigarettes/day, but greater than 25 per cent in those smoking more than 30 cigarettes/day. In a cross-sectional study Nórden and Nyberg (1984) analysed smoking habits in 47 matched pairs of patients with type 1 diabetes with and without nephropathy. Patients with nephropathy had a significantly higher smoking index (number of cigarettes smoked/day multiplied by number of years smoking) than control patients. There were also significantly more current smokers, more heavy smokers, and fewer individuals who had never smoked in the group with nephropathy compared to the group without nephropathy.

Since then a number of studies have confirmed an increased renal risk in patients with both types 1 and 2 diabetes who smoke, with an increase in risk of developing microalbuminuria, acceleration in the rate of progression from microalbuminuria to manifest proteinuria and an acceleration of progression to renal failure (Orth 2002).

An association between albuminuria/proteinuria and smoking has also been found among children with type 1 diabetes (Couper *et al.* 1994) and in patients with type 1 diabetes who had survived greater than 30–40 years (Borch-Johnsen *et al.* 1987; Mackin *et al.* 1996). A genetic predisposition of smokers to develop albuminuria is suggested by a strong association between the DD-genotype of the angiotensin-converting enzyme (ACE) gene and microalbuminuria in smokers (Perna *et al.* 2001). As in non-diabetics, microalbuminuria and overt nephropathy are independent and additive predictors of cardiovascular morbidity and mortality (Rossing *et al.* 1996).

The magnitude of this effect of smoking on the risk of diabetics developing microalbuminuria is by no means minor: Chase *et al.* (1991) reported that in young subjects with type 1 diabetes, the prevalence of borderline (>7.6 μg/min) and abnormal (>30 μg/min) urinary albumin excretion rate was 2.8-fold more in smokers than non-smokers. Similarly, the risk of having microalbuminuria shortly after diagnosis of type 2 diabetes is greatly increased in current smokers: the odds ratio for the presence of microalbuminuria was 26.3 for current smoking and 3.42 for a 1 per cent increment in glycosylated HbA_1 (Keller *et al.* 1996). Although the confidence intervals of these latter data were wide, the data indicate the importance of smoking compared to glycaemic control as a classic renal risk factor in diabetes mellitus.

A prospective study (Klein *et al.* 1993) with an observation time of 4 years in patients with type 2 diabetes reported a 2–2.5-fold increase in the relative risk of progression from microalbuminuria to gross proteinuria (>300 mg/day in heavy smokers than in those who had never smoked).

The acceleration of the progression of renal failure induced by smoking is dramatic. Sawicki *et al.* (1994) calculated the adjusted odds ratio for progression of nephropathy in patients with type 1 diabetes, defined as an increase in proteinuria greater than 20 per cent per year and/or a reduction of glomerular filtration rate (GFR) greater than 20 per cent. The odds ratio was 2.74 for each 10 cigarette pack-years. In this study all patients were on intensified insulin and antihypertensive therapy, so that confounding effects of hyperglycaemia and hypertension are minimized. In a study of Biesenbach *et al.* (1994), rate of loss of GFR rate was increased by a factor of 1.44 and 1.66 in smoking as compared to non-smoking patients with types 1 and 2 diabetes, respectively. Thus, the influence of smoking on renal functional decline is similar in types 1 and 2 diabetes.

Chuahirun and Wesson (2002) performed a prospective study to investigate the impact of smoking on progression of renal failure, in patients with type 2 diabetes and manifest nephropathy followed for a mean 5.3 years. The initial plasma creatinine was 93 ± 77 μmol/l in smokers (n = 13) and 95 ± 3 μmol/l in non-smokers (n = 20). At the end of observation time, the increase of serum creatinine was more pronounced in smokers as compared to non-smokers: 157 ± 18 versus 117 ± 4 μmol/l. This difference was not explained by potential confounding factors, and regression analysis revealed that smoking was the only parameter that significantly predicted renal functional decline. These data are of particular importance as BP had been treated according to contemporary standards, including an ACE inhibitor, achieving a mean arterial BP of 92 ±1 mmHg.

Although not comparable, a retrospective case–control study investigating patients with primary renal disease (Orth *et al.* 1998) had reported that ACE inhibitor treatment counteracts the deleterious effect of smoking on renal function. One potential mechanism of how ACE inhibition may protect against smoking-induced decline in renal function may be improvement of smoking-induced vascular dysfunction (Orth *et al.* 2001). Furthermore, despite low plasma renin concentrations there is good evidence that the intrarenal angiotensin II production in patients with type 2 diabetes mellitus is increased (Price *et al.* 1999). Thus, the finding of Chuahirun and Wessen (2002) is counter-intuitive and confirmation in a larger study is required.

That smokers are at greater risk of developing type 2 diabetes (Orth *et al.* 2001) presents a major clinical problem. In a prospective cohort study in non-diabetic males aged 35–59 years Nakanishi *et al.* (2000) found that the relative risk of developing impaired fasting glucose during 5 years of observation was increased 1.62-fold in those who had ever smoked as compared to those who had never smoked. The relative risk of developing type 2 diabetes was dose-dependent, and may be related to the fact that smoking aggravates insulin resistance in healthy smokers in some studies (Orth 2000).

In summary, there is clear evidence that smoking has adverse effects on the onset and evolution of diabetic nephropathy in types 1 and 2 diabetes mellitus. Moreover, the number of cigarettes smoked daily and the number of pack-years of exposure seem to be associated with development of impaired fasting glucose and type 2 diabetes.

Non-diabetic renal disease

There is no evidence in the literature that smoking *per se* induces any type of glomerulonephritis, or any systemic disease involving the kidney (Yaqoob *et al.* 1992; Merkel *et al.* 1994; Wakai *et al.* 1999; Hogan *et al.* 2001b). Good evidence has accumulated, however, that smoking is a major renal risk factor for progression of renal failure in patients with primary renal disease.

Smoking in primary renal disease

In patients with autosomal dominant polycystic kidney disease (ADPKD), Chapman *et al.* (1994) found that individuals with established proteinuria had a greater pack-year smoking history than did their non-proteinuric counterparts. We in turn performed a European retrospective matched case–control study (Orth *et al.* 1998), designed to assess whether smoking in patients with IgA-nephropathy and ADPKD increases the risk of progression to ESRF. Because analysis of smoking (given as pack-years on PY) was similar both these renal diseases, IgA-nephropathy and ADPKD were pooled for statistical analysis using data only from men (the sample size of females being to small). The crude estimators of different amounts of smoking document a dose-dependent increase for the risk of ESRF in male smokers compared to non-smokers or light smokers. After adjustment for possible confounders, multivariate analysis revealed that the risk of ESRF was substantially greater in male smokers without ACE inhibitor treatment, but in contrast the risk for smokers who had received ACE inhibitors was not significantly increased (Table 2). Another case–control study confirmed that male patients with glomerulonephritis who smoke are at increased risk of renal function impairment (Stengel *et al.* 2000), particularly prominent in elderly and hypertensive patients.

Prospective data to support these retrospective studies are needed, but the only data available are from a post hoc analysis of one prospective study (originally performed to evaluate the role of dyslipidaemia in progression of renal failure) in 73 patients with primary renal disease (Samuelsson and Attman 2000). Smoking status at entry was related to the decline in GFR after 3.2 years of follow-up in chronic glomerulonephritis; GFR—5.3 ml/min/year in heavy smokers but only 2.5 ml/min/year in non-smokers—which, however, did not reach significance at a 1 : 20 level.

Systemic diseases involving the kidney

Only a few data are available concerning the effect of smoking on renal function in one systemic disease involving the kidney, namely lupus nephritis. A retrospective cohort study (Ward and Studenski 1992) of 160 patients with a median follow-up of 6.4 years documented that smoking at the time of onset of lupus nephritis was an independent

Table 2 Smoking-associated risk of endstage renal failure in 144 male patients with IgA-glomerulonephritis or autosomal dominant polycystic kidney disease. (Data are stratified for ACE inhibitor treatment and adjusted for systolic blood pressure)

Pack-years	ACE inhibitor			No ACE inhibitor		
	Odds ratio	95% confidence interval	*p*-value	Odds ratio	95% confidence interval	*p*-value[a]
<5	1.0	—	—	1.0	—	—
>5	1.4	0.3–7.1	0.65	10.1	2.3–45	0.002

[a] (Wald χ^2).

Data from Orth *et al.* (1998).

risk factor for more rapid progression to ESRF (median time to ESRF 145 months in smokers and greater than 273 months in non-smokers). This effect was independent of hypertension and immunosuppressive treatment. These data have, however, not been confirmed in a recent prospective study on 70 patients with lupus nephritis (Font *et al.* 2001) compared to 70 age- and sex-matched lupus controls without nephropathy. After 10 years' follow-up, 67 per cent of lupus nephritis patients had normal plasma creatinine, 24 per cent had renal failure, and 9 per cent ESRF. Hyperlipidaemia and hypertension at study onset were the only factors associated with development of renal failure, and the influence of smoking on prognosis of lupus nephritis remains unclear.

The hypothesis that heavy smoking might be a risk factor for the development and/or progression of pauci-immune ANCA-positive extracapillary glomerulonephritis has been proposed (Sessa *et al.* 2000), and whilst plausible through damaging effects of smoking on the vascular endothelium leading to formation of antibodies against nuclear cell antigens extruded from endothelial cells, pertinent data are lacking.

Cigarette smoking appears to be a risk factor for pulmonary complications in two clinical situations of importance in nephrology. First, smoking increases the risk for fatal lung disease in hypocomplementaemic urticarial vasculitis syndrome (Wisnieski *et al.* 1995), a rare illness related to systemic lupus erythematosus (SLE). Second, the risk of pulmonary haemorrhage in antiglomerular basement membrane-disease, that is, for development of a full Goodpasture syndrome is greatly increased in smokers (Donaghy and Rees 1983) (see Chapter 3.11).

Smoking and atherosclerotic renal artery stenosis/ischaemic nephropathy

The prevalence of atherosclerotic renal artery stenosis is increasing in the ageing population, and ischaemic nephropathy is a significant cause of ESRF in patients over 65 years of age (Textor and Wilcox 2001) (see Chapters 9.5 and 14.2).

The incidence of renal vascular stenosis increases as the extent of peripheral vascular disease increases (Metcalfe *et al.* 1999). Since the latter is common in smokers, it is not surprising that smokers have a greater risk of critical atherosclerotic renal artery stenosis (Appel *et al.* 1995; Alcazar *et al.* 2001). Smoking is well known to promote atherogenesis. It is of interest that plasma total homocysteine concentration, a predictor of atherogenic risk, is strongly and dose-dependently related to cigarette smoking (Abdella *et al.* 2000; Jacques *et al.* 2001). There is, however, no doubt that other pathogenic mechanisms also play a role.

Hadj-Abdelkader *et al.* (2001) examined elderly hypertensive patients with renal failure by arteriography. Significantly, more patients with atherosclerotic renal artery stenosis were smokers compared to patients without atherosclerotic renal artery stenosis: (80.5 versus 44 per cent). A correlation was found also with the number of cigarettes smoked and the exposure time. The Spanish observational multicentre study of Alcazar *et al.* (2001) showed that 70 per cent of 156 elderly patients with bilateral atherosclerotic renal artery stenosis and elevated serum creatinine concentrations were smokers. As one would expect, the prevalence of smokers is increased both amongst patients with unilateral (Jaboureck *et al.* 2001) and bilateral (Shurrab *et al.* 2001) atherosclerotic renal artery stenosis.

In a group of 89 normotensive, non-diabetic elderly subjects with different degrees of peripheral atherosclerosis and no clinical signs of ischaemic nephropathy, renovascular hypertension, or other nephropathies, despite normal values for GFR, renal plasma flow declined progressively in parallel with the severity of peripheral atherosclerosis (Baggio *et al.* 2001). Stepwise multiple regression showed that the decrease in renal plasma flow was best explained by smoking and by serum LDL-cholesterol concentrations (Baggio *et al.* 2001). Since, there was a close association between the severity of extrarenal atherosclerosis and renal hypoperfusion, the authors proposed the existence of initial ischaemic nephropathy. These findings imply that renal function should be assessed in all patients with extrarenal atherosclerosis, particularly in those with classic cardiovascular risk factors.

Adverse effects of smoking in patients in renal replacement therapy

Regular dialysis

Baseline serum albumin is significantly lower in active as compared to non-smokers on haemodialysis (Leavey *et al.* 2000), and lower serum albumin concentrations are well known to predict increased mortality. Smoking is also a highly significant risk factor for death during the first 90 days on haemodialysis (Khan *et al.* 1995). Conversely, the prevalence of active smokers among long-term survivors on haemodialysis is low (11.8 per cent) (Owen *et al.* 1996).

The analysis of 936 patients enrolled in the baseline phase of the Hemodialysis Study (US National Institutes of Health) revealed that smoking and diabetes are strongly associated with cardiovascular disease (Cheung *et al.* 2000). In a national random sample of 4205 new ESRD in the United States, smoking was a significant risk factor for coronary artery disease, present in 38 per cent of patients (Stack and Bloembergen 2001).

Bypass surgery compared to angioplasty yields better results in patients with ESRF but it is important to be aware that smoking worsens outcome after bypass surgery. A retrospective study investigating 44 dialysis patients undergoing coronary artery bypass grafting from 1984 to 1997 reported a zero 5-year survival for smokers, but 84 ± 8 per cent for non-smokers (Franga *et al.* 2000).

Smoking further adds to the increased mortality in patients with diabetes mellitus on haemodialysis, being an independent risk factor contributing particularly to cardiovascular death (Akmal 2001; Orth *et al.* 2001). In one study, smoking and increasing age in patients with diabetes mellitus were the most important adverse features for outcome at the start of renal replacement therapy (McMillan *et al.* 1990). The relative risk for mortality in current cigarette smokers in this latter study, which did not exclusively include patients on haemodialysis, was 2.28. In another study of dialysed patients with type 1 diabetes, smoking was shown to confer a relative risk for lethal myocardial infarction of 2.6 (Koch *et al.* 1993). In another group of diabetic patients on haemodialysis (Biesenbach and Zazgornik 1996), smokers had higher fibrinogen and systolic BP values. The 5-year survival rate was lower (9 versus 37 per cent), and the incidence of myocardial infarction higher (77 versus 13 per cent) in the smoking versus the non-smoking patients. Cardiovascular events were the most frequent cause of death in both patient groups, but were more frequent in smokers (80 versus 63 per cent).

Smoking also confers a higher risk for atherosclerotic lesions outside the heart. In a study of dialysis patients, smoking correlated with the mean internal diameter of carotid arteries, the degree of carotid stenosis, and the number of plaques in the carotid arteries (Malatino *et al.* 1999). Data from the United States Renal Data System Dialysis Morbidity and Mortality Study documented that smoking is independently associated with peripheral vascular disease in haemodialysed patients (odds ratio up to 1.55) (O'Hare *et al.* 2002).

The risk of atrial fibrillation, a frequent arrythmia in haemodialysis patients, appears to be associated to coronary artery disease and may contribute to cardiovascular morbidity and mortality in ESRF (Fabbian *et al.* 2000). Smoking *per se* does, however, not seem to be of importance for ventricular premature beats or complex ventricular arrhythmia in haemodialysis patients (Blumberg *et al.* 1983; de Lima *et al.* 1999). Smoking contributes, at least partly, to the decreased heart rate variability observed in patients with ESRF (Steinberg *et al.* 1998) and furthermore is a risk factor for systolic dysfunction (Parfrey and Harnett 1994). As far as left ventricular function is concerned, a study of non-diabetic dialysis and transplant patients revealed that in addition to high alkaline phosphatase and high serum creatinine, smoking was the most significant and independent variable associated low-output left ventricular failure (Parfrey *et al.* 1987).

Rocco *et al.* (1996) investigated a cohort of patients who started haemodialysis in 1989 and found smoking to be amongst the strongest predictors of the number of days spent in hospital per year. The major part (64 per cent) of these patients were African-Americans and 33 per cent had diabetes mellitus as the primary cause of ESRF. Apart from cardiovascular and pulmonary complications, the increased number of hospital days per year in smokers on haemodialysis is probably also due to an increased risk of early and late fistula failure (Wetzig *et al.* 1985).

Little information about the adverse effects of smoking in patients on continuous peritoneal dialysis are available, but smoking increases the risk of permanent change to haemodialysis (Gokal *et al.* 1987). For non-diabetic patients, age, serum albumin during treatment, and current smoking were significant survival risk factors (Zimmerman *et al.* 1996). Whether smoking is a risk factor for the development of peripheral vascular disease in these patients is controversial (Webb and Brown 1993; Wakeen and Zimmerman 1998). Importantly, smoking is associated with non-compliance in both haemodialysis and peritoneal dialysis patients (Kutner *et al.* 2002).

Adverse effects of smoking in renal transplant recipients

Graft loss

Counter-intuitively, smoking does not appear to increase the risk of microalbuminuria in patients after transplantation (Halimi *et al.* 2001). Most studies indicate a lack of correlation of smoking with the development of progressive allograft dysfunction (Cho *et al.* 1995; Hegeman and Hunsicker 1995).

However, a recent study of adult renal allograft recipients evaluated the relationship between smoking and graft outcome (Sung *et al.* 2001). Patients who were smokers at operation had death-censored graft survivals of 84, 65, and 48 per cent at 1, 5, and 10 years, respectively, compared with non-smokers' 88, 78, and 62 per cent ($p = 0.007$), affecting both living and cadaver donor kidneys but not accounted for by differences in rejection episodes (64 versus 61 per cent). In a multivariate analysis, pretransplant smoking was associated with a relative risk of 2.3 for graft loss, and even among patients with a smoking history before transplantation who had stopped, death-censored graft survival was significantly greater. This suggests that cigarette smoking before kidney transplantation contributes significantly to censored allograft loss. In agreement with these data, a retrospective analysis of first-time kidney transplant recipients aged 60 years or more (Doyle *et al.* 2000) found current smoking to be a risk factor for decreased graft survival.

The finding that stopping smoking before renal transplantation improves graft survival has obvious major implications for the management of patients with ESRF who are considered for renal transplantation.

The effect of smoking on renal allograft function may depend on the renal disease that has led to ESRF. In patients who had reached ESRF as a result of lupus nephritis, the risk of renal transplant loss was substantially increased in smokers (Stone *et al.* 1998). In this study, smoking demonstrated both the strongest association and the highest RR for allograft loss (RR 2.5) as compared to the other factors such as delayed graft function, acute rejection episodes, and total HLA mismatches. Lupus nephritis as the reason for ESRF represents only a tiny subgroup of renal transplant patients, however, but the above results are of major clinical importance and point to the possibility that the alterations of the immune response reported in smokers (Orth *et al.* 1997) may be particularly detrimental in renal diseases related to major immune defects, such as in SLE.

It is of note that an investigation of kidney donor lifestyle factors, including smoking, as well as drinking, drug use, and sexual history, found no significant negative impact on renal allograft survival (Feduska 1993).

Death of the recipient

The evidence that the risk of death with a functioning graft is increased in patients with a history of cigarette smoking is beyond any doubt. The magnitude of the negative impact of smoking in renal transplant recipients is quantitatively similar to the presence of diabetes mellitus (Cosio *et al.* 1999). A retrospective analysis (Kasiske and Klinger 2000) found more cardiovascular deaths in smokers with a functioning graft. This has also been documented in first-time kidney transplant recipients aged 60 years or more (Doyle *et al.* 2000). Compared to never- or ex-smokers, the diabetic renal transplant recipient has a significantly increased risk of early death if he smoked during the predialysis phase or after having received his graft (Stegmayr 1990).

The increase in cardiovascular death arises from the well-known atherogenic effects of smoking (Ritz *et al.* 2000). Smoking appears to increase the risk for low-output left ventricular failure in patients with a renal transplant (Parfrey *et al.* 1987) and cigarette smoking at the time of transplantation is an independent risk factor for cerebrovascular and peripheral vascular disease in transplanted patients (Kasiske *et al.* 1996). Smoking post-transplantation is a risk factor for carotid plaques (Nankivell *et al.* 2000) and peripheral vascular occlusive disease (Sung *et al.* 2000). Diabetic transplant recipients are at an increased risk of peripheral vascular disease leading to amputation. Smoking has as profound negative effect on the amputation rate as an amputation prior to transplantation (Kalker *et al.* 1996).

Another clinically relevant aspect is the higher incidence of cancer in smokers. In one study, cigarette smoking was associated with an increased risk for cancer, with each 10 pack-years smoked at transplant increasing the risk by 1.12 (Danpanich and Kasiske 1999). It has also been reported that smoking increases the risk for squamous cell carcinoma of the skin (Ramsay *et al.* 2001). Furthermore, exposure to the sun and smoking are risk factors for dysplastic and malignant lip lesions in renal-transplant recipients (King *et al.* 1995).

Finally, smoking increases the risk for osteoporosis in corticosteroid-treated transplant patients (Joy *et al.* 2000) and favours the development of post-transplant erythrocytosis (Wickre *et al.* 1983).

Table 3 Potential pathomechanisms of smoking-induced renal injury

Increased sympathetic nerve activity
Increase in blood pressure and heart rate
Alteration of diurnal blood pressure rhythm
Increase in renal vascular resistance leading to decrease in glomerular filtration rate and renal plasma flow
Increase in intraglomerular capillary pressure
Aggravation of hyperfiltration in patients with diabetic nephropathy
Arteriosclerosis of the renal arteries and the intrarenal arteries and arterioles
Endothelin-1- and/or angiotensin II-mediated proliferation and matrix accumulation of vascular smooth muscle cells, endothelial cells, and mesangial cells
Tubulotoxicity
Direct toxic effects on endothelial cells Alteration of the prostaglandin/thromboxane metabolism Oxidative stress through generation of reactive oxygen species Nitric oxide depletion Impairment of endothelial cell-dependent vascular dilation Increased adhesion of monocytes to the endothelium Carbon monoxide-induced hypoxia
Increased platelet aggregation
Impaired lipoprotein and glycosaminoglycan metabolism
Modulation of the immune response
Antidiuresis (vasopressin-mediated)
Insulin resistance

Potential mechanisms of smoking-induced renal damage

The mechanisms by which smoking exerts its negative effects on the kidney are largely unknown. Several potential mechanisms of smoking-induced renal damage have been discussed in detail (Orth 2000) and a summary is given in Table 3. It is likely that the smoking-induced increase in BP is one of the most important mechanisms contributing to an adverse renal prognosis in smokers, particularly in those with hypertension and/or a diseased kidney (Orth 2002).

Pathological features of smoking-induced renal damage

An increase in thickness of walls of arterioles of organs not in direct contact with cigarette smoke, mainly due to fibroelastic intimal proliferation and hyaline thickening in the intima, has been observed in various organs of individuals without renal disease (Auerbach *et al.* 1968, 1976), including the kidney (Black *et al.* 1983; Oberai *et al.* 1984; Tracy *et al.* 1994).

In a renal biopsy study, the histological findings of 107 patients with chronic renal failure were assessed by investigating the possible effects of smoking on glomerulosclerosis and vascular damage (Lhotta *et al.* 2002). Most of these patients were suffering from glomerular disease with marked proteinuria. Only a minority had been treated with an ACE inhibitor at the time of biopsy and BP was not well controlled). Smoking was not associated with glomerulosclerosis. As compared to non-smokers, those who smoked at any time exhibited more severe myointimal hyperplasia, a finding particularly evident in patients more than 50 years of age. In younger patients, a trend toward arteriolar changes was evident for smoking, but it did not reach statistical significance. In females, no correlation was observed. This may be due to the fact that women were less likely to be smokers and smoked less than half as many pack-years than did men.

The above study is important, because it documents that in elderly male patients with renal disease ex-smokers as well current-smokers have myointimal hyperplasia. Since hypertension *per se* seems not to be related to myointimal hyperplasia of intrarenal arterioles (Bos *et al.* 2001), the effect of smoking has to be considered as major. The negative findings concerning glomerulosclerosis does not exclude a negative effect of smoking on glomerular structure. Using a more precise method for quantification of renal damage, our group found more severe glomerulosclerosis and tubulointerstitial fibrosis in a rat model of focal–segmental glomerulosclerosis (Odoni *et al.* 2002). Whether this is true for humans with non-inflammatory renal disease as well remains to be determined. An increase in the width of glomerular basement membrane in patients with type 2 diabetes who smoke has been reported in a preliminary study (Budakovic *et al.* 2001).

Reversibility of smoking-induced renal damage

The question arises whether cessation of smoking ameliorates adverse effects on renal prognosis. One study in patients with type 1 diabetes and nephropathy (Chase *et al.* 1991) showed that in patients with adequate control of BP and glycaemia, progression of renal failure was considerably less in patients who had stopped smoking than those who continued smoking. Furthermore, smoking cessation significantly decreased urinary albumin excretion in these patients. In another study, progression of diabetic nephropathy was found in 53 per cent of current smokers, but only in 33 per cent of ex-smokers and 11 per cent of non-smokers (Sawicki *et al.* 1994).

It is plausible to assume that this may also be true in non-diabetic renal disease. Concerning the general population, Pinto-Sietsma *et al.* (2000) found that the risk of microalbuminuria in non-diabetic subjects is only minor in ex-smokers, but not in current smokers. There is some evidence, however, that smoking-induced decrease in renal plasma flow is not completely reversible after smoking cessation (Gambaro *et al.* 1998).

The present data do not allow us to draw a definite conclusion about the magnitude of the renal benefit derived from smoking cessation. There is, however, good evidence indicating that this is one of the single most effective measures to retard progression of renal failure.

Conclusion

Smoking is one of the most important remediable renal risk factors. It has a negative impact on renal function even in subjects without apparent renal disease, but the adverse renal effects are particularly prominent in patients with a diseased kidney. Importantly, the increase in the rate of progression of renal failure attributable to smoking seems to be independent of the underlying renal disease. Some evidence suggests that men are more susceptible to the adverse renal effects of smoking than women, but this issue remains unresolved due to the limited data available in women.

Cessation of smoking undoubtedly improves cardiovascular prognosis in the renal patient. Thus, even if ESRF is reached smoking should be discontinued. Smoking is the strongest predictor of mortality in type 2 diabetes (Orth *et al.* 2001), and cessation prolongs the life of a 45-year-old smoking, hypertensive, diabetic male by 4–5 years; the treatment of hypertension is estimated to prolong the life of the same individual by only 1 year (Yudkin 1993). Of note, even among people who have a history of heavy smoking, the risk of coronary events can be halved by stopping the habit. This benefit from smoking cessation is seen regardless of how long or how much a person has previously smoked (Culleton and Wilson 1998). It is still true that '*persuading hypertensive patients not to smoke is the single most effective measure we can take to reduce their risk*' (Sleight 1993). It has been estimated that the risk of myocardial infarction can be reduced by 50–70 per cent as a consequence of smoking discontinuation. In contrast, the treatment of hypertension results in a reduction of risk of myocardial infarction of 'only' 2–3 per cent for each 1 mmHg decline in diastolic BP (Manson *et al.* 1992).

Major efforts have to be undertaken to help patients to quit smoking. These include the most effective pharmaceutical smoking cessation approaches known to date, that is, therapy with sustained-release bupropion and/or nicotine replacement therapy (Orth 2002).

Management of the renal patient requires information about (a) the magnitude of the renal and cardiovascular risk related to smoking including the benefits from smoking cessation and (b) application of the above modern therapeutic modalities to increase the success rate in patients willing to stop smoking. To the best of my knowledge, there is no detailed information on the pharmacokinetics of sustained-release bupropion in patients with impaired renal function, but the few data available indicate that it does not accumulate in renal failure. In contrast, nicotine does accumulate (Molander *et al.* 2000), which may limit the success rate of smoking discontinuation in patients with renal failure, because the patient is used to a higher level of 'intoxication'. Diabetic patients with nephropathy have smoked more and still smoke more than patients without nephropathy (Norden 1988). On the other hand, it is plausible to assume that more renal patients than individuals in the general population will stop smoking, because they are afraid of the prospect of progression to ESRF. This assumption of greater compliance in severely ill patients is based on the observation that in subjects receiving intervention to stop smoking one year smoking cessation rate is approximately 35 per cent in healthy subjects (Jorenby *et al.* 1999), but approximately 70 per cent in patients after a myocardial infarction (Cole 2001). It has to be pointed out that to date, no data are available about success rates of a modern smoking cessation strategy in renal patients.

Acknowledgement

The data given in Table 2 are reprinted by permission of Blackwell Science, Inc.

References

Abdella, N., Mojiminiyi, O. A., and Akanji, A. O. (2000). Homocysteine and endogenous markers of renal function in type 2 diabetic patients without coronary heart disease. *Diabetes Research and Clinical Practice* **50**, 177–185.

Akmal, M. (2001). Hemodialysis in diabetic patients. *American Journal of Kidney Diseases* **38**, S195–S199.

Alcazar, J. M. *et al.* (2001). Clinical characteristics of ischaemic renal disease. *Nephrology, Dialysis, Transplantation* **16** (Suppl. 1), 74–77.

Appel, R. G. *et al.* (1995). Renovascular disease in older patients beginning renal replacement therapy. *Kidney International* **48**, 171–176.

Auerbach, O., Hammond, E. C., and Garfinkel, L. (1968). Thickening of walls of arterioles and small arteries in relation to age and smoking habits. *New England Journal of Medicine* **278**, 980–984.

Auerbach, O. *et al.* (1976). Cigarette smoking and coronary artery disease. A macroscopic and microscopic study. *Chest* **70**, 697–705.

Baggio, B. *et al.* (2001). Renal involvement in subjects with peripheral atherosclerosis. *Journal of Nephrology* **14**, 286–292.

Biesenbach, G. and Zazgornik, J. (1996). Influence of smoking on the survival rate of diabetic patients requiring hemodialysis. *Diabetes Care* **19**, 625–628.

Biesenbach, G., Janko, O., and Zazgornik, J. (1994). Similar rate of progression in the predialysis phase in type I and type II diabetes mellitus. *Nephrology, Dialysis, Transplantation* **9**, 1097–1102.

Black, H. R. *et al.* (1983). Effect of heavy cigarette smoking on renal and myocardial arterioles. *Nephron* **34**, 173–179.

Bleyer, A. J. *et al.* (2000). Tobacco, hypertension, and vascular disease: risk factors for renal functional decline in an older population. *Kidney International* **57**, 2072–2079.

Blumberg, A. *et al.* (1983). Cardiac arrhythmias in patients on maintenance hemodialysis. *Nephron* **33**, 91–95.

Borch-Johnsen, K. *et al.* (1987). The natural history of insulin-dependent diabetes mellitus in Denmark: 1. Long-term survival with and without late diabetic complications. *Diabetic Medicine* **4**, 201–210.

Bos, W. J. *et al.* (2001). Renal vascular changes in renal disease independent of hypertension. *Nephrology, Dialysis, Transplantation* **16**, 537–541.

Budakovic, A. *et al.* (2001). Cigarette smoking and glomerular ultrastructure in type 2 diabetes. *Journal of the American Society of Nephrology* **12**, 143A.

Chapman, A. B. *et al.* (1994). Overt proteinuria and microalbuminuria in autosomal dominant polycystic kidney disease. *Journal of the American Society of Nephrology* **5**, 1349–1354.

Chase, H. P. *et al.* (1991). Cigarette smoking increases the risk of albuminuria among subjects with type I diabetes. *Journal of the American Medical Association* **265**, 614–617.

Cheung, A. K. *et al.* (2000). Atherosclerotic cardiovascular disease risks in chronic hemodialysis patients. *Kidney International* **58**, 353–362.

Cho, Y. W., Terasaki, P. I., and Cecka, J. M. (1995). New variables reported to the UNOS registry and their impact on cadaveric renal transplant outcomes—a preliminary study. *Clinical Transplantation* 405–415.

Christiansen, J. S. (1978). Cigarette smoking and prevalence of microangiopathy in juvenile-onset insulin-dependent diabetes mellitus. *Diabetes Care* **1**, 146–149.

Chuahirun, T. and Wesson, D. E. (2002). Cigarette smoking predicts faster progression of type 2 established diabetic nephropathy despite ACE inhibition. *American Journal of Kidney Diseases* **39**, 376–382.

Cole, T. K. (2001). Smoking cessation in the hospitalized patient using the transtheoretical model of behavior change. *Heart and Lung* **30**, 148–158.

Cosio, F. G. *et al.* (1999). Patient survival after renal transplantation: II. The impact of smoking. *Clinical Transplantation* **13**, 336–341.

Couper, J. J. *et al.* (1994). Relationship of smoking and albuminuria in children with insulin-dependent diabetes. *Diabetic Medicine* **11**, 666–669.

Culleton, B. F. and Wilson, P. W. (1998). Cardiovascular disease: risk factors, secular trends, and therapeutic guidelines. *Journal of the American Society of Nephrology* **9**, S5–S15.

Danpanich, E. and Kasiske, B. L. (1999). Risk factors for cancer in renal transplant recipients. *Transplantation* **68**, 1859–1864.

de Lima, J. J. *et al.* (1999). Blood pressure and the risk of complex arrhythmia in renal insufficiency, hemodialysis, and renal transplant patients. *American Journal of Hypertension* **12**, 204–208.

Donaghy, M. and Rees, A. J. (1983). Cigarette smoking and lung haemorrhage in glomerulonephritis caused by autoantibodies to glomerular basement membrane. *Lancet* **2**, 1390–1393.

Doyle, S. E. *et al.* (2000). Predicting clinical outcome in the elderly renal transplant recipient. *Kidney International* **57**, 2144–2150.

Fabbian, F. *et al.* (2000). Clinical characteristics associated to atrial fibrillation in chronic hemodialysis patients. *Clinical Nephrology* **54**, 234–239.

Feduska, N. J., Jr. (1993). Donor factors in cadaveric renal transplantation. *Clinical Transplantation* 351–357.

Font, J. *et al.* (2001). Cardiovascular risk factors and the long-term outcome of lupus nephritis. *Quarterly Journal of Medicine* **94**, 19–26.

Franga, D. L. *et al.* (2000). Early and long-term results of coronary artery bypass grafting in dialysis patients. *Annals of Thoracic Surgery* **70**, 813–818, discussion 9.

Gambaro, G. *et al.* (1998). Renal impairment in chronic cigarette smokers. *Journal of the American Society of Nephrology* **9**, 562–567.

Gerstein, H. C. *et al.* (2000). Prevalence and determinants of microalbuminuria in high-risk diabetic and nondiabetic patients in the Heart Outcomes Prevention Evaluation Study. The HOPE Study Investigators. *Diabetes Care* **23** (Suppl. 2), B35–B39.

Goetz, F. C. *et al.* (1997). Risk factors for kidney damage in the adult population of Wadena, Minnesota. A prospective study. *American Journal of Epidemiology* **145**, 91–102.

Gokal, R. *et al.* (1987). Multi-centre study on outcome of treatment in patients on continuous ambulatory peritoneal dialysis and haemodialysis. *Nephrology, Dialysis, Transplantation* **2**, 172–178.

Hadj-Abdelkader, M. *et al.* (2001). Tabac et stenoses atheromateuses des artères rénales. *Archives des Madies du Cœur et des Vaisseaux* **94**, 925–927.

Halimi, J. M. *et al.* (2000). Effects of current smoking and smoking discontinuation on renal function and proteinuria in the general population. *Kidney International* **58**, 1285–1292.

Halimi, J. M. *et al.* (2001). Micro-albuminurie chez le transplanté rénale hypertendu non proteinurique: influence des antecedents de rejet aïgu et le rapport de sode. *Archives des Maladies du Cœur et des Vaisseaux* **94**, 933–936.

Hays, J. T. *et al.* (1998). Trends in smoking-related diseases. Why smoking cessation is still the best medicine. *Postgraduate Medicine* **104**, 5–6, 56–62, 71.

Hegeman, R. L. and Hunsicker, L. G. (1995). Chronic rejection in renal allografts: importance of cardiovascular risk factors. *Clinical Transplantation* **9**, 135–139.

Hillege, H. L. *et al.* (2001). Microalbuminuria is common, also in a nondiabetic, nonhypertensive population, and an independent indicator of cardiovascular risk factors and cardiovascular morbidity. *Journal of Internal Medicine* **249**, 519–526.

Hogan, S. L. *et al.* (2001a). Association of smoking with albuminuria in a cross-sectional probability sample of U.S. adults. *Journal of the American Society of Nephrology* **12**, 209A.

Hogan, S. L. *et al.* (2001b). Silica exposure in anti-neutrophil cytoplasmic autoantibody-associated glomerulonephritis and lupus nephritis. *Journal of the American Society of Nephrology* **12**, 134–142.

Jaboureck, O. *et al.* (2001). Les characteristiques demographiques des hypertendus sont-elles differenetes en présence d'une sténose atheromateuse artérielle rénale? *Archives des Madies du Cœur et des Vaisseaux* **94**, 828–833.

Jacques, P. F. *et al.* (2001). Determinants of plasma total homocysteine concentration in the Framingham Offspring cohort. *American Journal of Clinical Nutrition* **73**, 613–621.

Janssen, W. M. *et al.* (2000). Low levels of urinary albumin excretion are associated with cardiovascular risk factors in the general population. *Clinical Chemistry and Laboratory Medicine* **38**, 1107–1110.

Jorenby, D. E. *et al.* (1999). A controlled trial of sustained-release bupropion, a nicotine patch, or both for smoking cessation. *New England Journal of Medicine* **340**, 685–691.

Joy, M. S., Neyhart, C. D., and Dooley, M. A. (2000). A multidisciplinary renal clinic for corticosteroid-induced bone disease. *Pharmacotherapy* **20**, 206–216.

Kalker, A. J. *et al.* (1996). Foot problems in the diabetic transplant recipient. *Clinical Transplantation* **10**, 503–510.

Kasiske, B. L. and Klinger, D. (2000). Cigarette smoking in renal transplant recipients. *Journal of the American Society of Nephrology* **11**, 753–759.

Kasiske, B. L. *et al.* (1996). Cardiovascular disease after renal transplantation. *Journal of the American Society of Nephrology* **7**, 158–165.

Keller, C. K. *et al.* (1996). Renal findings in patients with short-term type 2 diabetes. *Journal of the American Society of Nephrology* **7**, 2627–2635.

Khan, I. H. *et al.* (1995). Death during the first 90 days of dialysis: a case control study. *American Journal of Kidney Disease* **25**, 276–280.

King, G. N. *et al.* (1995). Increased prevalence of dysplastic and malignant lip lesions in renal-transplant recipients. *New England Journal of Medicine* **332**, 1052–1057.

Klag, M. J. *et al.* (1996). Blood pressure and end-stage renal disease in men. *New England Journal of Medicine* **334**, 13–18.

Klein, R., Klein, B. E., and Moss, S. E. (1993). Incidence of gross proteinuria in older-onset diabetes. A population-based perspective. *Diabetes* **42**, 381–389.

Koch, M. *et al.* (1993). Survival and predictors of death in dialysed diabetic patients. *Diabetologia* **36**, 1113–1117.

Kutner, N. G. *et al.* (2002). Psychosocial predictors of non-compliance in haemodialysis and peritoneal dialysis patients. *Nephrology, Dialysis, Transplantation* **17**, 93–99.

Leavey, S. F. *et al.* (2000). Cross-sectional and longitudinal predictors of serum albumin in hemodialysis patients. *Kidney International* **58**, 2119–2128.

Lhotta, K. *et al.* (2002). Cigarette smoking and vascular pathology in renal biopsies. *Kidney International* **61**, 648–654.

Lickint, F. *Tabak und Organismus. Handbuch der gesamten Tabakkunde.* Stuttgart: Hippocrates-Verlag, 1939.

Mackin, P. *et al.* (1996). Renal function in long-duration type I diabetes. *Diabetes Care* **19**, 249–251.

Malatino, L. S. *et al.* (1999). Smoking, blood pressure and serum albumin are major determinants of carotid atherosclerosis in dialysis patients. CREED Investigators. Cardiovascular Risk Extended Evaluation in Dialysis patients. *Journal of Nephrology* **12**, 256–260.

Manson, J. E. *et al.* (1992). The primary prevention of myocardial infarction. *The New England Journal of Medicine* **326**, 1406–1416.

McMillan, M. A., Briggs, J. D., and Junor, B. J. (1990). Outcome of renal replacement treatment in patients with diabetes mellitus. *British Medical Journal* **301**, 540–544.

Merkel, F. *et al.* (1994). Course and prognosis of anti-basement membrane antibody (anti-BM-Ab)-mediated disease: report of 35 cases. *Nephrology, Dialysis, Transplantation* **9**, 372–376.

Metcalfe, W., Reid, A. W., and Geddes, C. C. (1999). Prevalence of angiographic atherosclerotic renal artery disease and its relationship to the anatomical extent of peripheral vascular atherosclerosis. *Nephrology, Dialysis, Transplantation* **14**, 105–108.

Molander, L. *et al.* (2000). Pharmacokinetics of nicotine in kidney failure. *Clinical Pharmacology and Therapeutics* **68**, 250–260.

Nakanishi, N. *et al.* (2000). Cigarette smoking and risk for impaired fasting glucose and type 2 diabetes in middle-aged Japanese men. *Annals of Internal Medicine* **133**, 183–191.

Nankivell, B. J. *et al.* (2000). Progression of macrovascular disease after transplantation. *Transplantation* **69**, 574–581.

Norden, G. (1988). Diabetic nephropathy. A clinical study of risk factors in type-I diabetes mellitus. *Scandinavian Journal of Urology and Nephrology Supplement* **116**, 1–76.

Norden, G. and Nyberg, G. (1984). Smoking and diabetic nephropathy. *Acta Medica Scandinavica* **215**, 257–261.

Oberai, B., Adams, C. W., and High, O. B. (1984). Myocardial and renal arteriolar thickening in cigarette smokers. *Atherosclerosis* **52**, 185–190.

Odoni, G. *et al.* (2002). Cigarette smoke condensate aggravates renal injury in the renal ablation model. *Kidney International* **61** (in press).

O'Hare, A. M. *et al.* (2002). Peripheral vascular disease risk factors among patients undergoing hemodialysis. *Journal of the American Society of Nephrology* **13**, 497–503.

Orth, S. R. (2000). Smoking—a renal risk factor. *Nephron* **86**, 12–26.

Orth, S. R. (2002). Smoking and the kidney. *Journal of the American Society of Nephrology* **13** (in press).

Orth, S. R., Ritz, E., and Schrier, R. W. (1997). The renal risks of smoking. *Kidney International* **51**, 1669–1677.

Orth, S. R. *et al.* (1998). Smoking as a risk factor for end-stage renal failure in men with primary renal disease. *Kidney International* **54**, 926–931.

Orth, S. R., Viedt, C., and Ritz, E. (2001). Adverse effects of smoking in the renal patient. *Tohoku Journal of Experimental Medicine* **194**, 1–15.

Owen, W. F., Madore, F., and Brenner, B. M. (1996). An observational study of cardiovascular characteristics of long-term end-stage renal disease survivors. *American Journal of Kidney Diseases* **28**, 931–936.

Parfrey, P. S. and Harnett, J. D. (1994). Clinical aspects of cardiomyopathy in dialysis patients. *Blood Purification* **12**, 267–276.

Parfrey, P. S. *et al.* (1987). Low-output left ventricular failure in end-stage renal disease. *American Journal of Nephrology* **7**, 184–191.

Perna, A. *et al.* (2001). DD ACE genotype and smoking cluster with high-normal albuminuria: cross sectional analysis in 1209 normo-albuminuric type 2 diabetics enrolled in the BErgamo NEphrologic DIabetes Complications Trial (BENEDICT). *Journal of the American Society of Nephrology* **12**, 154A.

Perry, H. M., Jr. *et al.* (1995). Early predictors of 15-year end-stage renal disease in hypertensive patients. *Hypertension* **25**, 587–594.

Pinto-Sietsma, S. J. *et al.* (2000). Smoking is related to albuminuria and abnormal renal function in nondiabetic persons. *Annals of Internal Medicine* **133**, 585–591.

Price, D. A. *et al.* (1999). The paradox of the low-renin state in diabetic nephropathy. *Journal of the American Society of Nephrology* **10**, 2382–2391.

Ramsay, H. M. *et al.* (2001). Polymorphisms in glutathione S-transferases are associated with altered risk of nonmelanoma skin cancer in renal transplant recipients: a preliminary analysis. *Journal of Investigative Dermatology* **117**, 251–255.

Regalado, M., Yang, S., and Wesson, D. E. (2000). Cigarette smoking is associated with augmented progression of renal insufficiency in severe essential hypertension. *American Journal of Kidney Diseases* **35**, 687–694.

Ritz, E. *et al.* (2000). Atherosclerotic complications after renal transplantation. *Transplantation International* **13** (Suppl. 1), S14–S19.

Rocco, M. V. *et al.* (1996). Risk factors for hospital utilization in chronic dialysis patients. Southeastern Kidney Council (Network 6). *Journal of the American Society of Nephrology* **7**, 889–896.

Rossing, P. *et al.* (1996). Predictors of mortality in insulin dependent diabetes: 10 year observational follow up study. *British Medical Journal* **313**, 779–784.

Ruilope, L. M. *et al.* (2001). Renal function: the Cinderella of cardiovascular risk profile. *Journal of the American College of Cardiology* **38**, 1782–1787.

Samuelsson, O. and Attman, P. O. (2000). Is smoking a risk factor for progression of chronic renal failure? *Kidney International* **58**, 2597.

Sawicki, P. T. *et al.* (1994). Smoking is associated with progression of diabetic nephropathy. *Diabetes Care* **17**, 126–131.

Sessa, A. *et al.* (2000). Cigarette smoking and pauci-immune extracapillary glomerulonephritis with ANCA-associated idiopathic systemic vasculitis. A retrospective study. *Contributions to Nephrology* **130**, 103–108.

Shurrab, A. E. *et al.* (2001). Increasing the diagnostic yield of renal angiography for the diagnosis of atheromatous renovascular disease. *British Journal of Radiology* **74**, 213–218.

Sleight, P. (1993). Smoking and hypertension. *Clinical and Experimental Hypertension* **15**, 1181–1192.

Stack, A. G. and Bloembergen, W. E. (2001). Prevalence and clinical correlates of coronary artery disease among new dialysis patients in the United States: a cross-sectional study. *Journal of the American Society of Nephrology* **12**, 1516–1523.

Stegmayr, B. G. (1990). A study of patients with diabetes mellitus (type 1) and end-stage renal failure: tobacco usage may increase risk of nephropathy and death. *Journal of Internal Medicine* **228**, 121–124.

Steinberg, A. A. *et al.* (1998). Effect of end-stage renal disease on decreased heart rate variability. *American Journal of Cardiology* **82**, 1156–1158, A10.

Stengel, B. *et al.* (2000). Age, blood pressure and smoking effects on chronic renal failure in primary glomerular nephropathies. *Kidney International* **57**, 2519–2526.

Stone, J. H., Amend, W. J., and Criswell, L. A. (1998). Outcome of renal transplantation in ninety-seven cyclosporine-era patients with systemic lupus erythematosus and matched controls. *Arthritis and Rheumatism* **41**, 1438–1445.

Sung, R. S. *et al.* (2000). Peripheral vascular occlusive disease in renal transplant recipients: risk factors and impact on kidney allograft survival. *Transplantation* **70**, 1049–1054.

Sung, R. S. *et al.* (2001). Excess risk of renal allograft loss associated with cigarette smoking. *Transplantation* **71**, 1752–1757.

Telmer, S. *et al.* (1984). Smoking habits and prevalence of clinical diabetic microangiopathy in insulin-dependent diabetics. *Acta Medica Scandinavica* **215**, 63–68.

Textor, S. C. and Wilcox, C. S. (2001). Renal artery stenosis: a common, treatable cause of renal failure? *Annual Reviews of Medicine* **52**, 421–442.

Tracy, R. E. *et al.* (1994). Nephrosclerosis, glycohemoglobin, cholesterol, and smoking in subjects dying of coronary heart disease. *Modern Pathology* **7**, 301–309.

Wachtell, K. *et al.* (2002). Microalbuminuria in hypertensive patients with electrocardiographic left ventricular hypertrophy: the LIFE Study. *Journal of Hypertension* **20**, 405–412.

Wakai, K. *et al.* (1999). Risk factors for IgA nephropathy: a case–control study in Japan. *American Journal of Kidney Diseases* **33**, 738–745.

Wakeen, M. and Zimmerman, S. W. (1998). Association between human recombinant EPO and peripheral vascular disease in diabetic patients receiving peritoneal dialysis. *American Journal of Kidney Diseases* **32**, 488–493.

Ward, M. M. and Studenski, S. (1992). Clinical prognostic factors in lupus nephritis. The importance of hypertension and smoking. *Archives of Internal Medicine* **152**, 2082–2088.

Webb, A. T. and Brown, E. A. (1993). Prevalence of symptomatic arterial disease and risk factors for its development in patients on continuous ambulatory peritoneal dialysis. *Peritoneal Dialysis International* **13** (Suppl. 2), S406–S408.

Wetzig, G. A., Gough, I. R., and Furnival, C. M. (1985). One hundred cases of arteriovenous fistula for haemodialysis access: the effect of cigarette smoking on patency. *Australian and New Zealand Journal of Surgery* **55**, 551–554.

Whelton, P. K. *et al.* (1995). Cigarette smoking and ESRD incidence in men screened for the MRFIT. *Journal of the American Society of Nephrology* **6**, 408a.

Wickre, C. G. *et al.* (1983). Postrenal transplant erythrocytosis: a review of 53 patients. *Kidney International* **23**, 731–737.

Wisnieski, J. J. *et al.* (1995). Hypocomplementemic urticarial vasculitis syndrome. Clinical and serologic findings in 18 patients. *Medicine (Baltimore)* **74**, 24–41.

Yaqoob, M. *et al.* (1992). Primary glomerulonephritis and hydrocarbon exposure: a case–control study and literature review. *Quarterly Journal of Medicine* **83**, 409–418.

Yudkin, J. S. (1993). How can we best prolong life? Benefits of coronary risk factor reduction in non-diabetic and diabetic subjects. *British Medical Journal* **306**, 1313–1318.

Zimmerman, S. W. *et al.* (1996). Long-term outcome of diabetic patients receiving peritoneal dialysis. *Peritoneal Dialysis International* **16**, 63–68.

5

The patient with tubular disease

5.1 The structure and function of tubules

David G. Shirley and Robert J. Unwin

Brief overview of segmental transport along the nephron

Given the extent of filtration at the glomerulus (~180 l/day), the nephron is concerned largely with reabsorption, although secretion is important for a few solutes—notably K^+, H^+, NH_4^+, and some organic acids/bases. The bulk of reabsorption occurs in the proximal convoluted tubule (PCT) and loop of Henle. However, the various subsections of the distal tubule and collecting duct have an important role in determining the final excretion of solutes and water.

The PCT (the initial two-thirds of the proximal tubule) is responsible for the reabsorption of: sodium (~50 per cent of the filtered load), chloride (~45 per cent), potassium (~45 per cent), water (~50 per cent), glucose (~100 per cent), amino acids (~100 per cent), bicarbonate (~80 per cent), phosphate (~80 per cent), calcium (~50 per cent), magnesium (~15 per cent), urea (~45 per cent), urate (~90 per cent), and proteins (~100 per cent), as well as a number of solutes present in trace amounts.

The loop of Henle, which comprises the proximal straight tubule (pars recta), thin descending limb, and thin and thick ascending limbs, is responsible for the reabsorption of a further ~40 per cent of filtered Na^+, ~45 per cent of filtered Cl^-, ~45 per cent of filtered K^+, ~25 per cent of filtered water, and significant amounts of Ca^{2+} and Mg^{2+}.

In the distal tubule and collecting duct, Na^+ and Cl^- reabsorption continues (to the extent that excretion of both ions is usually <1 per cent of the filtered load), while net K^+ secretion occurs. Some reabsorption of Ca^{2+} and Mg^{2+} takes place in the distal tubule. Water reabsorption in the distal nephron is highly variable, dictated (through variations in vasopressin secretion) by the body's state of hydration. Significant urea reabsorption normally occurs in the inner medullary collecting duct (IMCD).

Most of the transport processes along the nephron are linked, directly or indirectly, to the reabsorption of Na^+. Throughout the nephron, Na^+ enters the epithelial cells from the lumen passively, down a large electrochemical gradient, using a series of transporters (cotransporters/exchangers) or Na^+ channels. Sodium exit through the basolateral membrane requires the 'sodium pump'—the Na^+,K^+-ATPase (Fig. 1). It is this pump that is ultimately responsible for most reabsorptive and secretory processes, although a few other pumps (transporting H^+ ions, Ca^{2+} ions, and H^+/K^+ exchange) play specific roles. The mechanism of Na^+ reabsorption is thus essentially the same throughout the nephron; only the route of entry into the cell varies from segment to segment.

Below we will describe the structure (morphology and transport proteins) and function of each nephron segment, focusing largely on the transport of Na^+, K^+, and Cl^-. A brief account of the factors controlling transport in each segment will also be given. We will then describe the urinary concentrating and diluting processes and, finally, the renal handling of specific solutes of particular interest.

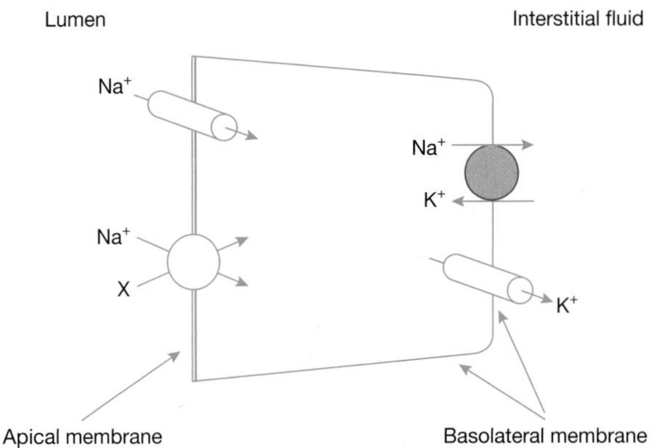

Fig. 1 *General features of transepithelial sodium transport in the nephron.* Intracellular Na^+ concentration is kept low through the action of the basolateral Na^+,K^+-ATPase, while the K^+ re-cycles through basolateral K^+ channels. Na^+ enters from the lumen down a large electrochemical gradient, using either Na^+ channels (in the distal nephron) or a series of cotransporters (or exchangers) that transport the non-sodium molecules or ions against their electrochemical gradients. In this and succeeding figures, red circles denote primary active transport whereas open circles denote cotransporters and exchangers; the stoichiometry of transporters is not shown. The Na^+,K^+-ATPase pumps out three Na^+ ions for every two K^+ ions pumped in.

Structure and function of each nephron segment

The accepted subdivisions of the nephron are indicated in Fig. 2. It is usually stated that each human kidney contains approximately one million nephrons, although the figure varies considerably between individuals. Broadly speaking, the deeper in the cortex that a nephron originates, the longer is the loop of Henle. Only deep (juxtamedullary) nephrons have loops that penetrate the inner medulla. In rodents, short loops of Henle (those present in superficial nephrons—the majority type in humans) all turn close to the outer medulla/inner medulla junction, whereas in humans short loops turn at various levels of the outer medulla, and some even remain within the cortex.

According to embryological criteria, the distal convoluted tubule (DCT), which is considered the final part of the nephron proper (those segments derived from the nephrogenic blastema), is joined to the collecting duct (derived from the ureteric bud) by a connecting

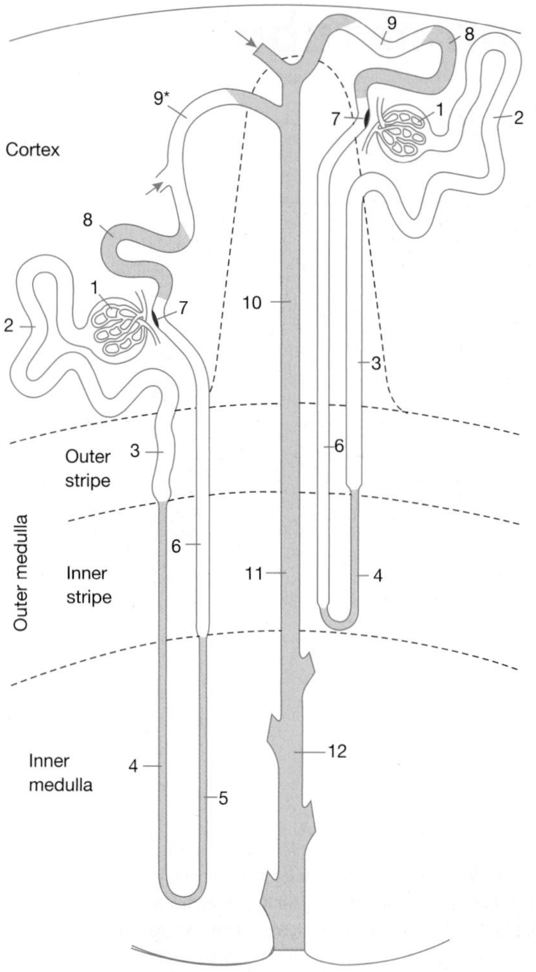

Fig. 2 *Anatomical divisions of the nephron.* The drawing (not to scale) depicts a short-looped (superficial) and a long-looped (juxtamedullary) nephron. Within the cortex, a dashed line delineates a medullary ray. Reproduced, with permission, from Kriz and Bankir (1988). 1, Renal corpuscle, including glomerulus and Bowman's capsule; 2, proximal convoluted tubule; 3, proximal straight tubule (pars recta); 4, thin descending limb; 5, thin ascending limb; 6, thick ascending limb; 7, macula densa; 8, distal convoluted tubule; 9, connecting tubule; 9*, connecting tubule of juxtamedullary nephron that forms an arcade; 10, cortical collecting tubule; 11, outer medullary collecting duct; 12, inner medullary collecting duct.

tubule (CNT) whose embryological origin is still disputed. In superficial nephrons the CNT is short and unbranched, whereas in deep nephrons the CNTs of a number of adjacent tubules may join together to form arcades. Arcades are less prevalent in humans than in other species. Within the cortex, collecting ducts accept fluid from approximately 10 nephrons, then descend, unbranched, to the inner medulla, where they fuse with other collecting ducts. In humans, usually eight fusions occur.

Proximal tubule

Structure

Histologically, the proximal tubule is divided into three subsegments (S_1, S_2, and S_3). S_1 cells make up the initial short segment of the PCT, and S_2 cells make up the remainder. The cortical segment of the proximal straight tubule (pars recta) also consists of S_2 cells, while S_3 cells

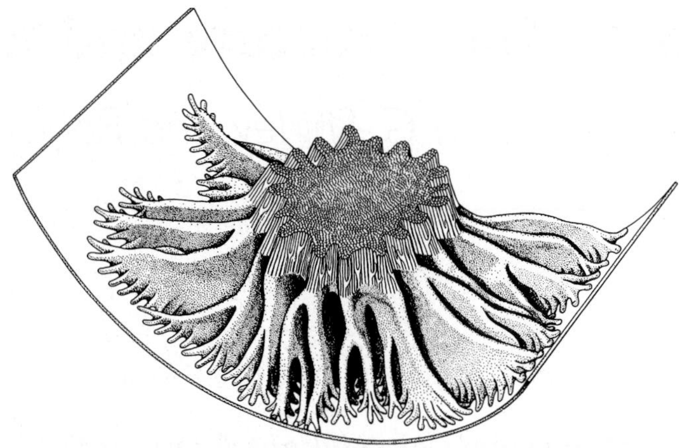

Fig. 3 *Diagram of three-dimensional structure of a proximal convoluted tubular cell.* The model illustrates the extensive surface area of both apical and basolateral membranes. The basolateral membranes of adjacent cells interdigitate with one another. Reproduced, with permission, from Welling and Welling (1976).

make up the medullary segment. The surface area available for transtubular transport is greatly increased by microvilli present on the apical membrane, the so-called 'brush border' seen under the light microscope, and by extensive infoldings of the basolateral membrane (Fig. 3). As befits the gradual decline in absolute reabsorptive load, the length of the apical microvilli and the degree of basolateral infolding both tend to decrease along the length of the proximal tubule (Fig. 4).

All proximal tubular cells have large numbers of mitochondria (packed close to the basal membrane) and lysosomal vacuoles. Contact between adjacent cells is restricted to a short region between the apical membrane and the basolateral membrane: the tight junction. In the proximal tubule, the tight junction is relatively permeable, providing a low-resistance pathway (paracellular shunt).

Membrane transport proteins

Some transporters are present throughout the length of the proximal tubule; others are restricted to particular regions (Table 1). The Na^+,K^+-ATPase pump is present in the basolateral membrane in the whole of the proximal tubule, as is a basolateral K^+ channel through which K^+ is 'recycled'. The water channel aquaporin-1 (AQP-1), present in both basolateral and apical membranes of the entire proximal tubule, largely accounts for the very high water permeability of this segment (Verkman 2002), although a proportion of water reabsorption may occur paracellularly. Because of the high water permeability, proximal tubular reabsorption is always isosmotic. The NHE-3 isoform of the Na^+/H^+ exchanger, located in the apical membrane throughout the proximal tubule, is the main transporter responsible for Na^+ entry into cells from the lumen.

In addition to transporters, the apical membrane (brush border) contains a range of enzymes (e.g. carbonic anhydrase, neutral endopeptidase) that may destroy or modify luminal compounds or indeed produce substances capable of modifying tubular function (see later sections).

Transport processes

Proximal convoluted tubule

S_1 segment In this segment, most of the filtered glucose and amino acids and a large proportion of phosphate and bicarbonate are reabsorbed.

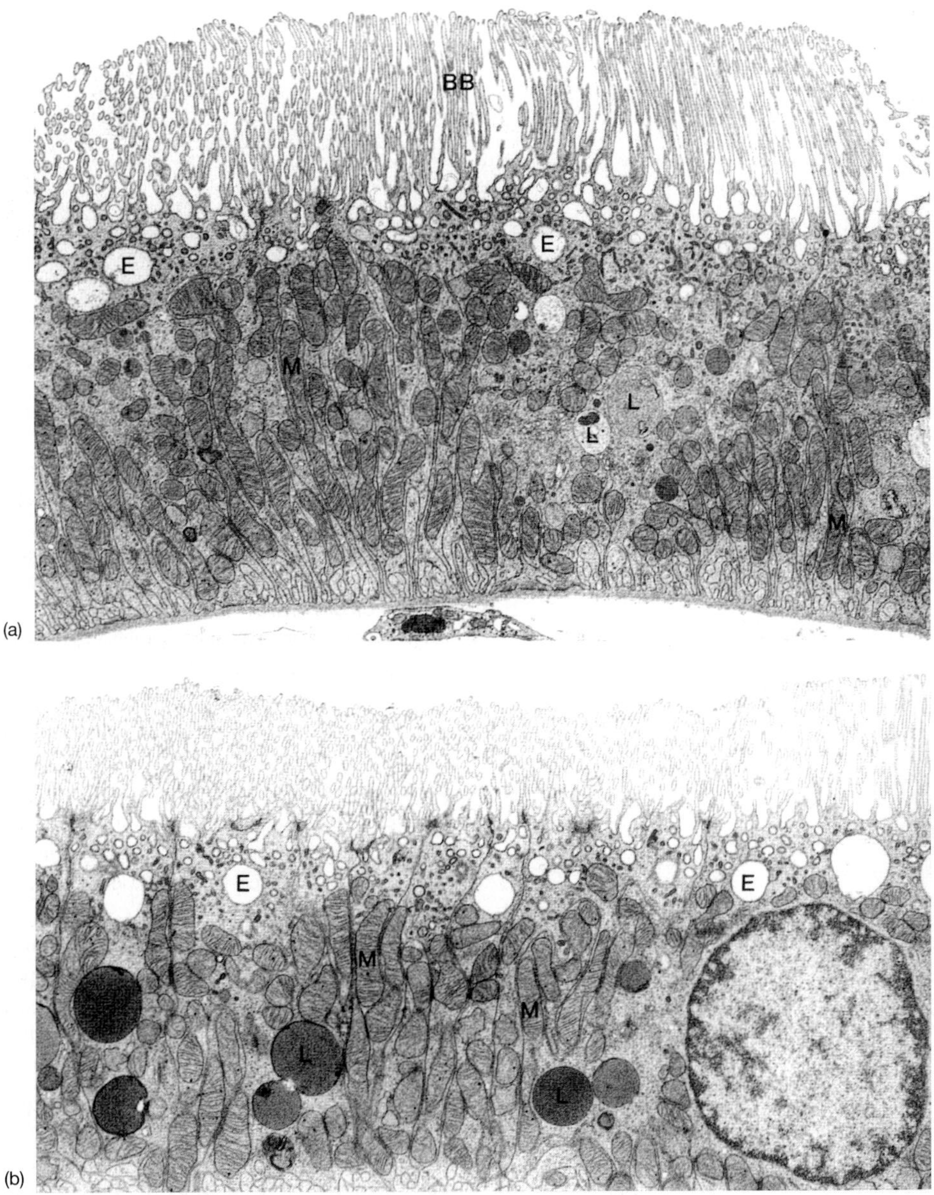

Fig. 4 *Electron micrographs of proximal convoluted tubular epithelium from rat kidney:* (a) S_1 segment; (b) S_2 segment (both 6200×). Reproduced, with permission, from Maunsbach and Christensen (1992). M, mitochondria; L, lysosomes; E, endosomes; BB, brush border. Note the taller brush border in S_1 than S_2.

Reabsorption is linked with Na^+: entry into the cell from the lumen relies on cotransporters or, in the case of bicarbonate, on the NHE-3 exchanger that secretes H^+ into the lumen where the proton combines with filtered HCO_3^- to convert it to H_2CO_3 and, ultimately, CO_2 and H_2O (see section on 'Bicarbonate'). In every case, the non-sodium ion or molecule moves against its electrochemical gradient, using the energy dissipated from the 'downhill' entry of Na^+ into the cell (Fig. 5). The Na^+ reabsorption that is associated with cotransport of neutral amino acids and glucose is electrogenic, creating a small lumen-negative transepithelial potential difference (PD) of ~−2 mV. (The paracellular shunt precludes the creation of large electrical gradients in the proximal tubule.) This PD drives the reabsorption of a certain amount of filtered Cl^- via the paracellular route. However, the permeability of the S_1 segment to Cl^- is relatively low, so Cl^- reabsorption lags behind that of Na^+ (and water), and consequently the Cl^- concentration of the tubular fluid rises slightly (by 10–20 per cent).

Micropuncture evidence indicates that, like Cl^-, K^+ reabsorption in the S_1 segment does not keep pace with Na^+ or water, leading to a slight elevation of its tubular fluid concentration (Le Grimellec 1975).

S_2 segment As indicated above, the intratubular Cl^- concentration at the start of the S_2 segment is greater than that of plasma [while, as a consequence of preferential HCO_3^- reabsorption in the S_1 segment, there is a HCO_3^- concentration gradient in the opposite direction (plasma to lumen)]. The tight junctions in the S_2 segment have a high permeability to Cl^- and low permeability to HCO_3^-, and passive

Table 1 Membrane transport proteins in the proximal tubule

Apical	Basolateral
Na^+–glucose cotransporter (SGLT2) [S_1 *and* S_2]	Na^+,K^+ATPase
$2Na^+$–glucose cotransporter (SGLT1) [S_3]	Glucose carrier proteins (GLUT-1 and GLUT-2)
Fructose transporter (GLUT-5)	
Na^+–amino acids cotransporter [S_1 *and* S_2]	Amino acid carrier proteins
Na^+–phosphate cotransporters: —type IIa (predominant) —type I	Na^+/phosphate cotransporter-type III Phosphate/anion exchanger Phosphate channel?
Na^+–citrate cotransporter	
Na^+–lactate cotransporter	Cl^- channel
$2Na^+$–sulfate cotransporter	Na^+–$3HCO_3^-$ cotransporter
Na^+/H^+ exchanger (NHE-3)	Na^+/H^+ exchanger (NHE-1)
H^+ATPase	Urate channel?
Urate/anion exchanger (URAT-1)	Urate/anion exchanger?
H^+/organic base exchanger	K^+Cl^- cotransporter
Anion/organic acid exchanger [*mainly* S_2 *and* S_3]	Organic base carrier protein
$Cl^-/HCOO^-$ exchanger	α-Ketoglutarate/organic anion exchanger [*mainly* S_2 *and* S_3]
H^+–$HCOO^-$ cotransporter	
Sulfate/oxalate exchanger	
Oxalate/Cl^- exchanger	
K^+ channel	
AQP-1	AQP-1

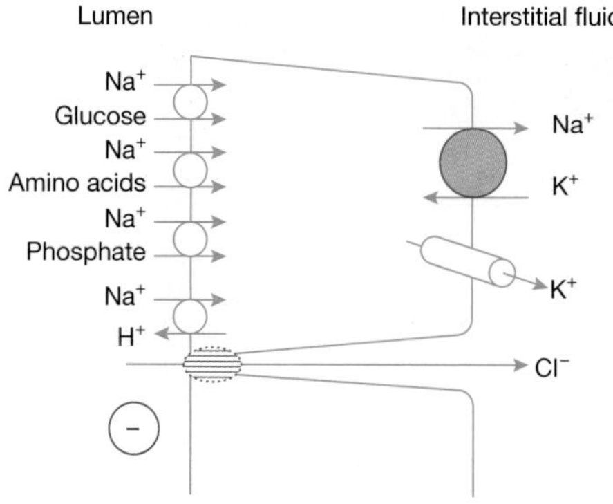

Fig. 5 *Major solute transport processes in the* S_1 *segment of the proximal convoluted tubule.* Cotransport of Na^+ with neutral amino acids and glucose creates a small lumen-negative transepithelial potential difference that drives some paracellular Cl^- reabsorption.

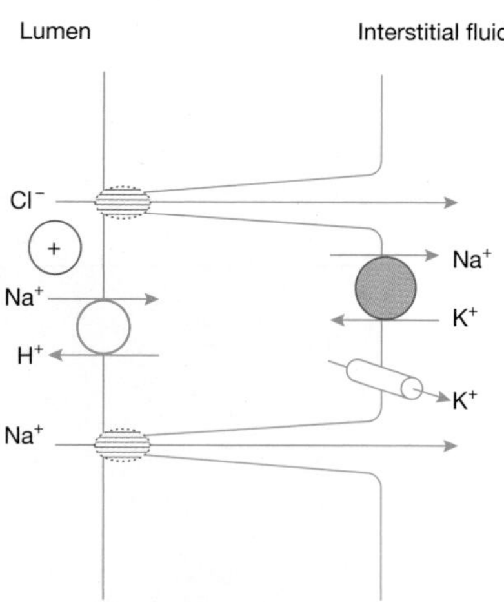

Fig. 6 *Major solute transport processes in the* S_2 *segment of the proximal convoluted tubule.* Passive paracellular Cl^- reabsorption down its concentration gradient creates a small lumen-positive transepithelial potential difference that provides a driving force for the reabsorption of some cations such as Na^+, K^+, and Ca^{2+}. However, most Na^+ reabsorption is transcellular, via apical Na^+/H^+ exchange.

paracellular Cl^- reabsorption therefore occurs down its concentration gradient. This Cl^- movement, together with a much reduced rate of electrogenic Na^+ transport (owing to the diminishing amounts of intratubular glucose and amino acids remaining to be cotransported), reverses the transepithelial PD, to ~+2 mV (Aronson and Giebisch 1997). The lumen-positive PD drives a certain amount of Na^+ reabsorption passively via the paracellular route (Fig. 6), but most Na^+ reabsorption is transcellular, via the apical NHE-3.

Not all Cl^- reabsorption is by simple diffusion, using the paracellular route. Some Cl^- is reabsorbed transcellularly, using transporters whose operation, in the final analysis, depends on the basolateral Na^+,K^+-ATPase (secondary or tertiary active transport). One of them involves a Cl^-/formate exchanger in the apical membrane, which is coupled with recycling of formate via either a formate–H^+ cotransporter or non-ionic diffusion of formic acid (Fig. 7). Another is believed to use oxalate in place of formate, the oxalate recycling via a sulfate/oxalate exchanger (Aronson and Giebisch 1997). In each case, Cl^- exit from the cell is via a basolateral K^+–Cl^- cotransporter or Cl^- channel (Fig. 7).

Potassium reabsorption in the PCT is incompletely understood, but there is little evidence for active transport. The raised tubular fluid/plasma K^+ concentration ratio achieved in the S_1 segment (see above), combined with the lumen-positive PD in the S_2 segment, may be sufficient to account for most, if not all, K^+ reabsorption paracellularly by simple diffusion (Fig. 8). The remainder is likely to be by solvent drag: fluid reabsorption will entrain any solute whose reflection coefficient is significantly less than unity (a reflection coefficient of unity signifies complete impermeability to the solute in question; a reflection coefficient of zero signifies that the solute is completely permeant); that of K^+ in the S_2 segment has been estimated at less than 0.4 (Wareing *et al.* 1995).

Together with the S_3 segment, the S_2 segment is the nephron site at which organic acids and organic bases are secreted into the lumen. For organic acids, the mechanism involves uptake at the basolateral membrane, using an α-ketoglutarate exchanger, and transport across the apical membrane using an anion exchanger. For organic bases, uptake is via a carrier unlinked to another ion, while luminal entry is via a H^+ exchanger (Fig. 9). A list of organic acids and bases using these systems is given in Table 2.

Pars recta

Although information on the function of the pars recta is limited, there is a consensus that this segment as a whole shares many of the characteristics of the PCT in terms of hydraulic and electrical conductivities, mechanisms of Na^+, Cl^-, and HCO_3^- reabsorption, and the isosmotic nature of reabsorption (Schafer and Barfuss 1982). Its intrinsic capacity for Na^+ and water reabsorption is about half that of the PCT (see Jacobson 1982), which accords with its lower basolateral

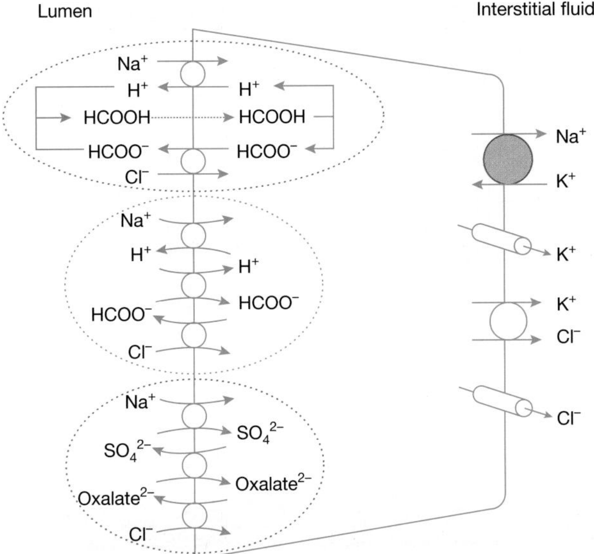

Fig. 7 *Transcellular chloride reabsorption in the S_2 segment of the proximal convoluted tubule.* Cl^- is believed to enter cells against its electrochemical gradient in two ways: (i) a Cl^-/formate exchanger, with the formate recycling across the apical membrane either by non-ionic diffusion of formic acid or on a H^+–formate cotransporter—in each case in parallel with Na^+/H^+ exchange; (ii) a Cl^-/oxalate exchanger, which works in conjunction with an oxalate/sulfate exchanger and a (2)Na^+–sulfate cotransporter. All entry mechanisms depend, in the final analysis, on the electrochemical gradient for Na^+ across the apical membrane, which in turn is dependent on the basolateral Na^+,K^+-ATPase. Cl^- exit across the basolateral membrane uses a Cl^- channel or a K^+–Cl^- cotransporter.

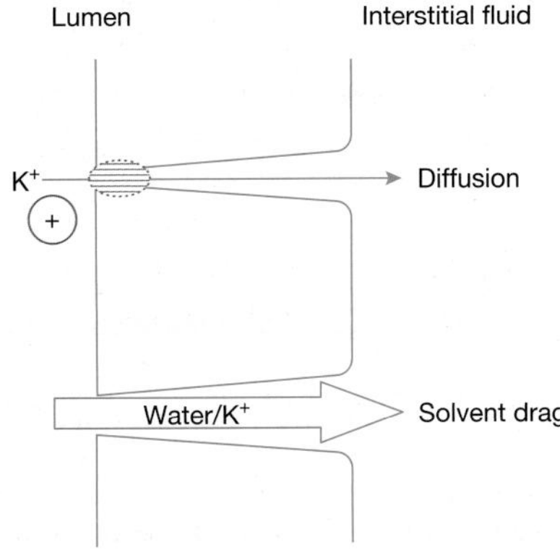

Fig. 8 *Mechanism of potassium reabsorption in the S_2 segment of the proximal convoluted tubule.* Most K^+ reabsorption is likely to result from simple diffusion, down small concentration and electrical gradients, through the paracellular pathway. A second possible component is solvent drag, K^+ being entrained in reabsorbed fluid.

Na^+,K^+-ATPase activity (per millimetre of tubule length). A major difference between the pars recta and PCT concerns K^+ handling. *In vitro* studies have consistently indicated K^+ *secretion* into the tubular fluid of the pars recta in both S_2 and S_3 segments.

It is generally believed that the pars recta is an important site of organic acid and organic base secretion, using mechanisms identical to those in the S_2 segment of the PCT.

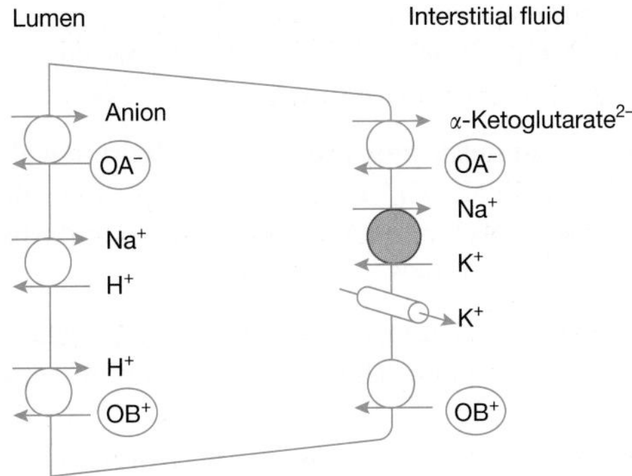

Fig. 9 The major *mechanisms of organic acid (OA^-) and organic base (OB^+) secretion in the S_2 and S_3 segments of the proximal tubule.* The operation of all the exchangers/cotransporters depends, in the final analysis, on the basolateral Na^+,K^+-ATPase. Thus, secretion of organic acids/bases is secondary active.

Table 2 Some of the physiologically and pharmacologically important substances transported by the proximal tubular organic acid and base transport systems

Organic acids	Organic bases
Para-Aminohippurate	Atropine
Acetazolamide	Cimetidine
Thiazide diuretics	Isoprenaline
Loop diuretics	Procaine
Penicillin	Amiloride
Probenecid	Acetylcholine
Salicylate	Histamine
Indomethacin	Creatinine
Bile acids	Dopamine
Corticosteroids	Adrenaline/noradrenaline
Sulfonamides	Quinolones
	Cephalosporins
	Paraquat

Major control mechanisms

- An intrinsic mechanism, referred to as *glomerulotubular balance*, normally ensures that any fluctuations in glomerular filtration rate (GFR) are accompanied by near-proportionate fluctuations in proximal tubular reabsorption, so that in the absence of other factors the fraction of glomerular filtrate reaching the end of the proximal tubule varies little (see later section).
- Acute increases in arterial blood pressure lead to a *pressure natriuresis*, caused largely by reduced proximal tubular reabsorption as a consequence of an increase in *renal interstitial hydrostatic pressure*. The latter, which is believed to depend on intrarenally produced *nitric oxide* (Nakamura *et al.* 1998), reduces net reabsorption by increasing paracellular backflux through the tight junctions.
- Increased *renal sympathetic nervous discharge* (following a reduction in effective circulating volume) directly stimulates proximal tubular reabsorption (DiBona 2000).
- Physiological increases in plasma *angiotensin II* (AII) concentrations, following stimulation of the renin–angiotensin–aldosterone

system, directly stimulate proximal tubular reabsorption through an effect on Na^+/H^+ exchange, although pharmacological concentrations can be inhibitory (Ichikawa and Harris 1991).

- *Glucocorticoids* stimulate proximal tubular reabsorption of HCO_3^-. They increase both Na^+/H^+ exchange at the apical membrane and the activity of the Na^+–(3)HCO_3^- cotransporter at the basolateral membrane (Ruiz *et al.* 1995).
- It is likely that several agents act *intraluminally* to influence proximal tubular reabsorption. Thus far, there is firm evidence for two such agents:
  —intraluminal *dopamine* contributes to the reduction in fractional proximal reabsorption seen during acute volume expansion (Reddy *et al.* 1991);
  —intraluminal *AII* (whose concentrations in the PCT exceed those in plasma by an order of magnitude) stimulates proximal tubular reabsorption (Navar *et al.* 1999).

Loop of Henle

The loop of Henle is defined anatomically as that segment of the nephron between the PCT and the macula densa (Kriz and Bankir 1988). It comprises the pars recta, the thin descending limb, the thin ascending limb (in deep nephrons), and the medullary and cortical thick ascending limb of Henle (TALH). The pars recta has already been discussed.

Structure

Thin limbs

Thin descending limbs differ between short and long loops. In short loops they consist of a simple epithelium of flat, non-interdigitating cells with very few, short microvilli and few mitochondria or other cell organelles. In long loops they are more complex: the upper segments have a greater diameter and thicker epithelium than seen in short loops, and have extensive basolateral interdigitations (Fig. 10), but as they descend through the inner medulla they gradually become thinner and simpler, a change delayed in the longest loops. The structural characteristics of thin descending limbs have been best defined in rodents; they have not, as yet, been described fully in humans.

The transition from descending limb to thin ascending limb epithelium (in long loops) occurs just before the bend of the loop. The cells of the thin ascending limb are flat, with extensive interdigitations (Fig. 10).

Thick ascending limb of Henle

The cells of the TALH in the outer medulla and cortex are similar, although those in the medulla are taller (Fig. 11). Unlike the thin limbs, the TALH cells contain a high density of mitochondria. The apical membrane has a number of short microvilli that increase in density as the TALH reaches the cortex. The TALH ends at the junction with the DCT, shortly after the *macula densa*. The latter comprises a plaque of specialized cells with relatively large, densely packed nuclei. Its basal surfaces about the extraglomerular mesangium between the afferent and efferent arterioles.

Membrane transport proteins

Thin limbs

The osmotic water permeability of each subsegment of thin descending limbs is high, owing to the abundance of AQP-1 water channels in both apical and basolateral membranes. The permeability to Na^+ varies among species; the channels/transporters/paracellular pathways have not been identified. A similar variability exists with respect to urea permeability. In this context, urea transporters (UT-A2) have been identified in types 1 and 3 thin descending limb (Smith and Rousselet 2001). There is some evidence for Cl^- and K^+ channels, as well as for a K^+–Cl^- cotransporter, in rabbit thin descending limb basolateral membranes. Only very low levels of basolateral Na^+,K^+-ATPase have been detected.

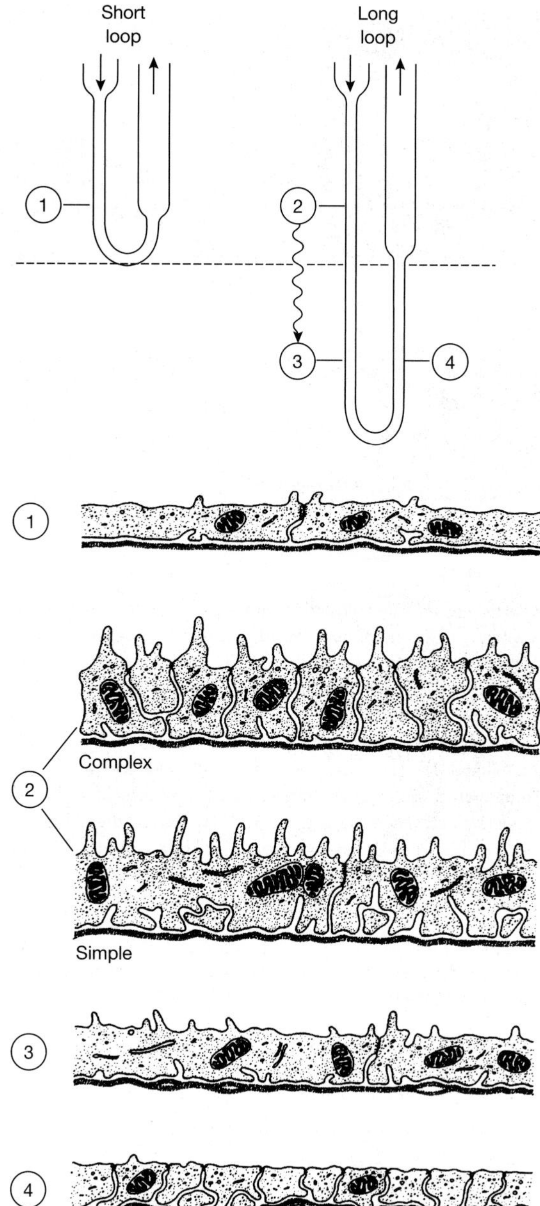

Fig. 10 *Diagram of the ultrastructure of the thin limbs of the loop of Henle.* Four types of epithelium have been described: (1) thin descending limb of short loops; (2) thin descending limb of upper part of long loops, which is either 'complex' (upper panel) or 'simple' (lower panel); (3) thin descending limb of lower part of long loops; and (4) thin ascending limb. Reproduced, with permission, from Kriz and Kaissling (2000).

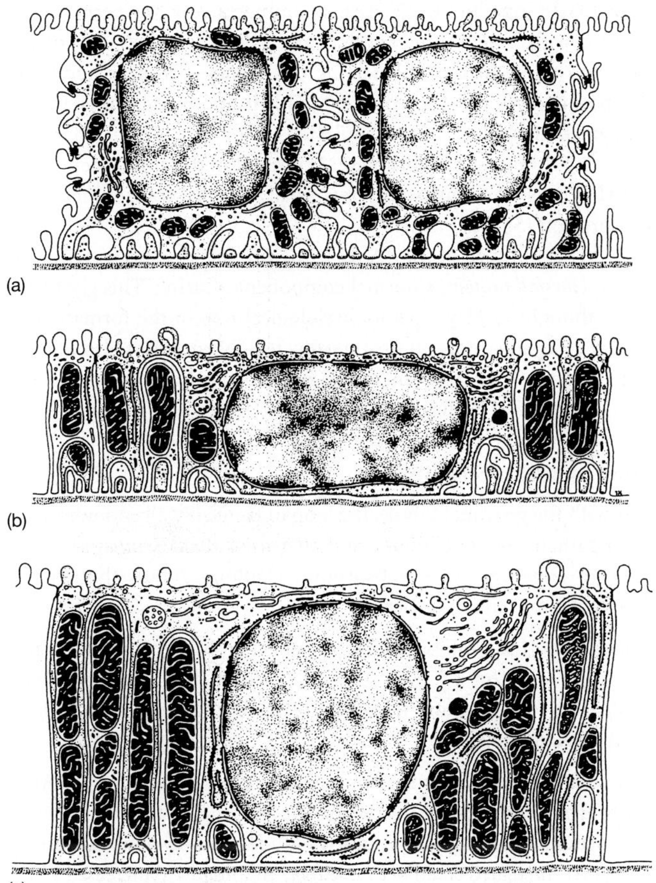

Fig. 11 *Diagram of cells of (a) macula densa, (b) cortical thick ascending limb, and (c) medullary thick ascending limb.* Reproduced, with permission, from Kaissling and Kriz (1992).

The thin ascending limb lacks AQPs and has a correspondingly low osmotic water permeability. Its permeability to Na^+ and Cl^- is relatively high. No Na^+ channels or transporters have been described, but a Cl^- channel has been identified in both apical and basolateral membranes (ClC-K1 in rodents, ClC-Ka in humans; Uchida and Marumo 2000). There is a significant permeability to urea. As in thin descending limbs, basolateral Na^+,K^+-ATPase activity is very low.

Thick ascending limb of Henle (see also Chapter 5.5, Fig. 1)

Like the thin ascending limb, the TALH has no AQPs and water permeability is essentially zero, but in other respects the TALH is markedly different. It is well endowed with a range of transporters in both apical and basolateral membranes. Basolateral Na^+,K^+-ATPase activity is high, while the major Na^+ entry step on the apical membrane is the bumetanide-sensitive Na^+–K^+–$2Cl^-$ cotransporter (BSC-1; otherwise known as NKCC-2) that is characteristic of this nephron segment. The apical membrane also contains Na^+/H^+ exchangers, H^+ATPase, and at least two K^+ channels through which K^+ ions that enter the cell on the Na^+–K^+–$2Cl^-$ cotransporter can recycle into the lumen (Giebisch 2001). The basolateral membrane contains K^+ and Cl^- (ClC-K2 or ClC-Kb) channels, as well as a K^+–Cl^- cotransporter. The transport characteristics of the macula densa region are similar to those of the TALH, although Na^+,K^+-ATPase activity is much lower.

Table 3 Membrane transport proteins in the loop of Henle (excluding pars recta)

Loop segment	Apical	Basolateral
Thin descending limb		Na^+,K^+-ATPase (extremely low levels)
	AQP-1	AQP-1
	Urea transporter (UT-A2)	Urea transporter (UT-A2)
		K^+ channel?
		Cl^- channel?
		K^+–Cl^- cotransporter?
Thin ascending limb		Na^+,K^+-ATPase (extremely low levels)
	Cl^- channel (ClC-Ka; ClC-K1)	Cl^- channel (ClC-Ka; ClC-K1)
Thick ascending limb	Na^+–K^+–$2Cl^-$ cotransporter (BSC-1; NKCC-2)	Na^+,K^+-ATPase
	K^+ channels (x3?)	K^+ channel
	Na^+/H^+ exchanger (NHE-3 and possibly NHE-2)	Na^+–$3HCO_3^-$ cotransporter
		Cl^-/HCO_3^- exchanger (AE-2)
	H^+ATPase	Na^+/H^+ exchanger (NHE-1)
	Cl^-/HCO_3^- exchanger	Cl^- channel (ClC-Kb; ClC-K2)
		K^+–Cl^- cotransporter
		Ca^{2+}ATPase

However, unlike TALH cells, macula densa cells do not elaborate Tamm–Horsfall protein (see below).

Table 3 lists those transport proteins in the loop of Henle that have been identified to date.

Transport processes

Thin limbs

Fluid within the descending limbs comes into osmotic equilibrium with the hypertonic medullary interstitium primarily by water abstraction, via the AQP-1 channels. There is general agreement that any Na^+ transport in the thin descending limbs is passive, but, as indicated above, the transepithelial pathways have not been identified. Although it might be presumed that Na^+ should enter the lumen from the interstitium (owing to the high interstitial Na^+ concentration in the medulla), there is some indirect evidence (from computer modelling) for significant Na^+ *reabsorption*. The latter would occur as a consequence of the water reabsorption, partly by solvent drag and partly by diffusion down a concentration gradient created by the water abstraction (Imai *et al.* 1987). The extent of any such Na^+ reabsorption will be greatly influenced by the length of the loop and by the precise permeability characteristics of the descending limbs, for which considerable interspecies variation has been described.

Computer modelling and experimental observations both point to significant secretion of K^+ ions and urea in the thin descending limbs (Taniguchi *et al.* 1987). Indeed, the delivery of K^+ to the tip of the loop sometimes exceeds the filtered load (Wright 1987). The secretory pathways have not been defined.

The thin ascending limb can dilute the tubular fluid as a result of NaCl reabsorption unaccompanied by water (Berliner 1982);

however, evidence for active transport is scant. Because of events in the descending limb, the NaCl concentration of fluid entering the thin ascending limb is thought to exceed that of the surrounding interstitium. This would allow NaCl reabsorption down its electrochemical gradient (see section on 'Countercurrent system'). Cl^- is probably reabsorbed transcellularly, through the Cl^- channels (ClC-Ka) in apical and basolateral membranes; the conductive pathway for Na^+ is unknown, but paracellular transport seems likely. The diluting effect of NaCl reabsorption in the water-impermeable thin ascending limb is blunted to some extent by the simultaneous entry of urea into the lumen, down its concentration gradient.

Thick ascending limb of Henle

The TALH is a major site of NaCl reabsorption, driven, ultimately, by the basolateral Na^+,K^+-ATPase. Sodium enters the TALH cells mainly via the apical Na^+–K^+–$2Cl^-$ cotransporter (BSC-1; NKCC-2), which is inhibited by loop diuretics such as frusemide and bumetanide; these compete with Cl^- for one of the carrier sites. Chloride exits the basolateral membrane via the Cl^- channel (ClC-Kb) and K^+–Cl^- cotransporter (Fig. 12).

It is thought that most K^+ that enters the cell on the Na^+–K^+–$2Cl^-$ cotransporter promptly diffuses back into the lumen ('recycles') through the apical K^+ channels. Potassium recycling has two consequences: (i) it ensures the availability of sufficient K^+ in the lumen to facilitate the continued operation of the Na^+–K^+–$2Cl^-$ cotransporter (the K^+ concentration in the fluid delivered to the TALH is an order of magnitude lower than that of Na^+ or Cl^-) and (ii) it effectively renders electrogenic the Na^+–K^+–$2Cl^-$ cotransporter (which is intrinsically electroneutral). The latter effect, coupled with the Cl^- conductance across the basolateral membrane, establishes a transepithelial PD that is lumen positive (Greger 1985), measured under *in vitro* conditions at ~+10 mV. In theory, this transepithelial PD can drive the reabsorption of cations or, alternatively, the secretion of anions. In practice, the tight junctions display selectivity to cations over anions; thus cations are reabsorbed passively through the paracellular route. (Tight junctions in the TALH combine a very low permeability to water with a high ionic conductance.) Approximately half of the Na^+ reabsorbed in the TALH is by this voltage-driven, paracellular transport (Reeves and Andreoli 2000). Other cations reabsorbed by this mechanism include K^+, Ca^{2+}, and Mg^{2+}.

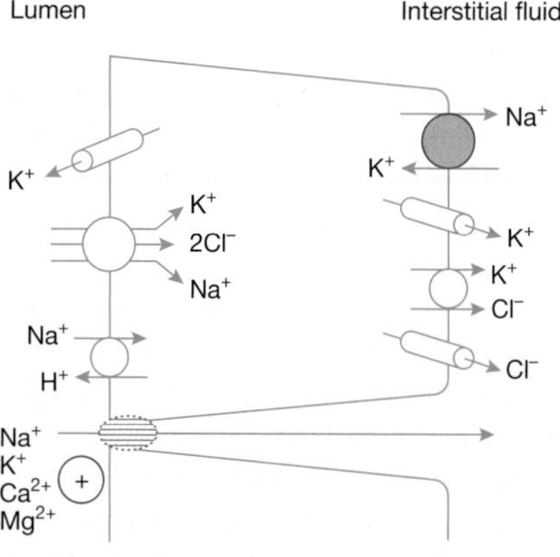

Fig. 12 *Major transport mechanisms in the thick ascending limb of Henle.* Transcellular Na^+ reabsorption is mediated largely by the apical Na^+–K^+–$2Cl^-$ cotransporter, although Na^+/H^+ exchange plays a minor role. Na^+,K^+-ATPase effects Na^+ exit across the basolateral membrane, while Cl^- exit is via the Cl^- channel and the K^+–Cl^- cotransporter. K^+ ions entering on the Na^+–K^+–$2Cl^-$ cotransporter recycle across the apical membrane through K^+ channels. This recycling, together with Cl^- exit across the basolateral membrane, creates a lumen-positive transepithelial potential difference which drives the paracellular reabsorption of cations.

The NHE-3 (and possibly NHE-2) present in the apical membrane of TALH cells contributes only marginally to total transcellular Na^+ reabsorption (Shirley *et al.* 1998).

A curious feature of the TALH is the production and secretion of *Tamm–Horsfall protein*, a normal component of urine. This glycoprotein is thought to play a pathophysiological role in the formation of urinary casts and, more controversially, renal stones. It is also implicated in renal defence mechanisms against infection, by interfering with adherence of bacteria to tubular cells (Kokot and Dulawa 2000).

Major control mechanisms

- As with the proximal tubule, the loop of Henle is well endowed with sympathetic nerve endings, and increased *renal sympathetic discharge* enhances Na^+ reabsorption (DiBona 2000), though the mechanisms remain unclear.
- *Aldosterone* has a minor stimulatory effect on Na^+ reabsorption and a major one on K^+ reabsorption in perfused loops of Henle (Stanton 1986). Again, the nature of the changes underlying these effects is unknown.
- Circulating *vasopressin* stimulates Na^+ reabsorption in the TALH through mechanisms initiated by the binding of the hormone to basolateral V_2 receptors coupled to adenylate cyclase activation. A cAMP-mediated chain of events then culminates in increased activity of apical K^+ channels and basolateral Cl^- channels and, in the long term, increased expression of the apical Na^+–K^+–$2Cl^-$ cotransporter (Kim *et al.* 1999).
- Some *eicosanoids*, produced intrarenally from arachidonic acid through the action of cyclooxygenase (e.g. prostaglandin E_2), inhibit Na^+ reabsorption in the TALH.
- *Intraluminal* factors influencing reabsorption in the loop are thought to include:
  —*atrial natriuretic peptide*, which inhibits Cl^- reabsorption in the TALH of the mouse, at least under *in vitro* conditions (Bailly 2000);
  —*endothelin*, which also inhibits Cl^- reabsorption in perfused mouse TALH (de Jesus Ferreira and Bailly 1997).

Distal tubule and collecting duct

The distal tubule is defined as that segment of the nephron between the macula densa and the point of confluence with another distal tubule to form a collecting duct. It incorporates several subsegments (see Fig. 2): the final (very short) part of the TALH, the DCT, the CNT, and a short section of cortical collecting tubule epithelium (often referred to as the *initial collecting tubule*). The collecting duct can be divided into cortical, outer medullary, and inner medullary regions. There are further differences between the outer and inner stripes of the outer medullary collecting duct (OMCD), while the IMCD can be divided into three zones. In addition to the cell type characteristic of each subsegment, *intercalated cells* are found in much of the distal nephron. Throughout the distal tubule and collecting duct the tight junctions between adjacent cells are deeper than in the proximal tubule and much less 'leaky'.

Structure

Distal convoluted tubule

This segment makes up approximately half of the total distal tubule. The first part (DCT_1) consists exclusively of DCT cells (Fig. 13). The second part (DCT_2), a transitional zone between DCT and CNT, includes a small proportion of intercalated cells (Tisher *et al.* 1968). The total surface area of the basolateral membrane of DCT cells is considerably greater than that of the apical membrane (referred to as 'amplification'), largely as a result of lateral cell processes that interdigitate with neighbouring cells. The density of mitochondria in these cells is the greatest along the nephron. The mitochondria line up along the basal membrane, whereas the cell nucleus is located close to the apical surface, which has large numbers of very short microvilli. There is a paucity of cell organelles between the nucleus and the apical surface, a characteristic feature of DCT cells.

Intercalated cells (Fig. 14) are of two types: α and β, both of which are found in the distal tubule and cortical collecting tubule, but only α-intercalated cells in the medullary collecting duct. Each type has a roundish appearance under the microscope, with the nucleus close to the basal surface. α-intercalated cells have many apical microvilli and their mitochondria are concentrated on the apical side, whereas β-intercalated cells have fewer apical microvilli, and their mitochondria are located mainly on the basal side.

Connecting tubule

The CNT comprises two cell types: CNT cells, the majority; and intercalated cells, the remainder (ranging from 25 to 45 per cent, depending on species). CNT cells (Fig. 13) have a similar structure regardless of whether they are located in superficial distal tubules or in the branched arcades of deep nephrons (see Fig. 2). They exhibit basolateral amplification, not as a result of lateral cell processes as in DCT cells, but from infolding of the basal membrane. Mitochondria are present along the basal membrane and also in the apical region. Microvilli are short and sparse.

Cortical collecting tubule

The 'initial collecting tubule' (the final segment of the distal tubule) and the CCT have the same epithelium, comprising mainly *principal* cells (Fig. 13), with intercalated cells making up the remaining 30–40 per cent.

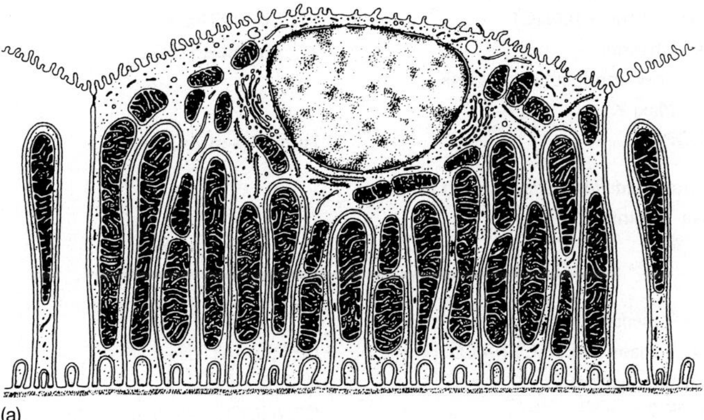

(a)

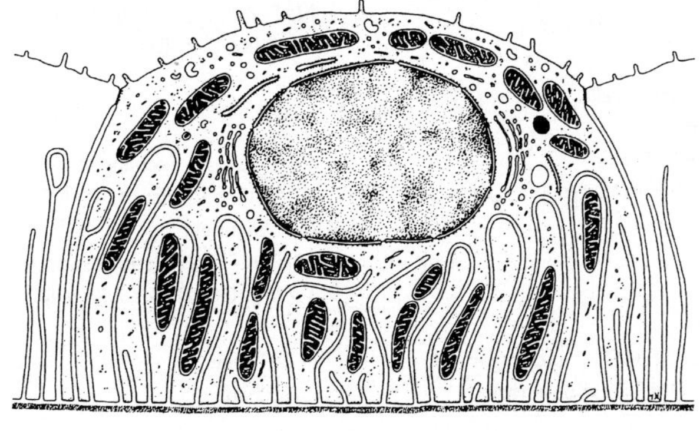

(b)

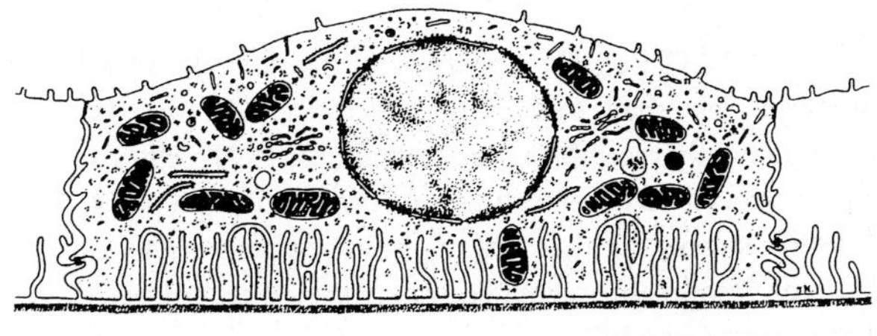

(c)

Fig. 13 *Diagram of (a) distal convoluted tubule cell, (b) connecting tubule cell, and (c) cortical collecting tubule principal cell.* Reproduced, with permission, from Kaissling and Kriz (1992).

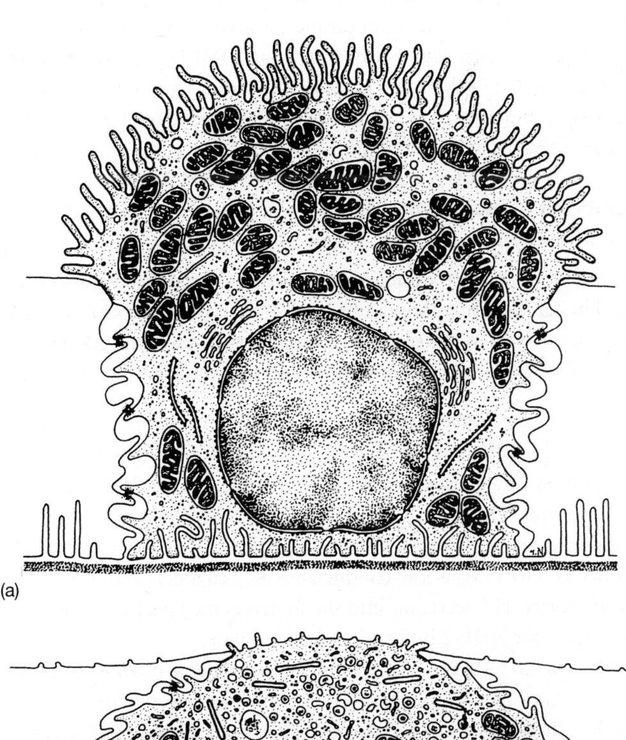

(a)

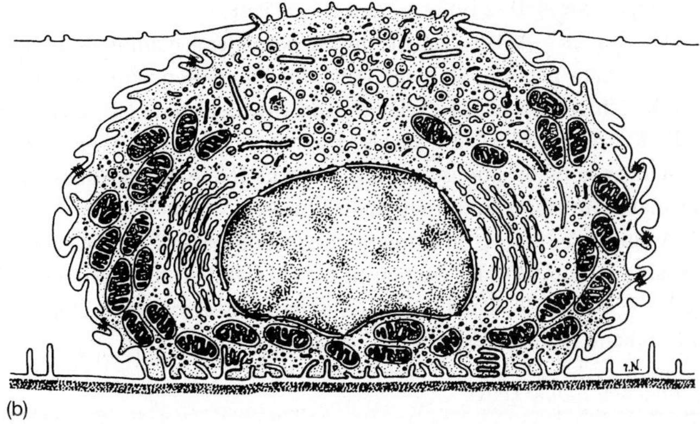

(b)

Fig. 14 *Diagram of (a) α-intercalated cell and (b) β-intercalated cell.* Reproduced, with permission, from Kaissling and Kriz (1992).

CCT principal cells are flatter, with more shallow basal infoldings, than CNT cells. Their apical side contains a meshwork of microtubules and microfilaments that includes small vesicles containing AQP channels that can be inserted into the apical membrane (see later).

Outer medullary collecting duct

The division of the outer medulla into outer and inner stripes is defined merely by the transition of pars recta to thin descending limb of Henle. It is therefore not surprising to find no sharp transition of the OMCD between the two stripes but instead a gradual change. In the outer stripe, the OMCD is very similar to CCT, both in the distribution of principal and α-intercalated cells, and in their appearance. In the inner stripe, there is a gradual diminution in the proportion of intercalated cells, and subtle changes in the appearance of 'principal' cells, including a reduction in the density of mitochondria (Kaissling and Kriz 1992).

Inner medullary collecting duct

As the IMCD progresses towards the papilla, its diameter and the height of its epithelium increase. In $IMCD_1$ (the outermost zone), a few α-intercalated cells (~10 per cent of the total cell population) are interspersed with collecting duct cells (modified principal cells), the latter being similar in appearance to those of the OMCD inner stripe. Intercalated cells are absent from $IMCD_2$ and $IMCD_3$. From $IMCD_2$, cells of somewhat different appearance, called IMCD cells, replace the collecting duct cells. These are larger than OMCD cells, their height increasing as the renal papilla is approached; they have numerous short microvilli; and they have extensively developed lateral intercellular spaces (Kaissling and Kriz 1992).

Membrane transport proteins (see also Chapter 5.5, Figs 2 and 3)

Membrane transport proteins identified in the distal nephron are listed in Table 4. Only those in the major cell type of each subsegment will be dealt with in this section; transport processes in the intercalated cells will be considered separately (see section on 'Bicarbonate').

Distal convoluted tubule cells

The distinguishing feature of DCT cells at the molecular level is the presence, in the apical membrane, of the thiazide-sensitive Na^+–Cl^- cotransporter (TSC; NCC). (Thiazide diuretics bind to its Cl^- site.) The apical membrane also contains a Ca^{2+} channel (ECaC; more recently known as TRPV-5), a low-conductance K^+ channel, and a K^+–Cl^- cotransporter. H^+ secretion into the lumen is mediated by a Na^+/H^+ exchanger (the NHE-2 isoform) and H^+ ATPase.

The Na^+,K^+-ATPase activity in the basolateral membrane is the highest of any nephron segment. It acts in conjunction with a basolateral K^+ channel, which recycles K^+ ions. A basolateral Cl^- channel (ClC-K2) and Ca^{2+}ATPase are also present. The basolateral Na^+/H^+ exchanger is of the 'housekeeping' isoform (NHE-1) and does not normally contribute to transepithelial fluxes.

As indicated above, in humans the second part of the DCT is a transitional zone (DCT_2) containing hybrid cells that share properties of DCT and CNT. Thus, DCT_2 cells have an apical Na^+ channel (ENaC) and basolateral Na^+/Ca^{2+} exchanger.

Connecting tubule cells

In CNT cells, the Na^+–Cl^- cotransporter entry route is largely replaced by the amiloride-sensitive epithelial Na^+ channel (ENaC), and the basolateral membrane contains the Na^+/Ca^{2+} exchanger (as well as Ca^{2+}ATPase). The activity of the basolateral Na^+,K^+-ATPase is somewhat less than that of the DCT. In rodents, whose distal nephron generally resembles that of humans, CNT cells also express AQP-2 water channels, as well as vasopressin V_2 receptors (Kishore *et al.* 1996), suggesting that this nephron segment is the most proximal site of vasopressin-regulated water reabsorption (see section on 'Countercurrent system').

Table 4 Membrane transport proteins in the distal tubule and collecting duct

Apical	Basolateral
Distal convoluted tubule cells	
Na^+–Cl^- cotransporter (NCC; TSC)	Na^+,K^+-ATPase
K^+ channel (ROMK?)	K^+ channel
K^+–Cl^- cotransporter	Cl^- channel (ClC-K2)
Na^+/H^+ exchanger (NHE-2)	Na^+/H^+ exchanger (NHE-1)
H^+ATPase	Ca^{2+}ATPase
Ca^{2+} channel (ECaC; TRPV-5)	Na^+/Ca^{2+} exchanger [DCT_2 *only*]
Na^+ channel (ENaC) [DCT_2 *only*]	
Connecting tubule cells	
Na^+ channel (ENaC)	Na^+,K^+-ATPase
K^+ channel (ROMK?)	K^+ channel
Na^+/H^+ exchanger (NHE-2)	Cl^- channel (ClC-K2)
Ca^{2+} channel (ECaC; TRPV-5)	Na^+/H^+ exchanger (NHE-1)
AQP-2	Ca^{2+}ATPase
	Na^+/Ca^{2+} exchanger
Cortical collecting tubule principal cells	
Na^+ channel (ENaC)	Na^+,K^+-ATPase
K^+ channels	K^+ channels (x3)
Low-conductance (ROMK)	
Maxi K	
AQP-2	AQP-3 (and AQP-4)
Outer medullary collecting duct cells	
Na^+ channel (ENaC)	Na^+,K^+-ATPase
AQP-2	AQP-3 (and AQP-4)
	K^+ channel?
Inner medullary collecting duct cells	
Na^+ channel (ENaC) [$IMCD_1$]	Na^+,K^+-ATPase
Cation channel?	K^+ channel
AQP-2	Cl^-/HCO_3^- exchanger (AE-2)
Urea transporter (UT-A1) [$IMCD_{2\ and\ 3}$]	AQP-4 (and AQP-3)
	Na^+–K^+–$2Cl^-$ cotransporter (NKCC-1; BSC-2)?
Intercalated cells	
Alpha	
H^+ATPase	Cl^-/HCO_3^- exchanger (AE-1)
H^+,K^+-ATPase	K^+–Cl^- cotransporter (KCC-4)
	Cl^- channel
	Na^+–K^+–$2Cl^-$ cotransporter (NKCC-1) [*Medulla only*]
Beta	
Cl^-/HCO_3^- exchanger (AE-4 or pendrin)	H^+ATPase
	Cl^- channel

Cortical collecting tubule principal cells

CCT principal cells contain apical ENaC and two types of apical K^+ channel: low-conductance (~35 pS) and high-conductance

(>100 pS; 'maxi-K') channels. Under basal conditions, basolateral Na^+,K^+-ATPase activity in CCT cells is lower than that of the CNT, but it is greatly influenced by prevailing mineralocorticoid levels (see later). The basolateral membrane also contains no fewer than three K^+ channels (Giebisch 2001).

Vasopressin-regulated AQP-2 channels are found in the apical membrane of principal-like cells throughout the collecting duct. AQPs are also present in the basolateral membrane; AQP-3 predominates in the CCT and OMCD, AQP-4 in the IMCD (Agre *et al.* 2000).

Outer medullary collecting duct cells

ENaC expression, present in the apical membrane, falls gradually from outer to inner stripe (Palmer and Garty 2000). From this segment onwards, no K^+ channels are found in the apical membrane. Na^+,K^+-ATPase is present in the basolateral membrane.

Inner medullary collecting duct cells

Apical ENaC has been identified only in the first segment of IMCD ($IMCD_1$), but there is evidence for a non-selective cation channel, inhibitable by amiloride, in the apical membrane of cultured IMCD cells (Light *et al.* 1988). An apical urea transporter (UT-A1) is present in the final segments of the IMCD ($IMCD_2$ and $IMCD_3$; Smith and Rousselet 2001).

The basolateral membrane contains Na^+,K^+-ATPase and a K^+ channel, but in addition there is some evidence (in the mouse) for a Na^+–K^+–$2Cl^-$ cotransporter of the secretory type (BSC-2; NKCC-1).

Transport processes

Distal convoluted tubule

The major transport processes in DCT cells are illustrated in Fig. 15. Sodium ions enter the cell on the apical Na^+–Cl^- cotransporter and are pumped across the basolateral membrane by the Na^+,K^+-ATPase. Potassium ions are recycled across the basolateral membrane. The apical Na^+–Cl^- cotransporter raises the intracellular Cl^- concentration above its electrochemical equilibrium; basolateral exit is via Cl^- channels (ClC-K2).

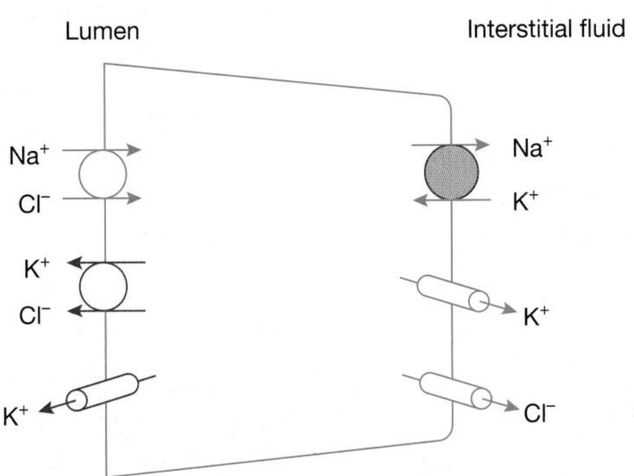

Fig. 15 *Major transport mechanisms in the distal convoluted tubule.* Na^+ and Cl^- ions enter cells across the apical membrane by means of the Na^+–Cl^- cotransporter. Na^+ ions exit the basolateral membrane using the Na^+,K^+-ATPase, while Cl^- ions use Cl^- channels. The K^+–Cl^- cotransporter in the apical membrane affords the possibility of K^+ secretion, but only if the luminal Cl^- concentration is unusually low. In the DCT_2 subsegment, some K^+ secretion takes place through the apical K^+ channel, facilitated by a small lumen-negative transepithelial potential difference.

The presence in the apical membrane of a K^+ channel and a K^+–Cl^- cotransporter allows the possibility of K^+ secretion into the DCT lumen. Any secretion using the K^+–Cl^- cotransporter requires Cl^- effectively to recycle across the apical membrane; such transport occurs only if the intraluminal Cl^- concentration is unusually low. Furthermore, little K^+ secretion normally occurs via the K^+ channels, at least in the early DCT (DCT_1), because there is no electrogenic Na^+ entry across the apical membrane; in this situation the magnitude of the PD across the apical membrane severely limits K^+ diffusion from the cell (Reilly and Ellison 2000). Lack of electrogenic Na^+ transport in DCT_1 is reflected by a transepithelial PD of essentially zero. However, in the transitional zone (DCT_2), the presence of ENaC allows partial depolarization of the apical membrane, resulting in the establishment of a small, lumen-negative PD (~10 mV). Accordingly, the DCT_2 subsegment sustains some K^+ secretion (Reilly and Ellison 2000).

Connecting tubule

The major route of Na^+ reabsorption in the CNT is apical entry via ENaC and basolateral exit via Na^+,K^+-ATPase. Therefore, the magnitude of the lumen-negative transepithelial PD in the CNT (30–40 mV in the rat) is greater than in DCT_2 (Reilly and Ellison 2000). The apical Na^+/H^+ exchanger (NHE-2) is also involved in transepithelial Na^+ transport; and, in the rabbit at least, there is functional evidence for a thiazide-sensitive component, although this does not tie in with the virtual absence of an apical Na^+–Cl^- cotransporter. The route of Cl^- transport is not clear. A basolateral Cl^- channel (ClC-K2) is available if Cl^- can enter the cell. Alternatively, Cl^- might be reabsorbed paracellularly. (Of note, Cl^- can be reabsorbed by β-intercalated cells—see section on 'Bicarbonate'.)

As already indicated, Na^+ entry via ENaC depolarizes the apical membrane. This, combined with the presence of apical K^+ channels and the high intracellular K^+ concentration (resulting from basolateral Na^+,K^+-ATPase activity), allows significant K^+ secretion in this nephron segment.

Cortical collecting tubule

Sodium reabsorption by CCT principal cells uses the same mechanism as in CNT cells: Na^+ entry via ENaC and exit via Na^+,K^+-ATPase (Fig. 16), generating a lumen-negative transepithelial PD. *In vitro* measurements in perfused tubules reveal that CCTs from rats pretreated with mineralocorticoids have transepithelial PDs nearly as great as those measured *in vivo* in CNT, whereas in the absence of mineralocorticoids the PD is much lower (Reif *et al.* 1986).

Evidence for Cl^- channels or cotransporters in either apical or basolateral membranes of principal cells is inconclusive; despite CCT being a 'tight' epithelium, transepithelial Cl^- reabsorption is thought to be mainly paracellular, driven by the lumen-negative PD. Additionally, some Cl^- reabsorption may take place through β-intercalated cells (see section on 'Bicarbonate').

Potassium transport by CCT principal cells has been studied extensively. Potassium enters the cell via the basolateral Na^+,K^+-ATPase and either recycles through K^+ channels in the basolateral membrane or exits into the lumen via apical K^+ channels. The latter process (K^+ secretion) predominates, owing to the depolarizing effect of apical Na^+ entry. As already indicated, low- and high-conductance K^+ channels are present in the apical membrane of principal cells. There is general agreement that the low-conductance K^+ channel mediates most K^+ secretion: it has a high open probability, and its activity

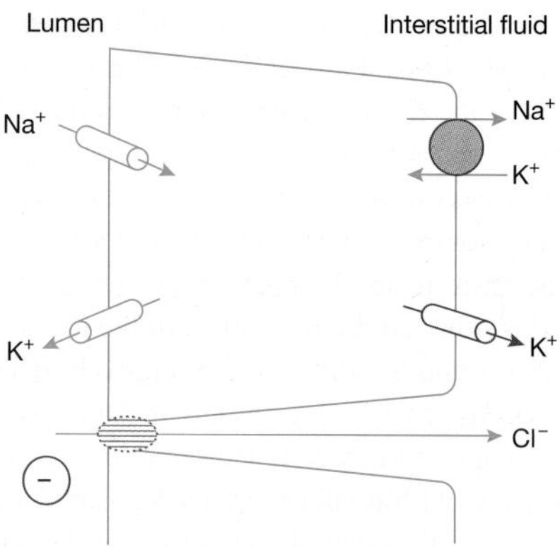

Fig. 16 *Major transport mechanisms in the principal cells of the cortical collecting tubule.* The apical membrane contains Na^+ channels through which Na^+ ions enter cells; the Na^+,K^+-ATPase then extrudes them across the basolateral membrane. Both apical and basolateral membranes contain K^+ channels, but the K^+ entering on the Na^+,K^+-ATPase leaves preferentially by the apical route owing to the depolarization of this membrane by apical Na^+ entry. Cl^- reabsorption is believed to be largely paracellular, driven by the transepithelial potential difference.

increases (due to insertion of additional channels) in response to a high K^+ diet or intracellular alkalosis, conditions known to stimulate K^+ secretion (Giebisch 1998).

Outer medullary collecting duct

In the outer stripe of the outer medulla, the collecting duct reabsorbs Na^+ through an amiloride-sensitive pathway, although at a lower rate than in the CCT. Net Na^+ transport in the inner stripe is undetectable (Stokes 1993), consistent with the gradual reduction in ENaC expression along the OMCD and the finding of a lumen-positive transepithelial PD in the inner stripe—due to electrogenic H^+ secretion by α-intercalated cells (see later) in the absence of electrogenic Na^+ transport in the opposite direction. Little information is available on Cl^- transport in the OMCD.

Little K^+ secretion normally occurs in any segment of the collecting duct beyond the CCT. In fact, there is usually net K^+ *reabsorption* in the OMCD (Stokes 1993).

Inner medullary collecting duct

There is *in vivo* evidence for amiloride-sensitive Na^+ reabsorption in the IMCD (Sonnenberg *et al.* 1987), whereas *in vitro* measurements have detected hardly any Na^+ reabsorption in this segment (Reeves and Andreoli 2000). Some Cl^- reabsorption occurs in the IMCD (Kokko and Baum 1992). Since the transepithelial PD is thought to be close to zero, a transcellular route is implied, but the mechanism is unknown.

Uncertainty also surrounds K^+ transport in the IMCD. In the absence of specific K^+ channels in the apical membrane, K^+ ions might use the apical non-selective cation channel described in these cells. Paracellular K^+ transport is also possible (Stanton and Giebisch 1992). However, neither the direction nor the mechanism of K^+ fluxes in this segment is clear. Likewise, the role, if any, of the basolateral Na^+–K^+–$2Cl^-$ cotransporter (see above) in IMCD transport processes remains speculative.

Major control mechanisms

- The major regulator of Na^+ reabsorption (and K^+ secretion—see Chapter 2.2) in the distal nephron is *aldosterone*, secreted from the zona glomerulosa of the adrenal cortex principally in response to raised plasma AII but also in response to increased plasma K^+ concentrations. Aldosterone binds to mineralocorticoid receptors within principal cells and initiates increased shuttling of ENaC to the apical membrane, followed by increased expression of ENaC and of basolateral Na^+,K^+-ATPase, thereby stimulating electrogenic Na^+ reabsorption. The depolarization of the apical membrane increases K^+ entry into the lumen. The apical low-conductance K^+ channels are also believed to be upregulated. Mineralocorticoid receptors are located throughout the distal nephron, including DCT and CNT, and there is evidence that aldosterone also stimulates thiazide-sensitive NaCl transport (Velazquez *et al.* 1996). Interestingly, the mineralocorticoid receptors in the distal nephron inherently have equal affinity for aldosterone and *glucocorticoids* (the latter having much higher plasma concentrations), yet *in vivo* they display specificity for aldosterone. This is due to the type 2 isoform of the enzyme 11β-hydroxysteroid dehydrogenase, which colocalizes with the mineralocorticoid receptors and inactivates glucocorticoids in their vicinity (see Chapter 5.5).
- *Atrial natriuretic peptide*, released from atrial myocytes in response to stretch, increases Na^+ excretion partly through suppression of the renin–angiotensin–aldosterone system and partly by a direct inhibitory effect on Na^+ reabsorption in the medullary collecting duct (Cogan 1990).`
- The neurohypophysial hormones *vasopressin* and *oxytocin* are both thought to influence Na^+ reabsorption in the collecting duct. Physiological concentrations of vasopressin stimulate Na^+ reabsorption in CCT (Inoue *et al.* 2001), although supraphysiological plasma concentrations are natriuretic. Oxytocin, even at physiological concentrations, is natriuretic; its likely site of action is the collecting duct (Walter *et al.* 2000).
- The role of *paracrine* factors on collecting duct function is increasingly recognized. In particular, *endothelin-1*, working through or in conjunction with *nitric oxide*, appears to reduce Na^+ reabsorption in IMCD (Kotelevtsev and Webb 2001).
- As in other nephron segments, *intraluminal factors* influence transport in the distal nephron:
  —*Angiotensin II*, acting from within the lumen, stimulates Na^+, HCO_3^-, and water reabsorption in distal tubules (Wang and Giebisch 1996);
  —Intraluminal *nucleotides*, acting on apical P2 receptors, inhibit ENaC-mediated Na^+ reabsorption in collecting ducts (Lehrmann *et al.* 2002);
  —The urinary content of *vasopressin* is surprisingly high, and apical V_{1a} receptors have been identified along the whole length of the collecting duct. Intraluminal vasopressin can inhibit the actions of basolateral vasopressin on ion and water transport (Inoue *et al.* 2001), although the physiological value of this effect is obscure.

Intrinsic control mechanisms

In addition to the numerous extrinsic (nerves, hormones) and autocrine/paracrine factors outlined above that influence tubular function, two major intrinsic mechanisms ensure that under normal circumstances the volume of glomerular filtrate delivered to the distal tubule is kept within fairly narrow limits. These are *glomerulotubular balance*, which automatically alters tubular reabsorptive rates to match changes in filtered load, and *tubuloglomerular feedback* (TGF), which adjusts the filtered load (i.e. GFR) appropriately if the amount of filtrate reaching the distal tubule is altered markedly.

Glomerulotubular balance

Fluctuations in GFR result in similar fluctuations in proximal tubular reabsorption. In other words, *fractional*, as opposed to absolute, reabsorption in the proximal tubule tends to remain constant. Indeed, an intrinsic feature of tubular function throughout the nephron is that in each segment the extent of Na^+ reabsorption is roughly proportional to Na^+ delivery (although the adjustment in reabsorption does not usually match the alteration in load). The mechanism of glomerulotubular balance is not understood but, as far as the proximal tubule is concerned, may involve GFR-induced changes in peritubular capillary oncotic pressure (which would influence capillary uptake of proximal tubular reabsorbate) and/or changes in the filtered load of glucose or amino acids, which could directly influence Na^+-coupled reabsorption (see Shirley *et al.* 2003).

Tubuloglomerular feedback

An increased tubular delivery of NaCl to the macula densa region of the nephron causes vasoconstriction of the afferent arteriole supplying that nephron's glomerulus and thus reduces both glomerular blood flow and glomerular capillary hydrostatic pressure. The resulting fall in the nephron's GFR normalizes the macula densa NaCl delivery (Schnermann 1998). The major mediator of TGF is thought to be adenosine, acting on adenosine A_1 receptors in the afferent arteriole. Raised NaCl delivery increases NaCl uptake (via NKCC-2) by macula densa cells, which stimulates the release of ATP into the adjacent extracellular space, where it is converted to adenosine (Thomson 2002). ATP itself may also constrict the afferent arteriole, via P2X purinoceptors. The sensitivity of TGF is enhanced by locally produced AII and blunted by nitric oxide, generated in macula densa cells by the type I isoform of nitric oxide synthase (Welch and Wilcox 2002).

Countercurrent system: urine concentration and dilution

The loop of Henle, while reabsorbing considerable amounts of filtered ions and water (see above), also functions as a *countercurrent multiplier*, generating and maintaining the osmotic gradient in the renal medullary interstitium. The ascending limb of Henle reabsorbs solute without water and thereby generates the so-called 'single effect', a small osmotic gradient (~200 mOsm/kg H_2O) between the lumen and interstitium. A 'single effect' also exists at any given level between the ascending and descending limbs as a consequence of the latter's high osmotic permeability. The U-shaped, countercurrent arrangement of the loop of Henle ensures that this single effect is multiplied so that a much larger osmotic gradient is generated along the length of the loop and within the medullary interstitium (Fig. 17). The result is the establishment of a corticomedullary osmotic gradient in the interstitium (ranging in humans from ~290 mOsm/kg H_2O in the cortex to as high as ~1200 mOsm/kg H_2O at the papillary tip) whilst hypotonic fluid (~100 mOsm/kg H_2O) is delivered from the TALH to the distal tubule.

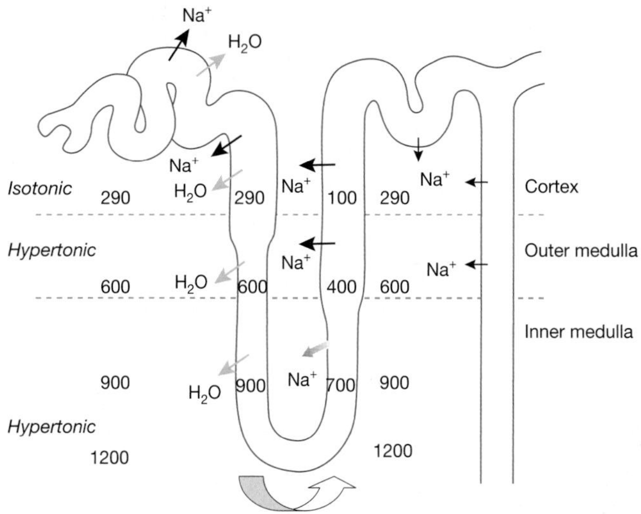

Fig. 17 *Countercurrent multiplication by the loop of Henle.* Fluid reabsorption in the proximal tubule is isosmotic. In the thin descending limb, osmotic water abstraction renders the tubular fluid hypertonic, while in the ascending limb NaCl is reabsorbed (passively in the thin ascending limb, actively in the TALH) without water until an osmotic gradient of ~200 mOsm/kg H_2O is achieved across the wall of the ascending limb at any given level. Countercurrent flow in the two limbs of the loop of Henle multiplies this small transverse osmotic gradient so that a much larger osmotic gradient, both within and without the tubule, is achieved longitudinally. The net result is the creation of a hypertonic medullary interstitium and the delivery of hypotonic fluid to the distal tubule. Thereafter, the tubular fluid can become even more dilute (in the absence of vasopressin), as a consequence of continued Na^+ reabsorption in the distal nephron, or it can become hypertonic, due to vasopressin-dependent water reabsorption in the late distal tubule and collecting duct. All figures are in mOsm/kg H_2O.

The countercurrent multiplier function of the loop of Henle means that it is possible to produce hypotonic or hypertonic urine simply by varying the secretion of vasopressin (antidiuretic hormone) from the hypothalamus (via the posterior pituitary). Vasopressin activates V_2 receptors in the basolateral membrane of the principal cells of the late distal tubule and collecting duct (and may additionally activate V_2 receptors in the CNT cells of the distal tubule), which results in the shuttling of AQP-2 water channels from intracellular vesicles to the apical membrane (see Chapter 2.1). Since the basolateral membrane contains AQP-3 and/or AQP-4 (constitutively expressed), the action of vasopressin renders this epithelium water permeable. At high plasma vasopressin concentrations, the hypotonic fluid delivered to the distal tubule becomes isotonic within the CCT and increasingly hypertonic (up to a maximum of ~1200 mOsm/kg H_2O) as it descends the medullary collecting duct. At low plasma vasopressin concentrations, much less water is reabsorbed in the distal nephron and the final urine is hypotonic (minimum value ~50 mOsm/kg H_2O, owing to the continued reabsorption of NaCl). Intermediate plasma vasopressin concentrations result in intermediate urine osmolalities.

Role of urea

As indicated earlier, NaCl reabsorption in the TALH depends on basolateral Na^+,K^+-ATPase. Ultimately, this active NaCl reabsorption is responsible for the 'single effect' not only in the TALH but also, indirectly, in the thin ascending limb, thanks partly to urea. The PCT reabsorbs (by passive diffusion) ~45 per cent of filtered urea, while the thin limbs of the loop of Henle secrete some urea. However, segments from the TALH to the initial IMCD are essentially impermeable to urea; the only segment of the distal nephron with significant urea permeability is the terminal IMCD ($IMCD_2$ and $IMCD_3$), where a vasopressin-sensitive urea transporter is present (Smith and Rousselet 2001). Vasopressin-stimulated water reabsorption in the cortical and outer medullary collecting ducts (which is dependent on the action of the TALH) therefore raises intraluminal urea concentrations and considerably enhances urea reabsorption into the interstitium across the terminal IMCD. This urea contributes significantly to the inner medullary interstitial osmolality, causing water abstraction from the thin descending limb. The fluid entering the thin ascending limb therefore has a higher NaCl concentration than that of the surrounding interstitium (Berliner 1982), and passive NaCl reabsorption in the thin ascending limb becomes possible.

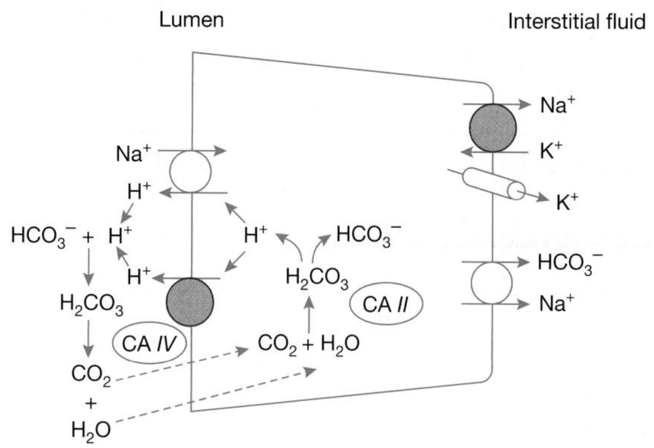

Fig. 18 *Bicarbonate reabsorption in the proximal tubule.* H^+ and HCO_3^- ions are generated from CO_2 and water, owing to the presence of the intracellular isoform of carbonic anhydrase (CA II). The H^+ ions are secreted into the lumen, mainly by Na^+/H^+ exchange but partly by H^+ATPase, while the HCO_3^- ions cross the basolateral membrane using the Na^+–(3)HCO_3^- cotransporter. The secreted H^+ ions react with filtered HCO_3^- ions to produce CO_2 and water [the reaction being catalysed by the type IV isoform of carbonic anhydrase (CA IV) present in the brush border], which can then diffuse into the cell. Thus, a filtered HCO_3^- ion is removed and another one replaces it in plasma.

Renal handling of specific solutes

Bicarbonate

In individuals on an acid-producing diet, the kidneys must reabsorb essentially all the filtered bicarbonate (>4000 mmol/day) and add sufficient extra bicarbonate to the plasma to regenerate the buffer anions consumed in buffering the daily acid load (normally ~50 mmol/day).

Bicarbonate reabsorption

The bulk of filtered bicarbonate (~80 per cent) is reabsorbed in the proximal tubule, largely in the S_1 and S_2 segments. About half of the remainder is reabsorbed in the loop of Henle, the rest in the distal tubule and collecting duct. Bicarbonate reabsorption is indirect: H^+ and HCO_3^- ions are generated in tubular cells [facilitated by intracellular carbonic anhydrase (type II)]; the H^+ ions are secreted into the lumen whereas the HCO_3^- ions enter the plasma (Fig. 18).

In the proximal tubule, H^+ is secreted mainly via the apical Na^+/H^+ exchanger (NHE-3) but also via apical H^+ATPase (Nakhoul and Hamm 2002). The secreted H^+ ions combine with filtered HCO_3^- ions to form H_2CO_3, which is rapidly converted to CO_2 and H_2O in the presence of apical carbonic anhydrase (type IV); CO_2 and H_2O diffuse into the cell. The HCO_3^- ions generated within the cell enter the interstitial fluid (and thence plasma) via the basolateral Na^+–HCO_3^- cotransporter, which carries three HCO_3^- ions to one Na^+ ion. The net result of these processes is that a filtered HCO_3^- ion is removed while another one replaces it in plasma.

Bicarbonate reabsorption in the loop of Henle takes place mainly in the TALH. Secretion of H^+ into the lumen is largely via the NHE-3 exchanger, although H^+ATPase makes a modest contribution. There is no apical carbonic anhydrase in the loop of Henle. Intracellularly generated HCO_3^- enters the interstitial fluid via a basolateral Na^+–$3HCO_3^-$ cotransporter, as in the proximal tubule, and possibly a Cl^-/HCO_3^- anion exchanger (AE-2). Interestingly, if loop H^+ secretion is inhibited by blockade of apical NHE-3 and H^+ATPase, net HCO_3^- secretion occurs, suggesting the existence of paracellular backflux of HCO_3^- (Capasso *et al.* 2002).

In the DCT, there is evidence for some H^+ secretion through apical NHE-2 and H^+ATPase, but the basolateral exit pathways for HCO_3^- are unknown. In nephron segments beyond the DCT, HCO_3^- handling is believed to be confined largely to the *intercalated cells*. These cells contain carbonic anhydrase (type II) and generate H^+ and HCO_3^- ions. α-intercalated cells reabsorb HCO_3^- ions, β-intercalated cells secrete them; α-intercalated cell activity usually predominates. Intercalated cells have the highest levels of H^+ATPase of any renal cells. It is found in the apical membrane of α-intercalated cells and in the basolateral membrane of β-intercalated cells. Some intercalated cells have diffuse cytoplasmic H^+ATPase distribution and may polarize their H^+ATPase expression according to the prevailing acid–base status.

α-Intercalated cells, scattered throughout the distal nephron from DCT_2 to $IMCD_1$, secrete H^+ ions into the lumen, predominantly through H^+ATPase. Basolateral HCO_3^- exit is via AE-1 (Fig. 19); the Cl^- entering the cell by this route is recycled through basolateral Cl^- channels and/or the K^+–Cl^- cotransporter (KCC-4). The basolateral membrane also contains NKCC-1, at least in rat medullary collecting ducts.

In addition to H^+ATPase, evidence exists for another type of proton pump in intercalated cells: apical H^+,K^+-ATPase, whose precise role is controversial. Two different H^+,K^+-ATPases have been detected in the mammalian distal nephron: a gastric-like isoform and a colonic-like isoform. During K^+ depletion, H^+,K^+-ATPase is upregulated, but evidence is conflicting as to whether it is expressed in the apical membrane of α-intercalated, principal, or even β-intercalated cells (Horisberger and Doucet 2000; Muto 2001; Wagner and Geibel 2002).

β-Intercalated cells, present only in the distal tubule and CCT, are essentially the reverse of α-intercalated cells: H^+ ions are pumped across the basolateral membrane via H^+ATPase, and HCO_3^- ions enter the lumen via an anion exchanger (Fig. 19). The molecular identity of the apical anion exchanger is not fully established, but it is likely to be 'pendrin'. Chloride ions entering the cell on this exchanger can exit the basolateral membrane through Cl^- channels, thus providing a mechanism for transepithelial Cl^- reabsorption.

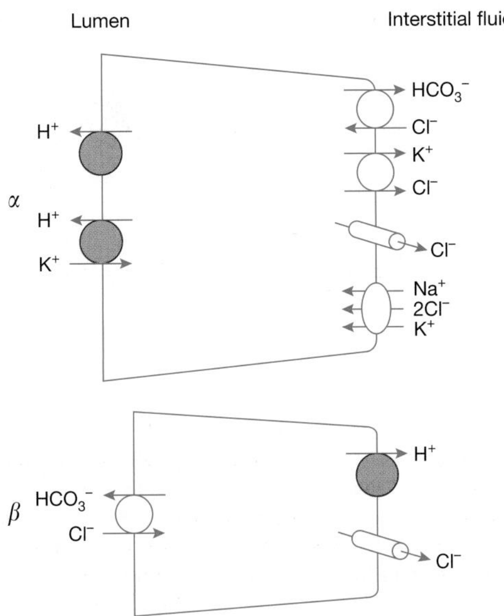

Fig. 19 *α- and β-intercalated cells of the distal nephron. Both types generate H^+ and HCO_3^- ions, owing to the presence of intracellular carbonic anhydrase (CA II).* In α-intercalated cells, the H^+ ions are secreted across the apical membrane, mainly using H^+ATPase but also, under certain circumstances (see text), using electroneutral H^+,K^+-ATPase; the HCO_3^- ions cross the basolateral membrane using a Cl^-/HCO_3^- anion exchanger, the Cl^- ions recycling via a Cl^- channel and K^+–Cl^- cotransporter. In β-intercalated cells, H^+ATPase transports the H^+ ions across the basolateral membrane, while the HCO_3^- ions are secreted across the apical membrane by a Cl^-/HCO_3^- exchanger. In this case, the Cl^- ions cross the basolateral membrane via Cl^- channels, thereby effecting net Cl^- reabsorption.

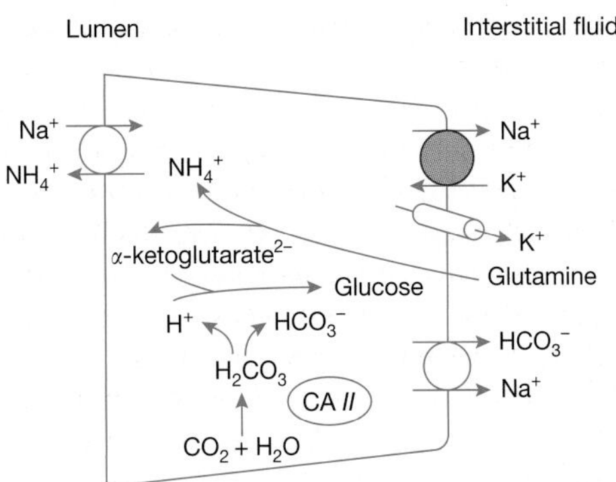

Fig. 20 *Ammonium secretion in the proximal tubule.* Glutamine is taken up by proximal tubular cells and deaminated, through a series of reactions (not shown), to NH_4^+ and α-ketoglutarate. The NH_4^+ ions are secreted into the lumen largely by substituting for H^+ on the apical Na^+/H^+ exchanger. [However, some NH_4^+ dissociates into NH_3 and H^+ inside the cells; the NH_3 is free to diffuse across the cell membrane into the lumen (not shown) where it reacts with H^+ to reform NH_4^+; the latter is trapped in the lumen, as the membrane is impermeable to NH_4^+.] Meanwhile, the cell generates H^+ and HCO_3^- ions from CO_2 and water (catalyzed by carbonic anhydrase type II; CA II); the HCO_3^- ions are transported across the basolateral membrane and contribute to the plasma's buffer reserves, while the H^+ ions are consumed in a series of reactions (not shown) that culminate in the conversion of α-ketoglutarate to glucose.

Addition of extra bicarbonate to plasma

As indicated above, the kidneys not only reabsorb virtually all filtered HCO_3^- but also add further HCO_3^- to the renal circulation. This is achieved by the generation of H^+ and HCO_3^- in tubular cells, by the same mechanism as for HCO_3^- reabsorption, and the addition of HCO_3^- to the peritubular plasma (again, as for HCO_3^- reabsorption). The problem then becomes how to deal with the extra H^+ ions generated simultaneously with the extra HCO_3^- ions. There are two principal means of doing so.

Titratable acid excretion

Some of the extra H^+ ions are secreted into the lumen (via Na^+/H^+ exchange and H^+ATPase), where they react with buffer anions (principally filtered HPO_4^{2-}); any buffer that escapes reabsorption effectively eliminates H^+ ions in the urine. The quantity of H^+ lost in this way, determined by back-titrating the urine with strong base to pH 7.4 (hence the term 'titratable acid'), normally amounts to approximately one-third of overall acid excretion. (Some free H^+ ions appear as such in the urine, but these are quantitatively insignificant since the minimum urine pH is ~4.5.)

Ammonium excretion

The other means of dealing with the extra H^+ ions requires the production of NH_4^+ ions in the proximal tubule (mainly S_1 and S_2 segments). Proximal tubular cells take up the amino acid glutamine and deaminate it, through reactions catalyzed by two enzymes (glutaminase and glutamate dehydrogenase), to NH_4^+ and α-ketoglutarate (Fig. 20). The NH_4^+ ions are secreted into the tubular lumen largely by substituting for H^+ on the NHE-3 transporter (although some intracellular NH_4^+ dissociates into NH_3, which diffuses across the apical membrane to be 'trapped' in the lumen by recombining with secreted H^+). The α-ketoglutarate is largely metabolized to glucose, through a series of reactions that consume H^+ ions.

Most (50–80 per cent) NH_4^+ ions secreted into the proximal tubule and delivered to the loop of Henle are reabsorbed in the TALH (for TALH cell model, see Fig. 12). This reabsorption is partly paracellular, driven by the lumen-positive transepithelial PD, and partly transcellular. For the latter, apical uptake is thought to involve two transporters: the Na^+–K^+–$2Cl^-$ cotransporter (NKCC-2), on which NH_4^+ can substitute for K^+, and a K^+/NH_4^+ exchanger (Karim *et al.* 2002). Uptake is partly opposed by NH_4^+ transport into the lumen on Na^+/H^+ exchangers (mainly, if not exclusively, NHE-3). Basolateral NH_4^+ exit into the interstitial fluid may use the K^+–Cl^- cotransporter (KCC-4), on which NH_4^+ substitutes for K^+.

As a result of events in the TALH, NH_4^+/NH_3 accumulates in the medullary interstitium, to be eventually transferred into the medullary collecting ducts. Entry into the tubular lumen from the cells lining the collecting duct occurs largely by simple diffusion of NH_3, followed by its reconversion to NH_4^+ within the lumen. However, the mechanisms of basolateral NH_4^+/NH_3 uptake from the interstitium into the cells are not yet clear.

Regulation of bicarbonate handling

- *Chronic acidosis* (of non-renal origin) enhances H^+ secretion/HCO_3^- addition to the plasma, while *chronic alkalosis* results in HCO_3^- excretion. A variety of mechanisms is involved:
  —Changes in systemic pH are paralleled by changes in renal intracellular pH which affect H^+ secretion directly.

—In chronic acidosis, NHE-3 activity in the apical membrane of proximal tubule and TALH cells is upregulated.

—In chronic acidosis, H^+ secretion in the collecting duct is enhanced by increased translocation of H^+ATPase from the cytoplasm of α-intercalated cells to the apical membrane, combined with increased translocation of AE-1 to the basolateral membrane, while β-intercalated cell activity is downregulated. In alkalosis, apical H^+ATPase of α-intercalated cells is internalized, while HCO_3^- secretion by β-intercalated cells increases, partly as a result of upregulation of the apical anion exchanger.

—In chronic acidosis, the enzymes responsible for ammoniagenesis in the proximal tubule are upregulated, and in this situation NH_4^+ excretion can account for 90 per cent of total urinary acid excretion.

The factors responsible for the adaptive responses to chronic acidosis are not completely understood but include: a direct effect of reduced intracellular pH; stimulation of the renin–angiotensin–aldosterone system (see below); increased plasma parathyroid hormone (PTH) and glucocorticoids, which stimulate ammoniagenesis; and increased intrarenal endothelin production, which stimulates H^+ secretion in the distal nephron.

- In addition to the factors described above, acid–base disorders of *respiratory* origin affect intracellular partial pressures of CO_2 and thereby influence the generation of H^+ and HCO_3^- within tubular cells, thus altering renal H^+ secretion/HCO_3^- reabsorption appropriately.
- Stimulation of the *renin–angiotensin–aldosterone system*, by extracellular volume depletion and/or acidosis, increases H^+ secretion in both the proximal tubule and distal nephron. Circulating AII stimulates Na^+/H^+ exchange in the proximal tubule and intraluminal AII stimulates HCO_3^- reabsorption in the distal tubule. Aldosterone stimulates H^+ secretion by α-intercalated cells in the distal tubule and collecting duct, partly through a direct action on the cells and partly through an enhanced lumen-negative transepithelial PD (in the distal tubule and CCT) resulting from increased electrogenic Na^+ reabsorption.
- The metabolic alkalosis resulting from *hypokalaemia* (see Chapter 2.2) is due to the combined effects of several factors:

—Hypokalaemia causes a compensatory loss of K^+ ions across the basolateral membrane of renal cells and a reciprocal movement of H^+ into the cells. The raised intracellular H^+ concentration leads to increased renal H^+ secretion.

—Hypokalaemia stimulates renal ammoniagenesis (possibly as a result of the lowered intracellular pH).

—Hypokalaemia induces increased insertion of apical H^+ATPase in α-intercalated cells. In addition, as indicated above, hypokalaemia increases the activity of apical H^+,K^+-ATPase in the distal nephron.

Phosphate (see also Chapter 2.4)

Inorganic phosphate (P_i) is filtered as HPO_4^{2-} and $H_2PO_4^-$, normally in the ratio 4 : 1. Micropuncture studies in superficial nephrons indicate that ~80 per cent of the filtered P_i is usually reclaimed in the proximal tubule. The urinary excretion of P_i normally amounts to ~10 per cent of the filtered load, suggesting that a small proportion is reabsorbed beyond he proximal tubule. There is some (controversial) evidence for

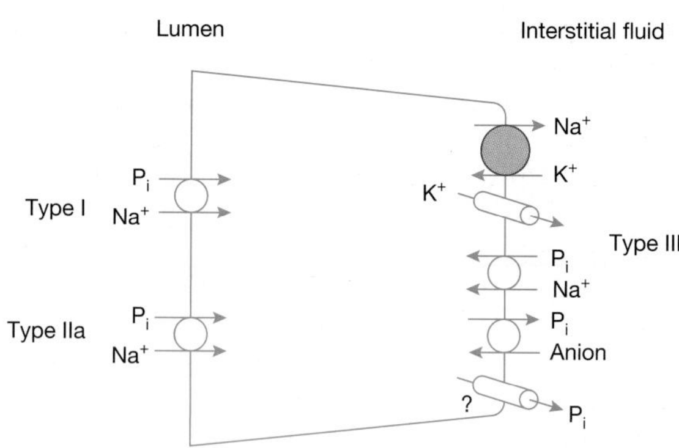

Fig. 21 *Mechanism of phosphate reabsorption in the proximal tubule.* Inorganic phosphate (P_i) enters the cell across the apical membrane using two Na^+–P_i cotransporters; type IIa ($3Na^+$: $1P_i$) predominates. The mechanism of basolateral exit is less clear. There is thought to be a P_i/anion exchanger and possibly a P_i channel. P_i reabsorption is opposed by P_i entry across the basolateral membrane by type III Na^+–P_i cotransporter.

P_i reabsorption in the distal tubule but an alternative possibility is that the proximal tubules of deep (micropuncture-inaccessible) nephrons may have higher reabsorption rates.

Proximal tubular reabsorption of P_i is transcellular (Fig. 21). Entry across the apical membrane uses well-defined Na^+–P_i cotransporters, which raise intracellular P_i above its electrochemical equilibrium; exit across the basolateral membrane is not so well understood (Murer *et al.* 2000). The apical membrane contains two Na^+–P_i cotransporters: type I, which appears to play only a minor role; and type IIa, the major player, whose expression is subject to physiological regulation. In the basolateral membrane, there is functional evidence for a Na^+–P_i cotransporter (type III), a P_i/anion exchanger, and possibly a P_i channel. The basolateral Na^+–P_i cotransporter drives P_i into the cell, a potentially important mechanism should apical P_i entry not meet the requirements of cell metabolism. However, this mechanism is usually masked by P_i efflux into the peritubular interstitial fluid via the P_i/anion exchanger and possibly the P_i channel.

Control of phosphate reabsorption

- *Dietary phosphate* is a major factor in the control of P_i reabsorption. A high phosphate intake lowers, and a low phosphate intake raises, the number of type IIa Na^+–P_i cotransporters in the apical membrane.
- *Parathyroid hormone* reduces the number of type IIa Na^+–P_i cotransporters in the apical membrane and thereby increases P_i excretion.
- The active metabolite of vitamin D, *calcitriol* (*1,25-dihydroxycholecalciferol*), is thought to increase proximal tubular P_i reabsorption.
- Disturbances of *acid–base balance* affect P_i excretion: alkalosis stimulates, whilst chronic acidosis inhibits, apical Na^+–P_i cotransporters, causing corresponding changes in P_i excretion rates.

Calcium (see also Chapter 2.3)

Most filtered calcium (Ca^{2+}) is reabsorbed in the proximal tubules (~60 per cent of the filtered load), mainly in the PCT but also in the pars recta. No significant Ca^{2+} transport occurs in the thin descending or thin ascending limbs of Henle, owing to their low permeability to Ca^{2+}, but the TALH normally reabsorbs ~25 per cent of the filtered load. Most of the remaining Ca^{2+} reabsorption takes place in the distal tubule (~10 per cent of the filtered load); very little is reabsorbed in the collecting duct (Friedman 2000a). Usually, 1–2 per cent of the filtered load of Ca^{2+} is excreted, the actual figure being closely regulated by the requirements for overall Ca^{2+} balance.

Proximal tubule

Micropuncture evidence indicates that in the S_1 segment the intratubular Ca^{2+} concentration increases slightly (by 10–20 per cent), so that throughout the S_2 segment a small concentration gradient obtains across the tubular epithelium. Together with the small lumen-positive transepithelial PD, this gradient is sufficient to drive most proximal Ca^{2+} reabsorption passively by the paracellular route, while a small proportion may be reabsorbed by solvent drag. The situation is analogous to that described for proximal tubular K^+ reabsorption (see Fig. 8). A small component of proximal Ca^{2+} reabsorption is active and transcellular, but little information is available on the possible mechanisms.

Thick ascending limb of Henle

At least half the Ca^{2+} reabsorption in the TALH is passive and paracellular, driven by the lumen-positive transepithelial PD (see Fig. 12). The remainder is transcellular, most likely due to passive entry through as-yet-unidentified apical Ca^{2+} channels, coupled with active exit across the basolateral membrane via Ca^{2+}ATPase (Friedman 2000a).

Distal tubule

Calcium is reabsorbed in both the DCT and CNT exclusively through a transcellular route (Fig. 22). Apical entry is down a large electrochemical gradient through a Ca^{2+} channel (ECaC; TRPV-5); basolateral exit is via Ca^{2+}ATPase or Na^+/Ca^{2+} exchange (Friedman 2000b). DCT cells exhibit the highest Ca^{2+}ATPase activity of any nephron segment, and in the DCT_1 region it is the sole mode of basolateral Ca^{2+} efflux, whereas in DCT_2 and in CNT cells the basolateral membrane also contains Na^+/Ca^{2+} exchangers. Transcellular Ca^{2+} reabsorption is facilitated by calbindin D28k, an intracellular Ca^{2+}-binding protein expressed predominantly in the DCT and CNT (Reilly and Ellison 2000). By binding Ca^{2+}, calbindins help to maintain the extremely favourable electrochemical gradient for apical entry; they are also thought to help 'shuttle' Ca^{2+} from apical to basolateral membrane.

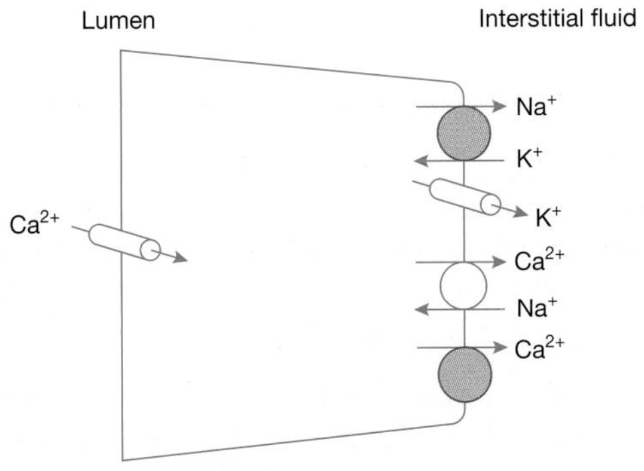

Fig. 22 *Mechanism of calcium reabsorption in the distal convoluted tubule and the connecting tubule.* Ca^{2+} enters the cell, down its electrochemical gradient, using the apical Ca^{2+} channel. In the DCT_1 subsegment, basolateral exit is solely via Ca^{2+}ATPase; in DCT_2 and CNT, both Ca^{2+}ATPase and the Na^+/Ca^{2+} exchanger are available. The large electrochemical gradient for apical Ca^{2+} entry is maintained partly by the binding of intracellular Ca^{2+} to calbindin D28k (not shown). Calbindin D28k is also thought to help 'shuttle' Ca^{2+} from apical to basolateral membrane.

Regulation of calcium reabsorption

Calcium reabsorption in the proximal tubule is essentially unregulated; physiological control of Ca^{2+} excretion is exerted at the TALH and the distal tubule:

- The principal hormone involved in the regulation of renal Ca^{2+} reabsorption is *PTH*. Although PTH may have a small inhibitory effect in the proximal tubule, it more than compensates for this by stimulating Ca^{2+} reabsorption in the TALH (at least in the cortical segment) and distal tubule. PTH appears to exert its effect on transcellular, rather than paracellular, reabsorption, by stimulating apical Ca^{2+} uptake and basolateral Na^+/Ca^{2+} exchange activity. See Chapter 2.3 for further information on PTH-regulated Ca^{2+} transport.
- The effects of the hormone *calcitonin* on renal Ca^{2+} reabsorption are somewhat paradoxical. Despite its generally hypocalcaemic action, calcitonin *stimulates* Ca^{2+} reabsorption in the TALH and distal tubule by cAMP-dependent mechanisms.
- *Calcitriol (1,25-dihydroxycholecalciferol)* targets mainly intestine and bone, but may also affect Ca^{2+} handling in the kidney: there is evidence that it can stimulate Ca^{2+} reabsorption in the distal tubule, either directly or by potentiating the effect of PTH (Friedman 2000a).
- A *Ca^{2+}/Mg^{2+}-sensing receptor* (which can also respond to other divalent cations) has been located in the basolateral membrane of the TALH and distal tubule (Riccardi *et al.* 1998). Stimulation by elevated plasma concentrations of Ca^{2+} or Mg^{2+} reduces the reabsorption of these ions.
- Renal Ca^{2+} excretion is influenced by *acid–base status*: acidosis increases, and alkalosis reduces, Ca^{2+} excretion rates. Although this can be attributed partly to changes in the filtered load of Ca^{2+} (acidosis reduces the proportion of plasma calcium bound to albumin and thereby increases ultrafilterable Ca^{2+}), and partly to nonspecific changes in proximal tubular reabsorption, these effects cannot account fully for the phenomenon. A specific inhibitory effect of acidosis on Ca^{2+} reabsorption in the distal tubule has been documented, and it is thought that the mechanism might involve pH sensitivity of the distal tubular apical Ca^{2+} channel.

Magnesium

Overall magnesium (Mg^{2+}) reabsorption normally amounts to ~97 per cent of the filtered load, leaving ~3 per cent to be excreted. Only a relatively small proportion (up to ~20 per cent of the filtered load) is reabsorbed in the proximal tubule. Most Mg^{2+} is reabsorbed in the loop of Henle (60–70 per cent of the filtered load), the remainder in the distal tubule. Mg^{2+} transport is detailed in Chapter 2.5; only a brief account will be presented here.

Magnesium reabsorption in the proximal tubule is not understood. In the S_2 segment, both concentration and electrical gradients favour Mg^{2+} reabsorption, but the paracellular permeability to Mg^{2+} is low.

In the loop of Henle, Mg^{2+} is reabsorbed at two major sites: the thin descending limb and the TALH. In the thin descending limb, reabsorption is thought to occur by simple diffusion, resulting from the concentration gradient caused by water reabsorption, analogous to the mechanism of Na^+ reabsorption in the thin descending limb described above. In the TALH, Mg^{2+} reabsorption is passive, driven through the cation-selective paracellular pathway by the lumen-positive PD, at least in the cortical segment (see Fig. 12).

Although reabsorption in the distal tubule is usually limited to no more than ~10 per cent of the filtered load, this is an important site of physiological control. Distal tubular Mg^{2+} reabsorption is transcellular. On the basis of studies using cell lines, Mg^{2+} is thought to enter DCT cells (down an electrochemical gradient) through a specific, apically located Mg^{2+} channel, and exit the basolateral membrane (against an electrochemical gradient) using a Na^+/Mg^{2+} exchanger (Quamme and de Rouffignac 2000).

Factors affecting magnesium reabsorption

Magnesium reabsorption in the TALH is modulated by factors that affect the transepithelial PD (e.g. loop diuretics) and/or paracellular permeability:

- Peptide hormones (*PTH, calcitonin, glucagon, vasopressin*), acting via basolateral receptors and cAMP-dependent mechanisms, stimulate Mg^{2+} reabsorption in the cortical TALH by increasing the transepithelial PD and the paracellular permeability. A protein expressed in the tight junctions of the TALH (*paracellin-1*) seems able to modulate selectively the barrier to divalent cations such as Ca^{2+} or Mg^{2+} (Yu 2000).
- *Plasma* Mg^{2+} *and* Ca^{2+} *concentrations* influence Mg^{2+} (and Ca^{2+}) reabsorption in the TALH through interaction with the Ca^{2+}/Mg^{2+}-sensing receptor located in the basolateral membrane, as described above.
- Changes in Mg^{2+} *intake* affect Mg^{2+} reabsorption in the appropriate direction, independently of changes in plasma Mg^{2+} concentration. Thus, Mg^{2+} reabsorption in the cortical TALH is more than doubled, in the absence of a change in transepithelial PD, in mice fed a Mg^{2+}-free diet (Quamme and de Rouffignac 2000).

Magnesium reabsorption in the distal tubule is affected by many of the factors that affect reabsorption in the TALH. Thus, peptide hormones stimulate apical Mg^{2+} uptake; raised plasma Mg^{2+} or Ca^{2+} concentrations, acting through the basolateral Ca^{2+}/Mg^{2+}-sensing receptor, inhibit hormone-stimulated apical Mg^{2+} uptake; and changes in dietary Mg^{2+} intake affect distal tubular Mg^{2+} reabsorption appropriately.

Urate

Renal urate transport is thought to be restricted to the proximal tubule, where both reabsorption and secretion take place, although in humans the degree of secretion is minor. The net result is that normally ~90 per cent of the filtered load is reabsorbed.

Apical entry is via urate/anion exchangers, one of which (URAT-1) has recently been identified in human proximal tubules. A variety of intracellular anions can act as substrate. Urate exit across the basolateral membrane (down its electrochemical gradient) is less well defined. There is functional evidence for a urate/anion exchanger and there may be another carrier protein allowing voltage-driven facilitated diffusion. A fuller account of urate transport is given in Chapter 6.4.

Proteins

Under normal circumstances, the filtered fraction of albumin and other high molecular weight proteins is slight. However, their total filtration is significant on a daily basis, owing to the high GFR. Low molecular weight proteins, such as β_2-microglobulin, pass freely through the filtration barrier. The fact that urine is normally virtually protein free is a consequence of uptake of proteins in the proximal tubule by endocytosis. This involves binding at the apical membrane, followed by internalization of protein-containing endosomes and subsequent fusion of endosomes with lysosomes, where the proteins are degraded.

The initial apical binding involves at least two membrane proteins, *megalin* and *cubilin*, each of which has multiligand properties and therefore deals with a wide variety of proteins (Verroust and Kozyraki 2001). Megalin and/or cubilin is released from its ligand in the endosomal vesicles and returned to the apical membrane for re-use. The overall process of endocytosis requires acidification of the endosomal vesicles, which is effected by vesicular membrane-bound H^+ATPase and a colocalized Cl^- channel (ClC-5), the latter acting as an electrical shunt (Gunther *et al.* 1998).

References

(Entries marked with an asterisk comprise useful general readings.)

Agre, P., Nielsen, S., and Knepper, M. A. Aquaporin water channels in mammalian kidney. In *The Kidney: Physiology and Pathophysiology* (ed. D. W. Seldin and G. Giebisch), pp. 363–377. Philadelphia, PA: Lippincott Williams and Wilkins, 2000.

*__Aronson, P. S. and Giebisch, G.__ (1997). Mechanisms of chloride transport in the proximal tubule. *American Journal of Physiology* **273**, F179–F192.

Bailly, C. (2000). Effect of luminal atrial natriuretic peptide on chloride reabsorption in mouse cortical thick ascending limb: inhibition by endothelin. *Journal of the American Society of Nephrology* **11**, 1791–1797.

*__Berliner, R. W.__ (1982). Mechanisms of urine concentration. *Kidney International* **22**, 202–211.

Capasso, G. *et al.* (2002). Bicarbonate transport along the loop of Henle: molecular mechanisms and regulation. *Journal of Nephrology* **15** (Suppl. 5), S88–S96.

Cogan, M. G. (1990). Atrial natriuretic peptide. *Kidney International* **37**, 1148–1160.

de Jesus Ferreira, M. C. and Bailly, C. (1997). Luminal and basolateral endothelin inhibit chloride reabsorption in the mouse thick ascending limb via a Ca^{2+}-independent pathway. *Journal of Physiology* **505**, 749–758.

DiBona, G. F. (2000). Neural control of the kidney: functionally specific renal sympathetic nerve fibers. *American Journal of Physiology* **279**, R1517– R1524.

Friedman, P. A. Renal calcium metabolism. In *The Kidney: Physiology and Pathophysiology* (ed. D. W. Seldin and G. Giebisch), pp. 1749–1789. Philadelphia, PA: Lippincott Williams and Wilkins, 2000a.

Friedman, P. A. (2000b). Mechanisms of renal calcium transport. *Experimental Nephrology* **8**, 343–350.

Giebisch, G. (1998). Renal potassium transport: mechanisms and regulation. *American Journal of Physiology* **274**, F817–F833.

*__Giebisch, G.__ (2001). Renal potassium channels: function, regulation, and structure. *Kidney International* **60**, 436–445.

Greger, R. (1985). Ion transport mechanisms in thick ascending limb of Henle's loop of mammalian nephron. *Physiological Reviews* **65**, 760–797.

Günther, W. *et al.* (1998). ClC-5, the chloride channel mutated in Dent's disease, colocalizes with the proton pump in endocytotically active kidney cells. *Proceedings of the National Academy of Sciences of the United States of America* **95**, 8075–8080.

Horisberger, J.-D. and Doucet, A. Renal ion-translocating ATPases: the P-type family. In *The Kidney: Physiology and Pathophysiology* (ed. D. W. Seldin and G. Giebisch), pp. 139–170. Philadelphia, PA: Lippincott Williams and Wilkins, 2000.

Ichikawa, I. and Harris, R. C. (1991). Angiotensin actions in the kidney: renewed insight into the old hormone. *Kidney International* **40**, 583–596.

Imai, M., Taniguchi, J., and Tabei, K. (1987). Function of thin loops of Henle. *Kidney International* **31**, 565–579.

Inoue, T., Nonoguchi, H., and Tomita, K. (2001). Physiological effects of vasopressin and atrial natriuretic peptide in the collecting duct. *Cardiovascular Research* **51**, 470–480.

Jacobson, H. R. (1982). Transport characteristics of *in vitro* perfused proximal convoluted tubules. *Kidney International* **22**, 425–433.

*__Kaissling, B. and Kriz, W.__ Morphology of the loop of Henle, distal tubule, and collecting duct. In *Handbook of Physiology, Section 8: Renal Physiology* (ed. E. E. Windhager), pp. 109–167. New York, NY: Oxford University Press, 1992.

Karim, Z., Attmane-Elakeb, A., and Bichara, M. (2002). Renal handling of NH_4^+ in relation to the control of acid–base balance by the kidney. *Journal of Nephrology* **15** (Suppl. 5), S128–S134.

Kim, G.-H. *et al.* (1999). Vasopressin increases Na–K–2Cl cotransporter expression in thick ascending limb of Henle's loop. *American Journal of Physiology* **276**, F96–F103.

Kishore, B. K. *et al.* (1996). Rat renal arcade segment expresses vasopressin-regulated water channel and vasopressin V_2 receptor. *Journal of Clinical Investigation* **97**, 2763–2771.

Kokko, J. P. and Baum, M. Chloride transport. In *Handbook of Physiology, Section 8: Renal Physiology* (ed. E. E. Windhager), pp. 739–765. New York, NY: Oxford University Press, 1992.

Kokot, F. and Dulawa, J. (2000). Tamm–Horsfall protein updated. *Nephron* **85**, 97–102.

Kotelevtsev, Y. and Webb, D. J. (2001). Endothelin as a natriuretic hormone: the case for a paracrine action mediated by nitric oxide. *Cardiovascular Research* **51**, 481–488.

*__Kriz, W. and Bankir, L.__ (1988). A standard nomenclature for structures of the kidney. *American Journal of Physiology* **254**, F1–F8.

Kriz, W. and Kaissling, B. Structural organization of the mammalian kidney. In *The Kidney: Physiology and Pathophysiology* (ed. D. W. Seldin and G. Giebisch), pp. 587–654. Philadelphia, PA: Lippincott Williams and Wilkins, 2000.

Le Grimellec, C. (1975). Micropuncture study along the proximal convoluted tubule. *Pflügers Archiv* **354**, 133–150.

Lehrmann, H. *et al.* (2002). Luminal $P2Y_2$ receptor-mediated Na^+ absorption in isolated perfused mouse CCD. *Journal of the American Society of Nephrology* **13**, 10–18.

Light, D. B. *et al.* (1988). Amiloride-sensitive cation channel in apical membrane of inner medullary collecting duct. *American Journal of Physiology* **255**, F278–F286.

*__Maunsbach, A. B. and Christensen, E. I.__ Functional ultrastructure of the proximal tubule. In *Handbook of Physiology, Section 8: Renal Physiology* (ed. E. E. Windhager), pp. 41–107. New York, NY: Oxford University Press, 1992.

Murer, H. *et al.* (2000). Proximal tubular phosphate reabsorption: molecular mechanisms. *Physiological Reviews* **80**, 1373–1409.

Muto, S. (2001). Potassium transport in the mammalian collecting duct. *Physiological Reviews* **81**, 85–116.

Nakamura, T. *et al.* (1998). Effects of renal perfusion pressure on renal interstitial hydrostatic pressure and Na^+ excretion: role of endothelium-derived nitric oxide. *Nephron* **78**, 104–111.

Nakhoul, N. L. and Hamm, L. L. (2002). Vacuolar H^+-ATPase in the kidney. *Journal of Nephrology* **15** (Suppl. 5), S22–S31.

Navar, L. G. *et al.* (1999). Concentrations and actions of intraluminal angiotensin II. *Journal of the American Society of Nephrology* **10** (Suppl. 11), S189–S195.

Palmer, L. G. and Garty, H. Epithelial Na channels. In *The Kidney: Physiology and Pathophysiology* (ed. D. W. Seldin and G. Giebisch), pp. 251–276. Philadelphia, PA: Lippincott Williams and Wilkins, 2000.

Quamme, G. A. and de Rouffignac, C. Renal magnesium handling. In *The Kidney: Physiology and Pathophysiology* (ed. D. W. Seldin and G. Giebisch), pp. 1711–1729. Philadelphia, PA: Lippincott Williams and Wilkins, 2000.

Reddy, S. *et al.* (1991). Transfer of Na transport inhibition in proximal tubules from saline volume-expanded to nonexpanded rats. *American Journal of Physiology* **260**, F69–F74.

*__Reeves, W. B. and Andreoli, T. E.__ Sodium chloride transport in the loop of Henle, distal convoluted tubule, and collecting duct. In *The Kidney: Physiology and Pathophysiology* (ed. D. W. Seldin and G. Giebisch), pp. 1333–1369. Philadelphia, PA: Lippincott Williams and Wilkins, 2000.

Reif, M. C., Troutman, S. L., and Schafer, J. A. (1986). Sodium transport by rat cortical collecting tubule. Effects of vasopressin and desoxycorticosterone. *Journal of Clinical Investigation* **77**, 1291–1298.

*__Reilly, R. F. and Ellison, D. H.__ (2000). Mammalian distal tubule: physiology, pathophysiology, and molecular anatomy. *Physiological Reviews* **80**, 277–313.

Riccardi, D. *et al.* (1998). Localization of the extracellular Ca^{2+}/polyvalent cation-sensing protein in rat kidney. *American Journal of Physiology* **274**, F611–F622.

Ruiz, O. S. *et al.* (1995). Regulation of renal $Na–HCO_3$ cotransporter: III. Presence and modulation by glucocorticoids in primary cultures of the proximal tubule. *Kidney International* **47**, 1669–1676.

Schafer, J. A. and Barfuss, D. W. (1982). The study of pars recta function by the perfusion of isolated tubule segments. *Kidney International* **22**, 434–448.

*__Schnermann, J.__ (1998). Juxtaglomerular cell complex in the regulation of renal salt excretion. *American Journal of Physiology* **274**, R263–R279.

Shirley, D. G., Capasso, G., and Unwin, R. J. Renal physiology. In *Comprehensive Clinical Nephrology* 2nd edn. (ed. R. J. Johnson and J. Feehally), pp. 13–26. Edinburgh: Mosby, 2003.

Shirley, D. G. *et al.* (1998). Contribution of $Na^+–H^+$ exchange to sodium reabsorption in the loop of Henle: a microperfusion study in rats. *Journal of Physiology* **513**, 243–249.

Smith, C. P. and Rousselet, G. (2001). Facilitative urea transporters. *Journal of Membrane Biology* **183**, 1–14.

Sonnenberg, H., Honrath, U., and Wilson, D. R. (1987). Effects of amiloride in the medullary collecting duct of rat kidney. *Kidney International* **31**, 1121–1125.

Stanton, B. A. (1986). Regulation by adrenal corticosteroids of sodium and potassium transport in loop of Henle and distal tubule of rat kidney. *Journal of Clinical Investigation* **78**, 1612–1620.

Stanton, B. A. and Giebisch, G. H. Renal potassium transport. In *Handbook of Physiology, Section 8: Renal Physiology* (ed. E. E. Windhager), pp. 813–874. New York, NY: Oxford University Press, 1992.

Stokes, J. B. (1993). Ion transport by the collecting duct. *Seminars in Nephrology* **13**, 202–212.

Taniguchi, J., Tabei, K., and Imai, M. (1987). Profiles of water and solute transport along long-loop descending limb: analysis by mathematical model. *American Journal of Physiology* **252**, F393–F402.

Thomson, S. C. (2002). Adenosine and purinergic mediators of tubuloglomerular feedback. *Current Opinion in Nephrology and Hypertension* **11**, 81–86.

Tisher, C. C., Bulger, R. E., and Trump, B. F. (1968). Human renal ultrastructure. III. The distal tubule in healthy individuals. *Laboratory Investigation* **18**, 655–668.

Uchida, S. and Marumo, F. (2000). Severely impaired urine-concentrating ability in mice lacking the CLC-K1 chloride channel. *Experimental Nephrology* **8**, 361–365.

Velazquez, H. *et al.* (1996). Adrenal steroids stimulate thiazide-sensitive NaCl transport by rat renal distal tubules. *American Journal of Physiology* **270**, F211–F219.

*__Verkman, A. S.__ (2002). Renal concentrating and diluting function in deficiency of specific aquaporin genes. *Experimental Nephrology* **10**, 235–240.

Verroust, P. J. and Kozyraki, R. (2001). The roles of cubilin and megalin, two multiligand receptors, in proximal tubule function: possible implication in the progression of renal disease. *Current Opinion in Nephrology and Hypertension* **10**, 33–38.

Wagner, C. A. and Geibel, J. P. (2002). Acid–base transport in the collecting duct. *Journal of Nephrology* **15** (Suppl. 5), S112–S127.

Walter, M. F., Forsling, M. L., and Shirley, D. G. (2000). Contribution of endogenous oxytocin to sodium excretion in anaesthetized, surgically operated rats. *Journal of Endocrinology* **165**, 19–24.

Wang, T. and Giebisch, G. (1996). Effects of angiotensin II on electrolyte transport in the early and late distal tubule in rat kidney. *American Journal of Physiology* **271**, F143–F149.

Wareing, M. *et al.* (1995). Estimated potassium reflection coefficient in perfused proximal convoluted tubules of the anaesthetized rat *in vivo*. *Journal of Physiology* **488**, 153–161.

Welch, W. J. and Wilcox, C. S. (2002). What is brain nitric oxide synthase doing in the kidney? *Current Opinion in Nephrology and Hypertension* **11**, 109–115.

Welling, L. J. and Welling, D. J. (1976). Shape of epithelial cells and intercellular channels in the rabbit proximal nephron. *Kidney International* **9**, 385–394.

Wright, F. S. (1987). Renal potassium handling. *Seminars in Nephrology* **7**, 174–184.

Yu, A. S. L. (2000). Paracellular solute transport: more than just a leak? *Current Opinion in Nephrology and Hypertension* **9**, 513–515.

5.2 Isolated defects of tubular function

George B. Haycock

Two-thirds of filtered salt and water is reabsorbed in the proximal tubule. Solutes such as bicarbonate, uric acid, glucose, phosphate, amino acids and certain organic anions, are reabsorbed completely or almost completely by means of specific, mostly sodium-coupled, epithelial transport systems. Proximal tubular handling of sodium, chloride, potassium, and bicarbonate are discussed elsewhere (Chapter 5.1), as is the renal Fanconi syndrome (Chapter 5.3) and renal tubular acidosis (Chapter 5.4). This chapter will describe defects of proximal tubular handling of glucose, amino acids, and phosphate.

Transport mechanisms in the proximal tubule—general aspects

Tubular epithelial cells are bounded by the plasma membrane, which separates the cell contents from the surrounding environment (the extracellular fluid, ECF). Movement of many substances between the ECF and the cytoplasm is mediated by specialized membrane proteins or transporters, each of which is specific for one or a few solute species. Some transporters are energy dependent while others are not; some require sodium as a cotransportate and some do not. Net, vectorial transport from one side of the intact epithelium to the other depends on asymmetric distribution of specific transporters between the apical (brush border or luminal) membrane which is bathed by tubular fluid and the basolateral membrane which is in contact with the ECF. The apical and basolateral membranes lie on either side of the *tight junction*, which is situated just below the site of apposition of the apical membranes of adjacent cells (Fig. 1). Therefore, the reabsorption of any substance from the glomerular filtrate perfusing the proximal tubule involves at least two steps: movement from lumen into the tubular epithelial cell (the entry step), and from the cell interior into the peritubular interstitial fluid (the exit step).

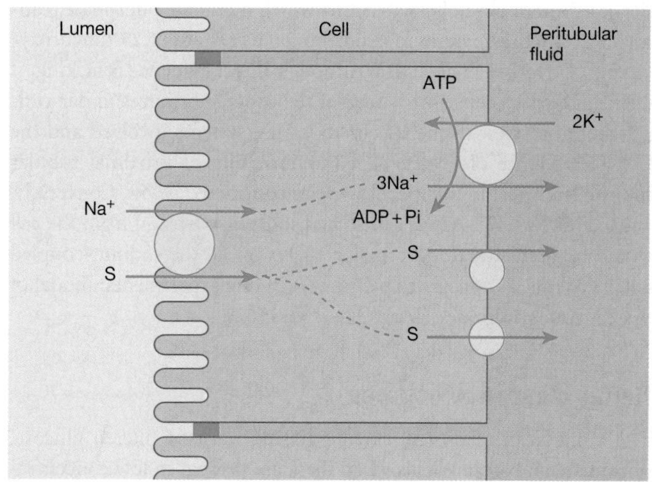

Fig. 1 Generalized scheme for sodium-coupled reabsorption of a solute, S, in the proximal tubule. The energy-consuming step is the extrusion of sodium across the basolateral membrane by sodium, potassium-ATPase (upper right in diagram). This creates a gradient favouring sodium entry across the luminal membrane via a sodium/S cotransporter (left): S is thus carried against its concentration gradient by secondary active transport.

The entry step

Many solutes enter the proximal tubular cell across the apical membrane by a series of cotransport systems, each of which binds one or more sodium ions and its specific substrate(s) and carries them across the cell membrane. These include glucose, some amino acids, phosphate, and organic anions, including citrate and lactate. The presence of sodium stimulates transport of the cotransportate and vice versa. The energy for sodium transport is provided by the lumen-to-cell interior concentration gradient, maintained in turn by removal of sodium from the cell across the basolateral cell membrane (Fig. 1). The energy for the transport of charged systems is provided by the membrane voltage. Thus, the cotransportate is transported against its own concentration gradient by a process of secondary active transport which may be electrogenic or electroneutral depending on the stoichiometry of the transport system and the charge on the cotransportate. The somewhat different, sodium-independent, system involved in entry of cystine, dibasic and neutral amino acids is discussed in the section on cystinuria (see below). Recently, the structure of many of these transporters has been elucidated and the corresponding genes mapped and cloned. Further details of some of these are given under the relevant sections below. There is evidence of more than one transport system for some substances. In general, the rule seems to be that the early, convoluted segments of the proximal tubule (S_1 and S_2) contain transporters of high capacity, broad specificity, and low affinity, while the more distal straight (S_3) segment contains transporters with low capacity, high affinity, and narrow specificity (Scriver and Tenenhouse 1985).

The exit step

Sodium ions are pumped out of the cell across the basolateral membrane against a steep concentration gradient by primary active transport.

The energy source is hydrolysis of ATP by the enzyme Na^+,K^+-ATPase, which also drives potassium into the cell with a stoichiometry of $3Na^+ : 2K^+$. The resulting very low intracellular concentration of Na^+ generates a Na^+ gradient across the apical membrane favouring entry of Na^+ and its various cotransportates. The cotransportates leave the cell across the basolateral membrane by transport systems that are generally different from those involved in the entry step. These are substrate-specific, mostly sodium-independent and are active processes in some cases (Na^+, Ca^{2+}) and facilitated diffusion pathways in others. As with entry step transporters, further details are given below in relation to the individual transported substances.

In the case of phosphate, the entry step (luminal sodium-phosphate cotransport) is thought to be rate limiting, and is the major site of action of physiological factors which modulate phosphate reabsorption, such as parathyroid hormone (PTH) and 1,25-dihydroxy-vitamin D (Murer *et al.* 2001). Although direct evidence is lacking, it seems likely that the same is true of the other substances under consideration, in view of the specificity of the systems involved and the lack of evidence of a generalized abnormality of proximal tubular sodium transport in the specific defects considered below. Conversely, a defect of Na^+,K^+-ATPase-mediated sodium extrusion from the cell would be predicted to have major effects on all the sodium-coupled entry systems, as appears to be the case in one experimental model of the Fanconi syndrome (Hong Que *et al.* 1982).

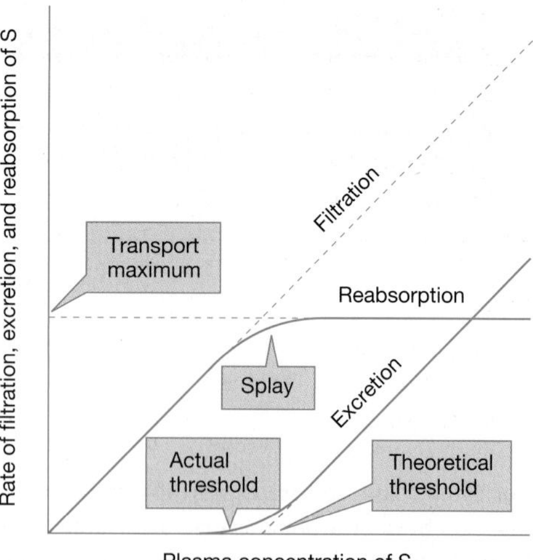

Fig. 2 'Family' of titration curves describing the reabsorption of a solute, S, by saturable active transport in the proximal tubule. The curve for excretion of S is plotted from direct measurements, that for filtration of S by multiplying plasma S by glomerular filtration rate, and that for reabsorption is obtained by subtracting the former from the latter. The terms transport maximum, splay and threshold are explained in the text.

Renal clearance studies

The kidney can reabsorb virtually 100 per cent of filtered glucose, phosphate and amino acids when these are present in low concentration. If the plasma concentration of such a solute (S) is manipulated by infusing it under controlled conditions it is possible to plot the excretion of S (E_S) against its plasma concentration. If inulin or an equivalent marker of glomerular filtration rate (GFR) is infused at the same time, the rate of filtration of S (F_S) can be calculated; by subtracting E_S from F_S, the rate of tubular reabsorption (R_S) may be derived. The resulting family of titration curves is shown in Fig. 2. The form of the curve for R_S indicates that above a certain value no more solute can be reabsorbed, despite a further increase in the filtered load. This limiting value for reabsorption is known as the tubular maximal reabsorptive capacity for the solute (T_MS). If the point of inflexion of the curve of R_S (the point at which the ascending part meets the horizontal part) were a sharp angle, T_MS would be reached at precisely the plasma concentration of the solute above which it begins to appear in the urine: the *renal threshold* for the given solute. In fact this angle is bridged by a curved *splay*, the degree of which varies with the solute, being large for glucose and small for some amino acids such as lysine. Where splay is significant, two threshold values can be quoted: an actual threshold, which will be somewhat lower than the plasma concentration at which T_MS is reached, and a theoretical threshold, which is the projection on the abscissa of the theoretical point of inflexion of the R_S curve if there were no splay. The theoretical threshold is obtained by dividing T_MS by GFR, and is commonly abbreviated to T_MS/GFR. It is convenient to factor individual values of E_S, F_S, and R_S by GFR before plotting the curves such that, for example, a given point would be expressed in milligram (or millimoles) of solute per 100 ml GFR; in this case, T_MS/GFR can be read off directly as the projection on the ordinate of the horizontal portion of the R_S curve. The alternative method, of plotting filtered load (GFR H plasma S) on the abscissa against E_S, F_S, and R_S on the ordinate is mathematically equivalent: glomerulotubular balance dictates that T_MS will change proportionately with changes in GFR, and either method of correcting for GFR will compensate for this effect. It is important to note that T_MS and T_MS/GFR, when experimentally derived, are in part determined by the conditions under which the measurements are made. In particular, changes in extracellular fluid volume alter the threshold value for all proximally reabsorbed solutes. If titration experiments are performed by a method which causes progressive volume expansion as a result of the infusion of the solute the threshold will progressively fall and it will prove impossible to demonstrate a T_MS.

Significance of T_M

If the reabsorption curve for a given solute exhibits a T_M, (i.e. eventually becomes parallel to the abscissa) the transporting mechanism is saturable. This means that all receptor sites for the solute on the luminal side of the carrier protein are occupied and the rate of transport is therefore limited by the next step in the process: the rate at which receptor sites can be vacated on the cytoplasmic side of the membrane and presented again to the luminal fluid for reuse. A T_M can be demonstrated for glucose, phosphate, and most amino acids, but it has not been possible to demonstrate a T_M for other substances, histidine for example, probably because it is so high that it is not attainable at non-toxic plasma concentrations. The kinetics of saturable proximal tubular reabsorption are described by the Michaelis–Menten equation:

$$T = \frac{T_M \times S}{K_M + S}$$

where T is the rate of transport, T_M the transport maximum, S the substrate concentration in glomerular filtrate and K_M the Michaelis–Menten constant for the transport system.

Significance of threshold

By definition, below the renal threshold value for a particular solute S the urine contains no S or only trace amounts. This can only occur if the solute is reabsorbed by active transport (either primary or secondary) since absorption of the last traces of the solute from the tubular fluid into the cell must take place against a concentration gradient unless its intracellular concentration is zero.

Significance of splay

The existence of splay can be explained in two ways. The first rests on the concept of nephron heterogeneity. If individual nephrons had slightly different thresholds for S, the urine would not be free of S unless its plasma concentration was below the lowest single nephron threshold value. Similarly, the whole kidney T_M would not be reached until the plasma concentration exceeded the highest single nephron threshold value. In this model the curve of the splay joins these two extreme threshold values, and its exact shape is a function of the distribution of single nephron threshold values in the total nephron population (Fig. 3) (Smith *et al.* 1943). The second explanation concerns the affinity of the carrier protein receptor for the solute: the combination of a solute with its receptor B is reversible and obeys the law of mass action:

$$K = \frac{[S] \times [B]}{[SB]}$$

where K is the dissociation constant and the terms in square brackets the activities of S, B, and the SB complex, respectively. The higher the value of K, the lower the affinity of B for S and the broader the splay; in the limiting case where $K = 0$ there would be no splay. The significance of splay is discussed further in the section on glycosuria.

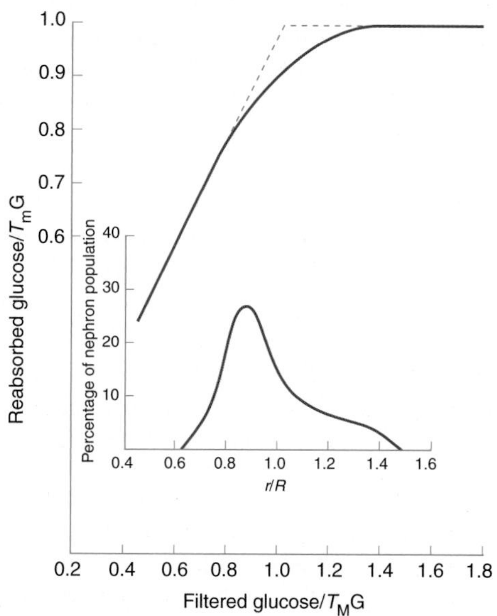

Fig. 3 Theoretical explanation of splay in the normal glucose reabsorption curve according to the nephron heterogeneity hypothesis. The term *r*/*R* is the ratio of GFR to glucose reabsorptive capacity for each individual nephron (*r*) factored by the ratio of whole kidney GFR to whole kidney glucose reabsorptive capacity (*R*). The extended right hand tail of the frequency distribution curve is due to the presence of a minority of nephrons with functional glomerular preponderance (glomerulotubular imbalance) (modified from Smith *et al.* 1943).

Glycosurias

Normal glucose reabsorption

Figure 4 depicts glucose titration studies in a normal human subject and in patients with types A and B renal glycosuria. A prominent feature of the normal curve is the considerable splay, such that actual or minimum threshold for glucose is 8–11 mmol/l (145–200 mg/dl). The T_M for glucose (T_MG) corrected for surface area (mmol or mg/min/1.73 m^2) is similar in children and adults but is significantly lower in infants: for example, Smith *et al.* (1943) obtained a value (mean $\pm$ SD) of 1.96 ± 0.45 mmol/min/1.73 m^2 in adults, while Brodehl *et al.* (1972) found corresponding values of 2.01 ± 0.53 in children but only 1.18 ± 0.39 in infants. Although this has been interpreted by some as evidence of tubular immaturity the discrepancy is entirely explicable as a consequence of the low GFR which is characteristic of the first few months of life. Thus values for T_MG/GFR (mmol/l) are 15.1 ± 2.5 in adults, 15.7 ± 2.6 in children, and 16.3 ± 4.1 in infants: there is no evidence of glomerulotubular imbalance for glucose even in premature neonates (Arant *et al.* 1974).

Causes of glycosuria

Small amounts of glucose are present in the urine of normal individuals: the definition of 'abnormal' glycosuria is somewhat arbitrary. Most agree that glucose excretion rates above about 2.75 mmol (500 mg)/day/1.73 m^2 are unequivocally abnormal, and this seems a reasonable criterion by which to define significant glycosuria. Glycosuria may be due to hyperglycaemia in the presence of normal renal glucose handling (overload or hyperglycaemic glycosuria), or to abnormalities of tubular glucose transport at normal blood glucose concentrations (renal glycosuria). Causes of hyperglycaemic and renal glycosurias are listed in Table 1. Hyperglycaemic glycosuria will not be further discussed here; the Fanconi syndrome is described in Chapter 5.3. The remainder of this section will deal with renal glycosurias.

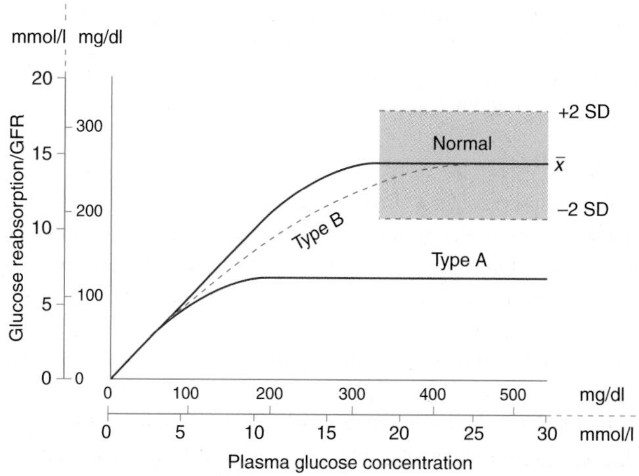

Fig. 4 Glucose reabsorption curves for normal subjects and patients with types A and B renal glycosuria (see text for details).

Table 1 Causes of glycosuria

Hyperglycaemic (overload) glycosuria
Diabetes mellitus
Type 1
Type 2
Iatrogenic
Drugs
Glucocorticoids
Catecholamines
Infusion fluids
Dextrose solutions
Total parenteral nutrition
Renal glycosuria
Type A (reduced T_MG/GFR)
Type B (increased splay)
Glycosuria of pregnancy
Glucose–galactose malabsorbtion
Fanconi syndrome
Drug induced
Unclassified
Raised intracranial pressure
Catabolic stress (burns, major trauma)
Endocrine causes
Infection
Malignancy

Primary (isolated) renal glycosurias

Definition and incidence

Primary renal glycosuria is defined as abnormal glucose excretion at normal plasma glucose concentrations, in the absence of other abnormalities of renal function. Its incidence varies markedly depending on the criteria used to define it. Transient glycosuria occurs during the course of a glucose tolerance test in up to 65 per cent of subjects investigated for glycosuria; this seems an excessively inclusive standard by which to define a 'disease' (high sensitivity, low specificity). Marble *et al.* (1939) required glycosuria to be present in all urine samples tested, including those obtained after an overnight fast: such a stringent test will be highly specific but relatively insensitive: many subjects with T_MG/GFR or a renal glucose threshold outside the normal range conventionally defined as mean ± 2SD will be missed. Defined by these criteria, isolated glycosuria was attributed to renal causes in less than 1 in 500 of a large series of cases.

Pathophysiology

Clearance studies suggest three types of renal glycosuria which show different abnormalities of the glucose titration curve. Type A is characterized by an abnormally low T_MG/GFR (low J_{max}) and a low glucose threshold (low K_m), although the general conformation of the curve is normal; in type B, T_MG and T_MG/GFR are normal but the splay is exaggerated (low K_m) (Fig. 4). The third, very rare, variant is designated type O and is associated with complete or nearly complete failure of reabsorption of filtered glucose (Bagga *et al.* 1991): the main transporter is either absent or mutated and thus essentially functionless. The physiological interpretation of type A glycosuria is relatively straightforward: the carrier mechanism is presumably defective in all nephrons, so that single nephron T_MG is uniformly subnormal. The explanation of type B glycosuria is less satisfactory; the exaggerated splay can be explained in one of two ways, as can the normal splay. The hypothesis of a nephron heterogeneity with variable degrees of internephron glomerulotubular imbalance failed to find morphological support in one study (Monasterio *et al.* 1964), in which the glomerular and tubular dimensions of 50 microdissected nephrons from two subjects with renal glycosuria were no more variable than those from normal individuals. The kinetic analysis of Woolf *et al.* (1966) is more satisfactory. According to conventional Michaelis–Menten kinetics (see above) both types of renal glycosuria can be explained by abnormalities of the carrier protein. If the number of carrier sites were reduced, but the affinity (K_M) of the carrier molecules for glucose was normal, a type A glucose reabsorption curve would be predicted. Conversely, if K_M were reduced but the number of carrier sites was normal, splay would be increased with a lowered actual glucose threshold but normal T_MG/GFR, although T_MG would only be achieved at a higher plasma glucose (and therefore filtered load) than normal: this is precisely the situation in type B renal glycosuria.

There are at least two Na^+-glucose transporters in the proximal tubule, with different stoichiometries and affinities in different segments (S1 and S3) of the proximal tubule. That which predominates in the early (S1) segment has high capacity but low affinity (K_M = 2–6 mM) and a stoichiometry of one Na^+ to one glucose molecule. It accounts for the reabsorption of the bulk of the filtered load of glucose. The other has low capacity but high affinity (K_M = 0.3 mM), transports two Na^+ with each glucose molecule and is responsible for recovering the last traces of glucose from the fluid traversing the late proximal tubule. The latter is identical to the main intestinal transporter SGLT1, transports galactose as well as glucose and is lacking or abnormal in glucose–galactose malabsorption (see below). The human SGLT1 is a protein of 664 amino acids whose gene has been mapped to 22q (Hediger *et al.* 1989). Abnormalities of the low affinity transporter, SGLT2, cause the primary renal glycosurias, since SGLT1 deficiency, even when severe or total as in glucose–galactose malabsorption, is associated with only mild glycosuria. SGLT2, has been characterized in pig but not yet in man. In the pig, SGLT1 and SGLT2 have 76 per cent amino acid sequence homology, suggesting a common evolutionary ancestry (Mackenzie *et al.* 1996). The isolation of a cDNA from human kidney that codes for a 672 residue protein with 59 per cent identity with SGLT1 at the amino acid level, not present in intestine, provides one candidate for the human SGLT2. Kinetic studies confirm that SGLT2 binds first one Na^+ ion and secondly one glucose molecule followed by simultaneous translocation of both across the cell membrane (Mackenzie *et al.* 1996).

The matter is complicated further by the finding of cases of both type A and type B glycosuria in the same family (Elsas *et al.* 1971). Furthermore, reported values for T_MG in patients with renal glycosuria appear to form a single distribution with no clear separation into two subgroups, as would be expected if types A and B really represented the consequences of two distinct abnormalities of glucose transport. Alternatively, the glucose titration curve observed in any individual, whether 'normal' or with renal glycosuria, might result from the interaction of several genetically determined characteristics, one (or more) determining T_MG and one (or more) determining splay. Thus subjects classified as having type A renal glycosuria (low T_MG/GFR) may independently have normal or increased splay.

Clinical features and diagnosis

Primary (isolated) renal glycosuria is a benign condition. It is usually detected accidentally, when a urine specimen is tested routinely (as for insurance purposes) or during investigation of an unrelated disorder. The amount of glycosuria varies from a minimum (by definition) of 500 mg/day to 100 g/day or more, with most subjects excreting 1–30 g/day. Even at the higher recorded levels of glucose excretion symptoms such as polyuria, polydipsia, and dehydration are rare. There is no treatment.

The diagnosis is established by exclusion of other causes of glycosuria, the most important of which is diabetes mellitus. The finding of normal random or fasting blood glucose concentrations in the presence of glycosuria excludes diabetes. The absence of aminoaciduria, phosphaturia, hypokalaemia, and the proximal type of renal tubular acidosis excludes the Fanconi syndrome. Glucose–galactose malabsorption with glycosuria presents acutely in infancy with intestinal symptoms; it does not arise in the differential diagnosis of the asymptomatic patient with glycosuria. The finding of glycosuria in asymptomatic first degree relatives of the patient supports the diagnosis but is not essential.

Genetics

Primary renal glycosuria is commonly familial and presumably inherited. The distinction between types A and B glycosuria is insecure and, at present, not helpful from the genetic point of view. Hjärne (1927) found vertical transmission of glycosuria through several generations in a large Swedish pedigree, and concluded that the disorder was autosomal dominant. However, in this study the magnitude of the glycosuria was not taken into account. Elsas *et al.* (1971) found that heavy, continuous glycosuria behaved as an autosomal recessive trait, in that heavy glycosuria was seen in some siblings of index cases but mild or no glycosuria was found in the parents. Given that mild glycosuria is found in some obligate heterozygotes it would be more satisfactory to classify familial renal glycosuria as partially recessive, in that some abnormality can be demonstrated in heterozygotes with much more marked abnormality in homozygotes. A boy with type O renal glycosuria was recently described in India, whose mother and younger brother had mild and severe type A renal glycosuria, respectively, while the father's glucose reabsorption was normal (Bagga *et al.* 1991). The most plausible explanation of these bewildering apparent inconsistencies is that the different subtypes of renal glycosuria represent the effect of different mutations of the gene for SGLT2, with mixed heterozygosity for different mutations producing form with mixed features of type A and type B glycosuria.

Other (secondary) renal glycosurias

Glucose–galactose malabsorption

This rare disease presents with severe fermentative diarrhoea in infancy, as soon as the child is given a feed containing glucose, galactose or any polysaccharide containing either or both of these hexoses—normally on the first day of life. It is recessively inherited, and due to functional absence or deficiency of the small intestinal glucose–galactose transporter SGLT1 (Turk *et al.* 1991). The fact that patients with this disease also have renal glycosuria, apparently of type B (Meeuwisse 1970), is of no clinical importance but confirms that the intestine and the renal tubule have this glucose transporter in common. Conversely, the fact that the great majority of subjects with renal glycosuria have no abnormality of intestinal sugar absorption excludes a role for abnormalities of SGLT1 in that condition. One specific mutation of the SGLT1 gene (D28N) has been identified in a consanguineous Syrian family (Turk *et al.* 1991). This is a G to A transition at base pair 92 of exon 1, which results in substitution of asparagine for aspartate at position 28. The mutant protein was incorporated successfully into *Xenopus* oöcytes but Na^+-dependent α-methyl-D-glucopyranoside transport was not induced as a result (in contrast to the effect of the intact SGLT1 gene). D28N is not present in all families with glucose–galactose malabsorption, indicating allelic heterogeneity in this disease.

Glucoglycinuria

Käser *et al.* (1962) described a boy with cystic fibrosis who also had type B renal glycosuria and glycinuria without generalized aminoaciduria. Thirteen of 45 relatives had both renal glycosuria and glycinuria, indicating an abnormality of a common transport mechanism or very close genetic linkage of two transport systems. The familial pattern suggested autosomal dominant inheritance. No further patients with this disorder have yet been described.

Glycosuria with hyperphosphaturia and glycinuria

The combination of severe hyperphosphaturic rickets, type A glycosuria with markedly depressed T_MG and increased urinary excretion of glycine and glycyl-proline was described by Scriver *et al.* (1964b). Absence of other features of the Fanconi syndrome suggest that this is a distinct genetic entity, whose underlying transport defect(s) is unknown.

Glycosuria of pregnancy

As with other glycosurias, the apparent incidence of glycosuria of pregnancy varies with the diagnostic criteria used. The most clinically relevant definition is a positive dip-stick test in the setting of a routine antenatal clinic. By this criterion Chen *et al.* (1976) reported an incidence of 1.7 per cent. Clearance studies have thrown light on the mechanism of this disorder. Christensen (1958) found a reduced actual glucose threshold with normal T_MG; however, the importance of relating T_MG to GFR is illustrated by the studies of Welsh and Sims (1960), who clearly showed that T_MG/GFR is lower in glycosuric pregnant women than in non-glycosuric pregnant women at all levels of GFR. They also showed that T_MG/GFR was lower even in non-glycosuric pregnant subjects that in non-pregnant controls. Davison and Hytten (1975) showed in addition that although glucose reabsorption had improved when their subjects were restudied 8–10 weeks after delivery, it remained less efficient in those who had been glycosuric when pregnant than in those who had not.

Two points emerge clearly from these results. First, T_MG/GFR falls during pregnancy in all women, as the well-known increase in GFR is not accompanied by a parallel increase in T_MG. The volume expansion associated with pregnancy inhibits proximal tubular sodium reabsorption. Coupling between reabsorption of sodium and its cotransportates (including glucose) in the proximal tubule might enforce the observed parallel reduction of fractional reabsorption of glucose. The increased urinary excretion of amino acids (Hytten and Cheyne 1972) and uric acid (Semple *et al.* 1974) observed during pregnancy supports this interpretation. There is considerable variation in renal glucose handling among the general population, with those heterozygous for primary renal glycosuria ('renal glycosuria trait': see above) having a T_MG/GFR lower than controls, although not always being clinically glycosuric. It may well be that women glycosuric in pregnancy are simply manifesting the physiological effect of pregnancy on a lower than average T_MG/GFR and that some of them represent mild (perhaps heterozygous) cases of primary renal glycosuria. The main importance of glycosuria of pregnancy is its distinction from diabetes mellitus by means of a glucose tolerance test. If this is normal, the condition should be regarded as benign.

Aminoacidurias

Normal amino acid reabsorption (see also Chapter 5.1)

With the exception of tryptophan, which is 60–90 per cent protein bound, amino acids are present in plasma in free solution and their concentrations in glomerular filtrate are the same as those in plasma water. In health, reabsorption is nearly complete, ranging from 97 to 99.9 per cent of the filtered load in adults and older children, with the exception of histidine which is only 90–95 per cent reabsorbed (Brodehl and Gellissen 1968). In infants aged less than 4 months, the fractional reabsorption of all amino acids is slightly lower than in children and adults, but is still more than 97 per cent except for histidine (mean ± SD, 86.6 ± 5.1 per cent), glycine (87.6 ± 6.4 per cent) and serine (93.4 ± 2.7 per cent). Premature infants have generalized aminoaciduria with fractional reabsorption of many amino acids below 90 per cent, presumably reflecting functional immaturity (O'Brien and Butterfield 1963). The resulting pattern of plasma concentrations and urinary excretion rates for the main amino acids in normal children is shown in Fig. 5. It is essentially identical in adults. Infants excrete significantly more threonine, asparagine, serine, proline, glycine, and alanine.

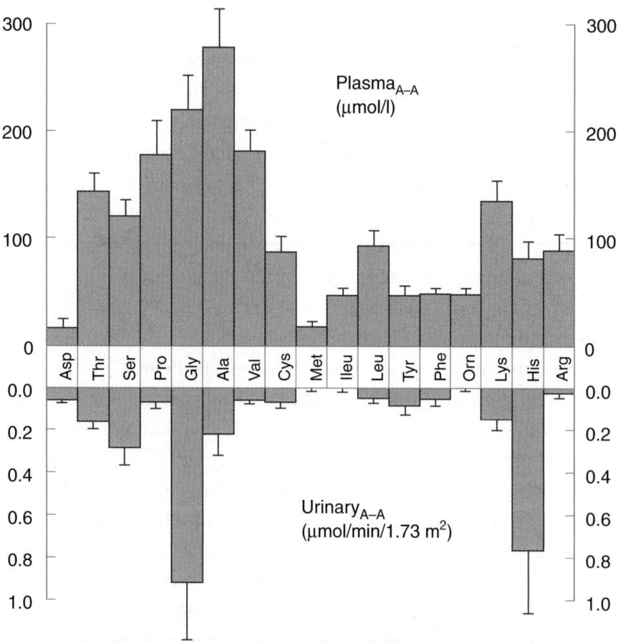

Fig. 5 Plasma concentrations and urinary excretion rates of free amino acids (A–A) measured in 12 normal children aged 2–13 years. The bars represent one standard deviation. Values in adults are essentially the same. Data from Brodehl and Gellison (1968).

The multiplicity and chemical diversity of amino acids are matched by their epithelial transport systems in the proximal tubule (Silbernagl 1988). Most amino acids are reabsorbed by more than one transporter: one which is specific to each amino acid and characterized by high specificity and affinity (K_M) and low maximal transport capacity (V_{MAX}), and one shared with other members of a group of chemically related amino acids, characterized by low K_M and high V_{MAX}. Membrane vesicle studies have identified five carrier systems in the latter, group-specific category (Sacktor 1978). These transport neutral and cyclic amino acids, glycine and imino acids, cystine and dibasic amino acids, dicarboxylic amino acids, and β-amino acids, respectively. The existence of transporters specific to single amino acids is suggested by inborn errors of metabolism in which there is excessive loss of an individual amino acid without increased excretion of the other amino acids normally reabsorbed by the corresponding group carrier. The best documented example is isolated hypercystinuria without increased excretion of dibasic amino acids (Brodehl *et al.* 1967): a specific cystine transporter has been found in isolated rat proximal tubules (Foreman *et al.* 1980). Recent studies indicate that the main amino acid transporters are heteromeric, consisting of a heavy chain and a light subunit, both of which are necessary for transport activity (Palacín *et al.* 2000). Furthermore, the transport of cystine and dibasic amino acids on the one hand, and neutral amino acids on the other, are intimately interconnected by transporters that act as exchangers at both the apical and the basolateral membranes, as discussed further in the sections on cystinuria and Hartnup disease.

Titration studies for individual amino acids show typical T_M-limited tubular reabsorption much as for glucose, but the degree of splay varies greatly. For example, lysine has almost no splay (Wright *et al.* 1947) while for glycine the splay extends over at least a six-fold range of filtered load (Pitts 1943).

Mechanisms of aminoaciduria

Theoretically, impaired tubular reabsorption of amino acids could result from abnormalities of any of the successive steps in the transport process. Possible defects include the following:

1. the transporter for the entry step (either the group transporter or the specific transporter) is absent or defective;
2. the luminal membrane is excessively leaky to the amino acids in question, leading to secondary back leak into the lumen;
3. the exit step is abnormal;
4. some metabolic process linking the entry step to the exit step is deficient, leading to accumulation of substrate within the cell and the generation of a lumen-to-cell gradient too steep for the entry process to surmount.

Recent evidence has identified abnormalities of the entry step in classical (type 1) cystinuria, iminoglycinuria and Hartnup disease, and of the exit step in non-type 1 cystinuria.

Non-renal (overflow) aminoacidurias

An amino acid whose plasma concentration exceeds the (normal) renal threshold is excreted in the urine, leading to overflow or non-renal aminoaciduria. Such aminoacidurias are not described further here since, by definition, renal function is normal. The interested reader is referred to standard textbooks of paediatrics (Behrman *et al.* 2000) and metabolic medicine (Scriver *et al.* 2001).

Renal aminoacidurias

Renal aminoacidurias imply, by definition, an increased loss of one or more amino acids due to a defect in renal tubular reabsorption. In accordance with the concept of group-specific and individual amino acid specific transporters discussed above, some diseases involve abnormal excretion of groups of amino acids while others are characterized by loss of an individual amino acid. Table 2 lists the major renal aminoacidurias classified according to the lost amino acid(s).

Classical cystinuria

The renal defect

Cystine stones were first identified in the urinary tract in the early nineteenth century. An inborn error of metabolism was postulated as early as 1908, but confirmed only in 1951 by the demonstration of defective renal tubular reabsorption of cystine and the dibasic amino acids arginine, lysine, and ornithine (Dent and Rose 1951). The consistent finding of increased excretion of all four acids in classical cystinuria together with their structural similarities led to the recognition that cystine and the dibasic amino acids share a common transport system. This insight was based first on the consistent finding of increased excretion of all four acids in classical cystinuria and, second, on the structural similarities between them. The finding that lysine infusion increases the urinary excretion of cystine, arginine, and ornithine in normal humans, suggests competition for tubular reabsorption: this effect is absent in patients with cystinuria, in whom the transporter is presumed to be non-functional (Robson and Rose 1957).

Cystine excretion may exceed GFR, indicating net secretion. This has been noted in cystinuric patients both spontaneously (Crawhall *et al.* 1967) and during lysine infusion (Lester and Cusworth 1973) as well as in dogs (Webber *et al.* 1961) perhaps as a consequence of the uptake of cystine into tubular cells across the peritubular (basolateral) membrane with secondary, probably passive, diffusion into the lumen.

The entry of cystine and dibasic amino acids across the apical membrane of proximal tubular cells is mediated by a heteromeric transporter, consisting of a heavy chain (rBAT, 90,000 kDa) and a light subunit ($b^{0,+}$AT, 40,000 kDa). When co-expressed, both moieties together comprise the $b^{0,+}$ amino acid transport system (Palacín *et al.* 2001b).

Table 2 Classification of renal aminoacidurias

A	Cystine and dibasic amino acids
	Classical cystinuria[a]
	Isolated hypercystinuria
	Dibasic aminoaciduria
	Type 1
	Type 2
	Lysinuria
B	Neutral amino acids
	Hartnup disease[a]
	Methionine malabsorption (oasthouse syndrome)
	Histidinuria
C	Glycine and imino acids
	Iminoglycinuria[a]
	Glycinuria
D	Dicarboxylic amino acids
	Dicarboxylic aminoaciduria[a]

[a] These disorders are believed to represent defects of group-specific amino acid transport systems.

The superscript (0,+) refers to transport of both neutral and dibasic amino acids. In the apical membrane, the $b^{0,+}$ system facilitates the entry of cystine and dibasic amino acids into the cell in exchange for exit of neutral amino acids into the lumen. The driving forces for this exchange are believed to be (i) intracellular reduction of cystine to cysteine and (ii) the presence of a high concentration of neutral amino acids in the cell interior due to the activity of another, sodium dependent, neutral amino acid specific transporter also present in the apical membrane. The dibasic amino acids leave the cell across the basolateral membrane by another heteromeric exchanger, system y^+L. The larger component of this is 4F2hc, the heavy chain of the surface antigen 4F2 (CD98). The light subunit is y^+LAT-1. This system facilitates the outward movement of dibasic amino acids and the inward movement of neutral amino acids in the presence of sodium. The interaction of these various transport systems is schematized in Fig. 6 (Palacín *et al.* 2000).

The intestinal defect

The polyamines cadaverine and putrescine, decarboxylation products of lysine and arginine, are present in greatly increased amounts in the

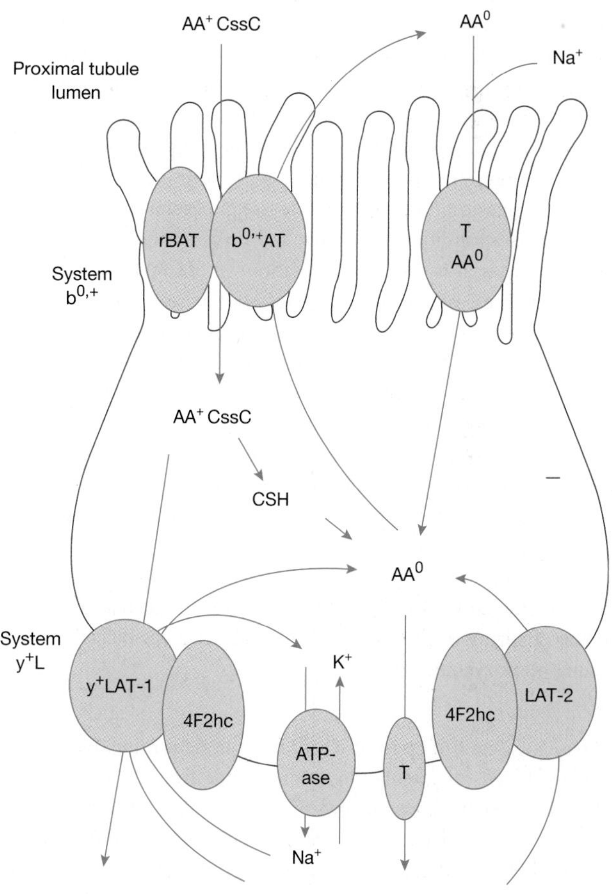

Fig. 6 Map of the main apical membrane (top of diagram) and basolateral membrane (bottom of diagram) amino acid transporters in proximal tubular epithelial cells. System $b^{0,+}$, system y^+L and system L are heterodimers. Mutations in the genes coding for rBAT, $b^{0,+}$AT and y^+LAT-1 cause type 1 cystinuria, non-type 1 cystinuria and lysinuric protein intolerance, respectively. Abbreviations: AA+, dibasic amino acids; AA^0, neutral amino acids; CssC, cystine; CSH, cysteine. Further details are given in the text. From Palacín *et al.* (2000), with permission.

urine of cystinuric patients. Their presence is due to bacterial degradation of unabsorbed lysine and arginine in the gut, as shown by increased urinary polyamine excretion following feeding of these amino acids (Milne *et al.* 1961; Asatoor *et al.* 1962). The intestinal absorption of cystine and dibasic amino acids is defective as demonstrated by direct measurement of uptake in jejunal and duodenal biopsy material (Furlong and Stiel 1993). The intestinal defect is of little or no clinical consequence, however. Sufficient cystine and dibasic amino acids for nutritional needs are probably absorbed as dipeptides: protein feeding, but not cystine feeding, is followed by increased urinary cystine excretion (Brand *et al.* 1935). Not surprisingly, the $b^{0,+}$ amino acid transport system is expressed in intestine as well as in kidney.

Genetics

The human rBAT gene, SLC3A1, has been localized to 2p16 (Calonge *et al.* 1995). Linkage analysis in families with type 1 cystinuria confirms inheritance on chromosome 2 (Pras *et al.* 1994). Over 60 mutations in SLC3A1 have been identified: they include missense, frameshift, nonsense, and splice site mutations as well as large deletions (Palacín *et al.* 2001b). The gene for $b^{0,+}$AT, SLC7A9, has been assigned to 19q12–13.1 and mutations in it have been identified in patients with non-type 1 cystinuria (Palacín *et al.* 2001b). As defined clinically, cystinuria is inherited as an autosomal recessive disease. Traditionally, it has been divided into three clinical subtypes on the basis of intestinal transport characteristics and whether or not obligate heterozygotes have measurably increased urinary excretion of cystine and dibasic amino acids. As classified by Rosenberg *et al.* (1966), type 1 (by far the most common) is characterized by the absence of *in vitro* intestinal uptake of cystine and dibasic amino acids and no rise in plasma cystine following oral administration in homozygotes, and no abnormal aminoaciduria in heterozygotes. It is caused by mutations in SLC3A1. Types 2 and 3 differ from type 1 in that heterozygotes have increased urinary excretion of cystine and dibasic amino acids, although these are well below homozygote levels. Type 2 is associated with some intestinal transport of cystine (less than normal but more than type 1) but not of dibasic amino acids, while in type 3 intestinal transport of cystine and dibasic amino acids is present and an oral cystine load is followed by a rise in its plasma concentration. At the molecular level, types 2 and 3 are now grouped together as non-type 1, and it appears likely that all non-type 1 cases of cystinuria are due to mutations in SLC7A9, with different specific mutations probably accounting for the minor differences in clinical expression. The three types are indistinguishable clinically, and the offspring of parents with different subtypes behave as stone forming homozygotes.

Clinical features

The true incidence of cystinuria is difficult to determine. Estimates of incidence based on population studies range from 1 : 100,000 to as high as 1 : 2500 in Sephardic Jews of Libyan origin (Weinberger *et al.* 1974). An even higher incidence of 1 : 1100 was claimed in a population of 70,000 newborns screened in Vienna (Thalhammer 1975), although the same author reported figures between 1 : 15,000 and 1 : 25,000 for newborns in Boston and Prague, similar to that found by in Sydney (Smith *et al.* 1979).

The symptomatology of cystinuria is entirely related to stone formation. Cystine stones may manifest themselves in any of the ways common to stones in the urinary tract: renal colic, haematuria, infections, or the urethral passage of stones. Urethral obstruction occurs occasionally, usually in males. If stones form bilaterally and are not adequately treated, chronic renal failure may ensue. Cystine lithiasis may present at any age, but most cases come to light in childhood or early adult life. The stones are radio-opaque, but typically less so than calcium stones, and often have a uniform 'ground-glass' appearance. They may become very large and can form complete 'staghorn' casts of the pelvicalyceal system.

Although it has been suggested that the incidence of mental handicap and psychiatric illness is higher in patients with cystinuria than in the general population, psychometric assessment failed to reveal any differences between a group of homozygous cystinurics and controls (Gold *et al.* 1977). The apparent high incidence in inmates of mental institutions might reflect the fact that such patients are often subjected to repeated metabolic investigation, and that the baseline prevalence of cystinuria in most populations is not known and probably underestimated.

Diagnosis

The diagnosis of cystinuria rests on the demonstration of increased urinary excretion of cystine. Cystine crystals may be seen on microscopy and are diagnostic. A simple, colorimetric screening test is available (the cyanide–nitroprusside test) and, if positive, should be confirmed by quantitation of the excretion rate of cystine and the dibasic amino acids. This is necessary since homocysteine gives a false positive cyanide–nitroprusside test and because some heterozygotes for non-type 1 cystinuria may also give a positive reaction. Normal individuals excrete less than 10 nmol cystine/mol creatinine (often expressed as $<$20 nmol 2-cystine, i.e. cysteine) while patients homozygous for cystinuria exceed this value at least 10-fold. Cystine excretion in heterozygotes is intermediate between that in normals and that in homozygotes.

Treatment

The objective of medical treatment is to prevent stone formation. Two strategies are employed: reduce the urinary concentration of cystine, and increase its solubility. At physiological urine pH (4.5–7.5) the upper limit of solubility is 1.0–1.25 mmol/l (240–300 mg/l); solubility increases progressively at pH above 7.5. Alkalinization of the urine is therefore desirable but difficult to achieve continuously. Alkali (sodium bicarbonate or equivalent) should be given in several divided doses to maintain pH above 7.5. A high water intake should also be encouraged. Quantitation of the cystine excretion rate in the individual patient provides a guideline for the minimum recommended water intake—1 l of water should be ingested daily for every millimole of cystine (2 mmol 2-cystine). This also is difficult to achieve, particularly at night, since it requires an intake of 4–10 l daily. A combination of alkali and high water intake is effective and safe. It remains the treatment of first choice.

Patients who are unable to comply with the above regimen may be treated with D-penicillamine by mouth in a dose of 30 mg/kg/day to a maximum of 2 g/day in adults. D-penicillamine reacts with cystine to produce a mixed penicillamine–cysteine disulfide which is much more soluble than cystine. The drug is highly effective but, unfortunately, causes many side-effects, including proteinuria with membranous glomerulonephritis and the nephrotic syndrome (Rosenberg and Hayslett 1967), rashes, arthralgia, bone marrow depression, epidermolysis, and loss of taste sensation. However, in one study of over 275 patient-years in 26 patients, D-penicillamine was generally well tolerated and no patient in this series needed to be switched to other thiol compounds (Combe *et al.* 1993). Pyridoxine supplements (10 mg/day) should be prescribed for patients on penicillamine, since the action of pyridoxine is antagonized by the drug. Other sulfydryl compounds have a similar effect. Mercaptopropionyl glycine was initially thought to be less toxic than penicillamine (Hautman *et al.* 1977) but subsequent experience suggests that it offers little, if any, advantage.

Recent observations by Jaeger *et al.* (1986) suggested a relationship between dietary sodium intake and urinary cystine excretion. In cystinuric patients, basal cystine excretion was lower on a low (150 mmol/day) than on a high (300 mmol/day) sodium diet and fell further when sodium intake was reduced to 50 mmol/day. The mechanism of this relationship is not known, but may implicate changes in extracellular fluid volume and their influence on proximal tubular reabsorption of sodium and other solutes. Another small study confirmed that dietary sodium restriction markedly reduces urinary excretion of cystine and lysine (but not ornithine or arginine) (Peces *et al.* 1991). The therapeutic consequences of this observation are obvious but the effect on the rate of stone formation, the key clinical purpose of treatment, has not yet been assessed. If a low-sodium diet is prescribed, any accompanying alkali therapy would presumably have to be given in a sodium-free form, such as potassium citrate.

Two studies have claimed that administration of captopril reduces cystine excretion. The first (Perazella and Buller 1993) described only two patients and both the methodology and conclusions were criticized by Coulthard (1995). The second (Cohen *et al.* 1995) found a significant reduction in cystine excretion in nine patients but not in the rate of stone formation. Coulthard (1995) pointed out that, on theoretical grounds, only a small reduction in cystine excretion could be expected from the administration of a clinically acceptable amount of captopril, assuming that the drug works by mixed disulfide formation. At present there is no good evidence that captopril has a place in the treatment of cystinuria.

Once stones have formed in the kidney they should be treated on their merits by a urological team experienced in the management of urolithiasis. Stone formation during medical treatment indicates either inadequate treatment or (commonly) non-adherence.

Other disorders of cystine and dibasic amino acid excretion

Isolated hypercystinuria

Two children, a brother and sister, have been described with excessive urinary cystine excretion without dibasic aminoaciduria (Brodehl *et al.* 1967). Neither had stone formation, and urine amino acid excretion was normal in both parents and another sibling. The molecular basis of this disease is not known, but it has been suggested that it may be an allelic form of the already identified cystinuria genes (Palacín *et al.* 2001b).

Lysinuric protein intolerance

Several individuals with increased urinary excretion of arginine, lysine, and ornithine without cystinuria, can be regrouped into two types. The first, called lysinuric protein intolerance (LPI) (Perheentupa and Visakorpi 1965), is characterized by dibasic aminoaciduria and intestinal malabsorption of dibasic amino acids, presumably due to a defect in a transport system common to the renal tubule and intestine. In this severe, autosomal recessive disease, protein loading produces hyperammonaemia with vomiting, weakness, and neurological symptoms including coma. Other manifestations include failure to thrive, hepatosplenomegaly, and occasionally a form of life-threatening pulmonary alveolar proteinosis. The mechanism is thought to be intracellular depletion of arginine and ornithine, which are important components of the urea cycle. Intravenous infusion of arginine prevents the acute adverse response to protein loading (Simell 2001). Oral supplementation with dibasic amino acids is helpful in some, but not all, patients: its effectiveness is presumably limited by the underlying intestinal defect. Citrulline supplementation has also been used and appears promising, since it is absorbed by a pathway independent of that for the dibasic amino acids and is converted to arginine and ornithine in the liver (Rajantie and Perheentupa 1980). A combination of oral supplementation with citrulline and lysine (which cannot be made from citrulline) and moderate protein restriction is the current treatment of choice. The disease is caused by mutations in the gene (SLC7A7) for y^+LAT-1, the light subunit of the basolateral transporter y+L that exchanges dibasic amino acid (out) for neutral amino acids and sodium (in) (see above). SLC7A7 is located at 14q11–13; more than 20 mutations have been found in different pedigrees with LPI (Palacín *et al.* 2001a). All Finnish patients with LPI, the most commonly affected population, have the same, presumably founder, mutation.

Autosomal dominant hyperdibasic aminoaciduria

A second type of dibasic aminoaciduria has been described in several individuals from two generations of a family (Whelan and Scriver 1968b). Dibasic aminoacidurias without cystinuria is not accompanied by hyperammonaemia, and affected individuals appeared clinically normal. Sporadic case reports may represent this second type or, possibly, new entities. They are extremely rare and the nature of the biochemical transport abnormality has not been elucidated.

Isolated lysinuria

A severely mentally retarded child with excessive urinary excretion of lysine but not arginine, ornithine, or cystine has been reported. He had an intestinal defect of absorption limited to lysine (Omura *et al.* 1976). Whether this is an allelic variant of one of the commoner conditions discussed above, or a mutation in a different, as yet uncharacterized, transport system is unknown.

Hartnup disease

The renal defect The tubular reabsorption of the neutral (monoamino, monocarboxylic) amino acids: alanine, asparagine, glutamine, histidine, isoleucine, leucine, methionine, phenylalanine, serine, threonine, tryptophan, tyrosine, and valine is incomplete. Only about 50 per cent of the filtered load of most of these amino acids is reabsorbed, apart from histidine of which virtually 100 per cent of the filtered load is excreted. Absorption of other amino acids is normal. The neutral amino acid group transporter is defective. It might possibly be the system labelled $T\,AA^0$ in Fig. 6.

The intestinal defect An abnormality of intestinal amino acid absorption was first suspected because indoles and indicans, products of the bacterial breakdown of tryptophan, were present in increased amounts in urine and faeces of affected patients (Baron *et al.* 1956), and subsequently confirmed by the finding of unabsorbed neutral amino acids in the stool, the pattern being similar to that in urine (Scriver and Shaw 1962), and by the demonstration of several abnormalities following an oral tryptophan load. These included: (i) a much smaller than normal rise in plasma tryptophan; (ii) an increase in faecal tryptophan; (iii) absent conversion of tryptophan to indolyl-3-pyruvic acid; and (iv) a further increase in the already high urinary and faecal excretion rate of indoles and indicans (Milne *et al.* 1960). The metabolic consequences of this absorptive defect are presumably ameliorated by the fact that dipeptides containing tryptophan, histidine, and phenylalanine are absorbed normally by patients with Hartnup disease (Asatoor *et al.* 1970).

Genetics Hartnup disease is inherited as an autosomal recessive trait. Its incidence has been estimated at about 1 : 20,000. A candidate gene, ASCT1, has been identified at 19q13.3 (Jones *et al.* 1994).

Clinical features The clinical features of Hartnup disease are due to deficiency of nicotinamide, which is partly derived from dietary tryptophan. The intestinal malabsorption of this amino acid, probably exacerbated by increased urinary losses, leads to a nicotinamide production that varies from borderline to inadequate, according to dietary intake and, perhaps, metabolic need. The major signs and symptoms of the disease are a scaly, photosensitive erythematous rash that is clinically identical to pellagra (niacin deficiency), cerebellar ataxia, psychiatric symptoms including emotional liability and confusional states, and occasional mental retardation. All these are intermittent and variable in severity except mental retardation, which affects only a minority of patients. Many patients remain completely asymptomatic, perhaps as a consequence of good dietary intake. Symptomatic patients tend to improve with age.

Diagnosis Diagnosis is straightforward and rests on the demonstration of an increased urinary excretion of all neutral amino acids but not the dibasic, dicarboxylic, or imino acids or glycine. This test should be performed in all patients presenting with a pellagra-like rash, otherwise unexplained cerebellar ataxia or intermittent 'psychiatric' symptoms, and in relatives of known cases. Some affected infants will be detected as a result of routine urine screening for phenylketonuria and other inborn errors of metabolism. Full chromatographic analysis of urinary amino acids is mandatory in all cases to avoid confusion with the renal Fanconi syndrome and the (even rarer) abnormalities of tubular reabsorption of individual neutral amino acids.

Treatment Nicotinamide supplementation reverses the cutaneous and neuropsychiatric features (Halvorsen and Halvorsen 1963): it should be prescribed for all affected subjects, even asymptomatic, since the treatment is harmless and since the possible effects of subclinical nicotinamide deficiency are unknown.

Other disorders of renal transport of neutral amino acids

Methionine malabsorption (oasthouse syndrome)

Two children with increased urinary excretion of methionine have been described (Smith and Strang 1958; Hooft *et al.* 1965). Both had large amounts of α-hydroxybutyric acid in the urine and, in one patient, methionine was present in the faeces, suggesting a specific defect of methionine transport in both intestine and renal tubule. Breakdown of methionine in the colon by bacterial degradation produces α-hydroxybutyric acid which is then absorbed into the bloodstream and excreted in the urine. Clinical features were similar in the two cases: white hair, oedema, mental retardation, and seizures. The urine had an offensive odour, said to be similar to that of an oasthouse (a building in which hops are dried for use in the brewing of beer)—hence the alternative name for the condition.

The presence of α-hydroxybutyric acid, rather than methionine deficiency, appears responsible for the clinical features, since a low methionine diet resulted in disappearance of α-hydroxybutyric acid from the urine and striking clinical improvement.

Histidinuria

Sabater *et al.* (1976) described two mentally retarded brothers with isolated histidinuria, accompanied by intestinal malabsorption of this amino acid. Consistent with recessive transmission, both parents had a mild intestinal absorptive defect for histidine but neither had histidinuria. This unique family provides direct evidence for a specific histidine transporter common to intestine and renal tubule.

Disorders of renal glycine and imino acid transport

Renal tubular reabsorption of glycine and the imino acids proline and hydroxyproline involves a group-specific carrier as well as specific systems for each amino acid (Silbernagl 1988). Indirect evidence for a group specific carrier was provided by Scriver *et al.* (1964a), who found that the (overflow) increase in urinary proline excretion observed in familial hyperprolinaemia was accompanied by increased excretion of hydroxyproline and glycine. In contrast, developmental studies in rats, dogs, and in man show that tubular reabsorption of imino acids matures more rapidly than that of glycine, suggesting that separate carrier systems are involved (Brodehl 1976). *In vitro* studies, reviewed by Foreman *et al.* (1980), suggest the existence of three carriers: one for imino acids, one for glycine, and a third, probably of lower affinity, that transports both.

Iminoglycinuria The first patient with increased urinary excretion of proline, hydroxyproline, and glycine without generalized aminoaciduria had early onset seizures (Joseph *et al.* 1958). Later reports suggest that iminoglycinuria is probably a benign condition, the apparent association with neurodevelopmental disease suggested by early reports being due to selection bias (Procopis and Turner 1971). The disease is inherited as an autosomal recessive trait with an estimated incidence of 1 : 20,000. Several allelic variants probably occur. In some, but not all patients, there is an associated defect of intestinal absorption of glycine and imino acids; furthermore, heterozygotes in some pedigrees excrete increased amounts of glycine (Whelan and Scriver 1968a) while those in other affected families do not (Bank *et al.* 1972). Although of no clinical importance, this genetic heterogeneity indicates that inheritance and molecular biology of glycine and imino acid transport is even more complex than the 'three transporter' model described above.

Isolated glycinuria Several patients have dominantly inherited hyperglycinuria without iminoaciduria occurring at normal plasma glycine concentrations. In the first pedigree, the abnormality was confined to females, and associated with calcium oxalate stone formation in three of four affected individuals (de Vries *et al.* 1957). The association of glycinuria with urolithiasis has not been observed in other affected families.

However, as already pointed out, some obligate heterozygotes for iminoglycinuria exhibit isolated glycinuria. Subjects with isolated, dominantly inherited glycinuria might be carriers of iminoglycinuria in families without a homozygous member: the heterozygous state would, of course, mimic a dominant mode of inheritance. This question cannot be resolved by the available evidence.

Glucoglycinuria Glucoglycinuria has been discussed in the section on glycosuria (above).

Disorders of renal dicarboxylic amino acid transport

Two patients with heavy dicarboxylic amino acid (aspartic and glutamic acid) excretion have been described: one was mentally retarded and hypothyroid (Teijema *et al.* 1974) but the other was clinically normal (Melancon *et al.* 1977). A causal link between the aminoaciduria and the abnormalities observed in the first case remains purely speculative. In both patients, the renal clearance of aspartic and glutamic acid exceeded the glomerular filtration rate, indicating net secretion. The apparent normality of both sets of parents, and the fact that one patient was male and the other female, suggests autosomal recessive inheritance.

Phosphaturias (see also Chapters 14.1 and 14.2)

Disorders of renal tubular phosphate transport

Familial X-linked hypophosphataemic rickets

Familial X-linked hypophosphataemic rickets (XLH), the most common inherited disorder of phosphate metabolism, has been claimed to be the leading cause of rickets in developed countries. It is known by several synonyms, of which the most widely used is vitamin D-resistant rickets (not to be confused with vitamin D-dependency rickets, see below). Two mutant strains of mice (the *Hyp* and *Gy* strains) exhibit an apparently identical, also X-linked, transport defect. These models have thrown much light on the human disease. The following description of the condition is based on both clinical studies in the human and experimental studies in the *Hyp* and *Gy* mouse. Extrapolation from mouse models is vindicated by the fact that the two models are now known to be caused by different mutations in the mouse PHEX gene, which is highly conserved between mouse and man (Tenenhouse 1999). The molecular biology of the corresponding PHEX gene in man is detailed in Chapter 2.4.

The renal defect

The characteristic abnormality in XLH is hypophosphataemia with urinary inorganic phosphate wasting, in the absence of other abnormalities of tubular reabsorption. Plasma inorganic phosphate is typically below 0.8 mmol/l (2.5 mg/dl) while T_MP/GFR is less than 0.56 mmol/l (1.8 mg/dl). Both plasma levels of inorganic phosphate and T_MP/GFR are somewhat higher in affected children than in adults, as is the case in normal subjects (Stickler *et al.* 1970).

Human disease (Anonymous 1995) and both murine models (Tenenhouse 1999) are caused by mutations in PHEX. The absorptive defect for phosphate was located in the apical membrane before identification of the genetic defect. In vitro uptake of inorganic phosphate by isolated brush border vesicles is markedly impaired, while uptake of glucose and amino acids is normal (Tenenhouse and Scriver 1978). In contrast, inorganic phosphate uptake by renal cortical slices from *Hyp* mice is normal, indicating normal transport in the basolateral membrane (Tenenhouse *et al.* 1978). Dietary inorganic phosphate restriction increases uptake by brush border membrane vesicles, but to a level well below that seen in similar vesicles from normal mice (Tenenhouse and Scriver 1979). Total parathyroidectomy does not improve phosphaturia in the *Hyp* mouse (Cowgill *et al.* 1979), nor does subtotal parathyroidectomy in human patients (Talwalkar *et al.* 1974). It is most likely that the mutated PHEX gene fails to inactivate FGF23 (phosphatonin), which inhibits Na/Pi II and causes phosphaturia.

The intestinal defect

The small intestinal absorption of calcium and inorganic phosphate is defective in both XLH and the *Hyp* mouse. Oral calcium loading produces only a minimal rise in plasma calcium concentration and urine calcium excretion in affected patients (Stickler 1963); balance and *in vitro* studies of isolated intestinal segments demonstrate calcium and inorganic phosphate malabsorption in juvenile, but not in adult, *Hyp* mice (Meyer *et al.* 1984, 1986). The mechanism of this malabsorption, and its link to the renal phosphate-losing abnormality, is not yet clear, but it is probably a consequence of the abnormality of vitamin D metabolism found in both the human disease and the *Hyp* mouse (see below).

Osteoblast function in XLH

Defective bone mineralization in XLH is not due solely to hypophosphataemia, and an abnormality of osteoblast function has been suggested (Hruska *et al.* 1995). Phosphate uptake into *Hyp* mouse osteoblasts is normal, but experiments in which periosteum is transplanted between normal and *Hyp* mice suggest that *Hyp* periosteum produces abnormal bone even in the environment of a normal host mouse (Ecarot *et al.* 1992). These findings require confirmation before their significance in the pathophysiology of murine or human XLH can be assessed.

Parathyroid hormone in XLH

Immunoreactive parathyroid hormone (iPTH) levels are normal in most patients with XLH, although slightly raised levels have been reported (Hahn *et al.*, 1975). These levels are much lower than those seen in dietary (vitamin D deficiency) rickets, untreated renal osteodystrophy, and vitamin D-dependent rickets. It is unlikely that PTH has an important primary role in XLH since iPTH levels are suppressed by calcium infusion without correction of the hyperphosphaturia or hypophosphataemia. As previously mentioned, parathyroidectomy also fails to return T_MP/GFR in *Hyp* mice to normal. Nocturnal hyperparathyroidism of moderate degree occurs in some patients with XLH (Carpenter *et al.* 1994), a phenomenon obviously missed by conventional daytime sampling. Autonomous (tertiary) hyperparathyroidism has been observed in adult patients (Knudtzon *et al.* 1995); whether this was due to the disease itself or a consequence of previous treatment is unclear.

Vitamin D metabolism in XLH

Plasma concentrations of calcitriol are normal to low in patients with XLH (Scriver *et al.* 1978). Despite hypophosphataemia, which should stimulate renal 1-α hydroxylase activity, phosphate deprivation lowers plasma levels of calcitriol in patients with XLH, as opposed to the rise seen in normal subjects. This adds further support to the contention that vitamin D metabolism is altered in the disease, and that calcitriol levels are lower than would be expected in a hypophosphataemic normal subject. The recent finding that *Hyp* and *Gy* mice have low levels of calcitriol, as in the human disease, whereas mice homozygous for null mutations in the gene for Na/Pi II have high levels despite comparable degrees of phosphaturia and hypophosphataemia (Beck *et al.* 1998), suggests an inhibitory action of phosphatonin on the enzyme 25-hydroxycholecalciferol 1 α-hydroxylase. The fact that calcitriol concentrations are also low in autosomal dominant hypophosphataemic rickets is consistent with this hypothesis.

Genetics

XLH is inherited as an X-linked dominant condition with variable expression. A recent study of genotype/phenotype correlations in

31 patients with different mutations of the PHEX gene found no consistent differences in clinical expression predicted either by the type or the location of the mutation (Holm *et al.* 2001). The gene has been mapped to Xp22.1 (Econs *et al.* 1997). Both mouse models of XLH, the *Hyp* and *Gy* (Gyro) strains, have mutations in the PHEX gene. *Gy* mice display a pattern of hypophosphataemic, phosphaturic rickets apparently identical to that in *Hyp* mice, but in addition have neurological abnormalities and cochlear deafness. An audiometric study of 22 patients with familial X-linked hypophosphataemic rickets revealed sensorineural deafness, which apparently bred true, in five: families were internally consistent with respect to the presence or absence of deafness (Boneh *et al.* 1987). Whether the deafness in these families is caused by the same mechanism as that in the *Gy* mouse is unknown.

Clinical features

The major clinical features of XLH are growth retardation and rickets, mainly affecting the legs. Affected infants appear normal at birth, but statural growth delay is usually evident by the age of 6 months to 2 years. The rickets becomes apparent after weight bearing, usually with smooth bowing of femur and tibia leading to genu valgum. Short stature is not due entirely to restricted growth of the lower limbs, as careful measurement shows that the arms are also short, although proportionately less so than the legs. Craniosynostosis affects some patients and dentition is abnormal in all, although the abnormality is different from the enamel hypoplasia characteristic of vitamin D-deficiency rickets, consisting of defective dentine maturation with enlarged pulp chambers; recurrent dental abscesses are common. Radiologically, the appearances are those of rickets: widening and fraying of the epiphyseal plates associated with coarse trabeculation and osteomalacia of the shafts of the long bones. Features of hyperparathyroidism (subperiosteal bone resorption, osteitis fibrosa cystica) are minimal or absent. The histomorphometric features of XLH are osteomalacia in both cortical and trabecular bone, decreased calcification rate and increased mineralization lag time, and reduction in the occurrence of bone remodelling units (Marie and Glorieux 1981).

After growth is complete, disabling bone pain and arthritis affecting the large limb joints are common. Ectopic ossification occurs at points of muscle attachment to the skeleton and in periarticular regions. Considerable disability may result from these late manifestations.

Skeletal features of the disease are highly variable, especially in females. Most, but not all, studies suggest that males are more severely affected than females. An analysis by Rasmussen and Tenenhouse (1989) of 143 patients, all (by definition) with hypophosphataemia, revealed 47 females but only two males without bone disease. Both *Hyp* and *Gy* mutant mice show the same sex difference in the gene expression. However, a recent study of patients with known mutations in the PHEX gene failed to confirm this sex difference, except for a trend ($P = 0.064$) towards more severe dental disease in prepubertal males (Holm *et al.* 2001). The effect of the disease on final height is also highly variable. In each of three series the mean adult height for both sexes lay between -2 and -3 population standard deviation scores (SDS), with a standard deviation of about 1.5 (Steendijk and Latham 1971; Stickler and Morgenstern 1989; Reusz *et al.* 1990). This distribution implies that about 40 per cent of patients have a final height within the lower half of the normal range, whereas the most severely affected 40 per cent will lie between -4 and -6 SDS, equivalent to 136–149 cm for men and only 129–140 cm for women.

Diagnosis

The characteristic diagnostic findings in XLH are phosphaturia in the presence of hypophosphataemia (low T_MP/GFR), normocalcaemia and low urinary calcium excretion, normal plasma iPTH and urinary cAMP, and normal or slightly reduced plasma calcitriol. The diagnosis of vitamin D-deficiency rickets (nutritional rickets) is usually apparent from the history of dietary vitamin D deficiency and lack of exposure to sunlight. Plasma total and ionized calcium concentration is reduced, iPTH levels are raised, and, by definition, plasma calcitriol level is very low. Prompt response to physiological doses of vitamin D confirms the diagnosis. The clinical features of autosomal dominant hypophosphataemic rickets overlap those of XLH considerably (see below), but there are some differences other than the pattern of inheritance (Econs and McEnery 1997). Vitamin D-dependent rickets mimics the biochemical changes of nutritional rickets closely but is unresponsive to physiological doses of vitamin D and a history of dietary deficiency and absence of exposure to sunlight is lacking. The rare disease hereditary hypercalciuric, hypophosphataemic rickets has many similarities with familial X-linked hypophosphataemic rickets but urinary calcium excretion is high: so far, it has only been clearly described in a few pedigrees. Tumour-induced osteomalacia (TIO) (see below) is biochemically indistinguishable from XLH, but is an acquired disease of adults: its clinical context prevents confusion between the two diseases.

There are no other abnormalities of tubular transport in either XLH or TIO. Patients with both vitamin D-deficiency and vitamin D-dependency rickets have a generalized aminoaciduria, secondary to hyperparathyroidism (Fraser *et al.* 1967), that resolves with treatment. Children with the Fanconi syndrome due to cystinosis may present in infancy with hypophosphataemic rickets but other components of the syndrome (glycosuria, aminoaciduria, proximal renal tubular acidosis, and hypokalaemia) are present by the second year of life; corneal and leucocyte accumulation of cystine is diagnostic. Plasma and urinary levels of inorganic phosphate may be normal in the first few months of life in patients with XLH; a child known to be genetically at risk for the disease must therefore be observed for at least a year from birth before reassurance can be given that he or she is not affected. Asymptomatic females may be difficult to diagnose: however, low fasting plasma inorganic phosphate in the presence of phosphaturia is invariably present in asymptomatic mothers of affected children, confirming that renal phosphate handling is abnormal, even in the absence of bone disease.

Treatment

Treatment of XLH remains unsatisfactory and difficult. Vitamin D_3 (cholecalciferol) in supraphysiological doses (10,000–300,000 U/day), frequently induces hypercalcaemia, with the attendant risks of hypercalciuria, nephrocalcinosis, and renal damage. In view of the primary role of renal phosphate wasting, oral phosphate supplements have been introduced (Frame *et al.* 1963). A combination of oral inorganic phosphate with vitamin D may result in a net positive balance of inorganic phosphate but large doses (2–4 g oral phosphate per day) and frequent administration (4–6 doses/day) are necessary, making adherence difficult. Diarrhoea is a frequent complication but may be overcome to some extent by starting with a small dose of oral phosphate which is then gradually increased.

The availability of synthetic calcitriol and calcidiol (1α- hydroxy-cholecalciferol) has led to numerous therapeutic trials, reviewed by

Latta *et al.* (1993). Both calcidiol and calcitriol improve intestinal absorption of calcium and inorganic phosphate, heal rachitic bone lesions, and improve linear growth. Petersen *et al.* (1992) found that calcitriol increased T_MP/GFR in those children who showed good growth in response to treatment, although not to the normal range. Dosage should be adjusted to the highest level attainable without hypercalcaemia and hypercalciuria: this is usually 25–100 ng/kg/day. Tubular inorganic phosphate wasting is not fully corrected so that phosphate supplements are usually added to maintain the plasma concentration as close to the normal range for age as possible. However, Seikaly *et al.* (1994) found no additional benefit of phosphate supplementation over calcitriol or dihydrotachysterol alone. If such is the case, withdrawal of phosphate supplements might avoid diarrhoea and thus improve patient compliance. More observations are needed on this point.

Stickler and Morgenstern (1989) sounded a cautionary note on the benefits of XLH treatment. In a retrospective review of 52 patients treated at the Mayo Clinic since 1934, and who had reached the age of 18 or over in 1989, they found no difference in final height and in bone, joint, and muscle symptom scores between patients treated with vitamin D_2 (calciferol), calcitriol and phosphate in various combinations and patients who had never been treated at all,. They also pointed out that previous studies were uncontrolled, and that claims of improved growth often rested on growth velocity analysis but not on improved final height SDS (*Z* score). Most importantly, three, treated patients developed end-stage renal failure in their twenties: medullary nephrocalcinosis had previously been noted in treated children by Goodyer *et al.* (1987). Several studies have now claimed to show improved growth from treatment in comparison with (usually) historical controls. Kooh *et al.* (1994) reported that, despite nephrocalcinosis, seen in 20 of 25 children treated with phosphate and calcitriol but absent in nine untreated patients, creatinine clearance and urine concentrating ability were normal in all. Still, the conclusion that treatment-induced nephrocalcinosis does not necessarily lead to loss of renal function remains questionable. At present, patients treated with vitamin D analogues and phosphate supplements should be monitored with regards to plasma and urine calcium levels, GFR and for the development of nephrocalcinosis.

A short (6 months) trial, in 11 children with XLH, concluded that recombinant human growth hormone (rHGH) raised the serum phosphate concentration in all patients, even in the absence of vitamin D or phosphate treatment. Triple therapy, given for 6 months to nine patients, improved growth velocity *Z* scores (Wilson *et al.* 1991). The biochemical improvement was recently confirmed (Darendeliler *et al.* 2001). Saggese *et al.* (1995) compared six patients treated for 3 years with rHGH and conventional therapy with six given conventional therapy alone. The height *Z* score, height velocity *Z* score, predicted adult height, plasma phosphate concentration, alkaline phosphatase, propeptides of type I and type III procollagen, PTH, 1,25-hydroxycholecalciferol, T_MP/GFR and radial bone density were improved in the former group. No adverse effects on renal function were observed. Exogenous rHGH may thus be indicated in XLH, even though endogenous HG secretion is normal in this condition (Saggese *et al.* 1995; Seikaly *et al.* 1997).

Autosomal dominant hypophosphataemic rickets

Autosomal dominant hypophosphataemic rickets (ADHR) was first demonstrated in a family in which a father, two of his three daughters and his only son were affected (Bianchine *et al.* 1971). The clinical features of the disease disclose two patterns of expression (Econs and McEnery 1997). In the first, patients have hypophosphaturia, hypophosphataemia and osteomalacia, but no limb deformity, either in adolescence or in adult life. In the second, hypophosphataemic rickets with lower limb deformity is evident in infancy or early childhood. The biochemical features are essentially those of XLH, including normal PTH and inappropriately greater than normal 1,25 DHCC levels. Surprisingly, some patients in the second group spontaneously lost the hyperphosphaturic defect after puberty. Since all patients in this study were from the same kindred, they presumably shared the same mutation. The variation in clinical features is presumably explained either by variable gene penetrance or by interaction with other, unknown genes. Positional cloning studies in four kindreds with ADHR identified several new genes at 12p13. One of these was found to be a member of the fibroblast growth factor family, subsequently named FGF23, and three mutations were found in four families (two unrelated families shared the same mutation) (Anonymous 2000). No mutations were found in a wide variety of control subjects, including normal individuals and some with other inherited bone diseases. The putative mechanism whereby FGF23 causes phosphaturia is discussed in Chapter 2.4.

Hereditary hypophosphataemic rickets with hypercalciuria

This rare, familial disease, despite some similarities, is distinct from XLH. In a large, consanguineous Arab pedigree, nine of 59 inter-related family members investigated had hereditary hypophosphataemic rickets with hypercalciuria and a further 21 had lesser degrees of biochemical abnormality but were clinically normal (Tieder *et al.* 1985a). A second kindred of Yemenite Jews has subsequently been described (Tieder *et al.* 1992). The unfathomable complexity of Bedouin tribal genealogy makes the genetics of the disease difficult to ascertain. Two apparent degrees of severity, the milder approximately twice as common as the more severe, within a multiply inbred family tree is suggestive of autosomal recessive inheritance with partial expression in the heterozygote, but the reported pattern is also compatible with a variably expressed dominant gene.

The clinical features are those of rickets and osteomalacia: short stature, bone deformity and pain with muscle weakness. Biochemical findings include phosphaturia with hypophosphataemia and reduced T_MP/GFR, normal plasma calcium and PTH concentrations, and increased plasma calcitriol and urinary calcium excretion. Those with the milder form of the disease (heterozygotes) are clinically normal but have plasma phosphate and calcitriol levels and urinary calcium excretion intermediate between those of fully affected patients and controls (Tieder *et al.* 1985b). Oral loading tests disclose increased intestinal absorption of calcium and phosphate, while oral phosphate administration also leads to endogenous PTH release and increased phosphaturia (lowered T_MP/GFR). Infusion of PTH increases phosphaturia and further depresses T_MP/GFR. Taken together, these findings indicate that the primary abnormality in hereditary hypophosphataemic rickets with hypercalciuria is a PTH-independent renal tubular phosphate leak, while the increased intestinal absorption of calcium and phosphate and resulting hypercalciuria are secondary to increased production of calcitriol appropriate to the degree of phosphate depletion. If this interpretation is correct, the key difference between hereditary hypophosphataemic rickets with hypercalciuria and familial X-linked hypophosphataemic rickets lies in the subnormal response of renal 1α-hydroxylase to phosphate depletion in the latter. Recent molecular studies have excluded mutations in the gene for NaPi-II as the cause of the disease (van den Heuvel *et al.* 2001).

The only available treatment is the oral administration of 1–2 g neutral phosphate in divided daily doses, which improves the clinical symptoms and signs of the disease, including growth rate, as well as the radiological and histological features of rickets and osteomalacia. It is important to distinguish this entity from classical X-linked hypophosphataemia since treatment with vitamin D metabolites is indicated in the latter but contraindicated in hypophosphataemic rickets with hypercalciuria (Tieder *et al.* 1992).

Tumour-induced osteomalacia

Tumour-induced osteomalacia (TIO), also known as oncogenic hypophosphataemic osteomalacia, is a paraneoplastic syndrome with biochemical features similar to those of XLH and ADHR, the main differences being that it is an acquired disease and that cure is effected by removal of the causative tumour. The tumour consists usually of connective tissue or bone, and may be benign or malignant: a list of more than a dozen tumour types has been associated with this syndrome (Chesney 1985). It has also been reported in syndromes of multiple epidermal naevi (Aschinberg *et al.* 1977). The disease may present at any age from childhood to old age, with insidious and progressive weakness, bone pain and, in children, growth failure and bony deformities. The radiological appearances are those of rickets and/or osteomalacia depending on the age of onset. TIO has recently been shown to be due to secretion of FGF23 by the tumour (see also Chapter 2.4).

Treatment of TIO relies on the identification and excision of the underlying tumour. If the tumour cannot be found or is inoperable, phosphate supplementation and administration of calcidiol or calcitriol may provide some symptomatic relief, but the results are often disappointing. Patients with the clinical and biochemical abnormalities of TIO, but in whom an exhaustive search fails to find a tumour, are sometimes said to have sporadic hypophosphataemic osteomalacia.

Hypophosphataemic non-rachitic bone disease

In this uncommon disease, affected individuals present with bowing of the legs, typically at 1–3 years of age (Scriver *et al.* 1977). Hyperphosphaturia and hypophosphataemia are present, but at any given plasma phosphate concentration phosphaturia is less marked than in XLH. The bone disease is generally less severe than in XLH, and active rickets is not seen. The main biochemical difference between this entity and XLH is that 1,25-DHCC levels are normal in the former but remain low in the latter, even with 25-HCC supplements. As already discussed, the low 1,25-DHCC levels in XLH and ADHR are thought to be due to inappropriately high levels of FGF23 (phosphatonin). The specific transport defect responsible for this condition has not been identified, but it is possible that renal phosphate loss with preserved capacity to synthesise 1,25-DHCC might account for the less severe phenotype than that usually seen in the commoner hereditary phosphaturias.

Hypophosphataemic rickets with hypercalciuria and microglobulinuria

Dent and Friedman (1964) described two children with a form of hypophosphataemic rickets accompanied by hypercalciuria with low to normal plasma calcium, moderate aminoaciduria, and 'tubular' proteinuria that appears to be distinct from both familial X-linked hypophosphataemic rickets and hereditary hypophosphataemic rickets with hypercalcaemia: an apparently identical case was investigated by Carey and Hopfer (1987). Unlike hereditary hypophosphataemic rickets with hypercalcaemia, the hypercalciuria appears to be due to a primary defect in tubular calcium reabsorption and not to excessive intestinal absorption. In agreement with this view, long-term hydrochlorothiazide administration reduces urinary calcium excretion by 60 per cent, with eventual healing of the rickets. The cause of this rarely recognized disease is unknown. There is no evidence as to whether it is inherited or acquired.

Rickets with low plasma 25-hydroxycholecalciferol

Two Japanese children have been described with typical clinical and radiological features of rickets, normocalcaemia, normophosphataemia and very low circulating levels of 25-hydroxycholecalciferol despite adequate nutritional status (Asami *et al.* 1995). Plasma 1,25-DHCC levels were normal. The low plasma 25-hydroxycholecalciferol was not corrected by physiological doses of vitamin D but rose when massive, pharmacological doses were given. The underlying cause is not known, but a defect of hepatic 25 hydroxylation of vitamin D seems likely.

Vitamin D-dependent rickets type I (VDDR-I)

VDDR-I is an autosomal recessive disorder which presents with severe rickets of early onset (3 months of age or less), hypocalcaemia with tetany and convulsions, hyperphosphaturia and hypophosphataemia, and dental enamel hypoplasia (Fraser and Salter 1958). Aminoaciduria is secondary to the associated severe hyperparathyroidism. In contrast to familial X-linked hypophosphataemic rickets, vitamin D in large doses (100,000 U/day) heals the rickets, restores plasma calcium and inorganic phosphate levels to normal and reverses hyperparathyroidism and its consequences (hyperphosphaturia, aminoaciduria). Physiological doses of 1α-hydroxycholecalciferol and calcitriol are curative. The disease is due to mutations in the gene for vitamin D $1\text{-}\alpha$ hydroxylase (mitochondrial P450c $1\text{-}\alpha$), the enzyme that converts 25-hydroxycholcalciferol to calcitriol (Wang *et al.* 1998). The structure of the gene, which maps to 12q13.3, has been elucidated and mutations have been identified in both alleles in all affected patients so far studied (Portale and Miller 2000). As would be predicted, circulating endogenous calcitriol levels are very low while those of 25-hydroxycholecalciferol, its immediate precursor, are normal in untreated patients and high in those treated with vitamin D.

Vitamin D-dependent rickets type II (VDDR-II)

The type II disease is clinically and biochemically similar to type I, with the important differences that endogenous levels of 25-hydroxycholecalciferol and calcitriol are high, and that it is resistant to doses of 1α-hydroxycholecalciferol and calcitriol that are curative in type I. More than one mechanism probably exists for end-organ resistance to the action of calcitriol. Point mutations in the gene for the human vitamin D receptor (VDR) have been identified in most studied pedigrees (Rut *et al.* 1994). The gene for the vitamin D receptor has been mapped to 12q13–14, close to the locus for VDDR-I (Labuda *et al.* 1992). However, no abnormalities were found in the nucleotide sequence of this gene in a large series of patients ($n > 200$) from an isolated rural community in Colombia (Giraldo *et al.* 1995). End-organ resistance to the action of calcitriol was evident: hypocalcaemia with normal phosphate, high alkaline phosphatase, high calcitriol and normal 25-hydroxycholecalciferol. Normal function of VDR depends on heterodimerisation with another protein, retinoid X receptor (RXR) (Whitfield *et al.* 1996). Different mutations in the VDR gene not only differentially affect vitamin D binding to the receptor, but also heterodimer formation. Whether the Colombian patients have mutations in the RXR gene is not known, although it is a plausible hypothesis. Resistance to calcitriol with normal binding of the hormone to fibroblasts has been reported in one case and attributed to a postreceptor abnormality (Griffin *et al.* 1982). End-organ resistance is indirectly suggested by a subnormal intestinal calcium absorption despite high levels of calcitriol (Marx *et al.* 1978). VDDR II is recessively inherited: affected members of some, but not all, pedigrees have alopecia and extreme growth retardation in addition to the other features of the disease (the Columbian patients did not). It must be presumed that the molecular basis for end-organ resistance to calcitriol differs in those with and those without these phenotypic features.

Treatment of VDDR-II is difficult. Patients with mutations in the ligand binding domain of the VDR gene show some response to high doses of calcium and calcitriol. Those with mutations in the DNA binding domain do not respond, since transcriptional regulation is absent. Recent *in vitro* studies suggest that synthetic analogues of calcitriol may be effective in subjects in the former category, probably by binding to a different part of the VDR molecule than the natural hormone (Gardezi *et al.* 2001). Alopecia, where present, is not improved and the effect on growth rate has not yet been evaluated.

References

Anonymous (1995). A gene (PEX) with homologies to endopeptidases is mutated in patients with X-linked hypophosphatemic rickets. A report of the HYP Consortium. *Nature Genetics* **11**, 130–136.

Anonymous (2000). Autosomal dominant hypophosphataemic rickets is associated with mutations in FGF23. A report of the ADHR Consortium. *Nature Genetics* **26**, 345–348.

Arant, B. S., Jr., Edelmann, C. M., Jr., and Nash, M. A. (1974). The renal reabsorption of glucose in the developing canine kidney: a study of glomerulotubular balance. *Pediatric Research* **8**, 638–646.

Asami, T., Kawasaki, T., and Uchiyama, M. (1995). Unique form of rickets with low serum 25-hydroxyvitamin D in two normally nourished children. *Acta Paediatrica Japonica* **37**, 182–188.

Asatoor, A. M., Cheng, B., Edwards, K. D., Lant, A. F., Matthews, D. M., Milne, M. D., Navab, F., and Richards, A. J. (1970). Intestinal absorption of dipeptides and corresponding free amino acids in Hartnup disease. *Clinical Science* **39**, 1P.

Asatoor, A. M., Lacey, B. W., London, B. R., and Milne, M. D. (1962). Amino acid metabolism in cystinuria. *Clinical Science* **23**, 285–304.

Aschinberg, L. C., Solomon, L. M., Zeis, P. M., Justice, P., and Rosenthal, I. M. (1977). Vitamin D-resistant rickets associated with epidermal nevus syndrome: demonstration of a phosphaturic substance in the dermal lesions. *Journal of Pediatrics* **91**, 56–60.

Bagga, A., Shankar, V., Moudgil, A., and Srivastava, R. N. (1991). Type O renal glucosuria. *Acta Paediatrica Scandinavica* **80**, 116–119.

Bank, H., Crispin, M., Ehrlich, D., and Szeinberg, A. (1972). Iminoglycinuria. A defect of renal tubular transport. *Israel Journal of Medical Sciences* **81**, 606–612.

Baron, D. N., Dent, C. E., Harris, H., Hart, E. W., and Jepson, J. B. (1956). Herediary pellagra-like skin rash with temporary cerebellar ataxia, constant renal amino-aciduria and other bizarre biochemical features. *Lancet* **1**, 421–428.

Beck, L., Karaplis, A. C., Amizuka, N., Hewson, A. S., Ozawa, H., and Tenenhouse, H. S. (1998). Targeted inactivation of Npt2 in mice leads to severe renal phosphate wasting, hypercalciuria, and skeletal abnormalities. *Proceedings of the National Academy of Science of the USA* **95**, 5372–5377.

Behrman, R. E., Kliegman, R. M., and Jenson, H. B., ed. *Nelson Textbook of Pediatrics*. Philadelphia, PA: W.B. Saunders Company, 2000.

Bianchine, J. W., Stambler, A. A., and Harrison, H. E. (1971). Familial hypophosphatemic rickets showing autosomal dominant inheritance. *Birth Defects Original Articles Series* **7**, 287–295.

Boneh, A., Reade, T. M., Scriver, C. R., and Rishikof, E. (1987). Audiometric evidence for two forms of X-linked hypophosphatemia in humans, apparent counterparts of Hyp and Gy mutations in mouse. *American Journal of Medical Genetics* **27**, 997–1003.

Brand, E., Cahill, G. H., and Harris, M. M. (1935). Cystinuria. II. The metabolism of cysteine, methionine and glutathione. *Journal of Biological Chemistry* **109**, 69–83.

Brodehl, J. Postnatal development of tubular amino acid transport. In *Amino Acid Transport and Uric Acid Transport* (ed. S. Silbernagl, F. Lang, and R. Greger), pp. 128–135. Stuttgart: Georg Thieme, 1976.

Brodehl, J. and Gellissen, K. (1968). Endogenous renal transport of free amino acids in infancy and childhood. *Pediatrics* **42**, 395–404.

Brodehl, J., Franken, A., and Gellissen, K. (1972). Maximal tubular reabsorption of glucose in infants and children. *Acta Paediatrica Scandinavica* **61**, 413–420.

Brodehl, J., Gellissen, K., and Kowalewski, S. (1967). Isolated cystinuria (without lysin-, ornithin- and argininuria) in a family with hypocalcemic tetany. *Monatsschrift Kinderheilkund* **115**, 317–320.

Calonge, M. J., Nadal, M., Calvano, S., Testar, X., Zlante, L., Zorzano, A., Estivill, X., Gasparini, P., Palacín, M., and Nunes, V. (1995). Assignment of the gene responsible for cystinuria (rBAT) and of markers D2S119 and D2S177 to 2p16 by fluorescence *in situ* hybridization. *Human Genetics* **95**, 633–636.

Carey, D. E. and Hopfer, S. M. (1987). Hypophosphatemic rickets with hypercalciuria and microglobulinuria. *Journal of Pediatrics* **111**, 860–863.

Carpenter, T. O., Mitnick, M. A., Ellison, A., Smith, C., and Insogna, K. L. (1994). Nocturnal hyperparathyroidism: a frequent feature of X-linked hypophosphatemia. *Journal of Clinical Endocrinology and Metabolism* **78**, 1378–1383.

Chen, W. W., L., S., Tankatsen, P., and Tricomi, V. (1976). Pregnancy associated with renal glycosuria. *Obstetrics and Gynecology* **47**, 37–40.

Chesney, R. W. Phosphaturic syndromes. In *Renal Tubular Disorders: Pathophysiology, Diagnosis and Management* (ed. H. C. Gonick and V. M. Buckalew), pp. 201–238. New York: Marcel Dekker, 1985.

Christensen, P. (1958). Tubular reabsorption of glucose during pregnancy. *Scandinavian Journal of Clinical and Laboratory Investigation* **10**, 364–373.

Cohen, T. D., Streem, S. B., and Hall, P. (1995). Clinical effect of captopril on the formation and growth of cystine calculi. *Journal of Urology* **154**, 164–166.

Combe, C., Deforges-Lasseur, C., Chehab, Z., de Precigout, V., and Aparicio, M. (1993). Cystine lithiasis and its treatment with d-penicillamine. The experience in a nephrology service in a 23-year period. Apropos of 26 patients. *Annales d'urologie* **27**, 79–83.

Coulthard, M. G., Richardson, J., and Fleetwood, A. (1995). The treatment of cystinuria with captopril. *American Journal of Kidney Diseases* **25**, 661–662.

Cowgill, L. D., Goldfarb, S., Lau, K., Slatopolsky, E., and Agus, Z. S. (1979). Evidence for an intrinsic renal tubular defect in mice with genetic hypophosphatemic rickets. *Journal of Clinical Investigation* **63**, 1203–1210.

Crawhall, J. C., Scowen, E. F., Thompson, C. J., and Watts, R. W. E. (1967). The renal clearance of amino acids in cystinuria. *Journal of Clinical Investigation* **46**, 1162–1170.

Darendeliler, F., Bas, F., Karaaslan, N., Hekim, N., Bundak, R., Saka, N., and Gunoz, H. (2001). The effect of growth hormone treatment on biochemical indices in hypophosphatemic rickets. *Hormone Research* **55**, 191–195.

Davison, J. M., and Hytten, F. E. (1975). The effects of pregnancy on the renal handling of glucose. *British Journal of Obstetrics and Gynaecology* **82**, 374–381.

de Vries, A., Kochwa, S., Lazebnik, J., Frank, M., and Djaldetti, M. (1957). Glycinuria, a hereditary disorder associated with nephrolithiasis. *American Journal of Medicine* **23**, 408–415.

Dent, C. E. and Friedman, M. (1964). Hypercalciuric rickets associated with renal tubular damage. *Archives of Disease in Childhood* **39**, 240–249.

Dent, C. E. and Rose, G. A. (1951). Amino acid metabolism in cystinuria. *Quarterly Journal of Medicine* **20**, 205–218.

Ecarot, B., Glorieux, F. H., Desbarats, M., Travers, R., and Labelle, L. (1992). Effect of dietary phosphate deprivation and supplementation of recipient mice on bone formation by transplanted cells from normal and X-linked hypophosphatemic mice. *Journal of Bone and Mineral Research* **7**, 523–530.

Econs, M. J. and McEnery, P. T. (1997). Autosomal dominant hypophosphatemic rickets/osteomalacia: clinical characterization of a novel renal phosphate-wasting disorder. *Journal of Clinical Endocrinology & Metabolism* **82**, 674–681.

Econs, M. J., McEnery, P. T., Lennon, F., and Speer, M. C. (1997). Autosomal dominant hypophosphatemic rickets is linked to chromosome 12p13. *Journal of Clinical Investigation* **100**, 2653–2657.

Elsas, L. J., Busse, D., and Rosenberg, L. E. (1971). Autosomal recessive inheritance of renal glycosuria. *Metabolism* **20**, 968–975.

Foreman, J. W., Hwang, S. M., and Segal, S. (1980). Transport interactions of cystine and dibasic amino acids in isolated rat renal tubules. *Metabolism* **29**, 53–61.

Frame, B., Smith, R. W., Jr., Fleming, J. L., and Hanson, G. (1963). Oral phosphates in vitamin D-refractory rickets and osteomalacia. *American Journal of Diseases of Children* **106**, 147–153.

Fraser, D., and Salter, R. B. (1958). The diagnosis and management of the various types of rickets. *Pediatric Clinics of North America* **5**, 417–441.

Fraser, D., Kooh, S. W., and Scriver, C. R. (1967). Hyperparathyroidism as the cause of hyperaminoaciduria and phosphaturia in human vitamin D deficiency. *Pediatric Research* **1**, 425–435.

Furlong, T. J. and Stiel, D. (1993). Decreased uptake of L-cystine by duodenal brush border membrane vesicles from patients with cystinuria. *Australian and New Zealand Journal of Medicine* **23**, 258–263.

Gardezi, S. A., Nguyen, C., Malloy, P. J., Posner, G. H., Feldman, D., and Peleg, S. (2001). A rationale for treatment of hereditary vitamin D-resistant rickets with analogs of 1 alpha,25-dihydroxyvitamin D(3). *Journal of Biological Chemistry* **276**, 29148–29156.

Giraldo, A., Pino, W., Garcia-Ramirez, L. F., Pineda, M., and Iglesias, A. (1995). Vitamin D dependent rickets type II and normal vitamin D receptor cDNA sequence. A cluster in a rural area of Cauca, Colombia, with more than 200 affected children. *Clinical Genetics* **48**, 57–65.

Gold, R. J., Dobrinski, M. J., and Gold, D. P. (1977). Cystinuria and mental deficiency. *Clinical Genetics* **12**, 329–332.

Goodyer, P. R., Kronick, J. B., Jequier, S., Reade, T. M., and Scriver, C. R. (1987). Nephrocalcinosis and its relationship to treatment of hereditary rickets. *Journal of Pediatrics* **111**, 700–704.

Griffin, J. E., Chandler, J. S., Haussler, M. R., and Zerwekh, J. E. (1982). Receptor-positive resistance to 1,25-dihydroxyvitamin D: a new case of osteomalacia associated with impaired induction of 24-hydroxylase in fibroblasts (abstract). *Clinical Research* **30**, 524.

Hahn, T. J., Scharp, C. R., Halstead, L. R., Haddad, J. G., Karl, D. M., and Avioli, L. V. (1975). Parathyroid hormone status and renal responsiveness in familial hypophosphatemic rickets. *Journal of Clinical Endocrinology and Metabolism* **41**, 926–937.

Halvorsen, K. and Halvorsen, S. (1963). Hartnup disease. *Pediatrics* **31**, 29–38.

Hautman, R., Terhorst, B., Stuhlsatz, H. W., and Lutzeyer, W. (1977). Mercaptopropionylglycine: a progress in cystine stone therapy. *Journal of Urology* **117**, 628–630.

Hediger, M. A., Budarf, M. L., Emanuel, B. S., Mohamdas, T. K., and M., W. E. (1989). Assignment of the human intestinal Na^+/glucose transporter gene (SGLT1) to the q11 > qter region of chromosome 22. *Genomics* **4**, 297–300.

Hjärne, U. (1927). A study of orthoglycaemic glycosuria with particular reference to its heritability. *Acta Medica Scandinavica* **67**, 422–571.

Holm, I. A., Nelson, A. E., Robinson, B. G., Mason, R. S., Marsh, D. J., Cowell, C. T., and Carpenter, T. O. (2001). Mutational analysis and genotype–phenotype correlation of the PHEX gene in X-linked hypophosphatemic rickets. *Journal of Clinical Endocrinology and Metabolism* **86**, 3889–3899.

Hong Que, N. T., Gmaj, P., and Angielski, S. (1982). Uncoupling of Na^+-dependent solute transport in renal brush border membranes of maleate-treated rats. *Acta Biochimica Polonica* **29**, 275–287.

Hooft, C., Timmermans, J., Snoeck, J., Antener, I., Oyaert, W., and van den Hende, C. (1965). Methionine malabsorption syndrome. *Annals of Pediatrics* **205**, 73–84.

Hruska, K. A., Rifas, L., Cheng, S. L., Gupta, A., Halstead, L., and Avioli, L. (1995). X-linked hypophosphatemic rickets and the murine Hyp homologue. *American Journal of Physiology* **268**, F357–F362.

Hytten, F. E. and Cheyne, G. A. (1972). The aminoaciduria of pregnancy. *Journal of Obstetrics and Gynaecology of the British Commonwealth* **79**, 424–432.

Jaeger, P., Portmann, L., Saunders, A., Rosenberg, L. E., and Thier, S. O. (1986). Anticystinuric effects of glutamine and of dietary sodium restriction. *New England Journal of Medicine* **315**, 1120–1123.

Jones, E. M., Menzel, S., Espinosa, R., III, Le Beau, M. M., Bell, G. I., and Takeda, J. (1994). Localization of the gene encoding a neutral amino acid transporter-like protein to human chromosome band 19q13.3 and characterization of a simple sequence repeat DNA polymorphism. *Genomics* **23**, 490–491.

Joseph, R., Ribierre, M., Job, J.-C., and Girault, M. (1958). Maladie, familiale associante des convulsions à début très précoce, une albuminorachie et une hyperaminoacidurie. *Archives Françaises de Pédiatrie* **15**, 374–387.

Käser, H., Cottier, P., and Antener, I. (1962). Glucoglycinuria: a new familial syndrome. *Journal of Pediatrics* **61**, 386–394.

Knudtzon, J., Halse, J., Monn, E., Nesland, A., Nordal, K. P., Paus, P., Seip, M., Sund, S., and Sodal, G. (1995). Autonomous hyperparathyroidism in X-linked hypophosphataemia. *Clinical Endocrinology* **42**, 199–203.

Kooh, S. W., Binet, A., and Daneman, A. (1994). Nephrocalcinosis in X-linked hypophosphataemic rickets: its relationship to treatment, kidney function, and growth. *Clinical and Investigative Medicine* **17**, 123–130.

Labuda, M., Fujiwara, T. M., Ross, M. V., Morgan, K., Garcia-Heras, J., Ledbetter, D. H., Hughes, M. R., and Glorieux, F. H. (1992). Two hereditary defects related to vitamin D metabolism map to the same region of human chromosome 12q13–14. *Journal of Bone and Mineral Research* **7**, 1447–1453.

Latta, K., Hisano, S., and Chan, J. C. (1993). Therapeutics of X-linked hypophosphatemic rickets. *Pediatric Nephrology* **7**, 744–748.

Lester, F. T. and Cusworth, D. C. (1973). Lysine infusion in cystinuria: theoretical renal thresholds for lysine. *Clinical Science* **44**, 99–111.

Mackenzie, B., Loo, D. D., Panayotova-Heiermann, M., and Wright, E. M. (1996). Biophysical characteristics of the pig kidney Na+/glucose cotransporter SGLT2 reveal a common mechanism for SGLT1 and SGLT2. *Journal of Biological Chemistry* **271**, 32678–32683.

Marble, A., Joslin, E. P., Dublin, L. I., and Marks, H. H. (1939). Studies in diabetes mellitus. VII. Non-diabetic glycosurias. *American Journal of Medical Sciences* **197**, 533–556.

Marie, P. J. and Glorieux, F. H. (1981). Histomorphometric study of bone remodeling in hypophosphatemic vitamin D-resistant rickets. *Metabolic Bone Disease and Related Research* **3**, 31–38.

Marx, S. J., Spiegel, A. M., Brown, E. M., Gardner, D. G., Downs, R. W., Jr., Attie, M., Hamstra, A. J., and DeLuca, H. F. (1978). A familial syndrome of decrease in sensitivity to 1,25-dihydroxyvitamin D. *Journal of Clinical Endocrinology and Metabolism* **47**, 1303–1310.

Meeuwisse, G. W. (1970). Glucose-galactose malabsorption. A study on the transfer of glucose across the red cell membrane. *Scandinavian Journal of Clinical and Laboratory Investigation* **25**, 145–149.

Melancon, S. B., Dallaire, L., Lemieux, B., Robitaille, P., and Potier, M. (1977). Dicarboxylic aminoaciduria: an inborn error of amino acid conservation. *Journal of Pediatrics* **91**, 422–427.

Meyer, M. H., Meyer, R. A., Jr., and Iorio, R. J. (1984). A role for the intestine in the bone disease of juvenile X-linked hypophosphatemic mice: malabsorption of calcium and reduced skeletal mineralization. *Endocrinology* **115**, 1464–1470.

Meyer, R. A., Jr., Meyer, M. H., Erickson, P. R., and Korkor, A. B. (1986). Reduced absorption of 45calcium from isolated duodenal segments in vivo in juvenile but not adult X-linked hypophosphatemic mice. *Calcified Tissue International* **38**, 95–102.

Milne, M. D., Asatoor, A. M., Edwards, K. D. G., and Loughridge, L. W. (1961). The intestinal absorption defect in cystinuria. *Gut* **2**, 323–337.

Milne, M. D., Crawford, M. A., Girao, C. B., and Loughbridge, L. (1960). The metabolic disorder in Hartnup disease. *Quarterly Journal of Medicine* **29**, 407–421.

Monasterio, G., Oliver, J., Muiesan, G., Pardelli, G., Marinozzi, V., and MacDowell, M. (1964). Renal diabetes as a congenital tubular dysplasia. *American Journal of Medicine* **37**, 44–61.

Murer, H., Hernando, N., Forster, L., and Biber, J. (2001). Molecular mechanisms in proximal tubular and small intestinal phosphate reabsorption. *Molecular Membrane Biology* **18**, 3–11 (plenary lecture).

O'Brien, D., and Butterfield, L. J. (1963). Further studies on renal tubular conservation of free amino acids in early infancy. *Archives of Disease in Childhood* **38**, 437–442.

Omura, K., Yamanaka, N., Higami, S., Matsuoka, O., and Fujimoto, A. (1976). Lysine malabsorption syndrome: a new type of transport defect. *Pediatrics* **57**, 102–105.

Palacín, M., Bertran, J., and Zorzano, A. (2000). Heteromeric amino acid transporters explain inherited aminoacidurias. *Current Opinion in Nephrology and Hypertension* **9**, 547–553.

Palacín, M., Borsani, G., and Sebastio, G. (2001a). The molecular bases of cystinuria and lysinuric protein intolerance. *Current Opinion in Genetics and Development* **11**, 328–335.

Palacín, M., Fernandez, E., Chillaron, J., and Zorzano, A. (2001b). The amino acid transport system b(o,+) and cystinuria. *Molecular Membrane Biology* **18**, 21–26.

Peces, R., Sanchez, L., Gorostidi, M., and Alvarez, J. (1991). Effects of variation in sodium intake in cystinuria. *Nephron* **57**, 421–423.

Perazella, M. A. and Buller, G. K. (1993). Successful treatment of cystinuria with captopril. *American Journal of Kidney Diseases* **21**, 504–507.

Perheentupa, J., and Visakorpi, J. K. (1965). Protein intolerance with deficient transport of basic aminoacids. Another inborn error of metabolism. *Lancet* **2**, 813–816.

Petersen, D. J., Boniface, A. M., Schranck, F. W., Rupich, R. C., and Whyte, M. P. (1992). X-linked hypophosphatemic rickets:a study (with literature review) of linear growth response to calcitriol and phosphate therapy. *Journal of Bone and Mineral Research* **7**, 583–597.

Pitts, R. F. (1943). A renal reabsorptive mechanism in the dog common to glycine and creatinine. *American Journal of Physiology* **140**, 156–167.

Portale, A. A. and Miller, W. L. (2000). Human 25-hydroxyvitamin D-1alpha-hydroxylase: cloning, mutations, and gene expression. *Pediatric Nephrology* **14**, 620–625.

Pras, E., Arber, N., Aksentijevich, I., Katz, G., Schapiro, J. M., Prosen, L., Gruberg, L., Harel, D., Liberman, U., Weissenbach, J., Pras, M., and Kastner, D. L. (1994). Localization of a gene causing cystinuria to chromosome 2p. *Nature Genetics* **6**, 415–419.

Procopis, P. G. and Turner, B. (1971). Iminoaciduria:a benign renal tubular defect. *Journal of Pediatrics* **79**, 419–422.

Rajantie, J. and Perheentupa, J. (1980). Lysinuric protein intolerance. *Lancet* **2**, 978.

Rasmussen, H. and Tenenhouse, H. S. Hypophosphatemias. In *The Metabolic Basis of Inherited Disease* (ed. C. R. Scriver, A. L. Beaudet, W. S. Sly, and D. Valle), pp. 2581–2604. New York: McGraw-Hill, 1989.

Reusz, G. S., Hoyer, P. F., Lucas, M., Krohn, H. P., Ehrich, J. H., and Brodehl, J. (1990). X linked hypophosphataemia: treatment, height gain, and nephrocalcinosis. *Archives of Disease in Childhood* **65**, 1125–1128.

Robson, E. B. and Rose, G. A. (1957). The effects of intravenous lysine on the renal clearances of cystine, arginine and ornithine in normal subjects, in patients with cystinuria and their relatives. *Clinical Science* **16**, 75–91.

Rosenberg, L. E. and Hayslett, J. P. (1967). Nephrotoxic effects of penicillamine in cystinuria. *Journal of the American Medical Association* **201**, 698–699.

Rosenberg, L. E., Downing, S., Durant, J. L., and Segal, S. (1966). Cystinuria: biochemical evidence for three genetically distinct diseases. *Journal of Clinical Investigation* **45**, 365–371.

Rut, A. R., Hewison, M., Kristjansson, K., Luisi, B., Hughes, M. R., and O'Riordan, J. L. (1994). Two mutations causing vitamin D resistant rickets: modelling on the basis of steroid hormone receptor DNA-binding domain crystal structures. *Clinical Endocrinology* **41**, 581–590.

Sabater, J., Ferre, C., Puliol, M., and Maya, A. (1976). Histidinuria: a renal and intestinal histidine transport deficiency found in two mentally retarded children. *Clinical Genetics* **9**, 117–124.

Sacktor, B. Mechanisms and specifications of amino acid transport in proximal tubule membrane vesicles. In *Renal Function* (ed. G. H. Giebisch and E. F. Purcell), pp. 221–229. New York: Josiah Macy Jr. Foundation, 1978.

Saggese, G., Baroncelli, G. I., Bertelloni, S., and Perri, G. (1995). Long-term growth hormone treatment in children with renal hypophosphatemic rickets: effects on growth, mineral metabolism, and bone density. *Journal of Pediatrics* **127**, 395–402.

Scriver, C. R. and Shaw, K. N. (1962). Hartnup disease: an example of genetically determined defective cellular amino acid transport. *Canadian Medical Association Journal* **86**, 232.

Scriver, C. R. and Tenenhouse, H. S. (1985). Genetics and mammalian transport systems. *Annals of the New York Academy of Science* **456**, 384–397.

Scriver, C. R., Baudet, A. L., Sly, W. S., and Valle, D., ed. *The Metabolic and Molecular Bases of Inherited Disease*. New York: McGraw-Hill, 2001.

Scriver, C. R., Efron, M. L., and Schafer, I. A. (1964a). Renal tubular transport of proline, hydroxyproline and glycine in health and in familial hyperprolinemia. *Journal of Clinical Investigation* **43**, 374–385.

Scriver, C. R., Goldbloom, R. B., and Roy, C. (1964b). Hypophosphatemic rickets with renal hyperglycinuria, renal glycosuria and glycylprolinuria. *Pediatrics* **34**, 357–371.

Scriver, C. R., MacDonald, W., Reade, T., Glorieux, R. H., and Nogrady, B. (1977). Hypophosphatemic nonrachitic bone disease: an entity distinct from X-linked hypophosphatemia in the renal defect, bone involvement, and inheritance. *American Journal of Medical Genetics* **1**, 101–117.

Scriver, C. R., Reade, T. M., DeLuca, H. F., and Hamstra, A. J. (1978). Serum 1,25-dihydroxyvitamin D levels in normal subjects and in patients with hereditary rickets or bone disease. *New England Journal of Medicine* **299**, 976–979.

Seikaly, M. G., Brown, R., and Baum, M. (1997). The effect of recombinant human growth hormone in children with X-linked hypophosphatemia. *Pediatrics* **100**, 879–884.

Seikaly, M. G., Browne, R. H., and Baum, M. (1994). The effect of phosphate supplementation on linear growth in children with X-linked hypophosphatemia. *Pediatrics* **94**, 478–481.

Semple, P. F., Carswell, W., and Boyle, J. A. (1974). Serial studies of the renal clearance of urate and inulin during pregnancy and after the puerperium in normal women. *Clinical Science and Molecular Medicine* **47**, 559–565.

Silbernagl, S. (1988). The renal handling of amino acids and oligopeptides. *Physiological Reviews* **68**, 911–1007.

Simell, O. Lysinuric protein intolerance and other cationic aminoacidurias. In *The Metabolic and Molecular Bases of Inherited Disease* Vol. 3 (ed. C. R. Scriver, A. L. Beaudet, W. S. Sly, and D. Valle), pp. 4933–4956. New York: McGraw-Hill, 2001.

Smith, A., Yu, J. S., and Brown, D. A. (1979). Childhood cystinuria in New South Wales. Results in children who were followed up after being detected by urinary screening in infancy. *Archives of Disease in Childhood* **54**, 676–681.

Smith, A. J. and Strang, L. B. (1958). An inborn error of metabolism with the urinary excretion of alpha-hydroxybutyric acid and phenyl-pyruvic acid. *Archives of Disease in Childhood* **33**, 109–113.

Smith, H. W., Goldring, W., Chasis, H., Ranges, H. A., and Bradley, S. E. (1943). The application of saturation methods to the study of glomerular and tubular function in the human kidney. *Journal of the Mount Sinai Hospital* **10**, 59–108.

Steendijk, R. and Latham, S. C. (1971). Hypophosphataemic vitamin D-resistant rickets; an observation on height and serum inorganic phosphate in untreated cases. *Helvetica Paediatrica Acta* **26**, 179–184.

Stickler, G. B. (1963). External calcium and phosphate metabolism in resistant rickets. *Journal of Pediatrics* **63**, 942–948.

Stickler, G. B. and Morgenstern, B. Z. (1989). Hypophosphataemic rickets: final height and clinical symptoms in adults. *Lancet* **2**, 902–905.

Stickler, G. B., Beabout, J. W., and Riggs, B. L. (1970). Vitamin D-resistant rickets: clinical experience with 41 typical familial hypophosphatemic patients and 2 atypical nonfamilial cases. *Mayo Clinic Proceedings* **45**, 197–218.

Talwalkar, Y. B., Musgrave, J. E., Buist, N. R., Campbell, R. A., and Campbell, J. R. (1974). Vitamin D-resistant rickets and parathyroid adenomas: renal transport of phosphate. *American Journal of Diseases of Children* **128**, 704–708.

Teijema, H. L., van Gelderen, H. H., Giesberts, M. A., and Laurent de Angulo, M. S. (1974). Dicarboxylic aminoaciduria:an inborn error of glutamate and aspartate transport with metabolic implications, in combination with a hyperprolinemia. *Metabolism* **23**, 115–123.

Tenenhouse, H. S. (1999). X-linked hypophosphataemia:a homologous disorder in humans and mice. *Nephrology, Dialysis, Transplantation* **14**, 333–341.

Tenenhouse, H. S. and Scriver, C. R. (1978). The defect in transcellular transport of phosphate in the nephron is located in brush-border membranes in X-linked hypophosphatemia (Hyp mouse model). *Canadian Journal of Biochemistry* **56**, 640–646.

Tenenhouse, H. S. and Scriver, C. R. (1979). Renal brush border membrane adaptation to phosphorus deprivation in the Hyp/Y mouse. *Nature* **281**, 225–227.

Tenenhouse, H. S., Scriver, C. R., McInnes, R. R., and Glorieux, F. H. (1978). Renal handling of phosphate *in vivo* and *in vitro* by the X-linked hypophosphatemic male mouse:evidence for a defect in the brush border membrane. *Kidney International* **14**, 236–244.

Thalhammer, O. (1975). Frequency of inborn errors of metabolism, especially PKU, in some representative screeing centers around the world:a collaborative study. *Humangenetik* **30**, 273–286.

Tieder, M., Arie, R., Bab, I., Maor, J., and Liberman, U. A. (1992). A new kindred with hereditary hypophosphatemic rickets with hypercalciuria: implications for correct diagnosis and treatment. *Nephron* **62**, 176–181.

Tieder, M., Modai, D., Samuel, R., Arie, R., Halabe, A., Bab, I., Gabizon, D., and Liberman, U. A. (1985a). Hereditary hypophosphatemic rickets with hypercalciuria. *New England Journal of Medicine* **312**, 611–617.

Tieder, M., Samuel, R., Liberman, U. A., Arie, R., Halabe, A., Gabizon, D., Maor, Y., Halperin, N., Capeliovitch, L., and Modai, D. (1985b). Hypercalciuric rickets:metabolic studies and pathophysiological considerations. *Nephron* **39**, 194–200.

Turk, E., Zabel, B., Mundlos, S., Dyer, J., and Wright, E. M. (1991). Glucose/galactose malabsorption caused by a defect in the Na^+/glucose cotransporter. *Nature* **350**, 354–356.

van den Heuvel, L., Op de Koul, K., Knots, E., Knoers, N., and Monnens, L. (2001). Autosomal recessive hypophosphataemic rickets with hypercalciuria is not caused by mutations in the type II renal sodium/phosphate cotransporter gene. *Nephrology, Dialysis, Transplantation* **16**, 48–51.

Wang, J. T., Lin, C. J., Burridge, S. M., Fu, G. K., Labuda, M., Portale, A. A., and Miller, W. L. (1998). Genetics of vitamin D 1alpha-hydroxylase deficiency in 17 families. *American Journal of Human Genetics* **63**, 1694–702.

Webber, W. A., Brown, J. L., and Pitts, R. F. (1961). Interaction of amino acids in renal tubular transport. *American Journal of Physiology* **200**, 380–386.

Weinberger, A., Sperling, O., Rabinovitz, M., Brosh, S., Adam, A., and De Vries, A. (1974). High frequency of cystinuria among Jews of Libyan origin. *Human Heredity* **24**, 568–572.

Welsh, G. W. and Sims, E. A. H. (1960). The mechanism of renal glycosuria in pregnancy. *Diabetes* **9**, 363–369.

Whelan, D. T. and Scriver, C. R. (1968a). Cystathioninuria and renal iminoglycinuria in a pedigree. *New England Journal of Medicine* **278**, 924–927.

Whelan, D. T. and Scriver, C. R. (1968b). Hyperdibasicaminoaciduria: an inherited disorder of amino acid transport. *Pediatric Research* **2**, 525–534.

Whitfield, G. K., Selznick, S. H., Haussler, C. A., Hsieh, J. C., Galligan, M. A., Jurutka, P. W., Thompson, P. D., Lee, S. M., Zerwekh, J. E., and Haussler, M. R. (1996). Vitamin D receptors from patients with resistance to 1,25-dihydroxyvitamin D3: point mutations confer reduced transactivation in response to ligand and impaired interaction with the retinoid X receptor heterodimeric partner. *Molecular Endocrinology* **10**, 1617–1631.

Wilson, D. M., Lee, P. D., Morris, A. H., Reiter, E. O., Gertner, J. M., Marcus, R., Quarmby, V. E., and Rosenfeld, R. G. (1991). Growth hormone therapy in hypophosphatemic rickets. *American Journal of Diseases of Children* **145**, 1165–1170.

Woolf, L. I., Goodwin, B. L., and Renold, A. E. (1966). Tm-limited reabsorption and the genetics of renal glycosuria. *Journal of Theoretical Biology* **11**, 10–21.

Wright, H. R., Russo, H. F., Skeggs, H. R., Patch, E. K., and Beyer, K. H. (1947). The renal clearance of essential amino acids: arginine, histidine, lysine and methionine. *American Journal of Physiology* **149**, 130–134.

5.3 Fanconi syndrome

William G. van't Hoff

Introduction

The renal tubule regulates the body's fluid, electrolyte, and acid–base balance (see Chapter 5.1). The handling of the glomerular filtrate by the proximal tubule is reviewed in Chapter 5.2 as well as in Chapters 5.1 and 2.4. Specific disorders of proximal tubular function result in a variety of hereditary and acquired diseases described in Chapter 5.2. Sometimes the coexistence of several such disorders mirror a generalized dysfunction of the proximal tubule resulting in the renal Fanconi syndrome, the topic of this chapter. The tubular transport dysfunction causes bicarbonaturia leading to hyperchloraemic metabolic acidosis, phosphaturia leading to hypophosphataemia, rickets, osteomalacia and growth retardation, abnormal urinary losses of proteins, hormones, and a variety of other compounds. The Fanconi syndrome may be congenital or acquired, primary or secondary, complete or incomplete. Several of these important disorders (e.g. cystinosis, Dent's disease) are described in detail in Chapters 2.4, 5.2, and 16.5.1. This chapter provides an overview of the Fanconi syndrome including developments in our understanding of its pathogenesis.

Table 1 Causes of the renal Fanconi syndrome: see text for details

Genetic/metabolic	Drugs/toxins	Acquired
Cystinosis	Aminoglycosides	Membranous nephropathy
Tyrosinaemia	Ifosfamide	Focal–segmental glomerulosclerosis
Mitochondrial disorders	Sodium valproate	Tubulointerstitial nephritis
Lowe's syndrome	Adefovir/cidofovir	Monoclonal gammopathies
Fanconi–Bickel syndrome	Ranitidine	Amyloidosis
Galactosaemia	Aristolochic acid (Chinese herbs)	Postrenal transplantation
Hereditary fructose intolerance	Colloidal bismuth subcitrate	Balkan nephropathy
ARC (arthrogryposis, renal tubular abnormalities and cholestasis) syndrome	Suramin	Vitamin D deficiency (nutritional or secondary to malabsorption)
Wilson's disease	Cadmium	
	Lead	
	Lysine	
	Fumarate	

Clinical features

The presentation of the renal Fanconi syndrome depends on the underlying cause, severity, and on the age of the patient. In children congenital, often metabolic causes, such as cystinosis and tyrosinaemia predominate. The clinical features consist of polyuria, polydipsia, dehydration, muscle weakness or delay in motor development, rickets (presenting as bone deformity or pain), and poor growth. Other features may be related to the underlying cause, such as symptoms of liver dysfunction in tyrosinaemia or to a history of exposure to drugs or toxins in older patients. Presentation is usually insidious and apparently non-specific. However, the pattern of biochemical abnormalities from a routine plasma and urine biochemical screen (hyperchloraemic metabolic acidosis, hypokalaemia, hypophosphataemia, glycosuria, and proteinuria) prompts the alert physician to consider the diagnosis. Confirmation, usually by the demonstration of generalized amino aciduria and tubular proteinuria, should be followed by the identification of the underlying cause, frequently an underlying metabolic disorder in children or, very often, toxic exposure in adults (see Table 1).

Biochemical abnormalities

Excessive urinary levels of a wide range of solutes and substances normally reabsorbed in the proximal tubule characterize the Fanconi syndrome. The most significant abnormalities are as follows:

1. *Proteinuria* is made up of albumin, low molecular weight proteins, and tubular enzymes, such as retinol binding protein (RBP), α1-microglobulin, β2-microglobulin, *N*-acetylglucoseaminidase, alanine aminopeptidase. The urinary level of these very sensitive markers of proximal tubular dysfunction is markedly elevated in Fanconi syndrome as shown in Fig. 1 (Norden *et al.* 2000). In Dent's disease, an X-linked Fanconi syndrome, median urinary RBP level in males is 2000 times higher than in healthy normal individuals. Similar increases in the level of other low molecular weight proteins are present in Fanconi syndrome of other causes such as multiple myeloma in adults (Leheste *et al.* 1999). Albuminuria precedes glomerular dysfunction in Fanconi syndrome and whilst significantly increased compared to normal, does not reach the levels observed in the nephrotic syndrome and does not lead to plasma deficiencies (Norden *et al.* 2001). However, tubular proteinuria, reflecting proximal tubular dysfunction, is also present in some forms of nephrotic syndrome, especially focal–segmental glomerulosclerosis and membranous nephropathy. Albuminuria is then much heavier, but the degree of tubular proteinuria may give some indication as to the underlying nature and prognosis of the nephropathy (Bazzi *et al.* 2000; Valles *et al.* 2000).
2. *Aminoaciduria* seen in Fanconi syndrome is generalized and reflects defective tubular reabsorption. Its pattern is influenced by plasma values, so that in rare situations of severe protein malnutrition,

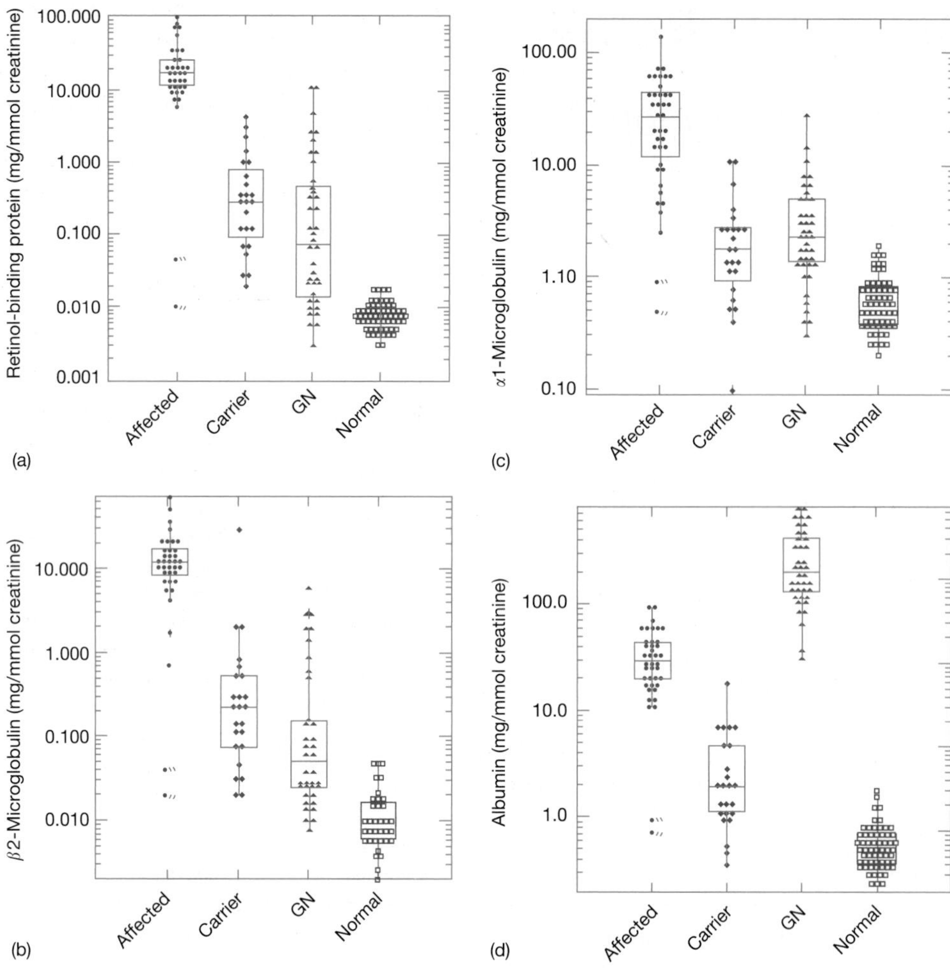

Fig. 1 Urinary excretion of (a) retinol binding protein, (b) β2-microglobulin, (c) α1-microglobulin, and (d) albumin in four groups of subjects: 'Affected': affected males with Dent's disease and autosomal Fanconi syndrome ('F'), and Lowe ('L') syndromes; 'Carrier': female carriers of Dent's disease; 'GN': patients with glomerulonephritis; and 'Normal adults'. Each point is the result of one patient. The 'box and whiskers' identify the middle 50th centile of results and the 25th and 75th centiles, respectively. The line bisecting the box indicates the median. (From Norden *et al.* 2000, permission sought.)

aminoaciduria as analysed on thin-layer chromatography, may be recorded as 'normal' or 'mild'. Quantitative analysis by ion-exchange chromatography should be used to determine the degree of aminoaciduria.

3. *Phosphaturia* is another hallmark of Fanconi syndrome but, just as with aminoaciduria, reflects the plasma phosphate level. Whereas tubular proteinuria and aminoaciduria are seen in virtually every case of Fanconi syndrome, phosphaturia leading to hypophosphataemia may not be observed in milder cases. Thus, infants with Lowe's syndrome rarely have hypophosphataemia whereas it is universal in similarly aged children with nephropathic cystinosis. Tubular handling of phosphate is characterized by the maximal phosphate reabsorption corrected for glomerular filtration rate (Tm_P/GFR) as described in Chapter 2.4. Hypophosphataemia is the most important causal factor of rickets and osteomalacia in the more severe forms of the Fanconi syndrome.

4. *Glycosuria* is variable and may not be detected using routine bedside urine labstix. In most cases it is mild but in patients with Fanconi–Bickel syndrome, it is very high and may contribute in part to the hypoglycaemia that these patients experience. Renal glycosuria in Fanconi syndrome is characterized by a low threshold, a low maximal glucose reabsorption at saturation glucose concentrations in blood, but normal values of maximal reabsorptive capacity (Tm_G) during excessive glucose loading (see also Chapter 5.2).

5. *Bicarbonaturia* reflects a reduced threshold for reabsorption and is again variable in extent, according to the underlying cause of Fanconi syndrome. In severe acidosis, filtered bicarbonate is reduced to a level below the threshold for proximal reabsorption and urine pH falls below 5.3. The attendant hyperchloraemic metabolic acidosis (type II renal tubular acidosis) requires treatment with large doses of alkali. It also contributes to loss of skeletal calcium and hypercalciuria.

6. *Electrolyte, fluid, and mineral losses* can be very severe. The excess urinary sodium loss underlies the other solute, electrolyte, and water losses, and is the leading cause of the clinical symptomatology. Increased urinary sodium increases potassium loss, in turn causing hypokalaemia. In rare cases, this can be so severe as to lead to a contraction (hypovolaemic) alkalosis (Houston *et al.* 1968). In addition, sodium wasting may contribute to hypercalciuria, a feature of some,

but not all cases of Fanconi syndrome. Excess water loss varies from mild (e.g. in cases with Lowe's syndrome) to severe (in cystinosis), when infants may pass 3–4 l of urine per day. It results from excessive solute loss (sodium and glucose) together with a defect in urinary concentrating ability. Maximal urinary concentration after DDAVP was impaired in five of seven patients with overt Fanconi syndrome following ifosfamide therapy (Rossi *et al.* 1995).

7. *Lactate and glyceraldehyde* levels in urine are increased in some patients with Fanconi syndrome, especially in those with mitochondrial disorders (Jonas *et al.* 1989; Niaudet and Rotig 1996). Likewise, urinary excretion of pyroglutamate (5-oxoglutarate) is elevated in cystinosis (Rizzo *et al.* 1999). These abnormalities probably reflect abnormal energy production and an altered redox potential in proximal tubular cells.

8. *Carnitine* is normally reabsorbed in the proximal tubule and is therefore lost in excess in Fanconi syndrome. Low plasma carnitine concentrations have been reported in children with cystinosis and tyrosinaemia (Gahl *et al.* 1993; Nissenkorn *et al.* 2001), leading to plasma and muscle deficiencies of carnitine, which could contribute to the myopathy in these disorders. Long-term oral carnitine supplementation increases plasma and muscle carnitine concentrations, but the clinical benefit of such therapy is uncertain (Gahl *et al.* 1993).

9. *Losses of vitamins, carrier proteins, chemokines* have all been described in Fanconi syndrome as shown in Fig. 2 (Moestrup and Verroust 2001; Norden *et al.* 2001). Children with cystinosis and adults with idiopathic Fanconi syndrome may have low circulating levels of vitamin D (Chesney *et al.* 1980; Colussi *et al.* 1985), possibly resulting from reduced proximal tubular uptake secondary to defects in the endocytic pathway (see below).

Pathogenesis

Megalin, cubulin, and the endocytic pathway

The proximal tubule transports large and small substances by different mechanisms. Small substances (ions, amino acids, monosaccharides, etc.) are transported by a variety of channels and transporters (see Chapter 5.1). Larger substances (proteins, lipoproteins, vitamins, etc.) are taken up by pinocytosis or bind to specific receptors and are endocytosed. The endocytic receptors are localized to clathrin-coated pits in the intermicrovillar regions of the apical membranes of proximal tubular epithelia. Ligands bind to these receptors and are internalized in clathrin-coated vesicles, which then uncoat delivering the ligand–receptor complex to endosomes (see Fig. 3; reviewed in Moestrup and Verroust 2001). ATP-dependent proton pumps acidify endosomes, leading to dissociation of the ligand–receptor complex. The receptors are recycled back to the apical membrane and the endosome fuses with lysosomes where ligands (such as proteins, complex carbohydrates, etc.) are usually degraded into their constituent parts (e.g. amino acids).

The major endocytic receptors are megalin (previously known as gp330) and cubilin [previously known as gp280 or intrinsic factor-Cobalamin (vitamin B_{12}) receptor]. Megalin is a member of the low-density lipoprotein (LDL) receptor family, characterized by a ligand-binding region consisting of a number LDL receptor type A repeats flanked by epidermal growth factor-type repeats (Moestrup and Verroust 2001). Ligands bind to the type A repeats which are negatively charged calcium binding protein molecules. Megalin has a single transmembrane domain and a short cytoplasmic tail, involved in binding to adaptor proteins and the clustering in coated pits. Cubilin consists of eight EGF repeats followed by 27 CUB (each made up of complement C1r/C1s, Uegf, and bone morphogenic protein-1 domains), responsible for ligand binding. There is no transmembrane domain, but the *N*-terminal cubilin region has a conserved amphipathic helix pattern (Lys^{74}–Glu^{109}) suitable for hydrophobic interactions, which would serve as a candidate site for membrane association (Kristiansen *et al.* 1999). Both cubilin and megalin are widely expressed but are most abundant in the visceral yolk sac and proximal renal tubule where they colocalize in the apical membrane (Moestrup and Verroust 2001). Megalin, but not cubilin, rapidly associates with receptor associated protein (RAP) which is involved in its processing to the apical membrane. The proteins are upregulated *in vitro* by vitamin D, retinoids, and cAMP but the relevance of this *in vivo* is unknown.

Cubilin and megalin interact in a process dependent on calcium, to achieve ligand uptake by the endocytic pathway. A large number of ligands are now known to bind to these receptors, some to one or the other and some to both (reviewed in Moestrup and Verroust 2001). A major group of ligands are carrier or binding complexes such as vitamin D-binding protein, vitamin D, RBP, vitamin A, lipoproteins, PTH, transthyretin, transferrin, thyroglobulin, and intrinsic factor-B_{12}. Drugs (e.g. aminoglycosides) and toxins also bind to megalin (see section on 'Acquired Fanconi syndrome').

A number of studies have shown that megalin and cubilin are the major receptors for urinary proteins reabsorbed in the proximal tubule:

1. *In vitro* uptake of albumin into proximal renal tubules is inhibited by RAP, a megalin inhibitor (Cui *et al.* 1996).

2. Megalin deficient mice have reduced numbers of clathrin-coated pits, endosomes and lysosomes (Leheste *et al.* 1999). They excrete several low molecular weight proteins, including albumin, RBP, and β2-microglobulins well as significant amounts of vitamin A and 25-OH vitamin D_3.

3. Dogs born with an inherited deficiency of cubilin have markedly deficient proximal tubule reabsorption and excrete large amounts of albumin (Birn *et al.* 2000).

4. Immunoblotting and immunohistochemical studies suggest that low-molecular weight albumin binding proteins are fragments of cubilin (Birn *et al.* 2000).

The urinary abnormalities observed in megalin or cubilin deficient animals are very similar to those of the human Fanconi syndromes. Dysfunction of the endocytic pathway in Fanconi syndromes has been further documented in Lowe's syndrome and in Dent's disease (further details are given in Chapters 2.4, 5.1, and 5.2):

1. CLC-5, a gated chloride channel, defective in Dent's disease, colocalizes with albumin-containing endocytic vesicles (Devuyst *et al.* 1999).

2. Mice in which the *clcn5* gene is deleted, have proteinuria, glycosuria, amino aciduria, and evidence of markedly impaired apical proximal tubular endocytosis (Piwon *et al.* 2000; Wang *et al.* 2000).

3. Patients with Lowe's syndrome and Dent's disease, two forms of Fanconi syndrome, have low molecular weight proteinuria and a marked deficiency of urinary megalin, see Fig. 4 (Norden *et al.* 2002).

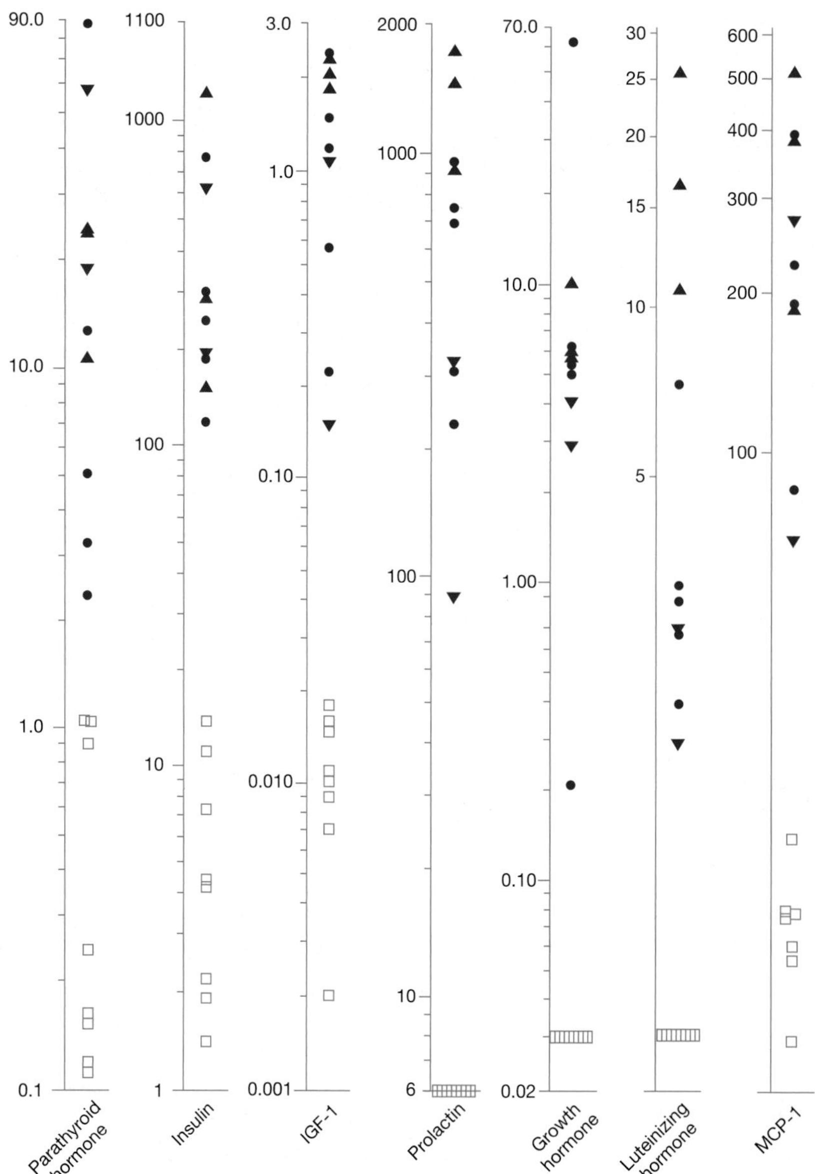

Fig. 2 Urinary excretion of hormones and chemokines (expressed per mmol creatinine) in patients with Fanconi syndromes: (●) Dent's disease; (▲) Lowe syndrome; (▼) autosomal dominant idiopathic Fanconi syndrome; (□) normal individuals. Units: parathyroid hormone, ng; insulin, pmol; IGF-1, nmol; prolactin, mIU; growth hormone, mIU; luteinizing hormone, mIU, MCP-1, ng. (Reproduced from Norden *et al.* 2001, permission sought.)

Intact endocytic function is thus required for normal proximal tubular protein reabsorption. Mutations affecting the CLC-5 chloride channel, in patients with Dent's disease, cause failure of endosomal acidification by as yet unknown mechanisms. Whatever the mechanisms, if trafficking of megalin from endosomes to the apical membrane was impaired, the endocytic pathway would be disrupted. This would explain the reduced apical expression of megalin seen in the knock-out *clc-5* mouse and the reduced urinary excretion seen in humans with Fanconi syndrome (Piwon *et al.* 2000; Wang *et al.* 2000; Norden *et al.* 2002). Since megalin also acts as a receptor for PTH and precursor 25(OH) vitamin D3, perturbation of these processes might explain the hypercalciuria that is characteristic of Dent's syndrome (Piwon *et al.* 2000). Furthermore, the low levels of 1,25-dihydroxy-vitamin D3, documented in many cases of Fanconi syndrome despite severe hypophosphataemia (that in normal individuals would be expected to stimulate 1-hydroxylation) might be explained by excess urinary losses secondary to defective endocytosis. Megalin-knockout mice have increased urinary losses of vitamins A and 25(OH) D3 (Leheste *et al.* 1999), markedly decreased plasma levels of 25(OH) D3, bone deformity and reduced bone density. Cubilin-deficient dogs exhibit similar biochemical abnormalities. It is likely that normal reabsorption and processing of vitamin D-D binding protein, requires both cubilin (as the ligand) and megalin (to internalize the complex).

Disruption of megalin/cubilin-mediated endocytosis thus occurs in a number of animal and human models of Fanconi syndrome. It accounts

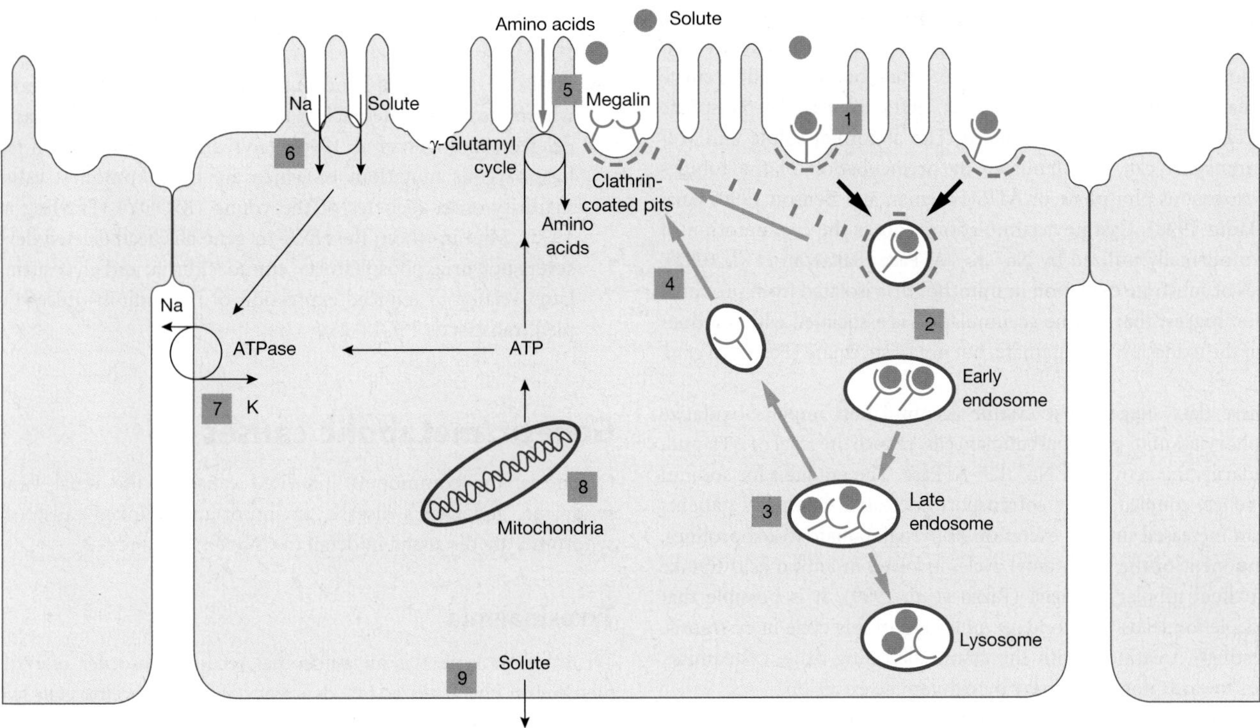

Fig. 3 Schematic drawing of proximal tubular cell showing the endocytic pathway (1–4), γ-glutamyl cycle (5), and sodium co-transport system (6–9). [Reproduced from van't Hoff, W.G. (2003).]

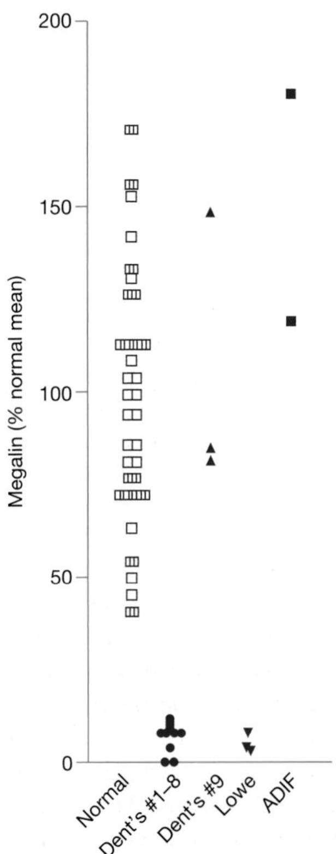

Fig. 4 Urinary excretion of total megalin in normal individuals and patients with Dent's disease (pedigrees 1–9), Lowe's syndrome and autosomal dominant Fanconi syndrome. (Reproduced from Norden *et al.* 2002, permission sought.)

not only for the characteristic low molecular weight proteinuria, but also for losses of vitamins, hormones, and other substances, the effects of which may contribute to the clinical heterogeneity of the syndrome.

Defective solute transport

Solute uptake in the proximal tubule is principally achieved by cotransport with sodium across the apical membrane. Extrusion of sodium across the basolateral membrane by the action of Na^+,K^+-ATPase, transfers three sodium ions out of the cell in exchange for the inward movement of two extracellular potassium ions, thus creating an electrochemical gradient which drives sodium-coupled solute cotransport. Na^+,K^+-ATPase function depends on the supply of ATP generated in mitochondria as a result of oxidative phosphorylation (see Fig. 3). Once in the cytosol, solutes move into the peritubular fluid mainly by facilitated diffusion (see Chapter 5.1). The phenotype of the Fanconi syndrome could be due to defects in any one or more of these stages of solute transport. Other mechanisms such as back-leakage of solutes and water across the intercellular tight junctions (similar to defective paracellin function in the hypomagnesaemia–hypercalciuria syndrome), or increased solute loss from the bloodstream across the tubular cells could further contribute to the problem.

The effect of accumulation or deficiency of a substrate has been investigated in the various metabolic disorders that can cause Fanconi syndrome, especially in cystinosis. To date, much of this work has been undertaken in animal models. Rats given intraperitoneal cystine dimethyl ester (CDME) have an increased urine volume and excretion of phosphate, glucose, and amino acids (Foreman *et al.* 1987). Isolated animal renal tubules loaded with cystine accumulate cystine within lysosomes, mimicking the human disorder (Sakarcan *et al.* 1990), have a decreased solute and volume transport (Foreman *et al.* 1987; Salmon and Baum 1990), with a significant reduction in oxygen consumption and in the oxidation of glucose, lactate, butyrate, and succinate (Foreman and Benson 1990; Coor *et al.* 1991). Intracellular phosphate and ATP concentration are reduced. The abnormal solute and volume transport can be attenuated by preincubation of the tubules with exogenous phosphate or ATP (Foreman and Benson 1990; Bajaj and Baum 1996). Cystine accumulation reduces the consumption of oxygen normally utilized by Na^+,K^+-ATPase (Sakarcan *et al.* 1992). Studies of substrate oxidation in mitochondria isolated from proximal tubules, suggest that cystine accumulation is associated with a reduction in the oxidation of glutamate, but not of succinate (Foreman *et al.* 1995).

These data suggest that cystine accumulation impairs oxidative phosphorylation in proximal tubular cells, reduce the level of ATP and, secondarily, the activity of Na^+,K^+-ATPase. The gradient for sodium and, hence, coupled solute cotransport decreases. Cystinosis patients have an increased urinary excretion of pyroglutamate (5-oxoproline), a component of the γ-glutamyl cycle, involved in amino acid uptake in proximal tubular epithelia (Rizzo *et al.* 1999). It is possible that ATP depletion leads to secondary inhibition of this cycle in cystinosis. Interestingly, treatment with the cystine-depleting drug, cysteamine, returns towards normal urinary pyroglutamate excretion.

An alternative mechanism of tubular cell dysfunction has been recently proposed (Ccetinkaya *et al.* 2002). Whole cell patch clamping, applied to human kidney (HK) epithelial cells, discloses that cystine loading with CDME rapidly alters basal membrane voltage, with an initial depolarization followed by a marked hyperpolarization (due to activation of K^+-channels). Prolonged cystine loading (>30 min) inhibits the activity of Na^+-alanine cotransporter and the Na^+/H^+ exchanger. The Na^+-phosphate (NaPi2) cotransporter was much more sensitive, with substantial inhibition occurring after very little exposure to cystine (1–2 min) (Ccetinkaya *et al.* 2002).

It is not yet clear whether these data, derived from animals with intact lysosomal cystine transport, can be extrapolated to the human disorder in which lysosomal cystine transport is defective. Reduced sodium-cotransporter activity is likely to be a key component of the generalized proximal tubular dysfunction seen in the Fanconi syndrome. Whether this is due to intracellular phosphate and ATP depletion with secondary inhibition of Na^+,K^+-ATPase or to reduced expression/activity of the transporters themselves, or to a combination of both mechanisms, requires further investigation.

Whereas, these aforementioned studies suggest transport dysfunction in intact epithelia, recent work has indicated the possibility that programmed tubular cell death may be an aetiological factor. The rate of apoptosis in nephropathic cystinosis fibroblasts is two to three times greater than controls (Park *et al.* 2002). Cystine loading of cultured normal renal tubular cells significantly increases the apoptotic rate, whereas cysteamine treatment of cystinosis fibroblasts decreases the rate (Park *et al.* 2002).

Other models/mechanisms

1. Drugs/toxins: Toxin-induced Fanconi syndrome is discussed below (section 'Acquired Fanconi syndrome').
2. Basenji dog: A spontaneous Fanconi syndrome develops in Basenji dogs (Bovee *et al.* 1978). Affected dogs have an alteration in brush border membrane fluidity, an increased cholesterol but normal phospholipid and total free fatty acid content of the brush border (Hsu *et al.* 1994).
3. HNF-1α: A Fanconi syndrome has been described in mice in whom the hepatocyte nuclear factor-1α (*HNF-1α*) gene has been deleted (Pontoglio *et al.* 1996). *HNF-1α* is a transcription factor, heterozygous mutations of which are the commonest cause of maturity-onset diabetes of the young (MODY) (Frayling *et al.* 1997). Mice in whom the *HNF-1α* gene has been deleted develop severe polyuria, phosphaturia, aminoaciduria, and glycosuria, the latter related to reduced expression of the sodium–glucose coupled transporter (SGLT-2).

Genetic/metabolic causes

Cystinosis, the commonest inherited cause of the renal Fanconi syndrome, and Dent's disease, an important X-linked cause of the syndrome, are discussed in detail in Chapters 2.4 and 5.2.

Tyrosinaemia

Tyrosinaemia type 1 is an autosomal recessive disorder of tyrosine metabolism, characterized by a deficiency of fumaryl acetoacetate hydrolase (FAH). Deficiency of FAH causes accumulation of metabolites, in particular succinylacteone (SA) and succinylacetoacetate (Lindblad *et al.* 1977). Affected children present with either the acute or the chronic form of the disease. Early features include fulminant liver disease with hepatomegaly, jaundice, ascites, and evidence of hepatic dysfunction. A more chronic form of liver disease leading to hepatic cirrhosis and with a risk of hepatocellular carcinoma can also occur. It is associated with a severe Fanconi syndrome with marked hypophosphataemia and rickets. The kidneys are enlarged and echobright on ultrasound; some may develop nephrocalcinosis, perhaps related to hypercalciuria (Forget *et al.* 1999). In the longer term, glomerular function deteriorates leading to chronic renal failure. There is a marked elevation of plasma tyrosine and the diagnosis is confirmed by an increased urinary SA. Accumulation of SA inhibits porphobilinogen synthetase, which in turn predisposes to acute and recurrent episodes of polyneuropathy (similar to hepatic porphyria) and cardiomyopathy.

The accumulated metabolite (SA) appears responsible for the Fanconi syndrome. SA reduces sodium-dependent uptake of sugar and amino acids across rat brush-border membranes (Spencer *et al.* 1988), inhibits sodium-dependent phosphate transport, decreases ATP production, and reduces mitochondrial respiration (Roth *et al.* 1991). Intraperitoneal injection of SA to rats induces a Fanconi syndrome (Wyss *et al.* 1992). Further evidence has come from a mouse model of tyrosinaemia. Mice in which the fumaryl acetoacetate hydrolase (*Fah*) gene is homozygously deleted (mimicking the human genotype) die in the newborn period. They are rescued by the simultaneous deletion of the 4-OH-phenylpyruvate dioxygenase (HPD) gene (Endo and Sun 2002). HPD is an enzyme proximal to FAH in the tyrosine pathway that converts 4-OH-phenylpyruvate to homogenisate. Tyrosine catabolism is thus blocked at a step higher than in tyrosinaemia type 1 so that nephrotoxic metabolites do not accumulate. Thus, mice with these two gene defects (*Fah* and 4-hydroxyphenylpyruvate dioxygenase, *Hpd*) grow normally without renal or liver phenotype. Administration of homogentisic acid to these mice leads to rapid apoptosis and, on electron microscopy, to distortion and enlargement of mitochondria and lysosomes in proximal tubules. The treated mice excrete more glucose and phosphate, mimicking the renal Fanconi syndrome (Endo and Sun 2002). These data underline to role of accumulated toxic metabolites in the pathogenesis of the renal tubular dysfunction.

Liver transplantation was undertaken as a form of enzyme replacement therapy, but a number of survivors developed chronic renal failure (Freese *et al.* 1991; Laine *et al.* 1995). Treatment with 2-(2-nitro-4-trifluoromethylbenzoyl)-1,3-cyclohexanedione (NTBC), which inhibits HPD, prevents the accumulation of SA and subsequent metabolic derangements (Lindstedt *et al.* 1992). Up to 90 per cent of patients with acute tyrosinaemia respond to NTBC therapy. Early treatment reduces the incidence of hepatocellular carcinoma and appears to prevent or even reverse the associated renal tubulopathy (Holme and Lindstedt 1998).

Lowe's (oculocerebrorenal) syndrome

The oculocerebrorenal syndrome is an X-linked disorder in which boys are born with severe bilateral cataracts, muscle hypotonia and later develop a renal Fanconi syndrome (reviewed in Nussbaum and Suchy 2001). In addition to the cataracts, other ocular manifestations such as buphthalmos and glaucoma can occur and generally vision is severely impaired. Neuromuscular involvement is usually severe with profound neonatal hypotonia, characteristic areflexia, seizures, behavioural disturbance (hyperactivity and obsessive–compulsive traits) and variable impairment of intellectual function.

The renal manifestations are initially mild but by the end of their first year of life, most affected boys have developed features of the renal Fanconi syndrome. Early tubular dysfunction is evidenced by aminoaciduria and tubular proteinuria; glycosuria is mild or may not be evident (Norden *et al.* 2000). Plasma chemistry is only mildly distributed in comparison with Fanconi syndromes of other origin. Hypercalciuria is severe, predisposing to nephrocalcinosis and occasionally renal stones. Glomerular filtration decreases progressively leading to chronic renal failure from late childhood onwards.

Lowe's syndrome is caused by mutations in an X-linked gene that encodes the OCRL protein (Attree *et al.* 1992). OCRL is an inositol polyphosphate 5-phosphatase responsible for hydrolysis of a number of enzymes and lipids including phosphatidylinositol 4,5-bisphosphate [PtdIns(4,5)P_2] and phosphatidylinositol 3,4,5-trisphosphate (Zhang *et al.* 1995). OCRL is found in the *trans*-Golgi network (Dressman *et al.* 2000). PtdIns(4,5)P_2 is localized on the cytoplasmic surface of plasma membrane and has a number of functions including vesicle trafficking (e.g. in the assembly of clathrin-coated pits) (Dressman *et al.* 2000). Patients with Lowe's syndrome, as well as those with some other forms of Fanconi syndrome, have a marked deficiency of urinary megalin, but not of cubilin, possibly due to defective trafficking of megalin (Norden *et al.* 2002). Disruption of the megalin pathway might explain defective proximal tubular transport, but it remains to be seen whether it is the sole mechanism of renal dysfunction and how other organs are involved. Plasma levels of several lysosomal enzymes are elevated in Lowe's patients. It has been speculated that excess PtdIns(4,5)P_2, secondary to a defect in OCRL, might lead to abnormal trafficking of lysosomal enzymes which in turn, might contribute to cytotoxicity (Ungewickell and Majerus 1999).

Fanconi–Bickel syndrome

The Fanconi–Bickel syndrome is a very rare autosomal recessive disorder of monosaccharide transport due to mutations in the GLUT-2 facilitative glucose transporter. GLUT-2 is expressed in hepatocytes, pancreatic β-cells, and the basolateral membranes of intestinal and renal tubular epithelia (Santer *et al.* 1997). Affected children present in the first year of life with symptoms of hypoglycaemia. There is hepatomegaly (due to glycogen storage) and rickets secondary to a severe Fanconi syndrome. Characteristically, there is preprandial hypoglycaemia and postprandial hyperglycaemia. Glucose homeostasis is disturbed as a consequence of defective transport of glucose out of the liver (in the fasting state) and into hepatocytes (after feeding). Impaired glucose-sensing with an attendant inappropriately low insulin secretion, exacerbates postprandial hyperglycaemia. Defective function of GLUT-2 in the proximal renal tubule leads to excessive urinary losses of glucose and galactose (far in excess of that seen in other causes of Fanconi syndrome) which contributes to hypoglycaemia (Manz *et al.* 1987; Santer *et al.* 1997, 1998). Renal glomerular hyperfiltration, microalbuminuria, and diffuse mesangial expansion have been reported in one child (Berry *et al.* 1995) and reduced GFR has been observed in some adults. In addition to standard measures to treat the Fanconi syndrome and rickets, children require frequent feeds and benefit from uncooked cornstarch supplements (Lee *et al.* 1995).

Mitochondrial disorders

Proximal renal tubular cells are rich in mitochondria in order to provide sufficient ATP to drive Na^+,K^+-ATPase, creating the sodium gradient upon which solute coupled transport depends (see section on 'Defective solute transport'). It is therefore not surprising that mitochondrial disorders may lead to Fanconi syndrome; indeed this is the commonest renal manifestation of these defects (Neiberger *et al.* 2002). Congenital mitochondrial disorders predominantly affect children, but acquired mitochondrial toxicity (e.g. secondary to drugs) can affect any age group (see section on 'Adefovir/cidofovir'). Mitochondrial defects causing Fanconi syndrome are manifest in the first 2 years, and often as early as the first few weeks of life (Niaudet and Rötig 1996). Often, these babies have multisystem dysfunction and the prognosis is poor. A variety of specific mitochondrial disorders have been associated with Fanconi syndrome, including deficiencies of respiratory chain complexes I, III, and IV (Luder and Barash 1994; Morris *et al.* 1995; Kuwertz-Broking *et al.* 2000). It has also been seen in a number of defined phenotypes of mitochondrial cytopathies such as Pearson's, Kearns Sayre, Leigh's, and MELAS syndromes (Ogier *et al.* 1988; Mori *et al.* 1991; Niaudet *et al.* 1994; Campos *et al.* 1995).

Mitochondrial disorders are often characterized by elevated blood lactate and pyruvate concentrations, although blood lactate levels may be misleadingly normal when the Fanconi syndrome induces profound urinary losses of lactate (Niaudet and Rötig 1996). Proximal tubular damage is evidenced by cell vacuolization and characteristic giant mitochondria (Niaudet and Rötig 1996). Definitive proof of a mitochondrial cytopathy rests on the determination of respiratory chain complex activities in biopsy tissue (frequently muscle). Genetic studies may show large rearrangements, specific point mutations or deletions.

ARC syndrome (arthrogryposis, renal tubular abnormalities and cholestasis)

Two siblings from a consanguineous family, with severe cholestasis, arthrogryposis, renal tubular disease and poor growth were reported in 1973 (Lutz-Richner and Landolt 1973). Approximately 30 further children have been reported, although some cases lack some features of the syndrome (reviewed in Eastham *et al.* 2001). The condition appears inherited in an autosomal recessive manner. Its major renal feature is a severe Fanconi syndrome, together, in some patients, with nephrogenic diabetes insipidus (Coleman *et al.* 1997; Eastham *et al.* 2001). The kidneys are generally small and possibly dysplastic. Individual cases of nephrocalcinosis, interstitial nephritis, and multicystic dysplasia have been described (Eastham *et al.* 2001). Cholestasis is severe but serum gamma glutamyltransferase values are normal. Histology of the liver shows cholestasis and hepatocyte multinucleate giant cell transformation and, in some cases, intrahepatic biliary hypoplasia and lipofuscin deposition. These latter differences may depend on the timing of the biopsy (Eastham *et al.* 2001). Additional features include ichthyosis, recurrent febrile illnesses, abnormally large platelets, and diarrhoea. Despite extensive metabolic evaluation, the underlying cause of this disorder is not yet known and no treatment is available; affected infants die within the first year.

Galactosaemia

An incomplete form of Fanconi syndrome is seen rarely in infants with the autosomal recessive disorder, galactosaemia, which is due to a deficiency of galactose 1-phosphate uridyl-transferase, involved in the conversion of galactose to glucose (reviewed in Holton *et al.* 2001). Affected children become unwell after galactose-containing feeds. The main extra-renal symptoms include jaundice, poor feeding and growth, vomiting, liver disease, cataracts, and subsequently, learning difficulties. Infants appear particularly prone to *Escherichia coli* sepsis. There is marked galactosuria, secondary to the increased blood galactose. The diagnosis is confirmed by the finding of increased blood levels of galactose 1-phosphate and by the demonstration of the enzyme deficiency. The renal Fanconi syndrome is reversible upon withdrawal of galactose and substitution with lactose feeds. The mechanism of the renal tubular dysfunction is uncertain but may be related to intracellular phosphate depletion.

Hereditary fructose intolerance

Hereditary fructose intolerance is an autosomal recessive disorder due to a deficiency of fructose 1,6-bisphosphate aldolase (also known as aldolase) (reviewed in Steinmann *et al.* 2001). Affected patients remain well unless given fructose or sucrose-containing foodstuffs. In babies, there are no ill effects during milk feeding but, at weaning, when fruits and vegetables are offered, they develop poor feeding, vomiting, and poor growth. More severe reactions include hypoglycaemia, liver dysfunction, and shock. There is laboratory evidence of an acute generalized proximal tubular dysfunction. Metabolic acidosis is due partly to proximal tubular dysfunction, but mainly to lactic acidosis (Richardson *et al.* 1979).

Fructose ingestion rapidly leads to accumulation of fructose 1-phosphate, which, in turn, causes further metabolic derangement, including marked hyperuricaemia due to the degradation of adenine nucleotides, a rapid fall in ATP levels and intracellular phosphate. These abnormalities are evident in hepatocytes, but are also seen in proximal tubular cells. Recently, another mechanism of proximal tubular cell dysfunction has been explored. Aldolase interacts with vacuolar H(+)-ATPases, responsible for acidification of intracellular compartments (e.g. endosomes) and for hydrogen ion secretion across the tubular epithelia (Lu *et al.* 2001). Aldolase deficiency as in hereditary fructose intolerance, could conceivably disrupt this interaction and lead to acidosis.

Acquired Fanconi syndrome

Aminoglycosides

Aminoglycosides are extensively used antibacterial agents whose nephrotoxicity is well known. Mild renal tubular toxicity (often subclinical) is common and rarely culminates in a Fanconi syndrome (Schwartz and Schein 1978; Gainza *et al.* 1997). Aminoglycosides are freely filtered by the glomerulus and largely excreted intact. A small proportion (approximately 5 per cent) is reabsorbed in the proximal tubule, where as a result of its long half-life, a number of deleterious effects can occur (Mingeot-Leclercq and Tulkens 1999). Early events include accumulation of polar lipids (myeloid bodies) leading to lysosomal enlargement. Subsequently, lysosomal rupture, mitochondrial swelling, and disruption of the brush border lead to apoptosis and focal necrosis (reviewed in Mingeot-Leclercq and Tulkens 1999).

Megalin acts as a receptor for aminoglycosides (Moestrup *et al.* 1995). Indeed, megalin-deficient mice do not accumulate [^{3}H]gentamicin in their kidneys (0.6 per cent), unlike the wild-type mice (11 per cent), although similar amounts are excreted in urine (Schmitz *et al.* 2002). These data suggest that megalin receptor antagonists might prevent aminoglycoside-induced nephrotoxicity in patients. However, gentamicin-induced nephrotoxicity is observed *in vitro* in LLC-PK(1) cells that do not express megalin (Girton *et al.* 2002). In this model, clusterin, a secreted glycoprotein normally upregulated after renal injury, had a protective effect in cells exposed to high levels of gentamicin, but not in ATP depleted cells (a model of hypoxic-ischaemic damage) (Girton *et al.* 2002). The clusterin protective effect therefore occurs independently of megalin.

Ifosfamide

Ifosfamide is commonly associated with proximal tubular dysfunction, but this is rarely clinically relevant (Skinner *et al.* 1993). Early (often subclinical) features include low molecular weight proteinuria and amino aciduria in approximately 65 per cent, phosphaturia in 40 per cent, generalized proximal dysfunction in 12 per cent, and a frank Fanconi syndrome in 5 per cent of the exposed patients (Rossi *et al.* 1994). Risk-factors for nephrotoxicity include the cumulative dose, use of other nephrotoxic agents (such as *cis*-platinum), unilateral nephrectomy, and possibly age (younger age being more susceptible) (Skinner *et al.* 1993; Rossi *et al.* 1994; Aleska *et al.* 2001). Whilst initial toxicity affects the proximal tubule, there is also a longer term risk of glomerular toxicity (reviewed in Skinner *et al.* 2000). Ifosfamide nephrotoxicity appears mediated by its toxic metabolite, chloroacetaldehyde (CAA). CAA, but not ifosfamide, is cytotoxic *in vitro*. It reduces markedly intracellular phosphate, ATP, coenzyme-A, and glutathione, increases lactate dehydrogenase and pyruvate with an attendant impaired lactate, and glucose metabolism (Dubourg *et al.* 2001). CAA is itself detoxified in the kidney to choroacetate. Its toxicity is also minimized, *in vitro*, by mesna and amifostine.

Sodium valproate

Sodium valproate therapy has been associated with proximal renal tubular dysfunction in a series of case reports. In several isolated cases, the Fanconi syndrome developed in children on long term valproate therapy and usually remitted upon discontinuation of the drug (Lenoir *et al.* 1981; Hawkins and Brewer 1993; Lande *et al.* 1993; Smith *et al.* 1995; Yoshikawa *et al.* 2002). Two children given valproate had a biopsy-proven tubulointerstitial nephritis, one presenting with a Fanconi syndrome and the other with haematuria and proteinuria (Lin and Chiang 1988; Yoshikawa *et al.* 2002).

Investigation of proximal tubular function in children on anticonvulsant therapies disclosed an increased excretion of *N*-acetylglucosaminidase (NAG) in patients on valproate, ethosuximide, or phenytoin and an increased α1-microglobulin in those on carbamazepine and phenytoin. Creatinine clearance and levels of Tam–Horsfall protein remained normal (Korinthenberg *et al.* 1994). Increased urinary NAG levels have been observed in up to 50 per cent of valproate-treated children, whereas other markers of proximal function (e.g. phosphate reabsorption, β2-microglobulin) or distal function (calcium excretion) were unaffected (Yuksel *et al.* 1999; Altunbasak *et al.* 2001). Overall, subclinical proximal tubular dysfunction appears quite common during valproate therapy but leads only very occasionally to a Fanconi syndrome.

Adefovir/cidofovir

Adefovir and cidofovir are nucleotide analogues with powerful antiviral activity, extensively used in HIV and CMV infections. Both are associated with considerable proximal tubular toxicity, but rarely with a frank Fanconi syndrome (Polis *et al.* 1995; Vittecoq *et al.* 1997; Bagnis *et al.* 1999; Fisher *et al.* 2001). In one study, seventeen of twenty-one patients with HIV, treated with cidofovir infusions for CMV infection, developed proteinuria and four had to stop therapy due to renal toxicity (Polis *et al.* 1995). A French review reported that most cidofovir-treated patients developed glycosuria, 40 per cent had proteinuria and 12 per cent progressed to acute renal failure (Bagnis *et al.* 1999). Patients were treated with hyperhydration and probenecid to limit toxicity. Proximal tubular dysfunction has been reported in 17 per cent of 253 patients with advanced HIV disease, treated with adefovir (Fisher *et al.* 2001).

Adefovir and cidofovir are transported into proximal tubular cells by the human renal organic anion transporter 1 (hOAT1). In an *in vitro* system, Chinese hamster ovary cells expressing hOAT1 accumulated both nucleotide analogues, leading to 4–500-fold increase in cytotoxicity (Ho *et al.* 2000). Accumulation and cytotoxicity were attenuated in presence of hOAT1 inhibitors such as the non-steroidal anti-inflammatory drugs (in particular, ketoprofen and naproxen) (Mulato *et al.* 2000). Severe acute degenerative changes affecting the proximal tubules with marked enlargement and distortion of mitochondria were observed in a patient with adefovir toxicity (Tanji *et al.* 2001). Immunostaining revealed a deficient mitochondrial enzyme cytochrome C oxidase, a finding supported by the demonstration of a significant reduction in mitochondrial DNA. Adefovir cytotoxity might thus be mediated by mitochondrial DNA depletion.

Aristolochic acid

Aristolochic acid, derived from *Aristolochia* plants, has been implicated as the causative toxin in Chinese herbs nephropathy, to the extent that the latter may be better termed aristolochic acid-associated nephropathy (Tanaka *et al.* 2000). It may also be involved in the pathogenesis of Balkan nephropathy (see Chapter 6.8). Chinese herbs nephropathy has been reported in a number of countries, notably Belgium and Japan, and is associated with marked proximal tubular dysfunction (low molecular weight proteinuria, glycosuria) and with the development of urothelial tumours (Cosyns *et al.* 1999). Histological examination has shown flattened proximal tubular epithelial cells and interstitial fibrosis. Aristolochic acid may be concentrated in proximal tubular cells by uptake through a basolateral organic anion cotransporter hOAT1, also implicated in adefovir-mediated nephrotoxicity (see above) (Lebeau *et al.* 2001). The toxic effects of aristolochic acid *in vitro* in opossum kidney (OK) cell include inhibition of cellular uptake of albumin and β2-microglobulin and decreased expression of megalin (Lebeau *et al.* 2001).

Other drugs/toxins

Several other drugs and chemicals have been occasionally associated with the Fanconi syndrome. Cadmium and maleate have both been extensively used to create experimental models of Fanconi syndrome. These toxins result in mitochondrial concentration, distortion and dysfunction. Maleate reduces ATP and phosphate concentrations, Na^+,K^+-ATPase activity, and coenzyme A (Eiam-Chong *et al.* 1995). Durable tubular dysfunction (e.g. phosphaturia) may result from the inhibition of Na-Pi mRNA and Na-Pi2 protein expression, with an attendant reduction in cotransport (Haviv *et al.* 2001). In rats, maleate also markedly reduces renal glutathione and glutathione peroxidase activity, thus impairing free radical inactivation (Mimic-Oka and Simic 1997). In addition maleate appears to disrupt the endocytic pathway and may inhibit receptor binding to megalin by chelation of calcium, which mediates this interaction (Christensen *et al.* 1992).

Suramin, an antiparasitic drug, caused profound hypophosphataemia in all 15 patients with advanced carcinoma in whom it was given as a chemotherapeutic agent (Rago *et al.* 1994). A muscle biopsy disclosed in one patient abnormal mitochondria and a cytochrome C oxidase deficiency, which resolved when suramin was discontinued. Ranitidine, lead, fumarate, colloidal bismuth subcitrate, and L-lysine have all been associated with the development of Fanconi syndrome with or without histological evidence of tubulo-interstitial nephropathy (Neelakantappa *et al.* 1993; Lo *et al.* 1996; Loghman-Adham 1998; Raschka and Koch 1999; Hruz *et al.* 2002).

Fanconi syndrome associated with renal glomerular diseases

Proximal tubular dysfunction is an additional feature of a number of glomerular diseases. Many patients with focal segmental glomerulosclerosis have increased low molecular weight proteinuria and enzymuria. This degree of proximal tubular dysfunction is usually subclinical, but may have prognostic importance (Valles *et al.* 2000; Bazzi *et al.* 2002; Mastroianni Kirsztajn *et al.* 2002). Overt Fanconi syndrome is seen in some patients with membranous nephropathy, often associated with tubulointerstitial disease and antitubular basement membrane antibodies (Dumas *et al.* 1982; Makker *et al.* 1996). Some affected children also develop non-renal manifestations such as autoimmune haemolytic anaemia, enteropathy, and lung disease (Levy *et al.* 1978; Griswold *et al.* 1997) and an X-linked inherited form has been described (Tay *et al.* 2000).

Monoclonal gammopathies

Some patients with monoclonal gammopathies also develop a Fanconi syndrome (reviewed in Lacy and Gertz 1999; Messiaen *et al.* 2000). A number of them have haematological malignancies (multiple myeloma, Waldenstrom's macroglobulinaemia) or other lymphoproliferative disorders. Current evidence suggests that monoclonal light chains are taken up by proximal tubular epithelia, but incompletely catabolized, leading to intracellular crystal formation and cytotoxicity. Nearly all such patients excrete kappa light chains (often of the V kappa I variability subgroup), but some lambda cases have been described. The kappa light chains also appear unusually resistant to cathepsin B proteolysis which may be a further factor in the pathogenesis of the Fanconi syndrome. Tubular dysfunction causes hypophosphataemia and osteomalacia, which contribute to chronic bone pain.

Idiopathic Fanconi syndrome

A few patients with Fanconi syndrome have no obvious underlying cause. The syndrome is thus designated as idiopathic. In a few families, the idiopathic Fanconi syndrome is clearly inherited in a dominant manner (Brenton *et al.* 1981; Chesney *et al.* 1981; Patrick *et al.* 1981; Tolaymat *et al.* 1992). In several families, tubular proteinuria in the first decade has preceded electrolyte abnormalities and has been eventually followed by progressive deterioration of glomerular filtration rate (Friedman *et al.* 1978; Brenton *et al.* 1981). Renal failure can, however, occur in childhood and several patients have been transplanted. A variety of other abnormalities have been described in some of these families, including diabetes mellitus (Friedman *et al.* 1978). A gene locus for idiopathic Fanconi syndrome has been identified on chromosome 15q15.3 in one extended pedigree (Lichter-Konecki *et al.* 2001). Interestingly, Norden *et al.* found a marked urinary megalin deficiency in Fanconi syndromes associated with Lowe's and Dent's diseases but normal values in two individuals with the idiopathic form, suggesting a different pathogenesis (Norden *et al.* 2002).

Balkan endemic nephropathy (see also Chapter 6.8)

This chronic tubulointerstitial nephropathy has some features of the Fanconi syndrome and progresses slowly to chronic renal failure. It is localized in specific areas of some Balkan states (Serbia, Bosnia, Croatia, Bulgaria, and Romania). The disease occurs in early to mid-adult life, affects both sexes, may be familial, and is associated with a history of farming. Its course is insidious with polyuria, polydipsia, symptoms of anaemia, and an increased incidence of urothelial tumours. Investigations show anaemia, tubular proteinuria, renal tubular acidosis, salt wasting, and impaired concentrating ability.

Its pathogenesis is still disputed. Environmental toxicity with trace metals such as lead, cadmium, manganese, and copper, or deficiency of selenium has been suggested. Aristolochic acid has been implicated as Chinese herbs nephropathy caused by aristolochic acid has many similarities with Balkan endemic nephropathy (BEN). Contamination of flour with *Aristolochia clematis* has been incriminated. Ochratoxin A is a mycotoxin responsible for porcine nephropathy, which is similar to BEN. It is found in higher concentrations in parts of Croatia but also in non-endemic areas. A chromosomal marker on 3q25-26 has been implicated. There is, as yet, no clear link between any pathogenetic factor and the proximal tubular dysfunction seen in these patients.

Other associations

Vitamin D deficiency is associated with aminoaciduria, phosphaturia leading to hypophosphataemia, and in some reports, metabolic acidosis (Huguenin *et al.* 1974; Chesney and Harrison 1975). This situation is usually accompanied by marked secondary hyperparathyroidism, a potential trigger for proximal tubular dysfunction.

Manz and colleagues described a single case of a child with neonatal onset Fanconi syndrome in whom a renal biopsy demonstrated a widespread absence of brush borders in proximal tubular cells (Manz *et al.* 1984). Two other young children with severe Fanconi syndrome, chronic renal failure, growth and developmental delay, were found to have marked thinning of brush border villi and glomerular capillary wall thickening on renal biopsy (Bartsocas *et al.* 1986). There are isolated reports of Fanconi syndrome associated with cryptogenic fibrosing pleuritis, pulmonary alveolar proteinosis, and with membranous lipodystrophy (Hishikawa *et al.* 1988; Garcia Rio *et al.* 1995; Hayes *et al.* 1995). Mild generalized proximal tubular dysfunction has been reported in a group of patients with idiopathic acquired sideroblastic anaemia (Hanson *et al.* 1995).

Treatment

The management of patients with Fanconi syndrome is based on general and specific measures. The multiple causes and degrees of severity of the syndrome call for a therapy tailored to individual needs. The first measure is to correct dehydration with the infusion of 0.9 per cent saline, in view of the considerable salt wasting. Historically, fatalities occurred during rehydration with glucose-containing solutions, which exacerbated the already profound hypokalaemia that many new patients exhibit. The next measure is to correct the major electrolyte and acid–base deficiencies. Once again, cautious, progressive correction is advised (especially for hypokalaemia and hypocalcaemia). Rapid correction of acidosis can precipitate hypocalcaemic seizures, the 'hungry bone' phenomenon (Frisch and Mimouni 1993).

Free access to water is essential and many severely affected children will consume 3–6 l per day. Once stabilized, many patients require large doses of alkali (3–20 mmol/kg/day) to be prescribed in the form of sodium or potassium bicarbonate or citrate, or as a compound preparation (e.g. Polycitra). Citrate is useful as a large proportion of patients are prone to hypercalciuria and subsequent development of nephrocalcinosis. Supplements of sodium chloride may also be needed. Rickets or osteomalacia requires phosphate supplementation and vitamin D, given in the form of 1α-calcidol or calcitriol, as there is some evidence of impaired renal hydroxylation in some Fanconi syndromes. Many children with severe Fanconi syndromes (especially cystinosis) require nutritional support. In some, provision of all the above supplements fails to correct the biochemical disturbances and growth suffers as a result. Indomethacin is widely used in such cases by many European paediatric nephrologists (Haycock *et al.* 1982). However, a double-blind trial in children with Fanconi syndrome due to cystinosis, failed to show a significant advantage of indomethacin, a finding, which, coupled with its potential gastrointestinal toxicity, explains why it has not found favour in North America (Clark *et al.* 1996). Chronic administration of thiazide diuretics may also provide symptomatic improvement by contracting extracellular volume. Carnitine supplements have been used to correct the plasma and muscle carnitine deficiencies that occur in cystinosis (see Chapter 16.5.1).

Specific therapy of Fanconi syndromes depends on the underlying cause. The tubulopathy of galactosaemia and hereditary fructose intolerance is reversible, once either galactose or fructose respectively, is withdrawn from the feeds. Likewise, NTBC reverses the Fanconi syndrome in tyrosinaemia (see section 'Tyrosinaemia' above). Cysteamine, used as a cystine-depleting agent in cystinosis, has a beneficial but not curative effect on proximal tubular function. Removal of the causative toxin or drug usually ameliorates the tubulopathy, although some drugs (e.g. ifosfamide) can cause long-term dysfunction.

References

Aleksa, K., Woodland, C., and Koren, G. (2001). Young age and the risk for ifosfamide-induced nephrotoxicity: a critical review of two opposing studies. *Pediatric Nephrology* **16**, 1153–1158.

Altunbasak, S. *et al.* (2001). Renal tubular dysfunction in epileptic children on valproic acid therapy. *Pediatric Nephrology* **16**, 256–259.

Attree, O. *et al.* (1992). The Lowe's oculocerebrorenal syndrome gene encodes a protein highly homologous to inositol polyphosphate-5-phosphatase. *Nature* **358**, 239–242.

Bagnis, C., Izzdine, H., and Deray, G. (1999). Renal tolerance of cidofovir. *Therapie* **54**, 689–691.

Bajaj, G. and Baum, M. (1996). Proximal tubule dysfunction in cystine-loaded tubules: effect of phosphate and metabolic substrates. *American Journal of Physiology* **271**, F717–F722.

Bartsocas, C. S. *et al.* (1986). A familial syndrome of growth retardation, severe Fanconi-type renal disease and glomerular changes—a new entity? *International Journal of Pediatric Nephrology* **7**, 101–106.

Bazzi, C. *et al.* (2000). A modern approach to selectivity of proteinuria and tubulointerstitial damage in nephrotic syndrome. *Kidney International* **58**, 1732–1741.

Bazzi, C. *et al.* (2002). Urinary *N*-acetyl-beta-glucosaminidase excretion is a marker of tubular cell dysfunction and a predictor of outcome in primary glomerulonephritis. *Nephrology, Dialysis, Transplantation* **17**, 1890–1896.

Berry, G. T. *et al.* (1995). Diabetes-like renal glomerular disease in Fanconi–Bickel syndrome. *Pediatric Nephrology* **9**, 287–291.

Birn, H. *et al.* (2000). Cubilin is an albumin binding protein important for renal tubular albumin reabsorption. *Journal of Clinical Investigation* **105**, 1353–1361.

Bovee, K. C., Joyce, T., Reynolds, R., and Segal, S. (1978). The Fanconi syndrome in Basenji dogs: a new model for renal transport defects. *Science* **201**, 1129–1131.

Brenton, D. P. *et al.* (1981). The adult presenting idiopathic Fanconi syndrome. *Journal of Inherited Metabolic Diseases* **4**, 211–215.

Campos, Y. *et al.* (1995). Mitochondrial DNA deletion in a patient with mitochondrial myopathy, lactic acidosis, and stroke-like episodes (MELAS) and Fanconi's syndrome. *Pediatric Neurology* **13**, 69–72.

Ccetinkaya, I., Schlatter, E., Hirsch, J. R., Herter, P., Harms, E., and Kleta, R. (2002). Inhibition of Na(+)-dependent transporters in cystine-loaded human renal cells: electrophysiological studies on the Fanconi syndrome of cystinosis. *Journal of the American Society of Nephrology* **13**, 2085–2093.

Chesney, R. W. and Harrison, H. E. (1975). Fanconi syndrome following bowel surgery and hepatitis reversed by 25-hydroxycholecalciferol. *Journal of Pediatrics* **86**, 857–861.

Chesney, R. W. *et al.* (1980). Serum 1,25-dihydroxyvitamin D levels in normal children and in vitamin D disorders. *American Journal of Diseases of Childhood* **134**, 135–139.

Chesney, R. W. *et al.* (1981). Metabolic abnormalities in the idiopathic Fanconi syndrome: studies of carbohydrate metabolism in two patients. *Pediatrics* **67**, 113–118.

Christensen, E. I., Gliemann, J., and Moestrup, S. K. (1992). Renal tubule gp330 is a calcium binding receptor for endocytic uptake of protein. *Journal of Histochemistry and Cytochemistry* **40**, 1481–1490.

Clark, K. F. *et al.* (1996). A comparative study of indomethacin for the treatment of the Fanconi syndrome in cystinosis. *Journal of Rare Diseases* **11**, 5–12.

Coleman, R. A. *et al.* (1997). Cerebral defects and nephrogenic diabetes insipidus with the ARC syndrome: additional findings or a new syndrome (ARCC–NDI)? *American Journal of Medical Genetics* **72**, 335–338.

Colussi, G. *et al.* (1985). Vitamin D metabolites and osteomalacia in the human Fanconi syndrome. *Proceedings of the European Dialysis and Transplant Association* **21**, 756–760.

Coor, C., Salmon, R. F., Quigley, R., Marver, D., and Baum, D. (1991). Role of adenosine triphosphate and NaK ATPase in the inhibition of proximal tubule transport with intracellular cystine loading. *Journal of Clinical Investigation* **87**, 955–961.

Cosyns, J. P. *et al.* (1999). Urothelial lesions in Chinese-herb nephropathy. *American Journal of Kidney Diseases* **33**, 1011–1017.

Cui, S. C. *et al.* (1996). Megalin/gp330 mediates uptake of albumin in renal proximal tubules. *American Journal of Physiology* **271**, F900–F907.

Devuyst, O. *et al.* (1999). Intra-renal and subcellular distribution of the human chloride channel, CLC-5, reveals a pathophysiological basis for Dent's disease. *Human Molecular Genetics* **8**, 247–257.

Dressman, M. A. *et al.* (2000). Ocrl1, a PtdIns(4,5)P(2) 5-phosphatase, is localized to the trans-Golgi network of fibroblasts and epithelial cells. *Journal of Histochemistry and Cytochemistry* **48**, 179–190.

Dubourg, L. *et al.* (2001). Human kidney tubules detoxify chloroacetaldehyde, a presumed nephrotoxic metabolite of ifosfamide. *Journal of the American Society of Nephrology* **12**, 1615–1623.

Dumas, R. *et al.* (1982). Membranous glomerulonephritis in two brothers associated in one with tubulo-interstitial disease, Fanconi syndrome and anti-TBM antibodies. *Archives Francaises de Pediatrie* **39**, 75–78.

Eastham, K. M. *et al.* (2001). ARC syndrome: an expanding range of phenotypes. *Archives of Disease in Childhood* **85**, 415–420.

Eiam-Chong, S. *et al.* (1995). Insights into the biochemical mechanism of maleic acid-induced Fanconi syndrome. *Kidney International* **48**, 1542–1548.

Endo, F. and Sun, M. S. (2002). Tyrosinaemia type I and apoptosis of hepatocyte and renal tubular cells. *Journal of Inherited Metabolic Disease* **25**, 227–234.

Fisher, E. J. *et al.* (2001). Terry Beirn Community Programs for Clinical Research on AIDS. The safety and efficacy of adefovir dipivoxil in patients with advanced HIV disease: a randomized, placebo-controlled trial. *AIDS* **15**, 1695–1700.

Foreman, J. W. and Benson, J. L. (1990). Effect of cystine loading and cystine dimethylester on renal brushborder membrane transport. *Pediatric Nephrology* **4**, 236–239.

Foreman, J. W. *et al.* (1987). Effect of cystine dimethyl ester on renal solute handling and isolated renal tubule transport in the rat: a new model of the Fanconi syndrome. *Metabolism* **36**, 1185–1191.

Foreman, J. W. *et al.* (1995). Metabolic studies of rat renal tubule cells loaded with cystine: the cystine dimethyl ester model of cystinosis. *Journal of the American Society of Nephrology* **6**, 269–272.

Forget, S. *et al.* (1999). The kidney in children with tyrosinemia: sonographic, CT and biochemical findings. *Pediatric Radiology* **29**, 104–108.

Frayling, T. M. *et al.* (1997). Mutations in the hepatocyte nuclear factor-1alpha gene are a common cause of maturity-onset diabetes of the young in the U.K. *Diabetes* **46**, 720–725.

Freese, D. K. *et al.* (1991). Early liver transplantation is indicated for tyrosinaemia type I. *Journal of Pediatric Gastoenterology and Nutrition* **13**, 10–15.

Friedman, A. L., Trygstad, C. W., and Chesney, R. W. (1978). Autosomal dominant Fanconi syndrome with early renal failure. *American Journal of Medical Genetics* **2**, 225–232.

Frisch, L. S. and Mimouni, F. (1993). Hypomagnesemia following correction of metabolic acidosis: a case of hungry bones. *Journal of the American College of Nutrition* **12**, 710–713.

Gahl, W. A. *et al.* (1993). Muscle carnitine repletion by long-term carnitine supplementation in nephropathic cystinosis. *Pediatric Research* **34**, 115–119.

Gainza, F. J., Minguela, J. I., and Lampreabe, I. (1997). Aminoglycoside-associated Fanconi's syndrome: an underrecognized entity. *Nephron* **77**, 205–211.

Garcia Rio, F. *et al.* (1995). Six cases of pulmonary alveolar proteinosis: presentation of unusual associations. *Monaldi Archives Chest Disease* **50**, 12–15.

Girton, R. A., Sundin, D. P., and Rosenberg, M. E. (2002). Clustering protects renal tubular epithelial cells from gentamicin-mediated cytotoxicity. *American Journal of Physiology* **282**, F703–F709.

Griswold, W. R. *et al.* (1997). The syndrome of autoimmune interstitial nephritis and membranous nephropathy. *Pediatric Nephrology* **11**, 699–702.

Hanson, B. *et al.* (1995). Phosphaturia, glycosuria and aminoaciduria associated with idiopathic acquired sideroblastic anemia. *Clinical Nephrology* **44**, 382–388.

Haviv, Y. S. *et al.* (2001). Late-onset downregulation of NaPi-2 in experimental Fanconi syndrome. *Pediatric Nephrology* **16**, 412–416.

Hawkins, E. and Brewer, E. (1993). Renal toxicity induced by valproic acid (Depakene). *Pediatric Pathology* **13**, 863–868.

Haycock, G. B. *et al.* (1982). Effect of indomethacin on clinical progress and renal function in cystinosis. *Archives of Disease in Childhood* **57**, 934–939.

Hayes, J. P. *et al.* (1995). Familial cryptogenic fibrosing pleuritis with Fanconi's syndrome (renal tubular acidosis). A new syndrome. *Chest* **107**, 576–578.

Hishikawa, R. *et al.* (1988). A case of membranous lipodystrophy complicated by Fanconi's syndrome. *Bone and Mineral* **5**, 99–105.

Ho, E. S. *et al.* (2000). Cytotoxicity of antiviral nucleotides adefovir and cidofovir is induced by the expression of human renal organic anion transporter 1. *Journal of the American Society of Nephrology* **11**, 383–393.

Holme, E. and Lindstedt, S. (1998). Tyrosinaemia type I and NTBC (2-(2-nitro-4-trifluoromethylbenzoyl)-1,3-cyclohexanedione). *Journal of Inherited Metabolic Diseases* **21**, 507–517.

Holton, J. B., Walter, J. H., and Tyfield, L. A. Galactosemia. In *The Metabolic and Molecular Bases of Inherited Disease* 8th edn. (ed. C. R. Scriver, A. L. Beaudet, W. S. Sly, D. Valle, B. Childs, K. W. Kinzler, and B. Vogelstein), pp. 1553–1587. New York: McGraw-Hill, 2001.

Houston, I. B., Boichis, H., and Edelmann, C. M., Jr. (1968). Fanconi syndrome with renal sodium wasting and metabolic alkalosis. *American Journal of Medicine* **44**, 638–646.

Hruz, P. *et al.* (2002). Fanconi's syndrome, acute renal failure, and tonsil ulcerations after colloidal bismuth subcitrate intoxication. *American Journal of Kidney Diseases* **39**, E18.

Hsu, B. Y. *et al.* (1994). Renal brush border membrane lipid composition in Basenji dogs with spontaneous idiopathic Fanconi syndrome. *Metabolism* **43**, 1073–1078.

Huguenin, M., Schacht, R., and David, R. (1974). Infantile rickets with severe proximal renal tubular acidosis, responsive to vitamin D. *Archives of Disease in Childhood* **49** (12), 955–959.

Jonas, A. J. *et al.* (1989). Urine glyceraldehyde excretion is elevated in the renal Fanconi syndrome. *Kidney International* **35**, 99–104.

Korinthenberg, R., Wehrle, L., and Zimmerhackl, L. B. (1994). Renal tubular dysfunction following treatment with anti-epileptic drugs. *European Journal of Pediatrics* **153**, 855–858.

Kristiansen, M. *et al.* (1999). Molecular dissection of the intrinsic factor—vitamin B12 receptor, cubilin, discloses regions important for membrane association and ligand binding. *Journal of Biological Chemistry* **274**, 20540–20544.

Kuwertz-Broking, E. *et al.* (2000). Renal Fanconi syndrome: first sign of partial respiratory chain complex IV deficiency. *Pediatric Nephrology* **14**, 495–498.

Lacy, M. Q. and Gertz, M. A. (1999). Acquired Fanconi's syndrome associated with monoclonal gammopathies. *Hematology/Oncology Clinics of North America* **13**, 1273–1280.

Laine, J. *et al.* (1995). The nephropathy of type I tyrosinaemia after liver transplantation. *Pediatric Research* **37**, 640–645.

Lande, M. B. *et al.* (1993). Reversible Fanconi syndrome associated with valproate therapy. *Journal of Pediatrics* **123**, 320–322.

Lebeau, C. *et al.* (2001). Aristolochic acid impedes endocytosis and induces DNA adducts in proximal tubule cells. *Kidney International* **60**, 1332–1342.

Lee, P. J., van't Hoff, W., and Leonard, J. V. (1995). Catch-up growth in Fanconi–Bickel syndrome with uncooked cornstarch. *Journal of Inherited Metabolic Diseases* **18**, 153–156.

Leheste, J. R. *et al.* (1999). Megalin knockout mice as an animal model of low molecular weight proteinuria. *American Journal of Pathology* **155**, 1361–1370.

Lenoir, G. R. *et al.* (1981). Valproic acid: a possible cause of proximal tubular renal syndrome. *Journal of Pediatrics* **98**, 503–504.

Levy, M. *et al.* (1978). Membranous glomerulonephritis associated with anti-tubular and anti-alveolar basement membrane antibodies. *Clinical Nephrology* **10**, 158–165.

Lichter-Konecki, U. *et al.* (2001). Genetic and physical mapping of the locus for autosomal dominant renal Fanconi syndrome, on chromosome 15q15.3. *American Journal Human Genetics* **68**, 264–268.

Lin, C.-Y. and Chiang, H. (1988). Sodium-valproate-induced tubulo-interstitial nephritis. *Nephron* **48**, 43–46.

Lindbladt, B., Lindstedt, S., and Steen, G. (1977). On the enzymic defects in hereditary tyrosinemia. *Proceedings of the National Academy of Sciences* **74**, 4641–4645.

Lindstedt, S. *et al.* (1992). Treatment of hereditary tyrosinaemia type I by inhibition of 4-hydroxyphenylpyruvate dioxygenase. *Lancet* **340**, 813–817.

Lo, J. C. *et al.* (1996). Fanconi's syndrome and tubulointerstitial nephritis in association with L-lysine ingestion. *American Journal of Kidney Diseases* **28**, 614–617.

Loghman-Adham, M. (1998). Aminoaciduria and glycosuria following severe childhood lead poisoning. *Pediatric Nephrology* **12**, 218–221.

Lu, M. *et al.* (2001). Interaction between aldolase and vacuolar H+-ATPase: evidence for direct coupling of glycolysis to the ATP-hydrolyzing proton pump. *Journal of Biological Chemistry* **276**, 30407–30413.

Luder, A. and Barash, V. (1994). Complex I deficiency with diabetes, Fanconi syndrome and mtDNA deletion. *Journal of Inherited Metabolic Diseases* **17**, 298–300.

Lutz-Richner, A.-R. and Landolt, R. F. (1973). Familiäre Gallengangmissbildungen mit tubulärere Niereninsufflizienz. *Helvetica Paeditrica Acta* **28**, 1–12.

Makker, S. P., Widstrom, R., and Huang, J. (1996). Membranous nephropathy, interstitial nephritis, and Fanconi syndrome—glomerular antigen. *Pediatric Nephrology* **10**, 7–13.

Manz, F. *et al.* (1984). Idiopathic de Toni–Debre–Fanconi syndrome with absence of proximal tubular brush border. *Clinical Nephrology* **22**, 149–157.

Manz, F. *et al.* (1987). Fanconi–Bickel syndrome. *Paediatric Nephrology* **1**, 509–518.

Mastroianni Kirsztajn, G. *et al.* (2002). Urinary retinol-binding protein as a prognostic marker in glomerulopathies. *Nephron* **90**, 424–431.

Messiaen, T. *et al.* (2000). Adult Fanconi syndrome secondary to light chain gammopathy. Clinicopathologic heterogeneity and unusual features in 11 patients. *Medicine (Baltimore)* **79**, 135–154.

Mimic-Oka, J. and Simic, T. (1997). Time course of renal glutathione levels in experimental Fanconi syndrome: an enzyme-based approach. *Renal Failure* **19**, 373–381.

Mingeot-Leclercq, M.-P. and Tulkens, P. M. (1999) Aminoglycosides: nephrotoxicity. *Antimicrobial Agents and Chemotherapy* **43**, 1003–1012.

Moestrup, S. K. and Verroust, P. J. (2001). Megalin- and Cubilin-mediated endocytosis of protein-bound vitamins, lipids, and hormones in polarised epithelia. *Annual Reviews of Nutrition* **21**, 407–428.

Moestrup, S. K. *et al.* (1995). Evidence that epithelial glycoprotein 330/megalin mediates uptake of polybasic drugs. *Journal of Clinical Investigation* **96**, 1404–1413.

Mori, K. *et al.* (1991). Renal and skin involvement in a patient with Kearns–Sayre syndrome. *American Journal of Medical Genetics* **38**, 583–587.

Morris, A. M. M. *et al.* (1995). Neonatal Fanconi syndrome due to a deficiency of complex III of the respiratory chain. *Pediatric Nephrology* **9**, 407–411.

Mulato, A. S., Ho, E. S., and Cihlar, T. (2000). Nonsteroidal anti-inflammatory drugs efficiently reduce the transport and cytotoxicity of adefovir mediated by the human renal organic anion transporter 1. *Journal of Pharmacology and Experimental Therapeutics* **295**, 10–15.

Neelakantappa, K., Gallo, G. R., and Lowenstein, J. (1993). Ranitidine-associated interstitial nephritis and Fanconi syndrome. *American Journal of Kidney Diseases* **22**, 333–336.

Neiberger, R. E. *et al.* (2002). Renal manifestations of congenital lactic acidosis. *American Journal of Kidney Diseases* **39**, 12–23.

Niaudet, P. and Rötig, A (1996). Renal involvement in mitochondrial cytopathies. *Pediatric Nephrology* **10**, 368–373.

Niaudet, P. *et al.* (1994). Deletion of mitochondrial DNA in a case of de Toni–Debré–Fanconi syndrome and Pearson syndrome. *Pediatric Nephrology* **8**, 164–168.

Nissenkorn, A. *et al.* (2001). Carnitine-deficient myopathy as a presentation of tyrosinemia type I. *Journal of Child Neurology* **16**, 642–644.

Norden, A. G. *et al.* (2000). Tubular proteinuria defined by a study of Dent's (CLCN5 mutation) and other tubular diseases. *Kidney International* **57**, 240–249.

Norden, A. G. *et al.* (2001). Glomerular protein sieving and implications for renal failure in Fanconi syndrome. *Kidney International* **60**, 1885–1892.

Norden, A. G. *et al.* (2002). Urinary megalin deficiency implicates abnormal tubular endocytic function in Fanconi syndrome. *Journal of the American Society of Nephrology* **13**, 125–133.

Nussbaum, R. L. and Suchy, S. F. The oculocerebrorenal syndrome of Lowe (Lowe syndrome). In *The Metabolic and Molecular Bases of Inherited Disease* 8th edn. (ed. C. R. Scriver, A. L. Beaudet, W. S. Sly, D. Valle, B. Childs, K. W. Kinzler, and B. Vogelstein), pp. 6257–6266. New York: McGraw-Hill, 2001.

Ogier, H. *et al.* (1988). de Toni–Debré–Fanconi syndrome with Leigh syndrome revealing severe muscle cytochrome *c* oxidase deficiency. *Journal of Pediatrics* **112**, 734–739.

Park, M., Helip-Wooley, A., and Thoene, J. (2002). Lysosomal cystine storage augments apoptosis in cultured human fibroblasts and renal tubular epithelial cells. *Journal of the American Society of Nephrology* **13**, 2878–2887.

Patrick, A., Cameron, J. S., and Ogg, C. S. (**1981**). A family with a dominant form of idiopathic Fanconi syndrome leading to renal failure in adult life. *Clinical Nephrology* **16**, 289–292.

Piwon, N. *et al.* (2000). ClC-5 Cl^--channel disruption impairs endocytosis in a mouse model for Dent's disease. *Nature* **408**, 369–373.

Polis, M. A. *et al.* (1995). Anticytomegaloviral activity and safety of cidofovir in patients with human immunodeficiency virus infection and cytomegalovirus viruria. *Antimicrobial Agents and Chemotherapy* **39**, 882–886.

Pontoglio, M. *et al.* (1996). Hepatocyte nuclear factor 1 inactivation results in hepatic dysfunction, phenylketonuria, and renal Fanconi syndrome. *Cell* **84**, 575–585.

Rago, R. P. *et al.* (1994). Suramin-induced weakness from hypophosphatemia and mitochondrial myopathy. Association of suramin with mitochondrial toxicity in humans. *Cancer* **73**, 1954–1959.

Raschka, C. and Koch, H. J. (1999). Longterm treatment of psoriasis using fumaric acid preparations can be associated with severe proximal tubular damage. *Human Experimental Toxicology* **18**, 738–739.

Richardson, R. M. *et al.* (1979). Pathogenesis of acidosis in hereditary fructose intolerance. *Metabolism* **28**, 1133–1138.

Rizzo, C. *et al.* (1999). Pyroglutamic aciduria and nephropathic cystinosis. *Journal of Inherited Metabolic Diseases* **22**, 224–226.

Rossi, R. *et al.* (1994). Unilateral nephrectomy and cisplatin as risk factors of ifosfamide-induced nephrotoxicity: analysis of 120 patients. *Journal of Clinical Oncology* **12**, 159–165.

Rossi, R. *et al.* (1995). Concentrating capacity in ifosfamide-induced severe renal dysfunction. *Renal Failure* **17**, 551–557.

Roth, K. S., Carter, B. E., and Higgins, E. S. (1991). Succinylacetone effects on renal tubular phosphate metabolism: a model for experimental renal Fanconi syndrome. *Proceedings of the Society of Experimental Biology and Medicine* **196**, 428–431.

Sakarcan, A., Timmons, C., and Baum, M. (1990). Intracellular distribution of cystine in cystine-loaded proximal tubules. *Pediatric Research* **35**, 447–450.

Sakarcan, A., Aricheta, R., and Baum, M. (1992). Intracellular cystine loading causes proximal tubule respiratory dysfunction: effect of glycine. *Pediatric Research* **32** (6), 710–713.

Salmon, R. F. and Baum, M. (1990). Intracellular cystine loading inhibits transport in the rabbit proximal convoluted tubule. *Journal of Clinical Investigation* **85**, 340–344.

Santer, R. *et al.* (1997). Mutations in *GLUT2*, the gene for the liver-type glucose transporter, in patients with Fanconi–Bickel syndrome. *Nature Genetics* **17**, 324–326.

Santer, R. *et al.* (1998). Fanconi–Bickel syndrome—the original patient and his natural history, historical steps leading to the primary defect, and a review of the literature. *European Journal of Pediatrics* **157**, 783–797.

Schmitz, C. *et al.* (2002). Megalin deficiency offers protection from renal aminoglycoside accumulation. *Journal of Biological Chemistry* **277**, 618–622.

Schwartz, J. H. and Schein, P. (1978). Fanconi syndrome associated with cephalothin and gentamicin therapy. *Cancer* **41**, 769–772.

Skinner, R., Cotterill, S. J., and Stevens, M. C. (2000). Risk factors for nephrotoxicity after ifosfamide treatment in children: a UKCCSG Late Effects Group study. United Kingdom Children's Cancer Study Group. *British Journal of Cancer* **82**, 1636–1645.

Skinner, R. *et al.* (1993). Ifosfamide, mesna, and nephrotoxicity in children. *Journal of Clinical Oncology* **11**, 173–190.

Smith, G. C., Balfe, J. W., and Kooh, S. W. (1995). Anticonvulsants as a cause of Fanconi syndrome. *Nephrology, Dialysis, Transplantation* **10**, 543–545.

Spencer, P. D. *et al.* (1988). Effects of succinylacetone on the uptake of sugars and amino acids by brush border vesicles. *Kidney International* **34**, 671–677.

Steinmann, B., Gitzelmann, R., and Van den Berghe, G. Disorders of fructose metabolism. In *The Metabolic and Molecular Bases of Inherited Disease* 8th edn. (ed. C. R. Scriver, A. L. Beaudet, W. S. Sly, D. Valle, B. Childs, K. W. Kinzler, and B. Vogelstein), pp. 1489–1520. New York: McGraw-Hill, 2001.

Tanaka, A. *et al.* (2000). Chinese herb nephropathy in Japan presents adult-onset Fanconi syndrome: could different components of aristolochic acids cause a different type of Chinese herb nephropathy? *Clinical Nephrology* **53**, 301–306.

Tanji, N. *et al.* (2001). Adefovir nephrotoxicity: possible role of mitochondrial DNA depletion. *Human Pathology* **32**, 734–740.

Tay, A. H. *et al.* (2000). Membranous nephropathy with anti-tubular basement membrane antibody may be X-linked. *Pediatric Nephrology* **14**, 747–753.

Tolaymat, A., Sakarcan, A., and Neiberger, R. (1992). Idiopathic Fanconi syndrome in a family. Part I. Clinical aspects. *Journal of the American Society of Nephrology* **2**, 1310–1317.

Ungewickell, A. J. and Majerus, P. W. (1999). Increased levels of plasma lysosomal enzymes in patients with Lowe syndrome. *Proceedings of the National Academy of Sciences USA* **96**, 13342–13344.

Valles, P. *et al.* (2000) Follow-up of steroid-resistant nephrotic syndrome: tubular proteinuria and enzymuria. *Pediatric Nephrology* **15**, 252–258.

van't Hoff, W. G. The tubule. In *The Kidney—From Normal Development to Congenital Disorders* (ed. P. D Vize, A. S Woolf, and J. B. L Bard), pp. 461–473. Amsterdam: Elsevier Press, 2003.

Vittecoq, D. *et al.* (1997). Fanconi syndrome associated with cidofovir therapy. *Antimicrobial Agents and Chemotherapy* **41**, 1846.

Wang, S. S. *et al.* (2000). Mice lacking renal chloride channel, CLC-5, are a model for Dent's disease, a nephrolithiasis disorder associated with defective receptor-mediated endocytosis. *Human Molecular Genetics* **9**, 2937–2945.

Wyss, P. A. *et al.* (1992). Physiological basis for an animal model of the renal Fanconi syndrome: use of succinylacetone in the rat. *Clinical Science* **83**, 81–87.

Yoshikawa, H., Watanabe, T., and Abe, T. (2002). Tubulo-interstitial nephritis caused by sodium valproate. *Brain Development* **24**, 102–105.

Yuksel, A. *et al.* (1999). *N*-acetyl-beta-glucosaminidase and beta-galactosidase activity in children receiving antiepileptic drugs. *Pediatric Neurology* **20**, 24–26.

Zhang, X. *et al.* (1995). The protein deficient in Lowe syndrome is a phosphatidylinositol-4,5-bisphosphate 5-phosphatase. *Proceedings of the National Academy of Sciences USA* **92**, 4853–4856.

5.4 Renal tubular acidosis

Horacio J. Adrogué and Nicolaos E. Madias

Renal tubular acidosis (RTA) defines a group of disorders in which tubular hydrogen ion secretion is impaired out of proportion to the prevailing glomerular filtration rate (GFR). These disorders result in a low plasma bicarbonate, hyperchloraemia, a normal anion gap, and distinct alterations in the plasma potassium. The defects responsible for impaired acidification are localized either to the proximal or the distal nephron, thereby, dividing RTA into two major types, proximal and distal, the latter type being subdivided into three distinct forms. Because the excretion of acid is a tubular function, all forms of renal acidosis are in fact 'tubular' in origin; yet, the acidosis of renal failure, characterized by decreased production/excretion of NH_4^+ and retention of organic and inorganic anions, is specifically excluded from the term RTA. Proper understanding of the clinical features of the various types and forms of RTA requires knowledge of the role of proximal and distal nephron segments in urinary acidification and potassium excretion. In this chapter, we first review the principles of renal acidification and potassium excretion, and examine the molecular basis of RTA; thereafter, we discuss the pathophysiological and clinical aspects of the various types and forms of RTA.

Principles of renal acidification and potassium excretion

Renal acidification (see also Chapters 2.6 and 5.1)

The kidney regulates acid–base balance by maintaining a normal plasma bicarbonate concentration. This task is achieved first by the excretion of an amount of acid, referred to as net acid excretion (NAE), that is equal to the extrarenal generation of acid by metabolism (net acid production); and second, by the complete reabsorption of the filtered bicarbonate load. Both processes are accomplished through renal hydrogen ion (H^+) secretion, namely the addition of H^+ by the renal tubule into the luminal fluid. NAE is estimated as follows:

$$\text{NAE} = U_{\text{NH}_4^+}V + U_{\text{TA}}V - U_{\text{HCO}_3^-}V$$

where V is the urinary volume in 24 h and U the urinary concentration of the substance listed in the subscript. Although ammonium (NH_4^+) is a weak acid ($pK_a = 9.0$), its urinary excretion is accompanied by the generation (neogenesis) of an equivalent amount of bicarbonate. Consequently, ammonium excretion represents renal acid excretion; it usually accounts for approximately two-thirds of the daily NAE, the remaining being attributed to titratable acid (TA). TA refers to closed buffers (those whose total concentration is constant within the solution) filtered at the glomerulus and titrated in the tubular lumen to a more acidic form by the low luminal pH, thereby, generating an equivalent amount of new bicarbonate for the body fluids. Normally, such buffers include phosphate, the principal moiety, and small amounts of creatinine and citrate. Urinary bicarbonate excretion is negligible under normal conditions considering the ordinarily acidic urinary pH.

Usual western diets generate approximately 0.4–1.6 mmol/kg body weight per day of a non-carbonic acid load in adult humans (Paillard 1998). Whereas meat-rich diets are replete with sulfur and phosphate that produce sulfuric and phosphoric acids, vegetarian diets contain organic anions that serve as alkali source. In young children, the acid load is larger, 1–3 mmol/kg body weight per day, as calcium deposition in bone generates an equimolar amount of acid (Paillard 1998).

Complete reabsorption of the filtered HCO_3^-, although of critical importance, does not contribute to the renal excretion of the metabolically produced acids. By far the bulk of the secreted H^+ is spent in reclaiming filtered bicarbonate; only a minute portion is spent in the production of urinary NH_4^+ and TA, which collectively represent renal H^+ excretion. Thus,

$$\text{Renal H}^+ \text{ secretion} = \text{HCO}_3^- \text{ reabsorption} + \text{NAE}$$

In a 70-kg adult with a GFR of 180 l/day, a plasma bicarbonate concentration of 24 mmol/l, and an endogenous acid load of 1 mmol/kg body weight per day, HCO_3^- reabsorption equals 4320 mmol/day (180×24), NAE 70 mmol/day, for a total renal H^+ secretion of 4390 mmol/day.

Acidification in the proximal nephron

Mechanism

The proximal tubule reabsorbs 70–90 per cent of filtered bicarbonate and reduces the luminal bicarbonate concentration from approximately 25 mmol/l in Bowman's space (equal to $[HCO_3^-]$ in plasma water corrected for Donnan factor because of the protein-free ultrafiltrate) to 5–10 mmol/l at the end of the proximal tubule. In addition, NH_3/NH_4^+ is transported into the tubular fluid and buffers (mainly phosphate) are titrated to their acidic forms as a result of the decrease in luminal pH from 7.4 to about 6.8 (range of 6.6–6.9).

$[H^+]$ is higher in the cytosol of renal tubule cells than in the extracellular fluid (e.g. 80 and 40 nmol/l, respectively) so that the chemical gradient favours the cellular exit of H^+. However, cell voltage in most cells is −30 to −80 mV (−70 mV in the proximal tubule cell) and represents an electric driving force that attracts H^+ into the cell, overpowering the chemical gradient. Consequently, H^+ transport out of renal tubule cells represents an active process, whereas transport of base (HCO_3^-, OH^-) out of cells can occur passively (Alpern 2000).

Approximately two-thirds of proximal H^+ secretion is achieved through a secondary active transport (Alpern and Chambers 1986). A Na^+–H^+ exchanger located in the apical (luminal) membrane takes advantage of the low intracellular Na^+ concentration established by the basolateral Na^+,K^+-ATPase to energize the countertransport of H^+ from the cytosol into the tubular fluid (Fig. 1). This Na^+–H^+ exchanger has been identified as the NHE-3 isoform, inhibitable by amiloride. The remaining one-third of proximal acidification relies on an apical membrane vacuolar H^+-ATPase (Fig. 1). In contrast with the Na^+–H^+ exchanger, the vacuolar ATPase represents primary active H^+ transport mediated by an electrogenic pump that derives energy directly from ATP hydrolysis (Stone and Xie 1988).

The proximal tubule is composed of an early segment (S_1), a mid-segment (S_2), and a terminal segment (S_3); the rate of bicarbonate reabsorption is highest in S_1 and lowest in S_3. As depicted in Fig. 1, H^+ secreted in the proximal tubule titrates filtered bicarbonate and generates carbon dioxide and water, a process accelerated by the presence of luminal carbonic anhydrase (type IV). Luminal carbon dioxide diffuses across the apical membrane into the proximal tubule cell where it reacts with cytosolic OH^- (derived from hydrolysis of water) regenerating bicarbonate, a process facilitated by cytosolic carbonic anhydrase (type II). Bicarbonate generated in the cytosol exits passively across the basolateral membrane driven by the cytosolic negative voltage via the *Na Bicarbonate Cotransporter* (actually a Na^+–HCO_3^-–CO_3^{2-} cotransporter), termed NBC. NBC is electrogenic, as it carries two negative charges (Akiba *et al.* 1986). In each cycle, this cotransporter moves passively out of the cell the equivalent of three HCO_3^- ions and

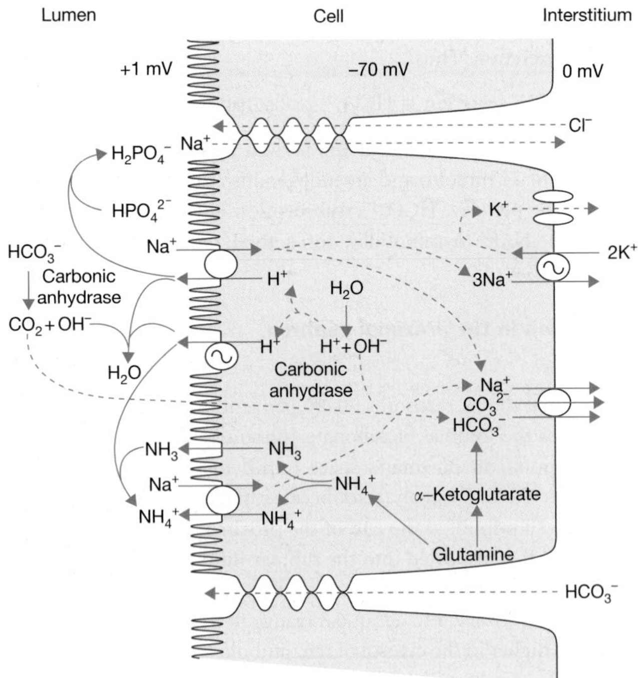

Fig. 1 Model of acidification by proximal tubule. Open circles represent secondary active transport. Sine waves within circles indicate primary active transport.

one Na^+, thereby, reducing the cellular concentration of both ions. Additional Na^+ is transported out of the cell across the basolateral membrane by the Na^+,K^+-ATPase, a process that is primarily active and consumes ATP. These two mechanisms of Na^+ transport are largely responsible for the low cytosolic Na^+ concentration, which provides the driving force for the apical membrane Na^+–H^+ exchanger to extrude H^+ into the lumen of the proximal tubule.

Proximal acidification (active H^+ secretion) titrates filtered bicarbonate, thereby, decreasing the luminal bicarbonate concentration and allowing passive diffusion of bicarbonate from the peritubular capillaries into the lumen via the paracellular pathway. Thus, active H^+ secretion exceeds net HCO_3^- reabsorption counterbalancing the passive HCO_3^- back-diffusion especially in the S_3 segment of the proximal tubule (that has the lowest luminal HCO_3^- concentration) (Alpern 1990).

The reabsorption of sodium and chloride in the proximal tubule is largely dependent on the magnitude of proximal acidification (Alpern and Hamm 2002). In the early proximal tubule, the Na^+–H^+ exchanger leads to a selective absorption of sodium and bicarbonate, which in turn increases luminal chloride concentration. In the late proximal tubule, the increased luminal chloride concentration drives chloride and sodium reabsorption through the paracellular pathway (Fig. 1).

Renal ammonia is mainly synthesized in the S_1 and S_2 segments. All the ammonium excreted in the final urine is already present in the luminal fluid by the end of the proximal tubule (Good and Knepper 1985; DuBose 1997). Excreted NH_4^+ returns an equal amount of bicarbonate to the blood (Alpern 2000). By contrast, retained NH_4^+ is transformed into urea by the liver with associated consumption of bicarbonate and without renal acid excretion.

The NH_3/NH_4^+ present in the medullary interstitium originates in the proximal tubule cell, which generates equal amounts of NH_4^+ and HCO_3^- from glutamine metabolism; whereas HCO_3^- is transported across the basolateral membrane towards the systemic circulation, NH_3/NH_4^+ is transported into the luminal fluid. Transport of NH_3/NH_4^+ occurs by non-ionic diffusion of NH_3 or ionic transport of NH_4^+ (Fig. 2). The high permeability for NH_3 of the apical membrane of the proximal tubule leads to non-ionic diffusion of sizeable amounts of this moiety. The lowered luminal pH due to proximal bicarbonate reabsorption transforms rapidly NH_3 to NH_4^+, thereby, enhancing the gradient for diffusion of NH_3 from the proximal tubular cell into the luminal fluid. In addition, NH_4^+ exits the proximal tubule cell by substituting for H^+ on the apical membrane Na^+–H^+ exchanger. The thick ascending limb subsequently transports NH_3/NH_4^+ out of the luminal fluid into the medullary interstitium, where they accumulate at high concentration. NH_3 added to the renal interstitium can re-enter the lumen of the proximal straight tubule to be reabsorbed again in the thick ascending limb of Henle. As a result, the NH_3/NH_4^+ concentration increases from the renal cortex to the medulla and promotes its entry into the medullary collecting duct.

Regulation

Luminal pH and [HCO_3^-] modulate both active cellular H^+ secretion and passive paracellular HCO_3^- backleak into the lumen. Their decrease lowers H^+ secretion. Conversely, increased luminal [HCO_3^-] augments net H^+ secretion as a result of stimulation of active cellular H^+ transport and concomitant reduction of passive paracellular HCO_3^- backleak into the lumen. Increases in GFR augment luminal flow and the filtered load of HCO_3^- and stimulate H^+ secretion (Alpern 2000).

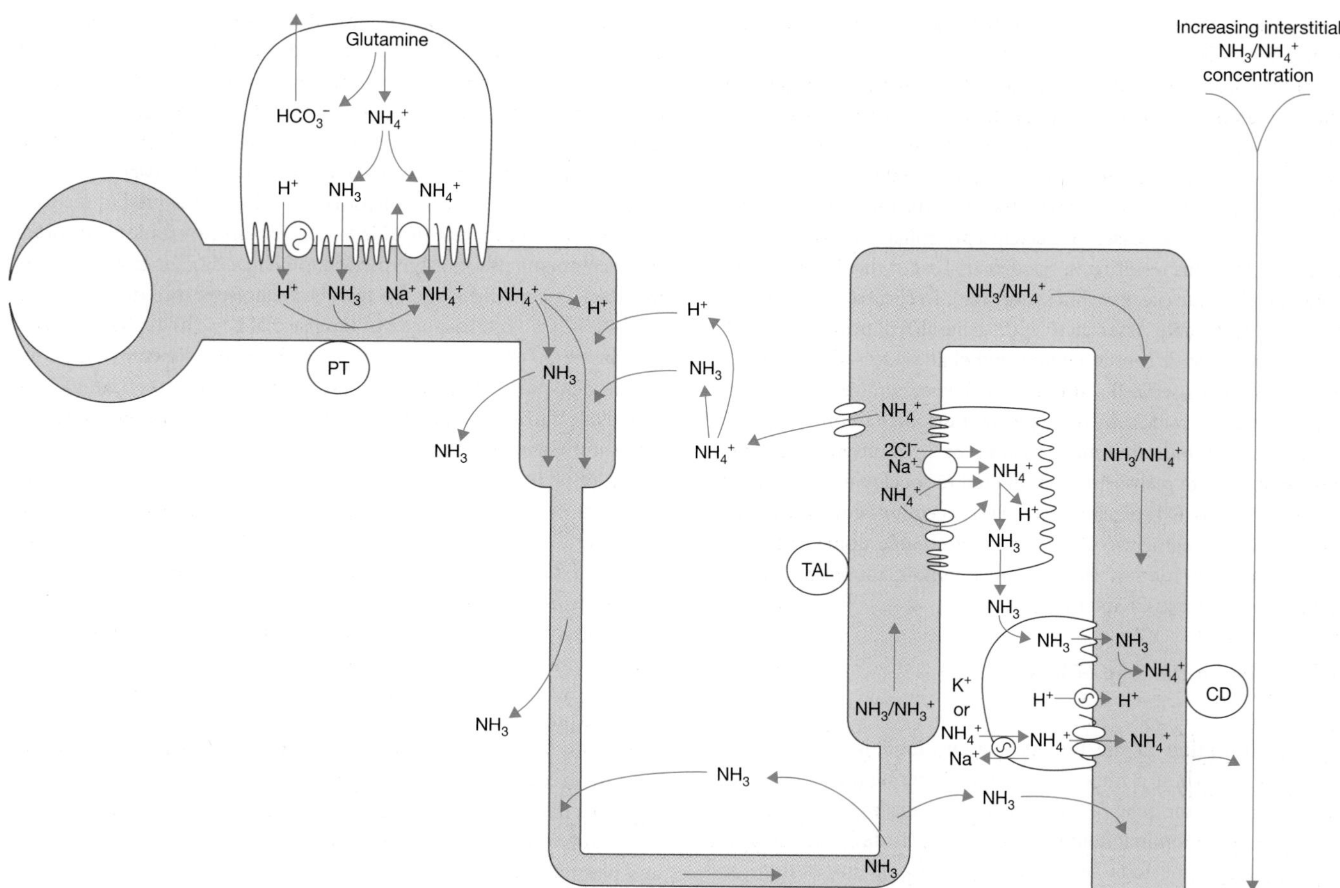

Fig. 2 Model of ammonia/ammonium (NH_3/NH_4^+) transport in the renal cortex and medulla. PT, proximal tubule; TAL, thick ascending limb of loop of Henle; CD, collecting duct.

Periluminal pH also influences proximal acidification, largely by modulating active H^+ secretion. Decreases in cell pH secondary to metabolic acidosis or respiratory acidosis instantly stimulate H^+ efflux by increasing the driving force across the transporter and by direct activation of the Na^+–H^+ exchanger. In addition, chronic metabolic acidosis and chronic respiratory acidosis progressively increase the activities of the apical Na^+–H^+ exchanger and the basolateral NBC (increases in V_{max} of each transporter). Augmented cortisol levels observed in acidosis also increase the Na^+–H^+ exchanger activity. Intracellular acidosis stimulates the vacuolar H^+ pump at the luminal membrane reflecting exocytotic insertion of H^+-ATPase-containing subapical vesicles to the membrane. Opposite changes occur in chronic metabolic alkalosis and chronic respiratory alkalosis, that is, parallel decreases in the activities of the apical Na^+–H^+ exchanger and the basolateral NBC (decreases in V_{max} of each transporter) and suppression of the vacuolar H^+ pump (endocytotic retrieval or H^+-ATPase pumps from the luminal membrane).

Potassium depletion stimulates proximal acidification by increasing the activities of the Na^+–H^+ exchanger and the NBC (Soleimani *et al.* 1990). In addition, ammoniagenesis as well as citrate absorption and metabolism to HCO_3^- are enhanced. These effects reflect the decreased cell pH characteristic of this derangement, and contribute to the pathophysiology of the commonly associated metabolic alkalosis.

Extracellular fluid volume participates in the control of proximal acidification largely by influencing passive paracellular HCO_3^- backleak (Alpern 2000). Volume expansion increases HCO_3^- backleak and thus decreases net HCO_3^- reabsorption; volume contraction has the opposite effects. In addition, Na^+–H^+ exchanger activity increases in states of volume depletion (Alpern and Hamm 2002).

Several hormones, including angiotensin II, catecholamines, and endothelin I stimulate Na^+–H^+ exchanger activity and active H^+ secretion. Conversely, dopamine and parathyroid hormone inhibit proximal acidification.

Defects (mechanisms and molecular basis of proximal RTA)

Because most of the filtered bicarbonate is reabsorbed in the proximal tubule, defective proximal acidification delivers large amounts of bicarbonate to distal nephron segments. Distal acidification has a limited capacity and, therefore, fails to compensate for faulty proximal acidification; the end result is substantial bicarbonaturia.

Certain clinical entities and experimental models of deranged proximal acidification have been linked with several potential defects (Adrogué and Madias 1999): (a) depressed function of luminal (type IV) or cytosolic (type II) carbonic anhydrase (CA) [e.g. acetazolamide, amiloride, families with deficient or abnormal red blood cell CA (type II)] (Sly *et al.* 1985); (b) impaired ability to maintain a low intracellular sodium concentration (resulting in generalized proximal tubular dysfunction, which is termed Fanconi syndrome); or (c) isolated defects of the luminal Na^+–H^+ exchanger (e.g. autosomal dominant proximal RTA), vacuolar H^+-ATPase, or the basolateral NBC (autosomal-recessive proximal RTA). Table 1 summarizes the molecular basis of proximal RTA (type 2 RTA or RTA-2).

An impaired ability to maintain a low intracellular sodium concentration decreases the gradient of sodium between the tubular fluid and the cytosol, thereby, reducing H^+ secretion by the luminal Na^+–H^+ exchanger (DuBose and McDonald 2002). In addition, all Na^+-coupled proximal transport processes are impaired, including the reabsorption of glucose, amino acids, phosphate, uric acid, and filtered proteins, thus resulting in the urinary loss of these substances as well as bicarbonate (i.e. Fanconi syndrome). In clinical practice, proximal RTA is usually associated with generalized proximal tubular dysfunction. Specific causes include epithelial cell loss, decreased ATP production, increased cell sodium permeability, and defects in membrane recycling, trafficking, or vacuolar transport (Coor *et al.* 1991). The proximal tubule dysfunction observed in multiple myeloma is likely secondary to reabsorption of filtered monoclonal immunoglobulin light chains (Messiaen *et al.* 2000); accumulation in proximal tubule cells of fragments of light chains (variable domain) that are resistant to degradation in lysosomes might cause the tubular dysfunction (see also Chapter 5.3).

Acidification in the loop of Henle

Mechanism

Water reabsorption in the thin descending limb increases luminal $[HCO_3^-]$ from about 8 mmol/l in the fluid entering the loop to about 22–24 mmol/l at the bend of the loop, thereby, alkalinizing the luminal fluid. The rise in luminal fluid pH promotes NH_3 diffusion out of the thin portion of the loop of Henle into the renal interstitium and finally into the medullary collecting duct. Luminal fluid $[HCO_3^-]$ returns to about 8 mmol/l in the fluid leaving the loop of Henle, a concentration similar to that of fluid entering the loop. The maintenance of similar $[HCO_3^-]$ in the fluid entering and exiting the loop occurs in association with substantial fluid removal and the absorption of 50–70 per cent of HCO_3^- delivered out of the proximal tubule. Bicarbonate reabsorption is very limited in the thin descending and ascending limbs but occurs mainly in the thick ascending limb via an apical Na^+–H^+ exchanger and a basolateral Na^+–HCO_3^- cotransporter (Good 1985; Krapf 1988) (Fig. 3). Up to 50–80 per cent of the NH_3/NH_4^+ secreted by the proximal tubule and delivered to the loop of Henle is reabsorbed in the thick ascending limb by ionic transport as its apical membrane is impermeable to NH_3. NH_4^+ is transported in the thick ascending limb by three mechanisms: (a) on the apical Na^+–K^+–$2Cl^-$ cotransporter in the place of K^+; (b) across the apical membrane K^+ channel; and (c) across the tight junction driven by the lumen-positive voltage (paracellular transport). The exit of NH_3/NH_4^+ from the thick ascending limb cell towards the medullary interstitium across the basolateral membrane occurs by non-ionic diffusion of NH_3 driven by the high cellular concentration and by ionic transport of NH_4^+ across basolateral K^+ channels. The recycling of NH_3/NH_4^+ due to the interaction of the thick ascending limb (absorption) and proximal straight tubule (re-entry followed by secretion) results in a countercurrent multiplier effect that leads to a corticomedullary axial gradient of these moieties (Good *et al.* 1987) (Fig. 2).

Regulation

As in the proximal tubule, acute and chronic metabolic acidosis stimulate HCO_3^- reabsorption in the loop of Henle, whereas, metabolic alkalosis has the opposite result. The effects of respiratory acid–base disorders have not been studied. Bicarbonate reabsorption is increased by aldosterone and frusemide and decreased by arginine vasopressin and plasma hyperosmolality.

Defect

The clinical significance of an altered acidification of the loop of Henle remains incompletely understood. Because urinary NH_4^+ excretion is

Table 1 Mechanisms and molecular basis of proximal RTA (RTA-2)

Defect	Clinical disorder
Carbonic anhydrase (CA), luminal (type IV), or cytosolic (type II)	
Inherited CA II deficiency	Autosomal-recessive proximal and distal RTA, with osteopetrosis and cerebral calcifications
Depression secondary to drugs	Acetazolamide, amiloride, sulfanilamide, mafenide acetate
Na^+–H^+ exchanger (luminal NHE-3)	
Inherited isolated defect	Autosomal-dominant RTA-2
Immaturity	Sporadic RTA-2 in infancy
$Na^+-HCO_3^--CO_3^{2-}$ cotransporter (basolateral NBC)	Autosomal-recessive RTA-2
Na^+,K^+-ATPase (basolateral)	
Inhibition due to ATP depletion	Fanconi syndrome of maleic acid nephropathy, cystinosis, hereditary fructose intolerance, galactosaemia, glycogen storage disease, mitochondrial diseases (cytochrome C oxidase deficiency)
Damage or loss in association with other cellular defects	Fanconi syndrome of most forms of acquired RTA-2
	Drugs (aminoglycosides, cisplatinum, ifosfamide, outdated tetracyclines)
	Chemical compounds (toluene, paraquat)
	Heavy metals (cadmium, mercury, lead, uranium, platinum)
	Paraproteinaemias (multiple myeloma)
	Renal transplantation
	Nephrotic syndrome
	Chronic tubulointerstitial nephritis

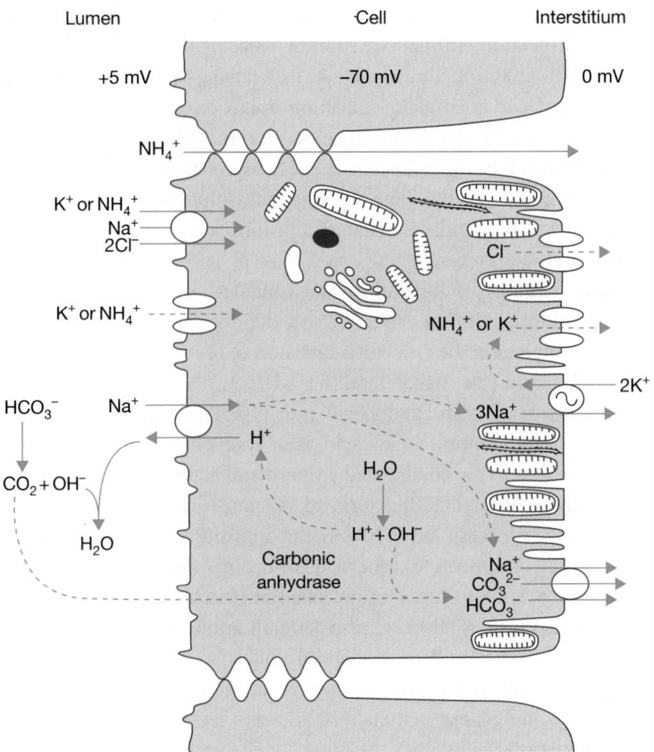

Fig. 3 Model of acidification by the thick ascending limb of loop of Henle. Open circles represent secondary active transport. Sine waves within circles indicate primary active transport.

determined by the build up of NH_3/NH_4^+ in the medullary interstitium, which in turn depends on NH_3/NH_4^+ transport by the loop of Henle, dysfunction of this nephron segment would lead to impaired NAE. In fact, the decreased urinary NH_3/NH_4^+ in some patients with RTA might well originate, at least in part, from an abnormal function of the loop of Henle.

Acidification in the distal nephron

Mechanism

Luminal acidification by the distal nephron (largely cortical and medullary collecting duct) traps most of the ammonium found in final urine, and completes the reabsorption of the remaining 5–10 per cent of the filtered load of bicarbonate, thus securing the final acidification of titratable buffers. The collecting duct has the ability to generate and maintain a highly acidic urine because its luminal membrane is relatively impermeable to the back-diffusion of H^+ ions and carbonic acid. If distal function is normal, acidaemia lowers urine pH to a level as low as 4.4, thereby, generating a 1000-fold transtubular gradient of H^+ (three pH units below the blood level) that secures trapping of ammonium and maximal titration of the urinary buffers. However, the overall capacity for H^+ secretion of the distal nephron is limited and substantially smaller than that of the proximal nephron.

H^+ secretion into the luminal fluid of the distal nephron is mediated by two pumps, a vacuolar H^+-ATPase and an H^+,K^+-ATPase, both localized to the apical membrane of type A (or α) intercalated cells (Caviston *et al.* 1999) (Fig. 4). The vacuolar H^+-ATPase, identical to the one present in the proximal nephron, is an electrogenic pump (it generates a positive lumen potential as H^+ ions are secreted into the lumen) responsible for most of the distal acidification (Brown and Breton 2000). It is also present in the membrane of intracellular endocytic vesicles and can be displaced towards the apical membrane by exocytosis following acidosis-induced stimulation. The H^+,K^+-ATPase is an electroneutral pump that secretes H^+ ions into the lumen

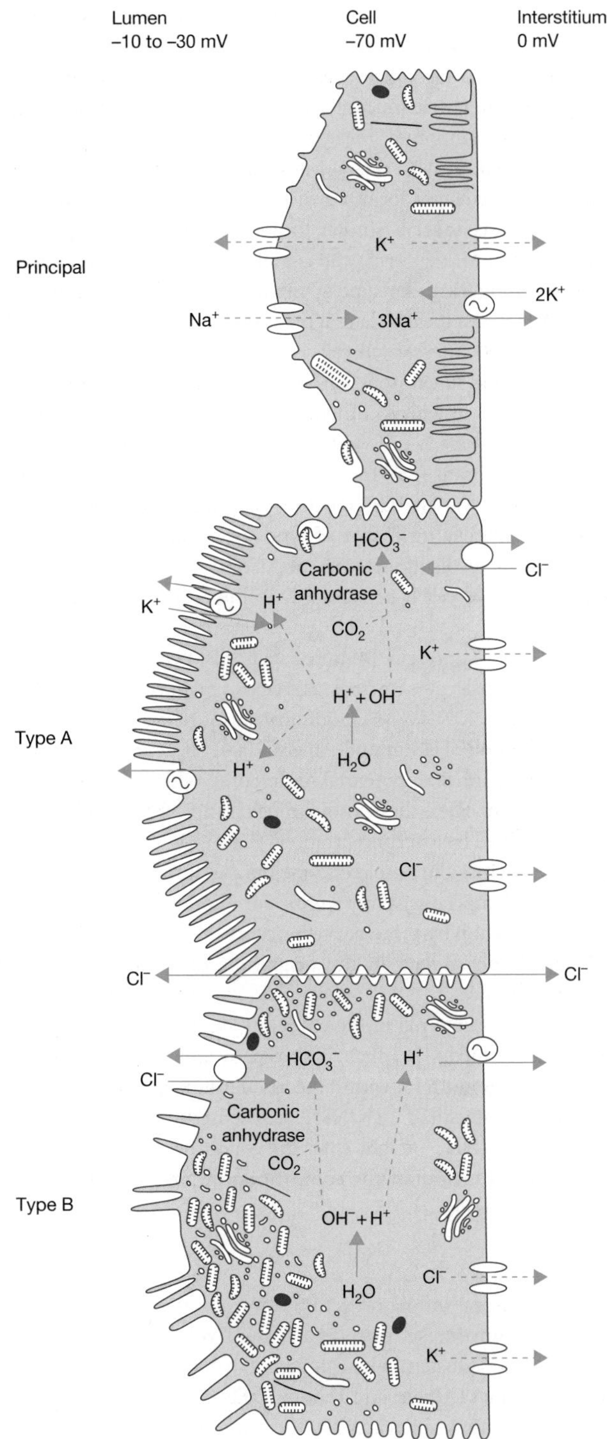

Fig. 4 Model of acidification by the cortical collecting duct including principal and intercalated (types A and B) cells. Open circles represent coupled passive transport. Sine waves within circles indicate primary active transport.

and absorbs potassium; its functional significance becomes manifest in states of potassium depletion, when its activity is enhanced (Caviston *et al.* 1999). The renal H^+,K^+-ATPase is similar to the pump present in gastric mucosa and is inhibited by omeprazole and the SCH 28080 compound. Bicarbonate generated within the type A intercalated cell, leaves the cytosol through the electroneutral Cl^-–HCO_3^- exchanger localized to the basolateral membrane; this Cl^-–HCO_3^- exchanger is similar to that present in red blood cells (band 3 protein, AE1 isoform) and is inhibited by disulfonic stilbenes. The chloride entering the type A intercalated cell in exchange for HCO_3^- exits across the basolateral membrane through a Cl^- channel.

Type B (or β) intercalated cells of the distal nephron are rich in mitochondria and in cytosolic CA, but secrete bicarbonate instead of H^+ ions. Consistent with its function, the type B intercalated cell is a mirror image of type A cell, with H^+-ATPase pump localized to the basolateral membrane, and the Cl^-–HCO_3^- exchanger to the apical membrane (Fig. 4). The Cl^-–HCO_3^- exchanger of type B cells is structurally different from that of type A cells and red blood cells, and is resistant to disulfonic stilbenes. Contrary to type A cell, the type B intercalated cell is present only in the cortical segment of the collecting duct.

Beyond type A and type B intercalated cells, two-thirds of cortical collecting duct cells are principal cells whose main role is to reabsorb Na^+ and secrete K^+ (Fig. 4). Sodium transport indirectly modifies distal acidification (Hamm and Alpern 2000). It generates a lumen-negative transepithelial potential difference, which promotes H^+ secretion; sodium enters the cytosol through an apical Na^+ conductance channel (inhibited by low concentrations—10^{-6} M—of amiloride) and exits the cell across the basolateral membrane through the Na^+,K^+-ATPase, the pump largely responsible for the low cytosolic $[Na^+]$. Potassium secretion by principal cells occurs by an apical K^+ channel and is largely dependent on the magnitude of the lumen-negative potential difference.

The acidic luminal pH of the collecting duct traps NH_4^+ derived from the renal medulla, which is driven by non-ionic diffusion of NH_3. The amount of NH_3 within the tubular lumen is determined by the medullary interstitial NH_3/NH_4^+ concentration and the luminal pH. In addition, NH_4^+ might enter the collecting duct cells through their basolateral membrane by competition of NH_4^+ for K^+ on the Na^+,K^+-ATPase (Fig. 2).

Regulation

Numerous factors influence acidification in the distal nephron, including sodium intake, extracellular fluid volume, mineralocorticoid hormones (aldosterone), acid–base status, potassium stores, and peptide hormones (Alpern and Hamm 2002).

A high NaCl intake increases Na^+ delivery to the cortical collecting duct, which, in the presence of high aldosterone levels, augments electrogenic Na^+ reabsorption and luminal electronegativity; consequently, it enhances the driving force for H^+ secretion (voltage sensitive). However, expansion of extracellular fluid volume caused by a high NaCl intake normally inhibits aldosterone secretion, which in turn reduces H^+ secretion; normal individuals receiving a high NaCl diet thus maintain a normal acid–base status. A low NaCl diet contracts the extracellular fluid volume and decreases distal sodium delivery, while stimulating aldosterone secretion. The counterbalancing effects of low distal sodium delivery and high aldosterone concentrations prevent substantial acid–base effects of a low sodium diet in normal subjects.

Aldosterone, the most important hormone in the regulation of distal acidification, influences sodium reabsorption and stimulates directly H^+ secretion by the H^+-ATPase in the type A intercalated cell (cortical and medullary collecting duct). A direct effect on the H^+-ATPase is of lesser importance, as clearance studies have shown that aldosterone has no substantial effect on renal acidification when distal Na^+ delivery is low. The negative potassium balance induced by aldosterone also stimulates distal acidification as a result of increased urinary NH_4^+ excretion.

Distal nephron acidification is stimulated by both acute and chronic acidosis. During acute acidosis the decreased cell pH stimulates simultaneously the exocytotic insertion of H^+ pumps in the apical membrane and the basolateral Cl^-–HCO_3^- exchange. Chronic acidosis further transforms type B into type A intercalated cells by altering the localization of its acid–base transporters, although this transformation has been disputed (Alpern and Hamm 2002). Luminal pH modifies distal acidification, an alkaline urine increasing H^+ secretion and an acidic urine having the opposite effect.

K^+ deficiency promotes exocytotic insertion of H^+ pumps into the apical membrane of type A intercalated cells in a manner similar to metabolic acidosis (Stetson *et al.* 1980). In addition, it increases the activity of H^+,K^+-ATPase. Enhanced collecting duct H^+ secretion together with increased ammoniagenesis in the proximal tubule augments NAE and generates metabolic alkalosis. Potassium supplementation or hyperkalaemia has the opposite effects, including decreased ammonium production in the proximal tubule, inhibition of ammonium absorption in the thick ascending limb of the Henle's loop, reduction of NH_3/NH_4^+ concentration in the medullary interstitium, and decreased entry of NH_3/NH_4^+ in the medullary collecting duct; the end result is hyperkalaemic RTA.

Defects (mechanisms and molecular basis of distal RTA)

A number of clinical entities and experimental models of disturbed distal acidification have been linked with several potential defects (Adrogué and Madias 1999): (a) decreased expression or impaired function of H^+-ATPase (e.g. acquired or inherited forms of classic distal RTA, also known as type I RTA or RTA-1); (b) impaired function of H^+,K^+-ATPase (e.g. chronic vanadate administration in rats); (c) carbonic anhydrase II deficiency (e.g. Sly syndrome); (d) impaired function of Cl^-–HCO_3^- exchanger or AE1 (e.g. inherited forms of RTA-1); (e) mineralocorticoid deficiency (e.g. 21-hydroxylase deficiency causing type 4 RTA or RTA-4); (f) mineralocorticoid resistance due to mutations of mineralocorticoid receptor gene in principal cells (pseudohypoaldosteronism type I, autosomal dominant) (Geller *et al.* 1998); (g) mineralocorticoid-independent reduction in distal sodium reabsorption (e.g. loss of function mutations in the epithelial Na^+ channel of pseudohypoaldosteronism type I, autosomal recessive); (h) enhanced Cl^- transport (chloride shunt) in the cortical collecting duct (e.g. pseudohypoaldosteronism type II or Gordon's syndrome); (i) H^+ backleak or permeability defect with decreased capacity to maintain steep pH gradients (e.g. amphotericin B toxicity); (j) buffer defect caused by impaired NH_3/NH_4^+ production or transport (e.g. chronic hyperkalaemia, RTA-4); (k) impaired function of Na^+,K^+-ATPase in principal cells (e.g. obstructive uropathy). Table 2 summarizes the molecular basis of all forms of distal RTA.

Impaired H^+ pump function caused by decreased expression of H^+-ATPase is likely the most common cause of classic hypokalaemic distal RTA or RTA-1 (Han *et al.* 2002). Complete absence of H^+-ATPase pump in the type A intercalated cell has been demonstrated by

Table 2 Mechanisms and molecular basis of distal RTA (all forms)

Defect	Clinical disorder
H^+-ATPase in type A intercalated cells	
Decreased expression	Acquired RTA-1, Sjögren's syndrome
Impaired function due to gene mutations	
α 4 Subunit	Inherited RTA-1 with normal hearing
β 1 Subunit	Autosomal-recessive RTA-1 with sensorineural deafness
Carbonic anhydrase II deficiency in type A intercalated cells	
Decreased expression	Inherited defect in red cells, bone, kidney
Autoantibodies	Acquired RTA-1
Cl^-/HCO_3^- (AE1 or band 3) in type A intercalated cells	
Impaired function due to gene mutations	Autosomal-dominant and autosomal-recessive RTA-1
Na^+ channel function in principal cells (CCD)	
Mutations with loss of Na^+ channel function	Pseudohypoaldosteronism type I, autosomal recessive
Interference with drugs	Amiloride, triamterene, trimethoprim, pentamidine
Reduced distal Na^+ delivery	Advanced cirrhosis
Mineralocorticoid deficiency	
21-Hydroxylase deficiency (adrenal cortex)	Combined glucocorticoid and mineralocorticoid deficiencies
3β-Hydroxydehydrogenase deficiency (adrenal cortex)	
Desmolase deficiency (adrenal cortex)	
Familial methyloxidase deficiency (adrenal cortex)	Isolated mineralocorticoid deficiency
Secondary to drugs	Heparin, angiotensin-converting enzyme inhibitors, AT1-receptor antagonists
Other defects (low renin release)	Hyporeninaemic hypoaldosteronism
Mineralocorticoid resistance	
Mutations of mineralocorticoid receptor gene (principal cell)	Pseudohypoaldosteronism type I, autosomal dominant
Enhanced Cl^- transport (distal nephron)	Pseudohypoaldosteronism type II
H^+ ion backleak (permeability defect in distal nephron)	Amphotericin B
NH_3/NH_4^+ production/transport deficiency	Chronic hyperkalaemia, chronic renal insufficiency
Na^+,K^+-ATPase in principal cells	
Interference with drugs	Cyclosporin A
Decreased function, damage, loss	Obstructive uropathy, sickle-cell disease, lupus nephritis

immunocytochemical analysis of renal biopsy specimens of patients with Sjögren's syndrome (Cohen *et al.* 1992). Mutations in the genes encoding the alpha 4 subunit or the B_1 subunit of the H^+-ATPase pump cause inherited forms of RTA-1, the latter being associated with sensorineural deafness (Karet *et al.* 1999). Chronic administration of vanadate in rats decreases H^+,K^+-ATPase activity and results in the RTA-1 phenotype. An endemic form of RTA-1 in Thailand has been associated with drinking water contaminated with vanadate. Gene mutations in the Cl^-–HCO_3^- exchanger (AE1 or band 3) localized to the basolateral membrane of the type A intercalated cells cause autosomal-dominant and autosomal-recessive RTA-1 (Bruce *et al.* 1997; Jarolim *et al.* 1998; Karet *et al.* 1998). Damage of the intercalated cells caused by autoantibodies directed against carbonic anhydrase II has been also implicated in the pathogenesis of distal RTA. Tubular injury in urinary tract obstruction, sickle-cell disease, and lupus nephritis can reduce the activity of the Na^+,K^+-ATPase in the principal cells, which in turn can depress H^+ secretion by the intercalated cells.

Amphotericin B therapy can increase the membrane permeability of the collecting duct, a defect that leads to reduced net H^+ secretion and potassium wasting (Sawaya *et al.* 1995). A lowered intracellular pH of the proximal tubule cells has been proposed as the primary defect in patients with the so-called incomplete RTA-1 (Donnelly et al. 1992). This condition is characterized by hypocitraturia (due to increased proximal reabsorption of filtered citrate), persistently high urinary pH, and normal systemic acid–base composition. The high urinary pH likely results from the increased ammonia production in the proximal tubule and its excretion in the urine. Some patients with incomplete RTA-1 progress to the complete form over a period of time.

Impaired distal sodium reabsorption can result from an inherited defect with loss of Na^+ channel function (pseudohypoaldosteronism type I, autosomal recessive); drugs impairing the function of the Na^+ channel (e.g. amiloride, trimethoprim, pentamidine), depressing the Na^+,K^+-ATPase (e.g. cyclosporin A); or antagonizing the action of aldosterone (e.g. spironolactone); or tubulointerstitial renal disease (e.g. obstructive nephropathy). A 'voltage defect' can also result from enchanced chloride transport (i.e. pseudohypoaldosteronism type II or Gordon's syndrome).

Renal potassium excretion (see also Chapters 2.2 and 5.5)

Mechanism

Almost all of filtered potassium is reabsorbed in the proximal tubule and loop of Henle. The H^+,K^+-ATPase pump localized to the luminal membrane of the type A intercalated cell (and presumably also in the type B intercalated cell) in the cortical and outer medullary collecting tubule further reabsorbs potassium and secretes H^+; its activity is increased in states of K^+ depletion. Thus, most of the potassium in the final urine derives from K^+ secretion by the principal cells in the cortical collecting tubule (Fig. 4). Potassium passively diffuses across the apical membrane into the urinary lumen through K^+ channels along an electrochemical gradient. The high cytosolic $[K^+]$ favours K^+ exit towards the lumen, opposing the electric gradient that tends to retain K^+ in the cytosol (cytosolic voltage is more negative than that of the urinary lumen). The lumen-negative potential is generated by the uptake of sodium into the cell by an apical sodium channel, while its accompanying anion (e.g. Cl^-, HCO_3^-, HPO_4^{2-}) is left in the lumen.

Regulation

Both luminal and periluminal factors modulate renal K^+ secretion.

Luminal factors

The electric profile of the distal nephron (i.e. degree of electronegativity of the tubule lumen compared with that of blood) is the single most important determinant of renal K^+ secretion. As noted, this profile is a function of sodium reabsorption. Because urinary K^+ excretion is determined by the product of urine $[K^+]$ and flow rate, the larger the diuresis, the greater the K^+ excretion. Rapid urine flow prevents a build up of luminal $[K^+]$ that opposes K^+ secretion by decreasing the chemical gradient between the cells and the lumen. Although any decrease in luminal $[K^+]$ tends to diminish kaliuresis, the overall effect of augmented diuresis is to increase potassium excretion. The increased urine flow observed in states of augmented natriuresis, including the administration of most diuretic agents (i.e. acetazolamide, loop diuretics, thiazides) and conditions of salt wasting partially explains the attendant increased kaliuresis (Schwalbe *et al.* 2002).

Kaliuresis is enhanced by an alkaline urine and decreased by an acidic urine, an effect due to changes in apical potassium conductance. A high $[Na^+]$ in the fluid of the distal nephron augments renal K^+ secretion by increasing the lumen-negative potential. This factor partially accounts for the increased kaliuresis engendered by diuretics (other than K^+-sparing agents). Conversely, a low luminal $[Na^+]$ limits the generation of a lumen-negative potential. At less than 30 mmol/l, it drastically diminishes K^+ secretion. In contrast to a low luminal $[Na^+]$, a low luminal $[Cl^-]$ stimulates distal K^+ secretion through either an electroneutral KCl symporter or parallel electrically coupled Cl^- and K^+ conductances (Schwalbe *et al.* 2002).

Periluminal factors

The extracellular $[K^+]$ ($[K^+]_e$) modulates urinary K^+ excretion in a parallel fashion, an effect mediated by changes in the chemical gradient between blood/distal tubule cells and urine. The $[K^+]$ of tubule cells increases in hyperkalaemia and magnifies the K^+ gradient between cells and urine. Hypokalaemia has the opposite effect.

A persistently high dietary K^+ intake enhances disposal of the K^+ load. This process, known as 'K^+ adaptation', increases the capacity of the cortical collecting tubule to secrete potassium (Schwalbe *et al.* 2002). Its mechanisms include a mild increase of $[K^+]_e$, which increases $[K^+]$ of tubular cells, and stimulation of aldosterone secretion (see Chapter 2.2 Potassium balance, Renal transport).

Aldosterone is the dominant regulatory hormone for K^+ excretion. Vasopressin (antidiuretic hormone or ADH) also stimulates Na^+ reabsorption and K^+ secretion in the distal convoluted tubule and cortical collecting duct. Their mechanism of action is further detailed in Chapter 2.2.

Finally, the systemic acid–base status influences importantly renal K^+ excretion. The immediate response to acidosis (respiratory or metabolic) is a decreased kaliuresis, and that to alkalosis (respiratory or metabolic) an increased kaliuresis. Both are short-lasting and reflect changes in the chemical gradient of K^+ between distal tubule cells and lumen. The sustained renal response to acidosis (respiratory or metabolic) is an increased kaliuresis that leads to a mild K^+ deficit in respiratory acidosis and a moderate deficit in metabolic acidosis. It is caused by an increased delivery of Na^+ to the distal nephron. In respiratory alkalosis, potassium excretion promptly returns to normal, thereby, preventing a significant K^+ deficit. By contrast, metabolic alkalosis features ongoing kaliuresis and therefore accrues a sizable K^+ deficit.

Effect of potassium intake and serum level on renal ammonium production and excretion

Dietary potassium loading and hyperkalaemia suppress NH_4^+ production and its reabsorption in the Henle's loop (DuBose and Good 1991). As a result, NH_3/NH_4^+ concentration in the medullary interstitium and urinary NH_4^+ excretion decrease. The hyperkalaemia-induced acidification defect can generate a hyperchloraemic metabolic acidosis known as hyperkalaemic distal RTA; the severity of the defect is aggravated by aldosterone deficiency/resistance or renal insufficiency. Conversely, chronic potassium deficiency increases renal NH_4^+ production and excretion, changes that can generate a metabolic alkalosis, the severity of which is augmented in the presence of NaCl restriction.

As already pointed out, potassium intake and serum level influence aldosterone secretion that exerts directional changes in distal acidification (DuBose 1997).

Defects

Potassium wasting and hypokalaemia (proximal RTA and classic distal RTA)

In proximal RTA (RTA-2), reduced proximal sodium reabsorption increases distal delivery of sodium (with sodium wasting) and causes secondary hyperaldosteronism; both these changes increase kaliuresis. Therefore, K^+ wasting in RTA-2 is secondary to the proximal renal acidification defect and does not reflect a distinct, K^+-specific renal lesion. In untreated RTA-2 with a stable low plasma bicarbonate, all filtered bicarbonate is reabsorbed, the final urine pH is acidic, and the serum K^+ is normal or only mildly decreased. Alkali therapy, initiated to correct acidaemia, augments distal sodium and water delivery, promoting a large kaliuresis and hypokalaemia (Sebastian *et al.* 1971; DuBose and McDonald 2002). Management of these patients with a combination of potassium and sodium bicarbonate (citrate) can help correct both metabolic acidosis and K^+ balance.

In untreated classic distal RTA (RTA-1), hypobicarbonataemia is commonly accompanied by symptomatic hypokalaemia, occasionally expressed by skeletal muscle paralysis, including respiratory failure. Kaliuresis in RTA-1 is due to an augmented K^+ secretion in the distal nephron, driven both by the electronegative luminal potential and the concomitant impairment of H^+ secretion. Consequently, K^+ wasting in RTA-1 is largely secondary to the renal acidification defect and, like in RTA-2, does not result from a distinct, K^+-specific renal lesion.

However, an additional mechanism might involve the absence of K^+ reabsorption by the H^+,K^+-ATPase pump of type A intercalated cells. Contrary to RTA-2, alkali therapy in RTA-1 has a salutary effect on K^+ wasting; by raising luminal pH, it allows more H^+ to be secreted without reaching the limiting gradient, thus decreasing renal K^+ secretion and excretion.

Potassium retention and hyperkalaemia (hyperkalaemic distal RTA)

Sodium reabsorption in the principal cells increases lumen electronegativity and promotes the secretion of both potassium and hydrogen ions (Kleyman *et al.* 1995). Impaired sodium reabsorption leads to metabolic acidosis and hyperkalaemia (Alappan *et al.* 1986). In turn, K^+ retention worsens NH_4^+ production and excretion and increases the severity of the hyperchloraemic metabolic acidosis. Hyperkalaemia and impaired distal acidification are commonly observed as a result of aldosterone deficiency or aldosterone resistance (pseudohypoaldosteronism), a condition known as type 4 RTA or RTA-4 (Bonny and Rossier 2002). A similar electrolyte pattern results from a 'voltage defect' caused by decreased sodium reabsorption in the collecting duct secondary to either low Na^+ delivery or inhibition of Na^+ reabsorption. In all forms of hyperkalaemic distal RTA, K^+ retention is the primary defect responsible for the altered renal acid excretion.

Proximal renal tubular acidosis

Proximal RTA (RTA-2) is characterized by hyperchloraemic metabolic acidosis with variable degrees of sodium and potassium wasting and a disordered renal acidification in the proximal tubule. The decreased plasma $[HCO_3^-]$ characteristically persists after correction of the prevailing salt and water deficit as well as of incidental extrarenal alkali losses (e.g. diarrhoea). In the great majority of patients, it is associated with other disorders of proximal tubular function, including abnormal urinary losses of glucose, phosphate, uric acid, citrate, low-molecular-weight proteins (tubular proteinuria), and amino acids. This composite disorder, known as the Fanconi syndrome (Madias and Perrone 1993) is detailed in Chapter 5.3.

Pathophysiology

Several defects listed in Table 1 impair proximal acidification (Kurtzman 2000) and augment distal tubular delivery of bicarbonate. The limited acidification capacity of the distal nephron results in bicarbonaturia and excessive natriuresis, causing lowered plasma $[HCO_3^-]$ and extracellular fluid volume depletion, respectively. Activation of the renin–angiotensin–aldosterone system promotes dietary NaCl retention and urinary K^+ loss leading to hyperchloraemic hypobicarbonataemia and hypokalaemia.

A stable, but diminished, plasma $[HCO_3^-]$ is reached in RTA-2 as a result of reduced filtered load of HCO_3^-; reduced HCO_3^- backleak due to the decreased plasma $[HCO_3^-]$; and stimulation of proximal HCO_3^- reabsorption secondary to K^+ and volume depletion. The reduced delivery of $NaHCO_3$ to the distal nephron permits full reclamation of luminal HCO_3^- and excretion of acidic urine with normal levels of TA and ammonium (Cogan and Morris 1988). Still, normal levels of NAE despite the prevailing metabolic acidosis are distinctly abnormal and indicate an impaired renal acidification even during the steady state. Retention of NaCl reduces the initial volume depletion and lowers plasma aldosterone levels and kaliuresis such that untreated patients with RTA-2 can be normokalaemic or only mildly hypokalaemic (Table 3). As previously pointed out, alkali therapy increases renal K^+ loss (see 'Treatment' section). Metabolic acidosis is usually mild to moderate (plasma $[HCO_3^-]$ 14–16 mmol/l) in RTA-2 and has a limited effect on skeletal buffers that release small amounts of Ca^{2+} into the extracellular fluid. The increased delivery of HCO_3^- to the distal nephron stimulates distal calcium reabsorption preventing hypercalciuria. Urinary citrate excretion is relatively high in most patients with RTA-2 despite metabolic acidosis and K^+ depletion, both of which reduce citrate production and excretion. The high urinary citrate excretion in RTA-2 is due to the frequent presence of an associated proximal defect in Na^+-coupled organic acid (including citrate) reabsorption. Therefore, RTA-2 is not associated with nephrocalcinosis or nephrolithiasis (Table 3).

When a generalized proximal tubule reabsorption defect is present—the Fanconi syndrome—phosphate wasting and vitamin D deficiency ensue, leading to the development of rickets and osteomalacia (Lemann *et al.* 2000) (Table 3). Vitamin D deficiency is caused by impaired 1α-hydroxylation of 25-hydroxy-vitamin D_3 by proximal tubule cells. Growth failure is commonly observed in all forms of chronic metabolic acidosis, including proximal and distal RTA. Acidosis impacts upon growth directly through effects on the skeleton (loss of mineral content due to buffering) and indirectly through reduction of growth hormone secretion and serum insulin-like growth factors (IGF) levels. In experimental animals, acidosis suppresses hepatic growth hormone receptor mRNA, hepatic IGF-1 mRNA, and gene expression of IGF at the growth plate of long bones (Challa *et al.* 1993).

Clinical features and causes

RTA-2 can develop in any age group, from the neonatal to the elderly, and results from multiple causes (Table 4). The clinical features vary according to the age at presentation and the possible presence of an underlying disease.

Patients with primary RTA-2 have no recognizable underlying condition and, therefore, exhibit clinical features that largely reflect the proximal tubular dysfunction (other concomitantly inherited defects can be present). Conversely, patients with secondary RTA-2 have additional manifestations related to the specific underlying disease. The primary forms occur much more frequently in children and the secondary forms mainly in adults. Both primary and secondary forms can present as an isolated proximal acidification defect or as a generalized proximal reabsorptive defect—the full-blown Fanconi syndrome (reviewed in Chapter 5.3).

The neonatal presentation of RTA-2 can be preceded by a history of polyhydramnios. Clinical manifestations include failure to thrive, increased thirst, polyuria, vomiting, and episodes of volume depletion. Renal salt wasting and, if present, renal glucosuria induce an excessive diuresis and negative fluid balance. The primary forms of infantile RTA-2 follow different inheritance patterns. Infants with isolated autosomal-recessive RTA-2 exhibit short stature, ocular abnormalities (glaucoma, cataracts, band keratopathy), and mental retardation. Infants with isolated autosomal-dominant RTA-2 have only short stature as an associated abnormality. Growth retardation and rickets are observed in children with the Fanconi syndrome. Bone abnormalities typical of rickets include low stature caused by bowing deformity

Table 3 Features of the renal tubular acidosis (RTA) syndromes

Feature	Proximal RTA (RTA-2)	Distal RTA		
		Type 1 (classic)	Type 4	Voltage-defect
Plasma bicarbonate concentration	14–16 mmol/l	Variable, may be <10 mmol/l	15–20 mmol/l	15–20 mmol/l
Plasma chloride concentration	Increased	Increased	Increased	Increased
Plasma potassium concentration	Mildly decreased	Mildly to severely decreased	Mildly to severely increased	Mildly to severely increased
Plasma anion gap	Normal	Normal	Normal	Normal
Glomerular filtration rate	Normal or slightly decreased	Normal or slightly decreased	Normal to moderately decreased	Normal to moderately decreased
Urine pH during acidosis	<5.5	>6.0	<5.5	>5.5
Urine pH after acid loading	<5.5	>6.0	<5.5	>5.5
$(U - B)\ P\text{CO}_2$ in alkaline urine	Normal	Decreased	Decreased	Decreased
Fractional excretion of HCO_3^- at normal $[HCO_3^-]_p$	>15%	<5%	<5%	<5%
$T_{max}\ HCO_3^-$	Decreased	Normal	Normal	Normal
Nephrolithiasis	Absent	Present	Absent	Absent
Nephrocalcinosis	Absent	Present	Absent	Absent
Rickets/osteomalacia	Present	Present	Absent	Absent
Fanconi syndrome[a]	Usually present	Absent	Absent	Absent
Alkali therapy	High dose	Low dose	Low dose	Low dose

[a] This syndrome signifies generalized proximal tubule dysfunction and is characterized by impaired reabsorption of glucose, amino acids, phosphate, and urate in addition to the proximal acidification defect.

$T_{max}\ HCO_3^-$, maximum reabsorption of bicarbonate; $U - B\ P\text{CO}_2$, difference between partial pressure of carbon dioxide values in urine and arterial blood.

Table 4 Causes of proximal renal tubular acidosis (RTA-2)

Selective defect (isolated bicarbonate wasting)

- Primary (no obvious associated disease)
  - Genetically transmitted
  - Transient (infants)
- Due to altered carbonic anhydrase activity
  - Acetazolamide
  - Sulfanilamide
  - Mafenide acetate
  - Genetically transmitted
  - Idiopathic
  - Osteopetrosis with carbonic anhydrase II deficiency (Sly syndrome)
- York-Yendt syndrome
- Cyanotic congenital heart disease

Generalized defect (associated with multiple dysfunctions of the proximal tubule: Fanconi syndrome)

- Primary (no obvious associated disease)
  - Sporadic
  - Genetically transmitted
- Genetically transmitted systemic disease
  - Tyrosinaemia
  - Wilson's disease
  - Lowe disease
  - Hereditary fructose intolerance (during administration of fructose)
  - Cystinosis
  - Pyruvate carboxylate deficiency
  - Metachromatic leukodystrophy
  - Methylmalonic acidaemia
- Conditions associated with chronic hypocalcaemia and secondary hyperparathyroidism
  - Vitamin D deficiency or resistance
  - Vitamin D dependence
- Dysproteinaemic states
  - Multiple myeloma
  - Light chain disease
  - Monoclonal gammopathy
- Drug-or-toxin-induced
  - Outdated tetracycline
  - 3-Methylchromone
  - Streptozotocin
  - Lead
  - Mercury
  - Glue (toluene)
  - Arginine
  - Valproic acid
  - Gentamicin
  - Ifosfamide
- Tubulointerstitial disease
  - Renal transplantation
  - Sjögren's syndrome
  - Medullary cystic disease
- Other renal diseases
  - Nephrotic syndrome
  - Amyloidosis
- Miscellaneous
  - Paroxysmal nocturnal haemoglobinuria
  - Hyperparathyroidism
  - Bone fibroma
  - Severe burns

of the lower extremities with metaphyseal widening of the proximal and distal tibia, distal femur, the ulna, and the radius (Gregory and Schwartz 1998).

Cystinosis, an autosomal-recessive disorder characterized by cystine accumulation within cell lysosomes, is the most common cause of Fanconi syndrome in children. The typical clinical form presents in the first year of life with increased thirst, polyuria, and failure to thrive. Progressive renal disease usually develops leading to endstage renal failure by the end of the first decade of life. Children with severe cystinosis have cystine accumulation in multiple organs, including the brain, liver, pancreas, kidney, and muscle, and die before reaching adolescence (Gahl *et al.* 1988). The diagnosis is made by measuring the cystine content of peripheral leucocytes or by recognizing the characteristic corneal crystals on slit-lamp examination (see also Chapter 16.5).

Multiple myeloma is the most common cause of non-familial Fanconi syndrome in adults (Maldonado *et al.* 1975). Diagnosis of the plasma cell dyscrasia might be evident at the time of diagnosis of the Fanconi syndrome or might lag behind by several years. Other dysproteinaemic states, including light chain disease, benign monoclonal gammopathy, and amyloidosis associated with Bence Jones proteinuria can also cause the Fanconi syndrome. Additional causes include malignancies (Hodgkin's disease and other lymphomas, leukaemias), interstitial renal disease (including kidney transplant rejection and Sjögren's syndrome), and rarely nephrotic syndrome (Table 4). Patients with adult-onset Fanconi syndrome develop osteomalacia manifested by severe bone pain and spontaneous fractures.

Hyperparathyroidism, primary or secondary, might produce proximal tubule dysfunction but rarely clinically significant metabolic acidosis (Hulter and Peterson 1985). Although high levels of parathyroid hormone decrease proximal HCO_3^- reabsorption, this effect is counterbalanced by the skeletal release of alkali and the stimulation of renal acidification associated with hypercalcaemia. In patients with vitamin D deficiency, secondary hyperparathyroidism contributes to a Fanconi syndrome. Several drugs and toxins have been implicated as causes of generalized proximal tubule defect (Table 4). Disorders of carbohydrate metabolism (glycogen storage diseases, galactosaemia, hereditary fructose intolerance) and copper homeostasis (Wilson's disease) as well as inherited CA defects are additional causes of RTA-2 (Table 4).

Diagnosis

The diagnosis of untreated RTA-2 rests on the presence of persistent hyperchloraemic metabolic acidosis associated with a relatively normal GFR, a urine pH below 5.5 in an early morning specimen (freshly voided urine collected under mineral oil in the fasting state), and the rapid excretion of administered bicarbonate (Madias and Perrone 1993) (Table 3). Most patients have additional signs of proximal tubular dysfunction (i.e. hypophophataemia, hypouricaemia, renal glucosuria, aminoaciduria). Formal bicarbonate reabsorption studies or acid-loading tests are not indicated unless diagnosis cannot be established on the above criteria. Sodium bicarbonate loading can be done orally or by intravenous infusion. Assuming an apparent space of distribution of retained HCO_3^- of 50 per cent body weight, a load of 1 mmol/kg body weight would increase plasma $[HCO_3^-]$ by approximately 2 mmol/l. An oral $NaHCO_3$ load of 3 mmol/kg is ingested in the morning of the study along with 500 ml of water after an overnight fast. A baseline blood sample is obtained for measurements of pH, $P\text{CO}_2$, and plasma $[HCO_3^-]$. All urine specimens voided during a 5-h period following $NaHCO_3$ administration are collected and immediately analysed for pH, $P\text{CO}_2$, and $[HCO_3^-]$. In RTA-2, urine pH rapidly increases following the alkali load as a result of substantial bicarbonaturia (Paillard 1998). As distal acidification is intact, urinary $P\text{CO}_2$ measured after bicarbonate loading is normal exceeding 70 mmHg (see below, RTA-1). Evaluation of the fractional HCO_3^- excretion requires clearance studies (measurement of GFR) and intravenous infusion of $NaHCO_3$ to increase plasma $[HCO_3^-]$ to 26–28 mmol/l. This is accomplished by infusing $NaHCO_3$ at a rate calculated to increase plasma $[HCO_3^-]$ by 2–3 mmol/l/h. During the test, timed urine (bladder catheterization) and venous blood samples are collected. The fractional excretion of filtered HCO_3^- is calculated as follows:

$$FE_{HCO_3} = \frac{[HCO_3]_u \times P\text{inulin}}{[HCO_3]_p \times U\text{inulin}} \times 100$$

and generally exceeds 15 per cent in RTA-2 (Table 3).

Therapy

Correction of the metabolic acidosis with sustained alkali therapy is mandatory in infants and children to allow normal growth (impaired by acidosis) and correct metabolic bone disease in the form of rickets or osteomalacia (McSherry 1981) (Table 3). Adults with RTA-2 have a plasma $[HCO_3^-]$ of 18 mEq/l or greater and are usually free of bone disease. They might not require alkali administration. The high fractional excretion of HCO_3^- in RTA-2 requires high doses of alkali, in the order of 10–15 mEq/kg/day, to secure a relatively normal plasma $[HCO_3^-]$. Alkali are conveniently given as sodium and potassium citrate to compensate for the enhanced urinary potassium wasting associated with alkali therapy (Sebastian *et al.* 1971) (Table 5). Large doses of alkali are not always well tolerated, so that addition of a thiazide diuretic can be beneficial: extracellular fluid volume is contracted, proximal bicarbonate reabsorption enhanced, and bicarbonaturia lowered (Donckerwolcke *et al.* 1970). Phosphate and vitamin D supplementation is required in patients with Fanconi syndrome.

Distal renal tubular acidosis

Distal RTA refers to a group of disorders impairing distal tubular acidification; it is characterized by hyperchloraemic metabolic acidosis in association with reduced NAE. Three distinct forms of distal RTA are currently recognized (Table 3): (a) type I RTA (classic distal RTA or RTA-1) characterized by hypokalaemia and the inability to lower urinary pH to less than 5.5 (pH usually above 6.0) during spontaneous acidaemia or after acid loading; it usually arises from a defect in the collecting-duct H^+ pump; (b) type 4 RTA (RTA-4) characterized by hyperkalaemia, impaired renal ammoniagenesis, and the capacity to lower urinary pH below 5.5 during acidaemia or after acid loading; it usually results from aldosterone deficiency or aldosterone resistance (pseudohypoaldosteronism); and (c) voltage-defect distal RTA characterized by hyperkalaemia and the inability to lower urinary pH to less than 5.5 (Batlle *et al.* 1987); it is due to low sodium delivery or inhibition of sodium reabsorption in the collecting duct. In contrast with proximal RTA, the metabolic acidosis of all forms of distal RTA is successfully treated with a small dose of alkali.

Table 5 Preparations of alkali replacement with and without potassium

Trade name/composition	Alkali equivalency	Indications
Shohl solution Sodium citrate and citric acid	1 mmol of $NaHCO_3$/ml	RTA-1 and RTA-4
Baking soda	60 mmol $NaHCO_3$/teaspoonful	RTA-1 and RTA-4
$NaHCO_3$ tablets	≅4 mmol/325 mg tablet ≅8 mmol/650 mg tablet	RTA-1 and RTA-4
Bicitra Sodium citrate and citric acid	≅1 mmol of $NaHCO_3$/ml	RTA-1 and RTA-4
Polycitra (K-Shohl solution) Na^+ citrate, K^+ citrate, and citric acid	Each ml is equivalent to 2 mmol of alkali (1 mmol of $NaHCO_3$ and 1 mmol of $KHCO_3$)	RTA-1 and RTA-2
Polycitra crystals K^+ citrate and citric acid	30 mmol $KHCO_3$/packet	Calcium stones Persistent hypokalaemia in RTA-1 or RTA-2
Urocit-K tablets K^+ citrate	5 or 10 mmol $KHCO_3$/tablet	Calcium stones Persistent hypokalaemia in RTA-1 or RTA-2

Classic distal RTA (RTA-1)

Typical features of RTA-1 include inability to lower urinary pH to less than 5.5 despite hyperchloraemic metabolic acidosis and adequate natriuresis (urinary [Na^+] exceeding 25 mmol/l), decreased urinary ammonium excretion (evaluated by urine anion gap or urine osmolal gap), and urinary potassium wasting.

Pathophysiology

RTA-1 is most commonly the result of an impaired H^+ pump function in the distal nephron and a lowered urinary ammonium excretion (Batlle and Kurtzman 1982). Its causes, summarized in Table 2, include a genetically transmitted disease (e.g. sickle-cell anaemia), structural abnormalities (e.g. obstructive uropathy), immunologically mediated conditions (e.g. renal transplant rejection), and drugs or toxins (e.g. lithium, analgesics) (Batlle and Flores 1996). Amphotericin B toxicity is the only established cause of RTA-1 in which the underlying abnormality is a permeability defect. The mechanisms and molecular basis of the various clinical disorders associated with RTA-1 are depicted in Table 2. The end result of the acidification defect observed in RTA-1 is an impaired urinary ammonium excretion. The prevailing acid–base status is variable ranging from a normal blood acid–base composition in the absence of acid loading (incomplete RTA-1) to severe acidaemia with plasma [HCO_3^-] lower than 10 mmol/l (Table 3).

As pointed out earlier, potassium wasting and hypokalaemia in RTA-1 are caused by the combined effects of secondary hyperaldosteronism and the resulting negative luminal potential that obligates a higher K^+ secretion in the presence of defective distal H^+ secretion (electrical vacancy) (Kurtzman 2000). They are ameliorated by the alkali correction of metabolic acidosis.

Metabolic acidosis-associated buffering decreases bone carbonate content and causes net calcium loss. Bone calcium efflux reflects the additive effects of physicochemical dissolution, inhibition of osteoblastic bone formation, and stimulation of osteoclastic bone resorption. The more severe the acidaemia, the worse the bone calcium efflux. In addition, metabolic acidosis impairs the hydroxylation of 25 (OH) vitamin D_3 to 1,25 $(OH)_2$ vitamin D_3, thus decreasing intestinal calcium absorption as well as tubular reabsorption of calcium. The end result is hypercalciuria, negative calcium balance, and secondary hyperparathyroidism with an additive deleterious effects on the skeleton.

The renal wasting of calcium and phosphorous is responsible for the nephrolithiasis and nephrocalcinosis frequently observed in RTA-1 (Coe *et al.* 1992) (Table 3). This effect is aggravated by the high urine pH and the low levels of citrate excretion (metabolic acidosis stimulates proximal citrate reabsorption) (Norman *et al.* 1978; Seikaly *et al.* 1996). In a minority of cases, however, hypercalciuria is the primary defect initiating nephrocalcinosis and secondary RTA-1. Such hypercalciuria can result from a variety of disorders, including intestinal hyperabsorption of calcium, primary hyperparathyroidism, hypervitaminosis D, or hyperthyroidism. Impaired renal concentration can develop as a result of nephrocalcinosis or tubulointerstitial disease.

Clinical features and causes

The dominant clinical manifestations of RTA-1 generally emanate either from bone or skeletal muscle (Caruana and Buckalew 1988) (Table 3). Impaired growth and rickets are common in children. Osteomalacia is characteristic in adults. Skeletal muscle weakness, paresis, or paralysis involving the limbs and trunk, including the respiratory muscles, can be observed in response to severe hypokalaemia (Poux *et al.* 1992). Associated polyuria secondary to nephrogenic diabetes insipidus and electrocardiographic abnormalities might be observed. Other major clinical features are nephrolithiasis, nephrocalcinosis, and consequent renal failure (Buckalew 1989). Variable degrees of volume depletion are encountered.

A large number of conditions, either primary (hereditary or sporadic) or acquired, can lead to RTA-1 (Table 6). Many have distinct clinical features superimposed on those strictly dependent on the distal acidification defect. The primary forms of RTA-1 are uncommon and occur in infants and children. Autosomal-recessive RTA-1 generally expresses itself in infants of families with parental consanguinity. Main features include severe growth impairment, mental retardation, deafness, rickets, pathological fractures, and hypokalaemia-induced muscle disease. Renal calculi, nephrocalcinosis, and secondary renal

Table 6 Causes of classic distal renal tubular acidosis (RTA-1)

Primary (no obvious associated disease)
Sporadic
Genetically transmitted
Autoimmune disorders
Hypergammaglobulinaemia
Hyperglobulinaemic purpura
Cryoglobulinaemia
Familial
Sjögren's syndrome
Thyroiditis
Pulmonary fibrosis
Chronic active hepatitis
Primary biliary cirrhosis
Systemic lupus erythematosus
HIV nephropathy
Vasculitis
Genetically transmitted systemic disease
Ehlers–Danlos syndrome
Hereditary elliptocytosis
Sickle-cell anaemia
Marfan syndrome
Carbonic anhydrase I deficiency or alteration
Osteopetrosis with carbonic anhydrase II deficiency (Sly syndrome)
Medullary cystic disease
Neuroaxonal dystrophy
Disorders associated with hypercalciuria and nephrocalcinosis
Primary or familial hyperparathyroidism
Vitamin D intoxication
Milk-alkali syndrome
Hyperthyroidism
Idiopathic hypercalciuria
Genetically transmitted
Sporadic
Hereditary fructose intolerance (after chronic fructose ingestion)
Medullary sponge kidney
Fabry's disease
Wilson's disease
Drug or toxin-induced
Amphotericin B
Toluene ('glue sniffing')
Analgesics
Lithium
Cyclamate
Vanadate
Ifosfamide
Foscarnet
Balkan nephropathy
Tubulointerstitial diseases
Chronic pyelonephritis
Obstructive uropathy
Renal transplantation
Leprosy
Hyperoxaluria
Miscellaneous
Hepatic cirrhosis
Empty sella syndrome

failure can be prominent. Autosomal-dominant RTA-1 generally manifests in childhood and leads to a milder syndrome than the autosomal-recessive form.

In some infants and young children (up to 6 years old) RTA-1 can feature renal bicarbonate wasting that resembles RTA-2, a syndrome previously referred to as type 3 or mixed RTA (Rodriguez Soriano 2002). At present, it is felt that the substantial bicarbonaturia is a feature of RTA-1 occurring at an early age, which then vanishes by age 4–6 years. Mixed RTA due to delayed renal maturation is seen during the first week of life in infants born with very low body weight. A persistent mixed RTA is observed in patients with CA II deficiency (Nagai *et al.* 1997).

In adults, RTA-1 is most commonly due to autoimmune disorders (e.g. Sjögren's syndrome), other causes including hypercalciuria/nephrocalcinosis, tubulointerstitial diseases, and drugs or toxins. Up to 50 per cent of patients with Sjögren's syndrome and hyperglobulinaemic purpura develop acquired RTA-1, which commonly presents with muscle dysfunction caused by profound hypokalaemia. RTA-1 secondary to hypercalciuria, such as in hyperparathyroidism, vitamin D intoxication, and milk-alkali syndrome, is usually associated with nephrocalcinosis. Transient RTA-2 occurs often immediately following renal transplantation, whereas RTA-1 can develop months to years after engraftment (e.g. chronic cellular rejection).

Incomplete RTA-1 is characterized by an impaired ability to lower urinary pH to less than 5.5 in response to acid loading but a normal acid–base balance sustained by a normal or only slightly reduced urinary ammonium excretion (Buckalew *et al.* 1968). This entity, described with both hereditary and acquired RTA-1, is sometimes recognized in patients evaluated for nephrolithiasis or nephrocalcinosis. Associated features include hypercalciuria, low urinary citrate excretion, and a family history of full-blown RTA-1.

Diagnosis

Hyperchloraemia together with low plasma [HCO_3^-] and hypokalaemia is consistent with the diagnosis of RTA-1, RTA-2, diarrhoea, chronic respiratory alkalosis, and other disorders (Table 7). The history, physical examination, and arterial blood gases help to rule out respiratory alkalosis (Adrogué and Madias 1998b). When RTA is the most likely diagnosis, evaluation of the response to sodium bicarbonate loading may be required to differentiate RTA-1 from RTA-2. The fractional excretion of bicarbonate is less than 5 per cent in RTA-1, but typically more than 15 per cent in RTA-2 (Table 3). Urinary pH values exceeding 6.0 in association with acidaemia are characteristic of RTA-1. Yet, the presence of bacteriuria or urinary tract infection can confound interpretation of urinary pH measurements as bacterial urease decomposes urea into NH_3 and increases the urinary pH. In the presence of urinary tract infection, urine stasis must be prevented by ensuring high urine flow, bactericidal agents must be added to the container, and urine samples must be analysed promptly after collection (Madias and Perrone 1993).

Urinary NH_4^+ excretion helps determine whether the acidosis is of renal or extrarenal origin; if extrarenal (e.g. diarrhoea), the urine is rich in ammonium. As most clinical laboratories do not measure it, urinary NH_4^+ can be estimated by calculating the urinary anion gap (the sum of sodium plus potassium minus chloride concentrations), which is an approximate index of urinary [NH_4^+] because its accompanying anion is largely chloride (Goldstein *et al.* 1986; Batlle *et al.* 1988). Consequently, in metabolic acidosis of extrarenal origin, the

Table 7 Conditions associated with hyperchloraemia and low plasma $[HCO_3^-]$

Chronic respiratory alkalosis
Bicarbonate (or potential HCO_3^-) wasting Diarrhoea Drainage/fistulas from small bowel, pancreas, bile ducts Ureterosigmoidostomy Renal ketone losses Drugs Calcium chloride Magnesium sulfate Cholestyramine
Acid gain Hyperalimentation Ammonium chloride Arginine hydrochloride Lysine hydrochloride Methionine sulfate
Renal tubular acidosis Proximal (RTA-2) Classic distal (RTA-1) RTA-4 Voltage-defect distal RTA
Dilutional acidosis
Metabolic acidosis of mild to moderate renal insufficiency

urinary anion gap exceeds −50 mmol/l (NH_4^+ representing the missing cation). When NH_4^+ excretion is impaired and urinary NH_4^+ levels are low, the urinary anion gap has a positive or only mildly negative value; this finding is characteristic of all forms of distal RTA. Interpretation of the urine anion gap is confounded if large quantities of bicarbonate or other organic anions (e.g. ketoanions) are present in the urine (Adrogué *et al.* 1984). An alternative method to estimate urinary NH_4^+ that is not significantly affected by the presence of ketonuria is the assessment of the urine osmolal gap (difference between measured and calculated osmolality) (Halperin 1995), as follows:

$$\text{urine osmolal gap} = \text{measured osmolality} - \text{calculated osmolality}$$

$$\text{calculated osmolality} = 2([Na^+] + [K^+]) + \text{urea} + \text{glucose}$$

$$\text{urinary } NH_4^+ = 0.5 \times \text{urine osmolal gap}$$

Each of the above urinary solutes is expressed in millimoles per litre.

The urine-minus-blood $P\text{CO}_2$—$(U - B)$ $P\text{CO}_2$—following an $NaHCO_3$ infusion (500 mmol/l infused at 3 ml/min) is helpful to establish the presence of a distal acidification defect (DuBose 1982). Secretion of H^+ in the distal nephron in the presence of high urinary $[HCO_3^-]$ forms carbonic acid followed by the slow release of CO_2 (absence of luminal CA in this nephron segment) and the subsequent generation of a high urinary $P\text{CO}_2$ in the CO_2 impermeable urinary tract. The magnitude of the $(U - B)$ $P\text{CO}_2$ is quantitatively related to distal nephron H^+ secretion. After 2–4 h of infusion, urinary pH exceeds 7.50 and the $(U - B)$ $P\text{CO}_2$ gradient rises above 20–30 mm Hg if distal acidification is normal. By contrast, virtually all patients with distal RTA, including incomplete RTA-1 but not amphotericin B-induced RTA-1, cannot generate a normal $(U - B)$ $P\text{CO}_2$ gradient (Halperin *et al.* 1974) (Table 3). In amphotericin B-induced RTA-1, urine $P\text{CO}_2$ rises normally because distal H^+ secretion remains intact, the acidification defect being due to backleak of H^+ (permeability defect).

An alternative test for the diagnosis of distal RTA in patients without spontaneous metabolic acidosis is the response to an acid load that reduces the plasma $[HCO_3^-]$ by 4–5 mmol/l. A single dose of NH_4Cl (100 mg/kg body weight dissolved in water) is ingested and sequential urine samples are collected over 6 h. The plasma $[HCO_3^-]$ is measured prior to and 3 h after the acid load to secure that its level has decreased by the amount noted above. Normally, urinary pH falls below 5.5; this response does not occur in RTA-1 (Table 3). When NH_4Cl loading is contraindicated (e.g. risk of hepatic encephalopathy), the alternative acid load is $CaCl_2$ (1 mmol/kg); it represents an HCl load because alkali binding in the intestinal lumen forms insoluble $CaCO_3$ and soluble HCl.

Other tests of distal acidification include the response to frusemide administration and the response to the infusion of neutral phosphate (Vallo and Rodriguez Soriano 1984). Frusemide (40–80 mg orally) given to normal individuals reduces urinary pH as a result of an increased delivery of NaCl to the distal nephron (Alvarado *et al.* 1991). Patients with RTA-1 (H^+-pump defect) fail to develop a normal response. Similarly, patients with RTA-1 do not properly lower urinary pH after sodium sulfate infusion. Administration of sodium with a non-reabsorbable anion, such as sodium sulfate, to sodium-avid subjects with normal distal acidification markedly lowers urinary pH and augments acid excretion (Morris *et al.* 1965).

The cause of the patient's hypokalaemia, whether renal or extrarenal, must be determined; the former is accompanied by urinary K^+ wasting, whereas the latter by urinary K^+ conservation. The ability of the cortical collecting tubule to secrete K^+ and maintain K^+ balance can be evaluated by the measurement of the fractional K^+ excretion or by the calculation of the transtubular potassium concentration gradient (TTKG) (Ethier *et al.* 1990). TTKG estimates the $[K^+]$ gradient between the lumen of the cortical collecting tubule and the peritubular capillaries. It relies on two assumptions: first, the osmolality of the luminal fluid at the end of the cortical collecting tubule is identical to that of plasma; and second, the medullary collecting duct does not transport K^+ in either direction. Consequently, the higher $[K^+]$ in final urine as compared with that of the cortical collecting tubule is due to water reabsorption from the medullary collecting duct. Dividing the urine $[K^+]$ by the ratio of the urine to plasma osmolality estimates the $[K^+]$ in the lumen of the cortical collecting tubule, and thus the TTKG, as follows:

$$\text{TTKG} = \frac{[K^+]_u/[K^+]_p}{U_{\text{OSM}}/P_{\text{OSM}}}$$

In normal K^+-replete subjects, the TTKG is approximately 6–9. It decreases to lower values in states of K^+ depletion if the renal response of K^+ conservation is appropriate. The finding of a TTKG in excess of 9 in hypokalaemia caused by K^+ depletion is indicative of renal K^+ wasting.

Therapy

Whenever feasible, management of RTA-1 should focus on the treatment of the underlying disorder (Rodriguez Soriano 2002). Otherwise, therapy centres on the administration of alkali to achieve a plasma [HCO_3^-] of 22–24 mmol/l. A dosage of approximately 1–2 mmol/kg/day is generally required in adults with RTA-1 to overcome the inability to excrete quantitatively the endogenous acid load and any element of bicarbonate wasting that might be present (Table 3). Young children might require 4–8 mmol/kg/day or even higher doses of alkali because urinary bicarbonate losses might be substantial. As children with the previously referred type 3 or mixed RTA mature, the bicarbonate wasting defect fades away and only the RTA-1 component persists. Alkali therapy should be maintained indefinitely, unless RTA-1 wanes with successful treatment or elimination of the underlying disorder.

Untreated patients with RTA-1, occasionally present with metabolic acidosis of extreme severity (i.e. plasma [HCO_3^-] < 5 mmol/l), profound hypokalaemia, and volume depletion (Adrogué and Madias 1998a). If respiratory failure prevents ventilatory adaptation or, worse, leads to CO_2 retention, severe acidaemia might ensue reflecting mixed metabolic and respiratory acidosis; in such cases, mechanical ventilation may be required. As acidosis correction with alkali worsens the hypokalaemia, potassium should be given prior to alkali administration. Potassium wasting is usually ameliorated by acidosis treatment because repair of the ECF volume deficit ameliorates the prevailing secondary hyperaldosteronism. However, as indicated above, early in the course of alkali therapy, plasma [K^+] can further decrease requiring substantial K^+ replacement.

Alkali therapy allows the resumption of normal growth in children and the correction of bone disease in adults (McSherry 1981). Urinary calcium excretion is reduced while urinary citrate excretion increases with an attendant improvement of nephrocalcinosis and of the risk of new stone formation (Brenner *et al.* 1982). Available products for therapy are listed in Table 5. Oral sodium citrate and citric acid contained in Shohl solution and Bicitra are usually well tolerated bicarbonate precursors. Most patients with RTA-1 do not require long-term K^+ supplementation; however, preparations of potassium citrate alone or with sodium citrate are indicated for persistent hypokalaemia (Table 5). In the presence of calcium stones, potassium citrate rather than sodium citrate should be administered, because the latter increases calciuria, thereby, promoting stone formation (Preminger *et al.* 1985). Alkali therapy with Na^+-containing preparations might result in oedema formation that can be managed with dietary NaCl restriction and diuretics.

Table 8 Causes of type 4 renal tubular acidosis (RTA-4)

Deficiency of aldosterone
Associated with glucocorticoid deficiency
Addison's disease
Adrenalectomy (bilateral)
Adrenal haemorrhage or carcinoma (bilateral)
Enzymatic defects
21-Hydroxylase deficiency
3-β-ol-Dehydrogenase deficiency
Desmolase deficiency
HIV nephropathy
Isolated aldosterone deficiency
Deficient renin secretion
(hyporeninaemic hypoaldosteronism)
Diabetic nephropathy
Tubulointerstitial renal disease
Nonsteroidal anti-inflammatory drugs
β-Adrenergic blockers
HIV nephropathy
Renal transplantation (early)
Obstructive uropathy
Amyloidosis
Multiple myeloma
Sickle cell nephropathy
Systemic lupus erythematosus
Normal or high renin secretion
Genetically transmitted
Corticosterone methyloxidase deficiency
Transient (infants)
Heparin therapy
Angiotensin-II-converting enzyme inhibitors
AT_1 receptor antagonists
Resistance to aldosterone action
Spironolactone
Pseudohypoaldosteronism type I—autosomal dominant (with salt wasting)

Type 4 RTA (RTA-4)

RTA-4 is a generalized distal nephron dysfunction characterized by hyperkalaemia associated with hyperchloraemic metabolic acidosis, a decreased NH_4^+ excretion and a urinary pH below 5.5 during acidaemia or after acid loading (DuBose 1997). The most common cause of RTA-4 encountered in clinical practice is mineralocorticoid (largely aldosterone) deficiency or resistance (pseudohypoaldosteronism) (Table 8). Hyporeninaemic hypoaldosteronism secondary to diabetes mellitus is distinctly frequent (DeFronzo 1980). The mechanisms and molecular basis of RTA-4 have been described in Table 2.

Pathophysiology

K^+ retention and hyperkalaemia are due to the lack of appropriate renal effects of aldosterone and, in turn, largely account for the decreased ammoniagenesis and ammonium excretion. Although aldosterone stimulates distal acidification, the defect in K^+ excretion is the main determinant of the hyperchloraemic metabolic acidosis of RTA-4. Indeed, correction of hyperkalaemia largely repairs the defect in NAE. The H^+ pump function and cellular membrane integrity are maintained, as evidenced by the capacity to lower urinary pH below 5.5 and a normal reduction of urinary pH in response to infusion of neutral phosphate or sulfate. However, urinary NH_4^+ and K^+ excretion in response to sodium sulfate infusion are reduced and the $(U - B)$ $P\text{CO}_2$ is decreased in akaline urine. Potassium retention is the dominant mechanism of impaired acidification in RTA-4 through the inhibition of NH_3/NH_4^+ production and excretion.

Mineralocorticoid deficiency is either a primary defect (impaired aldosterone production due to complete adrenal gland destruction, resection, damage limited to the zona glomerulosa, or enzymatic defects) or the result of reduced angiotensin II stimulation (hyporeninaemic hypoaldosteronism). Destruction of the adrenal cortex causes Addison's disease with both mineralocorticoid and glucocorticoid deficiencies. RTA-4 and renal salt wasting in Addison's disease result from aldosterone deficiency, whereas, weight loss, weakness, and hypoglycaemia are caused by glucocorticoid deficiency.

Congenital adrenal enzymatic defects, 21-hydroxylase deficiency being the most common, lead to combined glucocorticoid and mineralocorticoid deficiencies. In 21-hydroxylase deficiency, steroid synthesis is rerouted towards androgen synthesis and accounts for the development of an adrenogenital syndrome (premature virilization in males and ambiguous genitalia in females). Isolated mineralocorticoid deficiency can be idiopathic, familial, or caused by long-term heparin administration (Oster *et al.* 1995). Most patients with a primary mineralocorticoid deficiency have high plasma renin as a result of volume contraction, whereas, a low plasma renin activity is observed in hyporeninaemic hypoaldosteronism; in the latter group, decreased renin secretion and angiotensin II production lead to aldosterone deficiency. The underlying defect in hyporeninaemic hypoaldosteronism might reflect pharmacological inhibition of renin, volume expansion, specific damage of the juxtaglomerular apparatus, or generalized renal disease.

Diabetes mellitus is the most common cause of RTA-4. The determinants of this low-renin condition include damage (vascular disease) or dennervation (neuropathy) of the juxtaglomerular apparatus, production of inactive renin (known as 'big renin'), reduction of renal prostaglandin synthesis (with secondary impairment in renin secretion), aldosterone synthetic defects, and diminished overall renal function. Patients with hyporeninaemic hypoaldosteronism caused by diabetes mellitus and associated mild renal insufficiency develop asymptomatic hyperkalaemia; only half of them also feature hyperchloraemic metabolic acidosis.

Resistance to aldosterone action includes the administration of spironolactone (a competitive inhibitor of aldosterone) and pseudohypoaldosteronism type I—autosomal dominant (Table 8). The latter condition is characterized by renal-salt wasting, hypotension, RTA-4, and high renin and aldosterone levels.

Clinical features and causes

RTA-4 is most commonly observed in patients with diabetic nephropathy or interstitial nephritis and mild to moderate renal insufficiency, as well as those with primary adrenocortical insufficiency (Table 8). Relevant laboratory findings include clinically significant hyperkalaemia, mild hyperchloraemic metabolic acidosis ($[HCO_3^-]_p$ 15–20 mmol/l), and an appropriately acidic urine pH (Table 3). In contrast to aldosterone deficiency, patients with aldosterone resistance have normal or elevated plasma aldosterone.

Diagnosis

The diagnosis of RTA-4 is established in the presence of hyperkalaemia, hyperchloraemic metabolic acidosis, and a urinary pH less than 5.5. The diagnostic workup involves an evaluation of urinary K^+ excretion (as explained below), urinary NH_4^+ excretion (urinary anion or osmolar gap), and measurement of plasma renin activity, aldosterone, and cortisol. Demonstration of a low $(U - B)$ $P\text{CO}_2$ after alkali infusion establishes that a defect in distal acidification is present. Plasma aldosterone and cortisol measurements allow differentiation among combined glucocorticoid and mineralocorticoid deficiency, selective aldosterone deficiency, and aldosterone resistance (Table 8). Detection of normal plasma cortisol combined with a low aldosterone level establishes the diagnosis of selective aldosterone deficiency, a much more common condition than Addison's disease (combined glucocorticoid and mineralocorticoid deficiency). Because increased plasma $[K^+]$ stimulates aldosterone secretion, elevated aldosterone levels are usually observed in patients with aldosterone resistance. Occasionally, patients with aldosterone deficiency can have urine pH values exceeding 5.5 during spontaneous acidosis or acid loading, because of the simultaneous presence of a voltage-dependent defect (see below).

The TTKG is useful for assessing the appropriateness of the renal response in a hyperkalaemic patient (West *et al.* 1986). The TTKG is approximately 6–9 on a regular diet, but exceeds 11 following a potassium load in normal subjects. In a hyperkalaemic patient, a value below 6 suggests an abnormal renal response, whereas, a value below 5 is clearly abnormal. A reliable TTKG requires a concentrated urine (U_{OSM} higher than P_{OSM}) and a urinary sodium above 25 mmol/l.

Treatment

The severity of hyperkalaemia determines the need for therapy; elimination of K^+ retention tends to correct the RTA-4. Management of RTA-4 should focus on the identification of the underlying disorder as well as factors precipitating K^+ retention (DuBose and McDonald 2002). The patient's history with regard to K^+ intake and medication potentially leading to K^+ retention or metabolic acidosis must be investigated. Other precipitating factors include uncontrolled hyperglycaemia, volume depletion, and acute oliguric renal failure. A low K^+ intake should be prescribed and salt substitutes (K^+ salts) avoided. Potassium retaining medications, including angiotensin-converting enzyme inhibitors, AT1-receptor blockers, non-steroidal anti-inflammatory drugs, K^+-sparing diuretics (amiloride, triamterene, spironolactone), trimethoprim, and pentamidine, must be discontinued.

Patients with combined glucocorticoid and mineralocorticoid deficiency require replacement therapy. In these patients, as well as in those with selective mineralocorticoid deficiency, volume expansion, hypertension, and hypokalaemia can result from mineralocorticoid replacement (fludrocortisone, 0.1–0.3 mg/day). In the absence of a treatable primary disorder, therapy should increase distal Na^+ delivery to promote H^+ and K^+ excretion. In patients with diabetic nephropathy a higher NaCl intake (if tolerated) coupled with diuretic therapy (frusemide, bumetanide) generally overcomes the electrolyte disorder (Sebastian *et al.* 1984). Potassium exchange resins—sodium polystyrene sulfonate or Kayexalate—and alkali administration are necessary in some patients. As noted, mineralocorticoid administration, although effective, can precipitate sizable fluid retention, congestive heart failure, and hypertension. Mineralocorticoids are thus best avoided but, if necessary, they should be combined with loop diuretics. Patients with pseudohypoaldosteronism type I might respond to sodium supplements and K^+-binding resins.

Voltage-defect distal RTA

This condition is characterized by hyperchloraemic metabolic acidosis and hyperkalaemia. It is caused by decreased NaCl reabsorption in the collecting duct, secondary to either reduced NaCl delivery or inhibition of NaCl reabsorption in the principal cells. As a result, the lumen-negative transepithelial voltage decreases and both K^+ and H^+ secretion are inhibited. Hyperkalaemia, hyperchloraemic metabolic acidosis, and inability to decrease urinary pH below 5.5 ensue. The mechanisms and molecular basis of this form of distal RTA are depicted in Table 2.

Pathophysiology

A drastic reduction in distal sodium delivery with urine $[Na^+]$ less than 25 mmol/l (e.g. in severe volume depletion) or an impaired distal Na^+ transport reduces the lumen-negative potential of the collecting duct

(Golding 1975). Such a voltage defect is observed in pseudohypoaldosteronism type I—autosomal recessive, pseudohypoaldosteronism type II or Gordon's syndrome; in response to drugs that impair function of Na^+ channels (e.g. amiloride, triamterene, trimethoprim, pentamidine) or Na^+,K^+-ATPase (e.g. cyclosporin A); and in tubulointerstitial renal disease (e.g. obstructive nephropathy). Mutations with loss of Na^+ channels function in the apical membrane of principal cells of cortical collecting duct account for the voltage-defect RTA observed in pseudohypoaldosteronism type I—autosomal recessive. By contrast, a defect that accelerates distal nephron NaCl reabsorption and reduces or eliminates the lumen-negative voltage, thereby, decreasing K^+ and H^+ secretion, is observed in patients with Gordon's syndrome. This defect is termed 'chloride shunt' (Schambelan *et al.* 1981; Take *et al.* 1991).

Clinical features and causes

Diarrhoea with severe extracellular volume depletion, cirrhosis with ascites, or severe nephrotic syndrome reduce distal Na^+ delivery and lead to voltage-defect distal RTA (Table 9). The full-blown syndrome becomes apparent in the presence of a mild to moderate renal insufficiency. Pseudohypoaldosteronism type I—autosomal recessive—results in a salt-losing nephropathy. The Gordon's syndrome, by contrast, is characterized by NaCl retention, volume expansion, hypertension, and low to normal renin and aldosterone levels (Gordon 1986). Voltage-dependent defects due to drugs might be associated with the clinical features of the process responsible for the use of the drug (e.g. immunodeficiency syndrome). Tubulointerstitial disease can also lead to voltage-defect RTA as a result of impaired distal Na^+ reabsorption despite adequate sodium delivery and sufficiently high luminal $[Na^+]$ (in excess of 25 mmol/l) (Batlle *et al.* 1981).

Diagnosis

The diagnostic approach of RTA-4 applies to voltage-defect RTA. The patient's familial history can suggest that the voltage-defect RTA is inherited (e.g. a child with renal-salt wasting caused by pseudohypoaldosteronism type I—autosomal recessive, or an adult with hypertension caused by Gordon's syndrome). An acquired voltage-defect RTA is suggested by the use of certain drugs (amiloride, triamterene, pentamidine, trimethoprim). The possibility of tubulointerstitial renal disease should be investigated. Detection of a persistently elevated urinary pH in a patient with hyperkalaemic distal RTA indicates either low distal sodium delivery or impaired sodium transport (Batlle *et al.* 1987). Patients with a voltage-dependent defect have a urine pH greater than 5.5, a low $(U - B)$ $P\text{CO}_2$ with bicarbonate loading, and an abnormal acidification response to sulfate or frusemide administration.

Table 9 Causes of voltage-defect distal RTA

Decreased distal sodium delivery	Impaired distal sodium reabsorption
Diarrhoea with severe volume contraction	Pseudohypoaldosteronism type I—autosomal recessive
Advanced cirrhosis	Pseudohypoaldosteronism type II—Gordon's syndrome[a]
Severe nephrotic syndrome	Drugs impairing function of:
	Na^+ channels
	Amiloride
	Triamterene
	Trimethoprim
	Pentamidine
	Na^+,K^+-ATPase
	Cyclosporin A
	Tubulointerstitial renal disease
	Systemic lupus erythematosus
	Methicillin nephrotoxicity
	Obstructive nephropathy
	Kidney transplant rejection
	Sickle-cell disease

[a] Voltage-defect is presumed to be caused by increased chloride reabsorption in the distal tubule (chloride shunt).

Therapy

Voltage-defect RTA secondary to low distal Na^+ delivery requires NaCl repletion in low volume states (e.g. diarrhoea) or the administration of loop diuretics in conditions associated with fluid retention (e.g. congestive heart failure). Discontinuation of causal drugs reverses the electrolyte disorder. Patients with pseudohypoaldosteronism type I—autosomal recessive—should receive NaCl supplementation, whereas, those with Gordon's syndrome should receive a salt-restricted diet and thiazides.

Dietary K^+ restriction must be enforced in all patients with hyperkalaemic RTA, as K^+ retention and hyperkalaemia aggravate metabolic acidosis. Other therapeutic measures depend on the cause of voltage-defect RTA and can include alkali therapy, correction of extracellular fluid volume (if expanded, with the use of diuretics), and alkali therapy.

Simplified diagnostic approach to RTA (Tables 10 and 11)

A plasma electrolyte pattern of hyperchloraemia and hypobicarbonataemia is suggestive of RTA. If it persists and is accompanied by hyperkalaemia, the likelihood of hyperkalaemic RTA becomes substantial (Table 10). However, if serum $[K^+]$ is normal or low, conditions other than RTA are more likely, such as respiratory alkalosis or metabolic acidosis due to diarrhoea or other conditions (Adrogué and Madias 1995) (Table 11). The diagnosis of RTA cannot be established with certainty in acutely ill patients, in whom multiple alterations of fluid volume and composition might commonly lead to an electrolyte pattern resembling RTA. Persistence of high chloride and low plasma bicarbonate with acidaemia after restoration of plasma volume and the correction of extrarenal losses of alkali is consistent with a diagnosis of true RTA (Table 11). Patients in the recovery phase of diabetic ketoacidosis frequently develop a hyperchloraemic metabolic acidosis that resembles RTA but is caused by the renal loss of ketone salts (Adrogué *et al.* 1982).

A urinary pH persistently higher than 5.5 in a patient with hyperchloraemic metabolic acidosis and hypokalaemia who is not receiving alkali therapy, likely suggests RTA-1. The distal acidification defect can be confirmed by the failure of urinary $P\text{CO}_2$ to increase by at least 20–30 mmHg above that in arterial blood during bicarbonate infusion. Amphotericin B-induced RTA-1 is the only condition in which $(U - B)$ $P\text{CO}_2$ rises normally. Patients with incomplete RTA-1 have a similar abnormally low $(U - B)$ $P\text{CO}_2$ but urinary pH remains below 5.5. Conversely, if urinary pH is persistently lower than 5.5, alkali infusion can help establish the presence of RTA-2 by its prompt and

Table 10 Diagnostic approach to hyperchloraemia, hypobicarbonataemia, and hyperkalaemia

History, physical examination, ancillary studies	
Two or more disorders explain the electrolyte pattern (electrolyte disturbance is transient)	High $[K^+]_p$: K^+ loading, rhabdomyolysis, renal failure High $[Cl^-]$ and low $[HCO_3^-]_p$: intravenous saline infusion, respiratory alkalosis, diarrhoea, fistulas
A single disorder explains the electrolyte pattern (electrolyte disturbance is persistent)	RTA is likely: measure blood pH to document acidaemia present (not always required)
Urinary pH	
>5.5 (rule out infection with urea-splitting organisms)	Voltage-defect distal RTA likely: document a low urinary NH_4^+ with urinary anion gap/osmolar gap
Urinary $[Na^+] < 25$ mmol/l	Advanced cirrhosis, severe diarrhoea
Urinary $[Na^+] > 25$ mmol/l	Drugs (triamterene, pentamidine, trimethoprim, amiloride) Obstructive uropathy (renal ultrasound) Other causes
<5.5	RTA-4 is likely: document a low urinary NH_4^+ with urinary anion gap/osmolar gap
Diabetic nephropathy present	Hyporeninaemic hypoaldosteronism is likely: can be confirmed with serum hormonal levels
Diabetic nephropathy absent	
Low-plasma aldosterone with normal cortisol	Selective aldosterone deficiency
Low-plasma aldosterone and cortisol	Adrenal insufficiency, adrenogenital syndromes (congenital enzymatic defects)
Normal- or high-plasma aldosterone	Aldosterone resistance
Response to alkali load	
Slow elimination with fractional excretion <5% and decreased $(U - B)$ $P\text{CO}_2$ response	RTA-4 or hyperkalaemic distal RTA (this test is frequently not performed)
Urinary K^+ excretion	Low TTKG or fractional K^+ excretion observed in RTA-4 and voltage-defect distal RTA

Table 11 Diagnostic approach to hyperchloraemia, hypobicarbonataemia, and normal/low serum K^+ levels

History, physical examination, ancillary studies	
Two or more disorders explain the electrolyte pattern (electrolyte disturbance is transient)	Low $[K^+]_p$: stress hypokalaemia (β-adrenergic activation), negative K^+ balance High $[Cl^-]_p$ and low $[HCO_3^-]_p$: intravenous saline infusion, respiratory alkalosis, diarrhoea, fistulas
A single disorder explains the electrolyte pattern (electrolyte disturbance is persistent)	RTA is likely: measure blood pH to document acidaemia present (not always required especially when $[HCO_3^-]_p$ is below 15 mmol/l)
Significant acidaemia present (pH < 7.35)	
Urinary pH > 5.5 (rule out infection with urea-splitting organisms)	RTA-1 is likely: document a low urinary NH_4^+ with urinary anion gap/osmolar gap
Urinary pH < 5.5	RTA-2 is likely
Response to alkali load	
Rapid elimination with fractional excretion > 15% and normal $(U - B)$ $P\text{CO}_2$ response	RTA-2 (all elements of the response are not always evaluated)
Slow elimination with fractional excretion < 5% and decreased $(U - B)$ $P\text{CO}_2$ response	RTA-1 (all elements of the response are not always evaluated)
Significant acidaemia absent (pH > 7.35)	
Acid-loading test abnormal	RTA-1 is likely
Acid-loading test normal	RTA-2 is likely
Urinary K^+ excretion	High TTKG or fractional K^+ excretion with hypokalaemia observed in RTA-1
Urinary excretion of glucose, amino acids, phosphate, and urate	High exretion in RTA-2 with Fanconi syndrome

almost complete excretion while the initial hyperchloraemic hypobicarbonataemia remains largely unmitigated; in RTA-1, retention of a significant fraction of the alkali load corrects partially or fully (yet temporarily) the hyperchloraemic acidosis.

Patients with borderline hyperchloraemic metabolic acidosis are best evaluated by an acid loading test. Urinary pH falls below 5.5 in RTA-2 but not in RTA-1. The urine anion (or osmolar) gap contributes to the diagnosis of distal RTA. Detection of other clinical or laboratory derangements in the patient under evaluation can help establish the underlying disease responsible for the RTA.

References

(Entries marked with an asterisk comprise useful general reading.)

Adrogué, H. J. and Madias, N. E. Mixed acid–base disorders. In *The Principles and Practices of Nephrology* (ed. H. R. Jacobson, G. E. Striker, and S. Klahr), pp. 953–962. Philadelphia: B. C. Decker, 1995.

*__Adrogué, H .J. and Madias, N. E.__ (1998a). Management of life-threatening acid–base disorders. (First of two parts.) *New England Journal of Medicine* **338**, 26–34.

Adrogué, H. J. and Madias, N. E. Arterial blood gas monitoring: acid–base assessment. In *Principles and Practice of Intensive Care Monitoring* (ed. M. J. Tobin), pp. 217–241. New York: McGraw-Hill, Inc., 1998b.

Adrogué, H. J. and Madias, N. E. Disorders of acid–base balance. In *Atlas of Diseases of the Kidney* (ed. T. Berl and J. V. Bonventre), pp. 6.20–6.28. Boston: Current Medicine, Blackwell Science, 1999.

Adrogué, H. J., Eknoyan, E., and Suki, W. N. (1984). Diabetic ketoacidosis: role of the kidney in acid–base homeostasis re-evaluated. *Kidney International* **25**, 591–598.

*__Adrogué, H. J.__ *et al.* (1982). Plasma acid–base patterns in diabetic ketoacidosis. *New England Journal of Medicine* **307**, 1603–1610.

Akiba, T. *et al.* (1986). Electrogenic sodium/bicarbonate cotransport in rabbit renal cortical basolateral membrane vesicles. *Journal of Clinical Investigation* **78**, 1472–1478.

Alappan, R., Perazella, M. A., and Buller, G. K. (1986). Hyperkalaemia in hospitalized patients treated with trimethoprim-sulfamethoxazole. *Annals of Internal Medicine* **124**, 316–320.

Alpern, R. J. (1990). Cell mechanisms of proximal tubule acidification. *Physiological Reviews* **70**, 79–114.

Alpern, R. J. Renal acidification mechanisms. In *The Kidney* 6th edn. (ed. B. M. Brenner), pp. 455–519. Philadelphia: W. B. Saunders, 2000.

Alpern, R. J. and Chambers, M. (1986). Cell pH in the rat proximal convoluted tubule. Regulation by luminal and peritubular pH and sodium concentration. *Journal of Clinical Investigation* **78**, 502–510.

Alpern, R. J. and Hamm, L. L. Urinary acidification. In *Acid–Base and Electrolyte Disorders. A Companion to Brenner & Rector's The Kidney* (ed. T. D. DuBose, Jr. and L. L. Hamm), pp. 23–40. Philadelphia: Saunders, 2002.

Alvarado, L. C. *et al.* (1991). Urinary acidification by furosemide test. *Medicina (Buenos Aires)* **51**, 338–342.

*__Batlle, D. and Flores, G.__ (1996). Underlying defects in distal renal tubular acidosis: new understandings. *American Journal of Kidney Diseases* **27**, 896–915.

Batlle, D. C. and Kurtzman, N. A. (1982). Distal renal tubular acidosis: pathogenesis and classification. *American Journal of Kidney Diseases* **1**, 328–344.

Batlle, D. C., Arruda, J. A., and Kurtzman, N. A. (1981). Hyperkalaemic distal renal tubular acidosis associated with obstructive uropathy. *New England Journal of Medicine* **304**, 373–380.

*__Batlle, D. C., von Riotte, A., and Schlueter, W.__ (1987). Urinary sodium in the evaluation of hyperchloraemic metabolic acidosis. *New England Journal of Medicine* **316**, 140–144.

*__Batlle, D. C.__ *et al.* (1988). The use of the urinary anion gap in the diagnosis of hyperchloraemic metabolic acidosis. *New England Journal of Medicine* **318**, 594–599.

Bonny, O. and Rossier, B. C. (2002). Disturbances of Na/K balance: pseudohypoaldosteronism revisited. *Journal of the American Society of Nephrology* **13**, 2399–2414.

Brenner, R. J. *et al.* (1982). Incidence of radiographically evident bone disease, nephrocalcinosis, and nephrolithiasis in various types of renal tubular acidosis. *New England Journal of Medicine* **307**, 217–221.

Brown, D. and Breton, S. Structure, function, and cellular distribution of the vacuolar H^+ ATPase (H^+ V-ATPase) proton pump. In *The Kidney: Physiology and Pathophysiology* (ed. D. Seldin and G. Giebisch), pp. 171–191. Philadelphia: Lippincott, Williams & Wilkins, 2000.

Bruce, L. J. *et al.* (1997). Familial distal renal tubular acidosis is associated with mutations in the red cell anion exchanger (Band 3, AE1) gene. *Journal of Clinical Investigation* **100**, 1693–1707.

Buckalew, V. M., Jr. (1989). Nephrolithiasis in renal tubular acidosis. *Journal of Urology* **141**, 731–737.

Buckalew, V. M., Jr. *et al.* (1968). Incomplete renal tubular acidosis. Physiologic studies in three patients with a defect in lowering urine pH. *American Journal of Medicine* **45**, 32–42.

Caruana, R. J. and Buckalew, V. M., Jr. (1988). The syndrome of distal (type I) renal tubular acidosis. *Medicine (Baltimore)* **67**, 84–99.

Caviston, T. L. *et al.* (1999). Molecular identification of the renal H^+-K^+-ATPases. *Seminars in Nephrology* **19**, 431–437.

Challa, A. *et al.* (1993). Metabolic acidosis inhibits growth hormone secretion in rats: mechanism of growth retardation. *American Journal of Physiology* **265**, E547–E553.

Coe, F. L., Parks, J. H., and Asplin, J. R. (1992). The pathogenesis and treatment of kidney stones. *New England Journal of Medicine* **327**, 1141–1152.

Cogan, M. G. and Morris, R. C., Jr. Renal tubular acidosis. In *Textbook of Nephrology* Vol. 1, 2nd edn. (ed. S. G. Massry and R. J. Glassock), pp. 381–389. Baltimore: Williams & Wilkins, Co., 1988.

Cohen, E. P. *et al.* (1992). Absence of H^+-ATPase in cortical collecting tubules of a patient with Sjögren's syndrome and distal renal tubular acidosis. *Journal of the American Society of Nephrology* **3**, 264–271.

Coor, C. *et al.* (1991). Role of adenosine triphosphate (ATP) and Na^+K^+ ATPase in the inhibition of proximal tubule transport with intracellular cystine loading. *Journal of Clinical Investigation* **87**, 955–961.

DeFronzo, R. A. (1980). Hyperkalaemia and hyporeninemic hypoaldosteronism. *Kidney International* **17**, 118–134.

Donckerwolcke, R. A., van Stekelenburg, G. J., and Tiddens, H. A. (1970). Therapy of bicarbonate-losing renal tubular acidosis. *Archives of Disease in Childhood* **45**, 774–779.

Donnelly, S. *et al.* (1992). Might distal renal tubular acidosis be a proximal tubular cell disorder? *American Journal of Kidney Diseases* **19**, 272–281.

DuBose, T. D., Jr. (1982). Hydrogen ion secretion by the collecting duct as a determinant of the urine to blood $P\text{CO}_2$ gradient in alkaline urine. *Journal of Clinical Investigation* **69**, 145–156.

*__DuBose, T. D., Jr.__ (1997). Hyperkalaemic hyperchloraemic metabolic acidosis: pathophysiologic insights. *Kidney International* **51**, 591–602.

*__DuBose, T. D. and Good, D. W.__ (1991). Effects of chronic hyperkalaemia on renal production and proximal tubule transport of ammonium in rats. *American Journal of Physiology* **260**, F680–F687.

DuBose, T. D., Jr. and McDonald, G. A. Renal tubular acidosis. In *Acid–Base and Electrolyte Disorders. A Companion to Brenner & Rector's The Kidney* (ed. T. D. DuBose, Jr. and L. L. Hamm), pp. 189–206. Philadelphia: Saunders, 2002.

Ethier, J. H. *et al.* (1990). The transtubular potassium concentration in patients with hypokalaemia and hyperkalaemia. *American Journal of Kidney Diseases* **15**, 309–315.

Gahl, W. A. *et al.* (1988). Cystinosis: progress in a prototypic disease. *Annals of Internal Medicine* **109**, 557–569.

*__Geller, D. S.__ *et al.* (1998). Mutations in the mineralocorticoid receptor gene cause autosomal dominant pseudohypoaldosteronism type I. *Nature Genetics* **19**, 279–281.

Golding, P. L. (1975). Renal tubular acidosis in chronic liver disease. *Postgraduate Medical Journal* **51**, 550–556.

*__Goldstein, M. B.__ *et al.* (1986). The urine anion gap: a clinically useful index of ammonium excretion. *American Journal of the Medical Sciences* **292**, 198–202.

Good, D. W. (1985). Sodium-dependent bicarbonate absorption by cortical thick ascending limb of rat kidney. *American Journal of Physiology* **248**, F821–F829.

Good, D. W. and Knepper, M. A. (1985). Ammonia transport in the mammalian kidney. *American Journal of Physiology* **248**, F459–F471.

Good, D. W., Caflisch, C. R., and DuBose, T. D., Jr. (1987). Transepithelial ammonia concentration gradients in inner medulla of the rat. *American Journal of Physiology* **252**, F491–F500.

*__Gordon, R. D.__ (1986). Syndrome of hypertension and hyperkalaemia with normal glomerular filtration rate. *Hypertension* **8**, 93–102.

Gregory, M. J. and Schwartz, G. J. (1998). Diagnosis and treatment of renal tubular disorders. *Seminars in Nephrology* **18**, 317–329.

Halperin, M. L. (1995). Modified urine osmolal gap: an accurate method for estimating the urinary ammonium concentration. *Nephron* **69**, 100–101.

Halperin, M. L. *et al.* (1974). Studies on the pathogenesis of type I (distal) renal tubular acidosis as revealed by the urinary $P\text{CO}_2$ tensions. *Journal of Clinical Investigation* **53**, 669–677.

Hamm, L. L. and Alpern, R. J. Cellular mechanisms of renal tubular acidification. In *The Kidney: Physiology and Pathophysiology* 3rd edn. (ed. D. Seldin and G. Giebisch), pp. 1935–1979. Philadelphia: Lippincott, Williams & Wilkins, 2000.

Han, J. S. *et al.* (2002). Secretory-defect distal renal tubular acidosis is associated with transporter defect in H^+-ATPase and anion exhanger-1. *Journal of the American Society of Nephrology* **13**, 1425–1432.

Hulter, H. N. and Peterson, J. C. (1985). Acid–base homeostasis during chronic PTH excess in humans. *Kidney International* **28**, 187–192.

Jarolim, P. *et al.* (1998). Autosomal dominant distal renal tubular acidosis is associated in three families with heterozygosity for the R589H mutation in the AE1 (band 3) Cl^-/HCO_3^-exchanger. *Journal of Biological Chemistry* **273**, 6380–6388.

Karet, F. E. *et al.* (1998). Mutations in the chloride–bicarbonate exchanger gene AE1 cause dominant but not autosomal recessive distal renal tubular acidosis. *Proceedings of the National Academy of Sciences USA* **95**, 6337–6342.

Karet, F. E. *et al.* (1999). Mutations in the gene encoding B1 subunit of H^+-ATPase cause renal tubular acidosis with sensorineural deafness. *Nature Genetics* **21**, 84–90.

*__Kleyman, T. R., Roberts, C., and Ling, B. N.__ (1995). A mechanism for pentamidine-induced hyperkalaemia: inhibition of distal nephron sodium transport. *Annals of Internal Medicine* **122**, 103–106.

Krapf, R. (1988). Basolateral membrane $H/OH/HCO_3$ transport in the rat cortical thick ascending limb. Evidence for an electrogenic Na/HCO_3 cotransporter in parallel with a Na/H antiporter. *Journal of Clinical Investigation* **82**, 234–241.

Kurtzman, N. A. (2000). Renal tubular acidosis syndromes. *Southern Medical Journal* **93**,1042–1052.

Lemann, J., Jr. *et al.* (2000). Acid and mineral balances and bone in familial proximal renal tubular acidosis. *Kidney International* **58**, 1267–1277.

Madias, N. E. and Perrone, R. D. Acid–base disorders in association with renal disease. In *Diseases of the Kidney* 5th edn. (ed. R. W. Schrier and C. W. Gottschalk), pp. 2669–2699. Boston: Little Brown and Company, 1993.

Maldonado, J. E. *et al.* (1975). Fanconi syndrome in adults. A manifestation of a latent form of myeloma. *American Journal of Medicine* **58**, 354–364.

McSherry, E. (1981). Renal tubular acidosis in childhood. *Kidney International* **20**, 799–809.

Messiaen, T. *et al.* (2000). Adult Fanconi syndrome secondary to light chain gammopathy. Clinicopathologic heterogeneity and unusual features in 11 patients. *Medicine (Baltimore)* **79**, 135–154.

Morris, R. C., Piel, C. F., and Audioun, E. (1965). Renal tubular acidosis. Effects of sodium phosphate and sulfate on renal acidification in two patients with renal tubular acidosis. *Pediatrics* **36**, 899–904.

Nagai, R. *et al.* (1997). Renal tubular acidosis and osteopetrosis with carbonic anhydrase II deficiency: pathogenesis of impaired acidification. *Pediatric Nephrology* **11**, 633–636.

Norman, M. E. *et al.* (1978). Urinary citrate excretion in the diagnosis of distal renal tubular acidosis. *Journal of Pediatrics* **92**, 394–400.

Oster, J. R., Singer, I., and Fishman, L. M. (1995). Heparin-induced aldosterone suppression and hyperkalaemia. *American Journal of Medicine* **98**, 575–586.

Paillard, M. Renal tubular acidosis. In *Oxford Textbook of Clinical Nephrology* 2nd edn. (ed. A. M. Davison *et al.*), pp. 1063–1084. Oxford: Oxford University Press, 1998.

Poux, J. M. *et al.* (1992). Hypokalaemic quadriplegia and respiratory arrest revealing primary Sjögren's syndrome. *Clinical Nephrology* **37**, 189–191.

Preminger, G. M. *et al.* (1985). Prevention of recurrent calcium stone formation with potassium citrate therapy in patients with distal renal tubular acidosis. *Journal of Urology* **134**, 20–23.

Rodriguez Soriano, J. (2002). Renal tubular acidosis: the clinical entity. *Journal of the American Society of Nephrology* **13**, 2160–2170.

Sawaya, B. P., Briggs, J. P., and Schnermann, J. (1995). Amphotericin B nephrotoxicity: the adverse consequences of altered membrane properties. *Journal of the American Society of Nephrology* **6**, 154–164.

Schambelan, M, Sebastian, A., and Rector, F. C., Jr. (1981). Mineralocorticoid-resistant renal hyperkalaemia without salt-wasting (type II pseudohypoaldosteronism): role of increased renal chloride reabsorption. *Kidney International* **19**, 716–727.

Schwalbe, R. A., Weiner, I. D., and Wingo, C. S. Regulation of renal potassium transport. In *Acid-Base and Electrolyte Disorders. A Companion to Brenner & Rector's The Kidney* (ed. T. D. DuBose, Jr. and L. L. Hamm), pp. 365–380. Philadelphia: Saunders, 2002.

Sebastian, A., McSherry, E., and Morris, R. C., Jr. (1971). Renal potassium wasting in renal tubular acidosis (RTA): its occurrence in types 1 and 2 RTA despite sustained correction of systemic acidosis. *Journal of Clinical Investigation* **50**, 667–678.

Sebastian, A., Schambelan, M., and Sutton, J. M. (1984). Amelioration of hyperchloraemic acidosis with furosemide therapy in patients with chronic renal insufficiency and type 4 renal tubular acidosis. *American Journal of Nephrology* **4**, 287–300.

Seikaly, M., Browne, R., and Baum, M. (1996). Nephrocalcinosis is associated with renal tubular acidosis in children with X-linked hypophosphatemia. *Pediatrics* **97**, 91–93.

Sly, W. S. *et al.* (1985). Carbonic anhydrase II deficiency in 12 families with the autosomal recessive syndrome of osteopetrosis with renal tubular acidosis and cerebral calcification. *New England Journal of Medicine* **313**, 139–145.

Soleimani, M. *et al.* (1990). Potassium depletion increases luminal Na^+/H^+ exchange and basolateral $Na^+ : CO_3^{2-} : HCO_3^-$ cotransport in rat renal cortex. *Journal of Clinical Investigation* **86**, 1076–1083.

Stetson, D. L., Wade, J. B., and Giebisch, G. (1980). Morphologic alterations in the rat medullary collecting duct following potassium depletion. *Kidney International* **17**, 45–56.

Stone, D. K. and Xie, X. S. (1988). Proton translocating ATPases: issues in structure and function. *Kidney International* **33**, 767–774.

Take, C. *et al.* (1991). Increased chloride reabsorption as an inherited renal tubular defect in familial type II pseudohypoaldosteronism. *New England Journal of Medicine* **324**, 472–476.

Vallo, A. and Rodriguez Soriano, J. (1984). Oral phosphate-loading test for the assessment of distal urinary acidification in children. *Mineral and Electrolyte Metabolism* **10**, 387–390.

West, M. L. *et al.* (1986). New clinical approach to evaluate disorders of potassium excretion. *Mineral and Electrolyte Metabolism* **12**, 234–238.

5.5 Hypokalaemic tubular disorders

Nine V.A.M. Knoers, Patrick G.J.F. Starremans, and Leo A.H. Monnens

General introduction

Hypokalaemia is a frequent electrolyte disturbance in hospitalized patients. Its causes include inadequate dietary intake, increased renal or gastrointestinal losses, or an abnormal distribution of potassium in the body. Several genetic diseases are associated with hypokalaemia: disorders of mineralocorticoid synthesis or action (glucocorticoid-remediable hyperaldosteronism, apparent excess of mineralocorticoids, congenital adrenal hyperplasia), renal tubular disorders, or disorders of cellular transfer of potassium (hypokalaemic periodic paralysis) (see also Chapter 2.2).

This chapter concerns renal tubular disorders in which hypokalaemia associated with metabolic alkalosis is a prominent feature, such as in Bartter's syndrome (BS) and Gitelman's syndrome (GS), and in pseudoaldosteronism. Our understanding of the causes and pathophysiology of these tubular disorders has been recently enhanced by achievements in molecular genetics and cell physiology. The elucidation of the genetic and cellular defects involved in these disorders (Table 1) has improved the diagnosis, classification, and differential diagnosis of these disorders, and, thus, allowed accurate genetic counseling of patients and their family members.

Bartter's syndrome

In 1962, Bartter *et al.* described two individuals with hypokalaemic alkalosis, hyperaldosteronism with normal blood pressure, decreased pressor responsiveness to infused angiotensin II, and hyperplasia of the juxtaglomerular apparatus (Bartter *et al.* 1962). Additional clinical features included dehydration, tetany, convulsions, weakness, and fatigue. One of the two patients was clearly dwarfed (Bartter *et al.* 1962). In the subsequent 40 years more than 600 patients with the so-called BS have been reported. Before the identification of the causal gene defects, the syndrome was classified into distinct phenotypes, based on the age of onset and the severity of symptoms. The severe, potentially life-threatening antenatal variant was thus distinguished from the somewhat milder classic type of the syndrome with an onset later in infancy. In many cases it appeared difficult to distinguish the classic type of BS from GS observed mainly in adults. Difficulties regarding diagnosis and classification of these patients have now been overcome by molecular genetic studies.

Molecular genetics

Bartter's syndrome is inherited as an autosomal recessive trait. Linkage analysis in a large number of families, revealed that BS is genetically heterogeneous. Four different genetic defects have been identified that form the basis for a new classification of BS into four different phenotypes (type I-IV BS). Type I BS (OMIM 60083) is caused by mutations in the *SLC12A1* gene (Simon *et al.* 1996a), which maps to chromosome 15q12–q21. The *SLC12A1* gene consists of 26 exons and encodes the bumetanide-sensitive Na^+–K^+–$2Cl^-$ cotransporter (NKCC2), which is localized in the apical membrane of cells of the thick ascending limb of Henle's loop (TAL). NKCC2 mRNA is also expressed on the apical

Table 1 Genetic defects in inherited disorders with hypokalaemic alkalosis

Syndrome	Inheritance	Gene	Gene product
Bartter's syndrome type I	Autosomal recessive	*SLC12A1*	Na^+–K^+–$2Cl^-$ cotransporter (NKCC2)
Bartter's syndrome type II	Autosomal recessive	*KCNJ1*	Renal potassium channel ROMK
Bartter's syndrome type III	Autosomal recessive	*CLCNKB*	Renal chloride channel CLC-Kb
Bartter's syndrome type IV	Autosomal recessive	*BSND*	CLC-Kb/ClC-Ka subunit Barttin
Gitelman's syndrome	Autosomal recessive	*SLC12A3*	Na–Cl cotransporter NCC
Liddle's syndrome	Autosomal dominant	*SCNN1B* *SCNN1C*	Epithelial Na-channel β-subunit βENaC Epithelial Na-channel γ-subunit γENaC
Syndrome of apparent mineralocorticoid excess	Autosomal recessive	*HSD11B2*	11β-hydroxysteroid dehydrogenase type II
Hypertension exacerbated in pregnancy	Autosomal dominant	*NR3C2*	Mineralocorticoid receptor (S810L)

membrane of macula densa cells (Obermüller *et al.* 1996). NKCC2 is a protein of 1099 amino acid residues and its two dimensional (2-D) structure is predicted to contain 12 transmembrane domains flanked by intracellular amino- and carboxyterminal regions. Three human isoforms of NKCC2 (A, B, and F), which have risen from alternative splicing of three cassettes of exon 4 of the *SLC12A1* gene, have been identified. Although the exact localization of these isoforms in man is not known, it is likely that they are axially distributed along the nephron, as has been demonstrated for highly homologous NKCC2 isoforms in mouse, rat, and rabbit kidney. Thus, the F variant is expressed in the outer medulla, the A variant in the outer medulla and cortex and the B variant in the region of the macula densa (Obermüller *et al.* 1996). The three NKCC2 variants have dramatically different affinities for Na^+,K^+, and Cl^- (Gimenez *et al.* 2002). Kinetic properties of the NKCC2 splice variants are consistent with their spatial distribution along the TAL, as they are involved in the reabsorption of Na, K, and Cl from a progressively diluted fluid in the tubule lumen. Thus, the alternative mRNA splicing and distribution of these splice variants along the tubule represents functional specialization of NKCC2.

At least 20 different disease-causing mutations in *SLC12A1*, including non-conservative amino acid substitutions, non-sense- and frameshifts mutations, have been identified in BS patients.

Type II BS (OMIM 600359) is caused by mutations in the *KCNJ1* gene, which encodes the ATP-regulated, inwardly rectifying potassium channel ROMK. The genomic locus of *KCNJ1* has been mapped to chromosome 11q24–q25. The human *KCNJ1* gene contains five exons which, by alternative splicing, produce five distinct transcripts (Shuck *et al.* 1994). These transcripts produce three isoforms of ROMK proteins that share a highly conserved core sequence of 372 amino acids encoded by exon 5, but vary in length from 372 to 391 amino acids at their NH_2-termini. The secondary structure of these ROMK proteins is predicted to have an *N*-terminal cytoplasmic region, two transmembrane α-helices (M1 and M2) flanking a pore-forming H5 segment, and a long cytoplasmic *C*-terminal tail. The rat homologues of the human ROMK isoforms are differentially expressed along the loop of Henle and distal nephron, with ROMK2 and ROMK3 expressed in the TAL, and ROMK1 in the cortical collecting duct (CCD) (Boim *et al.* 1995). In patients with BS type II at least 23 different mutations in the *KCNJ1* gene, including frame-shift, missense and non-sense mutations, have been identified up to date. Most are located in the common exon 5, thus altering amino acid residues present in all isoforms of ROMK (Simon *et al.* 1996b; International Collaborative Study Group for Bartter-like Syndromes 1997). In addition, homozygous deletions of exons 1–2, which are likely to affect transcription and/or translation of ROMK, have been identified in a minority of patients. Based on functional studies and immunocytochemistry in *Xenopus leavis* oocytes expressing *KCNJ1* mutants, distinct groups of mutant ROMK proteins are distinguished: (a) mutants disturbed in their routing to the plasma membrane but endowed with channel activity when forced to the membrane upon over-expression; (b) mutants able to reach the plasma membrane at low expression levels but with impaired channel activity; and (c) mutants that do reach the plasma membrane and exhibit significant channel activity (Starremans *et al.* 2002). The impaired channel function of mutants in the second group might be due to a structural disturbance in the protein, which alters pH gating (Schulte *et al.* 2001). The elucidation of the underlying functional consequences of mutants in the third group requires their expression in a polarized cell system.

BS type III (OMIM 602023) is caused by mutations in the *CLCNKB* gene (Simon *et al.* 1997). This gene is located on chromosome 1p36 and consists of 19 exons. It encodes the kidney-specific voltage-gated chloride channel ClC-Kb, a protein of 687 amino acids that contains 12 transmembrane domains and intracellular amino- and carboxyterminal regions. In the rat, ClC-Kb is present in the basolateral membranes of the medullary and cortical thick ascending limbs, the distal convoluted tubule (DCT), and the CCD (Vandewalle *et al.* 1997). To date at least 25 different mutations, including missense, frame-shift, and splice-site mutations, have been identified in *CLCNKB*. These mutations are scattered throughout the channel protein. The most common mutation found in BS patients, however, is an homozygous deletion of the entire *CLCNKB* gene. These deletions have most likely arisen from unequal crossing-over between *CLCNKB* and the almost identical *CLCNKA* gene, located in close vicinity to *CLCNKB* on 1p36. *CLCNKA* encodes the related renal voltage-gated chloride channel ClC-Ka, which is expressed in the thin ascending limb of Henle's loop. Defects in ClC-Ka in humans have not yet been reported, but disruption of its mouse counterpart causes nephrogenic diabetes insipidus (Matsumura *et al.* 1999).

A fourth gene involved in BS has been recently identified. This gene, *BSND*, maps to chromosome 1p31, is mutated in a rare subset of BS associated with congenital sensorineural deafness and early renal failure (BS type IV, OMIM 602522). *BSND* contains four exons which encode a new integral membrane protein with two putative transmembrane α-helices, christened Barttin. As yet, seven different mutations have been identified in 10 families with type IV BS (Birkenhäger *et al.* 2001). Nine of these families were consanguineous and, as expected, the affected children were homozygous with respect to the mutations. The detected mutations are probably all loss-of-function mutations through deletion, loss of splice-site or loss of the initiation codon. Using immunohistochemistry, Estevez *et al.* (2001) have shown that Barttin colocalizes with ClC-K channels (both ClC-Ka and ClC-Kb) in the basolateral membranes of renal tubules and of dark cells of the stria vascularis of the inner ear. Barttin forms heteromers with both ClC-Ka and ClC-Kb that are crucial to the latter's function. Furthermore, specific mutations found in patients with BS type IV reduce the ability of Barttin to support the expression of the CLC-K channels. These data suggest that Barttin is an accessory subunit (β-subunit) of these chloride channels (Estevez *et al.* 2001).

The fact that a number of BS families does not show linkage to any of these four known genes, indicates that at least one other gene must be involved in the aetiology of BS.

Clinical features

The BS phenotype is very variable and relates in part to the gene defect involved (Peters *et al.* 2002). In patients with mutations in either the *SLC12A1* (NKCC2)- or the *KCNJ1* (ROMK) gene (BS types I and II, respectively), BS is manifest *in utero* with polyhydramnios due to fetal polyuria, and followed typically by premature delivery between 27 and 35 weeks of gestation. Neonates are extremely vulnerable as a consequence of pronounced salt and water wasting. The massive polyuria (12–50 mg/kg/h), with attendant periods of life-threatening dehydration, may persist for 4–6 weeks after birth. Virtually all patients with ROMK or NKCC2 mutations have nephrocalcinosis that may already be present *in utero*. Systemic symptoms seen in these patients such as fever, vomiting, and diarrhoea, although attributed by many authors to enhanced systemic prostaglandin formation, are in fact not fully explained. Fever is most likely due to dehydration. Since correction of hypokalaemia could stop vomiting in some BS patients (personal observation), we assume that a paralytic ileus due to hypokalaemia may be an underlying cause of vomiting. Failure to thrive and growth retardation are observed in all children with ROMK or NKCC2 mutations. The clinical phenotype in patients with mutations in the *CLCNKB* (ClC-Kb) gene (BS type III) is highly variable. In most patients, symptoms present later in infancy as compared to ROMK and NKCC2 patients. They include polyuria, polydipsia, vomiting, constipation, salt craving, failure to thrive, muscle weakness, and fatigue.

Some ClC-Kb patients have an antenatal presentation of BS, whereas others, at the other side of the spectrum, have a phenotype closely resembling GS, with only slight impairment of urinary concentration capacity and a tendency to hypomagnesaemia and hypocalciuria (Jeck *et al.* 2000). Nephrocalcinosis is observed in only a minority of ClC-Kb patients.

Patients with *BSND* (Barttin) mutations (BS type IV) have early signs of BS with polyhydramnios and premature delivery. The other hallmark of BS type IV, sensorineural deafness, is diagnosed as early as 1 month of age. The majority of the reported BS type IV patients develops chronic renal insufficiency during childhood, due to a predominant chronic interstitial fibrosis and atrophy.

Growth failure may occur in BS. At present, the limited available information precludes any general conclusion regarding growth. Of note, indomethacin treatment may lead to a significant catch-up growth in children with BS. Some BS patients, irrespective of the gene defect involved, develop endstage renal disease by an as yet unexplained mechanism.

A successful kidney transplantation fully corrects the abnormalities seen in BS indicating that the syndrome is due solely to renal abnormalities.

Biochemical features

The core biochemical manifestations seen in all BS variants are hypokalaemic metabolic alkalosis, hyperreninaemic hyperaldosteronism with normal blood pressure, and inappropriate excretion of urinary potassium. Urinary chloride excretion is increased when related to serum chloride. All patients with BS are normotensive despite elevated blood levels of renin. In a recent clinical study of 85 patients with BS, hypokalaemia is less severe in ROMK patients (serum potassium 2.9 ± 0.5 mmol/l) than in NKCC2- (serum potassium 2.6 ± 0.3 mmol/l) or ClC-Kb patients (2.4 ± 0.5 mmol/l) (Peters *et al.* 2002). Remarkably, the majority of ROMK patients show hyperkalaemia in the first days after birth, which is subsequently followed by hypokalaemia. This transient neonatal hyperkalaemia is not seen in NKCC2 patients.

Calcium excretion is very high in all NKCC2- and ROMK patients (>10 mg/kg/day and/or molar ratio of urinary calcium to creatinine >0.70). It corresponds to the high frequency of nephrocalcinosis seen in these patients. Hypercalciuria is also observed in about half of the ClC-Kb patients. Hypomagnesaemia (serum magnesium concentration <0.65 mmol/l) is found in about 50 per cent of the ClC-Kb patients but never in NKCC2-, or ROMK patients. In a few hypomagnesaemic ClC-Kb patients, hypocalciuria (urinary calcium excretion <1 mg/kg/day and or molar ratio of urinary calcium to creatinine <0.10) has been observed. These latter patients have biochemical features considered pathognomonic for GS. Renal functional studies in BS patients disclose a decreased urinary concentrating ability and a reduced distal fractional chloride reabsorption during hypotonic saline infusion. All BS patients exhibit blunted natriuretic and kaliuretic responses to loop diuretics, indicating that the defect in BS is located at the level of Henle's loop. Urinary prostaglandins (PGE_2 and $PGF_{2\alpha}$) are increased in the majority, but not in all BS patients. Prostaglandin production is stimulated by hypokalaemia and elevated plasma concentration of angiotensin II. Prostaglandin overproduction may cause defective platelet aggregation.

Apart from GS, a few other conditions need to be considered in the differential diagnosis of BS. Extrarenal forms of hypokalaemic metabolic alkalosis, for instance caused by vomiting, can be distinguished from the renal form, as present in BS, by measurement of urinary chloride excretion (Mersin *et al.* 1995). Abuse of loop diuretics and a rare entity called immune-related potassium nephritis (IRPLIN) can cause salt-wasting hypokalaemic alkalosis and thus mimic BS (Wrong *et al.* 1993). All three conditions are observed in older patients.

Pathophysiology

BS has long been suspected to result from impaired $Na^+/K^+/Cl^-$ transport at the level of the TAL. This hypothesis is now demonstrated by the recent molecular findings. Under normal circumstances, NaCl reabsorption in the TAL involves a complex interplay between co-transporters and channels in both the apical and basolateral membranes of TAL cells (Fig. 1). Thus, sodium chloride is reabsorbed together with potassium across the apical membrane by the activity of NKCC2. This cotransporter is driven by the low intracellular Na^+ and Cl^- concentrations, generated by the basolateral Na^+,K^+-ATPase and ClC-Kb channel, respectively. The apical ROMK channel is another important driving force for the function of NKCC2, by recycling K^+ entering the cell back into the tubular lumen. Impaired function of any of these proteins, as a result of mutations in their encoding genes, would be predicted to impair net reabsorption of NaCl in the TAL and result in increased NaCl delivery to the distal nephron with consequent salt wasting, volume contraction, and stimulation of the renin–aldosterone axis. An important alternative hypothesis to explain the stimulation of the renin–aldosterone axis is based on the presence of NKCC2 in the macula densa cells. In the normal situation, these specialized cells of the distal tubules control the secretion of renin from the nearby juxtaglomerular cells. When Na^+ and Cl^- enter the macula densa cells, renin secretion is inhibited. The genetic absence of Na^+ and Cl^- pathways in the macula densa cells might be responsible for the extreme elevations in plasma renin activity and the hypertrophy of the juxtaglomerular apparatus that occur in BS. Evidence confirming this latter hypothesis has been found in the recently generated NKCC2 knockout mice (Takahasi *et al.* 2000). Finally, prostaglandins may stimulate renin release.

The combination of increased distal flow of NaCl and hyperaldosteronism promotes potassium and hydrogen secretion in the CCD leading to hypokalaemic metabolic alkalosis.

Impaired reabsorption of NaCl at the level of the TAL will reduce the lumen-positive electrical transport potential that normally drives the paracellular reabsorption of calcium and magnesium through the tight-junction protein claudin-16 (paracellin-1). This explains the increased urinary calcium excretion found in BS. Hypermagnaesuria is not common in antenatal BS and absent in NKCC2 knockout mice.

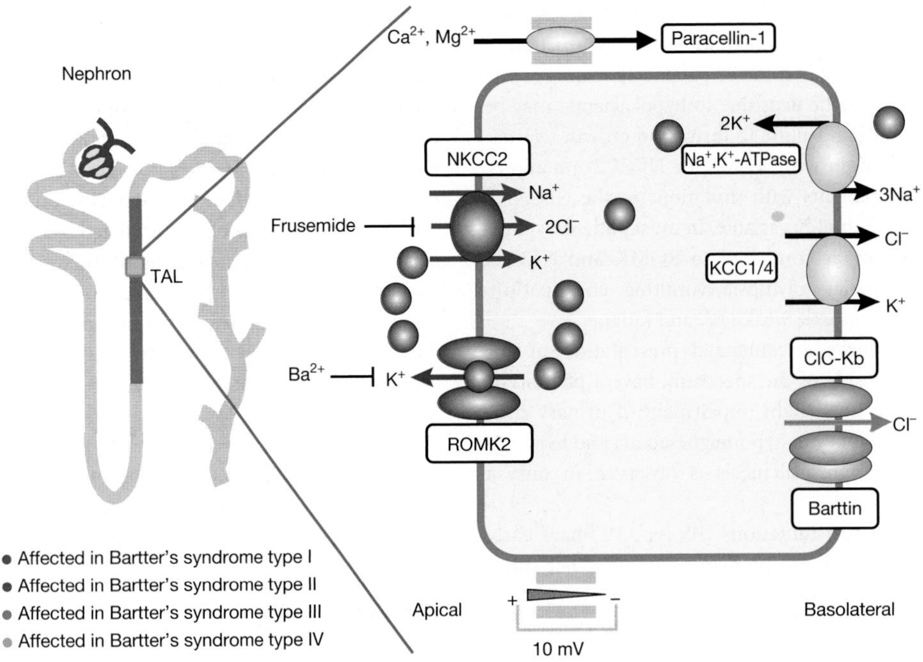

Fig. 1 Schematic model of transcellular and paracellular transport pathways in the thick ascending limb of Henle's loop (TAL). Sodium chloride (NaCl) enters the cell via the luminal frusemide-sensitive Na^+–K^+–$2Cl^-$ cotransporter (NKCC2). Potassium (K^+) is recycled into the lumen via the luminal ATP-regulated inwardly rectifying potassium channel (ROMK). Cl^- leaves the cell through the basolateral Cl^- channel (ClC-Kb/Barttin) and through the K^+–Cl^- cotransporter (KCC1/4). Na^+ exits the cell through the Na^+,K^+-ATPase system. The lumen-positive electrical potential, generated by Cl^- entry into the cell and recycling of K^+ across the luminal membrane, drives paracellular Ca^{2+} and Mg^{2+} transport via paracellin-1 (claudin-16).

A likely explanation for normal magnesium excretion in spite of reduced paracellular magnesium reabsorption in the TAL, is compensation of reabsorption in the DCT.

The impossibility to build up a hypertonic medullary interstitium due to impaired NaCl reabsorption in the TAL, accounts for the polyuria found in all patients with BS. In the neonatal period, polyuria may be massive as the immature proximal tubule is not yet able to retrieve water and salt. The inability of the TAL to compensate this proximal loss results in massive NaCl and water delivery to the distal tubule and collecting duct.

The initial hyperkalaemia found postnatally in some patients with BS type II, is explained by the fact that most mutations in *KCNJ1* also cause loss of function of the ROMK1-isoform, which is localized in the CCD and participates in net potassium secretion at that level of the nephron. Hyperkalaemia disappears within a few days and is followed by hypokalaemia. Is is likely that the developmental appearance and activity of other potassium-secreting mechanisms in the distal tubule underlies this shift from hyperkalaemia to hypokalaemia during the first week of life (Satlin 1999). The somewhat higher potassium levels observed in BS type II patients as compared to the other BS types, may also be explained by the expression of this ROMK1-isoform in the CCD.

It is now generally accepted that the increased prostaglandin production is secondary to the basic defect in NaCl reabsorption.

The phenotypic variability observed in patients with *CLCNKB* mutations, ranging from antenatal BS to a more Gitelman-like disorder, most likely reflects the wide distribution of ClC-Kb in the distal nephron. Thus, the Gitelman-like phenotype in some of these patients does not correspond to a TAL disorder, but rather to a disturbed function of ClC-Kb, with the secondary inhibition of apical sodium chloride reabsorption via NCC, in the DCT (Fig. 2). This indicates that ClC-Kb does not play an irreplaceable role in chloride reabsorption in the TAL. Other chloride transporting proteins in the basolateral membrane of TAL cells such as the K–Cl cotransporter KCC1 may compensate for the loss of the function of the ClC-Kb channel.

Ion transport processes of cells in the inner ear's striae vascularis are remarkably similar to those in the TAL. In the normal situation, the concerted action of the basolateral NKCC1(BSC2) and the Na^+, K^+-ATPase, raises intracellular K^+ concentration. This process is ensured by the basolateral chloride channels ClC-Ka and ClC-Kb (both with the same β-subunit Barttin), which recycle Cl^- ions for NKCC1. Potassium ions then leave the cell through the apical KCNQ1/KCNE1 potassium channel. The resulting high concentration of K^+ ions in the endolymph, aids in the mechanism whereby sound waves are converted to a voltage signal suitable for relay in the brain.

Patients with ClC-Kb mutations (type III BS) are not deaf. Deafness is also absent in ClC-K1 (the orthologue of ClC-Ka) knockout mice. This is probably due to the fact that both ClC-Ka and CLC-Kb are present in the cells of the striae vascularis, so that loss of function of one of the two chloride channels, as a result of mutations, can be compensated for by the other channel. However, mutational inactivation of the β-subunit of both chloride channels, Barttin, has a deleterious effect on their function and abolishes the recycling of chloride completely. This impairs K^+ secretion in the endolymph and as such explains the deafness found in BS type IV.

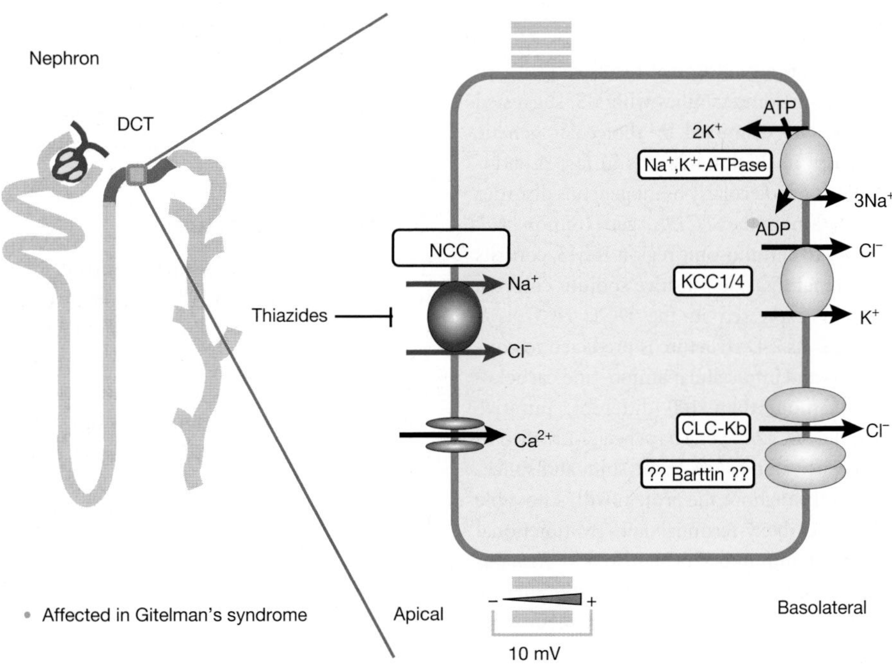

Fig. 2 Simplified schematic model of transport mechanisms in the distal convoluted tubule. Sodium chloride (NaCl) enters the cell via the luminal thiazide-sensitive Na^+–Cl^- cotransporter (NCC) and leaves the cell through the basolateral Cl^- channel (ClC-Kb) and the Na^+,K^+-ATPase. A K^+–Cl^- cotransporter is also present. Entry of Ca^{2+} occurs via luminal calcium channels.

Treatment and prognosis

The goal of the treatment is to restore the plasma potassium concentration to about 3.5 mmol/l. It is rarely reached. The treatment is based on dietary adaptation and the use of prostaglandin synthetase inhibitors. As a guideline, we double the normal potassium intake by giving KCl in 3–4 doses/day. Addition of magnesium salts should always be considered when hypomagnesaemia is present because magnesium deficiency may aggravate potassium wasting. Indomethacin is the most frequently used prostaglandin synthetase inhibitor (about 2 mg/day in 3–4 doses). It improves markedly the well being of BS children. Unfortunately, older children and adults may show signs of intolerance or toxicity such as nausea, anorexia, vomiting, abdominal pain, and gastroduodenal ulceration. Indomethacin can then be replaced by ibuprofen, which is better tolerated. Toxic complications of indomethacin include haematopoietic toxicity, skin reactions, liver damage, headache, and pseudotumour cerebri. In all children, it immediately decreases glomerular filtration rate. When glomerular filtration rate decreases slowly and progressively (months, years), our policy is to interrupt non-steroidal anti-inflammatory drugs (NSAID). The benefits of NSAIDS in BS may result from an increased reabsorption of NaCl and fluid in the proximal tubule and an attendant lower distal K^+ secretion due to a decreased plasma level of aldosterone. NSAIDS should not be given during the last trimester of pregnancy.

Indomethacin inhibits cyclo-oxygenase (COX) 1 and 2. The efficacy of selective COX-2 inhibitors is yet to be documented in BS.

Hypokalaemia may also benefit from a reduction of K^+ secretion in the distal nephron by the administration of either amiloride (or triamterene), which blocks the Na-channel ENaC or spironolactones which interfere with the mineralocorticoid receptor (MR). We avoid spironolactone, because of its promiscuous progestional and antiandrogenic action (gynaecomastia, irregular menstruation). The introduction of a selective aldosterone receptor antagonist such as eplerenone would increase our armamentarium. Inhibitors of the angiotensin converting enzyme carry the risk of symptomatic hypotension.

In the neonatal period NaCl and extra fluid is required usually by intravenous infusion.

Severe fatigue in some BS patients and poorly tolerated medication may markedly impair their quality of life (QOL). The pathogenesis of renal insufficiency due to interstitial nephritis remains to be elucidated. Finally, rational prevention is as yet not possible.

Gitelman's syndrome

Gitelman's syndrome, also referred to as familial hypokalaemia–hypomagnesaemia (GS; OMIM 263800) was first described in 1966 (Gitelman *et al.* 1966). Three adult individuals exhibited a syndrome characterized by hypomagnesaemia, hypokalaemia, and impaired renal conservation of potassium and magnesium, apparently unrelated to mineralocorticoid excess. The clinical symptoms consisted of transient episodes of muscle weakness and chronic non-specific dermatitis in two of the three patients. This syndrome was subsequently defined as the hypomagnesaemic and hypocalciuric variant of BS, or GS. Although extensive testing of tubular function helped differentiate the GS from the 'true' BS, a clear distinction between the two syndromes in an individual patient remained difficult and depends now on genetic analysis.

Molecular genetics

Gitelman's syndrome is inherited as an autosomal recessive trait. An autosomal dominant inheritance in some families with GS, suggested by Bettinelli *et al.* (1995) was later dismissed by molecular genetic analysis showing that inheritance in these families is in fact pseudo-dominant. In contrast to BS, GS is a molecularly homogeneous disorder caused by loss-of-function mutations in the *SLC12A3* gene (Simon *et al.* 1996c). The *SLC12A3* gene maps to chromosome region 16q13, consists of 26 exons, and encodes the renal thiazide-sensitive sodium chloride cotransporter NCC, specifically expressed in the DCT. NCC is a polypeptide of 1021 amino acids. Its 2-D structure is predicted to contain 12 transmembrane domains and intracellular amino- and carboxy-terminal regions. At present more than 100 different, putative loss-of-function mutations in the *SLC12A3* gene have been identified in GS patients. They include missense, non-sense, frame shift, and splice-site mutations and are scattered throughout the protein with a possible clustering of mutations in the carboxy-terminal tail. By functional expression studies and results of immunocytochemistry in *Xenopus leavis* oocytes, it was shown that most disease-causing NCC mutants are completely or partly impaired in their routing to the plasma membrane (Kunchaparty *et al.* 1999; deJong *et al.* 2002).

Clinical features

Patients with GS are diagnosed after 6 years of age and in many cases only at adult age. Most patients suffer from carpopedal spasms especially during periods of fever or when extra magnesium is lost by vomiting or diarrhoea. Paraesthesias, especially in the face, frequently occur. Some patients experience severe fatigue interfering with daily activities, while others never complain of tiredness. The severity of fatigue in GS is not related to the degree of hypokalaemia. In contrast to BS, polyuria is absent or only mild. Poor growth and short stature are only seen in a minority of cases. Some adult patients suffer from chondrocalcinosis, with swelling, local heat, and tenderness of the affected joints. There is ample evidence that hypomagnesaemia plays a role in the pathophysiology of chondrocalcinosis in GS. First, chondrocalcinosis also occurs in some patients with isolated magnesium loss (Meij *et al.* 1999). Second, joint cartilage lesions resembling chondrocalcinosis were induced by magnesium deficiency in juvenile rats. It is presumed that hypomagnesaemia induces chondrocalcinosis by reducing the activity of pyrophosphatase, thus promoting pyrophosphate crystallization (Calo *et al.* 2000).

Cruz and colleagues have recently challenged the generally accepted idea that GS is a mild disorder (Cruz *et al.* 2001a). They evaluated the symptoms and QOL in 50 adult patients with molecularly proven GS and compared them with 25 age- and gender-matched controls. GS patients were significantly more symptomatic than controls, suffering from salt craving, musculoskeletal symptoms such as cramps, muscle weakness and aches, and constitutional symptoms such as fatigue, generalized weakness and dizziness, and nocturia and polydipsia. QOL measurements were significantly lower in GS patients than in controls.

In general there is no correlation between the presence and severity of symptoms in GS and the type of mutation in the *SLC12A3* gene.

Progression to renal insufficiency is extremely rare in GS. As yet, only one patient developed chronic renal disease and progressed eventually to endstage renal failure (Bonfante *et al.* 2001).

Blood pressure in GS patients is lower than in the general population, indicating that even the modest salt wasting of this disease reduces blood pressure. Heterozygous mutation carriers remain normotensive, but consume larger quantities of salt, pointing to a compensated defect (Cruz *et al.* 2001b).

Biochemical features

Typical biochemical abnormalities in GS include hypokalaemia, hypomagnesaemia, and hypocalciuria. Hypokalaemia is similar (2.7 ± 0.4 mmol/l) to that of BS patients with *SCL12A1* or *CLCNKB* mutations. Serum magnesium concentration is uniformly low (<0.65 mmol/l). In a few patients, magnesium concentration initially remains easily within the normal range and drops only later below normal, leading to an early false diagnosis of BS (personal observation).

Urinary calcium excretion is always low (molar ratio of urinary calcium to urinary creatinine <0.1). It is the best parameter to differentiate GS from BS. Prostaglandin excretion is normal. Plasma renin activity and plasma aldosterone concentration are only slightly higher than in BS.

Functional studies have demonstrated a normal or slightly decreased urinary concentrating ability, but a clearly reduced distal fractional chloride reabsorption during hypotonic saline infusion. GS patients have a blunted natriuretic response to hydrochlorothiazide, but a prompt natriuresis after fursemide, indicating that the defect in GS is located at the level of the distal tubule.

Pathophysiology

Normally, about 7 per cent of the filtered load of sodium chloride is reabsorbed in the DCT. The disruption of NaCl reabsorption in the DCT, resulting from loss-of-function mutations in NCC, can explain most, but not all, features of GS (Fig. 2). Impaired NaCl reabsorption in the DCT, increases sodium delivery in the collecting duct and results in mild volume contraction. The vascular volume reduction increases renin activity, angiotensin, and aldosterone levels. Raised aldosterone levels increase electrogenic sodium reabsorption in the CCD via the epithelial sodium channel ENaC, maintain salt homeostasis at the expense of an increased secretion of potassium and hydrogen ions, and an attendant hypokalaemia with metabolic alkalosis.

The mechanisms of hypocalciuria and hypomagnesaemia in GS remain a matter of speculation. It has been suggested that mutations which inactivate NCC may cause hypocalciuria by the same mechanism as thiazides. According to this hypothesis, the reduced influx of NaCl in the DCT cells in combination with continued exit of intracellular chloride through basolateral chloride channels, causes hyperpolarization of the cell. This in turn increases calcium entry via apical calcium channels. The subsequent increase in intracellular calcium stimulates calcium efflux via the basolateral Na^+/Ca^{2+} exchanger and the Ca^{2+}-ATPase. The lowered intracellular sodium concentration facilitates calcium exit via the basolateral Na^+/Ca^{2+} exchanger. Hypomagnesaemia has been attributed to the associated hypokalaemia, a hypothesis disputed by studies in NCC-knockout mice which develop severe hypocalciuria and hypomagnesaemia despite the absence of hypokalaemia or alkalosis (Schultheis *et al.* 1998). Renal defects in Ca^{2+} and Mg^{2+} reabsorption might thus be a consequence of functional and/or structural alterations in the DCT caused by loss of NCC activity, rather than secondary to systemic metabolic disturbances such as hypokalaemia or alkalosis.

An alternative hypothesis is based on the possible existence of both an apical Mg^{2+} channel and a basolateral Mg^{2+} extrusion mechanism in DCT cells. These putative transporters could be affected by differences in NaCl homeostasis within these cells.

Treatment and prognosis

Most patients with GS remain untreated. The observation that chondrocalcinosis is due to magnesium deficiency, argues clearly in favour of magnesium supplementation. Normalization of serum magnesium is, however, difficult to achieve since high doses of magnesium cause diarrhoea. The bioavailability of magnesium varies according to the preparations. Magnesium oxide and magnesium sulfate have a significantly lower bioavailability than magnesium-chloride, magnesium lactate and magnesium aspartate (Firoz and Braber 2001). Hypokalaemia should be treated as described above for BS. We recommend the combination of amiloride with KCl but amiloride should be started with caution in order to avoid hypotension. In general, the long-term prognosis of GS is excellent.

Pseudoaldosteronism

Pseudoaldosteronism mimicks primary aldosteronism, except for very low levels of plasma renin and aldosterone. We now describe three different disorders characterized by pseudoaldosteronism.

Liddle's syndrome

Liddle's syndrome is characterized by low-renin, volume expanded, salt-sensitive hypertension associated with hypokalaemic metabolic alkalosis and lack of response to the administration of spironolactone, a blocker of the MR.

Molecular genetics

Liddle's syndrome (OMIM 177200) is inherited as an autosomal dominant trait with variable clinical expression. It is caused by constitutive activation of the amiloride-sensitive epithelial sodium channel ENaC. This channel is located in the apical membrane of Na^+-transporting epithelia in the kidney, colon, lung, and ducts of exocrine glands, and plays an essential role in Na^+ and fluid reabsorption. In the kidney, ENaC is found mainly in the connecting tubule and principal cells of the collecting duct (Fig. 3). The channel is composed of three homologous subunits, α, β, and γ, all of which are necessary for normal channel function. The subunits are encoded by separate genes, the α-subunit gene (*SCNN1A, OMIM 600278*) on chromosome 12, and the other two genes (*SCNN1B, OMIM 600760* and *SCNN1G, OMIM 600761*) very closely together on chromosome 16. The three subunits share 35 per cent identity in amino acid sequence. Each subunit has a large extracellular loop and two membrane-spanning domains with short amino- and carboxy termini. The carboxy-terminal end of each subunit contains two proline-rich regions, the second of which also includes a highly conserved sequence known as the PY motif. Normally, the PY motif binds to the tryptophan-rich WW domain of Nedd4, a ubiquitin protein ligase, that is expressed in ENaC-containing tissues. The binding of the PY motif to Nedd4 will lead to ubiquitination of the channel subunits, targeting ENaC for degradation by proteasomes. In this way Nedd4 regulates ENaC function by controlling the number of channels (as well as the open probability of single ion channels) at the cell surface. In Liddle syndrome, deletions or modifications of the PY-motifs in the β- or γ-subunits of ENaC

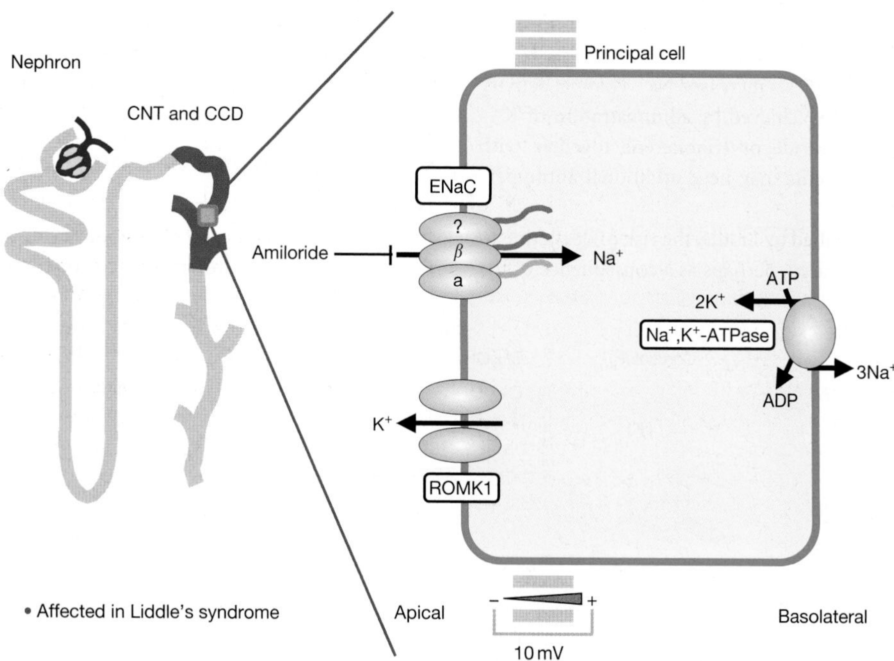

Fig. 3 Simplified schematic model of Na^+ transport pathways in a principal cell of the connecting tubule and cortical collecting duct. Na^+ is entering the principal cells via the apical amiloride-sensitive Na^+ channel (ENaC), a process driven by the basolateral Na^+,K^+-ATPase. Sodium uptake is coupled with secretion of positive charges (among which ROMK1 mediated K^+ exit) into the tubular lumen. In Liddle's syndrome, mutations are found in either the β- or the γ-subunit of ENaC. The specific mutations in the carboxy-terminal region of these subunits leads to a failure of Nedd4 binding.

have been identified. These mutations result in loss of Nedd4 binding sites in ENaC and subsequent reduced clearance of ENaC from the cell surface. The resulting increase in channel number and openings at the cell surface increases sodium reabsorption in the distal nephron (Warnock 2001).

Clinical symptoms and biochemical features

The clinical symptoms of Liddle's syndrome are related to hypokalaemia such as tiredness, polyuria, and polydipsia, and to hypertension, such as headache. These features may appear in infancy, but the diagnosis is often not made until later childhood or adolescence.

Classically, Liddle's syndrome is characterized by hypokalaemic metabolic alkalosis accompanied by low renin, low aldosterone, volume-expanded hypertension.

In the original family described by Liddle, the variable expression of the disorder is clearly exemplified: affected family members could be normokalaemic with hypertension, but also hypokalaemic without evidence of hypertension (Liddle *et al.* 1963). Hypokalaemia as well as hypertension may be mitigated by a restricted salt intake as increased distal delivery of Na^+ augments K^+ secretion.

Pathophysiology

Unregulated, continuing sodium reabsorption across the connecting and collecting tubules results in volume expansion with hypertension and inhibition of the renin–aldosterone axis. The increased lumen-negative transepithelial potential generated by augmented electrogenic Na^+ reabsorption provides the driving force for secretion of K^+ by the principal cells and of H^+ by the intercalated cells, resulting in hypokalaemia and metabolic alkalosis, respectively. K^+ depletion also stimulates renal acidification (Palmer and Alpern 1998).

Treatment and prognosis

The guidelines for treatment are clear: increased Na^+ channel activity should be inhibited. This can be achieved by administration of K^+-sparing diuretics, such as amiloride or triamterene together with a salt-restricted diet. Older patients may need additional antihypertensive drugs.

In the original kindred described by Liddle, the risk of death due to stroke or heart failure was increased, perhaps as a consequence of the lack of adequate treatment. Renal failure in patients with Liddle's syndrome has been rarely reported and remains as yet unexplained.

Syndrome of apparent mineralocorticoid excess

The syndrome of apparent mineralocorticoid excess (AME) is due either to a congenital or to an acquired deficiency of 11-β hydroxysteroid dehydrogenase type II (11βHDS-2). This enzyme activates the conversion of cortisol to cortisone (Fig. 4). *In vitro*, both cortisol and aldosterone are potent activators of the type 1 MR, but *in vivo* almost all MR activation is mediated only by aldosterone. This *in vivo* specificity of MR for aldosterone is mediated indirectly, with 11βHDS-2 'protecting' MR from cortisol by metabolizing it to cortisone, which does not activate MR. In AME, deficiency of 11βHDS-2 permits cortisol to exert its mineralocorticoid effect by binding to MR in the target tissues: distal nephron, colon, salivary gland, sweat gland, and placenta (Stewart 1999). The congenital form of AME is an autosomal recessive disorder (OMIM;218030) caused by loss-of-function mutations in the gene encoding 11βHDS-2. This gene, HSD11B2, is located on chromosome 16q22.

The acquired form of defective functioning of 11βHDS-2 is due to the intake of liquorice, which is a potent inhibitor of the enzyme. About 100 mg glycyrrhetinic acid, corresponding to 50 mg liquorice, already produce adverse effects (Frey and Ferrari 2000).

Pathophysiology

The pathophysiology of hypertension in AME is similar to that in Liddle's syndrome. In addition, AME interferes with a normal pregnancy. Placental 11βHDS-2 protects the fetus from the high concentration of cortisol in maternal blood by converting cortisol to inactive cortisone. Prenatal exposure to high concentrations of cortisol causes intrauterine growth retardation.

Clinical symptoms and biochemical features

In contrast to Liddle's syndrome, most patients are diagnosed in the first year of life or in early childhood. Symptoms consist of failure to thrive, with catch-up growth after treatment, polyuria, polydipsia, and

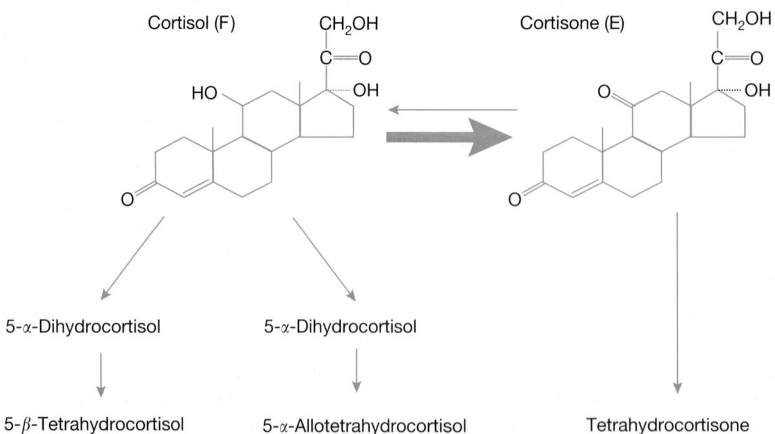

Fig. 4 Simplified scheme of cortisol metabolism. Cortisol is converted to cortisone by 11-β hydroxysteroid dehydrogenase type II.

muscle weakness. Hypertension is severe and sometimes complicated by retinopathy. Death may be caused by stroke or cardiac decompensation. Intrauterine growth retardation is characteristic for the disorder. Excess urinary excretion of the reduced metabolites of cortisol compared to cortisone (THF/THE ratio) confirms the diagnosis. In plasma, hypokalaemic alkalosis is present together with suppressed plasma renin activity and very low aldosterone concentration.

Treatment and prognosis

Dexamethasone is generally considered to be the treatment of choice. Dexamethasone, a mineralocorticoid less potent than cortisol, inhibits ACTH secretion and reduces cortisol concentration. The results reported in some patients, however, are not convincing. Treatment by amiloride (or triamterene) together with a low salt diet and combined, if necessary, with frusemide, appears effective (Mantero *et al.* 1996).

Clinical symptoms are more severe than in Liddle's syndrome. Early diagnosis and aggressive treatment are mandatory in order to prevent cerebral and cardiac complications.

Activating mineralocorticoid receptor mutation

A new autosomal dominant form of pseudoaldosteronism caused by a specific mutation in the gene (*NR3C2*) encoding the MR has been recently described (OMIM 600938; Geller *et al.* 2000). Although the phenotype resembles Liddle's syndrome with hypertension and suppressed renin activity and aldosterone secretion, it differs from it because hypertension is dramatically accelerated during pregnancy. The mutation involves a serine to leucine mutation (S810L) in the ligand-binding domain of MR which results in a constitutively activated receptor with altered specificity. Compounds which normally bind but do not activate MR, including progesterone and other steroids lacking 21-hydroxyl groups, are potent agonists for the mutant receptor. The increased activation of MR by progesterone explains the exarcerbation of hypertension during pregnancy.

References

Bartter, F. *et al.* (1962). Hyperplasia of the juxtaglomerular complex with hyperaldosteronism and hypokalemic alkalosis. A new syndrome. *American Journal of Medicine* **33**, 811–828.

Bettinelli, A. *et al.* (1995). Genetic heterogeneity in tubular hypomagnesemia-hypokalemia with hypocalciuria (Gitelman syndrome). *Kidney International* **47**, 547–551.

Birkenhäger, R. *et al.* (2001). Mutation of *BSND* causes Bartter syndrome with sensorineural deafness and kidney failure. *Nature Genetics* **29**, 310–314.

Boim, M. *et al.* (1995). ROMK inwardly-rectifying ATP-sensitive K^+ channel II. Cloning and distribution of alternate forms. *American Journal of Physiology* **268**, F1132–F1140.

Bonfante, L. *et al.* (2001). Chronic renal failure, end-stage renal disease, and peritoneal dialysis in Gitelman's syndrome. *American Journal of Kidney Diseases* **38**, 165–168.

Calo, L., Punzi, L., and Semplicini, A. (2000). Hypomagnesemia and chondrocalcinosis in Bartter's and Gitelman's syndrome: review of the pathogenetic mechanism. *American Journal of Nephrology* **20**, 347–350.

Cruz, D. N. *et al.* (2001a). Gitelman's syndrome revisited: an evaluation of symptoms and health-related quality of life. *Kidney International* **59**, 710–717.

Cruz, D. N. *et al.* (2001b). Mutations in the Na–Cl cotransporter reduce blood pressure in humans. *Hypertension* **37**, 1458–1464.

Estevez, R. *et al.* (2001). Barttin is a Cl^- channel β-subunit crucial for renal Cl^- reabsorption and inner ear K^+ secretion. *Nature* **414**, 558–561.

Firoz, M. and Braber, M. (2001). Bioavailability of U.S. commercial magnesium preparations. *Magnesium Research* **4**, 257–262.

Frey, F. J. and Ferrari, P. (2000). Pastis and hypertension—what is the molecular basis? *Nephrology, Dialysis, Transplantation* **15**, 1512–1514.

Geller, D. S. *et al.* (2000). Activating mineralocorticoid receptor mutation in hypertension exacerbated by pregnancy. *Science* **289**, 119–123.

Gimenez, I., Isenring, P., and Forbush, B. (2002). Spatially distributed alternative splice variants of the renal Na–K–Cl cotransporter exhibit dramatically affinities for the transported ions. *Journal of Biological Chemistry* **277**, 8767–8770.

Gitelman, H. J., Graham, J. B., and Welt, L. G. (1966). A familial disorder characterized by hypokalemia and hypomagnesemia. *Transactions of the Association of American Physicians* **79**, 221–235.

International Collaborative Study Group for Bartter-like Syndromes (1997). Mutations in the gene encoding the inwardly-rectifying renal potassium channel, ROMK, cause the antenatal variant of Bartter syndrome: evidence for genetic heterogeneity. *Human Molecular Genetics* **6**, 17–26.

Jeck, N. *et al.* (2000). Mutations in the chloride channel gene, *CLCNKB*, leading to a mixed Bartter-Gitelman phenotype. *Pediatric Research* **48**, 754–758.

deJong, J. C. *et al.* (2002). Functional expression of mutations in the human NaCl co-transporter (NCC): evidence for impaired routing mechanisms in Gitelman's syndrome. *Journal of the American Society of Nephrology* **13**, 1442–1448.

Kunchaparty, S. *et al.* (1999). Defective processing and expression of thiazide-sensitive Na–Cl cotransporter as a cause of Gitelman's syndrome. *American Journal of Physiology* **277**, F643–F649.

Liddle, G. W. *et al.* (1963). A familial renal disorder stimulating primary aldosteronism but with negligible aldosterone secretion. *Transactions of the Association of American Physicians* **76**, 199–213.

Mantero, F. *et al.* (1996). Apparent mineralocorticoid excess: type I and type II. *Steroids* **61**, 193–196.

Matsumura, Y. *et al.* (1999). Overt nephrogenic diabetes insipidus in mice lacking the ClC-K1 chloride channel. *Nature Genetics* **21**, 95–98.

Meij, I. C. *et al.* (1999). Hereditary isolated renal magnesium loss maps to chromosome 11q23. *American Journal of Human Genetics* **64**, 180–188.

Mersin, S. S. *et al.* (1995). Urinary chloride excretion distinguishes between renal and extrarenal metabolic alkalosis. *European Journal of Pediatrics* **154**, 979–982.

Obermüller, N. *et al.* (1996). Expression of the Na–K–2Cl cotransporter by macula densa and thick ascending limb cells of rat and rabbit nephron. *Journal of Clinical Investigation* **98**, 635–640.

Palmer, B. E. and Alpern, R. J. (1998). Liddle's syndrome. *American Journal of Medicine* **104**, 301–309.

Peters, M. *et al.* (2002). Clinical presentation of genetically defined patients with hypokalemic salt-loosing tubulopathies. *Amercian Journal of Medicine* **112**, 183–190.

Satlin, L. M. (1999). Regulation of potassium transport in the maturing kidney. *Seminars in Nephrology* **19**, 155–165.

Schulte, U. *et al.* (1999). PH gating of ROMK (Kir1.1) channels: control by an Arg–Lys–Arg triad disrupted in antenatal Bartter syndrome. *Proceedings of the National Academy of Sciences USA* **96**, 15298–15303.

Schultheis, P. J. *et al.* (1998). Phenotype resembling Gitelman's syndrome in mice lacking the apical Na^+Cl^- cotransporter of the distal convoluted tubule. *Journal of Biological Chemistry* **273**, 29150–29155.

Shuck, M. E. *et al.* (1994). Cloning and characterization of multiple forms of the human kidney ROM-K potassium channel. *Journal of Biological Chemistry* **269**, 24261–24270.

Simon, D. B. *et al.* (1996a). Bartter's syndrome, hypokalemic alkalosis with hypercalciuria, is caused by mutations in the Na–K–2Cl cotransporter NKCC2. *Nature Genetics* **13**, 183–188.

Simon, D. B. *et al.* (1996b). Genetic heterogeneity of Bartter's syndrome revealed by mutations in the K^+ channel, ROMK. *Nature Genetics* **14**, 152–156.

Simon, D. B. *et al.* (1996c). Gitelman's variant of Bartter syndrome, inherited hypokalaemic alkalosis, is caused by mutations in the thiazide sensitive Na–Cl cotransporter. *Nature Genetics* **12**, 24–30.

Simon, D. B. *et al.* (1997). Mutations in the chloride channel gene, *CLCNKB*, cause Bartter's syndrome type III. *Nature Genetics* **17**, 171–178.

Starremans, P. G. J. F. *et al.* (2002). Functional implications of mutations in the human renal outer medullary potassium channel (ROMK2) identified in Bartter syndrome. *Pflügers Archives* **443**, 466–472.

Stewart, P. M. (1999). Mineralocorticoid hypertension. *Lancet* **353**, 1341–1347.

Takahasi, N. *et al.* (2000). Uncompensated polyuria in a mouse model of Bartter's syndrome. *Proceedings of the National Academy of Sciences USA* **97**, 5434–5439.

Vandewalle, A. *et al.* (1997). Localization and induction by dehydration of ClC-K chloride channels in the rat kidney. *American Journal of Physiology* **272**, F678–F688.

Warnock, D. G. (2001). Liddle syndrome: genetics and mechanisms of Na^+ channel defects. *American Journal of Medical Science* **322**, 302–307.

Wrong, O. M., Feest, T. G., and Maciver, A. G. (1993). Immune-related potassium-losing interstitial nephritis: a comparison with distal renal tubular acidosis. *Quarterly Journal of Medicine* **86**, 513–534.

5.6 Nephrogenic diabetes insipidus

Daniel G. Bichet and Michael Zellweger

Nephrogenic diabetes insipidus (NDI), can be inherited or acquired. It is characterized by an inability to concentrate urine despite normal or elevated plasma concentrations of the antidiuretic hormone (ADH), arginine vasopressin (AVP). Polyuria, with hyposthenuria and polydipsia are its cardinal clinical manifestations.

A nephrogenic failure to concentrate urine maximally may be due to a defect in vasopressin-induced water permeability of the distal tubules and collecting ducts, insufficient build-up of the corticopapillary interstitial osmotic gradient, or a combination of both factors (Valtin and Schafer 1995). Thus, the broadest definition of the term 'nephrogenic diabetes insipidus' embraces any ADH resistant urinary concentrating defect, including medullary disease with low interstitial osmolality, renal failure, and osmotic diuresis. In its narrower sense, it describes only those conditions in which ADH release fails to induce the expected increase in water permeability of the cortical and medullary collecting duct (Table 1) (Magner and Halperin 1987).

Table 1 Causes of nephrogenic diabetes insipidus

Nephrogenic diabetes insipidus (restrictive definition): water permeability not increased by ADH
AVPR2 and *AQP2* mutations
Bartter's syndrome (*SLC12A1*, *KCNJ1*, and *Barttin* mutations)
Hypercalcaemia
Hypokalaemia
Drugs
Lithium
Demeclocycline
Amphotericin B (Canada *et al.* 2003)
Tenofovir (Verhelst *et al.* 2002)
Methoxyflurane
Diphenylhydantoin
Nicotine
Alcohol
Defective medullary countercurrent function
Renal failure, acute and chronic (especially interstitial nephritis and obstruction)
Medullary damage
Sickle-cell anaemia and trait
Amyloidosis
Sjögren's syndrome
Sarcoidosis
Hypercalcaemia
Hypokalaemia
Protein malnutrition
Cystinosis

Modified from Magner and Halperin (1987), with permission.

The various conditions in Table 1 are described in other parts of this book to which the reader is referred for further clinical discussion. This chapter concentrates upon the inherited forms of diabetes insipidus, but the discussion of the countercurrent system and the elaboration of concentrated urine described here are relevant to all these different clinical manifestations of diabetes insipidus in its widest sense.

Urine concentration and the countercurrent system (see also Chapters 2.1 and 5.1)

Urine is not concentrated by active transport of water from tubule fluid to blood, since such a system would require a tremendous expenditure of metabolic energy. It has been estimated that more than 300 times the energy needed by an active salt transport and passive water equilibration system would be required, as salt concentrations are about 0.15 mmol/l, whereas water concentrations are about 55 mmol/l. Instead, the urine is concentrated with relatively little expenditure of metabolic energy by a complex interaction between the loops of Henle, the medullary interstitium, the medullary blood vessels or vasa recta, and the collecting tubules. This mechanism of urine concentration is called the countercurrent mechanism because of the anatomical arrangement of the tubules and vascular elements. Tubular fluids move from the cortex towards the papillary tip of the medulla via the proximal straight tubule and the thin descending limbs. The tubules then loop back towards the cortex so that the direction of the fluid movement is reversed in the ascending limbs. Similarly, the vasa recta descend to the tip of the papilla and then loop back towards the cortex. This arrangement of tubule segments and vasa recta allows the two fundamental processes of the countercurrent mechanism to take place—countercurrent multiplication and countercurrent exchange (Jamison and Oliver 1982; Valtin and Schafer 1995).

ADH control of water transport (see also Chapter 2.1)

The ADH in man is AVP, a cyclic nonapeptide. In the presence of AVP, the entire collecting-tubule system becomes permeable to water and the kidney is able to take advantage of the osmotic pressure gradient between the hypertonic medullary interstitium and the dilute collecting-tubule fluid. In the human kidney, the maximum achievable osmolality is around 1200 mOsm/kg (see Chapter 5.1, Fig. 18) and since the obligatory excretion of waste products such as urea, sulfate, and phosphate amounts to about 600 mmol/day, at least 0.5 l of water per day must be excreted by the kidney.

Osmotic and non-osmotic stimulation

The regulation of AVP release from the posterior pituitary is dependent primarily on two mechanisms involving osmotic and non-osmotic pathways (Berl and Robertson 2000), described in detail in Chapter 2.1.

The osmotic regulation of AVP is dependent on 'osmoreceptor' cells in the anterior hypothalamus. The osmoreceptor cells are very sensitive to changes in osmolality of the extracellular fluid. With fluid deprivation a 1 per cent increase in that osmolality stimulates AVP release, whereas with water ingestion a 1 per cent decrease suppresses it.

AVP release can also be caused through a non-osmotic mechanism. Large decrements in blood volume or blood pressure (>10 per cent) sensed by stretch and baroreceptors in the central venous and arterial system stimulate AVP release.

The secretion of AVP is regulated by changes in blood osmolality, volume, and pressure (Berl and Robertson 2000). A variety of hypothalamic neurotransmitters, including monoamines and neuropeptides, is involved in the control of AVP release (Leibowitz 1988). Angiotensin II is a potent stimulant of AVP release (Fitzsimons 1998).

The osmotic stimulation of AVP release by dehydration or hypertonic saline infusion, or both, is regularly used to test the vasopressin secretory capacity of the posterior pituitary. This secretory capacity can be assessed directly by comparing the plasma AVP concentrations measured sequentially during the dehydration procedure with the normal values and then correlating the plasma AVP with the urinary osmolality measurements obtained simultaneously (Fig. 1) (Zerbe and Robertson 1981).

The AVP release can also be assessed indirectly by measuring plasma and urine osmolalities at regular intervals during the dehydration test (Miller *et al.* 1970). The maximal urinary osmolality obtained during dehydration is compared with the maximal urinary osmolality obtained after the administration of either pitressin or 1-desamino (8-D-arginine) vasopressin (dDAVP).

The non-osmotic stimulation of AVP release is used to assess the vasopressin secretory capacity of the posterior pituitary of a rare group of patients with the 'essential hyponatraemia and hypodipsia' syndrome (Howard *et al.* 1992). Although some of these patients may have partial central (neurogenic) diabetes insipidus, they respond normally to non-osmolar AVP release signals such as hypotension, emesis, and hypoglycaemia (Howard *et al.* 1992). In all other cases of suspected central (neurogenic) diabetes insipidus these non-osmotic stimulation tests will not give additional clinical information (Baylis *et al.* 1981).

Cellular actions of vasopressin and molecular biology of nephrogenic diabetes insipidus

The neurohypophyseal hormone AVP has multiple actions, including the inhibition of diuresis, contraction of smooth muscle, platelet aggregation, stimulation of liver glycogenolysis, modulation of ACTH release from the pituitary, and central regulation of somatic functions

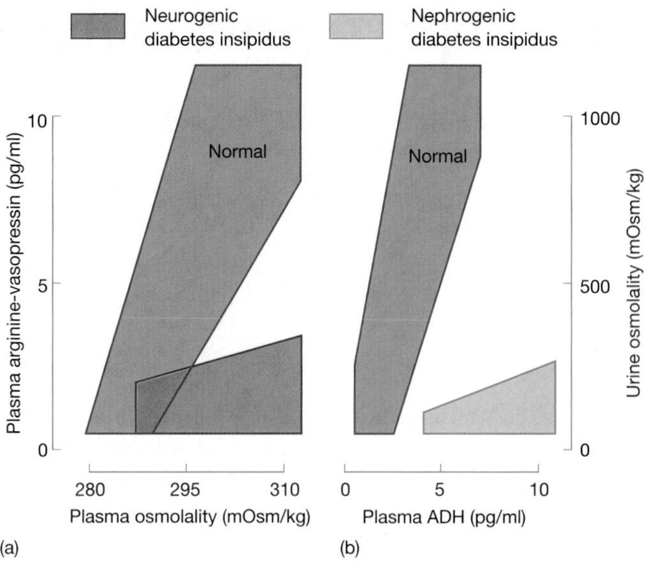

Fig. 1 Plasma AVP, plasma osmolality, and urine osmolality. (a) Relation between plasma AVP and plasma osmolality during hypertonic saline infusion. Patients with primary polydipsia and NDI have values within the normal range in contrast to patients with NDI who show subnormal plasma AVP responses. (b) Relation between urine osmolality and plasma AVP during dehydration and water loading. Patients with NDI and primary polydipsia have values within the normal range in contrast to patients with NDI who have hypotonic urine despite high plasma AVP. (Reproduced from Zerbe and Robertson 1984, with permission.)

(thermoregulation and blood pressure) (Jard 1985). These multiple actions of AVP could be explained by its interactions with at least three types of G protein-coupled receptors: the V_{1a} (vascular hepatic) and V_{1b} (anterior pituitary) receptors act through phosphatidylinositol hydrolysis to mobilize calcium (Nathanson *et al.* 1992), and the V_2 (kidney) receptor is coupled to adenylate cyclase (Jard 1985). The molecular identity of these three distinct vasopressin receptors has been established (Birnbaumer *et al.* 1992; de Keyzer *et al.* 1994; Sugimoto *et al.* 1994; Thibonnier *et al.* 1994).

The action of AVP on water excretion is described in Chapter 2.1, Fig. 4. Briefly, it is initiated by its binding to AVP type 2 receptors (V_2 receptors) on the basolateral membrane of the collecting-duct cells (Fig. 2). The human V_2 receptor gene, *AVPR2*, located in chromosome region Xq28, has three exons and two small introns (Birnbaumer *et al.* 1992; Seibold *et al.* 1992). The sequence of the cDNA predicts a polypeptide of 371 amino acids with a structure typical of guanine nucleotide (G) protein-coupled receptors with seven transmembrane, four extracellular, and four cytoplasmic domains (Watson and Arkinstall 1994) (see also Fig. 3). The activation of the V_2 receptor on renal collecting tubules stimulates adenylyl cyclase via the stimulatory G protein (G_s) and promotes the cAMP-mediated incorporation of water channels (aquaporins) into the luminal surface of these cells.

Aquaporin type 2 (AQP2), the vasopressin-regulated water channel, is exclusively present in principal cells of inner medullary collecting duct cells. It is diffusely distributed in the cytoplasm in the euhydrated condition, but concentrates in the apex in the dehydrated condition or after administration of dDAVP, a synthetic structural

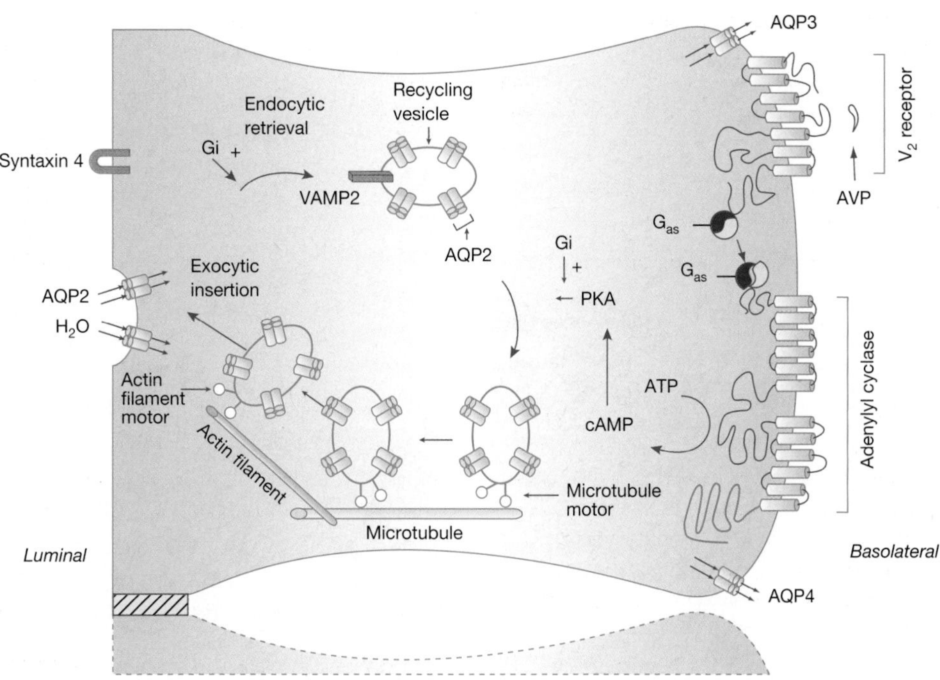

Fig. 2 Schematic representation of the effect of AVP to increase water permeability in the principal cells of the collecting duct. Please note that Na reabsorption, through the epithelial Na channel (ENaC) is not represented. AVP is bound to the V_2 receptor (a G-protein-linked receptor) on the basolateral membrane. The basic process of G-protein-coupled receptor signalling consists of three steps: a hepta-helical receptor that detects a ligand (in this case, AVP) in the extracellular milieu, a G-protein that dissociates into α subunits bound to GTP and $\beta\gamma$ subunits after interaction with the ligand-bound receptor, and an effector (in this case, adenylyl cyclase) that interacts with dissociated G-protein subunits to generate small-molecule second messengers. AVP activates adenylyl cyclase increasing the intracellular concentration of cAMP. The topology of adenylyl cyclase is characterized by two tandem repeats of six hydrophobic transmembrane domains separated by a large cytoplasmic loop and terminates in a large intracellular tail. Generation of cAMP follows receptor-linked activation of the heteromeric G-protein (G_s) and interaction of the free $G_{\alpha s}$-chain with the adenylyl cyclase catalyst. PKA is the target of the generated cAMP. Cytoplasmic vesicles carrying the water channel proteins (represented as homotetrameric complexes) are fused to the luminal membrane in response to AVP, thereby increasing the water permeability of this membrane. Microtubules and actin filaments are necessary for vesicle movement toward the membrane. The mechanisms underlying docking and fusion of AQP2 bearing vesicles are not known. The detection of the small GTP binding protein Rab3a, synaptobrevin 2, and syntaxin 4 in principal cells suggests that these proteins are involved in AQP2 trafficking (Valenti *et al.* 1998). When AVP is not available, water channels are retrieved by an endocytic process, and water permeability returns to its original low rate. AQP3 and AQP4 water channels are expressed on the basolateral membrane.

analogue of AVP. The short-term AQP2 regulation by AVP involves the movement of AQP2 from intracellular vesicles to the plasma membrane. In the long-term regulation, a sustained elevation of circulating AVP levels, for 24 h or more, increases the abundance of water channels. This is thought to be a consequence of increased transcription of the *AQP2* gene (Knepper 1997). Elevated effective osmolality is also crucial for the expression of AQP2 in primary cultured epithelial cells from the inner medulla of rat kidney (Storm *et al.* 2003). The activation of PKA leads to phosphorylation of AQP2 on serine residue 256 in the cytoplasmic carboxyl terminus. This phosphorylation step is essential for the regulated movement of AQP2-containing vesicles to the plasma membrane upon elevation of intracellular cAMP concentration (Fushimi *et al.* 1997; Katsura *et al.* 1997). A second G-protein (the first being the cholera-toxin sensitive G-protein G_s) has also been shown to be essential for the AVP-induced shuttling of AQP2. This G-protein is sensitive to pertussis toxin and is involved in the pathway downstream of the cAMP/cAMP-dependent protein kinase signal (Valenti *et al.* 1998). The molecular basis for the translocation of the AQP2-containing vesicles remains incompletely known, but it is thought to be analogous to neuronal exocytosis (Mandon *et al.* 1997). This is supported by the identification in the vesicles of various proteins known to be involved in regulated exocytosis, for example, Rab3a and synaptobrevin II (VAMP2) or synaptobrevin II-like protein (Jo *et al.* 1995; Liebenhoff and Rosenthal 1995; Nielsen *et al.* 1995). In contrast to neuronal exocytosis, which is triggered by Ca^{2+}, cAMP and PKA appear to be crucial for the translocation process (Star *et al.* 1988; Snyder *et al.* 1992). Vesicle trafficking probably involves the interaction of AQP2-containing vesicles with the cytoskeleton (Brown *et al.* 1998) (Fig. 2). Drugs that disrupt microtubules or actin filaments have long been known to inhibit the hormonally induced permeability response in target epithelia (Taylor *et al.* 1973).

AVP also increases the water reabsorptive capacity of the kidney by regulating the urea transporter UT-A1, which is present in the inner medullary collecting duct, predominantly in its terminal part (Shayakul *et al.* 1996; Sands 2002; Yang *et al.* 2002). AVP also increases the permeability of principal collecting duct cells to sodium (Ward *et al.* 1999).

In summary, as stated elegantly by Ward, Hammond, and Harris (Ward *et al.* 1999), in the absence of AVP stimulation, collecting duct epithelia exhibit very low permeabilities to sodium urea and water. These specialized permeability properties permit the excretion of large volumes of hypotonic urine formed during intervals of water diuresis.

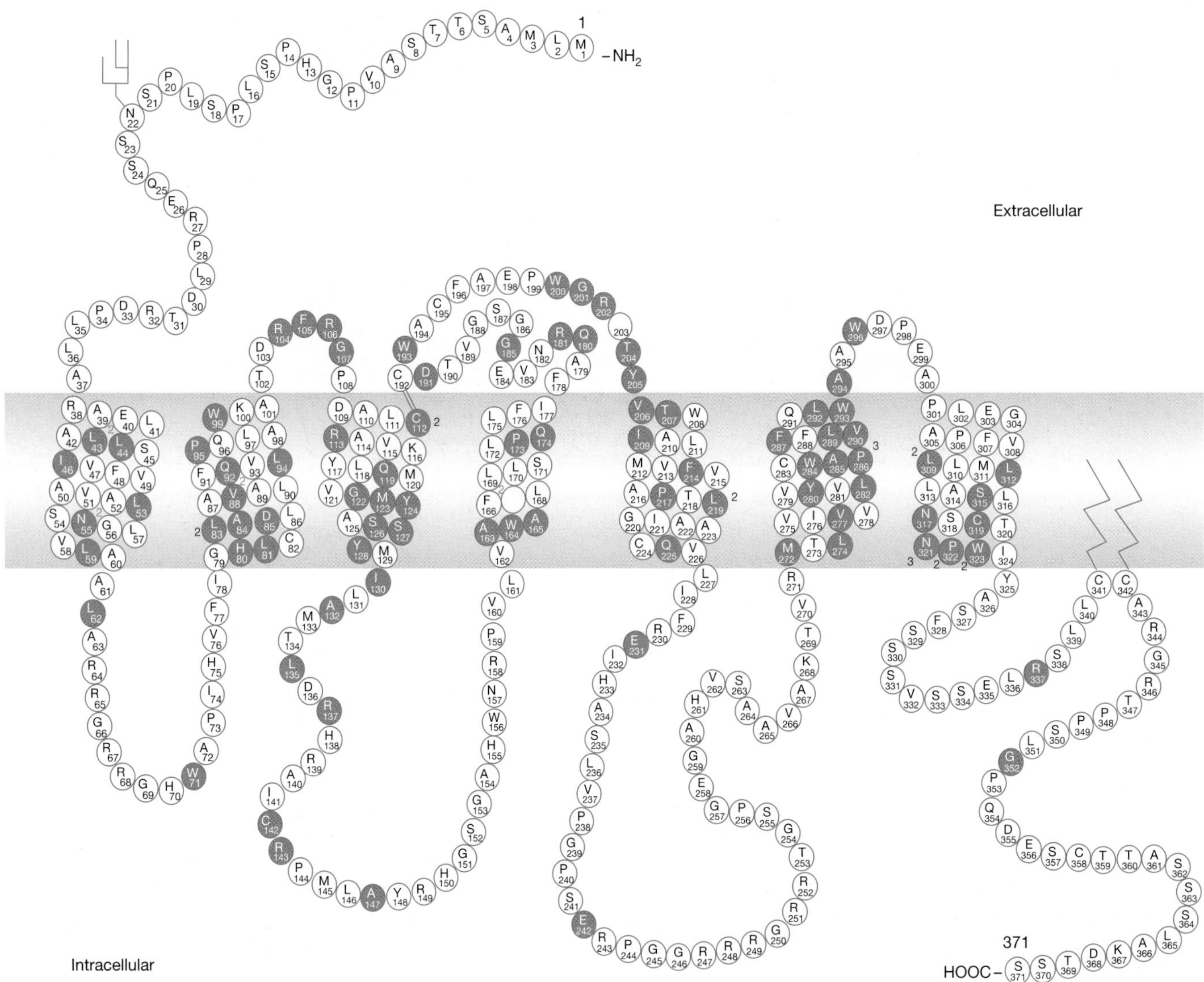

Fig. 3 Schematic representation of the V_2 receptor and identification of 183 putative disease-causing *AVPR2* mutations. Predicted amino acids are given as the one-letter code. Solid symbols indicate missense or nonsense mutations; a number indicates more than one mutation in the same codon. The names of the mutations were assigned according to recommended nomenclature (Antonarakis and the Nomenclature Working Group 1998). The extracellular, transmembrane, and cytoplasmic domains are defined according to Mouillac *et al.* (1995). The common names of the mutations are listed by type. *Eighty-nine missense, 18 nonsense mutations, 45 frameshift, seven inframe deletions or insertions, four splice-site* as well as 19 large deletions and one complex mutation have been identified.

In contrast, AVP stimulation of the principal cells of the collecting ducts leads to selective increases in the permeability of the apical membrane to water (P_f), urea (P_{urea}), and Na (P_{Na}).

The gene that codes for the water channel of the apical membrane of the kidney collecting tubule has been designated aquaporin-2 (*AQP2*) and was cloned by homology to the rat aquaporin of collecting duct (Fushimi *et al.* 1993; Deen *et al.* 1994a; Sasaki *et al.* 1994). The human *AQP2* gene is located in chromosome region 12q13 and has four exons and three introns (Deen *et al.* 1994a,b; Sasaki *et al.* 1994). It is predicted to code for a polypeptide of 271 amino acids that is organized into two repeats oriented at 180 degrees to each other and has six membrane-spanning domains, both terminal ends located intracellularly, and conserved Asn-Pro-Ala boxes (Fig. 4). These features are characteristic of the major intrinsic protein family (Sasaki *et al.* 1994). AQP2 is detectable in urine, and changes in urinary excretion of this protein can be used as an index of the action of vasopressin on the kidney (Kanno *et al.* 1995; Elliot *et al.* 1996; Saito *et al.* 1997).

Quantitating renal water excretion

Osmotic and non-osmotic polyuric states

Diabetes insipidus is characterized by the excretion of abnormally large volumes (>30 ml/kg body weight per day) of hypo-osmotic urine (<250 mOsm/kg). Polyuria occurs either with a normal solute excretion and a depressed water-retaining ability of the tubules or with a high solute excretion and a normal ability to retrieve filtered water.

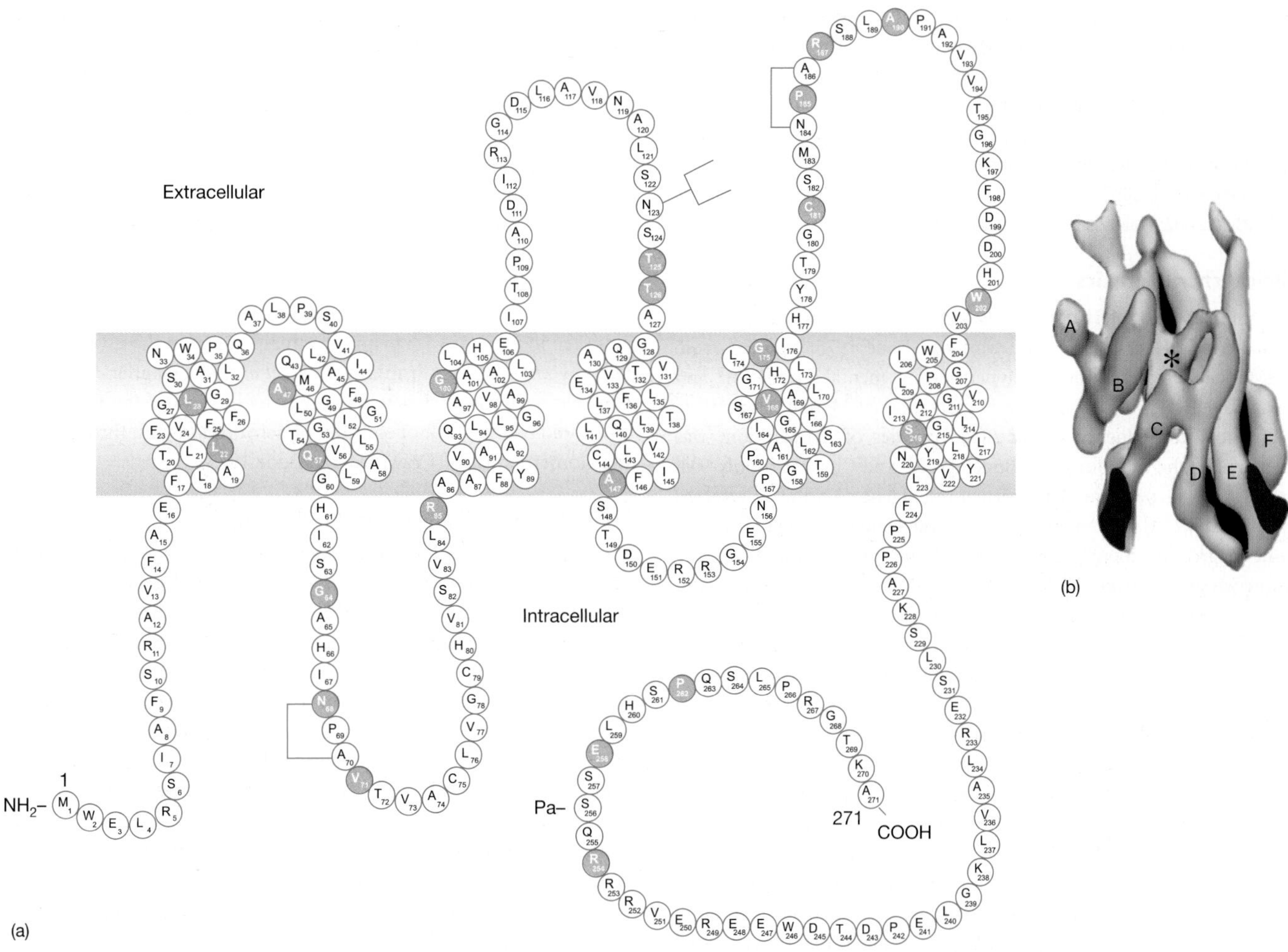

Fig. 4 A representation of the aquaporin-2 (AQP2) protein and identification of 32 putative disease causing *AQP2* mutations. A monomer is represented with six transmembrane helices. The location of the PKA phosphorylation site (Pa) is indicated. The extracellular, transmembrane, and cytoplasmic domains are defined according to Deen *et al.* (1994a). Solid symbols indicate the location of the mutations. The common names of the mutations are listed by type. *Twenty-two missense, two nonsense, six frameshift,* as well as *two splice-site* mutations have been identified.

The former is called diabetes insipidus, the latter osmotic diuresis. Osmotic diuresis occurs when excess solute is excreted, as with glucose in the polyuria of diabetes mellitus. Other agents that produce osmotic diuresis are mannitol, urea, glycerol, contrast media, and loop diuretics. Osmotic diuresis should be considered when solute excretion exceeds 60 mmol/h.

Osmolar clearance, free-water clearance, and tonicity balance

The quantitation of water excretion has been facilitated by the concept that urine flow can be divided into two components (Berl and Kumar 2000). One component is the urine volume needed to excrete solutes at the concentration of the solutes in the plasma. This isotonic component has been termed 'osmolar clearance' (C_{osm}). The other component is called 'free-water clearance' (C_{H_2O}) and is the theoretical volume of solute-free water that has to be added to (positive *C*) or removed from (negative C_{H_2O} or TC_{H_2O}) the isotonic portion of the urine (C_{osm}) to create either hypotonic or hypertonic urine, respectively. These calculations can be found in Berl and Kumar (2000). A tonicity balance calculation is an accurate way to understand the basis for the change in natraemia and the proper goals of therapy. This tonicity balance calculation allows the demonstration of iatrogenic sodium gains and their proper treatment (Carlotti *et al.* 2001).

Clinical and biochemical characteristics of nephrogenic diabetes insipidus

Congenital

About 90 per cent of patients with congenital NDI are males with X-linked recessive NDI (MIM 304800) (McKusick 2000), who have mutations in the arginine–vasopressin receptor 2 (*AVPR2*) gene that codes for the vasopressin V2 receptor (Bichet and Fujiwara 2001). The gene is located in the chromosome region Xq28.

In less than 10 per cent of the families studied, congenital NDI has an autosomal recessive or autosomal dominant mode of inheritance

(MIM 222000 and 125800) (McKusick 2000; Bichet and Fujiwara 2001). Mutations have been identified in the aquaporin-2 gene (*AQP2*), which is located in chromosome region 12q13 and codes for the vasopressin-sensitive water channel.

Other inherited disorders with mild, moderate, or severe inability to concentrate urine include Bartter's syndrome (MIM 601678) (McKusick 2000; Peters *et al.* 2002) and cystinosis (MIM 219800) (McKusick 2000; Gahl *et al.* 2002; Kalatzis and Antignac 2002).

Clinical characteristics

The clinical characteristics (Forssman 1942; Waring *et al.* 1945; Williams and Henry 1947; Crawford and Bode 1975; Niaudet *et al.* 1985) include hypernatraemia, hyperthermia, mental retardation, and repeated episodes of dehydration in early infancy. Mental retardation, a probable consequence of repeated episodes of dehydration, was prevalent in the Crawford and Bode (1975) study, in which only 9 of 82 patients (11 per cent) had normal intelligence. Of the 45 affected males that we examined in Montreal and Halifax, 70 per cent had some degree of mental retardation. More recent data from the Nijmegen group suggest that mental retardation is less prevalent and might have been overestimated in NDI patients (Hoekstra *et al.* 1996; van Lieburg *et al.* 1999). Early recognition and the subsequent treatment of congenital NDI with an abundant intake of water allows a normal lifespan with normal physical and mental development (Niaudet *et al.* 1985) (author's personal observations). Two characteristics suggestive of X-linked NDI are the familial occurrence and the confinement of mental retardation to male patients. It is then tempting to assume that the family described by McIlraith (1892) and discussed by Reeves and Andreoli (1995) was affected by congenital NDI. Lacombe (1841) and Weil (1884) described an autosomal-dominant type of transmission without any associated mental retardation. The descendants of the family originally described by Weil were later found to have autosomal-dominant central (neurogenic) diabetes insipidus (Weil 1908; Camerer 1935; Dölle 1951), a now well-characterized entity secondary to mutations in the *prepro-AVP-neurophysin II* gene, OMIM 192340 (McKusick 2000) (for review, see Fujiwara *et al.* 1995; Bichet and Fujiwara 2001). Patients with autosomal-dominant central (neurogenic) diabetes insipidus retain some limited capacity to secrete AVP during severe dehydration and the polyuro–polydipsic symptoms usually appear after the first year of life (Fujiwara *et al.* 1995; Rittig *et al.* 1996; Ito *et al.* 1999) when the ability of the infants to seek water is more likely to be understood by adults.

The early symptomatic pattern of the nephrogenic disorder and its severity in infancy is clearly described by Crawford and Bode (1975). Although the polydipsia and polyuria are often overlooked during infancy, the concentration defect is demonstrable within 6 days of birth, and parents aware of the disorder in the family have reported that their affected infants show a distinct preference for water over milk as early as 1 week of age. Pregnancies leading to the birth of affected infants are not complicated by polyhydramnios. Polyhydramnios is exclusively seen during the pregnancy leading to infants subsequently found to have Bartter's syndrome secondary to *KCNJ1*, *SLC12A1*, or *BSND* mutations (see Chapter 5.5). The infants are irritable, cry almost constantly, and, although eager to suck, will vomit milk soon after ingestion unless prefed with water. The history given by mothers often includes persistent constipation, erratic, unexplained fever, and failure to gain weight. Even though the patients characteristically show no visible evidence of perspiration, the increased water loss during fever or in warm weather exaggerates the symptoms. Unless the condition is recognized early, the children will experience frequent bouts of hypertonic dehydration, sometimes complicated by convulsions or death. Mental retardation is a frequent consequence of these episodes. The intake of large quantities of water combined with the patient's voluntary restriction of dietary salt and protein intake lead to hypocaloric dwarfism beginning in infancy. Affected children frequently develop dilatations and obstructions of the lower urinary tract, probably secondary to the large urinary volume (Streitz and Streitz 1988). Dilatation of the lower urinary tract is also seen in patients with primary polydipsia and in those with central (neurogenic) diabetes insipidus (Boyd *et al.* 1980; Gautier *et al.* 1981). Chronic renal insufficiency may occur by the end of the first decade and could be the result of episodes of dehydration with thrombosis of the glomerular tufts (Crawford and Bode 1975).

Clinical and biochemical diagnosis

The family history will usually provide the evidence for a presumptive diagnosis in an affected infant. However, several generations could have passed since the birth of the last affected male and a 'sporadic' case may then be diagnosed. Also, a number of *de novo* cases have now been described (for review see Fujiwara *et al.* 1995; Arthus *et al.* 2002). As a consequence, the absence of a family history of X-linked NDI does not rule out the disease, and the DNA of sporadic patients and their mothers should be analysed for *AVPR2* mutations (see 'Mutational analysis' below). The diagnosis of congenital NDI could be rapidly confirmed by a short dehydration test followed by vasopressin administration (see 'Investigation of a patient with polyuria' below) (Fig. 5). Measurements of plasma sodium, and plasma and urine osmolality should be immediately available at various intervals during dehydration procedures.

Urinary osmolalities are measured at the beginning of each dehydration procedure and at regular intervals (usually hourly) thereafter depending on the severity of the polyuric syndrome. For example, an 8-year-old patient (body weight 31 kg) with a clinical diagnosis of congenital NDI, later found to bear the *AVPR2 de novo* mutation 274insG (Bichet *et al.* 1994), continued to excrete large volumes of urine (300 ml/h) during a short, 4-h dehydration test. During this time, the patient was suffering from severe thirst, his plasma sodium 155 mmol/l, his plasma osmolality 310 mOsm/kg, and his urinary osmolality 85 mOsm/kg. The patient received 1 μg of dDAVP intravenously and was allowed to drink water. Repeated urinary osmolality measurements demonstrated a complete urinary resistance to dDAVP.

It would have been dangerous and unnecessary to prolong the dehydration further in this young patient. Thus, the usual prescription of overnight dehydration should not be used in patients, and especially children, with severe polyuria and polydipsia (>30 ml/kg body weight per day). Great care should be taken to avoid any severe hypertonic state, arbitrarily defined as a plasma sodium of more than 155 mmol/l.

Abnormal renal and extrarenal V_2 receptor responses in males with X-linked diabetes insipidus

In males with X-linked NDI, urinary osmolality does not change after administration of AVP or dDAVP—a selective V_2 agonist—and maximal urinary osmolality remains below 250 mOsm/kg (Fig. 6).

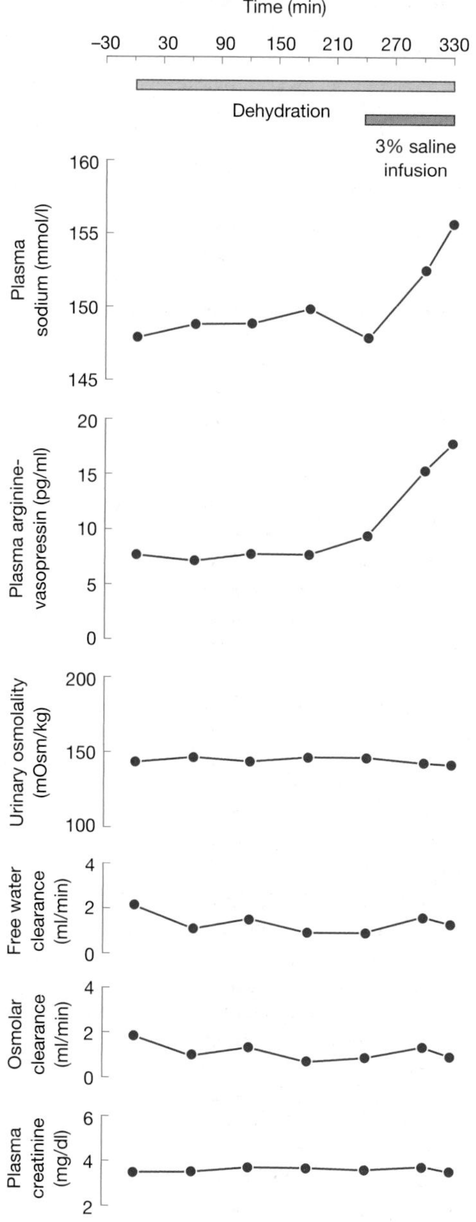

Fig. 5 The patient (age 45, weight 50 kg, height 1.6 m) had a personal and family history pathognomonic of hereditary NDI. His genealogical tree was published by Huard and Picard (1960). This patient was later found to have the 804delG mutation (Rosenthal *et al.* 1992). During the first years of his life he suffered repeated episodes of dehydration and is now mentally retarded. He has spent the past 20 years without medication but fitted with a permanent urinary catheter in a chronic care institution. During the past 5 years, he has had multiple episodes of urinary-tract infection and dehydration. At the time of this study, his serum creatinine was 3.5 mg/dl (309 μmol/l) with a creatinine clearance of 20 ml/min/1.73 m^2. This has been attributed to chronic pyelonephritis. The patient was dehydrated for a total of 330 min and received a 0.1 ml/kg body wt/min, 3 per cent saline infusion during the last 120 min of the test. Plasma sodium increased from 147 to 155 mmol/l and very high concentrations of plasma vasopressin were measured (from 7 to 15 pg/ml). However, urinary osmolality remained less than 150 mmol/kg and free-water clearance, osmolar clearance, and plasma creatinine were unchanged during the procedure.

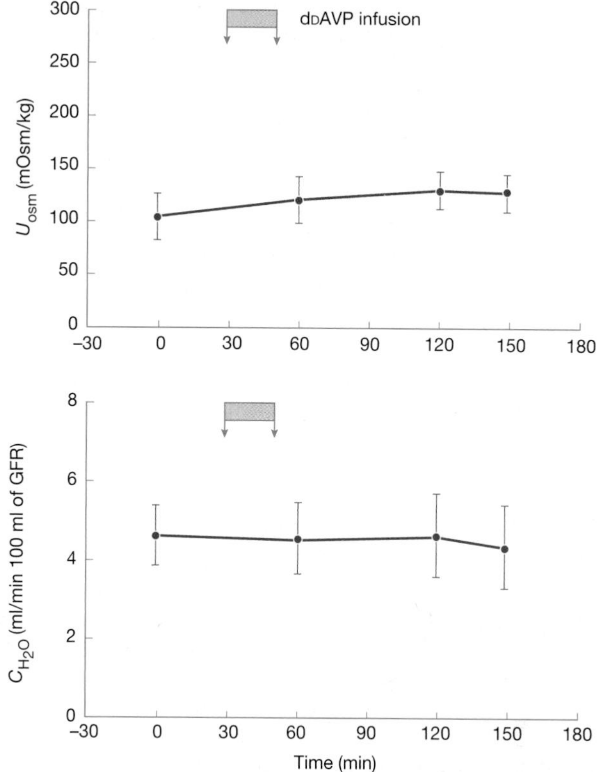

Fig. 6 Water-excretion characteristics after dDAVP infusion in six male patients with X-linked NDI. dDAVP (0.3 μg/kg body weight up to a maximum of 24 μg) was infused from 0 to 20 min. Urinary osmolality (U_{osm}), free-water clearance (C), and osmolar clearance (not shown) remained unchanged following the infusion. Mean ± SEM are represented.

Plasma endogenous vasopressin concentrations are initially within the normal range and increase normally during dehydration or hypertonic saline infusion (Fig. 7). These results indicate that the renal V_2-receptor responses are abnormal (Bichet *et al.* 1988, 1989).

Clinical evidence supports a concommitant abnormality of the extrarenal V_2 receptor influencing blood pressure and the level of coagulation factors.

Bichet *et al.* (1988, 1989) found that blood pressure did not decrease whereas plasma renin activity and the release of coagulation factors (factor VIIIc, von Willebrand factor, tissue plasminogen activator) failed to increase in response to the administration of dDAVP in 14 male patients with X-linked NDI, later found to have *AVPR2* mutations. These results, confirmed by other investigators (Derkx *et al.* 1987; Knoers *et al.* 1990), point to abnormal responses of the extrarenal V_2 receptors in patients with X-linked NDI (Kaufmann *et al.* 2000).

Mutational analysis of nephrogenic diabetes insipidus

The identification, characterization, and mutational analysis of two genes, the AVP receptor-2 gene (*AVPR2*) and the vasopressin-sensitive water-channel gene (aquaporin 2, *AQP2*), provide the basis for the understanding of three different forms of diabetes insipidus, X-linked NDI, autosomal-recessive NDI, and autosomal dominant NDI. The evolution of the molecular genetic techniques used for the analysis of

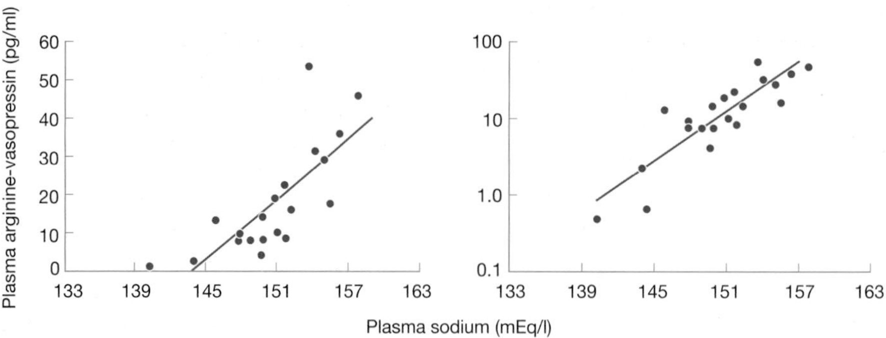

Fig. 7 Osmotic stimulation of AVP in five male patients with X-linked NDI. Plasma AVP was measured after various lengths of dehydration or during hypertonic saline infusion. Linear (left) and log linear (right) relations are represented.

patients with X-linked NDI have been reviewed by Hendy and Bichet (1995) and recent publications include details of the identified mutations (Arthus *et al.* 2000; Lin *et al.* 2002; Marr *et al.* 2002a,b). These advances provide additional diagnostic tools for physicians caring for these patients. Early molecular diagnosis of NDI is essential for early treatment of affected infants in order to avoid repeated episodes of dehydration.

X-linked nephrogenic diabetes insipidus and mutations in the *AVPR2* gene

The majority (approximately 90 per cent) of patients with congenital NDI have the X-linked form: affected male patients do not concentrate their urine after the administration of AVP. Because it is a rare, recessive X-linked disease, females are unlikely to be affected, but heterozygous females exhibit variable degrees of polyuria and polydipsia because of skewed X-chromosome inactivation. In Quebec, the incidence of this disease was estimated to be approximately 8.8 per million male live births for the 10-year period 1988–1997 (Arthus *et al.* 2000). A founder effect for a particular *AVPR2* mutation in Ulster Scot immigrants resulted in an increased prevalence of X-linked NDI in their descendants and we estimated the incidence in Nova Scotia and New Brunswick to be 58 per million male live births for the 10-year period 1988–1997 (Arthus *et al.* 2000). The W71X mutation was identified as the cause of NDI in the extended 'Hopewell' kindred (Bode and Crawford 1969) and in families in the Canadian Maritime provinces (Bichet *et al.* 1993; Holtzman *et al.* 1993). The W71X mutations of these patients are probably identical by descent, although a common ancestor has not been identified in all cases. Among patients with X-linked NDI in North America, the W71X mutation is more common than any other *AVPR2* mutation.

To date, 183 putative disease-causing *AVPR2* mutations have been identified in 284 NDI families (see Fig. 3) (additional information is available from the NDI Mutation Database at http://www.medicine.mcgill.ca/nephros/). Half of the mutations are missense mutations. Frameshift mutations due to nucleotide deletions or insertions (25 per cent), nonsense mutations (10 per cent), large deletions (10 per cent), inframe deletions or insertions (4 per cent), splice-site mutations, and one complex mutation account for the remainder. Mutations have been identified in every domain, of the AVPR2 receptor, but on a per nucleotide basis, about twice as many mutations occur in transmembrane domains compared with the extracellular or intracellular domains. We previously identified private mutations, recurrent mutations, and mechanisms of mutagenesis (Bichet *et al.* 1994; Fujiwara *et al.* 1996). The 10 recurrent mutations (D85N, V88M, R113W, Y128S, R137H, S167L, R181C, R202C, A294P, and S315R) were found in 35 ancestrally independent families (Arthus *et al.* 2000). The occurrence of the same mutation on different haplotype was considered evidence of recurrent mutation. In addition, the most frequent mutations—D85N, V88N, R113W, R137H, S167L, R181C, and R202C—occurred at potential mutational hot spots (a G-to-T or G-to-A nucleotide substitution occurred at a Cpg dinucleotide).

When studied *in vitro*, most *AVPR2* mutations lead to receptors that are trapped intracellularly and unable to reach the plasma membrane. A few mutant receptors reach the cell surface but are unable to bind AVP or to properly trigger an intracellular cAMP signal (for review, see Morello and Bichet 2001). *AVPR2* mutations are thus inducing a defective intracellular protein transport, an increasingly recognized anomally of hereditary disease-causing mutations (for review, see Kuznetsov and Nigam 1998; Aridor and Balch 1999).

Of clinical interest, non-peptide vasopressin V_2 receptor antagonists were recently found to facilitate the folding of mutant AVPR2 receptors and to increase urine osmolality in patients bearing the del62–64, R137H, and W164S mutations (Morello *et al.* 2000; Bichet *et al.* 2002).

Autosomal recessive and dominant nephrogenic diabetes insipidus and mutations in the *AQP2* gene

On the basis of desmopressin infusion studies and phenotypic characteristics of both males and females affected with NDI, a non-X-linked form of NDI with a postreceptor (post-cAMP) defect was suggested (Brenner *et al.* 1988; Knoers and Monnens 1991; Langley *et al.* 1991; Lonergan *et al.* 1993). A patient who presented shortly after birth with typical features of NDI but who exhibited normal coagulation and normal fibrinolytic and vasodilatory responses to desmopressin was shown to be a compound heterozygote for two missense mutations (R187C and S217P) in the *AQP2* gene (Deen *et al.* 1994a) (Fig. 4). To date, 32 putative disease-causing *AQP2* mutations have been identified in 40 NDI families (Fig. 4). By type of mutation, there are 69 per cent missense, 19 per cent frameshift due to small nucleotide deletions or insertions, 6 per cent nonsense, and 6 per cent splice-site mutations (additional information is available in the NDI Mutation Database at http://www.medicine.mcgill.ca/nephros/).

Reminiscent of expression studies done with AVPR2 proteins, misrouting of AQP2 mutant proteins has been shown to be the major cause underlying autosomal recessive NDI (Deen *et al.* 1995; Mulders *et al.* 1997; Tamarappoo and Verkman 1998). In contrast to the *AQP2* mutations in autosomal recessive NDI, which are located throughout the gene, the dominant mutations are predicted to affect the carboxyl terminus of AQP2 (van Os and Deen 1998; Kuwahara *et al.* 2001; Marr *et al.* 2002b; Kamsteeg *et al.* 2003). The autosomal dominant family described by Ohzeki *et al.* (1984) was found to be heterozygous for the 721delG mutation (Kuwahara *et al.* 2001). The dominant *AQP2-E258K* mutation was retained in the Golgi apparatus, which differs from mutants *AQP2* in recessive NDI that are retained in the endoplasmic reticulum. The dominant action of the *AQP2-E258K* mutation can be explained by the formation of heterotetramers of mutant and wild-type AQP2 that are impaired in their routing after oligomerization (Mulders *et al.* 1998; Kamsteeg *et al.* 1999). Hetero-oligomerization of AQP2-727delG with wt-AQP2 and consequent mistargeting of this complex to late endosomes/lysosomes results in the absence of AQP2 in the apical membrane, which can explain the dominant phenotype (Marr *et al.* 2002b).

Polyuria, polydipsia, electrolyte imbalance, and dehydration in cystinosis

Polyuria may be as mild as persistent enuresis or as severe as to contribute to death from dehydration and electrolyte abnormalities in infants with cystinosis who have acute gastroenteritis (Gahl *et al.* 2002).

Polyuria in hereditary hypokalaemic salt-losing tubulopathies (see Chapter 5.5)

Patients with polyhydramnios, hypercalciuria, and hypo- or isothenuria have been found to bear *KCNJ1* (ROMK) and *SLC12A1* (NKCC2) mutations. Patients with polyhydramnios, profound polyuria, hyponatraemia, hypochloraemia, metabolic alkalosis, and sensorineural deafness were found to bear *BSND* mutations. These observations demonstrate the critical importance of the proteins ROMK, NKCC2, and Barttin to transfer NaCl in the medullary interstitium and thereby to generate, together with urea, an hypertonic milieu.

Benefits of genetic testing

Prior knowledge of *AVPR2, AQP2*, or Bartter's syndrome mutations in NDI families and perinatal mutation testing is of direct clinical value because early diagnosis and treatment can avert the physical and mental retardation associated with repeated episodes of dehydration. Diagnosis of X-linked NDI was accomplished by mutation testing of chorionic villous samples ($n = 4$), cultured amniotic cells ($n = 5$), or cord blood ($n = 17$). Three infants who had mutation testing done on amniotic cells ($n = 1$) or chorionic villous samples ($n = 2$) also had their diagnosis confirmed by cord blood testing. Of the 23 offspring tested, 12 were found to be affected males, seven were unaffected males, and four were non-carrier girls (Bichet *et al.* unpublished). The affected males were immediately treated with abundant water intake, a low sodium diet, and hydrochlorothiazide. They have not experienced severe episodes of dehydration and their physical and mental development remains normal; however, their urinary output is only decreased by 30 per cent and a normal growth curve is still difficult to reach during the first 2–3 years of their life despite the above treatments and intensive attention.

Treatment

The treatment of congenital NDI has been reviewed (Knoers and Monnens 1992; Cheetham and Baylis 2002). An abundant, unrestricted water intake should always be provided and affected male patients should be carefully followed during their first years of life (Niaudet *et al.* 1984, 1985). Water should be offered every 2 h, day and night, and temperature, appetite, and growth should be monitored. The parents of these children easily accept to set their alarm-clock every 2 h during the night! Admission to hospital may be necessary for continuous gastric feeding. A low osmolar and sodium diet, hydrochlorothiazide (1–2 mg/kg/day), and indomethacin (1.5–3 mg/kg) substantially reduce water excretion (Blalock *et al.* 1977; Alon and Chan 1985; Libber *et al.* 1986; Knoers and Monnens 1990; Jakobsson and Berg 1994) and are helpful in the treatment of children. The voluminous amounts of water kept in patients' stomachs will exacerbate physiological gastro-oesophageal reflux as an infant and toddler, and many affected boys frequently vomit and have a strong positive 'Tuttle test' (oesophageal pH testing). These young patients often improve with the absorption of an H-2 blocker and with metoclopramide (which could induce extrapyramidal symptoms) or with domperidone, which seems to be better tolerated and efficacious. Many adult patients receive no treatment. In our experience, prior knowledge of the *AVPR2* mutation in families with NDI and perinatal mutational testing have been of direct clinical value for early treatment and prevention of dehydration episodes (Bichet *et al.* 1994). A vicious circle of dehydration leading to hospital admission and, possibly, less attention (in a non-familial environment) to fluid and solid intake is, in our experience, entirely preventable.

Acquired

The acquired form is much more common than the congenital form of NDI but it is rarely severe. The ability to elaborate a hypertonic urine is usually preserved, in spite of the impairment of the maximal concentrating ability of the nephrons. Polyuria and polydipsia are therefore moderate (3–4 l/day).

The more common causes of acquired NDI are listed in Table 1. Lithium administration has become the most frequent cause among them (see also Chapter 5.5). A review (Boton *et al.* 1987) reported this abnormality in at least 54 per cent of 1105 unselected patients on chronic lithium therapy. Nineteen per cent of these patients had polyuria, as defined by a 24-h urine output exceeding 3 l. Lithium inhibits adenylate cyclase in a number of cell types including renal epithelia (Christensen *et al.* 1985; Cogan *et al.* 1987). The concentration of lithium in the urine of patients on well-controlled lithium therapy (i.e. 10–40 mmol/l) is sufficient to exert this effect. Measurements of adenylate cyclase activity in membranes isolated from a cultured pig kidney cell line (LLC-PK_1) revealed that lithium in the concentration range of 10 mmol/l interfered with the hormone-stimulated guanyl nucleotide regulatory unit (G_s) (Goldberg *et al.* 1988). The effect of chronic lithium therapy on the expression of aquaporin 2 has been studied in rat kidney membranes prepared from the inner medulla; it caused a marked downregulation, only partially reversed by cessation of therapy, thirsting, or dDAVP treatment, consistent with clinical observations of slow recovery from lithium-induced urinary concentrating defects (Marples *et al.* 1995). Hypokalaemia, hypercalciuria, and the release of bilateral ureteral obstruction have also been shown to downregulate the expression of

Table 2 Differential diagnosis of diabetes insipidus

(1) Measure plasma osmolality and/or sodium concentration under conditions of *ad libitum* fluid intake. If they are greater than 295 mOsm/kg and 143 mmol/l, the diagnosis of primary polydipsia is excluded and the work-up should proceed directly to step (5) and/or (6) to distinguish between neurogenic and nephrogenic diabetes insipidus
Otherwise
(2) Perform a dehydration test. If urinary concentration does not occur before plasma osmolality and/or sodium reach 295 mOsm/kg or 143 mmol/l, the diagnosis of primary polydipsia is again excluded and the workup should proceed to step (5) and/or (6)
Otherwise
(3) Determine the ratio of urine to plasma osmolality at the end of the dehydration test. If it is less than 1.5 the diagnosis of primary polydipsia is again excluded and the workup should proceed to step (5) and/or (6)
Otherwise
(4) Perform a hypertonic saline infusion with measurements of plasma vasopressin and osmolality at intervals during the procedure. If the relation between these two variables is subnormal, the diagnosis of diabetes insipidus is established
Otherwise
(5) Perform a vasopressin infusion test. If urine osmolality increases by more than 150 mOsm/kg above the value obtained at the end of the dehydration test, NDI is excluded
Alternatively
(6) Measure urine osmolality and plasma vasopressin at the end of the dehydration test. If the relation is normal, the diagnosis of NDI is excluded

Data from Robertson (1987).

aquaporin 2 in rat kidney medulla (Frokiaer *et al.* 1996; Marples *et al.* 1996; Sands *et al.* 1998). In patients on long-term lithium therapy, amiloride has been proposed to prevent the uptake of lithium in the collecting ducts, thus preventing the inhibitory effect of intracellular lithium on water transport (Batlle *et al.* 1985).

Investigation of a patient with polyuria

Plasma sodium and osmolality are maintained within normal limits (136–143 mmol/l for plasma sodium, 275–290 mOsm/kg for plasma osmolality) by a thirst–AVP–renal axis. Thirst and AVP release, both stimulated by increased osmolality, have been termed a 'double negative' feedback system (Leaf 1979). Thus, even when the AVP limb of this 'double negative' regulatory feedback system is lost, the thirst mechanism still preserves the plasma sodium and osmolality within the normal range, but at the expense of pronounced polydipsia and polyuria. Thus, the plasma sodium concentration or osmolality of an untreated patient with diabetes insipidus may be slightly greater than the mean normal value, but, since the values usually remain within the normal range, these small increases have no diagnostic significance.

Theoretically, it should be relatively easy to differentiate between central (neurogenic) diabetes insipidus, NDI, and primary polydipsia. A comparison of the osmolality of urine obtained during dehydration from patients with central (neurogenic) diabetes insipidus or NDI with that of urine obtained after the administration of AVP should reveal a rapid increase in osmolality only in those with the central (neurogenic) type. Urinary osmolality should increase normally in response to moderate dehydration in patients with primary polydipsia.

However, these distinctions may not be as clear as one might expect, owing to several factors (Robertson 1985). First, chronic polyuria of any cause interferes with the maintenance of the medullary concentration gradient and this 'wash-out' effect diminishes the maximum concentrating ability of the kidney. The extent of the blunting varies in direct proportion to the severity of the polyuria and is independent of its cause. Hence, for any given basal urine output, the maximum urine osmolality achieved in the presence of saturating concentrations of AVP is depressed to the same extent in patients with primary polydipsia, central (neurogenic) diabetes insipidus, and NDI (Fig. 7). Second, most patients with central (neurogenic) diabetes insipidus maintain a small, but detectable, capacity to secrete AVP during severe dehydration and urinary osmolality may then increase to greater than the plasma osmolality. Third, many patients with acquired NDI have an incomplete deficiency in AVP action and concentrated urine could again be obtained during dehydration testing. Finally, all polyuric states [whether central (neurogenic), nephrogenic, or psychogenic] can induce large dilatations of the urinary tract and bladder (Boyd *et al.* 1980; Gautier *et al.* 1981). As a consequence, the urinary bladder of these patients has an increased residual capacity and changes in urinary osmolality induced by diagnostic manoeuvres might be difficult to demonstrate.

The methods of differential diagnosis are contained in Table 2.

Acknowledgements

The author's work cited in this chapter is supported by the Canadian Institutes of Health Research, the Canadian Kidney Foundation, and the Fonds de la recherche en santé du Québec. Danielle Binette provided secretarial and computer graphics expertise. DGB holds a Canada Research Chair in Genetics in Renal Diseases.

References

(Entries marked with an asterisk comprise useful general reading.)

Alon, U. and Chan, J. C. (1985). Hydrochlorothiazide-amiloride in the treatment of congenital nephrogenic diabetes insipidus. *American Journal of Nephrology* **5**, 9–13.

Antonarakis, S. and The Nomenclature Working Group (1998). Recommendations for a nomenclature system for human gene mutations. Nomenclature Working Group. *Human Mutation* **11**, 1–3.

*Aridor, M. and Balch, W. E. (1999). Integration of endoplasmic reticulum signaling in health and disease. *Nature Medicine* 5, 745–751.

*Arthus, M.-F. *et al.* (2000). Report of 33 novel *AVPR2* mutations and analysis of 117 families with X-linked nephrogenic diabetes insipidus. *Journal of the American Society of Nephrology* 11, 1044–1054.

Arthus, M.-F. *et al.* (2002). Thirteen large deletions/rearrangements of the AVPR2 gene causing X-linked nephrogenic diabetes insipidus. *Journal of the American Society of Nephrology* 13, 305A.

Batlle, D. C. *et al.* (1985). Amelioration of polyuria by amiloride in patients receiving long-term lithium therapy. *New England Journal of Medicine* 312, 408–414.

Baylis, P. H., Gaskill, M. B., and Robertson, G. L. (1981). Vasopressin secretion in primary polydipsia and cranial diabetes insipidus. *The Quarterly Journal of Medicine* 50, 345–358.

Berl, T. and Kumar, S. Disorders of water metabolism. In *Comprehensive Clinical Nephrology* (ed. R. J. Johnson and J. Feehally), pp. 9.1–9.20. London: Mosby, 2000.

Berl, T. and Robertson, G. L. Pathophysiology of water metabolism. In *Brenner and Rector's The Kidney* (ed. B. M. Brenner), pp. 866–924. Philadelphia: W.B. Saunders Company, 2000.

*Bichet, D. G. and Fujiwara, T. M. Nephrogenic diabetes insipidus. In *The Metabolic and Molecular Bases of Inherited Disease* (ed. C. R. Scriver *et al.*), pp. 4181–4204. New York: McGraw-Hill, 2001.

Bichet, D. G. *et al.* (1988). Hemodynamic and coagulation responses to 1-desamino[8-D-arginine]vasopressin (dDAVP) infusion in patients with congenital nephrogenic diabetes insipidus. *New England Journal of Medicine* 318, 881–887.

Bichet, D. G. *et al.* (1989). Epinephrine and dDAVP administration in patients with congenital nephrogenic diabetes insipidus. Evidence for a pre-cyclic AMP V2 receptor defective mechanism. *Kidney International* 36, 859–866.

*Bichet, D. G. *et al.* (1993). X-linked nephrogenic diabetes insipidus mutations in North America and the Hopewell hypothesis. *Journal of Clinical Investigations* 92, 1262–1268.

Bichet, D. G. *et al.* (1994). Nature and recurrence of AVPR2 mutations in X-linked nephrogenic diabetes insipidus. *American Journal of Human Genetics* 55, 278–286.

Bichet, D. G. *et al.* (2002). Decrease in urine volume and increase in urine osmolality after SR49059 administration in five adult male patients with X-linked nephrogenic diabetes insipidus. *Journal of the American Society of Nephrology* 13, 40A.

Birnbaumer, M. *et al.* (1992). Molecular cloning of the receptor for human antidiuretic hormone. *Nature* 357, 333–335.

Blalock, T. *et al.* (1977). Role of diet in the management of vasopressin-responsive and -resistant diabetes insipidus. *The American Journal of Clinical Nutrition* 30, 1070–1076.

Bode, H. H. and Crawford, J. D. (1969). Nephrogenic diabetes insipidus in North America: the Hopewell hypothesis. *New England Journal of Medicine* 280, 750–754.

Boton, R., Gaviria, M., and Batlle, D. C. (1987). Prevalence, pathogenesis, and treatment of renal dysfunction associated with chronic lithium therapy. *American Journal of Kidney Diseases* 10, 329–345.

Boyd, S. D., Raz, S., and Ehrlich, R. M. (1980). Diabetes insipidus and non-obstructive dilatation of urinary tract. *Urology* 16, 266–269.

Brenner, B., Seligsohn, U., and Hochberg, Z. (1988). Normal response of factor VIII and von Willebrand factor to 1-deamino-8D-arginine vasopressin in nephrogenic diabetes insipidus. *Journal of Clinical Endocrinology and Metabolism* 67, 191–193.

Brown, D., Katsura, T., and Gustafson, C. E. (1998). Cellular mechanisms of aquaporin trafficking. *American Journal of Physiology* 275, F328–F331.

Camerer, J. W. (1935). Eine ergänzung des Weilschen diabetes-insipidus-stammbaumes. *Archiv für Rassen-und Gesellschaftshygiene Biologie* 28, 382–385.

Canada, T. W., Weavind, L. M., and Augustin, K. M. (2003). Possible liposomal amphotericin B-induced nephrogenic diabetes insipidus. *Annals of Pharmacotherapy* 37, 70–73.

Carlotti, A. P. *et al.* (2001). Tonicity balance, and not electrolyte-free water calculations, more accurately guides therapy for acute changes in natremia. *Intensive Care Medicine* 27, 921–924.

Cheetham, T. and Baylis, P. H. (2002). Diabetes insipidus in children: pathophysiology, diagnosis and management. *Paediatric Drugs* 4, 785–796.

Christensen, S. *et al.* (1985). Pathogenesis of nephrogenic diabetes insipidus due to chronic administration of lithium in rats. *Journal of Clinical Investigations* 75, 1869–1879.

Cogan, E., Svoboda, M., and Abramow, M. (1987). Mechanisms of lithium-vasopressin interaction in rabbit cortical collecting tubule. *American Journal of Physiology* 252, F1080–F1087.

Crawford, J. D. and Bode, H. H. Disorders of the posterior pituitary in children. In *Endocrine and Genetic Diseases of Childhood and Adolescence* (ed. L. I. Gardner), pp. 126–158. Philadelphia: W.B. Saunders, 1975.

*Deen, P. M. T. *et al.* (1994a). Requirement of human renal water channel aquaporin-2 for vasopressin-dependent concentration of urine. *Science* 264, 92–95.

Deen, P. M. T. *et al.* (1994b). Assignment of the human gene for the water channel of renal collecting duct aquaporin 2 (AQP2) to chromosome 12 region q12→q13. *Cytogenetics and Cell Genetics* 66, 260–262.

Deen, P. M. T. *et al.* (1995). Water channels encoded by mutant aquaporin-2 genes in nephrogenic diabetes insipidus are impaired in their cellular routing. *Journal of Clinical Investigations* 95, 2291–2296.

de Keyzer, Y. *et al.* (1994). Cloning and characterization of the human V3 pituitary vasopressin receptor. *FEBS Letters* 356, 215–220.

Derkx, F. H. M. *et al.* (1987). Vasopressin V2-receptor-mediated hypotensive response in man. *Journal of Hypertension* 5, S107–S109.

Dölle, W. (1951). Eine weitere ergänzung des Weilschen diabetes-insipidus-stammbaumes. *Zeitschrift für Menschliche Vererbungs-und Konstitutionslehre* 30, 372–374.

Elliot, S. *et al.* (1996). Urinary excretion of aquaporin-2 in humans: a potential marker of collecting duct responsiveness to vasopressin. *Journal of the American Society of Nephrology* 7, 403–409.

Fitzsimons, J. T. (1998). Angiotensin, thirst, and sodium appetite. *Physiological Reviews* 78, 583–686.

Forssman, H. (1942). On the mode of hereditary transmission in diabetes insipidus. *Nordisk Medicine* 16, 3211–3213.

Frokiaer, J. *et al.* (1996). Bilateral ureteral obstruction downregulates expression of vasopressin-sensitive AQP-2 water channel in rat kidney. *American Journal of Physiology* 270, F657–F668.

Fujiwara, T. M., Morgan, K., and Bichet, D. G. (1995). Molecular biology of diabetes insipidus. *Annual Review of Medicine* 46, 331–343.

Fujiwara, T. M., Morgan, K., and Bichet, D. G. (1996). Molecular analysis of X-linked nephrogenic diabetes insipidus. *European Journal of Endocrinology* 134, 675–677.

Fushimi, K., Sasaki, S., and Marumo, F. (1997). Phosphorylation of serine 256 is required for cAMP-dependent regulatory exocytosis of the aquaporin-2 water channel. *Journal of Biological Chemistry* 272, 14800–14804.

Fushimi, K. *et al.* (1993). Cloning and expression of apical membrane water channel of rat kidney collecting tubule. *Nature* 361, 549–552.

*Gahl, W. A., Thoene, J. G., and Schneider, J. A. (2002). Cystinosis. *New England Journal of Medicine* 347, 111–121.

Gautier, B., Thieblot, P., and Steg, A. (1981). Mégauretère, mégavessie et diabète insipide familial. *La Semain des Hopitaux* 57, 60–61.

Goldberg, H., Clayman, P., and Skorecki, K. (1988). Mechanism of Li inhibition of vasopressin-sensitive adenylate cyclase in cultured renal epithelial cells. *American Journal of Physiology* 255, F995–F1002.

Hendy, G. and Bichet, D. G. Diabetes insipidus. In *Baillière's Clinical Endocrinology and Metabolism* (ed. R. V. Thakker), pp. 509–524. London: Baillière Tindall, 1995.

Hoekstra, J. A. *et al.* (1996). Cognitive and psychosocial functioning of patients with congenital nephrogenic diabetes insipidus. *American Journal of Medical Genetics* 61, 81–88.

Holtzman, E. J. *et al.* (1993). A null mutation in the vasopressin V2 receptor gene (AVPR2) associated with nephrogenic diabetes insipidus in the Hopewell kindred. *Human Molecular Genetics* **2**, 1201–1204.

Howard, R. L., Bichet, D. G., and Schrier, R. W. Hypernatremic and polyuric states. In *The Kidney: Physiology and Pathophysiology* (ed. D. W. Seldin and G. Giebisch), pp. 1753–1778. New York: Raven Press, 1992.

Huard, G. and Picard, J. L. (1960). Insuffisance congénitale du tubule rénal. *Union Médicale du Canada* **89**, 711–718.

Ito, M., Yu, R. N., and Jameson, J. L. (1999). Mutant vasopressin precursors that cause autosomal dominant neurohypophyseal diabetes insipidus retain dimerization and impair the secretion of wild-type proteins. *Journal of Biological Chemistry* **274**, 9029–9037.

Jakobsson, B. and Berg, U. (1994). Effect of hydrochlorothiazide and indomethacin treatment on renal function in nephrogenic diabetes insipidus. *Acta Paediatrica* **83**, 522–525.

Jamison, R. L. and Oliver, R. E. (1982). Disorders of urinary concentration and dilution. *American Journal of Medicine* **72**, 308–322.

Jard, S. Vasopressin receptors. In *Frontiers of Hormone Research* (ed. P. Czernichow and A. G. Robinson), pp. 89–104. Basel: S. Karger, 1985.

Jo, I. *et al.* (1995). Rat kidney papilla contains abundant synaptobrevin protein that participates in the fusion of antidiuretic hormone-regulated water channel-containing endosomes *in vitro*. *Proceedings of the National Academy of the Sciences of the United States of America* **92**, 1876–1880.

Kalatzis, V. and Antignac, C. (2002). Cystinosis: from gene to disease. *Nephrology, Dialysis, Transplantation* **17**, 1883–1886.

Kamsteeg, E.-J. *et al.* (1999). An impaired routing of wild-type aquaporin-2 after tetramerization with an aquaporin-2 mutant explains dominant nephrogenic diabetes insipidus. *The EMBO Journal* **18**, 2394–2400.

Kamsteeg, E.-J. *et al.* (2003). Reversed polarized delivery of an aquaporin-2 mutant causes dominant nephrogenic diabetes insipidus. *Journal of Cell Biology* **163**, 1099–1109.

Kanno, K. *et al.* (1995). Urinary excretion of aquaporin-2 in patients with diabetes insipidus. *New England Journal of Medicine* **332**, 1540–1545.

Katsura, T. *et al.* (1997). Protein kinase A phosphorylation is involved in regulated exocytosis of aquaporin-2 in transfected LLC-PK1 cells. *American Journal of Physiology* **272**, F817–F822.

Kaufmann, J. E. *et al.* (2000). Vasopressin-induced von Willebrand factor secretion from endothelial cells involves V2 receptors and cAMP. *Journal of Clinical Investigation* **106**, 107–116.

Knepper, M. A. (1997). Molecular physiology of urinary concentrating mechanism: regulation of aquaporin water channels by vasopressin. *American Journal of Physiology* **272**, F3–F12.

Knoers, N. and Monnens, L. A. (1990). Amiloride-hydrochlorothiazide versus indomethacin-hydrochlorothiazide in the treatment of nephrogenic diabetes insipidus. *Journal of Pediatrics* **117**, 499–502.

Knoers, N. and Monnens, L. A. (1991). A variant of nephrogenic diabetes insipidus: V2 receptor abnormality restricted to the kidney. *European Journal of Pediatrics* **150**, 370–373.

Knoers, N. and Monnens, L. A. (1992). Nephrogenic diabetes insipidus: clinical symptoms, pathogenesis, genetics and treatment. *Pediatric Nephrology* **6**, 476–482.

Knoers, N. *et al.* (1990). Fibrinolytic responses to 1-desamino-8-D-arginine-vasopressin in patients with congenital nephrogenic diabetes insipidus. *Nephron* **54**, 322–326.

Kuwahara, M. *et al.* (2001). Three families with autosomal dominant nephrogenic diabetes insipidus caused by aquaporin-2 mutations in the C-terminus. *American Journal of Human Genetics* **69**, 738–748.

Kuznetsov, G. and Nigam, S. K. (1998). Folding of secretory and membrane proteins. *New England Journal of Medicine* **339**, 1688–1695.

Lacombe, U. L. De la polydipsie. Thesis of Medicine, no. 99, Imprimerie et Fonderie de Paris: Rignoux, 1841.

Langley, J. M. *et al.* (1991). Autosomal recessive inheritance of vasopressin-resistant diabetes insipidus. *American Journal of Medical Genetics* **38**, 90–94.

Leaf, A. (1979). Neurogenic diabetes insipidus. *Kidney International* **15**, 572–580.

Leibowitz, S. F. Impact of brain monoamines and neuropeptides on vasopressin release. In *Vasopressin. Cellular and Integrative Functions* (ed. A. W. J. Cowley, J. F. Liard, and D. A. Ausiello), pp. 379–388. New York: Raven, 1988.

Libber, S., Harrison, H., and Spector, D. (1986). Treatment of nephrogenic diabetes insipidus with prostaglandin synthesis inhibitors. *Journal of Pediatrics* **108**, 305–311.

Liebenhoff, U. and Rosenthal, W. (1995). Identification of Rab3-, Rab5a- and synaptobrevin II-like proteins in a preparation of rat kidney vesicles containing the vasopressin-regulated water channel. *FEBS Letters* **365**, 209–213.

Lin, S. H. *et al.* (2002). Two novel aquaporin-2 mutations responsible for congenital nephrogenic diabetes insipidus in Chinese families. *Journal of Clinical Endocrinology and Metabolism* **87**, 2694–2700.

Lonergan, M. *et al.* (1993). Non-X-linked nephrogenic diabetes insipidus: phenotype and genotype features. *Journal of the American Society of Nephrology* **4**, 264A.

Magner, P. O. and Halperin, M. L. (1987). Polyuria—a pathophysiological approach. *Medicine North America* **15**, 2987–2997.

Mandon, B. *et al.* (1997). Expression of syntaxins in rat kidney. *American Journal of Physiology* **273**, F718–F730.

Marples, D. *et al.* (1995). Lithium-induced downregulation of aquaporin-2 water channel expression in rat kidney medulla. *Journal of Clinical Investigations* **95**, 1838–1845.

Marples, D. *et al.* (1996). Hypokalemia-induced downregulation of aquaporin-2 water channel expression in rat kidney medulla and cortex. *Journal of Clinical Investigations* **97**, 1960–1968.

Marr, N. *et al.* (2002a). Cell-biologic and functional analyses of five new aquaporin-2 missense mutations that cause recessive nephrogenic diabetes insipidus. *Journal of the American Society of Nephrology* **13**, 2267–2277.

*__Marr, N.__ *et al.* (2002b). Heteroligomerization of an aquaporin-2 mutant with wild-type aquaporin-2 and their misrouting to late endosomes/lysosomes explains dominant nephrogenic diabetes insipidus. *Human Molecular Genetics* **11**, 779–789.

McIlraith, C. H. (1892). Notes on some cases of diabetes insipidus with marked family and hereditary tendencies. *Lancet* **2**, 767–768.

McKusick, V. A. (2000). Online Mendelian Inheritance in Man OMIM, (TM). McKusick-Nathans Institute for Genetic Medicine, Johns Hopkins University (Baltimore, MD) and National Center for Biotechnology Information, National Library of Medicine (Bethesda, MD), 2000. World Wide Web URL: http://www.ncbi.nlm.nih.gov/omim/

Miller, M. *et al.* (1970). Recognition of partial defects in antidiuretic hormone secretion. *Annals of Internal Medicine* **73**, 721–729.

*__Morello, J.-P. and Bichet, D. G.__ (2001). Nephrogenic diabetes insipidus. *Annual Review of Physiology* **63**, 607–630.

Morello, J. P. *et al.* (2000). Pharmacological chaperones rescue cell-surface expression and function of misfolded V2 vasopressin receptor mutants. *Journal of Clinical Investigations* **105**, 887–895.

Mouillac, B. *et al.* (1995). The binding site of neuropeptide vasopressin V_{1a} receptor. Evidence for a major localization within transmembrane regions. *Journal of Biological Chemistry* **270**, 25771–25777.

Mulders, S. B. *et al.* (1997). New mutations in the AQP2 gene in nephrogenic diabetes insipidus resulting in functional but misrouted water channels. *Journal of the American Society of Nephrology* **8**, 242–248.

Mulders, S. M. *et al.* (1998). An aquaporin-2 water channel mutant which causes autosomal dominant nephrogenic diabetes insipidus is retained in the golgi complex. *Journal of Clinical Investigations* **102**, 57–66.

Nathanson, M. H. *et al.* (1992). Mechanisms of subcellular cytosolic Ca^{2+} signaling evoked by stimulation of the vasopressin V_{1a} receptor. *Journal of Biological Chemistry* **267**, 23282–23289.

Niaudet, P. *et al.* (1984). Nephrogenic diabetes insipidus: clinical and pathophysiological aspects. *Advances in Nephrology from the Necker Hospital* **13**, 247–260.

Niaudet, P. *et al.* Nephrogenic diabetes insipidus in children. In *Frontiers of Hormone Research* (ed. P. Czernichow and A. G. Robinson), pp. 224–231. Basel: Karger, 1985.

Nielsen, S. *et al.* (1995). Expression of VAMP-2-like protein in kidney collecting duct intracellular vesicles. Colocalization with Aquaporin-2 water channels. *Journal of Clinical Investigations* **96**, 1834–1844.

Ohzeki, T., Igarashi, T., and Okamoto, A. (1984). Familial cases of congenital nephrogenic diabetes insipidus type II: remarkable increment of urinary adenosine 3′,5′-monophosphate in response to antidiuretic hormone. *Journal of Pediatrics* **104**, 593–595.

*__Peters, M.__ *et al.* (2002). Clinical presentation of genetically defined patients with hypokalemic salt-losing tubulopathies. *American Journal of Medicine* **112**, 183–190.

Reeves, W. B. and Andreoli, T. E. Nephrogenic diabetes insipidus. In *The Metabolic and Molecular Bases of Inherited Disease* (ed. C. R. Scriver *et al.*), pp. 3045–3071. New York: McGraw-Hill, 1995.

Rittig, R. *et al.* (1996). Identification of 13 new mutations in the vasopressin-neurophysin II gene in 17 kindreds with familial autosomal dominant neurohypophyseal diabetes insipidus. *American Journal of Human Genetics* **58**, 107–117.

*__Robertson, G. L.__ Diagnosis of diabetes insipidus. In *Frontiers of Hormone Research* (ed. P. Czernichow and A. G. Robinson), pp. 176–189. Basel: Karger, 1985.

Robertson, G. L. (1987). Dipsogenic diabetes insipidus: a newly recognized syndrome caused by a selective defect in the osmoregulation of thirst. *Transactions of the Association of American Physicians* **100**, 241–249.

*__Rosenthal, W.__ *et al.* (1992). Molecular identification of the gene responsible for congenital nephrogenic diabetes insipidus. *Nature* **359**, 233–235.

Saito, T. *et al.* (1997). Urinary excretion of aquaporin-2 in the diagnosis of central diabetes insipidus. *Journal of Clinical Endocrinology and Metabolism* **82**, 1823–1827.

Sands, J. M. (2002). Molecular approaches to urea transporters. *Journal of the American Society of Nephrology* **13**, 2795–2806.

Sands, J. M. *et al.* (1998). Vasopressin-elicited water and urea permeabilities are altered in IMCD in hypercalcemic rats. *American Journal of Physiology* **274**, F978–F985.

Sasaki, S. *et al.* (1994). Cloning, characterization, and chromosomal mapping of human aquaporin of collecting duct. *Journal of Clinical Investigations* **93**, 1250–1256.

Seibold, A. *et al.* (1992). Structure and chromosomal localization of the human antidiuretic hormone receptor gene. *American Journal of Human Genetics* **51**, 1078–1083.

Shayakul, C., Steel, A., and Hediger, M. A. (1996). Molecular cloning and characterization of the vasopressin-regulated urea transporter of rat kidney collecting ducts. *Journal of Clinical Investigations* **98**, 2580–2587.

Snyder, H. M., Noland, T. D., and Breyer, M. D. (1992). cAMP-dependent protein kinase mediates hydrosmotic effect of vasopressin in collecting duct. *American Journal of Physiology* **263**, C147–C153.

Star, R. A. *et al.* (1988). Calcium and cyclic adenosine monophosphate as second messengers for vasopressin in the rat inner medullary collecting duct. *Journal of Clinical Investigations* **81**, 1879–1888.

Storm, R. *et al.* (2003). Osmolality and solute composition are strong regulators of AQP2 expression in renal principal cells. *American Journal of Physiology Renal Physiology* **284**, F189–F198.

Streitz, J. M. J. and Streitz, J. M. (1988). Polyuric urinary tract dilatation with renal damage. *Journal of Urology* **139**, 784–785.

Sugimoto, T. *et al.* (1994). Molecular cloning and functional expression of a cDNA encoding the human V1b vasopressin receptor. *Journal of Biological Chemistry* **269**, 27088–27092.

Tamarappoo, B. K. and Verkman, A. S. (1998). Defective aquaporin-2 trafficking in nephrogenic diabetes insipidus and correction by chemical chaperones. *Journal of Clinical Investigations* **101**, 2257–2267.

Taylor, A. *et al.* (1973). Vasopressin: possible role of microtubules and microfilaments in its action. *Science* **181**, 347–350.

Thibonnier, M. *et al.* (1994). Molecular cloning, sequencing, and functional expression of a cDNA encoding the human V_{1a} vasopressin receptor. *Journal of Biological Chemistry* **269**, 3304–3310.

Valenti, G. *et al.* (1998). A heterotrimeric G protein of the Gi family is required for cAMP-triggered trafficking of aquaporin 2 in kidney epithelial cells. *Journal of Biological Chemistry* **273**, 22627–22634.

Valtin, H. and Schafer, J. A. Concentration and dilution of urine: H_2O balance. In *Renal Function* (ed. H. Valtin and J. A. Schafer), pp. 151–182. Boston: Little Brown, 1995.

*__van Lieburg, A. F., Knoers, N. V. A. M., and Monnens, L. A. H.__ (1999). Clinical presentation and follow-up of 30 patients with congenital nephrogenic diabetes insipidus. *Journal of the American Society of Nephrology* **10**, 1958–1964.

van Os, C. H. and Deen, P. M. (1998). Aquaporin-2 water channel mutations causing nephrogenic diabetes insipidus. *Proceedings of the Association of American Physicians* **110**, 395–400.

Verhelst, D. *et al.* (2002). Fanconi syndrome and renal failure induced by tenofovir: a first case report. *American Journal of Kidney Diseases* **40**, 1331–1333.

Ward, D. T., Hammond, T. G., and Harris, H. W. (1999). Modulation of vasopressin-elicited water transport by trafficking of aquaporin2-containing vesicles. *Annual Review of Physiology* **61**, 683–697.

Waring, A. G., Kajdi, L., and Tappan, V. (1945). Congenital defect of water metabolism. *American Journal of Diseases in Childhood* **69**, 323–325.

Watson, S. and Arkinstall, S. *The G Protein Linked Receptor Factsbook*. London: Academic Press, 1994.

Weil, A. (1884). Ueber die hereditare form des diabetes insipidus. *Archives fur Pathologische Anatomie und Physiologie and fur Klinische Medicine (Virchow's Archives)* **95**, 70–95.

Weil, A. (1908). Ueber die hereditare form des diabetes insipidus. *Deutches Archiv fur Klinische Medizin* **93**, 180–290.

Williams, R. M. and Henry, C. (1947). Nephrogenic diabetes insipidus transmitted by females and appearing during infancy in males. *Annals of Internal Medicine* **27**, 84–95.

Yang, B. *et al.* (2002). Urea-selective concentrating defect in transgenic mice lacking urea transporter UT-B. *Journal of Biological Chemistry* **277**, 10633–10637.

*__Zerbe, R. L. and Robertson, G. L.__ (1981). A comparison of plasma vasopressin measurements with a standard indirect test in the differential diagnosis of polyuria. *New England Journal of Medicine* **305**, 1539–1546.

Zerbe, R. L. and Robertson, G. L. (1984). Disorders of ADH. *Medicine North America* **13**, 1570–1574.

6

The patient with chronic interstitial disease

6.1 Mechanisms of interstitial inflammation

Frank Strutz, Claudia A. Müller, and Gerhard A. Müller

Introduction

Interstitial inflammation is the hallmark of tubulointerstitial nephritis (TIN) both in its acute and chronic form. The term tubulointerstitial is preferred to interstitial since it emphasizes the frequent tubular involvement. TIN may affect the tubulointerstitial space primarily or can occur in the setting of primary glomerular or vascular disease (secondary TIN). All forms of interstitial disease are quite common. Up to 15 per cent of all cases of acute renal failure have been attributed to primary interstitial nephritis (Wilson *et al.* 1976), whereas, up to 25 per cent of all cases of endstage renal disease are caused by primary chronic TIN (Brunner *et al.* 1985). In 1998, 17 per cent of endstage renal diseases were caused in Germany by the combination of pyelonephritis and interstitial nephritis, both characterized by primary TIN (Frei and Schober-Halstenberg 1999) (Fig. 1). Secondary tubulointerstitial injury is one of the most important determinants for the outcome of primary glomerular and vascular disease (reviewed in Strutz and Müller 2001). Thus, interstitial nephritis is the common pathway of almost all forms of progressive renal disease and one of the most common lesions in nephrology (Neilson 1989).

The clinical and more specific aspects of TIN are discussed elsewhere in this section (analgesic nephropathy in Chapter 6.2, non-steroidal anti-inflammatory drugs in Chapter 6.3, the effects of uric acid in Chapter 6.4, nephrotoxic metals in Chapter 6.5, radiation nephritis in Chapter 6.6, Balkan nephropathy in Chapter 6.7, and Chinese herbs nephropathy and other rare causes of interstitial nephropathy in Chapter 6.8). This chapter discusses the principal mechanisms of interstitial inflammation in primary and particularly secondary interstitial nephritis and the significance of tubulointerstitial involvement for the progression to endstage renal failure.

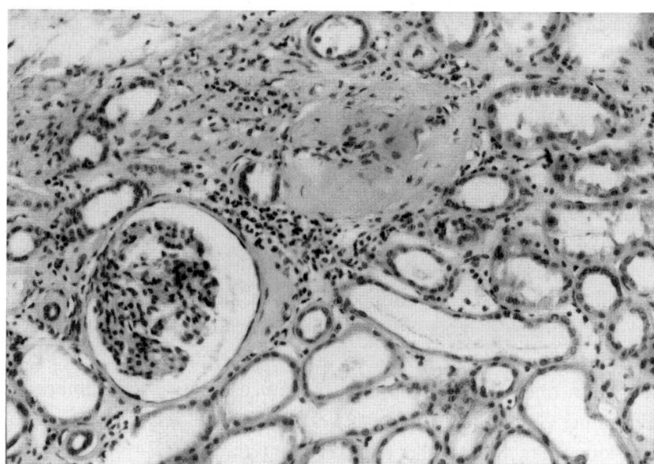

Fig. 1 Typical interstitial inflammation in a kidney from a patient with endstage renal failure due to recurrent urinary tract infections. Magnification 400×.

Primary tubulointerstitial nephritis

Primary interstitial nephritis is characterized by an inflammatory reaction that affects predominantly the tubulointerstitial space. Acute primary TIN can be divided into three forms: medication related TIN, TIN associated with infections, and idiopathic TIN (Michel and Kelly 1998) (Table 1). Accordingly, the mechanisms of acute TIN fall into three broad categories: (1) the administration of nephritogenic pharmaceuticals, (2) contact with infectious agents, and (3) the development of nephritogenic autoimmunity which is often the cause of idiopathic TIN (Neilson 1999). Nevertheless, as will be discussed below, the distinction between these three forms is somewhat artificial since immune mediated tubulointerstitial injury plays a major role even in TIN caused by pharmaceuticals and infection.

We will address first the nature of the immune response in TIN, describe the composition of interstitial infiltrating cells and then discuss briefly the two most common causes of TIN: the medication and the infection related forms.

Nature of the immune response in tubulointerstitial nephritis

An immune response to either foreign antigens or autoantigens may cause renal damage by predominantly humoral or cell-mediated reactions (O'Meara *et al.* 1992). In contrast with glomerular injury,

Table 1 Forms of primary acute tubulointerstitial nephritis

Form
Medication related form
Associated with infections (a) Direct invasion of micro-organisms (b) Immune mediated in remote infection
Idiopathic

cell-mediated reactions predominate over humoral mediated mechanisms in the pathogenesis of tubulointerstitial lesions (Strutz and Neilson 1994). Target antigens in human TIN remain poorly defined (Wilson 1991). In TIN only few antigens have been identified. The target antigen of experimental antitubular basement membrane (anti-TBM) disease in mice a glycoprotein (named 3M-1), is secreted by proximal tubular cells into the extracellular matrix (Haverty *et al.* 1988); antibodies against it are directed against an immunodominant epitope on 3M-1 (Clayman *et al.* 1988). Butkowski *et al.* (1990) also identified an antigen from rabbit TBM that reacts with human anti-TBM antibodies and termed it TIN antigen. This antigen is an extracellular matrix protein which has an important role in tubulogenesis (Yoshioka *et al.* 2002). A precise discussion of the various tubulointerstitial antigens is beyond the scope of this chapter but is available elsewhere (Wilson 2001).

Tubulointerstitial infiltrates

Tubulointerstitial infiltrates are the hallmark of any form of TIN. They include—to variable degrees—neutrophils, T- and B-lymphocytes, macrophages, natural killer, and plasma cells (Strutz and Neilson 1994). In all forms of primary TIN, $CD4^+$ and $CD8^+$ T-lymphocytes have been described: cell-mediated immunity is the predominant effector mechanism of acute TIN. The CD4/CD8 ratio of the interstitial infiltrate is usually equal to or above unity (Kelly *et al.* 1991) although a lower CD4/CD8 ratio has been observed in TIN due to non-steroidal anti-inflammatory drugs. The functional correlate of the CD4/CD8 ratio is rather low as it depends on the stage of the disease at the time of biopsy and on prior immunosuppressive treatment (Kelly *et al.* 1991).

Drug-induced forms

Several drugs can cause acute TIN, including antibiotics, diuretics, antiviral agents, and non-steroidal anti-inflammatory agents (see Chapters 6.2 and 6.3 for the clinical discussion). For methicillin alone, a semisynthetic penicillin no longer available, over 100 cases have been described (Appel 2001). The pathophysiology of drug-induced acute TIN remains poorly defined, despite evidence for immune-mediated reactions. The development is not dose dependent and recurrences or exacerbations may occur after re-exposure. The distal tubule is the focus of the greatest cellular infiltration. In several animal models, antigens such as dodecanoic acid-conjugated bovine serum albumin (BSA) may induce an allergic response of the delayed hypersensitivity reaction type making that a likely cause of drug-induced TIN (reviewed in Wilson 2001).

Infectious tubulointerstitial nephritis

Infectious TIN is usually caused by an ascending infection mostly with enterobacteriaceae (most commonly *Escherichia coli*) and *Streptococcus faecalis* in outpatients, and sometimes with *Serratia marcescens* or *Pseudomonas aeruginosa* in hospitalized patients exposed to instrumentation and antibiotic treatment. The development of infection is influenced by the presence of urinary reflux and by bacterial virulence factors best studied in *E. coli* (Hill 1994). The presence of fimbriae which enable the bacterium to adhere to epithelial cells, is an important virulence factor. P-fimbriae mediate adhesion to human P blood group receptors and play an important role in first attacks of pyelonephritis. Type 1 fimbriated bacteria cause a greater activation of polymorphonuclear neutrophils (PMN) and a larger scar formation than P-fimbriated organisms (Topley *et al.* 1989). Additional virulence factors include α-haemolysins. The importance of virulence factors is linked to their ability to activate neutrophils (Hill 1994). PMN may then activate fibroblasts and initiate chronic progressive disease (Strutz and Neilson 1994). The role of lymphocytes and cytokines in acute and chronic phases of infection is not as well defined as in other forms of TIN. Even in infectious TIN, T-lymphocytes accumulate within a few days (Wilz *et al.* 1993). $CD4^+$ lymphocytes propagated from lesions in experimental pyelonephritis display MHC-restricted proliferative responses to a variety of *E. coli* and related strains but not to other gram-negative bacteria. Many forms of chronic infectious TIN may thus be mediated by the same immune mechanisms as non-infectious forms. A number of cytokines have been implicated in infectious TIN: interleukin (IL)-1 and IL-6, granulocyte-colony stimulating factor (-CSF), granulocyte–monocyte-colony stimulating factor (GM-CSF), and tumour necrosis factor (TNF)-α. Obstruction, a common factor of chronic infection, plays an often underappreciated role as it may cause direct tubulointerstitial injury. Fibrogenic cytokines and transforming growth factor (TGF)-β1 mRNA expression increase in models of ureteral obstruction (Klahr 2001). Finally, sterile urine reflux causes cortical tubulointerstitial scarring in pigs potentially as a result of the extravasation of Tamm–Horsfall protein at high backflow pressures. Interestingly, expression of Epstein–Barr virus has been observed in the proximal tubules of kidneys with primary chronic interstitial nephritis (Becker *et al.* 1999), raising the possibility that an immune response to the virus was involved in the disease process. This hypothesis remains to be tested.

Secondary tubulointerstitial nephritis

Tubulointerstitial infiltrates

Almost all glomerulopathies are accompanied by interstitial infiltrates (reviewed in Strutz and Neilson 2002). An extensive study using monoclonal antibodies revealed the presence of infiltrating leucocytes in all forms of glomerulonephritis with the exception of minimal change disease (Hooke *et al.* 1987). Interstitial infiltrates are common in various forms of vasculitis, especially in Wegener's granulomatosis (Mignon *et al.* 1984). The majority of infiltrating cells in secondary human interstitial nephritis are $CD2^+$ T-lymphocytes most of which are $CD4^+$ helper cells (Markovic-Lipkovski *et al.* 1990). Conversely, $CD8^+$ T-cells predominate in allograft rejection, lupus nephritis, and in the nephrotic syndrome induced by PAN (Eddy and Michael 1988). The infiltrating cells often express activation markers such as IL-2 and transferrin receptors. They directly mediate the progression to organ fibrosis: injections of anti-$CD4^+$ or anti-$CD8^+$ antibodies significantly decrease fibrosis in a bleomycin-induced model of lung fibrosis as measured by pulmonary hydroxyproline content (Piguet *et al.* 1989). Depletion of both T-cell subsets in mice abrogates fibrosis. In human kidneys, the number of infiltrating $CD4^+$ (and somewhat weaker $CD8^+$) T-cells correlates well with kidney function (Müller *et al.* 1991). Infiltrating $CD14^+$ monocytes/macrophages usually accompany the infiltrating T-lymphocytes. Their importance, stressed by some authors (Eddy 1994b), remains controversial in the absence of correlation between $CD14^+$ monocytes/macrophages and renal function (Müller *et al.* 1991).

Factors involved in secondary interstitial inflammation and progression to renal fibrosis (Table 2)

Which factors cause the accumulation of lymphocytes in the tubulointerstitium in secondary TIN? Furthermore, how does tubulointerstitial infiltration lead to renal fibrosis?

Proteinuria

Persistent high-grade proteinuria is a bad prognostic sign in most human glomerulopathies with the exception of minimal change disease. It has been suggested that proteinuria itself causes tubulointerstitial inflammation and progression of renal disease. The extent of proteinuria correlates relatively well with the progression of glomerulopathies (Remuzzi and Bertani 1998), a more severe proteinuria being associated with an accelerated decline in renal function.

How could proteinuria cause tubulointerstitial damage? The increased glomerular permeability to proteins is associated with an augmented tubular reabsorption of proteins subsequently degraded through the lysosomal processing pathway. Excess reabsorption in the proximal tubule may cause lysosomal rupture and cellular self-injury. The activity of several lysosomal enzymes increases in proteinuric states in rats with PAN nephrosis: the activity of two proteases, cathepsin B and L, augment, particularly in the S2 segment of the proximal tubule. Not all proteins have the same capability to induce tubulointerstitial injury. In an *in vivo* study, using a tubular perfusion system, Sanders *et al.* (1988) found a great variability in the tubular toxicity of low molecular weight proteins. This may explain, at least in part, why albuminuria alone does not appear harmful for humans and why patients with the nephrotic syndrome and albuminuria rarely have tubulointerstitial disease (Eddy 1994a). Conversely, albuminuria in rats with Heymann nephritis increases the urinary excretion of lysozyme, a marker for tubular damage. In other experimental models, protein overload proteinuria results in interstitial inflammation (Eddy 1989) whereas protein restriction markedly decreases interstitial matrix accumulation (Eddy 1994a). Similarly, reduction of proteinuria, by dietary protein restriction or by the use of converting enzyme inhibitors lowers the urinary excretion of lysozyme and thus, probably, tubular damage (Hutchinson and Kaysen 1988). In adriamycin-induced glomerulosclerosis, the degree of proteinuria parallels the interstitial infiltrate (Bertani *et al.* 1986). Direct tubular toxicity is not the only effect of proteinuria. Kees-Folts *et al.* (1994) have described in BSA-induced overload proteinuria a novel chemotactic factor for macrophages that is generated in rat proximal tubule cells as a result of the metabolism of albumin-borne fatty acids but not if lipid-depleted BSA was used. Iron may also be released from filtered transferrin–iron complexes and promote tubular injury by the formation of hydroxyl radicals via the Haber–Weiss reaction. In one study, iron-deficient animals had significantly less tubulointerstitial injury than animals with normal iron stores (Alfrey *et al.* 1989). Filtration of complement may be also implicated in the pathogenesis of secondary TIN: the urine content of C5b-9 complex correlated well with the degree of proteinuria (Ogrodowski *et al.* 1991) but it remains to be seen whether the large-sized C5b-9 complex is filtered or rather formed by *in situ* complement activation. In IgA-nephropathy, Yoshioka *et al.* (1993) found a good correlation between the degree of proteinuria and the number of interstitial IL-6 positive cells. Finally, proteinuria enhances the tubular synthesis and secretion of endothelin-1 (ET-1) a strong chemoattractant for monocytes/macrophages.

Table 2 Factors involved in the formation of secondary interstitial infiltrates

Proteinuria
Immune deposits
Chemokines
Cytokines
Calcium phosphate
Metabolic acidosis
Lipids

Cytokines

Cytokines are important mediators of inflammation, tissue damage, and regeneration. They play a major role in primary and secondary TIN. Cytokines are generated first in infiltrating inflammatory cells and subsequently by renal somatic cells. Cytokines released in tubulointerstitial infiltrates include most notably IL-1 to IL-7, interferon (IFN)-α, -β, -γ, platelet-derived growth factor (PDGF)-A and -B, TNF-α and -β, epithelial growth factor (EGF), fibroblast growth factor (FGF)-2, and TGF-α and -β1–3 (Floege and Rees 1997). In some glomerulopathies, interstitial infiltrates are localized primarily around the glomeruli (Eddy 1994b). Eldredge *et al.* (1991) described an early periglomerular inflammation in a rabbit model of antiglomerular basement membrane (anti-GBM) disease, which, in the absence of extraglomerular immune deposits pointed to a possible role of chemotactic factors. Lan *et al.* (1993) localized the primary site of periglomerular infiltration to the perivascular sheath of hilar arterioles. The interstitial macrophage accumulation was reversed by the administration of an IL-1 receptor antagonist pointing to a critical role of IL-1. Similarly, IL-1 receptor antagonist treatment of rats with anti-GBM disease reduced neutrophil infiltration by 40 per cent and monocyte–macrophage infiltration by 30 per cent (Tang *et al.* 1994b).

Chemokines

Chemokines are a family of 8–10-kDa proteins involved in a variety of inflammatory reactions. They are subdivided into four subgroups, according to the position of conserved cysteine residues: C-, CC-, CXC-, and CX_3C-chemokines, and attract different subsets of leucocytes. Expression of chemokines is inducible by a variety of cytokines, lectins, bacterial products, and viruses in various renal cells, including tubular epithelial cells (Segerer *et al.* 2000). Chemokines have long been thought to be important for the pathogenesis of secondary interstitial nephritis in primary glomerular disease. Cytokine secretion by inflammatory cells within the glomerulus induces chemokine formation by tubular epithelial cells with an attendant secondary interstitial inflammation.

IL-8, a member of the CXC-subgroup, is a potent chemoattractant for neutrophils and some lymphocytes. It is synthesized in human tubular epithelial cells *in vitro* and *in vivo* and has been detected in normal as well as fibrotic kidney derived fibroblasts (Lonnemann *et al.*

1995). Platelet factor 4, another member of the CXC subgroup, is also a chemoattractant for neutrophils, monocytes, and fibroblasts. Conversely, members of the CC-subgroup mainly recruit mononuclear leucocytes and are thus, particularly attractive candidates as mediators of interstitial mononuclear infiltrates. Monocyte chemoattractant protein (MCP)-1, the prototype of this family, is chemotactic for monocytes but not for neutrophils. Its expression precedes the infiltration of mononuclear leucocytes (Tang *et al.* 1994a). Increased levels of MCP-1 protein have been demonstrated in experimental glomerulonephritis (Eddy 1994b) and in human tubular epithelial cells of various glomerulopathies (Prodjosudjadi *et al.* 1995). MCP-1 synthesis is upregulated by inflammatory cytokines such as IFN-γ, IL-1α, and TNF-α but downregulated by IL-15, which was shown recently to be tubuloprotective in interstitial nephritis (Shinozaki *et al.* 2002). However, not all data point to a decisive role for MCP-1 in the pathogenesis of secondary interstitial infiltrates. In the protein overload model, MCP-1 expression was not elevated until week 2, well after the accumulation of interstitial macrophages (Eddy *et al.* 1995). The number of infiltrating cells in the PAN nephrosis model was not reduced by MCP-1 neutralizing serum in one study (Eddy 1994b), whereas, in the same model, macrophage infiltration was reduced by 45 per cent by a neutralizing antibody (Tang *et al.* 1997). RANTES, another CC chemokine expressed in tubular epithelial cells robustly increases in allograft rejection and human immunodeficiency virus (HIV) nephropathy. Expression of MCP-1 and RANTES (and osteopontin) in kidney sections from patients with idiopathic membranous glomerulonephritis is well correlated with mononuclear infiltrates (Mezzano *et al.* 2000). The expression pattern of the various chemokines and in particular of CC chemokines may be disease specific, in experimental models, CC chemokine expression is upregulated only in rapidly progressive glomerulonephritis but not in PAN nephrosis (Ou and Natori 1999).

The role of chemokines in the formation of interstitial infiltrates is further supported by studies of chemokine receptors. The expression of CCR5, the receptor for RANTES, is restricted, in human renal disease, to infiltrating $CD3^+$ lymphocytes and is well correlated with renal function (Segerer *et al.* 1999). Similarly, expression of CCR4, which binds to MDC (macrophage-derived chemokine) increases in interstitial infiltrates in human renal allograft rejection. Finally, a new CCR1 receptor antagonist significantly reduced interstitial infiltration and ensuing fibrosis in the unilateral ureteral obstruction (UUO) model (Anders *et al.* 2002).

Expression of chemokines in tubular epithelial cells may be also induced by proteinuria. In confluent pig proximal tubule cells, BSA induced the expression of RANTES in a time- and dose-dependent manner dependent on the activation of NF-kappa B (Zoja *et al.* 1998). Interestingly, inhibition of NF-kappa B significantly decreased adriamycin-induced secondary interstitial nephritis (Rangan *et al.* 1999).

Lipid factors

Lipid factors are also involved in the pathogenesis of secondary TIN. Fatty acid depleted rats with PAN nephrosis do not develop an interstitial infiltrate (Diamond *et al.* 1989), whereas, lipid-lowering drugs, lovastatin and probucol, reduce the severity of tubulointerstitial infiltrates in experimental PAN nephrosis (Eddy 1994b). A cholesterol rich diet fed to uninephrectomized rats produces interstitial fibrosis within 12 weeks, perhaps as a consequence of lipid peroxidation since antioxidant therapy prevents it, possibly by increasing intrarenal metalloproteinase activity (Eddy 1998). The mechanism of cholesterol induced interstitial fibrosis is not entirely clear but may involve an increased expression of TGF-β1 in glomerular epithelial and possibly other kidney cells by oxidized low-density lipoprotein (LDL).

Increased serum triglycerides but not of LDLs and decreased high density lipoprotein (HDL) are risk factors for renal failure (Muntner *et al.* 2000). Hypertriglyceridaemia, also a risk factor for renal failure in patients with IgA nephropathy is often associated with diabetes mellitus and the nephrotic syndrome so that its significance as an independent risk factor remains to be proven. Further studies are needed to define the role of lipids in the formation of tubulointerstitial inflammation.

Immune deposits

Just as in several forms of glomerular disease and in the above described (rare) form of primary tubulointerstitial disease, deposition of antibodies or antibody–antigen complexes may play a role in the pathogenesis of secondary interstitial disease. In rats with classic anti-GBM disease, interstitial infiltrates are seen adjacent to linear TBM deposits of heterologous anti-GBM antibodies (Eddy 1991). A similar phenomenon is observed in passive Heymann nephritis where the common subepithelial GBM immune complexes are often accompanied by subepithelial TBM deposits in the close proximity of which interstitial infiltrates are often found, even after complement depletion (Eddy *et al.* 1992). Thus, just as in glomerular injury, interactions between the antibody and monocyte Fc receptors may lead to interstitial infiltration. In human disease, immune aggregates including antibodies and complement, have been described in types I and II membranoproliferative, in membranous and in poststreptococcal glomerulonephritis (Morel-Maroger 1974). It is however, unlikely that immune deposits play a major role in the induction of secondary TIN, since most interstitial immune deposits were noted only in single case reports except for the series of Lehman who found extraglomerular deposits in 30 per cent of patients with membranoproliferative (mesangiocapillary) disease type I (Lehman and Dixon 1975).

Tubular epithelial cells

Tubular epithelial cells, the vast majority of renal parenchymal cells, play a crucial role in primary and secondary TIN. In primary glomerulopathies, they are mediators between glomerular and interstitial inflammation (Fig. 2). As already stated, they are stimulated by various cytokines and proteinuria and, in response, express adhesion molecules and secrete cytokines and chemokines. IFN-γ, released by the first infiltrating leucocytes, is the most potent stimulator of tubular epithelial cells which, in an amplification cascade, activate adjacent tubular cells to release chemokines such as MCP-1. Intercellular adhesion molecule (ICAM)-1 and vascular cell adhesion molecule (VCAM)-1 are upregulated in many forms of glomerular and vascular disease (Müller *et al.* 1991) and, in part, mediate tubulointerstitial infiltration. ICAM-1 binds specifically to the CD11a/CD18 complex [formerly called lymphocyte function-associated antigen (LFA)-1], a β_2-integrin present on various leucocytes. Antibodies against ICAM-1 and LFA-1 significantly reduce injury in several models of glomerular disease and, presumably, in interstitial disease (Kawasaki *et al.* 1993). Tang *et al.* (1994c) found infiltrating $CD18^+$ leucocytes in a model of

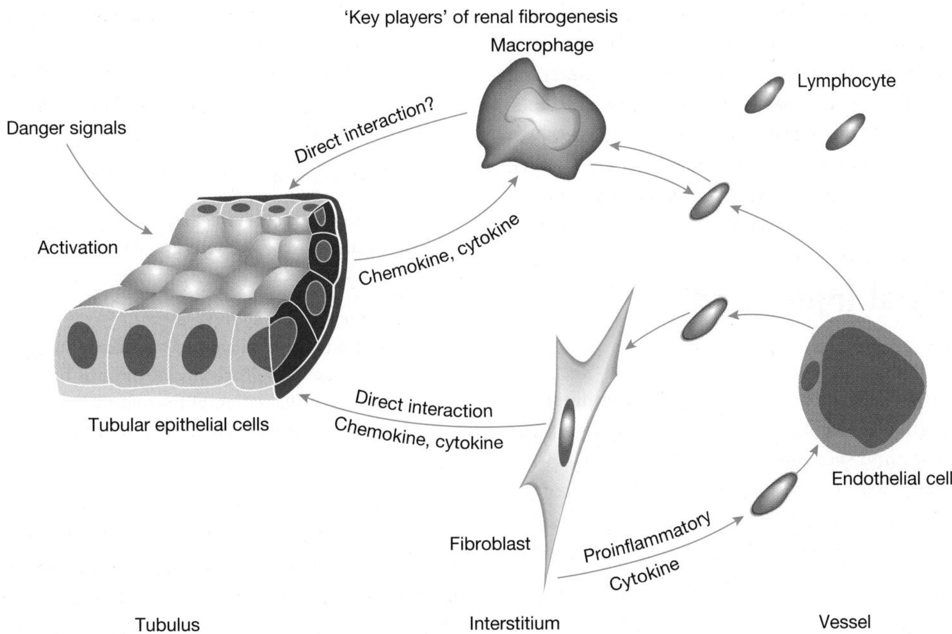

Fig. 2 Illustration of the central role of the tubular epithelial cell in the generation of interstitial infiltrates. The tubular cell becomes activated by a variety of signals including proteinuria, cytokines, and chemokines resulting in the subsequent activation of macrophages, lymphocytes, and fibroblasts.

anti-TBM nephritis, primarily in areas with increased ICAM-1 expression.

In TIN, certain cytokines are upregulated in human tubular epithelial cells. Frank *et al.* (1993) described a 29 per cent increase in PDGF mRNA expression and a 41 per cent rise in GM-CSF in tubular cells from patients with glomerulopathies compared to tubular cells from apparently normal cadaver kidneys. The increase is even higher, 54 and 72 per cent, respectively, when glomerular disease is accompanied by interstitial fibrosis. The expression of both cytokines is inducible by TNF-α and IL-1a. GM-CSF, a strong chemoattractant for recruitment and activation of leucocytes, induces fibroblast proliferation. Tubular epithelial cells also synthesize osteopontin, a cell–matrix adhesion molecule originally described in bone matrix. Upregulation of osteopontin has been demonstrated in anti-Thy-1 glomerulonephritis, PAN nephrosis, and Heymann nephritis as well as in glomerulosclerosis and angiotensin-II-induced tubulointerstitial fibrosis (Giachelli *et al.* 1994). In the latter study, osteopontin expression increased mostly in distal tubules and collecting ducts, mainly in the cortex and correlated with monocyte/macrophage accumulation.

Nephron structure is heterogenous in chronically diseased kidneys. Surviving nephrons increase oxygen consumption mainly as a result of an augmented rate of sodium reabsorption, with an attendant accentuation of ammonia and autoreactive oxygen radicals generation (Nath *et al.* 1990). The potential importance of reactive oxygen species for the development of tubulointerstitial injury was demonstrated by the development of acute TIN in rats fed a diet deficient in selenium and vitamin E, both scavengers of free oxygen radicals.

The direct stimulation by tubular epithelial cells of T-cell transformation into antigen-presenting cells seems rather exceptional. Whereas increased and aberrant expression of class II major histocompatibility complex (MHC) antigens has been described for a variety of glomerular diseases, the expression of required costimulatory molecules such as B7-1 or B7-2 is rare. Banu and Myers (1999) recently reported that stimuli such as IFN-γ and lipopolysaccharide induce B7-1 expression on tubular epithelial cells, at least *in vitro*. *In vivo* evidence for the role of direct T-cell stimulation stems from the model of cadmium induced renal injury in mice: tubular epithelial cells of damaged kidneys display *de novo* heatshock protein 70 expression resulting in interstitial infiltration. Passive transfer of these sensitized T-cells induce interstitial inflammation in unaffected kidneys. Conversely, in the chronic UUO-model, interstitial inflammation was unchanged in mice with severe combined immunodeficiency (Shappell *et al.* 1998), an observation questioning the concept of direct T-cell stimulation by tubular epithelial cells. Moreover, tubular epithelial cells express B7RP-1 *in vivo*, which inhibits T-cell activation (Wahl *et al.* 2002).

Of potential clinical significance is the correlation between tubular epithelial cell apoptosis and interstitial fibrosis, at least in some animal models. IL-15, has recently been shown to protect tubular epithelial cells against apoptosis and interstitial nephritis (Shinozaki *et al.* 2002).

Deposition of calcium phosphate

Phosphate retention complicates chronic renal failure. Calcium phosphate precipitates even at creatinine values of less than 1.5 mg/dl (132 mmol/l) and may result in interstitial inflammation (Loghman-Adham 1993). Dietary phosphorus restriction improves histological changes and preserves renal function in rats, after a 5/6-nephrectomy (Ibels *et al.* 1978). Thus, diets with very low phosphorus content have been advised in clinical practice but their clinical usefulness (apart from the reduction in total protein intake) remains to be demonstrated.

Metabolic acidosis

In chronic renal failure, each remaining nephron excretes more acid, mostly in the form of ammonium. Ammonium directly activates complement which, in turn, causes tubulointerstitial inflammation, at least in rats (Nath *et al.* 1985). Alkali therapy in these animals prevents the increase in ammonium production and decreases interstitial injury. A direct toxic effect of acidosis has also been described in rats, but its deleterious influence on disease progression has not been uniformly confirmed (Throssell *et al.* 1996). The beneficial effect of alkali therapy on disease progression remains unproven in humans.

Tubulointerstitial injury and renal function

The relationship between the integrity of the tubulointerstitial compartment and renal function, initially suspected in the 1840s was confirmed in both primary and secondary glomerulonephritis and in chronic tubulointerstitial diseases: tubulointerstitial scarring correlates much better with renal function than glomerular lesions (reviewed in Bohle *et al.* 1996). These conclusions were confirmed in nephrosclerosis and polycystic kidneys. The extent of interstitial infiltration and fibrosis further proved a rather accurate predictor of renal function 5 or more years later, a not surprising finding given the fact that the tubulointerstitial compartment corresponds to 80 per cent of the renal volume (Eddy 2000).

Tubulointerstitial fibrosis and progression to endstage renal failure

The mechanism of progressive renal deterioration is yet to be fully understood. The number of intertubular capillaries and their area is strongly correlated with the increase in serum creatinine. The mechanism whereby the loss of microvasculature results in progressive renal disease have been recently reviewed (Kang *et al.* 2002). The ensuing ischaemia might lead to tubular atrophy regularly found in interstitial fibrosis. Alternatively, tubular atrophy, might decrease glomerular filtration rate by two mechanisms. First, through the tubuloglomerular feedback mechanism. Second, through the formation of atubular glomeruli: up to 50 per cent of glomeruli are atubular in renal artery stenosis and chronic pyelonephritis (Marcussen 1995). However, there is as yet no experimental evidence that this latter factor plays a role in primary glomerular disease.

Renal interstitial fibrosis develops in three phases: induction, inflammatory matrix synthesis, and postinflammatory matrix synthesis (Strutz and Neilson 2002) summarized in Table 3.

Table 3 Phases of renal fibrogenesis

Induction phase
Release of chemokines by tubular epithelial cells
Infiltration of mononuclear cells
Release of profibrogenic cytokines
Activation and proliferation of resident fibroblasts
Inflammatory matrix synthesis
Increased matrix synthesis and deposition
Continued release of profibrogenic cytokines by infiltrating cells
Postinflammatory matrix synthesis
Cessation of the primary inflammatory stimulus
Secretion of profibrogenic cytokines by tubular epithelial cells
Autocrine proliferation of (myo)fibroblasts
Possible epithelial–mesenchymal transformation

Renal fibrosis: induction

During the induction phase, the proliferation and motility of fibroblasts is promoted. Renal fibroblasts are responsible for extracellular matrix synthesis in the kidney. Originally classified as type I interstitial cells, they are heterogeneous (Müller and Strutz 1995) and now classified according to growth potential and morphology into three mitotic and three postmitotic stages (Rodemann and Müller 1991). Fibroblasts from patients with tubulointerstitial fibrosis differ from those of normal kidneys: the relative percentage of fibroblasts growing out to confluency in primary culture increased from 7 to 47 per cent in cultures obtained from normal and fibrotic kidneys, respectively (Müller and Rodemann 1991). Clonal culture analysis revealed that the mitotic cell type MFI predominates in fibrotic kidneys (39 per cent of all fibroblasts) above the level of normal kidneys (2 per cent of all fibroblasts) (Rodemann and Müller 1991). The resistance to the cytostatic drug mitomycin C strongly increased in fibrosis-derived fibroblasts. Total collagen production, measured by [^{3}H] proline incorporation, increased in fibrosis-derived fibroblasts by a factor of 3–5 (Rodemann and Müller 1991). Besides these quantitative changes, fibroblasts from fibrotic kidneys display qualitative alterations. Their phenotype changes radically during fibrogenesis and wound repair (Grinnell 1994). Fibroblasts may differentiate into myofibroblasts which express certain smooth muscle proteins such as α-smooth muscle actin (Darby *et al.* 1990). Two-dimensional gel electrophoresis of [^{35}S]methionine-labelled intracellular proteins demonstrates that two proteins, absent from normal human fibroblasts, are expressed in human fibrosis-derived fibroblasts (Rodemann and Müller 1990). One of them is highly specific for fibrosis-derived fibroblasts and has been named 'fibrosin' (Müller *et al.* 1991). Its function is still unclear. Fibroblasts from fibrotic kidneys thus differ from their normal counterparts. Infiltrating cells in primary and secondary TIN may stimulate directly matrix-producing cells with eventual tubulointerstitial fibrosis.

Other cellular elements have been implicated in the production and deposition of interstitial matrix proteins including macrophages, endothelial cells, adventitial cells, and tubular epithelial cells (reviewed in Strutz and Muller 2000). Wiggins *et al.* (1993) used *in situ* hybridization with the α2-chain of collagen type I to localize collagen producing cells in a rabbit model of anti-GBM disease. They found that collagen production started in the perivascular adventitial compartment and extended only later throughout the interstitium. In rodents, tubular epithelial cells can secrete interstitial collagen types I and III (Haverty *et al.* 1988). Rat tubular epithelial cells stimulated with TGF-β express collagen (Creely *et al.* 1992). Tubular epithelial cells may also differentiate into α-smooth muscle actin positive mesenchymal cells (Strutz *et al.* 1995) which express *de novo* the fibroblast marker FSP-1 ('fibroblast specific protein'). In two mouse models of chronic progressive renal disease, interstitial staining for FSP-1 increased markedly (Strutz *et al.* 1995) a staining pattern reminiscent of that of collagen producing cells in the rabbit model of anti-GBM disease (Wiggins *et al.* 1993). The observation of *de novo* expression of FSP-1 in tubular epithelial cells, suggests a possible transformation of these cells into a mesenchymal phenotype. Tubular epithelial cells are particularly well suited to undergo phenotypic changes since they are derived (with the exception of collecting duct cells) from the metanephric mesenchyma. In addition to *de novo* expression of FSP-1, tubular epithelial cells also undergo epithelial–mesenchymal transformation (EMT). Rat tubular cells express *de novo* α-smooth muscle actin 3 weeks after 5/6-nephrectomy, lose their apical–basal polarity and migrate into the interstitium. Of particular note, the complete loss of epithelial characteristics occurs exclusively in areas of complete tubular disruption (Ng *et al.* 1998). The existence of EMT *in vivo* has recently been confirmed by Iwano *et al.* (2002).

What causes EMT? Okada *et al.* (1997) reported that a combination of TGF-β and epidermal growth factor *in vitro* strongly induces the expression of FSP-1 in tubular epithelial cells. TGF-β1 has a dose-dependant effect on EMT of a rat tubular epithelial cell line, indicated by an increase in the number of α-smooth muscle actin positive cells and a downregulated expression of the epithelial adhesion molecule E-cadherin (Fan *et al.* 1999). In a recent study, we have analysed the effects of FGF-2 on four aspects of EMT: expression of epithelial and/or mesenchymal cell markers, cell motility, secretion of matrix metalloproteinases (MMP), and matrix synthesis in two murine epithelial cell lines. FGF-2 had similar effects as EGF though its main impact was the potentiation of the induction of EMT by TGF-β1 (Strutz *et al.* 2002). Only TGF-β1 induced matrix synthesis whereas all tested cytokines induced expression of mesenchymal markers, cell motility, and MMP-2 and -9 secretion. In addition to cytokines, other stimuli are needed to induce complete EMT. The TBM has an essential function in stabilizing the epithelial phenotype (Zeisberg *et al.* 2001). Its disruption, by inhibition of collagen type IV assembly by soluble α1NC1-domains, leads to conversion to a mesenchymal phenotype. Complete EMT thus requires the disruption of the TBM integrity. Interestingly, this process of cellular differentiation can be blocked by addition of bone morphogenetic protein (BMP)-7, an antagonist of the effects of TGF-β1 (Zeisberg *et al.* 2002). It remains to be seen whether mesenchymal stem cells, recently described in the adult kidney (Poulsom *et al.* 2001), also have the potential to differentiate into interstitial fibroblasts. Figure 3 illustrates these (in part still hypothetical) mechanisms.

Inflammatory matrix synthesis

During this phase, fibroblasts are stimulated by cytokines from infiltrating inflammatory cells as well as from resident renal cells. One of the most relevant cytokines is angiotensin II which induces TGF-β synthesis in tubular epithelial cells and fibroblasts. A wealth of data support a beneficial role of blocking the effects of the renin–angiotensin system in models of progressive renal disease (summarized in Eddy 2000). Mice deficient in angiotensin II or its type I receptor develop less severe interstitial scarring than wild-type mice in the UUO model and anti-GBM disease (Hisada *et al.* 2001). Pharmacological blockade of the angiotensin system in patients with chronic allograft nephropathy or diabetes mellitus, reduces TGF-β and preserves renal function (Sharma *et al.* 1999). In addition, angiotensin II may induce *in vitro* collagen expression in interstitial fibroblasts and tubular epithelial cells.

TGF-β is currently viewed as the key cytokine promoting fibrosis. It mediates chemotaxis for fibroblasts, the transformation of fibroblasts to myofibroblasts and the synthesis of extracellular matrix proteins such as fibronectin and collagen type I. Its role in renal disease is supported by the demonstration that TGF-β transgenic mice develop glomerulosclerosis and interstitial fibrosis (Kopp *et al.* 1996). TGF-β1, the most extensively studied, is one of the three isoforms described in humans. It is a homodimer of two 112-amino acid polypeptides derived from proteolytic cleavage of a larger inactive precursor molecule. TGF-β1 expression is increased in models of renal, pulmonary, and hepatic fibrosis (Border and Noble 1994). In the kidney, increased TGF-β1 has been documented in anti-Thy 1.1 nephritis, Heymann nephritis, PAN nephrosis, anti-GBM disease,

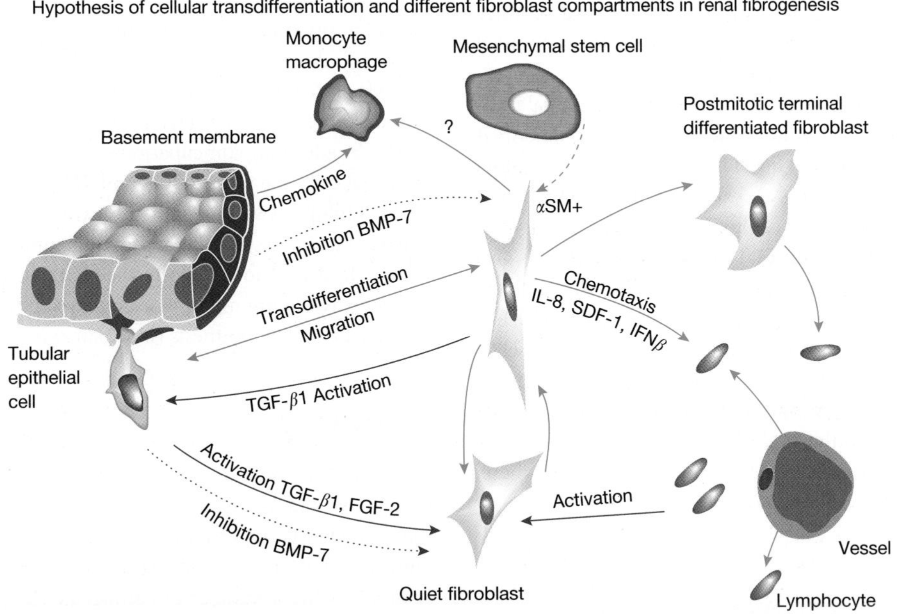

Fig. 3 Possible pathogenesis of tubular epithelial mesenchymal transformation via a transitional cell type. This process may be inhibited by bone morphogenetic protein-7 (BMP-7). The role of mesenchymal stem cells in the process of fibroblast generation is still unclear.

hypertensive and obstructive nephropathy. TGF-β1 is produced by resident as well as by inflammatory mononuclear cells, stimulated by a number of factors including angiotensin II, ET-1, glucose, insulin-like growth factor-1 (IGF-1), atrial natriuretic factor, platelet-activating factor, thromboxane, and drugs such as cyclosporin A. Autoinduction of TGF-β1 may also occur. TGF-β1 is secreted mainly in an inactive form necessitating extracellular activation by thrombospondin-1 or other mechanisms to release the active 25 kDa dimer. Thus, both upregulated thrombospondin-1 expression and increased TGF-β1 secretion are required for a biologic effect. In three different models of progressive renal disease in the rat, increased levels of thrombospondin-1 preceded the development of interstitial fibrosis (Hugo *et al.* 1998). Active TGF-β binds to its type II receptor that subsequently activates the type I receptor. The receptor complex then activates cytoplasmic proteins of the SMAD family by phosphorylation. Most cells express the TGF-β receptors indicating that receptor availability is not rate-limiting. The activity of TGF-β1 may be modified by a number of extracellular matrix molecules including the small proteoglycans decorin and biglycan. In decorin knock-out mice, interstitial matrix deposition was more severe than in wild-type mice (Schaefer *et al.* 2002).

TGF-β does not cause all its effects directly. Connective tissue growth factor (CTGF) is an important downstream mediator, originally isolated from endothelial cells. Its expression is strongly upregulated in human interstitial fibrosis and might mediate TGF-β-induced collagen synthesis (Duncan *et al.* 1999). Increased expression of CTGF has been also described in diabetic nephropathy and UUO models. Both cytokines may have synergistic effects: in a model of skin fibrosis, only combined injections of CTGF and TGF-β1 produced persistent scarring (Mori *et al.* 1999). The signalling events induced by CTGF are still unclear although they include the neutralization of the inhibitory BMP-4 (Abreu *et al.* 2002). Further studies are necessary to define the role of CTGF in renal fibrogenesis.

EGF might be another important cytokine for renal fibrogenesis but its role is still controversial. Whereas Chevalier *et al.* (1998) described an attenuation of renal fibrosis in the UUO model after administration of EGF, Terzi *et al.* (2000) using transgenic mice expressing a dominant negative form of the EGF receptor concluded that EGF is a strong profibrotic cytokine.

The relevance of ET-1 synthesis for the induction of interstitial infiltrates has already been discussed. Among the three isoforms described for ET, ET-1 is the most abundant in the kidney. Two types of receptors have been described: type A receptors are expressed mainly on vascular smooth muscle cells and type B receptors are present mainly on endothelial cells. ET, not only induces TGF-β1 production but also directly stimulates matrix synthesis and decreases collagenase activity. Transgenic mice overexpressing human ET-1 remain normotensive but display severe interstitial fibrosis and tubular cysts (Hocher *et al.* 1997). Addition of ET-1 type A receptor blockers decreases the severity of tubulointerstitial fibrosis in the chronic transplant nephropathy model and in lupus nephritis (Nakamura *et al.* 1995).

Additional factors implicated in inflammatory matrix synthesis include mast cell tryptase (Kondo *et al.* 2001), FGF-2, and PDGF as previously discussed.

Postinflammatory matrix synthesis

This phase differentiates fibrogenesis from regular wound healing characterized by resolution (Fig. 4). The primary inflammatory process, be it in the glomerulus, the interstitium, or the vasculature, subsides and interstitial inflammation is reduced to a few areas where matrix synthesis and deposition continues through different possible mechanisms. First, stimulation by the few remaining interstitial infiltrates is strong enough to sustain persisting myofibroblast proliferation. Second, autocrine loops result in autonomous stimulation of myofibroblasts. Lonnemann *et al.* (1995) observed that IL-1 secreted by fibrotic kidney derived fibroblasts led to a mitogenic response and to its autocrine stimulation. FGF-2 also affects autocrine fibroblast proliferation since its neutralization inhibits basal proliferation (Strutz *et al.* 2000). Furthermore, TGF-β1 induces the synthesis and secretion of FGF-2 from cortical fibroblasts (Strutz *et al.* 2001). Third, postinflammatory matrix synthesis results from the interaction between tubular epithelial cells and fibroblasts. PDGF levels are strongly upregulated in human tubular epithelial cells derived from fibrotic kidneys compared with cells from normal kidneys (Frank *et al.* 1993). In addition, coincubation of cortical fibroblasts with tubular epithelial cells enhances PDGF and TGF-β1 secretion (Johnson *et al.* 1998). Phillips *et al.* (1997) demonstrated that FGF-2 stimulates the release of latent TGF-β1 from proximal tubule cells indicating another positive feed-back loop. Finally, the progressive hypoxia due to the loss of microvasculature might worsen scarring through a direct effect on fibroblastic matrix synthesis (Norman *et al.* 1999).

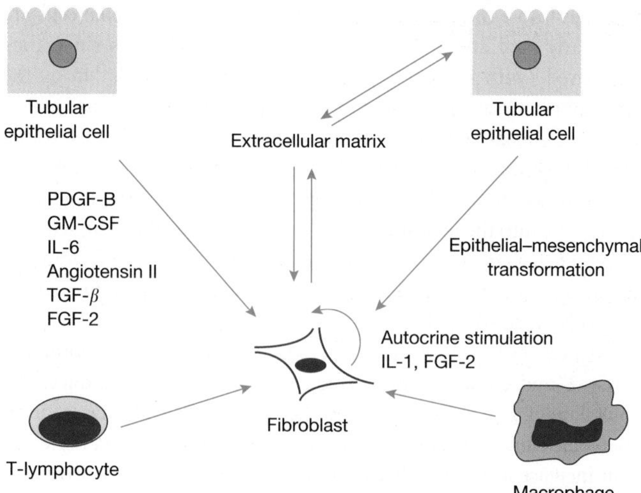

Fig. 4 Illustration of the possible mechanisms of postinflammatory phase of fibrogenesis. Tubular epithelial cells stimulate fibroblasts by secretion of profibrogenic cytokines and may participate in extracellular matrix synthesis directly (by direct synthesis of matrix proteins) or indirectly (by epithelial–mesenchymal transformation).

Summary

Tubulointerstitial inflammation is very common in renal disease both in primary and secondary interstitial forms. The significance of the tubulointerstitial compartment for renal function has been increasingly recognized in recent years. Interstitial fibrosis and tubular atrophy involve a number of pathogenic mechanisms leading to progressive renal disease. New forms of therapy to prevent progression of renal disease such as specific anti-inflammatory treatment or inhibition of fibrogenesis are expected to result from further research.

Acknowledgments

This work was supported in part by grants from the European Community (QLRT-2001-01215 and QOL-2001-14.4) to F. Strutz and G. A. Müller. We wish to thank Professor Van Ypersele for many helpful suggestions.

References

(Entries marked with an asterisk comprise useful general reading.)

Abreu, J. G., Ketpura, N. I., Reversade, B., and De Robertis, E. M. (2002). Connective-tissue growth factor (CTGF) modulates cell signalling by BMP and TGF-beta. *Nature Cell Biology* **4**, 599–604.

Alfrey, A. C., Fromment, D. H., and Hammond, W. S. (1989). Role of iron in tubulointerstitial injury in nephrotoxic serum nephritis. *Kidney International* **36**, 753–759.

Anders, H. J. *et al.* (2002). A chemokine receptor CCR-1 antagonist reduces renal fibrosis after unilateral ureter ligation. *Journal of Clinical Investigation* **109**, 251–259.

Appel, G. B. Acute interstitial nephritis. In *Immunologic Renal Disease* (ed. W. G. Couser and E. G. Neilson), pp. 1269–1281. Philadelphia, PA: Lippincott Williams and Williams, 2001.

Banu, N. and Meyers, C. M. (1999). IFN-gamma and LPS differentially modulate class II MHC and B7-1 expression on murine renal tubular epithelial cells. *Kidney International* **55**, 2250–2263.

Becker, J. L., Miller, F., Nuovo, G. J., Josepovitz, C., Schubach, W. H., and Nord, E. P. (1999). Epstein–Barr virus infection of renal proximal tubule cells: possible role in chronic interstitial nephritis. *Journal of Clinical Investigation* **104**, 1673–1681.

Bertani, T., Rocchi, G., Sacchi, G., Mecca, G., and Remuzzi, G. (1986). Adriamycin-induced glomerulosclerosis in the rat. *American Journal of Kidney Diseases* **7**, 12–19.

*__Bohle, A., Müller, G. A., Wehrmann, M., Mackensen-Haen, S., and Xiao, J. C.__ (1996). The pathogenesis of chronic renal failure in the primary glomerulopathies, renal vasculopathies, and chronic interstitial nephritides. *Kidney International* **49** (Suppl. 54), S2–S9.

*__Border, W. A. and Noble, N. A.__ (1994). Mechanisms of disease: transforming growth factor β in tissue fibrosis. *New England Journal of Medicine* **331**, 1286–1292.

Brunner, F. P., Broyer, M., and Brynger, H. (1985). Combined report on regular dialysis and transplantation in Europe XV, 1984. *Proceedings of the European Dialysis Transplant Association* **22**, 3–15.

Butkowski, R. J., Langeveld, J. P., Wieslander, J., Brentjens, J. R., and Andres, G. A. (1990). Characterization of a tubular basement membrane component reactive with autoantibodies associated with tubulointerstitial nephritis. *Journal of Biological Chemistry* **265**, 21091–21098.

Chevalier, R. L., Goyal, S., Wolstenholme, J. T., and Thornhill, B. A. (1998). Obstructive nephropathy in the neonatal rat is attenuated by epidermal growth factor. *Kidney International* **54**, 38–47.

Clayman, M. D., Sun, M. J., Michaud, L., Brul-Dashoff, J., Riblet, R., and Neilson, E. G. (1988). Clonotypic heterogeneity in experimental interstitial nephritis: restricted specificity of the antitubular basement membrane B cell repertoire is associated with a disease modifying cross-reactive idiotype. *Journal of Experimental Medicine* **167**, 1296–1313.

Creely, J. J., DiMari, S. J., Howe, A. M., and Haralson, M. A. (1992). Effects of transforming factor-β on collagen synthesis by normal rat kidney epithelial cells. *American Journal of Pathology* **140**, 45–55.

Darby, I., Skalli, O., and Gabbiani, G. (1990). α-Smooth muscle actin is transiently expressed by myofibroblasts during experimental wound healing. *Laboratory Investigation* **63**, 21–30.

Diamond, J. R., Pesek, I., Ruggeri, S., and Karnovsky, M. J. (1989). Essential fatty acid deficiency during acute puromycin nephrosis ameliorates late renal injury. *American Journal of Physiology* **257**, F798–F807.

Duncan, M. R., Frazier, K. S., Abramson, S., Williams, S., Klapper, H., Huang, X., and Grotendorst, G. R. (1999). Connective tissue growth factor mediates transforming growth factor beta-induced collagen synthesis: down-regulation by cAMP. *FASEB Journal* **13**, 1774–1786.

Eddy, A. A. (1989). Interstitial nephritis induced by protein-overload proteinuria. *American Journal of Pathology* **135**, 719–733.

Eddy, A. A. (1991). Tubulointerstitial nephritis during the heterologous phase of nephrotoxic serum nephritis. *Nephron* **59**, 304–313.

Eddy, A. (1994a). Protein restriction reduces transforming growth factor β and interstitial fibrosis in chronic purine aminonucleoside nephrosis. *American Journal of Physiology* **266**, F884–F893.

Eddy, A. A. (1994b). Experimental insights into the tubulointerstitial disease accompanying primary glomerular lesions. *Journal of the American Society of Nephrology* **5**, 1273–1287.

Eddy, A. A. (1998). Interstitial fibrosis in hypercholesterolemic rats: role of oxidation, matrix synthesis, and proteolytic cascades. *Kidney International* **53**, 1182–1189.

*__Eddy, A. A.__ (2000). Molecular basis of renal fibrosis. *Pediatric Nephrology* **15**, 290–301.

Eddy, A. A. and Michael, A. F. (1988). Acute tubulointerstitial nephritis associated with aminonucleoside nephrosis. *Kidney International* **33**, 14–23.

Eddy, A. A., Ho, G. C., and Thorner, P. S. (1992). The contribution of antibody-mediated cytotoxicity and immune-complex formation to tubulointerstitial disease in passive Heymann nephritis. *Clinical Immunology and Immunopathology* **62**, 42–55.

Eddy, A. E., Giachelli, C. M., McCulloch, L., and Liu, E. (1995). Renal expression of genes that promote interstitial inflammation and fibrosis in rats with protein-overload proteinuria. *Kidney International* **47**, 1546–1557.

Eldredge, C., Merritt, S., Goyal, M., Kulaga, H., Kindt, T. J., and Wiggins, R. (1991). Analysis of T cells and major histocompatibility complex class I and class II mRNA and protein content and distribution in antiglomerular basement membrane disease in the rabbit. *American Journal of Pathology* **139**, 1021–1035.

Fan, J. M., Ng, Y. Y., Hill, P. A., Nikolic-Paterson, D. J., Mu, W., Atkins, R. C., and Lan, H. Y. (1999). Transforming growth factor-beta regulates tubular epithelial-myofibroblast transdifferentiation *in vitro*. *Kidney International* **56**, 1455–1467.

Floege, J. and Rees, A. Growth factors and cytokines. In *Immunologic Renal Diseases* (ed. E. G. Neilson and W. G. Couser), pp. 417–588. Philadelphia, PA: Lippincott-Raven, 1997.

Frank, J., Engler-Blum, G., Rodemann, H. P., and Müller, G. A. (1993). Human renal tubular cells as a cytokine source: PDGF-B, GM-CSF and Il-6 mRNA expression *in vitro*. *Experimental Nephrology* **1**, 26–35.

Frei, U. and Schober-Halstenberg, H. J. (1999). Annual report of the German Renal Registry 1998. QuaSi-Niere Task Group for Quality Assurance in Renal Replacement Therapy. *Nephrology, Dialysis, Transplantation* **14**, 1085–1090.

Giachelli, C. M., Pichler, R., Lombardi, D., Denhardt, D. T., Alpers, C. E., Schwartz, S. M., and Johnson, R. J. (1994). Osteopontin expression in angiotensin II-induced tubulointerstitial nephritis. *Kidney International* **45**, 515–524.

Grinnell, F. (1994). Fibroblasts, myofibroblasts, and wound contraction. *Journal of Cell Biology* **124**, 401–404.

Haverty, T. P., Kelly, C. J., Hines, W. H., Amenta, P. S., Watanabe, M., Harper, R. A., Kefalides, N. A., and Neilson, E. G. (1988). Characterization of a renal tubular epithelial cell line which secretes the autologous target antigen of autoimmune experimental interstitial nephritis. *Journal of Cell Biology* **107**, 1359–1367.

Hill, G. S. (1994). Tubulointerstitial nephritis and vasculitis. *Current Opinion in Nephrology and Hypertension* **3**, 356–363.

*__Hisada, Y., Sugaya, T., Tanaka, S., Suzuki, Y., Ra, C., Kimura, K., and Fukamizu, A.__ (2001). An essential role of angiotensin II receptor type 1a in recipient kidney, not in transplanted peripheral blood leukocytes, in progressive immune-mediated renal injury. *Laboratory Investigation* **81**, 1243–1251.

Hocher, B. *et al.* (1997). Endothelin-1 transgenic mice develop glomerulosclerosis, interstitial fibrosis, and renal cysts but not hypertension. *Journal of Clinical Investigation* **99**, 1380–1389.

Hooke, D. H., Gee, D. C., and Atkins, R. C. (1987). Leukocyte analysis using monoclonal antibodies in human glomerulonephritis. *Kidney International* **31**, 964–972.

Hugo, C., Shankland, S. J., Pichler, R. H., Couser, W. G., and Johnson, R. J. (1998). Thrombospondin 1 precedes and predicts the development of tubulointerstitial fibrosis in glomerular disease in the rat. *Kidney International* **53**, 302–311.

Hutchinson, F. N. and Kaysen, G. A. (1988). Albuminuria causes lysozymuria in rats with Heymann nephritis. *Kidney International* **33**, 787–791.

Ibels, L. S., Alfrey, A. C., Haut, L., and Huffer, W. E. (1978). Preservation of function in experimental renal disease by dietary restriction of phosphate. *New England Journal of Medicine* **298**, 122–126.

Iwano, M., Plieth, D., Danoff, T. M., Xue, C., Okada, H., and Neilson, E. G. (2002). Evidence that fibroblasts derive from epithelium during tissue fibrosis. *Journal of Clinical Investigation* **110**, 341–350.

Johnson, D. W., Saunders, H. J., Baxter, R. C., Field, M. J., and Pollock, C. A. (1998). Paracrine stimulation of human renal fibroblasts by proximal tubule cells. *Kidney International* **54**, 747–757.

*Kang, D. H., Kanellis, J., Hugo, C., Truong, L., Anderson, S., Kerjaschki, D., Schreiner, G. F., and Johnson, R. J. (2002). Role of the microvascular endothelium in progressive renal disease. *Journal of the American Society of Nephrology* **13**, 806–816.

Kawasaki, K., Yaoita, E., Yamamoto, T., Tamatani, T., Miyasaki, M., and Kihara, I. (1993). Antibodies against intercellular adhesion molecule-1 and lymphocyte function-associated antigen-1 prevent glomerular injury in rat experimental crescentic glomerulonephritis. *Journal of Immunology* **150**, 1074–1083.

Kees-Folts, D., LevisSadow, J., and Schreiner, G. F. (1994). Tubular catabolism of albumin is associated with the release of an inflammatory lipid. *Kidney International* **45**, 1697–1709.

Kelly, C. J., Roth, D. A., and Meyers, C. M. (1991). Immune recognition and response to the renal interstitium. *Kidney International* **31**, 518–530.

*Klahr, S. (2001). Urinary tract obstruction. *Seminars in Nephrology* **21**, 133–145.

Kondo, S., Kagami, S., Kido, H., Strutz, F., Muller, G. A., and Kuroda, Y. (2001). Role of mast cell tryptase in renal interstitial fibrosis. *Journal of the American Society of Nephrology* **12**, 1668–1676.

Kopp, J. B., Factor, V. M., Mozes, M., Nagy, P., Sanderson, N., Bottinger, E. P., Klotman, P. E., and Thorgeirsson, S. S. (1996). Transgenic mice with increased plasma levels of TGF-beta 1 develop progressive renal disease. *Laboratory Investigation* **74**, 991–1003.

Lan, H. Y., Nikolic-Paterson, D. J., Zarama, M., Vannice, J. L., and Atkins, R. C. (1993). Suppression of experimental crescentic glomerulonephritis by the interleukin-1 receptor antagonist. *Kidney International* **43**, 479–485.

Lehman, D. H. and Dixon, F. J. (1975). Extraglomerular immunoglobulin deposits in human nephritis. *American Journal of Medicine* **58**, 765–796.

Loghman-Adham, M. (1993). Role of phosphate retention in the progression of renal failure. *Journal of Laboratory and Clinical Medicine* **122**, 16–26.

Lonnemann, G., Shapiro, L., Engler-Blum, G., Müller, G. A., Koch, K. M., and Dinarello, C. A. (1995). Cytokines in human renal interstitial fibrosis. I. IL-1 is an autocrine growth factor for cultured fibrosis-derived kidney fibroblasts. *Kidney International* **47**, 837–844.

Marcussen, N. (1995). Atubular glomeruli in chronic renal disease. *Current Topics in Pathology* **88**, 145–174.

Markovic-Lipkovski, J., Müller, C. A., Risler, T., Bohle, A., and Müller, G. A. (1990). Association of glomerular and interstitial mononuclear leucocytes with different forms of glomerulonephritis. *Nephrology, Dialysis, Transplantation* **5**, 10–17.

Mezzano, S. A., Droguett, M. A., Burgos, M. E., Ardiles, L. G., Aros, C. A., Caorsi, I., and Egido, J. (2000). Overexpression of chemokines, fibrogenic cytokines, and myofibroblasts in human membranous nephropathy. *Kidney International* **57**, 147–158.

*Michel, D. M. and Kelly, C. J. (1998). Acute interstitial nephritis. *Journal of the American Society of Nephrology* **9**, 506–515.

Mignon, F., Mery, J.-P., Morel-Maroger, L., Mougenot, B., Ronco, P., and Roland, J. (1984). Granulomatous tubulointerstitial nephritis. *Advcances in Nephrology* **13**, 219–245.

Morel-Maroger, L. (1974). Antitubular basement antibodies in rapidly progressive post-streptococcal glomerulonephritis. *Clinical Immunology and Immunopathology* **2**, 185–194.

Mori, T., Kawara, S., Shinozaki, M., Hayashi, N., Kakinuma, T., Igarashi, A., Takigawa, M., Nakanishi, T., and Takehara, K. (1999). Role and interaction of connective tissue growth factor with transforming growth factor-beta in persistent fibrosis: a mouse fibrosis model. *Journal of Cell Physiology* **181**, 153–159.

Müller, G. A. and Rodemann, H. P. (1991). Characterization of human renal fibroblasts in health and disease: I. Immunophenotyping of cultured tubular epithelial cells and fibroblasts derived from kidneys with histologically proven interstitial fibrosis. *American Journal of Kidney Diseases* **17**, 680–683.

Müller, G. A. and Strutz, F. (1995). Renal fibroblast heterogeneity. *Kidney International* **48** (Suppl. 50), S33–S36.

Müller, G. A., Markovic-Lipkovski, J., and Rodemann, H. P. (1991). The progression of renal diseases: on the pathogenesis of renal interstitial fibrosis. *Klinische Wochenschrift* **69**, 576–586.

Muntner, P., Coresh, J., Smith, J. C., Eckfeldt, J., and Klag, M. J. (2000). Plasma lipids and risk of developing renal dysfunction: the atherosclerosis risk in communities study. *Kidney International* **58**, 293–301.

Nakamura, T., Ebihara, I., Tomino, Y., and Koide, H. (1995). Effect of a specific endothelin A receptor antagonist on murine lupus nephritis. *Kidney International* **47**, 481–489.

Nath, K. A., Hostetter, M. K., and Hostetter, T. H. (1985). Pathophysiology of chronic tubulo-interstitial disease in rats. Interactions of dietary acid load, ammonia, and complement component C3. *Journal of Clinical Investigation* **76**, 667–675.

Nath, K. A., Croatt, A. J., and Hostetter, T. H. (1990). Oxygen consumption and oxidant stress in surviving nephrons. *American Journal of Physiology* **258**, F1354–F1362.

Neilson, E. G. (1989). Pathogenesis and therapy of interstitial nephritis. *Kidney International* **35**, 1257–1270.

*Neilson, E. G. (1999). Interstitial nephritis: another kissing disease? *Journal of Clinical Investigation* **104**, 1671–1672.

Ng, Y. Y., Huang, T. P., Yang, W. C., Chen, Z. P., Yang, A. H., Mu, W., Nikolic-Paterson, D. J., Atkins, R. C., and Lan, H. Y. (1998). Tubular epithelial-myofibroblast transdifferentiation in progressive tubulointerstitial fibrosis in 5/6 nephrectomized rats. *Kidney International* **54**, 864–876.

Norman, J. T., Orphanides, C., Garcia, P., and Fine, L. G. (1999). Hypoxia-induced changes in extracellular matrix metabolism in renal cells. *Experimental Nephrology* **7**, 463–469.

Ogrodowski, J. L., Hebert, L. A., Sedmak, D., Cosio, F. G., Tamerius, J., and Kolb, W. (1991). Measurement of SC5b-9 in urine in patients with nephrotic syndrome. *Kidney International* **40**, 1141–1147.

Okada, H., Danoff, T. M., Kalluri, R., and Neilson, E. G. (1997). Early role of Fsp1 in epithelial–mesenchymal transformation. *American Journal of Physiology* **273**, F563–F574.

O'Meara, Y. M., Natori, Y., Minto, A. W. M., Goldstein, D. J., and Salant, D. J. (1992). Nephrotoxic antiserum identifies a β1-integrin on rat glomerular epithelial cells. *American Journal of Physiology* **262**, F1083–F1091.

Ou, Z. L. and Natori, Y. (1999). Gene expression of CC chemokines in experimental acute tubulointerstitial nephritis. *Journal of Laboratory and Clinical Medicine* **133**, 41–47.

Phillips, A. O., Topley, N., Morrisey, K., Williams, J. D., and Steadman, R. (1997). Basic fibroblast growth factor stimulates the release of preformed transforming growth factor beta 1 from human proximal tubular cells in the absence of *de novo* gene transcription or mRNA translation. *Laboratory Investigation* **76**, 591–600.

Piguet, P. F., Collart, M. A., Grau, G. E., Kapanci, Y., and Vassalli, P. (1989). Tumor necrosis factor/cachectin plays a key role in bleomycin-induced pneumopathy and fibrosis. *Journal of Experimental Medicine* **170**, 655–663.

Poulsom, R. *et al.* (2001). Bone marrow contributes to renal parenchymal turnover and regeneration. *Journal of Pathology* **195**, 229–235.

Prodjosudjadi, W., Gerritsma, J. S. J., Klar-Mohamed, N., Gerritsen, A. F., Bruijn, J. A., Daha, M. R., and vanEs, L. A. (1995). Production and cytokine-mediated regulation of monocyte chemoattractant protein-1 by human proximal tubular epithelial cells. *Kidney International* **48**, 1477–1486.

Rangan, G. K., Wang, Y., Tay, Y. C., and Harris, D. C. (1999). Inhibition of nuclear factor-kappaB activation reduces cortical tubulointerstitial injury in proteinuric rats. *Kidney International* **56**, 118–134.

Remuzzi, G. and Bertani, T. (1998). Pathophysiology of progressive nephropathies. *New England Journal of Medicine* **339**, 1448–1456.

Rodemann, H. P. and Müller, G. A. (1990). Abnormal growth and clonal proliferation of fibroblasts derived from kidneys with interstitial fibrosis. *Proceedings of the Society of Experimental Biology and Medicine* **195**, 57–63.

Rodemann, H. P. and Müller, G. A. (1991). Characterization of human renal fibroblasts in health and disease: II. *In vitro* growth, differentiation, and collagen synthesis of fibroblasts from kidneys with interstitial fibrosis. *American Journal of Kidney Diseases* **17**, 684–686.

Sanders, P. W., Herrera, G. A., Chen, A., Booker, B. B., and Galla, J. H. (1988). Differential nephrotoxicity of low molecular weight proteins including Bence-Jones proteins in the perfused rat nephron *in vivo. Journal of Clinical Investigation* **82**, 2086–2096.

Schaefer, L. *et al.* (2002). Absence of decorin adversely influences tubulointerstitial fibrosis of the obstructed kidney by enhanced apoptosis and increased inflammatory reaction. *American Journal of Pathology* **160**, 1181–1191.

Segerer, S., Mac, K. M., Regele, H., Kerjaschki, D., and Schlondorff, D. (1999). Expression of the C-C chemokine receptor 5 in human kidney diseases. *Kidney International* **56**, 52–64.

*Segerer, S., Nelson, P. J., and Schlondorff, D.** (2000). Chemokines, chemokine receptors, and renal disease: from basic science to pathophysiologic and therapeutic studies. *Journal of the American Society of Nephrology* **11**, 152–176.

Shappell, S. B., Gurpinar, T., Lechago, J., Suki, W. N., and Truong, L. D. (1998). Chronic obstructive uropathy in severe combined immunodeficient (SCID) mice: lymphocyte infiltration is not required for progressive tubulointerstitial injury. *Journal of the American Society of Nephrology* **9**, 1008–1017.

*Sharma, K., Eltayeb, B. O., McGowan, T. A., Dunn, S. R., Alzahabi, B., Rohde, R., Ziyadeh, F. N., and Lewis, E. J.** (1999). Captopril-induced reduction of serum levels of transforming growth factor-beta1 correlates with long-term renoprotection in insulin-dependent diabetic patients. *American Journal of Kidney Diseases* **34**, 818–823.

Shinozaki, M., Hirahashi, J., Lebedeva, T., Liew, F. Y., Salant, D. J., Maron, R., and Kelley, V. R. (2002). IL-15, a survival factor for kidney epithelial cells, counteracts apoptosis and inflammation during nephritis. *Journal of Clinical Investigation* **109**, 951–960.

Strutz, F. and Muller, G. A. (2000). Transdifferentiation comes of age. *Nephrology, Dialysis, Transplantation* **15**, 1729–1731.

Strutz, F. and Müller, G. A. Mechanisms of renal fibrogenesis. In *Immunologic Renal Diseases* (ed. E. G. Neilson and W. C. Couser), pp. 73–104. Philadelphia, PA: Lippincott, Williams and Wilkins, 2001.

Strutz, F. and Neilson, E. G. (1994). The role of lymphocytes in the progression of interstitial disease. *Kidney International* **45** (Suppl. 45), S106–S110.

*Strutz, F. and Neilson, E. G.** (2002). New insights into mechanisms of fibrosis in immune injury. *Springer Seminars in Immunopathology* (in press).

Strutz, F., Okada, H., Lo, C. W., Danoff, T., Carone, B., Tomaszewski, J., and Neilson, E. G. (1995). Identification and characterization of fibroblast-specific protein 1 (FSP1). *Journal of Cell Biology* **130**, 393–405.

Strutz, F., Zeisberg, M., Hemmerlein, B., Sattler, B., Hummel, K., Becker, V., and Müller, G. A. (2000). Basic fibroblast growth factor (FGF-2) expression is increased in human renal fibrogenesis and may mediate autocrine fibroblast proliferation. *Kidney International* **57**, 1521–1538.

Strutz, F., Zeisberg, M., Renziehausen, A., Raschke, B., Becker, V., and Müller, G. A. (2001). Transforming growth factor (TGF)-β1 induces proliferation in human renal fibroblasts via induction of basic fibroblast growth factor (FGF-2). *Kidney International* **59**, 579–592.

Strutz, F., Zeisberg, M., Ziyadeh, F. N., Yang, C. Q., Kalluri, R., Muller, G. A., and Neilson, E. G. (2002). Role of basic fibroblast growth factor-2 in epithelial–mesenchymal transformation. *Kidney International* **61**, 1714–1728.

Tang, W. W., Feng, L., Mathison, J. C., and Wilson, C. B. (1994a). Cytokine expression, upregulation of intercellular adhesion molecule-1, and leucocyte infiltration in experimental tubulointerstitial nephritis. *Laboratory Investigation* **70**, 631–638.

Tang, W. W., Feng, L., Vannice, J. L., and Wilson, C. B. (1994b). IL-1 receptor antagonist ameliorates experimental anti-GBM antibody associated glomerulonephritis. *Journal of Clinical Investigation* **93**, 273–279.

Tang, W. W., Feng, L., Xia, Y., and Wilson, C. B. (1994c). Extracellular matrix accumulation in immune-mediated tubulointerstitial injury. *Kidney International* **45**, 1077–1084.

Tang, W. W., Qi, M., Warren, J. S., and Van, G. Y. (1997). Chemokine expression in experimental tubulointerstitial nephritis. *Journal of Immunology* **159**, 870–876.

Terzi, F., Burtin, M., Hekmati, M., Federici, P., Grimber, G., Briand, P., and Friedlander, G. (2000). Targeted expression of a dominant-negative EGF-R in the kidney reduces tubulo-interstitial lesions after renal injury. *Journal of Clinical Investigation* **106**, 225–234.

Throssell, D., Harris, K. P., Bevington, A., Furness, P. N., Howie, A. J., and Walls, J. (1996). Renal effects of metabolic acidosis in the normal rat. *Nephron* **73**, 450–455.

Topley, N., Steadman, R., Mackenzie, R., Knowlden, J. M., and Williams, J. D. (1989). Type 1 fimbriate strains of *Escherichia coli* initiate renal parenchymal scarring. *Kidney International* **36**, 609–616.

Wahl, P., Schoop, R., Bilic, G., Neuweiler, J., Le Hir, M., Yoshinaga, S. K., and Wuthrich, R. P. (2002). Renal tubular epithelial expression of the costimulatory molecule B7RP-1 (inducible costimulator ligand). *Journal of the American Society of Nephrology* **13**, 1517–1526.

Wiggins, R., Goyal, M., Merritt, S., and Killen, P. D. (1993). Vascular adventitial cell expression of collagen I mesenger ribonucleic acid in anti-glomerular basement membrane antibody-induced crescentic nephritis in the rabbit. *Laboratory Investigation* **68**, 557–565.

Wilson, C. B. (1991). Nephritogenic tubulointerstitial antigens. *Kidney International* **39**, 501–517.

Wilson, C. B. Immune models of tubulointerstitial injury. In *Immunologic Renal Diseases* (ed. E. G. Neilson and W. C. Couser), pp. 779–813. Philadelphia, PA: Lippincott-Raven, 2001.

Wilson, D. M., Turner, D. R., Cameron, J. S., Ogg, C. S., Brown, C. B., and Chantler, C. (1976). Value of renal biopsy in acute intrinsic renal failure. *British Medical Journal* **2**, 459–461.

Wilz, S. W., Kurnick, J. T., Pandolfi, F., Rubin, R. H., Warren, H. S., Goldstein, R., Kersten, C. M., and McCluskey, R. T. (1993). T lymphocyte responses to antigens of gram-negative bacteria in pyelonephritis. *Clinical Immunology and Immunopathology* **69**, 36–42.

Yoshioka, K., Takemura, T., and Murakami, K. (1993). *In situ* expression of cytokines in IgA nephritis. *Kidney International* **44**, 825–833.

Yoshioka, K., Takemura, T., and Hattori, S. (2002). Tubulointerstitial nephritis antigen: primary structure, expression and role in health and disease. *Nephron* **90**, 1–7.

Zeisberg, M., Bonner, G., Maeshima, Y., Colorado, P., Muller, G. A., Strutz, F., and Kalluri, R. (2001). Renal fibrosis: collagen composition and assembly regulates epithelial–mesenchymal transdifferentiation. *American Journal of Pathology* **159**, 1313–1321.

Zeisberg, M., Hanai, J.-I., Sugimoto, H., Strutz, F., and Kalluri, R. (2002). Bone morphogenic protein-7 is an antagonist of transforming growth factor β1 induced epithelial to mesenchymal transdifferentiation and reverses chronic renal injury. *Molecular Cell* (in revision).

Zoja, C., Donadelli, R., Colleoni, S., Figliuzzi, M., Bonazzola, S., Morigi, M., and Remuzzi, G. (1998). Protein overload stimulates RANTES production by proximal tubular cells depending on NF-kappa B activation. *Kidney International* **53**, 1608–1615.

6.2 Analgesic nephropathy

Wolfgang Pommer and Marc E. De Broe

Introduction and history

Analgesic nephropathy is the most widely known and widespread complication resulting from the chronic use of mixed analgesic preparations which include anilides, phenacetin or paracetamol, salicylates, and central acting substances such as coffeine or codeine. It is one of the few common renal diseases susceptible to primary prevention.

Three classes of potent analgesics, originally described in the second half of the nineteenth century (Haas 1983), were provided in combination in the early twentieth century to minimize their specific side-effects. Most analgesic mixtures also contained either caffeine or the potentially addictive codeine. Their popularity became rapidly exceptional (Carro-Ciampi 1978). The first class includes salicylates, the second anilide derivatives such as phenacetin and its metabolite acetaminophen (paracetamol), and the third pyrazolone derivatives (antipyrine, aminopyrine, or phenylbutazone). The latter class compounds were usually abandoned as a result of their haematological complications. Fixed combinations rested on the principle that two or more drugs with the same final effect have an additive and potentiating effect when their pharmacological mechanisms are different (Buergi 1927).

The nephrotoxicity of analgesic mixtures was recognized only after more than 50 years of current use, when Swiss pathologists recognized a changing pattern of chronic interstitial nephropathies at autopsy and suggested a relationship with the chronic use of analgesic mixtures (Spuehler and Zollinger 1953; Zollinger 1955). The hypothesis of a causal link between analgesic consumption and interstitial nephropathy was subsequently corroborated by several retrospective studies. Furthermore, urothelial malignancies were associated consistently with long-term analgesic abuse (Gloor 1978).

The main drug common to analgesic mixtures was phenacetin, hence the initial term phenacetin nephropathy. Phenacetin was therefore withdrawn or banned in the late 1960s and 1970s and usually replaced by acetaminophen (paracetamol). Subsequently, it has been argued on experimental and epidemiological grounds that analgesic mixtures without phenacetin are equally nephrotoxic (De Broe and Elseviers 1998). Restriction of over-the-counter sale of all analgesic mixtures in several countries has coincided with a significant decrease in analgesic associated kidney disease (Noels *et al.* 1995; Schwarz *et al.* 1999). The evidence supporting this latter view is further discussed. The all-inclusive name of analgesic nephropathy is now commonly used.

Definition

Analgesic nephropathy is a slowly progressive disease resulting from the daily use for many years of mixtures containing at least two antipyretics, anilides, and salicylates, usually together with caffeine or codeine (or both). It is characterized by renal papillary necrosis/calcifications and chronic interstitial nephritis, and is sometimes associated with transitional-cell carcinoma of the uroepithelium (Spühler and Zollinger 1953; Gloor 1961; Kincaid-Smith 1967; Mihatsch 1986, 1989; Kincaid-Smith and Nanra 1993; De Broe and Elseviers 1998). It has not been described after the intake of single analgesic substances. Analgesic nephropathy is part of a broad spectrum of clinical findings that is summarized as 'analgesic syndrome' (see below). In addition to the classical picture of analgesic nephropathy, excessive exposure to single or compound analgesics and non-steroidal anti-inflammatory drugs (NSAIDs) may contribute to the development or the progression of chronic renal disease of whatever aetiology towards endstage renal failure (Sandler *et al.* 1989; Morlans 1990; Pommer 1993; Perneger *et al.* 1994; Fored *et al.* 2001).

Epidemiology

Renal complications caused by analgesics have been reported worldwide, in countries in which mixed analgesics are available without prescription and are consumed in significant amounts. However, there are appreciable regional and local differences in the prevalence of endstage kidney damage due to analgesics for reasons which have so far not been clarified. Differences in consumption behaviour, in the frequency of other exogenous risk factors, pre-existent nephropathies, in the medical prejudice towards the analgesic syndrome, and in prevention policy may be responsible. Appreciation of the risks of renal complications resulting from chronic analgesic consumption has been controversial until very recently. This applies, in particular, to the substances responsible, the threshold dose for damage, and knowledge of additive risk factors. The psychosocial conditions of chronic analgesic consumption and their special regional features have rarely been characterized.

The proportion of the population that regularly takes analgesics is unknown in most countries. According to representative surveys in the general population, it is between 3 and 4 per cent in some European countries, with a greater prevalence in the middle-aged female population (reviewed in Gsell 1974; Buckalew and Schey 1986; Pommer *et al.* 1986). In some types of industry, the prevalence is much higher with a range from 8 to 30 per cent, according to the results of occupational medical investigation.

The definition of chronic analgesic consumption is variable; it is generally regarded as consumption daily or several times weekly. The assessment of a population-related dose, the per capita consumption, is almost impossible in many countries owing to the lack of published sales statistics, despite its importance to evaluate the effectiveness of legislative and preventive measures.

Patients with analgesic nephropathy have taken large amounts of analgesic mixtures over years or decades; however, only a small number of misusers develop clinically apparent disease. Dubach *et al.* (1991) reported, that after a 20-year follow-up of 576 cases (on phenacetin-containing analgesics) with complete observations, 16 had died from renal causes and four were on chronic dialysis for endstage renal disease. The absolute risk of developing endstage renal disease attributable to analgesic abuse can thus be calculated to be 1.7/1000/year. A similar 1.6/1000/year risk was calculated in a completely different study design by Elseviers (1994). This figure is in the same range as the risk of developing lung cancer in smokers.

The prevalence of analgesic nephropathy in patients with terminal kidney disease receiving renal replacement therapy differs greatly within and between countries both in and outside Europe (Buckalew and Schey 1986; Drukker *et al.* 1986; Brunner and Selwood 1994; Lawrence 1994; Elseviers *et al.* 1995a). Comparison between different countries is almost impossible, owing to the lack of age and gender standardization, the different rates of acceptance for inclusion in a renal replacement programme, and the diagnostic criteria. In the ANNE (Analgesic Nephropathy Network Europe) study, reliance on objectively well-established renal imaging criteria, identified analgesic nephropathy in 17.3 per cent of the included patients, in contrast to the 11.5 per cent incidence diagnosed by the attending nephrologists. In a representative sample of new dialysis patients in the Czech and Slovak Republics a prevalence of 9 per cent was found with the same criteria while the corresponding EDTA data never exceeded 5 per cent (Elseviers *et al.* 1995a).

The overall north–south gradient of endstage analgesic nephropathy existing in Europe in general as well as in Belgium (Elseviers and de Broe 1988) and in the former West Germany (Pommer *et al.* 1986) cannot be explained at present. Several studies indicate that during the last decade the incidence of analgesic nephropathy fell in the age group below 64 years but remained stable in the older group both in Europe (Brunner and Selwood 1994) and in Australia (Stewart *et al.* 1994). In Belgium, the incidence of analgesic nephropathy in the northern part of the country declined from 20 per cent in the mid-1980s to 8 per cent in 2001, earlier in the younger than in the older age categories (Michielsen and De Schepper 2001).

Autopsy studies, in which specific manifestations of chronic analgesic consumption are looked for, offer a good opportunity to investigate the long-term prevalence and incidence of the disease. Capillary sclerosis of the urinary tract has been attributed to the intake of analgesics containing phenacetin and paracetamol (Mihatsch *et al.* 1983). The prevalence of chronic analgesic intake in the general population is correlated with the frequency of capillary sclerosis in the autopsy material (Mihatsch *et al.* 1982, 1983; Ditscherlein *et al.* 1989). Other analgesic-associated lesions, such as renal papillary necrosis and interstitial nephritis, investigated in autopsy studies, are much more frequent than capillary sclerosis (Gloor 1961; Burry *et al.* 1966; Bethke and Schubert 1985; Marek 1987), but their specificity for analgesic misuse is lower.

The paucity, until the 1980s, of epidemiological studies with hard data on the relative risks of chronic kidney damage from regular analgesic intake has delayed appraisal of the aetiology of analgesic nephropathy and the introduction of adequate preventive measures (Christie 1978; Consensus Conference 1984; Lanes *et al.* 1986). Today, a number of case–control and cohort studies clearly indicate the detrimental effects of analgesic mixtures in the development of renal papillary necrosis or endstage renal disease (Table 1).

The risk of papillary necrosis after the intake of analgesic mixtures containing phenacetin and paracetamol has been investigated several times by an Australian group (McCredie *et al.* 1982; McCredie and Stewart 1988). They have shown dose-dependent risks at least after intake of mixed preparations containing phenacetin. In this population, no increase in risk could be demonstrated for an intake of paracetamol in a follow-up study (McCredie and Stewart 1988). However, the total exposure to analgesics containing paracetamol was far less than that to analgesics containing phenacetin. In the ANNE study, by contrast, among 226 subjects with progressive analgesic nephropathy diagnosed with validated criteria, 46 had reportedly used analgesics not containing phenacetin but acetaminophen, aspirin, pyrazolones, and others (Elseviers and De Broe 1996), a subsequently disputed finding (Feinstein *et al.* 2000a,b).

While Murray *et al.* (1983) were unable to demonstrate an increased risk of endstage renal disease after intake of either single substances or mixed analgesics in a population with a low prevalence of chronic intake of analgesics, four subsequent retrospective case–control studies demonstrated opposite results (Table 1). An increased dose-dependent risk of endstage renal failure for the use of mixed analgesics, containing phenacetin and in few cases paracetamol, was shown in a study carried out in West Berlin, a region with a high consumption of analgesics (Pommer *et al.* 1989). The risk was especially high for mixed analgesics containing caffeine (Table 1). A case–control study in patients with newly diagnosed renal insufficiency of various stages and types performed in North Carolina detected an increased risk for daily use of phenacetin- and paracetamol-containing mixtures, but not for acetylsalicylic acid taken alone (Sandler *et al.* 1989). Spanish investigators observed an increased risk of endstage renal failure for persons with different kidney diseases after regular consumption of analgesics (Morlans 1990). A dose-dependent risk of endstage renal failure after exposure to acetaminophen and NSAIDs were clearly demonstrated in the mid-Atlantic seaboard states of the United States (Perneger *et al.* 1994).

Two cohort studies substantiate the specific relation between analgesic exposure and renal disease. The dose-dependent risk of phenacetin-containing analgesics for the reduction of urinary concentrating capacity and renal insufficiency was shown in the Swiss cohort study of Dubach *et al.* (1983). In the Belgian cohort study, a sixfold increased risk of the development of renal insufficiency was demonstrated in cases with an abuse of different types of compound analgesics (Elseviers and De Broe 1995).

The regular use of analgesics also emerges as a significant risk factor for renal failure in several types of chronic renal disease such as diabetic nephropathy, nephrosclerosis, and others (Sandler *et al.* 1989; Pommer 1993; Fored *et al.* 2001) (Table 1). Recently, a Swedish study reported that the regular use of acetaminophen, aspirin, or both increased the risk for chronic renal failure in subjects with various renal diseases (Fored *et al.* 2001), none of whom had signs of the classical picture of analgesic nephropathy as detailed below. Risks described for the intake of single analgesic substances in this study are in contrast to other different studies (Akyol *et al.* 1982; Burry and Dieppe 1982; Pommer *et al.* 1989; Rexrode *et al.* 2001) but, in part of these studies, overall analgesic exposure was low.

To summarize, the assumption that the regular consumption of analgesic combinations with and possibly without phenacetin is associated with a significantly increased risk to develop the well-defined clinical

Table 1 Relative risks of chronic analgesic intake for analgesic-associated renal disease

Renal changes	Substance/dosage	RR (95% CI)	Reference
Urinary concentration diminished[a]	Mixtures containing phenacetin		
	>1.25 g/day[b]	4.2 (2.54–6.98)	(1)
		7.6 (4.81–12.04)	(1)
Serum creatinine elevated	>1.25 g/day[b]	8.08 (2.82–23.18)	(1)
		15.25 (5.25–44.48)	(1)
Renal papillary necrosis	Mixtures containing phenacetin	17.7 (9.0–35.1)	(2)
	Mixtures without phenacetin	3.0 (1.5–5.8)	
Renal papillary necrosis	Phenacetin		(3)
	>1 kg	19 (10–37)	
	>0.1 kg	15 (8–28)	
	Paracetamol		
	>1 kg[c]	0.5 (0.1–1.9)	
	>0.1 kg[c]	0.7 (0.3–1.9)	
Endstage renal failure	Single substance		(4)
	<1 kg	1.21 (0.63–2.31)	
	1–3 kg	0.88 (0.09–1.69)	
	>3 kg	0.30 (0.07–1.22)	
	Analgesic mixtures		
	<1 kg	1.39 (0.76–2.56)	
	1–3 kg	2.80 (0.98–8.40)	
	>3 kg	2.21 (0.5–9.68)	
Endstage renal failure	Single substance		(5)
	<1 kg	0.85 (0.49–1.48)	
	>1 kg	1.51 (0.40–5.37)	
	All analgesic mixtures		
	<1 kg	2.54 (1.83–3.54)	
	>1 kg	4.48 (2.61–7.68)	
	Mixtures		
	With phenacetin		
	<1 kg	2.08 (1.53–2.81)	
	>1 kg	4.48 (2.61–7.68)	
	With paracetamol		
	<1 kg	1.57 (1.90–4.23)	
	>1 kg	4.06 (1.32–12.43)	
	With acetylsalicyclic acid		
	<1 kg	1.93 (1.39–4.23)	
	>1 kg	2.42 (1.39–4.23)	
	With dipyrone		
	<1 kg	1.72 (1.08–2.74)	
	>1 kg	3.87 (0.40–37.88)	
	With phenazone		
	<1 kg	2.33 (1.69–3.20)	
	>1 kg	3.57 (2.26–5.64)	
	With caffeine		
	<1 kg	2.15 (1.61–2.87)	
	>1 kg	52.56 (6.83–402.8)	
Renal insufficiency	ASA		(6)
	Weekly	1.39 (0.95–2.04)	
	Daily	1.24 (0.62–2.45)	
	Paracetamol[c]		
	Weekly	1.26 (0.80–2.00)	
	Daily	4.97 (1.59–15.5)	
	Phenacetin mixtures		
	Weekly	1.74 (0.91–3.34)	
	Daily	6.06 (1.96–18.8)	

Table 1 Continued

Renal changes	Substance/dosage	RR (95% CI)	Reference
Endstage renal disease	All analgesics[c]	2.89 (1.78–4.68)	(7)
	<1 kg	3.09 (1.77–5.41)	
	1–3 kg	3.20 (1.00–10.26)	
	>3 kg	2.01 (0.39–10.28)	
Endstage renal failure	Acetaminophen		(8)
	<1000 pills	1.0	
	1000–4999 pills	2.0 (1.3–3.2)	
	>5000 pills	2.4 (1.2–4.8)	
	Aspirin		
	<1000 pills	1.0	
	1000–4999 pills	0.5 (0.3–0.7)	
	>5000 pills	1.0 (0.6–1.8)	
	NSAIDS		
	<1000 pills	1.0	
	1000–4999 pills	0.6 (0.3–1.1)	
	>5000 pills	8.8 (1.1–71.8)	
Decreased renal function[a]	Analgesic mixtures	6.1 (1.4–25.9)	(9)
	Analgesics (regular use)[d]		(10)
	Acetaminophen (without aspirin)		
	Regularly	2.5 (1.7–3.6)	
	1–99 g	1.2 (0.9–1.5)	
	100–499 g	1.3 (0.9–1.8)	
	>500 g	3.3 (2.0–5.5)	
	Aspirin (without acetaminophen)		
	Regularly	2.5 (1.9–3.3)	
	1–99 g	1.4 (1.1–1.7)	
	100–499 g	1.6 (1.2–2.1)	
	>500 g	1.9 (1.3–2.9)	
	Acetaminophen (regularly) plus aspirin	2.2 (1.4–3.5)	
	Aspirin (regularly) plus acetaminophen	1.6 (0.9–2.7)	

[a] Cohort study.

[b] Urinary NAPAP content related on daily ingestion of >1.25 g phenacetin.

[c] Ingested as single substances and mixtures.

[d] Regular use defined as intake of at least twice a week for 2 months.

References: (1) Dubach *et al.* (1983); (2) McCredie *et al.* (1982); (3) McCredie and Stewart (1988); (4) Murray *et al.* (1983); (5) Pommer *et al.* (1989); (6) Sandler *et al.* (1989); (7) Morlans (1990); (8) Perneger *et al.* (1994); (9) Elseviers (1994); (10) Fored *et al.* (2001).

entity of analgesic nephropathy is now substantiated by epidemiological findings. In addition, these epidemiologic studies generated the hypothesis that habitual analgesic use influences the progression of chronic renal disease in general. However, it is as yet impossible to determine whether exposure to analgesics is the initial cause of renal failure or a factor contributing to the progression of the renal disease, whether there is an interplay between the two possibilities, whether the association is non-causal, or whether analgesic consumption was triggered by predisposing conditions such as hypertension, chronic pain, etc., which are frequently observed in the context of chronic renal failure introducing protopathic bias (Barrett 1996).

The evidence derived from epidemiological studies is limited by the fact that association but no causal relationship is demonstrated by different types of biases, critically reviewed by Delzell and Shapiro (1998) and more recently by Feinstein *et al.* (2000a). Critical appraisal concerns the relationship of both, phenacetin- (Delzell and Shapiro 1998) and paracetamol-containing analgesics (Feinstein *et al.* 2000a), with renal and extrarenal complications. Improved epidemiological study design should include the following:

- patients with early stage disease should be included, avoiding the possibility that renal disease provoked analgesic use/abuse;
- explicit knowledge of both the time in which the drug was started and stopped, and the amount of drug ingested should be obtained;
- personal, not telephone, interviews should be performed, and must include visual (book with colour photographs) aids to obtain accurate information concerning the type of drug ingested;
- patients and control individuals should be drawn from the same population, and their number should be sufficient to reach statistical significance;

- an established set of clinical features characteristic of classical analgesic nephropathy should be used to define consequences of analgesic intake with respect to the development of specific analgesic kidney disease and the role of (single or combined) analgesic intake for the progression of kidney disease of other origin.

Pathophysiology

In spite of the clinically and epidemiologically well-documented association between analgesic consumption and kidney damage, the causative agents and the pathological mechanisms that lead to the development of analgesic nephropathy have not been completely elucidated.

Renal papillary necrosis (damage to the inner renal medulla that may be based on capillary sclerosis) is today regarded as the hallmark of analgesic nephropathy (Burry 1967; Gloor 1978; Mihatsch *et al.* 1978, 1983). Capillary sclerosis is especially pronounced in the vessels of the renal pelvis and ureteral mucosa. The interstitial lesions comprising the later morphological features of analgesic nephropathy are considered to be a consequence of the papillary necrosis (see below).

Analgesic mixtures very often consist of an anilide (traditionally phenacetin and, in recent years, more frequently paracetamol), a salicylate (most frequently acetylsalicylic acid, more rarely salicylamide), and, occasionally, a pyrazolone (phenazone or dipyrone) with, in addition, in most cases, a centrally acting agent (caffeine, barbiturate, codeine, or other sedatives). Three central questions concerning the aetiology and pathogenesis of analgesic nephropathy can be addressed:

1. What agent(s) are causally involved in the development of renal papillary necrosis? The following substances must be considered: phenacetin and paracetamol, acetylsalicylic acid or other salicylates, pyrazolone, caffeine, and other centrally acting agents.
2. What mechanisms result in papillary necrosis?
3. Are there predisposing factors that also affect the degree of medullary damage?

The agent(s) responsible

Although phenacetin was not initially mentioned by Spuehler and Zollinger (1953), it was readily apparent that this agent was common to all the analgesic preparations. Phenacetin was thus, quickly incriminated (Zollinger 1955) and the disease named 'phenacetin nephritis' (Gsell 1974). The phenacetin hypothesis was first questioned on the basis of epidemiological and clinical observations by Australian workers who noted that the replacement of phenacetin by other analgesics did not reduce appreciably the incidence of analgesic nephropathy (Nanra *et al.* 1978). In Flanders, Belgium, 30 years after withdrawal of phenacetin from the most popular analgesic mixtures and 20 years after its almost disappearance the incidence of analgesic nephropathy remained elevated. However, as pointed out by Michielsen and De Schepper (2001), it takes 20 years after withdrawal of phenacetin for analgesic nephropathy to subside as a cause of endstage renal failure and thus for the definition of the role of non-phenacetin containing analgesics in the development or progression of specific renal diseases.

Kidney damage caused by phenacetin alone is only sporadic in humans in the context of acute intoxications (Prescott 1982). For reasons that have not been clarified, phenacetin has practically never been available as a single substance on the pharmaceutical market. Long-term misuse of phenacetin without simultaneous intake of other analgesic agents has never been reported.

An important, as yet unsolved, question is the renal risk of monotherapy with acetaminophen (paracetamol), the primary metabolite of phenacetin which is now widely used as a minor analgesic. Acute renal failure with drugs including paracetamol has been reported (Kleinman *et al.* 1980; Björck *et al.* 1988). Four case–control studies suggest that acetaminophen alone is nephrotoxic (Segasothy *et al.* 1988; Sandler *et al.* 1989; Perneger *et al.* 1994; Fored *et al.* 2001), although its risk is probably below that of phenacetin–aspirin combinations (Sandler *et al.* 1989; Buckalew 1996).

Animal experiments are not helpful as the characteristic features of analgesic nephropathy cannot be induced. Renal papillary necrosis has been induced only in animals with either a genetic predisposition or a pre-existing disorder of kidney function (Bach and Hardy 1985). In dehydrated dogs, paracetamol and its glucuronide conjugate accumulate in the papilla after administration of phenacetin together with evidence of a cytotoxic action (Duggin and Mudge 1976; Duggin 1980). However, the doses of phenacetin or paracetamol necessary to induce papillary necrosis are not comparable to those used in man (Molland 1978).

As other analgesic acids, acetylsalicylic acid can cause functional and morphological kidney damage in humans, even with the acute administration of therapeutic doses. Papillary necrosis and analgesic nephropathy have been described in long-term therapy with acetylsalicylic acid in patients with rheumatic diseases, although prevalence in relation to consumption is low (Prescott 1982; Nanra 1983).

In animal experiments, acetylsalicylic acid and other salicylates are secreted in the proximal tubule and subsequently concentrated in the papilla (especially in dehydration), although to a lower extent than paracetamol (Duggin 1980). Chronic administration of acetylsalicylic acid in doses below the range of acute toxicity in humans causes a high incidence of necrosis in hydropenic rats (Molland 1978).

Pyrazolones can cause kidney damage (including papillary necrosis) after acute and chronic administration in man and also in animals (Prescott 1982).

Caffeine, codeine, and barbiturates have no nephrotoxic potential. Caffeine antagonizes the nephrotoxic action of phenacetin and acetylsalicylic acid (Molland 1978). Nevertheless, the central stimulant or sedative constituents of aspirin, phenacetin, codeine (APC) combinations can be important in the pathogenesis of analgesic nephropathy, as they are, in part, responsible for the behaviour that favours intake (duration and amount). The stimulating and addictive potential of caffeine has been proven in clinical and placebo-controlled human studies and in animals (Griffiths and Woodson 1988; Hughes *et al.* 1991; Silverman *et al.* 1992). Recently, however, it has been claimed that analgesics coformulated with caffeine in the absence of phenacetin do not stimulate or sustain overuse (Feinstein *et al.* 2000b).

Combination toxicity is an important issue in the pathogenesis of renal papillary necrosis. Molland (1978) showed that in the hydropenic rat the combination of acetylsalicylic acid with phenacetin or paracetamol caused severe medullary lesions more frequently than either of these agents alone (Table 2), a finding fitting with clinical and epidemiological observations in patients with analgesic nephropathy. To summarize, the causative agent of analgesic-associated papillary necrosis is probably not a uniform 'papillotoxin'. A combined action of

Table 2 Renal lesions in hydropenic rats. Comparison of different analgesics alone or in combination (Molland 1978)

Drug	Type of lesion (%)		
	Cortical	Intermediate RPN	Total RPN
Phenacetin	0	20	0
Acetaminophen	0	60	0
ASA	38	0	75
Phenacetin + ASA	100	20	80
Acetaminophen + ASA	80	20	80

RPN, renal papillary necrosis.

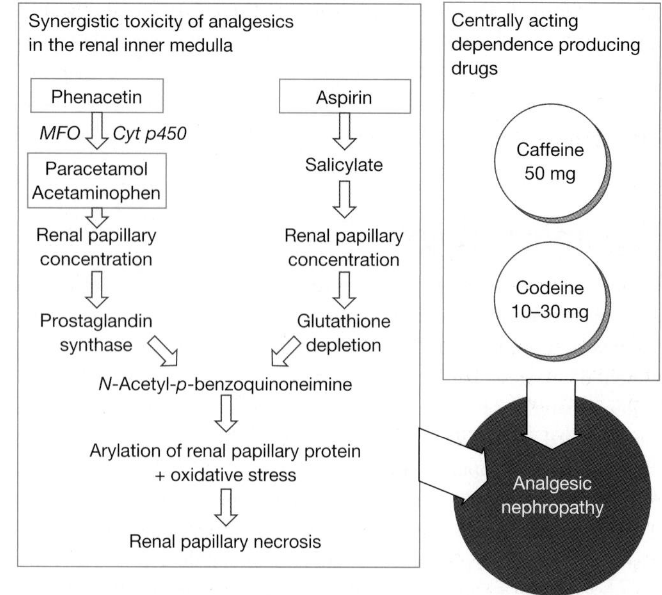

Fig. 1 Synergistic toxicity of analgesics in the renal inner medulla. Centrally acting dependence producing drugs [from Duggin, G.G. (1996). *American Journal of Kidney Diseases* **28** (Suppl. 1), S39–S47].

various agents with possibly different modes of insult and differing effects on predisposing factors is more probable.

Mechanisms of damage

Papillotoxins

The high medullary concentration of paracetamol after the administration of phenacetin initially led to the suggestion of a direct toxicity of this or other metabolites in the papilla. Chemical toxicity of acetylsalicylic acid may also result from its high concentration in the papilla. In experimental papillary necrosis in animals and analgesic nephropathy in man, however, urinary concentration is disturbed early, limiting this potential mechanism. Moreover, the patterns of localization of the substances vary among models and do not correlate with the actual damage (Bach and Hardy 1985).

The synergistic effect of acetylsalicylic acid and phenacetin or paracetamol (Molland 1978) in renal papillary necrosis is more complex. The cytochrome P_{450}-dependent activation of substrates to highly reactive metabolites is responsible for toxic effects of exogenous substances (e.g. drugs) such as the hepatotoxicity of paracetamol. This process might depend on dose and genetic predisposition. The potentiating effect of aspirin on both phenacetin and acetaminophen toxicity may be related to two factors.

Acetaminophen undergoes oxidative transformation by prostaglandin H synthase to reactive quinoneimine that is conjugated to glutathione. If acetaminophen is present alone, sufficient glutathione is generated in the papillae to detoxify the reactive intermediate. However, if acetaminophen is ingested with aspirin, the aspirin is converted to salicylate, which becomes highly concentrated and depletes glutathione in both the cortex and papillae of the kidney. Cellular glutathione depletion allows reactive metabolites of acetaminophen to produce lipid peroxides and arylation of tissue proteins, with eventual necrosis of the papillae (Fig. 1) (Bennett and De Broe 1989; Duggin 1996).

This mechanism, which might also explain the formation of cytotoxic substances and carcinogens from endogenous or exogenous substrates (Bach and Bridges 1984), has not so far been completely proven experimentally as the common cause of renal papillary necrosis in analgesic nephropathy. At present the pathogenesis of analgesic nephropathy in humans is not fully understood.

Haemodynamic factors

Many analgesics and NSAIDs inhibit prostaglandin synthesis. Since prostaglandins play an important part in the regulation of renal medullary blood flow as vasodilatory substances, medullary ischaemia has been considered as an explanation for the kidney damage (Garella and Matarese 1984; Carmichael and Shankel 1985). Papillary necrosis is associated with acetylsalicylic acid alone (Nanra and Kincaid-Smith 1970; Nanra *et al.* 1978) or with more recent substances from the NSAID series (Blackshear *et al.* 1985; Adams *et al.* 1986; Allen *et al.* 1986) might be interpreted in these terms. On the other hand, phenacetin and its main metabolite paracetamol modify prostaglandin synthesis only slightly (Bruchhausen and Baumann 1982; Clissold 1986), whereas paracetamol does not worsen the decreased renal excretion of prostaglandin E_2 induced by acetylsalicylic acid in healthy individuals (Froelich and Bippi 1989). Since phenacetin and paracetamol are causative agents (although not exclusively), it is evident that medullary ischaemia caused by inhibition of prostaglandin-mediated vasodilation is unlikely to be the sole cause of renal papillary necrosis in analgesic nephropathy.

Influence of risk factors

Genetic predisposition might be a risk factor for the development of kidney damage in users of analgesics. Familial incidences of analgesic nephropathy have occasionally been reported (Gsell 1974; Kincaid-Smith 1988). In almost all clinical descriptions, more women than men are reported (Prescott 1982). It is not possible to determine whether this reflects a genetic predisposition rather than psychosocial or cultural factors in analgesic intake. The higher prevalence of HLA-B12 in patients with analgesic nephropathy (Kincaid-Smith 1988) than in controls is compatible with a genetic predisposition, but more precise investigations are needed.

Dehydration is crucial for experimental induction of analgesic papillary necrosis (Molland 1978). The increased frequency of papillary necrosis observed in the northern, warmer parts of Australia, as well as the increased incidence in summer months, also suggest a role of dehydration in the development of analgesic nephropathy (Kincaid-Smith 1979).

Pathology

The pathological changes in analgesic nephropathy provide information on the lesions induced by the chronic ingestion of mixed analgesic preparations containing phenacetin. There are so far few reports on the renal pathology caused by the chronic intake of analgesic mixtures other than those containing phenacetin, single analgesic substances, and NSAIDs. The emphasis on the renal lesions attributed to phenacetin-containing analgesics changed over time: initially, interest concentrated on chronic interstitial nephritis (Spuehler and Zollinger 1953); later it focused on renal papillary necrosis (Gloor 1961, 1978; Burry *et al.* 1966), whereas, in recent years, capillary sclerosis and an equivalent alteration in the basement membrane of the tubules are at the forefront of interest in the pathogenesis of renal papillary necrosis and the consequent changes in the cortical parenchyma (Gloor 1978; Mihatsch *et al.* 1978, 1983). The following summary provides a dynamic developmental concept based on the studies of Zollinger and Mihatsch (Gloor 1978; Mihatsch *et al.* 1978; Mihatsch 1989).

According to this concept, the disease develops, from its earliest detectable lesions to the terminal stage with bilateral shrinkage of the kidneys, in three phases: (a) capillary sclerosis of the upper urinary tract; followed by (b) the stage of renal papillary necrosis; to undergo (c) consequent cortical parenchymal changes.

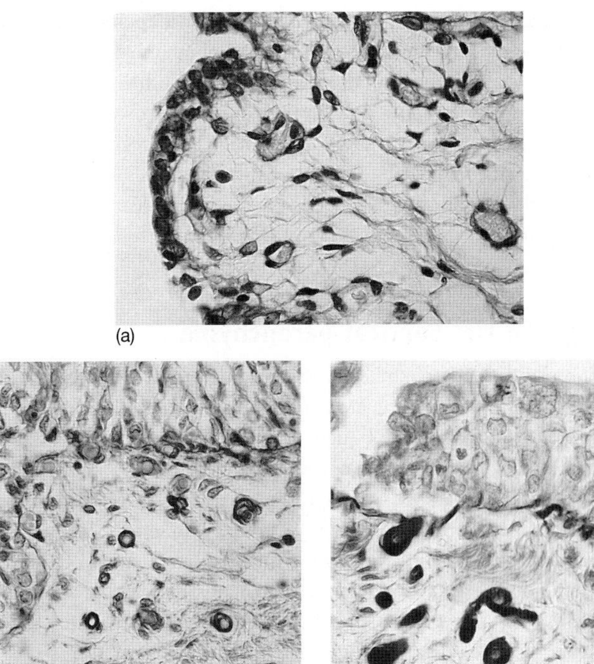

Fig. 2 Capillary sclerosis of the urinary-tract mucosa (periodic acid–Schiff, 620×): (a) normal mucosa with minimal capillary changes; (b) moderate capillary sclerosis; and (c) severe capillary sclerosis with narrowing of the vascular lumen (by courtesy of Professor Mihatsch, Basle).

Capillary sclerosis (Fig. 2)

Capillary sclerosis in the mucosa of the upper urinary tract is the earliest detectable alteration following prolonged exposure to analgesics. It is demonstrated in 80–90 per cent of all abusers of analgesics containing phenacetin. With increasing degrees of severity, there is an occlusive thickening of the basement membrane in the capillaries located below the unchanged urothelium. On electron microscopy, this thickening results from the deposition of a thin basement-membrane lamella with an onion skin-like arrangement. In some instances, appreciable deposition of lipids accounts for the occasional, macroscopically perceptible, brown discolouration of the mucosa of the urinary tract, which is absent in patients who have taken excess amounts of phenacetin-free analgesics. The severity of the capillary sclerosis increases from the mucosa of the renal pelvis to the pyeloureteral transition. The most pronounced capillary alteration is present in the proximal ureter, and decreases progressively towards the vesical mucosa. Nephropathy is absent in all patients with slight capillary sclerosis, as in 15 per cent of the patients with moderately severe or severe capillary changes.

Capillary sclerosis of the renal pelvis and the proximal urinary tract is attributed to a (so far unidentified) toxin that is eliminated by the kidney and diffuses back into the mucosa (Mihatsch *et al.* 1983). It is not known whether this involves metabolites generated during the metabolic activation of analgesic substances.

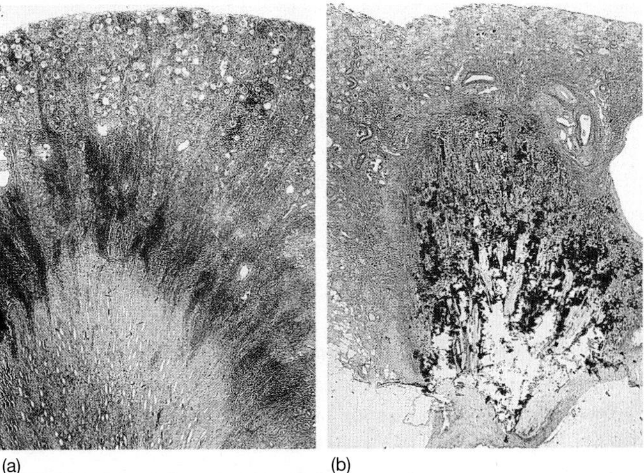

Fig. 3 Interstitial nephritis and renal papillary necrosis in analgesic nephropathy (haematoxylin and eosin): (a) severe cortical atrophy and marked non-destructive cellular infiltration in the cortical–medullary junction and (b) necrosis and calcification of the renal papilla (by courtesy of Professor Mihatsch, Basle).

Renal papillary necrosis (Fig. 3)

In the early stage of renal papillary necrosis, the kidney is macroscopically normal. After many years of exposure to analgesics containing phenacetin, the medullary pyramid displays a yellow-brown striation restricted to the central regions of the inner medullary zone. Outer parts of the medulla and the cortex are normal. A cross-section of the papillary tip shows macular lesions concentrated around the collecting tube. The matrix in the thickened interstitium is increased, and the peritubular capillaries and the ascending part of the loop of Henle show a capillary sclerosis or equivalent basement-membrane changes. Tubular epithelia of the ascending loop of Henle and the endothelial cells of the peritubular capillaries show degenerative alterations or are necrotic. Interstitial cells are also destroyed. Calcium salts may precipitate.

In the intermediate stage of renal papillary necrosis, the necrotic foci are confluent and extend as far as the outer medulla. The collecting ducts and the vasa recta are also destroyed in fully developed necrosis.

Changes in the cortical parenchyma

Necrotic papillae either remain *in situ* or are shed over a protracted period, or are rapidly demarcated and shed. The fate of the necrotic papilla is crucial for the subsequent cortical lesions. If there is rapid demarcation (which is rare), cortical changes may be completely absent. If the papilla is shed over a protracted period or remains *in situ* (partially ossified), progressive cortical atrophy with interstitial fibrosis and lymphohistiocytic inflammation ensue with an attendant chronic interstitial non-destructive nephritis. The relation between renal papillary necrosis and interstitial nephritis shows that the chronic interstitial nephritis is not the cause, but the result, of renal papillary necrosis.

The involvement of central parts of the papilla in the early stage of renal papillary necrosis explains two additional phenomena. The non-involvement of lateral parts of the papilla may lead to hypertrophy of the remaining lateral nephrons, which compensates for the loss of the suprapapillary parenchymal segments for a considerable period. On the one hand, this leads to a focal–segmental glomerulosclerosis and hyalinosis from presumed glomerular hyperfiltration in the affected hypertrophied regions. On the other hand, non-specific glomerular changes with periglomerular fibrosis, collapse, and complete obliteration occur in the atrophic cortical regions.

Clinical features

The multiple and variable clinical features of the analgesic syndrome (Duggan 1974) correspond to those of a multisystem disease. Women are affected five to seven times more often than men. The diagnosis, very rare in patients younger than 30 years, is made more frequently with increasing age.

Renal manifestations

Analgesic nephropathy is frequently asymptomatic for years until advanced renal insufficiency. The earliest renal manifestations such as impaired urinary concentration and acidification result from an altered tubular function. Renal salt losses and clinically manifest tubular acidosis occur in 10 per cent of the patients with advanced renal insufficiency (Nanra *et al.* 1978; Nanra 1992). Sterile leucocyturia and slight proteinuria may be present; a protein excretion above 3 g/24 h indicates a concomitant glomerular lesion. Haematuria indicates a fresh renal papillary necrosis with sequestration or a concomitant complication such as a urinary-tract infection, or (in later stages) a uroepithelial carcinoma.

Bacterial urinary-tract infections occur frequently, particularly in the later stages of the disease (Gsell 1974; Murray and Goldberg 1978; Nanra *et al.* 1978).

Arterial hypertension is present in about 50 per cent of patients, frequently in association with renal artery stenosis and a malignant course, which influences the clinical picture and rate of progression of the renal insufficiency. Acute papillary necrosis can elicit a hypertensive crisis with, occasionally, a paradoxical water and sodium depletion (Nanra *et al.* 1978).

Papillary necrosis is usually clinically silent. It causes symptoms when papillary tissue is shed into the urinary tract, giving rise to haemorrhage, ureteral colic, or ureteral obstruction. Calcified papillary necrosis may mimic urinary calculi.

As glomerular filtration rate falls, all the metabolic consequences of renal insufficiency become manifest. Kincaid-Smith (1988) estimated that only about 10 per cent of patients with manifest analgesic nephropathy reach the terminal stage of renal insufficiency. Progression is frequently slow and there is often no clinical difference from other kidney diseases with regard to individual symptoms. In patients with terminal renal insufficiency, complex urinary-tract infections may complicate the extrarenal manifestations of the 'analgesic syndrome'. A severe renal osteodystrophy and a carpal tunnel syndrome are more frequent than in controls (Schwarz *et al.* 1984).

Ureteral and renal-cell carcinomas

Uroepithelial carcinomas (Mihatsch 1986) of the renal pelvis, the ureters, the urinary bladder, and the proximal urethra occur with a latency of 21–30 years, frequently simultaneously at different sites of the urinary tract. Their increased incidence must be regarded as a late consequence of the analgesic intake. A relationship between phenacetin misuse and renal pelvic carcinoma (McCredie *et al.* 1986; McCredie 1993) as well as urinary bladder carcinoma in women (Piper *et al.* 1985) has been established in some but not all epidemiological studies (Linet *et al.* 1995). Studies on point mutations and polymorphism of carcinogenic-metabolizing enzymes in urothelial cancer of the renal pelvis suggest the implication of chronic tissue damage rather than a direct mutagenic effect of phenacetin (Bringuier *et al.* 1998).

After renal transplantation, despite intensive preoperative diagnostic procedures, urothelial tumours are significantly more frequent in patients with analgesic nephropathy than in those with other initial renal diseases (Vogt *et al.* 1990; Schwarz *et al.* 1992; Kliem *et al.* 1996). Therefore, even after termination of analgesic intake, regular cytological examinations of urine are necessary in patients on renal replacement therapy (Mihatsch 1986).

Two recent case–control studies indicate an association between analgesics, phenacetin, acetaminophen, and others, and renal-cell carcinoma (Gago-Dominguez *et al.* 1999; Kaye *et al.* 2001). They conflict with previous results of the International Renal-Cell Cancer Study (McCredie *et al.* 1995).

Extrarenal manifestations of the analgesic syndrome

The extrarenal complications of chronic analgesic consumption encompass a broad spectrum of manifestations that may obscure the relatively bland clinical course of the renal disease in individual cases and may lead to occasional misinterpretations of the underlying clinical picture. Most extrarenal findings were identified in clinical and autopsy studies of consumers of analgesics containing phenacetin and paracetamol. Very few of them have been verified in case–control studies. The extent to which these complications are also observed after the chronic intake of anilide-free and modern NSAIDs has not yet been established.

Cardiovascular complications

Accelerated atherosclerosis, arterial hypertension, renal artery stenosis, and increased cardiovascular mortality are frequently associated with chronic analgesic consumption (Kaladelfos and Edwards 1976; Kincaid-Smith 1979; Nanra 1980; Mihatsch *et al.* 1982; Dubach *et al.* 1983; Schwarz *et al.* 1984). Most of these studies are retrospective and individual findings have almost never been controlled for other cardiovascular risk factors. An increased cardiovascular mortality was demonstrated in the only prospective cohort study of female consumers of phenacetin-containing analgesics (Dubach *et al.* 1983), but the contribution of other additional risk factors was not investigated. While subjects were stratified by urine concentration of NAPAP, which may derive either from phenacetin or paracetamol, the aetiological role of the anilides (and other analgesic components) remains to be demonstrated. An autopsy study failed to confirm an increased prevalence of myocardial infarction in phenacetin misusers compared with a control population. Differences in the frequency of hypertension became less obvious when the degree of renal failure was considered (Mihatsch *et al.* 1982). An increased incidence of fatal cerebral haemorrhage was found in a controlled study of dialysis patients with analgesic nephropathy (Chachati *et al.* 1987).

Gastrointestinal complications

Peptic ulcers and erosive gastritis are the most common concomitant diseases in chronic analgesic consumption and are frequently related to the acetylsalicylic acid component of combination analgesics (Gsell 1974; Gault and Wilson 1978; Nanra 1980; Mihatsch *et al.* 1982; Prescott 1982). In the Basle autopsy study, gastric ulcers, but not duodenal ulcers, were more frequent in analgesic misusers (Mihatsch *et al.* 1982). In a prospective clinical investigation, chronic pancreatitis was found more frequently in patients with analgesic nephropathy than in a control group with other renal diseases (Hangartner *et al.* 1987).

Haematological complications

Ealier, haematological changes were an early manifestation of the analgesic syndrome (Sarre *et al.* 1958; Gsell 1974; Prescott 1982). Today, with the altered spectrum of analgesic preparations, they are less common. An anaemia inappropriate to the degree of renal insufficiency and mild haemolysis, partly in combination with splenomegaly and methaemoglobinaemia, was ascribed to phenacetin. In the comparative autopsy study mentioned above, however, the spleen was not significantly enlarged in phenacetin misusers (Mihatsch *et al.* 1982). Agranulocytosis due to pyrazolone derivatives is now very rare in chronic pyrazolone-free analgesic consumers. Chronic haemorrhagic anaemia due to the acetylsalicylic acid content of mixed analgesics has been reported, especially in English-speaking countries (Carro-Ciampi 1978) and is likely to be more frequent.

Skeletal complications

Skeletal problems are much more frequently symptomatic in analgesic misusers than in patients with other causes of renal insufficiency (Fellner and Tuttle 1969; Fassett *et al.* 1982; Jaeger *et al.* 1982). The causes appear complex: decreased plasma levels of vitamin D_3 and 1,25$(OH)_2$-vitamin D, metabolic acidosis and malabsorption, possibly in combination with laxative abuse.

Hypercalcaemia may be observed in analgesic nephropathy as a result of a carcinoma of the renal pelvis. It disappears after tumour nephrectomy (Derbyshire *et al.* 1989).

Psychosomatic aspects

A large number of psychopathological alterations has been described in chronic analgesic consumers (Gsell 1974; Carro-Ciampi 1978; Murray 1978; Prescott 1982). In one of the few controlled psychometric investigations of women from Swiss watch factories, heavy analgesic consumers were described by the Freiburg Personality Inventory as significantly more nervous and sensitive to irritation, depressive, more easily frustrated, and emotionally labile (Ladewig *et al.* 1979). Prior to analgesic dependence, disturbances of subjective well being are frequently associated with headaches, sleep disorders, gastrointestinal complaints, cardiac symptoms, and lumbar, as well as shoulder–neck pain. Factors giving rise to the intake of analgesics are emotional tension and overstrain. In addition, specific occupational demands resulting from shiftwork and piecework in various industrial production plants, as well as easy access to analgesics at the workplace, played a major part in the establishment of their misuse (Sarre *et al.* 1958; Gsell 1974). Traditional family habits are likely to be important for the inception of chronic analgesic consumption (Gsell 1974; Carro- Ciampi 1978; Murray 1978). The psychotropic effect of analgesic substances together with centrally active additives may perpetuate both the chronic intake and the chronic pain states (Prescott 1982; Woerz 1983; Diener 1988). Available results show that chronic consumers of analgesics are characterized less by a specific personality profile than by a restricted repertoire of reactions to situations of tension and a learned family pattern of analgesics use.

Diagnosis and differential diagnosis

Diagnosis

The diagnosis of analgesic nephropathy is not always easy. A large number of clinical signs has been associated with analgesic nephropathy (Kincaid-Smith 1986) but most are non-specific and their diagnostic value at different stages of renal failure has never been established. Papillary necrosis is admittedly the hallmark of the disease, but its demonstration is cumbersome particularly in the endstage renal disease patient (Gloor 1978).

Until recently, the most important argument in favour of analgesic nephropathy was a history of analgesic abuse in the absence of any other causes of renal disease. The history of analgesic misuse is frequently difficult to establish, since patients deny it or put it out of their mind when asked for the first time. In most cases, it is necessary to repeat the inquiry several times in a tension-free and private atmosphere. It is frequently more relevant to inquire initially about the reasons for taking analgesics for headaches or back pain. In suspicious cases, the current analgesic intake can be checked by investigating the urinary concentrations of paracetamol (Brodie and Axelrod 1949, 1950; Dubach 1967) and acetylsalicylic acid (Trinder 1954). The detection of analgesic agents from the serum of patients with

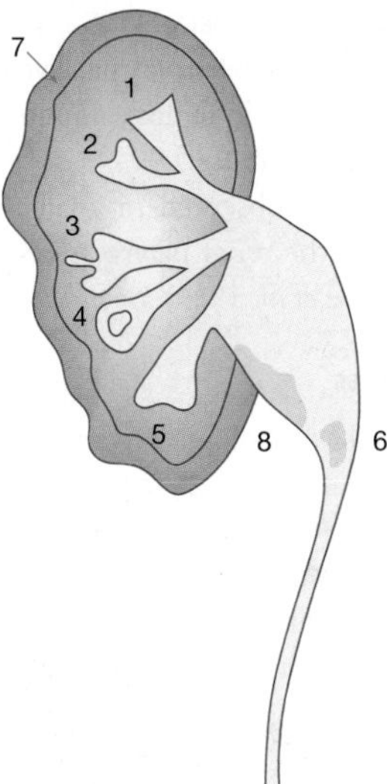

Fig. 4 Radiological signs of analgesic nephropathy: (1) normal calyx; (2) swollen papilla with reduced contrast and calyceal blunting; (3) partial papillary necrosis, central cavity, and fistula formation; (4) complete papillary necrosis—ring shadow; (5) papillary necrosis *in situ*; (6) sequestrated papilla with ureteral occlusion; (7) 'wavy' outline of the kidney by homogeneously thinned cortex with indentations over the necrotic papillae and bulging in the areas of hypertrophied Bertini's columnae; and (8) urothelial-cell carcinoma (taken from Schmitt 1986, with permission).

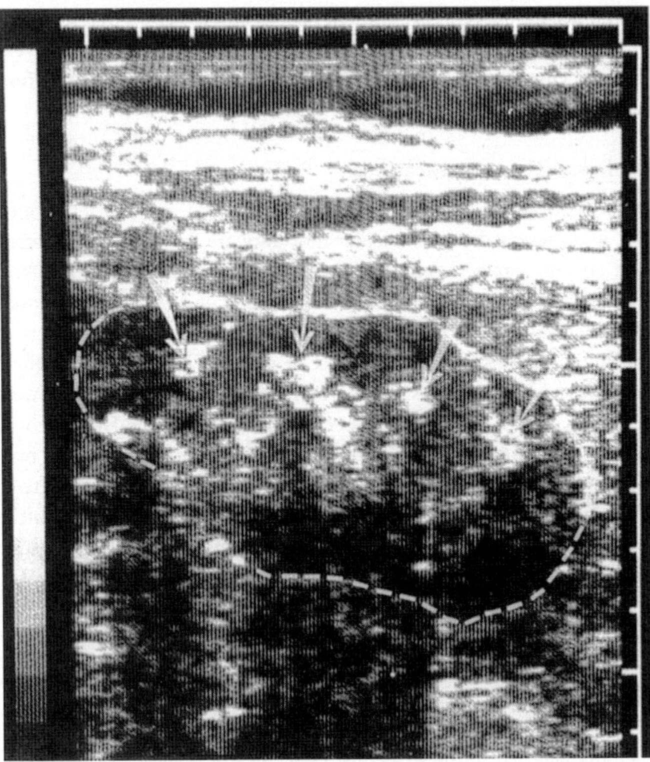

Fig. 5 Ultrasonogram of the left kidney in a patient with analgesic nephropathy and advanced renal failure: there is atrophic renal parenchyma with 'wavy' outline and a typical garland pattern of calcified renal papillae (arrow tips) with distal shadowing (by courtesy of Dr G. Schultze).

advanced renal failure is methodologically difficult, but possible with modified high-pressure liquid chromatographic procedures (Borner *et al.* 1986).

The suspicion of a tubulointerstitial disease is supported by the discovery of sterile leucocyturia, slight proteinuria, reduction of urinary osmolality in the morning urine, renal potassium and/or sodium wasting, and tubular acidosis. Renal papillary necrosis may be visualized in the early stages of analgesic nephropathy by intravenous pyelography or computed tomography (CT) scan (Fig. 4). Depending on the stage of the kidney disease, the kidney mass may be bilaterally shrunken, and the renal contour slightly irregular. The papillary deformations range from a swelling to defects of various size. Papillary necrosis can remain *in situ* and calcify or may be shed into the renal pelvis and manifest radiologically as radiolucent filling defects (Hartman *et al.* 1984; Davidson 1985). Today, real-time ultrasonographic investigation has gained acceptance in routine diagnostics, and also in late stages of renal insufficiency. This technique reveals a typical garland pattern of papillary calcifications surrounding the renal sinus. The kidney has an irregular outline and an increased echogenicity of the parenchyma (Weber *et al.* 1985; Segasothy *et al.* 1994) (Fig. 5).

The diagnostic performance of several clinical, laboratory, and radiological signs reported to be associated with analgesic nephropathy has been investigated in endstage renal disease patients. Renal imaging criteria showed a high diagnostic performance that was superior to other clinical signs as far as sensitivity and specificity were concerned (Elseviers *et al.* 1995a). In addition, the diagnostic value of different imaging methods—sonography, conventional tomography, and CT—was compared. In the detection of papillary calcifications, the CT scan was superior to the other methods (a sensitivity of 87 per cent and a specificity of 100 per cent). In patients with incipient and moderate renal failure (serum creatinine between 1.5 and 4 mg/dl), papillary calcifications were detected with a sensitivity of 92 per cent and a specificity of 100 per cent (Elseviers *et al.* 1995a).

A CT scan without contrast is therefore recommended in all patients, with an unclear diagnosis, in whom analgesic nephropathy might be the underlying renal disease even in the absence of reliable information on previous analgesic exposure. The demonstration of a bilateral decreased renal mass combined with bumpy contours and, in particular, papillary calcifications (Fig. 6) confirms the diagnosis of analgesic nephropathy even in advanced or endstage renal failure (Elseviers *et al.* 1995b).

Renal biopsy is of little use to confirm the diagnosis; the sample contains mainly cortical tissue so that the pathognomonic medullary alterations, renal papillary necrosis, and capillary sclerosis are detectable only in the few samples that contain medullary tissue. Biopsy is indicated in patients with analgesic nephropathy when there are simultaneous indications of a glomerular or vascular kidney disease. The histological identification of a shed and excreted papilla only very rarely verifies the diagnosis.

Differential diagnosis

Differential diagnosis of analgesic nephropathy initially includes all other chronic kidney diseases with a failing renal function. A review of the past history and clinical data still contributes to the identification

Analgesic nephropathy: measurement of diagnostic criteria

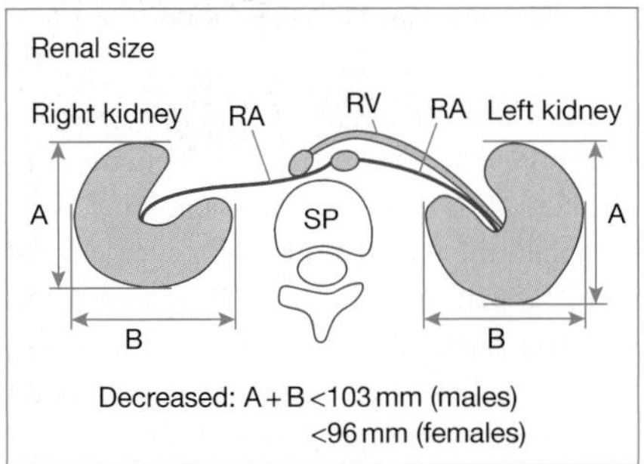

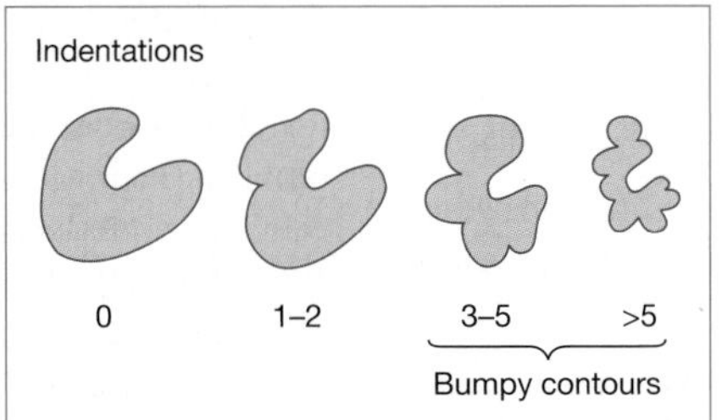

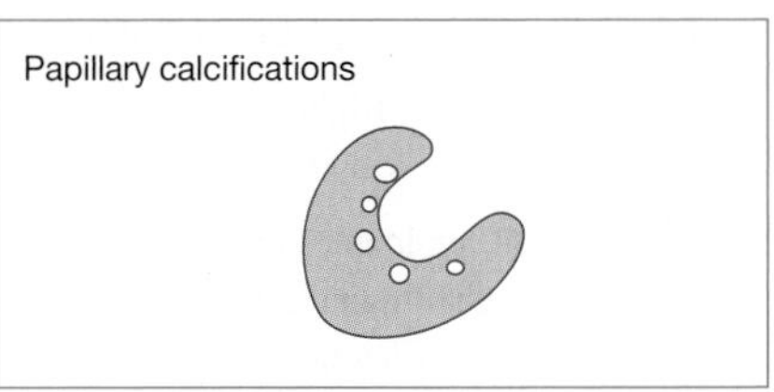

CT scans without contrast material

Normal kidney

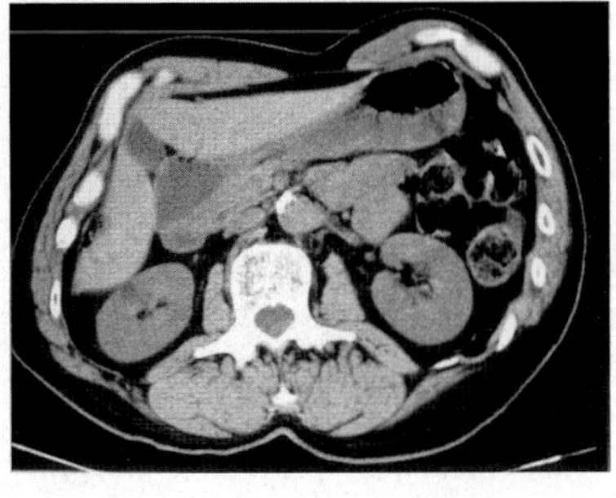

Moderate renal failure

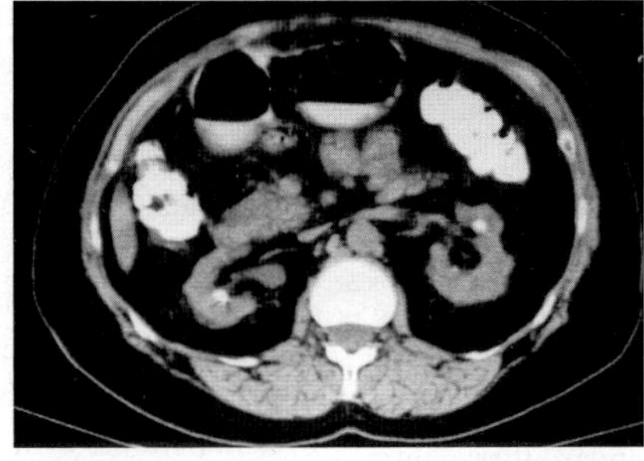

Belgian female, age 62 years, Scr 1.8 mg/dl.
Abuse: 20 years of mixture of pyrazolone derivatives

Endstage renal failure

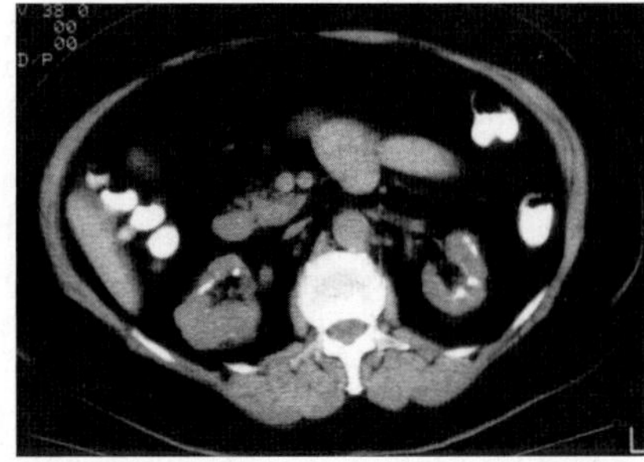

Belgian female, age 59 years, ESRF.
Abuse: 8 years of mixture of pyrazolone derivatives
26 years of mixture of aspirin + paracetamol

Fig. 6 CT scan with typical findings of papillary calcification and bumpy contours [from De Broe, M.E. and Elseviers, M.M. (1998). *New England Journal of Medicine* **338**, 446–452].

of analgesic nephropathy in patients whose renal disease has an unclear aetiology, even in the terminal stage.

Differential diagnosis of renal papillary necrosis comprises:

1. analgesic nephropathy,
2. diabetic nephropathy,
3. obstructive uropathy,
4. reflux nephropathy,
5. sickle-cell nephropathy.

As analgesic misuse and diabetes mellitus may coexist it is sometimes difficult to differentiate between both risk factors. Whereas the diagnosis of urinary-tract obstruction is not difficult, reflux nephropathy must be excluded in younger patients with renal papillary necrosis and renal insufficiency (Kincaid-Smith 1988).

Sickle-cell nephropathy is restricted to black patients and is easy to diagnose because of the numerous general symptoms of the underlying disease. Alcoholism and liver cirrhosis are other, albeit rare, causes of renal papillary necrosis (Pablo *et al.* 1986).

For differential diagnosis of tubulointerstitial nephritis see other chapters in this section.

Clinical course and prognosis

The clinical course of renal involvement in the analgesic syndrome is mostly protracted and undramatic. Many years of important use of analgesic mixtures are a prerequisite for development of clinically relevant renal symptoms (Dubach *et al.* 1983). The presence of relevant kidney damage is often obscured by cardiovascular consequences of hypertension or other extrarenal events such as gastrointestinal ulceration or haemorrhage. In many patients, analgesic misuse and nephropathy are only diagnosed in the terminal stage of renal insufficiency or following detection of a tumour of the urinary tract.

The prognosis of analgesic nephropathy largely depends on the stage of renal failure at the time of diagnosis and on the interruption of analgesics. Kidney function reportedly remains constant or improves in the early stages of renal insufficiency (Nanra *et al.* 1978; Brunner and Thiel 1986). Others (Schollmeyer and Ballé 1989; Schwarz *et al.* 1989), doubt that this optimistic assumption applies in the long term.

Patients with analgesic nephropathy rarely reach the terminal phase of renal insufficiency prior to age 40. On the average renal replacement therapy is initiated after age 60 (Wing *et al.* 1983).

The increased morbidity due to extrarenal components of the analgesic syndrome (Schwarz *et al.* 1984) suggests that the survival on renal replacement therapy of patients with analgesic nephropathy is poorer than in other groups of patients. However, appropriate data are not available.

Therapy

Interruption of analgesics and NSAIDs intake is the most important therapeutic measure in patients with confirmed analgesic nephropathy

(Consensus Conference 1984), even if it is doubtful that it always prevents the progression of renal insufficiency:

1. Headaches, frequently the cause of analgesic intake, may disappear after discontinuation (Prescott 1982; Woerz 1983; Diener 1988).
2. A substantial, avoidable, additional morbidity arises from analgesic-associated gastrointestinal ulceration and haemorrhage, even in stable renal insufficiency.
3. Although phenacetin-containing analgesics have been clearly associated with urological tumours, it is not clear, even today, which analgesics are responsible for this uroepithelial malignant degeneration. Hence, continued intake of analgesic mixtures, even without phenacetin, constitutes carcinogenic risk currently difficult to evaluate. Epidemiological data so far show no increased risk of acetaminophen (paracetamol) for ureteral or renal cancer although an experimental study has identified acetaminophen as more mutagenic than phenacetin (Sicardi *et al.* 1991).

Since dehydration favours the development of analgesic-associated papillary necrosis, it is not surprising that a high fluid intake reduces the progression of renal insufficiency. Control of the hydration state and maintenance of a urine volume of at least 2 l daily are necessary, unless there is a tendency to fluid overload. In patients with analgesic nephropathy, urological interventions may be required when shed papillae obstruct the ureters (Nanra *et al.* 1978). Standard therapeutic measures recommended in chronic renal failure patients include antihypertensive therapy, treatment of urinary-tract infections, correction of metabolic acidosis and electrolyte disturbances, and early therapy of disorders of calcium and phosphate metabolism.

Patients with analgesic nephropathy are suitable for dialysis and transplantation programmes just as patients with other renal diseases. Still they have a greater morbidity, and frequently indulge in self-medication with hypnotics, laxatives, and, unfortunately, sometimes analgesics. They have a lower motivation to undergo kidney transplantation (Schwarz *et al.* 1992). The incidence of urothelial carcinoma after renal transplanation is comparable to the general incidence of up to 10 per cent of urothelial carcinomas in endstage renal failure patients with analgesic nephropathy. Removal of the native kidneys prior to renal transplantation has also been suggested, but its efficacy is yet to be proven (Blohme and Johansson 1981).

Prevention

The present state of knowledge of the aetiology and pathogenesis of analgesic nephropathy indicates, as discussed above, that analgesic nephropathy is not caused by intake of phenacetin or any other substance exclusively. Analgesic nephropathy is related to the daily use, for many years, of mixtures containing at least two antipyretic analgesics and usually caffeine or codeine or both. Furthermore, increasing evidence derives that regular intake of analgesics is a risk factor for promoting chronic renal failure of different origin.

The centrally acting agents (caffeine, codeine, and barbiturates) included in APC mixtures contribute to the initiation and perpetuation of chronic analgesic consumption. The intake of mixed analgesics containing caffeine appears associated with major risks of serious kidney damage (Pommer *et al.* 1989). This finding correlates with the concomitant ingestion of very high doses of analgesic substances. The consumption of analgesic mixtures is oriented to stimulating effects of the centrally acting additives (Gsell 1974; Carro-Ciampi 1978; Murray 1978; Ladewig *et al.* 1979; Woerz 1983; Sandler *et al.* 1989).

Restriction of access to analgesics containing phenacetin or their withdrawal from the pharmaceutical market alone may not solve the problem (Pommer and Molzahn 1986). The restriction of phenacetin-containing products in the Scandinavian countries since the early 1960s does not adequately explain the reported declining incidence of analgesic-specific renal and extrarenal complications (Bengtsson 1979, 1989; Sillanpää *et al.* 1982). The Australian experience claims that a decisive effect is only to be expected from restriction of combination analgesics, at least with regard to renal complications (Kincaid-Smith 1986; McCredie *et al.* 1989). However, these observations are equally compatible with the long delay suggested for the decline of analgesic nephropathy (Michielsen and De Schepper 2001). Prevention of analgesic nephropathy and its extrarenal complications requires the end of abuse of both, phenacetin- and, perhaps of non-phenacetin-containing analgesic combinations. Legislative measures are necessary and information on the potential risks of these drugs must be made available. There is no strong evidence of a potentiation of analgesic effects or diminished risks from the combination of different peripheral analgesics. To date, few hard data substantiate the advantages of caffeine as an analgesic adjuvant. This also applies to the new generation of analgesics from the group of NSAIDs and their respective combinations with caffeine. The efficacy of preventive measures must be regularly controlled by monitoring the incidence of analgesic-associated diseases as well as the analgesic sales (Noels *et al.* 1995). It is our view that as long as analgesic mixtures containing centrally acting or dependence-producing drugs remain available over the counter, analgesic nephropathy will continue to be a problem.

References

Adams, D. H. A., Howie, A. J., Michael, J., McConkey, B., Bacon, P. A., and Adu, D. (1986). Non-steroidal antiinflammatory drugs and renal failure. *Lancet* **i**, 57–60.

Akyol, S. M., Thompson, M., and Kerr, D. N. S. (1982). Renal function after prolonged consumption of aspirin. *British Medical Journal* **284**, 631–632.

Allen, R. C., Petty, R. E., Lirenman, D. S., Malleson, P. N., and Laxer, R. M. (1986). Renal papillary necrosis in children with chronic arthritis. *American Journal of Diseases in Childhood* **140**, 20–22.

Bach, P. H. and Bridges, J. W. (1984). The role of metabolic activation of analgesics and non-steroidal anti-inflammatory drugs in the development of renal papillary necrosis and upper urothelial carcinoma. *Prostaglandins, Leukotrienes, and Medicine* **15**, 251–274.

Bach, P. H. and Hardy, T. L. (1985). Relevance of animal models to analgesic-associated renal papillary necrosis in humans. *Kidney International* **28**, 605–613.

Barrett, B. J. (1996). Acetaminophen and adverse chronic renal outcomes: an appraisal of the epidemiologic evidence. *American Journal of Kidney Diseases* **28** (Suppl. 1), S14–S19.

Bengtsson, U. (1979). Long-term pattern in pyelonephritis. *Contributions to Nephrology* **16**, 31–36.

Bengtsson, U. (1989). Analgetika-Nephropathie—Langfristige Erfahrungen aus Schweden. *Zeitschrift für Urologie und Nephrologie* **82** (Suppl.), 121–125.

Bennett, W. M. and De Broe, M. E. (1989). Analgesic nephropathy—a preventable renal disease. *New England Journal of Medicine* **320**, 1269–1271.

Bethke, B. A. and Schubert, G. E. (1985). Kapillarosklerose der ableitenden Harnwege als Indiz eines Analgetika-Abusus. Haeufigkeit bei unausgewaehlten Obduktionen in einer westdeutschen Grossstadt. *Deutsche Medizinische Wochenschrift* **110**, 343–346.

Björck, S., Svalander, C. T., and Aurell, M. (1988). Acute renal failure after analgesic drugs including paracetamol (acetaminophen). *Nephron* **49**, 45–53.

Blackshear, J. L., Napier, J. S., Davidman, M., and Stillman, M. R. (1985). Renal complications of nonsteroidal antiinflammatory drugs: identification and monitoring of those at risk. *Seminars in Arthritis and Rheumatism* **14**, 163–175.

Blohme, I. and Johansson, S. (1981). Renal pelvic neoplasms and atypical urothelium in patients with end-stage analgesic nephropathy. *Kidney International* **20** (5), 671–675.

Borner, K., Borner, E., Pommer, W., and Molzahn, M. (1986). Determination of paracetamol in serum of patients with terminal renal insufficiency. *Fresenius Zeitschrift fuer Analytische Chemie* **324**, 353.

Bringuier, P. P., McCredie, M., Sauter, G., Bilous, M., Stewart, J., Mihatsch, M. J., Kleihues, P., and Ohgaki, H. (1998). Carcinomas of the renal pelvis associated with smoking and phenacetin abuse: p53 mutations and polymorphism of carcinogen-metabolising enzymes. *International Journal of Cancer* **79**, 531–536.

Brodie, B. B. and Axelrod, J. (1949). The fate of acetophenetidin in man and methods for the estimations of acetophenetidin and its metabolites in biological material. *Journal of Pharmacology and Experimental Therapeutics* **97**, 58–67.

Brodie, B. B. and Axelrod, J. (1950). The fate of antipyrine in man. *Journal of Pharmacology and Experimental Therapeutics* **98**, 97–104.

Bruchhausen, F. and Baumann, J. (1982). Inhibitory actions and desacetylation products of phenacetin and paracetamol on prostaglandin synthetases in neuronal and glial cell lines and rat renal medulla. *Life Sciences* **30**, 1783–1791.

Brunner, F. P. and Selwood, N. H. (1994). End-stage renal failure due to analgesic nephropathy, its changing pattern and cardiovascular mortality. *Nephrology, Dialysis, Transplantation* **9**, 1371–1376.

Brunner, F. P. and Thiel, G. Klinik der Analgetikanephropathie. In *Das Analgetikasyndrom* (ed. M. J. Mihatsch), pp. 65–71. Stuttgart: Thieme, 1986.

Buckalew, V. M. (1996). Habitual use of acetaminophen as a risk factor for chronic renal failure: a comparison with phenacetin. *American Journal of Kidney Diseases* **28** (1, Suppl. 1), S7–S13.

Buckalew, V. M. and Schey, H. M. (1986). Renal disease from habitual antipyretic analgesic consumption: an assessment of the epidemiologic evidence. *Medicine* **65**, 291–303.

Buergi, E. (1927). Die Gelonida antineuralgica als Kombinationsmittel. *Muenchner Medizinische Wochenschrift* **16**, 673–674.

Burry, A. F. (1967). The evolution of analgesic nephropathy. *Nephron* **5**, 185–201.

Burry, H. C. and Dieppe, P. A. (1982). Renal function after prolonged consumption of aspirin. *British Medical Journal* **284**, 1117–1118.

Burry, A. F., de Jersey, P., and Weedon, D. (1966). Phenacetin and renal papillary necrosis: results of a prospective autopsy investigation. *Medical Journal of Australia* **53**, 873–879.

Carmichael, J. and Shankel, S. W. (1985). Effects of nonsteroidal antiinflammatory drugs on prostaglandins and renal function. *American Journal of Medicine* **78**, 992–1000.

Carro-Ciampi, G. (1978). Phenacetin abuse: a review. *Toxicology* **10**, 311–339.

Chachati, A., Dechenne, C., and Godon, J. P. (1987). Increased-incidence of cerebral hemorrhage mortality in patients with analgesic nephropathy on hemodialysis. *Nephron* **45**, 167–168.

Christie, D. (1978). The analgesic abuse syndrome: an epidemiological perspective. *International Journal of Epidemiology* **7**, 139–143.

Clissold, S. P. (1986). Paracetamol and phenacetin. *Drugs* **32** (Suppl. 4), 8–26.

Consensus Conference (1984). Analgesic-associated kidney disease. *Journal of the American Medical Association* **251**, 3123–3125.

Davidson, A. J. *Radiology of the Kidney.* Philadelphia, PA: Saunders, 1985.

De Broe, M. E. and Elseviers, M. M. (1998). Current concepts—analgesic nephropathy. *New England Journal of Medicine* **338**, 446–452.

Delzell, E. and Shapiro, S. (1998). A review of epidemiologic studies of nonnarcotic analgesics and chronic renal disease. *Medicine* **77**, 102–121.

Derbyshire, N. D., Asscher, A. W., and Matthews, P. N. (1989). Hypercalcemia as a manifestation of malignant urothelial change in analgesic nephropathy. *Nephron* **52**, 79–80.

Diener, H. C. (1988). Klinik des Analgetikakopfschmerzes. *Deutsche Medizinische Wochenschrift* **113**, 472–476.

Ditscherlein, G. *et al.* (1989). Kapillarosklerose der Nierenbecken und Harnleiterschleimhaut. Eine Multicenter-Studie in der DDR zur Frage der Analgetika-Nephropathie. *Zeitschrift für Urologie und Nephrologie* **82** (Suppl.), 37–40.

Drukker, W., Schwarz, A., and Vanherweghem, J. L. (1986). Analgesic nephropathy: an underestimated cause of end-stage renal disease. *International Journal of Artificial Internal Organs* **9**, 219–246.

Dubach, U. C. (1967). *p*-Aminophenol-Bestimmung im Urin als Routinemethode zur Erfassung der Phenacetineinnahme. *Deutsche Medizinische Wochenschrift* **92**, 211–215.

Dubach, U. C., Rosner, B., and Pfister, E. (1983). Epidemiologic study of abuse of analgesics containing phenacetin. Renal morbidity and mortality (1968–1979). *New England Journal of Medicine* **308**, 357–362.

Dubach, U. C., Rosner, B., and Stürmer, T. (1991). An epidemiologic study of abuse of analgesic drugs. Effects of phenacetin and salicylate on mortality and cardiovascular morbidity (1968 to 1987). *New England Journal of Medicine* **324**, 155–160.

Duggan, J. M. (1974). The analgesic syndrome. *Australian and New Zealand Journal of Medicine* **4**, 365–372.

Duggin, G. G. (1980). Mechanisms in the development of analgesic nephropathy. *Kidney International* **18**, 553–561.

Duggin, G. G. (1996). Combination analgesic-induced kidney disease: the Australian experience. *American Journal of Kidney Diseases* **28** (Suppl. 1), S39–S47.

Duggin, G. G. and Mudge, G. H. (1976). Analgesic nephropathy: renal distribution of acetaminophen and its conjugates. *Journal of Pharmacology and Experimental Therapeutics* **199**, 1–9.

Elseviers, M. M. (1994). Epidemiology of analgesic nephropathy. Thesis, Department of Nephrology, University of Antwerp.

Elseviers, M. M. and de Broe, M. E. (1988). Is analgesic nephropathy still a problem in Belgium? *Nephrology, Dialysis, Transplantation* **3**, 143–149.

Elseviers, M. M. and De Broe, M. E. (1995). A long-term prospective controlled study of analgesic abuse in Belgium. *Kidney International* **48**, 1912–1919.

Elseviers, M. M. and De Broe, M. E. (1996). Combination analgesics involvement in the pathogenesis of analgesic nephropathy: the European perspective. *American Journal of Kidney Diseases* **28**, S48–S55.

Elseviers, M. M. *et al.* (1995a). Evaluation of diagnostic criteria for analgesic nephropathy in patients with end-stage renal failure: results of the ANNE study. *Nephrology, Dialysis, Tranplantation* **10**, 808–814.

Elseviers, M. M. *et al.* (1995b). High diagnostic performance of CT scan for analgesic nephropathy in patients with incipient to severe renal failure. *Kidney International* **48**, 1316–1323.

Fassett, R. G., Lien, J. W. K., Mathew, T. H., and McClure, J. (1982). Bone disease in analgesic nephropathy. *Clinical Nephrology* **18**, 273–279.

Feinstein, A. R., Heinemann, L. A. J., Curhan, G. C., Delzell, E., DeSchepper, P. J., Fox, J. M., Graf, H., Luft, F. C., Michielsen, P., Mihatsch, M. J., Suissa, S., van der Woude, F., and Willich, S. (2000a). Relationship between nonphenacetin combined analgesics and nephropathy: a review. *Kidney International* **58**, 2259–2264.

Feinstein, A. R., Heinemann, L. A. J., Dalessio, D., Fox, J. M., Goldstein, J., Haag, G., Ladewig, D., and O'Brien, C. P. (2000b). Do caffeine-containing analgesics promote dependence? A review and evaluation. *Clinical Pharmacology Therapeutics* **68**, 457–467.

Fellner, S. K. and Tuttle, E. P. (1969). The clinical syndrome of analgesic abuse. *Archives of Internal Medicine* **124**, 379–382.

Fored, C. M., Ejerblad, E., Lindblad, P., Fryzek, J. P., Dickman, P. W., Signobello, L. B., Lipworth, L., Elinder, C.-G., Blot, W. J., McLaughlin, J. K., Zack, M., M., and Nyrén, O. (2001). Acetaminophen, aspirin, and chronic renal failure. *The New England Journal of Medicine* **345**, 1801–1808.

Froelich, J. C. and Bippi, H. (1989). Zur pathophysiologischen Bedeutung der renalen Eicosanoide. *Zeitschrift für Urologie und Nephrologie* **82** (Suppl.), 3–6.

Gago-Dominguez, M., Yuan, J. M., Castelao, J. E., Ross, R. K., and Yu, M. C. (1999). Regular use of analgesics is a risk factor for renal cell carcinoma. *British Journal of Cancer* **81**, 542–548.

Garella, S. and Matarese, R. A. (1984). Renal effects of prostaglandins and clinical adverse effects of nonsteroidal anti-inflammatory agents. *Medicine* **63**, 165–181.

Gault, M. H. and Wilson, D. R. (1978). Analgesic nephropathy in Canada: clinical syndrome, management, and outcome. *Kidney International* **13**, 58–63.

Gloor, F. (1961). Die doppelseitige chronische nichtobstruktive interstitielle Nephritis. *Ergebnisse der allgemeinen Pathologie und Pathologischen Anatomie* **41**, 63–207.

Gloor, F. (1978). Changing concepts in pathogenesis and morphology of analgesic nephropathy as seen in Europe. *Kidney International* **13**, 27–33.

Griffiths, R. R. and Woodson, P. P. (1988). Caffeine physical dependence: a review of human and laboratory anaimal studies. *Psychopharmacology* **94**, 437–451.

Gsell, O. (1974). Nephropathie durch Analgetika. *Ergebnisse der inneren Medizin und Kinderheilkunde* **35**, 68–175.

Haas, H. (1983). History of antipyretic analgesic therapy. *American Journal of Medicine* **75** (Suppl. 5A), 1–3.

Hangartner, P. J., Buehler, H., Muench, R., Zaruba, K., Stamm, B., and Ammann, R. (1987). Chronische Pankreatitis als wahrscheinliche Folge eines Analgetikaabusus. *Schweizerische Medizinische Wochenschrift* **117**, 638–642.

Hartman, G. W., Torres, V. E., Leago, G. F., Williamson, B., Jr., and Hattery, R. R. (1984). Analgesic-associated nephropathy. Pathophysiological and radiological correlation. *Journal of the American Medical Association* **251**, 1734–1738.

Hughes, J. R. *et al.* (1991). Caffeine self-administration, withdrawal, and adverse effects among coffee drinkers. *Archives of General Psychiatry* **48**, 611–617.

Jaeger, P., Burckardt, P., and Wauters, J. P. (1982). Ca, P metabolism is particularly disturbed in analgesic abuse nephropathy (AAN). *Kidney International* **21**, 903–904.

Kaladelfos, G. and Edwards, K. D. G. (1976). Increased prevalence of coronary heart disease in analgesic nephropathy: relation to hypertension, hypertriglyceridemia and combined hyperlipidemia. *Nephron* **16**, 388–400.

Kaye, J. A., Myers, M. W., and Jick, H. (2001). Acetaminophen and the risk of renal and bladder cancer in the general practice research database. *Epidemiology* **12**, 690–694.

Kincaid-Smith, P. (1967). Pathogenesis of the renal lesion associated with the abuse of analgesics. *Lancet* **i**, 859–862.

Kincaid-Smith, P. (1979). Analgesic nephropathy in Australia. *Contributions to Nephrology* **16**, 57–64.

Kincaid-Smith, P. (1986). Renal toxicity of non-narcotic analgesics. At-risk patients and prescribing applications. *Medical Toxicology* **1** (Suppl. 1), 14–22.

Kincaid-Smith, P. Analgesic-induced renal disease. In *Diseases of the Kidney* (ed. R. W. Schrier and C. W. Gottschalk), pp. 1202–1216. Boston: Little Brown, 1988.

Kincaid-Smith, P. and Nanra, R. S. Lithium-induced and analgesic-induced renal diseases. In *Diseases of the Kidney* 5th edn. (ed. R. W. Schrier and C. W. Gottschalk), pp. 1099–1129. Boston: Little Brown, 1993.

Kleinman, J. G., Breitenfield, R. V., and Roth, D. A. (1980). Acute renal failure associated with acetaminophen ingestion. *Clinical Nephrology* **14**, 201–205.

Kliem, V., Thon, W., Krautzig, S., Kolditz, M., Behrend, M., Pichlmayr, R. Koch, K. M., Frei, U., and Brunkhorst, R. (1996). High mortality from urothelial carcinoma despite regular tumor screening in patients with analgesic nephropathy after renal transplantation. *Transplantation International* **9**, 231–235.

Ladewig, D., Dubach, U. C., Ettlin, G., and Hobi, V. (1979). Zur Psychologie des Analgetikakonsums bei berufstaetigen Frauen. Ergebnisse einer epidemiologischen Perspektivstudie. *Nervenarzt* **50**, 219–224.

Lanes, S. F., Delzell, E., Dreyer, N. A., and Rothman, K. J. (1986). Analgesics and kidney disease. *International Journal of Epidemiology* **15**, 454–455.

Lawrence, J. R. (1994). The evolution of the end-stage renal disease program in Australia. *Renal Failure* **16**, 133–146.

Linet, M. S., Chow, W. H., McLaughlin, J. K., Wacholder, S., Yu, M. C., Schoenberg, J. B., Lynch, C., and Fraumeni, J. F., Jr. (1995). Analgesics and cancers of the renal pelvis and ureter. *International Journal of Cancer* **62**, 15–18.

McCredie, M. Analgesics as human carcinogens—clinical and epidemiological evidence. In *Analgesic and NSAID-induced Kidney Disease* (ed. J. H. Stewart), pp. 197–210. Oxford: Oxford University Press, 1993.

McCredie, M. and Stewart, J. H. (1988). Does paracetamol cause urothelial cancer or renal papillary necrosis? *Nephron* **49**, 296–300.

McCredie, M., Stewart, J. H., and Mahoney, J. F. (1982). Is phenacetin responsible for analgesic nephropathy in New South Wales? *Clinical Nephrology* **17**, 134–140.

McCredie, M., Stewart, J., Turner, J., and Mahoney, J. (1986). Phenacetin and papillary necrosis: independent risk factors for renal pelvic cancer. *Kidney International* **30**, 81–84.

McCredie, M., Stewart, J. H., Mathew, T. H., Disney, A. P. S., and Ford, J. M. (1989). The effect of withdrawal of phenacetin-containing analgesics on the incidence of kidney and urothelial cancer and renal failure. *Clinical Nephrology* **31**, 35–39.

McCredie, M. *et al.* (1995). International renal cell cancer study. II. Analgesics. *International Journal of Cancer* **60**, 345–349.

Marek, J. (1987). Vyskyt a morfologie analgeticke nefropatie 1972–1981. *Sbornik Lekarska* **89**, 33–40.

Michielsen, P. and De Schepper, P. (2001). Trends of analgesic nephropathy in two high-endemic regions with different legislation. *Journal of the American Society of Nephrology* **12**, 220–556.

Mihatsch, M. J. Analgetika-Abusus und Harnwegstumoren. In *Das Analgetikasyndrom* (ed. M. J. Mihatsch), pp. 86–93. Stuttgart: Thieme, 1986.

Mihatsch, M. J. (1989). Analgetika-Nephropathie und Harnwegstumoren. *Zeitschrift für Urologie und Nephrologie* **82** (Suppl.), 13–35.

Mihatsch, M. J., Hofer, H. O., Gudat, F., Knuesli, C., Torhorst, J., and Zollinger, H. U. (1983). Capillary sclerosis of the urinary tract and analgesic nephropathy. *Clinical Nephrology* **20**, 285–301.

Mihatsch, M. J., Kernen, R., and Zollinger, H. U. (1982). Phenacetinabusus VI: eine Autopsiestatistik unter besonderer Beruecksichtigung extrarenaler Befunde. *Schweizerische Medizinische Wochenschrift* **112**, 1383–1388.

Mihatsch, M. J., Torhorst, J., Amsler, B., and Zollinger, H. U. (1978). Capillarosclerosis of the lower urinary tract in analgesic (phenacetin) abuse. *Virchows Archiv A. Pathologisches Anatomie und Histologie* **381**, 41–47.

Molland, E. A. (1978). Experimental renal papillary necrosis. *Kidney International* **13**, 5–14.

Morlans, M. (1990). End-stage renal disease and non-narcotic analgesics: a case–control study. *British Journal of Clinical Pharmacology* **30**, 717–723.

Murray, R. M. (1978). Genesis of analgesic nephropathy in the United Kingdom. *Kidney International* **13**, 50–57.

Murray, T. G. and Goldberg, M. (1978). Analgesic-associated nephropathy in the U.S.A.: epidemiologic clinical and pathogenetic features. *Kidney International* **13**, 64–71.

Murray, T. G., Stolley, P. D., Anthony, J. C., Schinnar, R., Hepler-Smith, E., and Jeffreys, J. L. (1983). Epidemiologic study of regular analgesic use and end-stage renal disease. *Archives of Internal Medicine* **143**, 1687–1693.

Nanra, R. S. (1980). Clinical and pathological aspects of analgesic nephropathy. *British Journal of Clinical Pharmacology* **10**, 359–368S.

Nanra, R. S. (1983). Renal effects of antipyretic analgesics. *American Journal of Medicine* **75** (Suppl. 5A), 70–81.

Nanra, R. S. (1992). Pattern of renal dysfunction in analgesic nephropathy—comparison with glomerulonephritis. *Nephrology, Dialysis, Transplantation* **7**, 384–390.

Nanra, R. S. and Kincaid-Smith, P. (1970). Papillary necrosis in rats caused by aspirin and aspirin containing mixtures. *British Medical Journal* **3**, 559–561.

Nanra, R. S., Stuart-Taylor, J., de Leon, A. H., and White, K. (1978). Analgesic nephropathy: etiology, clinical syndrome, and clinicopathologic correlations in Australia. *Kidney International* **13**, 79–92.

Noels, L. N., Elseviers, M. M., and De Broe, M. E. (1995). Impact of legislative measures on the sales of analgesics and the subsequent prevalence of analgesic nephropathy: a comparative study in France, Sweden and Belgium. *Nephrology, Dialysis, Transplantation* **10**, 167–174.

Pablo, N. C., Churg, J., Needle, M. A., and Ganesharajah, M. (1986). Renal papillary necrosis: relapsing form associated with alcoholism. *American Journal of Kidney Diseases* **7**, 88–94.

Perneger, T. V., Whelton, P. K., and Klag, M. J. (1994). Risk of kidney failure associated with the use of acetaminophen, aspirin, and nonsteroidal anti-inflammatory drugs. *New England Journal of Medicine* **331**, 1675–1679.

Piper, J., Tonascia, J., and Matanoski, G. (1985). Heavy phenacetin use and bladder cancer in women aged 20 to 49 years. *New England Journal of Medicine* **313**, 292–295.

Pommer, W. Clinical presentation of analgesic-induced nephropathy. In *Analgesic and NSAID-induced Kidney Disease* (ed. J. H. Stewart), pp. 108–118. Oxford: Oxford University Press, 1993.

Pommer, W. and Molzahn, M. (1986). Banning phenacetin to prevent analgesic nephropathy. *Lancet* **i**, 40.

Pommer, W., Glaeske, G., and Molzahn, M. (1986). The analgesic problem in the Federal Republic of Germany: analgesic consumption, frequency of analgesic nephropathy and regional differences. *Clinical Nephrology* **26**, 273–278.

Pommer, W. *et al.* (1989). Regular analgesic intake and the risk of end-stage renal failure. *American Journal of Nephrology* **9**, 403–412.

Prescott, L. F. (1982). Analgesic nephropathy: a reassessment of the role of phenacetin and other analgesics. *Drugs* **23**, 75–149.

Rexrode, K. M., Buring, J. E., Glynn, R. J., Stampfer, M. J., Youngman, L. D., and Gaziano, J. M. (2001). Analgesic use and renal function in men. *Journal of the American Medical Association* **286**, 315–321.

Sandler, D. P. *et al.* (1989). Analgesic use and chronic renal disease. *New England Journal of Medicine* **320**, 1238–1243.

Sarre, H., Moench, A., and Kluthe, R. *Penacetinabusus und Nierenschaedigung*. Stuttgart: Thieme, 1958.

Schmitt, H. E. Bildgebende Verfahren bei Analgetikanephropathie. In *Das Analgetikasyndrom* (ed. M. J. Mihatsch), pp. 72–77. Stuttgart: Thieme, 1986.

Schollmeyer, P. and Ballé, C. (1989). Praevention und konservative Therapie der Analgetika-Nephropathie. *Zeitschrift für Urologie und Nephrologie* **82** (Suppl.), 101–108.

Schwarz, A., Pommer, W., Keller, F., Kuehn-Freitag, G., Offermann, G., and Molzahn, M. (1984). Morbidity of patients with analgesic-associated nephropathy and end-stage renal failure. *Proceedings of the European Dialysis and Transplant Association–European Renal Association* **21**, 311–316.

Schwarz, A., Kunzendorf, U., Keller, F., and Offermann, G. (1989). Progression of renal failure in analgesics-associated nephropathy. *Nephron* **53**, 244–249.

Schwarz, A., Offermann, G., and Keller, F. (1992). Analgesic nephropathy and renal transplantation. *Nephrology, Dialysis, Transplantation* **7**, 427–432.

Schwarz, A., Preuschoff, L., and Zellner, D. (1999). Incidence of analgesic nephropathy in Berlin since 1983. *Nephrology, Dialysis, Transplantation* **14**, 109.

Segasothy, M., Suleiman, A. B., Puvaneswary, M., and Rohana, A. (1988). Paracetamol: a cause for analgesic nephropathy and end-stage renal disease. *Nephron* **50**, 50–54.

Segasothy, M., Abdul Samad, S., Zulfiqar, A., Shaariah, W., Morad, Z., and Prasad Menon, S. (1994). Computed tomography and ultrasonography: a comparative study in the diagnosis of analgesic nephropathy. *Nephron* **66**, 62–66.

Sicardi, S. M., Martiarena, J. L., and Iglesias, M. T. (1991). Mutagenic and analgesic activities of anilide derivatives. *Journal of Pharmaceutical Sciences* **80**, 761–764.

Sillanpää, M., Kasanen, A., and Elonen, A. (1982). Changes of panorama in renal disease mortality in Finland after phenacetin restriction. *Acta Medica Scandinavica* **212**, 313–317.

Silverman, K., Evans, S. M., Strain, E. C., and Griffiths, R. R. (1992). Withdrawal syndrome after the double-blind cessation of caffeine consumption. *New England Journal of Medicine* **327**, 1109–1114.

Spuehler, O. and Zollinger, H. U. (1953). Die chronisch-interstitielle nephritis. *Zeitschrift fuer klinische Medizin* **151**, 1–50.

Stewart, J. H. *et al.* (1994). Trends in incidence of end-stage renal failure in Australia, 1972–1991. *Nephrology, Dialysis, Transplantation* **9**, 1377–1382.

Trinder, P. (1954). Rapid determination of salicylate in biological fluids. *Biochemical Journal* **57**, 301.

Vogt, P., Frei, U., Repp, H., Oldhafer, K., and Pichlmayr, R. (1990). Malignant tumours in renal transplant recipients receiving cyclosporin: survey of 589 first-kidney transplantations. *Nephrology, Dialysis, Transplantation* **5**, 282–288.

Weber, M., Braun, B., and Koehler, H. (1985). Ultrasonic findings in analgesic nephropathy. *Nephron* **39**, 216–222.

Wing, A. J. *et al.* (1983). Combined report on regular dialysis and transplantation in Europe XIII, 1982. *Proceedings of the European Dialysis and Transplant Association–European Renal Association* **20**, 5–71.

Woerz, R. (1983). Effects and risks of psychotropic and analgesic combinations. *American Journal of Medicine* **75** (Suppl. 5A), 139–140.

Zollinger, H. U. (1955). Chronische interstitielle Nephritis bei Abusus von phenacetinhaltigen Analgetica (Saridon usw.). *Schweizerische Medizinische Wochenschrift* **85**, 746.

6.3 Non-steroidal anti-inflammatory drugs and the kidney

Wai Y. Tse and Dwomoa Adu

Introduction

Non-steroidal anti-inflammatory drugs (NSAIDs) are not only one of the most commonly prescribed groups of drugs, but they are also available as over-the-counter drugs. Although uncommon, renal complications arising from their increasing use are likely to be seen more frequently. NSAIDs are potentially nephrotoxic and their renal side-effects include salt and water retention, acute tubular necrosis, acute interstitial nephritis, hyperkalaemia, and chronic renal failure (Clive and Stoff 1984; Blackshear *et al.* 1985).

The incidence of renal toxicity is unknown. A large hospital-based study of 41,000 inpatients, including 1222 who were taking NSAIDs, demonstrated no attributable increase in renal disease. Furthermore, long-term follow-up of 50,000 outpatient users of NSAIDs disclosed that none required hospital admission for acute renal disease (Fox and Jick 1984). By contrast, another study has suggested that NSAIDs accounted for 37 per cent of drug-associated acute renal failure and 7 per cent of all cases of acute renal failure (Kleinknecht *et al.* 1986). More recently, an increased risk of endstage renal failure has been reported in patients regularly taking NSAIDs (Sandler *et al.* 1991; Perneger *et al.* 1994).

Prostaglandin biochemistry

Pharmacokinetics

Most NSAIDs are metabolized by the liver either by hepatic oxidation or by glucuronidation, so that little active compound is eliminated into the urine (Verbeeck *et al.* 1983; Day *et al.* 1987). The aryl-propionic acids, however, are transformed into unstable acyl-glucuronide conjugates, readily cleaved back to the parent drug (Day *et al.* 1987). For example, ketoprofen and ketorolac are excreted predominantly as acyl-glucuronides by the kidney. In patients with renal insufficiency, the glucuronide conjugates accumulate and hydrolyze to reform the parent drug. As a result, the parent drug accumulates despite the fact that it is not eliminated as such by the kidney. Retention of the metabolites of NSAIDs, and to a degree of the parent compound, means that care should be taken when these drugs are prescribed in renal failure.

As NSAIDs are albumin bound, a decreased serum albumin increases the free plasma concentrations and, hence, increases their potential toxicity. This is observed in patients with hypoalbuminaemia or in uraemic subjects in whom raised NSAID metabolites compete with the parent drug for albumin binding. Free and total NSAIDs are also increased when impaired liver function prolongs the half-life and also after parenteral administration which leads to high peak concentrations.

Pharmacodynamics

The NSAIDs are a chemically heterogeneous group of compounds that were first reported to inhibit prostaglandin (PG) synthesis (Ferreira *et al.* 1971). Almost all are organic acids classified according to their chemical structure (Table 1). They share, to various degrees, analgesic, antipyretic, and anti-inflammatory properties. Most of their therapeutic and adverse effects are mediated through the inhibition of PG synthesis. PGs are

Table 1 Classification of NSAIDs according to chemical structure

Carboxylic acids
Acetic acid
Phenylacetates
Diclofenac
Carbo- and heterocyclic acetic acids
Indomethacin
Etodolac
Sulindac
Tolmetin
Fenamates
Mefenamic acid
Salicylates
Aspirin
Aloxiprin
Diflunisal
Salsalate
Benorylate
Choline magnesium trisalicylate
Propionates
Ibuprofen
Fenbufen
Fenoprofen
Flurbiprofen
Ketoprofen
Ketorolac
Nabumetone
Naproxen
Tiaprofenic acid
Enolic acids
Oxicams
Piroxicam
Tenoxicam
Pyrazolones
Phenylbutazone
Azapropazone

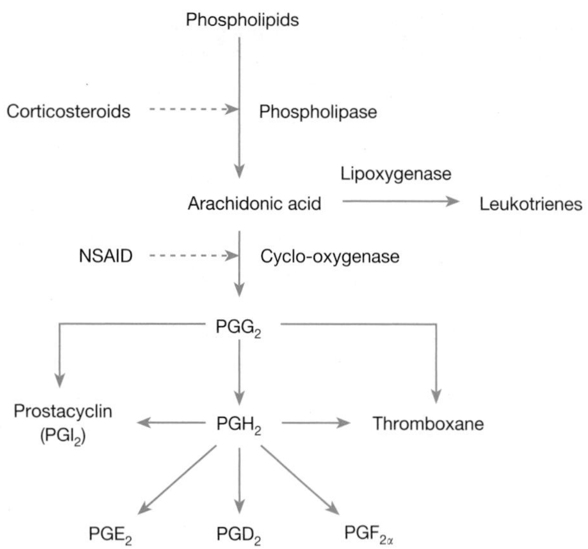

Fig. 1 The pathway of arachidonic acid metabolism. The lipoxygenase pathway results in the production of leukotrienes; the role of these compounds in the kidney is unclear. The cyclo-oxygenase pathway leads to the production of the unstable cyclic endoperoxidase PGG_2. Subsequent enzymatic conversion results in the production of the classical 2 series prostaglandins PGI_2, PGE_2, PGD_2, $PGF_{2\alpha}$, and thromboxane A_2.

synthesized close to the cells on which they act (autocoids). Their rapid inactivation in the circulation limits most of their effects to the site of synthesis.

PGs are unsaturated fatty acid compounds synthesized from cell membrane phospholipids. The enzyme phospholipase A_2 converts phospholipids into arachidonic acid which is the substrate for three different enzymes: cyclo-oxygenase (COX), which is inhibited by NSAIDs; cytochrome-P450 mono-oxygenase; and lipoxygenase. Phospholipase A_2, activated by kinins, vasopressin, angiotensin II, and extracellular hyperosmolarity, increases PG synthesis through the three pathways (Aiken and Vane 1973). The first product of the COX pathway is the cyclic endoperoxide PGG_2 subsequently converted to PGH_2. PGG_2 and PGH_2 are the key intermediates in the formation of the physiologically active PGs (PGD_2, PGE_2, $PGF_{2\alpha}$, and PGI_2) and thromboxane A_2 (Fig. 1). The lipoxygenase pathway leads to the formation of mono-, di-, and trihydroxyeicosatetraenoic acids (HETEs) and leukotrienes. The cytochrome-P450-mediated oxygenation is responsible for the formation of epoxyeicosatrienoic acids, their corresponding diols, HETEs, and mono-oxygenated amino acid derivatives. Each pathway influences some aspects of renal haemodynamics or tubular function. The blockade of COX by NSAIDs increases the substrate available to the other two pathways leading thus to possible adverse renal effects.

Cyclo-oxygenases in the kidney

Two isoforms of COX (COX-1 and COX-2) or endoperoxide H synthase (PGHS: PGHS-1 and PGHS-2) have been identified in mammalian cells and are encoded by genes sharing approximately 60 per cent homology in their coding regions (Kujubu *et al.* 1991; O'Banion *et al.* 1991). COX-1, constitutively expressed, mediates gastric cytoprotection and vascular homeostasis. COX-2, induced by proinflammatory cytokines, produces PGs in inflamed tissues (Jones *et al.* 1993). Its expression is regulated by salt and water intake, medullary tonicity, growth factors, cytokines, and adrenal steroids (Harris *et al.* 1994).

Selective blockade of pain and inflammation mediated by COX-2 stimulation without deleterious effects on homeostatic functions mediated by COX-1 activation should be useful. In the human kidney, COX-2 is present in podocytes, endothelium, proximal convoluted tubule and collecting duct, renal vasculature, the macula densa, and the medullary interstitial cells of the kidney (Komhoff *et al.* 1997), whereas COX-1 is found in the vasculature, the collecting ducts, glomeruli, and medullary interstitial cells (Nantel *et al.* 1999). It remains to be seen which of the two isoforms present in the vasculature is the predominant source of the increased production of vasodilator PGs that is critical to the preservation of renal blood flow when there is volume depletion. Inhibition of this homeostatic response accounts indeed for the most common renal side-effects associated with non-selective NSAID therapy. Many of the other renal effects of non-selective anti-inflammatory drugs (including sodium retention, decreased glomerular filtration rate, and effects on renin–angiotensin levels) appear mediated by the inhibition of COX-2 rather than COX-1 (Whelton 2001).

COX-2-dependent PG formation is also necessary for normal renal development. In mice, the complete absence of COX-2 resulted in severe renal dysplasia characterized by a postnatal arrest of maturation in the subcapsular nephrogenic zone and its progressive deterioration with increasing age (Dinchuk *et al.* 1995). Antenatal exposure of both mice and rats to an inhibitor of COX-2, but not of COX-1, had similar effects (Komhoff *et al.* 2000). In contrast, disruption of COX-1 gene expression failed to influence nephrogenesis (Langenbach *et al.* 1995).

In contrast to their gastrointestinal-sparing effects, the renal side-effects of COX-2-selective inhibitors (Simon *et al.* 1999; Bombardier *et al.* 2000) means that the same care should be taken for using COX-2-selective inhibitors as for the traditional non-selective NSAIDs. Still, the differential compartmental distribution of COX-1 and COX-2 might result in differences in renal effects of COX-2 inhibitors as compared with non-selective NSAIDs. The safety profile of COX-2-selective inhibitors will be discussed in a later section.

Renal prostaglandins

The kidney produces the vasodilator PGs: PGE_2, $PGF_{2\alpha}$, and PGI_2 and the vasoconstrictor thromboxane A_2. These autocoids, synthesized and metabolized by the kidney, autoregulate renal blood flow, renin release, tubular ion transport, and water metabolism (Table 2) (Henrich 1981; Dunn 1984). PGI_2, mainly present in the afferent arteriole and glomerulus, plays a major role in controlling glomerular haemodynamics. In contrast, PGE_2, predominantly produced in the collecting tubule and within the interstitium, regulates medullary haemodynamics (reviewed in Dunn 1984).

Actions of renal prostaglandins

Maintenance of renal blood flow and glomerular filtration rate

The major renal effects of PGs are summarized in Table 2. They maintain renal blood flow and glomerular filtration rate despite vasoconstrictor stimuli such as leukotrienes, thromboxane A_2, angiotensin II, vasopressin, endothelin, and catecholamines. Catecholamines also stimulate the local production of PGs, resulting in a feed-back loop between vasoconstrictors and vasodilatory PGs (Pelayo 1988). $PGF_{2\alpha}$-like peroxidation products also have major vasoconstrictive effects (Takahashi *et al.* 1992). Thus, in patients with underlying ischaemic or inflammatory renal injury and an attendant increased free oxygen radical production, the addition of NSAIDs not only decreases the production of vasodilatory PGs, but also results in the non-enzymatic formation of vasoconstrictor metabolites of arachidonic acid, which further jeopardize renal blood flow and glomerular filtration.

Renin release

PGE_2, PGI_2, and arachidonic acid are potent stimuli of renin release (Henrich 1981). NSAIDs thus inhibit renin secretion and, under some circumstances, lead to hyporeninaemia and hypoaldosteronism with an attendant hyperkalaemia, especially in patients with pre-existing renal impairment (Goldzer *et al.* 1980). NSAIDs have been used in the management of Bartter's syndrome where hypokalaemia is associated with increased PGs (see Chapter 5.5).

Potassium homeostasis

Inhibition of PG synthesis can also lead to hyperkalaemia by decreasing distal tubular flow rate and sodium delivery, both of which limit potassium secretion (see Chapter 2.2). Moreover, the action of antidiuretic hormone is enhanced with a further decrease in tubular flow and a lowered potassium secretion (Berl *et al.* 1977). A high-conductance potassium channel located on the luminal membrane of collecting tubular principal cells is regulated by intracellular calcium and arachidonic acid metabolites, including PGE_2 (Ling *et al.* 1992). Its modification by NSAIDs might also contribute to the development of hyperkalaemia.

Table 2 Effects of renal autocoids in the kidney

	Site of action	Effect
PGI_2	Intrarenal arterioles	Vasodilatation
	Afferent arteriole	Vasodilatation
	Efferent arteriole	Vasodilatation
	Capillary tuft	Vasodilatation
	Glomerular mesangium	Increased glomerular filtration rate
	Juxtaglomerular apparatus	Renin release
PGE_2	Afferent arteriole	Vasodilatation
	Glomerular mesangium	Increased glomerular filtration rate
	Thick ascending loop of Henle	Inhibition of Na^+,K^+-ATPase
	Collecting tubule, interstitium, and vasa recta	Inhibition of antidiuretic hormone
PGG_2	Thick ascending loop of Henle	Inhibition of Na^+,K^+-ATPase
PGH_2	Thick ascending loop of Henle	Inhibition of Na^+,K^+-ATPase
Thromboxane	Glomerular mesangium	Vasoconstriction
	Intrarenal arterioles	Vasoconstriction

Natriuresis and diuresis

Renal PGs are natriuretic and diuretic. They inhibit sodium and chloride reabsorption in the proximal and distal nephron and in the loop of Henle (Stokes 1979), reduce renal corticomedullary solute gradient, and antagonize the action of vasopressin *in vivo* (Lum *et al.* 1977). The complex mechanisms of these effects have been reviewed elsewhere (Dunn and Zambraski 1980). Whilst PGs acutely influence salt and water excretion they do not regulate it under normal conditions. Inhibition of renal PG synthesis causes only a transient salt and water retention except under circumstances such as heart failure, cirrhosis, or the nephrotic syndrome, which are already associated with sodium retention (Blackshear *et al.* 1985). NSAIDs have been incriminated in exacerbations of congestive cardiac failure sufficient to cause hospitalization (Oates *et al.* 1988). Their propensity to cause sodium retention is likely to be due to diminution of renal tubular synthesis of PGE_2 (Stokes and Kokko 1977).

Conditions in which renal prostaglandins are important (Table 3)

Under normal, euvolaemic conditions, NSAIDs produce negligible effects on renal haemodynamics (Dunn 1984). However, in the presence

Table 3 Conditions that predispose to NSAID-induced renal failure

Hypovolaemia
Haemorrhage
Septic shock
Congestive cardiac failure/heart disease
Nephrotic syndrome
Cirrhosis with ascites
Anaesthesia/surgery
Pre-eclampsia
Sodium depletion Diuretics Gastrointestinal losses
Renal artery stenosis
Glomerulonephritis
Urinary tract obstruction
Toxic injury Cyclosporin A Tacrolimus Gentamicin
Urinary tract infection
Advancing age
Chronic renal failure

of salt depletion, of an ineffective circulating plasma volume, or of conditions characterized by high circulating levels of vasoconstrictor hormones, NSAIDs may be nephrotoxic. Such conditions include cirrhosis, hypovolaemia, cardiac disease, renal disease, septic shock, advanced age, diuretic use, and postsurgery (Garella and Matarese 1984; Kleinknecht *et al.* 1986).

Cirrhosis

Hepatic cirrhosis is associated with several syndromes of renal dysfunction including alterations in renal PG synthesis (Epstein and Lifschitz 1987). It results in the accumulation of sodium and water, worsening ascites, and peripheral oedema. NSAIDs may decrease creatinine clearance in proportion with the degree of sodium retention. Boyer *et al.* (1979) reported that in cirrhotic patients indomethacin reduced the creatinine clearance from 74 to 60 ml per min and that this effect was most severe in the patients with ascites. Zipser *et al.* (1979) studied the effect of indomethacin or ibuprofen in 12 patients with cirrhosis and ascites during dietary sodium restriction (10 mmol/day). NSAID treatment decreased the glomerular filtration rate by 78 per cent in patients with a natriuresis below 1 mmol/day and only by 35 per cent in those with a natriuresis between 1 and 10 mmol/day.

Abnormalities of PG metabolism have also been postulated in the pathogenesis of the hepatorenal syndrome, that is, renal failure without specific cause developing in patients with liver disease. In such patients, urinary PGE_2 is decreased, as are the PG synthesizing enzymes in the renal medulla (Zipser *et al.* 1983; Govindarajan *et al.* 1987), and administration of NSAIDs leads to a reduction in glomerular filtration (Arroyo *et al.* 1983). Patients with cirrhosis and fluid retention often have reduced renal blood flow, usually associated with increased circulating angiotensin and vasopressin, frequently aggravated by treatment with diuretics. Maintenance of renal function depends on PGs, so that NSAIDs administration may precipitate acute renal failure (Epstein and Lifschitz 1987).

Sodium depletion

NSAIDs reduce glomerular filtration rate and renal blood flow in sodium depleted but not in euvolaemic subjects (Dunn 1984). Patients developing renal failure on NSAIDs frequently give a history of diuretic usage (Blackshear *et al.* 1985; Kleinknecht *et al.* 1986).

Heart failure

Patients with heart failure have increased levels of urinary PGs (Walshe and Venuto 1979). They may develop acute renal failure if treated with NSAIDs. Neonates with patent ductus arteriosus often have congestive cardiac failure and azotaemia. NSAIDs given in order to close the ductus may worsen azotaemia, sodium retention, and hyperkalaemia and result in oliguria (Heymann *et al.* 1976).

Chronic renal failure

Some patients with chronic renal failure rely on PG-mediated vasodilatation to maintain renal blood flow (Ciabattoni *et al.* 1984; Patrono and Pierucci 1986). Creatinine clearance is inversely correlated with urinary PGE_2 excretion. Addition of NSAIDs may further deteriorate renal function (Ciabattoni *et al.* 1984).

The elderly

Elderly people, particularly those with arterial disease, need renal PGs to sustain renal function. The majority of patients reported to have developed acute renal failure on NSAIDs were older than 60 years (Blackshear *et al.* 1985).

After surgery

NSAIDs are increasingly used in the perioperative period. However, they should be used with caution as they can precipitate acute, reversible renal failure or permanent renal toxicity, as well as a variety of effects on electrolyte and water homeostasis (Adverse Drug Reactions Advisory Committee 1993). Acute renal failure is the most important renal complication after surgery. A recent meta-analysis of eight trials showed that the postoperative use of NSAIDs in adults with normal preoperative renal function resulted in an 18 ml/min fall of creatinine clearance on the first day of surgery (Lee *et al.* 2001). Urine volume was maintained during the early postoperative period, and no patients required dialysis. Although the reviewers concluded that NSAIDs caused a clinically unimportant transient reduction in renal function in the early postoperative period, others have shown an overall incidence of postoperative renal insufficiency of 18 per cent after major surgery, with a subsequent hospital mortality rate of 13 per cent (Hou *et al.* 1983). NSAIDs should thus be used cautiously in the postoperative period in vulnerable patients with increased activation of the renin–angiotensin system and pre-existing impaired renal blood flow, such as the elderly, or those with heart failure, sepsis or volume depletion, or those concomitantly exposed to potentially nephrotoxic agents such as aminoglycoside antibiotics.

Clinical syndromes associated with NSAIDs

Acute renal impairment/acute tubular necrosis

The risk for adverse renal effects is largely dose dependent. It is increased in states of excess renin (discussed above). NSAID-induced reduction in glomerular filtration rate may result in acute renal failure with a fractional excretion of sodium less than 1 per cent, suggestive of prerenal azotaemia. This complication has been reported with most NSAIDs but only rarely with aspirin. Renal failure has also been described after topical and intramuscular NSAIDs (Pearce *et al.* 1993; O'Callaghan *et al.* 1994).

A multicentre study in France examined the incidence and subsequent outcome of patients with drug-induced acute renal failure (Kleinknecht *et al.* 1986). Out of 398 patients with acute renal failure, 147 (36.9 per cent) had taken NSAIDs. One-third of them required dialysis and 71.4 per cent recovered or regained previous renal function. Renal biopsies obtained in 25 patients with NSAID-associated renal failure disclosed acute tubular necrosis and acute interstitial nephritis in 21 patients and either minimal-change nephropathy or chronic renal damage in the last four. Predisposing factors included previous diuretic therapy, sodium depletion, congestive heart failure, underlying chronic renal failure, diabetes mellitus, and hepatocellular insufficiency. Thus, although renal side-effects from use of NSAIDs are relatively rare, acute renal failure may necessitate dialysis and permanent renal damage may ensue.

Acute tubulointerstitial nephritis

NSAIDs of different chemical classes have been associated with acute tubulointerstitial nephritis and renal failure. After its first description in 1979 (Brezin *et al.* 1979), this association has been repeatedly reported (Clive and Stoff 1984; Carmichael and Shankel 1985). The patients are often elderly and the drug may have been taken for months or years before the development of acute interstitial nephritis. Clinical evidence of an allergic reaction, such as fever, rash, arthralgia, eosinophilia, and eosinophiluria is uncommon. Of note, proteinuria, often in the nephrotic range, may occasionally appear, especially in fenoprofen-induced tubulointerstitial nephritis (Brezin *et al.* 1979; Finkelstein *et al.* 1982). NSAID-induced tubulointerstitial nephritis differs from that caused by other drugs which have an earlier onset and are often associated with clinical evidence of an allergic reaction. The insidious onset of NSAID-induced tubulointerstitial nephritis taken together with the wide use of NSAIDs warrants a careful drug history in all patients with unexplained acute renal failure.

NSAID-induced acute tubulointerstitial nephritis is formally diagnosed by renal biopsy (Figs 2 and 3). A patchy acute tubular damage coexists with tubulointerstitial infiltrates predominantly of T lymphocytes and, to a lesser extent of monocytes/macrophages, B lymphocytes, plasma cells, and eosinophils (Bender *et al.* 1984; Cameron 1988). Rarely, a granulomatous interstitial nephritis is seen (Schwartz *et al.* 1988). Immunofluorescence microscopy is usually negative or non-specific. The predominance of T lymphocytes in the interstitial infiltrate has been taken to indicate that T lymphocyte activation mediates this syndrome, rather than a humoral mechanism as in other forms of drug-induced acute interstitial nephritis (Finkelstein *et al.* 1982, see Chapter 6.1). Suggestions that the heavy proteinuria is due to an increased glomerular permeability caused by lymphokines released by activated T cells remains speculative. Inhibition of renal COX is associated with a stimulation of the lipoxygenase pathway of arachidonic acid metabolism and the production of leukotrienes, which are potent chemotactic factors for lymphocytes. PGs also have immunomodulatory functions whose inhibition might lead to an escape from immunological control (Torres 1982). Inhibition of PGs indeed leads to sustained or enhanced expression of proinflammatory and profibrogenic mediators, with eventual tubulointerstitial damage and fibrosis (Schneider *et al.* 1996).

In addition to renal failure, hyperchloraemic acidosis has been consistently noted (Baldwin *et al.* 1968), together with impaired concentrating ability, which last for many months despite recovery of renal function after the acute episode (Woodroffe *et al.* 1974). Renal failure may occasionally necessitate dialysis (Kleinknecht *et al.* 1986). After drug withdrawal, renal failure and proteinuria usually resolve although this may take up to a year or may be only partial (Cameron 1988) with chronic interstitial fibrosis progressing to chronic renal failure (Adams *et al.* 1986). Prednisolone has been successfully used in anecdotal reports without conclusive evidence that corticosteroids hasten the resolution of the renal lesion (Clive and Stoff 1984). Still, the fact that experimental acute interstitial nephritis typically precedes fibrogenesis by as short a time as 7–14 days (Neilson 1989) taken together with the potential for incomplete resolution leads us to advocate a 1 month course of prednisolone, starting at a dose of 30 mg daily, to be rapidly reduced as renal function improves. Although cross-reactivity among NSAIDs remains unknown, it is wise to avoid other NSAIDs in patients who have developed NSAID-induced acute interstitial nephritis. If impossible, a compound from a different structural class should be selected and the patient should be monitored closely.

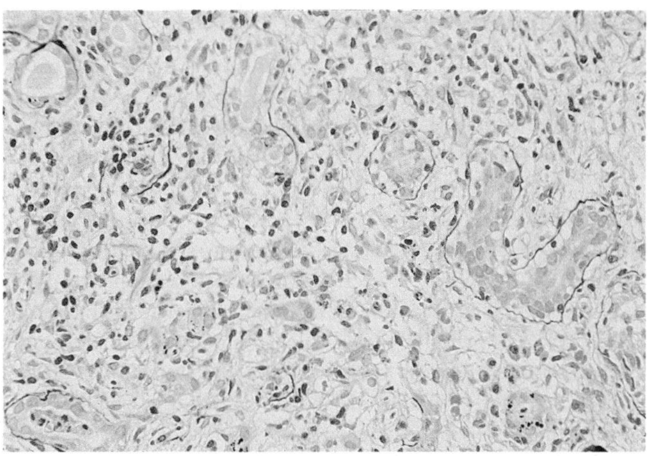

Fig. 2 Renal biopsy from a patient with NSAID-induced acute interstitial nephritis. There is an interstitial infiltrate of mononuclear cells and eosinophils which are entering and damaging tubules (PA—silver stain 100× magnification) (by courtesy of Dr A.J. Howie).

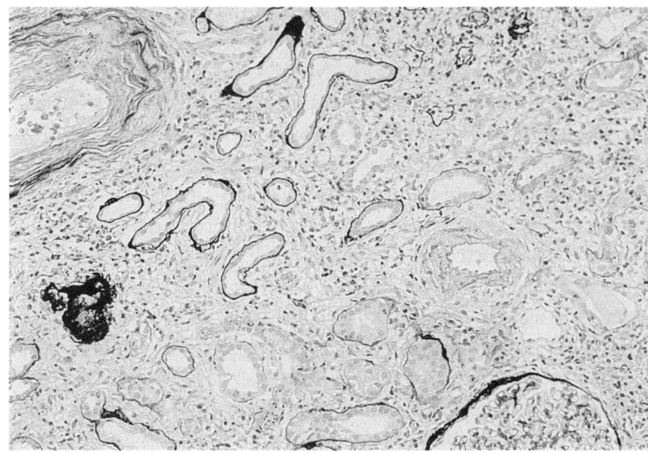

Fig. 3 Renal biopsy from a patient with late interstitial nephritis. There is fibrosis with tubular atrophy, intimal thickening in arteries, and a few mononuclear cells (PA—silver stain 50× magnification) (by courtesy of Dr A.J. Howie).

Vasculitis/glomerulonephritis

Membranous nephropathy with nephrotic syndrome may occur as idiosyncratic reaction to various classes of NSAIDs (Campistol *et al.* 1989; Grcevska *et al.* 1993). The temporal association with the intake of modest doses of NSAIDs, the prompt and complete recovery after drug discontinuation, and the absence of recurrent disease once the drug has been stopped may help distinguish NSAID-associated membranous nephropathy from the idiopathic form. Anecdotal reports of generalized vasculitis and glomerulonephritis in patients given NSAIDs include both thrombotic and non-thrombotic thrombocytopenic purpura (Carmichael and Shankel 1985) and vasculitis (Grennan *et al.* 1979; Mordes 1980). It is difficult to be certain of a causal relationship with NSAIDs in many of these cases, but generalized vasculitis has been reported after rechallenge with piroxicam (Goebal and Muellar-Brodmann 1982).

Renal papillary necrosis

Chronic and excessive ingestion of analgesic drugs may lead to papillary necrosis and chronic renal failure (see Chapter 6.2). Aspirin use is associated with a low risk of nephrotoxicity (Dubach *et al.* 1991; Sandler *et al.* 1991; Perneger *et al.* 1994), although this has been disputed (Pommer *et al.* 1989; Morlans *et al.* 1990). Renal papillary necrosis has been infrequently reported in patients treated with ibuprofen, indomethacin, phenylbutazone, fenoprofen, and mefenamic acid (Munn *et al.* 1976; Shah *et al.* 1981; Carmichael and Shankel 1985; Adams *et al.* 1986; Segasothy *et al.* 1987), and with paracetamol (Krikler 1967; Master 1973). Severe dehydration, coupled with massive NSAID ingestion, may lead to exceedingly elevated local concentrations of NSAIDs and/or metabolites within the papillae with eventual inhibition of the compensatory production of vasodilatory papillary PGs.

Chronic renal failure

Sandler *et al.* (1991) evaluated the risk for chronic renal disease associated with regular use of non-aspirin NSAIDs in 554 patients with newly diagnosed chronic renal dysfunction. They found a twofold increased risk for chronic renal disease in patients with a history of previous daily use of NSAIDs. The NSAID-associated risk was greater in older men (>65 years of age), and among those with conditions that might indicate an enhanced susceptibility to the effects of NSAIDs, including previous myocardial infarction, congestive heart failure, heavy alcohol consumption (as a surrogate for cirrhosis), or diuretic use. These observations were confirmed in a more recent case–control study of 716 patients with endstage renal failure and 361 controls (Perneger *et al.* 1994). A high cumulative intake of NSAIDs (>5000 tablets) was associated with a 4.5-fold excess risk of endstage renal failure. Adams *et al.* (1986) reported six patients with chronic renal failure associated with the use of NSAIDs, one of whom had renal papillary necrosis and five chronic tubulointerstitial fibrosis. In other reports of NSAID-induced acute tubulointerstitial nephritis, a proportion of patients showed moderate impairment of renal function after recovery (Cameron 1988). Other studies of NSAID usage in hospitalized patients failed to identify an increased incidence of renal failure (Fox and Jick 1984; Beard *et al.* 1988). On balance, however, it seems likely that chronic usage of NSAIDs may be associated with a slightly increased risk for the development of chronic renal failure.

Salt and water retention

NSAIDs therapy may aggravate the sodium retention induced by renal hypoperfusion in heart failure, cirrhosis, or the nephrotic syndrome (Blackshear *et al.* 1985). Hyponatraemia may occur if water retention is disproportionate to sodium retention (Blum and Aviram 1980) especially when thiazide diuretics are given simultaneously (Clive and Stoff 1984).

Hypertension

Two large meta-analyses encompassing more than 90 studies demonstrate that NSAIDs may increase blood pressure, especially in previously hypertensive patients (Johnson *et al.* 1994; Pope *et al.* 1994). NSAIDs elevate supine mean blood pressure by 5 mmHg, sufficient to increase hypertension-related morbidity and mortality (Collins *et al.* 1990). This complication is of importance in the elderly who are frequently prescribed NSAIDs for musculoskeletal disorders and also have a high prevalence of other chronic disorders, including hypertension.

Hyperkalaemia and hyporeninaemic hypoaldosteronism

NSAIDs may cause hyperkalaemia, more commonly in patients with chronic renal failure, diabetes mellitus, and type IV tubular acidosis (Kutyrina *et al.* 1979) through previously outlined mechanisms (see section 'Potassium homeostasis'). NSAIDs must be used with caution in patients taking other drugs known to decrease renal potassium excretion, such as potassium-sparing diuretics, angiotensin-converting enzyme inhibitors, and β-blockers.

Renal failure in neonates associated with the use of NSAIDs in pregnancy

NSAIDs, especially indomethacin, have been recommended as an effective treatment for preterm labour and polyhydramnios. Amniotic fluid originates, especially in the second half of pregnancy, in fetal urine; and the main mode by which NSAIDs reduce excess fluid in polyhydramnios is through the reduction of fetal urine production by an impaired renal function (Kirshon *et al.* 1990). Several cases of renal failure have been described in preterm infants as the result of prenatal maternal indomethacin treatment (Vanhaesebrouck *et al.* 1988). Renal failure in these infants is not always reversible, and the outcome can be fatal.

Flank pain syndrome

Suprofen was been associated with an unusual syndrome of flank pain and acute renal failure probably from an acute uric acid nephropathy, since this drug has uricosuric properties (Hart *et al.* 1987). Suprofen has now been withdrawn.

Drug interactions with NSAIDs

NSAIDs and diuretics

NSAIDs may blunt the natriuretic action of thiazides, aldosterone antagonists, and frusemide in patients with heart failure, the nephrotic syndrome, renal impairment, cirrhosis, and hypertension (Garella and Matarese 1984).

NSAIDs and antihypertensive drugs

The NSAID-induced retention of sodium impairs the effectiveness of hypotensive drugs such as diuretics (Lopez-Ovejero *et al.* 1978), β-blocking agents (Durao *et al.* 1977), and angiotensin-converting enzyme inhibitors (Witzgall *et al.* 1982).

NSAIDs and calcineurin inhibitors

NSAIDs can significantly worsen cyclosporin A nephrotoxicity (Berg *et al.* 1989; Altman *et al.* 1992). Acute renal failure has been reported after ibuprofen in liver allograft recipients treated by tacrolimus (Sheiner *et al.* 1994). NSAIDs and calcineurin inhibitor should not be coadministered, unless there is no other alternative. In the latter case, they should only be used with close monitoring of renal function.

Renal sparing NSAIDs

The growing awareness of the nephrotoxic potential of NSAIDs limits their use despite their clinical usefulness. Considerable efforts are being made to identify NSAIDs devoid of renal adverse side-effects.

Aspirin

Low-dose aspirin, an NSAID, is widely used as an antiplatelet drug in cardioprotection. It is approximately 50–100-fold more potent in inhibiting platelet COX-1 than monocyte COX-2 (Cipollone *et al.* 1997) and induces a permanent defect in thromboxane-dependent platelet function. Larger doses are required to inhibit COX-2-dependent pathophysiological processes such as hyperalgesia and inflammation. Low-dose aspirin has not been reported to adversely affect renal function or blood pressure control, consistent with its lack of effect on renal PG synthesis (Mené *et al.* 1995). Due to its selectivity, it is the drug of choice for the prevention of thrombotic events, even for patients with underlying renal disease, without the risk of jeopardizing PG-dependent renal function (Patrono 1994).

Sulindac and nabumetone

Sulindac and nabumetone were reported to have renal sparing properties (Ciabattoni *et al.* 1984; Boelaert *et al.* 1987) but this was never convincingly established (Whelton *et al.* 1990). These drugs are now only infrequently used.

Selective inhibitors of COX-2

NSAIDs selective towards COX-2 have been developed (see section 'Cyclo-oxygenase in the kidney'). COX-1 sparing should reduce drug-related gastrointestinal toxicity. Unfortunately, recent evidence suggests that COX-2 inhibitors are not devoid of renal effects. Published evidence is hampered by inadequate numbers, varied baseline patient characteristics, and different doses and lengths of drug treatment and do not allow definite conclusions.

Meloxicam

Compared with piroxicam, diclofenac, and naproxen, meloxicam produces significantly fewer total gastrointestinal side-effects (Distel *et al.* 1996). Comparison of meloxicam with diclofenac in 9323 symptomatic patients with osteoarthritis treated for 28 days showed significantly fewer increases in serum creatinine and urea with meloxicam (Hawkey *et al.* 1998). Urinary PGE_2 was not affected by meloxicam but reduced by indomethacin (de Meijer *et al.* 1999). However, another randomized crossover comparison of meloxicam and indomethacin showed that both NSAIDs inhibited frusemide-stimulated plasma renin activity and PGE_2 (Stichtenoth *et al.* 1984) and suggested that COX-2 is important for PGE_2 synthesis and renin release, implying that COX-2-selective inhibitors could have the same effects on renal function as conventional NSAIDs.

Rofecoxib and celecoxib

Efficacy

Rofecoxib and celecoxib are two newer COX-2-selective inhibitors with greater selectivity than meloxicam. Associated gastrointestinal toxicity (as measured by endoscopic studies and gastrointestinal ulcers and bleeding) is lower than with conventional NSAIDs but higher than with placebo (Simon *et al.* 1999; Bombardier *et al.* 2000). Pain relief and anti-inflammatory analgesic effect are equivalent to those of non-selective NSAIDs. Inhibition of the cytochrome-P450 enzyme system by celecoxib elevates plasma concentrations of drugs metabolized by this isoenzyme, such as some β-blockers, antidepressants, and antipsychotics. Rofecoxib does not inhibit this enzyme and has thus fewer metabolic interactions.

Effects on renal prostaglandins

The urinary excretion of PGE_2 and 6-keto-$PGF_{1\alpha}$ the stable metabolite of PGI_2, reflects the renal synthesis of PGE_2 and PGI_2, respectively. In healthy ageing adults, rofecoxib produced a 47 per cent decrease from baseline in urinary 6-keto-$PGF_{1\alpha}$, which was comparable to the 53 per cent reduction induced by indomethacin (Catella-Lawson *et al.* 1999). In another study, rofecoxib, meloxicam, and diclofenac reduced urinary PGE_2 and 6-keto-$PGF_{1\alpha}$ excretion by a similar 40–50 per cent (Van Hecken *et al.* 2000). Urinary 6-keto-$PGF_{1\alpha}$ was comparable in response to celecoxib and traditional NSAIDs (McAdam *et al.* 1999). In healthy elderly volunteers on a normal sodium intake, multiple doses of twice daily celecoxib reduced PGE_2 and 6-keto-$PGF_{1\alpha}$ excretion to the same extent as naproxen, by approximately 65 and 80 per cent, respectively (Whelton *et al.* 2000b). These data suggest that the COX-2 isoform plays an important role in renal PG biosynthesis and, thus, that their inhibitors will impact on renal function just as non-selective NSAIDs.

Effects on renal function

Sodium excretion and glomerular filtration rate

In the elderly, salt-replete subjects, both indomethacin and rofecoxib decreased sodium excretion but only indomethacin reduced glomerular filtration rate (Catella-Lawson *et al.* 1999). Celecoxib, like rofecoxib, affects renal function in selected groups of subjects at risk of NSAID-related renal effects. Celecoxib was compared with naproxen in a single-blind, randomized, crossover study involving 29 healthy elderly subjects given either celecoxib, 200 mg twice daily, for 5 days followed by celecoxib, 400 mg twice daily for the next 5 days, or naproxen, 500 mg twice daily, for 10 days (Whelton *et al.* 2000b). Glomerular filtration rate declined more with naproxen than with celecoxib, despite a comparable urinary excretion of PGE_2 and 6-keto-$PGF_{1\alpha}$ and sodium excretion. An early, transient, reduction in glomerular filtration rate induced by celecoxib might have been missed since glomerular filtration rate was measured only once, 3–5 h after drug administration. Rossat *et al.* (1999) found that in salt- depleted subjects, glomerular filtration rate fell to a nadir 60 or 120 min after celecoxib administration and returned to baseline shortly thereafter. The fall in glomerular filtration rate was significantly dose related. Celecoxib also promoted sodium and potassium retention. In another study involving salt-depleted elderly subjects, rofecoxib and indomethacin induced a comparable reduction of glomerular filtration rate (Swan *et al.* 2000). These studies illustrate that the effects of COX-2 inhibitors and non-selective NSAIDs on renal haemodynamics are similar. In patients with stable chronic renal insufficiency (glomerular filtration rate between 40 and 60 ml/min), celecoxib and naproxen both produced a small reduction in fractional sodium excretion and glomerular filtration rate [Celebrex (Celecoxib) Advisory Committee Briefing and Document 1998].

Renal failure

Acute renal failure and hyperkalaemia have been observed after the administration of COX-2-selective inhibitors to patients with risk factors for NSAID-induced acute renal insufficiency, including underlying chronic renal impairment and true or 'effective' volume depletion (Parazella and Eras 2000). Acute renal failure has also been reported in a patient with a renal transplant 4 weeks after starting rofecoxib (Wolf *et al.* 2000). COX-2-selective NSAIDs are thus similar to non-selective NSAIDs in their effects on both solute homeostasis and renal haemodynamics. A case of acute interstitial nephritis has been reported 3 weeks after the initiation of rofecoxib (Rocha and Fernandez-Alonso 2001).

Effects on oedema and blood pressure

A post hoc analysis of the renal safety of celecoxib based on more than 50 clinical studies including more than 13,000 subjects disclosed that the most common side-effects, peripheral oedema (2.1 per cent), hypertension (0.8 per cent), and exacerbation of pre-existing hypertension (0.6 per cent), were neither dose- nor time-related and that their incidence and profile were similar to those of non-selective NSAIDs. There was no evidence of drug–drug interactions between celecoxib and concomitant angiotensin-converting enzyme inhibitors, β-blockers, calcium channel blockers, or diuretics (Whelton *et al.* 2000a). Comparison of the side-effects of celecoxib 200 mg and rofecoxib 25 mg over a 6-week period in 810 hypertensive patients with osteoarthritis, aged over 65 years, demonstrated that oedema developed twice as frequently in rofecoxib-treated than in celecoxib-treated patients (9.5 versus 4.9 per cent, $p = 0.014$) and that systolic blood pressure increased significantly in 17 per cent of rofecoxib-compared with 11 per cent of celecoxib-treated patients ($p = 0.032$) (Whelton *et al.* 2001). Celecoxib induces thus less frequently oedema and blood pressure rises than rofecoxib.

Therapeutic use of NSAIDs in nephrotic syndrome

NSAIDs reduce proteinuria in patients with the nephrotic syndrome (Donker *et al.* 1978; Gansevoort *et al.* 1992) probably by reducing renal blood flow and glomerular filtration rate (Tiggeler *et al.* 1979). Apart from the effects on renal haemodynamics, Michielsen and Varenterghem (1983) have suggested that NSAIDs also alter capillary wall permeability. The occasional occurrence of irreversible renal failure in patients with a nephrotic syndrome treated with NSAIDs (Kleinknecht *et al.* 1986) suggests great caution in the use of these drugs.

Conclusion

The increasing use of NSAIDs both from prescription and from over-the-counter sales will increase the prevalence of nephrotoxicity. A history of NSAID use should be sought in all patients with unexplained impairment of renal function and or proteinuria. In patients at risk of developing NSAID-induced renal insufficiency, the use of NSAIDs should be avoided. NSAIDs should not be prescribed in patients with chronic renal impairment, or with a functioning renal transplant. Patients with an NSAID-induced, interstitial nephritis or papillary necrosis should not be given NSAIDs again. In some individuals who have developed NSAID-induced acute renal failure and who have recovered renal function, NSAIDs may be reintroduced, only if necessary, provided that the risk factors for enhanced susceptibility have been corrected and that renal function is closely monitored.

COX-2, constitutively expressed in renal tissues, is involved in PG-dependent homeostatic processes. Administration of COX-2-selective inhibitors produce qualitative changes in urinary PG excretion, glomerular filtration rate, sodium retention, and peripheral oedema similar to those associated with non-selective NSAIDs. Their use requires, therefore, the same precautions as with traditional NSAIDs.

References

Adams, D. H. *et al.* (1986). Non-steroidal anti-inflammatory drugs and renal failure. *Lancet* **i**, 57–60.

Adverse Drug Reactions Advisory Committee (1993). Ketorolac and renal failure. *Medical Journal of Australia* **159**, 488.

Aiken, J. W. and Vane, J. R. (1973). Intrarenal prostaglandin release attenuates the renal vasoconstrictor activity of angiotensin. *Journal of Pharmacology and Experimental Therapeutics* **184**, 678–687.

Altman, R. D., Perez, G. O., and Sfakianakis, G. N. (1992). Interaction of cyclosporin A and nonsteroidal anti-inflammatory drugs on renal function in patients with rheumatoid arthritis. *American Journal of Medicine* **93**, 396–402.

Arroyo, V. *et al.* (1983). Sympathetic nervous activation, renin-angiotensin system and renal excretion of prostaglandins E2 in cirrhosis: relationship to functional renal failure and sodium and water excretion. *European Journal of Clinical Investigation* **13**, 271–278.

Baldwin, D. S. *et al.* (1968). Renal failure and interstitial nephritis due to penicillin and methicillin. *New England Journal of Medicine* **279**, 1245–1252.

Beard, K., Perera, D. R., and Jick, H. (1988). Drug-induced parenchymal renal disease in outpatients. *Journal of Clinical Pharmacology* **28**, 431–435.

Bender, W. L. *et al.* (1984). Interstitial nephritis, proteinuria and renal failure caused by non-steroidal anti-inflammatory drugs. Immunological characterisation of the infiltrate. *American Journal of Medicine* **76**, 1006–1012.

Berg, K. J. *et al.* (1989). Renal side-effects of high and low cyclosporin A doses in patients with rheumatoid arthritis. *Clinical Nephrology* **31**, 225–231.

Berl, T., Raz, A., and Wald, H. (1977). Prostaglandin synthesis inhibition and the action of vasopressin: studies in man and rat. *American Journal of Physiology* **232**, 529–537.

Blackshear, J. L. *et al.* (1985). Renal complications of non-steroidal anti-inflammatory drugs: identification and monitoring of those at risk. *Seminars in Arthritis and Rheumatism* **14**, 163–175.

Blum, M. and Aviram, A. (1980). Ibuprofen-induced hyponatraemia. *Rheumatology Rehabilitation* **19**, 258–259.

Boelaert, J. R. *et al.* (1987). Nabumetone pharmacokinetics in patients with varying degrees of renal impairment. *American Journal of Medicine* **83**, 107–109.

Bombardier, C. *et al.* (2000). Comparison of upper gastrointestinal toxicity of rofecoxib and naproxen in patients with rheumatoid arthritis. VIGOR Study Group. *New England Journal of Medicine* **343**, 1520–1528.

Boyer, T. D., Zia, P., and Reynolds, T. B. (1979). Effect of indomethacin and prostaglandin A1 on renal function and plasma renin activity in alcoholic liver disease. *Gastroenterology* **77**, 215–222.

Brezin, J. H. *et al.* (1979). Reversible renal failure and nephrotic syndrome associated with nonsteroidal anti-inflammatory drugs. *New England Journal of Medicine* **310**, 1271–1273.

Cameron, J. S. (1988). Allergic interstitial nephritis: clinical features and pathogenesis. *Quarterly Journal of Medicine* **66**, 97–115.

Campistol, J. M. *et al.* (1989). Reversible membranous nephropathy associated with diclofenac. *Nephrology, Dialysis, Transplantation* **4**, 393–395.

Carmichael, T. and Shankel, S. W. (1985). Effects of non-steroidal anti-inflammatory drugs on prostaglandins and renal function. *American Journal of Medicine* **78**, 992–1000.

Catella-Lawson, F. *et al.* (1999). Effects of specific inhibition of cyclooxygenase-2 on sodium balance, hemodynamics, and vasoactive eicosanoids. *Journal of Pharmacology and Experimental Therapeutics* **289**, 735–741.

Celebrex (Celecoxib) Advisory Committee Briefing and Document (1998). Renal effects; www.fda.gov/cder/foi/adcomm/98/celebrex.htm.

Ciabattoni, G., Cinotti, G. A., and Pierucci, A. (1984). Effects of sulindac and ibuprofen in patients with chronic glomerular disease: evidence for the dependence of renal function on prostacyclin. *New England Journal of Medicine* **310**, 279–288.

Cipollone, F. *et al.* (1997). Differential suppression of thromboxane biosynthesis by indobufen and aspirin in patients with unstable angina. *Circulation* **96**, 1109–1116.

Clive, D. M. and Stoff, J. S. (1984). Renal syndromes associated with anti-inflammatory drugs. *New England Journal of Medicine* **310**, 563–572.

Collins, R. *et al.* (1990). Blood pressure, stroke, and coronary heart disease. Part 2. Short-term reductions in blood pressure: overview of randomised drug trials in their epidemiological context. *Lancet* **335**, 827–838.

Day, R. O. *et al.* (1987). Clinical pharmacology of non-steroidal anti-inflammatory drugs. *Pharmacology and Therapeutics* **33**, 383–433.

de Meijer, A. *et al.* (1999). Meloxicam, 15 mg/day, spares platelet function in healthy volunteers. *Clinical Pharmacology and Therapeutics* **66**, 425–430.

Dinchuk, J. E. *et al.* (1995). Renal abnormalities and an altered inflammatory response in mice lacking cyclooxygenase II. *Nature* **378**, 406–409.

Distel, M. *et al.* (1996). Safety of meloxicam: a global analysis of clinical trials. *British Journal of Rheumatology* **35**, 68–77.

Donker, A. J. M. *et al.* (1978). Treatment of the nephrotic syndrome with indomethacin. *Nephron* **22**, 374–381.

Dubach, U. C., Rosner, B., and Stürmer, T. (1991). An epidemiologic study of abuse of analgesic drugs-effects of phenacetin and salicylate on mortality and cardiovascular morbidity (1968–1987). *New England Journal of Medicine* **324**, 155–160.

Dunn, M. J. (1984). Nonsteroidal anti-inflammatory drugs and renal function. *Annual Review of Medicine* **35**, 411–428.

Dunn, M. J. and Zambraski, E. J. (1980). Renal effects of drugs that inhibit prostaglandin synthesis. *Kidney International* **18**, 609–622.

Durao, V., Prata, M., and Goncalves, L. (1977). Modification of anti-hypertensive effect of beta-adrenergic blocking agents by inhibition of endogenous prostaglandin synthesis. *Lancet* **2**, 1005–1007.

Epstein, M. and Lifschitz, M. (1987). Renal eicosanoids as determinants of renal function in liver disease. *Hepatology* **7**, 1359–1367.

Ferreira, S. H., Moncada, S., and Vane, J. R. (1971). Indomethacin and aspirin abolish prostaglandin release from the spleen. *Nature* **231**, 237–239.

Finkelstein, A. *et al.* (1982). Fenoprofen nephropathy: lipoid nephrosis and interstitial nephritis: a possible T lymphocyte disorder. *American Journal of Medicine* **72**, 81–87.

Fox, D. A. and Jick, H. (1984). Nonsteroidal anti-inflammatory drugs and renal disease. *Journal of the American Medical Association* **251**, 1299–1300.

Gansevoort, R. T. *et al.* (1992). Antiproteinuric drugs in patients with idiopathic membranous glomerulopathy. *Nephrology, Dialysis, Transplantation* **7**, 91–96.

Garella, S. and Matarese, R. A. (1984). Renal effects of prostaglandins and clinical adverse effects of non-steroidal anti-inflammatory drugs. *Medicine* **63**, 165–181.

Goebal, K. M. and Muellar-Brodmann, W. (1982). Reversible overt nephropathy with Henoch–Schönlein purpura due to piroxicam. *British Medical Journal* **284**, 311.

Goldzer, R. C. *et al.* (1980). Hyperkalaemia associated with indomethacin. *Archives of Internal Medicine* **141**, 802–804.

Govindarajan, S. *et al.* (1987). Immunohistochemical distribution of renal prostaglandin endoperoxidase synthase and prostacyclin synthase: diminished endoperoxidase synthase in the hepatorenal syndrome. *Hepatology* **7**, 654–659.

Grcevska, L. *et al.* (1993). Membranous nephropathy with severe tubulointerstitial and vascular changes in a patient with psoriatic arthritis treated with non-steroidal anti-inflammatory drugs. *Clinical Nephrology* **39**, 250–253.

Grennan, D. M. *et al.* (1979). Vasculitis in a patient receiving naproxen. *New Zealand Medical Journal* **89**, 48–49.

Harris, R. C. *et al.* (1994). Cyclo-oxygenase-2 is associated with the macula densa of rat kidney and increases with salt restriction. *Journal of Clinical Investigation* **94**, 2504–2510.

Hart, D., Ward, M., and Lifshitz, M. D. (1987). Suprofen-related nephrotoxicity. *Annals of Internal Medicine* **106**, 235–238.

Hawkey, C. *et al.* (1998). Gastrointestinal tolerability of meloxicam compared to diclofenac in osteoarthritis patients. International MELISSA Study Group. Meloxicam Large-scale International Study Safety Assessment. *British Journal of Rheumatology* **37**, 937–945.

Henrich, W. L. (1981). Role of the prostaglandins in renin secretion. *Kidney International* **19**, 822–830.

Heymann, M. A., Ruldolph, A. M., and Silverman, N. H. (1976). Closure of the ductus arteriosus in premature infancts by inhibition of prostaglandin synthesis. *New England Journal of Medicine* **295**, 530–533.

Hou, S. *et al.* (1983). Hospital-acquired renal insufficiency: a prospective study. *American Journal of Medicine* **1983**, 243–248.

Johnson, A. G., Nguyen, T. V., and Day, R. O. (1994). Do nonsteroidal anti-inflammatory drugs affect blood pressure? *Annals of Internal Medicine* **121**, 289–300.

Jones, D. A. *et al.* (1993). Molecular cloning of human prostaglandin endoperoxide synthase type II and demonstration of expression in response to cytokines. *Journal of Biological Chemistry* **268**, 9049–9054.

Kirshon, B., Mari, G., and Moise, J. K. L. (1990). Indomethacin therapy in the treatment of symptomatic polyhydramnios. *Obstetrics and Gynaecology* **75**, 202–205.

Kleinknecht, D., Landais, P., and Goldfarb, B. (1986). Analgesic and non-steroidal anti-inflammatory drug-associated acute renal failure: a prospective collaborative study. *Clinical Nephrology* **25**, 275–281.

Komhoff, M. *et al.* (1997). Localization of cyclooxygenase-1 and -2 in adult and fetal human kidney: implication for renal function. *American Journal of Physiology* **272**, F460–F468.

Komhoff, M. *et al.* (2000). Cyclooxygenase-2-selective inhibitors impair glomerulogenesis and renal cortical development. *Kidney International* **57**, 414–422.

Krikler, D. M. (1967). Paracetamol and the kidney. *British Medical Journal* **2**, 615–616.

Kujubu, D. *et al.* (1991). TIS 10, a phorbol ester tumor promoter-inducible mRNA from Swiss 3T3 cells, encodes a novel prostaglandin synthase/cyclooxygenase homologue. *Journal of Biological Chemistry* **266**, 12866–12872.

Kutyrina, I. M., Androsova, S. O., and Tareyeva, I. E. (1979). Indomethacin-induced hyporeninaemic hypoaldosteronism. *Lancet* **1**, 785.

Langenbach, R. *et al.* (1995). Prostaglandin synthesis I gene disruption in mice reduces arachidonic acid-induced inflammation and indomethacin-induced gastric ulceration. *Cell* **83**, 483–492.

Lee, A. *et al.* (2001). Effects of nonsteroidal anti-inflammatory drugs on post-operative renal function in normal adults. Review. *Cochrane Database Systemic Review* **2**, CD002765.

Ling, B. N., Webster, C. L., and Eaton, D. C. (1992). Eicosanoids modulate apical Ca^{2+}-dependent K^+ channels in cultured rabbit principal cells. *American Journal of Physiology* **263**, F116–F126.

Lopez-Ovejero, J. A. *et al.* (1978). Effects of indomethacin alone and during diuretic or beta-adrenoreceptor-blockade therapy on blood pressure and the renin system in essential hypertension. *Clinical Science and Molecular Medicine* **4** (Suppl.), 203s–205s.

Lum, G. M. *et al.* (1977). *In vivo* effect of indomethacin to potentiate the renal medullary cyclic AMP response to vasopressin. *Journal of Clinical Investigation* **59**, 8–13.

Master, D. R. (1973). Analgesic nephropathy associated with paracetamol. *Proceedings of the Royal Society of Medicine* **66**, 904.

McAdam, B. F. *et al.* (1999). Systemic biosynthesis of prostacyclin by cyclooxygenase (COX)-2: the human pharmacology of a selective inhibitor of COX-2. [Erratum appears in *Proceedings of the National Academy of Science, USA* 1999 May 11; **96** (10), 5890.] *Proceedings of the National Academy of Sciences of the United States of America* **96**, 272–277.

Mené, P., Pugliese, F., and Patrono, C. (1995). The effects of nonsteroidal anti-inflammatory drugs on human hypertensive vascular disease. *Seminars in Nephrology* **15**, 244–252.

Michielsen, P. and Varenterghem, Y. (1983). Proteinuria and nonsteroid anti-inflammatory drugs. *Advances in Nephrology from the Necker Hospital* **12**, 139–150.

Mordes, J. P. (1980). Possible naproxen associated vasculitis. *Archives of Internal Medicine* **140**, 985.

Morlans, M. *et al.* (1990). End-stage renal disease and non-narcotic analgesics: a case–control study. *British Journal of Clinical Pharmacology* **30**, 717–723.

Munn, E., Lynn, K. L., and Bailey, R. R. (1976). Renal papillary necrosis following regular consumption of NSAIDs. *New Zealand Journal of Medicine* **95**, 213–214.

Nantel, F. *et al.* (1999). Immunolocalization of cyclooxygenase 2 in the macula densa of human elderly. *FEBS Letters* **457**, 475–477.

Neilson, E. G. (1989). Pathogenesis and therapy of interstitial nephritis (clinical conference). *Kidney International* **35**, 1251–1270.

Oates, J. A. *et al.* (1988). Clinical implications of prostaglandin and thromboxane A2 formation. *New England Journal of Medicine* **319**, 689–698.

O'Banion, M. *et al.* (1991). A serum- and glucocorticoid-regulated 4-kilobase mRNA encodes a cyclooxygenase-related protein. *Journal of Biological Chemistry* **266**, 23261–23267.

O'Callaghan, C. A., Andrews, P. A., and Ogg, C. S. (1994). Renal disease and use of topical non-steroidal anti-inflammatory drugs. *British Medical Journal* **308**, 110–111.

Parazella, M. and Eras, J. (2000). Are selective COX-2 inhibitors nephrotoxic. *American Journal of Kidney Diseases* **35**, 937–940.

Patrono, C. (1994). Aspirin as an antiplatelet drug. *New England Journal of Medicine* **330**, 1287–1294.

Patrono, C. and Pierucci, A. (1986). Renal effects of nonsteroidal antiinflammatory drugs in chronic glomerular disease. *American Journal of Medicine* **82**, 71–83.

Pearce, C. J., Gonzalez, F. M., and Wallin, J. D. (1993). Renal failure and hyperkalemia associated with ketorolac tromethamine. *Archives of Internal Medicine* **153**, 1000–1002.

Pelayo, J. C. (1988). Renal adrenergic effector mechanisms: glomerular sites for prostaglandin interaction. *American Journal of Physiology* **254**, F184–F190.

Perneger, T. V., Whelton, P. K., and Klag, M. J. (1994). Risk of kidney failure associated with the use of acetaminophen, aspirin, and nonsteroidal anti-inflammatory drugs. *New England Journal of Medicine* **331**, 1675–1679.

Pommer, W. *et al.* (1989). Regular analgesic intake and the risk of end-stage renal failure. *American Journal of Nephrology* **9**, 403–412.

Pope, J. E., Anderson, J. J., and Felson, D. T. (1994). A meta-analysis of the effects of nonsteroidal anti-inflammatory drugs on blood pressure. *Archives of Internal Medicine* **21**, 289–300.

Rocha, J. L. and Fernandez-Alonso, J. (2001). Acute tubulointerstitial nephritis associated with the selective COX-2 enzyme inhibitor, rofecoxib. *Lancet* **357**, 1946–1947.

Rossat, J. *et al.* (1999). Renal effects of selective cyclooxygenase-2 inhibition in normotensive salt-depleted subjects. *Clinical Pharmacology and Therapeutics* **66**, 76–84.

Sandler, D. P., Burr, F. R., and Weinberg, C. R. (1991). Nonsteroidal anti-inflammatory drugs and the risk for chronic renal disease. *Annals of Internal Medicine* **115**, 165–172.

Schneider, A. *et al.* (1996). Prostaglandin G/H synthase (PGHS) inhibitors modulate glomerular MCP-1 mRNA expression in anti-Thy-1 antiserum (ATS) induced glomerulonephritis in rats. *Journal of the American Society of Nephrology* **7**, 1720.

Schwartz, A. *et al.* (1988). Granulomatous interstitial nephritis after non-steroidal anti-inflammatory drugs. *American Journal of Nephrology* **8**, 410–416.

Segasothy, M. *et al.* (1987). Mefenamic acid nephropathy. *Nephron* **45**, 156–157.

Shah, G. M., Muhalwas, K. K., and Winer, R. L. (1981). Renal papillary necrosis due to ibuprofen. *Arthritis and Rheumatism* **24**, 1208–1210.

Sheiner, P. A. *et al.* (1994). Acute renal failure associated with the use of ibuprofen in two liver transplant recipients on FK506. *Transplantation* **57**, 1132–1133.

Simon, L. S. *et al.* (1999). Anti-inflammatory and upper gastrointestinal effects of celecoxib in rheumatoid arthritis: a randomized controlled trial. *Journal of the American Medical Association* **282**, 1921–1928.

Stichtenoth, D. O., Wagner, B., and Frölich, J. C. (1984). Effect of selective inhibition of the inducible cyclooxygenase on renin release in healthy individuals. *Journal of Investigative Medicine* **46**, 290–296.

Stokes, J. B. (1979). Effect of prostaglandin E2 on chloride transport across the rabbit thick ascending limb of Henle. Selective inhibition of the medullary portion. *Journal of Clinical Investigation* **64**, 495–502.

Stokes, J. B. and Kokko, J. P. (1977). Inhibition of sodium transport by prostaglandin E2 across the isolated perfused rabbit collecting tubule. *Journal of Clinical Investigation* **59**, 1099–1104.

Swan, S. K. *et al.* (2000). Effect of cyclooxygenase-2 inhibition on renal function in elderly persons receiving a low-salt diet. A randomized, controlled trial. *Annals of Internal Medicine* **133**, 1–9.

Takahashi, K. *et al.* (1992). Glomerular action of a free radical-generated novel prostaglandin, 8-epi-prostaglandin F2 alpha in the rat. *Journal of Clinical Investigation* **90**, 136–141.

Tiggeler, R. G., Hulme, B., and Wijdeveld, P. G. (1979). Effect of indomethacin on glomerular permeability in the nephrotic syndrome. *Kidney International* **16**, 312–321.

Torres, V. E. (1982). Present and future of non-steroidal anti-inflammatory drugs in nephrology. *Mayo Clinic Proceedings* **57**, 390–393.

Vanhaesebrouck, P. *et al.* (1988). Oligohydramnios, renal insufficiency, and ileal perforation in preterm infants after intrauterine exposure to indomethacin. *Journal of Pediatrics* **113**, 738–743.

Van Hecken, A. *et al.* (2000). Comparative inhibitory activity of rofecoxib, meloxicam, diclofenac, ibuprofen and naproxen on COX-2 versus COX-1 in healthy volunteers. *Journal of Clinical Pharmacology* **40**, 1109–1120.

Verbeeck, R. K., Blackburn, J. L., and Loewen, G. R. (1983). Clinical pharmacokinetics of non-steroidal anti-inflammatory drugs. *Clinical Pharmacokinetics* **8**, 297–331.

Walshe, J. J. and Venuto, R. C. (1979). Acute oliguric renal failure induced by indomethacin: possible mechanism. *Annals of Internal Medicine* **91**, 47–49.

Whelton, A. (2001). Renal aspects of treatment with conventional nonsteroidal anti-inflammatory drugs versus cyclooxygenase-2 inhibitor. *American Journal of Medicine* **110**, 33–42.

Whelton, A. *et al.* (1990). Renal effects of ibuprofen, piroxicam, and sulindac in patients with asymptomatic renal failure: a prospective, randomized, crossover comparison. *Annals of Internal Medicine* **112**, 568–576.

Whelton, A. *et al.* (2000a). Renal safety and tolerability of celecoxib, a novel cyclooxygenase-2 inhibitor. *American Journal of Therapeutics* **7**, 159–175.

Whelton, A. *et al.* (2000b). Effects of celecoxib and naproxen on renal function in the elderly. *Archives of Internal Medicine* **160**, 1465–1470.

Whelton, A. *et al.* (2001). Cyclooxygenase-2—specific inhibitors and cardiorenal function: a randomized, controlled trial of celecoxib and rofecoxib in older hypertensive osteoarthritis patients. [Erratum appears in *American Journal of Therapeutics* 2001 May–June; **8** (3), 220.] *American Journal of Therapeutics* **8**, 85–95.

Witzgall, H. *et al.* (1982). Acute haemodynamic and hormonal effects of captopril are diminished by indomethacin. *Clinical Science* **62**, 611–615.

Wolf, G., Porth, J., and Stahl, R. A. K. (2000). Acute renal failure associated with rofecoxib. *Annals of Internal Medicine* **133**, 394.

Woodroffe, A. J. *et al.* (1974). Nephropathy associated with methicillin administration. *Australian and New Zealand Journal of Medicine* **4**, 256–261.

Zipser, R. D. *et al.* (1979). Prostaglandins: modulators of renal function and pressor resistance in chronic liver disease. *Journal of Clinical Endocrine Metabolism* **48**, 895–900.

Zipser, R. D. *et al.* (1983). Urinary thromboxane B2 and prostaglandin E2 in the hepatorenal syndrome. *Gastroenterology* **84**, 697–703.

6.4 Uric acid and the kidney

J. Stewart Cameron and H. Anne Simmonds

Uric acid

Uric acid, the end-product of purine metabolism in humans (see Chapter 16.5.3 for details), is 2,6,8-trihydroxypurine with a molecular weight of 168 (Stone and Simmonds 1991). At physiological pH, only one of the three hydroxyl groups dissociates to any significant extent (p*K* 5.44), so that *in vivo* it is effectively a monovalent organic acid. In solution, therefore, 99 per cent is in the form of urate but in urine, where the pH may range from 4.7 to 8.0 or beyond, the ratio of uric acid to urate varies with pH, being almost entirely undissociated uric acid at pH 5.0 and less.

Insolubility of uric acid and other purines

The solubility of urate in water at 37°C is only about 1 mmol/l at pH 5, but increases dramatically to 12 mmol/l at pH 8. However, solubility decreases as the ionic strength of a solution increases. This is important in urine (Shimizu *et al.* 1989) which may be concentrated or dilute, and is a factor in the formation of uric acid crystals or stones (see below). Also, urate/uric acid may remain in solutions which appear to be supersaturated, and thus metastable with regard to crystal or stone formation. Its metabolic precursor xanthine is even less soluble, and this varies little with pH (see Chapter 16.5.3). The uric acid analogue 2,8-dihydroxyadenine is the most insoluble purine (0.03 mmol/l at either pH 5 or pH 8). It is formed only in the congenital absence of the purine enzyme adenine phosphoribosyltransferase; its importance here is that it is easily mistaken for uric acid in chemical testing and is also radiolucent (see Chapter 16.5.3).

Interactions of urate/uric acid with cells

The clinical problems and pathological changes caused by urate/uric acid are due not only to its insolubility but also to the ability of the resultant crystals to initiate inflammation (Cameron and Simmonds 1981; Gresser and Zöllner 1991; Terkeltaub 1993). Phagocytosis or endocytosis of the negatively charged crystals activates the complement system and inflammatory cells, with release of cytokines and other mediators such as TNF from monocytes and IL-8 from polymorphonuclear leucocytes. Parenchymal cells of affected tissues, such as synovial cells and renal tubular cells (Emmerson *et al.* 1991) are capable of crystal endocytosis as well, and also of cytokine release, which amplifies the local inflammation. Crystals of uric acid are amorphous, whereas those of monosodium urate are acicular. This, together with a characteristic negative birefringence under polarized light aids their identification in body fluids and tissues. Recently it has been shown that soluble urate also has effects on renal and vascular cells (Mazzali *et al.* 2001a,b, 2002) (see below).

Relevant purine metabolism (see Chapter 16.5.3)

The reviews of purine metabolism of Stone and Simmonds (1991), and Becker (2001) are referred to throughout. The importance of purines in human metabolism as a whole is considerable. In addition to their role in the storage and transmission of genetic information (DNA, RNA), purines play a equally vital role in providing the energy (ATP) which drives many cellular reactions and also forms the basis of the coenzymes [nicotinamide adenine dinucleotide (phosphate) (NAD(P)), flavin adenine dinucleotide (FAD), etc.]. With guanine nucleotides, adenine nucleotides have separate functions in signal transduction and translation [guanosine triphosphate (GTP), cyclic adenosine monophosphate (cAMP), cyclic guanosine monophosphate (cGMP)]. Finally ATP, ADP, and UTP play a role in neurotransmission through the so-called purinergic fibres (Burnstock 2002).

Many of these functions are subserved by the main active form of purines, purine nucleotides (purine–ribose–phosphate). Nucleotides can be degraded to (or synthesized from) nucleosides (purine–ribose), which in turn can be deribosylated to give the purine bases hypoxanthine, guanine, and xanthine (Chapter 16.5.3, Fig. 1). These essential nucleotides may be synthesized by one of two routes: the energy expensive (5 mol ATP/mol purine) multistep synthetic route, or the single-step 'salvage' pathway, which requires only one mole of ATP per mole of purine synthesized (Becker 2001). Both routes require PP-ribose-P as a phosphate donor. In normal circumstances, salvage predominates over synthesis, but synthesis is particularly active in cells or tissues with a high rate of turnover or metabolism (e.g. bone marrow-derived cells, gut epithelium, skin, and gonadal epithelium).

Normally, only a small fraction of the purine turned over daily is actually degraded and lost to the body, the majority being recycled. In humans, the end-product of the non-recycled purine is uric acid, formed from the precursor bases xanthine and hypoxanthine by the action of xanthine oxidoreductase. Primates including humans lack the promoter of the gene for the hepatic enzyme uricase (Wu *et al.* 1992) and thus have appreciable concentrations of urate in their plasma and a continuous delivery of urate to their kidney. The biological value of failing to break down urate has been much debated (Ames *et al.* 1981; Hooper *et al.* 1998; Watanabe *et al.* 2002). Uric acid is a powerful antioxidant, providing more than half the antioxidant activity of primate and human plasma (Becker 1993; Rosell *et al.* 1999). Mice in which the uricase gene has been disrupted develop severe uric acid nephropathy, worsened by diabetes insipidus, and die before weaning with fibrotic kidneys—but of interest, without crystal deposition (Bradley and Caskey 1994; Kelly *et al.* 2001). In spiders, reptiles, snakes, and birds uric acid is the end-product of the whole of nitrogen metabolism (Danzler 1996), analogous to urea in mammals. The main advantage of this energy expensive end-product is that no obligatory water is required for its excretion as for urea, so that survival is ensured in arid environments or during long periods airborne.

Contribution of diet to uric acid excretion

Approximately two-thirds of uric acid is eliminated by the kidney and approximately one-third by the gut (Sorensen 1980), the ratio being reversed in renal failure. Basal renal uric acid excretion on a purine-free formula diet is as little as 2 mmol/24 h/70 kg body weight (Löffler *et al.* 1981). Purine-rich diets have been associated for millennia with 'primary' gout, a disorder of affluent societies. During times of food shortage, mean uric acid concentrations fell and 'primary' gout almost vanished (Gresser and Zöllner 1991). Humans have no requirement for dietary purines, since the intestine serves as an effective barrier capable of rapidly degrading dietary nucleotides, nucleosides, or bases to the metabolic end-product.

Normal ranges for plasma and urine uric acid in healthy populations

Effect of diet

Diet varies considerably between countries and cultures and thus there is geographical variation in expected values. Prior to 1990, the majority of adults in the United Kingdom ingested a relatively low purine diet, and urinary uric acid excretion greater than 3.5 mmol/day would be abnormal in a 70 kg man unless beer intake was high. At the other extreme in Australia, addicted to high beer and meat consumption, the limit is 7.0 mmol/day (Emmerson 1991). Increasing affluence in all developed countries, raises urate excretion especially in Japan, where gout was formerly uncommon (Johnson *et al.* 2004).

To assess the relative contributions of diet and syntheses to urate excretion, a purine-free diet is used for 5–7 days and urinary excretion of urate measured (Löffler *et al.* 1983). When specific methods (Simmonds *et al.* 1991) are used for uric acid estimation, the normal basic urate excretion is about 1.0–2.8 mmol/24 h; less than 1 per cent of adult males in any country are 'overproducers' in that they excrete more than 3.0 mmol/24 h (or >0.35 mmol/mmol creatinine). An underlying genetic metabolic defect generally explains this with normal feedback controls on *de novo* purine synthesis (Fig. 1) over-ridden, resulting in gross uric acid overproduction (Chapter 16.5.3).

Normal plasma urate concentrations vary also with the country and the method used: the mean plasma uric acid concentrations in the United Kingdom are 222 ± 42 μmol/l for females and 281 ± 41 μmol/l for males (±SD, specific enzymic method) (Simmonds *et al.* 1991). Non-specific methods give values greater than this, and unfortunately are used commonly in clinical practice.

Plasma urate concentrations in children and adolescents

Xanthine oxidoreductase-deficient females in whom blood urate concentrations are normally negligible (Chapter 16.5.3) indicate that fetal uric acid contributes to maternal plasma urate, which explains in part the increasing plasma urate in the later stages of pregnancy (Simmonds *et al.* 1984). Cord blood urate is from 460 μmol/l at 29–33 weeks' gestation to 310 μmol/l in the first day in full-term infants (Stapleton 1992). In neonates, problems associated with this hyperuricaemia and hyperuricosuria have been well documented (Stapleton 1992). These values decline rapidly to 140 μmol/l at 7 days postpartum resulting from marked temporary uricosuria, which may stain diapers pink and be mistaken for blood (Chapter 3.4). The fractional clearance of uric acid, fractional excretion of urate (FE_{ur}), the clearance of uric acid factored by creatinine clearance (100×) is a useful tool for examining the excretion of urate (see next section). The FE_{ur} in the first 24 h of life is particularly high (20–75 per cent) and is raised by hypoxia.

Plasma urate concentrations in older children are independent of gender and much lower than in adults. Throughout childhood however here is a linear fall in FE_{ur} and correspondingly an increase in plasma urate from infancy (Grivna *et al.* 1997) up to puberty (Sánchez-Bayle *et al.* 1992; Stapleton 1992). Normal population data for children vary slightly from country to country: in the United Kingdom values are from 100–230 μmol/l (McBride *et al.* 1998) but somewhat higher in the United States and Spain (Sánchez-Bayle *et al.* 1992). Plasma urate increases with a fall in FE_{ur} during puberty, more so in males than females, and remains relatively constant at these disparate concentrations from the age of 20 (Stapleton 1992). Less than 1.5 mmol/mmol creatinine are excreted by children at the age of 2, but this figure decreases slowly to less than 0.40 and 0.35 mmol/mmol in adult men and women respectively. The uric acid excretion/dl GFR is constant at all ages, about 0.34–0.40 ± 0.1 mg/dl.

Physiology and pharmacology of renal urate handling in humans

Overall renal handling of urate by the human kidney

Urate binding to protein *in vivo* is low (4–5 per cent) (Kovarsky *et al.* 1979) and hence urate is freely filterable. In adult humans, the renal tubule reabsorbs around 90 per cent of filtered urate, so that the FE_{ur} is about 10 per cent. Net reabsorption is slightly greater in males (92 per cent, FE_{ur} 8 per cent) than in younger females (88 per cent, FE_{ur} 12 per cent) and is less in children of either gender (70–85 per cent, FE_{ur} 11–30 per cent). Oestrogens increase FE_{ur} and lower plasma urate concentrations (Nicholls *et al.* 1972; Sumino *et al.* 1999). The differences in FE_{ur} between the sexes in adults decrease when postmenopausal females are compared to men of similar age (Mikkelsen *et al.* 1965) which may explain why postmenopausal females are much more prone to gout than young women. Others have stressed the role of diuretics use in older women (Lally *et al.* 1986). In addition to gender and age, race is an important factor to be taken into account when evaluating renal uric acid handling. Polynesians, both male and female, have much greater plasma urate concentrations than Caucasians, the result of a grossly reduced FE_{ur} compared with their age- and gender-matched Caucasian counterparts, although the same gender difference is still evident within the group (Gibson *et al.* 1984; Simmonds *et al.* 1994); hence the greater prevalence of gout in Polynesians of either gender.

Details of the tubular handling of urate which underlie these data are far from complete. Much of our knowledge derived in the past from micropuncture studies in the kidneys of other mammalian species

(Diamond 1989), demonstrating that transport of uric acid occurs predominantly, if not exclusively, in the proximal tubule, and is bidirectional with both reabsorptive and secretory components. The former has been located principally in the S_1 segment, and the latter in the S_2 segment of the proximal tubule (Maesaka and Fishbane 1998). The direction of net transport varies considerably with species (Danzler 1996). Even in humans, chimpanzees, and *Cebus* monkeys, which are all strong reabsorbers with a FE_{ur} of 5–15 per cent, a secretory flux is also present, and under some circumstances urate clearance can exceed the GFR (Diamond 1989; Maesaka and Fishbane 1998). This secretory flux predominates in species such as the pig and the rabbit, and in the pig always produces net secretion of urate (Simmonds *et al.* 1976). Earlier studies in man (in whom direct sampling of tubular fluid is not possible) relied on now suspect interpretations of pharmacological manipulation using pyrazinamide and uricosuric drugs (Colussi *et al.* 1987; Diamond 1989). Uric acid is, at physiological pH, an anion as outlined earlier in this chapter, and thus can compete for any system that will transport endogenous or exogenous (xenobiotic) anions, as well as for specific transmembrane transport systems for urate alone.

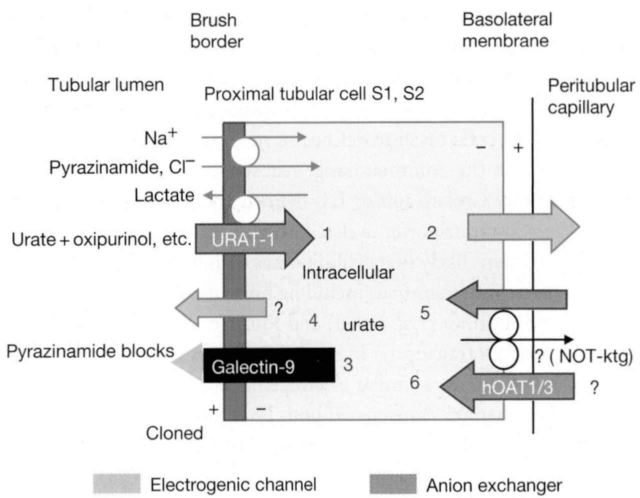

Fig. 1 A diagram of probable urate transport mechanisms in the early segments of the human proximal tubule. Reabsorption is mediated through the indirectly sodium-coupled brush-border anion exchanger URAT-1 (1), with subsequent efflux from the cell into the interstitium and peritubular capillaries probably via a voltage-driven transporter (2). Reabsorption of urate would be enhanced when more sodium is reabsorbed, or when anions with an affinity for the exchanger accumulate intracellularly: for example, lactate or ketones in diabetic ketoacidosis. Pyrazinoate also enters the cell coupled to sodium, and this allows entry of urate in exchange for its efflux. A putative apical electrochemical urate transporter which can explain secretion of urate has been described as galectin-9 and cloned (3); this is blocked by luminal pyrazinamide. Further similar channels have been described in other mammals (4) but their relationship to the galectin 'transporter' is not yet clear (see text). In humans, a convincing mechanism for entry of urate into the tubular cell from the peritubular capillaries and interstitium has not yet been described, since human tubular cells lack the basolateral α-ketoglutarate exchanger which will accept urate as well as PAH and other anions (5) which is present in the pig and other species with predominant secretion. The multispecific anion exchangers hOAT1 and hOAT3 could be one medium of transport into the cell (6), but this is uncertain. Resecretion of intracellular urate by the voltage-sensitive pathway is of course a possibility, without any entry into the peritubular interstitial fluid. Note that in humans intracellular urate is derived exclusively from ambient urate transported into the cell, whilst in other mammals, additional synthesis of urate dependent upon the presence of xanthine oxidoreductase also occurs within the cell.

Recent advances in understanding the transport of uric acid in the human kidney

Ideas of the handling of uric acid by the kidney have changed greatly during the past decade from the 'classical' four-component model: (Levinson and Sorensen 1980; Weiner 1979) filtration, reabsorption, secretion, and finally postsecretory reabsorption. These changes (Roch-Ramel and Dietzi 1997; Lipkowitz *et al.* 2001; Grassl 2002a,b) came about first, from studies of uric acid transport in the pig, and thereafter in membrane vesicles from the proximal tubule of a variety of species including human kidney specimens obtained at surgery; and second from the characterization, isolation, and cloning of transporters, as well as channels mainly or exclusively restricted to urate transport. This work is progressing rapidly but is still incomplete, so that a satisfactory account of urate transport in the renal tubule cannot yet be given (Fig. 1). Importantly, we do not know yet if all proximal tubular (S1–S3) cells express transporters equally, and are capable of both secreting and/or reabsorbing urate. Humans clearly retain an apical secretory flux of urate despite net reabsorption, probably because of ancestral transporters similar to those found in exclusively secreting species, as well in other urate-reabsorbing species.

Urate transport in the proximal tubular brush border

In isolated membrane vesicles from rat and dog urate reabsorptive transport across the brush-border membrane is indirectly coupled to sodium transport (Roch-Ramel and Diezi 1997), depending on the entry of sodium together with an anion (such as an organic acid) into the tubular cell, which in turn permits exit of the anion in exchange for entry of urate. The human anion exchanger has been cloned and characterized as a 40 kDa protein designated URAT-1 (Enomoto *et al.* 2002): the gene, SLC22A12 located at chromosome 11q13, is 42 per cent homologous to the already described organic ion transporter OAT4 (see below). On histochemistry, URAT-1 is present in the luminal brush border of human renal proximal tubules. As in the dog and rat vesicles (Roch-Ramel and Guisan 1999), the exchanger has a high affinity for urate together with lactate, ketones, ketoglutarate, and related compounds. However, in contrast to the rat and dog vesicle data [but in agreement with data from human tubular vesicles (Roch-Ramel *et al.* 1994)], hydroxyl and bicarbonate ions and *p*-aminohippurate (PAH) are not substrates. Pyrazinoate, probenecid, losartan, and benzbromarone all inhibit urate uptake in exchange for chloride at the luminal side of the cell by competition in both the human exchanger and mammalian vesicles. In the human exchanger, neither allopurinol nor xanthine/hypoxanthine are substrates, although the latter are in mammalian vesicles. Unique amongst mammals, the pig and the rabbit, like all birds (Grassl 2002a), completely lack this luminal anion exchanger (Roch Ramel and Diezi 1997) and are therefore net secretors of urate under all circumstances.

The presence of a luminal anion exchanger provides a new concept of the action of pyrazinamide (Roch-Ramel *et al.* 1994, 1997; Maesaka and Fishbane 1998; Enomoto *et al.* 2002). Pyrazinoic acid can accumulate in the cell by cotransport with Na^+ across the luminal membrane with other anions, and thus can serve as an exchange partner for urate and thereby stimulate urate reabsorption. The greater the intratubular concentration of pyrazinoic acid, the more it will displace urate from the external transport site on the anion exchanger. Ultimately, this competitive effect predominates and urate reabsorption is reduced.

Secretion of urate at the luminal brush border appears mediated principally by a voltage-sensitive transporter (or transporters). Obviously it has been easier to define this mechanism in urate-secreting species in whom the anion-exchange reabsorptive exchanger just described is absent. Grassl (2002a) has defined the functional characteristics of the avian transporter in detail using brush-border vesicles from the turkey. It seems likely that evolution has conserved many features of this transporter into mammals including humans, although this has yet to be shown. Martinez *et al.* (1990) and Knorr *et al.* (1994) described a voltage-dependent transporter in brush-border vesicles from the rabbit, and Krick *et al.* (2000) a similar electrogenic channel in the pig which, like the avian channel, transported both PAH and urate competitively. Urate transport via this channel was inhibited by losartan and probenecid but not pyrazinoate, as was the avian channel (Grassl 2002a). Unlike in rat, pig, and rabbit, in humans PAH does not appear to compete (Roch-Ramel and Diezi 1997).

In parallel with these studies of functional transport in kidney cells and membranes, the genomic sequence of a putative voltage-sensitive urate acid transporter (UAT) has been generated through screening of rat cortical cell membranes using a polyclonal antibody against uricase. Its gene has been described and cloned in rats (rUAT) (Leal-Pinto *et al.* 1997), subsequently in humans (hUAT) (Lipkowitz *et al.* 2001) and pigs (Spitzenberger *et al.* 2001) and is localized to the short arm of chromosome 17 in humans. The protein's urate-transporting function is suggested by its transmembrane structure, and demonstrated by insertion of the expressed protein into lipid bilayers. It is present throughout tissues, suggesting it may play a role in export of urate from cells. One isoform is also present in the intestine, and presumably could subserve urate secretion throughout the gut. The electronegativity of the cell interior with respect to the tubular lumen normally induces net secretion of urate from cells, and in theory could do so at either the luminal or the basolateral membrane of the renal proximal tubular cell. Pyrazinoate inhibits this voltage-sensitive carrier from the luminal side (Leal-Pinto *et al.* 1999), which suggests the action of this drug could be more complex than thought. Xanthine also competes. Despite early supposition from cross-immunoreactivity that the transporter was a uricase-like molecule (Knorr *et al.* 1994), its structure proved to be almost identical to that of galectin-9 (Lipkowitz *et al.* 2001).

At the moment the relationship between UAT and the electrogenic transporters described in renal proximal tubular vesicles from urate-secreting species remains unclear. Spitzenberger *et al.* (2000) cloned pig and human galectin-9, and were only able to demonstrate modest urate transport with one form of the porcine molecule transfected into HEK 293 cells, which however did not reproduce the transport characteristics previously described for the porcine apical electrogenic transporter (Krick *et al.* 2000), with zero transport under physiological conditions. Thus, the transport of urate via the cloned UAT has been demonstrated so far only in lipid bilayers, and not in renal tubular or other cells. Only the cloning of the human and or other mammalian apical electrogenic transporters can resolve these current difficulties of interpretation.

Urate transport in the basolateral membrane

Much less is known about basolateral urate transport, and almost nothing in humans. In species with net secretion, clearly urate transport into the tubular cell from peritubular capillaries must be predominant: Grassl (2002b) has described transport in turkey basolateral membrane vesicles as a chloride-dependent, ketoglutarate-coupled exchanger. In secreting mammalian species such as the pig anion exchanger is also present in the basolateral membrane with an affinity for urate and α-ketoglutarate, which permits transport of urate against a gradient into the cell. This exchanger seems absent in humans, however (Roch-Ramel and Diezi 1997). A suggested urate/chloride anion exchanger is probably an artefact of electrogenic transport. Recently, two members of the organic ion transporter (OAT) family, OAT1 and OAT3, have been characterized and are coded for at chromosome q11.7 (Sekine *et al.* 2000). The OAT family includes multispecific anion transporters, important in the excretion of many xenobiotics as well as endogenous anions. They are present in the basolateral membranes of proximal renal tubular cells in both animals and humans; in rats, Tojo *et al.* (1999) have shown rOAT1 to be basolaterally located and confined to the S2 segment. OAT1 mediates uptake of PAH in exchange for ketoglutarate and could be an important basolateral PAH transporter in reabsorbing mammals. However, there is controversy whether human hOATs are capable of facilitating uptake of urate into the tubular cell: hOAT1 inserted into mouse S_2 proximal tubular cells was reported by Ichida *et al.* (2000) to transport urate, whereas Hosoyamada *et al.* (1999) reported that high concentrations (2 mM) of urate inhibited PAH uptake by hOAT-1 in *Xenopus* oocytes; however, Race *et al.* (1999) reported that this was not so. Polkowski and Grassl (1993) described in the rat an additional voltage-sensitive pathway resulting in net urate transport from tubular cell into the interstitium, which could be the same transporter as present also in the luminal brush border, set to export urate by the negative charge within the cell relative to the outside. In urate-reabsorbing species such as rat and humans, this or a similar transporter could be the dominant mechanism of urate transport from cell to blood, but this is speculation.

Endogenous or exogenous factors affecting uric acid handling by the human kidney

Many factors (Table 1) alter renal tubular handling of urate/uric acid, and hence the plasma urate concentration. A number of pharmacological compounds in common use have a biphasic effect on urate excretion (Roch-Ramel and Weiner 1980): at low doses they lead to retention of urate, whereas at increased doses they are uricosuric. They include salicylate, phenylbutazone and other cyclo-oxygenase inhibitors, pyrazinamide, probenecid, and nicotinate. All uricosuric agents so far studied, except possibly benzbromarone and sulfinpyrazone, exhibit this biphasic response. In general this does not matter, because at the usually employed dosages they are always uricosuric. However salicylates are important in that low doses are often employed that can cause urate retention rather than uricosuria. The uricosuric effect of aspirin correlates closely with the urine salicylate concentration, which increases due to saturation of its metabolism to salicylurate (the principal metabolite at low doses) by the liver (Diamond 1989).

Factors which reduce the clearance of uric acid and induce hyperuricaemia

Several physiological and pathological agents reduce urate excretion and hence increase plasma urate concentration (Roch-Ramel and Diezi 1997) (Table 1). Any of these, therefore, may lead to an acute attack of gout in a susceptible individual whose plasma urate is already marginally increased by a reduced FE_{ur}.

Table 1 Substances that alter renal tubular handling of urate

Endogenous	Exogenous
Substances that decrease urate excretion	
Lactate	Salicylate (low doses)
β-Hydroxybutyrate	Pyrazinamide
Acetoacetate	Nicotinate
	Ethambutol
	Lead
	Beryllium
	Diuretics[a]
	Cyclosporin[a]
Substances that increase urate excretion	
Pregnancy[a]	Saline infusion[a]
	Sulfinpyrazone
	Benzbromarone
	Phenylbutazone
	Probenecid
	Radiocontrast agents
	Mega-dose vitamin C
	High-dose salicylate (>3 g)
	Fenofibrate
	Losartan

[a] Through effects on circulating volume and renal perfusion; diuretics are uricosuric initially, but lead to urate retention in chronic use.

Plasma volume contraction from inadequate intake, loss of fluid from diarrhoea or vomiting or administration of some diuretics increases fractional urate reabsorption, together with proximal tubular reabsorption of Na^+ and HCO_3^- (Cameron and Simmonds 1981) presumably due to the indirect sodium coupling of the urate anion exchanger. Repletion studies indicate that the major effector is the volume depletion, probably through physical factors resulting from renal vasoconstriction and a high filtration fraction, with consequent lower hydrostatic and higher oncotic pressures in blood traversing the peritubular capillaries. Thus, for example, severe gout and renal failure are a feature of chronic volume depletion in hereditary chloride-losing enteropathy, a recessive disorder found in Kuwait and Finland (Nuki *et al.* 1992). The appearance of gout in patients treated with diuretics (Kahn 1988) over long periods is well known, and currently accounts for over 50 per cent of new patients attending gout clinics (Meyers and Monteagudo 1985). The number of elderly females in this group is unusually high. The mode of clinical presentation is frequently atypical and leads to misdiagnosis (Platt and Dick 1985). In addition, renal vasoconstrictors such as adrenaline and noradrenaline, angiotensin, cyclosporin (see below) and some cyclo-oxygenase inhibitors as well as insulin (Muscelli *et al.* 1996) reduce urate clearance also.

The best-known physiological substances which decrease urate excretion and lead to hyperuricaemia are organic acids such as lactate, acetoacetate, and β-hydroxybutyrate; their overproduction explains in part the hyperuricaemia associated with status epilepticus or with excessive alcohol consumption (Faller and Fox 1982). The putative mechanisms of intracellular accumulation of these acids through the indirect sodium coupling and the anion transporter is discussed above. Chronic lead intoxication leads to a decrease in urate excretion by an undetermined mechanism as discussed in detail below and in Chapter 6.5; early renal failure is a prominent manifestation, but arthritis ('saturnine' gout) is usually mild. That the decrease in FE_{ur} in lead intoxication is reversible (at least initially) is shown by short-term studies involving chelation therapy (Lin *et al.* 2003).

The best-known pharmacological agents reducing urate excretion are the antituberculous drugs pyrazinamide and ethambutol; it is now believed that pyrazinoate stimulates uptake by the brush-border anion exchanger. Of the agents that are uricosuric at greater doses, benzbromarone was originally considered to be unique in that, unlike other agents, it was not carried by the proximal tubular organic acid transport system, and therefore did not appear to compete directly with urate for whatever carrier is present. However, excretion of benzbromarone and its metabolites *in vivo* is extremely low (Walter-Sack 1988), and urate retention with the drug has been described (Sommers and Schoenman 1987). It completely inhibits urate uptake by URAT-1 expressed into *Xenopus* oocytes (Enomoto *et al.* 2002), and is the most potent uricosuric agent available today, able to reduce plasma urate even in severe renal disease (Roch-Ramel *et al.* 1997; Grahame *et al.* 1998).

Factors which increase uric acid clearance and induce hypouricaemia

Causes of hypouricaemia include xanthine oxidoreductase deficiency, and acquired or inherited tubular defects leading to reduced urate reabsorption, discussed in Chapter 16.5.3. The circumstances that lead to an increase in uric acid excretion and a reduction of plasma urate are listed in Table 1 (Maesaka and Fishbane 1998; Sperling 2001). Excessive excretion of urate can uncommonly lead to crystalluria, colic stones and, rarely to acute obstructive renal failure.

Many states of circulatory volume expansion are associated with hyponatraemia and increased FE_{ur}. Such volume expansion—brought about by the inappropriate secretion of antidiuretic hormone (ADH) (Prospert *et al.* 1993)—may explain in part some of the hypouricaemias seen occasionally in patients with malignant disease. It may also explain the increased urate excretion and hypouricaemia during early pregnancy, by the converse of the explanation outlined in the previous section to account for the lowered urinary urate excretion in hypovolaemia. However, this simplistic view has been challenged recently (Maesaka and Fishbane 1998) since effects on FE_{ur} are modest or absent during acute or chronic studies of water infusion in normal subjects. Decaux *et al.* (1997, 2000) have suggested that the chronically low plasma sodium concentration present in many volume-expanded patients increases the FE_{ur} directly and independently of volume, perhaps through interactions with the V1 (but not the V2) receptor for ADH in the renal tubule (see Chapter 5.6).

On occasion the increased excretion of urate following administration of probenecid, sulfinpyrazone or benzbromarone may lead to acute renal failure, through precipitation of uric acid in the tubules (Keidar *et al.* 1982). Massive doses of vitamin C are also uricosuric and may lead to mixed crystalluria or stones from oxalate as a metabolic product of ascorbic acid together with urate. Other agents such as most radiocontrast media, warfarin, corticosteroids, and antibiotics such as ampicillin are also uricosuric (Sommers and Schoenman 1987). Their use in patients with genetic uric acid overproduction acutely exacerbated by excessive cell turnover such as in glandular fever (Dylewski and Gerson 1985) has also led to acute renal failure (Cameron *et al.* 1984).

Two agents have a potentially valuable uricosuric effect additive to their main effect: losartan and fenofibrate. Losartan, an angiotensin II (AT1) receptor blocker, is effective (Burnier *et al.* 1996) and safe

(Shahinfar *et al.* 1999) in lowering plasma urate concentrations although the effect may be slight (Puig *et al.* 1999). This effect is not shared with other AT1 antagonists and so must result from some aspect of the unique structure of losartan rather than a general effect of AT1 blockade, such as direct interaction with the brush-border anion transporter (Edwards *et al.* 1996). Losartan is effective in inhibiting urate uptake by URAT-1 in *Xenopus* oocytes (Enomoto *et al.* 2002). Fenofibrate is a hypolipidaemic agent often given to subjects with vascular disease; it strongly reduces plasma urate concentrations (Elisaf *et al.* 1999). Again, its action on tubular urate handling has not yet been explored fully. Some amino acids are uricosuric, particularly glycine, and this may account in part for the low plasma urate concentrations in patients receiving parenteral nutrition.

Hypouricaemia is found occasionally in many malignant disorders such as Hodgkin's disease (Tykarski 1988), leukaemias (Mir and Delamore 1974), and carcinomas (Mitnick and Beck 1979). In some cases it reversed following successful treatment but returned with relapse (Bennett *et al.* 1972). The exact mechanisms of this hypouricaemia remain obscure (Maesaka and Fishbane 1998). Hypouricaemia is seen also in patients with various intracranial lesions and with AIDS (Maesaka and Fishbane 1998), as well as in poisoning by *Amanita phalloides* (Zawadowski *et al.* 1993). Hyperuricosuria of obscure origin with visibly pink urine has been reported in morbidly obese patients following intestinal bypass surgery (Saran *et al.* 1998). Finally, the increased urate clearance in the Dalmatian dog, often attributed to the presence of a transport defect in kidney, has been attributed also to an abnormal metabolite produced in the liver (Briggs and Sperling 1982).

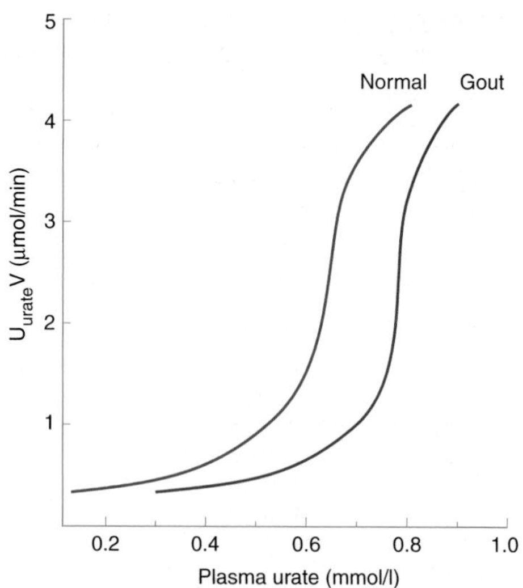

Fig. 2 The relationship between plasma urate at different purine intakes, at low and high fractional excretion of urate. The FE_{ur} 'sets' the plasma urate at different levels at a constant intake of purine, and, if low, renders the individual vulnerable to plasma urate concentrations that carry a high risk of an acute attack of gout. Thus typical middle-aged gout is fundamentally a disorder depending upon abnormal or unusual tubular urate transport, aggravated by a high purine intake.

Gout and renal failure

Urate handling in classical gout of middle age

In the overwhelming majority of middle-aged, predominantly male patients with gout, hyperuricaemia results from a polygenically inherited tendency to a reduced FE_{ur} (Short 1992) (Fig. 2), coupled almost always with a large intake of dietary purine. In middle-aged (42–57 years) male gouty patients, the mean tubular reabsorption is about 95 per cent (FE_{ur} of 5.4 per cent) compared with 91.9 per cent (FE_{ur} 8.1 per cent) in controls (Gibson *et al.* 1982). Plasma urate concentration is thus higher than in controls for the same level of uric acid excretion (Fig. 2). Production of urate, as judged by urate excretion on a purine-free diet is now known to be normal, despite earlier statements. In individuals without renal impairment the risk of attacks of gout is directly related to the urate concentration, from negligible at 300 µmol/l to almost certain, given time, at 600 µmol/l or greater.

A genetic basis for 'classical' gout is suggested by the strong family association amongst gouty patients, which has been known since antiquity and was emphasized by Thomas Sydenham in the seventeenth century. The high prevalence of hyperuricaemia and low FE_{ur} in some races such as Polynesians (Gibson *et al.* 1984; Simmonds *et al.* 1994) and Australian aboriginals, as well as studies of concordance in twins (Emmerson *et al.* 1992; Short 1992) (84 per cent in monozygotic and 43 per cent for dizygotic) supports this suggestion. Short (1992) suggests that segregation of a major dominant gene against a polygenic background best explains their critically evaluated data, a hypothesis obscured in some studies by diet, environmental factors such as obesity, alcohol and (probably) occult lead intoxication, and inclusion of some families with monogenic dominantly inherited familial juvenile hyperuricaemic nephropathy (FJHN). Plasma uric acid concentrations in gouty patients are smoothly distributed in a Gaussian fashion, with the mean shifted towards higher concentrations compared with normals (Fig. 2). Although large population studies are lacking, this is almost certainly true also for FE_{ur}. In view of the recent data outlined above it is likely to be the result of enhanced reabsorption. Few candidate genes are yet available for testing, as the renal tubular handling of urate is complex, still poorly understood, and the gene or genes in the monogenic dominant forms of renal hyperuricaemia such as FJHN are only now being identified and cloned (see Chapter 16.5.3).

Gout as a complication of renal failure

Clinical gout secondary to chronic renal failure is rare (Vecchio and Emmerson 1992). It was noted in only 17 of 1600 patients with uraemia even before allopurinol became available (Richet *et al.* 1965) and in only 13 of 201 patients on maintenance haemodialysis (Ifudu *et al.* 1994), despite greatly increased concentrations of urate in the plasma. It has been suggested that the uraemic environment inhibits the induction of inflammation (Buchanan *et al.* 1995; Schreiner *et al.* 2000). In agreement with this Ifudu *et al.* (1994) found that patients who had had gouty attacks before they entered end-stage renal disease no longer had attacks during dialysis, despite persisting or even greater plasma urate. This does not explain why the acute inflammation of pseudogout, arising from precipitation of calcium pyrophosphate, is common in untreated or poorly treated uraemia.

If a patient with chronic renal impairment or on dialysis *does* have a history of gout, or develops gout, three possibilities arise, namely that the patient may have:

(1) Evident or occult lead intoxication (see also Chapter 6.5).

(2) An inherited partial deficiency of hypoxanthine-guanine phosphoribosyltransferase (HPRT) (Chapter 16.5.3). These patients are generally young, or even children, and almost always male because

HPRT deficiency is an X-linked condition. However, they may present later in life only when renal failure has supervened.

(3) Inherited FJHN (Chapter 16.5.3)—again, these patients are invariably young adults or even children, and the male : female ratio is close to unity. The unusual finding of a young female with gout and renal failure is frequent in this group.

Effect of renal failure on renal handling of urate

In endstage uraemia, although the plasma concentrations of urea and creatinine may increase 30–40-fold, that of urate does not (Fig. 3a) which is fortunate since this would be fatal. Up to about twice the normal plasma concentration of creatinine, the plasma concentration of uric acid increases approximately in parallel with creatinine. Beyond this point, the concentration of urate in the plasma flattens off, despite a further reduction in the glomerular filtration rate, so that it remains twice normal in individuals with end-stage uraemia.

Total uric acid excretion in uraemia declines (Emmerson and Row 1975), raising the possibility of a decreased urate production, perhaps through feedback inhibition. Studies using [^{15}N] glycine plus [^{13}C] urate (Löffler *et al.* 1987) support this concept. In renal failure, in parallel with tubular rejection of sodium and a number of other solutes, FE_{ur} progressively increases from around 10 per cent to as much as 85 per cent in advanced renal failure (Danovitch *et al.* 1972; Colussi *et al.* 1987) (Fig. 3b). A consequence in patients with an initially subnormal FE_{ur} who develop renal failure, just at the point when their retention of urea and creatinine is barely evident FE_{ur} becomes, at least for a time, normal and diagnosis is thus rendered difficult (Calabrese *et al.* 1990). Precisely how adaptation in renal urate handling occurs is not clear. As a consequence of the increase in FE_{ur} normally uricosuric agents such as probenecid become ineffective as the plasma creatinine increases above 250 μmol/l (see below). However, benzbromarone can reduce plasma urate in subjects with a plasma creatinine as high as 500 mol/l (Grahame *et al.* 1998). Some compounds retained in uraemia appear uricosuric, for example, indoxyl sulfate or hippurates (Boumendil-Podevin *et al.* 1975). A role for increased flow rate in the tubular lumen has also been suggested (Löffler *et al.* 1983), implying that a combination of factors may be responsible for this adaptation to the uraemic state.

Finally, enhanced extrarenal secretion through the gut, from a normal one-third to two-thirds of total, is present in uraemia (Sorensen and Levinson 1975; Sorensen 1980) and contributes to the reduced urinary uric acid excretion in renal failure.

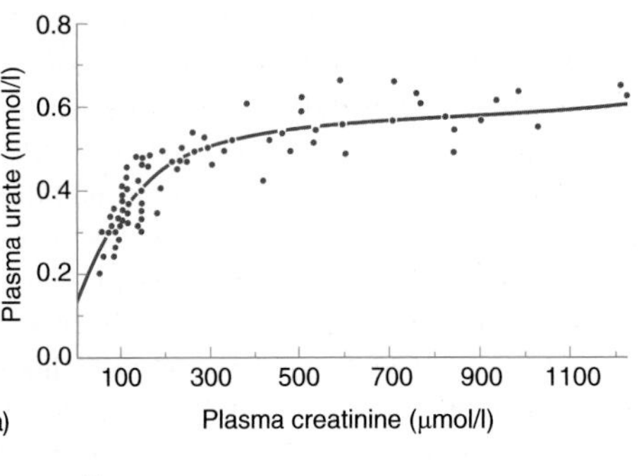

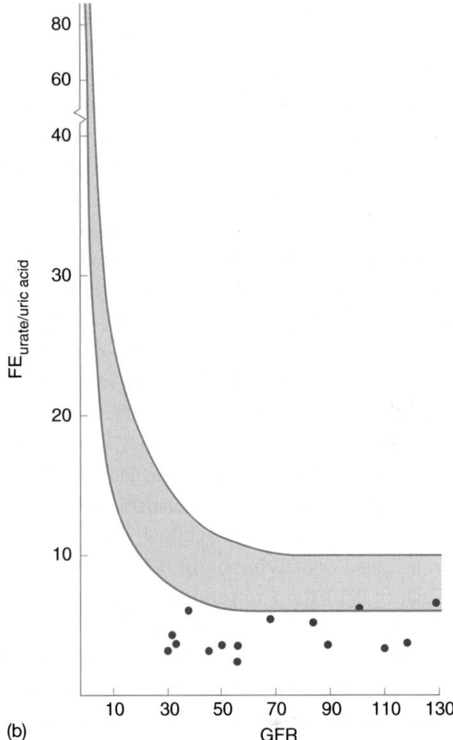

Fig. 3 (a) The relationship between plasma urate and plasma creatinine in patients with chronic renal failure. Initially the plasma urate increases at the same rate as the plasma creatinine, but as the plasma creatinine increases further the plasma urate concentration does not, because of an increase in FE_{ur}, increased excretion of urate, and uricolysis in the gut. (b) FE_{ur} at various degrees of renal insufficiency. The fractional excretion increases rapidly as glomerular filtration rate declines, in parallel with sodium and a number of other solutes, to reach 85 per cent or more of filtered urate in extreme renal failure (data of Danovitch *et al.* 1972). This, along with increased uricolysis in the gut, serves to limit the increase in plasma urate in uraemia. The points represent data from patients with familial juvenile gouty nephropathy, illustrating the very low FE_{ur} in these patients, especially in relation to their reduced renal function. (From Calabrese *et al.* 1990.)

'Gouty nephropathy': chronic renal disease in gout

The nature of 'gouty nephropathy'—or even its existence as such (Beck 1986; Nickeleit and Mihatsch 1997)—has been the subject of much debate in recent years. Part of the confusion relates to the fact that we can now recognize at least four main varieties of patients with gout, who were previously grouped together. In patients with 'classical' gout, normal urate production but a high purine intake and low FE_{ur} renal function is generally normal for age and remains so (Berger and Yü 1975; Gibson *et al.* 1982). In young patients or even children of either gender with familial gout there is a high incidence of rapidly progressive renal disease and a very reduced FE_{ur}; again production of uric acid is normal or low (see Chapter 16.5.3). Then there are patients with (usually occult) lead intoxication (Bennett 1985 and see Chapter 6.5). Finally, rare patients such as a partial deficiency of the salvage enzyme HPRT (see Chapter 16.5.3), have an increased production and excretion of uric acid. Their kidneys may show extensive crystal deposits. Undoubtedly, many cases of apparently 'primary' gout with severe renal involvement described in the past fell into one of the three last categories.

Renal disease in 'primary' gout

In the past, even in typical male gout of middle age, the incidence of renal involvement approached 100 per cent, and 20–80 per cent of patient deaths were recorded as the result of uraemia (Brown and Mallory 1950; Talbott and Terplan 1960; Barlow and Beilin 1968). Today, just as gout is rare in renal failure, it is equally true that renal failure is rare in patients aged about 50–60 years with 'primary' or classical gout (Berger and Yü 1975; Gibson *et al.* 1982; Nickeleit and Mihatsch 1997). In the absence of hypertension (Yü and Berger 1982), renal function remains stable, although abnormalities of urinary sediment and mild proteinuria are common. Reduced renal function has been reported in Taiwan in mixed groups of gouty patients, especially those with tophi or with hypertension (Tarng *et al.* 1995). However, the prevalence of occult lead intoxication is high in Taiwan (Lin *et al.* 2003). The only renal abnormality invariably present is the already mentioned low FE_{ur} (mean 5.4 per cent, Gibson *et al.* 1982).

The reason for this apparently much greater prevalence of renal failure in 'primary' gout in the past remains uncertain. Some suggest that *all* the renal damage followed the associated vascular disease of gout (Yü and Berger 1982) which is now more effectively treated, while others see a central role for the deposition of uric acid or urate crystals within the kidney (Emmerson and Row 1975; Cameron and Simmonds 1981). The background to the decline in the mortality from renal failure in gout is equally impossible to determine, but relates both to moderation of purine intake on the one hand, and the more effective treatment, first with uricosuric agents and then with allopurinol on the other. Another factor may be a decline in the incidence of chronic lead intoxication, which was undoubtedly a major factor in the 'epidemic' of gout in the eighteenth century England (see Chapter 6.5).

The origin of the renal lesion (Fig. 4) has also been the subject of debate. Some saw it as primarily due to interstitial sodium urate deposits (Barlow and Beilin 1968; Emmerson and Row 1975) others the erosion of precipitated uric acid crystals out of the tubules into the interstitium (Brown and Mallory 1950; Cameron and Simmonds 1981). In the interstitium of the kidney the ambient pH is that of plasma (around 7.37), the principal species of purine being the needle-shaped sodium urate monohydrate (Gresser and Zöllner 1991). However, within the tubules, where pH may be 5.0 or less, the predominant species will be amorphous uric acid, as in patients with acute overproduction of urate or hyperuricaemic nephropathy due to treatment of myeloid malignancies with cytotoxic drugs (see below). Both mechanisms could operate in chronic gouty nephropathy (Emmerson and Row 1975); both uric acid and sodium urate are able to generate inflammation with secondary scarring.

It is easy to miss the presence of uric acid crystals in the interstitium and tubules in histology specimens. Water-based fixatives wash out uric acid/urate, and the amorphous uric acid leaves no visible 'clefts' behind. Specimens need to be fixed in alcohol, or frozen and viewed under polarized light. Specific stains for urate are also available. Crystals may also disappear with time as shown in experimental studies of crystal nephropathy (Farebrother *et al.* 1975). Moreover, most needle biopsies contain only cortex, with little or no medulla, which is the predominant site of urate deposition. Non-crystal-dependent urate-mediated vascular and renal damage in a rat model of hyperuricaemia (Mazzali *et al.* 2001a, 2002) is discussed in more detail below.

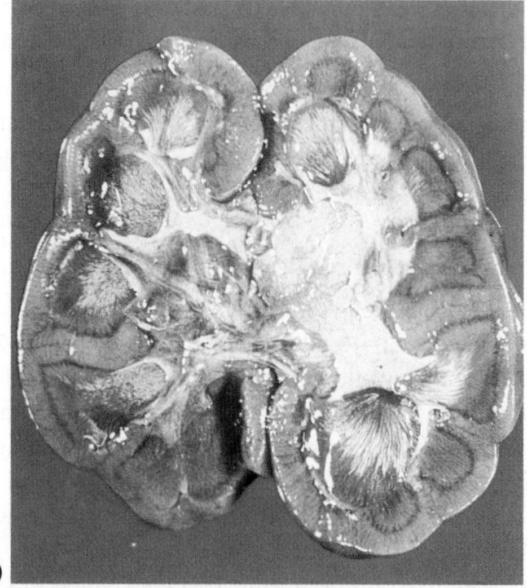
(a)

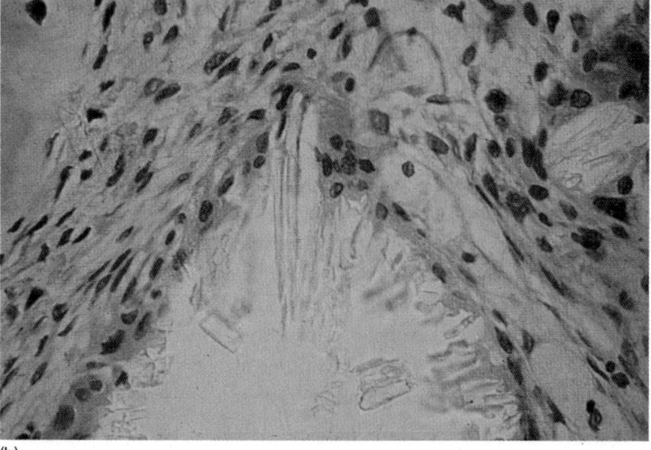
(b)

Fig. 4 (a) The typical appearance of the kidney in acute urate nephropathy, with linear streaks of uric acid/urate crystals outlining the cortical and medullary tubules, as first noted by Garrod in 1848. This appearance is today almost never seen, except in patients with overproduction of urate, either because of tumour lysis or inherited enzyme disorders such as deficiency of HPRT (see Chapter 16.5.3) (reproduced with permission from Mohr 1991). (b) At a microscopic level, crystals of monosodium urate can be seen within the renal parenchyma, surrounded by a cellular reaction, which may contain giant cells. Again, this appearance is now rarely seen except in gouty patients with overproduction, or in acute hyperuricaemic renal failure. Exactly how these renal tophi form has been the subject of controversy (see text).

How should we treat typical chronic gouty nephropathy?

The unresolved question as to whether urate or uric acid is implicated in the renal lesion has led to the belief that in gouty patients with renal impairment it is best to reduce urate production with allopurinol, which should be effective in either case. Whilst this is in general the right approach, two other important factors should be taken into consideration.

The first is that the active metabolite of allopurinol, oxipurinol, is handled by the human kidney in a fashion akin to uric acid (Graham *et al.* 1996; Roch-Ramel and Guisan 1999) and thus, unlike its parent drug which is freely filtered and excreted, is actively reabsorbed in the tubule by the brush-border anion exchanger. Therefore, even in patients with normal kidney function, it has a long half-life and its clearance is affected by all the events which affect urate clearance, including volume status (Hande 1986). Since it is also retained in renal failure (Fig. 5) and

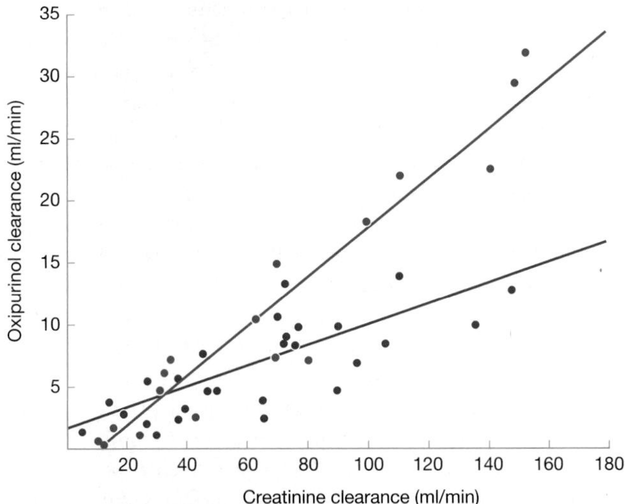

Fig. 5 The relationship between plasma oxipurinol and plasma creatinine in two groups of patients. Those with chronic renal failure from common causes (•) (data of Hande *et al.* 1984) show retention of oxipurinol in proportion to the degree of renal failure, and hence dosage of allopurinol must be reduced as renal function declines. However, our data from patients with a low FE_{ur} and familial juvenile hyperuricaemic nephropathy (•) (see Chapter 16.5.3) show even greater oxipurinol retention, because oxipurinol is reabsorbed, like urate, in the proximal tubule. The same effect is achieved as an unwanted side-effect in patients with a normal FE_{ur} by use of diuretics, which reduce plasma volume and lower FE_{ur} (see text).

in patients with a low FE_{ur}, and such retention is exaggerated by concomitant diuretics (Hande *et al.* 1984), the dose of allopurinol must be reduced to as little as 100 mg daily or even 100 mg three times weekly in advanced renal failure (Cameron and Simmonds 1987). The objective is to keep the plasma oxipurinol concentration around 100 μmol/l (Hande *et al.* 1984; Simmonds *et al.* 1986) well above the maximum inhibitory concentration for xanthine oxidoreductase (~20 mol/l) (Graham *et al.* 1996) and thus minimize the serious risk of bone marrow depression or other undesirable side-effects, which include epidermal necrolysis and hepatotoxicity. One study has pointed to the poor response to allopurinol in heavy drinkers (Ralston *et al.* 1988) and related this to the combined effect of ethanol in impairing urate excretion as well as increasing its production (Faller and Fox 1982).

Thus, agents such as benzbromarone (Perez-Ruiz *et al.* 2000)—might better serve the purpose of reducing the plasma urate in renal impairment. This strategy avoids allopurinol and its potentially serious side-effects. To complicate things further, uricosuric drugs such as probenecid may also interfere with the tubular transport of diuretics such as frusemide (Roch-Ramel and Diezi 1997).

Lead intoxication, saturnine gout, and renal failure

Hyperuricaemia and gout have long been recognized as complications following chronic lead intoxication (Bennett 1985, and see Chapter 6.5 for full discussion). The role of lead poisoning in the high incidence of renal disease associated with hyperuricaemia was described by Campbell and colleagues in 1977 (see Emmerson 1991). The reason for the reduced urate clearance is not established with certainty. Nolan and Shaik (1992) contend that lead interacts with renal membranes, ion transport and the renin–angiotensin system. Lin *et al.* (2003) demonstrated an increase in urate excretion after lead chelation therapy. It has also been related in part to extracellular fluid volume contraction (see above), since chronic lead intoxication may be accompanied by hyporeninaemic hypoaldosteronism.

The body burden of lead was shown to be greater in patients with gout as well as chronic renal failure submitted to an infusion of edetate, than that of age- and gender-matched controls with only renal failure (Colleoni and D'Amico 1986) and in patients submitted to lead chelation therapy, renal function improved (Lin *et al.* 2003). Most patients had no history of exposure to lead even on careful questioning. It seems likely that occult chronic lead poisoning plays a larger role in the genesis of otherwise obscure chronic renal failure than has been realized (Lin and Huang 1994) although this view has been contested (Nuyts *et al.* 1991). Exactly how the kidney is damaged in saturnine gout is not clear, but a direct toxic effect of lead on renal epithelia appears more likely than any role of uric acid/urate, whose increased reabsorption is probably a secondary phenomenon.

Gout in transplant recipients

Hyperuricaemia and gout were first noticed in renal transplant recipients before cyclosporin was introduced (Flury *et al.* 1977) but have become much more common since the use of this drug has become routine (Clive 2000). As many as 75–80 per cent of heart transplant recipients cumulatively suffer clinical gout while taking cyclosporin (Burack *et al.* 1992) and a similar but lower incidence (7–25 per cent) of gout has been noted in renal transplantation (Clive 2000), even in children (Laine and Holmberg 1996), the prevalence increasing with time. Although cyclosporin may inhibit secretion of urate (Marcén *et al.* 1995; Laine and Holmberg 1996) it is also a potent renal vasoconstrictor, inducing a fall in GFR and an increase in filtration fraction, perhaps the principal mechanism of action (Zürcher *et al.* 1996; Hansen *et al.* 1998). In addition, Mazzali *et al.* (2001b) showed that high urate concentrations worsened cyclosporin toxicity in the rat. In some (Noordzij *et al.* 1991; Marcén *et al.* 1995) but not in all studies, the effect of concomitant diuretic therapy is important. Allograft dysfunction with some degree of renal failure may have an additive role. Gout in transplant patients may be atypical, affecting proximal joints; combined deposition of urate and pyrophosphate may be observed (Cohen 1994). The body burden of urate may be large and tophi are relatively common, together with deposition of urate at extra-articular sites such as tendons, which may confuse and delay diagnosis. Tacrolimus, another calcineurin inhibitor, has been reported to cause hyperuricaemia as well (Ochiai *et al.* 1995) but actual gout seems not to be common.

Treatment of hyperuricaemia and gout following transplantation may not be easy, especially if there is graft dysfunction. In the acute attack the usual dose of colchicine (0.6 mg 6 hourly) is effective, but is slow to work and unpleasant to take because of the diarrhoea it induces. On occasion it provokes a neuromyopathy, which is more likely in the presence of diminished renal function so that dosage reduction is often needed (Clive 2000); a brief course of high-dose corticosteroids is better. Either are preferable to using conventional non-steroidal anti-inflammatory agents which can be used safely only if renal function is monitored closely. Cox-2 inhibitors may prove more satisfactory, but data are lacking so far. Diet may need attention in some indulgent patients to prevent further attacks, and diuretics should be avoided if at all possible. Obviously one would like to use allopurinol to inhibit urate formation and with careful attention to the white cell count it can be employed together with azathioprine (Chocair *et al.* 1993). However it is better to avoid allopurinol altogether under these circumstances, because severe or even fatal marrow depression can ensue because the active metabolite of azathioprine, 6-mercaptopurine, is also metabolized by xanthine oxidoreductase to 6-thiouric acid (Raman *et al.* 1990).

Another strategy is to modify the immunosuppressive regime, either by withdrawing cyclosporin or transferring the patient on to mycophenolate instead of azathioprine, which can be combined safely with allopurinol (Jacobs *et al.* 1997; Navascues *et al.* 2002). If one still wishes to continue with azathioprine then probenecid, or better benzbromarone (Zürcher *et al.* 1994; Perez-Ruiz *et al.* 2003) can be used as uricosuric agents. However, these are reportedly ineffective when the plasma creatinine exceeds 250–300 μmol/l (Flury *et al.* 1977; Zürcher *et al.* 1994) but others put the limit at 500 mol/l (Grahame *et al.* 1998). In addition losartan (but not other AT1 inhibitors, see above) as well as fenofibrate reduces urate concentrations and increases FE_{ur} in transplant recipients modestly (Kamper and Nielsen 2001), and might be preferred to lower blood pressure or lipids. In heart transplant recipients, injections of uricase have been used (Rozenberg *et al.* 1995). As discussed above, dosage of allopurinol must be adjusted for renal dysfunction (Cameron and Simmonds 1987).

In contrast, hypouricaemia and hyperuricosuria as well as uric acid stones (Norlén *et al.* 1995) and, in one case report acute hyperuricaemic nephropathy (Venkataseshan *et al.* 1990), have been noted in a few patients following transplantation (Schmidt *et al.* 1973).

Acute hyperuricaemic nephropathy

Acute hyperuricaemic nephropathy (Jones *et al.* 1995; Steele 1999) results from a large load of urate transiting through the kidney; volume contraction, a low urine flow rate or an acid urine decrease the solubility of uric acid within the tubular lumen. Thus precipitation of uric acid crystals occurs with tubular blockage; tubular ingestion of crystals leads to tubular necrosis, inflammation, and acute renal failure. Sludged uric acid may also fill the ureters. The kidneys are enlarged, very 'bright' on ultrasonography, the reduced urine volume contains massive amounts of uric acid crystals.

This syndrome is most commonly seen when tumours, almost always of myeloid origin (leukaemias, lymphomas, myeloma), undergo sudden lysis, usually under treatment, although it has been recorded occasionally following treatment of solid tumours. Large amounts of nucleic acid are released and rapidly degraded into urate, so that the plasma urate exceeds even 1000 μmol/l. In patients with tumour breakdown the plasma and urinary phosphate concentrations are also very high.

Acute uric acid nephropathy as well as a more chronic form of urate crystal nephropathy may be seen in the Lesch–Nyhan disease of complete HPRT deficiency, in which there is great overproduction of urate (Chapter 16.5.3). Gross overproduction of urate with hyperuricaemia and acute renal failure is also seen in rhabdomyolysis, such as from extreme exercise, use of 'angel dust' (phencylidine), crush injuries, epileptic fits, electrocution, metabolic muscle disorders, or prolonged immobilization, and here again plasma phosphate concentrations are increased. In these patients, the acute renal failure is associated with myoglobinuria, so that the role of hyperuricaemia is not clear. Finally, acute urate nephropathy can be precipitated by uricosuria from most of the uricosuric agents listed above (Keidar *et al.* 1982) (Table 1), but in the absence of urate overproduction this is very rare.

Treatment centres round prophylaxis during treatment of malignancies, with an adequate circulation and a diuresis established *before* treatment begins (Simmonds *et al.* 1986; O'Connor *et al.* 1989). Addition of either or both alkalinization and allopurinol (which again should be started before treatment) although theoretically attractive do not seem to make much difference. In addition, use of allopurinol runs the risk of inducing acute xanthine nephropathy or stones rather than urate nephropathy (Simmonds *et al.* 1986; Potter and Silvidi 1987) since xanthine is even more insoluble than uric acid and its solubility does not increase on increasing the urine pH. In the majority of treated patients the urinary concentration of xanthine exceeded its limit of solubility (Hande *et al.* 1981; Andreoli *et al.* 1986) (see Chapter 16.5.3 for xanthine nephropathy). Injections of encapsulated uricase, usually prepared from *Aspergillus* spp. have been used as acute treatment of severe hyperuricaemia in small series of patients (Jankovic *et al.* 1985; Chua *et al.* 1988; Ippoliti *et al.* 1990). However, low availability and solubility, rapid clearance and immunogenicity limited its use hitherto. Now that the mammalian gene has been cloned (Kelly et al. 2001), and recombinant PEG-uricase with a longer biological half-life (rasburicase) is more available (Ribiero and Pui 2003), it is likely that greater use will be made of this form of treatment. Dialysis will often be required to tide the patients over their renal failure, and should be by haemodialysis since urate is much less efficiently removed acutely by the peritoneal route.

Hyperuricaemia as a risk factor for hypertension, renal damage, and vascular disease

Hyperuricaemia, found in one-fourth to one-third of hypertensive subjects, is usually associated with both an increased purine intake and a reduced FE_{ur} (Culleton and Levy 2001; Johnson and Tuttle 2001). Correlations exist within and between families with alcohol intake, hyperlipidaemia, diabetes mellitus, insulin resistance, and obesity (Facchini *et al.* 1991). Changes in renal vascular resistance and perfusion may be responsible (Messerli *et al.* 1980) but the association is probably not specific, despite these authors' conclusions. Of relevance, however, urate concentrations tend to increase in patients with renal artery stenosis and improve after revascularization.

It has been suggested also that urate is an independent risk factor for vascular disease in general, and events such as strokes and myocardial infarcts, by a large—and controversial—literature beginning in the 1900s, which describes both general populations and those at high risk such as those with diabetes mellitus (Puig *et al.* 1999; Johnson *et al.* 1999; Waring *et al.* 2000; Culleton and Levy 2001). Uric acid concentrations predict the later appearance of hypertension, independent of renal function (Selby *et al.* 1990). In patients with hypertension, urate is a more powerful prognostic factor than blood glucose, lipids or even blood pressure (Alderman *et al.* 1999). However, in some studies the statistical association of urate with vascular events disappears when other risk factors such as hypertension, smoking, or hyperlipidaemia are taken into account (Culleton and Levy 2001). How these associations might be mediated is not known, but the close relationship between insulin resistance and hence high ambient insulin concentrations is worth noting; insulin causes a fall in both FE_{ur} and FE_{Na^+} and a rise in plasma urate concentrations in both hypertensive and normal individuals (Quinones *et al.* 1995; Muscelli *et al.* 1996). In this case, the increase in plasma urate would be an epiphenomenon. In contrast to other mammalian species, human vascular endothelium does not contain significant amounts of xanthine oxidoreductase [which is confined to jejunum and liver (Kooij *et al.* 1992)] and thus cannot synthesize urate from adenosine, secreted as a mediator of vascular tone in increased amounts during ischaemia (Raitikkainen *et al.* 1994) along with urate, atleast in experimental animals. Ischaemia also releases increased amounts of lactate, a powerful agent reducing FE_{ur} through its affinity for luminal URAT-1, thus creating a possible vicious cycle. In addition urate can promote LDL oxidation, at least *in vitro* (Schlotte *et al.* 1998) an important step in atherogenesis; and in microcrystalline form can promote endothelial damage by several mechanisms (reviewed in Waring *et al.* 2000).

Finally urate can induce hypertension directly in the rat (Mazzali *et al.* 2001b, 2002); treatment with low doses of the uricase inhibitor oxonic acid (Stavric *et al.* 1969), elevates uric acid concentrations modestly, and induces hypertension both systemic and glomerular (Sanchez-Lozada *et al.* 2002). Both were reversed by treatment with allopurinol, benziodarone, or oxonate withdrawal. No urate crystals were seen in the kidneys, but an ischaemic injury with hypertrophy of the juxtaglomerular apparatus and loss of NOS was present, which was inhibited by enalapril and losartan or L-arginine, but not a thiazide, even though this lowered blood pressure to a similar degree. The authors propose vascular damage by urate through a crystal- and hypertension-independent, angiotensin and NO-dependent mechanism. They also confirmed that urate in solution stimulates directly proliferation of arteriolar myocytes (Rao *et al.* 1991). In agreement with these findings, treatment of patients in heart failure with allopurinol restored endothelial cell function (Farquarson *et al.* 1999). In contrast, one must remember that as an antioxidant, urate has an important role in the neutralization of peroxynitrite which it converts to NO, thus promoting vasodilatation and protecting against oxidative damage simultaneously.

Hyperuricaemia has been incriminated as an important factor in the appearance and progression of renal impairment in general (Johnson *et al.* 1999; Kang *et al.* 2002), particularly in hypertensive patients with symptomless hyperuricaemia (Rosenfeld 1974) and in IgA nephropathy (Syrjanen *et al.* 2000; Ohono *et al.* 2001). In FJHN (see Chapter 16.5.3) and dominant MCDK (see Chapter 16.3) urate concentrations are raised while renal function is normal, as can occur in analgesic nephropathy also (Nanra *et al.* 1978). This suggestion was made more attractive by the old finding (Verger *et al.* 1967; Ostberg 1968) of urate crystals in the medulla of patients dying with uraemia from various renal disorders, not surprising since there is a normal corticomedullary gradient of urate concentration (Cannon *et al.* 1968), presumably the result of passive trapping of urate in the medulla. The studies of Mazzali *et al.* (2001a,b) in the rat, discussed above, showed that renal fibrosis in their model was dependent on hyperuricaemia and angiotensin II, but independent of crystal formation and of hypertension.

Whether in humans long-term reduction of plasma urate concentrations protects from, or reverses a fall in GFR in gout or symptomless hyperuricaemia is not known: data are scanty, generally uncontrolled and in conflict. Rosenfeld (1974) and Fessel (1979) failed to show any effect on renal function of reducing plasma urate using allopurinol in hyperuricaemic patients with hypertension or polycystic kidneys for periods of up to 2.5 years, and similar negative findings have been reported in patients with clinical gout (Berger and Yü 1975; Gibson *et al.* 1982). In contrast, Perez-Ruiz *et al.* (2000) report improvement in renal function in a group of 87 gouty patients treated with either allopurinol or benzbromarone for only a year, the improvement being particularly great in patients with a GFR less than 80 ml/min (mean 60–78 ml/min). An adequately-powered controlled trial of urate reduction in hypertensive subjects is needed rather urgently.

Uric acid stones

The aetiology, clinical features and management of uric acid stones are discussed in detail in Chapters 8.1–8.3. These need to be distinguished from the much more rare 2,8-dihydroxyadenine stones, which are also radiolucent and react in many chemical tests as urate (see Chapter 16.5.3). Both overproduction or diminished tubular reabsorption of urate will lead to urate lithiasis (see Chapter 16.5.3), as does the persistently acid urine of gout or idiopathic uricacid lithiasis (Sakhaee *et al.* 2002).

Xenotransplantation

The genetic absence of the urate exchanger on the brush border of the pig kidney (a net secretor of urate) (Simmonds *et al.* 1976) has important implications for the potential use of pig kidneys in human transplantation (Simmonds and Roch-Ramel 1994). In practical terms, this means that a human kidney, which reabsorbs around 90 per cent of filtered uric acid will be replaced by a kidney that clears uric acid in excess of the GFR. Consequently, the rapid elimination of any accumulated bolus of uric acid following successful renal transplantation could precipitate acute renal failure/uric acid nephropathy. Of even greater concern is the implication for therapeutic concentration of drugs (e.g. cyclosporin and thiazides) having affinities for this important luminal urate anion exchanger, which is absent in pig kidney.

References

Alderman, M. H., Cohen, H., Madhavan, S., and Kivlighn, S. (1999). Serum uric acid and cardiovascular events in successfully treated hypertensive patients. *Hypertension* **34**, 144–150.

Ames, B. N., Cathcart, R., Schwiers, E., and Hochstein, P. (1981). Uric acid provides an antioxidant defense in humans against oxygen- and radical-caused aging and cancer. A hypothesis. *Proceedings of the National Academy of Sciences of the USA* **78**, 6858–6862.

Andreoli, S. P., Clark, J. H., McGuire, W. A., and Bernstein, J. M. (1986). Purine excretion during tumor lysis syndrome children with acute lymphocytic leukemia receiving allopurinol: relationship to renal failure. *Journal of Pediatrics* **109**, 292–298.

Barlow, K. A. and Beilin, L. S. (1968). Renal disease in primary gout. *Quarterly Journal of Medicine* **37**, 79–96.

Beck, L. H. (1986). Requiem for gouty nephropathy. *Kidney International* **30**, 280–287.

Becker, B. F. (1993). Towards the physiological function of uric acid. *Free Radical Biology and Medicine* **14**, 615–631.

Becker, M. A. Hyperuricemia and gout. In *Metabolic and Molecular Basis of Inherited Disease* XXth edn. (ed. C. L. Scriver, A. L. Beauder, W. S. Sly, and W. D. Valle), pp. 2513–2535. New York: McGraw-Hill, 2001.

Bennett, J., Bond, J., Singer, I., and Gottlieb, A. (1972). Hypouricemia in Hodgkin's disease. *Annals of Internal Medicine* **76**, 751–756.

Bennett, W. M. (1985). Lead nephropathy. *Kidney International* **28**, 212–220.

Berger, L. and Yü, T.-F. (1975). Renal function in gout. An analysis of 524 gouty subjects including long term follow-up studies. *American Journal of Medicine* **59**, 605–613.

Boumendil-Podevin, E. F., Podevin, R. A., and Richet, G. (1975). Uricosuric agents in uremic sera. Identification of indoxyl sulfate and hippuric acid. *Journal of Clinical Investigation* **55**, 1142–1152.

Bradley, A. and Caskey, C. T. (1994). Hyperuricemia and urate nephropathy in urate oxidase deficient mice. *Proceedings of the National Academy of Sciences of the USA* **91**, 742–746.

Briggs, D. M. and Sperling, O. (1982). Uric acid metabolism in the Dalmatian coach hound. *Journal of the South African Veterinary Association* **53**, 201–204.

Brown, J. and Mallory, G. K. (1950). Renal changes in gout. *New England Journal of Medicine* **243**, 325–329.

Buchanan, W. W., Klinenberg, J. R., and Seegmiller, J. E. (1995). The inflammatory response to injected microcrystalline monosodium urate in normal, hyperuricemic, gouty and uremic subjects. *Arthritis and Rheumatism* **8**, 361–367.

Burack, D. A., Griffith, B. P., and Thompson, M. E. (1992). Hyperuricemia and gout amongst heart transplant recipients receiving cyclosporine. *American Journal of Medicine* **92**, 141–146.

Burnier, M., Roch-Ramel, F., and Brunner, H. R. (1996). Renal effects of angiotensin II receptor blockade in normotensive subjects. *Kidney International* **49**, 1787–1790.

Burnstock, G. (2002). Potential therapeutic targets in the rapidly expanding field of purinergic signalling. *Clinical Medicine: Journal of the Royal College of Physicians of London* **2**, 45–53.

Calabrese, G., Simmonds, H. A., Cameron, J. S., and Davies, P. M. (1990). Precocious familial gout with reduced fractional excretion of urate and normal purine enzymes. *Quarterly Journal of Medicine* **75**, 441–450.

Cameron, J. S. and Simmonds, H. A. (1981). Uric acid, gout and the kidney. *Journal of Clinical Pathology* **34**, 1245–1254.

Cameron, J. S. and Simmonds, H. A. (1987). Use and abuse of allopurinol. *British Medical Journal* **294**, 1504–1505.

Cameron, J. S. *et al.* (1984). Problems of diagnosis and *in vitro* enzyme instability in an adolescent with HGPRT deficiency presenting in acute renal failure. *Advances in Experimental Medicine and Biology* **165A**, 7–12.

Cannon, P. J., Symchych, P. S., and Demartini, F. E. (1968). The distribution of urate in human and primate kidney. *Proceedings of the Society for Experimental Biology and Medicine* **129**, 278–284.

Chocair, P. *et al.* (1993). Low-dose allopurinol plus azathioprine/cyclosporin/prednisolone, a novel immunosuppressive regimen. *Lancet* **342**, 83–84.

Chua, C. C. *et al.* (1988). Use of polyethyleneglycol uricase (PEG-uricase) to treat hyperuricemia in a patient with non-Hodgkin's lymphoma. *Annals of Internal Medicine* **109**, 114–117.

Clive, D. M. (2000). Renal transplant-associated hyperuricemia and gout. *Journal of the American Society of Nephrology* **11**, 974–979.

Cohen, M. R. (1994). Proximal gout following renal transplantation. *Arthritis and Rheumatism* **37**, 1709–1710.

Colleoni, N. and D'Amico, G. (1986). Chronic lead accumulation as a possible cause of renal failure in gouty patients. *Nephron* **44**, 32–35.

Colussi, G. *et al.* (1987). Pharmacological evaluation of urate handling in humans: pyrazinamide test vs combined pyrazinamide and probenecid administration. *Nephrology, Dialysis, Transplantation* **2**, 10–16.

Culleton, B. and Levy, D. (2001). Response: much ado about nothing, or much to do about something? The continuing controversy over the role of uric acid in cardiovascular disease. *Hypertension* **35**, E11.

Danovitch, G. M., Weinberger, J., and Berlyne, G. M. (1972). Uric acid in advanced renal failure. *Clinical Science* **43**, 331–341.

Danzler, W. H. (1996). Comparative aspects of renal urate transport. *Kidney International* **49**, 1549–1551.

Decaux, G., Prospert, F., Namais, B., and Soupart, A. (1997). Hyperuricemia as a clue for central diabetes insipidus. *American Journal of Medicine* **103**, 376–382. (See also discussion of this paper by **Sheikh-Hamad, D. and Ayus, C. J.** (1998). Journal club: Antidiuretic hormone and renal clearance of uric acid. *American Journal of Kidney Diseases* **32**, 692–697.)

Decaux, G., Prospert, F., Soupart, A., and Musch, W. (2000). Evidence that chronicity of hyponatraemia contributes to the high urate clearance observed in the syndrome of inappropriate antidiuretic hormone secretion. *American Journal of Kidney Diseases* **36**, 745–751.

Diamond, H. S. (1989). Interpretation of pharmacologic manipulation of urate transport in man. *Nephron* **51**, 1–5.

Dylewski, J. S. and Gerson, M. (1985). Hyperuricemia in patients with infectious mononucleosis. *Canadian Medical Association Journal* **132**, 1169–1170.

Edwards, R. M., Trizna, W., Stack, E. J., and Weinstock, J. (1996). Interaction of nonpeptide angiotensin II receptor antagonists with the urate transporter in rat renal brush-border membranes. *Journal of Pharmacology and Experimental Therapeutics* **276**, 125–129.

Elisaf, M., Tsimichodimos, V., Bairaktari, E., and Siamopoloulos, K. C. (1999). Effect of micronised fenofibrate and losartan combination on uric acid metabolism in hypertensive patients with hyperuricaemia. *Journal of Cardiovascular Pharmacology* **34**, 60–63.

Emmerson, B. T. (1991). Identification of the causes of persistent hyperuricaemia. *Lancet* **337**, 1461–1463.

Emmerson, B. T. and Row, G. (1975). An evaluation of the pathogenesis of the gouty kidney. *Kidney International* **8**, 65–71.

Emmerson, B. T., Cross, M., Osborne, J. M., and Axelsen, R. A. (1991). Ultrastructural studies of the reaction of urate crystals with a cultured renal tubular cell line. *Nephron* **59**, 403–408.

Emmerson, B. T., Nagel, S. L., Duffy, D. L., and Martin, N. G. (1992). Genetic control of the renal clearance of urate: a study of twins. *Annals of the Rheumatic Diseases* **51**, 375–377.

Enomoto, A. *et al.* (2002). Molecular identification of a renal urate-anion exchanger that regulates bood urate levels. *Nature* **417**, 447–452.

Facchini, F., Chen, Y.-D. I., Hollenbeck, C. B., and Reaven, G. M. (1991). Relationship between resistance to insulin-mediated glucose concentration uptake, urinary uric acid claearance, and plasma uric acid concentration. *Journal of American Medical Association* **266**, 3008–3011.

Faller, J. and Fox, I. H. (1982). Ethanol-induced hyperuricaemia. Evidence for increased urate production by activation of adenine nucleotide turnover. *New England Journal of Medicine* **307**, 1598–1602.

Farebrother, D. A., Hatfield, P., Simmonds, H. A., Cameron, J. S., Jones, A. S., and Cadenhead, A. (1975). Experimental cyrstal nephropathy (one year study in the pig). *Clinical Nephrology* **4**, 243–250.

Farquarson, C. A. J., Butler, R., Hill, A., Belch, J. J., and Struthers, A. D. (1999). Allopurinol improves endothelial dysfunction in patients with chronic heart failure. *Scottish Medical Journal* **44**, 24.

Fessel, W. J. (1979). Renal outcomes of gout and hyperuricemia. *American Journal of Medicine* **67**, 74–82.

Flury, W., Ruch, H. R., and Montandon, A. (1977). Zur Behandlung der Hyperurikämie nach Nierentransplantation. *Schweizer Medizinische Wochenschrift* **107**, 1339–1341.

Gibson, T., Rodgers, V., Potter, C., and Simmonds, H. A. (1982). Allopurinol treatment and its effect on renal function in gout: a controlled study. *Annals of Rheumatic Diseases* **41**, 59–65.

Gibson, T., Waterworth, P., Hatfield, P., Robinson, G., and Bremner, K. (1984). Hyperuricaemia, gout and kidney function in young New Zealand Maori men. *British Journal of Rheumatology* **23**, 276–282.

Graham, S., Day, R. O., Wong, H., McLachlan, A. J., Bergendal, L., Miners, J. O., and Birkett, D. J. (1996). Pharmacodynamics of oxypurinol after administration of allopurinol to healthy subjects. *British Journal of Clinical Pharmacology* **41**, 299–304.

Grahame, R., Simmonds, H. A., McBride, M. B., and Marsh, F. P. (1998). How should we treat tophaceous gout in patients with allopurinol hypersensitivity? *Advances in Experimental Medicine and Biology* **431**, 19–23.

Grassl, S. M. (2002a). Facilitated diffusion of urate in avian brush border membrane vesicles. *American Journal of Physiology, Cell Physiology* **283**, C1155–C1162.

Grassl, S. M. (2002b). Urate/ketoglutarate exchange in avian basolateral membrane vesicles. *American Journal of Physiology, Cell Physiology* **283**, C1144–C1154.

Gresser, U. and Zöllner, N., ed. *Urate Deposition in Man and its Clinical Consequences*. Berlin: Springer-Verlag, 1991.

Grivna, M., Průša, R., and Janda, J. (1997). Urinary uric acid excretion in healthy male infants. *Pediatric Nephrology* **11**, 623–624.

Hande, K. R. (1986). Evaluation of thiazide-allopurinol interaction. *American Journal of the Medical Sciences* **292**, 213–216.

Hande, K. R., Hixon, C. V., and Chabner, B. A. (1981). Postchemotherapy purine excretion in lymphoma patients receiving allopurinol. *Cancer Research* **41**, 2273–2279.

Hande, K. R., Noone, R. M., and Stone, W. E. (1984). Severe allopurinol toxicity. Description and guidelines for prevention in patients with renal insufficiency. *American Journal of Medicine* **76**, 47–56.

Hansen, J. M., Foch-Andersen, N., Leyssac, P. P., and Strandgaard, S. (1998). Glomerular and tubular function in renal transplant patients treated with and without cyclosporin A. *Nephron* **80**, 450–457.

Hooper, D. C. *et al.* (1998). Uric acid, a natural scavenger of peroxynitrite, in experimental allergic encephalomyelitis and multiple sclerosis. *Proceedings of the National Academy of Sciences of the USA* **95**, 675–680.

Hosoyamada, M., Sekine, T., Kanai, Y., and Endou, H. (1999). Molecular cloning and functional expression of a multispecific organic ion transporter from human kidney. *American Journal of Physiology* **276**, F122–F128.

Ichida, K., Hosoyamada, M., Kimura, H., Takeda, M., Endou, H., and Hosoya, T. Urate transport via human organic anion transporter 1. *10th International Symposium on Purines and Pyrimidines in Man*, Tel Aviv, 2000 (abstract).

Ifudu, O., Tan, C. C., Dulin, A. L., Delano, B. G., and Friedman, E. A. (1994). Gouty arthritis in end-stage renal disease: clinical course and rarity of new cases. *American Journal of Kidney Diseases* **23**, 347–351.

Ippoliti, G., Negri, M., Abelli, P., Martinelli, L., Minzioni, G., and Viganó, M. (1990). Urate oxidase in severe hyperuricaemia during acute renal failure after heart transplantation. *Haematologica* **75**, 487–488.

Jacobs, F., Mamzer-Bruneel, M. F., Skhiri, H., Rherevet, E., Legendre, C., and Kreis, H. (1997). Safety of the mycophenolate-allopurinol combination in kidney transplant recipients with gout. *Transplantation* **64**, 1087–1088.

Jankovic, M. *et al.* (1985). Urate oxidase as a hypouricaemic agent in a case of acute tumor lysis syndrome. *American Journal of Paediatric Hematology and Oncology* **7**, 202–204.

Johnson, R. J. and Tuttle, K. R. (2001). Much ado about nothing, or much to do about something? The continuing controversy over the role of uric acid in cardiovascular disease. *Hypertension* **35**, E10.

Johnson, R. J., Kivlighn, S. D., Kim, Y.-G., Suga, S., and Fogo, A. (1999). Reappraisal of the pathogenesis and consequences of hyperuricemia in hypertension, cardiovascular disease, and renal disease. *American Journal of Kidney Diseases* **33**, 225–234.

Johnson, R. J. *et al.* (2004). Uric acid evolution and primitive cultures. *Seminars in Nephrology* (in press).

Jones, D. P., Mahmoud, H., and Chesney, R. W. (1995). Tumor lysis syndrome: pathogenesis and management. *Pediatric Nephrology* **9**, 206–212.

Kahn, A. M. (1988). Effect of diuretics in the renal handling of urate. *Seminars in Nephrology* **8**, 305–314.

Kamper, A.-L. and Nielsen, A. H. (2001). Uricosuric effect of losartan in patients with renal transplants. *Transplantation* **72**, 671–674.

Kang, D. H. *et al.* (2002). A role for uric acid in the prognosis of renal disease? *Journal of the American Society of Nephrology* **13**, 2888–2897.

Keidar, S., Kohan, R., Levy, J., Grenadier, E., Palant, A., and Ben-Ari, J. (1982). Non-oliguric acute renal failure after treatment with sulfinpyrazone. *Clinical Nephrology* **17**, 266–267.

Kelly, S. J. *et al.* (2001). Diabetes insipidus in uricase-deficient mice: a model for evaluating therapy with poly (ethylene glycol)-modified uricase. *Journal of the American Society of Nephrology* **12**, 1001–1009.

Knorr, B. A., Beck, J. C., and Abramson, R. G. (1994). Classical and channel-like urate transporters in rabbit renal brush border membranes. *Kidney International* **45**, 727–736.

Kooij, A., Schijns, M., Fredricks, W. M., Van Noorden, C. J., and James, J. (1992). Distribution of xanthine oxidoreductase activity in human tissues—a histochemical and biochemical study. *Virchows Archiv B, Cell Pathology including Molecular Pathology* **63**, 17–23.

Kovarsky, J., Holmes, E., and Kelley, W. N. (1979). Absence of significant urate binding to plasma proteins. *Journal of Laboratory and Clinical Medicine* **93**, 85–91.

Krick, W., Wolff, N. A., and Burckhardt, G. (2000). Volatge-driven *p*-aminohippurate, chloride and urate transport in porcine renal brush border membrane vesicles. *European Journal of Physiology* **441**, 125–132.

Laine, J. and Holmberg, C. (1996). Mechanisms of hyperuricemia in cyclosporine-treated renal transplanted children. *Nephron* **74**, 318–323.

Lally, E. V., Ho, G., Jr., and Kaplan, S. R. (1986). The clinical spectrum of gouty arthritis in women. *Archives of Internal Medicine* **146**, 2221–2225.

Leal-Pinto, E., Cohen, B. E., and Abramson, R. G. (1999). Functional analysis and molecular modeling of a cloned urate transporter. *Journal of Membrane Biology* **169**, 13–27.

Leal-Pinto, E., Tao, W., Rappaport, J., Richardson, M., Knorr, B. A., and Abramson, R. G. (1997). Molecular cloning and functional reconstitution of a urate transporter/channel. *Journal of Biological Chemistry* **272**, 617–625.

Levinson, D. J. and Sorensen, L. B. (1980). Renal handling of uric acid in normal and gouty subjects: evidence for a 4-component system. *Annals of the Rheumatic Diseases* **39**, 173–179.

Lin, J. C. and Huang, P. T. (1994). Body lead and stores and urate excretion in men with chronic renal failure. *Journal of Rheumatology* **21**, 705–709.

Lin, J. L. *et al.* (2003). Environmental lead exposure and progression of chronic renal diseases in patients without diabetes. *New England Journal of Medicine* **348**, 277–286.

Lipkowitz, M. S., Leal-Pinto, E., Rappoport, J. Z., and Abramson, R. G. (2001). Functional reconstitution, membrane targeting, genomic structure, and chromosomal localization of a human urate transporter. *Journal of Clinical Investigation* **107**, 1103–1115.

Löffler, W., Gröbner, W., and Zöllner, N. (1981). Nutrition and uric acid metabolism. *Forschritte der Urologie und Nephrologie* **16**, 8–18.

Löffler, W., Simmonds, H. A., and Gröbner, W. (1983). Gout and uric acid nephropathy: some new aspects in diagnosis and treatment. *Klinische Wochenschrift* **61**, 1233–1239.

Löffler, W. *et al.* (1987). Uric acid production and turnover in patients with gout and renal insufficiency of rare origin. *Klinische Wochenschrift* **65**, 6–7.

Maesaka, J. K. and Fishbane, S. (1998). Regulation of renal urate excretion: a critical review. *American Journal of Kidney Diseases* **32**, 917–933.

Marcén, R. *et al.* (1995). Impairment of tubular secretion of urate in renal transplant patients on cyclosporine. *Nephron* **70**, 307–313.

Martinez, F., Manganel, M., Montrose-Rafidzadeh, C., Werner, D., and Roch-Ramel, F. (1990). Transport of urate and *p*-aminohippurate in rabbit renal brush border membranes. *American Journal of Physiology* **258**, F1145–F1153.

Mazzali, M. *et al.* (2001a). Elevated uric acid increases blood presure by a novel crystal-independent mechanism. *Hypertension* **38**, 1101–1106.

Mazzali, M. *et al.* (2001b). Hyperuricemia exacerbates chronic cyclosporine nephropathy. *Transplantation* **71**, 900–905.

Mazzali, M. *et al.* (2002). Hyperuricemia induces a primary renal arteriolopathy in rats by a blood-pressure independent mechanism. *American Journal of Physiology. Renal Physiology* **282**, F991–F997.

McBride, M. B. *et al.* (1998). Presymptomatic detection of familial juvenile hyperuricaemic nephropathy in children. *Paediatric Nephrology* **12**, 359–364.

Messerli, F. H., Frohlich, E. D., Dreslinski, G. R., Suraez, D. H., and Aristomuno, G. G. (1980). Serum uric acid in essential hypertension: an indicator of renal vascular involvement. *American Journal of Medicine* **93**, 817–821.

Meyers, O. L. and Monteagudo, F. S. E. (1985). Gout in females: analysis of 92 patients. *Clinical and Experimental Rheumatology* **3**, 105–109.

Mikkelsen, W. N., Dodge, H. J., and Valkenburg, H. (1965). The distribution of serum uric acid values in a population unselected as to gout and hypertension. *American Journal of Medicine* **39**, 242–251.

Mir, M. A. and Delamore, I. W. (1974). Hypouricemia and proximal renal tubular dysfunction in acute myeloid leukaemia. *British Medical Journal* **3**, 775–777.

Mitnick, P. D. and Beck, L. (1979). Hypouricemia and malignant neoplasm. *Archives of Internal Medicine* **139**, 186–187.

Mohr, P. Urate deposition in tissues. In *Urate Deposition in Man and its Clinical Consequences* (ed. U. Gresser and N. Zöllner), pp. 24–27. Berlin: Springer-Verlag, 1991.

Muscelli, E. *et al.* (1996). Effect of insulin on renal sodium and uric acid handling in essential hypertension. *American Journal of Hypertension* **9**, 746–752.

Nanra, R. S., Howard, M., and Daniel, V. (1978). Secondary gout in analgesic nephropathy. *Australian and New Zealand Journal of Medicine* **8**, 237.

Navascues, R. A. *et al.* (2002). Safety of allopurinol-mycophenolate mofetil combination in the treatment of hyperuricemia of renal transplant recipients. *Nephron* **91**, 173–174.

Nicholls, A., Snaith, M. L., and Scott, T. J. (1972). Effect of oestrogen therapy on plasma and urinary levels of uric acid. *British Medical Journal* **1**, 449–453.

Nickeleit, V. and Mihatsch, M. J. (1997). Uric acid nephropathy and end-stage renal disease—review of a non-disease. *Nephrology, Dialysis, Transplantation* **12**, 1832–1838.

Nolan, C. C. and Shaikh, Z. A. (1992). Lead nephrotoxicity and associated disorders: biochemical mechanisms. *Toxicology* **73**, 127–146.

Noordzij, T. C., Leunissen, K. M., and van Hooff, J. P. (1991). Renal handling of plasma urate and incidence of gouty arthritis during cyclosporine and diuretic use. *Transplantation* **52**, 64–67.

Norlén, B. J., Hellstrom, M., Nisa, M., and Robertson, W. G. (1995). Uric acid stone formation in a patient after renal transplantation: metabolic and therapeutic considerations. *Scandinavian Journal of Urology and Nephrology* **29**, 335–337.

Nuki, G., Watson, M. L., Williams, B. C., Simmonds, H. A., and Wallace, R. C. (1992). Congenital chloride losing enteropathy associated with tophaceous gouty arthritis. *Advances in Experimental Medicine and Biology* **309A**, 203–209.

Nuyts, G. D. *et al.* (1991). Does lead play a role in the development of chronic renal disease? *Nephrology, Dialysis, Transplantation* **6**, 307–315.

Ochiai, T., Ishibashi, M., Fukao, K., Takahashi, K., and Endo, T. (1995). Japanese muticenter studies of FK 506 in renal transplantation. *Transplantation Proceedings* **27**, 50–52.

O'Connor, N. T. J., Prentice, H. G., and Hoffbrand, A. V. (1989). Prevention of urate nephropathy in the tumour lysis syndrome. *Clinical and Laboratory Haematology* **11**, 97–100.

Ohono, I., Hosya, T., Gomi, H., Ichida, K., Okabe, H., and Hikita, M. (2001). Serum uric acid and renal prognosis in patients with IgA nephropathy. *Nephron* **87**, 333–339.

Ostberg, Y. (1968). Renal urate deposits in chronic renal failure. *Acta Medica Scandinavica* **183**, 197–201.

Perez-Ruiz, F., Calabozo, M., Herrero-Bietes, A. M., Garcia-Erauskin, G., and Pijoan, J. I. (2000). Improvement in renal function in patients with chronic gout after proper control of hyperuricemia and gout. *Nephron* **86**, 287–291.

Perez-Ruiz, F. *et al.* (2003). Long-term efficacy of hyperuricaemia treatment in renal transplant patients. *Nephrology, Dialysis, Transplantation* **18**, 603–606.

Platt, P. N. and Dick, W. C. (1985). Diuretic-induced gout: the beginnings of an epidemic. *The Practitioner* **229**, 281–284.

Polkowski, C. A. and Grassl, S. M. (1993). Uric acid transport in rat renal basolateral membrane vesicles. *Biochimica Biophysica Acta* **1146**, 145–152.

Potter, J. L. and Silvidi, A. A. (1987). Xanthine lithiasis, nephrocalcinosis and renal failure in a leukemia patients treated with allopurinol. *Clinical Chemistry* **33**, 2314–2316.

Prospert, F., Soupart, A., Brimioulle, S., and Decaux, G. (1993). Evidence of defective tubular reabsorption and normal secretion of uric acid in the syndrome of inappropriate secretion of antidiuretic hormone. *Nephron* **64**, 189–192.

Puig, J. G. *et al.* (1999). Effect of eprosartan and losartan on uric acid metabolism in patients with essential hypertension. *Journal of Hypertension* **17**, 1033–1039.

Quinones, G. A. *et al.* (1995). Effect of insulin on uric acid excretion in humans. *American Journal of Physiology* **268**, E1–E5.

Raatikainen, M. J., Peuhkurinen, K. J., and Hassinen, I. E. (1994). Contribution of endothelium and cardiomyocytes to hypoxia-induced adenosine release. *Journal of Molecular and Cellular Cardiology* **26**, 1069–1080.

Race, J. E., Grassl, S. M., Williams, W. J., and Holtzman, E. J. (1999). Molecular cloning and characterization of two novel human renal organic anion transporters (hOAT1 and hOAT3). *Biochemical and Biophysical Research Communications* **255**, 508–514.

Ralston, S. H., Capell, H. A., and Sturrock, R. D. (1988). Alcohol and response to treatment of gout. *British Medical Journal* **296**, 1641–1642.

Raman, V., Sharman, V. L., and Lee, H. A. (1990). Azathioprine and allopurinol: a potentially dangerous combination. *Journal of Internal Medicine* **228**, 69–71.

Rao, G. N., Corson, M. A., and Berk, B. C. (1991). Uric acid stimulates vascular smooth muscle cell proliferation by increasing platelet-derived growth factor A-chain. *Journal of Biological Chemistry* **266**, 8604–8608.

Ribiero, R. C. and Pui, C. H. (2003). Recombinant uric oxidase for prevention of hyperuricemia and tumor lysis syndrome in lymphoid malignancies. *Clinical Lymphoma* **3**, 225–232.

Richet, G., Mignon, F., and Ardaillou, R. (1965). Goutte secondaire des néphropathies chroniques. *Presse Médicale* **73**, 633–638.

Roch-Ramel, F. and Diezi, J. Renal transport of organic ions and uric acid. In *Strauss and Welt's Diseases of the Kidney* 7th edn. (ed. C. Gottschalk and R. W. Schrier), pp. 231–249. Boston: Little Brown, 1997.

Roch-Ramel, F. and Guisan, B. (1999). Oxypurine transport in human brush-border membrane vesicles (BBMV). *Cellular and Molecular Biology Letters* **4**, 443.

Roch-Ramel, F. and Weiner, I. M. (1980). Renal excretion of urate: factors determining the action of drugs. *Kidney International* **18**, 665–676.

Roch-Ramel, F., Guisan, B., and Diezi, J. (1997). Effect of uricosuric and antiuricosuric agents on urate transport in human brush-border membrane vesicles. *Journal of Experimental Pharmacology and Therapeutics* **280**, 839–845.

Roch-Ramel, F., Werner, D., and Guisan, B. (1994). Urate transport in brush-border membrane of human kidney. *American Journal of Physiology* **266**, F797–F805.

Rosell, M., Rennstrom, J., Kallner, A., and Hellenius, M. L. (1999). Serum urate determines antioxidant capacity in middle-aged men—a controlled, randomized diet and exercise study. *Journal of Internal Medicine* **246**, 219–226.

Rosenfeld, J. B. (1974). Effect of long term allopurinol administration on serial glomerular filtration rate in normotensive and hypertensive hyperuricemic subjects. *Advances in Experimental Medicine and Biology* **41B**, 581–596.

Rozenberg, S. *et al.* (1995). Urate oxidase for the treatment of tophaceous gout in heart transplant recipients. A report of three cases. *Revue du Rheumatisme* **62**, 392–394.

Sakhaee, K., Adams-Huet, B., Moe, O. W., and Pak, C. Y. K. (2002). Pathophysiologic basis for normouricosuric uric acid lithiasis. *Kidney International* **62**, 971–979.

Sánchez Bayle, M. *et al.* (1992). Uricosuria en la infancia y adolescencia. *Nefrología* **12**, 239–243.

Sanchez-Lozada, L. G. *et al.* (2002). Mild hyperuricemia induces glomerular hypertension in normal rats. *American Journal of Physiology. Renal Physiology* **283**, F1105–F1110.

Saran, R., Abdullah, S., Goel, S., Nolph, K. D., and Terry, B. E. (1998). An unusual case of pink urine. *Nephrology, Dialysis, Transplantation* **13**, 1579–1580.

Schlotte, V., Sevanian, A., Hochstein, P., and Weithmann, K. U. (1998). Effect of uric acid and chemical analogues on oxidation of human low density lipoprotein. *Free Radical Biology and Medicine* **25**, 839–847.

Schreiner, O., Wandel, E., Himmelbasch, F., Galle, P. R., and Marker-Hermann, E. (2000). Reduced secretion of proinflammatory cytokines of monosodium urate crystal-stimulated monocytes in chronic renal failure: an explanation for infrequent gout episodes in renal failure patients? *Nephrology, Dialysis, Transplantation* **15**, 644–649.

Sekine, T., Cha, S. H., and Endou, H. (2000). The multispecific organic ion transporter (OAT) family. *European Journal of Physiology* **440**, 337–350.

Selby, J. V., Friedman, G. D., and Queensbererry, C. P. J. (1990). Precursors of essential hypertension, pulmonary function, heart rate, uric acid, serum cholesterol and other serum chemistries. *American Journal of Epidemiology* **131**, 1017–1027.

Shahainfar, S. *et al.* (1999). For the Losartan uric acid study group. Safety of losartan in hypertensive patients with diuretic-induced hyperuricemia. *Kidney Intenational* **56**, 1879–1885.

Shimizu, T., Nishikawa, M., and Matsushige, H. (1989). The solubility of uric acid monosodium urate in urine. *Advances in Experimental Medicine and Biology* **253A**, 215–218.

Short, E. M. Hyperuricemia and gout. In *The Genetic Basis of Common Diseases* (ed. R. A. King *et al.*), pp. 482–566. Oxford: Oxford University Press, 1992.

Simmonds, H. A. and Roch-Ramel, F. (1994). Pigs aren't people. *New Scientist* **23**, 45–46.

Simmonds, H. A., Cameron, J. S., Morris, G. S., and Davies, P. M. (1986). Allopurinol in renal failure and the tumour lysis syndrome. *Clinica Chimica Acta* **160**, 189–195.

Simmonds, H. A., Duley, J. A., and Davies, P. M. Analysis of purines and pyrimidines in blood, urine and other physiological fluids. In *Techniques in Diagnostic Human Biochemical Genetics. A Laboratory Manual* (ed. F. Hommes), pp. 397–425. New York: Wiley-Liss, 1991.

Simmonds, H. A., Hatfield, P. J., Cameron, J. S., and Cadenhead, A. (1976). Uric acid excretion by the pig kidney. *American Journal of Physiology* **230**, 1654–1661.

Simmonds, H. A., McBride, M. B., Hatfield, P. J., Graham, R., McCaskey, J., and Jackson, M. (1994). Polynesian women are also at risk for hyperuricaemia and gout because of a genetic defect in renal urate handling. *British Journal of Rheumatology* **33**, 932–937.

Simmonds, H. A., Stutchbury, J. H., Webster, D. R., Spencer, R. E., Fisher, R. A., and Buckley, B. M. (1984). Pregnancy in xanthinuria: demonstration of fetal uric acid production? *Journal of Inherited Metabolic Diseases* **7**, 77–79.

Sommers, D. K. and Schoenman, H. S. (1987). Drug interactions with urate excretion in man. *European Journal of Pharmacology* **32**, 499–502.

Sorensen, L. B. (1980). Gout secondary to chronic renal disease: studies on urate metabolism. *Annals of Rheumatic Diseases* **39**, 424–430.

Sorensen, L. B. and Levinson, D. J. (1975). Origin and extrarenal elimination of uric acid in man. *Nephron* **14**, 7–20.

Sperling, O. Hereditary renal hypouricaemia. In *Metabolic and Molecular Basis of Inherited Disease* XX edn. (ed. C. L. Scriver, A. L. Beaudet, W. S. Sly, and W. D. Valle), pp. 5069–5083. New York: McGraw-Hill, 2001.

Spitzenberger, F., Graessler, J., and Schroeder, H. E. (2001). Molecular and functional characterization of galectin-9 mRNA isoforms in porcine and human cells and tissues. *Biochimie* **83**, 851–862.

Stapleton, F. B. Uric acid nephropathy. In *Pediatric Renal Disease* 2nd edn. (ed. C. M. Edelmann, Jr.), pp. 1647–1659. Boston: Little Brown, 1992.

Stavric, B., Johnson, W. J., and Grice, H. C. (1969). Uric acid nephropathy: an experimental model. *Proceedings of the Society for Experimental Biology and Medicine* **130**, 512–516.

Steele, T. H. (1999). Hyperuricemic nephropathies. *Nephron* **81** (Suppl. 1), 45–49.

Stone, T. W. and Simmonds, H. A. *Purines: Basic and Clinical Aspects*. London: Kluwer, 1991.

Sumino, H., Ichikawa, S., Kanda, T., Nakamura, T., and Sakamaki, T. (1999). Reduction of serum uric acid by hormome replacement therapy in post-menopausal women with hyperuricaemia. *Lancet* **354**, 650.

Syrjanen, J., Mustonen, J., and Pasternack, A. (2000). Hypertriglyceridemia and hyperuricaemia are risk factors for progression of IgA nephropathy. *Nephrology, Dialysis, Transplantation* **15**, 34–42.

Talbott, J. H. and Terplan, K. L. (1960). The kidney in gout. *Medicine (Baltimore)* **39**, 405–467.

Tarng, D. C., Lin, H. Y., Shyong, M. L., Wang, J. S., Yang, W. C., and Huang, T. P. (1995). Renal function in gout patients. *American Journal of Nephrology* **15**, 31–37.

Terkeltaub, R. A. (1993). Gout and mechanisms of crystal-induced inflammation. *Current Opinion in Rheumatology* **5**, 510–516.

Tojo, A. *et al.* (1999). Immunohistochemical localization of multispecific anion transporter 1 in rat kidney. *Journal of the American Society of Nephrology* **10**, 464–471.

Tykarski, A. (1988). Mechanism of hypouricemia in Hodgkin's disease. Isolated defect in post secretory reabsorption of uric acid. *Nephron* **50**, 217–219.

Vecchio, P. C. and Emmerson, B. T. (1992). Gout due to renal disease. *British Journal of Rheumatology* **31**, 63–65.

Venkataseshan, V. S., Feingold, R., Dikman, S., and Churg, J. (1990). Acute hyperuricemic nephropathy and renal failure after renal transplantation. *Nephron* **56**, 317–321.

Verger, D., Leroux-Robert, C., Ganter, P., and Richet, G. (1967). Les tophus goutteux de la médullaire rénale des urémiques chroniques. *Nephron* **4**, 356–370.

Walter-Sack, I. (1988). Benzbromarone disposition and uricosuric action: evidence for hydroxylation instead of debromination to benzarone. *Klinische Wochenschrift* **66**, 160–166.

Waring, W. S., Webb, D. J., and Maxwell, S. R. J. (2000). Uric acid as a risk for cardiovascular disease. *Quarterly Journal of Medicine* **93**, 707–713.

Watanabe, S. *et al.* (2002). Uric acid, hominoid evolution, and the pathogenesis of salt sensitivity. *Hypertension* **40**, 355–360.

Weiner, I. (1979). Urate transport in the nephron. *American Journal of Physiology* **237**, F85–F92.

Wu, X. W., Muzny, D. M., Lee, G. C., and Caskey, C. T. (1992). Two independent mutational events in the loss of urate oxidase during hominid evolution. *Journal of Molecular Evolution* **34**, 78–84.

Yü, T.-F. and Berger, L. (1982). Impaired renal function in gout. Its association with hypertensive vascular disease and intrinsic renal disease. *American Journal of Medicine* **72**, 95–99.

Zawadowski, J., Jankowska, I., Moszczynska, A., and Januszewicz, P. (1993). Hypouricemia due to increased secretion of urate in children with amanita phalloides poisoning. *Nephron* **65**, 375–380.

Zürcher, R. M., Bock, H. A., and Thiel, G. (1994). Excellent uricosuric efficacy of benzbromarone in cyclosporin-A-treated renal transplant patients: a prospective study. *Nephrology, Dialysis, Transplantation* **9**, 548–551.

Zürcher, R. M., Bock, H. A., and Thiel, G. (1996). Hyperuricaemia in cyclosporin-treated patients: a GFR-related effect. *Nephrology, Dialysis, Transplantation* **11**, 153–158.

6.5 Nephrotoxic metals

Richard P. Wedeen and Marc E. De Broe

Introduction

Kidney disease arising from exposure to environmental toxins plays a special role in nephrology because of the possibility of its prevention. Chronic renal disease caused by the heavy metals, lead, cadmium, mercury, uranium, arsenic, and germanium, as well as by the lightest metal lithium will be considered in this chapter. The immunologically mediated glomerular diseases associated with silica resemble that induced by mercury and will also be reviewed here. Chronic renal failure due to exposure to chromium, nickel, selenium, silver, and vanadium has not been reported; it may be more a testimony to the absence of careful investigation of the subject than to the safety of the metals. Iatrogenic renal diseases due to gold or copper are considered in Chapters 19.1 and 5.3. Occupational exposure is readily identified and is more intense than exposure in the general population; thus, information about environmental nephrotoxins usually originates with industrial reports. Occupational renal disease provides a clinical basis for the recognition of nephropathies induced by more subtle environmental exposure.

Heavy metals are ubiquitous in the environment created by contemporary society; of the thousands of chemicals which regularly enter the body, their nephrotoxic effects are best understood. Acute renal damage induced by the heavy metals is immediately apparent. High parenteral doses of inorganic lead, cadmium, and certain valance states of mercury, uranium, chromium, and bismuth regularly and rapidly induce acute renal failure. Acute tubular necrosis follows selective cellular accumulation and direct cytotoxic damage in the proximal tubule. Incomplete recovery and protracted low-grade exposure induce chronic tubulointerstitial nephritis and, occasionally, eventual chronic renal insufficiency.

Absorption of heavy metals in quantities insufficient to induce immediate toxic symptoms may also result in the insidious development of chronic renal failure. A causal relationship may be unclear: renal damage may not be evident for many years and relatively few exposed individuals develop clinically apparent renal failure. Multielemental exposure is frequent, making it difficult to analyse the role of individual metals. Confirmation of their nephrotoxicity is further obscured by the multifactorial nature of kidney disease, complex interactions with biologically essential metals (including calcium, zinc, iron, and magnesium), and genetically controlled differences in susceptibility. Advanced tubulointerstitial nephritis may be confused with glomerulonephritis as proteinuria increases with progressing renal failure.

Chronic renal disease caused by absorption of metals is readily misinterpreted in the elderly as the result of the ageing process or hypertension. The histological appearance of interstitial nephritis is easily confused with that of nephrosclerosis or pyelonephritis. Misdiagnosis in the elderly population is likely to continue unless accurate exposure histories are obtained and diagnostic tests reflecting cumulative lifetime absorption are more widely available, for example, *in vivo* X-ray fluorescence (XRF) and neutron activation analysis (Skerfving *et al.* 1987).

Urinary markers

Over 25 urinary proteins and biochemical markers (eicosanoids) have been measured in urine, with sensitive, specific immunoassays, in order to identify early stages of renal injury. The aim is to detect segment-specific damage before the reduction in glomerular filtration rate (GFR) becomes manifest clinically by an increase in serum creatinine. Fingerprints for specific environmental nephrotoxins have been partially characterized as the selected urinary markers reflect specific sites of renal injury:

(1) low molecular weight proteins and intracellular enzymes—proximal tubule damage;

(2) Tamm–Horsfall glycoprotein and kallikrein—distal tubule injury;

(3) high molecular weight proteins—increased glomerular permeability (if >200 mg/g creatinine);

(4) biochemical markers—eicosanoids suggesting vascular injury.

Comprehensive urinary profiles have been evaluated in cooperative studies conducted in Europe (Table 1; Mutti *et al.* 1992; Cardenas *et al.* 1993a,b; Roels *et al.* 1993; Fels *et al.* 1994; Nouwen and De Broe 1994). In order to achieve broad diagnostic value, the urinary markers are examined in subjects with known toxic exposures, over a wide range of dose rates and exposure times. Patients with clinical renal failure, glomerular disease, multinephrotoxin exposure, or systemic diseases that predispose to kidney damage (e.g. hypertension, diabetes mellitus, and gout) are excluded from these studies in order to reduce confounding variables. The specificity of tubular proteinuria may be lost once renal damage raises serum creatinine level.

A sampling of urinary markers is presented in order to illustrate how toxic nephropathies may be differentiated (Table 1). Intestinal alkaline phosphatase, tissue non-specific alkaline phosphatase, *N*-acetyl-β-D-glucosaminidase, and retinol binding protein reflect proximal tubular function. The isoenzyme intestinal alkaline phosphatase is a sensitive and specific indicator of S3 injury (Fig. 1) due to occupational exposure to mercury and cadmium (Nuyts *et al.* 1992; Cardenas *et al.* 1993a). Together with other markers of tubular and glomerular injury, it is increased in the ischaemic kidney and in hypertension and does not increase in analgesic abuse, lead, and perchloroethylene exposure (Verpooten *et al.* 1989; Mutti *et al.* 1992). In contrast to tissue non-specific alkaline phosphatase, *N*-acetyl-β-D-glucosaminidase is not elevated in the urine of workers exposed to perchloroethylene, but is minimally increased following exposure to lead or mercury (Mutti *et al.* 1992; Cardenas *et al.* 1993a,b). However, *N*-acetyl-β-D-glucosaminidase, intestinal alkaline phosphatase, and retinol binding protein are elevated after cadmium exposure (Mutti *et al.* 1985; Roels *et al.* 1993).

Table 1 Urinary markers in toxic nephropathies—European Cooperative Study (adapted from Mutti *et al.* 1992; Cardenas *et al.* 1993a,b; Roels *et al.* 1993; Fels *et al.* 1994)

Marker	Exposure to			
	Lead	Cadmium	Mercury	PCE[a]
Intestinal alkaline phosphatase		●●●	●●●	
Tissue non-specific alkaline phosphatase			●	●●●
N-Acetyl-β-D-glucosaminidase	●	●●●	●	
Retinol binding protein		●		
Tamm–Horsfall glycoprotein		●	●	○
β_2-Microglobulin		●		
Microalbuminuria		●●		●
Thromboxane B_2	●●			
6-Keto-prostaglandin $F_{1\alpha}$		●●		

[a] Perchloroethylene.

Tamm–Horsfall glycoprotein appears to be a marker of distal tubular injury. Although the pathophysiological significance of the urinary eicosanoids is unclear, measurement of urine PGE_2, $PGF_{2\alpha}$, and 6-keto-$PGF_{1\alpha}$ may provide insight into the mechanisms of hypertension, and injury to the glomerulus or renal medulla. The ability of these urinary markers to discriminate between various nephrotoxins increases with increasing exposure levels, but diminishes as renal failure supervenes.

Minor concentrations of urinary albumin may reflect either glomerular or tubular injury. Although generally considered to indicate early glomerular injury in patients with diabetes mellitus, the appearance of small quantities of albumin in the urine may sometimes result from the failure of the tubule to reabsorb/metabolize normally filtered albumin (Tucker *et al.* 1993). Microalbuminuria may thus represent proximal tubular dysfunction rather than increased glomerular permeability.

β_2-Microglobulin, the first tested low molecular weight protein, has largely been replaced for the characterization of tubular proteinuria. β_2-Microglobulin is dependent on the turnover of plasma membrane, which is influenced by several physiological and pathophysiological conditions, such as fever, infection, and neoplasia. Furthermore, its stability in urine is pH dependent so that alkalinization of the urine is necessary to obtain a valid determination.

A number of alternatives to the urinary markers shown in Table 1 are available. At present, they appear redundant (e.g. alanine aminopeptidase, α_1-microglobulin, γ-glutamyl transferase) or offer few advantages because their functional significance is unclear (e.g. fibronectin, glycosaminoglycans, kallikrein, sialic acid). Proximal tubule brush border antigens designated BB50, BBA, and HF5 may be sensitive indicators of proximal tubular injury (Mutti *et al.* 1985; Verpooten *et al.* 1989). However, standardization and quality control of these immunoassays are still lacking.

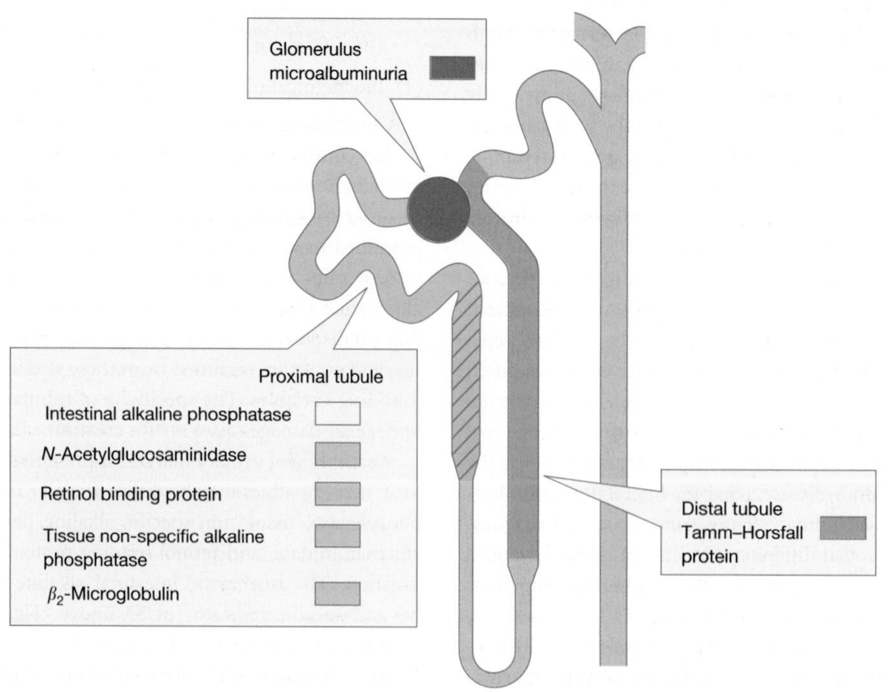

Fig. 1 Schematic representation of the nephron, showing site specificity of urinary protein markers.

Lead nephropathy

Three clinical forms of lead nephropathy are currently recognized. Acute lead nephropathy results from brief but massive lead absorption and is characterized by classical, symptomatic lead intoxication (colic, encephalopathy, peripheral neuropathy, and anaemia), and a transient Fanconi syndrome. It is frequently an incidental finding in children with overwhelming neurological symptoms. A chronic, slowly progressive interstitial nephritis results from cumulative excessive lead absorption, often in the absence of symptomatic acute lead poisoning. This nephropathy is associated with gout and/or hypertension, and is usually identified when a source of high exposure is known [occupational hazard, or consumption of illicitly distilled spirits (moonshine)]. The last form is hypertension arising from prolonged, low-level exposure to environmental lead. It develops in the absence of symptomatic lead intoxication before the clinical onset of renal failure.

Acute lead nephropathy

Acute lead poisoning occurs in children aged between 3 months and 6 years as a result of the habitual ingestion of non-food materials (pica), usually leaded paint chips. Encephalopathy and seizures bring the affected children to the attention of physicians. Blood lead concentrations uniformly exceed 4.83 μmol/l (100 μg/dl) (Piomelli *et al.* 1982). In the United States, the average blood lead in unexposed individuals has declined to about 0.14 μmol/l (3 μg/dl) in 1993 from about 0.63 μmol/l (13 μg/dl) in 1977 (Mahaffey *et al.* 1982; MMWR 1994). The concentration at which medical surveillance is recommended for children is currently 0.48 μmol/l (10 μg/dl) down from 1.21 μmol/l (25 μg/dl) in 1990. When the blood lead concentration exceeds 7.25 μmol/l (150 μg/dl), encephalopathy is common and fatal seizures may occur. In this setting, the appearance of the Fanconi syndrome, characterized by aminoaciduria, glycosuria, phosphaturia, and hypercalciuria, is of relatively minor importance (Wedeen 1984a). As with other forms of the Fanconi syndrome, vitamin D-resistant rickets may develop. Renal glycosuria may persist for over a decade following chelation therapy (Loghman-Adham 1998).

Acute elevations of blood lead concentrations result in selective accumulation of lead in the kidneys, where it is sequestered within characteristic acid-fast intranuclear inclusion bodies in proximal tubules (Goyer and Wilson 1975) (Fig. 2), and in bone. With prolonged excessive absorption, the kidney becomes only a minor storage site (Skerfving *et al.* 1983) and lead is retained primarily in bone. In acutely exposed children, about 75 per cent of the body burden is present in bone (Rosen *et al.* 1989) compared with over 90 per cent in adults (Barry 1975). Since more than 95 per cent of blood lead is bound to erythrocytes, clearance is difficult to measure, but like other cations, lead appears to undergo bidirectional transport across the tubular epithelium. Renal clearance ranges from about 1 to 3 ml/min and is relatively independent of renal failure (Behringer *et al.* 1986).

Removal of lead by chelation therapy reverses the proximal tubule reabsorptive defect and removes the intranuclear inclusion bodies of acute lead nephropathy (Goyer and Wilson 1975). If the child survives without chelation, chronic tubulointerstitial nephritis may develop several decades later (Emmerson 1973; Hu 1991). An epidemic of tubulointerstitial nephritis in young adults who had suffered from childhood lead poisoning was identified in Queensland, Australia, at the turn of the century. Studies of this 'Queensland nephritis' over

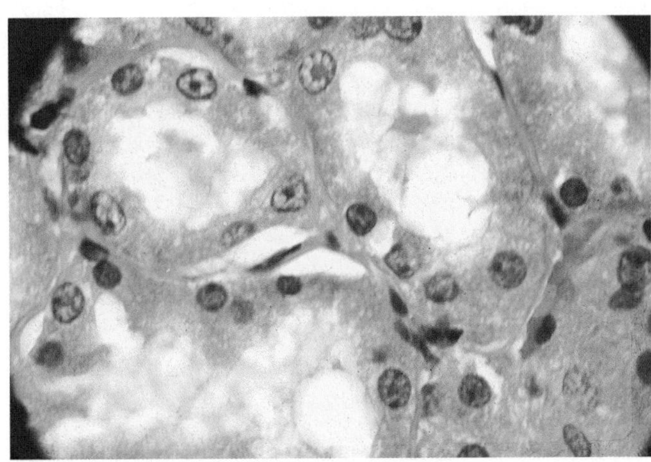

Fig. 2 Acid-fast intranuclear inclusion bodies induced by lead in human renal biopsy.

seven decades suggest that this delayed development of chronic renal failure corresponded to the lead nephropathy seen in occupationally exposed adults. Lead is gradually released into the bloodstream from bone storage sites for many years after cessation of exposure, and is thus believed to contribute to the delayed nephrotoxicity which follows childhood plumbism (Inglis *et al.* 1978).

Chronic lead nephropathy (see also Chapter 6.4)

Symptomatic lead poisoning in childhood led to the identification of the aetiology of Queensland nephritis. Similarly, symptomatic lead poisoning from occupational or non-occupational exposure, such as contaminated alcoholic beverages, has permitted the incrimination of lead as the cause of chronic interstitial nephritis (Wedeen 1984b). Typically, renal failure is evident only after years of excessive lead absorption, and is frequently associated with hypertension and/or gout (Batuman *et al.* 1981, 1983; Behringer *et al.* 1986; Colleoni and D'Amico 1986; Sánchez-Fructuoso *et al.* 1996). Fifty per cent of the patients with lead nephropathy suffer from gout, and although hyperuricaemia is universal in renal failure, gout is rare in renal disease unrelated to lead exposure. In the absence of renal failure, gout cannot usually be attributed to lead exposure, despite coexisting hypertension (Wright *et al.* 1984; Peitzman *et al.* 1985). As with other forms of interstitial nephritis, urinary protein excretion is initially meagre in lead nephropathy but increases as renal failure progresses.

In contrast to cadmium nephropathy, the excretion of urinary marker proteins such as intestinal alkaline phosphatase, tissue nonspecific alkaline phosphatase, Tamm–Horsfall glycoprotein, retinol binding protein, lysozyme, and β_2-microglobulin (Wedeen 1988; Cardenas *et al.* 1993b) are not increased in lead nephropathy. The increase in urinary *N*-acetyl-β-D-glucosaminidase reflect the Fanconi syndrome of acute lead poisoning rather than the chronic interstitial nephritis associated with occupational lead exposure (Endo *et al.* 1990; Verberk *et al.* 1996).

The kidney shows the characteristic morphology of relatively acellular, tubulointerstitial nephritis (Cramer *et al.* 1974; Wedeen *et al.* 1975; Inglis *et al.* 1978) (Fig. 3). Intranuclear inclusion bodies are not seen in the absence of current exposure. The appearance of arteriolar

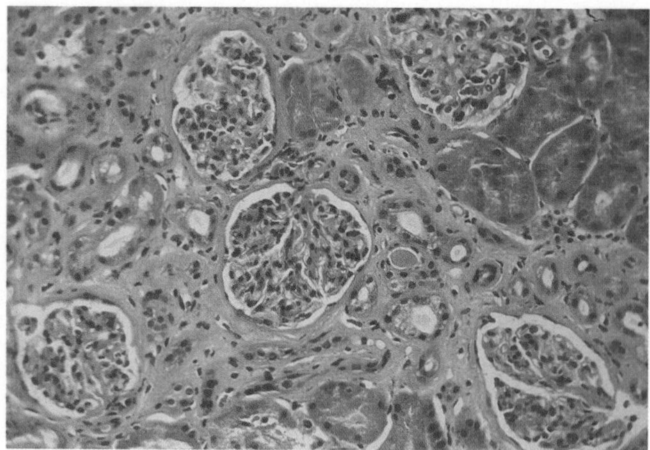

Fig. 3 Focal interstitial nephritis from a lead worker with chronic lead nephropathy and minimal renal dysfunction (from Wedeen *et al.* 1979, with permission).

nephrosclerotic lesions prior to the onset of hypertension and the relatively short duration of hypertension suggest that lead initially injures the microvascular endothelium (Wedeen *et al.* 1975; Batuman *et al.* 1983). This view is consistent with the finding that creatinine clearance decreases with increasing blood lead in the general population, an effect independent of blood pressure (Staessen *et al.* 1994).

There is no reason to believe that advanced chronic lead nephropathy is reversed by deleading with chelating agents; indeed, no improvement in renal function should be anticipated after the steady-state serum creatinine has exceeded about 266 mmol/l (3 mg/dl) (Germain *et al.* 1984). However, lead-induced focal interstitial nephritis may be accompanied by a reversible functional component that is, at least in part, prerenal in origin. Indeed, the mesenteric vasospasm of acute lead poisoning, which is believed to cause lead colic (Lilis *et al.* 1968), is associated with prerenal azotaemia. Chronic volume depletion and hyporeninaemic hypoaldosteronism may also contribute (Ashouri 1985). However, the effect of lead on the renin–angiotensin system remains controversial, because increased renin responsiveness has also been observed in lead-exposed experimental animals and humans (Campbell *et al.* 1985; Boscolo *et al.* 1988; Vander 1988).

In the absence of symptoms of acute plumbism or known excessive lead exposure, the diagnosis of lead nephropathy is more difficult. The blood lead concentration is inadequate for the detection of excessive body lead burdens after exposure has ceased. Because the biological half-life of lead in blood is approximately 30 days (Chamberlain 1985), blood concentrations reflect recent, rather than cumulative, lead exposure. However, the contribution of bone stores to the blood lead concentration increases as the blood lead decreases. In the past cumulative lead absorption is by the $CaNa_2EDTA$ (EDTA = ethylenediaminetetraacetic acid) lead mobilization test. $CaNa_2EDTA$ binds to lead in soft tissues and bone and the lead–chelate complex is cleared in the urine at the rate of glomerular filtration. Emmerson (1973) used the EDTA–lead mobilization test to demonstrate excessive body lead stores in young adults with Queensland nephritis. Chelatable lead correlates well with bone lead concentration (Inglis *et al.* 1978; Van de Vyver *et al.* 1988). Since renal failure reduces the rate of lead–chelate excretion, urine collections should be extended to 3 or 4 days after administration of $CaNa_2EDTA$. The EDTA–lead mobilization tests offers a better assessment of body lead stores than does a single blood lead measurement. However, because of the dramatic reduction in lead exposure in the general population, the standard for defining excessive lead absorption used decades ago is no longer valid. At present, there is no generally accepted value to define an abnormal EDTA–lead mobilization test. The cumulative blood lead index and *in vivo* K X-ray-induced X-ray fluorescence remain valuable tools for epidemiologic studies of lead absorption, but their role in diagnosis for individual patients has not been established.

Lead–chelate excretion over 3 days after the intramuscular injection of 2 g of EDTA demonstrated excessive body lead stores in the United States Armed Service veterans with renal failure and 'essential' hypertension or gout, who had never exhibited symptoms of acute lead poisoning (Batuman *et al.* 1981, 1983). At the time of examination, mean blood lead concentrations were less than 0.97 μmol/l (20 μg/dl). The patients' recall of lead exposure correlated poorly with the objective evidence of the EDTA test, and lead had not been suspected as the cause of the kidney disease. Elevated lead stores appeared to be the cause, rather than consequence, of the renal disease because control patients with comparable renal failure of non-lead aetiology had normal chelation tests. Similar findings have been reported from Spain (Sánchez-Fructuoso *et al.* 1996). Measurement of lead in transiliac bone biopsies by atomic absorption spectroscopy in patients with endstage renal disease confirmed that lead accumulation was not a consequence of renal failure (Van de Vyver *et al.* 1988). These direct bone measurements also demonstrated that a systematic increase in bone lead does not occur preferentially in interstitial, as compared to glomerular, disease.

In vivo tibial K XRF is a safe, non-invasive technique for measuring bone lead (Somervaille *et al.* 1988). Because lead is stored in bone for decades, bone lead provides more direct information on cumulative lead absorption than either the blood lead or chelatable lead. The relationship between these biological monitors of lead exposure is illustrated in Table 2. XRF is not as useful as the blood lead concentration or EDTA–lead mobilization test for the diagnosis of nephropathy. However, *in vivo* XRF measurements of bone lead have supported the notion that low-level lead exposure is a risk factor for hypertension (Korrick *et al.* 1999).

Low-level lead exposure and hypertension

The role of lead as a cause of hypertension has been the subject of controversy (Wedeen 1984a, 1992). Controversy stemmed, in part, from inadequate longitudinal clinical records in industry and the tendency for individuals with hypertensive cardiovascular disease to be lost from cross-sectional epidemiological studies. In addition, the high prevalence of hypertension in the general population makes it difficult to select appropriate controls because large study groups are necessary to assess statistically significant differences between occupational and ambient exposures. Nevertheless, mortality data support the notion that hypertensive cardiovascular disease is a more frequent cause of death among lead workers than among the general population (Fanning 1988; Wedeen 1988; Nuyts *et al.* 1991). A role for lead in the induction of hypertension with renal failure [serum creatinine > 133 μmol/l (>1.5 mg/dl)] was suggested by Batuman *et al.* (1983), who studied patients using the EDTA– lead mobilization test. Patients with elevated amounts of chelatable lead in this study would have been designated 'essential' hypertensives had the chelation test not been performed.

Table 2 Levels of lead exposure

Exposure	Symptoms	Blood Pb		EDTA test[a]		Tibial[b]		
		μg/dl	μmol/l	μg/3 days	μmol/3 days	[Pb]		Pb : Ca ratio[c]
						μg/g	nmol/g	
Low continuous (ambient)	Hypertension	<25	<1.21	<600	<2.90	<15	<72	<0.10
Moderate, occasional (intermittent)	Tubulointerstitial nephritis Hypertension Gouty kidney	20–50	0.97–2.42	>600	>2.90	15–40	72–193	0.10–0.35
High, persistent (chronic)	Tubulointerstitial nephritis Hypertension Gouty kidney	30–80	1.45–3.86	>1000	>4.83	>40	>193	>0.35
Massive, rapid (acute)	Transient Hypertension Fanconi syndrome	>60	>2.90	>1000	>4.83	Time-dependent		

[a] Values are for adults.

[b] Wet weight. Determined by *in vivo* tibial X-ray fluorescence.

[c] Ratio of fluorescent K X-rays to elastic scatter.

The role of lead in hypertension gains further credence from epidemiological studies. The Second National Health and Nutrition Examination Survey (NHANES II), performed between 1976 and 1980, included blood lead and blood pressure measurements in almost 10,000 non-institutionalized Americans aged between 6 months and 74 years (Mahaffey *et al.* 1982). The correlation between blood lead and blood pressure (after confounding variables were accounted for) indicated that blood lead predicts blood pressure even when both measurements are within the 'normal' range (Pirkle *et al.* 1985; Hu *et al.* 1996; Korrick *et al.* 1999; Cheng *et al.* 2001) (Fig. 4). An increase in blood lead from 0.68 to 1.45 μmol/l (14–30 μg/dl) resulted in an increase of 7 mmHg in mean systolic pressure and of 3 mmHg in diastolic pressure (Harlan 1988). Similar conclusions emerged from a British study of 7371 middle-aged men (Pocock *et al.* 1988) and a number of smaller studies performed throughout the world (Schwartz 1995; Korrick *et al.* 1999). Other epidemiological studies, however, have failed to demonstrate a robust relationship between lead and blood pressure (Elwood *et al.* 1988; Staessen *et al.* 1996). Epidemiologic investigations increasingly support the notion that lead may elevate blood pressure at blood lead concentrations below 20 μg/dl (Cheng *et al.* 2001; Rothenberg 2002; Munter 2003; Nash 2003; Vupputuri 2003). Although some doubts have been raised about the magnitude of the dose–response relationship, there is a growing consensus that lead contributes to hypertension in the general population. Other studies indicate that blood leads under 40 μg/dl impair renal function (Kim *et al.* 1996; Weaver *et al.* 2003).

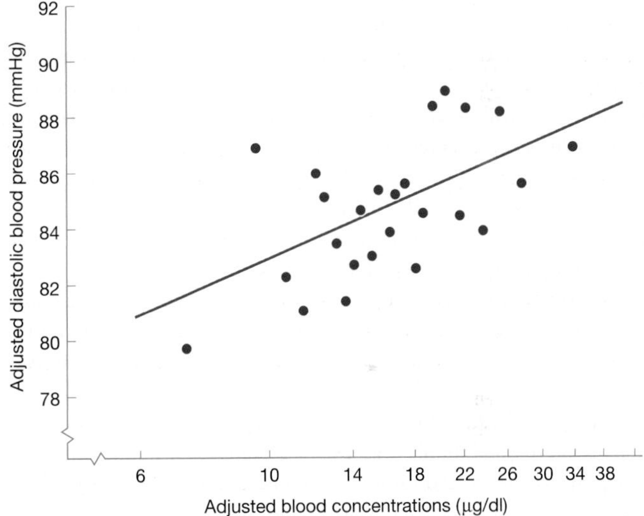

Fig. 4 Diastolic blood pressure and blood lead values for 564 Caucasian males aged 40–59 years from NHANES II. Values have been adjusted for age, age-squared, body mass index, and other potentially confounding variables and reduced to 25 points for illustrative purposes. These data show that blood lead predicts blood pressure even when both measurements are within the accepted 'normal' range (from Pirkle *et al.* 1985, with permission).

Management

Treatment of excessive lead absorption depends on the total amount of lead in the body, the rate of absorption, the age of the patient, and the degree of organ dysfunction. The method of assessing lead stores must be taken into account (blood lead, chelation test, or *in vivo* XRF), and the end-points of therapy determined before chelation therapy is undertaken. Lead removal from the body by chelation is not entirely innocuous: the toxicity of chelating agents in the presence of renal failure has not been systematically examined. $CaNa_2EDTA$ is safe as a diagnostic test (Wedeen *et al.* 1983), but the cumulative effect of repeated administration when renal function is compromised is not known. The efficacy and adverse effects of the promising new oral chelating agents, dimercaptopropanesulfonate, dimercaptosulfonic acid, and dimercaptosuccinic acid have not been examined in renal failure (Aposhian 1983; Twarog and Cherian 1984; Graziano *et al.* 1988).

Chelation therapy is indicated following acute massive exposure such as that encountered in childhood pica, after heavy occupational exposure, or following inadvertent poisoning from improperly glazed ceramics. Although chelation therapy can reverse the transient hypertension and Fanconi syndrome associated with massive, rapid lead absorption, treatment is primarily directed at preventing the life-threatening neurological complications of acute poisoning.

Low-level lead absorption can be minimized by environmental controls, avoiding excessive absorption from deteriorating lead-based paints, lead glazes, contaminated industrial sources, dust, and water.

The value of chelation therapy in chronic tubulointerstitial nephritis caused by chronic, moderate lead absorption is less clear. Although the prerenal component of acute exposure superimposed on chronic tubulointerstitial nephritis can be reversed by chelation therapy (Wedeen *et al.* 1979), there is no evidence that established interstitial fibrosis will be improved. The effectiveness of chelation therapy in reducing body lead stores can be monitored by repeated chelation testing or by *in vivo* K XRF (Batuman *et al.* 1989).

Cadmium nephropathy

An association between kidney disease and cadmium was first noted at the end of the nineteenth century, but the distinctive tubular proteinuria (Friberg 1948) and osteomalacia (Nicaud *et al.* 1942) were not recognized until the 1940s. Over the next 40 years, it remained unclear whether cadmium nephropathy was the result of concomitant nephrolithiasis or lead nephropathy. Until recently, few cases of progressive renal failure due to occupational exposure to cadmium had been identified; kidney stones are common among cadmium workers, and it was difficult to separate the effects of urinary tract obstruction from intrinsic renal parenchymal damage. In addition, workmen are frequently exposed to both lead and cadmium, each of which induces chronic tubulointerstitial nephritis whose clinical manifestations appear only years after the inception of exposure. The aetiological role of cadmium, therefore, was difficult to establish.

The differences between lead and cadmium nephropathies are, nevertheless, striking. Both metals are retained in the body with biological half-lives of about 10 years. In contrast to lead, cadmium is stored in the liver and kidney cortex, where it can be measured *in vivo* by neutron activation analysis. While both lead and cadmium accumulate in proximal tubule cells, lead is retained in intranuclear inclusion bodies, whereas cadmium is transported to lysosomes. Cadmium nephropathy is characterized by low molecular weight proteinuria due to diminished intrarenal uptake and catabolism of filtered proteins. In cadmium nephropathy, proximal tubular dysfunction persists until renal failure supervenes, whereas the Fanconi syndrome of acute lead poisoning is transient. The persistent hypercalciuria of cadmium nephropathy is responsible for characteristic clinical manifestations of kidney stones and osteomalacia.

Metabolism

Cadmium is widely used in the manufacture of plastics, pigments, glass, alloys, and electrical equipments. The greatest exposure occurs in smelting, electroplating, and welding operations; absorption is primarily by inhalation, but about 10 per cent is retained following ingestion. Inhalation of as little as 89–134 μmol (10–15 mg) causes severe gastrointestinal symptoms and may produce fatal acute pneumonitis or delayed chronic obstructive pulmonary disease (Nordberg *et al.* 1986). In experimental animals, high parenteral doses cause necrosis of the testes, sensory ganglia, and liver. An increased incidence of prostatic and lung cancer has been reported in cadmium workers, but the significance of these findings is questionable (Andersson *et al.* 1984; Waalkes and Rehm 1994).

Following absorption, cadmium is bound to albumin and transported to the liver where it induces the synthesis of a carrier protein, metallothionein, within 24 h. The cadmium–thionein complex is released from the liver into the blood, filtered in the glomerulus, and it accumulates in proximal tubules by pinocytosis and is transferred to lysosomes (Nordberg *et al.* 1986). Catabolism of the cadmium–thionein complex with release of unbound cadmium into the cytoplasm is believed to contribute to the proximal tubule injury together with the continuous resynthesis of metallothionein and prolonged organ retention. The cadmium–metallothionein complex has a biological half-life of several days (Elinder and Nordberg 1986) and is about 15 times more nephrotoxic than either cadmium alone or the zinc–thionein complex (Cherian 1984). Total body stores of cadmium in non-occupationally exposed adults range from 89 to 267 μmol (10–30 mg), with roughly one-third present in the kidneys and another third in the liver (Friberg 1984). Under steady-state conditions, red cell cadmium is 45–60 times that in the plasma.

Proximal tubule dysfunction

The kidney is considered the 'critical organ' for cadmium toxicity because the metal accumulates in the proximal tubule where it produces its most prominent toxic effect (Kjellstrom 1986a). In the absence of excessive exposure, cadmium accumulates in the kidney up to about 50 years of age, reaching a maximum concentration of 0.44–0.88 μmol/g kidney (50–100 μg/g kidney) and, although to a lower extent, in the liver up to about 80 years of age. At an intrarenal concentration of 1.78 μmol/g (200 μg/g) tubular injury becomes manifest by low molecular weight proteinuria, aminoaciduria, renal glucosuria, hypercalciuria, and increased urinary excretion of cadmium (Fig. 5).

Normal urinary cadmium excretion is lower than 2 μg/day. Once the critical intrarenal concentration is reached, urinary cadmium exceeds 10 μg/day. Above 30 μg/day, clinically important abnormalities of proximal tubular function ensue. The blood cadmium concentration is less reliable as an indicator of health effects. Although blood cadmium increases promptly following occupational exposure, blood is a poor indicator of cumulative absorption. Nevertheless, blood values greater than 0.089 μmol/l (1 μg/dl), as well as urine concentrations above 10 μg/g of creatinine, are considered evidence of excessive exposure.

Increased urinary excretion of low molecular weight proteins such as β_2-microglobulin or retinol binding protein is an early manifestation of the renal toxicity of cadmium (Table 1; Friberg 1986). Measurement of urinary retinol binding protein or *N*-acetyl-β-D-glucosaminidase is probably a more reliable indicator than β_2-microglobulin because these proteins are more stable in acid urine (Verschoor *et al.* 1987; Roels *et al.* 1993). Minor increases in the excretion of albumin and transferrin in cadmium workers with low molecular weight proteinuria and enzymuria raise the possibility of glomerular injury but are also compatible with an impaired tubular reabsorption/metabolism of these proteins that are normally filtered in small quantities. Proteinuria in cadmium workers rarely exceeds a few hundred milligrams per day and does not approach nephrotic levels (>2.5 g/day). The usual techniques for detecting albuminuria such as Albustix, heat and picric acid, or nitric acid are not sufficiently sensitive or specific to detect tubular proteinuria reliably. Although phosphotungstic, trichloroacetic, and sulfosalicylic

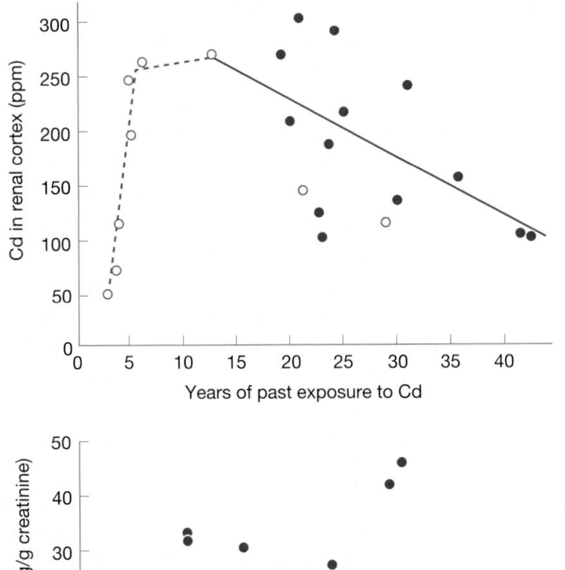

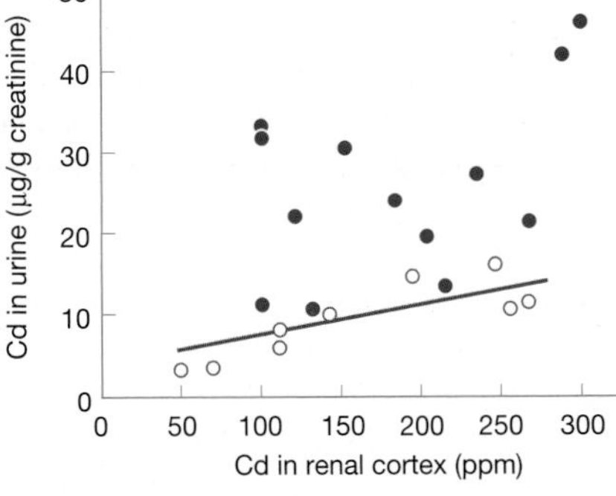

Fig. 5 The relationship of urinary cadmium excretion to renal cadmium content (determined by *in vivo* neutron activation analysis) and duration of past exposure. Open circles indicate no proteinuria, closed circles indicate increased urinary excretion of β_2-microglobulin (from Roels *et al.* 1981, with permission).

acids are more sensitive, immunological techniques are required for specific protein identification.

Renal calcium wasting raises the incidence of urinary tract stones up to 40 per cent among cadmium workers (Friberg 1986; Kjellstrom 1986b; Thun *et al.* 1989; Jarup and Elinder 1993). Osteomalacia with pseudofractures and severe bone pain was the major clinical manifestation of environmental cadmium poisoning identified in Japan after the Second World War (Nomiyama 1980; Friberg 1984). This syndrome, known as 'Itai–itai byo' ('ouch–ouch disease'), arose from consumption of rice contaminated by cadmium, derived from rivers polluted by metal-mining operations. The disease affected primarily postmenopausal, multiparous women who had subsisted on calcium- and vitamin D-deficient diets for decades. The victims developed a waddling gate, shortened stature, anaemia, glucosuria, and elevated serum alkaline phosphatase. Hypertension was absent. Excretion of β_2-microglobulin often exceeded the normal maximum (1 mg/g creatinine) 100-fold, and GFRs were substantially reduced in the most severely affected individuals. Mean serum creatinine increased from 106 to 149 µmol/l (1.19–1.68 mg/dl) in 21 individuals followed-up for 9–14 years after tubular proteinuria had been detected (Kido *et al.* 1990). This study was completed 5 years after cadmium had been removed from the environment, at which time the victims had reached an average age of 65 years. Japanese farmers appeared to be particularly vulnerable to cadmium-induced renal calcium wasting because of malnutrition, chronic calcium depletion, and the severity of the environmental contamination.

Chronic interstitial nephritis

The relative mortality from kidney disease is increased among cadmium workers (Andersson *et al.* 1984). Tubulointerstitial nephritis was reported in 23 occupationally exposed and in 26 environmentally exposed individuals in whom postmortem tissue or renal biopsies were examined (Kjellstrom 1986a).

In the United States, Thun *et al.* (1989) examined 45 current and retired non-ferrous smelter workers exposed to cadmium for a mean of 19 years. Blood and urine cadmium concentrations averaged 0.70 µmol/l (7.9 µg/dl) and 0.085 µmol/mol creatinine (9.3 µg/g creatinine), respectively. Excretion of β_2-microglobulin correlated significantly with serum creatinine values in these workers, three of whom had serum creatinines greater than 160 µmol/l (1.8 mg/dl). The cumulative cadmium dose estimated from air measurements correlated significantly with β_2-microglobulin and retinol binding protein excretion, and with fractional tubular reabsorption of phosphate and calcium. The cadmium workers had significantly more kidney stones, prostatic disease, diabetes mellitus, and hypertension than did local hospital workers who served as controls. The correlations between renal function and cadmium exposure, however, were independent of the latter medical conditions. The relationship between cadmium dose and serum creatinine persisted even when the smelter workers with hypertension, kidney stones, or diabetes mellitus were excluded from the analysis, and when blood lead concentrations were taken into consideration. This study indicates that the current US permissible exposure limit for cadmium of 200 µg/m^3 air in industry would result in renal disease after about 4.3 years of usual employment.

A longitudinal study of occupational cadmium nephropathy by Roels *et al.* (1989) further supports that clinical renal disease results from excessive cadmium absorption and that low molecular weight proteinuria predicts the adverse outcome. Twenty-three male workers with a mean age of 58.6 years, exposed to cadmium dust in a non-ferrous smelter up to 5 years previously, were examined annually for 5 years. They had been selected because their initial β_2-microglobulin or retinol binding protein excretion exceeded 0.3 mg/g creatinine. None had a history of hypertension, gout, kidney stones, or analgesic abuse. At the outset, urinary β_2-microglobulin averaged 1.8 mg/l, and urine cadmium 0.20 µmol/l (22.2 µg/l). Serum creatinine exceeded 177 µmol/l (2 mg/dl) in two workers. Cadmium concentrations ranged from 24 to 158 µg/g (mean 61 µg/g) in the liver and from 133 to 355 µg/g (mean 231 µg/g) in the kidney, as determined by *in vivo* neutron activation at the first examination. Subsequently, serum creatinine increased from a mean of 106 µmol/l (1.2 mg/dl) to a mean of 133 µmol/l (1.5 mg/dl) 5 years later. The estimated reduction in GFR averaged 30 ml/min/1.73 m^2 body surface area, about five times the anticipated age-adjusted reduction for males over 5 years. The predictive value of tubular proteinuria for progression of renal failure in cadmium-exposed workers does not hold for very low level exposures. A 5-year follow-up of 593 subjects with low-level environmental exposure to cadmium (urine cadmium $<$ 0.1 nmol/g creatinine) in the Cadmibel study in Belgium disclosed no reduction of renal function despite tubular proteinuria (Hotz *et al.* 1999). Nevertheless, even low-level exposure to cadmium may contribute to the progression of renal disease due to other causes (Hellström *et al.* 2001).

The effect of cadmium on blood pressure remains controversial because, in experimental animals, a hypertensive effect has been found after low dosage which disappears after high dosage (Elinder 1986). Evidence of a hypertensive effect of cadmium in humans is meagre (Staessen *et al.* 1991; Nakagawa and Nishijo 1996).

Diagnosis

In vivo measurement of liver and kidney cadmium content by neutron-capture γ-ray analysis is a safe, accurate, non-invasive, and portable method to assess cumulative cadmium retention. Once renal failure is clinically apparent, the renal cortex loses cadmium, so that neutron activation shows stable, rather than increasing cadmium levels, even when exposure is continued (Roels *et al.* 1981). Concomitant with the reduction in renal cadmium, urinary cadmium excretion increases, generally exceeding 0.09 μmol/l (10 μg/l), but liver cadmium may continue to increase. Liver cadmium concentrations greater than 0.54 μmol/g (60 μg/g) may therefore indicate cadmium nephrotoxicity even if renal cadmium declines to less than 1.79 μmol/g (200 μg/g) (Gompertz *et al.* 1983). Normally, urine contains less than 18 nmol/l (2 μg/l) and the whole blood concentration is less than 9 nmol/l (1 μg/l). Urine cadmium concentrations in excess of 0.09 μmol/l (10 μg/l; or 10 μg/g creatinine) are generally considered indicative of nephrotoxicity.

Management

Cadmium nephropathy cannot be reversed once tubulointerstitial disease has produced clinical renal failure. There is evidence that even the early cadmium-induced renal injury characterized by isolated tubular proteinuria may progress after termination of exposure (Roels *et al.* 1989; Thun *et al.* 1989). Chelation therapy with EDTA is ineffective after cadmium has accumulated in the kidney (Cantilena and Klassen 1982).

Mercury nephrotoxicity

The principal symptoms following environmental or occupational exposure to mercury are neurological, although acrodynia is still occasionally encountered in infants following the application of mercurial ointments for skin rashes. In the nineteenth century, tremors were present in up to 80 per cent of workers in the felt-hat industry (Wedeen 1989), a universally accepted risk to assume for the privilege of employment. Towards the end of the nineteenth century, elemental mercury lost favour among gilders and mirror manufacturers, only to find new uses in the production of scientific instruments. Proteinuria was first noted in 1916 as an uncommon accompaniment to the mercurial tremors (Teleky 1916). Occupational exposure to elemental mercury for a decade, with urine concentrations exceeding 2.5 μmol/l (50 μg/dl), is associated with increased intestinal alkaline phosphatase excretion but little increase in urinary tissue non-specific alkaline phosphatase, *N*-acetyl-β-D-glucosaminidase, retinol binding protein, Tamm–Horsfall glycoprotein, β_2-microglobulin, or microalbumin (Table 1; Nuyts *et al.* 1992; Cardenas *et al.* 1993a). There is as yet no evidence that enzymuria from mercury exposure predicts the development of renal failure as it does for cadmium.

Metabolism

Inorganic mercury selectively accumulates in the kidney, where it is retained with a half-life of about 2 months (Clarkson *et al.* 1988). The effect of mercury on the kidney is determined by its chemical form and the genetic background that modulates susceptibility to autoimmune disease. Neither elemental mercury nor the mercurous salt (Hg_2Cl_2, calomel) produces sustained renal tubular injury despite induction of tubular low molecular weight proteinuria, manifested by increased excretion of β_2-microglobulin, γ-glutamyl transferase, α_1-microglobulin, and *N*-acetyl-β-D-aminoglucosaminidase (Stonard *et al.* 1983). Tubular proteinuria occurs only after more than 0.5 μmol/l (100 μg/l) of mercury appears in the urine (Himeno *et al.* 1986). Biotransformation of inorganic mercury to mercuric ions is believed to account for renal accumulation. Mercury dichloride ($HgCl_2$), on the other hand, at parenteral doses of over 1 mg/kg, regularly produces acute tubular necrosis. Divalent mercury binds avidly to metallothionein and sulfydryl groups within the kidney. Recovery from tubular necrosis may be incomplete, leaving calcified tubular remnants, persistent tubulointerstitial nephritis, and chronic renal insufficiency.

A more complex picture emerges when one examines the renal effects of organomercurials. On the one hand, some organomercurials, including mercuhydrin and chlormerodrin, two diuretics, are avidly accumulated in the proximal tubule. Other organomercurials, such as *p*-chloromercuribenzoate, a compound devoid of diuretic effect but able to block mercurial diuresis, also accumulate within the proximal tubule (Wedeen and Goldstein 1963).

Inorganic and organic mercurials bind avidly to sulfydryl groups in circulating proteins and amino acids as well as intracellular glutathione, cysteine, and metallothionein. Selective accumulation in the pars recta of proximal tubules is achieved by absorptive endocytosis from the luminal side of mercury bound to amino acids or proteins. Mercury is released into the cytosol by intralysosomal enzymatic degradation (Zalups and Lash 1994). Excretion is primarily through bile in the faeces.

Industrial effluents containing mercury undergo biotransformation in aquatic reservoirs and are accumulated by both freshwater and saltwater fish as methylmercury, which induces neurological disease and is teratogenic. Methylmercury does not accumulate in the human kidney (Clarkson *et al.* 1988) and has not been reported to produce either acute or chronic renal failure (Iesato *et al.* 1977). Tubular proteinuria occurs after excessive methylmercury absorption, but total proteinuria is trivial. Phenylmercury is less neurotoxic than methylmercury but also induces tubular proteinuria (Clarkson *et al.* 1988); long-term intake can induce renal failure in experimental animals. Enzymuria from elemental, methyl, or phenylmercury is useful as an indicator of exposure for the prevention of the neurological effects, but whether such low molecular weight proteinuria signifies clinically important renal damage remains to be determined. A 40-year case–control follow-up study of patients with Minimata Disease due to environmental exposure to methylmercury found no increase in the incidence of renal disease despite evidence of the methylmercury-induced neurologic disease (Futatsuka *et al.* 2000).

Immunologically mediated glomerulonephritis

Case reports of the nephrotic syndrome (albuminuria >3.5 g/day) developing after occupational or therapeutic exposure to mercury have been taken to indicate idiosyncratic allergic reactions in humans. Kidney biopsies frequently reveal immune complex deposits in glomerular basement membranes indicative of membranous glomerulonephritis (Tubbs *et al.* 1982). A specific antigen has not been identified within the immune complexes. Normal glomeruli or antiglomerular basement membrane antibody disease have also been reported (Goldman *et al.* 1988).

The nephrotic syndrome is so uncommon in humans after exposure to mercury that the aetiological role of mercury has sometimes been doubted. Surveys of urinary protein excretion in occupationally exposed workers have shown only minimal increases in total protein excretion. Low molecular weight proteinuria (Buchet *et al.* 1980; Stonard *et al.* 1983), even when accompanied by minimal albuminuria, should not be confused with the massive albuminuria of the nephrotic syndrome, since very different pathophysiological mechanisms appear to be involved in both.

Genetic heterogeneity has made it difficult to study genetic susceptibility in humans. Immunological dose–response relationships cannot easily be discerned in genetically diverse populations. Consequently, inbred rodents have been used to identify a heightened immune response to chemical agents. Multiple small doses of $HgCl_2$ have been shown to induce membranous glomerulonephritis in certain inbred strains of rats (Bariety *et al.* 1971). This immunologically mediated glomerulonephritis may serve as a model for understanding human mercury-induced glomerulonephritis. The disease has also been produced in rabbits and mice using various forms of mercury, different routes of administration, and doses as low as 0.005 mg/l00 g body weight.

Druet and his associates have shown that the autoimmune response is under precise genetic control and is actually biphasic (Goldman *et al.* 1988). Antiglomerular basement membrane antibodies are found in glomeruli after 1 week. These autoantibodies are directed primarily against laminin in rats and against fibrillarin, a nucleolar protein, in mice (Hultman *et al.* 1998). Antifibrillarin antibodies are diagnostic of scleroderma in humans. Antibodies to these nucleolar proteins are also elicited by silver in susceptible mice (Hultman 1995). The initial linear deposits of antibasement glomerular membrane antibodies elicited by mercury in rats are replaced by granular IgG deposits in the arteriolar walls and mesangium, as well as in the glomerular basement membrane, 2 and 3 weeks after disease onset (Fig. 6). Immunoglobulin localization in the glomeruli is associated with heavy proteinuria, circulating immune complexes, and polyclonal B-cell activation due to anti-self Ia autoreactive T-cells. The glomerular disease can be transferred to T-cell-depleted rats by T-cells and T-helper cells taken from $HgCl_2$-treated rats of the same genetic background (Pelletier *et al.* 1988). Weening *et al.* (1981) found evidence that the autoimmune process is initiated by mercury inhibition of T-suppressor cell functions.

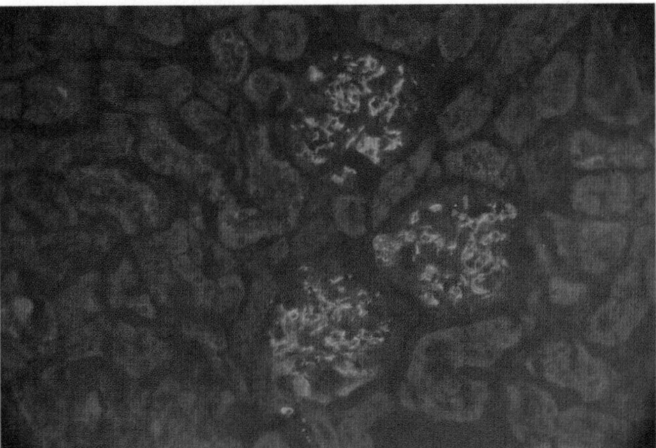

Fig. 6 Mercuric chloride-induced immune complex glomerulonephritis. IgG deposition is present in glomerular capillaries and mesangium of a Lewis/Brown Norway rat 4 weeks after intraperitoneal injection of $HgCl_2$, 0.1 mg/kg, three times a week for 2 weeks (from Wedeen 1984b, with permission).

The extremely low dose of mercury that elicits an autoimmune response in rodents makes an immune response to the minute doses of mercury absorbed from dental amalgams in humans (about 8 μg/day) plausible (Hultman *et al.* 1995). Although controversial, the possible relevance of these observations to human disease has stimulated extensive investigations of immune responses to a variety of metals in susceptible strains of rodents. Silver, gold, and cadmium have been shown to induce autoimmune responses in animals, but kidney disease has not developed in these models. Immune responses include the production of antinuclear antibodies in mice by minute doses of gold, silver, cadmium, and D-penicillamine. These responses to environmental agents are similar to the lupus- and scleroderma-like reactions in humans from hydralaizine, isoniazid, gold salts, and other xenobiotics (Ohsawa *et al.* 1988; Bigazzi 1999; Mayes 1999). Although the contribution of environmental agents to autoimmune disease in humans has not been convincingly established, the impact of these toxins on autoimmunity in humans may become clearer as the genetic basis of immune susceptibility is unravelled in the future.

Diagnosis

Blood mercury is a helpful indicator of the body burden of methylmercury, but is inappropriate for biological monitoring of inorganic mercury. While the presence of any mercury in urine is consistent with the diagnosis of mercury-induced nephrotic syndrome, individual susceptibility appears to be critical in determining the renal response. In the rodent model, genetic control of the autoimmune response to mercury has been demonstrated. It is not yet known whether specific genetic characteristics can be identified which will predict the induction of similar immunologically mediated glomerular disease by mercury in humans.

Management

The mercury-induced nephrotic syndrome disappears spontaneously after termination of exposure. British Antilewisite is an effective chelating agent for mercury when administered at an initial dose of 5 mg/kg intramuscularly, followed by 2.5 mg/kg for 10 days. The chelator of choice for mercury is generally considered to be DMPS (sodium-2-3-dimercapto-1-propane sulfonate) (Nerudova 2000).

Silicon

Crystalline silicon has a metallic lustre and greyish sheen and is therefore sometimes considered metallic, although with a specific gravity of only 2.3 it is not a heavy metal. Silicosis, the major adverse health effect of inhalation of silicon dusts, which occurs in miners, sandblasters, and glass manufacturers, for example, stimulates an autoimmune response characterized by the presence of circulating antinuclear antibodies, rheumatoid factor, and immune complexes (Stratta *et al.* 2001). In its severe form, nodular pulmonary fibrosis occurs, often complicated by tuberculosis and systemic manifestations of connective tissue disease simulating scleroderma or lupus erythematosus. Focal glomerulosclerosis and glomerular immune complex deposition have been described (Hauglustaine *et al.* 1980). Rapidly progressive crescentic glomerulonephritis in association with elevated antinuclear antibodies may complicate a fulminant form of silicosis known as silicoproteinosis (Bolton *et al.* 1981). Rapidly progressive glomerulonephritis has been reported in 11 coal miners with silicosis (Dracon *et al.* 1990) and a case–control study has shown an association between silica exposure and antineutrophil cytoplasmic antibody (ANCA)-positive rapidly progressive glomerulonephritis (Gregorini *et al.* 1993). Case–control studies have confirmed the association of silica exposure with ANCA-positive small vessel vasculitis (Hogan *et al.* 2001).

A case–control study of 272 patients with chronic renal failure confirmed the association of renal disease with exposure to silicon-containing compounds, as well as with exposure to lead, cadmium, and mercury (Nuyts *et al.* 1995a,b). In addition, grain dust and flour appeared to be significant risk factors for chronic renal disease. The possible role of these dusts in the induction of renal disease gains credence from a report indicating that grain dust and flour contain large amounts of silicon (Epstein 1994).

An association has also been found between the inhalation of silicon-containing compounds such as silica and grain dust and Wegener's granulomatosis in a case–control study (Nuyts *et al.* 1995a,b). The odds ratio for patients with endstage renal disease who worked as sandblasters is 3.8 compared to matched controls (Steenland *et al.* 1990). Linking data from 4626 silica-exposed workers with the US Endstage Renal Disease Registry (USRDS 1999) an excess of endstage renal disease (standardized incidence ratio = 1.97) and an excess of glomerulonephritis (standardized incidence ratio = 3.85) was found compared to the US population as a whole (Steenland *et al.* 2001). Silica appears to act as an adjuvant in stimulating the immune response (Parks *et al.* 1999).

Renal disease associated with silicon exposure may not be restricted to autoimmune manifestations: in one patient, electron-dense concentric lamellar cytoplasmic inclusions were found in glomerular epithelium, proximal, and distal tubules, simulating the fine structural alterations of Fabry's disease (Banks *et al.* 1983). In at least three cases, silicon-associated glomerulopathy, with silicon deposition in the kidneys, has been reported in the absence of pulmonary disease (Osorio *et al.* 1987). However, other potential aetiologies for glomerular disease were present, suggesting that silicon may interact with other causes of glomerular injury. It is, nevertheless, possible that silicates exert a direct nephrotoxic effect on the kidney: interstitial nephritis can be induced in guinea-pigs by the oral administration of silicates, and silicon calculi have been identified in the urinary tracts of both humans and animals (Dobbie and Smith 1986). Tubular proteinuria is found in workers exposed to silica dust (Dobbie and Smith 1982; Ng *et al.* 1993; Boujemaa *et al.* 1994; Hotz *et al.* 1995). These observations indicate that occupational exposure to silica in the absence of silicosis may lead to subclinical renal effects in less than 2 years.

Lithium

Lithium is used extensively in the treatment of manic-depressive psychosis. Different forms of renal effects/injury have been described: nephrogenic diabetes insipidus, the most frequent one, may lead to acute renal failure due to volume depletion. Chronic interstitial nephritis, nephrotic syndrome, and focal segmental glomerular sclerosis may lead to endstage renal disease with global glomerular sclerosis. Hyperparathyroidism is observed in lithium-treated patients.

Aetiology, pathogenesis, and pathology

Lithium is eliminated almost entirely by the kidney, through glomerular filtration followed by reabsorption in the proximal tubule, its renal clearance reaching one-third of the creatinine clearance. It moves slowly in and out of the intracellular compartment. Its accumulation in the collecting duct cells, through sodium channels of the luminal membrane (Boton *et al.* 1987), disrupts distal tubular function (resistance to antidiuretic hormone). Polyuria and polydipsia observed in lithium-treated patients is due to nephrogenic diabetes insipidus. Lithium inhibits adenylate cyclase and the generation of cyclic AMP with an attendant downregulation of aquaporin-2, the collecting tubule water channel (Marples *et al.* 1975) and a decrease in ADH receptor density (Hensen *et al.* 1996). The low intracellular level of cyclic AMP is also responsible for the increased cellular levels of glycogen observed in the kidney biopsy of patients given lithium.

The tubular defect in the distal nephron also impairs the ability to maximally acidify the urine, perhaps as a consequence of the lithium-induced decrease in the activity of the H ATPase pump in the collecting tubule (Dafnis *et al.* 1992). Lithium treatment has been aetiologically related to parathyroid hypertrophy and hyperfunction. Parathyroid hyperfunction seems due to an upward resetting of the level at which the plasma calcium concentration depresses parathyroid hormone (PTH) release. Persistent hypercalcaemia (5–10 per cent of the patients) may exacerbate both the concentrating defect and the interstitial nephritis of lithium-treated patients.

Biopsies in man show a specific histological lesion in the distal tubule and collecting duct. On light microscopy, considerable accumulation of periodic acid–Schiff (PAS)-positive glycogen is associated with swelling and vacuolization of the cells. This lesion, present in all renal biopsies from patients taking lithium, appears within days after administration of lithium and disappears when lithium ingestion is ceased (Walker *et al.* 1983).

Hestbech *et al.* (1977) were the first to suggest that progressive chronic interstitial lesions occurred in the kidneys of patients receiving lithium. A controlled study of renal biopsies, however, disclosed little difference between patients on lithium and patients with affective disorders but not given lithium (Walker *et al.* 1982a,b). There was, however, a significant increase in microcyst formation in the lithium-treated patients. Tubulointerstitial nephritis has been most frequently described in the presence of lithium-induced renal failure. Glomerular disease with the nephrotic syndrome has also been reported (Bosquet *et al.* 1997). On renal biopsy, foot process effacement, minimal change disease, or focal and segmental glomerulosclerosis have been observed. In 4 of 21 cases, the nephrotic syndrome regressed after withdrawal of lithium therapy but returned when lithium was reinstated (Bosquet *et al.* 1997). Bendz *et al.* (1994) found that 21 per cent of 142 patients treated with lithium for at least 15 years had significant reductions in age-adjusted GFR compared to a demographically matched control population. More recently, Markowitz *et al.* (2000) evaluated 24 patients with renal insufficiency (mean creatinine 2.8 mg/dl) who had received lithium for 2–25 years. They report in all cases a chronic tubulointerstitial nephropathy, associated with cortical and medullary tubular cysts or dilatation. There was a surprisingly high (50 per cent) prevalence of focal segmental glomerulosclerosis and global glomerulosclerosis, sometimes of a severity equivalent to the chronic tubulointerstitial disease.

Despite discontinuation of lithium, seven of nine patients with initial serum creatinine values greater than 2.5 mg/dl progressed to endstage renal disease. Nevertheless, the question whether chronic lithium therapy causes chronic interstitial nephritis, still needs more hard data.

Clinical expression

Next to the acute lithium intoxication (Timmer and Sands 1999), chronic toxicity can occur in patients with an elevated serum lithium level due to increased dosage, or to a decreased renal clearance induced by a lowered effective circulating volume, sodium intake, or by gastroenteritis, renal failure, and diabetes mellitus. Lithium alters glucose metabolism perhaps through the release of glucagon (Waziri and Nelson 1978). Symptoms associated with poisoning include lethargy, drowsiness, coarse hand tremor, muscle weakness, nausea, vomiting, loss polyuria, and polydipsia. Severe toxicity is associated with increased deep tendon reflexes, seizures, syncope, renal insufficiency, and coma. The common manifestation is altered mental status. Lithium chronic poisoning is frequently associated with electrocardiogram changes including ST-segment depression and inverted T-waves in the lateral precordial leads. Lithium is concentrated within the thyroid and inhibits thyroid synthesis and release that can go along with hypothyroidism and hypothermia (Lazarus 1986). It may also cause thyrotoxicosis and hyperthermia. Hypercalcaemia may coexist and exacerbate the urine concentration defect already present in these patients.

In the presence of glomerular lesions proteinuria may be present within 1.5–10 months after the onset of therapy, but resolves in most patients, completely or partially within 1–4 weeks after lithium is discontinued.

Diagnosis and treatment

The hyperparathyroidism observed in patients under lithium treatment is characterized with elevated PTH levels, hypercalcaemia, hypocalciuria, and normal serum phosphate levels in contrast to primary hyperparathyroidism in which hypophosphataemia and hypercalciuria are seen (Wolf *et al.* 1997).

The severity of chronic lithium intoxication correlates directly with the serum lithium concentration and may be categorized as mild (1.5–2.0 mmol/l), moderate (2.0–2.5 mmol/l), or severe (>2.5 mmol/l). Therapeutic serum lithium concentrations should be maintained below 1 mmol/l.

The symptoms of nephrogenic diabetes insipidus as well as the other acute manifestations of lithium renal toxicity usually disappear rapidly after lithium withdrawal. Life-threatening hypernatraemia related to diabetes insipidus has been successfully treated with indomethacin (Lam and Kjellstrand 1997). Prescription of Li should consider the benefits of controlling and preventing the manifestation of manic-depressive psychosis as well as the disadvantage to the patient of lithium's major side-effect, polyuria. Lithium is so clearly beneficial in most cases that the polyuria is accepted as a side-effect and lithium is usually continued. Serum concentration of lithium is important as renal damage is more likely to occur if the serum concentration is consistently high or if episodes of lithium toxicity recur. The serum lithium concentration should thus be maintained at the lowest level compatible with an adequate control of the manic-depressive psychosis. Episodes of toxicity should be prevented by a careful monitoring of serum lithium levels and by the avoidance of clinical conditions such as dehydration or medications such as diuretics reducing Li clearance.

Uranium

Uranyl nitrate injected into experimental animals consistently induces acute tubular necrosis. Extensive experiments in both animals and humans, connected with development of the atomic bomb during the Second World War, made it clear that the kidney is the primary site of acute toxicity (Dounce 1949). Hexavalent uranium readily enters the bloodstream after inhalation and is filtered at the glomerulus as a bicarbonate complex. The bicarbonate complex breaks down to UO_2^{2+}, which binds to intracellular proteins and produces necrotic lesions in the second and third parts of the proximal tubule. Uranyl nitrate has also been reported to induce intrarenal cyst formation in rats (Haley *et al.* 1982). Catalase, alkaline phosphatase, and β_2-microglobulin excretion are increased in uranium workers, but chronic renal failure has not been described in humans.

Arsenic and chromium

Chronic renal disease has not been reported after industrial exposure to arsenic or chromium. However, acute tubular necrosis may result from arsine gas (AsH_3) in industrial accidents. Arsine, used as a poison gas in the First World War, is a colourless and odourless gas, produced when arsenicals are mixed with acid. Inhalation produces massive haemolysis, haematuria, jaundice, and abdominal pain within a few hours and acute tubular necrosis within a few days. Haemodialysis is required. Removal of arsenic–haemoglobin complex from the circulation by exchange transfusion may be lifesaving. Incomplete recovery from acute tubular necrosis has resulted in persisting chronic tubulointerstitial nephritis in surviving victims (Muehrcke and Pirani 1968). Incomplete recovery from patchy cortical necrosis following consumption of 'moonshine' (illicitly distilled spirit) contaminated with arsenic may also result in persisting renal disease (Gerhardt *et al.* 1977).

Acute oliguric renal failure and tubular necrosis occur following massive absorption of hexavalent chromium as chromate or dichromate (Kaufman *et al.* 1970). Renal failure is not produced by trivalent chromium. Minimal tubular proteinuria in the absence of reduced glomerular filtration has been reported in chromeplaters (Lindberg and Vesterberg 1983), but the implications of this finding for clinically relevant renal disease remain speculative. Like other heavy metals, chromium selectively accumulates in the proximal tubule, but there is little evidence of chronic renal disease resulting from usual occupational exposure (Mutti *et al.* 1985; Verschoor *et al.* 1988; Wedeen and Qian 1991; Vyskocil *et al.* 1992; Wang *et al.* 1994). The finding of an odds ratio of 2.7 (confidence interval 1.2–6.3) for occupational exposure to chromium in a case–control study of chronic renal failure warrants further evaluation of the association of environmental exposure to chromium with chronic renal disease (Nuyts 1995a).

Germanium

Falling just below silica in Group IVA in the Periodic Table, which includes tin and lead, germanium has a specific gravity of 5.23. Like silicon, it has semiconductor properties. It has been used in the treatment of cancer, a variety of medical ailments, and in unproven remedies for conditions such as arthritis, AIDS, and the chronic fatigue syndrome. Germanium-containing elixirs and health foods were reported to cause chronic tubulointerstitial nephritis, first in Japan and subsequently in Europe and the United States (Okada *et al.* 1989; Takeuchi *et al.* 1992; Hess *et al.* 1993). Most cases are due to the ingestion of germanium oxide (GeO_2), but germanium–lactate–citrate, and the organic germanium compound, carboxyethylgermanium sesquioxide (Ge-132), have also been implicated. The tubulointerstitial nephritis is insidious; widening of the interstitium and tubular atrophy (apparently distal tubular) is evident after prolonged (6–36 months), high-dose (16 to hundreds of grams) consumption. The disease is slowly progressive even after exposure has been terminated. Fatal outcomes have been reported. The pathophysiological mechanism of tubular damage is unclear because selective accumulation in the kidney does not occur and immunological mechanisms have not been implicated. There is no evidence of primary proximal tubular injury. Proteinuria is absent. Electron-dense, PAS reagent-positive granules (containing germanium in the experimental rat) are found in distal tubular mitochondria (Sanai *et al.* 1991). Vacuolization is present in proximal and distal tubular epithelia. Prolonged consumption of germanium compounds also induces severe hepatic steatosis, polymyositis, and peripheral neuropathy. Acute lactic acidosis has been reported from germanium–lactate–citrate (Krapf *et al.* 1992; Hess *et al.* 1993).

References

(Entries marked with an asterisk comprise useful general reading.)

Andersson, K., Elinder, C. G., Hogstedt, Nuyts, G. D., and Van Viem, E. (1984). Mortality among cadmium and nickel-exposed workers in a Swedish battery factory. *Toxicological and Environmental Chemistry* **9**, 53–62.

Aposhian, H. V. (1983). DMSA and DMPS-water soluble antidotes for heavy metal poisoning. *Annual Review of Pharmacology and Toxicology* **23**, 193–197.

Ashouri, O. S. (1985). Hyperkalemic distal tubular acidosis and selective aldosterone deficiency: combination in a patient with lead nephropathy. *Archives of Internal Medicine* **145**, 1306–1307.

Banks, D. E. *et al.* (1983). Silicon nephropathy mimicking Fabry's disease. *American Journal of Nephrology* **3**, 279–284.

Bariety, J., Druet, P., Laliberte, F., and Sapin, C. (1971). Glomerulonephritis with gamma- and beta-1C-globulin deposits induced in rats by mercuric chloride. *American Journal of Pathology* **65**, 293–302.

Barry, P. S. I. A. (1975). A comparison of concentrations of lead in human tissues. *British Journal of Industrial Medicine* **32**, 119–139.

Batuman, V., Maesaka, J. K., Habbad, B., Tepper, E., Landy, E., and Wedeen, R. P. (1981). The role of lead in gout nephropathy. *New England Journal of Medicine* **304**, 520–523.

***Batuman, V., Landy, E., Maesada, J. K., and Wedeen, R. P.** (1983). Contribution of lead to hypertension with renal impairment. *New England Journal of Medicine* **309**, 17–21.

Batuman, V., Wedeen, R. P., Bogden, J., Balestra, D. J., Jones, K., and Schidlovsky, G. (1989). Reducing bone lead content by chelation treatment in chronic lead poisoning. An *in vivo* X-ray fluorescence and bone biopsy study. *Environmental Research* **48**, 70–75.

Behringer, D., Craswell, P., Mohl, C., Stoeppler, M., and Ritz, E. (1986). Urinary lead excretion in uremic patients. *Nephron* **42**, 323–329.

***Bendz, H., Aurell, M., Balldin, J., Mathé, A. A., and Sjödin, I.** (1994). Kidney damage in long-term lithium patients: a cross-sectional study of patients with 15 years or more on lithium. *Nephrology, Dialysis, Transplantation* **9**, 1250–1254.

***Bigazzi, P. E.** (1999). Metals and kidney autoimmunity. *Environmental Health Perspectives* **107**, 753–765.

Bolton, W. K., Suratt, P. M., and Stingill, A. (1981). Rapidly progressive silica nephropathy. *American Journal of Medicine* **71**, 823–828.

Boscolo, P., Galli, G., Iannaccone, A., Martino, F., Porcelli, G., and Troncone, L. (1988). Plasma renin activity and urinary kallikrein excretion in lead-exposed workers as related to hypertension and nephropathy. *Life Science* **28**, 175–184.

Bosquet, S., Gauthier, T., Fellay, G., and Regamey, C. (1997). Nephrotic syndrome during lithium therapy. *Nephrology, Dialysis, Transplantation* **12**, 2728–2731.

Boton, R., Gaviria, M., and Battle, C. D. (1987). Prevalence, pathogenesis, and treatment of renal dysfunction associated with chronic lithium therapy. *American Journal of Kidney Diseases* **10**, 329–345.

Boujemaa, W., Lauwerys, R., and Bernard, A. (1994). Early indicators of renal dysfunction in silicotic workers. *Scandanavian Journal of Work and Environmental Health* **20**, 181–191.

Buchet, J. P., Roels, H., Bernard, A., Jr., and Lauwerys, R. (1980). Assessment of renal function of workers exposed to inorganic lead, cadmium or mercury vapor. *Journal of Occupational Medicine* **22**, 741–750.

Campbell, B. C., Meredith, P. A., and Scott, J. J. G. (1985). Lead exposure and changes in the renin–angiotensin–aldosterone system in man. *Toxicology Letters* **55**, 25–32.

Cantilena, L. R. and Klassen, C. D. (1982). The effect of repeated administration of several chelators on the distribution and excretion of cadmium. *Toxicology and Applied Pharmacology* **66**, 361–367.

***Cardenas, A.** *et al.* (1993a). Markers of early renal changes induced by industrial pollutants. I. Application to workers exposed to mercury vapour. *British Journal of Industrial Medicine* **50**, 17–27.

***Cardenas, A.** *et al.* (1993b). Markers of early renal changes induced by industrial pollutants. II. Application to workers exposed to lead. *British Journal of Industrial Medicine* **50**, 28–36.

Chamberlain, A. C. (1985). Prediction of response of blood lead to airborne and dietary lead from volunteer experiments with lead isotopes. *Proceedings of the Royal Society, London* **B244**, 149–182.

Cheng, Y., Schwartz, J., Sparrow, D., Aro, A., Weiss, S. T., and Hu, H. (2001). Bone lead and blood lead levels in relation to baseline blood pressure and the prospective development of hypertension: the normative aging study. *American Journal of Epidemiology* **153** (2), 164–171.

Cherian, M. G. (1984). Chelation of cadmium without increased renal cadmium deposition. *Environmental Health Perspectives* **54**, 175–179.

Chisolm, J. J., Mellits, E. D., and Barrett, M. B. Interrelationships among blood lead concentration, quantitative daily ALA-U and urinary lead output following calcium EDTA. In *Effects and Dose–Response Relationships of Toxic Metals* (ed. G. F. Nordberg), pp. 416–433. Amsterdam: Elsevier, 1976.

Clarkson, T. W., Hursh, J. B., Sager, P. R., and Suversen, T. L. M. Mercury. In *Biological Monitoring of Heavy Metals* (ed. T. W. Clarkson, L. Friberg, G. F. Norberg, and P. R. Sager), pp. 199–247. New York, NY: Plenum Press, 1988.

***Colleoni, N. and D'Amico, G.** (1986). Chronic lead accumulation as a possible cause of renal failure in gouty patients. *Nephron* **44**, 32–35.

Cramer, K., Goyer, R. A., Jagenberurg, R., and Wilson, M. H. (1974). Renal ultrastructure, renal function, and parameters of lead toxicity in workers with different periods of lead exposure. *British Journal of Industrial Medicine* **31**, 113–127.

Dafnis, E., Kurtzman, N. A., and Sabatini, S. (1992). Effects of lithium and amiloride on collecting tubule transport enzymes. *Journal of Pharmacology and Experimental Therapeutics* **261**, 701–706.

Dobbie, J. W. and Smith, M. J. B. (1982). Silicate nephropathy in the experimental animal: the missing factor in analgesic nephropathy. *Scottish Medical Journal* **27**, 10–16.

Dobbie, J. W. and Smith, M. J. B. (1986). Urinary and serum silicon in normal and uraemic individuals. *Ciba Foundation Symposium* **12**, 194–213.

Dounce, A. L. The mechanism of action of uranium compounds in the animal body. In *Pharmacology and Toxicology of Uranium Compounds* Division VI, Vol. 1 (ed. C. Voegtlin and H. C. Hodge), pp. 951–991. New York, NY: McGraw-Hill, 1949.

Dracon, M., Noel, C., Wallaert, B., Dequiet, P., and Tacquet, A. (1990). Glomerulonephrites rapidement progressives chez les mineurs de charbon pneumoconiotiques. *Néphrologie* **11**, 61–65.

Elinder, C.-G. Other toxic effects. In *Cadmium and Health: A Toxicological and Epidemiological Appraisal* Vol. II (ed. L. Friberg, C.-G. Elinder, T. Kjellstrom, and G. F. Nordberg), pp. 159–204. Boca Raton, FL: CRC Press, 1986.

Elinder, C.-G. and Nordberg, M. Metallothionein. In *Cadmium and Health: A Toxicological and Epidemiological Appraisal* Vol. I (ed. L. Friberg, C.-G. Elinder, T. Kjellstrom, and G. F. Nordberg), pp. 159–204. Boca Raton, FL: CRC Press, 1986.

Elwood, P. C., Davey-Smith, G., Oldham, P. D., and Toothill, C. (1988). Two Welsh surveys of blood lead and blood pressure. *Environmental Health Perspectives* **78**, 119–122.

*Emmerson, B. T. (1973). Chronic lead nephropathy. *Kidney International* **4**, 1.

Endo, G., Horiguchi, S., and Kiyota, I. (1990). Urinary *N*-acetyl-β-D-glucosaminidase activity in lead-exposed workers. *Journal of Applied Toxicology* **10**, 235–238.

Epstein, E. (1994). The anomaly of silicon in plant biology. *Proceedings of the National Academy of Sciences, USA* **96**, 11–17.

Fanning, D. (1988). A mortality study of lead workers, 1926–1985. *Archives of Environmental Health* **43**, 247–251.

Fels, L. M., Bundschuh, I., Gwinner, W., Jung, K., Pergande, M., and Graubaum, H.-J. (1994). Early urinary markers of target nephron segments as studied in cadmium toxicity. *Kidney International* **46** (Suppl. 47), S-81–S-88.

Friberg, L. (1948). Proteinuria and kidney injury in workman exposed to cadmium and nickel dust. *Journal of Industrial Hygiene* **30**, 32–36.

Friberg, L. (1984). Cadmium and the kidney. *Environmental Health Perspectives* **54**, 1–11.

Friberg, L. Introduction. In *Cadmium and Health: A Toxicological and Epidemiological Appraisal* Vol. I (ed. L. Friberg, C.-G. Elinder, T. Kjellstrom, and G. F. Nordberg), pp. 1–6. Boca Raton, FL: CRC Press, 1986.

Futatsuka, M. *et al.* (2000). Health surveillance in the population living in a methyl mercury-polluted area over a long period. *Environmental Research* **83**, 83–92.

Gerhardt, R. E., Crecelis, E. A., and Hudson, J. B. (1977). Moonshine-related arsenic poisoning. *Archives of Internal Medicine* **140**, 211–213.

Germain, M. J., Braden, G. L., and Fitzgibbons, J. P. (1984). Failure of chelation therapy in lead nephropathy. *Archives of Internal Medicine* **144**, 2419–2420.

*Goldman, M., Baran, D., and Druet, P. (1988). Polyclonal activation and experimental nephropathies. *Kidney International* **34**, 141–150.

Gompertz, D. *et al.* (1983). Renal dysfunction in cadmium smelters: relation to *in-vivo* liver and kidney cadmium concentrations. *Lancet* **i**, 1185–1187.

Goyer, R. A. and Wilson, M. H. (1975). Lead-induced inclusion bodies: results of ethylenediaminetetraacetic acid treatment. *Laboratory Investigation* **32**, 149–156.

Graziano, J. H., Lolacono, N. J., and Meyer, P. (1988). Dose–response study of oral 2,3-dimercaptosuccinic acid in children with elevated blood lead concentrations. *Journal of Pediatrics* **113**, 751–757.

Gregorini, G., Ferioli, A., Donato, F., Tira, P., Morassi, L., and Taranico, R. Association between silica exposure and necrotizing crescentic glomerulonephritis with *p*-ANCA and with anti-MPO antibodies: a hospital based case control study. In *ANCA-Associated Vasculitides. Immunological and Clinical Aspects. Advances in Experimental Medicine and Biology* Vol. 336 (ed. W. Gross), pp. 435–439. New York, NY: Plenum Press, 1993.

Haley, D. P., Bulger, R. E., and Dobyan, D. C. (1982). The long-term effects of uranyl nitrate on the structure and function of the rat kidney. *Virchows Archiv (Cellular Pathology)* **41**, 181–192.

Harlan, W. R. (1988). The relationship of blood lead levels to blood pressure in the U.S. population. *Environmental Health Perspectives* **78**, 9–14.

Hauglustaine, D., Van Damme, B., Baenens, P., and Michielsen, P. (1980). Silicon nephropathy: a possible occupational hazard. *Nephron* **26**, 219–224.

Hensen, J., Haenelt, M., and Gross, P. (1996). Lithium induced polyuria and renal vasopressin receptor density. *Nephrology, Dialysis, Transplantation* **11**, 622–627.

*Hess, B. *et al.* (1993). Tubulointerstitial nephropathy persisting 20 months after discontinuation of chronic intake of germanium lactate citrate. *American Journal of Kidney Diseases* **21**, 548–557.

Hestbech, J., Hansen, H. E., Amdisen, A., and Olsen, S. (1977). Chronic renal lesions following long-term treatment with lithium. *Kidney International* **12**, 205–213.

*Hellström, L. *et al.* (2001). Cadmium exposure and end-stage renal disease. *American Journal of Kidney Diseases* **38**, 1001–1008.

Himeno, S., Watanabe, C., and Suzuki, T. (1986). Urinary biochemical changes in workers exposed to mercury vapor. *Industrial Health* **24**, 151–155.

*Hogan, S. I. *et al.* (2001). Silica exposure in anti-nuclear cytoplasmic antibody-associated glomerulonephritis and lupus nephritis. *Journal of the American Society of Nephrology* **12**, 134–142.

Hotz, P., Lorenzo, J., Fuentes, E., Cortes, G., Lauwerys, R., and Bernard, A. (1995). Subclinical signs of kidney dysfunction following short exposure to silica in the absence of silicosis. *Nephron* **70**, 438–442.

*Hotz, P., Buchet, J. P., Bernard, A., Lison, D., and Lauwerys, R. (1999). Renal effects of low-level environmental cadmium exposure: 5-year follow-up from the Cadmibel study. *Lancet* **354**, 1508–1513.

*Hu, H. (1991). A 50-year follow-up of childhood plumbism. Hypertension, renal function, and hemoglobin levels among survivors. *American Journal of Diseases of Children* **145**, 681–687.

Hu, H. *et al.* (1996). The relationship of bone and blood lead to hypertension. *Journal of American Medical Association* **275** (15), 1171–1176.

Hultman, P., Ganowiak, K., Turley, S. J., and Pollard, K. M. (1995). Genetic susceptability to silver-induced autoantibodies in mice. *Clinical Immunology and Immunopathology* **77**, 291–297.

*Hultman, P., Lindh, U., and Horsted-Bindslev, P. (1998). Activation of the immune system and systemic immune-complex deposits in Brown Norway rats with dental amalgam restorations. *Journal of Dental Research* **77**, 1415–1425.

Iesato, K., Wakashin, M., Wakashin, Y., and Tojo, S. (1977). Renal tubular dysfunction in Minimata disease. Detection of renal tubular antigen and beta-2-microglobulin in the urine. *Annals of Internal Medicine* **86**, 731–737.

Inglis, J. A., Henderson, D. A., and Emmerson, B. T. (1978). The pathology and pathogenesis of chronic lead nephropathy occurring in Queensland. *Journal of Pathology* **124**, 65–76.

Jarup, L. and Elinder, C. G. (1993). Incidence of renal stones among cadmium exposed battery workers. *British Journal of Industrial Medicine* **50**, 598–602.

Kaufman, D. B., DiNickola, W., and McIntosh, R. (1970). Acute potassium dichromate poisoning. *American Journal of Diseases of Children* **119**, 374–376.

*Kido, T., Nogawa, K., Ishizaki, M., Honda, R., Tsuritani, I., and Yamada, Y. (1990). Long-term observation of serum creatinine and arterial blood pH in persons with cadmium-induced renal dysfunction. *Archives of Environmental Health* **45**, 35–43.

Kim, R. *et al.* (1996). A longitudinal study of low-level lead exposure and impairment of renal function: The Normative Aging Study. *Journal of the American Medical Association* **275**, 1177–1181.

Kjellstrom, T. Renal effects. In *Cadmium and Health: A Toxicological and Epidemiological Appraisal* Vol. II (ed. L. Friberg, C.-G. Elinder, T. Kjellstrom, and G. F. Nordberg), pp. 21–110. Boca Raton, FL: CRC Press, 1986a.

Kjellstrom, T. Effect on bone, vitamin D and calcium metabolism. In *Cadmium and Health: A Toxicological and Epidemiological Appraisal* Vol. II (ed. L. Friberg, C.-G. Elinder, T. Kjellstrom, and G. F. Nordberg), pp. 111–158. Boca Raton, FL: CRC Press, 1986b.

Korrick, S. A., Hunter, D. J., Rotnitzky, A., Hu, H., and Speizer, F. E. (1999). Lead and hypertension in a sample of middle-aged women. *American Journal of Public Health* **89**, 330–335.

Krapf, R., Schaffner, T., and Iten, P. X. (1992). Abuse of germanium associated with fatal lactic acidosis. *Nephron* **62**, 351–356.

Lam, S. S. and Kjellstrand, C. (1997). Emergency treatment of lithium-induced diabetes insipidus with non-steroidal anti-inflammatory drugs. *Renal Failure* **19**, 183–188.

Lazarus, J. H. *Endocrine and Metabolic Effects of Lithium*. New York, NY: Plenum Medical, 1986.

Lilis, R., Gavrilescu, N., Nestorescu, B., Dumitriu, C., and Roventa, A. (1968). Nephropathy in chronic lead poisoning. *British Journal of Industrial Medicine* **25**, 196–202.

Lindberg, E. and Vesterberg, O. (1983). Urinary excretion of proteins in chromeplaters, exchromeplaters and referents. *Scandinavian Journal of Work, Environment and Health* **9**, 505–510.

Loghman-Adham, M. (1998). Aminoaciduria and glycosuria following severe childhood lead-poisoning. *Pediatric Nephrology* **12**, 218–221.

Mahaffey, K. R., Annest, J. L., Roberts, J., and Murphy, R. A. (1982). National estimates of blood lead levels, 1976–1980: association with selected demographic and socioeconomic factors. *New England Journal of Medicine* **307**, 573–579.

*Markowitz, G. S., Radhakrishnan, J., Kambham, N., Valeri, A. M., Hines, W. H., and D'Agati, V. D. (2000). Lithium nephrotoxicity: a progressive combined glomerular and tubulointerstitial nephropathy. *Journal of the American Society of Nephrology* **11**, 1439–1448.

Marples, D., Christensen, S., Christensen, E. I., Ottosen, P. D., and Nielsen, S. (1975). Lithium-induced down regulation of aquaporin-2 water channel expression in rat kidney medulla. *Journal of Clinical Investigation* **95**, 1838–1845.

Mayes, M. D. (1999). Epidemiologic studies of environmental agents and systemic autoimmune diseases. *Environmental Health Perspectives* **107**, 743–748.

MMWR (1994). Blood lead levels—United States, 1988–1991. *Morbidity and Mortality Weekly Report* **43**, 545–548.

*Muehrcke, R. C. and Pirani, C. L. (1968). Arsine-induced anuria. A correlative clinicopathological study with electron microscopic observations. *Annals of Internal Medicine* **68**, 853–866.

Munter, P., Vupputyuri, S., Coresh, J., and Batuman, V. (2003). Blood lead and chronic kidney disease in the general United States population: results from NHANES III. *Kidney International* **63**, 104–150.

Mutti, A., Valcavi, P., Fornari, M., Lucertini, S., Neri, T. M., and Alinivi, R. (1985). Urinary excretion of brush-border antigen revealed by monoclonal antibody: early indicator of toxic nephropathy. *Lancet* **ii**, 914–917.

*Mutti, A. *et al.* (1992). Nephropathies and exposure to perchloroethylene in dry cleaners. *Lancet* **340**, 189–193.

Nakagawa, H. and Nishijo, M. (1996). Environmental cadmium exposure, hypertension and cardiovascular risk. *Environmental Monitoring and Human Health* **3**, 11–17.

Nash, D., Magder, L., Lustberg, M., Sherwin, R., Rubin, R., Kaufmann, R., and Silbergeld, E. (2003). Blood lead, blood pressure, and hypertension in perimenopausal and postmenopausal women. *Journal of the American Medical Association* **289** (12), 1523–1531.

Nerudova, J., Cabelkova, Z. A., Frantik, E., Lukas, E., Urban, P., Blaha, K., Pelclova, D., Lebedova, D., and Cikrt, M. (2000). Mobilization of mercury by DMPS in occupationally exposed workers and in model experiments on rats: evaluation of body burden. *International Journal of Occupational Medicine and Environmental Health* **13**, 131–146.

Ng, T. P., Lee, H. S., and Phoon, W. H. (1993). Further evidence of human silica nephrotoxicity in occupationally exposed workers. *British Journal of Industrial Medicine* **50**, 907–912.

Nicaud, P., Lafitte, A., and Gross, A. (1942). Les troubles de l'intoxication chronique par le cadmium. *Archives des Maladies Professionelles de Medecine du Travail et de Scienité* **1**, 192–202.

Nomiyama, K. (1980). Recent progress and perspectives in cadmium health effects studies. *Science of the Total Environment* **14**, 199–232.

Nordberg, G. F., Kjellstrom, T., and Nordberg, M. Kinetics and metabolism. Other toxic effects. In *Cadmium and Health: A Toxicological and Epidemiological Appraisal* Vol. I (ed. L. Friberg, C.-G. Elinder, T. Kjellstrom, and G. F. Nordberg), pp. 103–178. Boca Raton, FL: CRC Press, 1986.

Nouwen, E. J. and De Broe, M. E. (1994). Human intestinal versus tissue-nonspecific alkaline phosphatase as complementary urinary markers for the proximal tubule. *Kidney International* **46** (Suppl. 47), S-43–S-51.

Nuyts, G., Dalemans, R. A., Jorens, G., Elseviers, M. M., Van de Vyver, E., and De Broe, M. E. (1991). Does lead play a role in the development of chronic renal disease? *Nephrology, Dialysis, Transplantation* **6**, 307–315.

Nuyts, G. D., Roels, H. A., Verpooten, G. F., Bernard, A. M., Lauwerys, R. R., and De Broe, M. E. (1992). Intestinal-type alkaline phosphatase in urine as an indicator of mercury induced effects on the S3-segment of the proximal tubule. *Nephrology, Dialysis, Transplantation* **7**, 225–229.

Nuyts, G. D. *et al.* (1995a). New occupational risk factors for chronic renal failure. *Lancet* **346**, 7–11.

*Nuyts, G. D. *et al.* (1995b). Wegener granulomatosis is associated to exposure to silicon compounds: a case control study. *Nephrology, Dialysis, Transplantation* **10**, 1162–1165.

Ohsawa, M., Takaha hi, K., and Osuka, F. (1988). Induction of antinuclear antibodies in mice orally exposed to cadmium at low concentrations. *Clinical and Experimental Immunology* **73**, 98–102.

Okada, K. *et al.* (1989). Renal failure caused by long-term use of a germanium preparation as an elixir. *Clinical Nephrology* **31**, 219–224.

Osorio, A. M., Thun, M. J., Novak, R. F., van Cura, J., and Avner, E. D. (1987). Silica and glomerulonephritis: a case report and review of the literature. *American Journal of Kidney Diseases* **9**, 224–230.

Parks, C. G., Conrad, K., and Cooper, G. S. (1999). Occupational exposure to crystalline silica and autoimmuune disease. *Environmental Health Perspectives* **107**, 793–802.

Peitzman, S. J., Bodison, W., and Ellis, I. (1985). Moonshine drinking among hypertensive veterans in Philadelphia. *Archives of Internal Medicine* **145**, 632–634.

Pelletier, L., Pasquier, R., Rossert, J., Vial, M.-C., Mandet, C., and Druet, P. (1988). Autoreactive T cells in mercury-induced autoimmunity. Ability to induce the autoimmune disease. *Journal of Immunology* **140**, 750–754.

Piomelli, S., Seaman, C., Zuillow. D., Curran, A., and Davidoff, B. (1982). Threshold for lead damage to heme synthesis in urban children. *Proceedings of the National Academy of Sciences USA* **79**, 3335–3339.

*Pirkle, J. L., Schwartz, J., Landis, J. R., and Harlan, W. R. (1985). The relationship between blood lead levels and blood pressure and its cardiovascular risk implications. *American Journal of Epidemiology* **121**, 246–258.

Pocock, S. J., Shaper, A. G., Ashby, D., Delves, H. T., and Clayton, B. E. (1988). The relationship between blood lead, blood pressure, stroke, and heart attacks in middle-aged British men. *Environmental Health Perspectives* **78**, 23–30.

Roels, H. A., Lauwerys, R. R., Buchet, J. P., Bernard, A. M., Vos, A., and Oversteyns, M. (1989). Health significance of cadmium-induced renal dysfunction: a five-year follow-up. *British Journal of Industrial Medicine* **46**, 755–764.

Roels, H. A. *et al.* (1981). *In vivo* measurement of liver and kidney cadmium in workers exposed to this metal: its significance with respect to cadmium in blood and urine. *Environmental Research* **26**, 217–240.

*Roels, H. *et al.* (1993). Markers of early renal changes induced by industrial pollutants. III. Application to workers exposed to cadmium. *British Journal of Industrial Medicine* **50**, 37–48.

Rosen, J. F. *et al.* (1989). L-line X-ray fluorescence of cortical bone lead compared with CaNa:2EDTA test in lead-toxic children: public health implications. *Proceedings of the National Academy of Sciences USA* **86**, 685–689.

Rothenberg, S.J., Kondrashov, V., Manalo, M., Jiang, J., Cuellar, R., Garcia., M., Reynoso, B., Reyes, S., Diaz, M., and Todd, A.C. (2002). Increases of hypertension and blood pressure during pregnancy with increased bone lead. *American Journal of Epidemiology* **156** (12), 1079–1087.

Sanai, T. *et al.* (1991). Chronic tubulointerstitial changes induced by germanium dioxide in comparison with carboyxethyl sesquioxide. *Kidney International* **40**, 882–890.

*Sánchez-Fructuoso, A. I., Torralbo, A., Arroyo, M., Luque, M, Ruilope, L. M., Santos, J. L., Crucyra, A., and Barrientos, A. (1996). Occult lead intoxication as a cause of hypertension and renal failure. *Nephrology, Dialysis, Transplantation* **11**, 1775–1780.

*Schwartz, J. (1995). Lead, blood pressure, and cardiovascular disease in man. *Archives of Environmental Health* **50**, 31–37.

Skerfving, S. *et al.* (1983). Metabolism of inorganic lead in occupationally exposed humans. *Arhiv za Higijenu Rada I Toksikologiju* **34**, 341–350.

Skerfving, S. *et al.* (1987). Biological monitoring, by *in vivo* XRF measurements, of occupational exposure to lead, cadmium, and mercury. *Biological Trace Element Research* **13**, 241–251.

Somervaille, L. J. *et al.* (1988). *In vivo* tibia lead measurements as an index of cumulative exposure in occupationally exposed subjects. *British Journal of Industrial Medicine* **45**, 174–181.

Staessen, J. *et al.* (1991). Blood pressure, the prevalence of cardiovascular disease, and exposure to cadmium: a population study. *American Journal of Epidemiology* **134**, 257–267.

Staessen, J. *et al.* (1994). Renal function is inversely correlated with lead exposure in the general population. *New England Journal of Medicine* **327**, 151–156.

Staessen, J., Roels, H., Fagard, R. for the PheeCad Investigators (1996). Lead exposure and conventional and ambulatory blood pressure. *Journal of the American Medical Association* **275**, 1563–1570.

Steenland, N. K., Thun, M. J., Ferguson, C. W., and Port, F. K. (1990). Occupational and other exposures associated with male end-stage renal disease; a case–control study. *American Journal of Public Health* **80**, 153–159.

***Steenland, K., Sanderson, W., and Calvert, G. M.** (2001). Kidney disease and arthritis in a cohort study of workers exposed to silica. *Epidemiology* **12**, 405–412.

Stonard, M. D., Chater, B. V., Duffield, D. P., Nevitt, A. L., Sullivan, J. J. O., and Steel, G. T. (1983). An evaluation of renal function in workers occupationally exposed to mercury vapour. *International Archives of Occupational and Environmental Health* **52**, 177–189.

***Stratta, P., Carnavese, C., Messuerotti, A., Fenoglio, I., and Fubini, B.** (2001). Silica and renal disease: no longer a problem in the 21st century? *Journal of Nephrology* **14**, 228–247.

Takeuchi, A. *et al.* (1992). Nephrotoxicity of germanium compounds: report of a case and review of the literature. *Nephron* **60**, 436.

Teleky, L. Mercury poisoning. In *Diseases of Occupation and Occupational Hygiene* (ed. G. M. Kober and W. C. Hanson), pp. 126–135. Philadelphia, PA: P. Blakiston's Sons, 1916.

***Thun, M. J., Osorio, A. M., Schober, S., Hannon, W. H., and Halperin, W.** (1989). Nephropathy in cadmium workers—assessment of risk from airborne occupational cadmium exposure. *British Journal of Industrial Medicine* **46**, 689–697.

Timmer, R. T. and Sands, J. M. (1999). Lithium intoxication. *Journal of the American Society of Nephrology* **10**, 666–674.

Tubbs, R. R. *et al.* (1982). Membranous glomerulonephritis associated with industrial mercury exposure. *American Journal of Clinical Pathology* **77**, 409–413.

Tucker, B. J., Rasch, R., and Blantz, R. C. (1993). Glomerular filtration and tubular reabsorption of albumin in preproteinuric and proteinuric diabetic rats. *Journal of Clinical Investigation* **92**, 686–694.

Twarog, T. and Cherian, M. G. (1984). Chelation of lead by dimercaptopropane sulfonate and a possible diagnostic use. *Toxicology and Applied Pharmacology* **72**, 550–556.

Vander, A. J. (1988). Chronic effects of lead on the renin–angiotensin system. *Environmental Health Perspectives* **78**, 77–84.

Van de Vyver, F. L. *et al.* (1988). Bone lead in dialysis patients. *Kidney International* **33**, 601–607.

Verberk, M. M., Willems, T. E. P., Verplanke, A. J. W., and De Wolff, F. A. (1996). Environmental lead and renal effects in children. *Archives of Environmental Health* **51**, 83–87.

Verpooten, G. F., Nouwen, E. J., Hoylaerts, M. F., Hendrix, P. G., and De Broe, M. E. (1989). Segment-specific localization of intestinal-type alkaline phosphatase in human kidney. *Kidney International* **36**, 617–625.

Verschoor, M. A., Herber, R., van Hemmen, J., Wibow, A., and Zielhuis, R. (1987). Renal function of workers with low-level cadmium exposure. *Scandinavian Journal of Work, Environment and Health* **13**, 232–238.

Verschoor, M. A., Bragt, P. C., Herber, R. M. F., Zielhuis, R. L., and Zwennis, W. C. M. (1988). Renal function of chrome-plating workers and welders. *International Archives of Occupational and Environmental Health* **60**, 67–70.

Vupputuri, S., He, J., Munter, P., Bazzano, L., Whelton, P. K., and Batuman, V. (2003). Blood lead level is associated with elevated blood pressure in blacks. *Hypertension* **41** (3), 463–468.

Vyskocil, A. *et al.* (1992). Lack of renal changes in stainless steel welders exposed to chromium and nickel. *Scandinavian Journal of Work, Environment and Health* **18**, 252.

Waalkes, A. P. and Rehm, S. (1994). Cadmium and prostate cancer. *Journal of Toxicology and Environmental Health* **43**, 251–269.

Walker, R. G., Bennett, W. M., Davies, B. M., and Kincaid-Smith, P. (1982a). Structural and functional effects of long-term lithium therapy. *Kidney International* **21** (Suppl. 11), S13–S19.

Walker, R. G., Davies, B. M., Holwill, B. J., Dowling, J. P., and Kincaid-Smith, P. (1982b). A clinicopathological study of lithium nephrotoxicity. *Journal of Chronic Diseases* **35**, 685–695.

Walker, R. G. *et al.* (1983). Renal pathology associated with lithium therapy. *Pathology* **15**, 403–411.

Waziri, R. and Nelson, J. (1978). Lithium in diabetes mellitus: a paradoxical response. *Journal of Clinical Psychology* **39**, 623–625.

Wang, X. *et al.* (1994). Chromium-induced early changes in renal function among ferrochromium-producing workers. *Toxicology* **90**, 93–101.

Weaver, B. M. *et al.* (2003). Associations of renal function with polymorphisms in the δ-aminolevulinic dehydratase, vitamin D receptor, and nitric oxide synthase genes in Korean lead workers. *Environmental Health Perspectives* **111**, 1613–1619.

Wedeen, R. P. *Poison in the Pot: The Legacy of Lead.* Carbondale, IL: Southern Illinois University Press, 1984a.

Wedeen, R. P. (1984b). Occupational renal disease. *American Journal of Kidney Diseases* **3**, 241–257.

Wedeen, R. P. (1985). Blood lead levels, dietary calcium, and hypertension. *Annals of Internal Medicine* **102**, 403–404.

Wedeen, R. P. (1988). Occupational and environmental renal diseases. *Current Nephrology* **11**, 65–106.

Wedeen, R. P. (1989). Were the hatters of New Jersey 'mad'? *American Journal of Industrial Medicine* **16**, 225–233.

***Wedeen, R. P.** Lead, the kidney, and hypertension. In *Human Lead Exposure* (ed. H. Needleman), pp. 170–189. Boca Raton, FL: CRC Press, 1992.

Wedeen, R. P. Occupational diseases of the kidney and urinary tract. In *The Identification and Control of Environmental and Occupational Diseases* Vol. 23 (ed. M. A. Mehlman and A. Upton), pp. 387–423. Princeton, NJ: Princeton Scientific Publishing, 1994.

Wedeen, R. P. and Goldstein, M. H. (1963). Renal tubular localization of chlormerodrin labelled with mercury-203 by autoradiography. *Science* **141**, 438–441.

Wedeen, R. P. and Qian, L. (1991). Chromium-induced kidney disease. *Environmental Health Perspectives* **92**, 71–74.

Wedeen, R. P., Batuman, V., and Landy, E. (1983). The safety of the EDTA lead-mobilization test. *Environmental Research* **30**, 58–62.

***Wedeen, R. P., Mallik, D. K., and Batuman, V.** (1979). Detection and treatment of occupational lead nephropathy. *Archives of Internal Medicine* **139**, 53–57.

Wedeen, R. P. *et al.* (1975). Occupational lead nephropathy. *American Journal of Medicine* **59**, 630–641.

Weening, J. J., Fleuren, G. J., and Hoedemaeker, P. J. (1981). Demonstration of antinuclear antibodies in mercuric-chloride-induced glomerulopathy in the rat. *Laboratory Investigation* **39**, 405–411.

Weiler, E., Khalil-Manesh, F., and Gonick, H. (1988). Effects of lead and natriuretic hormone on kinetics of sodium–potassium-activated adenosine triphosphatase: possible relevance to hypertension. *Environmental Health Perspectives* **78**, 113–118.

Wolf, M. E., Moffat, M., Mosnaim J., and Dempsey, S. (1997). Lithium therapy, hypercalcemia, and hyperparathyroidism. *American Journal of Therapeutics* **4**, 323–325.

Wright, L. F., Saylor, R. P., and Cecere, F. A. (1984). Occult lead intoxication in patients with gout and kidney disease. *Journal of Rheumatology* **11**, 517–520.

Zalups, R. K. and Lash, L. H. (1994). Advances in understanding the renal transport and toxicity of mercury. *Journal of Environmental Toxicology and Health* **42**, 1–44.

6.6 Radiation nephropathy

Eric P. Cohen

Introduction

Sufficient local kidney or total body irradiation (TBI) will injure kidneys, resulting in radiation nephropathy. The older term of 'nephritis' may imply an inflammatory condition, but radiation nephropathy does not have major inflammatory features. The classically described form is caused by local kidney irradiation, but TBI or radionuclide isotope therapy may also result in radiation nephropathy.

Historical aspects

That kidneys might be injured by X-ray therapy was first described in 1906, a little more than 10 years after the discovery of X-rays (Edsall 1906). Domagk, who later pioneered sulfa antibiotics, clearly documented in 1927 renal damage due to radiation. By the mid-twentieth century, the clinical features were well known and the dose limits of fractionated local kidney irradiation were also well described (Luxton 1953). This contributed to a declining use of radiation therapy when kidneys might be in the field of irradiation, so that by 1970, radiation nephropathy was a clinical rarity. The increasing use of chemotherapy instead of radiotherapy also contributed to this decline, as exemplified by the use of *cis*-platinum, and other cytotoxic chemotherapies, in the treatment of seminoma (Duchesne *et al.* 1997). Since 1980, radiation nephropathy has been increasingly reported in patients who have undergone TBI in preparation for bone marrow transplantation (BMT), the so called BMT nephropathy (Chappell *et al.* 1988; Antignac *et al.* 1989; Cohen 2000). Within the past several years, the use of yttrium^{90} radionuclide therapy for neuroendocrine malignancies has been recognized as a cause of radiation nephropathy (Cohen *et al.* 2001; Moll *et al.* 2001). Other radionuclides have been associated with radiation nephropathy (Giralt *et al.* 2003).

Pathogenesis

Two theories, the vascular and the parenchymal, have been proposed for the pathogenesis of radiation nephropathy. Both rest on the generally accepted mechanism of radiation induced cell death, which is the induction of double stranded DNA breaks. Both potentially apply to either external irradiation of kidneys or the whole body, as well as to internal irradiation by an isotope that reached the kidney after parenteral injection. The vascular theory posits that radiation causes a primary vascular lesion with subsequent ischaemic injury to the rest of the kidney. The parenchymal theory holds that cell loss in the kidney, particularly epithelial cell loss, is the direct and essential effect of irradiation. In favour of the vascular theory is the acknowledged early endothelial injury, the occurrence of intimal and medial thickening, and the clinical feature of hypertension. But radiation nephropathy is not merely ischaemic, and its arteriolar and arterial lesions are not primary in a chronological sense. In the dog model, for instance, they appear to have causal importance but only after the loss of tubular cells (Hoopes *et al.* 1985) and in a mouse model, the vascular abnormalities are late and unimpressive (Glatstein 1977). The parenchymal theory rests on an *in vitro* kidney epithelial cell radiation sensitivity that is comparable to that of other cell types, and on the epithelial cell depletion that has been well documented in several studies (Hoopes *et al.* 1985; Withers *et al.* 1986). It does not, however, account for the unusual glomerular injury of radiation nephropathy, and does not easily explain the hypertension, which can be a major feature. In addition, mere cellular depletion probably does not account for the enhanced glomerular permeability observed as early as one hour after irradiation in laboratory rats (Sharma *et al.* 2001). Both theories largely ignore the potential contribution of apoptosis to radiation injury, as opposed to necrotic cell death. This may be relevant, because unlike necrosis, apoptosis does not beget inflammation, and radiation nephropathy is not an inflammatory condition.

Endothelial injury appears to be an important feature of classical radiation nephropathy as well as its modern congener, BMT nephropathy. Glomerular capillary thromboses are described in each, and, on a molecular level, enhanced expression of plasminogen activator inhibitor type one (PAi-1) has been found in the glomeruli of irradiated rat kidneys (Oikawa *et al.* 1997). Tubular injury and interstitial fibrosis are undeniable additional features that are not easily explained by glomerular damage alone.

It appears more likely that although irradiation reaches simultaneously all kidney cells, the expression of the injury is influenced by the balance between necrotic and apoptotic cell death, and by the different time lag at which irradiated cells manifest injury. Thus, glomerular preceeds tubular injury, but both are probably of equal importance in determining organ failure. It is possible, for instance, that glomerular damage, via proteinuria, causes more downstream tubulointerstitial damage when there is downstream tubulolysis or atrophy. Simply put, the proteins that leak from the damaged glomerulus would have an easier egress into the interstitium, and could more readily start the scarring process (Fig. 1).

External irradiation causes radiation nephropathy when it exceeds 10 Gy in a single dose, or 20 Gy, fractionated in 20 doses over 4 weeks. Lower doses may cause injury after a longer interval. Generally, more than 50 per cent of the renal volume needs to be irradiated to result in radiation nephropathy. Of course, scarring of a smaller irradiated

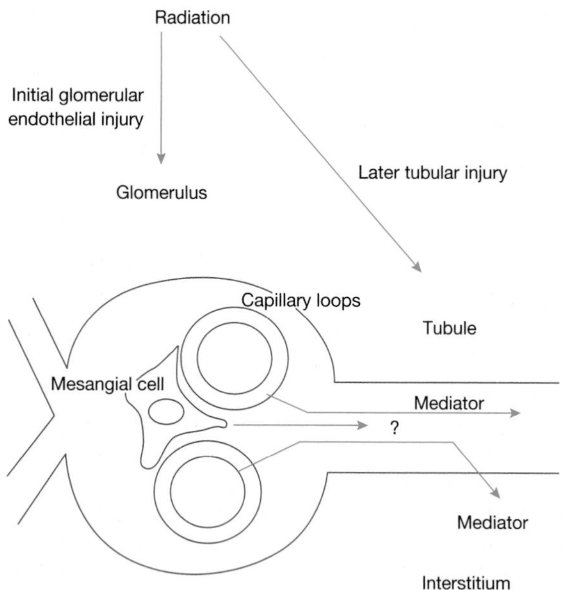

Fig. 1 Schematic view of radiation nephropathy. The initial glomerular injury is endothelial. Fibrin and other mediators are generated and lead to glomerular scarring. The same mediators leave the glomerulus via the tubule, and contribute to interstitial scarring, especially if there is subsequent tubular epithelial injury and death. The latter is a correlate and predictor of organ failure in many forms of kidney disease. Reproduced by permission, from Cohen E.P. and Lawton C.A. Pathogenesis, prevention, and management of radiation nephropathy. In *Current Radiation Oncology* Vol. 3 (ed. J.S. Tobias and P.R.M. Thomas). E. Arnold Ltd., 1997.

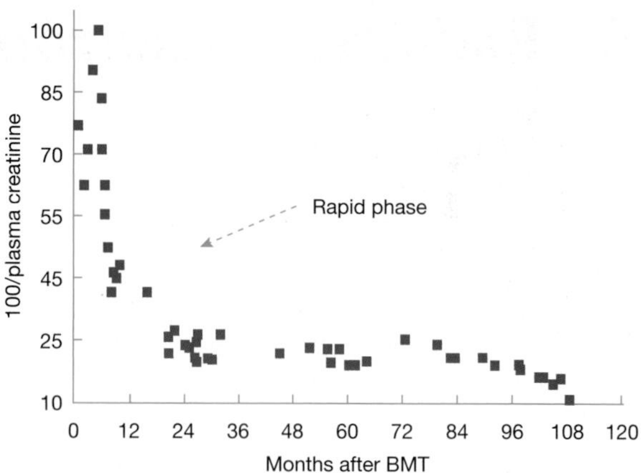

Fig. 2 Evolution of renal function in a patient with bone marrow transplant nephropathy, shown as 100/plasma creatinine versus time. The pattern is biphasic: an initial rapid decline ('rapid phase'), followed by a plateau culminating in endstage renal disease 9 years after bone marrow transplantation. Reproduced by permission, from Cohen, E.P. (2000). Radiation nephropathy after bone marrow transplantation. *Kidney International* **58**, 903–918.

volume could result in hypertension, perhaps mediated by renin, with subsequent hypertensive injury. Cytotoxic chemotherapy potentiates the effects of irradiation, in kidney as in other tissues (Arneil *et al.* 1974; Phillips *et al.* 1975). This probably explains why a total kidney dose of 14 Gy, fractionated in nine doses over three days, may cause radiation nephropathy in cancer patients undergoing BMT. Such patients have, indeed received substantial previous cytotoxic chemotherapy.

The beneficial effects of angiotensin-converting enzyme (ACE) inhibitors and angiotensin II blockers in experimental radiation nephropathy have suggested to some that the renin–angiotensin system is activated by renal irradiation. Although older data are compatible with this hypothesis (Fisher and Hellstrom 1968), current studies show that neither the systemic nor the intrarenal renin–angiotensin system is activated in radiation nephropathy (Cohen *et al.* 2002). The benefit of ACE inhibitors or angiotensin II blockers in radiation nephropathy appears to occur via blockade of a normally active renin–angiotensin system.

Clinical features

In the cases of local kidney irradiation, TBI, or radionuclide therapy, signs or symptoms of radiation nephropathy appear only several months after the incident irradiation: radiation-induced cell and organ injury is a delayed phenomenon. Three or more months after irradiation, symptoms and signs include fluid retention with oedema and hypertension, disproportionately severe anaemia, and azotaemia. The more severe cases may present as an haemolytic uraemic syndrome or thrombotic thrombocytopenic purpura (HUS/TTP). Such syndromes are well documented in BMT nephropathy (Chappell *et al.* 1988; Cohen 2000), and are associated with a rapid loss of kidney function. In most cases of BMT nephropathy, there is a biphasic loss of kidney function, well illustrated on a graph of 100/plasma creatinine versus time (Fig. 2) (Cohen *et al.* 1993). The initial loss of kidney function is rapid (5 ml/min/month or more) up to five times faster than in usual chronic renal failure (from 0.5 to 1 ml/min/month). Thus, unless interrupted by treatment, complete renal failure may ensue in a year or even less. Hypertension may be severe, and in some cases even malignant with altered mental status or seizures. Anaemia and its attendant symptoms complicate both classical radiation nephropathy and BMT nephropathy. It is more severe than expected for the degree of renal impairment, as shown on Fig. 3, for radiation and BMT nephropathy. Proteinuria is usually modest, at least in BMT nephropathy, being 2.5 g/day on the average (Cohen *et al.* 1993). Hyperkalaemia may occur, even in the absence of ACE inhibitors or angiotensin II blockers.

The urine sediment shows granular casts. Red blood cell casts were seen in one case, and haemoglobin casts in another.

Control of the blood pressure with ACE inhibitors or angiotensin II blockers may stabilize glomerular filtration rate (GFR) for months or years. Despite appropriate therapy, endstage renal failure sometimes ensues and imposes dialysis or kidney transplantation. The symptoms and signs of uraemia are no different in these patients than they are in others with endstage renal failure.

Differential diagnosis

Sufficient local kidney irradiation, usually greater than 2000 cGy (rads) fractionated over several weeks, encompassing more than 50 per cent of the total kidney volume, is a necessary feature of suspected radiation nephropathy. In the case of BMT nephropathy, one must confirm the use of TBI at the time of pre BMT 'conditioning'. In the case of radiation nephropathy related to use of radio-isotopes, there is a history of therapeutic doses of this isotope, often in excess of 200 mCi/m^2. An interval—usually months—separates the ionizing radiation and the occurrence of kidney disease. These patients may have other causes for

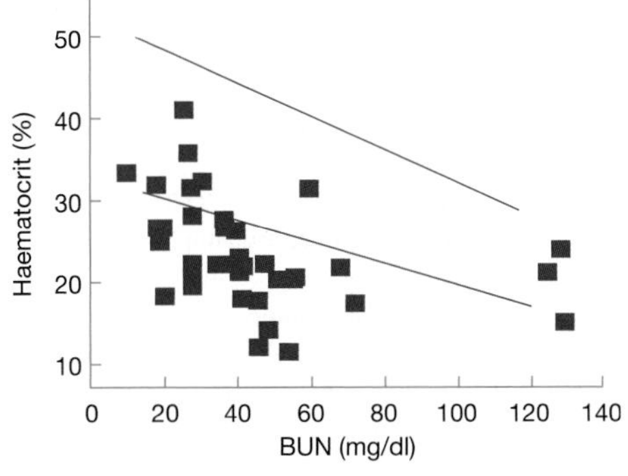

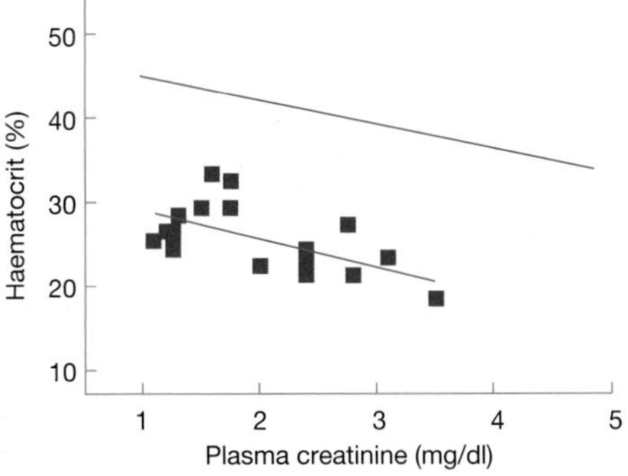

Fig. 3 Relationships between azotaemia, as BUN (top panel) and as plasma creatinine (bottom panel), and haematocrit, in classical radiation nephropathy (top panel) and in BMT nephropathy (bottom panel). The expected range of these relationships is shown by the upper and lower lines in each panel. The actual data from individual cases are shown as black squares. Anaemia of radiation and BMT nephropathy is relatively more severe than expected for the degree of concurrent azotaemia. Adapted from Cohen, E.P. and Lawton, C.A. Pathogenesis, prevention, and management of radiation nephropathy. In *Current Radiation Oncology* Vol. 3 (ed. J.S. Tobias and P.R.M. Thomas). E. Arnold Ltd., 1997, and reproduced by permission.

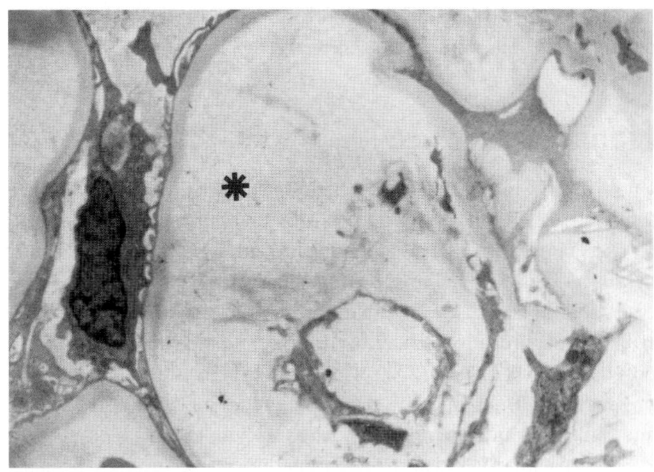

Fig. 4 Electron micrograph of a kidney biopsy in a case of BMT nephropathy, 6000×. There is a wide space between the endothelium and the glomerular basement membrane, indicated with an asterisk. The amorphous material accumulating in the gap contains non-specific plasma proteins and, sometimes, red cells or platelet fragments. There are no electron-dense deposits.

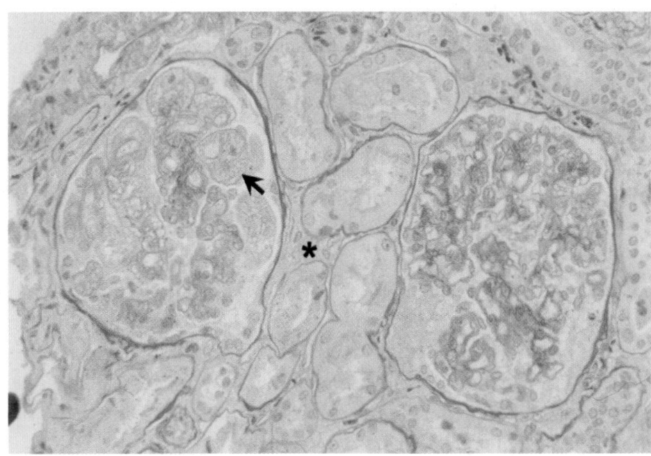

Fig. 5 Light micrograph of a kidney biopsy in a case of BMT nephropathy, 160×, PAS stain. There is mesangial cell dropout, that is, mesangiolysis, with ballooning out of the glomerular capillaries as a microaneurysm and extreme widening of the subendothelial space (arrow), interstitial fibrosis and tubular basement membrane thickening (asterisk).

renal injury. Use of *cis*-platinum, for instance, cause chronic interstitial nephritis. The magnesium wasting induced by *cis*-platinum may differentiate it from other causes of renal failure. Use of pamidronate, a bisphosphonate that may reduce bone mineral loss or reduce hypercalcaemia, has been associated with nephrotic syndrome and focal glomerulosclerosis in subjects with multiple myeloma who have undergone BMT (Barri *et al.* 2001; Markowitz *et al.* 2001). In such cases, proteinuria may exceed 10 g/day, which is much more than the average of 2.5 g/day in BMT nephropathy. BMT patients may be treated with nephrotoxins, such as cyclosporin, the effects of which may be hard to distinguish from radiation. Adjustment of the cyclosporin A (CSA) dose may improve kidney function in cases of CSA nephrotoxicity, but not in BMT nephropathy. The course of a BMT patient may be complicated by graft versus host disease (GVHD), a condition associated with membranous nephropathy and a nephrotic syndrome (Barbara *et al.* 1992).

Histology

Glomerular, tubular, vascular, and interstitial changes each occur in radiation nephropathy. In experimental radiation nephropathy, the glomerular endothelium appears to be the first site of injury, with leucocyte attachment and endothelial swelling occurring at 3 weeks after single dose 9.8 Gy local kidney irradiation (Jaenke *et al.* 1993).

Subsequently, in both experimental and clinical radiation nephropathy, there is a wide separation between the damaged endothelium and the glomerular basement membrane (Fig. 4). Mesangiolysis is a prominent feature. It may cause the formation of microaneurysms, with ballooning—out of the capillary loops (Fig. 5). Podocytes are not greatly affected. Glomerular capillary loops may show fibrin deposits with eventual thrombosis. Fibrinoid necrosis may be seen in arterioles. Intimal hyperplasia and medial thickening are seen. Glomerular changes preceed chronologically the vascular changes. Tubulolysis, a dropout of tubular epithelial cells leaving a denuded basement membrane, is observed in some experimental models of radiation nephropathy (Robbins and Bonsib 1995) but it is as yet unknown whether it preceeds the tubular atrophy seen in human radiation nephropathy. Interstitial fibrosis is a non-specific finding common to most chronic progressive kidney diseases. There is generally little inflammation in classical radiation nephropathy, or its modern congener, BMT nephropathy.

Management

Until recently, management of radiation nephropathy was only symptomatic. The beneficial effects of ACE inhibitors or angiotensin II blockers in experimental radiation nephropathy amply justify their use in clinical radiation nephropathy, much as in any chronic kidney disease. Clinical experience in subjects with BMT nephropathy or with radiation nephropathy related to yttrium^{90} radionuclide therapy support this view (Fonck *et al.* 2000). Control of hypertension, almost always present in BMT nephropathy, requires diuretics in 75 per cent of cases and sometimes antihypertensives such as calcium channel blockers.

The anaemia of radiation nephropathy can be reversed by parenteral erythropoietin. In some cases, the hyperkalaemia of BMT nephropathy has been associated with aldosterone deficiency necessitating the use of fludrocortisone.

Despite optimal management, some patients with BMT or radioisotope induced radiation nephropathy may eventually need dialysis or kidney transplantation. In the case of BMT nephropathy, survival on long-term dialysis is poor (Cohen *et al.* 1998), probably as a consequence of the associated cancer treatment, with bone marrow suppression, and increased susceptibility to infection. Kidney transplantation is possible, and may benefit from a special situation of immunological tolerance, especially if the marrow donor is also the kidney donor (Sayegh *et al.* 1991). The kidney would be tolerated, because the host's marrow/immune system would not view it as foreign. In such a situation, there is no need for immunosuppressive medication. While such a situation is fairly straightforward in the case of sib-to-sib transplants, it raises significant ethical questions when the marrow transplant originates from an unrelated donor. Specifically, can one ask, let alone obligate, the unrelated marrow donor to donate a kidney to his/her unrelated marrow recipient? Cadaveric transplantation for ESRD after BMT remains an option, but because of the not-fully-normal immune system of the recipient, immunesuppression should be reduced by about 50 per cent (Butcher *et al.* 1999).

Acknowledgements

This work was supported in part by a grant from the National Institutes of Health, CA 24652, and by a grant from the American Cancer Society, ROG 00-350-01.

References

Antignac, C. *et al.* (1989). Delayed renal failure with extensive mesangiolysis following bone marrow transplantation. *Kidney International* **35**, 1336–1344.

Arneil, G. C. *et al.* (1974). Nephritis in two children after irradiation and chemotherapy for nephroblastoma. *Lancet* **1**, 960–963.

Barbara, J. A. J. *et al.* (1992). Membranous nephropathy with graft versus host disease in a bone marrow transplant recipient. *Clinical Nephrology* **37**, 115–118.

Barri, Y. M. *et al.* (2001). Pamidronate induced FSGS in patients with multiple myeloma. *Journal of the American Society of Nephrology* **12**, 92a.

Butcher, J. A. *et al.* (1999). Renal transplantation for end-stage renal disease following bone marrow transplantation: a report of six cases, with and without immunosuppression. *Clinical Transplantation* **13**, 1–6.

Chappell, M. E., Keeling, D. M., Prentice, H. G., and Sweny, P. (1988). Haemolytic uraemic syndrome after bone marrow transplantation: an adverse effect of total body irradiation. *Bone Marrow Transplantation* **3**, 339–347.

Cohen, E. P. (2000). Radiation nephropathy after bone marrow transplantation. *Kidney International* **58**, 903–918.

Cohen, E. P., Fish, B. L., and Moulder, J. E. (2002). The renin angiotensin system in experimental radiation nephropathy. *Journal of Laboratory and Clinical Medicine* **139**, 251–257.

Cohen, E. P., Moulder, J. E., and Robbins, M. E. C. (2001). Radiation nephropathy caused by Yttrium 90. *Lancet* **358**, 1102–1103.

Cohen, E. P., Piering, W. F., Kabler-Babbitt, C., and Moulder, J. E. (1998). End-stage renal disease after bone marrow transplantation: poor survival compared to other causes of ESRD. *Nephron* **79**, 408–412.

Cohen, E. P. *et al.* (1993). Clinical course of late onset bone marrow transplant nephropathy. *Nephron* **64**, 626–635.

Domagk, G. (1927). Röntgenstrahlenschädigungen der niere beim menschen. *Medizinische Klinik* **23**, 345–347.

Duchesne, G. M. *et al.* (1997). Radiotherapy after chemotherapy for metastatic seminoma—a diminishing role. MRC Testicular Tumour Working Party. *European Journal of Cancer* **33**, 829–835.

Edsall, D. L. (1906). The attitude of the clinician in regard to exposing patients to the X-ray. *Journal of the American Medical Association* **47**, 1425–1429.

Fischer, E. R. and Hellstrom, H. R. (1968). Pathogenesis of hypertension and pathologic changes in experimental renal irradiation. *Laboratory Investigation* **19**, 530–538.

Fonck, C. *et al.* (2001). Glomérulopathie apres radiothérapie métabolique pour insulinome métastatique. *Néphrologie* **21**, 206.

Giralt, S. *et al.* (2003). ^{166}Ho-DOTMP plus melphalan followed by peripheral blood stem cell transplantation in patients with multiple myeloma: results of two phase 1/2 trials. *Blood* **102**, 2684–2691.

Glatstein, E., Fajardo, L. F., and Brown, J. M. (1977). Radiation injury in the mouse kidney. *International Journal of Radiation Oncology, Biology, Physics* **2**, 933–943.

Hoopes, P. J., Gillette, E. L., and Benjamin, S. A. (1985). The pathogenesis of radiation nephropathy in the dog. *Radiation Research* **104**, 406–419.

Jaenke, R. S. *et al.* (1993). Capillary endothelium: target site of renal radiation injury. *Laboratory Investigation* **68**, 396–405.

Luxton, R. W. (1953). Radiation nephritis. *Quarterly Journal of Medicine* **22**, 215–242.

Markowitz, G. S. *et al.* (2001). Collapsing focal segmental glomerulosclerosis following treatment with high dose pamidronate. *Journal of the American Society of Nephrology* **12**, 1164–1172.

Moll, S. *et al.* (2001). A new cause of renal thrombotic microangiopathy: Yttrium 90-DOTATOC internal radiotherapy. *American Journal of Kidney Diseases* **37**, 847–851.

Oikawa, T. *et al.* (1997). Modulation of plasminogen activator inhibitor 1 *in vivo*: a new mechanism for the antifibrotic effect of renin–angiotensin inhibition. *Kidney International* **51**, 164–172.

Phillips, T. L., Wharam, M. D., and Margolis, L. W. (1975). Modification of radiation injury to normal tissues by chemotherapeutic agents. *Cancer* **35**, 1678–1684.

Robbins, M. E. C. and Bonsib, S. M. (1995). Radiation nephropathy: a review. *Scanning Microscopy* **9**, 535–560.

Sayegh, M. H. *et al.* (1991). Immunologic tolerance to renal allografts after bone marrow transplants from the same donors. *Annals of Internal Medicine* **114**, 954–955.

Sharma, M., Sharma, R., Ge, X. L., Fish, B. L., McCarthy, E. T., Savin, V. J., Cohen, E. P., and Moulder, J. E. (2001). Early detection of radiation-induced glomerular injury by albumin permeability assay. *Radiation Research* **155**, 474–480.

Withers, H. R., Mason, K. A., and Thames, H. D. (1986). Late radiation response of kidney assayed by tubule cell survival. *The British Journal of Radiology* **59**, 587–595.

6.7 Balkan nephropathy

Vladisav Stefanović and J.P. Cosyns

Balkan nephropathy (BN) is a familial chronic tubulointerstitial disease with insidious onset and slow progression to terminal renal failure. It was first described in Serbia (Danilović *et al.* 1957) and in Bulgaria (Tanchev *et al.* 1956). It affects people living in the alluvial plains along the tributaries of the Danube River in Serbia, Bosnia, Croatia, Bulgaria, and Rumania (Fig. 1).

Epidemiological characteristics

The disease usually affects adults in their fourth/fifth decade with eventual endstage renal failure in their sixth decade. No case has been documented in children and adolescents. The age distribution is increasingly skewed towards the elderly (Radovanović 1991). The median age of incident cases has increased by 5.5 years between the 70s and 80s, and by another 7.5 years between the 80s and 90s, a trend paralleled by the associated urothelial carcinoma (Radovanović 2002). The incidence of terminal renal failure and BN death rates has decreased between 1978 and 1997 in the South Morava region as well as in some areas in Serbia, Bosnia, Croatia, and Bulgaria (Stefanović *et al.* 2000). Extension of this trend might lead to the disappearance of BN and to a reduction of urothelial cancer incidence in endemic area compared to that observed in non-endemic areas (Čukuranović *et al.* 2002). Both genders are almost equally affected, with only a slight

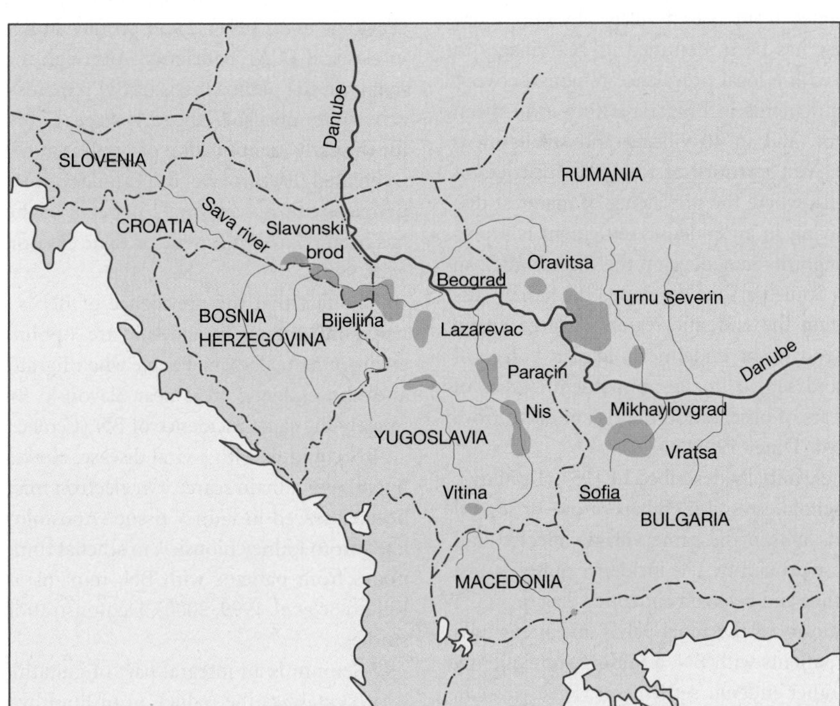

Fig. 1 Distribution map of Balkan nephropathy. On the west, endemic regions are distributed along the River Sava and its tributaries (14 villages in Croatia, near Slavonski Brod; 54 villages in the flood areas of Bosnia, near Bijeljina); in Serbia, 24 villages in the Kolubara valley, and 15 villages in the flood areas of Podrinje and Mačva with five adjacent villages in Vojvodina. Further endemic regions in Serbia are situated along the River Morava and its tributaries (nine villages in the middle section of the Morava; 14 villages around the South Morava; one village around the West Morava; and five villages along the River Binačka Morava). In Bulgaria, the endemic region lies in the north-western part of the country in the foothills of the Balkan mountains, with 33 endemic settlements in the Vratsa District and seven in the Mikhaylovgrad District. In Rumania, almost all cases are encountered in a limited south-west territory (districts of Mehedinti and Caras Severin), in about 40 villages and small towns.

Table 1 Epidemiological, clinical, and functional characteristics of Balkan nephropathy[a]

Epidemiological characteristics
Residence in an endemic settlement
Family history of renal disease and of renal deaths
Family history of urothelial tumours
Occupational history of farming
Clinical characteristics
Progressive renal insufficiency
Anaemia—normochromic or slightly hypochromic
Polyuria, polydipsia, nocturia
Hypertension—rare
Urothelial tumours—common
Abnormalities on urinalysis
Small or shrunken kidneys
Functional changes
Tubular proteinuria
Impaired urinary acidification
Glycosuria
Increased uric acid clearance
Renal salt wasting
Impaired concentrating capacity

[a] According to Stefanović (1983).

predominance of females. Occupational history usually reveals farming, at least for some period of time (Table 1).

BN occurs in some but not all villages in the endemic area. Affected villages are sometimes separated from spared villages by only a few kilometres. So far the disease has been identified in 142 villages in Bosnia, Croatia, and Serbia with a local prevalence ranging between 0.5 and 4 per cent, in 40 settlements in Bulgaria with a local mean morbidity rate of 3 per cent, and in 40 villages and small towns clustered in a limited south-west territory of Rumania (districts of Mehedinti and Caras-Severin), where the prevalence of manifest disease was over 2 per cent. Living in an endemic settlement is a prerequisite for diagnosis. Immigrants may develop the disease after an exposure of at least 25 years. Some persons developed the kidney disease several years after leaving the endemic region. A large group of inhabitants left simultaneously the endemic Bulgarian village of Karash during 1961/1962, and settled in the non-endemic areas of Sofia and Pleven. After 19 years of observation the risk of death from BN and morbidity diminished (Dinev 1983).

BN has a familial character, initially described in 1957 (Danilović *et al.* 1957). In a single household, several members of one or several generations may be affected. Within the same village, affected and spared households live in close proximity. The incidence of BN is thus very heterogeneous both within and between endemic villages.

A high prevalence of tumours of the renal pelvis and ureter was first described in Bulgarian patients with BN, a finding subsequently confirmed in inhabitants of other endemic settlements (Petković *et al.* 1971) and in affected families (Čukuranović *et al.* 1991).

Aetiological factors

The aetiology of BN is still debated. Hereditary factors, infectious agents, environmental toxic compounds, and trace element deficiencies have been considered.

The familial clustering of the disease has prompted genetic studies. Structural changes have been described in the third chromosome at the band 3q25 of patients with BN (Toncheva and Dimitrov 1996). A higher incidence of antigen HLA-B18 has been reported in people living in endemic areas (Minev *et al.* 1978), whereas no correlation with HLA A, B, and DR antigens was found in the Croatian and Serbian population (Djurinović-Bello *et al.* 1979). Susceptibility to toxic and/or carcinogenic substances is partially determined by the genetic polymorphism of cytochrome-P450-dependant mono-oxygenases involved in the metabolic activation of toxic compounds. The higher capacity of BN patients to hydroxylate debrisoquine (Ritchie *et al.* 1983) suggests such a genetic polymorphism. The enzyme debrisoquine 4-hydroxylase (CYP2D6), a part of the cytochrome-P450 enzyme family, is important in the activation of diverse procarcinogens and in the metabolism of a wide spectrum of drugs. It is highly polymorphic. The CYP2D6 allele distribution proved different in BN patients and in healthy individuals and has been suggested as a possible marker for BN susceptibility (Atanasova *et al.* 2002a). *N*-acetyltransferases (NATs) also activate several procarcinogens and chemicals whereas the multidrug resistance gene (MDR), which codes for P-glycoprotein, is associated with xenobiotic resistance. A study of their polymorphisms in 96 Bulgarian BN patients suggested that NAT2 and MDR variants are part of the genetic background of BN (Atanasova *et al.* 2002b). Genetic variants in xenobiotic metabolizing enzymes and transporters might thus augment the susceptibility of BN patients to exogenous factors.

A partial deficit of lecithin–cholesterol acyltransferase (LCAT) has been described in clinically healthy members of affected families (Pavlović *et al.* 1991). Lipid profiles in BN patients differ from those in classical LCAT deficiency. Although the role of this LCAT abnormality in the pathogenesis of BN remains unknown, decreased LCAT activity, found also in the early stages of BN, has been used as a marker for the early identification of persons at risk of developing the disease. Decreased erythrocyte δ-aminolaevulinate dehydratase activity in patients with BN and in 32 per cent of their healthy family members has been related to genetic or toxic environmental factors (Djordjević *et al.* 1991).

The fact that the prevalence of BN is similar in immigrants and native inhabitants in endemic areas points to a predominant role of environmental factors. People who migrated from Ukraine to endemic and non-endemic areas near Slavonski Brod (Croatia) have approximately the same incidence of BN (Čeović *et al.* 1985).

BN could fit with a viral disease. However, data substantiating this hypothesis remain scarce. On electron microscopy, viral particles have been observed in kidney tissue (Apostolov *et al.* 1975). A virus, isolated from kidney biopsies, urothelial tumours, and metastatic lymph nodes from patients with BN, remains as yet unidentified (Uzelac-Keserović *et al.* 1999, 2000). Demonstration of its role requires further studies.

Selenium is an integral part of glutathione peroxidase, an enzyme which catalyzes the reduction of lipid hydroperoxides and hydrogen peroxide and protects against the damaging effect of free radicals. The selenium level is low in soils and cereals from both endemic and non-endemic areas and is correlated with the levels detected in plasma and hair samples of inhabitants, irrespective of their area of origin (Maksimović 1991). Se-dependant glutathione peroxidase activity is the same in BN patients, their healthy relatives and in a control group (Čukuranović *et al.* 1992; Mihailović *et al.* 1992). In uraemic patients, glutathione peroxidase activity is lowered to levels observed in other renal failure patients. Selenium deficiency is thus an unlikely aetiological factor of BN.

Long-term exposure to polycyclic aromatic hydrocarbons and amines leaching into well drinking water from low rank Pliocene-age coals below or proximal to endemic settlements has recently been incriminated (Feder *et al.* 1991). However, a recent study of water samples from regional distribution systems or local springs and wells in Bulgaria failed to detect significant differences in the presence of coal-derived compounds between endemic and spared settlements (Voice *et al.* 2002).

Pathological features of BN are reminiscent of those observed in cadmium (Yasuda *et al.* 1995), lead (Wedeen 1991), ochratoxin A (OTA) (Krogh 1992), and aristolochic acid (AA) nephropathies (Ivić 1970; Cosyns *et al.* 1994, 2001). They include mainly subcapsular, hypocellular interstitial fibrosis associated with flattened proximal tubular cells. Coexistence of mild tubular proteinuria, glucosuria, and aminoaciduria is compatible with a toxic injury of the proximal tubule with ensuing progressive interstitial fibrosis. At present, no evidence points to an aetiological role of cadmium or lead. In contrast, OTA, a mycotoxin produced by several species of *Aspergillus* and *Penicillium*, are found in samples of staple foods more frequently in affected families or in endemic areas than in unaffected families or non-endemic areas (Petkova-Bocharova and Castegnaro 1985). High blood levels of the toxin are found more frequently in patients with BN and/or urinary tract tumours than in unaffected people from endemic or in subjects from control areas (Petkova-Bocharova and Castegnaro 1991). AA alkaloids, found in the plant *Aristolochia*, have been incriminated many years ago (Ivić 1970).

Both OTA and AA are nephrotoxic and carcinogenic substances contributing potentially to the development of both the renal interstitial fibrosis and the urothelial malignancies characteristic of BN. At high dosage, both drugs cause acute tubular necrosis in animals and man (Di Paolo *et al.* 1994). They both react with cellular DNA and form premutagenic DNA adducts in mice and man (Pfohl-Leszkowicz *et al.* 1991, 1993; Stiborova *et al.* 1994, 1999; Arlt *et al.* 2000, 2001). AA–DNA adducts are yet to be demonstrated in DNA extracted from kidney tissue of patients with BN. The role of OTA has been questioned because of its high toxicity (Mantle 2002). Another experimental mycotoxic nephropathy has been observed in rats. It is due to the water extract of a food-spoilage mould, *Penicillium polonicum*, which is common in the Balkans. Extensive apoptosis, noted in tubular epithelia (Mantle *et al.* 1998) might play a role in the silent development of BN. Interestingly, increased apoptosis has been reported in nine out of 10 patients with BN (Savin *et al.* 2001).

Clinical characteristics

BN is a chronic tubulointerstitial disease with insidious onset and slow progression to endstage renal failure associated with urothelial malignancies. Its clinical presentation is that of chronic interstitial nephritis of any cause (Table 1): asymptomatic, for years or decades, and manifest only at the stage of advanced renal failure. Anaemia, a constant and early feature of BN, is usually normocytic, normochromic, or slightly hypochromic and non-regenerative. Its severity worsens with the impairment of renal function and does not differ from that observed in chronic pyelonephritis (Pavlović-Kentera *et al.* 1991). Serum erythropoietin is within the normal range but inappropriately low for the degree of anaemia.

Mild and labile hypertension is occasionally observed in the early stage of the disease but becomes more frequent, 30–40 per cent of cases, in patients with advanced renal failure.

Urinary tract infection is observed in 13.5 per cent of patients in the early stage of the disease, and in 16.7 per cent of patients in asymptomatic renal failure (Stefanović *et al.* 1979). It may further compromise renal function and should be sought in every patient.

Salt retention with oedema does not occur. Lumbar or back pain are absent. There is no evidence of extrarenal involvement: pulmonary and hepatic functions remain normal.

There is no evidence of immune abnormalities. Serum immunoglobulins and complement are normal. Neither the classical nor the alternative pathway of the complement system is activated. Cryoglobulins, antiglomerular, and antitubular basement membrane antibodies are absent (Stefanović and Polenaković 1991). Proteinuria is initially intermittent and mild but increases up to 1 g/l in advanced renal failure. In the early stages, it is of the tubular type, including β_2-microglobulin, the most readily recognizable low molecular weight protein (Hall *et al.* 1972) and cystatin C (Begić *et al.* 1987). Urinary β_2-microglobulin excretion increases not only in patients but also in some clinically healthy relatives and can thus serve as a marker for early tubular damage in BN (Stefanović *et al.* 1991).

Urinary sediment is usually normal with a few red and white blood cells per high power field. Macroscopic haematuria usually indicates an associated urinary tract tumour. Uric acid, urate, and some other crystal formations are frequent, especially during summer months.

Imaging studies disclose normal-sized kidneys in the early stages. When renal failure develops, the kidneys are bilaterally, symmetrically small with a smooth outline.

Uric acid clearance and uric acid/creatinine clearance ratio are increased perhaps as a result of decreased proximal tubular reabsorption or altered distal tubular secretion. Glycosuria is present in about 40 per cent of BN patients without renal failure, and in 64 per cent of patients with chronic renal failure. A distal tubular acidifying defect with impaired ammonia excretion has also been described (Hall *et al.* 1972).

An early renal salt wasting has been occasionally observed. Global renal insufficiency develops slowly in late adulthood and progresses relentlessly to endstage renal failure. A rapid deterioration in renal function raises the possibility of complicating factors such as urinary tract infections, water and salt depletion, or drug nephrotoxicity.

Urothelial malignancies of the pelvis and ureter are significantly more frequent, up to 100 times, in endemic than in non-endemic areas (Čukuranović *et al.* 1991; Djokić *et al.* 1999). They tend to cluster in families affected with BN, indicating an association between both diseases and, probably, a common aetiologic agent (Radovanović *et al.* 1990; Čukuranović *et al.* 1991). Tumours develop usually later than the interstitial nephropathy. Their incidence increases with age at the time of diagnosis, with the female sex, and with a longer survival (Janković *et al.* 1988; Djokić *et al.* 1999). Tumours are multifocal and bilateral (Djokić *et al.* 1999) and have a transitional cell differentiation similar to that reported in the general population. In endemic areas, however, they are located more frequently in the renal pelvis and the proximal ureter. Urinary bladder tumours are also more frequent, up to 12 times, than in non-endemic villages (Čukuranović *et al.* 1991). The presenting symptom is usually a painless haematuria. Imaging studies (intravenous urography, retrogade ureteropyelography) and/or ureteroscopy, cystoscopy, and bladder biopsy are used. In addition, sonography and voided urine cytology have been used in the diagnosis and follow-up of urothelial carcinoma. The cytologic detection requires more than a single urine specimen, and a continued follow-up is indicated.

Pathological characteristics (Table 2)

A typical, though not pathognomonical, pathological picture of BN emerged only after the precise description of the clinical and epidemiological diagnostic criteria (Danilović *et al.* 1974; Stefanović 1983). BN is a chronic, paucicellular, sclerosing interstitial nephritis predominating in the superficial cortex (Nikulin and Rotter 1964; Hall *et al.* 1965; Sindjić *et al.* 1979; Dojčinov *et al.* 1979a; Ferluga *et al.* 1991, 2002; Čukuranović *et al.* 1998; Savić *et al.* 2002). At advanced stages, the kidneys are symmetrically shrunken with smooth outlines and weigh only about 10 g. On light microscopy there is a diffuse cortical, mainly subcapsular, hypocellular interstitial fibrosis with tubular atrophy (Fig. 2). The columns of Bertin and the medulla are usually spared. Most glomeruli show obsolescence of the collapsing type and are packed together in the outer cortex. Preserved glomeruli are ischaemic. Glomerular lesions similar to thrombotic microangiopathy (TMA) or focal–segmental sclerosis are occasionally found. Vascular lesions, present in most cases, include multifocal arteriolar hyalinosis, mainly interlobular arterial mural sclerosis and thickened peritubular capillary basement membranes. At early stages, the above-mentioned changes are multifocal, mainly in medullary rays and outer medulla. They are associated with areas of interstitial oedema together with peritubular capillary wall thickening as well as proximal tubule epithelial cell degenerative lesions.

Findings on immunofluoresce microscopy are non-specific (Vizjak *et al.* 1991). Glomerular immune deposits are either absent or limited to scanty, non-significant, granular segmental deposits of mainly IgM and/or C3. In a few cases, tubular basement membranes displaying granular or linear deposits of C3 have been reported. Damaged proximal tubule epithelial cells overexpress cytokeratin and vimentin (Stefanović *et al.* 1996). Collagen IV and laminin deposits have been observed in tubular basement membranes. Arterial walls frequently contain C3 deposits associated sometimes with IgM and peritubular capillaries contain laminin (Čukuranović *et al.* 1995; Vizjak *et al.* 2002).

Electron microscopy studies (Dojčinov *et al.* 1979b; Ferluga *et al.* 1991) reveal increased interstitial bundles of cross-banded collagen fibers and a slightly increased number of elongated, stellate fibroblast-like cells. Tubular changes, mainly in proximal tubules, include frequent widening of intercellular junctions, separation of the basal labyrinth from the tubular basement membrane, and condensation or cavitation of the mitochondrial matrix with disorganized cristae and occasional myelin-like figures. Glomerular basement membranes show occasionally either a mild thickening, or the deposition of a pale subendothelial fluffy material with an occasional double contour appearance similar to TMA lesions. Peritubular capillary endothelial cell swelling and reduced electron density of the basement membrane is an early finding.

Altogether, these lesions are consistent with a primary toxic insult of the proximal tubule cell leading to a slowly progressive, hypocellular, mainly subcapsular interstitial fibrosing nephropathy. A primary vascular injury cannot be excluded. It is suggested by the fact that, in early stages, peritubular capillaries exhibit an increased thickness and laminin expression above that noted in tubular basement membranes as well as by the occasional finding of TMA-like lesions.

Table 2 Renal morphological changes in Balkan nephropathy

Gross morphology
Symmetric, small kidneys with smooth outlines in advanced stages
Presence of upper urinary tract tumours
Microscopic findings
Early stages
Medullary rays and outer medulla
Focal interstitial oedema and hypocellular fibrosis
Proximal tubule epithelial cell degeneration
Peritubular capillaries with swollen endothelial cells and thickened basement membranes
Late stages
Mainly outer cortex
Diffuse interstitial hypocellular fibrosis
Flattened proximal tubule epithelial cells
Tubular atrophy
Glomerular ischaemia or obsolescence of collaptic type
Occasional thrombotic microangiopathy- or focal–segmental sclerosis-like lesions
Severe arteriolar hyalinosis
Intimal and medial fibrous hyperplasia of inter-lobular arteries
Thickened peritubular capillary basement membranes

Differential diagnosis

Chronic interstitial fibrosis is associated with urothelial malignancy in BN, in analgesic nephropathy (AN) (see Chapter 6.2), and in Chinese herbs (CHN) or aristolochic acid nephropathy (AAN) (see Chapter 6.8). All three diseases share a usually normal blood pressure, early and severe anaemia, low molecular weight tubular proteinuria (Kabanda *et al.* 1995), glycosuria, and the absence of recurrence after renal transplantation (Cosyns 2002; Stefanovic 2002). AN is characterized a.o. by a history of analgesic abuse, and medullary and papillary calcification or necrosis. CHN (or AAN) has a much more rapid progression rate towards endstage renal failure (Reginster *et al.* 1997). BN is characteristically circumscribed to endemic areas.

Prevention and treatment

In the absence of an identified aetiological factor, effective prevention of BN is not yet possible. Improved living conditions, water supply from distant sources, and migration of affected families outside the endemic region may have contributed to the decreasing incidence of the disease (Stefanović *et al.* 1999). Marriage with healthy partners might improve genetic predisposition (if any) in younger individuals.

Treatment of BN is similar to that of all chronic interstitial nephropathies: detection and treatment of potentially reversible aggravating factors, limited protein intake, and kidney replacement therapy. Hypertension, if present, should be treated with angiotensin-converting enzyme inhibitors. Diuretics should be added only in the advanced stage with special attention to avoid salt depletion. Haemo- and peritoneal dialysis as well as kidney transplantation have been

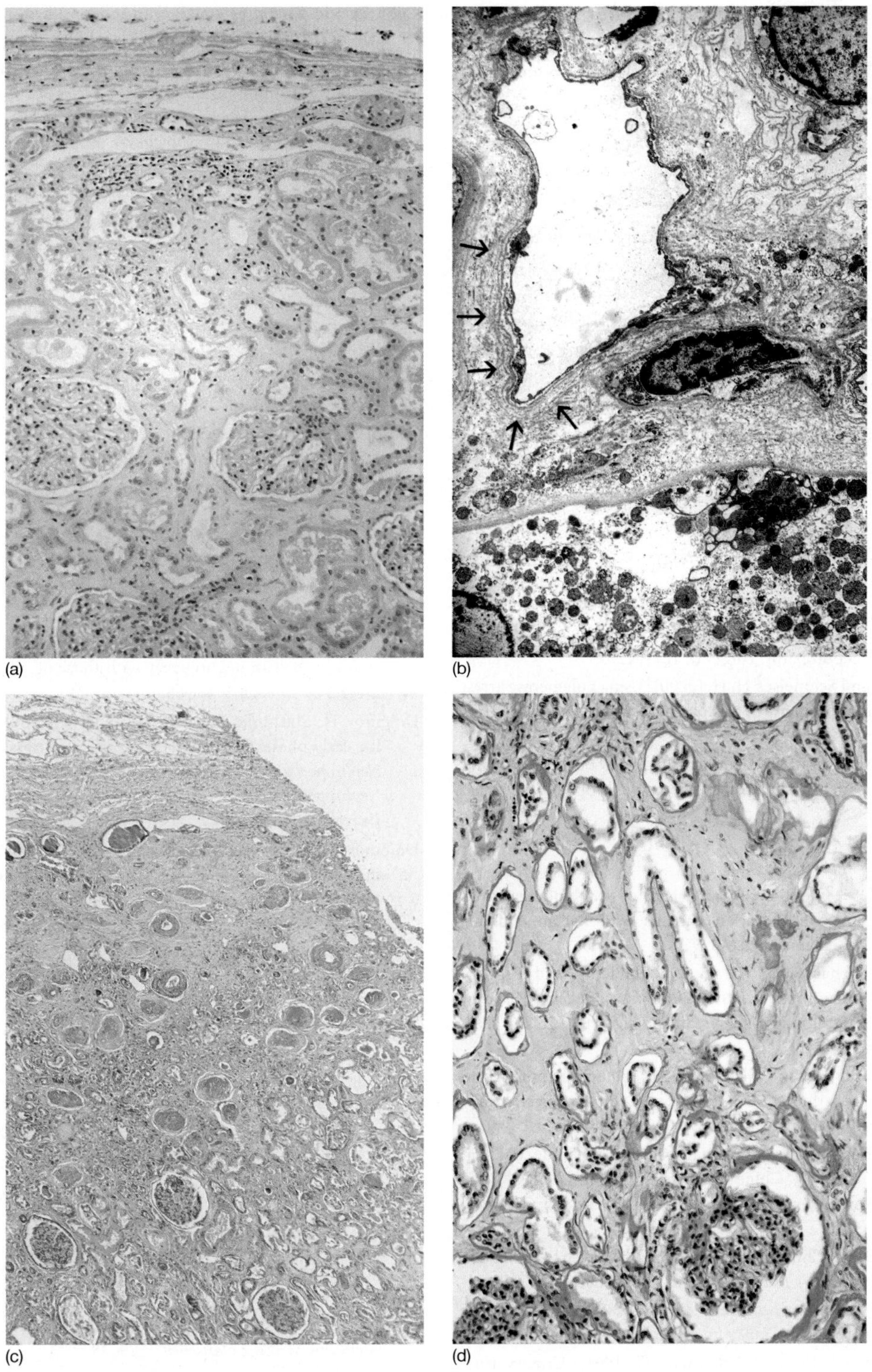

Fig. 2 Morphology of Balkan nephropathy. Early stage: (a) normal glomeruli surrounded by focal interstitial oedema and sclerosis with flattened tubular epithelia. HE. 100×; (b) electron micrograph showing thickening and splitting up of peritubular capillary basement membranes. 7235×. Advanced stage: (c) decreasing intensity from the upper to the inner cortex of interstitial sclerosis, tubular atrophy, and collapsing glomerular obsolescence. PAS. 50×; (d) hypocellular interstitial sclerosis surrounding proximal tubules with flattened epithelial cells. Ischaemic glomeruli and tubular atrophy. PAS. 165×. (By courtesy of Prof. D. Ferluga, Dr A. Hvala, and Dr A. Vizjak.)

used with success. BN does not recur after renal transplantation (Touraine *et al.* 1979). With longer survival on renal replacement therapy, patients develop tumours of the renal pelvis or ureter which should continuously be searched for.

Future studies

Research on BN is hampered by the lack of pathognomonical clinical and pathological characteristics. There is at present no specific biological marker of the disease.

Epidemiological studies point to the causal role of still to be identified environmental factors although genetic, predisposing abnormalities are not ruled out.

In the absence of a specific marker of the disease, it is impossible to state whether or not BN is confined to the Balkans (Stefanović and Polenaković 1991).

References

(Entries marked with an asterisk comprise useful general reading.)

Apostolov, K., Spasić, P., and Bojanić, N. (1975). Evidence of a viral aetiology in endemic (Balkan) nephropathy. *Lancet* **ii**, 1271–1273.

Arlt, V. M., Wiessler, M., and Schmeiser, H. H. (2000). Using polymerase arrest to detect DNA binding specificity of aristolochic acid in the mouse H-ras gene. *Carcinogenesis* **21**, 235–242.

Arlt, V. M. *et al.* (2001). Analyses of DNA adducts formed by ochratoxin A and aristolochic acid in patients with Chinese herbs nephropathy. *Mutation Research* **494**, 143–150.

Atanasova, S. *et al.* (2002a). Genotyping of CYP2D6 mutant alleles in BEN patients. *Facta Universitatis* **9**, 125–126.

Atanasova, S. *et al.* (2002b). Genetic polymorphisms of xenobiotic enzymes and transporter proteins in Bulgarian patients with Balkan endemic nephropathy. *Facta Universitatis* **9**, 126–127.

Begić, L., Halilbašić, A., Trnačević, S., Brzin, J., Mehikić, S., and Turk, V. Cystatin C in endemic nephropathy. In *Current Topics in Endemic (Balkan) Nephropathy* (ed. S. Strahinjić and V. Stefanović), pp. 25–29. Niš: University Press, 1987.

*__Čeović, S., Hrabar, A., and Radonić, M.__ (1985). An etiological approach to Balkan endemic nephropathy based on the investigation of two genetically different populations. *Nephron* **40**, 175–179.

Cosyns, J. P. (2002). Human and experimental features of aristolochic acid nephropathy (AAN; formerly Chinese herbs nephropathy—CHN): are they relevant to Balkan endemic nephropathy (BEN)? *Facta Universitatis* **9**, 49–52.

*__Cosyns, J. P.__ *et al.* (1994). Chinese herb nephropathy: a clue to Balkan endemic nephropathy. *Kidney International* **45**, 1680–1688.

Cosyns, J. P. *et al.* (2001). Chronic aristolochic acid toxicity in rabbits: a model of Chinese herbs nephropathy? *Kidney International* **59**, 2164–2173.

*__Čukuranović, R., Ignjatović, M., and Stefanović, V.__ (1991). Urinary tract tumors and Balkan nephropathy in the South Morava River basin. *Kidney International* **40** (Suppl. 34), S80–S84.

Čukuranović, R., Nikolić, J., and Stefanović, V. (1992). Erythrocyte glutathione peroxidase activity in patients with Balkan endemic nephropathy and in their healthy family members. *Archives of Biological Sciences, Belgrade* **44**, 23–30.

Čukuranović, R. *et al.* (1995). Immunohistochemical localization of laminin in renal lesions of Balkan nephropathy. *Nephron* **70**, 504–505.

Čukuranović, R. *et al.* (1998). Quantitative analysis of the renal changes in Balkan endemic nephropathy. *International Urology and Nephrology* **30**, 229–236.

Čukuranović, R. *et al.* (2002). Balkan endemic nephropathy and upper urothelial cancer in the South Morava River basin. *Facta Universitatis* **9**, 104–107.

Danilović, V., Naumović, T., and Velimirović, D. Endemic nephropathy in the Lazarevac community. In *Endemic Nephropathy. Proceedings of the 2nd International Symposium on Endemic Nephropathy* (ed. A. Puchlev, I. Dinev, B. Milev, and D. Dojcinov), pp. 281–283. Sofia: Bulgarian Academy of Sciences, 1974.

Danilović, V. *et al.* (1957). Néphrites chroniques provoquées par l'intoxication au plomb par voie digestive (farine). *La Presse Médicale* **65**, 2039–2040.

Dinev, I. Results of long-term observations of patients and healthy individuals who emigrated from the village of Karash and settled in villages near Sofia. In *Current Research in Endemic (Balkan) Nephropathy. Proceedings of the 5th Symposium on Endemic (Balkan) Nephropathy* (ed. S. Strahinjić and V. Stefanović), pp. 279–281. Niś: University Press, 1983.

Di Paolo, N. *et al.* (1994). Inhaled mycotoxins lead to acute renal failure. *Nephrology, Dialysis, Transplantation* **9**, 116–120.

Djordjević, V. B. *et al.* (1991). Erythrocyte δ-aminolevulinate dehydratase measurements in Balkan endemic nephropathy. *Kidney International* **40** (Suppl. 34), S93–S96.

Djurinović-Bello, I. *et al.* A study of endemic (Balkan) nephropathy with a view to association with histocompatibility (HLA) antigens. Population and family studies. In *Endemic (Balkan) Nephropathy. Proceedings of the 4th Symposium on Endemic (Balkan) Nephropathy* (ed. S. Strahinjić and V. Stefanović), pp. 69–76. Niś: University Press, 1979.

Djokic, M. *et al.* (1999). Comparison of upper urinary tract tumors in the region of Balkan nephropathy with those of other regions of Yugoslavia. *Progrès en Urologie* **9**, 61–68.

Dojčinov, D., Strahinjić, S., and Stefanović, V. Pathohistology of the kidney in the early phases of endemic *(Balkan)* nephropathy. In *Endemic (Balkan) Nephropathy. Proceedings of the 4th Symposium on Endemic (Balkan) Nephropathy* (ed. S. Strahinjić and V. Stefanović), pp. 91–104. Niś: University Press, 1979a.

Dojčinov, D., Strahinjić, S., and Stefanović, V. Ultrastructure of the kidney in the early phases of endemic (Balkan) nephropathy. In *Endemic (Balkan) Nephropathy. Proceedings of the 4th Symposium on Endemic (Balkan) Nephropathy* (ed. S. Strahinjić and V. Stefanović), pp. 105–112. Niś: University Press, 1979b.

Feder, G., Radovanović, Z., and Finklelman, R. B. (1991). Relationship between weathered coal deposits and the etiology of Balkan endemic nephropathy. *Kidney International* **40** (Suppl. 34), S9–S11.

*__Ferluga, D.__ *et al.* (1991). Renal function, protein excretion, and pathology of Balkan endemic nephropathy. III. Light and electron microscopic studies. *Kidney International* **40** (Suppl. 34), S57–S67.

Ferluga D. *et al.* (2002). Pathology of Balkan endemic nephropathy. A correlation with established kidney disease entities. *Facta Universitatis* **9**, 82–87.

Hall, P. W., III *et al.* (1965). Investigation of chronic endemic nephropathy in Yugoslavia. II. Renal pathology. *American Journal of Medicine* **39**, 210–217.

Hall, P. W. *et al.* (1972). Renal function studies in individuals with the tubular proteinuria of endemic Balkan nephropathy. *Quarterly Journal of Medicine* **41**, 385–393.

Ivić, M. (1970). The problem of etiology of endemic nephropathy. *Acta Facultatis Medicae Naissensis* **1**, 29–38.

Janković, S., Marinković, J., and Radovanović, Z. (1988). Survival of the upper-urothelial-cancer patients from the Balkan nephropathy endemic and nonendemic areas. *European Urology* **15**, 59–61.

Kabanda, A. *et al.* (1995). Low molecular weight proteinuria in Chinese herbs nephropathy. *Kidney International* **48**, 1571–1576.

Krogh, P. (1992). Role of ochratoxin in disease causation. *Food and Chemical Toxicology* **30**, 213–224.

Maksimović, Z. (1991). Selenium deficiency and Balkan endemic nephropathy. *Kidney International* **40** (Suppl. 34), S12–S14.

Mantle, P. G. (2002). Experimental mycotoxic nephropathies and Balkan endemic nephropathy. *Facta Universitatis* **9**, 64–65.

Mantle, P. G. *et al.* (1998). Does apoptosis cause renal atrophy in Balkan endemic nephropathy? *Lancet* **352**, 1118–1119.

Mihailovic, M. *et al.* (1992). Selenium status of patients with Balkan endemic nephropathy. *Biological Trace Elements Research* **33**, 71–77.

Minev, M. *et al.* (1978). HLA system and Balkan endemic nephropathy. *Tissue Antigens* **11**, 50–54.

Nikulin, A. and Rotter, W. (1964). Über das morphologische Substrat der in Semberien (Jugoslavien) endemischen 'chronischen Nephritis' (sog. Jugoslawien-Nephritis). *Frankfurter Zeitschrift für Pathologie* **73**, 668–688.

Pavlović, N. M. *et al.* (1991). Partial lecithin: cholesterol acyltransferase (LCAT) deficiency in Balkan endemic nephropathy. *Kidney International* **40** (Suppl. 34), S101–S104.

*__Pavlović-Kentera, V.__ *et al.* (1991). Anemia in Balkan endemic nephropathy. *Kidney International* **40** (Suppl. 34), S46–S48.

Petkova-Bocharova, T. and Castegnaro, M. (1985). Ochratoxin A contamination of cereals in an area of high incidence of Balkan endemic nephropathy in Bulgaria. *Food Additives and Contamination* **2**, 267–270.

Petkova-Bocharova, T. and Castegnaro, M. Ochratoxin A in human blood in relation to Balkan endemic nephropathy and urinary tract tumours in Bulgaria. In *Mycotoxins, Endemic Nephropathy and Urinary Tract Tumors* (ed. M. Castegnaro, R. Plestina, G. Dirheimer, I. N. Chernozemsky, and H. Bartsch), IARC Scientific Publications, No. 115, pp. 135–137. Lyon: International Agency for Research on Cancer, 1991.

*__Petković, S.__ *et al.* (1971). Les tumeurs du bassinet et de l'uretere. Recherches cliniques et étiologiques. *Journal d'Urologie et de Néphrologie* **6**, 429–439.

Pfohl-Leszkowicz, A. *et al.* DNA adduct formation in mice treated with ochratoxin A. In *Mycotoxins, Endemic Nephropathy and Urinary Tract Tumors* (ed. M. Castegnaro, R. Plestina, G. Dirheimer, I. N. Chernozemsky, and H. Bartsch), IARC Scientific Publications, No. 115, pp. 245–253. Lyon: International Agency for Research on Cancer, 1991.

Pfhol-Leszkowicz, A. *et al.* Ochratoxin A-related DNA adducts in urinary tract tumours of Bulgarian subjects. In *Postlabelling Methods for Detection of DNA Adducts* (ed. D. H. Phillips, M. Castegnaro, and H. Bartsch), IARC Scientific Publications, No. 124, pp. 141–148. Lyon: International Agency for Research on Cancer, 1993.

Radonić, M. *et al.* Odredjivanje antitjela protiv bazalne membrane tubula u bolesnika s endemskom nefropatijom. In *Proceedings of the 3rd Symposium on Endemic Nephropathy* p. 196. Documenta Galenika, Belgrade, 1977.

Radovanović, Z. Epidemiological characteristics of Balkan endemic nephropathy in eastern regions of Yugoslavia. In *Mycotoxins, Endemic Nephropathy and Urinary Tract Tumors* (ed. M. Castegnaro, R. Plestina, G. Dirheimer, I. N. Chernozemsky, and H. Bartsch), IARC Scientific Publications, No. 115, pp. 11–20. Lyon: International Agency for Research on Cancer, 1991.

Radovanović, Z. (2002). Balkan endemic nephropathy in Serbia: current status and future research. *Facta Universitatis* **9**, 26–30.

Radovanović, Z., Velimirović, D., and Naumović, T. (1990). Upper urothelial tumours and the Balkan nephropathy. Inference from the study of a family pedigree. *European Journal of Cancer* **26**, 391–392.

Reginster, F. *et al.* (1997). Chinese herbs nephropathy presentation, natural history and fate after transplantation. *Nephrology, Dialysis, Transplantation* **12**, 81–86.

Ritchie, J. C. *et al.* Evidence for an inherited metabolic susceptibility to endemic (Balkan) nephropathy. In *Current Research in Endemic (Balkan) Nephropathy. Proceedings of the 5th Symposium on Endemic (Balkan) Nephropathy* (ed. S. Strahinjić and V. Stefanović), pp. 23–27. Niś: University Press, 1983.

Savić, V. *et al.* (2002). Damage to kidney in Balkan endemic nephropathy: initial lesion, target structures and pathomorphogenesis. *Facta Universitatis* **9**, 92–94.

Savin, M. *et al.* (2001). The significance of apoptosis for early diagnosis of Balkan nephropathy. *Nephrology, Dialysis, Transplantation* **16** (Suppl. 6), S30–S32.

Sindjić, M. *et al.* Renal vascular changes and their possible role in the pathogenesis and morphogenesis of endemic Balkan nephropathy. In *Endemic (Balkan) Nephropathy. Proceedings of the 4th Symposium on Endemic (Balkan) Nephropathy* (ed. S. Strahinjić and V. Stefanović), pp. 113–122. Niś: University Press, 1979.

Stefanović, V. Diagnostic criteria for endemic (Balkan) nephropathy. In *Current Research in Endemic (Balkan) Nephropathy. Proceedings of the 5th Symposium on Endemic (Balkan) Nephropathy* (ed. S. Strahinjić and V. Stefanović), pp. 351–363. Niś: University Press, 1983.

*__Stefanović, V.__ (1998). Balkan endemic nephropathy: a need for novel aetiological approaches. *Quarterly Journal of Medicine* **9**, 457–463.

Stefanović, V. (2002). Analgesic nephropathy, Balkan endemic nephropathy and Chinese herbs nephropathy: separate tubulointerstitial kidney diseases associated with urothelial malignancy. *Facta Universitatis* **9**, 1–6.

*__Stefanović, V. and Polenaković, M. H.__ (1991). Balkan nephropathy. Kidney disease beyond the Balkans? *American Journal of Nephrology* **11**, 1–11.

Stefanović, V. *et al.* Urinary-tract infection in patients with endemic (Balkan) nephropathy. In *Endemic (Balkan) Nephropathy. Proceedings of the 4th Symposium on Endemic (Balkan) Nephropathy* (ed. S. Strahinjić and V. Stefanović), pp. 31–34. Niś: University Press, 1979.

*__Stefanović, V.__ *et al.* (1991). B2-microglobulin in patients with Balkan nephropathy and in healthy members of their families. *Kidney International* **40** (Suppl. 34), S97–S101.

Stefanović, V. *et al.* (1996). Coexpression of vimentin and cytokeratin in damaged tubular epithelia of kidney in Balkan nephropathy. *Nephron* **72**, 119–120.

Stefanović, V. *et al.* (1999). Balkan endemic nephropathy: slowed progression of kidney disease by avoidance of aetiological factors. *Nephron* **83**, 85–86.

Stefanović, V. *et al.* (2000). Balkan endemic nephropathy: a decreasing incidence of the disease. *Pathologie Biologie* **48**, 558–561.

Stiborova, M. *et al.* (1994). Characterization of DNA adducts formed by aristolochic acids in the target organ (forestomach) of rats by ^{32}P-postlabelling analysis using different chromatographic procedures. *Carcinogenesis* **15**, 1187–1192.

Stiborova, M. *et al.* (1999). Aristolactam I a metabolite of aristolochic acid I upon activation forms an adduct found in DNA of patients with Chinese herbs nephropathy. *Experimental and Toxicologic Pathology* **51**, 421–427.

Tanchev, I. *et al.* (1956). Prouchavaniia na nefrititev v vrachanska okolia. *Savremenaja Medizina* **9**, 14–29.

*__Toncheva, D. and Dimitrov, T.__ (1996). Genetic predisposition to Balkan endemic nephropathy. *Nephron* **72**, 564–569.

Touraine, J. L. *et al.* Kidney transplantation in endemic nephropathy. In *Endemic (Balkan) Nephropathy. Proceedings of the 4th Symposium on Endemic (Balkan) Nephropathy* (ed. S. Strahinjić and V. Stefanović), pp. 177–184. Niś: University Press, 1979.

Uzelac-Keserović, B. *et al.* (1999). Isolation of a coronavirus from kidney biopsies of endemic Balkan nephropathy patients. *Nephron* **81**, 141–145.

Uzelac-Keserović, B. *et al.* (2000). Isolation of a coronavirus from urinary tract tumours of endemic Balkan nephropathy patients. *Nephron* **86**, 93–94.

Vizjak, A. *et al.* (1991). Renal function, protein excretion, and pathology of Balkan endemic nephropathy. IV. Immunohistology. *Kidney International* **40** (Suppl. 34), S68–S74.

Vizjak, A. *et al.* (2002). Immunohistologic kidney biopsy study of Balkan endemic nephropathy. *Facta Universitatis* **9**, 88–91.

Voice, T. C. *et al.* (2002). Evaluation of coal leachate contamination of water supplies as a hypothesis for the occurrence of Balkan endemic nephropathy in Bulgaria. *Facta Universitatis* **9**, 128–129.

Wedeen, R. P. (1991). Environmental renal disease: lead, cadmium and Balkan endemic nephropathy. *Kidney International* **40** (Suppl. 34), S4–S8.

Yasuda, M. *et al.* (1995). Morphometric studies of renal lesions in Itai–Itai disease: chronic cadmium nephropathy. *Nephron* **69**, 14–19.

6.8 Chinese herbs (and other rare causes of interstitial nephropathy)

J.P. Cosyns and Charles van Ypersele

Chinese herbs nephropathy: aristolochic acid nephropathy and phytotherapy associated nephropathy

An epidemic of chronic interstitial nephritis, reported in more than 100 patients attending a Brussels outpatient clinic specialized in slimming cures, was attributed first to a Chinese herbs phytotherapy (Vanherweghem *et al.* 1993) and eventually to its aristolochic acid (AA) content (But *et al.* 1993; Van Haelen *et al.* 1994; Cosyns *et al.* 2001; Debelle *et al.* 2002). Pathognomonic characteristics included paucicellular interstitial fibrosis with a corticomedullary gradient of decreasing intensity (Cosyns *et al.* 1994a; Depierreux *et al.* 1994), a usually relentless progression despite withdrawal of the offending compound (Reginster *et al.* 1997) and a high prevalence of urothelial malignancies (Cosyns *et al.* 1999; Nortier *et al.* 2000). Similar cases were subsequently published throughout the world, outside the epidemic, some of which were clearly due to AA, some others possibly related to other phytotoxins (Cosyns 2003). Identification of AA as the cause of the so-called Chinese herbs nephropathy described in the Belgian epidemic dictated a switch in terminology to aristolochic acid nephropathy (AAN): first, the term CHN was resented as derogatory for Chinese medicine and second, the term AAN identified a precise clinicopathological entity to be distinguished from phytotherapy-associated interstitial nephritis (PAIN), regrouping the other cases of interstitial nephritis possibly caused by other phytotoxins (Chen *et al.* 2001; Gillerot *et al.* 2001; Solez *et al.* 2001; Cosyns *et al.* 2002). Hence the use of AAN and PAIN in this chapter.

Aristolochic acid nephropathy

Clinical presentation

Patients usually become symptomatic only when renal failure is advanced (Reginster *et al.* 1997). They complain of tiredness and polyuria of recent onset. Clinical examination is usually normal. The discovery of heart murmurs due to aortic valve abnormalities, described in some patients on the slimming regimen, has now been ascribed to the concommitant intake of fenfluramine and is therefore not part of the clinical picture of AAN (Connolly *et al.* 1997). Blood pressure is normal in half of the patients despite severe renal failure. Laboratory tests reveal renal failure. The urine sediment is virtually normal except for mild aseptic leucocyturia. Normoglycaemic glucosuria is often present. Proteinuria is usually mild (<2 g/day) but characteristically of the tubular type (Kabanda *et al.* 1995; Nortier *et al.* 1997). On X-ray irradiation, kidneys have a symmetric, reduced size with a smooth outline.

After (often repeated) questioning, the patients reveal the intake of Chinese herbs, which, after examination, contain AA.

Evolution and treatment

When renal failure is present at the time of diagnosis, progression is usually relentless over a period of months, sometimes years, even if the phytotoxin is interrupted. In the Belgian epidemic, progression rate proved related to the amount of ingested AA as evaluated either by the duration of the slimming regimen (Reginster *et al.* 1997) or by the cumulative dose of *Stephania tetrandra* the prescribed Chinese herb assumed to have been replaced by the AA-containing species (Martinez *et al.* 2002).

Urothelial malignancies have developed up to several years after exposure to AA (Cosyns *et al.* 1994b; Cosyns *et al.* 1999; Nortier *et al.* 2000) some of which have proven fatal. They remain a cause of major concern in the follow-up of these patients. Bilateral nephroureterectomy should be performed at least at the time of transplantation. The urine sediment should be regularly checked for malignant cells and, in case of doubt or in the presence of microscopic haematuria, cystoscopy is advised. Interestingly, nephrotoxicity and urothelial malignancies have been observed in only 3–5 per cent of the patients who followed the Brussels slimming regimen, an observation compatible with a variable individual susceptibility (Cosyns 2003).

Steroid therapy has been claimed to slow the deterioration of renal function (Vanherweghem *et al.* 1996), but definitive evidence is still missing (van Ypersele de Strihou and Jadoul 2002). Angiotensin converting inhibitors have also been advocated. Renal replacement therapy followed by renal transplantation has been successfully undertaken in over half the patients of the Belgian epidemic.

Pathology

On gross morphological examination, endstage kidneys are severely shrunken, weighing only about 10 g, with smooth outlines and only some retracted areas (Fig. 1a) (Cosyns *et al.* 1994a). The peripheral and interpyramidal cortex stand out as a diffuse, rather homogeneous, pale, granular, thin rim, only a few millimetres thick, against the dark relatively well-preserved medullae. Pelves and ureters have a normal gross appearance except in a single case with severe periureteral fibrosis (Jadoul *et al.* 1993). On light microscopy, an extensive, dense, almost

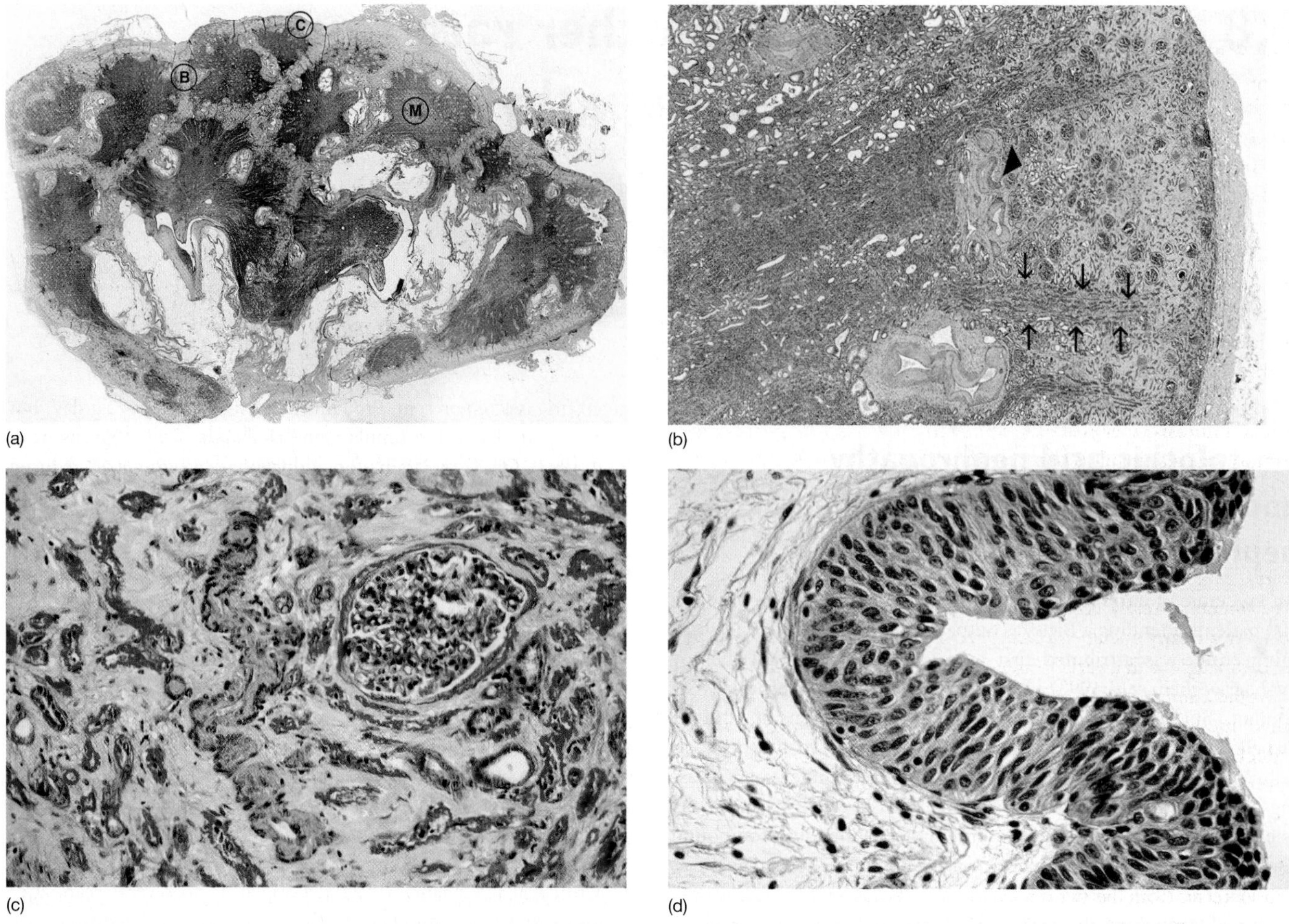

Fig. 1 Kidney (a–c) and ureteric (d) section of patient with endstage Chinese herbs nephropathy. (a) Diffuse atrophy of cortex (C) including columns of Bertin (B) down to the renal sinus. Slight involvement of the pyramids (M) (haematoxylin and eosin stain, 4×). (b) Hypocellular interstitial fibrosis and tubular atrophy are more marked in medullary rays (MR) (arrows) and the outer cortical labyrinth. Tubules are still visible in the inner cortical labyrinth (arrowhead). (Periodic acid–schiff stain, 30×.) (c) Severe fibrous intimal thickening of interlobular artery. Acellular interstitial sclerosis with few atrophic tubules (haematoxylin and eosin stain, 280×) [reproduced from Cosyns *et al.* with permission. *Kidney International* (1994) **45**, 1680–1688. *Kidney International* (2001) **59**, 2164–2173]. (d) Diffuse mild urothelial atypia (haematoxylin and eosin stain, 150×).

acellular interstitial fibrosis (Fig. 1c) decreases in intensity from the upper to the inner cortex (Fig. 1b). This decreasing corticomedullary gradient of interstitial fibrosis and its hypocellularity are the most striking histologic features of AAN (Cosyns *et al.* 1994a; Depierreux *et al.* 1994). Medullary rays and, to some extent, the outer stripe of outer medulla are severely involved, whereas the inner stripe of outer medulla and the inner medulla are usually less damaged. The associated tubular atrophy and global glomerular obsolescence of the collaptic type have a severity and topographic distribution similar to that of the interstitial fibrosis. Interlobular arteries show prominent intimal fibrosis, whereas larger arteries display usually mucoid fibrous hyperplasia. Non-specific, mild, granular deposits of IgM and C3 are present in the glomerular mesangium, along some glomerular capillaries and in small arterial walls and along the basement membranes of atrophic cortical tubules and of peritubular capillaries. On electron microscopy non-specific changes include scanty, segmental, subendothelial immune deposits or translucent zones, segmental glomerular basement membrane thickening, wrinkling or duplication, thickened tubular basement membranes and Bowman's capsules, and reduced tubular epithelial cells with loss of microvilli (Depierreux *et al.* 1994).

In the epithelial lining of collecting ducts and along the pelviureteric urothelium multifocal atypia are constantly found (Fig. 1d) (Cosyns *et al.* 1994a; Cosyns *et al.* 1999; Nortier *et al.* 2000). In about 50 per cent of the patients, they are associated as soon as 1 year after cessation of the toxic exposure with the development of multifocal transitional cell carcinoma *in situ* (CiS) mainly in the upper urinary tract (Cosyns *et al.* 1999; Nortier *et al.* 2000).

The role of aristolochic acid

The Chinese herbs content of the slimming pills was immediately suspected (Vanherweghem *et al.* 1993). Eventually it was found that one included herb, *S. tetrandra*, had been inadvertently replaced by another one, *Aristolochia fangchi*, containing AA (But *et al.* 1993; Van Haelen *et al.* 1994). Confirmation of AA intake by the patients was obtained by the discovery of AA-DNA adducts in their kidneys and ureters (Bieler *et al.* 1997; Nortier *et al.* 2000).

Experimental evidence of the nephrotoxicity of aristolochic acid

High doses of AA induce acute tubular necrosis in various species including man (Cosyns 2003). Low doses result in chronic nephrotoxicity in NZW rabbits. Tubular proteinuria with glucosuria is followed by a decreased glomerular filtration. The kidney damage closely resembles that observed in patients with AAN, that is, extensive hypocellular interstitial fibrosis with a characteristic corticomedullary gradient of decreasing severity, cellular atypia of the urothelium, the presence of AA-DNA adducts, and the development of urothelial malignancy. Of note, the predominance of fibrosis in the medullary rays and in the superficial cortex fits well with the hypothesis of a primary toxic insult of the S3 segment of the proximal tubules of mainly superficial nephrons (Cosyns *et al.* 2001). It has been hypothesized that chronic proximal tubular epithelial cell damage leads to interstitial inflammation and fibrosis (Joekes *et al.* 1958). Alternatively, the hypothesis of a primary vascular insult is hampered by the absence of vascular lesions in patients with AAN at early stages (Depierreux *et al.* 1994) as well as in the kidneys of rabbits given AA (Cosyns *et al.* 2001).

Low doses of AA are not nephrotoxic in rats (Cosyns *et al.* 1998) unless the animals are dehydrated (Debelle *et al.* 2002). In the latter experiments a mildly cellular interstitial fibrosis is observed without, however, a clearly documented corticomedullary gradient. These results are compatible with a variable interspecies susceptibility.

At the cellular level, '*in vitro*' exposure to AA of OK cells, an established model of proximal tubular cells, induces rapidly AA-DNA adducts followed by a decreased cellular expression of megalin and a permanent inhibition of protein absorption (Lebeau *et al.* 2001).

The carcinogenicity of aristolochic acid

AA is not only the nephrotoxic, but also the carcinogenic active principle extracted from the *Aristolochia* species. It is a mixture of structurally related nitrophenanthrene carboxylic acids. Its major components, AAI and AAII, bind covalently both *in vitro* and *in vivo* to the exocyclic amino group of DNA purine nucleotides and generate AA-DNA adducts (Stiborova *et al.* 1994) which were indeed found in patients with AAN (Bieler *et al.* 1997; Nortier *et al.* 2000). AA-DNA adducts provide a clue to understand the mutagenic and carcinogenic effects of AA. Their long-term persistence suggests non-reparable genomic lesions (Bieler *et al.* 1997). Overexpression of p53 by atypical and malignant urothelial cells in AAN patients suggests the mutation of this tumour suppressor gene (Cosyns *et al.* 1999). The mutagenic activity of AA is strongly suggested by the activation of Ha-ras protooncogene by an A→T transversion mutation in codon 61 from CAA to CTA in the DNA of AAI-induced forestomach carcinomas in rats (Schmeiser *et al.* 1990).

Aristolochic acid nephropathy outside the Belgian epidemic

The original description of AAN prompted the report of a number of cases in which phytotherapy was associated with a chronic nephropathy whose clinical presentation, evolution and pathology, characterized by hypocellular interstitial fibrosis, appeared similar to AAN. In approximately 65 patients (Cosyns 2003), AA intake was documented, occasionally with the presence of AA-DNA adducts in the kidneys. Urothelial malignancies were documented only in the few patients in whom nephroureterectomy specimens were examined (Gillerot *et al.* 2001; Lord *et al.* 2001). Of note, a Fanconi syndrome has been reported in a few of these patients (Ubara *et al.* 1999; Krumme *et al.* 2001; Tanaka *et al.* 2001; Yang *et al.* 2001, 2002).

The worldwide distribution of AAN suggests that only the tip of the iceberg of AA nephrotoxicity has been recognized. As a result of these observations, AA containing substances have been banned. In 2001, unfortunately, they were still available in several countries including China and The Netherlands.

Relationship between aristolochic acid nephropathy and Balkan nephropathy

Balkan nephropathy (BN) (see Chapter 6.7) has a clinical presentation (including urothelial malignancies) and pathologic features (a paucicellular interstitial fibrosis with a decreasing corticomedullary gradient and urothelial atypia) very close to those of AAN. AA has been incriminated in its genesis, a hypothesis still to be fully explored.

Still BN differs from AAN in several aspects. BN is characterized by a familial and environmental clustering, affects equally both genders and runs a very slow, decade long course. AAN by contrast has been reported throughout the world, mainly in females and runs a more rapid, often subacute course. On morphological grounds, the columns of Bertin are more constantly and extensively involved in AAN than in BN (Cosyns *et al.* 1994a).

Phytotherapy-associated interstitial nephritis

Clinical presentation, pathology, and evolution

Traditional medicine including phytotherapy (Seedat 1993) is a well-known cause of acute renal failure, mainly in the developing world. Several causes have been incriminated including adulteration of the remedies with toxic compounds, the inclusion of hepatotoxic herbs with eventual multiorgan failure and, finally, the substitution of one herb for the other.

Phytotherapy has also been associated worldwide with chronic interstitial nephritis whose clinical presentation and pathologic features are similar to those of AAN (Cosyns 2003). In these cases ingested herbs came from different sources, were prescribed for a variety of indications and were not analysed for the presence of AA or other toxic substances (Yang *et al.* 2000; Chang *et al.* 2001). The similarity of the clinical and pathological features with those of AAN suggests that these medications might have contained various phytotoxins yet to be identified. Of course, the nephrotoxicity associated with the consumption of these herbal remedies might result from adulteration by other toxic constituents deliberately added or spuriously contaminating the preparations (Firooz *et al.* 1998). In the absence of more information, it seems helpful to regroup them under the heading PAIN.

Prevention of phytotherapy-associated interstitial nephritis

The discovery of PAIN and AAN has drawn public attention to the possible harmful consequences of the various, traditional or non-traditional phytotherapies whose increasing worldwide use stems from the false belief that 'natural' compounds are necessarily harmless as well as from a certain dissatisfaction with Western medicine. Intervention of public authorities to regulate this market has been urgently called for (van Ypersele de Strihou and Vanherweghem 1995; Kessler *et al.* 2000).

Ochratoxin nephropathy

A chronic form of interstitial nephritis characterized by clinical and morphological features similar to those observed in endemic areas of the Balkan region have been reported together with high blood levels of ochratoxin A (OTA) after food contamination with this substance in Tunisia (Maaroufi *et al.* 1995) or without identified source of exposure in France (Godin *et al.* 1997).

OTA is a mycotoxin made of 7-carboxyl-5-chloro-8-hydroxyl-3,4-dihydro-3-methyl isocoumarinic acid bound by a peptidic bond to L-phenylalanine. Produced by several species of *Aspergillus* and *Penicillium*, it is nephrotoxic. Pigs fed OTA develop proteinuria and normoglycaemic glucosuria associated with polyuria and loss of concentrating capacity. Injury to tubular epithelial cells is suggested by *N*-acetyl glucosaminidase, leucine aminopeptidase, and lactate deshydrogenase enzymuria. Renal lesions include flattened proximal tubular epithelial cells renal interstitial fibrosis with tubular atrophy (Godin *et al.* 1997).

OTA has been incriminated in BN (see Chapter 6.7) for several reasons: samples of staple foods more frequently contain high levels of OTA in affected families or in endemic areas than in unaffected families or non-endemic areas. The number of blood samples with high levels of the toxin is higher in patients with nephropathy and/or urinary tract tumours than in unaffected people from endemic and control subjects from control areas.

Although urothelial malignancies have not been reported, it is noteworthy that OTA has mutagenic and tumorigenic effects in *Salmonella typhimurium* strains (Hennig *et al.* 1991) and in rodents (Huff *et al.* 1991), respectively. It reacts with cellular DNA to form premutagenic DNA adducts. OTA-related DNA adducts have been identified in kidney tissue obtained from mice given OTA (Pfohl-Leszkowicz *et al.* 1991) as well as in urinary tract tumours removed from Bulgarian subjects living in endemic areas of BN.

Rare forms of chronic interstitial nephritis

Beside the chronic interstitial nephropathy induced by the abuse of analgesics (see Chapter 6.2), a number of toxic compounds or drugs have been associated not only with acute renal failure but also with chronic interstitial renal disease. Most of these compounds and their clinical complications are described elsewhere.

Heavy metals (see Chapter 6.5)

Chronic lead intoxication produces a hypocellular interstitial fibrosis irregularly distributed throughout the cortex, without mention of predominance in any kidney compartments. Medulla is usually spared except in cases with concomitant uric acid microtophi.

Chronic lithium exposure may result in variable degrees of usually multifocal interstitial areas of fibrosis infiltrated mainly with lymphocytes and plasma cells, without evidence a corticomedullary gradient (Hestbech *et al.* 1977).

Chronic cadmium intoxication is characterized by a hypocellular interstitial fibrosis with flattened tubular epithelia predominating in the outer cortex and decreasing in intensity in the columns of Bertin or in the medullae (Yasuda *et al.* 1995).

Chronic arsenic intoxication is a very rare cause of interstitial nephritis characterized by a cellular interstitial fibrosis (Prasad *et al.* 1995).

Drugs

A number of drugs, introduced in the last 30 years, may induce a severe interstitial nephritis leading occasionally to endstage renal failure. Prevention requires minimal dosage and constant monitoring of renal function and, whenever feasible, prevailing serum drug levels.

Immunosuppressive agents (see Chapter 13.2.2)

Cyclosporin may induce a hypocellular interstitial fibrosis with a typical striped pattern extending from the corticomedullary junction. It is thought to be initiated by intrarenal angiotensin-mediated vasoconstriction. Tacrolimus (FK-506) induced nephropathy has similar characteristics.

Antineoplastic agents

Ifosfamide is an alkylating agent used in the treatment of several malignancies. After one to two courses of therapy, susceptible patients develop an increase in serum creatinine levels leading to endstage renal failure within a few months to years (Berns *et al.* 1995; Friedlaender *et al.* 1998; Hill *et al.* 2000). Adults appear more susceptible than children who develop Fanconi syndrome without renal failure. Renal biopsies disclose the development of moderate, diffuse acellular or hypo cellular interstitial fibrosis and tubular atrophy associated with degenerative and regenerative tubular epithelial cells. Glomeruli are normal except for a few which are sclerotic. There is mild to severe arteriosclerosis. Immunofluorescent microscopy shows virtually no immune deposits. The pathogenesis of ifosfamide-related nephrotoxicity and of its unabated progression despite drug discontinuation is unknown.

cis-Diamminodichloride platinum (CDDP) is an antitumour agent used in the treatment of several types of cancer, especially testicular dysgerminomas. Two cures of CDDP are followed after 6 months by an irreversible, 40 per cent decrease in renal function (Dentino *et al.* 1978). From the fifth month of treatment onwards, focal tubular dilation and flattened proximal and distal epithelia are associated with tubular atrophy and interstitial fibrosis without mention of its cellularity or location in the renal compartments. Susceptibility to CDDP is enhanced by the simultaneous administration of other potentially nephrotoxic drugs. Experimentally, rats given a single intraperitoneal dose of 6 mg CDDP/kg body weight develop early epithelial necrosis of the S3 segment of proximal tubules in the corticomedullary junction (Dobyan 1985). This is followed by inflammatory interstitial fibrosis and tubular atrophy predominating in the inner cortex and in the outer stripe of the outer medulla. It is suggested that macrophages induce the development of muscle actin-positive myofibroblasts producing interstitial fibrosis (Yamate *et al.* 1995, 1996).

Nitrosoureas are alkylating agents used in the treatment of malignant brain tumours. After six courses of therapy, nearly all patients develop progressive irreversible impaired renal function in the absence of significant urinary abnormalities or signs of hypersensitivity (Schacht *et al.* 1981). Endstage uraemia developed in a few cases. Of note, clinical evidence of nephrotoxicity appeared in all patients several months after the nitrosoureas were discontinued. Light microscopy reveals focal, mild to severe interstitial fibrosis infiltrated by chronic inflammatory cells and tubular atrophy without mention of its location in the parenchyma. It is associated with usually mild sclerosis of glomeruli, mild medial arterial hypertrophy and, in a few cases, atypical caryomegaly of tubular cells. Immunofluorescent microscopy shows no immune deposits. The pathogenesis of this nephrotoxicity awaits further elucidation.

Pamidronate

Renal lesions due to the administration of Pamidronate disodium, a biphosphonate used to combat osteolysis or osteoporosis, have been reported in a few patients. In addition to seven cases of nephrotic syndrome with collapsing focal segmental sclerosis, two cases of interstitial fibrosis displaying various degrees of cellularity and flattened tubular epithelia, one of whom also had a Fanconi syndrome has been described (Janssen van Doorn *et al.* 2001; Buysschaert *et al.* 2003). Advanced age and low body mass appear to be risk factors.

Conclusions

The chronic interstitial renal lesions induced by most toxic compounds are characterized by intense interstitial fibrosis. Still they can be differentiated by the cellularity of the fibrotic component and by its diffuseness as summarized in Table 1. Like AAN, several nephropathies (BN, Cad) have in common a diffuse, pauci- or acellular interstitial fibrosis with a corticomedullary gradient. By analogy with AAN, the possibility of a primary injury of the S3 segment of the proximal tubule might therefore be considered. Of interest, once renal function is reduced, most of these nephropathies progress relentlessly despite withdrawal of the offending drug. In several other toxic interstitial nephropathies the fibrotic process is also paucicellular, but available data do not permit the evaluation of a possible corticomedullary gradient. Finally, in four nephropathies (analgesics, nitrosoureas, lithium, and arsenic), interstitial fibrosis is invaded by several cellular types, a finding suggesting a possibly different pathogenesis.

Table 1 Pathological characteristics of various toxic-induced chronic interstitial nephropathies in man

	Interstitial fibrosis	
	Cellularity	**Existence of a decreasing corticomedullary gradient**
Cadmium	−	+
Aristolochic acid (AA)	−	+
Ochratoxin A (OTA)	−	+
Balkan nephropathy (BN)	?	?
Lead	−	?
Cyclosporin A	−	?
Ifosfamide	−	?
Phytotherapy-associated interstitial nephropathy (PAIN)	−	?
Pamidronate	±	?
Analgesics	+	−
Lithium	+	?
Arsenic	+	?
Nitrosoureas	+	?
Tacrolimus (FK506)	?	?
cis-Diamminedichloride platinum (CDDP)	?	?

A question mark (?) is indicated when available data are too scarce to assess the cellularity or the existence of a corticomedullary gradient.

References

Berns, J. S. *et al.* (1995). Severe, irreversible renal failure after Ifosfamide treatment. *Cancer* **76**, 497–500.

Bieler, C. A. *et al.* (1997). ^{32}P-post-labelling analysis of DNA adducts formed by aristolochic acid in tissues from patients with Chinese herbs nephropathy. *Carcinogenesis* **18**, 1063–1067.

But, P. P. H. (1993). Need for correct identification of herbs in herbal poisoning. *Lancet* **341**, 637 (letter).

Buysschaert, M. *et al.* (2003). Pamidronate-induced tubulointerstitial nephritis with Fanconi syndrome in a patient with primary hyperparathyroidism. *Nephrology, Dialysis, Transplantation* **18**, 826–829.

Chang, C. H. *et al.* (2001). Rapidly progressive interstitial renal fibrosis associated with Chinese herbal medications. *American Journal of Nephrology* **21**, 441–448.

Chen, H. Y. *et al.* (2001). Time to abandon the term 'Chinese herbs nephropathy'. *Kidney International* **60**, 2039–2040.

Connolly, H. M. *et al.* (1997). Valvular heart disease associated with fenfluramine–phentermine. *New England Journal of Medicine* **337**, 581–588.

Cosyns, J. P. (2002). When is 'aristolochic acid nephropathy' more accurate than 'Chinese herbs nephropathy'? *Kidney International* **61**, 1178–1181.

Cosyns, J. P. (2003). Aristolochic acid and 'Chinese herbs nephropathy': a review of the evidence to date. *Drug Safety* **26**, 33–48.

Cosyns, J. P. *et al.* (1994a). Chinese herbs nephropathy: a clue to Balkan endemic nephropathy? *Kidney International* **45**, 1680–1688.

Cosyns, J. P. *et al.* (1994b). Urothelial malignancy in nephropathy due to Chinese herbs. *Lancet* **344**, 188 (letter).

Cosyns, J. P. *et al.* (1998). Chinese herbs nephropathy-associated slimming regimen induces tumours in the forestomach but no interstitial nephropathy in rats. *Archives of Toxicology* **72**, 738–743.

Cosyns, J. P. *et al.* (1999). Urothelial lesions in Chinese-herb nephropathy. *American Journal of Kidney Diseases* **33**, 1011–1017.

Cosyns, J. P. *et al.* (2001). Chronic aristolochic acid toxicity in rabbits: a model of Chinese herbs nephropathy? *Kidney International* **59**, 2164–2173.

Debelle, F. D. *et al.* (2002). Aristolochic acids induce chronic renal failure with interstitial fibrosis in salt-depleted rats. *Journal of the American Society of Nephrology* **13**, 431–436.

Dentino, M. *et al.* (1978). Long term effect of *cis*-diamminedichloride platinum (CDDP) on renal function and structure in man. *Cancer* **41**, 1274–1281.

Depierreux, M. *et al.* (1994). Pathologic aspects of a newly described nephropathy related to the prolonged use of Chinese herbs. *American Journal of Kidney Diseases* **24**, 172–180.

Dobyan, D. C. (1985). Long-term consequences of *cis*-platinum-induced renal injury: a structural and functional study. *The Anatomical Record* **21**, 239–245.

Firooz, P. and James, P. L. (1998). Herbs and kidney disease: a review. *Kidney* **7**, 185–189.

Friedlaender, M. M. *et al.* (1998). End-stage renal interstitial fibrosis in an adult ten years after Ifosfamide therapy. *American Journal of Nephrology* **18**, 131–133.

Gillerot, G. *et al.* (2001). Aristolochic acid nephropathy in a Chinese patient: time to abandon the term 'Chinese herbs nephropathy'? *American Journal of Kidney Diseases* **38**, E26.

Godin, M. *et al.* (1997). Is ochratoxin a nephrotoxic in human beings? *Advances in Nephrology from the Necker Hospital* **26**, 181–206.

Hennig, A., Fink-Gremmels, J., and Leistner, L. Mutagenicity and effects of ochratoxin A on the frequency of sister chromatid exchange after metabolic activation. In *Mycotoxins, Endemic Nephropathy and Urinary Tract Tumors* Vol. 115 (ed. M. Castegnaro, R. Pleština, G. Dirheimer, I. N. Chernozemsky, and H. Bartsch), pp. 255–260. *IARC Scientific Publications*, 1991.

Hestbech, J. *et al.* (1977). Chronic renal lesions following long-term treatment with lithium. *Kidney International* **12**, 205–213.

Hill, P. A., Prince, H. M., and Power, D. A. (2000). Tubulointerstitial nephritis following high dose Ifosfamide in three breast cancer patients. *Pathology* **32**, 166–170.

Huff, J. E. Carcinogenicity of ochratoxin A, in experimental animals. In *Mycotoxins, Endemic Nephropathy and Urinary Tract Tumors* Vol. 115 (ed. M. Castegnaro, R. Pleština, G. Dirheimer, I.N. Chernozemsky, and H. Bartsch), pp. 229–244. *IARC Scientific Publications*, 1991.

Jadoul, M. *et al.* (1993). Adverse effects from traditional Chinese medicine. *Lancet* **341**, 892–893.

Janssen van Doorn, K. J. *et al.* (2001). Pamidronate-related nephrotoxicity (tubulointerstitial nephritis) in a patient with osteolytic bone metastases. *Nephron* **89**, 467–468.

Joekes, A. M., Heptinstall, R. H., and Porter, K. A. (1958). The nephrotic syndrome: a study of renal biopsies in 20 adult patients. *Quarterly Journal of Medicine* **27**, 495–516.

Kabanda, A. *et al.* (1995). Low molecular weight proteinuria in Chinese herbs nephropathy. *Kidney International* **48**, 1571–1576.

Kessler, D. A. (2000). Cancer and herbs. *New England Journal of Medicine* **342**, 1742–1743.

Krumme, B. *et al.* (2001). Reversible Fanconi syndrome after ingestion of a Chinese herbal 'remedy' containing aristolochic acid. *Nephrology, Dialysis, Transplantation* **16**, 400–402.

Lebeau, C. *et al.* (2001). Aristolochic acid impedes endocytosis and induces DNA adducts in proximal tubule cells. *Kidney International* **60**, 1332–1342.

Lord, G. M. *et al.* (2001). Urothelial malignant disease and Chinese herbal nephropathy. *Lancet* **358**, 1515–1516.

Maaroufi, K. *et al.* (1995). Foodstuffs and human blood contamination by the mycotoxin ochratoxin A: correlation with chronic interstitial nephropathy in Tunisia. *Archives of Toxicology* **69**, 552–558.

Martinez, M. C. *et al.* (2002). Progression rate of Chinese herb nephropathy: impact of *Aristolochia fangchi* ingested dose. *Nephrology, Dialysis, Transplantation* **17**, 408–412.

Nortier, J. L. *et al.* (1997). Proximal tubular injury in Chinese herbs nephropathy: monitoring by neutral endopeptidase enzymuria. *Kidney International* **51**, 288–293.

Nortier, J. L. *et al.* (2000). Urothelial carcinoma associated with the use of a Chinese herb (*Aristolochia fangchi*). *The New England Journal of Medicine* **342**, 1686–1692.

Pfohl-Leszkowicz, A., Chakor, K., Creppy, E. E., Dirheimer, G. DNA adduct formation in mice treated with ochratoxin A. In *Mycotoxins, Endemic Nephropathy and Urinary Tract Tumors* Vol. 115 (ed. M. Castegnaro, R. Pleština, G. Dirheimer, I.N. Chernozemsky, H. Bartsch), pp. 245–253. *IARC Scientific Publications*, 1991.

Prasad, G. V. R. and Rossi, N. F. (1995). Arsenic intoxication associated with tubulointerstitial nephritis. *American Journal of Kidney Diseases* **26**, 373–376.

Reginster, F., Jadoul, M., and van Ypersele de Strihou, C. (1997). Chinese herbs nephropathy presentation, natural history, and fate after transplantation. *Nephrology, Dialysis, Transplantation* **12**, 81–86.

Schacht, R. G. *et al.* (1981). Nephrotoxicity of nitrosoureas. *Cancer* **48**, 1328–1334.

Schmeiser, H. H. *et al.* (1990). Aristolochic acid activates *ras* genes in rat tumors at deoxyadenosine residues. *Cancer Research* **50**, 5464–5469.

Seedat, Y. K. (1993). Acute renal failure in the black population of South Africa. *The International Journal of Artificial Organs* **16**, 801–802.

Solez, K. *et al.* (2001). Is 'Chinese herbs nephropathy' a prejudicial term? *Kidney International* **38**, 1141–1142 (letter).

Stiborova, M. *et al.* (1994). Characterization of DNA adducts formed by aristolochic acids in the target organ (forestomach) of rats by ^{32}P-postlabelling analysis using different chromatographic procedures. *Carcinogenesis* **15**, 1187–1192.

Tanaka, A. *et al.* (2000). Chinese herb nephropathy in Japan presents adult-onset Fanconi syndrome: could different components of aristolochic acids cause a different type of Chinese herb nephropathy? *Clinical Nephrology* **53**, 301–306.

Tanaka, A. *et al.* (2001). Outbreak of Chinese herb nephropathy in Japan: are there any differences from Belgium? *Internal Medicine* **40**, 296–300.

Ubara, Y. *et al.* (1999). A case of Chinese herbs-induced renal interstitial fibrosis associated with fibrosis of salivary glands. *American Journal of Kidney Diseases* **33**, E6.

Van Haelen, M., Vanhaelen-Fastre, R., But, P., and Vanherweghem, J. L. (1994). Identification of aristolochic acid in Chinese herbs. *Lancet* **343**, 174 (letter).

van Ypersele de Strihou, C. and Jadoul, M. (2002). Progression rate of Chinese herb nephropathy: impact of *Aristolochia fangchi* ingested dose. *Nephrology, Dialysis, Transplantation* **17**, 1852–1861.

van Ypersele de Strihou, C. and Vanherweghem, J. L. (1995). The tragic paradigm of Chinese herbs nephropathy. *Nephrology, Dialysis, Transplantation* **10**, 157–160.

Vanherweghem, J. L. *et al.* (1993). Rapidly progressive interstitial renal fibrosis in young women: association with slimming regimen including Chinese herbs. *Lancet* **341**, 387–391.

Vanherweghem, J. L. *et al.* (1996). Effects of steroids on the progression of renal failure in chronic interstitial renal fibrosis: a pilot study in Chinese herbs nephropathy. *American Journal of Kidney Diseases* **27**, 209–215.

Yamate, J. *et al.* (1995). Immunohistochemical observations on the kinetics of macrophages and myofibroblasts in rat renal interstitial fibrosis induced by *cis*-diamminedichloroplatinum. *Journal of Comparative Pathology* **112**, 27–39.

Yamate, J. *et al.* (1996). Immunohistochemical study of rat renal interstitial fibrosis induced by repeated injection of cisplatin, with special reference to the kinetics of macrophages and myofibroblasts. *Toxicologic Pathology* **24**, 199–206.

Yang, C. S. *et al.* (2000). Rapidly progressive fibrosing interstitial nephritis associated with Chinese herbal drugs. *American Journal of Kidney Diseases* **35**, 313–318.

Yang, S. S. *et al.* (2001). Two clinical variants of Chinese-herb nephropathy: case reports and review of the literature. *Journal of Medical Sciences* **21**, 217–224.

Yang, S. S. *et al.* (2002). Aristolochic acid-induced Fanconi's syndrome and nephropathy presenting as hypokalemic paralysis. *American Journal of Kidney Diseases* **39**, E14.

Yasuda, M., Miwa, A., and Kitagawa, M. (1995). Morphometric studies of renal lesions in Itai–Itai disease: chronic cadmium nephropathy. *Nephron* **69**, 14–19.

7

The patient with urinary tract infection

7

The patient with urinary tract infection

7.1 Lower and upper urinary tract infections in the adult

W.R. Cattell

Infection of the urinary tract is common, distressing, and occasionally life-threatening. Infection may extend throughout part or all of the urinary tract and, more rarely, may involve the perinephric tissues. The clinical features, diagnosis, treatment, complications, and long-term significance of infection vary depending on the site of infection and the presence or absence of structural or functional abnormality within the system. This chapter addresses separately the problems of bacterial infection of the lower and upper urinary tract, and the perinephric tissues. It does not deal with the microbiology or pathogenesis of urinary tract infection which are reviewed in depth by Andriole and others (1997).

Definitions

Bacteriuria

Bacterial infection may be defined as that condition in which bacteria are established and multiplying within the urinary tract. Diagnosis requires demonstration of bacteriuria. Exceptions to this include patients with pyogenic abscess of the kidney or perinephric tissues, obstructed pyonephrosis, or bacterial prostatitis, in whom the urine may be sterile.

Contamination of samples of urine by bacteria normally present in the anterior urethra or periurethral area is common, especially in women. To solve this problem, Kass reintroduced quantitative culture of clean-catch midstream urine samples (Kass 1956) and demonstrated that a threshold bacterial count of more than 10^5/ml of the same bacterial species distinguished genuine bladder bacteriuria from contamination. 'Significant bacteriuria' was therefore defined as the presence of 10^5 or more of the same organism per millilitre of urine.

Rigid adherence to the Kass criteria for significant bacteriuria, particularly in symptomatic young women, has been questioned for some time. Thus, it seemed odd that in domiciliary studies of women with otherwise typical cystitis 'significant bacteriuria' was found in less than 50 per cent (Gallagher *et al.* 1965). Sequential studies of recurrently symptomatic women also showed that on occasion they had significant bacteriuria but on other occasions did not (O'Grady *et al.* 1973). From these and other observations there developed a concept of low-count bacteriuria. Stamm and colleagues have provided impressive evidence for diagnosing urinary tract infection in symptomatic young women on the basis of bacterial counts of 10^2 or more organisms/ml, particularly when accompanied by pyuria (>10 white blood cells/mm^3) (Stamm *et al.* 1982). The Infectious Disease Society of America (IDSA) gave a slightly more relaxed consensus definition, requiring 10^3 organisms/ml to diagnose cystitis and 10^4/ml for pyelonephritis. This has the advantage that such bacterial counts can be recorded by standard microbiological techniques in most laboratories (Hooton and Stamm 1997).

Low-count bacteriuria may be especially common in infections with organisms such as *Staphylococcus saprophyticus*, which have longer generation times in urine than enteral bacteria. This is supported by the finding of low numbers (10^2–10^4/ml) of *S. saprophyticus* in bladder urine obtained by suprapubic aspiration from symptomatic women (Hovelius *et al.* 1979).

Contamination of carefully collected urine samples in men is less common, and a count of 10^3/ml or more of the same organism is probably an appropriate level for diagnosing bladder bacteriuria in males (Lipsky 1989). The IDSA have gone for a count of 10^4/ml (Rubin *et al.* 1992).

Complicated and uncomplicated urinary tract infection

There is general agreement that for the best management of patients with urinary infection, it is important to distinguish between complicated and uncomplicated infection. However, there is no general agreement on the definition of complicated infection. In part, this relates to differing objectives in making the distinction.

In the American literature, there is a very wide ranging definition of complicated infection to include all those conditions which increase the risk of acquiring infection or failing treatment (Tables 1 and 2) (Hooton and Stamm 1997; Ronald and Harding 1997). The merit in this approach is that it focuses attention on the known or suspected presence of these conditions in deciding the type and duration of treatment, the need for further investigation and future preventive

Table 1 Factors predisposing to infection

Urinary infection in childhood
New sexual partner
Use of spermicide
Recent antibiotic treatment
Postmenopausal vaginal atrophy
Impaired bladder emptying
Diabetes
Male
Recent urinary tract instrumentation
Indwelling urethral catheter

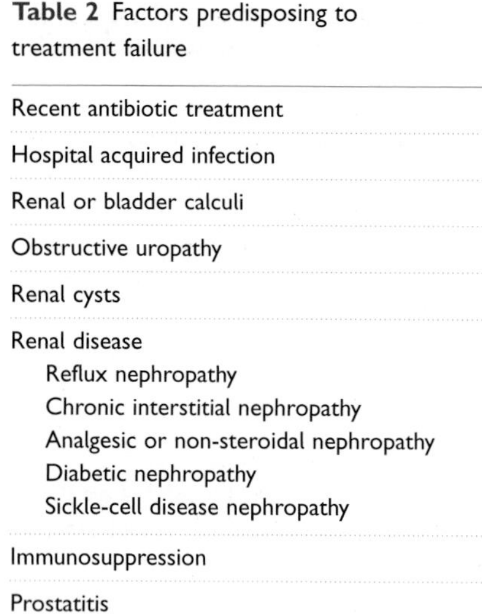

Table 2 Factors predisposing to treatment failure

Recent antibiotic treatment
Hospital acquired infection
Renal or bladder calculi
Obstructive uropathy
Renal cysts
Renal disease Reflux nephropathy Chronic interstitial nephropathy Analgesic or non-steroidal nephropathy Diabetic nephropathy Sickle-cell disease nephropathy
Immunosuppression
Prostatitis

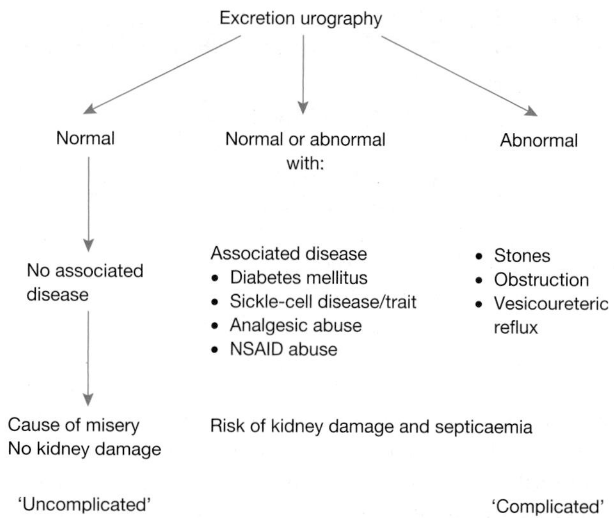

Fig. 1 Classification of 'complicated' and 'uncomplicated' urinary tract infection.

measures. The definition is, however, so wide ranging that it may be simpler to define *uncomplicated* infection as that occurring in young non-pregnant women with no previous urinary or vaginal infection, no family history, no anatomical or functional abnormality of the urinary tract, no associated disease such as diabetes, analgesic abuse, sickle-cell disease or trait, or AIDS, who are not immunosuppressed, do not use spermicidal jellies and in whom infection is unrelated to coitus. All the rest have complicated infection!

In previous editions of this textbook, the author has distinguished between complicated and uncomplicated infection on the basis of whether or not infection was likely to cause permanent kidney damage. In this context, time and extensive study have shown that persistent or recurrent infection in adults with anatomically and functionally normal urinary tracts rarely leads to significant kidney damage (Kunin 1985). The presence of obstruction, stones, or high pressure vesicoureteric reflux predispose to kidney damage, perinephric abscess, life-threatening septicaemia or a combination of these (Huland and Busch 1984). The potential for kidney damage and the response to treatment may also be conditioned by the presence of renal complications of systemic disease such as diabetes mellitus, sickle-cell disease or trait, analgesic abuse, or immunosuppression. It is on the basis of these observations that a different definition of complicated versus uncomplicated infection has been produced (Fig. 1).

There are merits in both approaches, but one or other is necessary when assessing management requirements and prognosis. Failure to do so confuses the interpretation of published data on the treatment and long-term sequelae of persistent or recurrent infection.

Recurrent infection—reinfection, relapse, and treatment failure

An isolated uncomplicated urinary infection rarely poses a treatment problem or results in significant morbidity. Recurrent infection is more troublesome. Failure to identify the nature and cause of the recurrence creates anxiety in the patient, confuses the management of the case, and makes the interpretation of antibacterial trials impossible.

Recurrent infection is of two types—reinfection and relapse (Kunin 1962)—which can only be distinguished by properly timed sequential urine cultures (Cattell *et al.* 1973). Contrary to popular belief, it is unusual for bacteria within the kidney or urinary tract to remain latent in some nidus of infection for any length of time. Thus, if there are bacteria within the kidney parenchyma, these will, in the absence of antibacterial therapy, enter the urinary system, multiply, and produce bladder bacteriuria. Exceptions to this general rule are infected renal cysts, bacterial prostatitis, and pyogenic abscesses.

Relapsing infection

This is defined as recurrence of bacteriuria with the same organism within 3 weeks of completing treatment, which, during treatment, rendered the urine sterile. It can only be diagnosed by obtaining urine samples before, during, and at between 10 and 21 days after treatment or on recurrence of symptoms.

Relapse implies that there has been a failure to eradicate the infection. This most often occurs in association with renal scars, stones, cystic disease, or prostatitis (Cattell *et al.* 1973), and in patients with chronic interstitial disease, or in those who are immunocompromised. Patients who relapse should undergo clinical review and have renal imaging to detect stones, renal scars, or other factors which make eradication of infection difficult (Table 2). An exception may be patients given single-dose therapy, in whom persistent vaginal and periurethral colonization may lead to rapid reinfection with the same organism.

Reinfection

This is much more common than relapse and accounts for some 80 per cent of recurrent infections (Stamey 1972). It is defined as eradication of bacteriuria by appropriate treatment, followed by infection with a different organism after 7–10 days. Reinfection with the same bacterial species may occur if colonization of the periurethral area has persisted or been re-established from persistence of the same organism in the faecal reservoir. Distinction from relapse may then be difficult, but relapsing infection is unlikely if the patient has remained abacteriuric and without pyuria for 21 days after completing treatment (Stapleton and Stamm 1997).

Unlike relapse, reinfection does not represent failure to eradicate infection from the urinary tract but is due to reinvasion of the system. Prophylactic measures must be initiated.

Treatment failure

There is considerable confusion regarding the definition of treatment failure, particularly in reports of antibacterial drug trials. The term has been used to describe failure to eradicate bacteriuria during treatment; failure to prevent relapse or, even more confusing, failure to prevent reinfection. In the two former cases, treatment failure correctly defines failure of the drug to eliminate bacteria from the urinary tract. Failure of a short course of antibacterial therapy to prevent reinfection should not be defined as treatment failure: the reinfection is due to persistence of factors predisposing to reinvasion of the system. To allow evaluation of the published results of treatment, it is essential that authors clearly define the criteria used for defining success or failure.

Failure to eradicate bacteriuria during treatment with an appropriate antibacterial drug, as defined by laboratory sensitivity testing, is unusual. It may be due to failure of the patient to take the drug or loss of the drug due to vomiting. Alternatively, there may be inadequate concentrations of the drug in the urine due to poor renal function, or there may have been an error in laboratory sensitivity testing. Failure to absorb antibacterial drugs is uncommon.

Diagnosis

With the exceptions already mentioned, definitive diagnosis of urinary tract infection requires the demonstration of bladder bacteriuria. It is important for clinicians to instruct patients carefully on the methods for collecting midstream urine samples (Table 3) and the desirability, where possible, of obtaining early morning urine samples when low bacterial counts are less likely to be found.

Suprapubic aspiration of urine

Where it is impossible to obtain uncontaminated samples, or in symptomatic patients with low (10^2–10^4/ml) bacterial counts, bladder bacteriuria should be diagnosed by the culture of urine obtained by suprapubic aspiration (Table 4). This is a simple procedure and, provided the bladder is full, urine samples are easily obtained, and should normally be sterile. Rarely, and especially in obese subjects, aspiration of urine may have to be guided by ultrasound. It is the author's belief that persistently or recurrently symptomatic patients should not be labelled abacteriuric without culture of urine obtained by suprapubic aspiration.

Catheter samples of urine

It should rarely be necessary to catheterize patients for the collection of urine samples for diagnostic culture. Catheterization itself introduces bacteria into the bladder, resulting in false-positive cultures and leading to infection in 1 per cent of patients.

Pyuria

Aside from its role in the diagnosis of urinary tract infection, persisting pyuria is of importance as an indicator of possible stone disease, papillary necrosis, interstitial nephritis, or tuberculous disease. In symptomatic, abacteriuric women it should also alert to the possibility of genital infection such as *Chlamydia* (Stamm *et al.* 1980).

Table 3 Collection of midstream specimens of urine

Female
1. Patient must have a full bladder
2. Patient removes underclothing and STANDS legs either side of the toilet
3. Separate labia with left hand
4. Cleanse vulva front to back with sterile swab
5. Void downward into toilet until 'half done'
6. Without interrupting stream, catch urine in sterile pot
7. The patient then completes voiding

Male
1. Patient must have a full bladder
2. Retract foreskin if present
3. Cleanse glans penis with a sterile swab
4. Void into toilet with foreskin retracted until 'half done'
5. Without interrupting stream catch sample in sterile pot
6. Complete voiding

Elderly female patients may need nursing assistance.

Table 4 Suprapubic aspiration of urine

1. Patient must have a full bladder which can be percussed. If not percussible or if in doubt, give 300 ml fluid and 20 mg frusemide orally and wait 1 h. If still in doubt and especially in obese subjects, localize bladder using ultrasound
2. With patient supine, choose site in midline 2.5 cm above symphysis pubis. Clean skin with spirit impregnated sterile gauze
3. Insert a 21 gauge 1 $^1/_2$" needle, attached to a 10 ml syringe, directly downwards and aspirate urine
4. Withdraw needle and collect midstream specimen of urine

The use of local anaesthetic is optional but usually unnecessary.

Diagnosis of upper versus lower tract infection

A diagnosis of upper urinary tract infection is usually based on clinical symptoms and signs. However, many studies in which the site of infection has been identified by one of a variety of techniques have shown that diagnosing the site of infection on the basis of symptoms and signs can be quite inaccurate. Using ureteral catheterization, Stamey *et al.* (1965) showed that approximately 50 per cent of women with asymptomatic bacteriuria had infection in their upper tracts, and that a small but significant proportion of women with primarily bladder symptoms also had upper tract infection. Conversely, loin pain and tenderness with fever may be present in 15–30 per cent of patients with infection confined to the bladder (Busch and Huland 1984).

These observations led to the introduction of various techniques for more accurate localization of the site of infection. The need to identify the site was based on the belief that renal infection, especially if repeated, led to kidney damage, and that treatment of upper tract infection differed from that of cystitis. Given the limitation of the various localization techniques and recognition that uncomplicated renal infection rarely led to kidney damage, localization tests are now rarely used.

Treatment of upper versus lower urinary tract infection does indeed differ (see below) but response to treatment is now used to distinguish between the two. This is based on the observation that many women with symptoms of cystitis shown by localization studies to be confined to the bladder can be cured by a single dose of antibiotic (Bailey 1983). Recurrence of bacteriuria with the same species within

7 days of single-dose therapy was reported to be most often associated with upper tract infection. However, some doubt has been cast on this with the observation that single-dose therapy has little effect on urethral, vaginal, and rectal colonization (Fihn *et al.* 1988). Persistence of bacteria in these sites may predispose to reinfection of the bladder within 10–14 days of treatment, when a distinction between relapse and reinfection cannot be made.

Special investigations

Urinary tract imaging in urinary tract infection

The indications for and choice of imaging remain slightly controversial. In general, imaging is done 3–6 weeks after cure of the infection to identify abnormalities predisposing to infection or renal damage or which may affect management (Cattell *et al.* 1989). Rarely, imaging is carried out in the acute phase, particularly where there is severe loin pain, to identify possible sepsis (pyonephrosis or abscess) or to differentiate acute pyelonephritis from ureteric colic.

Factors influencing a decision to undertake imaging and the choice of technique include recognition that abnormalities will be found in less than 5 per cent of unselected cases (Fowler and Polaski 1981), the need to minimize radiation and to avoid adverse reactions to contrast media, convenience, and cost.

Given these observations, it is best to examine the strengths and weaknesses of the different imaging techniques in the management of urinary infection before suggesting the indications for and choice of imaging.

Plain abdominal radiographs

These are used to show the presence and extent of calcification in the urinary tract. Their sensitivity for detecting opaque renal calculi is increased by supplementing them with plain tomography, especially when bowel overlies the kidneys or low-density stones are being sought (Fig. 2a and b). Intravenous urography (IVU) is required to localize calculi within the calyces or pelvis. Plain films are less sensitive in the detection of ureteric calculi, and IVU is needed to determine whether calcification along the line of the ureter is within it. Plain films are of value in monitoring change in position, size, and number of calculi.

Ultrasound

Ultrasonography combined with plain radiographs has become the imaging method of choice in patients with recurrent infection. Advantages compared to IVU include availability, cost, reduction in radiation exposure, and the avoidance of contrast media.

Ultrasonography is a sensitive detector of pelvicalyceal dilatation indicative of possible obstruction. Echoes within a dilated pelvicalyceal system, either diffuse or layered, suggest the presence of pyonephrosis. Drainage of an obstructed kidney can be guided by ultrasonography.

Ultrasonography provides accurate renal length measurements and identifies the majority of renal scars, abscesses, and perinephric fluid collections. It shows many renal calculi, but is less sensitive in detecting opaque calculi than a combination of plain radiographs and plain tomography (Vrtiska *et al.* 1992). In acute pyelonephritis, ultrasonography may show either diffuse or focal parenchymal swelling, with compression and attenuation of the sinus echoes. Ultrasonography can also assess the bladder for wall thickness, calculi, diverticula and emptying, as well as assess prostatic size.

Ultrasonography may show short segments of a dilated ureter adjacent to the renal pelvis, at pelvic brim level or behind the full bladder, but does not show the remainder of the ureter. It cannot identify medullary sponge kidney or papillary necrosis and is insensitive in the detection of calyceal clubbing, conditions which can affect the course and treatment of infection. Given these latter limitations, ultrasonography cannot allow reassurance of the patient that 'the urinary tract is normal' with the degree of confidence that is possible following a well-conducted IVU.

Ultrasonography combined with plain radiography is especially valuable for emergency imaging in patients presenting with a first infection with severe loin pain and fever (Fig. 3).

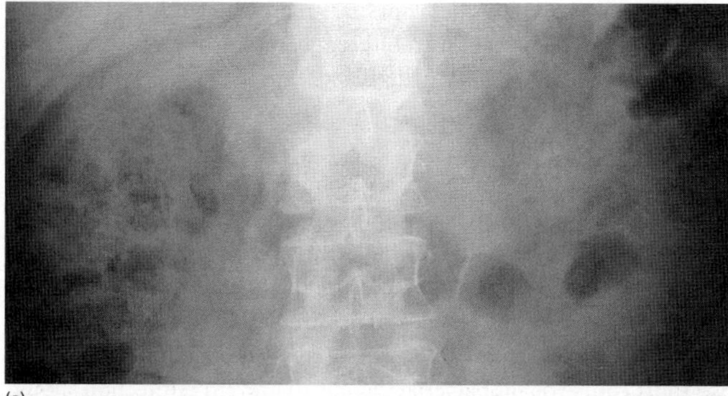

(a)

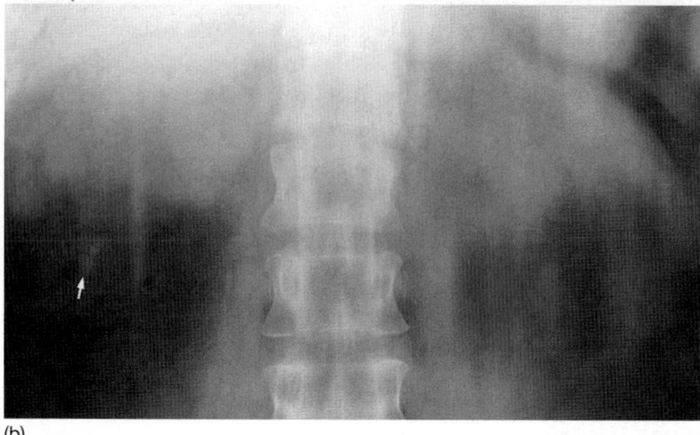

(b)

Fig. 2 (a) Right kidney obscured by bowel gas and faeces. (b) Tomography shows low density stone (arrow).

Intravenous urography

IVU provides anatomical detail of the calyces, pelvis, and ureter not obtained from ultrasonography. Calyceal detail is essential to diagnose papillary necrosis and medullary sponge kidney, and careful assessment of the calyces and overlying parenchyma is necessary to diagnose reflux nephropathy. IVU supplemented with intravenous frusemide can usually identify obstruction at the pelviureteric junction or more distally. It allows measurement of kidney length and identifies most scars. It also shows bladder diverticula and impaired bladder emptying.

The disadvantages of IVU compared to ultrasonography are the need for radiation, possible adverse reactions to contrast media, cost, and relative inconvenience. IVU is best avoided in acute pyelonephritis, as reduced function and renal swelling often lead to poor images. It should be avoided for the first six weeks after pregnancy to allow resolution of the physiological dilatation of the pelvicalyceal system and ureter. IVU is no longer used in renal failure, where a combination

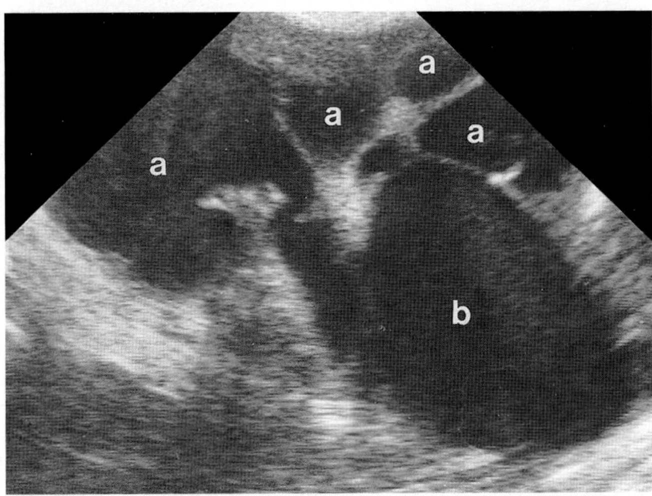

Fig. 3 Ultrasound picture of obstructed pyonephrosis. Dilated calyces (a) and pelvis (b) have contained echoes suggesting pus.

of ultrasonography and plain films provides the necessary diagnostic information (Cattell *et al.* 1989).

A potential problem in clinical practice is the casual, unnecessary repetition of IVUs in patients with recurrent infection previously shown to have a normal urinary tract and who do not have a condition predisposing to papillary necrosis: the likelihood of their acquiring some new abnormality is small. Urography should only be repeated if the clinical picture changes—for example, haematuria in the absence of bacteriuria.

Computed tomography

Computed tomography (CT) has many strengths for the evaluation of urinary tract infection. It is the most sensitive method of detecting renal and ureteric calculi, including calculi, such as urate stones, which are 'lucent' on plain radiographs. It is a sensitive detector of pelvicalyceal dilatation. CT is more sensitive than ultrasonography for the detection of renal abscesses (Soulen *et al.* 1989) and can show perinephric collections and their relationship to the perinephric fascial planes better than ultrasonography. Contrast-enhanced CT is a very sensitive detector of acute pyelonephritis. Typically, there are wedge- and band-shaped areas of reduced enhancement in a lobar distribution in the affected areas. The abnormal enhancement pattern may persist for months and, on CT follow-up, scars are seen in some patients (Meyrier *et al.* 1989).

However, CT involves more radiation than IVU, the potential risks of contrast media and is more expensive and less readily available than ultrasonography. It is therefore reserved as a second-line investigation for patients with severe infection not responding to appropriate treatment or for diagnostic problems not resolved by IVU or ultrasonography.

Static renal scintigraphy

Di-mercapto-succinic acid (DMSA) scintigraphy is a sensitive detector of renal parenchymal infection in children, but has been less evaluated in adults. It has recently been shown that CT is more sensitive than DMSA for detecting pyelonephritis in adults (Sattari *et al.* 2000). DMSA scans are unable to distinguish reduced uptake of radionuclide due to pyelonephritis from abscess and do not provide anatomical information about the pelvicalyceal system and perinephric space.

Indications for and choice of renal imaging

Acute infection

Patients who have severe loin pain or whose infection does not settle on treatment should have ultrasonography and plain radiographs to exclude pyonephrosis, intrarenal or perinephric sepsis or calculi. Renal or perinephric abnormalities seen on ultrasonography may require elucidation by CT. CT may also be undertaken if no abnormality is seen on ultrasonography.

Imaging may also be indicated if ureteric colic is suspected when IVU or spiral unenhanced CT should be used (Smith *et al.* 1996).

Imaging after treatment of infection

In *women*, there is no indication for imaging following a single or infrequent infection. Recurrent attacks more often than 2 per 6 months should be investigated by ultrasonography and plain radiographs.

In *men*, urinary infection is so much less common than in women that imaging is indicated after the first documentation of bacteriuria to exclude predisposing factors, especially impaired bladder emptying. Ultrasonography and plain radiographs are the best first choice (Andrews *et al.* 2002).

Imaging should be considered if urinary infection is slow to resolve; if there is relapse—especially if accompanied by pyuria—or if there are risk factors for papillary necrosis. IVU is the method of choice to check for papillary necrosis, medullary sponge kidney, or reflux nephropathy. IVU is also indicated in all patients over the age of 40 who have gross haematuria because of the risk of associated cancer.

Micturating cystourography and videourodynamics

Micturating cystography is not usually indicated in adults with urinary infection unless they have loin or abdominal pain during voiding, suggestive of reflux, or as part of the investigation of impaired bladder emptying.

Videourodynamic studies may be necessary in patients with unexplained impairment of bladder emptying.

Cystoscopy

This is rarely indicated in patients with isolated or recurrent infections who have normal results on IVU. It should always be performed in older patients with severe haematuria, in whom bladder cancer may be suspected, and must be undertaken in patients with recurrent or persistent unexplained frequency and dysuria who have no bacteriuria on repeated testing.

Asymptomatic bacteriuria

Numerous population studies have been carried out on the prevalence of asymptomatic bacteriuria, defined as the presence of greater than or equal to 100,000/ml of the same bacterial species in two consecutive midstream urine samples. These studies have been principally on women. The prevalence is strikingly similar in the United States, Jamaica, Wales, and Japan, varying between 3 and 7 per cent of women aged 16–65 years, compared to less than 0.1 per cent of men (Kunin and McCormack 1968; Evans *et al.* 1982). Prevalence increases with age: Gaymans *et al.* (1976) reported an increase in prevalence from 2.7 per cent of women aged 15–24, to 9.3 per cent of women aged 65 years or older. Kunin and McCormack (1968) also observed an increase in prevalence with age in nuns, who have a lower incidence of bacteriuria than matched controls. Over the age of 65 the prevalence increases markedly, especially in males.

The significance of asymptomatic bacteriuria and indications for treatment remain controversial. There is, however, considerable agreement on certain points. A distinction should be made between non-pregnant women with normal urinary tracts (uncomplicated) and pregnant women and patients who have bacteriuria associated with obstruction, stones, diabetes mellitus, or other complicating factor.

Uncomplicated asymptomatic bacteriuria

Longitudinal studies have shown that many non-pregnant women with uncomplicated asymptomatic bacteriuria spontaneously rid themselves of bacteriuria or change the bacterial species. However, most studies indicate that up to 30 per cent of those patients will develop symptomatic infection within 1 year (Gaymans *et al.* 1976). It has been proposed that transient bacteriuria merely reflects colonization of the bladder without tissue invasion. Stamm (1983) suggested that the presence of pyuria indicated infection and its absence indicated simple colonization. Recent studies showed a high incidence of symptomatic infections in women previously shown to have asymptomatic bacteriuria and pyuria (Hooton *et al.* 2000). It may be that those patients with pyuria were 'incubating' a typical attack of symptomatic infection. Aside from the potential for developing a symptomatic infection, uncomplicated asymptomatic bacteriuria is believed to be a benign condition which does not lead to renal damage or hypertension and only rarely to infected stone formation.

Treatment

There is no good evidence to suggest that treatment is required for uncomplicated asymptomatic bacteriuria in non-pregnant women. Patients should be warned that they may develop acute symptoms in the future and should be educated in prophylactic measures.

Complicated asymptomatic bacteriuria

Asymptomatic bacteriuria is less benign in patients with abnormal urinary tracts. Thus, patients with asymptomatic bladder bacteriuria or an infected ileal conduit who have some element of upper tract obstruction, such as pelviureteric junction narrowing or stenosis of the ureteroileal anastomosis, are at risk of ascending infection leading to a high-pressure infected system. This increases the likelihood of renal damage and septicaemia. The development of renal stones constitutes a further risk factor: the role of infection with urea-splitting organisms, particularly *Proteus mirabilis*, in the development of calcium, magnesium, and ammonium phosphate (triple) stones is well recognized (Griffith 1978). This is more likely in the presence of a dilated, poorly draining pelvicalyceal system. Ascent of infection may also result in infection of pre-existing metabolic stones, accelerating stone growth. Impaired bladder emptying or bladder diverticulae predispose to bladder stone formation.

Patients with asymptomatic bacteriuria who have conditions predisposing to papillary necrosis—diabetes mellitus, sickle-cell disease or trait, abuse of analgesics or non-steroidal anti-inflammatory drugs—must be considered at risk of potentially harmful extension of infection to the kidney, which may accelerate interstitial damage.

Immunosuppressed patients with asymptomatic bacteriuria run an increased risk of bacteraemia if renal infection develops. However, asymptomatic bacteriuria may be relatively benign in patients with kidney transplants on long-term immunosuppressive therapy, after the first few months (Griffin and Salaman 1979). Treatment is similar to that used for symptomatic patients (see below).

Asymptomatic bacteriuria in pregnant women

This is dealt with in Section 15.

Lower urinary tract infection—cystitis and urethritis

Incidence

Infection of the bladder is among the most common of all bacterial infections. Between the age of 20 and 40 years, 25–35 per cent of women give a history of symptoms diagnosed as being due to urinary infection, and some 20 per cent of women between the ages of 24 and 64 have at least one episode of dysuria per year, mostly due to bacterial infection (Sanford 1975). Urinary tract infection is reputed to result in some 6,000,000 outpatient visits per year in the United States (National Center for Health Statistics 1977) and in the United Kingdom, Asscher (1980) has quoted a figure of 12 per 1000 general practitioner consultations for cystitis.

During their reproductive years, women are 20–50 times more likely to acquire an infection than are men. It is more common in sexually active women and the incidence increases with age. Differences in incidence between the sexes diminish in later life.

Pathogens

In over 95 per cent of urinary infections a single bacterial species is responsible: 80 per cent of community-acquired acute infections are due to *Escherichia coli*, and *S. saprophyticus* is now recognized to be the second most common pathogen, accounting for some 10 per cent of infections overall and 15–30 per cent of acute infections in sexually active young women (Mabeck 1969; Wallmark *et al.* 1978). *Klebsiella*, *Proteus*, and enterococci are much less common. The aetiology of urinary pathogens in hospital-acquired infections is different, with a reduction in *E. coli* infection and an increase in *Klebsiella*, *Proteus*, *Pseudomonas aeruginosa*, and other enterobacteria.

The presence of more than one bacterial species in bladder urine is uncommon (3–5 per cent) except in catheterized patients. In non-catheterized patients it is usually associated with recurrent infection and repeated courses of antibacterial therapy, or impaired bladder emptying.

Histopathology

Acute bacterial infection of the bladder is associated with inflammation limited to the superficial mucosal layer of the bladder.

Clinical presentation and natural history

Patients with lower urinary tract infection may be symptomatic or asymptomatic. Asymptomatic bacteriuria has already been dealt with. Symptoms of bladder infection relate to inflammation—frequency, urgency, and dysuria. Dysuria usually describes pain in the urethra during voiding. It may be worse or only present at the end of voiding. Occasionally pain is described as being over the perineum. Typically, small volumes of urine are passed and a sensation of incomplete bladder emptying is common. Nocturia is a regular feature. Urge incontinence is not uncommon, especially in older women. There is often a feeling of lower abdominal discomfort or heaviness. The urine may have an offensive smell and haematuria occurs in approximately one-third of acute cases. In patients with recurrent infection, and especially the elderly, symptoms may be much less marked, with only a slight change in frequency, smelly urine, the development of incontinence, or vague abdominal pain.

In many young women, symptoms may disappear spontaneously or as a result of a high fluid intake. The response to antibacterial treatment is usually prompt, acute symptoms disappearing within 24–72 h. In some, if untreated, symptoms progress with features suggestive of extension of infection to the upper tract—loin pain, fever, rigors, and vomiting.

Single isolated infection

In the majority of women, acute cystitis is an isolated event, never or very infrequently repeated. It may coincide with the onset of sexual activity or change of sexual partner. Although acutely distressing, it does not constitute a long-term problem and rarely leaves any sequelae.

Recurrent infection

In a small proportion of women, infection is recurrent, with attacks occurring in clusters of two or three at intervals of a few months, or separate attacks spread throughout the year. They may always follow coitus, occur occasionally after intercourse, or be quite unrelated. Many studies have found an increased incidence in women using a cervical cap plus a spermicidal cream, the use of a sheath plus a spermicidal foam or the use of a spermicide alone (Hooten *et al.* 1991). It is suggested that the spermicidal agent may be the causal factor facilitating *E. coli* colonization of the vagina. In postmenopausal women, vaginal atrophy due to hormone deficiency facilitates colonization of the vagina with uropathogens, so leading to recurrent infection. This can be reversed by intravaginal oestrogen (Raz and Stamm 1993).

Infection confined to the lower tract does not predispose to kidney damage, except on the rare occasions when it contributes to bladder outflow obstruction and obstructive nephropathy. This may be due to the development of infected bladder stones or to bacterial prostatitis superimposed on benign prostatic hypertrophy. Although not altering life expectancy, recurrent frequency, and dysuria can be a cause of great misery and distress. It can lead to significant loss of time at work, make normal social and sexual activity impossible, and result in very considerable physical and psychological debility. All too often, if casually or inadequately treated, the quality of life of affected women can be seriously impaired. Conversely, when successfully managed, they are the most grateful of patients.

The urethral syndrome

This label has been used to describe women with persistent or recurrent frequency and dysuria in whom urine culture yields fewer than 10^5 organisms/ml. As previously discussed, rigid adoption of this criterion for the diagnosis of infection in acutely symptomatic women is incorrect. Stamm *et al.* (1982) and Kunin *et al.* (1993) have clearly shown that the majority of women diagnosed as having the urethral syndrome have low-count bacteriuria. Careful longitudinal study of such patients, with collection of midstream samples at the commencement of symptoms, preferably on waking, or collection of urine by suprapubic aspiration, shows that the majority of patients with the urethral syndrome have bacteriuria on some occasions while at other times have low-count bacteriuria (O'Grady *et al.* 1973).

Urethritis and vaginitis

Between 10 and 20 per cent of women with sexually transmitted genital infection due to *Chlamydia trachomatis*, *Neisseria gonorrhoeae*, or herpes simplex virus complain of frequency and dysuria due to urethritis. Stamm *et al.* (1980) investigated 59 young sexually active women with frequency and dysuria whose bladder urine was sterile by conventional microbiological methods: 11 had *Chlamydia* infection and 10 of these 11 women had pyuria. Others have reported symptoms suggestive of urinary tract infection in 30 per cent of women with gonorrhoea. Thus, urethritis accounts for a proportion of symptomatic, sexually active women with sterile bladder urine. The diagnosis may be suggested by an insidious onset of symptoms over some weeks, urethritis in a partner or vaginal discharge.

Patients with vaginal infection due to *Candida albicans* or *Trichomonas* spp. may also complain of dysuria. On careful questioning, the discomfort is described as being felt externally when urine flows over the inflamed labia. Vulval soreness with or without a malodorous discharge is usually present. Increased frequency and urgency are unusual.

Infection of the bladder by microorganisms with fastidious culture requirements not routinely used in the laboratory has been proposed to account for a proportion of symptomatic women with 'sterile' bladder urine. These organisms include *Ureaplasma urealyticum*, *Microplasma hyminis*, lactobacilli, and other anaerobic or microaerophylic bacteria (Maskell 1989). Their role as urinary pathogens remains controversial.

Bladder or genital infection having been excluded, 10–15 per cent of women with symptoms of persistent or recurrent frequency and dysuria still require a diagnosis. In postmenopausal women, such symptoms may be associated with hormone-deficient atrophy of the vulva or urethra. This is usually clinically evident and symptoms improve with the use of hormone replacement creams (Raz and Stamm 1993).

Interstitial cystitis of the bladder (Hunner's ulcer) may account for a few, and persistence of symptoms demands cystoscopy. Careful history taking will identify a number of women in whom the main problem is frequency rather than dysuria. Typically such patients do not have nocturia. If careful record is kept of the time and volume of all fluid consumed and the time and volume of all urine passed, these women are shown not to be polydypsic and to be capable of retaining and then voiding a large volume of urine on waking. Throughout the day they frequently pass small volumes of urine. Such patients have 'irritable bladders' and, not uncommonly, they also have symptoms of 'irritable bowel'. Symptoms usually improve on reassurance and small doses of sedative drugs such as diazepam.

Cold weather, tight clothing, allergies, stress, and psychosexual disturbances have all been incriminated as possible causes of frequency and dysuria. Their precise role is unclear and the management of these patients can be extremely difficult.

Treatment of lower tract infection

Symptomatic infection of the lower tract should be treated with antibacterial therapy. While many young women self-treat successfully with a high fluid intake, possibly combined with alkali therapy, a proportion of these will develop upper tract infection, possibly requiring hospital admission. In women with recurrent attacks, failure to eradicate infection, and especially vaginal or periurethral colonization, leads to increasingly frequent attacks and increasing morbidity.

For the discussion of management strategies it is convenient to subdivide patients into those with their first or only very occasional infection and those with recurrent infection.

Single infection

Previous studies have suggested that some 50 per cent of young women presenting with symptoms of lower tract infection do not have significant bacteriuria. Redefinition of what constitutes significant bacteriuria indicates that the majority of this 'abacteriuric' group have low bacterial counts and are indeed infected. It is therefore reasonable to diagnose bladder infection on the basis of acute symptoms in young women presenting for the first time. Further evidence of infection as a cause of symptoms can be provided by a positive sticks test for nitrite and leucocyte esterase, or by the finding of 10 leucocytes/mm^3 of unspun urine. A negative sticks test or the absence of pyuria is an indication for obtaining a urine culture. Routinely sending a sample for urine culture in all cases is not justified because of the highly predictable range of organisms causing urinary infection and their antimicrobial resistance patterns in the community (Hooton and Stamm 1997).

Choice of antibiotics

In the absence of sensitivity testing, the choice of antibiotic must be based on its probable effectiveness against uropathogenic bacteria, lack of side-effects (including disturbance of normal gut and vaginal flora), acceptability to the patient, and cost. This must be set against a background of increasing antimicrobial resistance among urinary pathogens causing community-acquired infection (Gupta *et al.* 2001a).

Sulfonamides have been used extensively, but with increasing *in vitro* resistance in *E. coli* and the advent of drugs with a wider antibacterial spectrum they are now seldom prescribed.

Ampicillin and amoxycillin are widely used and effective, although there is an increasing prevalence of drug-resistant *E. coli*. Amoxycillin is rather better absorbed from the gut but there is evidence that neither it or ampicillin is very effective in eliminating vaginal and periurethral flora (Fihn *et al.* 1988).

Clavulanic acid–amoxycillin (Augmentin®) is effective in treating infections due to β-lactamase-producing *E. coli* resistant to ampicillin. Its pharmacokinetics are similar to those of amoxycillin but it is more expensive and in general is not a first-line drug.

Nitrofurantoin is usually effective against most strains of *E. coli*, but is inactive against *Proteus* and *Pseudomonas* species. Its bactericidal effect is confined to the urine, tissue, and blood concentrations being subinhibitory. It is the drug of choice in pregnant women. It should not be used in patients with renal impairment as effective urine concentrations are less likely to be reached and peripheral neuropathy may develop, particularly with prolonged administration. Nausea is encountered in a significant number of patients but is less likely with macrocrystalline preparations (Macrodantin®).

Trimethoprim–sulfamethoxazole was originally produced as a combined drug in the belief that trimethoprim on its own was less effective. There is now little evidence to support this, and since most of the adverse side-effects relate to the sulfamethoxazole many now choose to use trimethoprim alone. Several studies have indicated superiority of this drug to ampicillin, possibly because it is more effective in reducing faecal, vaginal, and periurethral colonization (Fihn *et al.* 1988). Unfortunately, bacterial resistance to trimethoprim and trimethoprim–sulfamethoxazole is increasing in various communities.

Fluoroquinolones are an extremely valuable group of antibiotics for the treatment of urinary infection. Like trimethoprim they are concentrated in vaginal secretions and reduce vaginal and periurethral colonization. However, because they are expensive and have a special role in the oral treatment of *Pseudomonas* infections, many have been loath to advise their use as first-line drugs. Nevertheless, they are being increasingly used, the increased cost being justified by high cure rates with reduced costs for further care (Hooten and Stamm 1997).

Other antibiotics, including the cephalosporins and fosfomycin, may be chosen but, in general, have no special advantage as first-line drugs.

Duration of treatment

Controversy reigns regarding the appropriate duration of treatment. Some years ago, there was considerable interest in the use of single-dose therapy on the basis of convenience, cost, compliance, and reduction in side-effects. Trimethoprim–sulfamethoxazole in a dose of 320 mg trimethoprim and 1600 mg sulfamethoxazole, amoxycillin 3 g, cephaloridine 2 g, intramuscular kanamycin 500 mg, gentamicin 5 mg/kg, doxycycline 300 mg, ciprofloxacin 500 mg, and norfloxacin 800 mg have been used. Many studies have shown a cure rate greater than 85 per cent, but others have been less successful.

The suggestion that single-dose therapy was not only successful but distinguished lower from upper tract infection has been questioned, particularly because of the difficulty in distinguishing rapid reinfection from true relapse due to the persistence of periurethral colonization (Fihn *et al.* 1988; Stamm *et al.* 1989).

Most trials have shown 3-day therapy to be more effective than single-dose treatment (Warren *et al.* 1999). With the exception of nitrofurantoin, there is now little justification for 7-day or longer courses of treatment. There is considerable evidence in favour of 3-day treatment with either trimethoprim (200 mg twice daily), trimethoprim–sulfamethoxazole (160 mg/800 mg twice daily), ciprofloxacin (250 mg twice daily), or amoxycillin (250–500 mg thrice daily). Nitrofurantoin (Macrodantin®) (100 mg thrice daily) should be given for 7 days (Warren *et al.* 1999) (Table 5). Trimethoprim and fluoroquinolones which concentrate in vaginal secretion are especially effective in eradicating vaginal colonization with uropathogenic organisms, so reducing the potential for reinfection (Hooton and Stamm 1991).

Supportive measures

All patients must be encouraged to maintain a high fluid intake (2 l daily) and to void completely at 2- or 3-hourly intervals by day. Alkalinization of the urine with potassium citrate or sodium bicarbonate may give symptomatic relief and enhances the effectiveness of aminoglycosides and erythromycin.

Table 5 Antibacterial treatment for 'acute cystitis'

Trimethoprim 200 mg twice daily for 3 days
Trimethoprim–sulfamethoxazole (Septrin) 160/800 mg twice daily for 3 days
Nitrofurantoin (Macrodantin) 100 mg thrice daily for 7 days
Amoxycillin 500 mg thrice daily for 3 days
Ciprofloxacin 250 mg twice daily for 3 days

Table 6 Prophylactic regime

1. Drink sufficient fluid to void 2 l per day
2. Void 2–3 hourly with double micturition if reflux present
3. Void at bedtime and after intercourse
4. Avoid bubble baths and chemical additives in bath water
5. Avoid constipation which may impair bladder emptying

Follow-up

Patients should be warned that recurrence of infection may occur within the next few weeks and should be encouraged to practise prophylactic measures (Table 6) for several weeks or months. A urine culture may be obtained 7–10 days post-treatment to ensure there is no persisting pyuria or asymptomatic bacteriuria, but is unnecessary if symptoms resolve completely on treatment. Persistence of pyuria requires further investigation by IVU.

Recurrent infection

Some 20–40 per cent of women with an initial urinary infection will have recurrence (Stapleton and Stamm 1997). It is critical to distinguish between relapse and reinfection (see above). In women, recurrent infection is most often due to reinfection. The presence of complicated or uncomplicated disease must be ascertained in order to define the hazards and prognosis. If there is reinfection, the treatment of the acute attack is the same as for a single infection.

The essential problem in women with recurrent reinfection is the ease of vaginal colonization with uropathogenic organisms and their establishment within the bladder (Stapleton and Stamm 1997). The nature of the problem must be explained and a prophylactic regimen established (Table 6). Although this is difficult to subject to controlled trial, we have found it extremely effective over 30 years of experience: many women established on this regimen have no further problems. The maintenance of a high urine output is most important. Care should also be taken to identify and treat hormone-deficient atrophic vulval vaginitis in the elderly and to exclude the use of spermicidal cream or foam.

Given that colonization of the vagina and periurethral area with uropathogenic organisms is a critical step in the development of urinary infection, various measures are being explored to prevent this and so reduce the potential for recurrent infection. Since the presence of vaginal lactobacilli appears to reduce colonization with uropathogens, the intravaginal application of exogenous lactobacilli (probiotic therapy) has been investigated but with limited success (Reid and Bruce 2001). Vaginal mucosal immunization against uropathogenic organisms has also been studied (Uehling *et al.* 2001). Measures such as these which might successfully block the development of urinary infection in susceptible women are the logical next step in prophylaxis.

A significant number of women, and especially those with impaired bladder emptying, cannot be maintained free of infection. Impairment of bladder emptying requires careful urological examination to establish whether it can be improved surgically.

Patients with infrequent reinfection (once or twice a year) may be treated with single short courses of drugs, as described for isolated infections, and may be encouraged to self-treat (see below). If attacks occur more often than twice in 6 months, low-dose prophylaxis is usually required.

Low-dose prophylaxis

The introduction of low-dose prophylactic therapy in the 1960s (O'Grady *et al.* 1969) revolutionized the management and quality of life of thousands of women. The original philosophy of low-dose treatment was that a high fluid intake and frequent voiding could maintain bacterial clearance by day, but overnight this effect was lost. For this reason, a single dose of antibacterial was prescribed last thing at night. Trimethoprim (100 mg), trimethoprim–sulfamethoxazole (160 mg/800 mg), and nitrofurantoin (50–100 mg) have all been shown to be very effective (Nicolle *et al.* 1988; Stapleton 1999). Trimethoprim–sulfamethoxazole or trimethoprim alone may have a special role in reducing the level of periurethral colonization. Side-effects with low-dose therapy are unusual, as is the emergence of resistant strains. Superinfection with an organism resistant to the prophylactic agent can occur, when short-term treatment with an alternative appropriate antibacterial should be given. Then it is usually possible to return successfully to the original prophylactic drug.

Postcoital treatment

In a number of women recurrence of infection occurs only after sexual intercourse. In such patients, the use of spermicidal agents should be reviewed. Where this does not apply, patients may be controlled by taking a single dose of antibacterial after intercourse. This can significantly reduce the load of antibacterial agent administered.

Duration of treatment

In general, prophylactic treatment should be continued for 12 months from the time of the last infection as recurrence rates are significantly greater after shorter periods of treatment. Even so, some patients may have recurrence of infection and may require very long prophylaxis.

Self-treatment

While long-term low-dose prophylaxis has been very successful, there has been some concern as to whether this is *over-treatment*. Thus, the nature of recurrent infection is for attacks to occur in clusters, often at intervals of some months, or as random single attacks separated by long periods. It has therefore been suggested that *continuous* low-dose treatment may be unnecessary. From this evolved the concept of self-treatment when attacks occurred. This could reduce the inconvenience for the patient in attending her physician, the load of antibiotic taken and cost. To be successful it requires accuracy in self diagnosis, responsible use of antibiotics and proof of effectiveness.

Two well-conducted studies have shown that these objectives can be achieved in well-motivated women who have previously experienced culture proven infection. Thus, between 86 and 94 per cent of suspected infections were confirmed bacteriologically and clinical and bacteriological cure achieved in over 90 per cent of cases (Schaeffer and Stuppy 1999; Gupta *et al.* 2001b). Treatment in both studies was with a quinolone (Norfloxacin 400 mg twice daily and Levofloxacin 250 mg daily) for 3 days. It is concluded that motivated women who are familiar with the symptoms of acute cystitis can accurately diagnose infection and self-treat responsibly and effectively. All must be advised that frequent recurrences require review and a probable switch to continuous low-dose prophylaxis.

Recurrence of lower urinary tract infection due to relapse is uncommon, except in men with bacterial prostatitis. It is more often found in patients with upper tract disease and will be dealt with under this heading.

Lower tract infection—prostatitis

While urinary tract infection is much less common in males than in females, it may be associated with infection in the prostate which can be difficult to eradicate and a source of chronic disability.

Definitions

A useful working classification of prostatitis is to divide it into acute and chronic bacterial prostatitis, chronic non-bacterial prostatitis and chronic pelvic pain syndrome (Lipsky 1999). Both acute and chronic bacterial prostatitis are associated with urinary infection; prostatic secretions contain an excess of leucocytes and macrophages and bacteria can be cultured from the secretions. Urinary infection does not occur in non-bacterial prostatitis and bacteria cannot be recovered from prostatic secretions although these do contain an excess of leucocytes and macrophages. Patients with the pelvic pain syndrome do not have urinary infections and prostatic secretions show no abnormality.

Acute and chronic bacterial prostatitis

Pathogenesis

The causal organisms are the same as those causing urinary tract infection in general. *E. coli* is most common but *Klebsiella*, *Enterobacter*, *Pseudomonas*, and other less common uropathogenic Gram-negative bacteria may also cause infection. With the exception of enterococci, it is doubtful if infection occurs with Gram-positive bacteria. The role of *C. trachomatis* and *Ureaplasma urealyticum* in causing prostatitis is disputed, as is that of other fastidious bacteria.

The probable route of infection is via the urethra, facilitated by reflux of urine into the prostatic ducts during voiding (Kirby *et al.* 1982). There is some evidence to support sexual transmission, the same bacterial species having been recovered from prostatic and vaginal secretions of sexual partners (Stamey 1972). Indwelling urethral catheters facilitate prostatic infection, as may bladder outflow obstruction. Direct extension of infection from the rectum or haematogenous infection is speculative.

Normal prostatic secretion contains a factor (prostatic antibacterial factor) which is bactericidal to most uropathogenic species (Fair *et al.* 1976) and may be part of the normal defence against ascending infection. Prostatic antibacterial factor is present in low concentration in the prostatic secretion of patients with chronic bacterial prostatitis, but whether this is a primary event predisposing to infection or a consequence of infection is unknown.

Diagnosis

A diagnosis of prostatic infection is most often made on the basis of symptoms—frequency, dysuria, perineal or groin pain, difficulty in voiding—and the finding of an enlarged, tender prostate. However, similar symptoms and signs may be present in the absence of demonstrable bacterial infection in the gland. Relapsing urinary tract infection in men is highly suggestive of chronic bacterial prostatitis, but may also be due to infection in bladder or renal stones or scarred kidneys.

A diagnosis of bacterial prostatitis has been based on microscopy and culture of 'split urine samples' and expressed prostatic secretion (Stamey 1972).

Evidence of prostatic *inflammation* is based on the leucocyte count in expressed prostatic secretion compared with that in a first urethral sample and midstream urine sample. If the prostatic secretion contains more than 15 leucocytes per high power field, and there are fewer than three to five in the other two samples, inflammation of the prostate is present. More definite evidence is the presence of fat-laden macrophages in the prostatic secretion as these are rarely found in normal prostatic secretion. The leucocyte count in prostatic secretion increases following sexual intercourse and ejaculation. Patients should therefore abstain prior to any planned collection of split urine samples. Microscopy and culture of semen are unsatisfactory.

Evidence of prostatic *infection* is based on quantitative culture of the split samples and expressed prostatic secretion. If there is bladder bacteriuria, bacterial prostatitis cannot be diagnosed. Such patients should be treated with an antibiotic that does not penetrate the prostate—nitrofurantoin or ampicillin—and studies carried out when the midstream urine specimen is sterile. Prostatic infection is indicated by a 10-fold increase in bacterial counts in expressed prostatic secretion compared with the bacterial count in the first urethral sample. Bacterial counts in the postprostatic massage urine sample usually also exceed those in the first urethral sample by a factor of 10, but are not as great as those in expressed prostatic secretion.

Collection of split samples requires skill and careful laboratory examination. Serious limitations to the test have been reported (Lipsky 1999) and its use has declined. It has been suggested that demonstration of increased leucocyte counts and bacteria in urine samples obtained before and after prostatic massage may be just as reliable (Nickel 1997).

Inflammation of the prostate may be associated with an increase in serum prostate-specific antigen (PSA), causing some difficulty in the differential diagnosis of prostatic cancer. If an elevated PSA is due to inflammation it should fall following 4–6 weeks of antibacterial therapy, although the timescale may be more prolonged. Persisting elevation of PSA must be treated with suspicion and requires careful transrectal prostatic ultrasound examination and follow-up.

Radiography has little value in the diagnosis of prostatitis. Excretion urography may show slight impairment of bladder emptying. Prostatic calculi are often found in normal males and are of no diagnostic value, although their presence may make the eradication of infection more difficult.

Ultrasound examination of the prostate has become more satisfactory with the advent of single biplanar rectal transducers but detailed evaluation of transrectal ultrasound in the diagnosis of bacterial prostatitis is limited. In acute prostatitis the gland is typically enlarged, with uniformly decreased echogenicity. Abscesses may be seen as fluid collections. In chronic prostatitis, the gland is inhomogeneous with peripheral areas of reduced echogenicity, especially posteriorly. These are indistinguishable from carcinoma of the prostate so any focal lesion should be biopsied. Calculi are common. The absence of any abnormality makes chronic prostatic infection unlikely.

Urethroscopy may show an inflamed or swollen prostatic urethra. It is of most value in defining possible causes of impaired bladder emptying which may contribute to prostatic infection. Cystoscopy should be undertaken in symptomatic patients with no evidence of prostatic inflammation to exclude bladder cancer, particularly carcinoma *in situ*.

Acute bacterial prostatitis

Typically this presents as an acute illness with fever, rigors, and perineal or low back pain, frequency, dysuria, and difficulty in voiding. This is occasionally associated with acute epididymitis which may be the dominant feature. In young males, epididymitis is more likely to be due to gonococcal or chlamydial urethritis; in middle-aged men it is more likely to be due to bacterial prostatitis. On rectal examination the prostate is acutely tender and swollen. Massage of the prostate in patients with acute bacterial prostatitis may result in bacteraemia and is best avoided. However, if it is performed, the expressed prostatic secretion contains large numbers of leucocytes and macrophages, and culture yields high numbers of uropathogenic bacteria. Acute bacterial prostatitis is usually associated with bladder bacteriuria with the same causal organism.

Pathology

The prostate shows diffuse inflammation with large numbers of macrophages and other inflammatory cells within and around acini. There is diffuse hyperaemia and oedema of the gland. Microabscesses occasionally develop.

Treatment

Acutely ill, febrile patients, particularly those with difficulty in voiding, require admission to hospital. Intravenous gentamicin (3–5 mg/kg/day divided into three 8-hourly doses) should be administered with intravenous ampicillin (2 g 6-hourly). Treatment with a lipid-soluble drug with an appropriate pK_a is less necessary for penetration of the acutely inflamed prostate. If the clinical response is satisfactory, or in patients who are less severely ill, co-trimoxazole (trimethoprim– sulfamethoxazole: Septrin®) in a dose of 960 mg twice daily (160 mg trimethoprim + 800 mg sulfamethoxazole) or trimethoprim (200 mg twice daily) is the treatment of choice. Alternative drugs may be dictated by sensitivity testing. Treatment should be continued for 4–6 weeks.

The advent of fluoroquinolones has dramatically affected the treatment of both acute and chronic bacterial prostatitis. These agents have a broad spectrum of activity and penetrate the prostate well. Cure rates of 60–90 per cent have been reported with both ciprofloxacin (250–500 mg twice daily for 6 weeks) and norfloxacin (400 mg twice daily for 6 weeks). At present, in terms of cost, the use of quinolones is best reserved for those patients who fail to respond to trimethoprim or co-trimoxazole.

Urethral catheterization or instrumentation should be avoided. Retention should be treated by suprapubic drainage.

Chronic bacterial prostatitis

Presentation

Patients may present with a history of relapsing urinary tract infection with frequency and dysuria, or with symptoms more specifically related to prostatic inflammation—perineal, suprapubic, groin, or low back pain with variable frequency or difficulty in voiding. Perineal pain after ejaculation or pain in the glans penis is not unusual. Intermittent haemospermia may occur. Very occasionally, patients are asymptomatic, and the diagnosis is made following the finding of asymptomatic bacteriuria or the investigation of oligospermia.

On rectal examination the prostate is usually, but not always, tender and may feel slightly irregular or 'boggy'.

Pathology

There is non-specific, diffuse or, more usually, focal infiltration with chronic inflammatory cells in and around acini. The peripheral part of the gland is more severely affected. The findings are non-specific and may be found in the prostate of patients with no history or other evidence of bacterial infection.

Diagnosis is based on evidence of prostatic inflammation—increased white cells plus macrophages in expressed prostatic secretion—and recovery of a uropathogenic bacterium on culture of prostatic secretion.

Treatment

The choice of antibiotic is conditioned by pH changes which occur in the prostatic secretion in chronic bacterial prostatitis and on the presence of lipid-containing epithelial membranes. The prostatic fluid is distinctly more alkaline than normal. Animal and human studies suggest that entry of antibacterial agents into prostatic fluid depends on non-ionic diffusion from plasma across the lipid-containing prostatic epithelium. Effective penetration of prostatic fluid can therefore be achieved only by antibacterial drugs with a pK_a in plasma which allows accumulation of a significant concentration of non-ionized drug (Meares 1982). Antibiotics shown to have high concentration in prostatic fluid include trimethoprim, fluoroquinolones, erythromycin, and clindamycin. Conversely, drugs such as ampicillin, nitrofurantoin, and nalidixic acid penetrate prostatic fluid poorly.

The drug of choice in chronic bacterial prostatitis is trimethoprim or trimethoprim–sulfamethoxazole (co-trimoxazole). Treatment with co-trimoxazole (960 mg twice daily) or trimethoprim (200 mg twice daily) should be continued for 6 weeks and may be required for longer. Six weeks at full dosage may be followed by long-term, low-dose (suppressive) treatment with one dose of co-trimoxazole or trimethoprim (100 mg) nightly for 6–12 months.

Fluoroquinolones (ciprofloxacin and norfloxacin) are more effective than trimethoprim or co-trimoxazole but, in terms of cost, are usually reserved for the treatment of patients failing to respond to the latter. Alternative antibiotics, including erythromycin, minocycline, or doxycycline, may be required, depending on the results of sensitivity testing. Prolonged (6 weeks) treatment is recommended.

Non-bacterial prostatitis

This is the most common condition associated with intermittent or persistent symptoms of prostatitis. It is much more common than bacterial prostatitis and tends to occur in younger men (Lipsky 1999). The symptoms, clinical signs, and findings in prostatic secretion mimic those of bacterial prostatitis except that patients do not develop relapsing urinary infection and uropathogenic bacteria cannot be recovered from expressed prostatic secretion. Dysuria is unusual. The search for a causal infectious agent has been largely fruitless. The role of *C. trachomatis* and *U. urealyticum* remains controversial (Lipsky 1999) but at this time demonstration of these organisms in expressed prostatic secretion probably merits treatment.

Treatment

In the absence of an identifiable causal organism, treatment is by explanation and reassurance. A trial of terodiline hydrochloride (12.5–25 mg twice daily), prazosin hydrochloride (500 μg twice daily), or non-steroidal anti-inflammatory drugs (indomethacin, naproxen, or ibuprofen) may occasionally be helpful. Some recommend a single 4-week course of a quinolone, but repeated courses of antibacterial drugs are of no value. Many patients respond to amitriptyline (25–50 mg at night).

Chronic pelvic pain syndrome

This is the most difficult to manage of the prostatic syndromes. Typically, patients are aged between 20 and 50 and give no history of previous urinary tract infection or sexually transmitted disease. Symptoms are similar to those of chronic bacterial prostatitis but there is no evidence of *inflammation* or *infection* on examination of split urine samples and expressed prostatic secretion. Symptoms are often exacerbated by activity and are sometimes stress related. The cause is unknown. Urodynamic studies have suggested a functional disturbance in the pelvic sympathetic nervous system but neurological examination, including electrophysiological testing, shows no abnormality. Not uncommonly, patients are concerned that the syndrome may lead to impotence or infertility.

Treatment is by reassurance and trials of α-adrenergic blocking agents such as prazosin or the use of psychotropic drugs such as amitriptyline or diazepam.

Surgical treatment of chronic prostatitis

Surgery has a very limited role in the treatment of chronic bacterial prostatitis and carries the risk of serious complications. Since surgery will only be curative if all foci of infection are removed, and since most of the infection is in the peripheral zone of the prostate, a radical resection is required. Such a resection carries a significant risk of incontinence and damage to the adjacent sacral nerves. Such aggressive treatment is rarely justified. Conventional transurethral resection of the prostate, in the author's experience, rarely alters the natural history of prostatitis, although it improves the ease of voiding in patients with benign prostatic hypertrophy.

Upper urinary tract infection

Incidence

Since a differential diagnosis of upper or lower tract infection can only be made accurately by localization studies, which have limitations, the true incidence of acute symptomatic upper tract infection is unknown. It is, however, much less common than bladder infection. Pregnancy, associated severe illness, or immunosuppression all increase the likelihood of ascending infection.

Pathogenesis

With the exception of renal or perirenal abscess due to bacteraemia, infection of the upper tract is secondary to bladder infection. Acquisition of bladder bacteriuria is therefore the first step in the development of renal infection. The reasons for spread of infection to the upper tract are multiple including urodynamic factors, virulence factors, medullary susceptibility, obstruction, and vesicoureteric reflux.

Of special concern are conditions such as diabetes mellitus, analgesic nephropathy, and sickle-cell disease or trait. These are all conditions associated with disturbance of medullary blood flow predisposing to papillary necrosis. With the exception of diabetes, there is little evidence that there is an increased risk of acquiring bladder infection in these conditions. However, the medullary disease predisposes to infection within the kidney and makes eradication of infection more difficult. These conditions are also associated with an increased risk of permanent kidney damage (Fig. 1).

The bacterial species causing ascending urinary tract infection are similar to those causing lower tract infection, with the exception that it is doubtful whether *S. saprophyticus* causes renal infection. The virulence characteristics of bacteria are different.

Acute pyelonephritis

This is a time-honoured clinical diagnosis applied to patients with bacteriuria who have loin pain, fever, and flank tenderness, and are presumed to have renal infection. It may involve one or both kidneys.

Histopathology

Typically there is patchy infection of the kidney with wedge-shaped areas of intense inflammation extending from the medulla outwards into the cortex. These areas may be sharply demarcated from areas of normal kidney. There is intense infiltration with polymorphonuclear leucocytes within and around the tubules. Microabscess formation may occur and bacteria can be demonstrated within areas of suppuration. Glomeruli are usually spared.

Clinical presentation

In uncomplicated pyelonephritis, the onset is commonly acute and may or may not be preceded by bladder symptoms. Alternatively the patient may develop frequency and dysuria which is either ignored or self-treated with a high fluid intake and patent medicines, often with apparent improvement, only for symptoms to later progress to loin pain and fever. Many patients will give a history of cystitis within the previous 6 months. Bladder symptoms occasionally develop after the onset of loin pain. Severe renal infection may cause chills, rigors, and high fevers and also systemic symptoms of anorexia, nausea, vomiting, and general myalgia. Loin pain may be unilateral or bilateral and there may be exquisite tenderness over the kidneys posteriorly and anteriorly. Pain may radiate to the epigastrium or lower abdomen. Severe loin pain and tenderness in a febrile patient with minimal or no bladder symptoms should alert the clinician to the possibility of an infected obstructed upper tract or an infected renal cyst. Bacteraemia and septic shock may occur and is more common with complicated infection. Positive blood cultures have been reported in between 10 and 25 per cent of patients with acute pyelonephritis (Bryan and Reynolds 1984).

Renal conditions that may simulate acute pyelonephritis include obstructive uropathy, acute glomerulonephritis, renal infarction, and renal vein thrombosis. The differential diagnosis may also include conditions above or below the diaphragm, including pneumonia or lung abscess, cholecystitis, appendicitis, acute pancreatitis, or acute pelvic infection.

In patients with obstructive uropathy, infection may result in an infected pyonephrosis with severe loin pain, fever, septic shock, and oliguric renal failure.

Patients with persisting bacteriuria in association with stones, ileal conduits, or neurogenic bladders are often asymptomatic for long periods of time, only to have acute episodes of fever with or without loin pain and tenderness, when it is presumed renal infection has occurred.

Patients with diabetes mellitus, or those who are immunosuppressed, may have renal infection with minimal localizing symptoms or signs (Cattell *et al.* 1985). A diagnosis of renal infection should be suspected when relapse of infection occurs following appropriate antibacterial therapy.

Focal or multifocal acute bacterial interstitial nephritis

Severe renal infection may result in severe focal or multifocal inflammation within the kidney which, if untreated, may lead to abscess formation. This is usually, but not always, associated with severe vesicoureteric reflux, renal stones, papillary necrosis, or obstructive uropathy (Rosenfield *et al.* 1979). Healing may be associated with the development of cortical scars (Meyrier *et al.* 1989). Abscesses are more common in patients with diabetes mellitus and are reported to be more common in patients with primary hyperparathyroidism.

Incidence

The frequency with which either condition develops is unknown since diagnosis depends on renal imaging, with the use of contrast media, during the acute phase of infection. It appears to be uncommon but incidence increases with advancing age. It affects males and females equally. Multifocal bacterial nephritis is more common in diabetes mellitus.

Presentation

Patients are usually acutely ill, with high fever, rigors, and loin or abdominal pain (Corriere and Sandler 1982). On examination most have pain on deep palpation in the costovertebral angle or over the kidneys anteriorly. In some, a large, tender kidney may be felt.

Diagnosis

The diagnosis can only be made by renal imaging (Rosenfield *et al.* 1979). It is probable that many patients with severe ascending infection have some degree of focal or multifocal bacterial nephritis which is undiagnosed because imaging has not been deemed necessary. The diagnosis is usually made when renal imaging has been carried out to exclude an obstructed pyonephrosis.

On renal ultrasound, part or all of the kidney may appear enlarged. The involved area typically shows a focal mass or masses of reduced echogenicity. It is unusual to identify microabscesses on ultrasound.

CT with intravenous contrast clearly identifies focal and multifocal bacterial nephritis (Meyrier *et al.* 1989). In focal nephritis, a poorly demarcated, wedge-shaped area of reduced enhancement extending from the papillae outwards into the cortex can be seen. Microabscesses can be identified as small areas of fluid attenuation. In multifocal bacterial nephritis, enhancement is streaky with wedge-shaped areas of reduced enhancement throughout the kidney (Fig. 4a and b). There may be small fluid collections indicating microabscess formation. CT without contrast only shows a large kidney and is of limited diagnostic value.

Excretion urography shows local or diffuse enlargement of the kidney. Contrast enhancement may show focal or diffuse diminution in the nephrogram with diminished and delayed excretion. In patients with multifocal bacterial nephritis and oliguric renal failure, an immediate persisting nephrogram with no pelvicalyceal filling may be observed and may persist for 24 h (Rosenfield *et al.* 1979).

Gallium scintigraphy shows focal or diffuse diminution in uptake of the tracer. It is less specific than enhanced CT but may be the investigation of choice in patients with diabetes mellitus, who are at risk of developing contrast nephrotoxicity.

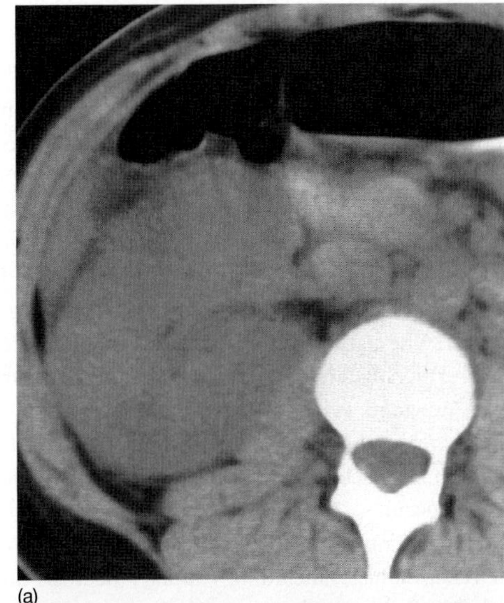

(a)

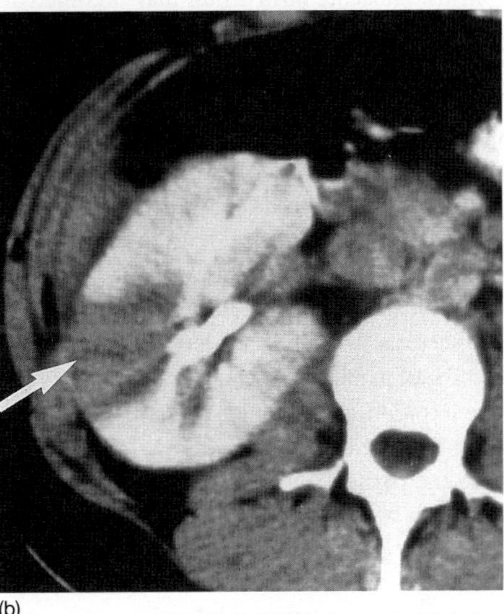

(b)

Fig. 4 CT scan showing (a) swollen left kidney. After contrast (b) there is focal failure of opacification (arrow) due to acute bacterial interstitial nephritis; 'lobar nephronia'.

Chronic pyelonephritis

Chronic pyelonephritis or reflux nephropathy is a radiological diagnosis based on the demonstration of clubbed calyces associated with focal or diffuse renal scarring (Cattell *et al.* 1989). This may be unilateral or bilateral and mild or severe. It a result of infection and vesicoureteric reflux in early childhood, and is usually present by the age of 4 years. It is doubtful whether it ever develops in adult life. The presence of reflux nephropathy does not predispose to the acquisition of infection, but it may predispose to extension of infection to the upper tract, especially if reflux persists. Reflux may be associated with ipsilateral loin pain during voiding in infected patients. Otherwise symptoms of acute renal infection are usually the same as in patients with normal kidneys. Many adults with reflux nephropathy are asymptomatic and abacteriuric, presenting with hypertension or renal impairment.

Natural history and sequelae of upper tract infection

The natural history and sequelae of upper tract infection are heavily conditioned by the presence or absence of complicating factors. Renal infection in patients with normal upper tracts and no associated disease is usually easily treated with a standard course of antibiotics and leaves no residual damage. Studies using CT imaging (Meyrier *et al.* 1989) indicate that patients with severe focal or multifocal infection may develop cortical scars, but the long-term functional significance of this is unclear. The natural history depends on the potential for acquisition of further bladder bacteriuria with ascent to the upper tract. There is no good evidence that a previous attack of acute pyelonephritis increases the likelihood of further renal infection if the patient again becomes bacteriuric. Relapsing infection is unusual but does occasionally occur.

Upper tract infection associated with obstruction increases the potential for renal damage, including papillary necrosis and severe bacterial nephritis. Subacute obstruction may become complete due to the inflammatory oedema associated with infection. An obstructed and infected system predisposes to life-threatening septicaemia and may lead to perinephric abscess.

Stones may cause obstruction and may be due to recurrent infection, particularly with *P. mirabilis*. Alternatively, an infected stone may be grafted on a metabolic stone. Large staghorn calculi obstruct or destroy the kidney tissue by their size (Griffith 1978).

Diabetes mellitus, sickle-cell disease or trait, analgesic abuse, or abuse of non-steroidal anti-inflammatory drugs may all be associated with papillary necrosis. Upper tract infection increases the potential for this. Sloughing of papillae may lead to obstruction.

In all of these complicated situations, it is more difficult to eradicate infection, and relapse may occur within 7–10 days of completing a course of treatment, particularly when stones are present. Bacteria that penetrate stones can be impossible to eradicate except by eliminating the stones.

Renal impairment due to urinary infection

There is now considerable evidence that recurrent uncomplicated symptomatic or asymptomatic urinary infection does not result in significant impairment of excretory function. Many studies in asymptomatic women have shown reversible impairment of urine concentrating ability associated with upper tract infection (Ronald *et al.* 1969). This is rarely severe—at most causing troublesome frequency and especially nocturia.

Reports of the development or progression of chronic pyelonephritic damage in adults almost certainly reflect a failure to distinguish the radiological features of reflux nephropathy from those of papillary necrosis or postobstructive atrophy (Cattell *et al.* 1989). This distinction is critical since the presence of papillary necrosis should stimulate a search for a treatable cause—for example, analgesic abuse or treatment with non-steroidal anti-inflammatory drugs. Evidence of papillary necrosis should also alert the clinician to the potential for further damage if infection persists or recurs.

Acute oliguric or non-oliguric renal failure is an uncommon complication of ascending infection, most often occuring in patients with pre-existing tubulointerstitial disease or with complicating factors such as stones, obstructive uropathy, diabetes mellitus, or chronic alcoholism (Cattell 1992). The picture is usually that of severe multifocal bacterial interstitial nephritis with or without septicaemia. Very occasionally it may present with more insidious loss of function, particularly in patients with diabetes mellitus (Cattell *et al.* 1985).

Reflux nephropathy (see also Chapter 17.2)

Reflux nephropathy accounts for between 12 and 15 per cent of patients with endstage renal failure accepted into renal replacement programmes. In such patients, extensive renal damage has occurred by the age of 4 years, and most reach endstage renal failure in their second or third decade. The prognosis is worse in patients with heavy (>2 g) proteinuria. The role of recurrent infection in the progression of renal damage in adults with reflux nephropathy remains slightly controversial. Most believe it plays little part. The degree of initial damage and the development of hypertension seem to play the major roles in determining the degree or progression of kidney failure.

Hypertension

Hypertension in patients with recurrent infection relates to the presence and extent of kidney scarring, whether due to reflux nephropathy, obstructive nephropathy, or other complicating conditions. In patients with uncomplicated urinary infection, the prevalence of hypertension does not differ from that in the general population (Parker and Kunin 1973).

Bacteraemia and metastatic infection

Infection in the urinary tract accounts for some 15–20 per cent of all cases of bacteraemia (Bryan and Reynolds 1984). Bacteraemia originating in the urinary tract is more common in hospital patients than in patients in the community. It is commonly associated with complicated upper tract infection or catheterization. Rarely, urinary tract infection may result in metastatic infection in bone, the heart, or other sites. Gram-negative osteomyelitis of the spine is the most common metastatic infection, usually presenting several weeks after the urinary infection. Endocarditis is most often due to Gram-positive bacteria and is usually superimposed on abnormal valves. Metastatic infection is more common in elderly males and may relate to prostatic infection.

Diagnosis of upper tract infection

Although known to be inaccurate, the diagnosis of upper tract infection is usually based on symptoms and clinical signs in a patient shown to have bacteriuria and pyuria. The presence in the urine of white cell casts adds clinical support. Localization studies are rarely necessary or carried out. Where symptoms are severe and no previous renal imaging has been done, plain abdominal radiographs and ultrasound examination should be carried out to exclude stones and obstruction.

IVU is rarely indicated during acute infection; the results are usually of poor quality and there may be an increased risk of contrast nephrotoxicity. If carried out, some 25–30 per cent of acutely infected kidneys appear swollen with compression and poor filling of the pelvicalyceal system. If infection is particularly severe in one part of the kidney—focal bacterial nephritis or acute lobar nephronia—localized reduced opacification during the nephrogram phase may suggest a space-occupying lesion. This can be shown more clearly on CT examination after intravenous administration of contrast medium.

Treatment

The treatment must be conditioned by the severity of the illness. Acutely ill patients with high fever, severe loin pain, and vomiting must be admitted to hospital. Patients with less severe symptoms may be managed on an outpatient basis with oral antibacterial therapy.

The acutely ill patient commonly requires intravenous fluids and analgesia. Pending urine culture and sensitivity testing initial therapy with intravenous gentamicin (1.5 mg/kg initially followed by 1 mg/kg 8-hourly) combined with intravenous ampicillin (1 g 6-hourly) is an effective combination. In recent years intravenous fluoroquinolones (e.g. ciprofloxacin, 100–200 mg twice daily) have been shown to be equally effective.

Serum creatinine must be measured to identify patients with renal impairment in whom dose schedules must be modified. In the presence of renal impairment, gentamicin blood concentration must be measured: trough levels should not exceed 2 μg/ml. An intravenous cephalosporin may be administered instead of ampicillin—cefuroxime (1.5 g 6-hourly) or ceftazidime (2 g 8-hourly). A fluid intake of 2 l daily should be achieved orally or intravenously. Intravenous drug treatment and fluids should be continued until fever and acute symptoms have been controlled for 24 h, when a switch may be made to oral treatment. This is usually possible within 24–48 h. A percutaneous nephrostomy must be established immediately in patients shown to have obstructed upper tracts on ultrasound examination.

In patients with symptoms and signs of renal infection who are not acutely ill, oral antibacterial therapy may be prescribed from the outset. Again, a high fluid intake must be encouraged. The choice of antibiotics is similar to that for a lower urinary tract infection (Table 5). However, it is essential to employ drugs which achieve significant blood and tissue concentrations. Nitrofurantoin, which does not, is not of value for renal infection. The development of L forms of bacteria in the hyperosmolar medulla with the use of drugs such as ampicillin has been postulated as a reason for treatment failure with subsequent relapse. This is unproven.

Duration of treatment

The duration of treatment is more controversial than the choice of antibiotic. In practice patients with clinical evidence of uncomplicated renal infection are best treated with a 2-week course of antibacterial drugs. Some will have recurrence of infection. A urine culture 10–14 days after initial treatment is essential. Relapse is commonly treated with more prolonged treatment (6 weeks).

In patients with infection complicated by stones, renal scars, diabetes mellitus, or drug-related interstitial nephritis, prolonged (6 weeks) treatment is commonly recommended. In practice, such patients are best given treatment for 2 weeks and only given more prolonged therapy if shown to relapse on completing the initial treatment.

Persistently relapsing infection

Contributing factors must be sought in patients who relapse even after 6 weeks' treatment. Prevention of further relapse is unlikely in patients with stones, unless the stones can be removed (Griffith 1978). If this is not possible, and in patients with cystic disease or renal scars, consideration must be given to long-term, low-dose suppressive treatment, in the hope that the patient's intrinsic defence mechanism will eradicate infection.

Follow-up

As with patients suffering lower tract infection, all those with kidney infection must be advised to follow prophylactic regimens designed to reduce the potential for recurrence of bladder bacteriuria (Table 6). If not previously performed, IVU should be carried out 4 or more weeks after recovery.

When not to treat

In patients with ileal conduit or multiple renal stones not amenable to removal, it may be impossible to eradicate infection or prevent reinfection. In such patients, provided they do not have obstructive uropathy, it is best to avoid repeated or prolonged courses of antibiotics. Rather, the nature of the problem should be explained to the patient and treatment restricted to acute episodes of loin pain and fever.

Xanthogranulomatous pyelonephritis (see also Chapter 18.1)

Xanthogranulomatous pyelonephritis is an uncommon but distinct form of chronic kidney infection (Malek and Elder 1978) that predominantly affects women. It may occur at any age but is more frequent in the elderly. The condition is commonly associated with renal calculi or obstructive uropathy, but may occur without either; it rarely affects both kidneys. Most often, infection is caused by *P. mirabilis*, but *E. coli*, *Klebsiella* spp., and *Staphylococcus aureus*, or a mixture of organisms, may be present.

Pathology

The kidney is enlarged, with either local or diffuse involvement. The cut surface appears yellow and there are often multiple abscesses. Perirenal fat is usually inflamed and adherent to the kidney. Inflammation may extend to the retroperitoneal space. Histologically there is diffuse replacement of renal parenchyma with large, foamy lipid-containing macrophages (xanthoma cells), neutrophils, plasma cells, and necrotic debris. Foreign-body giant cells are frequently present. Precisely why this form of chronic renal infection occurs is unclear, but it may be associated with a lysosomal defect in macrophages, which prevents complete digestion of the bacteria.

Clinical presentation

Xanthogranulomatous pyelonephritis usually presents with loin pain, intermittent fever, weight loss, general malaise, and symptoms of anaemia. Many patients have a history of recurrent infection with or without renal stones. The condition is frequently only diagnosed after a prolonged period of progressive ill health. A renal mass is palpable in more than 50 per cent of patients. Urine microscopy shows pyuria and often microscopic haematuria. Urine culture is usually positive but very occasionally may be negative. Anaemia, leucocytosis, and disturbed liver function tests are usual.

The most common differential diagnoses are renal carcinoma or renal tuberculosis. In the past, a correct diagnosis was seldom made preoperatively, many kidneys being removed in the belief that the lesion was a cancer. With modern imaging techniques and fine-needle aspiration, the diagnosis, if suspected, should not be difficult (Solomon *et al.* 1983).

Diagnosis

The suspicion of xanthogranulomatous pyelonephritis is usually raised when IVU shows focal or diffuse enlargement of a kidney with appearances suggestive of focal or multiple space-occupying lesions in association with renal calculi. There is little or no excretion of contrast in the affected area. If there is filling of the calyces, these are usually distorted or displaced.

Ultrasound shows dilated calyces containing low-level echoes surrounded by thickened hypoechoic parenchyma. CT shows multiple low-attenuation areas of soft tissue density within the kidney, surrounded by thickened parenchyma, and may also demonstrate associated perinephric collections (Solomon *et al.* 1983).

A combination of these investigations usually makes the diagnosis obvious where there is also bacteriuria. If doubt remains, fine-needle aspiration of a low-attenuation area with positive culture of the aspirate will confirm the diagnosis.

Angiography, which shows hypovascular renal masses with neovascularization, is now rarely required.

Treatment

Antibacterial agents rarely eradicate infection, and as extensive irreversible renal damage has usually occurred prior to the diagnosis, nephrectomy is the treatment of choice. Rarely, partial nephrectomy with removal of calculi may be possible. Happily, the condition rarely involves both kidneys and does not recur after treatment. Subsequent involvement of the contralateral kidney following removal of one kidney has not been reported.

Renal cortical abscess (renal carbuncle)

Cortical abscesses are a result of haematogenous infection, usually by *S. aureus*, from a primary focus elsewhere in the body. The most common sources of infection are skin furuncles, paronychia, or boils. Less commonly the primary infection may be in bone or infected heart valves. The interval between a known primary infection—for example, in the skin—and the onset of symptoms of renal abscess may be days or several weeks, when the original lesion may no longer be present.

Pathology

Infection begins with a group of cortical microabscesses which coalesce to form a larger, thick-walled abscess. Rarely the abscess may rupture into the perinephric space. Abscesses do not usually communicate with the collecting system and are usually single and unilateral. For reasons which are unclear, they are more common in the right kidney.

Clinical presentation

Renal cortical abscess is some three times more common in men than women. It occurs at all ages but is more common in the second and third decades. Presentation is most often with rigors, fever, and loin or hypochondrial pain. Localizing symptoms may be absent, the patient presenting with pyrexia of unknown origin. Bladder symptoms are unusual.

There is usually loin tenderness with pain, particularly on percussion over the costovertebral angle. Careful inspection of the lumbar region reveals fullness over the kidney area compared to the contralateral side. There is often loss of the normal concavity of the lumbar spine. In some patients a mass may be felt in the upper lateral abdomen. Not uncommonly, there are signs of collapse or consolidation in the lower chest on the same side.

Most patients have a modest neutrophil leucocytosis but urine microscopy and culture are usually negative. On rare occasions the abscess may rupture into the collecting system leading to pyuria, microhaematuria, and bacteriuria. Blood culture is usually negative.

When renal disease is suspected, the differential diagnosis is between an obstructed pyonephrosis, infected renal cysts, a perinephric abscess, or a renal tumour. With modern imaging techniques, a correct diagnosis should be possible in most cases.

Renal ultrasound is now the investigation of first choice because of its sensitivity in identifying fluid collections, its immediate availability, and its non-invasive nature (Andriole 1983). When a cortical abscess is fully developed, ultrasound will show a fluid collection which may have a thick wall, contained echoes, or a level. This should be aspirated to confirm the presence of pus and to allow culture. In the early stage of abscess formation, before liquefaction, the ultrasound appearances are those of a solid or semisolid mass.

If renal ultrasound is negative or equivocal, CT with intravenous contrast should be carried out. The typical appearance of an abscess is a fluid collection with a thick wall which enhances after contrast. A mass with an atypical appearance should be subject to needle aspiration. CT can be used to follow the response to treatment.

Intravenous urography is now seldom used. The appearances are those of a mass lesion with reduced nephrographic density which may or may not cause a bulge on the renal outline and distortion of the calyceal system. IVU cannot distinguish an abscess from a tumour or a cyst.

Angiography is now very rarely, if ever, necessary. Typically, an abscess appears avascular with displacement of vessels around it. The abscess wall may enhance or show neovascularity. However, all of these appearances may be present with necrotic or hypovascular tumours.

Isotope scanning using gallium-67 citrate has been used to locate renal abscesses, but has little advantage over ultrasound or CT (Dembry and Andriole 1997). False-positive results may be obtained in patients with acute focal bacterial nephritis or with renal carcinoma.

Treatment

Ultrasound or CT scanning with aspiration of pus from the abscess confirms the diagnosis and permits culture to identify the causal organism. An attempt should be made to aspirate as much as possible of the pus or to insert a drainage catheter if the collection is large. The most common infecting organism is *S. aureus*. Treatment is with intravenous vancomycin (1 g 12-hourly) or flucloxacillin (1 g 6-hourly), but the use of alternative antibacterial agents may be dictated by bacterial sensitivity testing. Parenteral therapy should be continued for at least 7 days. Vancomycin blood levels should be measured, particularly if there is renal impairment. Oral antistaphylococcal treatment should be continued for at least 4 weeks. Clinical improvement with gradual resolution of fever usually occurs over 2–3 days. Failure to do so requires review of the diagnosis and bacterial sensitivities. A percutaneous drain should be inserted into the abscess if this has not already been done. Resolution of the abscess should be monitored by serial ultrasound or CT scanning. Operative drainage of renal carbuncles is now seldom necessary.

Infected renal cysts

Infection of solitary cysts, or of one or more cysts in patients with polycystic disease, usually occurs as a complication of ascending infection. It is most often manifest as relapsing infection.

It is impossible to distinguish between an infected solitary cyst and a cortical renal abscess on the basis of symptoms, signs, and renal imaging. Patients with infected cysts usually give a history of prior urinary tract infection and are more likely to have bladder symptoms and bacteriuria. Fluid aspirated from the lesion usually yields an enterobacterium from infected cysts and a staphylococcus from a cortical abscess. Ultrasound shows a fluid collection which may have contained echoes: the features of a 'complicated solitary cyst'. Diagnosis is confirmed by fine-needle aspiration and culture of the fluid. CT scanning shows a localized area of reduced attenuation which does not enhance after intravenous contrast.

Diagnosis is difficult in patients with polycystic kidney disease in whom bleeding into a cyst may have occurred. The differentiation between this and an infected cyst may be impossible on ultrasound or CT examination. If only one cyst is atypical, this may be aspirated to give the diagnosis. Commonly, however, two or more cysts may be involved, when needling of each is impractical.

Treatment

This is by aspiration of pus from the cyst and aggressive antibacterial therapy, as for focal bacterial nephritis.

Perinephric abscess

Infection and abscess formation within the perirenal space is most often due to extension or rupture of an intrarenal abscess (Corriere and Sandler 1982). Rarely, there may be primary bloodborne infection of this space or spread of infection from adjacent viscera or from osteomyelitis of the spine. Causative bacteria are most often *S. aureus*, *E. coli*, *P. mirabilis*, or *Klebsiella* spp., but other enterobacteria may be recovered. Intrarenal abscesses rupturing into the perinephric space may be either a renal carbuncle or abscess formation secondary to severe bacterial nephritis. Infection is usually confined to the perinephric space bounded by Gerota's fascia. It may, however, spread: cephalic extension may result in a subphrenic abscess, empyema, or even a nephrobronchial fistula. Caudal extension may present as a groin or pelvic abscess. Infection may extend through the renal fascia to involve the psoas muscle and even present as a draining abscess in the flank. Rarely, it ruptures into the large bowel or peritoneum.

Clinical presentation

A perinephric abscess usually presents more insidiously than a renal carbuncle or severe bacterial nephritis (Saiki *et al.* 1982). Patients commonly give a history of several weeks of progressive ill health and intermittent fever. Depending on the underlying cause, symptoms may be mainly loin pain, rigors, and fever without urinary symptoms (renal carbuncle) or there may be a previous history of urinary infection. Pain may be referred to the lower abdomen, the ipsilateral hip, or thigh.

The most common findings are costovertebral angle tenderness with fullness in the flank. There may be scoliosis of the spine, concave to the affected side. Pain may be made worse by extension of the thigh or lateral flexion of the spine to the contralateral side. A flank or abdominal mass may be found. Pyuria and bacteriuria are present when the cause of the abscess is complicated urinary infection but are usually absent with renal carbuncle. Blood cultures are positive in less than 50 per cent of patients.

Diagnosis

Careful history-taking and constant awareness of this diagnosis are essential. Most difficulty arises in patients with non-specific symptoms and signs who present with vague ill health and pyrexia of unknown origin. Historically, some 25–30 per cent of cases have been first diagnosed at autopsy (Thorley *et al.* 1974), but the availability of new imaging techniques such as ultrasound, CT scanning, and gallium scintigraphy make the diagnosis less likely to be missed. Plain abdominal radiographs may show an upper abdominal mass, loss of the renal outline, vertebral scoliosis, and absence of the lateral psoas margin, but all of these are unreliable diagnostic signs. Very occasionally, gas bubbles in the retroperitoneal space outside the renal area may result from infection with gas-forming bacteria.

On IVU, a perinephric abscess is most often suggested by medial and anterior displacement of the kidney by a soft tissue mass inferolateral to it. There may be evidence of a renal mass if there is an associated renal abscess. Ultrasound shows a perinephric fluid collection with or without renal displacement or evidence of intrarenal abscess formation. CT scanning following the administration of contrast has the advantage of defining the relationship of the perinephric collection with the fascial planes and showing any extension into other perirenal tissues, including muscles (Fig. 5a and b). CT scanning is especially helpful when planning drainage.

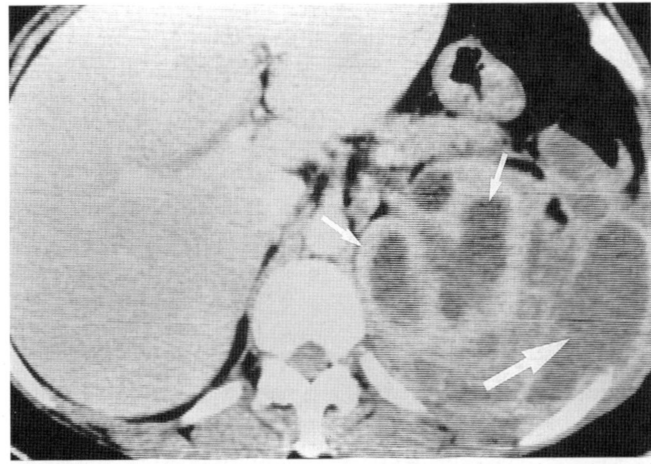

(a)

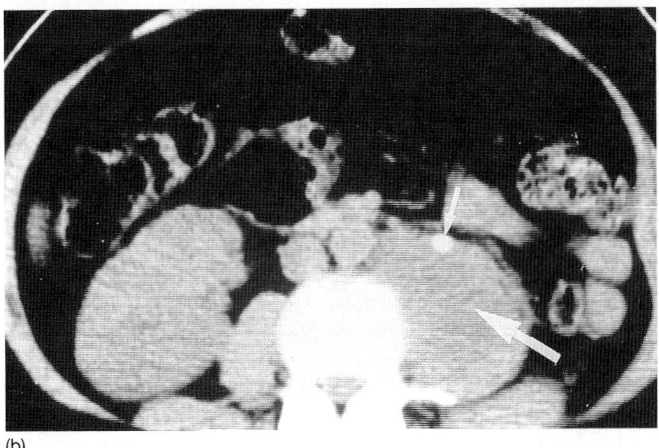

(b)

Fig. 5 CT scan of a patient with obstructive pyonephrosis and perinephric abscess. (a) Shows the dilated collecting system (small arrows) and perinephric abscess (large arrow). (b) Shows a radiodense stone (small arrow) in the ureter lying on the front of a grossly swollen psoas muscle (large arrow) containing pus.

Treatment

All perinephric abscesses require drainage. This may be done percutaneously under ultrasonography or CT control (Dembry and Andriole 1997) or surgically (Saiki *et al.* 1982). Antibacterial therapy should commence prior to the drainage procedure but will not control perinephric abscesses on its own. Unless the perinephric abscess is unequivocally secondary to ascending renal infection, initial treatment, pending the results of fluid culture, should aim to deal both with normal uropathogenic bacteria and *S. aureus*. Gentamicin (1 mg/kg 8-hourly) combined with cefuroxime (1.5 g 6-hourly) or ceftazidime (2 g 8-hourly) intravenously is a satisfactory combination. Therapy may be modified when the results of bacterial sensitivity testing are available. Parenteral treatment should continue until fever has been controlled for 24 h, when oral therapy can be substituted and must be continued for at least 4 weeks. Many patients will subsequently require nephrectomy for removal of badly damaged obstructed kidneys.

Bibliography

Anderson, K. A. and McAninch, J. W. (1980). Renal abscesses: classification and review of 40 cases. *Urology* **16**, 333–338.

Andriole, V. T. (1997). Urinary tract infections. *Infectious Disease Clinics of North America* **11** (Multiple Author Review).

Latham, R. H. and Stamm, W. E. (1984). Urethral syndrome in women. *Urological Clinics of North America* **11**, 95–101.

Roland, A. R. (1987). Optimal duration of treatment for kidney infection. *Annals of Internal Medicine* **106**, 467–468.

Stamm, W. E. (1982). Recent development in the diagnosis and treatment of urinary tract infections. *Western Journal of Medicine* **137**, 213–220.

References

Andrews, S. J. *et al.* (2002). Ultrasonography and abdominal radiography versus intravenous urography in investigation of urinary tract infection in men: prospective incident cohort study. *British Medical Journal* **324**, 454–456.

Andriole, V. (1983). Renal carbuncle. *Medical Grand Rounds* **2**, 250–261.

Asscher, A. W. *The Challenge of Urinary Tract Infection*. London: Academic Press, 1980.

Bailey, R. R. *Single-dose Therapy of Urinary Tract Infection*. Balgowlah, Australia: ADIS Health Science Press, 1983.

Bryan, C. S. and Reynolds, K. L. (1984). Community acquired bacteraemic urinary tract infections: epidemiology and outcome. *Journal of Urology* **132**, 490–493.

Busch, R. and Huland, H. (1984). Correlation of symptoms and results of direct bacterial localization in patients with urinary tract infections. *Journal of Urology* **132**, 282–285.

Cattell, W. R. Urinary tract infection and acute renal failure. In *Advanced Renal Medicine* (ed. A. E. G. Raine), pp. 302–313. Oxford: Oxford University Press, 1992.

Cattell, W. R., Greenwood, R. N., and Baker, L. R. I. Reversible renal failure due to interstitial infection of the kidney. In *Recent Advances in Chemotherapy* (ed. J. Ishigami), pp. 225–228. Tokyo: University of Tokyo Press, 1985.

Cattell, W. R., Webb, J. A. W., and Hilson, A. J. *Clinical Renal Imaging*. Chichester: John Wiley and Sons, 1989.

Cattell, W. R. *et al.* The localisation of urinary tract infection and its relationship to relapse, reinfection and treatment. In *Urinary Tract Infection* (ed. W. Brumfitt and A. W. Asscher), pp. 206–214. London: Oxford University Press, 1973.

Corriere, J. N., Jr. and Sandler, C. M. (1982). The diagnosis and immediate therapy of acute renal and perirenal infections. *Urological Clinics of North America* **9**, 219–228.

Dembry, L.-M. and Andriole, V. T. (1997). Renal and perirenal abscesses. *Infectious Disease Clinics of North America* **11**, 663–680.

Evans, D. A. *et al.* (1982). Bacteriuria and subsequent mortality in women. *Lancet* **i**, 156–158.

Fair, W. R., Couch, J., and Wehner, N. (1976). Prostatic antibacterial factor. Identity and significance. *Urology* **7**, 169–177.

Fihn, S. D. *et al.* (1988). Trimethoprim–sulfamethoxazole for acute dysuria in women—a single dose or 10-day course. *Annals of Internal Medicine* **108**, 350–357.

Fowler, J. E. and Polaski, E. T. (1981). Excretory urography, cystography and cystoscopy in the evaluation of women with urinary tract infection. *New England Journal of Medicine* **304**, 462–465.

Gallagher, D. J. A., Montgomerie, J. Z., and North, J. D. K. (1965). Acute infection of the urinary tract and the urethral syndrome in general practice. *British Medical Journal* **1**, 622–626.

Gaymans, R. *et al.* (1976). A prospective study of urinary tract infection in a Dutch general practice. *Lancet* **ii**, 674–677.

Griffin, P. J. A. and Salaman, J. (1979). Urinary tract infections after renal transplantation: do they matter? *British Medical Journal* **1**, 710–711.

Griffith, D. P. (1978). Struvite stones. *Kidney International* **13**, 372–382.

Gupta, K., Hooton, T. M., and Stamm, W. E. (2001a). Increasing antimicrobial resistance and the management of uncomplicated community acquired urinary tract infections. *Annals of Internal Medicine* **135**, 41–50.

Gupta, K. *et al.* (2001b). Patient-initiated treatment of uncomplicated recurrent urinary tract infections in young women. *Annals of Internal Medicine* **135**, 9–16.

Hooton, T. M. and Stamm, W. E. (1991). Management of acute uncomplicated urinary tract infection in adults. *Medical Clinics of North America* **75**, 339–357.

Hooton, T. M. and Stamm, W. E. (1997). Diagnosis and treatment of uncomplicated urinary tract infection. *Infectious Disease Clinics of North America* **11**, 551–581.

Hooton, T. M. *et al.* (1991). *Escherischia coli* bacteriuria and contraceptive method. *Journal of the American Medical Association* **265**, 64–69.

Hooton, T. M. *et al.* (2000). A prospective study of asymptomatic bacteriuria in sexually active young women. *New England Journal of Medicine* **343**, 992–997.

Hovelius, B., Mardh, P. A., and Byrgen, P. (1979). Urinary tract infections caused by *Staphylococcus saprophyticus*: recurrence and complications. *Journal of Urology* **122**, 645–647.

Huland, H. and Busch, R. (1984). Pyelonephritic scarring in 213 patients with upper and lower urinary tract infections: long-term follow-up. *Journal of Urology* **132**, 936–939.

Kass, E. H. (1956). Asymptomatic infections of the urinary tract. *Transactions of the Association of American Physicians* **69**, 56–64.

Kirby, R. S. *et al.* (1982). Intraprostatic urinary reflux: an aetiological factor in abacterial prostatitis. *British Journal of Urology* **54**, 729–731.

Kunin, C. M. (1962). Microbial persistence versus reinfection in recurrent urinary tract infection. *Antimicrobial Agents and Chemotherapy* 21–25.

Kunin, C. M. (1985). Does kidney infection cause renal failure? *Annual Review of Medicine* **36**, 165–176.

Kunin, C. M. and McCormack, R. C. (1968). An epidemiological study of bacteriuria and blood pressure among nuns and working women. *New England Journal of Medicine* **278**, 635–642.

Kunin, C. M., White, L. V., and Hua, T. H. (1993). A reassessment of the importance of 'low count' bacteriuria in young women with acute urinary symptoms. *Annals of Internal Medicine* **119**, 454–460.

Lipsky, B. A. (1989). Urinary tract infection in men. *Annals of Internal Medicine* **110**, 138–150.

Lipsky, B. A. (1999). Prostatitis and urinary tract infection in men: what's new; what's true. *American Journal of Medicine* **106**, 327–334.

Mabeck, C. D. (1969). Significance of coagulase-negative staphylococcal bacteriuria. *Lancet* **ii**, 1150–1152.

Malek, R. S. and Elder, J. S. (1978). Xanthogranulomatous pyelonephritis: a critical analysis of 26 cases and of the literature. *Journal of Urology* **119**, 589–593.

Maskell, R. (1989). A new look at the diagnosis of infection of the urinary tract and its adjacent structures. *Journal of Infection* **19**, 207–217.

Meares, E. M., Jr. (1982). Prostatitis: review of pharmacokinetics and therapy. *Review of Infectious Diseases* **4**, 475–483.

Meyrier, A. *et al.* (1989). Frequency of development of early cortical scarring in acute primary pyelonephritis. *Kidney International* **35**, 696–703.

National Center for Health Statistics (1977). Ambulatory medical care rendered in physicians' offices—United States—1975. *Advanced Data* **12**, 1.

Nickel, J. C. (1997). The pre and post massage test (PPMT): a simple screen for prostatitis. *Techniques in Urology* **3**, 38–43.

Nicolle, L. E. *et al.* (1988). Efficacy of five years of continuous low-dose trimethoprim–sulfamethozole prophylaxis for urinary tract infection. *Journal of Infectious Diseases* **157**, 1239–1242.

O'Grady, F. *et al.* (1969). Long-term low dosage trimethoprimsulphonamide in the control of chronic bacteriuria. *Postgraduate Medical Journal, Supplement* **45**, 61–64.

O'Grady, F. W. *et al.* Natural history of intractable 'cystitis' in women referred to a special clinic. In *Urinary Tract Infection* (ed. W. Brumfitt and A. W. Asscher), pp. 81–91. London: Oxford University Press, 1973.

Parker, J. and Kunin, C. (1973). Pyelonephritis in young women. *Journal of the American Medical Association* **244**, 585–590.

Raz, R. and Stamm, W. E. (1993). A controlled trial of intravaginal estriol in post-menopausal women with recurrent urinary tract infection. *New England Journal of Medicine* **329**, 753–756.

Reid, G. and Bruce, A. W. (2001). Selection of lactobacillus strains for urogenital probiotic applications. *Journal of Infectious Diseases* **183** (Suppl. 1), S77–S80.

Ronald, A. R. and Harding, G. K. M. (1997). Complicated urinary tract infection. *Infectious Disease Clinics of North America* **11**, 583–592.

Ronald, A. R., Cutler, R. E., and Truck, M. (1969). The effect of bacteria on the renal concentrating mechanism. *Annals of Internal Medicine* **70**, 723–733.

Rosenfield, A. T. *et al.* (1979). Acute focal bacterial nephritis (acute lobar nephronia). *Radiology* **132**, 553–561.

Rubin, R. H. *et al.* (1992). Evaluation of new anti-infective drugs for the treatment of urinary tract infection. *Clinical Infectious Diseases* **15** (Suppl. 4), S216–S227.

Saiki, J., Vaziri, N. D., and Barton, C. (1982). Perinephric and intranephric abscess: a review of the literature. *Western Journal of Medicine* **136**, 95–109.

Sanford, J. P. (1975). Urinary tract symptoms and infections. *Annual Review of Medicine* **26**, 485–498.

Sattari, A. *et al.* (2000). CT and 99m Tc-DMSA scintigraphy in adult acute pyelonephritis: a comparative study. *Journal of Computer Assisted Tomography* **24**, 600–604.

Schaeffer, A. J. and Stuppy, B. A. (1999). Efficacy and safety of self-start therapy in women with recurrent urinary tract infections. *Journal of Urology* **161**, 207–211.

Smith, R. C. *et al.* (1996). Diagnosis of acute flank pain; value of unenhanced helical CT. *American Journal of Roentgenology* **166**, 97–101.

Solomon, A. *et al.* (1983). Computerized tomography and xanthogranulomatous pyelonephritis. *Journal of Urology* **130**, 323–325.

Soulen, M. C. *et al.* (1989). Bacterial renal infection; role of CT. *Radiology* **171**, 703–707.

Stamey, T. A. *Pathogenesis and Treatment of Urinary Tract Infections*. Baltimore: Williams and Wilkins, 1972.

Stamey, T. A., Govan, D. E., and Palmer, J. M. (1965). The localisation and treatment of urinary tract infection: the role of bactericidal urine levels as opposed to serum levels. *Medicine* **44**, 1–36.

Stamm, W. E. (1983). Measurement of pyuria and its relation to bacteriuria. *American Journal of Medicine* **75** (July Suppl.), 53–57.

Stamm, W. E. *et al.* (1980). Causes of the acute urethral syndrome in women. *New England Journal of Medicine* **303**, 409–415.

Stamm, W. E. *et al.* (1982). Diagnosis of coliform infection in acutely dysuric women. *New England Journal of Medicine* **307**, 463–468.

Stamm, W. E. *et al.* (1989). Urinary tract infection: from pathogenesis to treatment. *Journal of Infectious Diseases* **159**, 400–406.

Stapleton, A. (1999). Prevention of recurrent urinary tract infections in women (Commentary). *Lancet* **353**, 7–8.

Stapleton, A. and Stamm, W. E. (1997). Prevention of urinary tract infection. *Infectious Disease Clinics of North America* **11**, 719–733.

Thorley, J. D., Jones, S. R., and Sanford, J. P. (1974). Perinephric abscess. *Medicine* **53**, 441–451.

Uehling, D. T., Hopkins, W. J., and Beierle, L. M. (2001). Vaginal mucosal immunization for recurrent urinary tract infection: extended Phase II clinical trial. *Journal of Infectious Diseases* **183** (Suppl. 1), S81–S83.

Vrtsika, T. J. *et al.* (1992). Role of ultrasound in medical management of patients with renal stone disease. *Urological Radiology* **14**, 131–138.

Wallmark, G., Arremark, I., and Telander, B. (1978). *Staphylococcus saprophyticus*; a frequent cause of urinary tract infection among female outpatients. *Journal of Infectious Diseases* **138**, 791–797.

Warren, J. W. *et al.* (1999). Guidelines for antimicrobial treatment of uncomplicated acute bacterial cystitis and acute pyelonephritis in women. *Clinical Infectious Diseases* **29**, 745–758.

7.2 Urinary tract infections in infancy and childhood

Heather J. Lambert and Malcolm G. Coulthard

Urinary tract infection (UTI) in childhood is a common problem, which is frequently dismissed as trivial. However, UTI is an important cause of acute illness in children and may be a marker of an underlying urinary tract abnormality. UTI may cause significant long-term morbidity, particularly renal scarring, hypertension, and renal impairment, which may not present until adult life. The risk of renal scarring is greatest in infants, the very group in whom diagnosis is often overlooked or delayed because clinical features are frequently non-specific. Thus, diagnosis of UTI requires a very high index of suspicion particularly in the youngest. *Accurate* diagnosis is essential because of the need for imaging, and the risks associated with over- or under-investigation.

Long-term sequelae of childhood urinary tract infection

It should be remembered that each adult presenting with reflux nephropathy had the origin of his or her problem in early childhood or even antenatally. There is good evidence that UTI in childhood is associated with renal scarring, the risk being highest in the youngest infants.

Scarring, once present, is irreversible and if severe may lead to chronic renal failure (CRF). This usually presents many years (sometimes, several decades) later. Renal scarring is probably the most important aetiological factor in the development of hypertension in children and young adults. However, there is no way of quantifying the long-term risk of CRF or hypertension resulting from an individual episode of UTI in childhood. Nor is there good evidence of the extent of long-term risk associated with minor degrees of scarring. One major problem is time scale. Adults presenting now with reflux nephropathy may not have access to details of medical problems in early childhood, many decades ago. In addition, many will not have had UTI in early childhood correctly diagnosed or appropriately investigated. Children with reflux nephropathy may not present in renal failure or with hypertension until very many years later, making prospective studies difficult to perform. Many existing studies are of small numbers or are retrospective. Ideally, cohorts of children need following prospectively for 40 or 50 years to determine more accurate estimates of adverse outcomes in adulthood.

The terms renal scarring, reflux nephropathy, and chronic pyelonephritis are often used loosely and, sometimes, interchangeably which leads to confusion. Focal renal scarring is usually associated with previous UTI, and is normally inferred from investigation findings, for example, the photon deficient areas on a radioisotope dimercaptosuccinic acid (DMSA) scan or the appearance of an ultrasound or intravenous urogram. Reflux nephropathy refers to a spectrum of renal diseases associated with vesicoureteric reflux (VUR), which include renal scarring, dysplasia of various degrees, and *in-utero* renal damage. It is often difficult to distinguish between antenatal and postnatal reflux nephropathy as the two frequently coexist. Pyelonephritis is perhaps strictly a histological diagnosis but is often used to describe a clinical pattern.

Hypertension

There are numerous retrospective and prospective studies linking the development of hypertension with renal scarring (Goonasekera and Dillon 1998; Jacobson *et al.* 1999). There is very good evidence that there is a substantially increased risk, which is worse for those with more severe and bilateral scarring (Smellie *et al.* 1998). The size and duration of risk for any individual or for those with less severe scarring is difficult to enumerate. The data depend on the population studied, as one small population-based follow-up study 16–26 years after childhood UTI found no difference in blood pressure between those with or without renal scarring (Wennerström *et al.* 2000b). What appears to be a small or scarred kidney on imaging may actually represent a number of different or combined underlying pathologies, for example, dysplasia or hypoplasia. Not all of these may be associated with a greater risk of hypertension but in cases of doubt regular long-term monitoring of blood pressure is required. It is currently recommended that children with scars have their blood pressure monitored on at least a yearly basis for life in order to detect presymptomatic hypertension.

Renal failure

The published incidence of endstage renal failure (ESRF) secondary to renal scarring varies. Pyelonephritic renal scarring was reported to be the primary renal diagnosis in 39 per cent of children undergoing renal transplantation in Ireland from 1980–1990 (Thomas *et al.* 1992). In Wales, between 1994 and 1997, 30 per cent of CRF [glomerular filtration rate (GFR) less than one-third of normal] in childhood has been attributed to reflux nephropathy (Imam 1998). In Australia and New Zealand from 1971 to 1998 reflux nephropathy was the primary diagnosis in 13 per cent of patients entering the dialysis and transplantation programme between the ages of 5 and 44 years, with no clear trend or change (Craig *et al.* 2000). In one part of France, pyelonephritis with reflux accounted for 12 per cent of CRF (Deleau *et al.* 1994). North American and European registries do not code specifically for renal scarring. Thus, it is difficult to distinguish between those reaching renal failure due to scarring of normal kidneys (i.e. possibly preventable reflux nephropathy) and those in whom the underlying diagnosis is reflux associated dysplasia. Nor is it possible to discern the role of UTI in deterioration of renal function in those with dysplasia (who also have a high incidence of VUR putting them at risk of possible damage from UTI). Hopefully, prospective studies will clarify issues. The most compelling data come from Sweden where the incidence of ESRF in childhood caused by non-obstructive reflux nephropathy has reduced from 6 per cent in 1978–1985 to zero in 1986–1994 (Esbjorner 1997). The Swedish data suggest that increased awareness and improved diagnosis of UTI in young children has been important (Esbjorner 1997; Jakobsson *et al.* 1999).

Pregnancy related complications

Pregnant women have an increased risk of cystitis and UTI if they had UTI and VUR in childhood. However, ureteric reimplantation in childhood does not necessarily protect against symptomatic UTI in pregnancy and may be associated with increased risk (Mansfield *et al.* 1995). There is controversy about the role of UTI in pregnancy and risk of preterm delivery or poor fetal outcome (Davison 2001). The risk of hypertension (Martinell *et al.* 1990) and pre-eclampsia (McGladdery *et al.* 1992) is higher in women with renal scarring. Fetal and maternal outcome are worse if the mother has severe renal impairment or established hypertension prior to the pregnancy (Lindheimer *et al.* 2001).

Challenges

Most children who are going to acquire renal scars already have them at the time they are investigated for the first time following UTI. Current management and investigation strategies for childhood UTI in the United Kingdom detect renal scarring but do little to prevent it (Coulthard 2002). If long-term outcome is to be improved, there are many challenges. These include improvement of diagnosis and early management of acute UTI; identification of those at high risk of sustaining renal damage; and increased awareness amongst healthcare professionals and the public of the importance of UTI.

Incidence of urinary tract infection in childhood

Urinary tract infection in childhood is very common. The true incidence of UTI is uncertain but is reported in Sweden as 2.2 per cent in boys and 2.1 per cent in girls cumulative incidence by age 2 years (Jakobsson *et al.* 1999). Cumulative referral rates in northern England are similar, rising to 2.8 per cent of boys and 8.2 per cent of girls by the age of 7 years and 3.6 per cent and 11.3 per cent, respectively, by the age of 16 years (Coulthard *et al.* 1997). It is generally accepted that the true rates are higher than those reported in earlier epidemiological studies from the 1970s and 1980s (Hellström *et al.* 1991; Marild and Jodal 1998). It is not known whether this represents a true rise in incidence or difference in rates of ascertainment. Some under-diagnosis is likely as there is evidence from Scandinavia that, even when strict diagnostic criteria are applied, rates vary between regions and are higher from centres with special interest (Jakobsson *et al.* 1999).

Large numbers of children with UTI are seen in the community by general practitioners and primary care physicians but there is frequently delay in treatment and not all are referred for further investigation (Vernon *et al.* 1997b). There are considerable problems in the diagnosis of UTI especially in younger patients, including: lack of awareness, non-specific symptoms, and difficulties collecting and analysing specimens. There is evidence that many cases are misdiagnosed in the community and it is our experience that diagnosis and referral of cases increase dramatically when there is targeted information and education (Coulthard 2003). Correct diagnosis is fundamental in directing subsequent management and investigation. UTI may be recurrent; about one-third of girls having a further UTI within a year. The recurrence rate in boys is much less.

Management of childhood UTI

Though UTI is a common problem there is no established consensus on investigation and management in childhood. Some inconsistencies may arise because of limited knowledge of basic pathophysiology and lack of evidence comparing long-term outcomes with different intervention strategies as well as problems associated with investigating young children.

Management and investigation of children with UTI consumes considerable healthcare resources in the United Kingdom and the rest of the world. It is important to optimize management strategies. The aim should be recognition of the child at risk of UTI, definitive early diagnosis, and prompt treatment. Those found to have a UTI should be referred appropriately for evaluation so that underlying renal tract abnormalities and renal damage can be identified; thus, aiming to prevent further renal damage. Some children will require long-term follow-up but it is equally important to avoid over-investigation and unnecessary follow-up.

Clinical presentation

Clinical features of UTI in childhood are often different to those found in adults and are frequently non-specific. Without a high index of suspicion many UTIs, especially in the very young, will be missed. *Classical* symptoms of lower UTI (dysuria, frequency, and incontinence) and upper UTI (fever, systemic upset, loin pain, and renal tenderness) are frequently not seen in paediatric practice. Attempts to distinguish between upper and lower UTI on clinical grounds are unreliable and clinical history is not closely related to findings on imaging. UTI can occasionally produce life-threatening illness, especially in very young infants, who may present severely unwell with shock or septicaemia. Boys and girls are equally affected in infancy but after that the ratio of girls to boys progressively increases (Fig. 1). After puberty the incidence of UTI is low in both sexes, but increases in females who are sexually active.

Preschool children

In general terms, the younger the child the more diverse and less specific are the symptoms and signs. Thus, evaluation of any unwell or febrile young child must include examination of urine. Sometimes there is a history of smelly urine or of crying on passing urine. Children may have an altered pattern of micturition and day or night-time

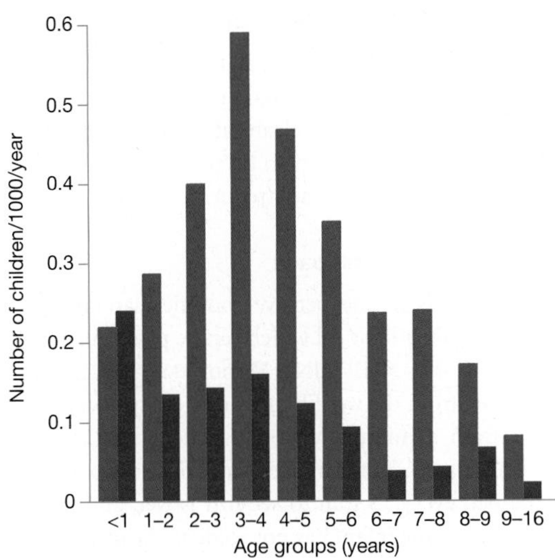

Fig. 1 UTI incidence in boys/girls with age (Newcastle data).

wetting may recur. Dysuria, urgency, frequency, or hesitancy may occur even in young children but is difficult to recognize in children who are still wearing nappies and who have limited means of communication. Non-specific manifestations such as poor feeding, vomiting, irritability, abdominal pain, failure to thrive, lethargy, restlessness should always lead to a suspicion of UTI but there are no data that assess sensitivity, specificity, or predictive value of these symptoms.

Fever is frequent but not always present and UTI should be suspected in any young child with unexplained fever. There is evidence that UTI is found in around 5 per cent of under 2 year olds with unexplained fever (American Academy of Pediatrics 1999b). The risk of UTI in uncircumcised boys under the age of one is reported to be increased between 3 and 15 times compared to those who are circumcised (Schoen *et al.* 2000; Wiswell 2000). However, the increased risk, when countered against the risks of circumcision, is not considered sufficient to recommend it as a routine preventative measure (American Academy of Pediatrics 1999a; Walsh 1999).

Older children

Older children may have more typical signs and symptoms localizing to the urinary tract including dysuria, frequency, urgency, hesitation, and enuresis. Some may have loin pain but absence of loin pain does not exclude upper urinary tract involvement. Generalized symptoms are common including fever, lethargy, anorexia, abdominal pain, nausea, and vomiting.

Whilst there is some evidence that patients with a clinical picture of pyelonephritis may be at more risk of sustaining permanent renal scars the converse is not true. A UTI can cause systemic upset and fever without classical lower urinary tract symptoms. Patients with lower urinary tract symptoms only (or no symptoms) can still sustain renal scarring.

Not all children with dysuria have a UTI. Dysuria may be associated with localized skin conditions such as candidiasis, vulvitis, or excoriation secondary to thread worms or other irritation. Febrile or mildly dehydrated children may complain of pain, stinging, or discomfort on passing concentrated or what they term 'strong' urine. Children with quite minor degrees of haematuria, for example, from glomerulonephritis, may present with dysuria.

Recurrent infections

About one-third of girls will have a further UTI within a year and some go on to have repeated infections. Recurrent infections may be associated with an underlying urinary tract abnormality or renal scarring (Wennerström *et al.* 2000a), but in practice a significant number of girls with non-scarred and non-refluxing urinary tracts have recurrent symptomatic UTI. This may cause considerable distress, anxiety, and frustration to the child and family. UTI may be associated with dysfunctional voiding and bladder instability (Koff *et al.* 1998). There has long been evidence that UTI is more common in children with constipation (Shopfner 1968; Blethyn *et al.* 1995). A history of constipation should be sought, and may be suspected on abdominal palpation. Bowel loaded with faeces may be seen on abdominal X-ray. UTI may be more frequent in girls suffering sexual abuse and this diagnosis should not be overlooked during assessment. Teenage girls may be sexually active and this may be a contributing factor in a recent onset of recurrent UTI. Boys seldom get recurrent UTI in the absence of urinary tract abnormalities (Wennerström *et al.* 2000a).

Assessment

Clinical history and appropriate examination are important including examination of the urine. Details should be sought of family history of urinary infection, VUR, renal disease, or hypertension; antenatal and perinatal history; drinking, voiding pattern, and bowel habits. Examination should include measurement of blood pressure; abdominal palpation for masses (bladder, kidney); inspection of external genitalia and lower back; assessment of lower limb sensation and reflexes. When UTI is recurrent, it is particularly important that bladder and bowel habits are evaluated.

Some centres attempt to distinguish between upper and lower UTI. Indicators such as temperature, C-reactive protein, and loin pain have been used. However, although there is some evidence that those with classical pyelonephritis may have an increased risk of scarring there is no convincing evidence that any particular clinical pattern is associated with an 'uncomplicated or lower' UTI. Renal scarring may occur in association with few or no symptoms.

Antibacterial defence mechanisms

Neonates, with immature immune systems, are particularly susceptible to *Escherichia coli* infection. Colonization of the newborn gut with bacteria including *E. coli* is thought to start rapidly. It is possible that this is influenced by factors such as breast feeding, location of delivery, maternity unit procedures, and use of antibiotics. It is not known whether these influence later development of UTI though it has long been thought, and has now been confirmed, that UTI may be caused by bacteria from the child's own gut (Jantunen *et al.* 2000).

After the first year of life there is a marked gender difference in incidence of UTI, with girls being far more susceptible. This is usually explained by difference in urethral length; the short female urethra providing easy access to the bladder for bacteria. Whilst urine provides a good culture medium for bacteria, the bladder normally provides some resistance to infection. Repeated voiding and complete emptying of the bladder helps remove bacteria. Increasing the fluid intake is often helpful in encouraging regular voiding, if the child and family understand the rationale. Incomplete emptying of the bladder may have an important role to play in recurrent UTI. Infection may affect normal ureteric peristalsis. Children with VUR, bladder outlet obstruction, constipation, neuropathic bladder, and dysfunctional voiding may have significant residual urine in the bladder limiting the ability to reduce bacterial colonization by simple washout.

The bladder epithelium may also have some antibacterial activity. Many uropathogentic *E. coli* strains have surface structures called type 1 pili that can facilitate both attachment to and invasion of bladder mucosal cells. There are numerous defence mechanisms which may be provoked in response including cytokine production, inflammation and exfoliation of superficial bladder cells which are removed in the flow of urine. Studies in animals have shown some strains of *E. coli* may form a persistent quiescent bacterial reservoir in deeper layers of the bladder mucosa, despite sterilization of the urine with antibiotics, which could theoretically lead to recurrent infection (Mulvey *et al.* 2000).

Making the diagnosis of UTI; urine collection and testing

It is easy to under- or overestimate the incidence of UTI in children if it is assumed that the diagnosis can be made on symptoms alone, and that it is unnecessary to examine the urine. Infants with UTI but only non-specific symptoms are frequently under-diagnosed (Mond *et al.* 1970; Royal College of Physicians Research Unit Working Group 1991), whereas girls with vulvitis, and febrile anorexic children who produce a highly concentrated urine and complain of dysuria are often falsely diagnosed as having a UTI. It is important to be certain of the diagnosis if children at risk of scarring are to be appropriately treated and investigated, whilst those without UTI are to be spared unnecessary antibiotics, tests, and radiation.

Unfortunately, it is common for some children to receive an antibiotic for a presumed UTI without a urine sample being either collected or tested (Jadresic *et al.* 1993; van der Voort *et al.* 1997; Vernon *et al.* 1997c). Once this has happened, it is not possible to reach a certain diagnosis, and the decision whether to investigate the child is very difficult. Frequently, urine is not collected because doctors imagine that uncontaminated samples are practically difficult to obtain in the very young, or difficult to transport to the laboratory quickly enough. These practical issues can be minimized, and are addressed below.

Collecting urines in children

Background

Ideally, urine collection would be inexpensive, quick, and easy for parents to manage at home with a child of any age, and would have zero contamination. Sadly, no such technique exists. Instead, there is a range of methods, and the best choice for a particular child will depend on the clinical setting, and the child's age. Every method produces some contaminated samples, and opinions as to which is best differ between units and families. Unfortunately, the very young children whose urine is most difficult to collect are the same ones that are at the greatest risk of scarring. Commonly, parents are asked to collect a child's urine at home, but are given no guidance on how to do it (Vernon *et al.* 1997c).

Collecting urine in infants; clean catch

Clean catch collection is convenient, if the infant voids quickly and it has a low contamination rate (Macfarlane *et al.* 1999). However, most parents are unenthusiastic about clean catch collections at home (Liaw *et al.* 2000). They consider them to be time consuming, messy, and difficult, and collection failures are frequent.

Collecting urine in infants; pads

Urine collection pads are inexpensive, modified sanitary towels without antiseptics or absorbent gel which can be placed inside the nappy (Ontex UK Ltd, Corby, NN17 4JN) (Vernon *et al.* 1994). The urine can then be aspirated from the wet fibres using a syringe without a needle, or squeezed from a minimally wetted pad by placing some fibres within a syringe barrel. To minimize contamination, parents are asked to check the pad every 15 min to see if it is wet, and to replace it if soiled, or after 2 h if the infant has not voided. The urine has only brief skin contact time. Parents like pads because they are easy to use and do not cause the baby any discomfort, though some find the urine extraction difficult (Liaw *et al.* 2000). Some white cells are retained by the pad, but we argue that this is unimportant. We advise having the sterile bottle ready when the pad is being placed inside the nappy so a clean catch can be collected if the baby happens to void at the time.

Collecting urine in infants; sterile adhesive bags

These bags can be stuck to the skin around the genitalia. In practice, it is often helpful to then replace the nappy to prevent the child from pulling at the bag. Most parents are upset by the redness and discomfort that the bags cause, and many find decanting the urine into the sterile bottle to be difficult (Liaw *et al.* 2000). Some general practitioners consider them to be too costly to use (Vernon *et al.* 1997c).

Collecting urine in infants; suprapubic aspiration

It is generally regarded that if *any* bacteria at all are grown from a suprapubic aspiration (SPA) urine, it *always* indicates a definite UTI. This assumes an infallibility, with no chance of contamination; a 100 per cent sensitivity and specificity. Hence, the SPA has the status of being the 'gold standard' collection method. However, this has not been rigorously tested, and some evidence suggests it is not the case.

The technique is to aspirate the bladder with a syringe and needle after thorough cleaning of the suprapubic skin. This is relatively easier in infants than older children because their bladders extend into the abdomen even when they are only partially full (Pryles *et al.* 1959; Nelson and Peters 1965). It is made easier by locating the bladder with ultrasound (Ramage *et al.* 1999).

SPA urines undoubtedly have less contamination than voided ones (Nelson and Peters 1965; Wettergren *et al.* 1985; Hansson *et al.* 1998). However, up to 16 per cent of SPA samples yield just one species of organism at very low colony counts (Nelson and Peters 1965) that would be considered evidence of contamination in voided urine. Further evidence of contamination is seen when two urines collected sequentially from the same infant produce a positive culture from the SPA, and a sterile bag sample (Aronson *et al.* 1973; Ramage *et al.* 1999). These authors state that the voided urine samples were falsely negative without justification. If the same definitions for contamination and false-positive results were applied to SPA and voided samples, the SPA failure rates would be between 11 per cent (Ramage *et al.* 1999) and 29 per cent (Aronson *et al.* 1973).

To clarify this important issue, it would be necessary to design a study in which the SPA was repeated in every apparently positive case. It is of interest that many authors fail to consider the possibility of contaminated SPA urine despite extensive clinical experience of contamination of blood culture samples (which essentially uses a similar collection technique of needle puncture of skin). Also, the needle frequently does not enter the bladder immediately during SPA, and it is easy to advance it too far initially; clearly it might enter the bowel transiently during this process (Weathers and Wenzl 1969).

Whilst the SPA is undoubtedly valuable in ill infants in whom it is unacceptable to delay starting antibiotic treatment, and where suprapubic pressure fails to induce voiding, it has no role in collecting urine at home or in the community, where most infant urine collections are made. Its use in non-emergency hospital cases is debatable. The main disadvantage of using non-invasive collection methods is the greater risk of obtaining contaminated samples, and this largely disappears if fresh urine can be screened by phase-contrast microscopy, and repeat samples collected if necessary.

Collecting urine in toddlers

Some toddlers will refuse to void into a sterile bottle, despite being potty trained. The choice then lies between putting them back into a nappy and using a collection pad, or using a potty with a sterile container in, or a carefully cleaned potty. Though some general practitioners advise preparing the potty by steeping it in bleach or household antiseptic, or rinsing it with boiling water (Vernon *et al.* 1997c), these methods are inadequate in removing contaminating organisms. However, potties can be quickly, easily, and effectively sterilized by simply washing them up in hot water and detergent which reliably removes the bacteria with the biofilm (Rees *et al.* 1996).

Collecting urine in older children

Older children can usually void directly into a sterile collection bottle after gently washing the genitalia with cotton wool and water. Disposable plastic funnels make this easier in girls. It is ideal to collect only the middle part of the urine stream after the contaminating periurethral bacteria have been washed off by the initial flow, but this is often impractical in younger children. However, cleanly caught complete samples have relatively little contamination (Macfarlane *et al.* 1999). The glans should be washed in those boys whose foreskin retracts easily. In girls, bacterial contamination may occur from the labia, or from urine flowing into the vagina before being collected. If this happens, most girls can produce a urethral stream by voiding into a bath whilst sitting on the side with their legs and labia parted.

Collecting urine by urethral catheterization

Occasionally, it may be necessary to obtain a diagnostic urine sample from an older child who is too ill to be able to cooperate. An SPA is usually difficult because in older children the bladder remains pelvic until it is very full. Under these circumstances brief urethral catheterization may be justified.

Testing urines for UTI in children

General principles

Although the diagnosis of a UTI in childhood is universally defined as the culture of more than 10^5 colonies/ml of a single bacterial species from urine, most authors also consider that the number of urinary white cells is important. We reconsider both of these assumptions.

An instant near-patient diagnostic test would be a major advantage. It would allow children to be confidently treated without delay, or for treatment to be safely withheld. In positive cases, treatment would begin with the 'best guess' antibiotic, but culture would still be necessary to allow it to be adjusted later according to the bacterial sensitivities. Negative samples could be discarded. The reason for minimizing treatment delay is not just to allow children to recover rapidly from their acute symptoms, but also to reduce the risk of scarring which may occur within a few days. Without an immediate and certain diagnosis, the options are to delay treatment pending the culture results (increasing the risk of scarring), or start treatment on clinical suspicion, and stop if the culture is negative (risking the overuse of antibiotics). The younger the child, the greater the risk of initiating a new scar, and therefore the stronger the argument for immediate treatment.

Bacteria in UTI

Organisms that cause UTI

About 85 per cent of urine samples from boys and girls with a first UTI grow *E. coli* on culture (Winberg *et al.* 1974; Jodal 1987). *Klebsiella*, *Proteus*, and *Streptococcus faecalis* are responsible for most of the rest. Children with abnormal urinary tracts are much more likely to have UTI due to less virulent organisms such as *Pseudomonas* or *Staphylococcus aureus*. These bacteria often contribute to the flora which may cause contamination from the genitalia and skin. Suspicions that bacteria that cause urine infections derive from the child's own bowel have been confirmed by genetic 'fingerprinting' of the bacteria (Jantunen *et al.* 2000).

Proteus spp. metabolize urea to produce ammonia, and the increased urinary pH tends to make calcium and magnesium phosphate salts precipitate, and thereby produce a risk of stone formation. This occurs especially if there is mucus and cellular debris from the inflammatory process. A thick sludge is created that takes up the shape of the drainage tract, and further chemical precipitation may make it more solid. Thus, stag-horn shaped calculi develop in the pelvicalyceal system, and date-stone shaped ones form in the ureter.

Bacterial numbers in a UTI

Kass provided the now universally accepted diagnostic criterion of a UTI in the middle of the last century, in a paper in which he made it very clear that he was aware that it was a compromise, and not the ideal definition (Kass 1956). Despite that, his definition of at least 10^5/ml colony forming units (cfu) of one bacterial species on culture has been treated ever since as if it was certain and uncontroversial. In his introduction, Kass recognized that the concentration of bacteria in the urine in most UTI was of the order of 10^9/ml, yet instead of choosing a slightly lower threshold for a cut-off he chose one more than a thousand times lower. He chose to continue to use the traditional inoculation technique for urine culture, with a wire-loop of urine being applied to the agar of a Petri dish. This method limits the concentration of cfu that can be counted; 10^5/ml bacteria produce confluent colonies, so no more can be counted without predilution. Thus, bacterial numbers lower than 10^5/ml can be counted, but concentrations tens of thousands higher will all be reported as greater than 10^5/ml.

Whilst fewer than 10^5 bacterial colonies/ml or a light mixture of organisms are generally regarded as indicating contamination (Kass 1956), it might be predicted that setting such a low threshold concentration would sometimes lead to minor contamination resulting in the culture of a pure growth of greater than 10^5/ml cfu. That is, false-positive results would be expected to be a common problem. There is clear evidence that this is the case. Kass himself reported apparent positive culture rates among asymptomatic adult outpatients of 4 per cent in men and 6 per cent in women (Kass 1956). We have found similar false-positive rates of 8 per cent in infants (Liaw *et al.* 2000) and 6.6 per cent in children (Vickers *et al.* 1991). Others have reported growing greater than 10^5 coliforms/ml in bag or clean catch samples from preterm (Nelson and Peters 1965) and term neonates (Nelson and Peters 1965; Hardy *et al.* 1976), infants (Shannon *et al.* 1969; Hardy *et al.* 1976), and older children (Shannon *et al.* 1969) who did not have urine infections (confirmed by sterile SPAs). These figures have major implications if we use urine culture as the primary definition of a UTI in children, because about 8 per cent of children without an infection may be subjected to antibiotics and imaging investigations. Many agree that all infants with an unexplained fever above 38.5°C should have a urine cultured (Mond *et al.* 1970; Royal College of Physicians Research Unit Working Group 1991; American Academy of Pediatrics 1999b). It is not uncommon for children to have three or more febrile illnesses in the first year or two of life, which would give at least a one in five chance of acquiring a false diagnosis of UTI.

Laboratory culture for bacteria

Culture has an inherent delay. It takes up to 24 h to grow the bacterial colonies, and traditionally the organisms on positive plates are then identified and subcultured with antibiotic-impregnated discs to determine their sensitivity to guide treatment. In practice, 4 or 5 days may easily elapse between a doctor seeing a child and receiving the laboratory report. This is a major disadvantage, given that children with a UTI may acquire their first scar quicker than that. Occasionally, standard culture fails to identify the causative organism and produces a false-negative result because it requires anaerobic culture conditions.

It is important to minimize the overgrowth of contaminating organisms during storage and transfer to the laboratory. Refrigeration provides highly effective storage for 72 h (Watson and Duerden 1977), but is not always convenient. Collection bottles containing boric acid are widely used, but may produce false-negative results (Watson and Duerden 1977; Jewkes *et al.* 1990). They are designed to be completely filled with urine to produce bacteriostatic concentrations, so small paediatric samples may result in bactericidal levels. Smaller borate bottles are available. Perceptions about storage and transport difficulties undoubtedly contribute to the fact that children suspected of having a urine infection during an evening or weekend are less likely to have their urine cultured by their general practitioners (Jadresic *et al.* 1993; Vernon *et al.* 1997c).

Bacterial culture on dipslides

A dipslide consists of a sterile bottle with a miniature agar-covered culture plate attached to the inside of the lid. The plate may be dipped in urine and allowed to drain. There may be problems with agar detachment if the sample is small and the plate shaken (Jewkes *et al.* 1990). To avoid this, urine can easily be applied to the plate using a sterile swab (Liaw *et al.* 2000).

The great advantage of the dipslide method is that urine can be cultured at any time, anywhere, and can be posted to the laboratory for incubation.

Phase-contrast microscopy of urine for bacteria

Unstained bacteria in fresh undiluted urine are difficult to see using standard light microscopy as they do not contrast greatly against the background glare. In the laboratory they are readily identified by Gram staining, but this technique is time consuming, and unsuitable for routine side-room urine screening (Kass 1956). However, bacteria can be identified very easily in unprepared urine by phase-contrast microscopy (Vickers *et al.* 1991), when they appear as clearly defined black organisms against a light background (Fig. 2). Therefore, phase-contrast microscopy can provide a fast, reliable, efficient, and economic near-patient UTI diagnostic service.

In our experience, the phase-contrast microscope becomes a convenient tool if it is kept in the clinical area (e.g. out patients, ward, day-unit) and is dedicated for use with urine only. We use 400× magnification and a slide with two counting chambers, each 0.1 mm deep, and with a grid etched on a lightly mirrored surface. This provides a clear point of focus so that it is certain that the microscope is correctly adjusted when inspecting a sterile urine which itself has no features to see. Urine can be introduced into the chamber by capillary action by using a test-strip for blood, protein, etc. and touching its wet tip on the edge of the cover slip. Reliable diagnosis depends on maintaining practice and experience. Using a double-viewing head so that the sample can be examined by two people is an invaluable tool to teach the skill. We recommend recording each examination in the case notes using adhesive results labels.

When an infected urine is examined by phase-contrast microscopy there will typically be tens, hundreds, or thousands of identical rods per high power field, equivalent to bacterial counts of between

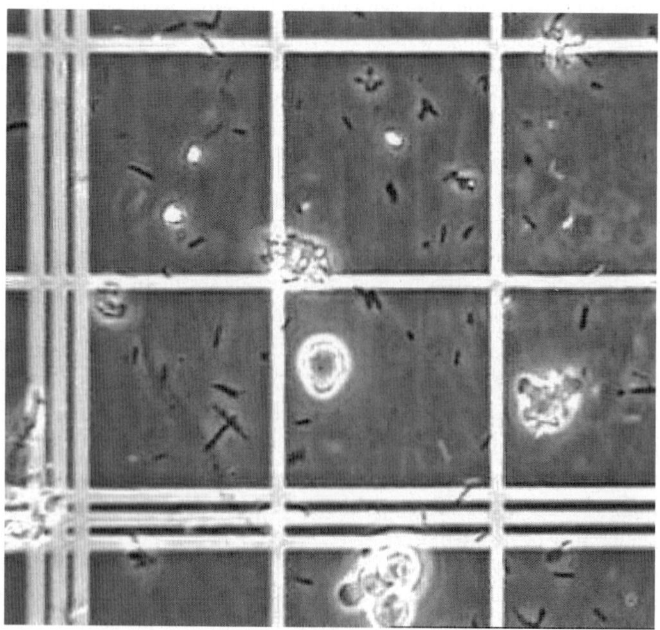

Fig. 2 Phase contrast microscopy of urine at 400×, showing myriad rods of similar length against the counting grid. Note the presence of some white blood cells.

10^6 and 10^9/ml (all reported identically as $> 10^5$/ml on culture). Occasionally, UTIs are caused by *S. faecalis* which are easily recognized as chains of cocci. These must not be confused with phosphate crystals, which are of a similar size, and seen individually or in clumps, but not chains. The fact that small particles shimmer due to Brownian motion can be misleading and suggest bacteria swimming to the unwary. Rarely, a UTI is diagnosed by phase-contrast but the culture is negative; typically this is because standard culture fails if the organism is anaerobic. Antibiotics can be commenced immediately after an infected urine is identified, but culture and sensitivity testing is also needed to guide treatment.

Uninfected urine simply has no organisms to see at all. The urine from a child with a UTI will almost invariably have many rods visible per high-power field, so a completely empty field virtually guarantees an uninfected sample. However, we advise inspecting about five fields (about 0.02 l of urine) to be certain. A completely clear urine can be discarded without being cultured, thus saving money.

Some urine samples will give uncertain results, either because just one or two bacteria are seen, or rods and streptococci are present together, or there is amorphous debris, cotton strands, etc., present. If these urine samples are cultured, some will be negative, some will have a low bacterial count and be reported as uninfected, some will grow a heavy mixture of organisms and be considered uncertain, and some will produce a pure growth of one organism at greater than 10^5/ml; the false positives described above (Vickers *et al.* 1991). However, these diagnostic difficulties can be avoided if microscopy is used because the uncertain nature of the sample is immediately apparent, and a repeat sample can be collected at once. This means that every child will receive a confident diagnosis at the time of presentation, if necessary by voiding two or more specimens. The majority of repeat specimens are completely clear, indicating that the first was contaminated. It is this facility that makes it relatively unimportant that some urine collection techniques have an intrinsic contamination rate, and eliminates the need for invasive methods such as SPA or urethral catheterization except in the most urgent cases.

Phase-contrast is also better than standard microscopy for examining other elements in the urine. White cells can be seen in detail. Red cell morphology is clear, and can differentiate glomerular from lower tract bleeding. The content of casts is clearly visible. Many older girls have vaginal epithelial cells in the urine, and occasionally long rods which are anaerobic vaginal lactobacilli. Children with metabolic stones may have identifiable crystals. Phosphate crystals are common in normal concentrated urine.

Identifying bacteria with nitrite stick tests

Most uropathogens produce nitrite as a result of their metabolism. A sufficient concentration of bacteria in urine for a sufficient period of time will produce quantities of nitrite that can be detected with a test-strip. Uninfected urine samples, or ones contaminated during collection, do not contain nitrite, so the specificity is about 100 per cent (American Academy of Pediatrics 1999b); a positive test therefore allows the child to be confidently treated without delay.

However, it often takes hours for the bacteria to produce detectable quantities of nitrite (Powell *et al.* 1987). Given that children with UTI tend to void frequently, it is unfortunate but inevitable that the test sensitivity is low (53 per cent, range 15–82) (American Academy of Pediatrics 1999b). If samples test negative for nitrite, this adds nothing to the diagnostic process, and they should all be cultured or examined by microscopy. In practice, some doctors interpret nitrite-negative tests as if they can reliably exclude a UTI, and use this as the basis of a screening test, only culturing ones that test positive (Vernon *et al.* 1997c). This practice will ensure that about half the children presenting with a UTI will be missed.

Urinary white blood cells in UTI

Background

Typically, children with UTI have an increased number of white blood cells (WBCs) in the urine, and this is widely considered to be an important diagnostic feature. However, the evidence does not support this.

First, infected urine often has little or no excess of WBCs. Sometimes this is because children did not void many WBCs. This is especially common in girls with asymptomatic bacteriuria. Sometimes a fresh sample will have a huge excess of cells, but the laboratory will report there being few or none a short while later, because some WBCs do not survive intact for very long (Vickers *et al.* 1991), perhaps related to factors such as pH (Stansfeld 1962). Rarely, a young child with an overwhelming infection may be unable to maintain a urinary WBC response (Kumar *et al.* 1996). Similarly, children being treated with immunosuppressant drugs may be unable to produce a pyuria.

Second, there can be an excess of urinary WBC in the absence of infection. The most common reason is that children with a pyrexia from any cause tend to have increased urinary WBC numbers, sometimes up to concentrations of several hundreds per microlitre (Turner and Coulthard 1995). Presumably this reflects an increase in the mobility and number of circulating white cells in the blood. In addition, girls may have moderately high urine WBC numbers from the vagina. This occurs in the absence of a recognizable discharge. It is probably because the urinary stream in many girls is deflected into the vagina by the labia before being collected.

Testing for urinary WBC

Though urine WBC are frequently raised in childhood UTI, the lack of concurrence makes the urine WBC count unreliable as a discriminating feature (Kass 1956; Royal College of Physicians Research Unit Working Group 1991; American Academy of Pediatrics 1999b). The slight reduction in WBC numbers in urine samples collected by pad (Vernon *et al.* 1994) is therefore unimportant.

Urine stick tests are available to detect leucocyte esterase concentrations which reflect an excess of WBC. They are more reliable than microscopy if there is any delay in reaching the laboratory because fragmented WBC are still detected. However, this does not make their presence or absence any easier to interpret. This is not the common view. In our experience, many doctors are less likely to accept the bacteriological diagnosis of a UTI if the laboratory does not report an excess of white cells.

Treatment

The primary treatment goals are twofold: elimination of symptoms associated with an acute UTI together with prevention of renal injury. In animal models, there is evidence of scarring of susceptible kidneys occurring if infection lasts more than a few days before treatment (Miller and Phillips 1981; Ransley and Risdon 1981). From retrospective studies in children there is an association between delayed treatment and increased risk of renal scarring (Smellie *et al.* 1985, 1994; Dick and Feldman 1996). Because of this, in practice, if UTI is suspected, a 'best guess' antibiotic should be started whilst awaiting results of the urine culture. This is particularly important in younger children. This does, however, present the primary care doctor with a dilemma in that the ideal of treating UTI very quickly, to prevent long-term sequelae, may cause overuse of antibiotics in cases where the urine is eventually found not to be infected. Judicious use of near-patient tests may reduce this problem. Sensitivities should be available within 48–72 h and antibiotics can be changed if indicated. It is important that procedures are implemented for obtaining reports on urine cultures quickly and that, for patients at home, information is rapidly conveyed to parents. Cephalexin, trimethoprim, or nitrofurantoin are frequently used, but discussion with the local microbiologist should help guide general advice about resistance patterns in community acquired infection in the local paediatric population. Recent antibiotic use by the patient should also be taken into account when prescribing. It is common practice to encourage increased intake of fluids when treating UTI.

Children, particularly infants, who are clinically dehydrated, toxic, or unlikely to retain oral fluids, should be referred to hospital for parenteral antibiotics initially. Fever should settle within about 48 h in the majority of infants treated with parenteral antibiotics. However, if the clinical condition does not improve within this time a repeat urine specimen should be obtained and further urgent investigation should be considered, for example, renal tract ultrasound to look for dilatation related to obstruction. Normally, there should be an aim for discharge on appropriate oral antibiotics once the child is improving and sensitivities are known. There is no clear evidence about the ideal length of therapy to eradicate acute infection in children. In adults, studies suggest improved efficacy of a 3-day treatment versus a one-dose treatment. In children, longer courses of antibiotics (5–10 days) achieve better results than short courses (one dose or up to 3 days) (American Academy of Pediatrics 1999b; Tran *et al.* 2001). Because of the association between recurrent UTI and scarring (Jodal 1987), after the acute course of antibiotics a urine specimen should be checked and a low dose of a suitable antibiotic should be continued until investigations are completed and assessed (Royal College of Physicians 1991; American Academy of Pediatrics 1999b).

In children with a normal urinary tract, but recurrent UTI, there is evidence that a long course of antibiotics (6 months) is associated with not only a reduced frequency of UTI whilst the antibiotics are being taken but also for the subsequent 2 years (Smellie 1978). Rotation of prophylactic antibiotics is sometimes advocated. Cranberry juice has been used for many years for prevention of UTI in adults based largely on folklore and anecdotal reports (Jepson *et al.* 2000). Whilst there is no evidence supporting its use in childhood it may be helpful though some children dislike the taste. Clinical experience suggests simple measures such as increasing fluid intake, regular voiding, and avoiding perineal irritants such as bubble-bath may be helpful in prevention of recurrent UTI in some girls.

Constipation and dysfunctional voiding are associated with recurrent UTI. Active treatment of constipation may reduce recurrent UTI in patients with normal urinary tracts (Loening-Bauche 1997). Postmicturition residue and upper tract dilatation has been found to be increased in children with constipation and improved after treatment (Dohil *et al.* 1994). UTI may be associated with dysfunctional voiding and bladder instability (Koff *et al.* 1998), and it is important that bladder and bowel habits are evaluated especially when UTI is recurrent. There is, however, little evidence regarding efficacy of interventions like bladder training, behaviour modification, or anticholinergic drugs in affected individuals. Clinical experience suggests these approaches may be effective and they warrant further study.

Treatment of children known to have VUR is addressed later. Children with complex urinary tract problems, who require interventions such as intermittent catheterization, frequently have both asymptomatic bacteriuria and symptomatic UTI. These children should all be managed in conjunction with a specialist paediatric centre and decisions on management and treatment will vary depending on the individual circumstances and underlying problems. There is no evidence of benefit from treatment of asymptomatic bacteriuria in girls with normal urinary tracts. They do not therefore require routine screening of urine when well.

Investigation

The general aim of investigation is to identify those with an underlying renal tract abnormality or predisposition to UTI such as structural abnormality of urinary tract, urinary tract obstruction, VUR, or abnormal bladder emptying. Those who have sustained damage to their kidneys or who are likely to do so should be identified. Unfortunately, current investigation strategies in the United Kingdom tend to identify those who have already scarred their kidneys rather that identifying those at high risk in whom renal damage may be prevented. There is considerable controversy about the appropriate investigation of the child with UTI, and no perfect solution. Investigation needs to be tailored to the individual patient in many cases and new developments in techniques will change current investigation schemes. Some understanding of the pathophysiology and an appreciation of some current hypotheses are essential in developing a pragmatic approach to investigation of UTI.

Renal scarring

Risk factors for development of renal scarring include young age (Berg and Johansson 1983), delay in antibiotic treatment of UTI (Smellie *et al.* 1985), recurrent infections (Winter *et al.* 1983; Wennerström *et al.* 2000a), VUR (Stokland *et al.* 1998), and obstruction of urinary tract.

Vesicoureteric reflux

VUR is the retrograde flow of urine from the bladder into the upper urinary tract. It is usually congenital but may occasionally be acquired, for example, after surgery. VUR is a major risk factor for progressive renal damage associated with UTI. Because of the difficulties and ethics of studies, the true incidence of VUR in the normal population at various ages is not known but is in the order of 1 per cent in infants (Coulthard 2002) and is increased in certain risk groups. VUR is found in up to one-third of children and in up to 50 per cent of infants investigated after UTI (Jacobson *et al.* 1999). Babies in whom there is an antenatal identification of renal pelvis dilatation have an increased risk of VUR. The figures depend on the population investigated postnatally but are in the region of 10–40 per cent (Zerin *et al.* 1993; Anderson *et al.* 1997). It remains to be demonstrated whether the increased risk of VUR will necessarily be associated with an increased incidence of renal scarring. VUR is found in association with congenital abnormalities of the urinary tract such as ureteric duplication, contralateral multicystic dysplastic kidney, or renal agenesis. There is evidence of a 20–50-fold increased risk of VUR in children with a family history of VUR (Scott *et al.* 1997; Jacobson *et al.* 1999). There is good evidence that VUR is a genetic disorder (Feather 2000). Different modes of inheritance have been proposed including dominant and polygenic inheritance (Feather 2000).

Grading of VUR

Grades of severity of VUR are recognized, designated grades I–V by the International Reflux Study Committee in 1981 and still generally accepted world-wide (Fig. 3).

Grades of VUR

I Into ureter only.
II Into ureter, pelvis and calyces with no dilatation.
III With mild to moderate dilatation; slight or no blunting of fornices.
IV With moderate dilatation of ureter and/or renal pelvis and/or tortuosity of ureter; obliteration of sharp angle of fornices.
V Gross dilatation and tortuosity; no papillary impression visible in calyces.

VUR is well described to be intermittent and variable in grade at different times during an examination and is not an 'all or none' phenomenon (Hellström and Jacobsson 1999). VUR in both humans and animals can be influenced by variations in urine flow (Zinner and Jr 1963; Ekman *et al.* 1966), which may be related to changes in ureteric peristalsis. Despite that, grading of VUR remains important because higher grades of reflux are associated with increased chance of renal scarring (Smellie *et al.* 1992; Stokland *et al.* 1998), of reflux associated dysplasia, and with less chance of spontaneous resolution (Elder *et al.* 1997).

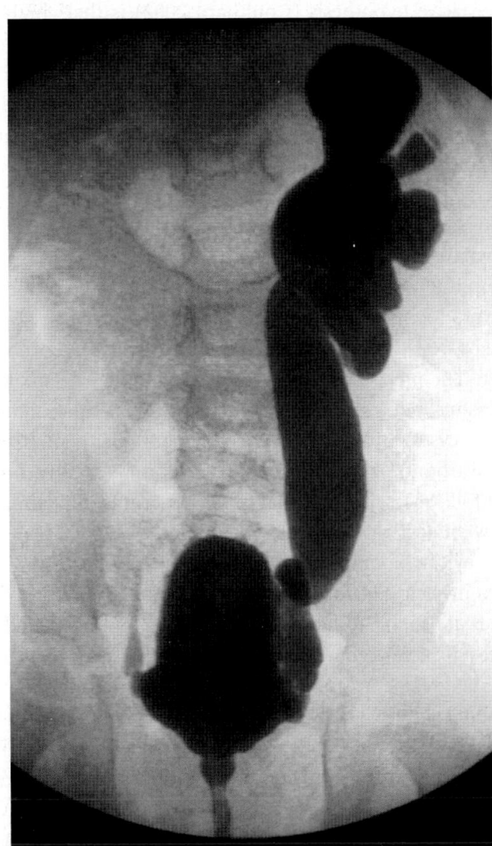

Fig. 3 MCUG showing unilateral grade IV/V plus contralateral grade I reflux.

VUR and altered bladder function

Bladder dysfunction may predispose to infection. Urodynamic dysfunction, bladder instability or high intravesical pressures are commonly found in infants, especially boys, with severe VUR (Yeung *et al.* 1998; Sillen 1999; Chandra and Maddix 2000; Willemsen and Nijman 2000). Urodynamics in normal infants are not easily studied for comparison and the relationship of abnormal urodynamic patterns to the pathogenesis or resolution of VUR is not known. In the growing pig, sterile VUR has been shown not to affect renal growth or uptake of DMSA, even in the presence of raised voiding pressures and abnormal bladder function (Godley *et al.* 1989).

Relationship of VUR, renal scarring, and reflux nephropathy

An association between VUR and scarring has been recognized since the 1960s but details of these relationships are far from clear. VUR is thought to predispose to renal damage by facilitating passage of bacteria from the bladder to the upper urinary tract. An immunological and inflammatory reaction is caused by renal infection leading to renal injury and scarring. Extensive renal scarring causes reduced renal function, reduced renal growth, renal failure, hypertension, and increased incidence of pregnancy related hypertension. Whilst these sequelae may occur in childhood, patients frequently do not present until many years or decades later.

Our understanding of the mechanism of focal scarring has been greatly advanced by the piglet model developed by Ransley and Risdon (1978, 1981). In their studies they found that neither VUR alone (with sterile urine) nor lower UTI alone (with no VUR) led to scarring. However, scars developed in some segments of kidneys when there was VUR and UTI, leaving the adjacent segments unaffected. They found that the scarred and unscarred segments had different shaped papillae. The scarred segments had compound papillae that were flat or concave in shape whereas the unscarred segments had simple cone shaped papillae. Compound papillae with open gaping orifices allow intrarenal reflux whereas simple papillae with slit-like orifices do not (Ransley and Risdon 1974) (Fig. 4).

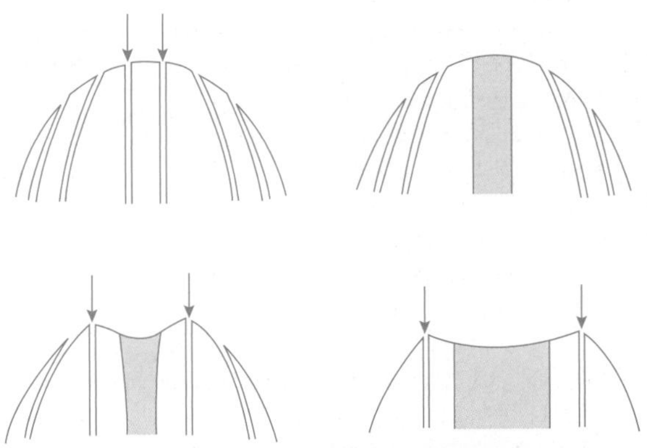

Fig. 4 Diagram of intrarenal reflux/papillae morphology. From Ransley and Risdon (1978). *British Journal of Radiology* (Fig. 33). Permission received from publishers.

Postmortem examination of kidneys from young children dying of a non-renal cause reveals similar variation in papillary form, likely to lead to intrarenal reflux in about two-thirds of kidneys (Ransley and Risdon 1975). This means that more than 90 per cent of children are likely to have at least one compound papillus capable of intrarenal reflux. This figure is higher than can be demonstrated radiologically in children with VUR (Rolleston *et al.* 1974; Uldall *et al.* 1976). A number of factors may interfere with demonstration of intrarenal reflux including timing of films, back flow of urine, or details obscured by bowel shadows. It is thus suggested that intrarenal reflux may be present more often than can be demonstrated (Ransley and Risdon 1975). There is good evidence in humans that the reflux of infected urine into the kidney in the presence of compound papillae can cause acute pyelonephritis and subsequent renal parenchymal scarring (Rolleston *et al.* 1974). The presence of both types of papillae in one kidney explains why scarring is segmental and why adjacent areas can remain pristine (Ransley and Risdon 1978) (Fig. 5). It is possible that the development of a scar can distort the intrarenal architecture to such an extent that adjacent papillae may develop intrarenal reflux leading to extension of scarring with subsequent infections. The absence of refluxing papillae may explain why some kidneys with a refluxing ureter do not scar even in the presence of infection.

Some babies born with VUR have associated dysplastic or hypoplastic renal malformations or *in utero* damage, all of which may impair renal function (Hinchcliffe *et al.* 1992; Risdon 1993). These abnormalities are usually associated with severe grades of VUR and sometimes with obstruction. It is not clear whether severe VUR is simply associated with renal abnormalities or whether there is a causal link. There is some evidence from animal work that fetal sterile reflux may impair GFR (Gobet *et al.* 1999) as well as concentrating ability (Ransley *et al.* 1987). Thus, renal abnormalities may be found on imaging, associated with VUR *in utero* but in the absence of any history of UTI. Confusingly these abnormalities may often also be referred to as scars. Therefore, when a child being investigated following a UTI is found to have abnormalities on DMSA scan it may be difficult to distinguish whether this is scarring caused by UTI or a congenital renal abnormality or both. Progressive renal impairment from dysplasia is probably not preventable and presumably results from lack of normal growth potential of abnormal renal tissue. Development of new or additional renal scarring secondary to UTI may be preventable and it is to this end that investigation and management strategies should be aimed.

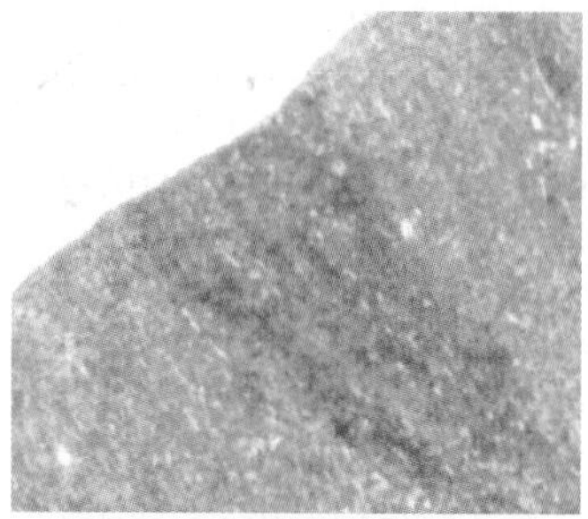

Pig kidney at low power showing a (darker staining) scarred segment reaching the renal capsule

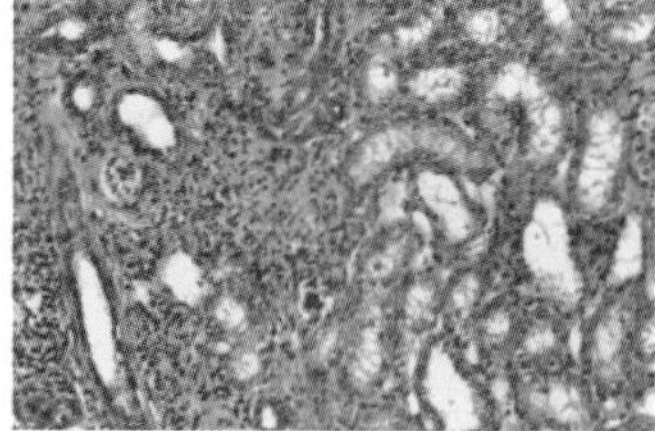

Pig kidney at high power showing the sharp junction between the scarred area on the left, and the normal tissue on the right

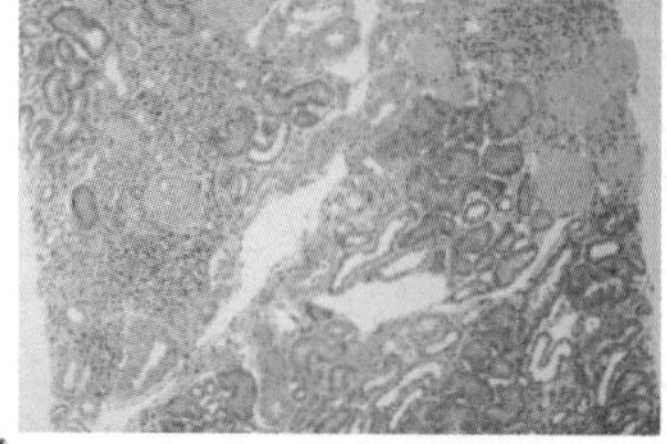

Biopsy specimen from a human kidney also showing a sharp distinction between scarred tissue to the left, and normal kidney on the right

Fig. 5 Histology of a focal scar in pig kidney and in human kidney.

Timing of scarring

The risk of scarring following a UTI varies with age, but the precise details of this are not clear. In clinical situations it is often very difficult to know at what age an individual child acquired their scars. Young children appear to be at most risk (Berg and Johansson 1983). In one study, children with normal DMSA scans after UTI were reinvestigated 2–11 years later. There were very few first scars found in children who had been older than 3 years at the time of their original DMSA, and none in those who had been older than 4 (Vernon *et al.* 1997a). The reasons for this are not clear. It has been suggested, and is widely assumed, that children's kidneys may mature, or 'grow out' of their tendency to scar. It is notable that the frequency of renal scars in children presenting with their first *documented* UTI is not related to age (Benador *et al.* 1997; Coulthard *et al.* 1997). This apparent paradox may be explained by scarring having occurred during an earlier undiagnosed UTI.

An alternative hypothesis (Coulthard 2002) is that children who are born with risk factors for developing focal renal scarring (i.e. with VUR and compound papillae that allow intrarenal reflux) are at such high risk of developing a scar that they are overwhelmingly likely to have done so by the age of 4. Currently in the United Kingdom, UTI in young children are frequently missed or treatment delayed. According to this model, most children who reach 4 years without scarring do so only by virtue of never having possessed the risk factors; hence they have no future risk.

One implication of this hypothesis is that the same proportion of children would be expected to be found to be scarred in population studies are born with risk factors. How many infants are born with risk of scarring? The precise number of babies with VUR is unknown for obvious reasons, but a summation of past studies of normal newborns subjected to cystography suggests it is about 1 per cent (Coulthard 2002). Since around 90 per cent of children have at least one compound papillus, it follows that approximately 0.9 per cent of children are born at risk. Few studies have been designed to assess population scarring rates, but they can be estimated from some. In Newcastle, 11.3 per cent of girls are investigated for a UTI by the age of 16 years, of whom 4.8 per cent are found to have focal scarring (Coulthard *et al.* 1997). Thus, at least 0.54 per cent of Newcastle girls have scars; the true figure is likely to be greater because diagnosis and referral rates are incomplete (Vernon *et al.* 1997a). This figure confirms that most girls born at risk of developing a scar do acquire one. It stands as an indictment of the past management of UTI that few children, if any, are prevented from developing a scar; it is easier to identify damage than prevent it.

Another implication of this hypothesis is that kidneys that have risk factors for scarring, but which are unscarred beyond 4 years (perhaps because of prompt treatment of UTI or use of prophylactic antibiotics) will remain at risk of developing a new scar later. There is some support for this hypothesis from animal work. Normal adult pigs whose kidneys have been protected from damage by having a non-refluxing ureter have been shown to be as vulnerable to acute segmental scarring as piglets if they are exposed experimentally to VUR and UTI (Coulthard *et al.* 2002). A parallel to this animal evidence is that unscarred adult human kidneys can acquire segmental scars after being grafted into a recipient (child or adult) who has a reflux into their transplant and develops a UTI (Howie *et al.* 2002).

These observations have important implications for infants known to have VUR but no scarring, such as babies identified by screening because of a family history of VUR (Scott *et al.* 1997). The 90 per cent of these children who are likely to have compound papillae would be expected to remain at risk of scarring until they outgrow their VUR. If correct, this theory suggests that children with VUR should be protected from scarring until they outgrow their reflux, rather than up to an arbitrary age. This would have major implications for clinical practice.

Practicalities of investigation

Preschool children

Younger children appear to be at greater risk of sustaining renal damage associated with UTI. In addition, UTI is more likely to be a marker of underlying urinary tract abnormality like severe VUR or obstruction in the very young children who therefore warrant intensive investigation. Because of the non-specific symptoms in this age group there is more likely to be a delay in treatment and diagnosis of UTI.

Older children

Older children warrant investigation after their first documented UTI because the detection of scarring does not appear to be related to age (Stokland *et al.* 1996b; Benador *et al.* 1997; Coulthard *et al.* 1997). In the United Kingdom, there is clinical experience that the first diagnosed UTI is often not the first. It is possible that UTI in later childhood may be a marker of previous risk of UTI.

Which investigations?

An intensive investigation programme, for example, of abdominal X-ray, DMSA scan, renal ultrasound, and micturating cystourethrogram (MCUG) for all children with a UTI would identify those with renal damage and risk factors like VUR or urethral abnormalities. However, UTI is so common that many children with no urinary tract abnormalities would be subjected to invasive investigations without benefit. Therefore, ideally one would like to be able to identify children who are at high risk of renal damage and thus of long-term sequelae, and only investigate them. Some units try to identify those with *upper* versus *lower* UTI. However clinical features are non-specific and not closely related to findings on imaging particularly in younger children. There is also conflicting evidence on the association of parameters such as C-reactive protein with scarring (Jakobsson *et al.* 1994; Stokland *et al.* 1996b).

There is an association, which is widely accepted, between renal scarring and VUR. The more severe the VUR the more likely the chance of finding scarring. However, the converse is not true. Renal scarring is widely found in kidneys drained by a ureter not found to be refluxing. The evaluation and investigation of VUR and its relationship to scarring is problematic. There are anomalies that are difficult to explain. There may be renal involvement on early DMSA (done at the time of infection) that does not go on to leave a permanent scar. However, when permanent scars do form, they do localize to the same site as the acute involvement. We do not fully understand what factors are involved in resolution of acute renal involvement as opposed to progression to permanent scarring. There may be renal involvement on acute DMSA but no evidence of VUR. This is one of the many unresolved questions surrounding the relationship of VUR, UTI, and scarring. However, both research and clinical evaluation and management are hampered by the nature of the techniques available to study it and by the intermittent, fluctuating nature of VUR itself.

Techniques commonly used for investigating the renal tract may have particular problems when used in children.

Ultrasonography

Ultrasound is widely available and has the advantage of involving no ionizing radiation. Because differences in density are clearly demonstrated, it is good for detecting structural abnormalities (e.g. dilated kidneys and ureters, cysts in kidneys). It can be used to detect parenchymal abnormalities but in childhood scars are often small and frequently missed. The main disadvantage is that the technique is very operator and situation dependant so what can theoretically be detected in a research centre under optimal conditions may not be replicated in practice particularly if the subject is not cooperative. Colour flow imaging may prove useful in detection of VUR. The findings on ultrasound cannot easily be reviewed retrospectively from still pictures.

DMSA scan

DMSA renal scans are very useful for detection of scarring (Fig. 6). Differential renal function is provided (though this is proximal tubular function, it corresponds well with GFR). Original data can be easily reviewed for second opinions, reporting of difficult studies, and comparison with previous or later studies. The technique can be standardized. The main disadvantages are that an intravenous injection is required and the patient receives a dose of ionizing radiation. The dose is small compared to the background radiation dose. Timing is important: a DMSA scan during or soon after acute infection may show areas of reduced uptake, which may not be permanent scars but may be mistakenly interpreted as scars. Thus, most units advise delaying DMSA scan for 2–3 months postacute UTI, though some suggest longer. DMSA scans are sometimes difficult to interpret especially in babies or if the position of the kidney is abnormal.

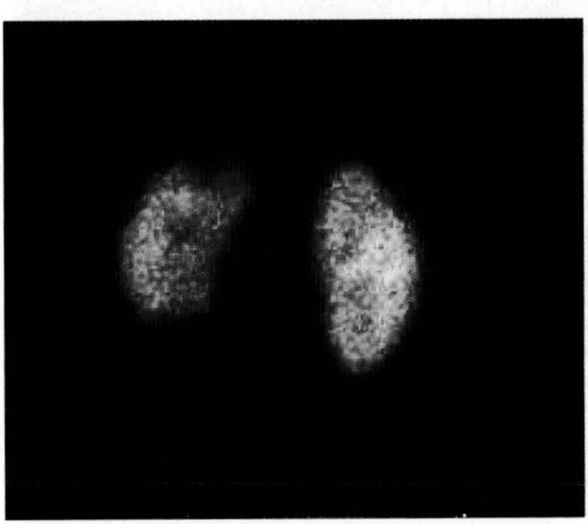

Fig. 6 DMSA scan showing unilateral focal scarring.

MCUG direct-contrast study

This investigation shows details of anatomy including bladder, urethra, and ureters, which may be of particular importance in excluding bladder outflow obstruction in male infants with UTI. Timing and grade of VUR are demonstrated and intrarenal reflux may be seen (Fig. 7). The main disadvantage is that it requires the insertion of a bladder catheter, and delivers ionizing radiation to the gonads. The test may fail to demonstrate intermittent VUR and many units advocate filling the bladder twice. Children dislike catherization and many find it difficult to micturate on demand during the investigation.

MCUG direct radioisotope study

This investigation delivers a lower radiation dose than contrast MCUG; prolonged imaging can be performed and therefore this procedure may detect intermittent VUR. Unfortunately, the investigation still requires the insertion of a bladder catheter. In addition, the anatomy is not defined, grading of reflux not possible, dilatation of ureters not easily seen and reflux into a ureter but not up to the kidney may be missed.

Indirect radioisotope study

This study is appealing because no bladder catheter is required, though an intravenous injection is, and there is a lower radiation dose than contrast MCUG. However, there is a substantial false-negative rate; no anatomical information is provided. Filling phase reflux (which occurs in some patients without micturition reflux) cannot be assessed.

Abdominal X-ray

Abdominal X-ray is useful for localization of stones in selective cases (e.g. *Proteus* infection) or where there is a suggestive history. In addition, spinal defects may be identified and constipation demonstrated.

Intravenous urography

Intravenous urography (IVU) can be useful for distinguishing anatomy when this is unclear from DMSA and ultrasonography, for example, in the demonstration of a scar in a duplex or horseshoe kidney. However, there is the radiation dose associated with multiple X-rays; scars are only demonstrated a number of months or years after occurrence. Scars on anterior and posterior surfaces of the kidney are often missed. The injection of contrast is unpleasant (metallic taste, flushing, etc.), and there is a small anaphylaxis risk. Acute tubular necrosis can occur if the patient is prepared by withholding fluids but poor pictures obtained if the patient is not prepared. Whilst IVU was previously a common investigation, it should not now be routinely used for investigation of children after a UTI. It may be useful in rare specific cases.

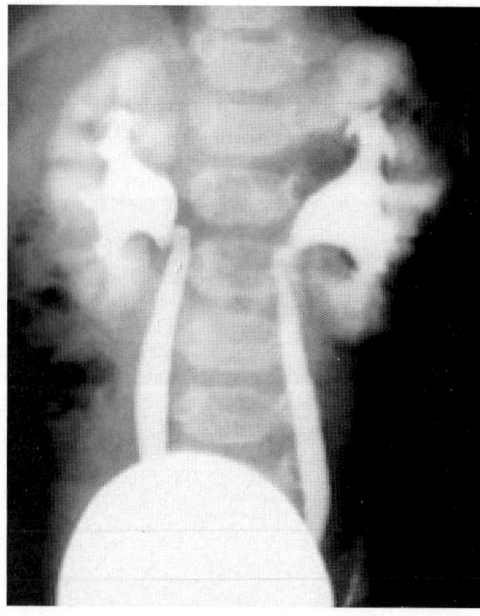

Fig. 7 MCUG showing intrarenal reflux.

General comments

Improved imaging and resolution as well as reductions in radiation doses are resulting from technological advances. Transfer of results and images between centres is frequently required for 'second opinions' and shared care. Increasingly, this can be done electronically. Images are susceptible to change by alteration of settings and use of different equipment. For example, interpretation of DMSA scans done in different centres with unfamiliar formats is sometimes difficult. In that situation it is often necessary to return to the raw data of the test. Ease of review of investigations varies. For example, the image obtained during a DMSA scan reflects the full examination whereas ultrasound is reported in real-time and mostly the pictures obtained only reflect 'highlights' of the examination.

Anatomical variants may yield misleading results which are difficult to interpret and may require comparison of more than one investigation. For example, horseshoe kidney may not be detected on ultrasound but is clearly seen on DMSA; a duplex kidney on DMSA may simply be reflected by an abnormal split function on DMSA but the anatomy will often be clarified on ultrasonography. Occasionally, additional investigations such as IVU or magnetic resonance imaging (MRI) may be useful to aid diagnosis.

A pragmatic approach to planning investigations

Clinicians need to be aware of the limitations of any combination of tests in order to interpret them intelligently. It is also important to acknowledge there is no single test that answers all the essential questions in a child who has had a UTI.

Detection of scars by DMSA scan or ultrasonography

There are several comparisons of DMSA scan and ultrasonography for detecting scars which report a widely varying degree of concurrence (Roebuck *et al.* 1999). The overall view, for which there is much evidence, is that there is good agreement for widespread and diffuse scarring but that ultrasonography misses focal scars (Tasker *et al.* 1993; Smellie *et al.* 1995). Ultrasonography is extremely operator dependent. However, under research conditions, in experienced hands with the best equipment and sufficient time, and with a cooperative subject, ultrasonography can detect scars as well as a DMSA scan (Barry *et al.* 1998). Routine clinical settings do not usually recreate these conditions in practice. Currently, DMSA should be used in most units for detection of scars in children.

Detection of reflux

There is no ideal test for detection of VUR. The contrast MCUG is often described as the gold standard but it has limitations. It only shows whether VUR exists over a very short period of time; it is unphysiological because of the presence of a catheter; and the child is unlikely to be relaxed. The use of general anaesthetics or sedatives for insertion of the catheter is controversial, but is likely to make the test less physiological unless the effect of drugs used has worn off. Since VUR is known to be a fluctuating and intermittent phenomenon, repeat filling of the bladder is often advocated. Contrast MCUG is the only study to give good anatomical details and should be the investigation of choice in young babies especially males to exclude urethral abnormalities. It is the only technique providing information on the grade of VUR. This is an important consideration since the risk of renal scarring and probability of resolution of VUR can be predicted from the grade at the outset (Elder *et al.* 1997). Thus, the grade may alter subsequent management.

Direct radionuclide cystography has the main advantage of being able to scan the child over a longer period of time with less radiation than a contrast MCUG. It may therefore detect intermittent VUR more often but may miss lower grades of VUR (Poli-Merol *et al.* 1998). These studies require bladder catheterization and the child to micturate on demand in a strange environment without privacy which may cause considerable problems. Attempts to quantify VUR detected on nuclear cystography have shown it not to predict outcome (Barthold *et al.* 1999). The arguments for using indirect radionuclide cystography are compelling because of the major advantage of not requiring bladder catheterization. However, it has a number of drawbacks and is generally considered less reliable. The test is unable to assess filling phase reflux which occurs in some patients without micturition reflux. Studies showing high sensitivity and specificity have been done on highly selected patients (Gordon *et al.* 1990) and other units have found difficulty reproducing these results when applied to the general population of patients with UTI. It has been shown to have a high false-negative rate (DeSadeleer *et al.* 1994). It is therefore considered useful if VUR is demonstrated but does not reliably exclude it. Modifications of technique and careful selection of patients may improve reliability.

Contrast enhanced ultrasonography is a new technique which still requires bladder catheterization for introduction of sonicated albumin or saline but avoids a radiation dose. Controversial results have been reported using colour flow Doppler to detect VUR. Neither of these ultrasound techniques has been fully evaluated.

Suggested investigation scheme

Aged 0–1 year

There is general consensus about investigation of these children (Royal College of Physicians 1991; American Academy of Pediatrics 1999b; Pilling and Postlethwaite 1996). They should have an early ultrasonography to detect anatomical detail; an MCUG for detection and grading of VUR and anatomical detail of bladder and urethra, together with a DMSA scan after at least a 2-month interval for detection of renal scarring. The detection of abnormalities of the urinary tract is higher, the younger the child. Very young children appear to be at highest risk of sustaining permanent renal damage. Therefore, the opportunities for prevention of initial or extending damage are high.

Aged 1–5 years

There is no clear consensus on investigation of this age group. The Guidelines issued by the Royal College of Physicians (1991) did not give clear advice and since then a consensus has not been established. Most centres would agree that all children in this age group with a proven UTI should be investigated because UTI may be a marker of underlying urinary tract abnormality and is associated with renal scarring. Ultrasonography and DMSA are the most widely used and logical tests. Ideally, one would like to know if these children have VUR (and intrarenal reflux). However, the only test currently available which has been shown to reliably demonstrate VUR in this age group is the contrast or direct isotope cystogram. Both of these involve catheterization and thus most centres are selective, reserving it for those with recurrent UTIs or those with scarring or other abnormalities seen on DMSA or ultrasonography, or those with a family history of VUR, or a personal history of antenatal renal dilatation.

This selective investigation plan has much to recommend at the present state of knowledge. It can, however, be criticized for not identifying children at risk of scarring kidneys at a subsequent UTI. Thus, if this selective approach is adopted it is essential that the families and their primary healthcare providers understand they should maintain a high index of suspicion for subsequent UTI and if another occurs further investigation in the form of a further DMSA and/or MCUG considered. The younger the child the more important it is to consider performing an MCUG.

Older children

One of the problems in investigating older children is judging whether the first *recognized* UTI is actually the first; often it is not. In children presenting with their first diagnosed UTI the rate of discovery of scars is similar at all ages (Coulthard *et al.* 1997). Thus, a test for scarring would seem to be the logical starting point for investigation of these children. Many people have suggested there is only the need to perform an ultrasonography. However, as already discussed, this misses scars in many situations and should not be relied on as the sole investigation (Smellie and Rigden 1995; Smellie *et al.* 1995). Thus, we would recommend a DMSA scan and an ultrasonography, unless routine ultrasonography in a particular unit or centre has been shown not to miss scars.

There is some evidence that if children get to the age of four without scarring their urinary tracts then they are statistically unlikely to develop first scarring after that age (Vernon *et al.* 1997a). In older children, it therefore makes sense to only look for VUR in those who have evidence of scarring. This is important because scarring may lead to local distortion of the intrarenal architecture predisposing adjacent areas to intrarenal reflux. Thus, children with renal scarring who have VUR may be at risk of extending the scar, if they develop a UTI.

The child with evidence of scarring diagnosed at any age

When scarring is first detected it is not possible to determine at what age that scar occurred. There is, as discussed above, evidence that the vast majority of novel scarring takes place within the first 4 years of life. There is also evidence that once a scar is present, progression of that scarring may develop at any age. Progression of scarring is presumed to occur because the conditions of intrarenal reflux and VUR are still present and in the face of infection further renal damage may occur. In addition, scarring itself distorts the intrarenal architecture and may make it more likely that adjacent areas of the kidney will have intrarenal reflux and be susceptible to scarring in the face of infection. Thus, it is logical to need to know whether there is still VUR present, with the intention of trying to prevent further damage from UTI in those with VUR. However, many shy away from this approach because of the nature of current methods of assessing or testing for reflux.

What is clear is that if there was a less invasive, low radiation, and reliable technique for detecting VUR, children would be investigated in a more logical way and also our ignorance about the natural history of VUR and it relationship to scarring would be improved.

The child with scarring but no VUR

Whilst it is clear that VUR is a major risk factor for the development of renal scarring, many children are found to have a scarred kidney but no evidence of VUR (Rushton *et al.* 1992).

A number of theories are proposed to explain this. In many cases the child had VUR but has now grown out of it. In a few cases the child has VUR but the test may fail to detect it. The diagnosis may be wrong, the child having dysplasia or hypoplasia rather than reflux. It is possible that infection can ascend in the absence of demonstrable VUR or that scarring can be caused by some mechanism other than ascending infection, for example, blood-borne infection, local toxin release. Resolution of reflux with time may be the correct explanation in many cases when scarring is discovered at initial investigation but the timing of the development of scarring is not known. However, there are sufficient anomalies, for example, when there is evidence of acute involvement of the kidney in the absence of VUR (Rushton *et al.* 1992), to require an open mind to be kept about the nature of the relationship of VUR and scarring.

Suggested simplified investigation scheme

Aged 0–1 year

- Ultrasonography
- DMSA
- MCUG

Aged over 1 year

- DMSA
- Ultrasonography

with urinary surveillance and/or high index of suspicion for UTI over the following 1–2 years

Plus

perform a locally reliable test for VUR if

- renal scar (any age)
- more than one UTI (aged under 4 years)
- family history of VUR (aged under 4 years)

In addition

- consider repeat DMSA scan if further UTI (if aged under 4 years at initial investigation)

In addition, consider performing an abdominal X-ray if

- history suggests stones
- proteus infection

Timing of Investigations

Ultrasonography

Ultrasonography can be performed in the acute phase or subsequently. Severe acute pyelonephritis may cause the kidney to appear 'bright' and/or enlarged on ultrasonography. These changes may be focal.

MCUG

There is no need to delay MCUG once the initial UTI is treated. There is suggestion but no good evidence that there is an increased detection of VUR at the time of UTI. Even if this hypothesis was correct then the patient is at risk of VUR at the very time it may be important. MCUG should often be arranged before discharge in those admitted for UTI to reduce non-attendance (McDonald *et al.* 2000).

DMSA

The question of timing of the DMSA scan is interesting. If DMSA is performed at the time of UTI then a large proportion will show some defects (Jakobsson *et al.* 1992; Rosenberg *et al.* 1992; Stokland *et al.* 1996a). However, only about 50 per cent of those defects will be still there more than 2 months later (Jakobsson *et al.* 1992; Benador *et al.* 1994). It is important therefore that the clinician is aware of the timing of the DMSA scan in relation to the acute infection in any individual case. In the piglet model of acute pyelonephritis, DMSA is highly specific and sensitive in diagnosing pathologically proven pyelonephritis (Rushton *et al.* 1988; Parkhouse *et al.* 1989). Whilst if permanent scars occur they localize to the site of the acute defect, acute defects do not predict for those with VUR, and we do not understand the factors involved in resolution of acute changes versus progression to permanent scarring. Whilst acute DMSA is clearly useful in a research setting, its place in the routine clinical investigation of children with UTI is not yet established. In order to show *permanent* scarring reliably, DMSA should be performed at least 2–3 months after a UTI, though some suggest a longer interval (Jakobsson and Svensson 1997).

The child with a family history of VUR

This is a very important group of children, who are at high risk of developing UTI and reflux nephropathy, in whom there is the possibility of preventative management. VUR is a genetic disorder (Feather 2000) and there is evidence of a 20–50 times increased risk of VUR in children with a family history of VUR (Scott *et al.* 1997; Jacobson *et al.* 1999). Children with UTI who have a family history of VUR probably warrant more intensive investigation than those without. Routine screening for VUR in asymptomatic siblings or offspring of individuals with VUR would appear to be justified to identify those at greatest risk of subsequent renal damage. As well as offering an opportunity to prevent renal damage in this group, careful surveillance may provide further information and insight into the natural history of VUR and the relationship of UTI, VUR, and scarring. Currently, our own policy is to offer investigation, with MCUG and DMSA scan, to newborn siblings or offspring of patients with VUR or reflux nephropathy. Older children, over 4 years, with a similar family history are offered a DMSA scan, with an ultrasonography and MCUG only for those who have been symptomatic or who have an abnormality on DMSA scan. Those with ages in between have a variable investigation plan.

Whilst it is obvious that early detection and treatment of UTI in this high-risk group is important in preventing renal scarring, the ideal form of management is not known. It is clear that increased knowledge and awareness through education of parents and healthcare attendants is important. However, it remains to be shown whether screening first-degree relatives for VUR offers advantages over increasing awareness of parents and healthcare professionals that first-degree relatives are a high-risk group in whom there should be a high index of suspicion for UTI. When asymptomatic children are found to have VUR through screening because of family history, it is not known whether treatment with prophylactic antibiotics offers any advantage over high index of suspicion and prompt treatment, nor how long antibiotics should be continued for. It has been suggested that early surgical treatment of severe VUR detected on screening may prevent renal damage but prospective studies are required to confirm this (Sweeney *et al.* 2001).

Long-term management

A culture of education and partnership with families should be encouraged. Parents generally want the best for their children and this motivation can be harnessed by increasing their understanding of the medical issues.

Information and education of families is important in suspicion and detection of UTI, and with compliance with treatment. It is therefore important within organizations to develop systems that empower parents. Parents will often be more assiduous at tasks like urine collection than healthcare professionals.

Important points about issues such as investigation plans or VUR should be backed up with written information whenever feasible, since it is well recognized that people absorb only a fraction of a clinic discussion.

Management of VUR

Historically, both medical and surgical management strategies for VUR have been introduced without controlled studies documenting long-term benefit.

Resolution of VUR with time

Resolution of VUR over time with medical treatment is related to the grade of VUR and the age of the patient. In general, a lower grade of reflux has a better chance of spontaneous resolution. A review of studies on nearly 2000 patients suggests that for children with grades I or II reflux there is resolution in about 50 per cent after 2 years and in about 80–90 per cent after 5 years. For grade III reflux increasing age at presentation and bilateral reflux decrease the probability of resolution. Bilateral grades IV and V refluxes have the poorest chance, with spontaneous resolution in less than 20 per cent of patients after 5 years (Elder *et al.* 1997). It is not known whether urine infection affects resolution of VUR but in monkeys there is some evidence it may delay normal resolution (Roberts 1992).

Medical management

Since it is known that in the vast majority of cases VUR will resolve with time, the aim in medical management of VUR, with prophylactic antibiotics, is to prevent recurrent (or sometimes first) UTI and consequent renal scarring, whilst waiting for resolution of VUR. There is some evidence that antibiotic prophylaxis does provide protection against recurrent UTI, with less than 50 per cent having a recurrence in a 5-year follow-up (Lohr *et al.* 1977; Smellie 1978; Jodal 1992; Olbing *et al.* 1992; Weiss *et al.* 1992). However, there is still uncertainty as to the effectiveness of prophylaxis (Williams *et al.* 2001) and there are no prospective randomized trials of prophylaxis compared to controls receiving no medication but supervision and urinary surveillance. Breakthrough infections may be problematic and may be due to non-compliance or true bacterial resistance. Trimethoprim, nitrofurantoin, or cephalexin are frequently used for prophylaxis.

Probably only between one-third and two-thirds of patients are compliant with prophylaxis (Smyth and Judd 1993). Patient and family understanding of the underlying reasoning and purpose of prophylaxis are essential in encouraging compliance. Non-compliance should be suspected when the infecting organism is sensitive to the prophylactic antibiotic prescribed.

Whilst the aim of prophylaxis is to obtain high concentration of the antibiotic in the urine with minimal effect on normal body flora, there is little data on the effect of long-term antibiotic prophylaxis on bowel and periurethral flora or on drug resistance in the community.

Optimum duration of prophylaxis is not known; some propose a fixed time period or up to a certain age. However, new evidence about the continued susceptibility of vulnerable kidneys to scarring suggests that active medical treatment, whether antibiotic prophylaxis or close urinary surveillance, should continue as long as VUR persists. There are small reports and clinical experience of antibiotic prophylaxis being successfully discontinued in some highly selected groups of children with persistent VUR (Cooper *et al.* 2000). However, there is no real evidence that helps in answering the difficult and important question of how long to continue antibiotic prophylaxis when VUR does not resolve.

Surgical management

There are two main forms of surgical treatment of VUR, endoscopic subureteric injection and reimplantation.

Endoscopic subureteric injection

Injection of tissue-augmenting substances is done under general anaesthetic and requires only a short stay (or day case) in hospital. The success rate in abolition of VUR varies with the centre, the material used, the timing of re-evaluation, and test used in re-examination.

Use of polytetraflouroethylene (teflon) or silicon has a success rate of 70–90 per cent (Elder *et al.* 1997) and a recurrence rate of 5–10 per cent. Use of collagen has a success rate of around 60 per cent and dextranomer, 60–90 per cent (Lackgren *et al.* 1999). The term STING (initially referring to the technique when Teflon is injected) is frequently used generically to refer to this type of procedure. The technique is very operator dependent. There is a lack of controlled studies of the technique and studies have included large numbers of grades I and II VUR which tend to have spontaneous resolution of VUR. There are concerns regarding long-term effects including migration of foreign materials. The longevity of the treatment and need for repeat are not fully known.

Reimplantation

Surgical success in curing VUR with reimplantation is high, greater than 95 per cent overall. The success rate is greater than 98 per cent in grades of reflux I–IV but dropping to 80 per cent with grade V (Elder *et al.* 1997). This is, however, a major operation requiring a stay of several days in hospital with the associated risks and costs. The likelihood of obstruction following reimplantation surgery is in the region of 2 per cent (Elder *et al.* 1997).

Comparison of medical versus surgical treatment for VUR

Two large multicentre prospective trials of medical versus surgical treatment for children with severe VUR do not show superiority of either treatment (International Reflux Study Committee 1981; Birmingham Reflux Study Group 1987; Olbing *et al.* 1992; Smellie *et al.* 1992; Weiss *et al.* 1992). Neither surgical nor medical treatment appears to completely protect against progression of scarring, though apparent progression may result from contraction of a scar or a differential rate of growth of normal versus scarred kidney tissue. Although the incidence of further UTI was similar in the medically and surgically treated groups there was a reduction in clinical pyelonephritis in the surgical group, though no difference in renal scarring. Surgical correction of VUR does not appear to improve the outcome for renal function in children with severe VUR and bilateral nephropathy (Smellie *et al.* 2001). There is little evidence regarding the optimum management in cases where severe VUR is detected by screening. Retrospective data suggest that the outcome might be better for infants with grades IV or V reflux detected without UTI and treated surgically, though there are no prospective randomized studies on this subgroup yet (Sweeney *et al.* 2001).

The choice of treatment therefore remains an individual judgement that will be based on a number of factors. Breakthrough infection, despite medical treatment or because of non-compliance, remains a commonly used factor for consideration of surgical treatment, as does deterioration of DMSA appearance. There is an understandable reluctance to continue prophylactic antibiotics indefinitely and a finality about successful surgical treatment of VUR which is appealing if VUR does not resolve spontaneously. Where there is no clear evidence of superiority of one treatment then patient and parental preference will clearly be a major factor.

Management plan for a child found to have a scar

- Establish whether they have VUR.
- Prevent UTI (and extension of scarring) whilst VUR persists, for example, antibiotic prophylaxis.
- Consider surgical treatment in some situations, for example, if medical management fails; breakthrough infections; non-compliance.
- Initiate lifetime blood pressure monitoring.
- Discuss familial nature of VUR and increased risk in siblings; future siblings; parents; future offspring.

Conclusion

UTI is common and may be associated with renal abnormalities and significant long-term sequelae in a minority of cases. There are many unanswered questions about the relationship of VUR, UTI, and scarring and there is debate about the best investigation and management strategies. Since currently in the United Kingdom most children with scarring already have it at the time of first investigation, it is likely that the greatest potential for prevention of renal damage lies in increased awareness. This should lead to improved diagnosis and more urgent treatment of young children with UTI in primary healthcare. Children with a family history of reflux or reflux nephropathy are at high risk of developing UTI and renal scarring. Therefore, increased awareness amongst adult physicians and nephrologists is important in education of patients of the risks to their offspring and the potential for preventative action.

Key points

- Childhood UTI is associated with significant long-term sequelae in some individuals.
- Increased awareness, early diagnosis, and rapid treatment of childhood UTI is essential in preventing renal damage.
- Accurate diagnosis of UTI is vital.
- All urine collecting methods may result in contamination.
- Antibiotics should be started as soon as a suitable urine sample has been collected.
- Children should be investigated after a first UTI.
- VUR is familial.

References

American Academy of Pediatrics (1999a). Circumcision policy statement. *Pediatrics* **103**, 686–693.

American Academy of Pediatrics (1999b). Practice parameter: the diagnosis, treatment, and evaluation of the initial urinary tract infection in febrile infants and young children. *Pediatrics* **103**, 843–852.

Anderson, N. *et al.* (1997). Vesicoureteric reflux in the newborn: relationship to fetal renal pelvic diameter. *Pediatric Nephrology* **11**, 610–616.

Aronson, A. S., Gustafson, B., and Svenningsen, N. W. (1973). Combined suprapubic aspiration and clean-voided urine examination in infants and children. *Acta Paediatrica Scandinavica* **62**, 396–400.

Barry, B. *et al.* (1998). Improved ultrasound detection of renal scarring in children following urinary tract infection. *Clinical Radiology* **53**, 747–751.

Barthold, J. *et al.* (1999). Quantitative nuclear cystography does not predict outcome in patients with primary vesicoureteral reflux. *Journal of Urology* **162**, 1193–1196.

Benador, D. *et al.* (1994). Cortical scintigraphy in the evaluation of renal parenchymal changes in children with pyelonephritis. *Journal of Pediatrics* **124**, 17–20.

Benador, D. *et al.* (1997). Are children at highest risk of renal sequelae after pyelonephritis? *Lancet* **349**, 17–19.

Berg, U. and Johansson, S. (1983). Age as a main determinant of renal functional damage in urinary tract infection. *Archives of Disease in Childhood* **58**, 963–969.

Birmingham Reflux Study Group (1987). Prospective trail of operative versus non-operative treatment of severe vesicoureteric reflux in children: five years' observation. *British Medical Journal* **295**, 237–241.

Blethyn, A. *et al.* (1995). Radiological evidence of constipation in urinary tract infection. *Archives of Diseases in Childhood* **73**, 534–535.

Chandra, M. and Maddix, H. (2000). Urodynamic dysfunction in infants with vesicoureteral reflux. *Journal of Pediatrics* **136** (6), 754–759.

Cooper, C. *et al.* (2000). The outcome of stopping prophylactic antibiotics in older children with vesicoureteral reflux. *Journal of Urology* **163**, 269.

Coulthard, M. G. (2002). Do kidneys outgrow the risk of reflux nephropathy? *Pediatric Nephrology* **17**, 477–480.

Coulthard, M., Lambert, H., and Keir, M. (1997). Occurence of renal scars in children after their first referral for urinary tract infection. *British Medical Journal* **315**, 918–919.

Coulthard, M. G., Flecknell, P., Orr, H., Manas, D., and O'Donnel, M. (2002). Renal scarring caused by vesicoureteric reflux and urinary infection: a study in pigs. *Pediatric Nephrology* **17**, 481–484.

Coulthard, M. G., Vernon, S. J., Lambert, H. J., and Matthews, J. N. S. (2003). A nurse led education and direct access service for the management of urinary tract infections in children: prospective controlled trial. *British Medical Journal* **327**, 656–659.

Craig, J. *et al.* (2000). Does treatment of vesicoureteric reflux in childhood prevent end-stage renal disease attributable to reflux nephropathy. *Pediatrics* **105**, 1236–1241.

Davison, J. (2001). Renal disorders in pregnancy. *Current Opinion in Obstetrics and Gynaecology* **13**, 109–114.

Deleau, J. *et al.* (1994). Chronic renal failure in children: an epidemiological survey in Lorraine (France) 1975–1990. *Pediatric Nephrology* **8**, 472–476.

DeSadeleer, C. *et al.* (1994). How good is technetium-99m mercaptoacetyltriglycine indirect cystography? *European Journal of Nuclear Medicine* **21**, 223–227.

Dick, P. and Feldman, W. (1996). Routine diagnostic imaging for childhood urinary tract infections: a systematic overview. *Journal of Pediatrics* **128**, 15–22.

Dohil, R. *et al.* (1994). Constipation and reversible urinary tract abnormalities. *Archives of Diseases in Childhood* **56**, 56–57.

Ekman, H. *et al.* (1966). High diuresis, a factor in preventing vesicoureteric reflux. *Journal of Urology* **95**, 511–515.

Elder, J. *et al.* (1997). Pediatric vesicoureteral reflux guidelines panel summary report on the management of primary vesicoureteral reflux in children. *Journal of Urology* **157**, 1846–1851.

Esbjorner, E. (1997). Epidemiology of chronic renal failure in children: a report from Sweden 1986–1994. *Pediatric Nephrology* **11**, 438–442.

Feather, S. (2000). Primary, nonsyndromic vesicoureteric reflux is genetically heterogeneous with a locus on chromosome 1. *American Journal of Human Genetics* **66**, 1420–1425.

Gobet, R. *et al.* (1999). Experimental fetal vesicoureteral reflux induces renal tubular and glomerular damage and is associated with persistant bladder instability. *Journal of Urology* **162**, 1090–1095.

Godley, M., Risdon, R., and Ransley, P. (1989). Effect of unilateral vesicoureteric reflux on renal growth and the uptake of 99mTc DMSA by the kidney. An experimental study in the minipig. *British Journal of Urology* **63**, 340–347.

Goonasekera, C. and Dillon, M. (1998). Reflux nephropathy and hypertension. *Journal of Human Hypertension* **12**, 497–504.

Gordon, I., Peters, A., and Morony, S. (1990). Indirect radionuclide cystography: a sensitive technique for the detection of vesico-ureteral reflux. *Pediatric Nephrology* **4**, 604–606.

Hansson, S. *et al.* (1998). Low bacterial counts in infants with urinary tract infection. *Journal of Pediatrics* **132**, 180–182.

Hardy, J. D., Furnell, P. M., and Brumfitt, W. (1976). Comparison of sterile bag, clean catch and suprapubic aspiration in the diagnosis of urinary infection in early childhood. *British Journal of Urology* **48**, 279–283.

Hellström, A.-L. *et al.* (1991). Association between urinary symptoms at 7 years old and previous urinary tract infection. *Archives of Disease in Childhood* **66**, 232–234.

Hellström, M. and Jacobsson, B. (1999). Diagnosis of vesico-ureteric reflux. *Acta Paediatrica* **88** (Suppl.), 3–12.

Hinchcliffe S. A. *et al.* (1992). Renal hypoplasia and postnatally acquired loss in children and vesicoureteral reflux. *Pediatric Nephrology* **6**, 439–444.

Howie, A. J., Buist, L. J., and Coulthard, M. G. (2002). Reflux nephropathy in transplants. *Pediatric Nephrology* **17**, 485–490.

Imam, A., Roberts E., Verrier Jones, K., and Jenkins, H. R. (1998). Chronic renal failure in children in Wales: a prospective epidemiological study 1994–1997. *Pediatric Nephrology* **12**, C182.

International Reflux Study Committee (1981). Medical versus surgical treatment of primary vesico-ureteral reflux. *Pediatrics* **67**, 392–400.

Jacobson, S., Hansson, S., and Jakobsson, B. (1999). Vesico-ureteric reflux: occurence and long-term risks. *Acta Paediatrica* **431** (Suppl.), 22–33.

Jadresic, L. *et al.* (1993). Investigation of urinary tract infection in childhood. *British Medical Journal* **307**, 761–764.

Jakobsson, B. and Svensson, L. (1997). Transient pyelonephritic changes on 99m technetium-dimercaptosuccinic acid scan for at least five months after infection. *Acta Paediatrica* **86**, 803–807.

Jakobsson, B., Soderlundh, S., and Berg, U. (1992). Diagnostic significance of 99mTc-dimercaptosuccinic acid (DMSA) scintigraphy in urinary tract infection. *Archives of Diseases of Childhood* **67**, 1338–1342.

Jakobsson, B., Berg, U., and Svensson, L. (1994). Renal scarring after acute pyelonephritis. *Archives of Diseases in Childhood* **70**, 111–115.

Jakobsson, B., Esbjorner, E., and Hansson, S. (1999). Minimum incidence and diagnostic rate of first urinary tract infection. *Pediatrics* **104**, 222–226.

Jantunen, M. E. *et al.* (2000). Genomic identity of pyelonephritic *Escherichia coli* isolated from blood, urine and faeces of children with urpsepsis. *Pediatric Nephrology* **14**, C42.

Jepson, R. G., Mihaljevic, L., and Craig, J. (2001). Cranberries for preventing urinary tract infections. *Cochrane Database of Systematic Reviews* (3), CD001321.

Jewkes, F. E. M. *et al.* (1990). Home collection of urine specimens-boric acid bottles or dipslides? *Archives of Disease in Childhood* **65**, 286–289.

Jodal, U. (1987). The natural history of bacteruria in childhood. *Infectious Disease Clinics of North America* **1**, 713–729.

Jodal, U., Koskimies, O., Hanson, E., Lohr, G., Olbing, H., Smellie, J., and Tamminen-Mobius, T. (1992). Infection pattern in children with vesicoureteral reflux randomly allocated to operation or long-term antibacterial prophylaxis. The International Reflux Study in Children. *Journal of Urology* **148**, 1650–1652.

Kass, E. H. (1956). Asymptomatic infections of the urinary tract. *Transactions of the Association of American Physicians* **69**, 65–63.

Koff, S., Wagner, T., and Jayanthi, V. (1998). The relationship among dysfunctional elimination syndromes, primary vesicoureteral reflux and urinary tract infections in children. *Journal of Urology* **160**, 1019–1022.

Kumar, R. K., Turner, G. M., and Coulthard, M. G. (1996). Don't count on urinary white cells to diagnose childhood urinary tract infection. *British Medical Journal* **312**, 1359.

Lackgren, G., Wahlin, N., and Stenberg, A. (1999). Endoscopic treatment of children with vesico ureteric reflux. *Acta Paediatrica* **431** (Suppl.), 62–71.

Liaw, L. C. T. *et al.* (2000). Home collection of urine for culture from infants by three methods: survey of parents' preferences and bacterial contamination rates. *British Medical Journal* **320**, 1312–1313.

Lindheimer, M., Davison, J., and Katz, A. (2001). The kidney and hypertension in pregnancy: twenty exciting years. *Seminars in Nephrology* **21**, 173–189.

Loening-Bauche, V. (1997). Urinary incontinence and urinary tract infection and their resolution with treatment of chronic constipation of childhood. *Pediatrics* **100**, 228–232.

Lohr, J. *et al.* (1977). Prevention of recurrent urinary tract infections in girls. *Pediatrics* **59**, 562–565.

Macfarlane, P. I., Houghton, C., and Hughes, C. (1999). Pad urine collection for early childhood urinary-tract infection. *Lancet* **354**, 571.

Mansfield, J. *et al.* (1995). Complications of pregnancy in women after childhood reimplantation for vesicoureteral reflux: an update with 25 years of followup. *Journal of Urology* **154**, 787–790.

Marild, S. and Jodal, U. (1998). Incidence rate of first-time symptomatic urinary tract infection in children under 6 years of age. *Acta Paediatrica* **87**, 549–552.

Martinell, J., Jodal, U., and Lindin-Janson, G. (1990). Pregnancies in women with and without renal scarring and urinary infections in childhood. *British Medical Journal* **300**, 840–844.

McDonald, A. *et al.* (2000). Voiding cystourethrograms and urinary tract infections: how long to wait? *Pediatrics* **105**, 851–852.

McGladdery, S. *et al.* (1992). Outcome of pregnancy in an Oxford–Cardiff cohort of women with previuos bacteriuria. *Quarterly Journal of Medicine* **84**, 533–539.

Miller, T. and Phillips, S. (1981). Pyelonephritis: the relationship between infection, renal scarring and antimicrobial therapy. *Kidney International* **19**, 654–662.

Mond, N. C., Grüneberg, R. N., and Smellie, J. M. (1970). Study of childhood urinary tract infection in general practice. *British Medical Journal* **i**, 602–605.

Mulvey, M. *et al.* (2000). Bad bugs and beleaguered bladders: interplay between uropathogenic *Escherichia coli* and innate host defenses. *Proceedings of the National Academy of Sciences of the United States of America* **97**, 8829–8835.

Nelson, J. D. and Peters, P. C. (1965). Suprapubic aspiration of urine in premature and term infants. *Pediatrics* **36**, 132–134.

Olbing, H. *et al.* (1992). Renal scars and parenchymal thinning in children with vesicoureteral reflux: a 5-year report of the International Reflux Study in Children (European branch). *Journal of Urology* **148**, 1653–1656.

Parkhouse, H. *et al.* (1989). Renal imaging with Tc99m labeled DMSA in the detection of acute pyelonephritis: an experimental study in the pig. *Nuclear Medicine Communications* **10**, 63–70.

Pilling, D. and Postlethwaite, R. (1996). *Clinical Opinion-Imaging in Urinary Tract Infection*. British Paediatric Association Standing Committee on Paediatric Practice Guidelines.

Poli-Merol, M. *et al.* (1998). Interest of direct radionuclide cystography in repeated urinary infection exploration in childhood. *European Journal of Pediatric Surgery* **8**, 339–342.

Powell, H. R., McCredie, D. A., and Ritchie, M. A. (1987). Urinary nitrite in symptomatic and asymptomatic urinary infection. *Archives of Disease in Childhood* **62**, 138–140.

Pryles, C. V. *et al.* (1959). Comparative bacteriologic study of urine obtained from children by percutaneous suprapubic aspiration of the bladder and by catheter. *Pediatrics* **24**, 983–991.

Ramage, I. J. *et al.* (1999). Accuracy of clean-catch urine collection in infancy. *Journal of Pediatrics* **135**, 765–767.

Ransley, P. G. and Risdon, R. A. (1974). Renal papillae and intrarenal reflux in the pig. *Lancet* **2** (7889), 1114.

Ransley, P. and Risdon, R. (1975). Renal papillary morphology in infants and young children. *Urological Research* **3**, 111–113.

Ransley, P. G. and Risdon, R. A. (1978). Reflux and renal scarring. *British Journal of Radiology* **51** (Suppl. 14), 1–35.

Ransley, P. G. and Risdon, R. A. (1981). Reflux nephropathy: effects of antimicrobial therapy on the evolution of the early pyelonephritic scar. *Kidney International* **20**, 733–738.

Ransley, P., Risdon, R., and Godley, M. (1987). Effects of vesicoureteric reflux on renal growth and function as measured by GFR, plasma creatinine, and urinary concentrating ability. *British Journal of Urology* **60**, 193.

Rees, J. *et al.* (1996). Collecting urine from washed-up potties. *Lancet* **348**, 197.

Risdon, R. A., Yeung, C. K., and Ransley, P. G. (1993). Reflux nephropathy in children submitted to unilateral nephrectomy: a clinopathological study. *Clinical Nephrology* **40**, 308–314.

Roberts, J. (1992). Vesicoureteral reflux and pyelonephritis in the monkey: a review. *Journal of Urology* **148**, 1721–1725.

Roebuck, D., Howard, R., and Metreweli, C. (1999). How sensitive is ultrasound in the detection of renal scars? *British Journal of Radiology* **72**, 345–348.

Rolleston, G., Maling, T., and Hodson, C. (1974). Intrarenal reflux and the scarred kidney. *Archives of Diseases in Childhood* **49**, 531–539.

Rosenberg, A. *et al.* (1992). Evaluation of acute urinary tract infection in children by dimercaptosuccinic acid scintigraphy: a prospective study. *Journal of Urology* **148**, 1746–1749.

Royal College of Physicians (1991). Guidelines for the management of acute urinary tract infection in childhood. *Journal of the Royal College of Physicians of London* **25**, 36–42.

Royal College of Physicians Research Unit Working Group (1991). Guidelines for the management of acute urinary tract infection in childhood. *Journal of the Royal College of Physicians of London* **25**, 36–42.

Rushton, H. *et al.* (1988). Evaluation of sup 99m technitium-dimercaptosuccinic acid renal scans in experimental acute pyelonephritis in piglets. *Journal of Urology* **140**, 1169–1174.

Rushton, H. *et al.* (1992). Renal scarring following reflux and nonreflux pyelonephritis in children: evaluation with 99m technitium-dimercaptosuccinic acid scintigraphy. *Journal of Urology* **147**, 1327–1332.

Schoen, E., Colby, C., and Ray, G. (2000). Newborn circumcision decreases incidence and costs of urinary tract infections during the first year of life. *Pediatrics* **105**, 789–793.

Scott, J. *et al.* (1997). Screening of newborn babies for familial ureteric reflux. *Lancet* **350**, 396–400.

Shannon, F. T., Sepp, E., and Rose, G. R. (1969). The diagnosis of bacteriuria by bladder puncture in infancy and childhood. *Australian Paediatric Journal* **5**, 97–100.

Shopfner, C. (1968). Urinary tract pathology associated with constipation. *Radiology* **90**, 865–877.

Sillen, U. (1999). Bladder dysfunction in children with vesico-ureteric reflux. *Acta Paediatrica* **431** (Suppl.), 40–47.

Smellie, J. (1978). Controlled trial of prophylactic treatment in childhood urinary tract infection. *Lancet* **ii**, 175–178.

Smellie, J. and Rigden, S. (1995). Pitfalls in the investigation of children with urinary tract infection. *Archives of Diseases of Childhood* **72**, 251–258.

Smellie, J., Poulton, A., and Prescod, N. (1994). Retrospective study of children with renal scarring associated with reflux and urinary infection. *British Medical Journal* **308**, 1193–1196.

Smellie, J., Rigdon, S., and Prescod, N. (1995). Urinary tract infection: a comparison of four methods of investigation. *Archives of Diseases in Childhood* **72**, 247–250.

Smellie, J. *et al.* (1992). Five year study of medical or surgical treatment in children with severe reflux: radiological renal findings. *Pediatric Nephrology* **6**, 223–230.

Smellie, J. *et al.* (1998). Childhood reflux and urinary infection: a follow-up of 10–41 years in 226 adults. *Pediatric Nephrology* **12**, 727–736.

Smellie, J. *et al.* (2001). Medical versus surgical treatment in children with severe bilateral vesicoureteric reflux and bilateral nephropathy: a randomised trial. *Lancet* **357**, 1329–1333.

Smellie, J. M. *et al.* (1985). Development of new renal scars: a collaborative study. *British Medical Journal* **290**, 1957–1960.

Smyth, A. and Judd, B. (1993). Compliance with antibiotic prophylaxis in urinary tract infection. *Archives of Diseases in Childhood* **68**, 235–236.

Stansfeld, J. M. (1962). The measurement and meaning of pyuria. *Archives of Disease in Childhood* **37**, 257–262.

Stokland, E. *et al.* (1996a). Early 99mTc dimercaptosuccinic acid (DMSA) scintography in symptomatic first time urinary tract infection. *Acta Paediatrica* **85**, 430–436.

Stokland, E. *et al.* (1996b). Renal damage one year after first urinary tract infection: role of dimercaptosuccinic acid scintography. *Journal of Pediatrics* **129**, 815–820.

Stokland, E. *et al.* (1998). Evaluation of DMSA scintigraphy and urography in assessing both acute and permanent renal damage in children. *Acta Radiologica* 447–452.

Sweeney, B. *et al.* (2001). Reflux nephropathy in infancy: a comparison of infants presenting with and without urinary tract infection. *Journal of Urology* **166**, 648–650.

Tasker, A., Lindsell, D., and Moncrieff, M. (1993). Can ultrasound reliably detect renal scarring in children with urinary tract infection? *Clinical Radiology* **47**, 177–179.

Thomas, G. *et al.* (1992). Paediatric renal transplantation in Ireland: 1980–1990. *Irish Journal of Medical Sciences* **161**, 487–489.

Tran, D., Muchant, D., and Aronoff, S. (2001). Short-course versus conventional length antimicrobial therapy for uncomplicated lower urinary tract infection in children: a meta-analysis of 1279 patients. *Journal of Pediatrics* **139**, 93–99.

Turner, G. M. and Coulthard, M. G. (1995). Fever can cause pyuria in children. *British Medical Journal* **311**, 924.

Uldall, P., Frokjaer, O., and Kaas, K. (1976). Intrarenal reflux. *Acta Paediatrica Scandinavica* **65**, 711–715.

van der Voort, V. *et al.* (1997). The struggle to diagnose UTI in children under two in primary care. *Family Practice* **14**, 44–48.

Vernon, S. *et al.* (1994). Urine collection on sanitary towels. *Lancet* **344**, 612.

Vernon, S. *et al.* (1997a). New renal scarring in children who at age 3 and 4 years had had normal scans with dimercaptosuccinic acid: follow up study. *British Medical Journal* **315**, 905–908.

Vernon, S., Foo, C., and Coulthard, M. (1997b). How general practitioners manage children with urinary tract infection: an audit in the former Northern Region. *British Journal of General Practice* **47**, 297–300.

Vernon, S., Foo, C. K., and Coulthard, M. G. (1997c). How general practitioners manage children with urinary tract infection: an audit in the former Northern Region. *British Journal of General Practice* **47**, 297–300.

Vickers, D., Ahmad, T., and Coulthard, M. G. (1991). Diagnosis of urinary tract infection in children: fresh urine microscopy or culture? *Lancet* **338**, 767–770.

Walsh, P. (1999). Editorial comment. *Journal of Urology* **162**, 1562.

Watson, P. G. and Duerden, B. I. (1977). Laboratory assessment of physical and chemical methods of preserving urine specimens. *Journal of Clinical Pathology* **30**, 532–536.

Weathers, W. and Wenzl, J. (1969). Suprapubic aspiration of the bladder: perforation of a viscus other than the bladder. *American Journal of Disease in Childhood* **117**, 590–592.

Weiss, R., Duckett, J., and Spitzer, A. (1992). Results of a randomized clinical trial of medical versus surgical management of infants and children with grade III and IV primary vesicoureteral reflux (United States). *Journal of Urology* **148**, 1667–1673.

Wennerström, M. *et al.* (2000a). Primary and aquired renal scarring in boys and girls with urinary tract infection. *Journal of Pediatrics* **136**, 30–34.

Wennerström, M. *et al.* (2000b). Ambulatory blood pressure 16–26 years after the first urinary tract infection in childhood. *Journal of Hypertension* **18**, 485–491.

Wettergren, B., Jodal, U., and Jonasson, G. (1985). Epidemiology of bacteriuria during the first year of life. *Acta Pediatrica Scandinavica* **74**, 925–933.

Willemsen, J. and Nijman, R. (2000). Vesicoureteral reflux and videourodynamic studies: results of a prospective study. *Urology* **55**, 939–943.

Williams, G., Lee, A., and Craig, J. (2001). Antibiotics for the prevention of urinary tract infection in children: a systematic review randomized controlled trials. *Journal of Paediatrics* **138**, 868–874.

Winberg, J. *et al.* (1974). Epidemiology of symptomatic urinary tract infection in childhood. *Acta Paediatrica Scandinavica* **252** (Suppl.), 1–20.

Winter, A. L. *et al.* (1983). Acquired renal scars in children. *Journal of Urology* **129**, 1190–1194.

Wiswell, T. E. (2000). The prepuce, urinary tract infections, and the consequences. *Pediatrics* **105**, 860–862.

Yeung, C. *et al.* (1998). Urodynamic patterns in infants with normal lower urinary tracts or primary vesico-ureteric reflux. *British Journal of Urology* **81**, 461–467.

Zerin, J., Ritchey, M., and Chang, A. (1993). Incidental vesicoureteral reflux in neonates with antenatally detected hydronephrosis and other renal abnormalities. *Radiology* **187**, 157–160.

Zinner, N. R. and Paquin, A. J. J. (1963). Experimental vesicoureteral reflux: III. Role of hydration in vesicoureteral reflux. *Journal of Urology* **90**, 713–718.

7.3 Renal tuberculosis and other mycobacterial infections

John B. Eastwood, Catherine M. Corbishley, and John M. Grange

The genus *Mycobacterium*

The principal characteristic of members of the genus *Mycobacterium* is their elaborate lipid-rich cell walls which impart the property of acid-fastness; namely, the ability to retain colouring by arylmethane dyes after treatment with dilute mineral acids.

The genus contains two major pathogens, the *Mycobacterium tuberculosis* complex and *Mycobacterium leprae*. The former contains several named species, although they are really variants of a single species. These variants are *M. tuberculosis* (the human tubercle bacillus), *Mycobacterium bovis* (the bovine tubercle bacillus, also a cause of human disease), and *Mycobacterium africanum* (a heterogeneous group of strains mostly isolated from human beings in Equatorial Africa). Rarely encountered variants are *Mycobacterium microti* (a cause of tuberculosis in small mammals such as the vole but attenuated in humans) and *Mycobacterium canetti* (a rare variant of *M. tuberculosis* forming smooth colonies on culture media). This complex also contains the living attenuated vaccine strain, Bacille Calmette-Guérin (BCG), which was derived from *M. bovis*. Intravesical instillation of this vaccine in the treatment of superficial bladder cancer has led to the development of renal lesions (Lamm 1992).

In addition to the major pathogens, many mycobacterial species live freely in the environment as saprophytes and some are able to cause opportunist human disease. Currently, there are about 100 named species but many are rarely encountered. These species are termed environmental mycobacteria (EM) and sometimes, particularly in the United States, non-tuberculous mycobacteria (NTM). In the older literature they were termed atypical mycobacteria and MOTT (mycobacteria other than typical tubercle) bacilli.

The natural habitats of the EM are watery—marshes, mud, ponds, lakes, rivers, and estuaries (Collins *et al.* 1984). Some species colonize water-pipes and thus gain access to water used for washing and bathing. Accordingly, they frequently contaminate the lower urethra and external genitalia and care is required in the interpretation of the microscopic detection of acid-fast bacilli in, and cultures of EM from, urine. Likewise, collection of urine into non-sterile containers has led to misdiagnosis of urinary infection by EM (Collins *et al.* 1984).

The EM are divided into two main groups, rapid and slow growers. The more frequently isolated EM responsible for human disease are listed in Table 1. Most are slow growing, although among the rapid growers *Mycobacterium chelonae*, *Mycobacterium abscessus*, *Mycobacterium fortuitum*, and *Mycobacterium peregrinum* are well-recognized pathogens. Among the slow-growing opportunist pathogens, the most frequently encountered are *Mycobacterium avium*, the avian tubercle bacillus, and the closely related *Mycobacterium intracellulare* which are often grouped together as the *M. avium* complex (MAC). This complex is a common cause of opportunist infection in patients with AIDS although the number of cases seen in industrialized countries has declined since the introduction of highly active antiretroviral therapy (HAART).

Tuberculosis

Epidemiology (Fig. 1)

Tuberculosis is on the increase worldwide. Skin testing surveys have shown that one-third of the world's human population, approximately 2000 million people, have been infected by tubercle bacilli and that approximately 1 per cent of the population is newly infected each year. The disease is principally transmitted by those with cavitary postprimary pulmonary tuberculosis. Children with primary tuberculosis are rarely infectious. In some regions, infection is the result of drinking milk contaminated by *M. bovis* and primary skin lesions are the result of traumatic inoculation.

The number of people infected by a source case depends on many factors including crowding and ventilation. On average, an untreated source case infects between 10 and 15 people every year but the range is very large.

Only a minority of infected persons develop active tuberculosis. About 5 per cent of those infected develop primary tuberculosis within 3 years of infection and a further 5 per cent develop postprimary tuberculosis later in life: a total risk of 10 per cent. While many cases of postprimary tuberculosis are the result of endogenous reactivation, DNA fingerprinting has revealed that exogenous reinfection also occurs.

In the year 2000 there were around 8 million new cases of tuberculosis, 95 per cent occurring in developing nations. Each year, between 2 and 3 million people, mostly young adults, die of tuberculosis, 98 per cent of the deaths being in developing nations.

A principal reason for the increase in the prevalence of tuberculosis is the adverse impact of HIV/AIDS. The risk of a person coinfected with the tubercle bacillus and HIV developing tuberculosis is around 20 times greater than that of someone not immunocompromised. Thus a coinfected person has around an 8 per cent chance of developing tuberculosis each year. The risk of a person with AIDS developing tuberculosis after exposure to a source case is extremely high, approaching 100 per cent. Also, the progress of the disease is very rapid—severe and widespread tuberculosis may develop within a few months of infection.

In the year 2000, there were an estimated 35 million HIV positive persons worldwide. One-third were coinfected with tubercle bacilli and, as they had an 8 per cent chance of developing overt tuberculosis

Table 1 The more frequently encountered environmental mycobacteria

M. abscessus	A rapid grower, previously regarded as a subspecies of *M. chelonae*
M. avium	Usually included with *M. intracellulare* in the *M. avium* complex (MAC). A common cause of disseminated AIDS-related disease
M. celatum	Principally a pulmonary pathogen
M. chelonae	A rapid grower. A cause of some cases of disseminated disease in renal transplant recipients and the most common cause of mycobacterial peritonitis in CAPD patients
M. fortuitum	A rapid grower. An occasional cause of peritonitis in CAPD patients
M. gordonae	A common isolate from water (hence the old name *M. aquae*). A frequent contaminant of urine. A very rare pulmonary pathogen
M. haemophilum	An occasional cause of skin lesions in renal transplant patients
M. intracellulare	Usually included with *M. avium* in the (MAC)
M. kansasii	Principally a pulmonary pathogen
M. malmoense	A species isolated with increasing frequency in Europe. Principally a pulmonary pathogen
M. marinum	Found in water and as a cause of cutaneous granulomas resembling lupus vulgaris ('swimming pool or fish tank granuloma'). A rare cause of disseminated disease in immunosuppressed patients
M. peregrinum	A rapid grower, previously regarded as a subspecies of *M. fortuitum*
M. scrofulaceum	A cause of cervical lymphadenopathy (scrofula) and also, occasionally, pulmonary disease
M. simiae	Principally a pulmonary pathogen
M. szulgai	Principally a pulmonary pathogen
M. ulcerans	A cause of increasingly common massive skin ulcers ('Buruli ulcer') in some tropical countries. No known association with renal disease or immunosuppression
M. xenopi	A species of limited geographical distribution. A frequent contaminant of urine in South England

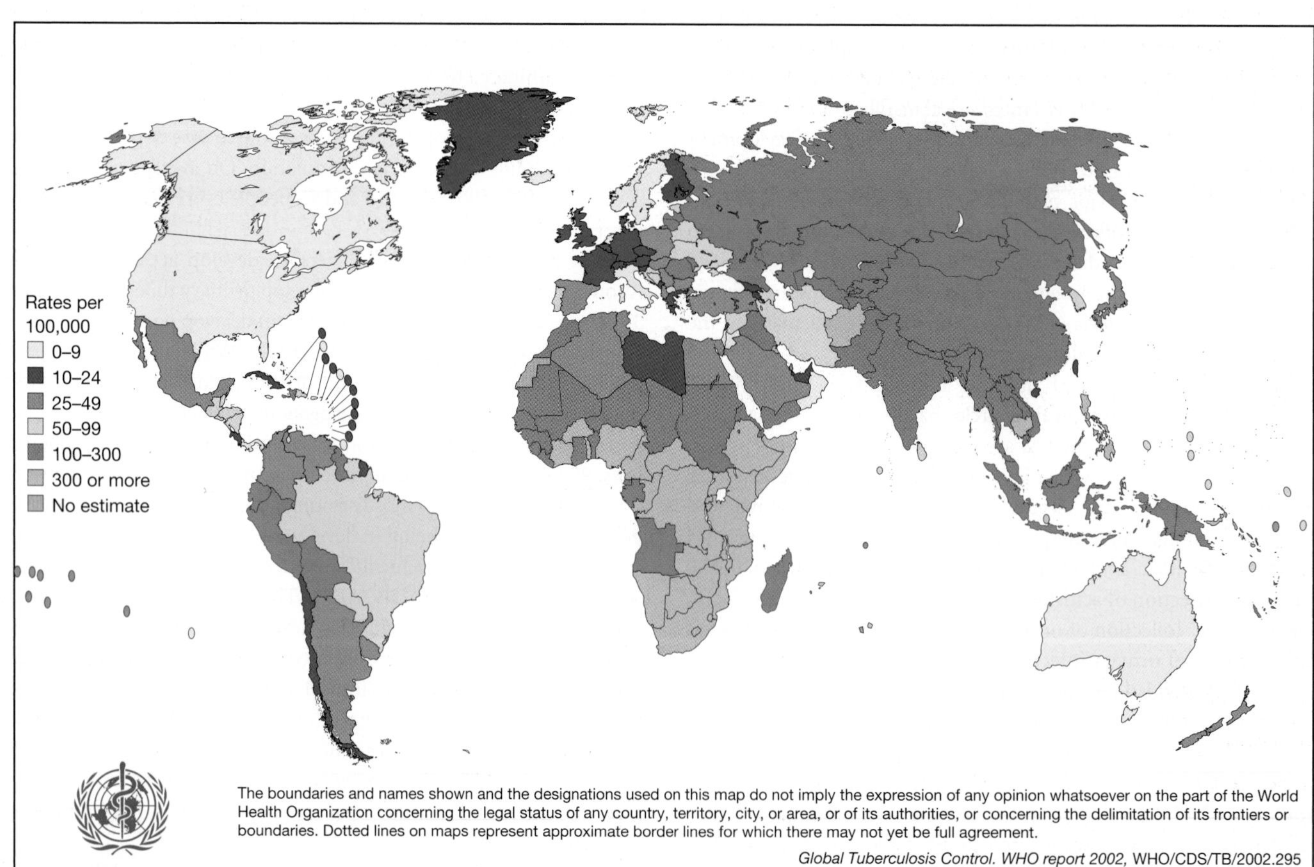

Fig. 1 Estimated tuberculosis incidence rates, 2000.

annually, HIV infection was responsible for an additional million cases of tuberculosis during that year. In the same year, tuberculosis was responsible for almost one-third of the estimated 3 million AIDS-related deaths. Also in that year, 70 per cent of cases of HIV-related tuberculosis occurred in subSaharan Africa but HIV infection is spreading rapidly in the Indian subcontinent and South East Asia where most of the world's cases of tuberculosis occur.

Another worrying trend in the epidemiology of tuberculosis is the increasing prevalence of drug resistance, including 'multidrug resistance' defined as resistance to at least rifampicin and isoniazid. A survey covering 72 countries (World Health Organization/International Union Against Tuberculosis and Lung Disease 2000) showed that, while on average only 1 per cent of new cases of tuberculosis were multidrug resistant, there were local areas of very high prevalence, such as the Henan province of China (35 per cent), the Ivanovo Oblast (district) in the Russian Federation (32.4 per cent), and Latvia (29.9 per cent).

The prevalence of genitourinary tuberculosis relative to the total burden of this disease is not easily estimated as it is under-diagnosed and under-notified in many parts of the world. An analysis of 13,634 cases of non-pulmonary tuberculosis aggregated from five studies in the United States and United Kingdom showed that genitourinary disease comprised 27 per cent of cases (range 14–41 per cent). It was thus the second most frequent form of non-pulmonary tuberculosis, after tuberculous lymphadenopathy (32 per cent, range 22–46 per cent) (Kennedy 1989).

The relative incidence of genitourinary tuberculosis also varies within a region or country according to the ethnic origin of the patients. Reports from a number of industrially developed countries show a higher than expected incidence of non-pulmonary tuberculosis in ethnic minority groups but a less than expected incidence of genitourinary tuberculosis. A survey in south-eastern England showed that extrapulmonary forms of tuberculosis were more common in patients of Indian subcontinent ethnic origin than in ethnic Europeans but that genitourinary disease occurred less frequently than in the latter (Table 2). In contrast to other forms of non-pulmonary tuberculosis, genitourinary disease occurred more frequently in males than in females in both ethnic groups.

One study indicated that the low prevalence of genitourinary tuberculosis in individuals in the United Kingdom who were from the Indian subcontinent was similar in all age groups (Ormerod 1993). Another indicated that the difference between this group and the indigenous group is age-related (Grange *et al.* 1995).

Tuberculosis due to *M. bovis* is now rare in industrially developed nations and most cases occur in elderly people due to reactivation of dormant infection acquired before the disease was controlled in the cattle population. Between 1977 and 1988, a quarter of cases of tuberculosis due to *M. bovis* in south-eastern England involved the genitourinary system (Yates and Grange 1988). This is relevant to tuberculosis control in cattle as farm workers with genitourinary tuberculosis due to *M. bovis* have infected cattle by urinating in cowsheds: one worker infected 48 cows in four different herds (Schliesser 1974).

Pathogenesis

The primary site of infection by the tubercle bacillus is usually the lung, with involvement of the hilar lymph nodes. Some bacilli are disseminated further via the blood stream and lodge in distant structures and organs where they may cause non-pulmonary manifestations of primary tuberculosis. In immunocompetent individuals, about 95 per cent of primary infections resolve.

Primary tuberculosis usually develops within 3 years of infection (Wallgren 1948) but renal tuberculosis is an exception and often only develops 8 or more years after the initial infection (Ustvedt 1947). If a tuberculous lesion erodes the wall of a major blood vessel large numbers of bacilli are released into the bloodstream leading to miliary tuberculosis, which is characterized by the development of millet seed-like granulomas throughout the body, including the kidney (Latin: *milium*—a millet seed).

In the majority who successfully overcome their primary infection, some tubercle bacilli enter a poorly understood latent or 'persister' state and may undergo reactivation years or even decades later. It is usually assumed that persisters are confined to old tuberculous scars, but the use of an *in situ* polymerase chain reaction (PCR) indicates that DNA of *M. tuberculosis* is widely distributed in the lung, including

Table 2 Non-pulmonary tuberculosis in indigenous European and Indian subcontinent ethnic groups in south-eastern England—1977–1991[a] (all values in percentage except 'total individuals')

	European		Indian subcontinent	
	1977–1983	1984–1991	1977–1983	1984–1991
Genitourinary	37.6	27.2	6.8	8.4
Lymphadenopathy	30.3	36.6	55.6	59.6
Bone and joint	19.5	19.7	24.7	19.2
Abdomen	5.1	7.8	7.8	8.3
Central nervous system	6.7	4.4	4.3	3.7
Disseminated	0.8	4.2[b]	0.7	0.6
Total individuals	1470	861	1914	1794
Non-pulmonary as % of all cases of tuberculosis	21.3	18.9	49.5	45.1

[a] Data from Yates and Grange (1993).

[b] Increase related to emergence of HIV.

histologically normal regions (Hernandez-Pando *et al.* 2000). It remains to be determined if this DNA is associated with viable tubercle bacilli and whether such DNA is regularly present in other organs including the kidney.

Primary tuberculous lesions, whether self-limiting or progressive, result in the development of tuberculin reactivity 3–10 weeks after infection. About 5 per cent of infected, tuberculin positive, persons eventually develop postprimary tuberculosis in which the principal characteristic is the extensive immune-mediated tissue necrosis responsible for pulmonary cavitation and infectivity.

Granulomas resulting from the implantation of tubercle bacilli in the kidney during haematogenous dissemination following primary infection usually appear first near glomeruli. The situation may be a consequence of the high blood flow and relatively high oxygen tension. These cortical granulomas, often bilateral, remain dormant until unknown factors permit the bacilli to proliferate. It is not known why there is often an interval of several years between this initial infection and the development of renal tuberculosis. If enlarging granulomas rupture into the proximal tubule live bacilli reach the loop of Henle where they tend to survive well, possibly on account of impaired phagocytosis in the hypertonic environment. Granulomas can then develop in the medulla, a process sometimes sufficiently destructive to cause papillary necrosis with rupture into the pelvicalyceal system. Bacilli can then enter the renal pelvis, ureters, bladder, prostate, and epididymis. Bacilli may also reach these structures by dissemination via the local lymphatics, or by direct haematogenous spread from the lung or other site of primary infection.

Clinical manifestations

'Classical' urinary tract tuberculosis

Urinary tract tuberculosis is a relatively late manifestation of disease. In developed nations, it typically presents in the fourth to sixth decade (Kennedy 1989), and in an insidious manner. It is therefore easily overlooked.

There may be lower urinary symptoms typical of infection of the urine with a common pathogen; yet routine urine culture will be sterile. The finding of significant numbers of white blood cells yet negative culture (Table 3) in a patient with urinary tract symptoms should alert the clinician to the possibility of tuberculosis of the urinary tract. Another indicator is failure of the patient's symptoms to respond to conventional antibacterial treatment.

Table 3 Causes of a 'sterile' pyuria

Tuberculosis of the urinary tract
Chlamydia trachomatis, *Mycoplasma*, or *Ureaplasma* infection
Chemically induced cystitis
Renal calculi, prostatitis
Coliform (or other pathogen) urinary tract infection but antibiotic inhibiting growth
Failure to realize that low numbers of organisms can indicate infection
WBC from outside urinary tract, e.g. from foreskin or vulva
Renal parenchymal cause—acute tubulointerstitial nephritis, glomerular disease

In addition to dysuria, frequency, and suprapubic pain there may be malaise, fever, night sweats, nocturia, and weight loss—but these are unusual. Indeed, constitutional symptoms should lead to a search for other foci of tuberculosis. In some patients there is back, flank or abdominal pain, and occasionally macroscopic haematuria. Renal colic occurs in up to 10 per cent of patients (Pasternack and Rubin 1993). Only about one-third of patients have an abnormal chest X-ray (Simon *et al.* 1977).

Lattimer (1965) described 25 physicians with renal tuberculosis, 18 presenting only after advanced cavitating disease had developed. Most had not considered the diagnosis. Indeed, in the past it was not uncommon for the diagnosis to be made either at operation or on postmortem examination.

When renal tuberculosis is advanced and bilateral, a reduction in glomerular filtration rate (GFR) due to generalized destruction of the parenchyma is likely and in some patients this progresses to endstage renal failure. A more common cause for loss of GFR is ureteric and bladder involvement due to seeding of *M. tuberculosis* into the urine. This can lead to ureteric scarring with distortion and urinary tract obstruction. Similarly, there can be considerable fibrosis and contraction of the bladder—'thimble bladder'.

Tuberculous interstitial nephritis

In recent years, it has become clear that there is another more insidious form of renal tuberculosis. In 1981, three patients were described (two from the Indian subcontinent and one from West Africa) with advanced renal failure in whom imaging revealed equal-sized smooth kidneys without evidence of calcification or gross anatomical distortion (Mallinson *et al.* 1981). Renal histology revealed interstitial infiltrates with chronic inflammatory cells and granulomas in all three patients, caseation in two and acid-fast bacilli in two. In two patients there was radiological evidence of pulmonary tuberculosis and one patient had tuberculous peritonitis. This report emphasizes that there can be tuberculous involvement of the kidneys, sufficient to cause renal failure, in the absence of either the typical renal destruction with calcification and fibrosis, or urinary tract obstruction. Indeed, in these three cases tubercle bacilli were neither seen in the urine nor grown from it. In a review of 3500 renal biopsies carried out in Paris over a 14-year period (Mignon *et al.* 1984), interstitial granulomas were found in 24. Three of these patients had tuberculosis and in one acid-fast bacilli were found in the kidney.

Benn *et al.* (1988) reported a Ugandan Asian woman (urea, 13.3 μmol/l; creatinine, 260 μmol/l; creatinine clearance, 17 ml/min) with equal-sized smooth kidneys on intravenous urography (IVU) in whom renal biopsy showed interstitial fibrosis with epithelioid and giant cell granulomas, one showing caseation. Acid-fast bacilli were not seen in, nor was *M. tuberculosis* grown from, biopsy material or urine. Her Mantoux test was strongly positive and antituberculosis therapy for 12 months led to improvement in GFR (creatinine, 223 μmol/l; creatinine clearance, 39 ml/min) over the next 3 years (Fig. 2). Tuberculosis had not been considered before the biopsy because, unlike some other reported cases (Mallinson *et al.* 1981), there was no other evidence of tuberculosis and five of the six midstream samples of urine were free of leucocytes.

Tuberculosis and glomerular disease

No firm link has been established between tuberculosis and glomerulonephritis although there are a number of case reports including

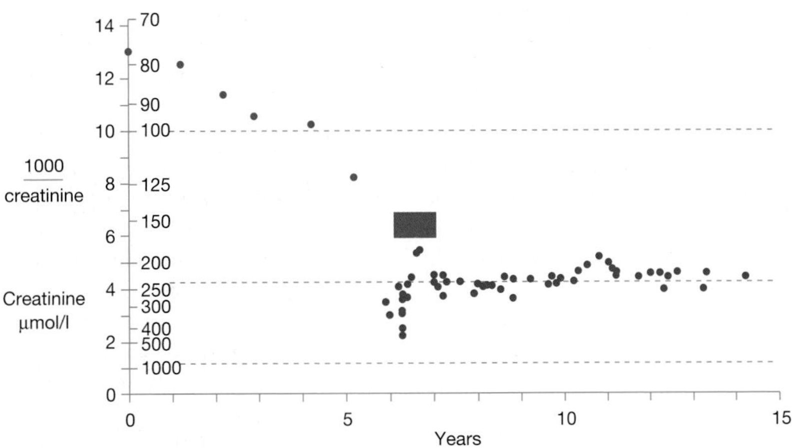

Fig. 2 Graph of reciprocal creatinine plot against time. Illustrates arrest of decline of renal function after treatment of renal tuberculosis. Bar indicates treatment with antituberculosis drugs and prednisolone for 6 months. Vertical axis: numbers to the left refer to 1000/creatinine, numbers to the right are measured plasma creatinine values.

a patient with dense deposit disease and tuberculosis (Hariprasad *et al.* 1979) and another with miliary tuberculosis who had focal proliferative glomerulonephritis (Shribman *et al.* 1983). In the latter case, there was granular staining for IgA, IgM, and C3 in the mesangium and around capillary loops but granulomas were not seen. Interestingly, similar renal histology has been documented in lepromatous leprosy (Iveson *et al.* 1975).

Chronic tuberculosis sometimes leads to amyloidosis and in India is a not uncommon cause of renal amyloid and renal failure (Chugh *et al.* 1981).

Tuberculosis in patients with chronic renal failure

It has been suggested that tuberculosis is more common in patients with renal failure than in the general population. In a study in west London where there were significant numbers of refugees and asylum-seekers, many of whom came from countries where tuberculosis is endemic, three factors were considered to be of importance (Moore *et al.* 2002), namely, being born overseas, the immunosuppressive effect of uraemia and the association between diabetes mellitus and tuberculosis in patients with renal failure.

There is evidence for a state of relative immunological anergy in uraemia—as indicated by skin testing—but the incidence of tuberculin anergy is difficult to assess unless data on tuberculin reactivity before the onset of renal failure is available (Woeltje *et al.* 1998). On the other hand, use of common antigens such as tetanus, candida, and mumps revealed anergy in 32 per cent of dialysis patients in one study (Woeltje *et al.* 1998) and in 40 per cent in another (Smirnoff *et al.* 1998). A further study showed that 69 per cent of uraemic patients commencing haemodialysis were anergic but that reactivity to common antigens was partly restored by haemodialysis, affecting 50 and 24 per cent of patients on dialysis for 1–8 and 9–69 months respectively (Kaufmann *et al.* 1994). The incidence of anergy increased by 46 per cent in those on dialysis for 6 years or more. Diabetes is a major cause of endstage renal disease, about 20 per cent of patients starting dialysis in the United Kingdom being diabetic. Another factor is that many patients with renal failure have low circulating 25-OH-vitamin D (Eastwood *et al.* 1979).

Endstage renal disease

Tuberculosis is an important cause of progressive renal failure as, unlike many other causes of renal failure, it is potentially preventable and treatable (Benn *et al.* 1988). In 1991, the European Dialysis and Transplant Association (EDTA) registry reported that 195 (0.65 per cent) of 30,064 new patients (from 35 European countries) assigned a renal diagnosis had renal failure due to tuberculosis, an incidence similar to that of earlier years (Eastwood *et al.* 1994). A report from Portugal showed that there may be local areas of high incidence (Neves *et al.* 1993). Over a 10-year period in the Algarve, tuberculosis caused renal failure in 12 of 345 patients (3.5 per cent) starting haemodialysis. In some instances, the patients presented terminally without having had any symptoms of tuberculosis. From published data on primary renal diagnosis, it is clear that tuberculosis is more common in Europe as a primary renal diagnosis [2247 cases (0.7 per cent)] than in either the United States (0.004 per cent) or Australasia (0.16 per cent) (Maissonneuve *et al.* 2000).

The incidence of urinary tract tuberculosis as a cause of endstage renal disease is probably being underestimated as, although many individuals with classical urinary tract tuberculosis are identified, the interstitial form is easily overlooked. Hence, it is important that the diagnosis is considered in all patients with equal-sized smooth kidneys without a clear-cut renal diagnosis, especially in high-risk groups (Mallinson *et al.* 1981; Morgan *et al.* 1990). In such patients renal biopsy should always be considered.

Dialysis patients

Haemodialysis

Tuberculosis is a problem in haemodialysis patients, in whom it often presents in an insidious manner with anorexia, low-grade fever and weight loss. In some reports the majority of cases have been extrapulmonary or, occasionally, miliary (Sasaki *et al.* 1979; Hussein *et al.* 1990). Tuberculosis appears to be much more common among haemodialysis patients than in the general population (Smith 1982) and the type of presentation suggests that dialysis is associated with reactivation of quiescent disease. Among predominantly Caucasian dialysis populations ethnic minorities may be over-represented (Pazianas *et al.* 1991; Roderick *et al.* 1994), and they may have a higher incidence of tuberculosis (Kwan *et al.* 1991). Recently, Moore *et al.* (2002) described 11 cases, all born overseas, among dialysis patients at the Hammersmith Hospital, London. The incidence equates to an annual rate of 1187 per 100,000. In England and Wales in 1998 the overall rate was 12 per 100,000; among Black Africans and individuals from the Indian subcontinent incidence rates were at the most 210 and 132 cases per 100,000 of the population. Clearly, renal physicians should look carefully for tuberculosis in immigrants who have renal failure.

Peritoneal dialysis

There are fewer reports of tuberculosis among patients undergoing CAPD (continuous ambulatory peritoneal dialysis) but there is no reason why reactivation of tuberculosis is any less likely in these patients. There have been a number of reports of tuberculous peritonitis in CAPD patients (Cheng *et al.* 1989; Ahijado *et al.* 1991; Tan *et al.* 1991; Ong *et al.* 1992). Most recently, Quantrill *et al.* (2001) reported eight cases of peritoneal tuberculosis occurring over a 13-year period. All were patients on CAPD rather than the automated form (APD), and in six cases the organism was grown, usually from the peritoneal fluid itself. The disease presented soon after starting dialysis and was indistinguishable clinically from bacterial peritonitis.

Transplant patients

Tuberculosis should always be considered when a renal transplant patient develops fever, especially when the patient is from a high-risk group, such as immigrants or refugees from regions with a high incidence of tuberculosis. Until recently tuberculosis received less attention than opportunist infections such as those caused by *Pneumocystis carinii*, Epstein–Barr virus, and cytomegalovirus. Indeed, when the literature was reviewed in 1983, when renal transplantation had been a part of nephrological practice for 30 years, only 42 cases of tuberculosis in patients with renal transplants were found (Lichtenstein and MacGregor 1983). Subsequently, in Saudi Arabia, 14 cases were found among 403 renal transplant patients and the annual incidence of tuberculosis in these patients was about 50 times that of the general population (Qunibi *et al.* 1990). A particular finding in these patients and in published reports totalling 130 Saudi Arabian patients was a high proportion of miliary disease (64 per cent in the series of 14 patients, and 38 per cent of the total of 130). No difference in the risk of developing tuberculosis was found between those who did or did not have a positive tuberculin test. One of the patients acquired tuberculosis from the transplanted kidney as had been described in an earlier report (Peters *et al.* 1984).

There are few data on the prevention of tuberculosis in renal transplant patients. Accordingly, the desirability of prescribing tuberculosis preventive therapy to renal transplant patients is controversial and until recently there has been no consensus on such prevention. With modern post-transplant immunosuppressive regimes a basal level of immunosuppression is often reached by 6 months post-transplant. For this reason some transplant units have given at-risk patients prophylactic isoniazid in a dose of 100 mg daily for 1 year.

Recently, the European Best Practice Guidelines for Renal Transplantation (2002) have been published. The guidelines recommend that all renal transplant candidates and recipients considered to have latent tuberculosis be treated with isoniazid 300 mg daily for 9 months. Such patients are defined as those with one or more of the following: induration after Mantoux testing of 5 mm (transplant recipients) or 10 mm (transplant candidates on dialysis); a history of inadequately treated tuberculosis; a chest X-ray suggestive of old tuberculosis; and close contact with a person with tuberculosis. Preventive therapy should also be given to tuberculin-negative patients who receive a kidney from a tuberculin-positive donor.

It is widely believed that treatment with corticosteroids predisposes to reactivation of tuberculosis but, surprisingly, there is little published supporting evidence for this belief. Nevertheless, the American Thoracic Society recommends that patients with healed pulmonary tuberculosis who have respiratory disease requiring long-term corticosteroid therapy should be given isoniazid chemoprophylaxis for one year (American Thoracic Society 1974). As renal transplant patients usually have more pronounced depression of their immunity than those with respiratory disease, this recommendation would appear to be suitable for the former as well.

Tuberculosis of the genital tract

In the male, genital tuberculosis is acquired by seeding from infected urine or via the bloodstream. The most common manifestation is epididymo-orchitis; less common is tuberculous prostatitis. Tuberculosis of the urethra and penis are much less common but, like tuberculous prostatitis (O'Flynn 1970; Symes and Blandy 1973), can present with papulonecrotic skin lesions, fistulae, and genital ulceration. Although infection usually results from direct seeding from infected urine, penile tuberculosis can be acquired by direct inoculation from contaminated surgical instruments or clothing following ritual circumcision (Annobil *et al.* 1990). The urinary tract should be fully investigated in any patient found to have genital tuberculosis since 75 per cent of patients with epididymo-orchitis or prostatitis have evidence of urinary tract involvement (Ferric and Rundle 1983).

Tuberculosis of the female genital tract is accompanied by urinary tract tuberculosis in less than 5 per cent of cases—far less commonly than in the male. Presumably, this is because the genital and urinary tracts in the female are separate so avoiding the possibility of direct infection of the genital tract from the urine. Thus tuberculosis of the female genital tract is probably almost always the result of haematogenous spread (Pasternack and Rubin 1993).

Hypercalcaemia and tuberculosis

There have been reports of hypercalcaemia in patients on chronic haemodialysis with either disseminated or genitourinary tuberculosis (Felsenfeld *et al.* 1986; Peces and Alvarez 1987; Peces *et al.* 1998). In one case, hypercalcaemia was not observed until the patient had been on dialysis for 8 months and its onset coincided with the development of widely disseminated tuberculosis presenting with persistent fever (Felsenfeld *et al.* 1986). Circulating calcitriol levels were elevated but those of parathyroid hormone were not. Hypercalcaemia has also been reported in a CAPD patient with tuberculous peritonitis (Lye and Lee 1990).

Hypercalcaemia has been described in patients with disseminated tuberculosis who had neither renal failure nor renal involvement. Levels of calcitriol [1,25-$(OH)_2D_3$] are elevated in such patients as a result of increased synthesis of this active form of vitamin D by activated macrophages within the granulomas (Rook 1988).

Tuberculosis and HIV positivity

The kidney is often involved in the disseminated tuberculosis characteristic of those infected with HIV but only a minority of patients have clinical features such as sterile pyuria or haematuria (Marques *et al.* 1996). In south-eastern England between 1984 and 1992 *M. tuberculosis* was isolated from the genitourinary system of only seven of 167 HIV positive tuberculosis patients (Yates *et al.* 1993), but the low incidence may indicate a failure to cultivate relevant specimens from such patients in the absence of specific clinical symptoms. In a study in India, 17 of 35 patients dying of AIDS were found to have tuberculous lesions in their kidneys, with this disease being more common than fungal infections (five cases) and CMV (two cases) (Lanjewar *et al.* 1999). The isolation of EM from urine of HIV positive patients is described below.

Imaging (Figs 3–8)

Intravenous urography is the most useful imaging investigation for diagnosing urinary tract tuberculosis because of its ability to detect calcification, to provide images of detailed anatomy and to show the commonly occurring multiple lesions.

Renal tuberculosis may be unilateral or bilateral. Calcification is seen in about 30 per cent of cases (Roylance *et al.* 1970). It may have a variety of patterns—punctate, speckled, or hazy. In advanced tuberculosis the whole pelvicalyceal system and ureter may be outlined by calcification—the so-called tuberculous autonephrectomy.

Early tuberculosis is seen as irregularity of the papillary margins with reduced density of contrast medium in the affected areas. Cavities, either smooth or irregular, then develop and communicate with the pelvicalyceal system. As destruction progresses there is associated parenchymal loss. Fibrosis leads to strictures. When these affect the calyceal infundibula there is no calyceal filling at urography and the infundibulum shows a typical 'pinched-off' appearance. Fibrosis at the pelviureteric junction causes obstruction at this level. Local granuloma formation or dilated obstructed calyces that do not fill with contrast medium may produce a mass effect. Extension of infection into the perinephric space may lead to abscess formation. Fistulae may develop, particularly to the skin and gut. To show them fully, retrograde ureterography or sinography may be required.

Ureteric and bladder tuberculosis are usually secondary to renal tuberculosis and there is commonly evidence of renal involvement. The earliest ureteric change is ulceration but this is rarely demonstrated radiologically. Strictures develop and there may be filling defects on IVU if there is florid granuloma formation. As fibrosis progresses the ureter shortens and becomes thick-walled. Sometimes incompetence at the vesicoureteric junction leads to reflux. The bladder wall tends to thicken and granulomas may cause filling defects. With generalized involvement, bladder capacity is reduced. Calcification in the ureters and bladder only occurs with advanced disease. Calcification may also occur in the seminal vesicles, vas, and prostate if these are involved.

Ultrasonography shows many of the changes of advanced disease such as pelvicalyceal dilatation, local collections, and calcification (Schaffer *et al.* 1983), but is less sensitive than urography, even in advanced disease (Premkumar *et al.* 1987).

Computed tomography is useful for demonstrating the many changes in advanced disease: calcification, pelvicalyceal dilatation, scars, strictures, and extrarenal spread (Goldman *et al.* 1985; Premkumar *et al.* 1987). Its sensitivity in early disease has not been assessed, but is likely to be less than urography because detailed pelvicalyceal anatomy is less well shown.

Follow-up studies of patients on antituberculosis drugs show that ureteric strictures can develop during treatment. They may occur at sites apparently normal on the IVU obtained at presentation, presumably because mucosal ulceration at the affected site was not visualized. A limited IVU is the best method of looking for ureteric strictures and their effects on the upper tracts. As yet, there are few reports on the place of ultrasonography in detecting strictures and obstruction during treatment with antituberculosis drugs.

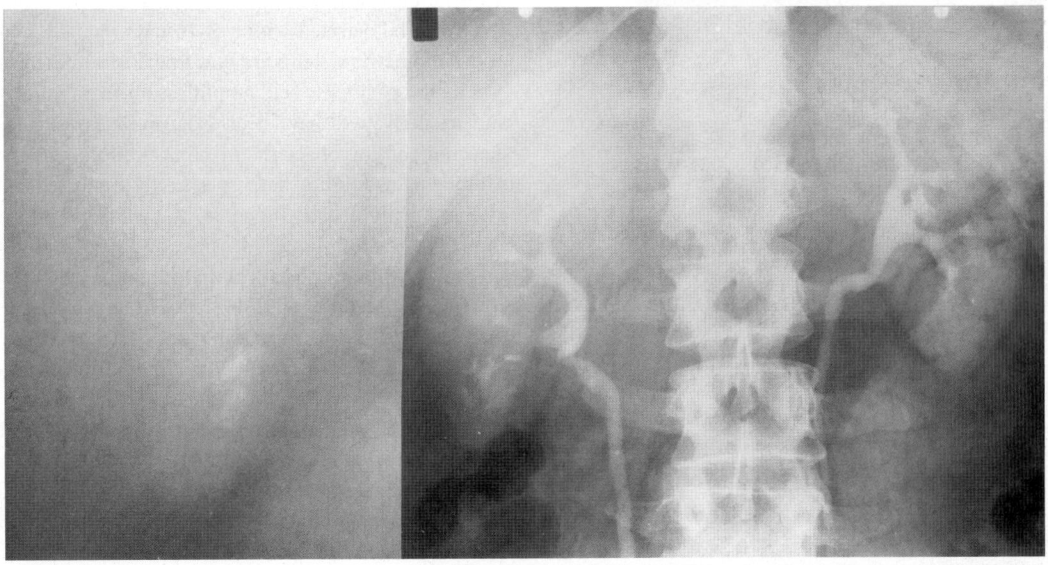

Fig. 3 Early focal renal tuberculosis. Plain film shows calcification in the lower pole of the right kidney. The 5-min IVU film shows the abnormal lower pole calyx with loss of adjacent parenchyma. There was sterile pyuria and *M. tuberculosis* was cultured from the urine.

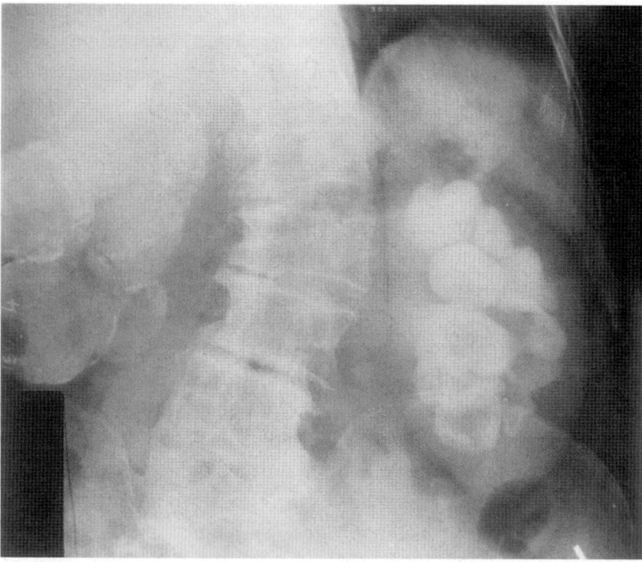

Fig. 4 Late bilateral renal tuberculosis. IVU film shows bilateral calyceal dilatation, calcified on the right.

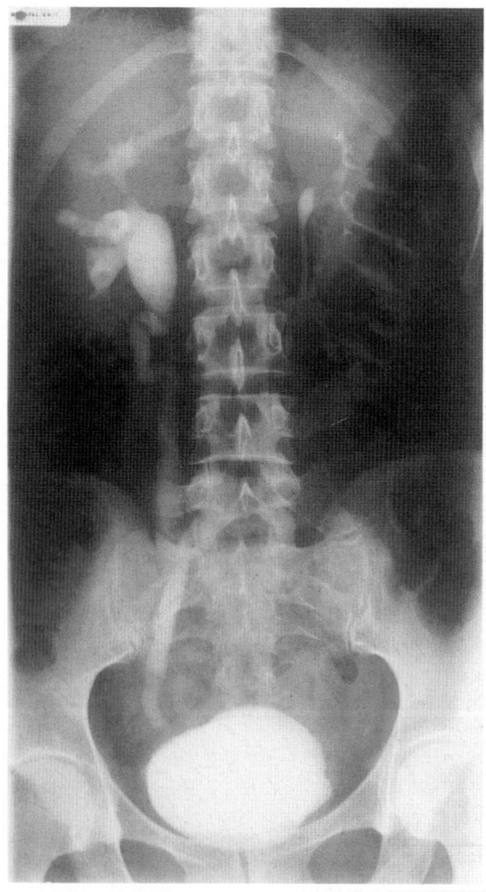

Fig. 5 Early changes of renal tuberculosis on 20-min IVU film. There are cavities in the parenchyma adjacent to the right upper and interpolar calyces; there is dilatation of the right ureter. The left kidney is normal.

Bacteriological diagnosis

The diagnosis of genitourinary tuberculosis and disease due to EM is made or confirmed by bacteriological examination of urine or tissue biopsies. Ideally, early morning midstream urine specimens collected on three successive days are examined. The most suitable containers are sterile 28 ml glass or plastic screw-capped bottles (Universal Containers). If the patient cannot void urine directly into the container, the collecting vessel must be sterile. Specimens should be delivered to the laboratory as quickly as possible to prevent replication of bacterial and fungal contaminants. When delays are unavoidable, the urine samples should be refrigerated but not frozen.

Urine samples are centrifuged and deposits examined microscopically after staining by the Ziehl–Neelsen or similar acid-fast techniques. As contamination by EM is common, genitourinary tuberculosis should never be diagnosed on the basis of microscopical evidence *alone*. Tissue biopsies reveal the characteristic histological appearances associated with mycobacterial disease and can be stained for acid-fast bacilli. Failure to detect acid-fast bacilli on microscopic examination does not rule out their presence in the specimen. Tissue must contain 10^4–10^5 acid-fast bacilli per gram for them to be detected with confidence.

Mycobacterial culture is usually carried out by inoculating deposits of urine or homogenized tissue on to solid media. As urine contains contaminating microorganisms which may overgrow the culture medium, deposits for culture must first be 'decontaminated', usually by treating the deposits with dilute sulfuric or oxalic acid, neutralizing and recentrifuging before inoculating the medium. Alternatively, a 'cocktail' of antibiotics that kill virtually all microorganisms other than mycobacteria can be added to the medium. Aspirated pus and caseous material generally contain few viable mycobacteria so it is more rewarding to examine biopsies of the surrounding tissue.

Egg-based media, such as Löwenstein–Jensen medium have been the mainstay of mycobacterial culture but colonies of *M. tuberculosis* take 2–8 weeks to appear. More rapid culture systems have therefore been introduced, the first being a radiometric system (BACTEC) based on the detection of radioactive CO_2 released by viable mycobacteria from radiolabelled palmitic acid. This method allows mycobacterial growth to be detected within 2–10 days. Equally rapid and sensitive non-radiometric systems are now available commercially.

The use of nucleic acid amplification techniques, such as the PCR and its derivatives have been extensively investigated for the rapid detection of mycobacteria in clinical specimens, notably sputum. Although few studies have specifically evaluated PCR for the diagnosis of genitourinary tuberculosis, the limited information available shows that the technique is sensitive and specific although some urine specimens contain substances that inhibit the PCR (van Vollenhoven *et al.* 1996; Sechi *et al.* 1997). PCR has also been used to detect mycobacterial DNA in urine in cases of disseminated tuberculosis in HIV-positive persons (Aceti *et al.* 1999). Test kits are commercially available.

Mycobacterial identification is usually undertaken in central reference laboratories by means of cultural and biochemical tests or more rapid nucleic acid-based methods. Drug susceptibility testing is usually based on growth inhibition on drug-containing solid media but results are not available for several weeks. Radiometry and the newer non-radiometric systems provide a more rapid means for achieving such information. Rapid techniques for the detection of mutations in the *RpoB* gene responsible for resistance to rifampicin are commercially available and are around 95 per cent accurate.

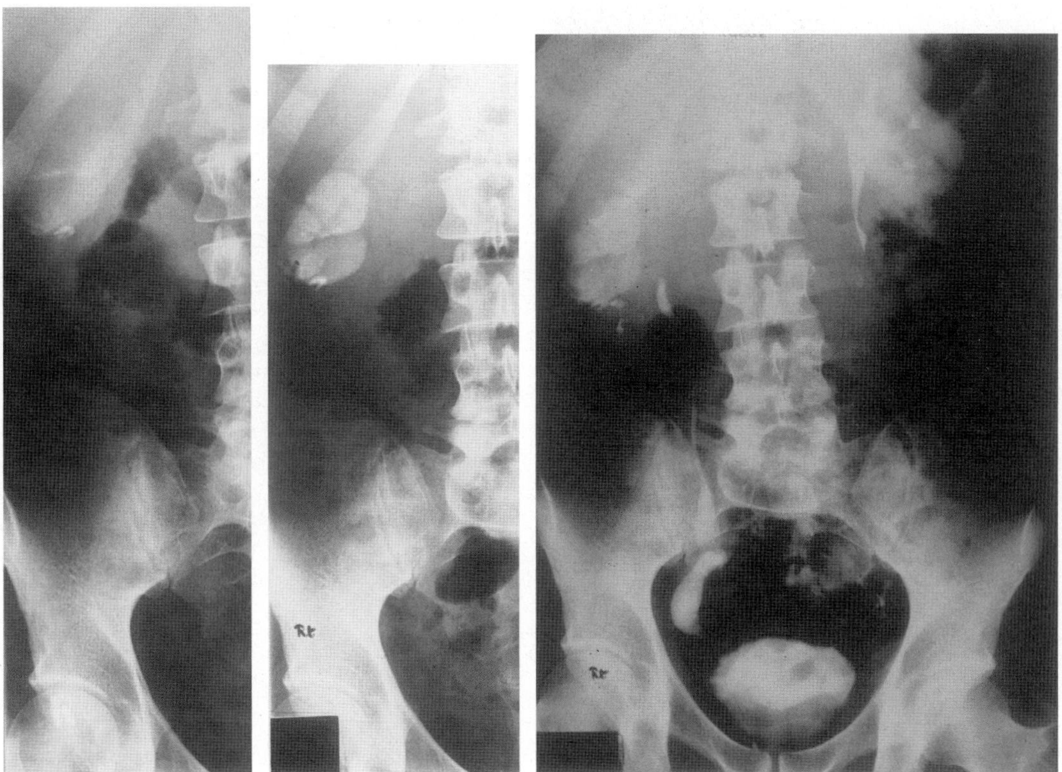

Fig. 6 Left-hand panel shows calcification in the right hypochondrium. Middle panel shows more pronounced calcification in the same area 9 years later. The 20-min IVU film (right-hand panel) shows calyceal distortion and stricture, these appearances being typical of tuberculosis. The multifocal strictures and dilated segments of the ureter are typical late features of tuberculosis; there is also irregularity of the bladder wall. The left kidney is normal.

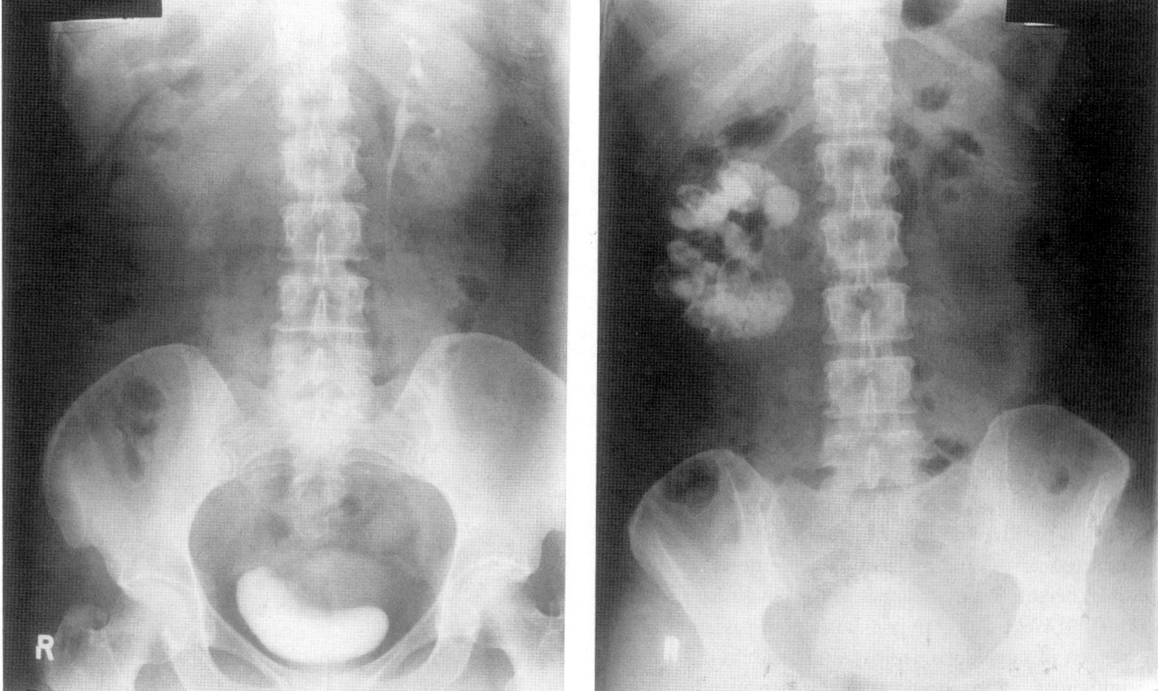

Fig. 7 Left-hand panel shows 30-min IVU film—normal left kidney and ureter with lack of excretion on the right. Right-hand panel shows 1-h film. Contrast is no longer seen in the collecting system on the left side but there is opacification of a grossly distorted kidney on the right side. This appearance is typical of the eventual tuberculous 'autonephrectomy' that sometimes occurs. The lack of calcification is unusual.

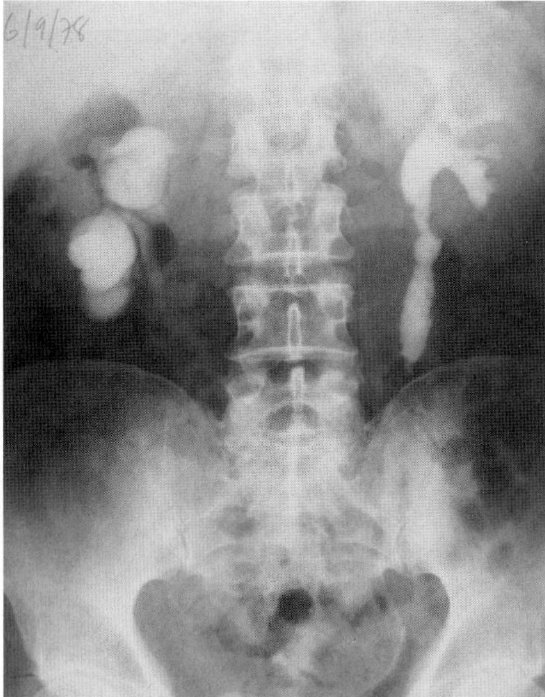

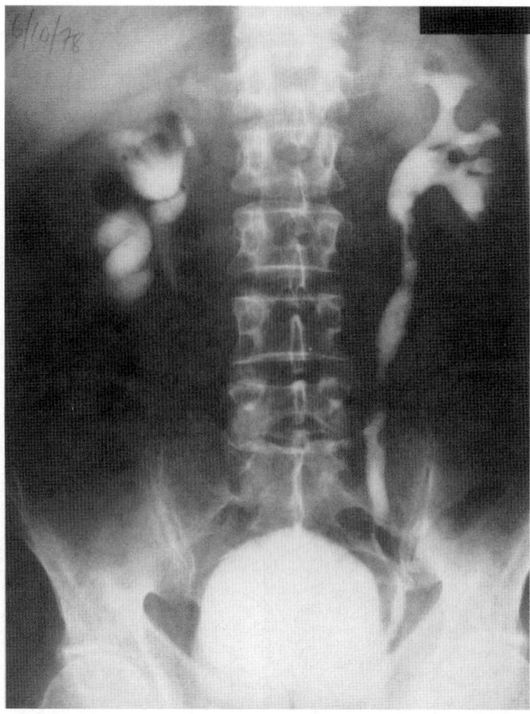

Fig. 8 Two 10-min IVU films taken 1 month apart. Note the mural abnormalities in the ureter (left-hand panel) that have progressed to frank strictures 1 month later. The right kidney shows global calyceal dilatation.

Laboratory procedures for isolation, identification, and drug susceptibility testing of mycobacteria are described in detail by Collins *et al.* (1997).

Histopathology

Tuberculosis may involve the kidney as part of generalized disseminated infection or as localized genitourinary disease. The morphology of the lesions depends on the type of infection, the virulence of the organism, and the immune status of the patient. The characteristic microscopic lesion of mycobacterial infection is the caseating epithelioid granuloma (Fig. 9), but caseation may not always be apparent, notably in overwhelming or miliary infections, environmental mycobacteria, BCG-related lesions and in leprosy. Although acid-fast bacilli may often be demonstrated in early active disease and in lesions in the immunosuppressed (Ridley and Ridley 1987) (Fig. 10), they may be difficult or impossible to identify in immunocompetent or treated patients and in old lesions. Fluorescent methods of identification in tissue sections are more sensitive and molecular methods such as *in situ* PCR are becoming more widely used. However, PCR on formalin-fixed and paraffin-processed tissue sections may be misleading, producing both false-positive and false-negative results.

Healing produces scarring and frequently calcification. The differential diagnosis of necrotizing granulomas in the renal tract includes fungal infections and Wegener's granulomatosis. Non-caseating granulomas may be seen in sarcoidosis, leprosy, and brucellosis. 'Foreign body type' granulomas, which are occasionally seen in response to amyloid, ruptured tubules, myeloma protein, and therapeutic embolization, are usually readily distinguishable from those caused by infection.

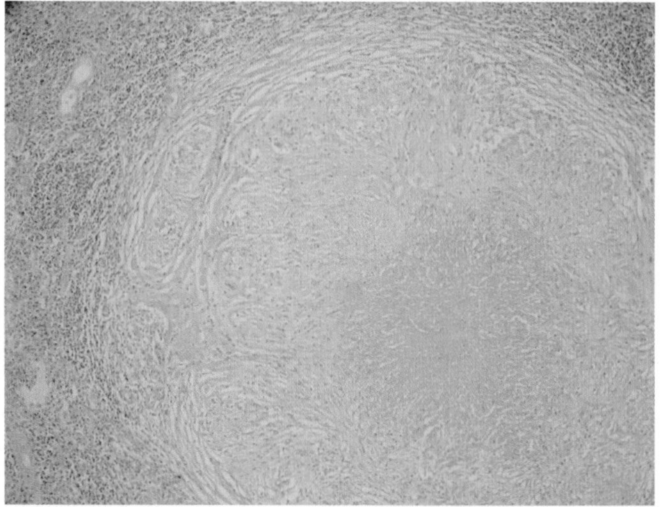

Fig. 9 Caseating epithelioid granuloma, the histological hallmark of classical tuberculosis.

Patterns of renal tuberculosis

Disseminated infection

The kidney is frequently involved in miliary ('septicaemic') tuberculosis where blood borne miliary tubercles are seen throughout the renal substance, most noticeably in the cortex (Fig. 11). The lesions measure up to 3 mm in size and are usually pale or white. Histologically, they consist of epithelioid granulomata, with or without caseation, and often contain Langhans type giant cells. Organisms can usually be demonstrated within these lesions, but are often difficult to find. Renal function usually remains normal.

In immunosuppressed patients the granulomas may be less well formed and organisms more readily demonstrated. Caseous necrosis, which is the result of cell-mediated hypersensitivity and therefore dependent on an effective immune response, is less frequently seen. When immunosuppression is severe, and in cases where the infective organism is an environmental mycobacterium, such as a member of the MAC (Horsburgh 1991), the lesions may be more diffuse and poorly formed than the usual miliary lesions and the granulomatous response consists of histiocytic cells with abundant pale cytoplasm packed with organisms ('multibacillary histiocytosis'). Necrosis is not a feature.

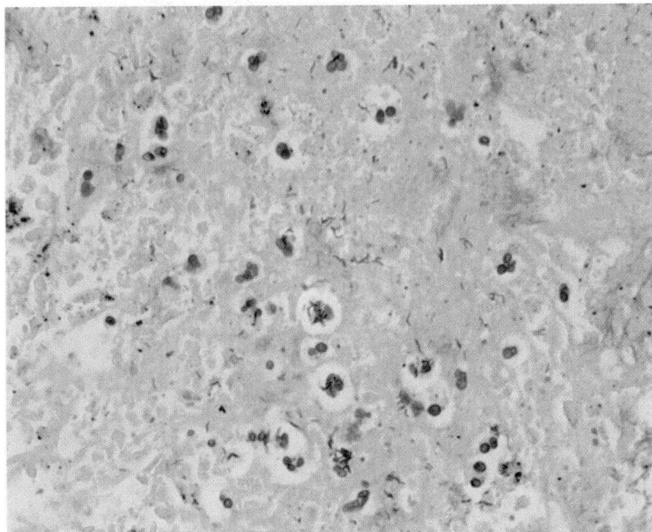

Fig. 10 Large numbers of acid-fast bacilli in a caseating granuloma in an immunosuppressed patient with overwhelming infection. Ziehl–Nielsen stain.

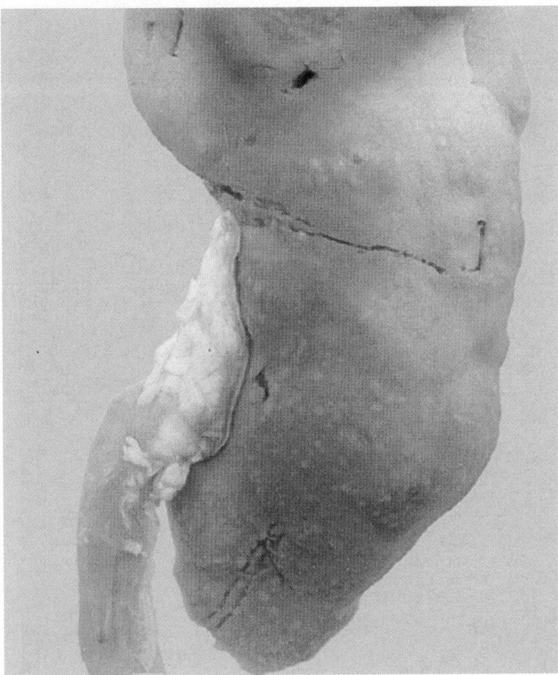

Fig. 11 Miliary tuberculosis involving the renal cortex. Typical tubercles are seen on the cortical surface; they were also present within the renal parenchyma.

In some patients with pulmonary or disseminated tuberculosis there is evidence of renal failure without typical miliary involvement or localized genitourinary lesions. In these cases biopsy has shown interstitial nephritis, usually, but not in all cases, with granulomata (Fig. 12). The evidence that the renal malfunction is due to a combination of infection and immunological renal damage is the recovery of function with a combination of antituberculosis treatment and corticosteroids (Mallinson *et al.* 1981). Proliferative glomerulonephritis due to immune complex disease has also been reported (Shribman *et al.* 1983).

Localized infection

The kidney is usually infected by haematogenous spread from a focus of infection in the lung, but it is unusual for there to be evidence of active pulmonary disease when renal involvement becomes manifest. There may be clinical or radiological evidence of past infection indicating that the renal component arises as a result of reactivation rather than as a new infection (Christensen 1974; Narayana 1982). Clinically, renal tuberculosis usually presents as unilateral involvement but studies undertaken in the prechemotherapeutic era indicate that the disease is frequently bilateral at autopsy (Kretschmer 1930; Greenberger *et al.* 1935).

If a tuberculous lesion in the lung gains access to the vascular system by erosion of the wall of a vessel, usually a vein, emboli containing organisms may be disseminated throughout the body. However, they generally only proliferate in a small number of sites including kidney, epididymis, fallopian tube, bone marrow, brain (particularly the hindbrain) and adrenal. In the kidney, the site of preference is the renal medulla where the lesions produced are confluent epithelioid granulomata with caseous necrosis leading to local tissue destruction. The infection may cause vascular insufficiency of the papillae by damaging blood

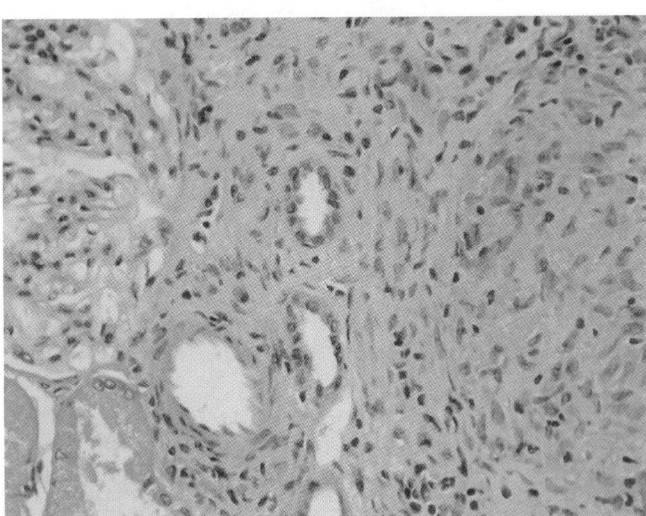

Fig. 12 Granulomatous interstitial nephritis; note that the glomerulus is normal.

vessels, and papillary necrosis may ensue (Fig. 13). Spread to the renal pelvis produces tuberculous pyelonephritis and may even progress to a pyonephrosis-like lesion, also known as a 'cement' or 'putty' kidney (Fig. 14). Scarring develops within the renal pelvis with calcification in 24 per cent, identifiable as renal or ureteric stones in up to 19 per cent (Ross 1970), and infection frequently spreads down the ureters into the bladder producing mucosal and mural granulomatous lesions associated with scarring, dilatation, and obstruction. The clinical consequences of an extensive renal lesion include autonephrectomy. The destructive renal lesions occasionally spread outside the renal capsule and produce a mass lesion that can mimic a neoplasm (Njeh *et al.* 1993).

Lower urinary tract involvement

Ureteric involvement may also produce irregular ureteric strictures (Fig. 15), segmental dilatation, obstruction, and/or reflux. Recognition that the ureteric obstruction and reflux may sometimes be due to tuberculosis may help avoid unnecessary nephrectomy if active treatment including relief of obstruction is instituted early (Christensen 1974; Ramanathan *et al.* 1998). Secondary bacterial infection of the urinary tract is common. Keratinizing squamous metaplasia (previously known as leukoplakia) may develop as a late complication of chronic inflammation and infection of the renal pelvis or bladder (Fig. 16), and may persist after treatment of the active tuberculous lesion (Byrd *et al.* 1976). Keratinizing squamous metaplasia is a risk factor for the development of squamous carcinoma. Treatment of the tuberculosis leading to reduction in the inflammation lowers this risk but the metaplasia may persist. Long-term follow up is therefore required so that any tendency to malignant transformation can be

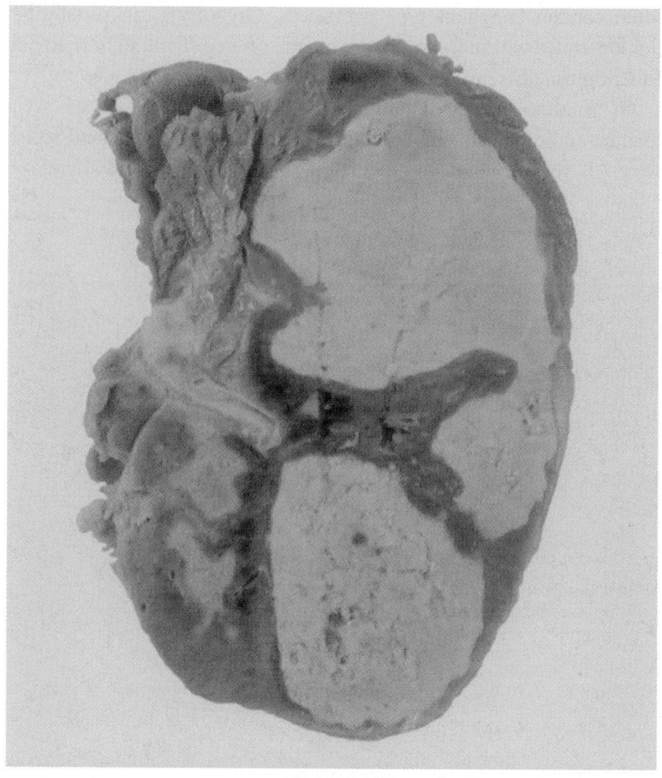

Fig. 14 Tuberculous 'pyonephrosis' with extensive caseous necrosis and renal parenchymal destruction. 'Cement' or 'putty' kidney.

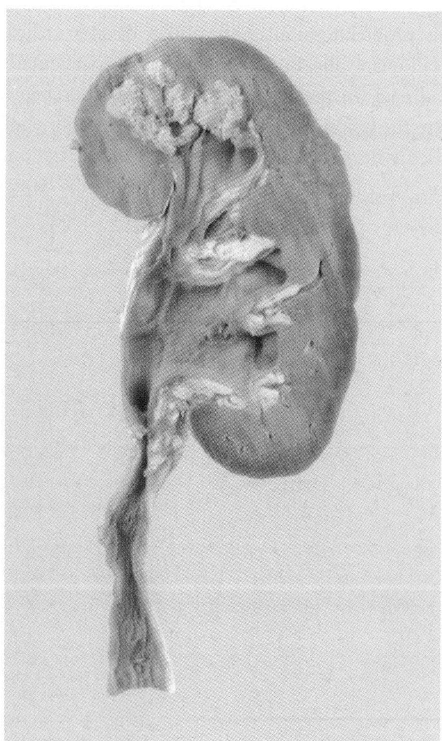

Fig. 13 Widespread tuberculous involvement of the renal papillae with papillary necrosis. The ureter is also involved and shows mucosal irregularity and dilatation.

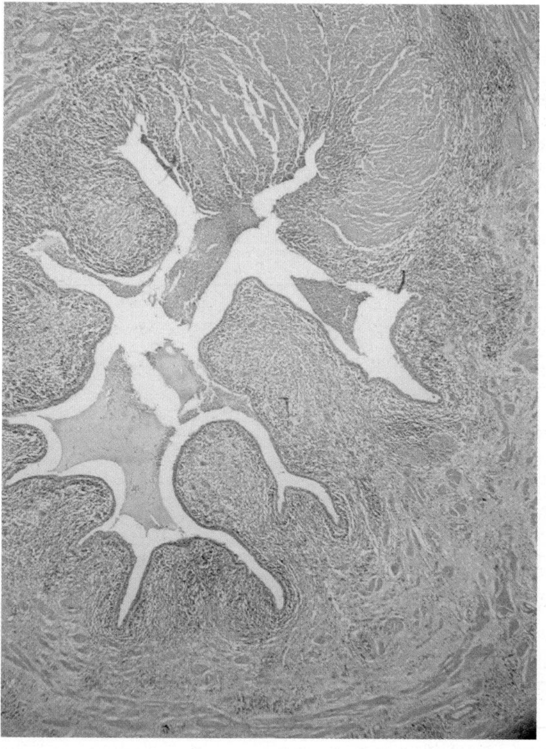

Fig. 15 Tuberculous stricture of the ureter with mucosal and mural inflammation and thickening.

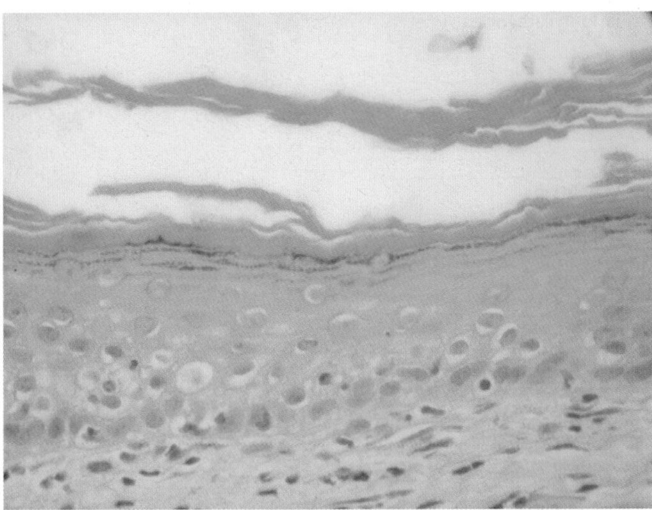

Fig. 16 Keratinizing squamous metaplasia of the bladder. There is no epithelial dysplasia but such cases carry an increased risk of developing squamous cell carcinoma.

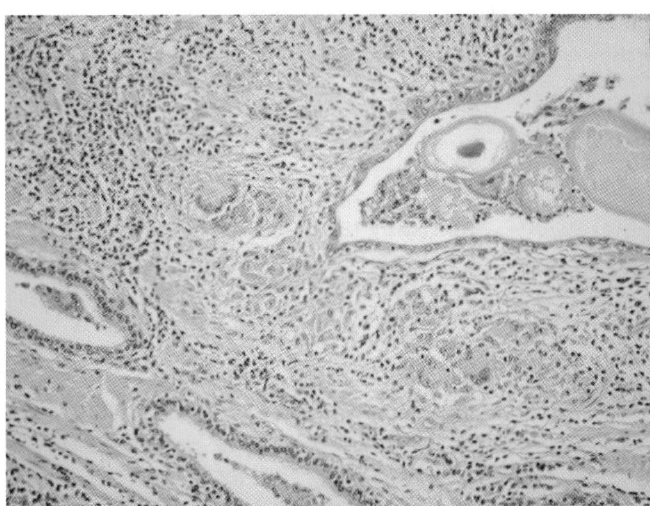

Fig. 17 BCG-induced granulomatous prostatitis in a cystoprostatectomy specimen. Patient had been treated with intravesical BCG for transitional carcinoma-*in situ* of the bladder.

detected. Sometimes, the large masses of keratin produced by metaplastic lesions in the renal pelvis produce renal colic.

Up to three-quarters of cases of bladder tuberculosis are associated with renal tuberculosis, although some cases are due to spread from the epididymis. The bladder capacity may be severely reduced due to scarring and contraction (Laidlaw 1976) making cystectomy or bladder augmentation necessary even in fully treated cases.

BCG-induced urinary tract infection

The use of intravesical BCG has improved the prognosis of both transitional carcinoma-*in situ* and superficial bladder cancer. This usually causes only a self-limiting low-grade superficial cystitis, but sometimes the inflammatory reaction is more severe. There are reports of both disseminated infection with BCG and reflux of the organisms up the ureter causing ureteric obstruction, the latter occurring in 0.3 per cent of 2602 patients (Lamm 1992). Renal involvement was recorded in 0.1 per cent of these patients and is presumed to have arisen from ascending infection rather than haematogenous spread. The infection frequently involves the prostate, but this is often asymptomatic. Histologically, the lesions caused by BCG are indistinguishable from those seen in classical tuberculosis (Fig. 17) and caseation may be present, more frequently in the prostate than in the bladder. Organisms may sometimes be demonstrated by standard acid-fast staining techniques.

Treatment

Although principally evaluated in clinical trials in patients with pulmonary tuberculosis, extensive clinical experience indicates that short-course treatment regimens are suitable for all forms of the disease. Most modern regimens are based on an intensive phase, usually lasting 2 months, during which time virtually all the tubercle bacilli in the lesions are killed, followed by a 4-month less intensive phase designed to kill any remaining organisms. The drugs used in the intensive phase are rifampicin (rifampin), isoniazid, pyrazinamide, ethambutol, and under some circumstances, streptomycin. The principal drug used in the continuation phase is rifampicin that has the unique ability to kill near-dormant tubercle bacilli, although in some regimens ethambutol replaces rifampicin, with therapy being extended for an additional two months. Isoniazid is also given during the continuation phase to kill any mutants resistant to the principal drug that arise and commence replication.

The regimens currently recommended by the World Health Organization (1997) are listed in Table 4. Most patients with newly diagnosed genitourinary tuberculosis will be in Treatment Category I. Ideally, the drugs are given daily but if this is difficult to organize, the drugs may be administered thrice weekly, either throughout or just in the continuation phase.

The single most important reason for treatment failure is non-adherence to therapy by the patient. There are many causes for such non-adherence and the fault usually lies with the health services rather than the patient. As a result, the World Health Organization has stressed the importance of directly observed therapy as a key component of effective tuberculosis control.

In cases of multidrug resistance, other agents including ethionamide, prothionamide, thiacetazone, cycloserine, capreomycin, *p*-amino salicylic acid, fluoroquinolones, such as ofloxacin and sparfloxacin, and the newer macrolides including clarithromycin and azithromycin are used. Limited evidence indicates that the antileprosy drug clofazimine and combinations of aminopenicillins and β-lactamase inhibitors, such as amoxycillin with sulbactam, are also of use. These drugs are generally more toxic, more expensive and less active than the first-line drugs and treatment is often prolonged and costly. Such therapy should, whenever possible, be guided by rigorously controlled drug susceptibility testing and single drugs should never be added blindly to failing treatment regimens. For details of the management of multidrug resistant tuberculosis see World Health Organization (1999).

Three of the first-line drugs used to treat tuberculosis—rifampicin (rifampin), isoniazid, pyrazinamide—and also ethionamide and prothionamide—are either eliminated in the bile or metabolized and may be given in the usual recommended doses to patients with impaired renal function. Isoniazid is the exception as the risk of neurological toxicity, particularly peripheral neuropathy, but also encephalopathy

Table 4 The WHO-recommended short-course antituberculosis drug regimens in four categories of patients

Treatment category	Definition	Initial intensive phase (daily or three times each week)	Continuation phase[a]
I	New smear positive pulmonary TB; new smear negative pulmonary TB with extensive lung involvement; new severe forms of extrapulmonary (including genitourinary) TB	2 EHRZ (SHRZ) 2 EHRZ (SHRZ) 2 EHRZ (SHRZ)	4 HR 4 H_3R_3 6 HE
II	Smear positive pulmonary TB: relapse, treatment failure or treatment after interruption	2 SHRZE/1 HRZE 2 SHRZE/1 HRZE	5 HRE 5 $H_3R_3E_3$
III	New smear negative pulmonary TB (other than Category I); new less severe forms of extrapulmonary TB	2 HRZ 2 HRZ 2 HRZ	4 HR 4 H_3R_3 6 HE
IV	Chronic cases, that is, still bacteriologically positive after supervised retreatment	Second line drugs required according to WHO guidelines in specialized centres	

[a] Subscript '3' indicates thrice weekly dosing.

H = isoniazid; R = rifampicin (rifampin); Z = pyrazinamide; E = ethambutol; S = streptomycin.

(see below), appears to be higher in patients with impaired renal function. Accordingly, in Appendix 3 of the British National Formulary, an adult dose of 200 mg rather than 300 mg is recommended.

The limited data on isoniazid-induced hepatotoxicity in renal transplant recipients is reviewed in the European Best Practice Guidelines for Renal Transplantation (2002). It is concluded that the incidence of serious hepatotoxicity is low when isoniazid is given alone, as in preventive therapy, but is more common when given with other antituberculosis drugs. It is therefore recommended that renal transplant recipients receiving multidrug antituberculosis therapy should be closely monitored for hepatotoxicity. Notably, the risk of isoniazid hepatotoxicity does not appear to be enhanced in those infected with hepatitis B or C viruses.

Ethambutol is eliminated principally by the kidney and reduced doses should be given according to GFR: 25 mg should be given three times weekly if the GFR is between 50 and 100 ml/min and twice weekly if it is between 30 and 50 ml/min (Mitchison and Ellard 1980; Girling 1989). Aminoglycosides including streptomycin are excreted entirely by the kidney and are a cause of serious ototoxicity as well as renal toxicity. They should therefore be used with caution in patients with renal failure, whether on dialysis or not. In practice, the drugs should only be given if frequent plasma measurements of the drugs can be carried out so that a safe dose can be established.

In general, the occurrence of toxic side-effects with modern antituberculosis therapy is uncommon. The major adverse effects of the first-line drugs are listed in Table 5.

Encephalopathy, normally a rare complication of isoniazid therapy, can occur in patients with renal failure, although its incidence is reduced by the prescription of pyridoxine, 25–50 mg/day. Cases have been reported in dialysis patients even though they were receiving pyridoxine; the encephalopathy has resolved on stopping isoniazid (Cheung *et al.* 1993).

In renal transplant patients, care should be taken with rifampicin (rifampin) as it increases the catabolism of many drugs, including corticosteroids, azathioprine, cyclosporin, sirolimus, and tacrolimus, as well as other important drugs used in transplant patients such as diazepam, digoxin, opioids, oral contraceptives, phenytoin, and warfarin (Finch *et al.* 2002). Streptomycin is contraindicated in patients on cyclosporin as it increases the level of this agent and can lead to cyclosporin nephrotoxicity.

Particular problems are encountered in the treatment of tuberculosis in HIV-positive patients receiving antiretroviral agents. Protease inhibitors and non-nucleoside reverse transcriptase inhibitors interfere with the metabolism of rifampicin (rifampin) and, by inducing hepatic cytochromes, rifampicin enhances the metabolism of antiretroviral agents, the serum levels of which may become subtherapeutic. Adverse interactions are lower with rifabutin. Guidelines and advice on this problem change from time to time and clinicians should seek specialist advice or consult up-to-date guidelines issued by the Centers for Disease Control and Prevention, Atlanta, Georgia or the World Health Organization (see, e.g. Centers for Disease Control and Prevention 1998).

There were initial concerns that the use of prophylactic isoniazid in transplant patients might increase the plasma cyclosporin level and induce cyclosporin nephrotoxicity. A recent detailed study, however, on seven renal transplant recipients with slow isoniazid acetylation status showed that the pharmacokinetics of cyclosporin were unaffected by isoniazid and it was concluded that concomitant administration of these agents is safe (Sud *et al.* 2000). As yet, there are insufficient data to draw

Table 5 Adverse effects of first-line antituberculosis agents

Agent	Adverse effects
Isoniazid	
Uncommon	Hepatitis, cutaneous hypersensitivity reactions including erythema multiforme, peripheral neuropathy
Rare	Vertigo, convulsions, optic neuritis and atrophy, psychiatric disturbance, haemolytic anaemia, aplastic anaemia, dermal reactions including pellagra, purpura and lupoid syndrome, gynaecomastia, hyperglycaemia, arthralgia
Rifampicin (rifampin)	
Uncommon	Hepatitis, flushing, itching with or without a rash, gastrointestinal upsets, 'flu-like' syndrome, headache
Rare	Dyspnoea, hypotension with or without shock, Addisonian crisis, haemolytic anaemia, acute renal failure, thrombocytopenia with or without purpura, transient leucopenia or eosinophilia, menstrual disturbances, muscular weakness, pseudomembranous colitis
Pyrazinamide	
Common	Anorexia
Uncommon	Hepatitis, nausea and vomiting, urticaria, nausea, arthralgia
Rare	Sideroblastic anaemia, photosensitization, gout, dysuria, aggravation of peptic ulcer
Ethambutol	
Uncommon	Optic neuritis, arthralgia
Rare	Hepatitis, cutaneous hypersensitivity including pruritis and urticaria, photosensitive lichenoid eruptions, paraesthesia of the extremities, interstitial nephritis
Streptomycin	
Uncommon	Vertigo, ataxia, deafness, tinnitus, cutaneous hypersensitivity
Rare	Renal damage, aplastic anaemia, agranulocytosis, peripheral neuropathy, optic neuritis with scotoma, severe bleeding due to antagonism of Factor V, neuromuscular blockade in patients receiving muscle relaxants or with myaesthenia gravis

any firm conclusions as to the effect of isoniazid on the metabolism of tacrolimus or sirolimus.

The role of preventive antituberculosis therapy in renal transplant patients is controversial and has been discussed earlier.

Leprosy

The global distribution of leprosy is shown in Fig. 18.

Leprosy and renal disease

Direct involvement of the kidney by *M. leprae* is unusual, possibly because renal tissue is more resistant than other organs to invasion by this bacillus (Gupta *et al.* 1977). While epithelioid granulomas consistent with lepromas have been seen in the kidney, acid-fast bacilli have not been reported (Al-Mohaya *et al.* 1988). Despite the rarity of direct bacillary invasion, renal damage is a major cause of morbidity and mortality in patients with leprosy, in whom cases of interstitial nephritis, secondary amyloidosis, and most histological forms of glomerulonephritis have been reported (Mittal *et al.* 1972; Iveson *et al.* 1975; Ng *et al.* 1981; Date *et al.* 1985; Chopra *et al.* 1991). Between 11 and 38 per cent of leprosy patients die of renal failure due to glomerulonephritis or amyloidosis (Ridley 1988) but the incidence of milder or resolving renal disease detectable by percutaneous renal biopsy is higher (Date and Johny 1975).

The relative incidence of the various types of renal disease in leprosy patients varies from region to region. In an autopsy study in Brazil of 199 leprosy patients dying between 1970 and 1986, renal lesions were found in 144 (72 per cent) (Nakayama *et al.* 2001). Renal amyloidosis was detected in 61 patients (42.7 per cent of those with renal lesions), glomerulonephritis in 29 (20.2 per cent), nephrosclerosis in 22 (15.3 per cent), tubulointerstitial nephritis in 18 (12.5 per cent), granulomas in two and other lesions in 12 patients. For unknown reasons, renal amyloidosis is less frequent in the Indian subcontinent (Chugh *et al.* 1981; Nigam *et al.* 1986; Jayalakshmi *et al.* 1987) and Japan (Ozaki and Furuta 1975).

Glomerulonephritis occurs most frequently in patients with multibacillary (lepromatous and borderline lepromatous) leprosy and is due to deposition of immune complexes in the glomeruli (Date and Johny 1975; Ng *et al.* 1981; Date *et al.* 1985). Thus deposits of immunoglobulin in the IgG and IgM classes, and the C3 component of complement, have been seen in the renal lesions although it is uncertain whether the antigen responsible for the immune complex formation is mycobacterial (Date *et al.* 1977). Impairment of renal function, sometimes significant, commonly occurs during acute episodes of erythema nodosum leprosum (ENL) but, in the absence of complicating conditions such as amyloidosis, renal function improves during periods of quiescence (Bajaj *et al.* 1981a; Kanwar *et al.* 1984). Opinions differ as to whether glomerulonephritis is more common in patients with ENL than in other forms of leprosy (Drutz and Gutman 1973; Ng *et al.* 1981; Al-Mohaya *et al.* 1988).

Amyloidosis also is associated with multibacillary leprosy and its geographical incidence varies considerably. In the Brazilian autopsy study referred to above (Nakayama *et al.* 2001), amyloidosis was more common in those with lepromatous leprosy (36 per cent) than in those with tuberculoid or borderline disease (5 per cent), and occurred most frequently in patients with recurrent ENL and trophic ulcers. In the same report, 95 per cent of the patients with renal amyloid had proteinuria and 88 per cent renal failure, with the latter being a common

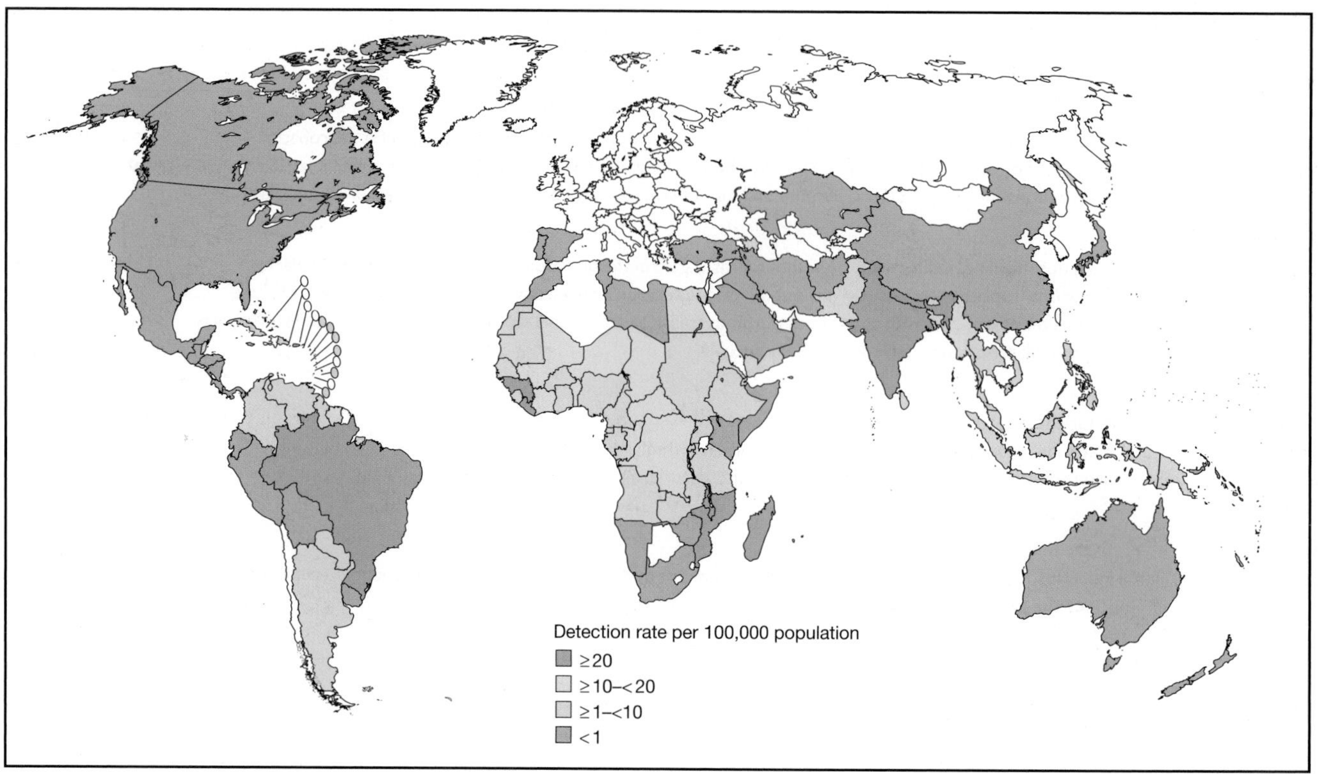

Fig. 18 Global detection of leprosy, 1996 (World Health Organization, 1997).

cause of death. Repeated flare-ups of ENL appear to be an important factor in the development of amyloidosis (McAdam *et al.* 1975).

In a search for sensitive and early markers for renal damage in leprosy patients, haematuria, microalbuminuria, and elevation of urinary β_2-microglobulin were found in 22, 16, and 20 per cent, respectively, of 96 leprosy patients with normal serum creatinine levels (Kirsztajn *et al.* 1993). In India, significant impairment of renal function was common in a group of 122 patients with lepromatous leprosy, notably in those with ENL (Bajaj *et al.* 1981b). Although many patients had diminished endogenous creatinine clearance and proteinuria, serum creatinine levels were significantly increased only in patients with active ENL.

There have been a few reports of renal failure in leprosy patients as a complication of rifampicin therapy (Gupta *et al.* 1992).

Leprosy has been described in renal transplant patients. In one report of four patients (Roselino *et al.* 1993), two who had the disease before the transplant did not relapse but two presented with new disease (one lepromatous, one borderline) after the transplant. In another report, from the Indian subcontinent (Date *et al.* 1998), three of nine renal transplant patients were known to have leprosy before transplantation. After transplant one had an exacerbation of previously unrecognized leprosy and five developed new disease 22 months to 12 years later. The immunosuppressive drugs taken by the patients seemed to have no adverse effect on treatment of the disease.

Leprosy and genital lesions

While direct invasion of the kidney by *M. leprae* is rare, bacillary invasion of the testis is common in multibacillary leprosy. Patients with lepromatous or, less often, borderline lepromatous leprosy may present with painful swollen testes, sometimes associated with ENL reactions. Such a presentation is rarely the first indication of leprosy, but leprosy should be considered in the differential diagnosis of orchitis in at-risk populations (Akhtar *et al.* 1980).

In addition to orchitis, chronic testicular involvement in leprosy may lead to small soft testicles with impaired testicular sensation, oligospermia, and aspermia (Nigam *et al.* 1988). Hormonal changes, including reduction of the level of testosterone and elevation of luteinizing hormone, follicle stimulating hormone, and oestradiol levels (Saporta and Yuksel 1994), may result in gynaecomastia and reduction of sexual function. Infertility is common. The epididymis may also be involved and in some cases aspermia and infertility is due to fibrous obstruction in the ducts of the epididymis in patients with relatively normal testes (Ibrahiem *et al.* 1979). The lack of testosterone resulting from testicular atrophy may lead to osteoporosis, bone density showing a correlation with free testosterone levels (Ishikawa *et al.* 1997, 2000).

Histological examination of the testis and epididymis reveals typical lepromatous lesions or a very variable and poorly defined pattern of vascular and obliterative changes (Kumar *et al.* 1982; Nigam *et al.* 1988).

By contrast, information on the effect of leprosy on the female genital tract is limited and contradictory. In one study, no pathological evidence of leprosy, and no dysfunction, was found (Sharma *et al.* 1981). On the other hand, in a study of 86 women with multi-bacillary leprosy, 30 gave a history of irregular periods; half the 24 married women with irregular periods were infertile and had hormonal evidence of ovarian dysfunction (Neena *et al.* 2003).

Treatment

Treatment is with standard antileprosy drugs (World Health Organization 1994), making allowance for the degree of renal dysfunction.

Environmental mycobacterial disease

Urinary tract involvement

Disease of the genitourinary system due to EM is exceedingly rare. Diagnosis poses serious problems in view of the frequency with which such bacteria are harmless contaminants of urine. Between 1980 and 1989, 572 EM cultured from urine in south-east England were submitted to the regional mycobacterium reference centre but, with five dubious exceptions, all appeared to be contaminants (Grange and Yates 1992). Brooker and Aufderheide (1980) proposed six criteria for the diagnosis of such disease:

- symptoms of chronic or recurrent genitourinary infection
- radiological or endoscopic evidence of genitourinary disease
- abnormalities on urine analysis
- failure to isolate other urinary tract pathogens
- repeated isolations of the same mycobacterial species
- histological demonstration of granulomas and, preferably, acid-fast bacilli.

The first four criteria should alert the clinician to the possibility of a mycobacterial aetiology, the fifth strongly suggests the diagnosis, but only the sixth is confirmatory. A retrospective application of these criteria failed to confirm the diagnosis in 19 supposed cases (Brooker and Aufderheide 1980).

The few confirmed cases of renal disease were caused by *M. intracellulare*, termed the 'Battey bacillus' in the older literature. Two such patients were treated successfully by nephrectomy (Faber *et al.* 1965; Pergament *et al.* 1974) and one by nephroureterectomy (Newman 1970). A further patient with pulmonary disease due to a slow-growing, non-chromogenic mycobacterium (a description compatible with *M. intracellulare*) developed a renal abscess due to an identical strain (Tsai *et al.* 1968). Three cases of epididymitis have been reported, one due to *Mycobacterium xenopi* (Engbeck *et al.* 1967) and two to *Mycobacterium kansasii* (Wood *et al.* 1956; Hepper *et al.* 1971). Both *M. xenopi* and *M. fortuitum* were isolated from a case of prostatitis with a granulomatous appearance compatible with mycobacterial disease (Lee *et al.* 1977).

In a study of the isolation of mycobacteria from HIV-positive patients in south-eastern England, EM were isolated relatively infrequently from the urine and genitourinary tract compared with other sites (Yates *et al.* 1993). EM were isolated from 616 patients but from the urine of only 21 of them. In 15 cases the EM (12 MAC and three *M. kansasii*) were isolated from several other sites and in six cases they were single isolates (two *M. chelonae*, two *M. fortuitum*, one *Mycobacterium gordonae*, and one *M. xenopi*) and were probably casual contaminants. The low isolation rate of mycobacteria from urine in HIV/AIDS patients may be artefactual as, owing to the high incidence of contaminating EM, many centres may not examine urine for mycobacteria when there is evidence of mycobacterial disease involving other sites.

Treatment of disease due to EM depends on the causative species and specialist reference centres should be consulted. *In vitro* drug susceptibility tests are used to select suitable regimens but the results of these tests do not always correlate with clinical response. Owing to their rarity, there is no reliable information on therapy of genitourinary disease due to EM and treatment should therefore be based on drug regimens evaluated for pulmonary and disseminated disease. These include a newer macrolide (azithromycin, 600 mg daily or clarithromycin, 500 mg twice daily), in combination with ethambutol for disease due to MAC (Dunne *et al.* 2000). Limited evidence indicates that such therapy is suitable for other slowly growing species.

Treatment of disease caused by the rapid growers *M. chelonae*, *M. abscessus*, and *M. fortuitum* is largely based on anecdotal experience, but the outcome of therapy is unpredictable and the duration of therapy is based on clinical response. Therapeutic success has been reported with various combinations of trimethoprim, doxycycline, amikacin, gentamicin, cephalosporins, imipenem, erythromycin, and the newer macrolides (e.g. clarithromycin) and quinolones (e.g. ciprofloxacin).

Complicating endstage renal disease and its treatment

Dialysis patients

Haemodialysis

Small clusters and isolated cases of disseminated disease due to *M. chelonae* have occurred in patients on haemodialysis (Lowry *et al.* 1990). In some cases, the cause was contamination of the dialysis machine by *M. chelonae*. In one case (Azadian *et al.* 1981), isolates from the patient and from the water-softener resin used to purify the water in a hospital haemodialysis unit were shown by isoelectric focusing patterns of mycobacterial enzymes to be identical (Sparks and Ross 1981).

Peritoneal dialysis

Environmental mycobacterial disease can be a complication of intermittent chronic peritoneal dialysis. Band *et al.* (1981) reviewed 17 cases, all due to *M. chelonae*. As in the case of haemodialysis, the cause appeared to be use of contaminated equipment. This complication is less frequently encountered with CAPD. Dunmire and Breyer (1991) reviewed nine cases: four due to *M. fortuitum*; three to *M. chelonae*, and one each to *M. gastri* and MAC. *M. gastri* is not a known mycobacterial pathogen and raises the question, to which there is no clear answer, of whether a mycobacterium isolated from CAPD fluid is a pathogen or behaving as a saprophyte. *M. gordonae*, a common isolate from water but rarely implicated as a pathogen, has also been isolated from peritoneal fluid from a CAPD patient with peritonitis and was probably the cause of the infection (London *et al.* 1988).

Other reported cases of mycobacterial peritonitis include one due to *M. kansasii* (Giladi *et al.* 1992) and two due to *M. fortuitum* (LaRocco *et al.* 1986; Choi *et al.* 1993). These reports emphasize the need to culture for mycobacteria in cases of CAPD-related peritonitis when 'routine' cultures are repeatedly negative.

Treatment, which is usually successful, involves drainage of residual fluid, removal of the catheter (essential for success), and appropriate chemotherapy. Complications include abdominal abscesses, fistulae, and adhesions. Most patients with mycobacterial peritonitis need to be transferred to haemodialysis (White *et al.* 1993).

Transplant patients

Renal transplantation and the accompanying iatrogenic immunosuppression predispose the patient to mycobacterial disease (Sinnott and Emmanuel 1990). The incidence of such disease in these patients is much higher than in the general population and in 25–40 per cent of cases the cause is an EM. The development of clinical tuberculosis is usually the result of reactivation of dormant foci; the disease may be confined to the lung or involve many organs. Disease due to EM may also be localized to the lung or disseminated, but is often a cutaneous problem, typical organisms being *Mycobacterium haemophilum*, *Mycobacterium marinum*, *M. chelonae*, and *M. fortuitum*. The great majority of reports of *M. haemophilum* infection have been of cases of cutaneous involvement in renal transplant recipients.

Two different mycobacterial diseases may occur in the same patient. Koizumi and Sommers (1980) described a patient with culture-positive *M. tuberculosis* 4 years after renal transplantation. The following year, after an episode of transplant rejection treated with methylprednisolone, the patient developed a radiological opacity in the left lower lobe of the lung which, on excision and culture, yielded a heavy growth of *M. xenopi*.

Symptoms of mycobacterial disease in transplant patients are often masked by the immunosuppression so diagnosis is not easy and thus often delayed; mortality is around 30 per cent. Therapy of diseases caused by EM is by agents appropriate to the species, modified by sensitivity testing.

Conclusion

The association of disease of the kidneys and urinary tract with mycobacterial infection is of two kinds. First, mycobacteria (especially *M. tuberculosis*) may cause renal and urinary tract disease which, occasionally, leads to renal failure. Second, patients with renal failure, especially when treated by dialysis or transplantation, are more susceptible both to reactivation of latent mycobacterial disease (usually tuberculosis) or to new infection, especially by EM, but also sometimes tuberculosis. A further association is that some patients with renal disease, notably vasculitides and certain forms of glomerulonephritis, require treatment with immunosuppressive drugs that render them more susceptible to mycobacterial disease. The development of unexplained fever, malaise, and weight loss in these patients, especially during treatment with immunosuppressive drugs, and in renal transplant recipients should lead to a suspicion of mycobacterial disease.

Patients with chronic renal failure, including those treated by haemodialysis or CAPD need careful attention to drug dosages when treatment for mycobacterial disease is indicated. A further complication in renal transplant patients is the interaction between cyclosporin, tacrolimus and other immunosuppressive drugs with some of the antibacterial agents used in the treatment of mycobacterial disease.

Acknowledgements

We thank Dr Sandra Gibson for taking the photographs of the macroscopic specimens from the St George's Hospital Medical School Pathology Museum. We are grateful to Dr Uday Patel for assistance in selecting suitable X-ray images. Mara Radjenovic, of Audiovisual Services, St George's Hospital Medical School, kindly reconfigured Fig. 2.

References

Aceti, A. *et al.* (1999). Identification of HIV patients with active pulmonary tuberculosis using urine based polymerase chain reaction assay. *Thorax* **54**, 145–146.

Ahijado, F. *et al.* (1991). Tuberculous peritonitis on CAPD. *Contributions to Nephrology* **89**, 79–86.

Al-Mohaya, S. A. *et al.* (1988). Renal granuloma and mesangial proliferative glomerulo-nephritis in leprosy. *International Journal of Leprosy and Other Mycobacterial Diseases* **56**, 599–602.

Akhtar, M., Ali, M. A., and Mackey, D. M. (1980). Lepromatous leprosy presenting as orchitis. *American Journal of Clinical Pathology* **73**, 712–715.

American Thoracic Society (1974). Preventative therapy of tuberculosis infection. *American Review of Respiratory Disease* **110**, 371–374.

Annobil, S. H., Al Hilfi, A., and Kazi, T. (1990). Primary tuberculosis of the penis in an infant. *Tubercle* **71**, 229–230.

Azadian, B. S. *et al.* (1981). Disseminated infection with *Mycobacterium chelonei* in a haemodialysis patient. *Tubercle* **62**, 281–284.

Bajaj, A. K. *et al.* (1981a). Sequential renal functions in leprosy. *Leprosy in India* **53**, 185–189.

Bajaj, A. K. *et al.* (1981b). Renal functional status in lepromatous leprosy. *International Journal of Leprosy and Other Mycobacterial Diseases* **49**, 37–41.

Band, J. D., Ward, J. I., and Fraser, D. W. (1981). Peritonitis due to a *Mycobacterium chelonei*-like organism associated with intermittent chronic peritoneal dialysis. *Journal of Infectious Diseases* **145**, 9–17.

Benn, J. J. *et al.* (1988). Cryptogenic tuberculosis as a preventable cause of end-stage renal failure. *American Journal of Nephrology* **8**, 306–308.

Brooker, W. J. and Aufderheide, A. C. (1980). Genitourinary tract infections due to atypical mycobacteria. *Journal of Urology* **124**, 242–244.

Byrd, R. B. *et al.* (1976). Leukoplakia associated with renal tuberculosis in the chemotherapeutic era. *British Journal of Urology* **48**, 377–381.

Centers for Disease Control and Prevention (1998). Prevention and treatment of tuberculosis among patients infected with human immunodeficiency virus: principles of therapy and revised recommendations. *Morbidity and Mortality Weekly Report* **47** (RR-20), 1–58.

Cheng, I. K., Chan, P. C., and Chan, M. K. (1989). Tuberculous peritonitis complicating long-term peritoneal dialysis. *American Journal of Nephrology* **9**, 155–161.

Cheung, W. C. *et al.* (1993). Isoniazid induced encephalopathy in dialysis patients. *Tubercle and Lung Disease* **74**, 136–139.

Choi, C. W. *et al.* (1993). *Mycobacterium fortuitum* peritonitis associated with continuous ambulatory peritoneal dialysis. *Korean Journal of Internal Medicine* **8**, 25–27.

Chopra, N. K. *et al.* (1991). Renal involvement in leprosy. *Journal of the Association of Physicians of India* **39**, 165–167.

Christensen, W. I. (1974). Genitourinary tuberculosis: review of 102 cases. *Medicine* **53**, 377–390.

Chugh, K. S. *et al.* (1981). Pattern of renal amyloidosis in Indian patients. *Postgraduate Medical Journal* **57**, 31–35.

Collins, C. H., Grange, J. M., and Yates, M. D. (1984). Mycobacteria in water. *Journal of Applied Bacteriology* **57**, 193–211.

Collins, C. H., Grange, J. M., and Yates, M. D. *Tuberculosis Bacteriology. Organisation and Practice* 2nd edn. Oxford: Butterworth Heinemann, 1997.

Date, A. and Johny, K. V. (1975). Glomerular subepithelial deposits in lepromatous leprosy. *American Journal of Tropical Medicine and Hygiene* **24**, 853–855.

Date, A., Haribar, S., and Jeyavarthini, S. E. (1985). Renal lesions and other major findings in necropsies of 133 patients with leprosy. *International Journal of Leprosy and Other Mycobacterial Diseases* **53**, 455–460.

Date, A. *et al.* (1977). Glomerular pathology in leprosy. An electron microscopic study. *American Journal of Tropical Medicine and Hygiene* **26**, 266–272.

Date, A. *et al.* (1998). Leprosy and renal transplantation. *Leprosy Review* **69**, 40–45.

Drutz, D. J. and Gutman, R. A. (1973). Renal manifestations of leprosy: glomerulonephritis a complication of erythema nodosum leprosum. *American Journal of Tropical Medicine and Hygiene* **22**, 496–502.

Dunmire, R. B. and Breyer, J. A. (1991). Non-tuberculous mycobacterial peritonitis during chronic ambulatory peritoneal dialysis: case report and review of diagnostic and therapeutic strategies. *American Journal of Kidney Diseases* **18**, 126–130.

Dunne, M. *et al.* (2000). A randomized, double-blind trial comparing azithromycin and clarithromycin in the treatment of disseminated *Mycobacterium avium* infection in patients with human immunodeficiency virus. *Clinical Infectious Diseases* **31**, 1245–1252.

Eastwood, J. B. *et al.* (1979). Plasma 25-hydroxyvitamin D in normal subjects and patients with terminal renal failure, on maintenance haemodialysis and after transplantation. *Clinical Science* **57**, 473–476.

Eastwood, J. B. *et al.* (1994). Tuberculosis as primary renal diagnosis in end-stage uremia. *Journal of Nephrology* **7**, 290–293.

Engbeck, H. C., Vergmann, B., and Baess, I. (1967). *Mycobacterium xenopi*: a bacteriological study of *M. xenopi* including case reports of Danish patients. *Acta Pathologica et Microbiologica Scandinavica* **69**, 576–594.

European Best Practice Guidelines for Renal Transplantation (Part 2) (2002). Tuberculosis. *Nephrology, Dialysis, Transplantation* **17** (Suppl. 4), 39–43.

Faber, D. R., Lasky, I. I., and Goodwin, W. E. (1965). Idiopathic unilateral renal hematuria associated with atypical acid-fast bacillus, Battey type: cure by partial nephrectomy. *Journal of Urology* **93**, 435–439.

Felsenfeld, A. J., Drezner, M. K., and Llach, F. (1986). Hypercalcaemia and elevated calcitriol in a maintenance dialysis patient with tuberculosis. *Archives of Internal Medicine* **146**, 1941–1945.

Ferric, B. G. and Rundle, J. S. H. (1983). Tuberculous epididymo-orchitis. A review of 20 cases. *British Journal of Urology* **55**, 437–439.

Finch, C. K. *et al.* (2002). Rifampin and rifabutin drug interactions: an update. *Archives of Internal Medicine* **162**, 985–992.

Giladi, M. *et al.* (1992). Peritonitis caused by *Mycobacterium kansasii* in a patient undergoing continuous ambulatory peritoneal dialysis. *American Journal of Kidney Diseases* **19**, 597–599.

Girling, D. J. The chemotherapy of tuberculosis. In *The Biology of the Mycobacteria* Vol. 3 (ed. C. Ratledge, J. L. Stanford, and J. M. Grange), pp. 285–323. London and New York: Academic Press, 1989.

Goldman, S. M. *et al.* (1985). Computed tomography of renal tuberculosis and its pathological correlates. *Journal of Computer Assisted Tomography* **9**, 771–776.

Grange, J. M. and Yates, M. D. (1992). Survey of mycobacteria isolated from urine and the genito-urinary tract in South-East England from 1980 to 1989. *British Journal of Urology* **69**, 640–646.

Grange, J. M., Yates, M. D., and Ormerod, L. P. (1995). Factors determining ethnic differences in the incidence of bacteriologically confirmed genitourinary tuberculosis in South East England. *Journal of Infection* **30**, 37–40.

Greenberger, M. E., Wershub, L. P., and Auerbach, O. (1935). The incidence of renal tuberculosis in five hundred autopsies for pulmonary and extrapulmonary tuberculosis. *Journal of the American Medical Association* **104**, 726–730.

Gupta, J. C. *et al.* (1977). A histopathological study of renal biopsies in 50 cases of leprosy. *International Journal of Leprosy and Other Mycobacterial Diseases* **45**, 167–170.

Gupta, A. *et al.* (1992). Intravascular hemolysis and acute renal failure following intermittent rifampin therapy. *International Journal of Leprosy and Other Mycobacterial Diseases* **60**, 185–188.

Hariprasad, M. K. *et al.* (1979). Dense deposit disease in tuberculosis. *New York State Journal of Medicine* **79**, 2084–2085.

Hepper, N. G., Karlson, A. G., and Leary, F. J. (1971). Genito-urinary infection due to *Mycobacterium kansasii*. *Mayo Clinic Proceedings* **446**, 387–390.

Hernandez-Pando, R. *et al.* (2000). Persistence of DNA from *Mycobacterium tuberculosis* in superficially normal lung tissue during latent infection. *Lancet* **356**, 2133–2138.

Horsburgh, C. R. (1991), *Mycobacterium avium* complex infection in the acquired immunodeficiency syndrome. *New England Journal of Medicine* **324**, 1332–1338.

Hussein, M. M., Bakir, N., and Roujouleh, H. (1990). Tuberculosis in patients undergoing maintenance dialysis. *Nephrology, Dialysis, Transplantation* **5**, 584–587.

Ibrahiem, A. A. *et al.* (1979). Pathologic changes in testis and epididymis of infertile leprotic males. *International Journal of Leprosy and Other Mycobacterial Diseases* **47**, 44–49.

Ishikawa, S. *et al.* (1997). Osteoporosis due to testicular atrophy in male leprosy patients. *Acta Medica Okayama* **51**, 279–283.

Ishikawa, S. *et al.* (2000). Leydig cell hyperplasia and the maintenance of bone volume: bone histomorphometry and testicular histopathology in 29 male leprosy autopsy cases. *International Journal of Leprosy and Other Mycobacterial Diseases* **68**, 258–266.

Iveson, J. M. *et al.* (1975). Lepromatous leprosy presenting with polyarthritis, myositis and immune-complex glomerulonephritis. *British Medical Journal* **3**, 619–621.

Jayalakshmi, P. *et al.* (1987). Autopsy findings in 35 cases of leprosy in Malaysia. *International Journal of Leprosy and Other Mycobacterial Diseases* **55**, 510–514.

Kanwar, A. J., Bharija, S. C., and Belhaj, M. S. (1984). Renal functional status in leprosy. *Indian Journal of Leprosy* **56**, 595–599.

Kaufmann, P. *et al.* (1994). Impact of long-term hemodialysis on nutritional status in patients with end-stage renal failure. *Clinical Investigation* **72**, 754–761.

Kennedy, D. H. Extrapulmonary tuberculosis. In *The Biology of the Mycobacteria* Vol. 3 (ed. C. Ratledge, J. L. Stanford, and J. M. Grange), pp. 245–284. London and New York: Academic Press, 1989.

Kirsztajn, G. M. *et al.* (1993). Renal abnormalities in leprosy. *Nephron* **65**, 381–384.

Koizumi, J. H. and Sommers, H. M. (1980). *Mycobacterium xenopi* and pulmonary disease. *American Journal of Clinical Pathology* **73**, 826–830.

Kretschmer, H. L. (1930). Tuberculosis of the kidney, a critical review based on a series of 221 cases. *New England Journal of Medicine* **202**, 660–671.

Kumar, B. *et al.* (1982). Clinico-pathological study of testicular involvement in leprosy. *Leprosy in India* **54**, 48–55.

Kwan, J. T. *et al.* (1991). Mycobacterial infection is an important infective complication in British Asian dialysis patients. *Journal of Hospital Infection* **19**, 249–255.

Laidlaw, M. (1976). Renal tuberculosis. In *Scientific Foundations of Urology* Vol. 1, Chapter 30 (ed. D. Innes Williams and G. D. Chisholm), pp. 211–217. London: Heinemann.

Lamm, D. L. (1992). Complications of Bacille Calmette-Guérin immunotherapy. *Urological Clinics of North America* **19**, 565–572.

Lanjewar, D. N. *et al.* (1999). Renal lesions associated with AIDS—an autopsy study. *Indian Journal of Pathology and Microbiology* **42**, 63–68.

LaRocco, M. T., Mortensen, J. E., and Robinson, A. (1986). *Mycobacterium fortuitum* peritonitis in a patient undergoing chronic peritoneal dialysis. *Diagnostic Microbiology and Infectious Disease* **4**, 161–164.

Lattimer, J. K. (1965). Renal tuberculosis. *New England Journal of Medicine* **273**, 208–212.

Lee, L. W. *et al.* (1977). Granulomatous prostatitis: association with isolation of *Mycobacterium fortuitum*. *Journal of the American Medical Association* **237**, 2408–2409.

Lichtenstein, I. H. and MacGregor, R. R. (1983). Mycobacterial infections in renal transplant recipients: report of five cases and review of the literature. *Reviews of Infectious Diseases* **5**, 216–226.

London, R. D. *et al.* (1988). *Mycobacterium gordonae*: an unusual peritoneal pathogen in a patient undergoing continuous ambulatory peritoneal dialysis. *American Journal of Medicine* **85**, 703–704.

Lowry, P. W. *et al.* (1990). *Mycobacterium chelonei* infections among patients receiving high-flow dialysis in a haemodialysis clinic in California. *Journal of Infectious Diseases* **161**, 85–90.

Lye, W. C. and Lee, E. J. (1990). Tuberculous peritonitis in CAPD—a cause of hypercalcaemia. *Peritoneal Dialysis International* **10**, 307–308.

Maisonneuve, P. *et al.* (2000). Distribution of primary renal diseases leading to end-stage renal failure in the United States, Europe, and Australia/New Zealand: results from an international comparative study. *American Journal of Kidney Diseases* **35**, 157–165.

Mallinson, W. J. W. *et al.* (1981). Diffuse interstitial renal tuberculosis—an unusual cause of renal failure. *Quarterly Journal of Medicine* **50**, 137–148.

Marques, L. P. *et al.* (1996). AIDS-associated renal tuberculosis. *Nephron* **74**, 701–704.

McAdam, K. P. W. J. *et al.* (1975). Association of amyloidosis with erythema nodosum leprosum reactions and recurrent neutrophil leucocytosis in leprosy. *Lancet* **3**, 572–576.

Mignon, F. *et al.* Granulomatous interstitial nephritis. In *Advances in Nephrology* Vol. 13 (ed. J. F. Bach, J. Grosnier, J. L. Funch-Brentano, J. P. Grönfeld, and W. H. Maxwell), pp. 218–245. Chicago: Year Book Publishers, 1984.

Mitchison, D. A. and Ellard, G. A. (1980). Tuberculosis in patients having dialysis. *British Medical Journal* **1**, 1186 and 1533.

Mittal, M. M. *et al.* (1972). Renal lesions in leprosy. *Archives of Pathology* **93**, 8–12.

Moore, D. A. J. *et al.* (2002). High rates of tuberculosis in end-stage renal failure: the impact of international migration. *Emerging Infectious Diseases* **8**, 77–78.

Morgan, S. H., Eastwood, J. B., and Baker, L. R. I. (1990). Tuberculous interstitial nephritis—the tip of an iceberg. *Tubercle* **71**, 5–6.

Nakayama, E. E. *et al.* (2001). Renal lesions in leprosy: a retrospective study of 199 autopsies. *American Journal of Kidney Diseases* **38**, 26–30.

Narayana, A. S. (1982). Overview of renal tuberculosis. *Urology* **19**, 231–237.

Neena, K. *et al.* (2003). Ovarian function in female patients with multibacillary leprosy. *International Journal of Leprosy and Other Mycobacterial Diseases* **71**, 101–105.

Neves, P. L. *et al.* (1993). Unusual presentation of renal tuberculosis: end-stage renal disease. *Nephrology, Dialysis, Transplantation* **8**, 288–289.

Newman, H. (1970). Renal disease associated with atypical mycobacteria, Battey type: case report. *Journal of Urology* **103**, 403–405.

Ng, W. L., Scollard, D. M., and Hua, A. (1981). Glomerulonephritis in leprosy. *American Journal of Clinical Pathology* **76**, 321–329.

Njeh, M. *et al.* (1993). La tuberculose renale a forme pseudo tumorale. *Journal d'urologie (Paris)* **99**, 150–152.

Nigam, P. *et al.* (1986). Histo-functional status of kidney in leprosy. *Indian Journal of Leprosy* **58**, 567–575.

Nigam, P. *et al.* (1988). Male gonads in leprosy—a clinico-pathological study. *Indian Journal of Leprosy* **60**, 77–83.

O'Flynn, D. (1970). Treatment of genito-urinary tuberculosis. *British Journal of Urology* **42**, 667–671.

Ong, A. C. *et al.* (1992). Tuberculous peritonitis complicating peritoneal dialysis: a case for early diagnostic laparotomy. *Nephrology, Dialysis, Transplantation* **7**, 443–446.

Ormerod, L. P. (1993). Why does genito-urinary tuberculosis occur less often than expected in the ethnic Indian subcontinent population living in the United Kingdom? *Journal of Infection* **27**, 27–32.

Ozaki, M. and Furuta, M. (1975). Amyloidosis in leprosy. *International Journal of Leprosy and Other Mycobacterial Diseases* **43**, 116–124.

Pasternack, M. S. and Rubin, R. H. Urinary tract tuberculosis. In *Diseases of the Kidney* 5th edn. (ed. R. W. Schrier and C. W. Gottschalk), p. 915. London: Churchill Livingstone, 1993.

Pazianas, M. *et al.* (1991). Racial origin and primary renal diagnosis in 771 patients with end-stage renal disease. *Nephrology, Dialysis, Transplantation* **6**, 931–935.

Peces, R. and Alvarez, J. (1987). Hypercalcemia and elevated 1,25$(OH)_2D_3$ levels in a dialysis patient with disseminated tuberculosis. *Nephron* **46**, 377–379.

Peces, R. *et al.* (1998). Genitourinary tuberculosis as the cause of unexplained hypercalcaemia in a patient with pre-end-stage renal failure. *Nephrology, Dialysis, Transplantation* **13**, 488–490.

Pergament, M., Gonzalez, R., and Fraley, E. E. (1974). Atypical mycobacterioses of the urinary tract: a case report of extensive disease caused by the Battey bacillus. *Journal of the American Medical Association* **229**, 816–817.

Peters, F. T., Reiter, C. G., and Boswell, R. L. (1984). Transmission of tuberculosis by kidney transplantation. *Transplantation* **38**, 514–516.

Premkumar, A., Latimer, M., and Newhouse, J. H. (1987). CT and sonography of advanced urinary tract tuberculosis. *American Journal of Roentgenology* **148**, 65–69.

Quantrill, S. J. *et al.* (2001). Peritoneal tuberculosis in patients receiving continuous ambulatory peritoneal dialysis. *Nephrology, Dialysis, Transplantation* **16**, 1024–1027.

Qunibi, W. Y. *et al.* (1990). Mycobacterial infection after renal transplantation—a report of 14 cases and review of the literature. *Quarterly Journal of Medicine* **77**, 1039–1060.

Ramanathan, R. *et al.* (1998). Relief of urinary tract obstruction in tuberculosis to improve renal function. Analysis of predictive factors. *British Journal of Urology* **81**, 199–205.

Ridley, D. S. *Pathogenesis of Leprosy and Related Diseases* pp. 89–90. London: John Wright, 1988.

Ridley, D. S. and Ridley, M. J. (1987). Rationale for the histological spectrum of tuberculosis. A basis for classification. *Pathology* **19**, 186–192.

Roderick, P. J. *et al.* (1994). Population need for renal replacement therapy in Thames regions: ethnic dimension. *British Medical Journal* **309**, 1111–1114.

Rook, G. A. W. (1988). The role of vitamin D in tuberculosis. *American Review of Respiratory Disease* **138**, 768–770.

Roselino, A. M. *et al.* (1993). Renal transplantation in leprosy patients. *International Journal of Leprosy and Other Mycobacterial Diseases* **61**, 102–105.

Ross, J. C. (1970). Calcification in genito-urinary tuberculosis. *British Journal of Urology* **42**, 656–660.

Roylance, J. *et al.* (1970). The radiology of tuberculosis of the urinary tract. *Clinical Radiology* **21**, 163–170.

Saporta, L. and Yuksel, A. (1994). Androgenic status in patients with lepromatous leprosy. *British Journal of Urology* **74**, 221–224.

Sasaki, S. *et al.* (1979). Ten years' survey of dialysis-associated tuberculosis. *Nephron* **24**, 141–145.

Schaffer, R., Becker, J. A., and Goodman, J. (1983). Sonography of tuberculous kidney. *Urology* **22**, 209–211.

Schliesser, T. (1974). Die Bekämpfung der Rindertuberkulose-Tierversuch der Vergangenheit. *Praxis der Pneumonologie vereinigt mit der Tuberkulosearzt* **28** (Suppl.), 870–874.

Sechi, L. A. *et al.* (1997). Detection of *Mycobacterium tuberculosis* by PCR analysis of urine and other clinical samples from AIDS and non-HIV-infected patients. *Molecular and Cellular Probes* **11**, 281–285.

Sharma, S. C. *et al.* (1981). Leprosy and female reproductive organs. *International Journal of Leprosy and Other Mycobacterial Diseases* **49**, 177–179.

Shribman, J. H., Eastwood, J. B., and Uff, J. S. (1983). Immune-complex nephritis complicating miliary tuberculosis. *British Medical Journal* **287**, 1593–1594.

Simon, H. B. *et al.* (1977). Genito-urinary tuberculosis: clinical features in a general hospital population. *American Journal of Medicine* **63**, 410–420.

Sinnott, J. T. and Emmanuel, P. J. (1990). Mycobacterial infections in the transplant patient. *Seminars in Respiratory Infections* **5**, 65–71.

Smirnoff, M. *et al.* (1998). Tuberculin and anergy skin testing of patients receiving long-term hemodialysis. *Chest* **113**, 25–27.

Smith, E. C. (1982). Tuberculosis in dialysis patients. *International Journal of Artificial Organs* **5**, 11–12.

Sparks, J. and Ross, G. W. (1981). Isoelectric focusing studies on *Mycobacterium chelonei*. *Tubercle* **62**, 289–293.

Sud, K. *et al.* (2000). Isoniazid does not affect bioavailability of cyclosporine in renal transplant recipients. *Methods and Findings in Experimental and Clinical Pharmacology* **22**, 647–649.

Symes, J. M. and Blandy, J. P. (1973). Tuberculosis of the male urethra. *British Journal of Urology* **45**, 432–436.

Tan, D. *et al.* (1991). Successful treatment of tuberculous peritonitis while maintaining patient on CAPD. *Advances in Peritoneal Dialysis* **7**, 102–104.

Tsai, S. H., Yuc, W. Y., and Duthoy, E. J. (1968). Roentgen aspects of chronic pulmonary mycobacteriosis. An analysis of 18 cases including one with renal involvement. *Radiology* **90**, 306–310.

Ustvedt, H. J. (1947). The relationship between renal tuberculosis and primary infection. *Tubercle* **28**, 22–25.

van Vollenhoven, P. *et al.* (1996). Polymerase chain reaction in the diagnosis of urinary tract tuberculosis. *Urological Research* **24**, 107–111.

Wallgren, A. (1948). The 'timetable' of tuberculosis. *Tubercle* **29**, 245–251.

White, R. *et al.* (1993). Non-tuberculous mycobacterial infections in continuous ambulatory peritoneal dialysis patients. *American Journal of Kidney Diseases* **22**, 581–587.

Woeltje, K. F. *et al.* (1998). Tuberculosis infection and anergy in hemodialysis patients. *American Journal of Kidney Diseases* **31**, 848–852.

Wood, L. E., Buhler, V. B., and Pollak, A. (1956). Human infection with the 'yellow' acid fast bacillus. A report of fifteen additional cases. *American Review of Tuberculosis and Pulmonary Diseases* **73**, 917–929.

World Health Organization. *Chemotherapy of Leprosy*. Technical Report Series No. 847. Geneva: World Health Organization, 1994.

World Health Organization (1997). Leprosy situation in the world in 1997. *Weekly Epidemiological Record* **72**, 293–295.

World Health Organization. *Treatment of Tuberculosis: Guidelines for National Programmes* 2nd edn. Geneva: World Health Organization, 1997.

World Health Organization. Multidrug resistant tuberculosis (MDRTB). Basis for the development of an evidence-based case-management strategy for MDRTB within the WHO's DOTS strategy. Geneva: World Health Organisation (Communicable Diseases), 1999.

World Health Organization/International Union Against Tuberculosis and Lung Disease. *Global Project on Anti-tuberculosis Drug Resistance Surveillance. Anti-tuberculosis Drug Resistance in the World*. Report No. 2. Geneva: World Health Organization, 2000.

Yates, M. D. and Grange, J. M. (1988). Incidence and nature of human tuberculosis due to bovine tubercle bacilli in South East England: 1977–1987. *Epidemiology and Infection* **101**, 225–229.

Yates, M. D. and Grange, J. M. (1993). A bacteriological survey of tuberculosis due to human tubercle bacillus (*Mycobacterium tuberculosis*) in South-East England: 1984–1991. *Epidemiology and Infection* **110**, 609–619.

Yates, M. D., Pozniak, A., and Grange, J. M. (1993). Isolation of mycobacteria from patients seropositive for the human immunodeficiency virus (HIV) in South East England: 1984–1992. *Thorax* **48**, 990–995.

7.4 Schistosomiasis

Rashad S. Barsoum

Introduction

Schistosomes are highly conserved flat worms that seem to have emerged with the existence of man. The Pharos blamed them for causing haematuria in the Royal servants collecting the sacred Papyrus leaves from the Nile. The disease, which they called *âââ*, was well described in the Ebers Papyrus (sixteenth century BC), which also referred to its known response to antimony. Material evidence of the identity of *âââ* with schistosomiasis was provided for the first time by Ruffer in 1910, who discovered schistosomal ova in the bladder of a rehydrated Egyptian mummy, over 3000 years old. Ova were subsequently identified in the livers and bladders of other mummies, more recently examined in the Manchester Museum Department of Egyptology.

It remained for Theodore Bilharz to rediscover *Schistosoma hematobium* in 1852, hence, the alternative name 'bilharziasis', and for Sonsino to describe its lifecycle about 40 years later. Different species of the parasite were subsequently identified in Africa, Latin America, and the Far East, with the most recent being *Schistosoma mekongi* discovered in Malaysia in 1974.

Renal disease associated with schistosomiasis remained within the surgical domain for many decades, ever since the syndromes of lower urinary tract (LUT) involvement with *S. hematobium* were described by Egyptian pioneers around the middle of the past century (Badr 1986). The observation of proteinuria, without any LUT pathology in *Schistosoma mansoni* infection (Andrade and Rocha 1979; Houba 1979), introduced schistosomiasis to nephrology as a major cause of glomerulonephritis of considerable global epidemiological, clinical, and academic impact.

Epidemiology

The parasite

Schistosomes are bisexual trematodes with a highly sophisticated genome (Le *et al.* 2000). Seven species affect man as a definitive host, namely *S. hematobium*, *S. mansoni*, *S. japonicum*, *S. mekongi*, *S. intercalatum*, *S. mattheei*, and *S. bovis*.

Lifecycle

Infection is acquired through contact with contaminated fresh water in relatively stagnant small rivers and canals. The parasite's infective stage, the cercaria, penetrates the skin and mucous membranes, a process that is completed in about 30 s. The cercariae lose their bifid tails and are transformed into 'skin-stage schistosomulae' that stay in the dermis for 1–3 days during which they change their surface structure and antigenicity. They eventually migrate by the regional lymphatics to the bloodstream and ultimately are trapped in the pulmonary capillaries. Some 10–40 per cent of the 'lung-stage schistosomulae' manage to escape from this sieve and find their way to the hepatic sinusoids, where they increase in size and differentiate into males and females. The male is larger, measuring about 15 mm × 2 mm × 3 mm, and has a mammillated surface and two suckers that help to fix it to the venous walls. The longer and more slender female has a smooth surface and two tapered ends, and also has two suckers.

The worms then migrate to their eventual habitat, that is, the mesenteric veins for all species except *S. hematobium*. The latter resides in the perivesical venous plexus, which it reaches through retroperitoneal venous communications between the mesenteric, perivesical, and pudendal veins. One or more pairs live for some 3–8 years, but prolonged survival for up to 30 years has been reported.

The worms live in almost continuous copulation (Fig. 1). The female leaves the male's 'gynaecophoric canal' for a few hours every day and travels against the bloodstream to reach the mucosa of the colon, rectum, or LUT where it lays its eggs, starting 8–10 weeks after infection. The daily production of ova varies from 300 with *S. hematobium*

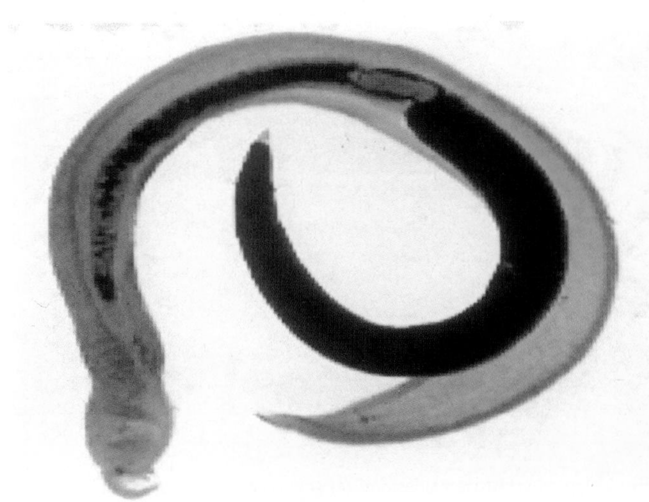

Fig. 1 Adult schistosomes in copulation.

and *S. mansoni* to 3000 with *S. japonicum*. Some ova remain trapped in the submucosa leading to a local granulomatous reaction (Fig. 2). Yet, the majority are able to find their way to the rectal or bladder lumena 10–12 days after being laid. Exteriorization is facilitated by the spines, which are characteristic of *Schistosoma* eggs. The position of the spine helps to differentiate species, as it is located terminally in *S. hematobium* eggs or laterally in all other species.

The eggs that reach fresh water hatch, releasing mature miracidia. These are ciliated organisms, which can survive for up to 8 h while searching for the appropriate intermediate host. This is a snail, specific for each species of schistosomes, within which the miracidium grows and multiplies, producing large numbers of cercariae. The latter are subsequently shed into the fresh water and remain viable for up to 72 h searching for their definitive host to complete the lifecycle, or they die.

The host

Schistosomiasis affects people of all ages but is usually acquired during childhood, reaching a peak during the second decade. Significant morbidity occurs two or three decades later. Males are more frequently affected, presumably because of socially imposed increased exposure.

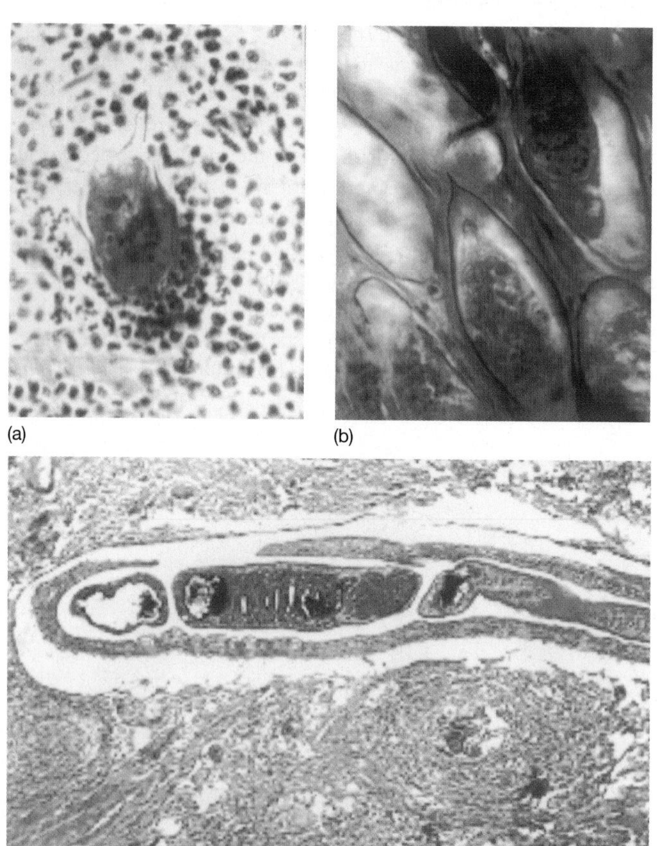

Fig. 2 Typical schistosomal lesions: (a) granuloma with a damaged *S. mansoni* ovum in the middle (note the lateral spike); (b) conglomeration of *S. hematobium* eggs (with characteristic terminal spikes) in the bladder submucosa; (c) adult worm in a venule with adjacent multiple granulomata around deposited ova.

Innate host immunity is of major importance in limiting the acquisition of infection and consequent morbidity. In humans, these mechanisms are capable of killing at least 60 per cent of migrating schistosomulae. Racial variation in ensuing morbidity may be due to genetically determined differences in innate immunity. The Black population of Brazil appears to be less susceptible to the sequelae of chronic schistosomiasis, while Caucasians seem to be more vulnerable to acute presentations of the disease.

Genetic factors seem to play an important role in individual variations in the susceptibility to infection and morbidity. Specific HLA-haplotypes, for example, HLA-Dw12-DR2-DQwl, are required for the *in vitro* proliferative response of T-lymphocytes to schistosomal antigens (Hirayama *et al.* 1987). The development of intestinal polyposis in infected Egyptians has been linked with HLA-B5, glomerulopathy with HLA-A28 (Barsoum 1987), and hepatic fibrosis in a Chinese population with certain HLA-DRB1 and HLA-DQB1 alleles (McManus *et al.* 2001). However, these data are based on relatively small cohorts and require confirmation in larger population studies.

Active infection confers partial protection against reinfection by the same and, to a lesser extent, other species. Living mature worms, attenuated larvae, as well as individual recombinant parasitic antigens are protective, an effect that is augmented by advancing host's age. Undernutrition impairs the acquired immunity of the host, but it also reduces the resistance of the worm to treatment and to the host's immune defence.

Natural world

Prevalence

According to recent WHO estimates, about 600 million of the world's population are at risk, with documented infection in at least 200 million inhabitants of 76 countries in five continents. About 120 million infected subjects are symptomatic, while 20 million suffer from serious sequelae of the disease, particularly those living in China, the Philippines, Egypt, Brazil, northern Senegal, and Uganda, with an estimated directly related annual mortality of 20,000.

Many factors influence the intensity of infestation including the prevailing parasitic strains, host susceptibility, and extent of exposure, as well as climatic factors that influence snail and animal reservoir kinetics. Natural and man-made ecological changes resulting from the construction of dams and artificial lakes have a major impact.

The most widely spread species is *S. hematobium*, which is endemic in most of Africa, Mauritius, Madagascar, the Near East, and Iraq, with a few foci in India and Portugal. *S. mansoni* is also prevalent, mainly along the Nile Valley and in the Near East, Yemen, South America, and the Caribbean. *S. japonicum* is endemic in Japan, China, and the Philippines. *S. intercalatum*, which is closely related to *S. mansoni*, is localized to a small area in Central Africa including Zaire, the Gabon, and the Cameroon. *S. mekongi*, which is related to *S. japonicum*, is mainly seen in Laos, Thailand, and Malaysia. Much less frequently encountered are *S. mattheei*, in South, Central, and Western Africa, and *S. bovis*, essentially an infection of cattle and higher primates, which very rarely affects humans.

Morbidity increases with the intensity of infection, host susceptibility and, delay of primary treatment. The virulence of certain parasitic species and strains also seems to play a significant role. Other factors include associated nutritional deficiency and other endemic diseases such as salmonella, mycobacteria, staphylococci, hepatitis viral infection, and human papilloma virus.

Immunology

Over several thousand years, schistosomes learnt to live and let live. It is not in their favour to overwhelm the host, nor to be vulnerable to the host's immunological artillery. Accordingly, successful infection requires a delicate balance between the parasite's antigenic challenge, its own immune system, and the host's immune response. This balance is known as 'concomitant immunity'.

Antigens

A large number of schistosomal antigens have been identified *in vitro* and in infected humans and experimental animals. Antigenicity varies with different species and strains and declines with ageing of the parasite.

Four groups of antigens have been isolated *in vitro*:

Tegument-associated antigens are a complex set of proteins and glycoproteins on the surface of cercariae, schistosomulae, and adult worms. Many such antigens have been characterized, encoded, sequenced, and prepared by recombinant techniques (Bashir *et al.* 1994). They are distinguished according to their sources (e.g. Sm for *S. mansoni*, Sj for *S. japonicum*, etc.) suffixed by their molecular weights. Tegument-associated antigens appear to have a limited role in the pathogenesis of host morbidity, yet they are of crucial importance in immunity to infection and reinfection. The 23, 26, and 28 kDa antigens are isoenzymes of tegument-associated glutathione-*S*-transferase (GST), one of the most promising vaccine candidates.

Adult worm tissue antigens include those associated with microsomes, smooth muscles, and others. The microsomal antigens are specific for the genus *Schistosoma*, with distinct species differences (MAMA, HAMA, and JAMA for *S. mansoni*, *S. hematobium*, and *S. japonicum* adult microsomal antigens, respectively). Hence, they are of particular epidemiological importance as markers of active infection (Al-Sherbiny and Osman 1995).

Gut-associated antigens are released by regurgitation of the worm's digestive juices, and constitute the main part of circulating schistosomal antigens *in vivo*. Of those antigens identified *in vitro*, at least two are involved in the pathogenesis of immune-complex-mediated lesions (de Water *et al.* 1988). These are a proteoglycan that migrates to the anode in an electrical field, hence the name 'circulating anodic antigen' (CAA) and a glycoprotein that migrates to the cathode, 'circulating cathodic antigen' (CCA).

Soluble egg antigens are released by diffusion through micropores in the eggshell into the surrounding tissue fluids. A few have been purified and shown to be protein or glycoprotein in nature. The most immunogenic are a peptide called Sm-p40, which induces a predominantly TH1 response, and two more recently identified antigens, *S. mansoni* phosphoenolpyruvate carboxykinase (Sm-PEPCK) and thioredoxin peroxidase-1 (Sm-TPx-1), which induce a balanced TH1/TH2 response (Stadecker *et al.* 2001). Egg antigens are mainly involved in the pathogenesis of local granulomas and may be carcinogenic.

The majority of the circulating schistosomal antigens are gut-derived. Seropositivity varies in different reports, with increased frequency among the older population and with longer duration of infection. Patients with hepatosplenic schistosomiasis are usually seropositive, which is attributed to the intensity and longevity of infection. Circulating antigens are not detectable a few weeks after successful treatment.

The immune response

The host's complex immune response to schistosomiasis (Fig. 3) can be classified into the phases of antigen presentation, immune activation, and parasite elimination. Evasive mechanisms modulate the immune response in all three phases.

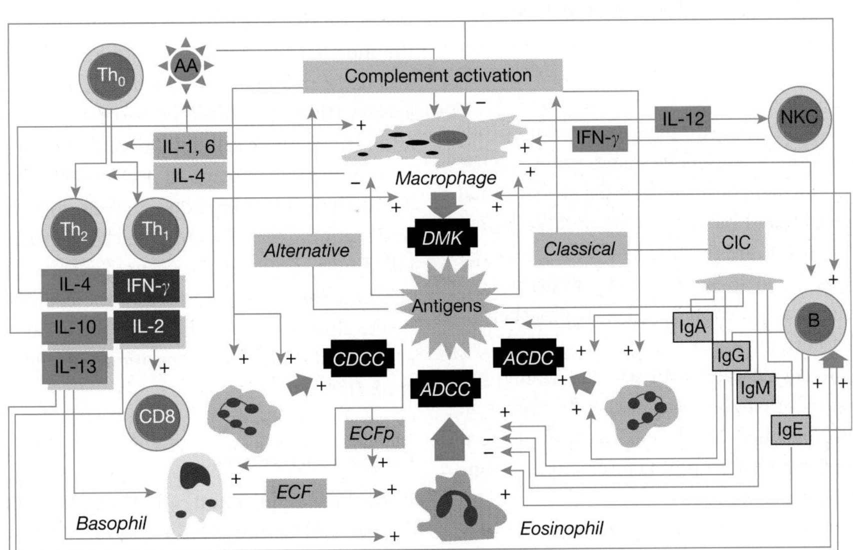

Fig. 3 The immune response to schistosomiasis. AA, amyloid A protein; ACDC, antibody- and complement-dependent cytotoxicity; ADCC, antibody-dependent cell-mediated cytotoxicity; CDCC, complement-dependent cell-mediated cytotoxicity; CIC, circulating immune complexes; DMF, direct macrophage killing; ECF, eosinophil chemotactic factor; ECF-p, eosinophil chemotactic factor of parasitic origin.

Antigen presentation

The cells principally involved in early schistosomal antigen presentation are dendritic cells of the skin during the invasion stage, the circulating monocytes and B-lymphocytes during the migration stage and the hepatic macrophages in established infection.

Schistosomal antigens are expressed at the surfaces of these cells in conjunction with class II MHC antigens. Antigen presentation is initially associated with the synthesis and release of interleukins-1, -6, -12, G-CSF, GM-CSF, and tumour necrosis factor (TNF)-α, which is known as the 'classical activation' (Stadecker 1999). This is amplified by a positive feedback loop generated by interferon-γ (IFG), secreted by activated lymphocytes, and modulated by the negative autocrine influence of somatostatin. The latter is secreted by active monocytes in response to IFG, and acts through SSTR2 receptors on the same cells. Somatostatin has a wide spectrum of paracrine immunomodulatory function including down regulation of inflammatory cells and fibroblasts in the schistosomal granuloma, which also express the SSTR2 receptor (Chatterjee and Van Marck 2001).

Later, the antigen-presenting cells (APCs) undergo a phenotypic and functional change, known as the 'alternative activation', which is maintained by TH2 cytokines (Stadecker 1999), transforming growth factor-β (TGF-β) (Omer *et al.* 2000), as well as inhibitory proteins of parasitic origin (Pemberton *et al.* 1994).

Immune activation

The first lymphocyte subset that responds to schistosomal antigen presentation, mainly under the influence of IL-12, is the natural killer cells. These have a major role in parasite elimination, and help to upregulate the APCs through the secretion of IFG.

Further immune activation (Wahl *et al.* 1997) occurs largely under the influence of 'classical' APC secretory products. These lead to proliferation of antigen-specific TH1 clones, which are responsible for the major proinflammatory host response that *contains* the infection.

With the gradual switching of APCs to the 'alternative' activation mode, IL-4 becomes its predominant cytokine product. This leads to proliferation of TH2 clones that *complement*, but also *modulate* the initial predominance of the TH1 clones. The principal outcome of this change is the predominance of IL-4, -10, -13, and TGF-β (McKenzie 2000).

TH1 and TH2 clones work in concert with parasite secretory products to recruit and regulate other lymphocytes and granulocytes. Although CD8 cells are an important constituent of the schistosomal granuloma, they seem to be of limited capacity in the parasite killing process. Similarly, mast cells, which are recruited by TH2 cytokines and certain parasitic antigens, seem to be mostly catalytic for the inflammatory response through the secretion of an eosinophil chemotactic factor (Owhashi *et al.* 1996).

Eosinophils, the principal cells charged with parasite killing, are recruited by chemotactic factors of parasitic origin (Pemberton *et al.* 1994) as well as TH2- (Brombacher 2000) and basophil-derived cytokines (Cutts and Wilson 1997). Eosinophil cytotoxicity is essentially antibody-dependent (Capron *et al.* 1983).

Neutrophils are also important for parasite killing, particularly during the early phases of infection. They are mostly seen in young granulomata. Their function requires the presence of complement as well as IgG antibodies (Capron *et al.* 1987).

While the major expression of the immune response in schistosomiasis is cellular, concomitant humoral response is of fundamental importance. B-lymphocytes are committed by reading the antigen, either directly or upon expression on the macrophages. They proliferate under the influence of TH1 cytokines, IL-2, and IL-6. Their subsequent antibody production depends on the supervening cytokine profile. They tend to produce IgM, IgG1, and IgG2 under the influence of IL-2, IgG3, IgG4, and IgA under the influence of IL-10, and IgE under the influence of IL-13. The impact of individual immunoglobulin classes is different. While IgE interacts with the monocytes and eosinophils in the process of parasite elimination, IgM, IgA, IgG2, and IgG4 seem to have an immunomodulatory effect, largely by inhibiting antibody-mediated cytotoxicity (Dunne *et al.* 1987).

Several studies have demonstrated the presence of circulating anti-DNA, idiotypic antiphospholipid antibodies, rheumatoid factor, and antinuclear factor in association with schistosomiasis (Thomas *et al.* 1989). The pathogenesis and clinical significance of these antibodies are unclear. Although they may represent a non-specific polyclonal response associated with advanced hepatic fibrosis, they may also indicate a significant role of autoimmunity in the pathogenesis of certain schistosoma-associated lesions.

Both classical and alternative pathways of the complement cascade are activated in the immune response against schistosomiasis. While the classical pathway is activated by circulating immune complexes, parasitic toxins directly activate the alternative pathway. The latter is magnified by the effect of associated bacterial endotoxins, for example, salmonella.

Parasite elimination

The process of parasite killing involves four cytotoxic cells, monocytes/macrophages, neutrophils, basophils, and eosinophils, interacting with appropriate immunoglobulins and complement (Fig. 3). Each is mostly active during a particular phase of the parasite's life cycle in the host. Monocytes and basophils are mainly active against the schistosomulae, neutrophils against the ova, and eosinophils against the ova and adult worms. This distinction is related to declining vulnerability of the parasite along with its maturity. Schistosomulae are the most fragile, being susceptible to phagocytosis by the monocytes and tissue macrophages as well as to the lethal effect of reactive oxygen species (ROS) produced by basophils and neutrophils. For killing an adult worm, these cells join forces with the monocytes and eosinophils in producing a stream of ROS that punches the parasite's cuticle. Through the resulting holes, the eosinophils pour a lethal dose of their basic cationic protein. Ova, which are protected by a resistant shell, are killed by a similar mechanism. That the Eosinophil Cationic Protein (ECT) is the main parasiticidal molecule in schistosomiasis is shown by the close correlation between the inflammatory lesions in the urinary tract and the urinary excretion of that protein (Jyding Vennervald *et al.* 2000).

Escape mechanisms

In established infection, adult worms seem to escape recognition by the host's APCs and specific effector pathways. This tolerance is specific for a particular host, the parasite being rapidly killed if transferred to another. The mechanism is uncertain but it may be related to the capacity of the parasite's tegument to mop up native host molecules, thereby being recognized as self, such as H blood group substance, immunoglobulins (mainly IgG), and the MHC antigens.

Live adult worms also have the capacity of suppressing the host's immune response, an effect that increases with their ageing. This is achieved by suppressing macrophages and promoting anti-idiotypic T-cell clones (Lima *et al.* 1986). Preferential production of IgG4, IgG2c, and circulating IgM immune complexes leads to blockade of T-cell and eosinophil receptors (Dunne *et al.* 1987). Other potential mechanisms include clonal exhaustion and/or deletion by persistent antigenic stimulation and 'diversion' of the immune system by polyclonal activation of the lymphocytes. These effects are blamed in the pathogenesis of schistosoma-associated amyloidosis.

Basic pathology

The pathological lesions in schistosomiasis mirror the progression of the host–parasite interaction all the way from infection to outcome, which may be spontaneous cure, adaptation, or overt disease.

Initial invasion

Local reaction

Cercarial penetration of the skin is associated with an immediate local reaction characterized by an innate response of the local dendritic (Langerhan's) cells. Chemokines and proinflammatory cytokines are released, leading to a dermal inflammatory response. This is expressed as a transient, hardly visible, wheal composed of oedema, dilated capillaries, and a few eosinophils. The duration and severity of this reaction depend on the length of schistosomular stay in the dermis. The lesion is most pronounced in infections with non-human-pathogenic species of the parasite, whose schistosomulae cannot migrate. An Arthus skin reaction has been occasionally described in expatriates acquiring infection in endemic areas.

Systemic response

A systemic serum sickness-like syndrome, comprising polyarthritis and skin vasculitis, may be encountered in expatriates who acquire new infection with *S. japonicum* or *S. mansoni* in endemic areas. It occurs about 7 weeks after exposure when the worms have reached sexual maturity. IgM immune complexes have been consistently identified in the sera of such patients. Cryoglobulins may be occasionally detected (Atkin *et al.* 1986).

Established infection

Granuloma

A delayed cellular reaction is, by far, the most important type of immune response in schistosomiasis, the hallmark of which being the granuloma. This is usually formed around tissue-trapped single (*S. hematobium* and *S. mansoni*) or multiple (*S. japonicum*) ova, schistosomulae, or even adult worms (Fig. 2). All cells involved in the immune reaction participate in the granuloma. Neutrophils are also seen during the initial phases, but suppuration does not occur. Macrophages frequently coalesce to form giant cells. Fibroblasts eventually shell off the periphery of the granuloma leading to progressive fibrosis.

The evolution of cellular into fibrotic granulomata constitutes the essence of progression of schistosomiasis in different organs. With the possible exception of the spleen, all tissues may be affected. The most frequently involved are the LUT and the seminal vesicles, the colon, rectum, hepatic portal tracts, and the lungs. Lesions in the brain, spinal cord, skin, kidneys, pancreas, prostate, vagina, uterine cervix, and adnexae are less common. Calcifications are common, particularly in the LUT with *S. hematobium* and the central nervous system with *S. japonicum*.

The extent of fibrosis induced by healing granulomata can be appreciated by considering the millions of ova produced by even one pair of worms during their lifespan of several years. Indeed, most of the clinical features of schistosomiasis are attributed to healed rather than active granulomata.

Glomerulonephritis

Mesangial and subendothelial deposits of schistosoma-specific immune complexes are detected in the glomeruli within a few weeks of experimental infection (Houba 1979). They have also been demonstrated in asymptomatic patients with *S. mansoni* infection (Sobh *et al.* 1988a) and subjects recently infected with *S. hematobium* (Ezzat *et al.* 1974). The glomerular response is mainly mesangioproliferative. Endothelial swelling and proliferation are more frequently seen in experimental models than in humans.

These lesions may be subsequently modified by associated infections or complications. Concomitant infection with salmonella adds an exudative element to the glomerular lesions of schistosomiasis. Associated hepatitis C virus leads to prominent mesangial matrix expansion and fibrin deposition. The presence of significant hepatic fibrosis and porta-systemic shunts may be associated with mesangial and subendothelial IgA deposits, which alter the glomerular histology and lead to progressive glomerulosclerosis.

The different histopathological lesions encountered in schistosomiasis are categorized into five classes (Fig. 4), which have distinct clinical and prognostic features (described later).

Late sequelae

Amyloidosis

Secondary amyloidosis has been reported in patients with long-standing infection with *S. mansoni*, *S. hematobium*, or both (Barsoum *et al.* 1979). Whenever specified, amyloid protein was of the AA type, usually restricted to the kidneys, and associated with the conventional schistosoma-associated glomerular and interstitial lesions (Fig. 4).

It is believed that schistosoma-associated amyloidosis results from an imbalance between the formation of AA protein by the monocytes and hepatocytes, mainly under the influence of IL-6, and its re-uptake by the monocytes. IL-10, which supervenes in late stages of the infection, is blamed for such monocyte dysfunction (Flores-Villanueva *et al.* 1996). The retained AA protein would then deposit as typical beta pleated fibrils in areas of chronic inflammation where the appropriate P substance is abundant.

Malignancy

Schistosomiasis has been associated with malignancy of the bladder (Ghoneim *et al.* 1997), rectum (Matsuda *et al.* 1999), and spleen (Chirimwami *et al.* 1991); the pathogenetic link being most firmly established with the former.

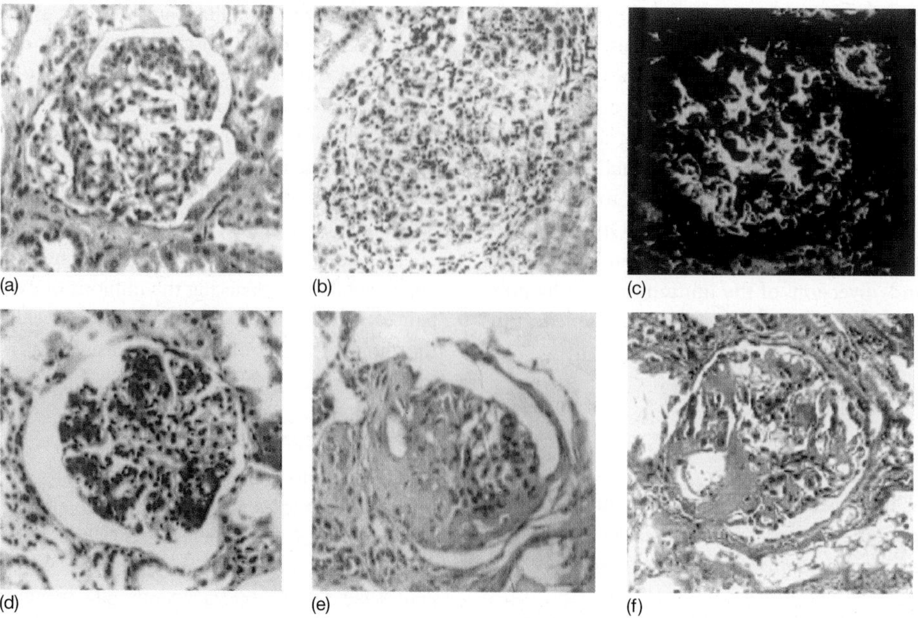

Fig. 4 Histopathological lesions in schistosomal glomerulopathy: (a) Class I, axial mesangial proliferative glomerulonephritis; (b) Class II, exudative glomerulonephritis; (c) mesangial IgA deposits in Class III disease; (d) Class III, mesangiocapillary (membranoproliferative) glomerulonephritis; (e) Class IV, focal and segmental glomerulosclerosis (Masson trichrome stain); (f) Class V, amyloidosis.

Bladder neoplasia can be experimentally induced in baboons by *S. hematobium* infections (Hicks *et al.* 1980). Its reported incidence in patients may be as much as 4.5 per cent of those with urinary bilharziasis (Chugh *et al.* 1986). The histological type is squamous cell in roughly 60 per cent, transitional cell carcinoma in 20 per cent, adenocarcinoma in 10 per cent, and mixed in the rest. Schistosomal ova were detected in more than 85 per cent of bladder cancers in an Egyptian series of 1026 cases subjected to surgical cystectomy (Ghoneim *et al.* 1997). The tumour, particularly when of the squamous-cell type, remains localized for a long time before spreading to the surrounding pelvic tissues or distant site, thanks to the occlusion of lymphatics by the preceding fibrotic process.

Associated bacterial and viral infections, rather than parasitic products, are suggested to be the main pathogenetic factors. Associated infection with Human Papilloma Virus has received considerable recent attention in this respect (el-Mawla *et al.* 2001), being encountered in about one-fourth of cases. Specific p53 gene mutations were detected in one-third of cases (Warren *et al.* 1995). This may be attributed to neutrophil-generated reactive oxygen molecules, cleavage of conjugated urinary carcinogens, or the production of nitrosamines by bacterial enzymes (Mostafa *et al.* 1999).

Clinical syndromes

The clinical evolution of schistosomiasis includes four successive phases: invasion, migration, established infection, and late stage. The initial two phases usually pass unnoticed except in expatriates who may develop schistosomal dermatitis (swimmer's itch) during the invasion phase, transient pneumonitis or bronchial asthma during the migration phase, and/or acute schistosomiasis (Katayama fever) simultaneously with worm maturation.

Syndromes of established infection

About 3 months after initial infection, 10–20 per cent of subjects develop one of the two principal clinical syndromes characteristic of schistosomiasis, namely the urinary or the hepatointestinal. An occasional patient may also suffer from the effects of metastatic granulomata, particularly in the central nervous system.

Urinary schistosomiasis

Urinary schistosomiasis is the classical expression of *S. hematobium* infection. It involves the bladder, the lower ureters, the seminal vesicles, and, less frequently, the vas deferens, prostate, and the female genital system. The typical presentation is terminal haematuria, usually associated with increased frequency of micturition and occasional dysuria. Diagnosis is made by finding characteristic ova in the urine. Cystoscopic examination (Fig. 5), which is usually unnecessary during this stage, may show mucosal oedema, congestion, and erythema, together with schistosomal pseudotubercles (to be distinguished from those of tuberculosis), granulation tissue, polyps, or nodules. Superficial ulcerations may occur. These lesions are completely reversible with treatment.

Hepatointestinal schistosomiasis

This syndrome involves the colon, rectum, and hepatic portal tracts.

The usual clinical presentation is dysenteric. Chronic spastic colitis, the irritable colon syndrome, and colonic polyposis are also frequently encountered. Rarely, large pericolic or perirectal masses may be formed, which may be confused with malignancy.

The liver is involved in the majority of patients. Initially, it is mildly to moderately enlarged and tender with transient elevation of serum aspartate aminotransferase and alanine aminotransferase, but hepatocellular functions are not impaired. A few weeks to months later, the spleen is also enlarged due to the lymphoid hyperplasia featuring the host's immune response.

The diagnosis is made by finding schistosoma ova in stools, rectal scrapings, or rectal snips. Proctocolonoscopic examination helps to establish the diagnosis and to categorize the histopathological patterns, which include ulcers, polyps, and sessile granulomas. Liver biopsy is rarely needed, though it may provide conclusive tissue diagnosis based on the finding of schistosomal granulomata around ova, egg remnants, or 'pigments'.

'Metastatic' syndromes

Granulomas may develop around metastatic ova in different organs. At this stage, they are not associated with any significant manifestations except in the central nervous system. Brain granulomas present with recurrent seizures, usually without notable neurological deficit. Those in the spinal cord present as transverse myelitis. Both lesions usually respond to early treatment.

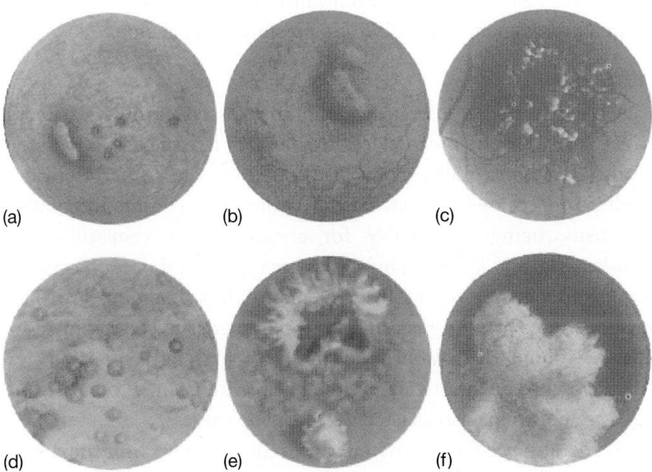

Fig. 5 Cystoscopic appearances in urinary schistosomiasis: (a) bilharzial pseudotubercles adjacent to an acute ulcer; (b) pseudotubercles covering a chronic inflammatory mass; (c) bilharzial 'sandy patches'; (d) bilharzial 'cystitis cystica'; (e) malignant ulcer eroding streaky calcifications with an adjacent calcified chronic inflammatory mass; (f) fungating bladder carcinoma. (Courtesy of Professor Naguib Makar.)

Late-stage syndromes

Chronic sequelae of schistosomiasis constitute the main direct causes of morbidity and mortality. They usually develop insidiously several years after the earlier manifestations of established infection have burnt out. The proportion of patients who progress to late-stage syndromes varies widely in different geographical regions (Barsoum 1993), depending on genetic factors, intensity of infestation, and timely therapy.

Practically every organ may be involved in this stage. The urinary, hepatosplenic, and cardiopulmonary syndromes are of major epidemiological importance.

Renal and urinary tract syndromes

Lower urinary tract

The spectrum of healed lesions in the urinary bladder includes 'sandy patches', 'ground-glass mucosa', chronic ulcers, mucosal pseudocysts, and 'cystitis glandularis' (islands of glandular tissue within the fibrotic background). The main symptoms are increased frequency of micturition, dysuria, pyuria, and haematuria. These symptoms are considerably modified by associated bacterial infections, calcular disease, urodynamic disturbances, and complicating malignancy.

The functional reflection of bilharzial cystitis depends on the extent of fibrosis. On the one hand, there is a large proportion of asymptomatic patients with normal bladder function, in whom the only evidence of bladder fibrosis is radiological (Fig. 6) or endoscopic. Wall trabeculations are detected in the majority of patients without demonstrable outflow obstruction. They seem to result from patchy compensatory hypertrophy of the detrusor associated with focal fibrosis.

At the other end of the spectrum, the fibrotic process may completely destroy the bladder mucosa and detrusor. The bladder is eventually turned into a small non-compliant organ (bilharzial contracted bladder) or a dilated virtually non-contractile viscus (bilharzial atonic bladder).

The development of malignancy is characterized by an appreciable change in symptoms. Severe dysuria, a persistent dull deep perineal ache, and passage of clots and necrotic tissues (necroturia) with urine

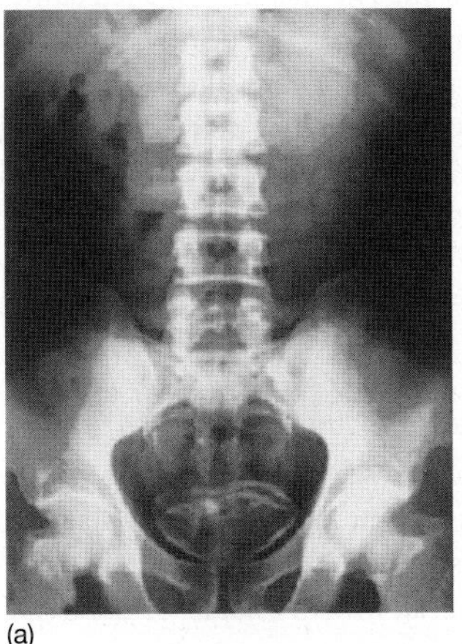

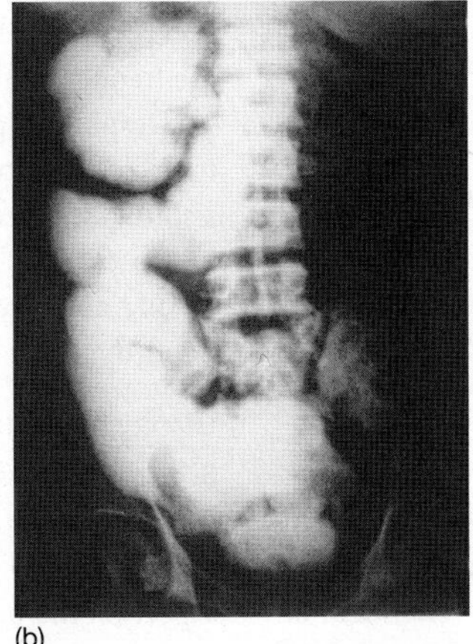

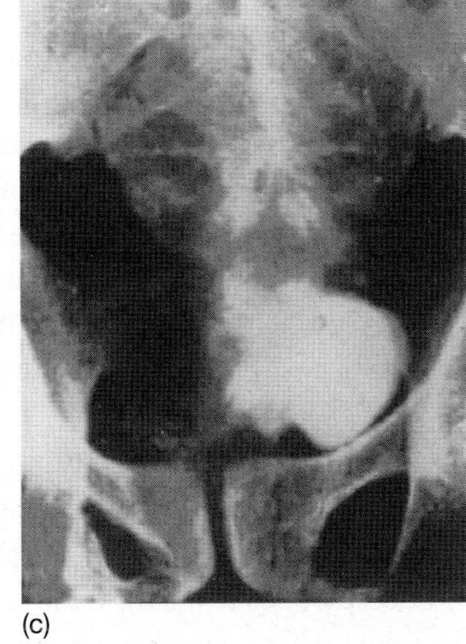

Fig. 6 Characteristic radiological appearances in urinary schistosomiasis: (a) plain radiogram showing faint linear calcification of the urinary bladder; (b) retrograde urogram showing grade IV right vesicoureteric reflux; (c) plain X-ray showing bilharzial cancer eroding dense bladder calcification.

are highly suggestive. Malignancy is also suspected when diffuse bladder calcifications are 'eaten up', or when isolated dirty blotches of calcification are seen in a plain radiological examination. The tumour is usually readily felt by rectal or bimanual examination, and can be shown by various imaging techniques (Fig. 6). Final diagnosis is made by cystoscopy (Fig. 5) and biopsy.

Bilharzial urethral fistulas are of historic interest. These used to be the outcome of periuretheral granulomas, without any obstruction to urine flow. Uretheral strictures are very rare in schistosomiasis.

Ureteric obstruction

Obstructive uropathy is the most common urological syndrome caused by schistosomiasis with a reported frequency of up to 9.1 per cent (Chugh *et al.* 1986) in adequate field studies, although higher figures are often reported in hospital series. Endstage renal disease attributed to bilharzial ureteric obstruction accounts for 6.7 per cent of the dialysis population in Egypt (Egyptian Registry 2000). The observation that a considerable proportion of autopsy-detected obstructions are clinically silent suggests that some potentially obstructive lesions are either missed or are functionally insignificant. Indeed, the bilharzial ureter enjoys an outstanding urodynamic adaptability. In the majority of cases, the dilated ureter above an obstructed segment retains its capacity of generating and perpetuating a high-pressure urinary bolus that readily overcomes the potential obstruction. Many patients maintain this 'active dilatation' without any renal back-pressure for several decades.

In contrast, other subjects may develop massive ureteric dilatation, which cannot be explained by any contemporary distal obstruction. The pathology seems to be largely dominated by neuromuscular dysfunction, and correlates with the severity of fibrosis (passive dilatation). The syndrome frequently follows surgical interventions for the correction of distal pathology. Despite the striking ureteric dilatation, back-pressure effects on the kidneys are minimal.

When back-pressure occurs, it is usually bilateral but asymmetrical, with the left side being more frequently affected, for anatomical reasons (see above). The kidneys may become extremely large unless their distensibility is limited by chronic interstitial lesions. The main symptoms are renal aches, colics, and abdominal distention. Some patients remain asymptomatic owing to the slow evolution of obstruction. In those, the diagnosis is often made during assessment for other reasons or, unfortunately, during evaluation of established chronic renal failure.

Functional consequences are typical of chronic partial obstructive nephropathy (see Chapter 17.2). Impaired urinary concentrating ability with defective generation of free water is a common early feature. Urinary sodium conservation is impaired, and most patients are chronically salt depleted unless the glomerular filtration rate is critically reduced. Although type I (distal) renal tubular acidosis (RTA) can be demonstrated by an acid load test, clinically significant disturbances in acid–base balance are infrequent. Hypocitriuria, as a manifestation of incomplete distal RTA, may be responsible for the increased incidence of stones.

The diagnosis of obstruction is established by appropriate imaging techniques, which also help to localize the site of ureteric obstruction. This is usually the lower third, mainly the intramural part. Less frequently, strictures may be seen opposite the third lumbar vertebra or at the level of the sacroiliac joints, where extensive periureteric fibrosis may occur. These are sites of rich venous plexuses, which provide optimal conditions for oviposition. However, adequate care must be taken not to confuse an atonic dilated urinary system in schistosomiasis with an organically obstructed system. Several techniques, including radioisotopic studies, diuresis urography and ultrasonography, and invasive pressure studies, have been used to make this distinction. Although these tests may be of considerable value in making the diagnosis, the ambiguity of some cases may remain unresolved owing to the lack of adequately standardized criteria for the interpretation of the test results.

Vesicoureteric reflux

Transient reflux may occur during active disease and with moderate to severe secondary bacterial infection. Reflux in late-stage schistosomiasis is usually iatrogenic, being induced by surgical or endoscopic manipulations. It should be suspected when the ureters and/or pelvicalyceal system are dilated without an obviously obstructive lesion (Fig. 6). Reflux should also be considered when chronic interstitial nephropathy is associated with hypertension and/or nephrotic range proteinuria. In such cases it may be confused with immune-complex-mediated schistosomal glomerulopathy, from which it should be distinguished by adequate assessment of the LUT and possibly by renal biopsy.

Infection

Bacterial infection is extremely common in association with urinary schistosomiasis. The mucosal lesions, blood and tissue debris, and the urodynamic consequences of schistosomiasis seem to be important predisposing causes. *Escherichia coli* is the most common causative organism, being responsible for about 70 per cent of cases. *Pseudomonas* and *Klebsiella* infections are typical in those subjected to diagnostic or therapeutic instrumentation. As mentioned earlier, various strains of *Salmonella* are commonly associated with schistosomiasis. Although occasionally silent, these may be responsible for relentless chronic cystitis or pyelonephritis. Resistant Proteus infections are notoriously associated with struvite stones.

In the absence of obstruction and reflux, urinary infection may remain restricted to the bladder for many decades, where it contributes significantly to symptoms and to progression of the mucosal pathology, and may be involved in the pathogenesis of bladder malignancy.

Calcular disease

Mixed stones are common among patients with chronic urinary infection, mainly with Proteus. Very low urinary citrate levels are often encountered in such cases due to associated RTA as well as consumption by the organism. The majority of such stones are formed in the renal pelvis or lower calyces, but primary ureteric and bladder stones are frequently formed on bilharzial lesions.

Despite the greater frequency of hyperoxaluria, hypercalciuria, and hyperphosphaturia often associated with hepatosplenic schistosomiasis, the incidence of primary oxalate and calcium stones is not increased. This is probably attributed to the impaired urinary concentrating ability characteristic of the associated obstructive and reflux nephropathies.

Glomerulonephritis (see also Chapter 3.14)

Schistosoma-associated glomerulonephritis has been reported from Africa (Egypt, The Sudan, Algeria, Nigeria, Madagascar), Latin America (Brazil, Peru, Costa Rica), and South East Asia (Thailand). Clinical aspects of this are dealt with in Chapter 3.14. Its epidemiological impact is uncertain. While it was reported in autopsy and clinical studies to affect 12–15 per cent of patients with schistosomal hepatic fibrosis in Brazil (Andrade and Rocha 1979), it was considered to have a potential pathogenetic role in up to 74 per cent of patients with proliferative glomerulonephritis in Egypt (Ezzat *et al.* 1974; Barsoum 1993).

The disease is encountered clinically as occult, overt, or endstage glomerulopathy (Barsoum 1993). Among the factors that define the severity of glomerular lesions are species and strains of the parasite, associated infections, racial and genetic host factors, and the degree of associated hepatic involvement.

Five distinct clinicopathological patterns (Fig. 4) are identified (Barsoum 1993).

Class I is species-independent. It is characterized by focal or diffuse mesangioproliferative glomerular lesions with mesangial IgM, C3, and other schistosomal gut antigen deposits. It is often subclinical, or may be associated with mild proteinuria and/or haematuria. Renal function is preserved.

Class II occurs when hepatosplenic schistosomiasis is associated with *Salmonella* infection (Barsoum *et al.* 1977). The typical lesion is an exudative glomerulonephritis with subendothelial C3 deposits. Such patients are quite ill, pyrexial, and very anaemic. Their hair becomes brittle, thin, and depigmented. They develop a characteristic skin rash, mainly on the flexor surfaces of the forearms and the front of the chest and abdomen. The spleen is moderately enlarged, soft, and tender. Acute-onset nephrotic syndrome is characteristic, with gross proteinuria and severe hypoalbuminaemia.

Classes III and IV occur in patients with advanced *S. mansoni* hepatosplenic disease with impaired macrophage function (Barsoum *et al.* 1988), thereby allowing schistosomal antigens and mucosal IgA to pour in large quantities into the systemic circulation. Class III lesions are consistent with either Type I or Type III mesangiocapillary (membranoproliferative) glomerulonephritis (see also Chapter 3.9). Class IV lesions, which are more often encountered in black patients (Lopes *et al.* 1999), are characterized by focal and segmental glomerulosclerosis. Mesangial and subendothelial IgA glomerular deposits are detected in the majority of patients in either class, together with IgG, C3, and occasionally IgM (Barsoum *et al.* 1996).

The clinical picture in both classes is identical, being characterized by proteinuria, microhaematuria, and progressive renal insufficiency. The nephrotic syndrome is encountered in over two-thirds of patients during evolution of the disease, and hypertension occurs in one-third. Nutritional deficiency and/or associated infection often confound the clinical syndrome. Associated hepatitis C viral infection is commonly encountered in these classes, leading to typical vasculitis, glomerular thrombosis, and rapid progression of the renal disease.

Class V, like Class I, is species-independent, though it requires prolonged active infection. Its distinctive feature is the deposition of amyloid A material amidst other glomerular schistosomal glomerular lesions (Barsoum *et al.* 1979). The usual presentation is nephrotic, with gross proteinuria that continues until very late in the evolution of the disease. Hypertension is encountered in 10–15 per cent of patients. The kidneys are enlarged in only 25 per cent of cases, being checked by associated interstitial fibrosis.

Extraurinary syndromes

Hepatosplenic schistosomiasis

With the progressive portal fibrosis of schistosomal granulomata, the liver becomes firm and shrunken. Presinusoidal portal hypertension develops and is clinically manifested by splenomegaly, portasystemic collaterals, and ascites.

The diagnosis can be readily made by clinical examination at the bedside. Ultrasonography is extremely helpful in showing the specific pattern of hepatic fibrosis and in demonstrating portal dilatation, splenomegaly, and ascites. Liver biopsy confirms the diagnosis and helps to exclude associated diseases, particularly concomitant active hepatitis.

The tests of hepatocellular function are not significantly affected until very late in the disease. Disturbance of hepatocellular function usually indicates concomitant bacterial or viral infection or other associated conditions.

Cardiopulmonary schistosomiasis

Schistosomal cor pulmonale is mainly seen in males in their third decade with long-standing *S. mansoni* or *S. hematobium* infection, who usually present with manifestations of right ventricular failure. The physical signs are dominated by those of right ventricular hypertrophy, pulmonary dilatation and hypertension, tricuspid incompetence, and eventually severe and sustained systemic venous congestion.

A restrictive pattern of right ventricular dysfunction was observed in some of these patients. Endomyocardial biopsy showed considerable subendocardial fibrosis, which is thought to represent a diffuse form of the cellular response to schistosomiasis. The specificity of this lesion has yet to be confirmed.

Other extraurinary syndromes

S. hematobium infection is occasionally associated with a number of extraurinary manifestations of little clinical importance. The male genital system is most commonly involved. Schistosomiasis of the seminal vesicles is seen almost as frequently as that of the bladder. Although it may lead to transient haemospermia in early stages, it usually has no clinical sequelae. Healing by fibrosis and extensive calcification produces a pathognomonic radiological picture of the disease. Involvement of the vas deferens, prostate, and testicles is rare and is usually clinically insignificant. An occasional patient may develop sterility due to extensive fibrosis of the vas deferens.

Involvement of the female genital system is less frequent. The vagina is the most common site. The lesions are basically the same as those of the bladder, being dominated by a granulomatous reaction with superficial ulcerations and progressing to fibrosis and formation of sandy patches. The usual clinical presentation is dyspareunia associated with a vaginal discharge. The uterine cervix may be affected, with the formation of polypoid granulomas that protrude from the internal os and bleed on touch. Involvement of the Fallopian tubes is rare. It leads to fibrosis that usually does not interrupt the patency of the tubes, so that sterility is rare. Involvement of the ovaries is usually a histopathological finding of little clinical interest.

Apart from swimmer's itch and occasional generalized allergic manifestations during the invasion stage of schistosomiasis, involvement of the skin is rare. The most common sites are genital, where nodular lesions develop in the skin of the scrotum, penis, and vulva. They are usually asymptomatic, being non-tender, non-itchy, and non-ulcerative. Very rarely, similar lesions have been reported to occur around the umbilicus and overlying the scapulae and shoulders.

Nodular lesions have also been described in the palpebral conjunctiva in patients with extensive *S. hematobium* disease. However, no effects on the eyeball have been reported.

Treatment

Primary prevention of schistosomiasis is largely a matter of education and sanitation. Simple measures to interrupt the parasite's lifecycle by avoiding human contact with contaminated water have been remarkably successful. Mass treatment, which has become possible since the introduction of effective and safe oral chemotherapy, has also been very effective in China and Egypt.

Several vaccines using whole or parts of adult worms, cercariae, or egg antigens have been tested in rats, mice, baboons, and cattle. Induction of resistance to infection, sterilization of the worms or reduction of their fecundity, and amelioration of egg-induced pathology have been targets of vaccination research over the past few decades. With the recent establishment of the schistosoma gene library, mapping of potent antigen epitopes, and identification of particular antibody specificities, rational models for the development of a vaccine have been developed and tested with considerable success in animals. Human trials are under way (Katz 1999).

Active lesions

Active lesions readily respond to antischistosomal chemotherapy. Antimony preparations, used since the Pharaonic era, are no longer prescribed mainly because of their toxicity.

The drug of choice today is praziquantel, a pyrazinoisoquinoline derivative (Mahmoud 1987). It is effective against all species of human pathogenic schistosomes with a cure rate of 80 per cent. However, it cannot be used for chemoprophylaxis, since it is active only against mature worms. The recommended therapeutic dose is 40 mg/kg body weight as a single morning dose for *S. hematobium* and *S. mansoni*. For *S. japonicum*, the dose should be increased to 60 g/kg body weight given in two divided doses on the same day. The same dose is used for *S. mekongi*, preferably divided into three doses given in the same day. The drug is safe, but a few side-effects have been reported including abdominal pains, headaches, dizziness, and skin rash.

The organophosphorus preparation metrifonate is effective only against *S. hematobium* infections. The drug is safe and can be used in mass treatment. The recommended dose is 10 mg/kg body weight as a single dose, which may be repeated twice at fortnightly intervals in order to achieve a high cure rate.

Oxamniquine is a quinoline derivative (2-aminomethyl-tetrahydroquinoline), which is effective only against *S. mansoni* infections. The recommended single-dose treatment is 20 mg/kg body weight.

Artemether, a derivative of the Chinese antimalarial Quyinghaosu alkaloids, is a promising new agent that can effectively kill the invading cercariae, maturing schistosomulae, as well as the mature adult worms by interfering with the parasite's glycolytic pathways (Shuhua *et al.* 2000).

Adjuvant treatment with colchicine has been successful in reducing fibrosis in experimental murine schistosomiasis (Badawy *et al.* 1999) and the development of amyloidosis in Syrian Hamsters (Sobh *et al.* 1995). It has been widely used in patients with hepatosplenic schistosomiasis, yet without conclusive therapeutic benefit.

Results of treatment

Antischistosomal chemotherapy leads to parasitological cure in 40–80 per cent of cases, depending on the drug used, the parasite species and strains, the host's nutritional state, and other factors. Even without such a cure, the intensity of infection is significantly reduced (Mahmoud 1987). The effectiveness of treatment can be tested by the progressive decline in the number of eggs excreted in urine and stools; to disappear within 3–4 months. Tissue biopsy from the bladder or rectal mucosa after effective treatment may still show trapped dead ova for many years. The titres of circulating gut and egg antigens rapidly decline with effective treatment. Persistence of the former after the disappearance of eggs from the excreta usually indicates the survival of sterile or single-sex worms. This outcome has the advantage of possibly conferring active immunity against reinfection, so much so that it is considered the aim of certain mass treatment programmes. Owing to the absence of ova, such a setting is certainly harmless from the point of view of granulomatous lesions. However, its effect on the development and propagation of immune-complex-mediated glomerular injury has not yet been elucidated.

The reversibility of established lesions after effective antischistosomal therapy depends on the species, the organ(s) affected, the duration of infection, and the degree of damage already sustained.

S. hematobium lesions are the simplest to eradicate. Since the associated granulomas are often small and mainly affect the LUT, early treatment is usually rewarded by very limited residual pathology. It may be surprising to see extensive radiological lesions resolving under antischistosomal chemotherapy. It is a golden rule not to proceed to any surgical intervention for the correction of LUT pathology unless active infection has been completely eradicated.

S. mansoni lesions in the gut are also reversed by antischistosomal therapy. Residual colonic lesions usually have little or no functional consequences.

The size of hepatic granulomas is reduced by treatment, which explains the reversibility of hepatic enlargement noticed in early stages of infection. Development of subsequent portal hypertension depends on the residual portal fibrosis. The majority of patients who are treated sufficiently early are left with mild hepatosplenomegaly but no functional impairment.

S. japonicum is more difficult to treat, but the outcome of the lesions that it induces is similar to that described for *S. mansoni*. Many of the neurological lesions seen with *S. japonicum* infection are reversible, but cord lesions may need early surgical intervention in order to avoid permanent neurological deficit.

Fibrotic lesions

Many of the residual healed lesions need no surgical correction. Examples are colonic submucosal and pericolic fibrosis sparing motility, hepatosplenic schistosomiasis without portal hypertension, lower ureteric fibrosis without pelvicalyceal dilatation even when associated with mild to moderate reflux, and bladder fibrosis and calcification without significant urodynamic disturbances.

In certain instances, however, extreme degrees of portal hypertension may necessitate shunting procedures. Prominent oesophageal varices may require sclerotherapy. LUT lesions are frequently treated by urological manoeuvres that include percutaneous nephrostomies for the temporary relief of obstruction, endoscopic dilatation of stenosed ureters, subureteric silicone injection for the amelioration of reflux, ureterovesical implantation, ureteroplasty and cystoplasty, and the use of ileal loops for restoration of adequate urodynamic function.

Owing to the silence of cardiopulmonary lesions, the diagnosis is usually delayed beyond the point of any reversibility. Patients with schistosomal cor pulmonale tend to have progressive right ventricular failure, which is barely affected by any form of treatment.

Schistomal glomerulopathy

The effect of treatment on glomerular lesions is questionable. Regression of proteinuria has been reported following the administration of niridazole, oxamniquine, or praziquantel, with and without the use of corticosteroids and immunosuppressive agents. These observations have not been confirmed by histopathologically documented longitudinal studies (Sobh *et al.* 1988b). It is difficult, however, to integrate the available data since most reports lack standardization of the pattern and duration of glomerular injury. A notable exception to this controversy is the usual response of Class II disease to combined antischistosomal and antibacterial treatment. Complete recovery is expected in those patients by 6–8 weeks of treatment.

No adequate data are available on the progress of renal amyloidosis after effective antischistosomal chemotherapy. Improvement or mere stability of the lesions have been described in different reports. Results of clinical trials with colchicine are awaited. The drug is known to be clinically effective in amyloidosis associated with Familial Mediterranean Fever, and to prevent the development of amyloidosis when used in conjunction with Praziquantel in Syrian Golden Hamsters (Sobh *et al.* 1995).

Renal replacement therapy

Dialysis

The treatment of endstage renal failure associated with schistosomiasis is basically the same as that of other aetiologies. Special problems are encountered in patients with hepatosplenic schistosomiasis, who have considerable oesophageal or gastric varices and/or ascites. These are particularly risky candidates for peritoneal dialysis, owing to the excessive loss of protein, and for haemodialysis, owing to the regular need for anticoagulation. In our experience, it was possible to achieve a 1-year survival of 67 per cent in those treated by haemodialysis following prophylactic sclerotherapy of their varices (unpublished data).

Transplantation

The overall results of renal transplantation in patients with healed schistosomal lesions are not different from those with other renal disorders. However, gross bladder fibrosis may lead to a greater incidence of surgical complications, mainly urinary fistulas, during the early postoperative period (Mahmoud *et al.* 2001). Pretransplant intervention may be needed for correction of disturbed bladder urodynamics or removal of persistent infection. The latter frequently necessitates bilateral nephrectomy.

Uncomplicated residual hepatic fibrosis in the recipient does not seem to significantly modify the pharmacokinetics of the immunosuppressive agents used in transplanted patients. However, variations in cyclosporin blood concentrations have been noticed by certain groups (Mahmoud *et al.* 2001) and attributed to altered absorption of the drug. Associated viral hepatitis may have a considerable impact on the protocols of donor selection and prophylactic immunosuppression, and on the eventual outcome (Section 11).

Recurrence of schistosomal glomerulopathy has been described in a few patients (Azevedo *et al.* 1987), suggesting the persistent release of antigens from living worms. Reinfection with *S. hematobium*, without evidence of recurrence of glomerular pathology, has also been described in patients living in an endemic area (Mahmoud *et al.* 2001). In view of these observations, prophylactic antischistosomal chemotherapy has been recommended for recipients known to have been previously infected with the parasite.

References

Al-Sherbiny, M. and Osman, A. (1995). Field application method for detection of antibodies to schistosoma species and genus-specific antigens using dipsticks (abstract). *SRP International Conference on Schistosomiasis*, Cairo, p. 154.

Andrade, Z. A. and Rocha, H. (1979). Schistosomal glomerulopathy. *Kidney International* **16**, 23–29.

Atkin, S. L. *et al.* (1986). Schistosomiasis and inflammatory polyarthritis: a clinical, radiological and laboratory study of 96 patients infected by *S. mansoni* with particular reference to the diarthrodial joint. *Quarterly Journal of Medicine* **59**, 479–487.

Azevedo, L. S. *et al.* (1987). Renal transplantation and schistosomiasis *mansoni*. *Transplantation* **44**, 795–798.

Badawy, A. A. *et al.* (1999). Colchicine therapy for hepatic murine schistosomal fibrosis: image analysis and serological study. *International Journal of Experimental Pathology* **80**, 25–34.

Badr, M. M. Surgical management of urinary Bilharziasis. In *Rob and Smith's Operative Surgery* (ed. H. Dudley, W. J. Pories, D. C. Carter, and W. S. McDougal). London: Butterworth, 1986.

Barsoum, R. S. (1987). Schistosomal glomerulopathy: selection factors. *Nephrology, Dialysis, Transplantation* **2**, 488–497.

Barsoum, R. S. (1993). Schistosomal glomerulopathies. *Kidney International* **44**, 1–12.

Barsoum, R. S. *et al.* (1977). Renal disease in hepatosplenic schistosomiasis: a clinicopathological study. *Transactions of the Royal Society of Tropical Medicine and Hygiene* **71**, 387–391.

Barsoum, R. S. *et al.* (1979). Renal amyloidosis and schistosomiasis. *Transactions of the Royal Society of Tropical Medicine and Hygiene* **73**, 367–374.

Barsoum, R. S. *et al.* (1988). Hepatic macrophage function in schistosomal glomerulopathy. *Nephrology, Dialysis, Transplantation* **3**, 612–616.

Barsoum, R. S. *et al.* (1996). Immunoglobulin A and the pathogenesis of schistosomal glomerulopathy. *Kidney International* **50**, 920–928.

Bashir, M. *et al.* (1994). Evaluation of defined antigen vaccines against *Schistosoma bovis* and *S. japonicum* in bovines. *Tropical and Geographical Medicine* **46**, 255–258.

Brombacher, F. (2000). The role of interleukin-13 in infectious diseases and allergy. *BioEssays* **22**, 646–656.

Capron, A. *et al.* (1983). Macrophages as effector cells in helminthic infections. *Transactions of the Royal Society of Tropical Medicine and Hygiene* **77**, 631–635.

Capron, A. *et al.* (1987). Immunity to schistosomes; progress toward vaccine. *Science* **238**, 1065–1072.

Chatterjee, S. and Van Marck, E. (2001). The role of somatostatin in schistosomiasis: a basis for immunomodulation in host–parasite interactions? *Tropical Medicine and International Health* **6**, 578–581.

Chirimwami, B., Okonda, L., and Nelson, A. M. (1991). Lymphoma and *Schistosoma mansoni* schistosomiasis. Report of 1 case. *Archives D Anatomie et de Cytologie Pathologiques* **39**, 59–61.

Chugh, K. S. *et al.* (1986). Urinary schistosomiasis in Maiduguri, north east Nigeria. *Annals of Tropical Medicine and Parasitology* **80**, 593–599.

Cutts, L., and Wilson, R. A. (1997). Elimination of a primary schistosome infection from rats coincides with elevated IgE titres and mast cell degranulation. *Parasite Immunology* **19**, 91–102.

deWater, R. *et al.* (1988). *Schistosoma mansoni*: ultrastructual localization of the circulating anodic antigen and the circulating cathodic antigen in the mouse kidney glomerulus. *American Journal of Tropical Medicine and Hygiene* **38**, 118–124.

Dunne, D. W. *et al.* (1987). The blocking of human antibody-dependent, eosinophil-mediated killing of *Schistosoma mansoni* schistosomula by monoclonal antibodies which cross-react with a polysaccharide-containing egg antigen. *Parasitology* **94**, 260–280.

Egyptian society of Nephrology Registry. Annual Report 2000. http://www.idsc.gov.eg/health/esn/esn.htm.

el-Mawla, N. G., el-Bolkainy, M. N., and Khaled, H. M. (2001). Bladder cancer in Africa: update. *Seminars in Oncology* **28**, 174–178.

Ezzat, E. *et al.* (1974). The association between *Schistosoma hematobium* infection and heavy proteinuria. *Transactions of the Royal Society of Tropical Medicine and Hygiene* **68**, 315–317.

Flores-Villanueva, P. O. *et al.* (1996). Recombinant IL-10 and IL-10/Fc treatment down-regulate egg antigen-specific delayed hypersensitivity reactions and egg granuloma formation in schistosomiasis. *Journal of Immunology* **156**, 3315–3320.

Ghoneim, M. A., El-Mekresh, M. M., and El-Baz, M. A. (1997). Radical cystectomy for carcinoma of the bladder, critical evaluation of the results in 1026 cases. *Journal of Urology* **158**, 393–399.

Hicks, R. V., James, C., and Webbe, G. (1980). Effect of *Schistosoma hematobium* and *N*-butyl-*N*-14-hydroxybutylnitrosamine on the development of urothelial neoplasia in the baboon. *British Journal of Cancer* **42**, 730–755.

Hirayama, K. *et al.* (1987). HLA-DQ is epistatic to HLA-DR in controlling the immune response to schistosomal antigen in humans. *Nature* **327**, 426–430.

Houba, V. (1979). Experimental renal disease due to schistosomiasis. *Kidney International* **16**, 30–43.

Jyding-Vennervald, B., Kahama, A. I., and Reimert, C. M. (2000). Assessment of morbidity in *Schistosoma hematobium* infection: current methods and future tools. *Acta Tropica* **77**, 81–89.

Katz, N. (1999). Problems in the development of a vaccine against schistosomiasis *mansoni. Revista da Sociedade Brasileira de Medicina Tropical* **32**, 705–711.

Le, T. H., Blair, D., and McManus, D. P. (2000). Mitochondrial DNA sequences of human schistosomes: the current status. *International Journal of Parasitology* **30**, 283–290.

Lima, M. S. *et al.* (1986) Immune responses during human Schistosomiasis *mansoni*. Evidence for antiidiotypic T lymphocyte responsiveness. *Journal of Clinical Investigation* **78**, 983–988.

Lopes, A. A. *et al.* (1999). Racial differences between patients with focal segmental glomerulosclerosis and membranoproliferative glomerulonephritis from the State of Bahia. *Revista da Associacao Medica Brasileira* **45**, 115–120.

Mahmoud, A. A. F. (1987). Praziquantel for the treatment of helminthic infections. *Advances in Internal Medicine* **32**, 193–206.

Mahmoud, K. M. *et al.* (2001). Impact of schistosomiasis on patient and graft outcome after renal transplantation: 10 years' follow-up. *Nephrology, Dialysis, Transplantation* **16**, 2214–2221.

Matsuda, K. *et al.* (1999). Possible associations of rectal carcinoma with *Schistosoma japonicum* infection and membranous nephropathy: a case report with a review. *Japanese Journal of Clinical Oncology* **29**, 576–581.

McKenzie, A. N. (2000). Regulation of T helper type 2 cell immunity by interleukin-4 and interleukin-13. *Pharmacology and Therapeutics* **88**, 143–151.

McManus, D. P. *et al.* (2001). HLA class II antigens positively and negatively associated with hepatosplenic schistosomiasis in a Chinese population. *International Journal of Parasitology* **31**, 674–680.

Mostafa, M. H., Sheweita, S. A., and O'Connor, P. J. (1999). Relationship between schistosomiasis and bladder cancer. *Clinical Microbiology Reviews* **12**, 97–111.

Omer, F. M., Kurtzhals, J. A., and Riley, E. M. (2000). Maintaining the immunological balance in parasitic infections: a role for TGF-beta? *Parasitology Today* **16**, 18–23.

Owhashi, M., Maruyama, H., and Nawa, Y. (1996). Kinetic study of eosinophil chemotactic factor production with reference to eosinophilia and granuloma formation in mice infected with *Schistosoma japonicum. International Journal of Parasitology* **26**, 705–711.

Pemberton, R. M. *et al.* (1994). Cell-mediated immunity to schistosomes. Evaluation of mechanisms operating against lung-stage parasites which might be exploited in a vaccine. *Tropical and Geographical Medicine* **46**, 247–254.

Ruffer, M. A. (1910). Note on the presence of 'Bilharzia haematobia in Egyptian mummies of the Twentieth Dynasty (1250–1000 BC). *British Medical Journal* **1**, 1–16.

Shuhua, X., Hotez, P. J., and Tanner, M. (2000). Artemether, an effective new agent for chemoprophylaxis against shistosomiasis in China: its *in vivo* effect on the biochemical metabolism of the Asian schistosome. *Southeast Asian Journal of Tropical Medicine and Public Health* **31**, 724–732.

Sobh, M. A. *et al.* (1988a). Nephropathy in asymptomatic patients with active *Schistosoma mansoni* infection. *International Urology and Nephrology* **22**, 37–43.

Sobh, M. A. *et al.* (1988b). Effect of antischistosomal treatment on schistosoma-specific nephropathy. *Nephrology, Dialysis, Transplantation* **3**, 744–751.

Sobh, M. *et al.* (1995). Effect of colchicine on schistosoma-induced renal amyloidosis in Syrian golden hamsters. *Nephron* **70**, 478–485.

Stadecker, M. J. (1999). The regulatory role of the antigen-presenting cell in the development of hepatic immunopathology during infection with *Schistosoma mansoni. Pathobiology* **67**, 269–272.

Stadecker, M. J., Hernandez, H. J., and Asahi, H. (2001). The identification and characterization of new immunogenic egg components: implications for evaluation and control of the immunopathogenic T cell response in schistosomiasis. *Memórias do Instituto Oswaldo Cruz* **96** (Suppl.), 29–33.

Thomas, M. A. *et al.* (1989). A common anti-DNA antibody idiotype and anti-phospholipid antibodies in sera from patients with schistosomiasis and filariasis with and without nephritis. *Journal of Autoimmunity* **2**, 803–811.

Wahl, S. M. *et al.* (1997). Cytokine regulation of schistosome-induced granuloma and fibrosis. *Kidney International* **51**, 1370–1375.

Warren, W. *et al.* (1995). Mutations in p53 gene in schistosomal bladder cancer. *Carcinogenesis* **16**, 1181–1189.

7.5 Fungal infections and the kidney

Krishan Lal Gupta

Introduction

As a result of the increased number of immunocompromised patients and increased use of multiple antibiotics, fungal infections have assumed a greater role as opportunistic infections. Different fungi produce characteristic patterns of tissue injury, which are modified by the special structures of the tissues in which they invade. The genitourinary system is a potential site for primary, invasive, or disseminated fungal infection. Angioinvasive fungal infections such as aspergillosis and mucormycosis are associated with severe renal lesions and renal failure with high morbidity and mortality (Raghavan *et al.* 1987; Gupta 2001). They are also seen with increased frequency in patients with renal failure and following renal transplantation with ominous complications. As these infections are frequently subtle in presentation, a high index of clinical suspicion, a thorough understanding of epidemiology, and appropriate utilization of investigations including tissue biopsy, and other invasive procedures are essential for early diagnosis and adequate management.

Pathogenic fungi

Fungi involving the kidneys may be classified as primary, opportunistic, or unusual pathogens (Table 1). Primary pathogens are indigenous to the environment and exposure to their germ spores may cause infection in apparently healthy individuals or patients who have defective cell-mediated immunity. Examples of primary pathogens are *Blastomyces*, *Coccidioides*, and *Histoplasma* species. On the other hand, opportunistic pathogens such as *Candida*, *Cryptococcus*, and *Aspergillus* may be found in the environment or as commensal organisms in humans. They cause infections in patients who have defective phagocytic function due to a variety of causes that include metabolic dysfunction, chronic disease, or steroid or immunosuppressive therapy. Some of the pathogens described earlier as rare and unusual as *Zygomycetes* (Wise and Silver 1993) have been seen more frequently in recent years, and are known to cause serious infections.

Table 1 Pathogenic fungi affecting genitourinary system

Common pathogens	Rare and unusual pathogens (Wise and Freyle 1997)
Primary	*Geotrichum candidum*
Histoplasma capsulatum	*Paecilomyces*
Coccidioides immitis	*Paracoccidioides brasilensis*
Blastomyces dermatidis	*Penicillium glaucum*
Opportunistic	*Penicillium ciftrinum*
Candida albicans	*Trichosporon*
Aspergillus species	*Fusarium*
Cryptococcus neoformans	*Pseudallescheria boydii*
Zygomycetes fungi	*Cunninghamella*
	Rhinosporidium seeberi
	Sporothrix schenckii

Opportunistic infections

Candidiasis

Candidiasis refers to a range of infections caused by species of the fungal genus Candida. These infections can be acute or chronic, localized or systemic. Disseminated candidiasis is frequently life-threatening.

Mycology

The genus *Candida* encompasses more than 160 species. The organisms can be found widely among animal and plant kingdom, associated with naturally occurring high-sugar substrates (honey, nectar) and fermentation products, dairy products, and in the air (Meyer *et al.* 1998). Candida can exist in two morphological states including yeast (cellular) and filamentous (hyphal or mycelial) forms. It has been postulated that the hyphal form can cause invasive infection although not definitely documented (Wise and Silver 1993).

Torulopsis glabrata is similar to candida species in morphology, growth characteristics, and clinical manifestation. However, *T. glabrata* does not develop pseudohyphae or produce germ tubes (Fidel *et al.* 1999). It represents 5–21 per cent of the isolates from positive fungal cultures and is the second most common genitourinary fungal pathogen with more pathogenicity and worse prognosis compared to other candida species (Frye *et al.* 1988).

Pathophysiology

Candida albicans is a normal inhabitant of human gastrointestinal tract, female genital tract, and frequently the oropharynx. Intact skin and gastrointestinal mucosa provide a powerful barrier to infections by candida. Any break in the above barriers may lead to a possible invasion by the fungi. Polymorphonuclear neutrophils with their various intracellular enzymes constitute the primary defence to candida. The role of humoral immunity is complex. While the antibodies are incapable of killing the fungi, the observation that complement deficient humans are more susceptible to candidiasis indicates a possible role of the complement system in the host defence against candida (Han and Cutler 1997).

The fungus usually gains access to the kidney through the blood. In experimental candidiasis attachment of the blastospores to the glomerular and peritubular capillary endothelium takes place through surface fibrils immediately after localization in the kidney (Barnes *et al.* 1983). Host cell necrosis and abscess formation ensue within 24 h. These microabscesses have a predilection for the medullary region and the tips of the papillae, which may result in papillary necrosis and pyonephrosis.

Lower urinary tract involvement

Most lower urinary tract infections are caused by retrograde spread from indwelling catheters, perineal colonization, or intertriginous infection. Candidal cystitis may occur in patients who require long-term urinary catheter drainage. They present with recurrent episodes of urinary frequency, urgency, and bladder discomfort. Cystoscopy may reveal grey-white patches on the bladder that are mixed with areas of mucosal oedema and erythema and may also show 'snow storm effect' obscuring visualization (Zincke *et al.* 1973). Accretions of the candidal pseudohyphae may develop with the formation of fungus ball that may require a surgical removal. There also have been reports of *perivesical infection* of the bladder as well as emphysematious cystitis (Sheynkin and Wise 1995), emphysematous prostatitis and prostatic abscesses (Wise and Freyle 1997), and candidal epididymo-orchitis (Jenkin *et al.* 1998).

The presence of candiduria (*C. albicans* accounts for 52 per cent of the cases) has diverse pathological significance. It may be asymptomatic or indicate acute haematogenous dissemination or even be the source of subsequent dissemination in critically ill, neutropenic patients, low birth weight infants, renal allograft recipients, and patients likely to undergo surgical manipulations (Nossoura *et al.* 1993). Urinary colony counts of more than 10,000–15,000/ml, and urinary casts containing fungal material as demonstrated by Papanicolaus' stain (Argyle 1985), may suggest infection of the urinary tract rather than mere colonization of bladder.

Upper tract involvement

Candidal infection of the upper tract, that is, of the collecting system or ureter can be caused by direct ascent from lower urinary tract or disseminated infection. Indwelling urinary catheter, diabetes mellitus, immunosuppression, or obstructive uropathy enhance vulnerability to upper tract infection by a non-haematogenous route (Shelp *et al.* 1966). In a study of 50 patients with candiduria, Wainstain *et al.* (1995) classified infections as *complex* (upper tract or disseminated) and *simple* (confined to bladder). The incidence of obstructive uropathy (88 versus 20 per cent), malnutrition (88 versus 48 per cent), malignancy (56 versus 16 per cent), renal failure (24 versus 8 per cent), and prolonged antibiotic use (60 versus 32 per cent) were higher in patients with complex infection. In the absence of systemic involvement ascending infection was considered to be the most likely source.

Fungal accretions, known as fungal balls, are known to cause ureteral obstruction or renal pelvic obstruction (Stein *et al.* 1993; Scerpella and Alhalel 1994). They can occur secondary to either ascending funguria or haematogenous dissemination with renal parenchymal involvement. Once the collecting system has been invaded, candida has the ability to proliferate in spite of acidity, forming masses of pseudohyphal elements mixed with mucoid debris and sloughed papillary epithelium. *C. albicans* and *Candida tropicalis* have been commonly associated with fungal balls but other organisms including *Candida glabratra*, *Aspergillus*, *Pencillium*, and *Mucor* have been reported as causal (Irby *et al.* 1990). Patients usually present with ureteral obstruction (Fig. 1) and are often clinically ill with fever or flank pain. Oliguria and anuria have also been known to occur (Scerpella and Alhalel 1994).

Renal candidiasis

Renal involvement occurs in 82 per cent of patients with disseminated disease as a result of haematogenous spread and it is usually bilateral (Myerowitz *et al.* 1977). Infection of the kidneys should be assumed whenever candida is recovered from blood.

Clinical manifestations are those of pyelonephritis, that is, fever with chills, flank, and/or abdominal pain, costoverteberal angle tenderness, or hypertension. Urine may reveal pyuria or haematuria. Oliguria and anuria may also occur. Imaging studies may demonstrate filling defect compatible with fungal accretions. Computed tomography (CT) scans or sonography may show typical appearance of kidneys studded with microabscesses.

Pathological findings include multiple small abscesses in the interstitium and glomeruli, as well as large abscesses resulting in pyonephrosis. Budding yeast and pseudomycelia in peritubular vessels and collecting tubules have been demonstrated. Emphysematous pyelonephritis (Johnson *et al.* 1986) and renal papillary necrosis (Tomashefski and Abramowsky 1981) have also been reported. In a recent analysis of 30 patients with renal candidiasis, papillary necrosis was noted in half of them (Gupta 2001).

Blood and serologic tests

In patients with histologically proven renal candidiasis, fungaemia could be detected in fewer than 50 per cent (Meunier-Carpentier *et al.* 1981). Whole cell agglutination, agar cell diffusion, latex agglutination, and counter-immune electrophoresis are not reliable tests for candidal infection (de Repentigny 1992). Circulating candida enolase by immunoassay can detect parenchymal candidal infection (Walsh *et al.* 1991).

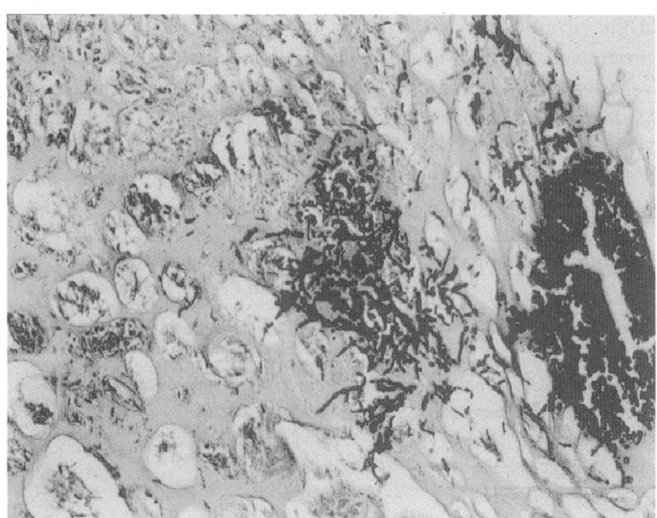

Fig. 1 Microsection of the kidney showing colonies of yeast and filament forms of *Candida* in necrosed papilla (PAS, 550×) (reproduced from Gupta 2001, with permission).

Polymerase chain reaction (PCR) technique has provided 100 per cent sensitivity and specificity for the detection of candiduria.

Management

Candiduria Treatment depends upon the site of infection, for example, bladder versus renal. Improvement of the host's nutritional status and an early removal of the indwelling catheter (if present) are important considerations in ameliorating the potential for persistent candidal infection or colonization. Simply changing a Foley's catheter in candiduric individuals results in eradication of candiduria in almost 40 per cent of patients (Sobel *et al.* 2000). Antifungal therapy for 7–14 days is warranted in patients at risk of dissemination of infection (Rex *et al.* 2000). Fluconazole (200 mg/day PO or IV) achieves high urinary concentrations and it was effective in 19 of 20 critically ill patients (Nossoura *et al.* 1993). Other drugs such as amphotericin B at widely ranging doses of 0.3–1 mg/kg/day and in the absence of renal insufficiency, oral flucytosine 25 mg/kg/QID may be effective in eradicating candiduria. The latter drug, administered especially in those with *non-albicans Candida species*, is associated with a high rate of drug resistance when used alone.

Persistence of candiduria after the removal of local factors may be treated by irrigation of the bladder with amphotericin B (Occhipinti *et al.* 1993) provided there is no invasive parenchymal disease. The role of bladder irrigation has been questioned recently (Sobel *et al.* 2000). Jacobs *et al.* (1996) had also observed that 1-month mortality rate was greater among patients who were treated with amphotericin B bladder irrigation than those who received oral fluconazole therapy even when eradication of funguria was similar in the two treatment groups.

Renal/disseminated candidiasis As renal infection is indicative of parenchymal and or disseminated disease, systemic therapy should be continued until the patient becomes clinically well, with normal counts and negative cultures. Adults are usually treated with an amphotericin B dose of 0.6 mg/kg/day administered over several weeks (Solomkin *et al.* 1982). However, total cumulative dose of up to 1 g has been advocated for renal candidiasis by some authors.

Fluconazole has also been used successfully in renal candidiasis. In a randomized trial, Rex *et al.* (1994) compared amphotericin B (0.5–0.6 mg/kg/day) and oral fluconazole 400 mg/day in the treatment of candidaemia in non-neutropenic patients, and found them equally effective. Because many *C. glabrata* strains are resistant to fluconazole, the most conservative approach is to treat fungaemia due to this species with amphotericin B till a total dose 600–2000 mg is given (Fidel *et al.* 1999). For local infection, amphotericin B irrigation and oral 5,flurocytosine (5-FC) have been found to be successful. Modification of flucytosine as well as that of fluconazole is required in renal insufficiency (Table 2).

Fungal bezoar Access to the upper tract is necessary in all cases of fungal bezoar to relieve obstruction, establish drainage, and apply antifungal medication directly to the diseased site (Irby *et al.* 1990). This can be achieved by a percutaneous nephrostomy tube or irrigation through a ureteral catheter. Surgical debulking is required in the absence of improvement. Systemic amphotericin therapy is given prior to surgery to avoid potential dissemination and is continued postoperatively till absence of fungaemia is ensured. Systemic medical treatment should also be instituted immediately when disseminated infection is suspected or evidenced (fungaemia, retinitis/endophthalmitis, radiological stigmata including pulmonary infiltration, diffuse mucocutaneous mycosis).

Table 2 Dose modification of antifungals in renal failure

Drug (normal dosage)	Creatinine clearance (ml/min)			Supplemental dose after dialysis
	>50	10–50	<10	
Fluconazole (100–200 mg/day)	100%	50%	25%	HD—full dose CAPD—quarter dose
Itraconazole (200–400 mg/day)	100%	100%	50%	HD/CAPD—full dose
5-Flucytosine 12.5–37.5 mg/kg q6h (0.5–1 g/day)	No change	q12–24h	q24–48h	HD—full dose CAPD—0.5–1 g/day

HD, haemodialysis; CAPD, continuous ambulatory peritoneal dialysis; q, dose interval.

For disease limited to the collecting system intravenous amphotericin B is of negligible benefit.

Zygomycosis

Zygomycosis (also earlier called phycomycosis and mucormycosis) is a rare mycotic infection caused by the angioinvasive fungi belonging to the class *Zygomycetes* (Benbow and Stoddart 1986). The most common pathogenic species including *Rhizopus oryzae*, *Rhizomucor pusillus*, and *Absidia corymbifera* as well as others implicated in the systemic infection, usually initiate a serious disease in immunocompromised patients although rarely apparently healthy subjects may also be affected (Blodi *et al.* 1969; Gupta *et al.* 1999).

Different species of the *Zygomycetes* produce virtually identical disease and do not influence the diagnosis and management. They are opportunistic organisms with ubiquitous distribution in soil, decaying organic matter, and air. They have minimal intrinsic pathogenicity but may initiate an aggressive and often fatal infection in patients with diabetic ketoacidosis, lymphoproliferative disorders, renal failure, viral hepatitis, burns, and severe malnutrition (Gupta *et al.* 1990; Sugar 1992). The list of predisposing conditions continues to grow, the latest additions being desferrioxamine therapy for iron/aluminium overload in dialysis patients (Boelaert *et al.* 1993) and intravenous drug abuse particularly in those with HIV infection (Weng *et al.* 1998). Whereas acidosis, seen in diabetic ketoacidosis, may interfere with neutrophil-mediated chemotaxis and phagocytosis thus impairing killing of the fungus, the Mucorales, being siderophores, on the other hand, have been demonstrated to have augmented growth in the presence of iron chelated in patients on desferrioxamine therapy (Boelaert *et al.* 1993).

Clinical manifestations of the disease are dependent on the portal of entry (inhalation, ingestion, or direct inoculation) of the fungus as well as the underlying health status of the affected individual. In humans the four main presentation of zygomycosis are the rhinocerebral, pulmonary, gastrointestinal, and disseminated forms (Benbow and Stoddart 1986). Following infection in the immunocompromised host, *Zygomycetes*, being facultative necrotrophs, invade and kill the living tissue, drawing nutrition in the process. They have a predilection for invading blood vessels, with resultant ischaemia and necrosis associated with acute inflammatory infiltrate in the affected organ. The pathological manifestations following infection are similar regardless of the anatomical site.

Renal involvement occurs both as a part of disseminated infection (Ingram *et al.* 1989; Gupta *et al.* 1999) as well as in isolated disease

(Levy and Bia 1995; Williams 1997). In an autopsy series of disseminated disease, the kidneys were involved in up to 22 per cent of patients (Ingram *et al.* 1989). Isolated renal involvement in the absence of an underlying predisposing factor is rare and the disease is often unilateral (Levy and Bia 1995). However, Gupta *et al.* (1999) in a series of 18 patients observed that half the patients had isolated renal zygomycosis and all of them except one had bilateral involvement and did not have any predisposing condition. In patients without identifiable focus, the occurrence of isolated renal involvement may be attributed to a subclinical pulmonary infection with subsequent haematogenous dissemination to the kidney, akin to renal tuberculosis.

Most patients with renal zygomycosis present with fever, flank pain, and oligoanuria. A very high incidence of renal failure (up to 95 per cent) is encountered in patients with bilateral involvement (Gupta 2001). Renal failure results from occlusion of the renal arteries or their branches (Fig. 2). Histologically, the kidneys reveal an extensive cortical and medullary involvement with evidence of infarction and necrosis associated with neutrophilic infiltrate. The characteristics fungal hyphae may be also seen in the infiltrate along with granulomas and Langhan's type multinucleated giant cells (Davila *et al.* 1990). Glomerular as well as tubular hyphal invasion may be seen (Fig. 3).

Up to now, there are no features on intravenous pyelography or ultrasonography that distinguish zygomycosis from other diseases producing abcesses in the kidney. However, there may be characteristic findings on CT (Chugh *et al.* 1993). These include diffuse enlargement of the kidney with absence of contrast excretion and presence of multiple low-density areas in the renal parenchyma representing fungal abscesses. Rupture of such an abscess may result in perinephric collection. Nosher *et al.* (1988) have also described areas of low attenuation with diminished enhancement referred as a 'diffuse patchy nephrogram'. Magnetic resonance imaging (MRI) may be preferred for the diabetic patient in whom intravenous contrast agents may be contraindicated.

The 'gold standard' for diagnosis remains the morphological identification of mycotic elements in biopsy tissue. Demonstration of irregularly shaped, broad (10–20 mm in diameter), aseptate hyphae with right angle branching invading endothelial surface with very little surrounding inflammation is very important. Cultures of blood and bodily secretions or infected tissues rarely detect these fungi. Unfortunately more than 90 per cent of the patients with disseminated zygomycosis, have been diagnosed at autopsy and in addition these organisms become non-viable due to damage to their wall during grinding because they lack septae (Ingram *et al.* 1989). Unlike renal candidiasis fungal hyphae may be identified in urine only exceptionally (Florentine *et al.* 1997). Serology has been useful only in isolated cases. A sensitivity of 73 per cent and a specificity of 100 per cent have been reported in immunodiffusion tests for specific *Absidia*, *Mucor*, and *Rhizopus* species (Wise *et al.* 1999).

Successful therapy of renal zygomycosis involves a coordinated surgical and medical approach (Parfrey 1986; Williams 1997). Extensive debridement of the infected and necrotic tissue, administration of amphotericin B (0.6–1 mg/kg/day up to a total of 2–3 g), and the reversal of the underlying condition form the triad of therapy. There are reports of survival following amphotericin B therapy without nephrectomy in patients with unilateral renal disease (Levy and Bia 1995; Weng *et al.* 1998). Recently the unilamellar liposomal formulation of amphotericin B, has been also recommended for use in view of its lesser side effects (Saltoglu *et al.* 1998; Weng *et al.* 1998).

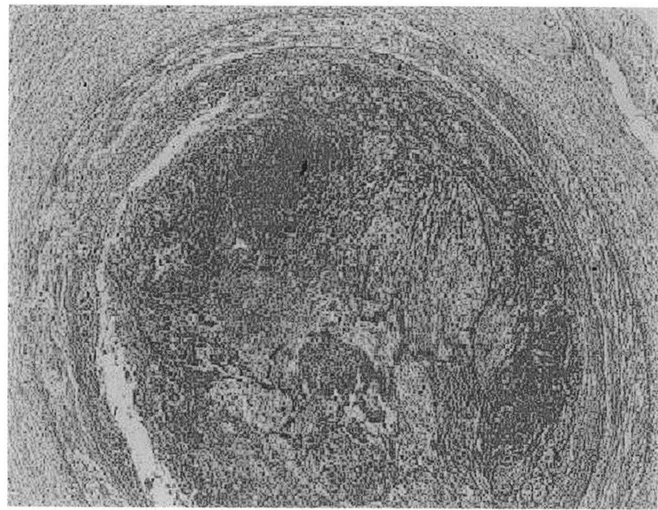

Fig. 2 Photomicrograph of renal artery at the hilum showing transmural arteritis and subtotal occlusion of the lumen by a thrombus (H&E, 55×) (reproduced from Gupta 2001, with permission).

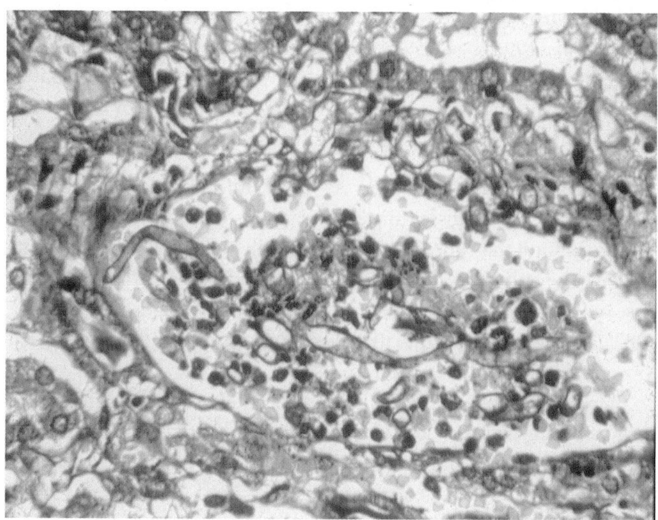

Fig. 3 Section of a renal tubule showing aseptate, broad hyphae of zygomycetes in the lumen (Grocott's stain, 1375×) (reproduced from Gupta 2001, with permission).

Aspergillosis

Invasive aspergillosis is caused by fungi of the genus *Aspergillus*. Of the several hundred species described about 20 are pathogenic to human beings. Among them *Aspergillus fumigatus* is the most common followed by *A. flavus*, *A. terreus*, *A. nidulans*, and *A. niger* species (Rippon 1988). These fungi have characteristic septate hyphae with dichotomous branching which can easily distinguish them from aseptate irregular branching hyphae of *Mucor*. Aspergilli are ubiquitous in distribution and can be found in the soil, dust, vegetation, and decaying organic matter. Hospital outbreaks have occurred due to contaminated air-conditioning ducts and ventilators.

Aspergillosis is primarily a pulmonary infection, which can present with allergic alveolitis and bronchopulmonary aspergillosis. Disseminated infection can occur following a haematogeous spread in patients with debilitating diseases such as diabetes mellitus, tuberculosis, cirrhosis, obstructive uropathy, or in patients receiving steroid and cytotoxic therapy (Rippon 1988).

Aspergillosis of the kidneys has been reported in 8–13 per cent of patients with disseminated disease (Young *et al.* 1970), but primary renal aspergillosis is rare (Hadaya *et al.* 1998). Renal involvement is usually unilateral involvement but sometimes bilateral renal disease may also occur (Sud *et al.* 1998). Clinical features include proteinuria, pyuria, haematuria, and sometimes oliguric renal failure. Most patients have fungal bezoars producing hydronephrosis, and less infrequently they have single or multiple abscesses. Because of angioinvasion, vascular thrombosis and areas of infarction in the kidney may occur, although not as severe as in the case of zygomycosis. Renal papillary necrosis and isolated prostatic infection may occasionally occur (Madge and Lombardias 1973; Hood *et al.* 1998). Clinical presentation of renal aspergillosis may fall in one of the following categories (Flechner and McAninch 1987):

1. *Disseminated aspergillosis* with renal involvement. It results from haematogenous spread of fungi to the kidneys leading to formation of multiple focal abscesses. Infection of the renal vessels in some cases also results in multiple areas of infarction which is more common in the medulla than cortex. This may result in papillary necrosis.
2. *Aspergillus cast of renal pelvis.* It results in obstructive uropathy which may present with urinary retention or anuria and can be diagnosed by demonstration of filling defects on ultrasonography.
3. *Ascending pan-urothelial aspergillosis.* It refers to the ascending infection involving the urethra, bladder, ureters, and the kidney. Such patients may present with symptoms of systemic infection as well as renal colic caused by fungal ball or renal papillary tissue.

Among the 27 cases of renal aspergillosis recently analysed at a tertiary centre in India, 15 of 17 (88 per cent) autopsied cases had disseminated infection involving lungs, brain, heart, gastrointestinal tract, and liver (Gupta 2001). Pathological lesions included microabscesses, vasculitis with infarction, and papillary necrosis (Fig. 4). Renal failure occurred in 15 (55 per cent) patients.

Diagnosis of renal aspergillosis is usually difficult. Clinical features of renal involvement are either absent or non-specific. Radiological investigations including ultrasonography and/or CT scan can lead towards renal localization. Fungus is difficult to culture from midstream urine samples and the diagnosis is usually made from the identification and culture of the organism from percutaneous drainage of the abscesses or obstructed urinary tract. In systemic aspergillus infections, blood cultures are usually negative.

Serological studies using late agglutination, immuno-diffusion or radioimmunoassay can be helpful in the diagnosis. Of particular importance is the detection of Aspergillus antigen (galactomannan) in plasma or serum samples by the commercially available enzyme-linked immunosorbent assay (ELISA) which had high sensitivity (67–100 per cent) and specificity (81–98 per cent) when performed with sera from patients receiving treatment for haematological malignancies (Verweij *et al.* 1996). A positive ELISA galactomannan test may occur early in the infection, sometimes 6–13 days before clinical features. PCR methodology may also detect Aspergillus DNA fragments in urine, bronchoalveolar lavage, serum, and plasma thus helping in diagnosing invasive infections, although later than ELISA (Bretagne *et al.* 1998).

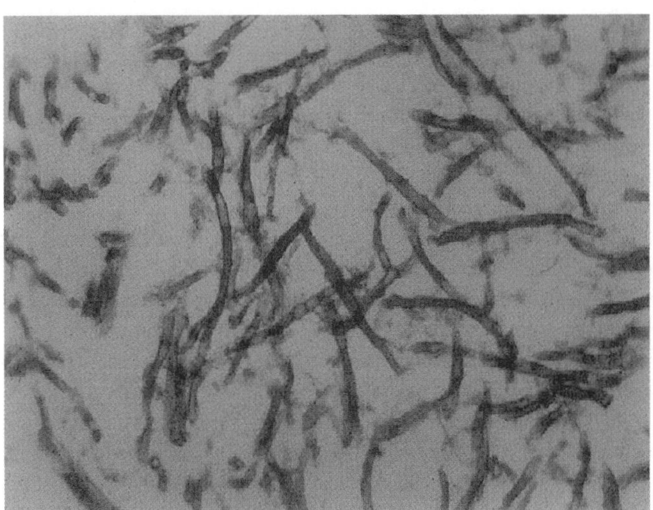

Fig. 4 High-power magnification of septate hyphae of aspergillus identified in sloughed papillary tissue (PAS, 1375×).

Treatment

Early recognition, aggressive pharmacotherapy and prompt urological intervention are necessary for the control of renal aspergillus infection (Denning 1998). Patients with aspergillus bezoars in the renal pelvis require management as discussed under candidiasis. Large and solitary renal abscesses require surgical drainage. Nephrectomy can be resorted to in patients not responding to the above measures if the disease is unilateral (Irby *et al.* 1990).

Medical therapy includes amphotericin B and itraconazole. The overall success rate of amphotericin B is 34 per cent. Itraconazole at a dose of 200 mg three times a day has been found to be equally effective. In patients who are critically ill or immunosuppressed, intravenous amphotericin B is usually preferred (dose 0.8–1 mg/kg/day). A total cumulative dose of 2–2.5 g is usually recommended to arrest disease progression. Lipid preparations of amphotericin B (dose of 4–5 mg/kg/day) may be preferred if there is evidence of pre-existing renal failure. Amphotericin B is followed by oral therapy with itraconazole for a prolonged period (Denning 1998). Newer azoles voriconazole and posaconazole, as well as echinocandins, capsofungin have also been used in the treatment of resistant aspergillosis as discussed later in the chapter.

Cryptococcosis

Cryptococcosis, also known as Torulopsis, is caused by basidiomycetous, encapsulated yeast, *Cryptococcus neoformans*. This fungus has also been isolated from roosting sites of pigeons and in association with rotting vegetation, eucalyptus trees, and soil infested with bird guano (Ellis and Pfeiffer 1990). Heavy fungal growth can be found in old buildings and barn lofts. After inhalation, the fungus causes a pulmonary infection which may be asymptomatic or may develop into a virulent respiratory infection with dissemination to other organs in an immunocompromised host (Rippon 1988).

The central nervous system (CNS) is the primary target of haematogenous spread. Genitourinary involvement usually follows the neurological manifestations but it may sometime precede or occur alone (Randall *et al.* 1968). In an autopsy series of 39 patients, Salyer and Salyer (1973) observed renal involvement in 51 per cent, while prostate was involved in 26 per cent of male patients. Urine cultures were positive in 40 per cent of isolates. Clinical presentation of renal involvement may be cystitis, pyuria, haematuria, moderate proteinuria, and laboratory evidence of mild renal insufficiency. Renal failure is uncommon in renal cryptococcosis.

Analysis of the renal lesions suggests that the fungal organisms may lodge within glomeruli (Fig. 5) and possibly within the postglomerular vasculature, with the formation of small abscesses. In addition granulomas containing giant cells, papillary necrosis, tubular obstruction, dilatation and atrophy may result, along with intense interstitial and glomerular fibrosis in some patients.

In AIDS patients, the prostate may be the main reservoir of genitourinary infection in patients with disseminated cryptococcosis and sometimes even after successful treatment of meningitis (Larsen *et al.* 1989). Fungi were observed in the expressed prostate secretions in four of these patients. The prostatic lesions vary from small, chronic inflammatory changes to large granulomas with caseation and retention of urine may be the presenting feature.

Diagnosis is established by examination or culture of infected secretions. India ink preparation, best used for CNS infection, may demonstrate large clear capsules surrounding yeast cells. Mucicarmine stain can identify the capsule and wall of the fungus. Standard mycological techniques using Saboraud's agar yields the fungus from blood, pulmonary secretions, cerebrospinal fluid, and in rare instances the urine. Assessment of cryptococcal antigen titre in the blood, urine, or cerebrospinal fluid by a latex agglutination system may be helpful in establishing infection (Jaye *et al.* 1998).

The choice of treatment depends on the host's immune status, the severity of the disease, and the presence of meningitis (Van des Horst *et al.* 1997). For patients with prostatic infection or isolated urinary tract infection, fluconazole at a dose of 200–400 mg/day for 3–6 months is recommended. For those patients who are unable to tolerate fluconazole, itraconazole 200–400 mg/day for 6–12 months is an acceptable alternative (Denning *et al.* 1989).

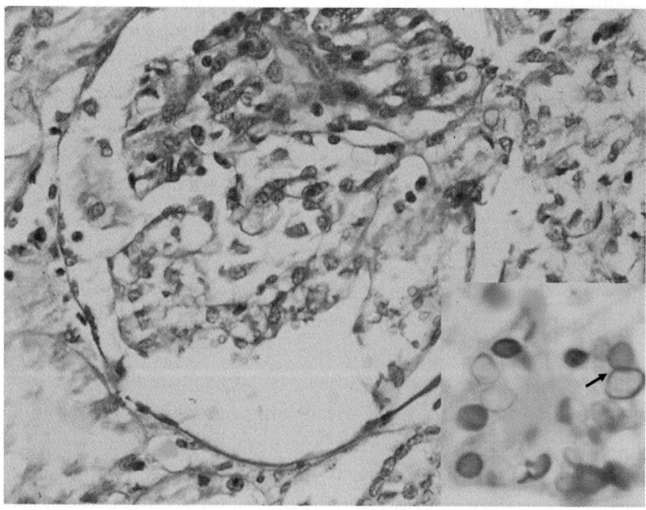

Fig. 5 Photomicrograph of a glomerulus, showing partial destruction and infiltration by many cryptococcus spores (PAS, 550×). The inset at higher magnification with arrow showing budding spores (PAS–Alcian blue, 1375×) (reproduced after modification from Gupta 2001, with permission).

Primary infections

Histoplasmosis

Histoplasma capsulatum is a dimorphic fungus that grows readily in soil high in nitrogen content that has been enriched by the guano of birds (including chickens, pigeons, and especially starlings) or bats. It often causes infection among spelunkers exploring bat-infested caves, and urbanites exposed to construction sites and tree removal. Inhalation of fungal conidia may result in asymptomatic self-limiting pulmonary infection. Diagnosis is made by chest X-ray findings of small pulmonary granulomas and calcification and a positive skin test. Approximately one in 2000 individuals exposed to *H. capsulatum* goes on to develop disseminated disease (Wheat 1994). This variability in outcome of infection appears to depend on inoculum size and the strength of host cell-mediated immune defence mechanisms (Goodwin *et al.* 1980).

Renal involvement in patients with disseminated disease varies widely. In a series of 46 patients with disseminated histoplasmosis, Wheat *et al.* (1981) described one patient who had interstitial nephritis with *H. capsulatum* identified in a renal hilar lymph node. Goodwin *et al.* (1980) noted fungus in macrophages in glomerular capillaries or the interstitial tissues of the cortex or medulla in 40 per cent of patients with disseminated histoplasmosis. Nephrotic range proteinuria with preserved renal function has been reported in a patient of disseminated histoplasmosis associated with advanced HIV disease (Burke *et al.* 1997). Renal biopsy tissue has revealed immune complexes and *H. capsulatum* antigen within the mesangium. There may also, sometime, be evidence of non-caseating granuloma and cutaneous fistula formation (Kedar *et al.* 1988). Transplant recipients are at continued risk for disseminated infection (2.1 per cent, Wheat *et al.* 1983), obstructive uropathy (Superdock *et al.* 1994), or graft loss (Sridhar *et al.* 1991).

Diagnosis of histoplasmosis is dependent on clinical suspicion and identification of the fungus in urine, semen, and tissue. New molecular techniques that use radioimmunoassay and enzyme-linked assays can detect histoplasma antigen in serum and urine (Durkin *et al.* 1997). In disseminated infection in addition to antigen demonstration of intraleucocytic budding yeast in Wright–Giemsa stained peripheral blood smears may also lead to definite diagnosis (Wise and Silver 1993).

As genitourinary infection is generally associated with disseminated disease administration of intravenous amphotericin B (>2 g of total dose) followed by long-term itraconazole (200 mg once or twice a day for 3–6 months) is the therapy of choice (Wheat 1994). Fluconazole (200–800 mg/day) has been tried in non-HIV patients but response was only moderate. Its use has been advocated only in those who cannot take itraconazole.

Blastomycosis

Blastomycosis is a systemic pyogranulomatous infection, caused by *Blastomyces dermatidis*. It primarily involves the lungs with frequent dissemination to other organs. The exact prevalence of the disease is unknown, but rates range between 0.5 and four cases per 100,000 population per year in vulnerable geographic regions including Mississippi and Ohio River basins, South America, Africa, and Middle East (Chapman *et al.* 1997).

Two serotypes of *B. dermatidis* have been identified based upon the presence or absence of A antigen and these have been, respectively, associated with isolates from America and Africa (Kaufman *et al.* 1983). The fungus exhibits thermal dimorphism, growing as mycelial phase at room temperature (25°C) and as the yeast phase at 37°C. Humidity is important in promoting growth of the organism. Its habitat is possibly rotting or damp wood or soil containing decaying vegetation.

Inhalation of the spores initiates an acute or chronic pulmonary infection. Clinical manifestations range from asymptomatic illness detected only by screening to chronic respiratory illness mimicking tuberculosis or cancer (Davies and Sarosi 1997). Patients with AIDS more often present with fulminant infections. Infection has also been reported following sexual exposure and inoculation accidents (Craig *et al.* 1970).

Pulmonary infection may be followed by haematogenous dissemination in adult males, pregnant women, and their unborn children as well as patients with endstage AIDS and transplant recipients (Pappas 1997). Skin, bone, and CNS are common sites of extrapulmonary blastomycosis. Genitourinary disease has also been reported in as many as 20–30 per cent of patients with disseminated disease (Witorsch and Utz 1968; Eickenberg *et al.* 1975). There is predominant involvement of the prostate, epididymis and testis whereas kidney and ureters are less frequently involved. In a retrospective review of 51 patients with systemic blastomycosis, Eickenberg *et al.* (1975) found that the prostate was involved in eight (16 per cent) and the epididymis in 10 (20 per cent). The kidney, testis, and prepuce were involved in 1 (2 per cent) each. Patient may present with symptoms suggestive of prostatitis. Pyuria and haematuria are found in the majority. Infection of the female genital tract is uncommon.

Infection is usually diagnosed by identification of the fungus in urine. Semen and tissue infection of prostate and epididymis can be confirmed by detection of blastomyces A antigen by immunodiffusion. Serological tests such as enzyme immunoassay and radioimmunoassay have a sensitivity of up to 90 per cent and specificity of up to 100 per cent.

Systemic amphotericin B is recommended for patients who are immunocompromised or who have disseminated infection as well as pregnant females. Itraconazole has been found to be useful in focal uncomplicated disease. The azoles have embryotoxic and teratogenic properties and are *contraindicated* in pregnancy.

Coccidiomycosis

Coccidioidomycosis is the infection caused by the dimorphic fungus, *Coccidioides immitis*, which is endemic to the semi-arid sub-Sonoran regions of the Western Hemisphere (Drutz and Cantanzaro 1978). The saprophytic mycelial phase of this fungus exists in the soil and, under proper environmental conditions, it releases the infectious arthrospores (3–5 μm in size) into the air. When inhaled by the animal host, arthrospores evolve into large spherules (>70 μm in diameter). The cytoplasm of the enlarging spherule undergoes cleavage to produce endospores that are released into the infected tissue when the mature spherule ruptures. The endospore can develop into a spherule and continue the cycle. Specimens from patients show a reversion to mycelia on most laboratory media (Cole and Sun 1985). The mycelial phase is extremely infectious while the endospore phase is not. The disease is not transmissible from person to person. Direct infection through cutaneous inoculation is rare and usually self limited (Drutz and Cantanzaro 1978).

Following inhalation, an asymptomatic and transient pulmonary infection ensues. Of the infected persons, 60 per cent have subclinical disease. Most of the remainder will have a mild to severe respiratory illness with complete resolution, although around 5 per cent will have residual pulmonary infection (Stevens 1995). The patient may manifest high fever, cough, night sweats, or pleuritic chest pain. An allergic reaction to the infection may develop with manifestation of erythema nodosum, also known as 'valley fever'.

Less than 1 per cent of patients develop extrapulmonary multiorgan dissemination. Patients with dark skin, pregnant women (usually in the third trimester), immunosuppressed patients including solid organ transplant recipients, age less than 5 or greater than 50 are risk factors in the development of disseminated disease (Stevens 1995). Preferred sites of dissemination include the meninges, bone, joints, skin, and soft tissue.

Postmortem studies of patients with disseminated infection have noted involvement of kidney (46–60 per cent), adrenals (16–22 per cent), prostate (3–6 per cent), retroperitonum (up to 3 per cent), and scrotum (1.5 per cent) (Forbus and Besterbreurtje 1946; Huntington *et al.* 1967). Renal involvement may manifest as *micro-abscesses* or granulomas (Kuntze 1988). Bladder infection may present with haematuria, pnematuria (caused by vesicocolic fistula) and concomitant bacilluria (Conner *et al.* 1975). Prostate infection may present with symptoms suggestive of a bladder outflow tract obstruction (Price *et al.* 1982).

Diagnosis of renal infection is difficult. Up to one third of patients with coccidioiduria had proven genitourinary pathology. Radiographic findings are akin to tuberculosis, and may include moth-eaten calyces, infundibular stenosis, ureteral stricture and renal calcification (Kuntze *et al.* 1988). Diagnosis of bladder infection is established by tissue biopsy and serological studies. Infection of tissues such as prostatitis and epididymitis can be diagnosed by tissue biopsy. The mycelial form of the fungus will grow on standard microbiological fungal media but definitive diagnosis is dependent on specialized techniques, such as using DNA probes. Serological tests measuring IgA and IgM antibodies to coccidiodin antigen are useful clinical tools to assess the degree of infection (Wise *et al.* 1999).

Treatment is dependent on the degree of infection. Patients who have inactive pulmonary infection do not require therapy. Clinical or laboratory evidence of active or disseminated infection requires systemic antifungal therapy in the form of amphotericin B at a dose of 1.0–1.5 mg/kg/day for at least 2–3 months. Lipid formulations of amphotericin B provide higher dosage with less toxicity. The triazoles, itraconazole (200 mg/day), or fluconazole (400–600 mg/day) given for arbitrary time of 6 months, are useful for chronic systemic infection, although the relapse rate may be high (Stevens 1995).

Fungal peritonitis

Fungal peritonitis occurs at a rate of 0.01–0.19 episodes per dialysis year in patients performing continuous ambulatory peritoneal dialysis (CAPD) and accounts for 15 per cent of all episodes (Goldie *et al.* 1996). Risk factors include use of immunosuppressive drugs, frequent episodes of bacterial peritonitis, and antecedent antibiotic therapy. Candida is responsible for 90 per cent of cases with fungal peritonitis and among these most common organisms are *C. albicans* and *C. parapsilosis* (Johnson *et al.* 1985). Besides these other yeasts and filamentous fungi including *C. tropicalis*, *T. glabrata*, *Rhadotorula*, *Geotrichum*, *Aspergillus*, *Trichosporon*, *Paecilomyces*, and *Mucor* have also been reported as causal (Holley *et al.* 1994).

The patient with fungal peritonitis may not have any specific signs or he may be acutely ill and deteriorate rapidly to death. Findings include low-grade fever, abdominal pain, and cloudy dialysate. Catheter outflow malfunction may occur in up to 50 per cent (Johnson *et al.* 1985). Neutrophil predominance is seen in peritoneal fluid but the fluid may also show eosinophilia. Gram stain of peritoneal fluid is often negative. Fungal cultures are usually positive within 3–5 days, whereas species such as *Aspergillus* may be difficult to grow and identify in the culture.

As soon as a diagnosis of fungal peritonitis is made, immediate catheter removal is suggested, although some have advised a conservative approach (Chan *et al.* 1994; Goldie *et al.* 1996). According to latest International Society for Peritoneal Dialysis (ISPD) guidelines for adult PD-related peritonitis (Keane *et al.* 2000) imidazole/triazoles—5-FC combinations in retrospective analysis have been found to be as effective as amphotericin B, particularly for non-filamentous fungi. It is advised to start with a loading dose of 2 g of flucytosine given orally and fluconazole 200 mg given orally or intraperitoneally, followed by maintenance dose of 1 g of flucytosine and 200 mg of fluconazole. If the organism is resistant, consider itraconozole. If a patient shows clinical improvement at 4–7 days continue therapy for 4–6 weeks. If there is no improvement, remove catheter and continue therapy for the next 7 days after catheter removal.

In case of filamentous fungi, catheter is removed immediately and the patient is treated with amphotericin B, which may also be used to treat cases with non-filamentous fungi not responding to treatment with other drugs. Catheter can be reinserted 4–6 weeks later, at least 1 week after all clinical evidence of peritonitis has subsided. However, not many patients are able to continue CAPD or have the technique re-established because of peritoneal adhesions, abscess formation, or progressive sclerosing peritonitis (Kapan *et al.* 2000).

Fungal infections following renal transplantation

Fungal infections remain a significant challenge after solid organ transplantation. Recipients of renal transplants also have a 24–40 per cent incidence of opportunistic fungal infections which are associated with very high mortality in them (Reis *et al.* 1995; Patel and Paya 1997; Fishman and Rubin 1998). This is related to the environmental exposure and net state of immunosuppression. Most fungi cause disease within the first 6 months when the intensity of immunosuppression is maximum; Cryptococcal infection usually develops later (John *et al.* 1994). In an analysis of 850 renal transplant recipients from a tertiary care centre in North India, Gupta (2001) described systemic fungal infections in 83 patients (9.8 per cent). These were candidiasis in 25 (2.8 per cent), cryptococcosis in 16 (1.9 per cent), aspergillosis in 20 (2.3 per cent), zygomycosis in 17 (2.0 per cent), and rare fungal infections in five others including pheohyphomycosis in three and disseminated histoplasmosis in two patients. This analysis compared with earlier studies from the same centre (Chugh *et al.* 1992), showed a significant increase in the occurrence of angioinvasive infections after the addition of cyclosporin and other potent drugs in the immunosuppressive regimen. These infections may be caused by multiple organisms (Zazgornik *et al.* 1979), and that makes the management more difficult particularly in presence of fungi such as *Aspergillus* and *Mucor* (Varma *et al.* 1993; Gupta *et al.* 1998). Serious fungal infections may involve the gastrointestinal tract (Gupta *et al.* 1994; Kathuria *et al.* 1995), lungs (Jha *et al.* 1999), or CNS (Sakhuja *et al.* 2001).

While treating fungal infections in renal transplant recipients due consideration should be given to interaction between the immunosuppressive therapy and some of the antifungal drugs. Levels of calcineurin inhibitors, cyclosporin and tacrolimus, increase after administration of azole derivatives (ketoconazole, fluconazole, and itraconazole) due to altered hepatic metabolism of the former hence requiring dose modification and monitoring of their levels. Similarly the nephrotoxicity of both the cyclosporin and tacrolimus may be augmented by concurrent administration of amphotericin B and it should be watched for by regular check on renal function. The role of prophylaxis or pre-emptive antifungal therapy following renal transplantation is still not defined, although clinical evidence supports such strategies in lung, heart, and liver transplant recipients (Singh *et al.* 2001). In addition emerging fungal pathogens may be resistant to conventional antifungal agents, and specific microbiological diagnosis is important.

Newer antifungal agents and strategies

In addition to amphotericin B, fluconazole, and itraconazole various antifungal agents are now available. Lipid formulations of amphotericin B have been found to be as effective but considerably less toxic than conventional amphotericin (Arikan and Rex 2001). They offer the ability to administer and deliver high doses of amphotericin B (1–5 mg/kg/day) before toxicity develops. Infusion-related events are also less common in liposomal amphotericin compared with other formulations.

Among the newer azole antifungal agents (Walsh *et al.* 2000), intravenous itraconazole has become a new modality for treating patients with invasive fungal infections with response rates of about 50 per cent. The main problem with its use is drug interactions at the cytochrome P-450 level, as well as limited pharmacokinetic knowledge of its carrier molecule: cyclodextrin. There is also a theoretical concern for antagonism between itraconazole and amphotericin B (Schaffner and Bohler 1993). Voriconazole, ravuconazole, and posaconazole are other azole derivatives having excellent activity against *Aspergillus* and many other fungi including *Scedosporium* and *Fusarium*, which have been found difficult to treat in the past.

The newly FDA-approved echinocandin antifungal, caspofungin, a beta 1–3 glucan synthase inhibitor, has activity against virtually all *Candida* sp. including azole-resistant species, and *Aspergillus* sp. but not *Cryptococcus* (Keating and Jarirs 2001). Main utility of this as well as other echinocandins (micafungin and anidulafungin) is their administration in form of combination antifungal therapy, which has been advocated recently in patients with resistant fungal infections, in view of possible synergism between the echinocandins and amphotericin B (Sugar 1998). Other combinations of particular interest are lipid-based amphotericin B with echinocandins, lipid-based amphotericin B with the new azoles, and echinocandins with the new azoles. Echinocandins do not require dose modification in renal failure.

Adjunctive immunomodulatory therapy is an area of interest. Granulocyte colony-stimulating factor, granulocyte–macrophage colony-stimulating factor, and interferon gamma have been used to augment neutrophil-mediated killing of filamentous fungi; interferon-γ appeared to have the broadest effect (Gaviria *et al.* 1999). Current research focuses on stem cell content of grafts, lymphoid progenitor transfusions, and the use of other cytokines, such as Th-1 effectors (Roilides *et al.* 1998).

References

Argyle, C. (1985). The identification of fungal casts: a new method for diagnosing visceral candidiasis. *Clinical Laboratory Medicine* **5**, 331–354.

Arikan, S. and Rex, J. H. (2001). Lipid-based antifungal agents: current status. *Current Pharmaceutical Design* **7**, 393–415.

Barnes, J. L. *et al.* (1983). Host parasite interactions in the pathogenesis of experimental renal candidiasis. *Laboratory Investigation* **49**, 460–467.

Benbow, E. W. and Stoddart, R. W. (1986). Systemic zygomycosis. *Postgraduate Medical Journal* **62**, 985–986.

Blodi, P. C., Hunnah, F. T., and Wadsworth, J. A. C. (1969). Lethal orbitocerebral phycomycosis in otherwise healthy children. *American Journal of Opthalmology* **67**, 698–705.

Boelaert, J. R. *et al.* (1993). Mucormycosis during desferroxamine therapy is a siderophone mediated infection: *in vitro* and *in vivo* animal studies. *Journal of Clinical Investigation* **91**, 1979–1996.

Bretagne, S. *et al.* (1998). Comparison of serum galactomannan antigen detection and competitive polymerase chain reaction for diagnosing invasive aspergillosis. *Clinical Infectious Diseases* **26**, 1407–1421.

Burke, P. G. *et al.* (1997). Histoplasmosis and kidney disease in patients with, AIDS. *Clinical Infectious Diseases* **25**, 281–284.

Chan, T. M. *et al.* (1994). Treatment of fungal peritonitis complicating continuous ambulatory peritoneal dialysis with oral fluconazole: a series of 21 patients. *Nephrology, Dialysis, Transplantation* **9**, 539–542.

Chapman, S. W. *et al.* (1997). Endemic blastomycosis in Mississippi: epidemiological and clinical studies. *Seminars in Respiratory Infections* **12**, 219–228.

Chugh, K. S. *et al.* (1992). Fungal infections in renal allograft recipients. *Transplantion Proceedings* **24**, 1940–1942.

Chugh, K. S. *et al.* (1993). Renal mucormycosis: computerized tomographic findings and their diagnostic significance. *American Journal of Kidney Diseases* **22**, 393–397.

Cole, G. T. and Sun, S. H. Arthroconidium—spherule—endospore transformation in *Coccidioides immitis*. In *Fungal Dimorphism* (ed. P. J. Szaniszlo), p. 281. New York, NY: Plenum Publishing Corperation, 1985.

Connor, W. T., Drach, G. W., and Bucher, W. C., Jr. (1975). Genitourinary aspects of disseminated coccididiodomycosis. *Journal of Urology* **147**, 1116–1117.

Craig, M. W., Davey, W. N., and Green, R. A. (1970). Conjugal blastomycosis. *American Reviews of Respiratory Diseases* **102**, 86.

Davies, S. F. and Sarosi, G. A. (1997). Epidemiological and clinical features of pulmonary blastomycosis. *Seminars in Respiratory Infections* **12**, 206–218.

Davila, R. M., Moser, S. A., and Arosso, L. E. (1990). Renal mucormycosis: a case report and review of the literature. *Journal of Urology* **145**, 1242–1244.

de Repentigny, L. (1992). Serodiagnosis of candidiasis aspergillosis and cryptococcosis. *Clinical Infectious Diseases* **1** (Suppl.), 511–522.

Denning, D. W. (1998). Invasive aspergillosis. *Clinical Infectious Diseases* **26**, 781–803.

Denning, D. W. *et al.* (1989). Itraconazole therapy for cryptococcal meningitis and cryptococcosis. *Archives of Internal Medicine* **149**, 2301–2308.

Drutz, D. J. and Cantanzaro, A. (1978). Coccidiodomycosis Part I. *American Journal of Respiratory Diseases* **711**, 559–585.

Durkin, M. M., Connolly, P. A. and Wheat, L. J. (1997). Comparison of radio immunoassay and enzyme linked immuno assay methods for detection of histoplasma capsulatium var capsulatium antigen. *Journal of Clinical Microbiology* **35**, 2252–2255.

Eickenberg, H. U., Amin, M., and Lich, R., Jr. (1975). Blastomycosis of the genitourinary tract. *Journal of Urology* **113**, 650–652.

Ellis, D. H. and Pfeiffer, T. J. (1990). Natural habitat of *Cryptococcus neoformans* var. *gattii*. *Journal of Clinical Microbiology* **28**, 1642–1644.

Fidel, P. L., Vaquez, J. A., and Sobel, J. D. (1999). *Candida glabrata*, Review of epidemiology, pathogenesis, and clinical disease with comparison to *C. albicans*. *Clinical Microbiology Reviews* **12**, 80–96.

Fishman, J. A. and Rubin, R. H. (1998). Infection in organ-transplant recipients *New England Journal of Medicine* **338**, 741–751.

Flechner, S. M. and McAninch, J. W. (1987). Aspergillosis of the urinary tract, ascending route of infection and evolving patterns of disease. *Journal of Urology* **125**, 598–601.

Florentine, B. D., Carriere, C., and Abdul Karim, F. W. (1997). *Mucor* pyelonephritis. Report of a case diagnosed by vein cytology with diagnostic consideration in the work up of funguria. *Acta Cytologica* **41**, 1797–1800.

Forbus, W. D. and Besterbreurtje, A. M. (1946). Coccidioidomycosis, a study of 95 cases of the disseminated type with special reference to the pathogenesis of the disease. *Military Surgeon* M 46 **99**, 653.

Frye, K. R., Donovan, J. M., and Drach, G. W. (1988). *Torulopsis glabrata* urinary infections: a review. *Journal of Urology* **139**, 1245–1249.

Gaviria, J. M. *et al.* (1999). Comparison of interferon-gamma, granulocyte colony-stimulating factor, granulocyte-macrophage colony-stimulating factor for priming leukocyte-mediated hyphal damage of opportunistic fungal pathogens. *Journal of Infectious Diseases* **179**, 1038–1041.

Goldie, S. J. *et al.* (1996). Fungal peritonitis in a large chronic peritoneal dialysis population: a report of 55 episodes. *American Journal of Kidney Diseases* **28**, 86–91.

Goodwin, R. A. *et al.* (1980). Disseminated histoplasmosis clinical and pathologic correlations. *Medicine (Baltimore)* **59**, 1–33.

Gupta, K. L. (2001). Fungal infections and the kidney. *Indian Journal of Nephrology* **11**, 147–154 (review).

Gupta, K. L. *et al.* (1990). Mucormycosis in patients with renal failure. *Renal Failure (USA)* **11**, 195–199.

Gupta K. L. *et al.* (1994). Esophageal candidiasis after renal transplantation: comparative study in patients on different immunosuppressive protocols. *American Journal of Gastroenterology* **89**, 1062–1065.

Gupta, K. L. *et al.* (1998). Pulmonary mucormycosis presenting as fatal massive haemoptysis in a renal transplant recipient. *Nephrology, Dialysis, Transplantation* **13**, 3258–3260.

Gupta, K. L. *et al.* (1999). Renal zygomycosis an underdiagnosed cause of acute renal failure. *Nephrology, Dialysis, Transplantation* **14**, 2720–2725.

Hadaya, K. *et al.* (1998). Isolated primary aspergillosis in a renal transplant recipient. *Nephrology, Dialysis, Transplantation* **13**, 2382–2384.

Han, Y. and Cutler, J. E. (1997). Assessment of a mouse model of neutropenia and the effect of an anti-candidiasis monoclonal antibody in these animals. *Journal of Infectious Diseases* **175**, 1169–1175.

Holley, J. L., Bernandini, J., and Poraino, B. (1994). Infecting organisms in continuous ambulatory peritoneal dialysis patient on the Y-set. *American Journal of Kidney Diseases* **23**, 569–573.

Hood, S. V. *et al.* (1998). Prostatic and epididymo-orchitis due to Aspergillus fumigatus in a patient with AIDS. *Clinical Infectious Diseases* **26**, 229–231.

Huntington, R. W., Jr. *et al.* Pathologic and clinical observations on 142 cases of fatal coccidioidomycosis with necropsy. In *Coccidioidomycosis* (ed. L. Agello), pp. 148–167. Tucson: The University of Arizona Press, 1967.

Ingram, C. W. *et al.* (1989). Disseminated zygomycosis. Report of four cases and review. *Reviews of Infectious Diseases* **11**, 741–754.

Irby, P. B., Stoller, M. L., and Mc Aninch, J. W. (1990). Fungal bezoars of the upper urinary tract. *Journal of Urology* **143**, 447–451.

Jacobs, L. G. *et al.* (1996). Oral fluconazole compared with bladder irrigation with amphotericin B for treatment of fungal urinary tract infections in elderly patients. *Clinical Infectious Diseases* **22**, 30–35.

Jaye, D. L. *et al.* (1998). Comparison of two rapid latex tests for detection of cryptococcal capsular polysaccharide. *American Journal of Clinical Pathology* **109**, 634–641.

Jenkin, G. A., Choo, M., and Johnson, P. D. R. (1998). Candidal epidididymo-orchitis: case report and review. *Clinical Infectious Diseases* **26**, 942–945.

Jha, V. *et al.* (1999). Successful management of pulmonary tuberculosis in renal allograft recipients in a single center. *Kidney International* **56**, 1944–1950.

John, G. T. *et al.* (1994). Cryptococcosis in renal allograft recipients. *Transplantation (United States)* **58**, 855–856.

Johnson, J. R., Ireton, R. C., and Lipsky, B. A. (1986). Emphysematous pyelonephritis caused by *Candida albicans*. *Journal of Urology* **136**, 80–82.

Johnson, R. J. *et al.* (1985). Fungal peritonitis in patients on peritoneal dialysis: incidence, clinical features and prognosis. *American Journal of Nephrology* **5**, 169–175.

Kapan, H. T. *et al.* (2000). The rate, risk factors, and outcome of fungal peritonitis in CAPD patients: experience in Turkey. *Peritoneal Dialysis International* **20**, 338–341.

Kathuria, P. *et al.* (1995). Gastro-intestinal complications after renal transplantation; 10-year data from a North Indian transplant centre. *American Society for Artificial Internal Organs Journal* **41**, M698–M703.

Kaufman, L. *et al.* (1983). Detection of two *Blastomyces dermatitidis* serotypes by exoantigen analysis. *Journal of Clinical Microbiology* **18**, 110–114.

Keane, W. F. *et al.* (2000). The International Society for Peritoneal Dialysis (ISPD) recently published new recommendations for the treatment of adult PD-related peritonitis. *Peritoneal Dialysis International* **20**, 396–411.

Keating, G. H. and Jarirs, B. (2001). Capsofungin. *Drugs* **61**, 121–129.

Kedar, S. S. *et al.* (1988). Histoplasmosis of kidneys presenting as chronic recurrent renal disease. *Urology* **31**, 490–494.

Kuntze, J. R., Herman M. H., and Evans, G. S. (1988). Genitourinary coccidioidomycosis. *Journal of Urology* **140**, 370–374.

Larsen, R. A. *et al.* (1989). Persistent *Cryptococcus neoformans* infection of the prostate after successful treatment of meningitis. *Annals of Internal Medicine* **111**, 125–128.

Levy, E. and Bia, M. J. (1995). Isolated renal mucormycosis, case report and review. *Journal of the American Society of Nephrology* **5**, 2014–2019.

Madge, G. E. and Lombardias, S. (1973). Chronic liver disease and renal papillary necrosis with Aspergillus. *Southern Medical Journal* **66**, 486–488.

Meunier-Carpentier, F., Kiehn, T. E., and Armstrong, D. (1981). Fungemia in the immunocompromised host. Changing patterns, antigenemia, high mortality. *American Journal of Medicine* **71**, 363–370.

Meyer, S. A., Payne, R. W., and Yarrow, D. Candida Berkhout. In *The Yeasts, a Taxonomic Study* (ed. C. P. Kurtzman and J. W. Fell), pp. 454–473. Amsterdam: Elsevier, 1998.

Myerowitz, R. L., Pazin, C. J., and Allen, C. M. (1977). Disseminated candidiasis. Changes in incidence, underlying diseases and pathology. *American Journal of Pathology* **68**, 29–38.

Nosher, J. L. *et al.* (1988). Acute focal bacterial nephritis. *American Journal of Kidney Diseases* **11**, 36–42.

Nossoura, Z. *et al.* (1993). Candiduria as an early marker of disseminated infection in critically ill surgical patients. *Journal of Trauma* **35**, 290–294.

Occhipinti, D. J., Schoonover, L. L., and Danziger, L. H. (1993). Bladder irrigation with amphotricin B for treatment of patients with candiduria. *Clinical Infectious Diseases* **17**, 812–813.

Pappas, P. G. (1997). Blastomycosis in the immunocompromised patient. *Seminars in Respiratory Infections* **12**, 243–251.

Parfrey, N. A. (1986). Improved diagnosis and prognosis of mucor mycosis, a clinico pathologic study of 33 cases. *Medicine (Baltimore)* **65**, 113–123.

Patel, R. and Paya, C. V. (1997). Infections in solid-organ transplant recipients. *Clinical Micrbiology Reviews* **10**, 86–124.

Price, M. J., Lewis, E. L., and Carmalt, J. E. (1982). Coccidioidomycosis of prostate gland. *Urology* **19**, 653.

Raghavan, R., Date, A., and Bhaktaviziam, A. (1987). Fungal and nocardial infections of the kidney. *Histopathology* **11**, 9–20.

Randall, R. E. *et al.* (1968). Cryptococcal pyelonephritis. *New England Journal of Medicine* **279**, 60–65.

Reis, M. A., Costa, R. S., and Ferraz, A. S. (1995). Causes of death in renal transplant recipients, a study of 102 autopsies from 1968 to 1991. *Journal of the Royal Society of Medicine* **88**, 24–27.

Rex, J. H. *et al.* (1994). A randomized trial comparing fluconazole with amphotericin B for the treatment of candidemia in patients with out neutropenia. *New England Journal of Medicine* **331**, 1325–1330.

Rex, J. H. *et al.* (2000). Practice guidelines for the treatment of candidiasis. *Clinical Infectious Diseases* **30**, 662–675.

Rippon, J. W. The pathogenic fungi and the pathogenic actinomycetes. *Medical Mycology* 3rd edn., p. 588. Philadelphia, PA: W.B. Saunders, 1988.

Roilides, E. *et al.* (1998). The role of immunoreconstitution in the management of refractory opportunistic fungal infections. *Medical Mycology* **36**, 12–25.

Sakhuja, V. *et al.* (2001). Central nervous system complications in renal transplant recipients in a tropical environment. *Journal of Neurologic Sciences* **183**, 89–93.

Saltoglu, N. *et al.* (1998). Rhinocerebral zygomycosis treated with amphotericin B and surgery. *Mycoses* **41**, 45–49.

Salyer, W. R. and Salyer, D. C. (1973). Involvement of the kidney and prostate in cryptococcosis. *Journal of Urology* **109**, 695–698.

Scerpella, E. G. and Alhalel, R. (1994). An unusual cause of acute renal failure: bilateral ureteral obstruction due to *Candida tropicalis* fungus balls. *Clinical Infectious Diseases* **18**, 440–442.

Schaffner, A. and Bohler, A. (1993). Amphotericin B refractory aspergillosis after itraconazole: evidence for significant antagonism. *Mycoses* **36**, 421–424.

Shelp, W. D., Wen, S. F., Weinstein, A. B. (1966). Uretero pelvic obstruction caused by candida pyelitis in the homotransplanted kidney. *Archives of Internal Medicine* **117**, 401–404.

Sheynkin, Y. R. and Wise, G. J. (1995). Fungal infections of the perivesical space. *Journal of Urology* **153**, 722–724.

Singh, N. *et al.* (2001). Preemptive prophylaxis with a lipid preparation of amphotericin B for invasive fungal infections in liver transplant recipients requiring renal replacement therapy. *Transplantation (United States)* **71**, 910–913.

Sobel, J. D. *et al.* (2000). Candiduria, a randomised, double blind study of treatment with fluconazole and placebo. *Clinical Infectious Diseases* **30**, 19–24.

Solomkin, J. S., Flohr, A., and Simmons, R. L. (1982). Candida infection in surgical patient: dose requirements and toxicity of amphotericin B. *Annals of Surgery* **195**, 177–185.

Sridhar, R. N. *et al.* (1991). Disseminated histoplasmosis in a renal transplant recipient: a cause of renal failure several years following transplantation. *American Journal of Kidney Diseases* **6**, 719–721.

Stein, H. *et al.* (1993). Unusual case of renal candida fungus balls. *Urology* **41**, 49–51.

Stevens, D. A. (1995). Coccidioidomycosis. *New England Journal of Medicine* **332**, 1677–1682.

Sud, K. *et al.* (1998). Isolated bilateral renal aspergillosis, an unusual presentation in an immunocompetent host. *Renal Failure* **20**, 839–843.

Sugar, A. M. (1992). Mucormycosis. *Clinical Infectious Diseases* **14** (Suppl. 1), S-126–S-129.

Sugar, A. M. (1998). Antifungal combination therapy: where we stand. *Drug Resistance Updates* **1**, 89–92.

Superdock, K. R. *et al.* (1994). Disseminated histoplasmosis presenting as urinary tract obstruction in a renal transplant recipient. *American Journal of Kidney Diseases* **4**, 600–604.

Tomashefski, J. F., Jr. and Abramowsky, C. R. (1981). *Candida*—associated renal papillary necrosis. *American Journal of Clinical Pathology* **75**, 190–194.

Van des Horst *et al.* (1997). Treatment of cryptococcal meningitis associated with the acquired immunodeficiency syndrome. *New England Journal of Medicine* **337**, 15–21.

Varma, P. P. *et al.* (1993). Invasive pulmonary aspergillosis and nocardiosis in an immunocompromised host. *Journal of the Association of Physicians of India* **41**, 237–238.

Verweij, P. E. *et al.* (1996). Prospects for the early diagnosis of invasive aspergillosis in the immunocompromised patient. *Reviews of Medical Microbiology* **7**, 105–113.

Wainstain, M. A. *et al.* (1995). Predisposing factors of systemic fungal infection of the genitourinary tract. *Journal of Urology* **154**, 160–163.

Walsh, T. J. *et al.* (1991). Detection of circulating by immunoassay in patient with cancer and invasive candidiasis. *New England Journal of Medicine* **324**, 1026–1031.

Walsh, T. J. *et al.* (2000). New targets and delivery systems for antifungal therapy. *Medical Mycology* **38**, 335–347.

Weng, D. E. *et al.* (1998). Successful medical management of isolated renal zygomycosis; case report and review. *Clinical Infectious Diseases* **26**, 601–605.

Wheat, J. (1994). Histoplasmosis: recognition and treatment. *Clinical Infectious Diseases* **19** (Suppl. 1), S19–S27.

Wheat, L. J. *et al.* (1981). A large urban outbreak of histoplasmosis clinical features. *Annals of Internal Medicine* **94**, 331–337.

Wheat, L. J. *et al.* (1983). Histoplasmosis in renal transplant recipients—two large urban outbreaks. *Archives of Internal Medicine* **143**, 703–707.

Williams, J. C. (1997). Mucormycosis of the genitourinary tract. *Infections in Urology* **10**, 178–182.

Wise, G. J. and Silver, D. A. (1993). Fungal infections of the genitourinary system. *Journal of Urology* **149**, 1377–1388.

Wise, G. J. and Freyle, J. (1997). Changing patterns in genitourinary fungal infections. *American Urological Association Update Series* **16**, 1–7.

Wise, G. J., Talluri, G. S., and Marella, V. K. (1999). Fungal infections of the genitourinary system; manifestations, diagnosis and treatment. *The Urologic Clinics of North America* **26**, 701–718.

Witorsch, P. and Utz, J. P. (1968). North American blastomycosis, a study of 40 patients. *Medicine* **47**, 169–200.

Young, R. C. *et al.* (1970). Aspergillosis, the spectrum of disease in 98 patients. *Medicine (Baltimore)* **49**, 147–173.

Zazgornik, J. *et al.* (1979). 'Triple infections' (fungal, bacterial and viral) in immunosuppressed renal transplant recipients. *International Urology and Nephrology* **11**, 145–150.

Zincke, H., Furlow, W. L., and Barnow, G. H. (1973). *Candida albicans* cystitis: report of a case with special emphasis on diagnosis and treatment. *Journal of Urology* **109**, 612–614.

8

The patient with renal stone disease

8.1 Aetiological factors in stone formation

Hans-Göran Tiselius

It is estimated that at least 10 per cent of the population in the industrialized part of the world is afflicted by urinary tract stone disease. In some geographical areas the prevalence is even greater, for instance, in the Arabian countries. The formation of urolithiasis occurs in both men and women but the risk is generally higher in men. There appears, however, to be a changing pattern inasmuch as stone disease now is becoming more common in young women (Robertson *et al.* 2000). With its multifactor aetiology and high rate of recurrences, urinary tract stone disease provides a medical challenge. It is roughly estimated that the annual incidence of stones amounts to around 2000 per million inhabitants in Europe and North America. For a group of first time calcium stone formers, the expected risk of recurrent stone formation during a 10-year period was estimated to 30 per cent and in those who had formed at least two stones at the start of follow-up the corresponding figure was as high as 70 per cent (Tiselius 2000). For patients with certain other types of stone the recurrence risk might be even more.

An acute episode of renal stone colic or the mere demonstration of one or several stones in the urinary tract raise a number of questions: Does the stone(s) require active removal and if so, how should this procedure be carried out? Why did stone formation occur? What is the risk of further stone problems for this individual patient? What can be done to prevent recurrent stone formation?

The first question, which is a matter of surgical concern, is beyond the scope of this chapter, but it is noteworthy that the modern non-invasive or low-invasive techniques for stone removal undoubtedly has caused at least some urologists to spend too little efforts in considering the other two questions. There is, however, no logical reason for such an attitude, because although up to 75 per cent of the patients pass their stones without active stone removal, several of them may suffer from severe and recurrent stone formation. Moreover, a substantial fraction of patients are left with residual fragments in their kidneys after the stone treatment. Not all residual fragments will develop into new stones, but the presence of fragments in the kidney might provide a nidus for new stone formation.

In view of the high risk of recurrences in patients with stone disease, it is necessary to identify risk factors that might be of aetiological importance and thus get some clues for predicting the further course of the disease. Only in this way is a ground provided for appropriate medical advice and treatment.

The direction in which the search for risk factors should be made is facilitated by information on the stone composition. In Northern Europe and North America, roughly 75 per cent of the stones are composed of calcium oxalate with or without an admixture of calcium phosphate. Approximately 5 per cent of the stones are composed of pure calcium phosphate, 5–15 per cent of uric acid/urate, 10 per cent of infection stone material, such as struvite and carbonate apatite (CarbAp), and 1 per cent of cystine (Herring 1962; Leusmann *et al.* 1995; Tiselius 1996). There is a geographical variation in stone composition. In some regions, the occurrence of uric acid stones is very high and figures up to 40 per cent have been reported. Stones with other constituents are only rarely encountered.

Formation of stones in the urinary tract is the result of a pathological crystallization (Finlayson 1974; Robertson 1976; Nancollas 1983; Tiselius 1996). The principles of this process are discussed in the Appendix. (The different physical–chemical parameters and expressions used are summarized in Tables 1 and 2.)

Aspects on the process of stone formation

For non-calcium stones, that is, stones composed of uric acid, urate salts, cystine, and struvite, the supersaturation of each one of the salts under physiological conditions also might exceed its formation product. This situation most certainly makes a homogeneous nucleation possible. Continuously high levels or peaks of supersaturation, therefore, is the most likely explanation for the risk of precipitation of these salts and subsequent stone formation.

It is possible that the precipitation of calcium phosphate in urine also can occur as the result of a supersaturation that is above the formation product of homogeneous nucleation. It is reasonable to assume, however, that nucleation of calcium phosphate most commonly is the result of heterogeneous crystallization.

In terms of calcium oxalate crystallization the situation has proved to be much more complex and the various parts of this process are schematically summarized in Fig. 1. *Crystal nucleation, crystal growth, crystal aggregation*, and *crystal retention* are considered to be the fundamental steps in stone formation. The last step in the process is poorly understood, but most certainly an *assembling* of crystalline material is necessary to build up a stone.

Nucleation of calcium oxalate is assumed to be induced by one or several promoters. Growth and aggregation of calcium oxalate crystals can proceed as long as the ion-activity product of calcium oxalate exceeds the solubility product (SP). All these processes are counteracted by inhibitors. The inhibition is accomplished by either large or small molecules which are further discussed below.

Whether the initial crystallization takes place as free or fixed particles has been a matter of debate over the years and it has generally been assumed that the precipitation of calcium oxalate is too slow to give

Table 1 Overview and definition of physical–chemical parameters discussed in this chapter

Physical–chemical parameter	Definition
Activity of an ion	The activity of an ion is the product of the free concentration C of that ion and its activity coefficient (f_z). For an ion A^+ the activity is $C_{A+} \times f_1$ and for an ion B^{3-} the activity is $C_{B3-} \times f_3$
AP_{AB}	This is ion-activity product (AP) of a specific salt AB. That is the product of the activities of the two ions A and B
$FP_{heterogeneous}$	Formation product of heterogeneous nucleation is the ion-activity product at which facilitated crystal formation occurs
$FP_{homogeneous}$	Formation product of homogeneous nucleation is the ion-activity product required for spontaneous (non-facilitated) formation of a solid crystal phase
f_z	Activity coefficient of an ion with the charge Z
$K_{stability}$	The stability constant gives a value of the stability of a certain ion complex. A high value of the constant means that the complex has a high stability and does not easily dissociate
Nucleation	Formation of a solid crystal phase in the solution/urine
Solubility product (SP)	The solubility product (SP) of a salt is the ion-activity product at which the solution/urine is in equilibrium with the solid crystal phase
Supersaturation (SS)	The ratio between the actual ion-activity product of a salt and its solubility product
Z	Z is the charge of an ion. For the ions Ca^{2+} and Cl^-, Z takes the value of 2 and 1, respectively

Table 2 Various expressions of ion-activity products mentioned in the text

Expressions of ion-activity products	Definition
AP_{CaOx}	The ion-activity product of calcium oxalate
AP(CaOx)-index	A simplified estimate of the ion-activity product of calcium oxalate
AP(CaOx)-index$_s$	A standardized simplified estimate of the ion-activity product of calcium oxalate, calculated for a 24-h urine volume of 1500 ml
AP_{CaP}	The ion-activity product of calcium phosphate
AP(CaP)-index	A simplified estimate of the ion-activity product of calcium phosphate
AP(CaP)-index$_s$	A standardized simplified estimate of the ion-activity product of calcium phosphate, calculated for a 24-h urine volume of 1500 ml and a pH of 7.0
AP_{H_2U}	The ion-activity product of uric acid
AP_{NH_4U}	The ion-activity product of ammonium urate
AP_{NaHU}	The ion-activity product of sodium urate
AP_{MAP}	The ion-activity product of magnesium ammonium phosphate
$AP_{Cystine}$	The ion-activity product of cystine

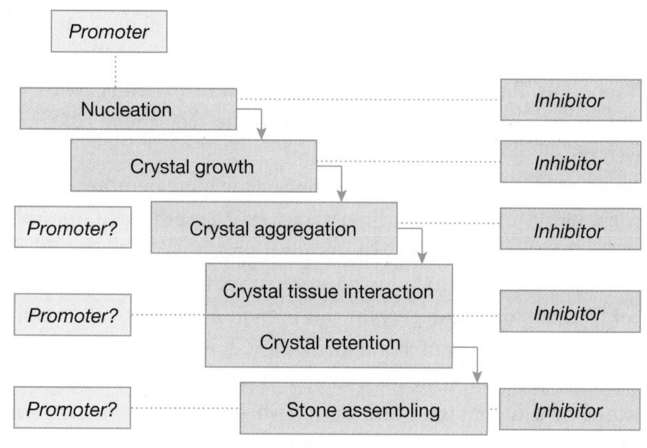

Fig. 1 Major steps in calcium salt crystallization.

crystals of sufficient size to be trapped in the tubular system unless there is some kind of fixation of the crystalline material (Finalyson and Reis 1978). Recalculation of old data has, however, indicated that free particles of calcium phosphate as well as of calcium oxalate might form at the levels of supersaturation that occasionally are built up in nephron urine (Kok and Khan 1994). In this way crystals might become large enough to be trapped intratubularly. Irrespective of whether the initial crystallization is the result of free or fixed particles, stone formation cannot occur unless crystal material is retained in the renal collecting system. Retention of crystal material can, however, also be the result of interaction between the crystals and the cells and such a mechanism is assumed to play an important role (Mandel 1994; Khan 1996; Verkoelen *et al.* 1995, 1997; Lieske *et al.* 1999).

It needs to be emphasized again that if the urine is not sufficiently supersaturated, there will be no salt precipitation and accordingly, under such conditions, the fundamental prerequisite for stone formation is lacking. This important fact is the theoretical basis for most of the recurrence preventive treatment regimens that are used today clinically in patients with urinary tract stone disease.

Inasmuch as recurrence preventive treatment ideally should be as selective as possible, there are two steps that are necessary to enable such an action. First, to decide whether the patient has a high supersaturation level or may be at risk of forming a critically supersaturated urine. Thereby the supersaturation or the ion-activity product is the *effective* or *secondary risk factor*. Second, it is necessary to identify those factors that in an important way contribute to the supersaturation and the risk of crystallization. These latter variables can thus be considered as *primary risk factors*.

There is evidence that the process of calcium stone formation starts as a precipitation of calcium phosphate either in the loop of Henle or in the distal part of the distal tubule (Luptak *et al.* 1994; Tiselius *et al.* 1996; Asplin *et al.* 1996a; Kok 1997; Höjgaard and Tiselius 1999). Although the urine at these levels of the nephron might be critically supersaturated with calcium oxalate in patients with hyperoxaluria and in experimental animals following administration of ethylene glycol, the ion-activity product of calcium oxalate is usually too low to result in calcium oxalate crystal formation (Luptak *et al.* 1994). Any crystallization that occurs in this part of the nephron most certainly is facilitated by promoters (Fig. 2) and it has been suggested that lipoprotein membranes from the brush border of proximal tubular cells might serve this purpose (Khan *et al.* 2000). Experimental research has shown that the brush border membrane might be injured by free radicals formed as the result of toxic effects on the cell (Scheid *et al.* 1996). This might lead to lipid peroxidation and cell death (Thamilselvan and Khan 1998). The released membrane fragments that are transported down the nephron thereby can supply a suitable surface for deposition of both calcium oxalate and calcium phosphate.

There are also other less specific constituents of nephron urine that have the capacity to induce nucleation of calcium salts, such as, for instance, blood cells, crystals of sodium urate, cholesterol, or other intratubular particles.

Crystals of calcium phosphate that form at a high nephron level (Tiselius 1997b) (Fig. 2) might be dissolved when they are exposed to the acid urine in the collecting duct (Höjgaard and Tiselius 1999). Dissolution of calcium phosphate causes a high level of supersaturation with calcium oxalate by increased urine concentration of calcium. Nucleation of calcium oxalate can thus take place either by epitaxis on the surface of the dissolving calcium phosphate crystal or by nucleation, with or without the contribution of a promoter, or by nucleation in the macromolecular environment that surrounds the calcium phosphate crystals. The latter process might take place either freely in the tubular lumen or more likely at tubular wall.

Under normal conditions, the crystals of calcium oxalate and calcium phosphate that form are small and well protected from crystal growth and crystal aggregation by a cover of inhibitory macromolecules. The negatively charged macromolecules have a high affinity to the positively charged surface of calcium salt crystals. The aggregation inhibiting properties of small as well as of large molecules are related to their electronegativity which establishes repulsive forces between adjacent crystals and between the crystals and the similarly negatively charged macromolecular layer on the surface of tubular cells (Fig. 3). In this way, it is likely that small crystals are fast and can easily move through the tubular system and be excreted with urine. It is possible that small calcium phosphate crystals are completely dissolved during their transport through the collecting duct. Under appropriate conditions primary nucleation of calcium oxalate might occur in collecting duct urine. As long as these crystals remain small and are well protected from growth and aggregation they leave the tubular system without problems.

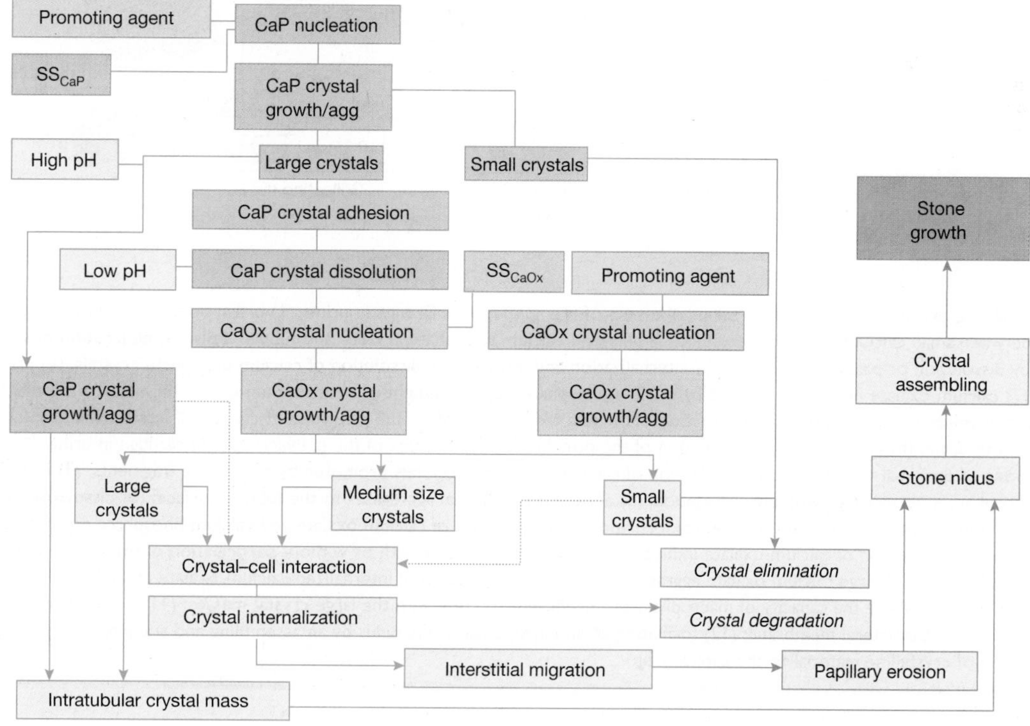

Fig. 2 Overview of the various possible steps in calcium stone formation. SS, supersaturation.

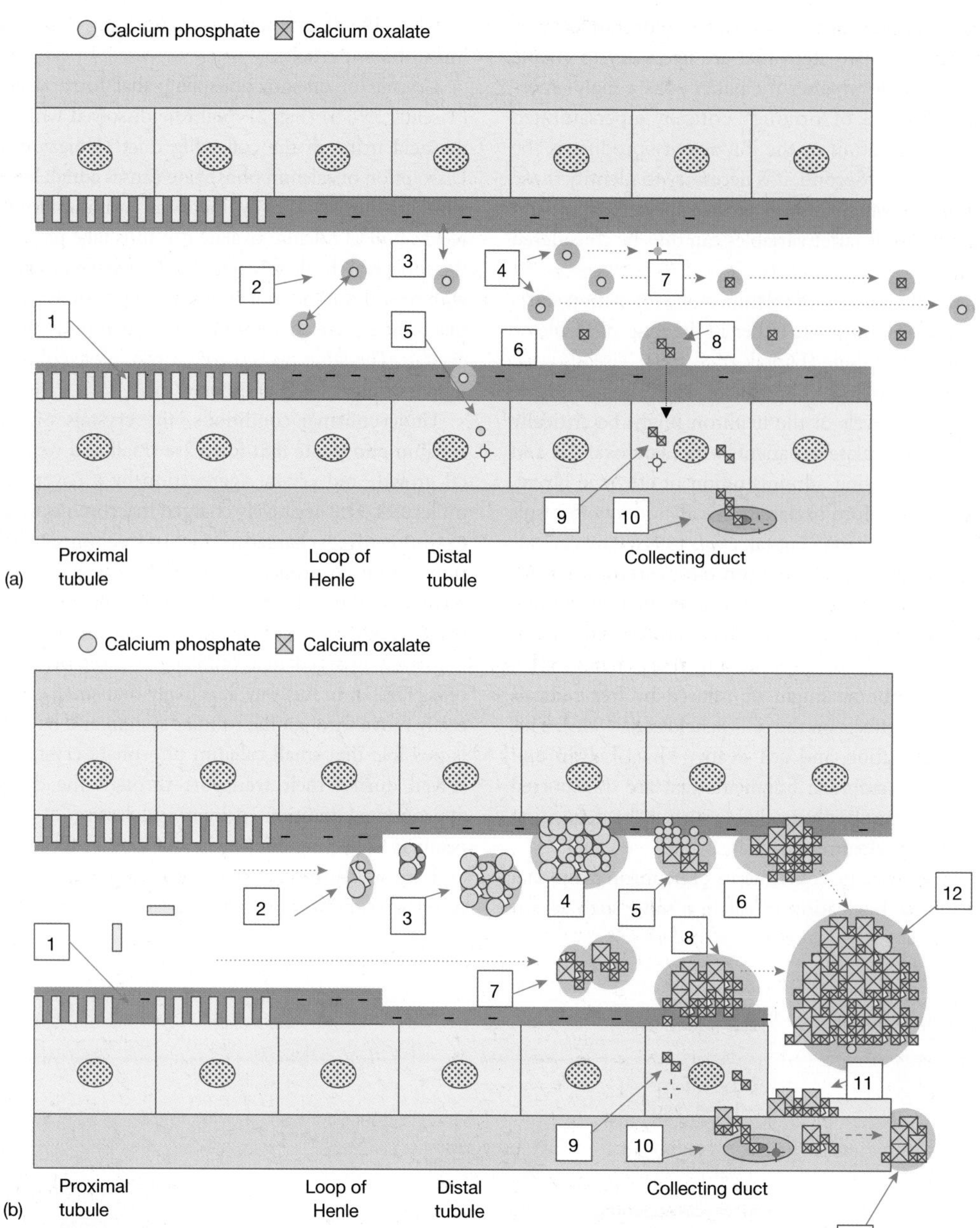

Fig. 3 (a) Hypothetical interpretation of the possible series of events of the *normal crystallization* in urine: (1) brush-border membrane of proximal tubular cells; (2) repulsion between small calcium phosphate crystals; (3) between calcium phosphate crystals and tubular cells; (4) elimination of small calcium phosphate crystals by dissolution or passage with urine; (5) internalization and intracellular dissolution of calcium phosphate crystals; (6) primary nucleation of calcium oxalate; (7) calcium oxalate nucleation induced by calcium phosphate; (8) attachment of small calcium oxalate crystals to the tubular cell; (9) internalization and dissolution; (10) macrophage destruction of calcium oxalate crystals in the interstitial tissue, small intraluminal crystals of calcium oxalate are excreted with urine. (b) Hypothetical interpretation of the possible series of events of the *pathological crystallization* in urine: (1) destruction of the brush-border membrane of proximal tubular cells; (2) nucleation of calcium phosphate crystals promoted by membrane fragments; (3) formation of large masses of calcium phosphate crystals by growth and aggregation; (4) adherence of crystal aggregates to the tubular surface; (5) dissolution of calcium phosphate in acid urine and nucleation of calcium oxalate; (6) formation of a large mass of calcium oxalate and calcium phosphate crystals attached to the tubular wall; (7) primary nucleation of calcium oxalate induced by membrane fragments with or without participation of urinary macromolecules; (8) attachment to the tubular cell of large calcium oxalate aggregates; (9) partial dissolution of internalized calcium oxalate crystal material; (10) migration of crystals to the interstitial tissue where the capacity of macrophages is insufficient to cope with the large crystal masses; (11) destruction of tubular cells with binding of crystals to the basolateral membrane; (12) formation of an intratubular stone nidus by an assembling and trapping of crystal aggregates; (13) interstitial migration of crystalline material to the papillary tip.

The interaction between the tubular cells and crystals are modified by several macromolecules excreted with urine or secreted by the tubular cells (Verkoelen *et al.* 1997; Lieske *et al.* 1997c).

Experimental studies with cell cultures have shown that calcium oxalate monohydrate crystals adhere to tubular cells in a specific and rapid way (Lieske *et al.* 1996). The cellular affinity for brushite (Bru) crystals was much less pronounced. It has, moreover, been shown that a number of polyanions might prevent the adherence of crystals to cells. Such an effect, accordingly, was recorded for glycosaminoglycans (heparin, heparan sulfate, hyaluronic acid, and chondroitin sulfate), citrate, nephrocalcin, and uropontin. Tamm–Horsfall protein (THP), on the other hand, did not counteract the adherence of crystals to the cells, but inhibited crystal endocytosis. It was concluded that crystals of calcium oxalate binds to sialic acid residues on cell surface glycoproteins. Also, the lipids of the plasma membrane appear to be of great importance for the adherence of crystals (Bigelow *et al.* 1997). Normally, cells lining the tubular system are well protected from crystal adherence, but the situation alters dramatically following cell injury.

The same principles for crystal attachment as for calcium oxalate is applicable to crystals of hydroxyapatite (HAP) (Lieske *et al.* 1997b). Crystals of calcium oxalate monohydrate (COM), calcium oxalate dihydrate (COD), and HAP that have adhered to the cell surface might be internalized by endocytosis (Lieske *et al.* 1992; Lieske and Deganello 1999). Some of these crystals might be dissolved by the action of lysosomal enzymes within the tubular cell, whereas others might be transported to the basolateral membrane and expelled into the interstitial tissue where macrophages and other inflammatory cells can take care of the crystals and destroy them (Khan 1996). In this way, a substantial amount of crystalline material might be removed from the tubular system and it is likely that this is one of the defence systems that the kidney has developed to protect from intratubular crystallization and obstruction. In response to high concentrations of oxalate or calcium oxalate crystals tubular cells might proliferate and thus increase the capacity to eliminate crystals.

The risk of crystal adherence is certainly greatest for calcium phosphate and calcium oxalate crystals that are large and thus move slowly through the nephron. For very large crystals and crystal masses the repulsive forces described above are probably insufficient to counteract both crystal aggregtion and crystal–cell adherence. It is also well recognized that patients with calcium stone disease excrete in their urine larger crystals and crystal aggregates than normal subjects.

Given these principles for the normal crystallization in the nephron, a pathological crystallization leading to stone formation might be the net result of one or several abnormalities or defects in the control of this process (Fig. 3). Low concentrations or structural abnormalities of crystallization modifying macromolecules or small molecules will cause increased growth and aggregation of crystals so that large crystal masses form either of calcium phosphate or of calcium oxalate (Coe and Parks 1990). Large crystal masses with or without insufficient protection by macromolecules will adhere to the tubular cell. The crystals might alter the plasma membrane so that endocytosis occurs; whereas crystals of reasonable size can be taken care of and destroyed by the cell, larger crystal agglomerates might cause cell death (Koul *et al.* 1996; Khan *et al.* 2000). When the crystals that are bound to the basolateral membrane or deposited interstitially are too large, the capacity of macrophages and inflammatory cells will probably be insufficient to cope with the crystals. Such crystal material might accordingly be transported within the interstitial tissue down to the papilla where it can provide a basis for crystal deposition and growth following erosion of the epithelial surface.

It is understood that the insufficient or defect control of the crystallization process also will result in development of large crystals or crystal agglomerates that remain within the tubular lumen. Under such conditions crystals of calcium oxalate or calcium phosphate might be trapped at the lower and narrow end of the collecting duct and thereby serve as a nidus for further crystal deposition in the supersaturated urine.

Figure 4 summarizes the various possibilities of calcium salt crystalluria and calcium stone formation. Small crystals of calcium oxalate or calcium phosphate that might have formed in the nephron can disappear either by intraluminal dissolution or by cellular action. These crystals can also be excreted with urine as microscopic crystalluria, which is a common finding in both stone formers and normal subjects. A primary precipitation of calcium phosphate and subsequent dissolution in acid collecting duct urine can give rise to crystal aggregates containing calcium oxalate and calcium phosphate or, in case of complete dissolution, pure calcium oxalate. Pure calcium oxalate aggregates also might form when calcium oxalate is primarily precipitated in the nephron unrelated to a calcium phosphate crystal phase (Lieske *et al.* 1998). In patients with a constantly high pH, calcium phosphate crystals will not dissolve and inasmuch as calcium phosphate is the favoured crystal phase in alkaline urine, pure calcium phosphate crystals and stones will be the result. Such crystals most commonly consist of HAP, but might occasionally be composed of Bru, particularly at a lower pH.

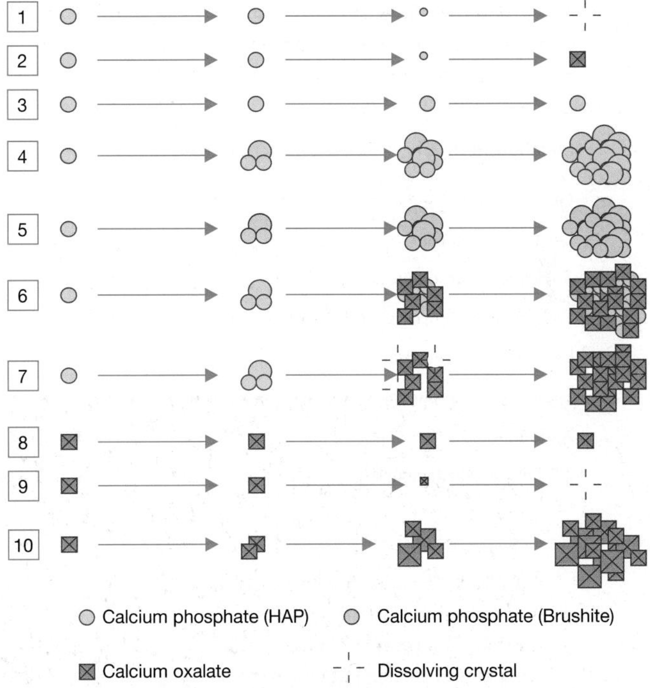

Fig. 4 Possible outcomes of calcium salt crystallization in the urinary tract. Small crystals of calcium phosphate or calcium oxalate can disappear by dissolution (1, 9) or remain small (3, 8). Nucleation of calcium oxalate might be induced by calcium phosphate (2, 6, 7). Following complete dissolution of calcium phosphate pure calcium oxalate aggregates can form (7). In constantly alkaline urine there is no precipitation of calcium oxalate and the result will be pure calcium phosphate aggregates, either in the form of hydroxyapatite (4) or brushite (5). A primary nucleation of calcium oxalate results in small crystals (8) or crystal aggregates (10).

Primary risk factors

Uric acid/urate stones

Precipitation of uric acid can occur at a normal excretion of urate if the urine volume and the urine pH are low (Sperling 1990). This is seen in patients living in a hot climate with excessive insensible loss, small urine volumes, and, accordingly, also an acid urine. This is one explanation for the much greater frequency of uric acid stones seen in Israel, the Arabian countries, and Australia compared with Northern Europe (Sperling 1990; Tiselius 1996).

An increased excretion of urate is, however, often the cause of uric acid stone formation. Several diseases are associated with an increased purine metabolism and an increased urate excretion. Treatment with cytotoxic agents have the same effect. Conditions with an increased urinary excretion of urate are summarized in Table 3. Ingestion of a purine-rich diet sometimes results in a supernormal excretion of urate. Table 4 gives examples of food stuffs that are particularly rich in purine (Hesse *et al.* 1997).

Patients with an ileostomy form stones of uric acid rather than calcium oxalate because of a small urine volume and a low pH attributable to losses of fluid and bicarbonate from the stoma.

The ammonium (NH_4) ions required for precipitation of ammonium urate most commonly is the result of a urinary tract infection with urease producing microorganisms (Griffith and Klein 1983; Lerner *et al.* 1989). With a concomitant high concentration of urate, crystals and stones of ammonium urate might form. It has also been shown that ammonium urate stones are also seen as a consequence of laxative abuse (Polykoff and Dretler 1993).

Table 3 Clinical conditions with a disturbed purine metabolism or an increased production urate

Gout
Leukaemic disorders
Treatment with cytotoxic agents
Treatment with uricosuric agents
Lesch–Nyhan syndrome
Superactivity of phosphoribosylpyrophosphate synthetase
Xanthinuria
2,8-Dihydroxyadeninuria

Table 4 Food stuffs with a high content of purines (adapted from Hesse *et al.* 1997). The content of purines is as expressed as mmol of uric acid per 100 g

Calf thymus	5.4
Liver	1.5–2.1
Kidney	1.3–1.5
Skin of poultry	1.8
Herring with skin	1.9
Sardines, sprats, anchovies	1.5–3.0
Soy beans	1.3

There are a few very rare genetic defects of purine metabolism which result in urinary tract stone formation (Danpure 2000). Figure 5 gives an overview of purine metabolism.

In the Lesch–Nyhan syndrome there is a deficient synthesis of the enzyme hypoxanthine guanine phosphoribosyl transferase (HPRT). This metabolic defect causes a pronounced over-production of urate and an increased risk of uric acid stone formation. The use of xanthine oxidase inhibitors in the treatment of this abnormality reduces urinary urate but can occasionally increase xanthine excretion with xanthine stone formation as a result (Rossiter and Caskey 1995). The genetic defect is on chromosome Xq 26-q27 and the disease, moreover, is associated with mental retardation and spastic cerebral palsy.

One condition with gout and uric acid stone formation is caused by superactivity of the enzyme phosphoribosylpyrophosphate synthetase (PRPS). This enzyme is responsible for conversion of ribosyl-5-phosphate to 5-phosphoribosyl-1-pyrophosphate. The enzyme is encoded by a gene on chromosome Xp 22.3-p22.2 (Zoref *et al.* 1997).

The formation of xanthine stones is seen in patients with a deficiency of xanthine oxidase (also called xanthine dehydrogenase). The conversions of xanthine to urate and that of hypoxanthine to xanthine are blocked and the urinary excretion of xanthine is increased as a result of guanine conversion to xanthine (Dent and Philpot 1954). The genetic defect has been localized to chromosome 2p 22.3-p 22.2.

A deficient production of adenine phosphoribosyl transferase (APRT) brings about an increased synthesis of 2,8-dihydroxyadenine (Kelly *et al.* 1968). This substance is poorly soluble in urine and forms crystals and stones. The disease might end up with renal failure. APRT catalyzes the conversion of adenine to AMP, but when this enzyme is lacking 2,8-dihydroxyadenine forms. The APRT gene is found on chromosome 16q 22.2-23.2.

It is generally considered that a 24-h excretion of urate greater than 4 mmol/l (1997a) or an ion-activity product of uric acid greater than 3.0−4.5 mmol/4 (Tiselius 1997c) is abnormal; and it is noteworthy that whereas *uric acid* can successfully be dissolved by alkalinization of urine, dissolution with this method is not possible for neither ammonium urate nor sodium urate. We also lack methods for dissolution of xanthine and 2,8-dihydroxyadeneine.

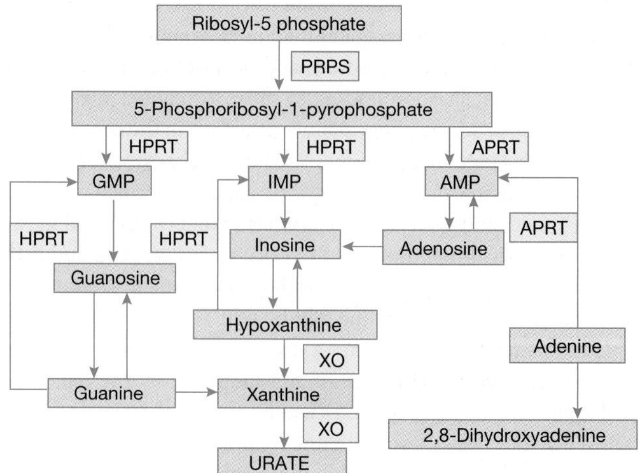

Fig. 5 Pathways of the metabolism of purines (adapted from Danpure 2000). The following enzymes are indicated in the diagram: phosphoribosylpyrophosphate synthetase (PRPS), hypoxanthine guanine phosphoribosyl transferase (HPRT), adenine phosphoribosyl transferase (APRT), and xanthine oxidase (XO).

In terms of uric acid, ammonium urate, and sodium urate, urinary pH is an important discriminating determinant (see Fig. 11). At a low pH, precipitation of uric acid might occur at normal urine urate concentrations. Inasmuch as urine pH decreases when the urine concentration is reduced, episodes of excessive fluid loss or reduced intake might be associated with an obvious risk of uric acid crystallization. This is a major explanation why patients with ileostomies easily form uric acid stones.

Ammonium urate and sodium urate, on the other hand, precipitate at high pH. These stone constituents that are relatively rare do not usually form unless urinary urate is increased together with high concentrations of NH_4 or sodium, respectively.

Infection stone disease

Magnesium ammonium phosphate (MAP; stuvite) and CarbAp precipitate in urine at a *high pH*, usually greater than 7.2. It is generally considered that this combination of salts, with a few exceptions, is the result of urinary urease activity. Catalysed by urease, urea is degraded to *ammonia* and *carbonate*. *Proteus* is the most common urease-producing microorganism. Other urease-producing microorganisms often present in stones are *Staphylococcus*, *Enterobacter*, *Providencia*, *Haemophilus*, *Mycoplasma* (*Ureaplasma urealyticum*), *Pseudomonas*, *Corynebacterium*, *Klebsiella*, *Bacteroides*, and *Micrococci* (Griffith and Klein 1983). Urease production is, however, not a consistent finding in these microorganisms and it is necessary to analyse for urease production in order to definitely establish the aetiological importance of the isolated strain.

Although both MAP and CarbAp can precipitate by a homogeneous nucleation, it is likely that the mucoid matrix substances secreted by the urothelium as a result of the infection act by providing a scaffold for the crystallization (Griffith and Klein 1983). Such a mechanism helps to explain why infection-associated stones rapidly increase in size.

Stagnation of urine increases the risk of maintaining bacteria in the calices, the renal pelvis, and the collecting ducts. Such a condition also significantly contributes to a rapid stone development. Anatomical abnormalities leading to retention of urine and crystals are common in patients with infection stones, but are of aetiological importance also in non-infection stone disease. Table 5 summarizes some anatomical abnormalities that might be encountered in patients with stone disease.

Both MAP and CarpAp can be dissolved in acid solutions and the combined use of ESWL and percutaneous chemolysis with Renacidin® provides a low-invasive and gentle therapeutic option for removal of large infection stones (Tiselius *et al.* 1999).

Table 5 Anatomical abnormalities associated with an increased risk of stone formation

Calix diverticulum
Caliectasis
Tubular ectasia (medullary sponge kidneys)
Obstruction of the pelvo–ureteric junction
Horseshoe kidney
Malrotated kidney
Pelvic kidney
Ureteral stricture
Megaureter
Vesicoureteral reflux
Ureterocele

Although infection stones very often have a complete or partial staghorn morphology, not all staghorn stones are caused by infection. Staghorn stones composed of calcium oxalate are thus not uncommon in certain parts of the world, for example, in the Arabian countries and in the Balkan area.

It is of importance to distinguish between *infection stones* and *stones associated with infection*. In the first type of stone an infection with urease producing microorganisms is the cause of stone formation, in the latter type infection with non-urease producing bacteria is a secondary event. Stones associated with infection can have any stone composition. In this regard it is important to note that the common urine pathogen *Escherichia coli* almost never produces urease.

Cystine stone disease

Cystinuria is a genetic defect in which there is an increased excretion of the four dibasic amino acids cystine, ornithine, lysine, and arginine, of which only cystine has a poor solubility. In urine with pH 7.2 the solubility of cystine is about 300 mg or 1.25 mmol/l, and at higher concentrations cystine will precipitate (Ettinger and Kolb 1971; Nakagawa *et al.* 2000). There is, however, a pH-dependent increase in the solubility of cystine particularly at pH greater than 7.2. For a pH of 8 the solubility per litre is approximately 4 mmol (1000 mg). Moreover, the solubility of cystine increases in the presence of urinary macromolecules and with increasing ion strength (Pak and Fuller 1983). The SP of cystine is approximately 1×10^{-3} $(\text{mol/l})^3$, but clinical observations indicate that no crystal formation takes place in urine with an ion-activity product less than $1.3\text{–}1.6 \times 10^{-3}$ $(\text{mol/l})^3$ (Marshall and Robertson 1976).

In heterozygous cystinuria there is a low risk of cystine stone formation, but an increased formation of calcium stones has been demonstrated (Nancollas 1983). Mixtures of cystine and calcium salts are also frequently encountered in patients with homozygous cystinuria.

The abnormality in cystinuric patients is a defect or deficient production of the amino acid transporter necessary for uptake of the four basic amino acids from the tubular lumen (International Cystinuria Consortium 1999, 2001; Bisceglia *et al.* 2001). Recently, several abnormal alleles have been demonstrated as responsible for the reabsorptive defect. Three genetically different types of cystinuria have been described: Types 1, 2, and 3. Type 1 is inherited in an autosomal recessive way whereas Types 2 and 3 have an incomplete recessive trait. The gene that is affected in cystinuria Type 1 is SLC3A1, whereas cystinuria Types 2 and 3 apparently are associated with mutations in SLC7A9 (International Cystinuria Consortium 2001).

Cystinuria has been reported to occur in between 0.07 and 0.40‰ of the population. The diagnosis is established by demonstration of an excessive excretion of cystine in urine. Quantitative amino acid chromatography and the presence of the typical hexagonal cystine crystals in the sediment are necessary for this diagnostic step. A qualitative analysis with the cyanide nitroprusside test gives a red colour at cystine concentrations greater than 75 mg/l (0.3 mmol/l). Stones composed of cystine have a low density on the X-ray film.

Two types of cystine stones have been described, one with a smooth and one with a rough surface (Bhatta *et al.* 1989). They respond differently to disintegration by shock wave lithotripsy. It has also been noted that treatment with citrate changes the appearance of cystine stones to less solid structures (Tiselius *et al.* 2002).

Calcium oxalate stone disease

Calcium oxalate stones are either composed of pure calcium oxalate or of mixtures of calcium oxalate and calcium phosphate. The formation of this type of stone is apparently much more complex than that of the non-calcium stones discussed above. The possible steps in the process of calcium oxalate stone formation has been outlined above. It is important to emphasize, however, that despite considerable research efforts in order to increase our knowledge of calcium stone formation several fundamental details of the process are still poorly understood. Due to these shortcomings our therapeutic tools to prevent recurrent stone formation are less powerful than desirable.

The tentative model presented in Figs 2 and 3 has been derived from clinical as well as from experimental data and although some steps in the stone forming process are reasonable assumptions without definite proof, the possible series of events in the nephron nevertheless might be helpful in the management of the patients.

Calcium

A high urinary excretion of calcium is one important factor that contributes to a high supersaturation with both calcium oxalate and calcium phosphate. Hypercalciuria is accordingly a common finding in patients with calcium stone formation and frequencies of hypercalciuria up to or more than 50 per cent have been reported. The actual occurrence of hypercalciuria, however, depends on how the normal value is chosen and there is no real consensus on the definition of a normal calcium excretion (Pak 1981; Buck 1990). The most commonly used upper normal limits for 24-h excretion of calcium are 7.5 mmol for men and 6.25 mmol for women, or 0.10 mmol/kg body weight (Breslau 1994; Jaeger 1998; Polito *et al.* 2000). With a 24-h excretion above 10 mmol there is a marked increase in the risk of stone formation (Robertson *et al.* 1978; Coe and Bushinsky 1984).

There are three different types of hypercalciuria recorded in stone formers: *absorptive*, *renal*, and *resorptive hypercalciuria* (Pak 1981; Buck 1990). Absorptive hypercalciuria is the most common form of what is commonly termed idiopathic hypercalciuria (Peacock and Robertson 1979). The major explanation for this abnormality is an overproduction of 1,25-dihydroxy-vitamin D_3 [$1,25(OH)_2D_3$]. This active form of vitamin D is responsible for the transport of calcium ions from the lumen of the gut through the brush border membrane into the intestinal cell. $1,25(OH)_2D_3$ also controls the transport of calcium through the cell, as well as the exit of calcium from the enterocyte at the basolateral membrane (Buck 1990; Breslau 1994; Jaeger 1998). All three processes act in concert to accomplish the active absorption of dietary calcium.

Vitamin D_3 is supplied by dietary intake of vitamin D and by synthesis in the liver from the provitamin that forms in the skin as a result of exposure to ultraviolet light. There is a dominance in the body of $25(OH)D_3$ and this form of the vitamin is converted to $1,25(OH)_2D_3$ by 1α-hydroxylase in the proximal renal tubular cells. Several factors regulate the activity of 1α-hydroxylase. A low serum concentration of calcium increases the production of 1α-hydroxylase. This effect most certainly is accomplished by a direct effect of parathyroid hormone (PTH) on the tubular cells. Reduced serum concentrations of phosphate (PO_4) also stimulates the production of $1,25(OH)_2D_3$. An increased rate of hydroxylation is seen as a result of prostaglandin PGE2 stimulation. It has, moreover, been demonstrated that the production of $1,25(OH)_2D_3$ and consequently the absorption of calcium is related to the size of the kidneys (Hess *et al.* 1995b). An excessive intake of protein was one factor that explained the development of large kidneys.

Pak (1981) identified and described three different forms of absorptive hypercalciuria. In Type I, there is increased urinary calcium irrespective of the dietary intake. Patients with Type II absorptive hypercalciuria have an increased excretion of calcium only following a calcium load and with a normal intake of calcium the urinary excretion is normal. Type III absorptive hypercalciuria is characterized by a low serum PO_4 which thus stimulates the renal synthesis of 1α-hydroxylase. A clinical distinction between these three types of absorptive hypercalciuria can be made by assessing serum PO_4 and the creatinine-related urinary excretion of calcium following a fasting period and following an oral load of calcium (usually 1 g) (Pak 1981; Hesse *et al.* 1997). Today, the clinical importance of distinguishing between these different types is, however, limited.

Of the calcium that is filtered through the glomerulus the vast majority is reabsorbed by the tubular cells. Renal loss of calcium due to impaired tubular reabsorption of filtered calcium gives a negative calcium balance with reduced bone density. Dietary sodium causes an increased renal excretion of calcium (Jaeger 1994).

The most common pathological condition with resorptive hypercalciuria is hyperparathyroidism. In this disease calcium is mobilized from the skeleton by excess PTH (Smith and Werness 1983; Silverberg *et al.* 1990; Mollerup *et al.* 1994).

Several pharmacological agents can contribute to an excessive calcium excretion, such as corticosteroids, frusemide, as well as supplements of calcium and vitamin D (Hess 1998). Pharmacological effects on urine composition, pathological crystallization, and stone formation are further discussed below.

The exact role of calcium in the calcium stone forming process is currently under debate, since it was noted that the occurrence of stone disease in a large population was inversely related to the dietary intake of calcium (Curhan 1999). This was an observation that suddenly turned matters related to recurrence prevention upside down, because one of the most common recommendations given to calcium stone formers had so far been to reduce the intake of calcium (Robertson 1999). To uncritically reduce the intake of calcium is obviously not the right way to go and such therapeutic measures might not only worsen the disease, but may also cause a negative calcium balance and further loss of bone tissue (Lemann 1992).

Measurements of the skeletal mineral content have subsequently shown a lower than average bone density in patients with calcium stone disease (Jaeger *et al.* 1994; Zanchetta *et al.* 1996). It is essential not to reduce the daily calcium intake less than 800–1000 mg (20–25 mmol) to maintain a positive calcium balance (Hesse *et al.* 1997; Robertson 1999). The question now is whether an increased intake of calcium generally will be of benefit to these patients. No such studies have been carried out, but it is of note that supplements of calcium given between meals were associated with an increased risk of stone formation (Curhan and Curhan 1997). A high urinary calcium is, however, necessary for establishing high levels of supersaturation with calcium oxalate as well as with calcium phosphate and the inverse relationship between calcium intake and stone formation does not allow us to ignore dietary calcium. For patients with an absorptive hypercalciuria an *excessive* intake of calcium undoubtedly will increase urinary calcium and accordingly the ion-activity products of both calcium phosphate and calcium oxalate.

The observed inverse relationship between dietary calcium and calcium stone formation can be explained by complex formation between calcium and oxalate in the intestine and the ensuing reduction in oxalate absorption when the free oxalate concentration is decreased. The normal absorption of oxalate is, however, only in the range of 10–15 per cent (Tiselius 1981; von Unruh *et al.* 2000) and a pronounced reduction in urinary oxalate by an excessive intake of calcium, therefore, should not be expected. Based on this argument calcium stone formers should be adviced to have a daily intake of 20–25 mmol of calcium but to avoid excessive intake of dairy products. In Table 6, the calcium content of some common calcium-rich products is summarized (from Hesse *et al.* 1997).

In a number of patients a high urinary excretion of calcium is the result of a state of hypercalcaemia. Diseases and some other conditions associated with high serum or plasma levels of calcium are listed in Table 7.

In a few patients with calcium stone formation the reason is an increased secretion of PTH. A parathyroid adenoma or hyperplasia is usually the explanation for PTH overproduction, hypercalcaemia, and hypercalciuria. Surgical removal of the adenoma or of surplus parathyroid tissue in most cases results in cure. Patients with *hyperparathyroidism* develop urinary tract stones in 50–80 per cent of cases and in approximately 5 per cent of the patients there is also nephrocalcinosis. Inasmuch as urinary pH is high, as a result of renal bicarbonate loss, in these patients there is commonly a dominance of calcium phosphate in the stones that develop.

The diagnosis of hyperparathyroidism is confirmed by a high total serum calcium (corrected for the albumin concentration), a high ionized calcium, usually a low serum PO_4, and a high plasma PTH. It is the author's routine to assess plasma PTH in patients with a total serum/plasma calcium greater than 2.60 or an ionized calcium greater than 1.30.

Table 6 Food stuffs with a high content of calcium (adapted from Hesse *et al.* 1997). The content of calcium is expressed in mmol per 100 g

Milk	3
Yoghurt	3
Cream	2
Soft cheese	10–15
Hard cheese	20–30

Table 7 Clinical diseases and conditions with hypercalcaemia and hypercalciuria

Hyperparathyroidism
Hyperthyroidism
Renal tubular acidosis (distal type)
Sarcoidosis
Immobilization
Hypertension
Dent's disease
Familial idiopathic hypercalciuria

Patients with *distal renal tubular acidosis* (dRTA) have a defect in tubular handling of hydrogen ions (Backman *et al.* 1980). This abnormality results in systemic metabolic acidosis, *alkaline urine*, *hypercalciuria*, and *hypocitraturia*. The abnormalities in urine composition favour the precipitation of calcium phosphate rather than of calcium oxalate. There are complete and incomplete forms of dRTA. The complete form is uncommonly seen whereas incomplete dRTA occurs more frequently. The diagnosis of dRTA is established by demonstrating an inability of the kidney to acidify urine to less than pH 5.3–5.4. The fasting morning pH is usually not less than 6.0–6.1 and repeated pH measurements never give values below 5.8. In the complete form of dRTA blood bicarbonate and blood pH are reduced, but in incomplete dRTA these variables are normal. Patients with complete dRTA usually have both nephrocalcinosis and urolithiasis. There is also a proximal type of renal tubular acidosis, but this condition is not associated with stone formation.

Several diseases and toxic agents might cause a disturbed handling of hydrogen ions because of damage to the distal tubular cells. Such an effect is seen in patients suffering from *Wilson's disease, the Fanconi syndrome*, and *hyperglobulinaemia*. It is also observed following administration of some nephrotoxic agents, for instance, *amphotericin B* (Smith 1974) and regularly accompanies treatment with the carbonic anhydrase inhibitors *acetazolamide* and *topiramate* (Ahlstrand and Tiselius 1987; Higashihara *et al.* 1991).

Both nephrocalcinosis and formation of renal stones occur in patients with *sarcoidosis*. These patients usually have hypercalciuria, but not always hypercalcaemia. Hypercalciuria in these patients is attributable to an increased intestinal absorption of calcium (Rodman and Mahler 2000).

Immobilized patients have an increased bone resorption and consequently elevated serum and urine calcium.

The *milk-alkali syndrome* is not very common today because of improvements in the treatment of patients with peptic ulcers. The pathophysiology of this syndrome is a combination of a high urine pH, as a result of ingestion of absorbable alkali, and a high urinary concentration of calcium from an excessive intake of milk. Thereby the prerequisites for calcium phosphate precipitation are met.

Dent's disease is a rare X-linked recessive genetic abnormality with urinary tract stone formation and hypophosphataemic richets (Dent and Friedman 1964). The abnormality has been localized to the CLCN5 gene in chromosome Xp11.12. The defect results in disturbed function of the tubular chloride transporting system with decreased reabsorption of calcium. The exact mechanism by means of which this occurs is, however, unknown.

Familial idiopathic hypercalciuria is an autosomal inherited disease. The genetic defect has not been identified and the mechanism that leads to hypercalciuria is not completely understood.

Oxalate

Beside the urine volume, urinary oxalate is the most powerful determinant of the ion-activity product of calcium oxalate and even very small increments in oxalate result in pronounced changes in terms of supersaturation and driving force of the crystallization (Finlayson 1974; Robertson *et al.* 1981; Tiselius 1982).

Eighty to ninety per cent of urinary oxalate is derived from the endogenous synthesis, most of which takes place in the liver (Menon and Mahle 1982).

The upper normal limit of 24-h urinary oxalate excretion is around 0.4–0.5 mmol. There is no absolute consensus in the literature whether patients with so-called idiopathic calcium stone disease have an oxalate excretion that is greater than that in normal subjects. Several authors report a slightly higher excretion in stone formers whereas others do not (Tiselius 1996). Methodological inconsistencies and a geographical variation can, however, probably explain the discrepancies that exist. Irrespective of the variable results, it can, nevertheless, be stated that the differences in oxalate excretion between stone formers and normal subjects usually are small. In view of the pronounced effect that oxalate has on the supersaturation, however, *mild hyperoxaluria* also appears to be an important factor in patients with calcium oxalate stone disease (Hatch 1993; Holmes *et al.* 1998; Trinchieri *et al.* 1998; Robertson 1999).

Although most oxalate excreted in urine is derived from the endogenous metabolism, small changes in dietary oxalate might be important from a recurrence preventive point of view and Table 8 shows some products with a particularly high content of oxalate (Hesse *et al.* 1997).

Primary hyperoxaluria

The most serious abnormality of the metabolism of oxalate is *primary hyperoxaluria.* Primary hyperoxaluria occurs in two different forms: Type 1 and Type 2 and the 24-h excretion in these patients is usually greater than 1.0–1.5 mmol. Patients with Type 1 hyperoxaluria have a deficiency of alanine-glyoxylate aminotransferase (AGT), which is a pyridoxal phosphate-dependent enzyme (Danpure 2000). This enzyme is responsible for the conversion of glyoxylate to glycine (Fig. 6). The deficiency or insufficient synthesis of AGT results in an increased supply of glyoxylate. In this way increased amounts of oxalate are synthesized from glyoxalate by the action of peroxisomal glyoxylate oxidase (XO) and cystosolic lactate dehydrogenase (LD).

Moreover, increased amounts of glyoxylate are reduced to glycolate by the action of glyoxylate reductase (GR), which works normally in Type 1 hyperoxaluria, and the urinary excretion of glycolate increases. The high production of oxalate leads to stone formation in the urinary tract and deposition of calcium oxalate crystals in renal tissue as well as other organs (Holmes 1998; Petrarulo *et al.* 1998). The enzyme AGT is synthesized in the liver where it is localized to the peroxisomes. It is encoded by the AGXT gene on the 2q 37.3 chromosome. Several mutations have been identified (Danpure 2000).

Primary hyperoxaluria Type 1 usually starts early in life and might result in renal failure already in childhood. There is, however, a wide variability in the production of AGT, which accordingly influences the clinical presentation and the course of the disease. In extreme cases, the patients might be without symptoms through their whole lifetime despite the genetic defect.

The analytical findings in patients with primary hyperoxaluria Type 1 are increased urinary excretion of *oxalate* and *glycolate.* The stones are in most cases composed of COM. Liver biopsy and assessment of the AGT activity is required for a reliable diagnosis. A definite cure for these patients cannot be obtained unless liver transplantation is carried out.

The abnormality behind primary hyperoxaluria Type 2 is a deficient production of GR. This enzyme is responsible for conversion of glyoxylate to glycolate. A deficient function of GR leads to an accumulation of glyoxylate with an increased conversion to oxalate. Inasmuch as GR also is responsible for conversion of hydroxypyruvate to D-glycerate, surplus amounts of hydroxypyruvate give an excessive production of L-glycerate by the action of LD. The genetic defect has been localized to chromosome 9q11 (Danpure 2000).

Primary hyperoxaluria Type 2 usually has a milder clinical course than hyperoxaluria Type 1 and renal failure is less commonly seen in patients with the Type 2 disease. Clinically, these patients have an increased urinary excretion of *oxalate* and *L-glycerate* and it has been stated that stone formation is a more typical entity in hyperoxaluria Type 2 than is nephrocalcinosis.

Enteric hyperoxaluria

A marked increase in oxalate absorption is seen in patients with disturbed intestinal function and malabsorption. This *enteric hyperoxaluria*, or *hyperoxaluria Type 3*, brings about an increased absorption of oxalate by removal of calcium ions through complex formation with fatty acids (McLeod and Churchill 1992). Enteric hyperoxaluria is seen in patients with Crohn's disease, particularly following intestinal resection, with jejuno-ileal bypass for obesity, or with any other condition associated with fat and bile acid malabsorption such as pancreatic insufficiency.

Only a minor fraction of dietary calcium is normally absorbed from the gut because of the intraluminal complex formation between oxalate and calcium (Fig. 7). In conditions with disturbed absorption of fatty acids, calcium might preferably form soaps with fatty acids

Table 8 Food stuffs with a high content of oxalate (adapted from Hesse *et al.* 1997). The content of oxalate is expressed as mmol of oxalic acid per 100 g

Rhubarb	6.0
Spinach	6.3
Tea leaves	4.2–16.1
Cocoa	6.9
Nuts	2.2–6.7
Beetroot	1.2

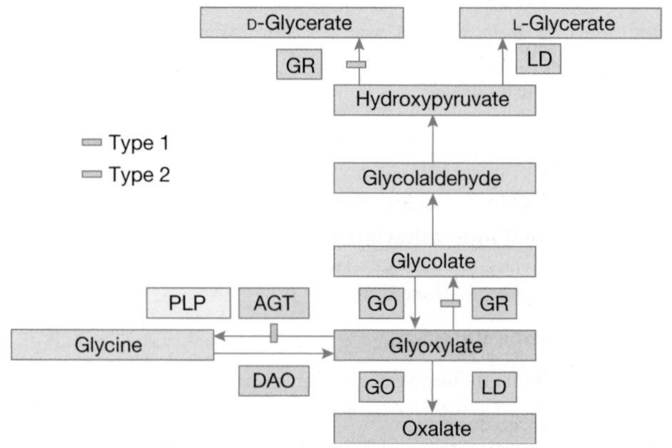

Fig. 6 Metabolic pathways leading to the formation of oxalate. The various interconversions are catalyzed by the enzymes alanine glyoxylate aminotransferase (AGT), D-amino acid oxidase (DAO), glycolate oxidase (GO), glyoxylate reductase (GR), and lactate dehydrogenase (LD). The defects in hyperoxaluria Types 1 and 2 are indicated.

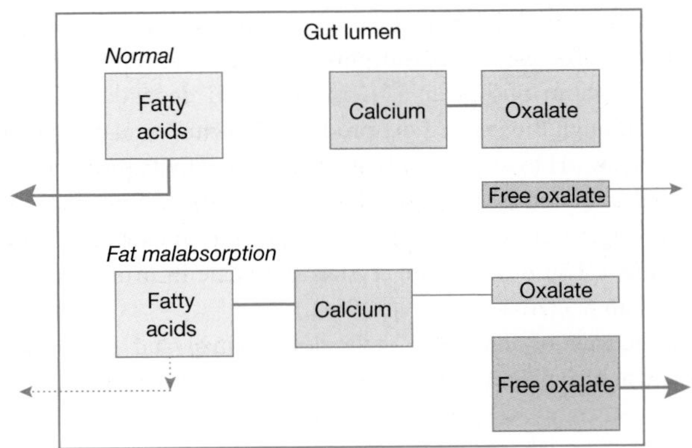

Fig. 7 Intestinal absorption of oxalate under normal conditions and in patients with enteric hyperoxaluria.

and much less calcium is left for the normal calcium–oxalate complex formation. The increased concentration of free oxalate results in an excessive absorption. It has, moreover, been suggested that bile acids, which are present at high concentrations throughout the intestinal tract because of the malabsorption, increase the permeability of the colon mucosa (Dobbins and Binder 1976). This mechanism might thus further augment the intestinal absorption of oxalate. The importance of the colon for oxalate absorption is further supported by the fact that patients with an ileostomy usually form uric acid and not calcium oxalate stones.

Patients with enteric hyperoxaluria usually have a 24-h excretion of oxalate in the range 0.5–1.0 mmol.

Oxalobacter formigenes

There is recent evidence that the intestinal bacteria *Oxalobacter formigenes*, by its capacity to degrade oxalate, plays an important role in oxalate metabolism. Patients with a high rate of stone recurrences to a large extent were lacking this microorganism (Hoppe *et al.* 2000; Sidhu *et al.* 2000).

Citrate

A low urinary citrate is reported in between 13 and 63 per cent of calcium stone formers (Pak 1978; Nicar *et al.* 1983; Pattaras and Moore 1999). It is seen in patients with dRTA, intestinal diseases with malabsorption and diarrhoea, hypokalaemia induced by treatment with thiazides, excessive intake of animal proteins, and following extreme physical exercise. The reduced excretion of citrate reflects an intracellular acidosis and this abnormality can be corrected or modified by administration of alkali (Coe 1994; Pak 1994; Győry and Ashby 1999; Pattras and Moore 1999; Tiselius *et al.* 2001). A low urinary citrate also is seen in patients treated with carbonic anhydrase inhibitors (Ahlstrand and Tiselius 1987; Higashihara *et al.* 1991).

Citric acid is a tricarboxylic acid with pK values of 2.9, 4.3, and 5.6. This means that in urine citric acid usually is highly or fully dissociated. The power of citrate as a modifier of the calcium salt crystallization process is linked to the negatively charged molecule which has the capacity to both form complexes with positively charged ions and to bind or adhere to the positively charged surface of calcium oxalate and calcium phosphate crystals.

According to these properties citrate plays a crucial role in modifying the formation and development of calcium oxalate and calcium phosphate crystals and stones. Citrate thereby influences the ion-activity products of both calcium oxalate and calcium phosphate. Urinary citrate also acts as an inhibitor of calcium oxalate as well as of calcium phosphate crystal growth and aggregation (Tiselius *et al.* 1993; Bek-Jensen *et al.* 1996; Schwille *et al.* 2001). Moreover, it counteracts the heterogeneous growth of calcium oxalate on calcium phosphate and the calcium phosphate-induced nucleation of calcium oxalate. The increased aggregation of crystals that is caused by polymerization of THP at a low urine pH and high concentrations of calcium is counteracted by administration of alkaline citrate (Hess *et al.* 1993; Hess 1994). There is also some experimental evidence that intestinal complex formation between Ca^{2+} and Cit^{3-} is one factor in explanation of the reduced excretion of calcium seen in patients treated with alkaline citrate.

Treatment of patients with alkaline citrate before and after extracorporeal shock wave lithotripsy indicated that both sodium potassium citrate (Cicerello *et al.* 1994) and potassium citrate (Cicerello *et al.* 2000) increased the clearance of stone fragments from the kidney.

Administration of alkaline citrate (potassium citrate, sodium potassium citrate, and magnesium potassium citrate) *increases both urinary citrate* and *pH*. In contrast, treatment with acetazolamide results in a *reduced excretion of citrate* and *a high pH*, similar to the situation in patients with renal tubular acidosis. The low citrate is the effect of an intracellular acidosis in the tubular cells. Most citrate that is administered is metabolized in Kreb's cycle and only a small fraction is directly excreted in urine. The increased excretion of citrate that follows administration of alkaline citrate is caused by the increased pH in the tubular cells.

The wide range of hypocitraturia that has been reported in stone formers is explained by the lack of consensus on the normal urinary excretion of citrate. A lower limit for the 24-h excretion of between 0.6 and 3.5 mmol is found in the literature (Menon and Mahle 1983; Klocke *et al.* 1989; Hess *et al.* 1994; Pak 1994; Hesse *et al.* 1997; Tiselius 1997c; Marangella *et al.* 1999; Pattaras and Moore 1999). With a lower excretion limit of 2.0 mmol during 24 h the author recorded hypocitraturia in approximately 30 per cent of the patients with recurrent calcium stone formation. For a 24-h excretion of 2.5 mmol the corresponding figure was between 40 and 50 per cent.

One factor that has been used to describe the risk of crystallization and the severity of stone formation is the ratio between calcium and citrate (Schwille 1985; Höbart and Hofbauer 1991; Tiselius 1997c). Among the patients seen by the author a ratio greater than 3.0 was recorded in less than 10 per cent of the normal subjects but in as much as 40 per cent of recurrent stone formers. In addition to an increased excretion of citrate, urinary calcium is reduced during administration of alkaline citrate. Administration of alkaline citrate thus favourably affects the calcium/citrate ratio and thereby probably the risk of stone formation.

Citrate has the capacity to inhibit crystal growth and crystal aggregation also at very low concentrations. Although it is difficult to prove, citrate possibly exerts the most powerful effect in the diluted urine that is present in the proximal part of the collecting ducts, the distal tubules, and the loops of Henle.

In most clinical studies of stone formers treated with alkaline citrate in prevention of recurrent calcium stone formation, the annual rates of stone formation have been reduced significantly (Leumann *et al.* 1993; Pak 1994; Whalley *et al.* 1996; Ettinger *et al.* 1997; Lee *et al.* 1999). It is noteworthy in this respect that potassium citrate appears to be superior to that of sodium potassium citrate (Preminger *et al.* 1988). The load of sodium in a long-term perspective probably counteracts the reduced calcium excretion that otherwise is seen.

Despite the lack of a generally accepted lower normal 24-h excretion limit of urinary citrate, it is reasonable to assume that treatment with alkaline citrate is most beneficial for patients with a low or low normal urinary citrate. A lower 24-h urinary citrate excretion of 2.0–2.5 mmol, therefore, might be a clinically useful limit (Hesse *et al.* 1997).

Magnesium

There are usually no major differences reported in magnesium (Mg) excretion between stone formers and normal subjects (Evans *et al.* 1967; Johansson 1979). Low blood and urinary Mg are almost only observed in patients with disturbed intestinal function and malabsorption. The inhibitory properties of Mg are mainly related to the growth of calcium phosphate crystals. In terms of calcium oxalate a reduced magnesium slightly increases the ion-activity product of the salt. Mg also reduces the rate of conversion of amorphous calcium phosphate (ACP) to octacalcium phosphate (OCP) and HAP. It should also be noted that a reduced calcium/Mg quotient counteracts the formation of Bru. Although the risk of stone formation probably cannot be eliminated by such a shift in urine composition, the formation of a calcium phosphate crystal phase other than Bru is favourable because of its high recurrence risk and shock wave resistant structure.

Phosphate

Information on PO_4 excretion in stone formers and normal subjects is scarce. PO_4 is directly dependent on the type of diet ingested and it is accordingly subject to huge variations. For the latter reason urinary PO_4 usually has been ascribed a small and less important role in stone formation. Nevertheless, urinary PO_4 is of importance for establishing a sufficient degree of supersaturation with the various calcium phosphate crystal phases.

The excretion of pyrophosphate which parallels urinary PO_4 is of importance for inhibition of calcium oxalate and calcium phosphate crystal growth (Kok *et al.* 1988; Schwille 1988; Baumann *et al.* 1989; Sharma *et al.* 1992).

An above-normal 24-h excretion of PO_4 can be set to 35 mmol and Table 9 gives examples of particularly phosphate-rich foodstuffs (Hesse *et al.* 1997).

pH

Urinary pH is highly dependent on the intake of fluids and foodstuffs and on the metabolic state. A pH range between 4.9 and 7.5 is normal for most persons. The pH is the most important determinant of the ion-activity product of calcium phosphate and the solubility of the different calcium phosphate salts is highly pH dependent (Tiselius 1996). Although the ion-activity product of calcium oxalate is usually influenced by pH to a very small extent, the ion-activity product might nevertheless be reduced in alkaline urine as a result of calcium phosphate precipitation. Whereas crystals of calcium oxalate are found in acid urine, calcium phosphate crystals dominate in urine with a pH greater than 6.5 (Ahlstrand *et al.* 1984).

The activity of inhibitory molecules of small and large sizes is increased at high pH because of an increased dissociation (Tiselius 1981).

Table 9 Food stuffs with a high content of phosphate (adapted from Hesse *et al.* 1997). The content of phosphate is expressed as mmol of phosphorous per 100 g

Soft cheese	30
Hard cheese	16–28
Nuts	13–19
Beans	14–19
Cocoa	24
Liver	11–12

Urate

Urate has no direct influence on the ion-activity products of calcium phosphate or calcium oxalate and its role in calcium stone formation has been a matter of debate for decades. It has thus been suggested that sodium urate might serve as a nidus for calcium oxalate precipitation (Coe *et al.* 1975; Pak *et al.* 1976; Koutsoukos *et al.* 1980; Tiselius 1984b), that colloidal urate might interfere with the activity of crystallization inhibitors (Robertson *et al.* 1981; Zerwekh *et al.* 1983), or that calcium oxalate is precipitated as a result of a salting-out effect (Kallistratos *et al.* 1970; Grover and Ryall 1994). Of these alternatives the last one presently appears most plausible.

A uricosuric calcium oxalate stone syndrome was described by Coe and coworkers (Coe and Kavalach 1974; Coe 1983), but there is no information available on how common this syndrome is. Geographical and dietary factors might explain the variability by means of which hyperoxaluric calcium oxalate stone formation obviously occurs in different populations of the world. In some groups of stone-formers urinary urate is increased compared with normal subjects, in others it is not. It is noteworthy that an increased excretion of urate usually accompanies several of the other changes in urine composition that are associated with excessive dietary habits.

Macromolecules and their role in calcium stone formation

It is well recognized that differences in supersaturation alone cannot explain why some people develop stones whereas others do not. Although crystal nucleation, crystal growth, and to some extent, crystal aggregation also depend on the driving force and the ion composition of urine, macromolecular modifiers of the various steps of calcium salt crystallization and stone formation are considered to play an important role.

From a theoretical point of view, the formation of crystalluria with aggregates of large crystals, which is typical for stone formers, can be explained by an abnormal promotion of crystal nucleation and/or an insufficient inhibition of crystal growth, crystal aggregation, and crystal retention.

Urinary macromolecules usually exert their effects on crystallization by binding or adhering to crystals. Inasmuch as urinary macromolecules have an anionic character they have a high affinity to the positive surface of calcium oxalate and calcium phosphate crystals.

It is possible that certain macromolecules by exposing nucleating sites to supersaturated urine can induce and control crystal nucleation. In that way crystal formation might occur at specific domains of the molecule where high levels of supersaturation are established when ions accumulate. In the presence of high concentrations of macromolecules or otherwise a high availability of nucleation sites, the crystals might be small whereas with few sites larger crystals will form.

A great number of macromolecules, glycosaminoglycans, glycoproteins, and proteins, have been demonstrated in stones and isolated from both stones and urine in a more or less pure form. The literature on urinary macromolecules and their role in stone formation accordingly is both huge and confusing. Although various crystallization modifying properties of macromolecules have been shown in numerous crystallization experiments, it is very difficult to draw definite conclusions on the *in vivo* effects of the compounds. It is also technically impossible to develop crystallization systems that appropriately reflect the intratubular conditions. For detailed information on the macromolecules and their possible role in stone formation the reader is referred to excellent reviews on the subject (Ryall 1996, 1997).

Calcium stones usually contain an organic matrix constituting 1–3 per cent of the stone weight. The following compounds extracted from the stone matrix need to be mentioned: albumin and globulins (Boyce *et al.* 1962; Boyce 1968), THP (Melick *et al.* 1980), nephrocalcin (Nakagawa *et al.* 1987), α-1-microglobulin (Morse and Resnick 1988), elastase (Petersen *et al.* 1989), transferrin (Fraij 1989), osteopontin/uropontin (Shiraga *et al.* 1992), α-1-antitrypsin (Umekawa *et al.* 1993), protein (Binette and Binette 1993), superoxide dismutase (Binette and Binette 1994), β_2-microglobulin, α-1-acidic glycoprotein, apolipoprotein AI, retinol-binding protein and renal lithostatine (Dussol *et al.* 1995), urinary prothrombin fragment 1, UPTF1 (Stapleton *et al.* 1996), inter-α-trypsin inhibitor (Dawson *et al.* 1998), calprotectin (Umekawa and Kurita 1994), heparan sulfate (Nishio *et al.* 1985), hyaluronic acid (Roberts and Resnick 1986), fibronectin (Masao *et al.* 2000), calgranulin (Pillay *et al.* 1998), and nucleoline-like protein (Sorokina and Kleinman 1999).

For only few of these compounds have effects on the calcium salt crystallization that might be of importance for stone formation been demonstrated. The main interest thus has been focused on *heparan sulfate, hyaluronic acid, nephrocalcin, bikunin, inter-α-inhibitor, UTPF1, uropontin*, and *THP*.

The glycosaminoglycans excreted in urine are chondroitin sulfate, heparan sulfate, and hyaluronic acid, but the major glycosaminoglycans in stones are heparan sulfate and hyaluronic acid (Nishio *et al.* 1985; Roberts and Resnick 1986). Glycosaminoglycans inhibit calcium oxalate crystal growth and crystal aggregation, but their definite role in stone formation is not known and there are usually no differences in the total excretion of glycosaminoglycans between stone formers and normal subjects (Ryall 1996).

Nephrocalcin, which is secreted from the proximal tubules and the thick ascending loop of Henle, occurs in urine in mono-, di-, tri-, and tetrameric forms and the range of molecular weight varies between 14 and 68 kDa (Nakagawa *et al.* 1987; Coe *et al.* 1991; Berland and Dussol 1994; Ryall 1997; Parkinson 1998). It has been claimed that the deficient crystallization inhibitory function of nephrocalcin, which is found in stone formers, is related to a low content of γ-carboxyglutamic acid residues in the molecule. A high concentration of γ-carboxyglutamic acid gives the molecule a high capacity to bind or attract calcium ions. It has recently been suggested that nephrocalcin is related to bikunin which is the light chain of inter-α-inhibitor (Ryall 1997; Atmani *et al.* 1999; Iida *et al.* 1999; Médetognon-Benissan *et al.* 1999; Suzuki *et al.* 2001).

Uropontin is the form of osteopontin excreted in urine (Hoyer *et al.* 1995; Soerensen *et al.* 1995; Asplin *et al.* 1996b; deBruijn *et al.* 1997; Iguchi *et al.* 1999). Uropontin inhibits crystal nucleation, growth, and aggregation (Shiraga *et al.* 1992) as well as the crystal attachment to tubular cells (Lieske *et al.* 1997a). The effect of uropontin most certainly is related to its high content of aspartic acid residues.

The matrix protein of calcium oxalate stones has been identified as UPTF1. It is a protein with inhibitory properties, but its exact role for the crystallization or the stone formation is not known (Grover and Ryall 1996; Ryall 1997). It has recently been suggested that the matrix stucture within the crystals facilitates crystal dissolution following internalization by giving better access to the lysosomal enzymes (de Warter *et al.* 1999; Fleming *et al.* 2000; Ryall *et al.* 2000). UPTF1 has a high content of γ-carboxyglutamic acid residues and favours the formation of COD over COM. This effect might be clinically important because the cell affinity for the dihydrate crystal phase is less than that for the monohydrate.

THP (Rose and Sulaiman 1982; Scurr and Robertson 1986; Yoshioka *et al.* 1989; Coe *et al.* 1991; Hess *et al.* 1991; Tiselius 1997a; Siddiqiu *et al.* 1999) has effects on both crystal growth and crystal aggregation. In alkaline solution THP inhibits and in acid solution it promotes aggregation of calcium oxalate crystals (Hess 1992). The latter effect is caused by self-polymerization in acid urine. Urinary citrate counteracts this polymerization (Hess *et al.* 1993).

Nucleation of calcium oxalate and probably also of calcium phosphate is regulated by promoters (Parkinson 1998; Atmani and Khan 2000; Khan *et al.* 2000) and it is possible that certain macromolecules can act as both inhibitors and promoters.

The macromolecular effects on nucleation, growth, and aggregation of calcium salt crystals is summarized in Table 10.

It can be concluded that the exact role of the various macromolecules in the sequence of events that leads to stone formation has not been established so far. Neither are we in possession of any effective tools by means of which the excretion of inhibitory macromolecules can be increased. The only clinical way to increase the potential of their crystallization potential is to make the urine alkaline or to modify the structure of the inhibitors by changing urine composition.

Urine volume

Small urine volumes are of great importance for establishing high levels of supersaturation with calcium oxalate. The increased concentration of crystallization driving urine constituents, caused by a low urine flow, is often the only abnormality in stone formers. In a recent randomized study it was shown that patients who increased their fluid intake were able to reduce the stone forming activity significantly better than patients who maintained their normal drinking habits (Borghi *et al.* 1999).

One problem for conclusions on a person's urine volume is that the situation during urine collection commonly makes the patients drink more than they normally do. The recorded volume might, therefore, not be representative for the average-day urine flow. In order to compensate for such errors a standardized estimate of the ion-activity product of calcium oxalate was designed for the clinical routine work, in which the 24-h urine volume was set to 1.5 l (Tiselius 1989). This step makes it possible to compare patients in terms of the ionic effects on the risk that the patient has to form a urine that is critically supersaturated with calcium oxalate.

Calcium phosphate stones

As mentioned above, stones composed of pure calcium phosphate are relatively uncommon and form mainly in patients who produce a constantly alkaline urine (Marshall and Robertson 1976; Pak 1978). This type of stone is thus seen in association with dRTA (Backman *et al.* 1980;

Table 10 Effects of large and small molecules on the crystallization of calcium salts

Urine component	Effects on the crystallization of calcium oxalate/calcium phosphate			
	Nucleation	**Growth**	**Aggregation**	**Cell adherence**
Nephrocalcin	INH	INH	INH	—
Bikunin	—	INH	INH	INH
THP	PRO	INH?	INH/PRO	—
Uropontin	INH	INH	INH	INH
UPTF1	?	INH	INH	INH
Glycosaminoglycans	INH	INH	INH	INH
Citrate	—	INH	INH	—
Pyrophosphate	—	INH	—	—
Magnesium	—	INH	—	—

INH, inhibition; PRO, promotion; THP, Tamm–Horsfall protein; UPTF1, urinary prothrombin fragment 1.

Hesse *et al.* 1997; Penney and Oleesky 1999), primary hyperparathyroidism (Buck 1990; Hess and Jaeger 1993; Fliser and Ritz 1999), and during treatment with acetazolamide and other carbanhydrase inhibitors (Ahlstrand and Tiselius 1987; Higashihara *et al.* 1991). Typical for these conditions is a high urine pH and a low urine citrate. There is a fear that treatment with alkali in prevention of recurrent calcium oxalate stone formation should lead to the development of calcium phosphate stones, but the authors have not seen this complication and the risk is probably very small. Although the ion-activity product of calcium phosphate is increased, it is likely that the concomitant increment in citrate concentration prevents the formation of large crystals and crystal aggregates (Tiselius 1984c).

Hydroxyapatite is the thermodynamically most stable calcium phosphate crystal phase and it is also the major crystal phase in mixed calcium oxalate/calcium phosphate stones. Under certain conditions brushite (Bru; calcium hydrogen phosphate) is formed (Leusmann *et al.* 1995; Győry and Ashby 1999; Hesse and Heimbach 1999). This salt precipitates at a lower pH than that required for HAP. The conversion of ACP to OCP is counteracted by Mg. Bru is of particular interest because of the very high recurrence rate in patients with this stone-type (Leusmann *et al.* 1995). In addition, it has a very solid structure and is accordingly difficult to break with shock waves. Both HAP and Bru are soluble in acid solutions, which thus can be used for percutaneous chemolysis.

The macromolecular modifiers of calcium oxalate crystallization (Romberg *et al.* 1986) are also active in the corresponding steps of calcium phosphate crystallization. There is, however, evidence that Mg, citrate, and pyrophosphate are the most important inhibitors of calcium phosphate crystal growth.

In order to enable conclusions on the relative risk for a patient to form a urine that is critically supersaturated with calcium phosphate, a standardized form of the *AP(CaP)-index* was developed in which the 24-h urine volume set to 1.5 l and the pH to 7.0 (Tiselius 1997b). Similar to the standardized *AP(CaOx)-index*, the standardized *AP(CaP)-index* is clinically useful for roughly estimating the risk of forming a urine critically supersaturated with calcium phosphate. In addition to doubts regarding how well the recorded urine volume reflects everyday conditions, it is usually also difficult to correctly assess pH in a urine sample that is collected during a longer period of the day and subsequently stored. Moreover, an adequate analysis of both calcium and phosphate cannot be obtained unless the urine has been acidified (Tiselius *et al.* 2001).

Dietary effects on urine composition

Some food stuffs that are directly related to the excretion of important urine variables have already been discussed and summarized in Tables 4, 6, 8, and 9. The effects of diet on urine composition has been the subject of several recent publications (Curhan and Curhan 1997; Hesse *et al.* 1997; Hess *et al.* 1999; Assimos and Holmes 2000; Borghi *et al.* 2002) and in this section only a few aspects are discussed.

It is of interest to note that there has been an increased incidence of stone formation in the European population after the Second World War and it is likely that this effect is related to an increased affluence and altered dietary habits (Buck 1996). One factor that is considered of great importance for the increased occurrence of calcium stones is the excessive intake of animal protein, an issue that has been addressed by many authors (Robertson and Peacock 1982; Kok *et al.* 1990; Tiselius *et al.* 2001). Trinchieri *et al.* (1991) found that their patients with calcium stone disease had an increased intake of both animal and vegetable protein. A high intake of animal protein during the evening was observed in a group of Japanese stone patients. In addition to a higher intake of animal protein than that recorded in normal subjects, these patients also had a higher intake of carbohydrates (Iguchi *et al.* 1990).

The protein intake brings about a number of changes in urine composition. There is an acid load that gives rise to a metabolic acidosis whereby the urinary excretion of citrate is reduced and the excretion of calcium increased by bone resorption. There is also an inhibition of calcium reabsorption in the distal renal tubules caused by the acidosis.

Phenylalanine and tyrosine in protein diets are converted to oxalate with ensuing mild hyperoxaluria. Animal protein also increases urinary urate and can accordingly increase the risk of both calcium oxalate and uric acid crystallization. The precipitation of uric acid is further augmented by the reduced pH. The most likely explanation for the facilitated precipitation of calcium oxalate in urine with a high concentration of urate is a salting-out effect (Kallistratos *et al.* 1970; Grover and Ryall 1994).

An excessive intake of animal protein increases the glomerular filtration rate and this hyperfiltration contributes to an increased urinary excretion of oxalate, calcium, and urate. Moreover, the high protein intake might be responsible for the larger kidney volumes seen in stone formers and for the consequently increased production of 1α-hydroxylase and intestinal calcium absorption (Hess *et al.* 1995b). It is generally considered that a daily intake of protein greater than 1–2 g per kg body weight should be avoided.

Food stuffs rich in oxalate (Table 8) causes an oxalate load to the intestine and an increased risk of oxalate absorption particularly for an oxalate intake that occurs unrelated to regular meals. In this respect, the intake of dark chocolate and nuts as snacks without the simultaneous ingestion of calcium might result in a pronounced absorption of oxalate and peaks of oxalate concentration in urine. The dietary oxalate load varies considerably from one geographic or cultural area to another.

Not only dietary protein but also dietary fat is increased as a result of affluence (Iguchi *et al.* 1990). Based on experimental studies Baggio formulated the hypothesis that abnormalities in urine composition among idiopathic calcium stone formers might be related to an increased content of arachidonic acid and a higher arachidonic/linoleic acid ratio of the cell membranes (Baggio and Gambaro 1996). This abnormality was corrected by fish oil. It is of great interest that urinary stone disease does not occur among Inuits or in the Japanese population living in the coast area. It has been assumed that this is an effect of the rich supply of fish oil. It is suggested that eicosapentaenoic acid might favourably affect the composition and ion-exchange in the plasma membranes of tubular cells and in that way cause a reduction in calcium as well as oxalate excretion (Baggio and Gambaro 1996; Buck 1996).

An excessive intake of sodium increases urinary excretion of calcium and it has been recommended that the daily sodium intake should not exceed 100 mmol.

There is experimental support for a beneficial effect of phytate, but only a minor fraction of ingested phytate is excreted in urine (Grases *et al.* 1998).

From a clinical point of view the most attractive way of influencing the risk of crystallization and stone formation is by modifying the dietary and drinking habits. Although this sometimes is a very difficult process for the patient it is usually the first therapeutic step. There are several interesting observations that show the importance of dietary factors on urine composition. In a recent randomized study it was concluded that dietary recommendations on a diet low in animal protein and salt but normal in its content of calcium resulted in a significantly reduced rate of stone formation compared with that recorded for patients taking a diet with a low content of calcium (Borghi *et al.* 2002).

The important conclusion derived from the physical–chemical considerations discussed above is that by a sufficient intake of fluids, the urine will be diluted to a level below the critical supersaturation. Although this dilution also reduces the concentrations of inhibitors of crystallization, it is generally considered far more important to eliminate the prerequisite of crystal nucleation by lowering supersaturation. From a clinical point of view this goal is usually reached with a 24-h urine volume of 2000–2500 ml, for which a daily intake of more than 3000 ml is necessary.

Various beverages have constituents that might affect urine composition in a positive or a negative way. The calcium content of tap water or mineral water varies considerably, but at least in terms of calcium oxalate crystallization and stone formation, this factor is usually not very important. The alkalinizing effect of water with a high content of bicarbonate is, however, of much greater interest for patients with calcium oxalate and uric acid stone formation, because of its favourable effects on urine pH and citrate. For patients who form pure calcium phosphate stones and in whom alkalization should be avoided, water with a low content of bicarbonate and calcium might be a better choice.

Juices of citrus fruits are useful for calcium oxalate stone patients because of the high content of citrate, but it needs to be emphasized that a high content of oxalate in some fruits might counteract this beneficial effect.

Although alcoholic beverages increase the urine flow temporarily, this effect is followed by a period of antidiuresis. Moreover, an excessive intake of wine and beer is associated with an increased excretion of urate and a reduced pH. Beverages with a rich content of sugar such as cola drinks and lemonades can bring about an increased urinary excretion of calcium. Coffee in large quantities increases urinary urate and black tea gives an oxalate load.

Pharmacological effects on urine composition

Treatment with different pharmacological agents can cause stone formation either by direct precipitation of the excreted compound or its metabolites, or by effects of the treatment on urine composition in a way that favours crystallization and stone formation (Hess 1998). Pharmacological agents and their effects on urine composition are summarized in Table 11.

Megadoses of ascorbic acid theoretically might increase the excretion of oxalate as a consquence of oxidation of ascorbate to oxalate (Hatch *et al.* 1980; Traxer *et al.* 2001). Based on several recent clinical observations it is, however, generally considered that a significant increase in urinary oxalate does not occur with a daily ascorbic acid intake of less than 4 g (Tiselius *et al.* 2001).

Table 11 Pharmacological agents with risk of stone formation because of effects on urine composition

Calcium supplement	U-Calcium ↑	U-Oxalate ↓
Prostaglandins	U-Calcium ↑	
Testosterone	U-Oxalate ↑	
Gentamycin	U-Calcium ↑	
D-Penicillamine	U-Oxalate ↑	
Vitamin D	U-Calcium ↑	
Acetazolamide	U-Citrate ↓	U-pH ↑
Topiramate	U-Citrate ↓	U-pH ↑
Thyroid hormone	U-Calcium ↑	
Corticosteroids	U-Calcium ↑	
Ascorbic acid	U-Oxalate ↑	U-Urate ↑
Salicylates	U-Urate ↑	

When Daudon *et al.* (1995) reported analytical findings in more than 10,000 stones, 0.44 per cent of the stones constituted precipitated pharmacological compounds. Protease inhibitors used in the treatment of patients with HIV infection have a low solubility in urine and crystallization and stone formation accordingly is a common complication. Most reports in the literature are on patients treated with *indinavir*, but there are also other protease inhibitors on the market with similar properties such as *acyclovir*, *ritonavir*, and *saquinavir*. The solubility of these substances increases with increasing acidity of the urine. There is a pronounced risk of precipitation when the urinary concentration of indinavir exceeds 0.3 mg/l.

Other pharmacological compounds that can form precipitates and stones in urine because of limited solubility are: *triamterene*, *sulfadiazine*, *sulfametoxazol*, *cephalexin oxipurinol* (which is the main metabolite of allopurinol), *penicillin*, *oxytetracycline*, *barbiturates*, and *silicate*. There are also some other rare pharmaceutical substances that can be found in stones. For detailed information on these compounds the reader is referred to the original work by Daudon *et al.* (1995).

Intoxication with ethylene glycol leads to an increased excretion of oxalate and calcium oxalate precipitation.

Clinical aspects

An understanding of the mechanisms responsible for or contributing to stone formation in the individual patient is essential for design of an appropriate recurrence preventive treatment. In a great number of patients one or several risk factors can be identified, the elimination or correction of which will be an important part of the clinical management.

As stated above, the risk of stone formation is related to an imbalance between supersaturation, modifiers of the crystallization, and factors that determine crystal–cell interaction. Although with reasonable efforts we can get estimates of the supersaturation or the risk of forming a critically supersaturated urine, it is much more difficult to assess the inhibitory or promoting properties and there are no methods by means of which the *in vivo* interaction between cells and crystals can be assessed (Hess *et al.* 2001).

Because of the variable course of stone disease it is desirable to offer specific recurrence preventive treatment only to those who will benefit from such measures. There are, however, no methods by means of which the further course of the disease reliably can be predicted. It is well recognized that patients who have formed stones composed of uric acid/urate, cystine, and struvite/CarbAp have a high recurrence risk. These patients, therefore, always will benefit from active preventive treatment unless the responsible risk factor or risk factors have been eliminated.

Although an extensive metabolic risk evaluation might give important information in first time as well as recurrent stone formers, it is of major interest to search for risk factors primarily in patients with a severe disease as well as in those who have residual stones or fragments in their kidneys. The patient's age, gender, occupation, and genetic status are important determinants of the risk of stone formation. Also important is the presence of anatomical abnormalities as well as diseases and pharmacological treatment with effects on urine composition and crystallization properties. It has, therefore, been recommended that an analysis of urine composition, in addition to the risk groups mentioned above, should be undertaken in those patients who present with stone formation before the age of 25, or when there is a heavy family history of stone formation. Risk evaluation is also advised in patients with diseases and pharmacological treatment known to be associated with stone formation. The presence of Bru in the stone is another reason for risk evaluation because of the high recurrence risk in these patients. Inasmuch as anatomical abnormalities, which have not been surgically corrected, increase the risk of new stone formation, assessment of metabolic risk factors is motivated in this group as well.

By tradition, stone formers usually are classified according to one or several biochemical abnormalities that have been demonstrated and linked to the disease. Although an isolated abnormality might suggest a specific aetiology, it should be pointed out that one or several abnormalities in urine composition does not necessarily indicate an increased risk of salt precipitation or stone formation. It is the combined effect of all urine constituents as expressed by the level of supersaturation that makes sense (Tiselius 1996; Parks and Coe 1997). This means that the aim of the therapeutic corrections of individual biochemical abnormalities always should be to significantly reduce the risk of forming a urine that is critically supersaturated with the salt.

One important question related to the interpretation of the clinical risk evaluation of patients with calcium stone disease is to what extent there are differences between stone formers and normal subjects.

There are numerous reports in the literature on differences in individual urine variables such as calcium, oxalate, citrate, Mg, phosphate, pH, sodium, potassium, sulfate, urine volume, and crystallization inhibiting or promoting properties. Table 12 gives an example of the average urine composition and crystallization properties in stone formers and normal subjects.

Figure 8 shows the cumulative frequency distributions of the standardized *AP(CaOx)-index*$_s$ in stone formers and normal subjects. There is indeed a considerable overlapping between the two distributions and it is in several respects difficult to decide on the clinical significance of a specific ion-activity product. Most biochemical data are derived from 24-h urine samples or urine samples collected during other defined periods of the day (Tiselius 1997c; Tiselius *et al.* 2001), which only give an average information on urine composition during the whole collection period. Peak values of supersaturation will not be disclosed.

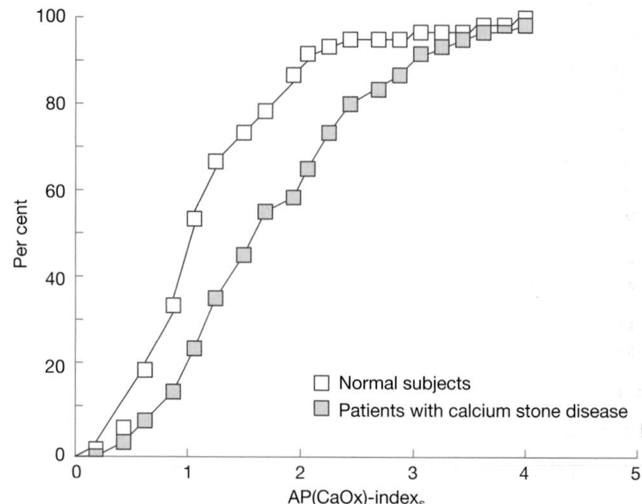

Fig. 8 Cumulative frequency distributions of standardized AP(CaOx)-index in normal subjects and patients with calcium stone disease.

Table 12 Composition of 16-h urine (06.00–22.00) in stone-forming men (SFM), stone-forming women (SFW), normal men (NM), and normal women (NW) (Tiselius 1997c)

Variable	Men, mean (SD)			Women, mean (SD)		
	SFM $n = 102$	NM $n = 51$	p-Value	SFW $n = 51$	NW $n = 50$	p-Value
Calcium, mmol	4.7 (2.5)	3.5 (1.9)	<0.01	4.0 (1.8)	3.1 (1.4)	<0.01
Oxalate, mmol	0.29 (0.10)	0.27 (0.07)	n.s	0.25 (0.09)	0.22 (0.05)	<0.05
Citrate, mmol	1.96 (0.90)	2.18 (1.08)	n.s	2.17 (1.01)	2.63 (0.89)	<0.02
Magnesium, mmol	3.0 (1.2)	3.4 (1.3)	<0.10	2.5 (1.1)	2.8 (1.0)	n.s
Phosphate, mmol	22.5 (7.1)	24 (8)	n.s	17.4 (6.0)	19.0 (5.0)	n.s
Volume, ml	1285 (648)	1054 (448)	<0.05	1135 (498)	1223 (595)	n.s
Ca/Cit	3.08 (3.9)	1.89 (1.26)	<0.05	2.73 (4.4)	1.25 (0.49)	<0.02
AP(CaOx)-index	1.82 (1.56)	1.37 (0.63)	<0.05	1.49 (0.86)	0.95 (0.49)	<0.001
AP(CaOx)-index$_S$	1.99 (1.06)	1.41 (0.83)	<0.05	1.49 (0.80)	0.99 (0.44)	<0.001
AP(CaP)-index$_S$	5.13 (20.5)	49.1 (35.7)	<0.05	44.2 (24.4)	34.2 (17.7)	<0.05
Inhib. CaOx-growth 2% urine	49 (12) $n = 56$	54 (13) $n = 49$	<0.01	55 (13) $n = 28$	47 (10) $n = 38$	n.s
Inh. CaOx-aggr. 3.5% urine	67 (14) $n = 69$	83 (12) $n = 26$	<0.001	63 (12) $n = 30$	78 (13) $n = 22$	<0.007

AP, ion-activity product; Inh, inhibition; Ca, calcium; Cit, citrate.

Table 13 Different parameters reflecting the risk of crystallization in urine of stone formers and normal subjects reported in the literature

Urine variable	Normal subjects	Stone formers	p-Value	Reference
APR[a]	1.45	2.34	<0.001	Pak and Holt (1976)
FPR[b]	11.1	8.71	<0.01	Pak and Holt (1976)
Probability index	0.001–0.34	0.28–0.99	<0.001	Robertson *et al.* (1978)
Discriminant score, men	−0.45	0.48	<0.001	Parks and Coe (1986)
Discriminant score, women	−1.02	1.20	<0.001	Parks and Coe (1986)
Oxalate tolerance high risk	31%	60%	—	Briellman *et al.* (1985)
Calcium oxalate crystallization risk, men	1.13	1.31	<0.05	Tiselius (1996)
Calcium oxalate crystallization risk, women	0.98	1.24	<0.02	Tiselius (1996)
V_{kr} (gel crystallization)[c]	0.47	0.78	<0.01	Achilles and Ulshöfer (1985)
Discrimination index	1.38	0.48	<0.001	Sarig *et al.* (1982)
Bonn risk index	0.94	2.51	—	Laube *et al.* (1999)
Metastable limit	0.33	0.24	<0.001	Walton *et al.* (2000)
Turbidity index	0.023	0.030	<0.01	Walton *et al.* (2000)

[a] Activity product ratio.

[b] Formation product ratio.

[c] Estimate of the rate of crystallization in a gel system.

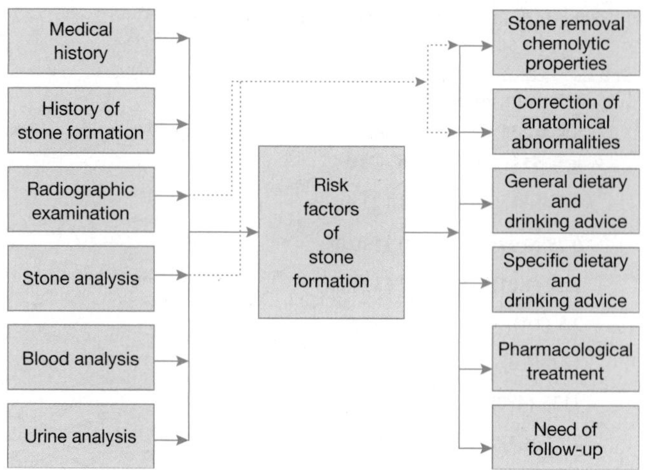

Fig. 9 Overview of diagnostic procedures necessary for identification of risk factors of stone formation and for prediction of the future course of the disease. Based on these findings an individualized clinical management can be designed.

Unfortunately, it has not been definitely established when during the 24-h period the risk of abnormal crystal formation is greatest. Analysis of urine composition has disclosed a great risk of forming a critically supersaturated urine during the late night and early morning hours. There was, however, also high levels of inhibitors at that time of the day. In another study there were indications that certain risk periods might occur during the day as a result of a dietary load and variations in urine flow and pH. Most certainly risk periods differ from one patient to another. Ideally, therefore, the risk of crystallization should be assessed in repeated urine samples during the day in order to identify individual risk periods. Unfortunately, such an approach is not easily accomplished on a large scale partly because of difficulties for the patient to comply with such collection instructions and partly because the sampling procedure probably will alter the normal dietary and drinking habits.

Moreover, the initial steps in the crystallization most certainly very often occur at a nephron level where we have no exact information on the urine composition (Luptak *et al.* 1994; Asplin *et al.* 1996a; Kok 1997; Höjgaard and Tiselius 1999).

Inasmuch as the risk of pathological crystallization apparently depends not only on supersaturation, but also on the crystallization modifying properties, several methods have been developed to assess the combined effect of the driving force of supersaturation and the inhibiting/promoting activity in urine. Such studies have generally demonstrated pronounced differences between stone formers and normal subjects and some of these estimates are summarized in Table 13.

Whatever analytical method that is used it is usually not possible to predict further cause of the disease. But there are some very useful measures. The 10-year recurrence risk obviously was greater in those patients who had a high risk of forming a urine critically supersaturated with calcium oxalate (Tiselius 1999). Another useful predictor was the numbers of stones in the patient's history (Parks and Coe 1994; Strohmaier 2000). Stones composed of calcium oxalate dihydrate have a tendency to recur more frequently than monohydrate stones (Leusmann *et al.* 1995).

For many patients no clues to the stone formation is obtained despite an extensive search for risk factors. Such an outcome most certainly reflects our incomplete understanding of the stone formation or the way that we usually collect and analyse urine.

Despite the obvious shortcomings it is important to emphasize that by addressing the various risk factors obtained by a careful medical history, a radiographic examination as well as an analysis of stone, blood, and urine composition, an effective individualized treatment and/or a follow-up programme can usually be designed (Fig. 9).

Acknowledgement

The expert secretarial assistance by Marie Karlsson is highly appreciated.

References

Achilles, W. and Ulshöfer, B. Die GKV-Messung relativer Kristallwachtumsgeschwindigkeit von Kalziumoxalat in 24-Stunden Sammelurinen von Normalpersonen und Steinträgern mit rezidivierender Kalzium Urolithiasis. In *Pathogenese und Klinik der Harnsteine XI. Fortschritte Urologie und Nephrologie* Vol. 23 (ed. G. Gasser and W. Vahlensieck), pp. 261–266. Dramstadt: Steinkopff, 1985.

Ahlstrand, C. and Tiselius, H. G. (1987). Urine composition and stone formation during treatment with acetazolamide. *Scandinavian Journal of Urology and Nephrology* **21**, 225–228.

Ahlstrand, C., Tiselius, H. G., and Larsson, L. (1984). Studies on crystalluria in calcium oxalate stone formers. *Urolological Research* **12**, 103–106.

Asplin, J. R., Mandel, N. S., and Coe, F. L. (1996a). Evidence for calcium phosphate supersaturation in the loop of Henle. *American Journal of Physiology* **270**, F604–F613.

Asplin, J. R., Hoyer, J., Gillespie, C., and Coe, F. L. Uropontin inhibits aggregation of calcium oxalate monohydrate crystals. In *Urolithiasis 1996* (ed. C. Y. C. Pak, M. Resnick, and G. M. Preminger), pp. 303–304. Dallas: Millet the Printer Inc., 1996b.

Assimos, D. G. and Holmes, R. P. (2000). Role of diet in the therapy of urolithiasis. *Urologic Clinics of North America* **27**, 269–273.

Atmani, F. and Khan, S. R. (2000). Effects of an extract from Herniari hirsuta on calcium oxalate crystallization *in vitro*. *BJU Internationa*l **85**, 621–625.

Atmani, F., Glenton, P. A., and Khan, S. R. (1999). Role of inter-α-inhibitor and its related proteins in experimentally induced calcium oxalate urolithiasis. Localization of proteins and expression of bikunin gene in rat kidney. *Urological Research* **27**, 63–67.

Backman, U. *et al.* (1980). Incidence and clinical importance of renal tubular defects in recurrent renal stone formers. *Nephron* **25**, 96–101.

Baggio, B. and Gambaro, G. (1996). Nutrition and calcium nephrolithiasis: the lipid hypothesis. *Italian Journal of Mineral and Electrolyte Metabolism* **10**, 119–129.

Bhatta, K. M., Prien, E. L., Jr., and Dretler, S. P. Cystine calculi: two types. In *Shock Wave Lithotripsy 2* (ed. J. E. Lingeman and D. M. Newman), pp. 55–59. New York: Plenum Press, 1989.

Baumann, J. M., Ackermann, D., and Affolter, B. (1989). The influence of hydroxyapatite and pyrophosphate on the formation product of calcium oxalate at different pHs. *Urological Research* **17**, 153–155.

Bek-Jensen, H. *et al.* (1996). Is citrate an inhibitor of calcium oxalate crystal growth in high concentrations of urine? *Urological Research* **24**, 67–71.

Berland, Y. and Dussol, B. (1994). New insights into renal stone formation. *Mineral Metabolism* **3**, 417–423.

Bigelow, M. W. *et al.* (1997). Surface exposure of phosphatidylserine increases calcium oxalate crystal attachment. *American Journal of Physiology* **272**, F55–F62.

Binette, J. P. and Binette, M. B. (1993). A cationic protein from a urate–calcium oxalate stone: isolation and purification of a shared protein. *Scanning Microscopy* **7**, 1107–1110.

Binette, J. P. and Binette, M. B. (1994). Sequencing of proteins extracted from stones. *Scanning Microscopy* **8**, 233–239.

Bisceglia, L. *et al.* (2001). Cystinuria type I: identification of eight new mutations in SLC3A1. *Kidney International* **59**, 1250–1256.

Borghi, L. *et al.* (1999). Urine volume: stone risk factor and preventive measure. *Nephron* **81** (Suppl. 1), 31–37.

Borghi, L. *et al.* (2002). Comparison of two diets for the prevention of recurrent stones in idiopathic hyper calciuria. *New England Journal of Medicine* **346**, 77–84.

Boyce, W. H. (1968). Organic matrix of human urinary concretions. *American Journal of Medicine* **45**, 673–683.

Boyce, W. H., King, J., and Fielden, M. (1962). Total non-dialyzable solids (TNDS) in human urine XIII. Immunological detection of a component peculiar to renal calculous matrix and to urine of calculous patients. *Journal of Clinical Investigation* **41**, 1180–1189.

Breslau, N. A. (1994). Pathogenesis and management of hypercalciuric nephrolithiasis. *Mineral and Electrolyte Metabolism* **20**, 328–339.

Briellman, T. *et al.* (1985). The oxalate-tolerace-value: a whole urine method to discriminate between calcium oxalate stone formers and others. *Urological Research* **13**, 291–295.

Buck, A. C. Hypercalciuria in idiopathic calcium oxalate urolithiasis. In *Renal Tract Stone. Metabolic Basis and Clinical Practice* (ed. J. E. A. Wickham and A. C. Buck), pp. 239–251. Edingburgh: Churchill Livingstone, 1990.

Buck, A. C. Is marine oil and evening primrose oil the treatment for nephrolithiasis? In *Renal Stones—Aspects on their Formation, Removal and Prevention. Proceedings of the Sixth Symposium on Urolithiasis* (ed. H. G. Tiselius), pp. 49–57. Stockholm, 1995. Edsbruk: Akademitryck AB, 1996.

Cicerello, E. *et al.* (1994). Effect of alkaline citrate therapy on clearance of residual fragments after extracorporeal shock wave lithotripsy in sterile calcium and infection stone patients. *Journal of Urology* **151**, 5–9.

Cicerello, E. *et al.* In *Urolithiasis 2000* (ed. A. L. Rodgers, B. E. Hibbert, B. Hess, S. R. Khan, and G. M. Preminger), pp. 592–593. Cape Town, South Africa: University of Cape Town, 2000.

Coe, F. L. (1983). Uric acid and calcium oxalate nephrolithiasis. *Kidney International* **24**, 392–403.

Coe, F. L. (1994). Calcium restriction, thiazide, citrate, and allopurinol in calcium oxalate nephrolithiasis. *Acta Urologica Belgica* **62**, 25–29.

Coe, F. L. and Bushinsky, D. A. (1984). The pathophysiology of hypercalciuria. *American Journal of Physiology* **247**, F1–F13.

Coe, F. L. and Kavalach, A. G. (1974). Hypercalciuria and hyperuricosuria in patients with calcium nephrolithiasis. *New England Journal of Medicine* **291**, 1344–1350.

Coe, F. and Parks, J. H. (1990). Defenses of an unstable compromise: crystallization inhibitors and the kidney's role in mineral regulation. *Kidney International* **38**, 625–631.

Coe, F. L., Lawton, R. L., Goldstein, R. B., and Tembe, V. (1975). Sodium urate accelerates precipitation of calcium oxalate *in vitro*. *The Society for Experimental Biology and Medicine* **149**, 926–929.

Coe, F. L., Parks, J. H., and Nakagawa, Y. (1991). Protein inhibitors of crystallization. *Seminars in Nephrology* **11**, 98–109.

Curhan, G. C. (1999). Epidemiologic evidence for the role of oxalate in idiopathic nephrolithiasis. *Journal of Endourology* **13**, 629–631.

Curhan, G. C. and Curhan, S. G. (1997). Diet and urinary stone disease. *Current Opinion in Urology* **7**, 222–225.

Danpure, C. J. (2000). Genetic disorders and urolithiasis. *Urologic Clinics of North America* **27**, 287–299.

Daudon, M. *et al.* (1995). Sex and agerelated composition of 10617 calculi analysed by infrared spectroscopy. *Urological Research* **23**, 319–326.

Dawson, C. J. *et al.* (1998). Inter-α-inhibitor in calcium stones. *Clinical Science* **95**, 187–193.

de Bruijn, W. C. *et al.* (1997). Ultrastructural osteopontin localization in papillary stones induced in rats. *European Urology* **32**, 360–367.

Dent, C. E. and Philpot, G. R. (1954). Xanthinuria: an inborn error of metabolism. *Lancet* **i**, 182.

Dent, C. E. and Friedman, M. (1964). Hypercalciuric rickets associated with renal tubular damage. *Archives of Diseases of Children* **39**, 240.

de Water, R. *et al.* (1999). Calcium oxalate nephrolithiasis: effect of renal crystal deposition on the cellular composition of the renal interstitium. *American Journal of Kidney Diseases* **33**, 761–771.

Dobbins, J. W. and Binder, H. J. (1976). Effect of bile salts and fatty acids on the colonic absorption of oxalate. *Gastroenterology* **70**, 1096–1100.

Dussol, B. *et al.* (1995). Analysis of the soluble matrix of five morphologically different kidney stones. *Urological Research* **23**, 45–51.

Erwin, C.-Y. L. and Nancollas, G. H. (1981). The crystallization and dissolution of sodium urate. *Journal of Crystal Growth* **53**, 215–223.

Ettinger, B. and Kolb, F. O. (1971). Factors involved in crystal formation in cystinuria. *In vivo* and *in vitro* crystallisation dynamics and a simple quantitative colorimetric assay for cystine. *Journal of Urology* **106**, 106–110.

Ettinger, B. *et al.* (1997). Potassium-magnesium citrate is an effective prophylaxis against recurrent calcium oxalate nephrolithiasis. *Journal of Urology* **158**, 2069–2073.

Evans, R. A. *et al.* (1967). Urinary excretion of calcium and magnesium in patients with calcium containing renal stones. *Lancet* **2**, 958–961.

Finlayson, B. (1974). Renal lithiasis in review. *Urologic Clinics of North America* **1**, 181–212.

Finlayson, B. and Reis, S. (1978). The expectation of free and fixed particles in urinary stone disease. *Investigative Urolology* **15**, 442–448.

Fleming, D. E. *et al.* An unexpected role of urinary proteins in the prevention of calcium oxalate urolithiasis. In *Urolithiasis 2000* (ed. A. L. Rodgers, B. E. Hibbert, B. Hess, S. R. Khan, and G. M. Preminger), pp. 169–171. Cape Town, South Africa: University of Cape Town, 2000.

Fliser, D. and Ritz, E. (1999). Störungen des Kazium- und Phosphathaushalts. *Urologe A* **38**, 285–295.

Fraij, B. M. (1989). Separation and identification of urinary proteins and stone-matrix proteins by mini-slab sodium dodecyl sulfate-polyacrylamide gel electrophoresis. *Clinical Chemistry* **35**, 652–662.

Grases, F. *et al.* (1998). Effects of phytic acid on renal stone formation in rats. *Scandinavian Journal of Urology and Nephrology* **32**, 261–265.

Griffith, D. P. and Klein, A. S. Infection-induced urinary stones. In *Stones—Clinical Management of Urolithiasis* (ed. R. A. Roth and B. Finlayson), pp. 210–227. Baltimore: Williams & Wilkins, 1983.

Grover, P. K. and Ryall, R. L. (1994). Urate and calcium oxalate stones: from repute to rhetoric to reality. *Mineral and Electrolyte Metabolism* **20**, 361–370.

Grover, P. K. and Ryall, R. L. Inhibition of calcium oxalate crystal aggregation and growth *in vitro*: a comparison of four human proteins. In *Urolithiasis 1996* (ed. C. Y. C. Pak, M. Resnick, and G. M. Preminger), pp. 271–272. Dallas: Millet the Printer Inc., 1996.

Győry, A. Z. and Ashby, R. (1999). Calcium salt urolithiasis—review of theory for diagnosis and management. *Clinical Nephrology* **51**, 192–208.

Hatch, M. (1993). Oxalate status in stone formers. Two distinct hyperoxaluric entites. *Urological Research* **21**, 55–59.

Hatch, M. *et al.* (1980). Effect of megadoses of ascorbic acid on serum and urinary oxalate. *European Urology* **6**, 166–169.

Herring, L. C. (1962). Observations on the analysis of ten thousand urinary calculi. *Journal of Urology* **88**, 545–562.

Hess, B. (1992). Tamm–Horsfall glycoprotein—inhibitor or promoter of calcium oxalate monohydrate crystallization processes? *Urological Research* **20**, 83–86.

Hess, B. (1994). Tamm–Horsfall glycoprotein and calcium nephrolithiasis. *Mineral and Electrolyte Metabolism* **20**, 393–398.

Hess, B. (1998). Drug-induced urolithiasis. *Current Opinion in Urology* **8**, 331–334.

Hess, B. and Jaeger, P. (1993). The tale of parathyroid function in idiopathic hypercalciuria. *Scanning Microscopy* **7**, 403–408.

Hess, B. *et al.* (1991). Molecular abnormality of Tamm–Horsfall glycoprotein in calcium oxalate nephrolithiasis. *American Journal of Physiology* **260**, F569–F578.

Hess, B., Zipperle, L., and Jaeger, P. (1993). Citrate and calcium effect on Tamm–Horsfall glycoprotein as a modifier of calcium oxalate crystal aggregation. *American Journal of Physiology* **265**, F784–F791.

Hess, B. *et al.* (1994). Risk factors for low urinary citrate in calcium nephrolithiasis: low vegetable fibre intake and low urine volume to be added to the list. *Nephrology, Dialysis, Transplantation* **9**, 642–649.

Hess, B. *et al.* (1995). Renal mass and serum calcitriol in male idiopathic calcium renal stone formers: role of protein intake. *Journal of Clinical Endocrinology and Metabolism* **80**, 1916–1921.

Hess, B. *et al.* (1999). Effects of a 'common sense diet' on urinary composition in patients with idiopathic calcium urolithiasis. *European Urology* **36**, 136–143.

Hess, B. *et al.* (2001). Methods for measuring crystallization in urolithiasis research: why, how and when? *European Urology* **40**, 220–230.

Hesse, A. and Heimbach, D. (1999). Causes of phosphate stone formation and the importance of metaphylaxis by urinary acidification: a review. *World Journal of Urology* **17**, 308–315.

Hesse, A., Tiselius, H. G., and Jahnen, A., ed. *Urinary Stones, Diagnosis, Treatment and Prevention of Recurrence.* Basel: Karger, 1997.

Higashihara, E. *et al.* (1991). Calcium metabolism in acidotic patients induced by carbonic anhydrase inhibitors: responses to citrate. *Journal of Urology* **145**, 942–948.

Höbarth, K. and Hofbauer, J. (1991). Value of routine citrate analysis and calcium/citrate ratio in calcium urolithiasis. *European Urology* **19**, 165–168.

Höjgaard, I. and Tiselius, H. G. (1999). Crystallization in the nephron. *Urological Research* **27**, 397–403.

Holmes, R. P. (1998). Pharmacological approaches in the treatment of primary hyperoxaluria. *Journal of Nephrology* **11** (Suppl. 1), 32–35.

Holmes, R. P., Assimos, D. G., and Goodman, H. O. (1998). Genetic and dietary influences on urinary oxalate excretion. *Urological Research* **26**, 195–200.

Hoppe, B. *et al.* Risk of urolithiasis in cystic fibrosis patients in due to persistent hyperoxaluria. In *Urolithiasis 2000* (ed. A. L. Rodgers, B. E. Hibbert, B. Hess, S. R. Khan, and G. M. Preminger), pp. 474–476. Cape Town, South Africa: University of Cape Town, 2000.

Hoyer, J. R., Otvos, L., and Urge, L. Osteopontin in urinary stone formation. In *Osteopontin. Role in Cell Signalling and Adhesion* Vol. 760 (ed. D. T. Denhart, W. T. Butler, A. F. Chamber, and D. R. Senger), pp. 257–265. New York: Annals New York Academy of Sciences, 1995.

Iguchi, M. *et al.* (1990). Dietary intake and habits of Japanese patients. *Journal of Urology* **143**, 1093–1095.

Iguchi, M. *et al.* (1999). Inhibitory effects of female sex hormones on urinary stone formation in rats. *Kidney International* **56**, 479–485.

Iida, S. *et al.* (1999). Expression of bikunin mRNA in renal epithelial cells after oxalate exposure. *Journal of Urology* **162**, 1480–1486.

International Cystinuria Consortium (1999). Non-type I cystinuria by mutations in SLC7A9, encoding a subunit ($b^{0,+}AT$) of rBAT. *Nature Genetics* **23**, 52–57.

International Cystinuria Consortium: Font, M., Feliubadalo, L., Estivill, X., Bisceglia, L., D'Adamo, A. P., Zelante, L., Gasparini, P., Bassi, M. T., George, A. L., Jr., Manzoni, M., Riboni, M., Ballabio, A., Borsani, G., Reig, N., Fernandez, E., Zorzano, A., Bertran, J., and Palacin, M. (2001). Functional analysis of mutations in SLC7A9 and genotype–phenotype correlation in non-Type I cystinuria. *Human Molecular Genetics* **10**, 305–316.

Jaeger, Ph. (1994). Prevention of recurrent calcium stones: diet versus drugs. *Mineral and Electrolyte Metabolism* **20**, 410–413.

Jaeger, Ph. (1998). Pathophysiology of idiopathic hypercalciuria: the current concept. *Current Opinion in Urology* **8**, 321–325.

Jaeger, Ph. *et al.* (1994). Low bone mass in idiopatic renal stone formers: magnitude and significance. *Journal of Bones Mineral Research* **9**, 1525–1532.

Johansson, G. (1979). Magnesium metabolism. Studies in health, primary hyperparathyroidism and renal stone disease Dissertation. Uppsala, Almqvist & Wiksell, Stockholm.

Kallistratos, G., Timmermann, A., and Fenner, O. (1970). Zum Einfluß des Aussalzeffektes. *Naturwissenschaften* **57**, 198.

Kelley, W. N. *et al.* (1968). Adenine phosphoribosyltransferase deficiency: a previously undescribed genetic defect in man. *Journal of Clinical Investigation* **47**, 2281–2289.

Khan, S. R. (1996). Calcium oxalate crystal interaction with renal epithelium, mechanism of crystal adhesion and its impact on stone development. *Urological Research* **23**, 71–79.

Khan, S. R., Maslamani, S. A., Atmani, F., Glenton, P. A., Opalko, F. J., Thamilselvan, S., and Hammet-Stabler, C. (2000). Membranes and their constituents as promoters of calcium oxalate crystal formation in human urine. *Calcified Tissue International* **66**, 90–96.

Klocke, K. *et al.* Citrate excretion and stone formation: the prevalence of hypocitraturia in stone formers and its dependence on age and sex. In *Urolithiasis* (ed. V. R. Walker, R. A. L. Sutton, E. C. B. Cameron, C. Y. C. Pak, and W. G. Robertson), p. 503. New York: Plenum Press, 1989.

Kok, D. J. (1997). Intratubular crystallisation events. *World Journal of Urolology* **15**, 219–228.

Kok, D. J. and Khan, S. R. (1994). Calcium oxalate nephrolithiasis, a free or fixed particle disease. *Kidney International* **46**, 847–854.

Kok, D. J. *et al.* (1988). Modulation of calcium oxalate monohydrate crystallization kinetics *in vitro*. *Kidney International* **34**, 346–350.

Kok, D. J. *et al.* (1990). *Journal of Clinics of Endocrinology and Metabolism* **71**, 861–867.

Koul, H. *et al.* (1996). Activation of the c-myc gene mediates the mitogenic effects of Ox in LLC-PK1 cells, a line of renal epithelial cells. *Kidney International* **50**, 1525–1530.

Koutsoukos, P. G., Lam-Erwin, C. Y., and Nancollas, G. H. (1980). Epitaxial considerations in urinary stone formation. I. The urate-oxalate-phosphate system. *Investigative Urology* **18**, 178–184.

Laube, N., Schneider, A., and Hesse, A. A new calcium oxalate risk-index? In *Kidney Stones. Proceedings of the 8th European Symposium on Urolithiasis* (ed. L. Borghi, T. Meschi, A. Briganti, T. Schianchi, and A. Novarini), pp. 279–281. Parma. Cosenza: Editoriale Bios, 1999.

Lee, Y. H. *et al.* (1999). The efficacy of potassium citrate based medical prophylaxis for preventing upper urinary tract calculi: a midterm followup study. *Journal of Urology* **161**, 1453–1457.

Lemann, J., Jr. Pathogenesis of idiopathic hypercalciuria and nephrolithiasis. In *Disorders of Bone and Mineral Metabolism* (ed. F. L. Coe and M. J. Favus), pp. 685–706. New York: Raven Press, 1992.

Lerner, S. P., Gleeson, M. J., and Griffith, D. P. (1989). Infection stones. *Journal of Urology* **141**, 753–758.

Leumann, E., Hoppe, B., and Neuhaus, T. (1993). Management of primary hyperoxaluria: efficacy of oral citrate administration. *Pediatric Nephrology* **7**, 207–211.

Leusmann, D. B. *et al.* (1995). Recurrence rates and severity of urinary calculi. *Scandinavian Journal of Urology and Nephrology* **29**, 279–283.

Lieske, J. C. and Coe, F. L. Urinary inhibitors and renal stone formation. In *Kidney Stones—Medical and Surgical Management* (ed. F. L. Coe, M. J. Favus, C. Y .C. Pak, J. H. Parks, and G. M. Preminger), pp. 65–113. Philadelphia: Lippincott-Raven, 1996.

Lieske, J. C. and Deganello, S. (1999). Nucleation, adhesion and internalization of calcium-containing urinary crystals by renal cells. *Journal of American Nephrology Society* **10**, 422–429.

Lieske, J. C., Walsh-Reitz, M. M., and Toback, F. G. (1992). Calcium oxalate monohydrate crystals are endocytosed by renal epithelial cells and induce proliferation. *American Journal of Physiology* **262**, 622–630.

Lieske, J. C., Toback, F. G., and Deganello, S. (1996). Phase-selective adhesion of calcium oxalate dihydrate crystals to renal epithelial cells. *Calcified Tissue International* **58**, 195–200.

Lieske, J. C., Norris, R., Swift, H., and Toback, F. G. (1997a). Adhesion, internalization and metabolism of calcium oxalate monohydrate crystals by renal epithelial cells. *Kidney International* **52**, 1291–1301.

Lieske, J. C., Norris, R., and Toback, F. G. (1997b). Adhesion of hydroxyapatite crystals to anionic sites on the surface of renal epithelial cells. *American Journal of Physiology* **273**, 224–233.

Lieske, J. C. *et al.* (1997c). Renal cell osteopontin production is stimulated by calcium oxalate monohydrate crystals. *Kidney International* **51**, 679–686.

Lieske, J. C., Toback, F. G., and Deganello, S. (1998). Direct nucleation of calcium oxalate dihydrate crystals onto the surface of living renal epithelial cells in culture. *Kidney International* **54**, 796–803.

Lieske, J. C., Deganello, S., and Toback, F. G. (1999). Cell–crystal interactions and kidney stone formation. *Nephron* **81** (Suppl. 1), 8–17.

Lupták, J. *et al.* (1994). Crystallisation of calcium oxalate and calcium phosphate of supersaturation levels corresponding to those in different parts of the nephron. *Scanning Microscopy* **8**, 47–62.

Mandel, N. (1994). Crystal–membrane interaction in kidney stone disease. *Journal of the American Society of Nephrology* **5**, 37–45.

Marangella, M. *et al.* (1999). Idiopathic calcium nephrolithiasis. *Nephron* **81** (Suppl. 1), 38–44.

Marshall, R. W. and Robertson, W. G. (1976). Nomograms for the estimation of the saturation of urine with calcium oxalate, calcium phosphate, magnesium ammonium phosphate, uric acid, sodium acid urate, ammonium acid urate and cystine. *Clinica Chimica Acta* **72**, 253–260.

Masao, T. *et al.* (2000). Fibronectin is a potent inhibitor of calcium oxalate urolithiasis. *Nephron* **164**, 1718–1723.

McLeod, R. S. and Churchill, D. N. (1992). Urolithiasis complicating inflammatory bowel disease. *Journal of Urology* **148**, 974–978.

Médetognon-Benissan, J. *et al.* (1999). Inhibitory effect of bikunin on calcium oxalate crystallisation *in vitro* and urinary decrease in renal stone formers. *Urological Research* **27**, 69–75.

Melick, R. A., Quelch, K. J., and Rhodes, M. (1980). The demonstration of sialic acid in kidney stone matrix. *Clinical Science* **59**, 401–404.

Menon, M. and Mahle, C. J. (1982). Oxalate metabolism and renal calculi. *Journal of Urology* **127**, 148–151.

Menon, M. and Mahle, C. J. (1983). Urinary citrate excretion in patients with renal calculi. *Journal of Urology* **192**, 1158–1168.

Mollerup, C. L., Bollerslev, J., and Blichert-Toft, M. (1994). Primary hyperparathyroidism: incidence and clinical and biochemical characteristics. *European Journal of Surgery* **160**, 485–489.

Morse, R. and Resnick, M. I. (1988). A new approach to the study of urinary macromolecules as a participant in calcium oxalate crystallization. *Journal of Urology* **139**, 869–873.

Nakagawa, Y. *et al.* (1987). Isolation from human calcium oxalate renal stones of nephrocalcin, a glycoprotein inhibitor of calcium oxalate crystal growth. Evidence that nephrocalcin from patients with calcium oxalate nephrolithiasis is deficient in γ-carboxyglutamic acid. *Journal of Clinical Investigation* **79**, 1782–1787.

Nakagawa, Y. *et al.* (2000). Clinical use of cystine supersaturation measurements. *Journal of Urology* **164**, 1481–1485.

Nancollas, G. H. (1983). Crystallization theory relating to urinary stone formation. *World Journal of Urology* **1**, 131–137.

Nicar, M. J. *et al.* (1983). Low urinary citrate excretion in nephrolithiasis. *Urology* **21**, 8–14.

Nishio, S. *et al.* (1985). Matrix glycosaminoglycan in urinary stones. *Journal of Urology* **134**, 503–505.

Pak, C. Y. C. *Urolithiasis-Pathogenesis, Diagnosis and Treatment.* New York: Plenum Medical Book Company, 1978.

Pak, C. Y. C. (1981). The spectrum and pathogenesis of hypercalciuria. *Urologic Clinics of North America* **8**, 245–252.

Pak, C. Y. C. (1994). Citrate and renal calculi: an update. *Mineral and Electrolyte Metabolism* **20**, 371–377.

Pak, C. Y. C. and Holt, K. (1976). Nucleation and growth of brushite and calcium oxalate in urine of stone formers. *Metabolism* **25**, 665–673.

Pak, C. Y. C. and Fuller, C. J. (1983). Assessment of cystine solubility in urine and of heterogeneous nucleation. *Journal of Urology* **129**, 1066–1070.

Pak, C. Y. C., Hayashi, Y., and Arnold, L. H. (1976). Heterogenous nucleation between urate, calcium phosphate and calcium oxalate. *Proceedings of the Society of Experimental Biology and Medicine* **153**, 83–87.

Parkinson, G. M. (1998). Crystal–macromolecule interactions in urolithiasis: lessons from healthy biomineralizations systems. *Current Opinion in Urology* **8**, 301–308.

Parks, J. H. and Coe, F. L. (1986). A urinary calcium-citrate index for the evaluation of nephrolithiasis. *Kidney International* **30**, 85–90.

Parks, J. H. and Coe, F. L. (1994). An increasing number of calcium stone events worsens treatment outcome. *Kidney International* **45**, 1722–1730.

Parks, J. H. and Coe, F. L. (1997). Correspondence between stone composition and urine supersaturation in nephrolithiasis. *Kidney International* **51**, 894–900.

Pattaras, J. G. and Moore, R. G. (1999). Citrate in the management of urolithiasis. *Journal of Endourology* **13**, 687–692.

Peacock, M. and Robertson, W. G. The biochemical aetiology of renal lithiasis. In *Urinary Calculus* (ed. J. E. A. Wickham), pp. 69–95. London: Churchill Livingstone, 1979.

Penney, M. D. and Oleesky, D. A. (1999). Renal tubular acidosis. *Annals of Clinical Biochemistry* **36**, 408–422.

Petersen, T. E., Thørgesen, I., and Petersen, S. E. (1989). Identification of hemoglobin and two serine proteases in acid extracts of calcium containing kidney stones. *Journal of Urology* **142**, 176–180.

Petrarulo, M. *et al.* (1998). Biochemical approach to diagnosis and differentation of primary hyperoxalurias: an update. *Journal of Nephrology* **11** (Suppl. 1), 23–28.

Pillay, S. N., Asplin, J. R., and Coe, F. L. (1998). Evidence that calgranulin is produced by kidney cells and is an inhibitor of calcium oxalate crystallization. *American Journal of Physiology* **275**, F255–F261.

Polito, C. *et al.* (2000). Clinical presentation and natural course of idiopathic hypercalciuria in children. *Pediatric Nephrology* **15**, 211–214.

Polykoff, G. I. and Dretler, S. P. (1993). Ammonium urate calculi: review of 26 cases. *The Journal of Stone Disease* **5**, 208–212.

Preminger, G. M., Sakhaee, K., and Pak, C. Y. C. (1988). Alkali action on the urinary crystallisation of calcium salts: contrasting responses to sodium citrate and potassium citrate. *Journal of Urology* **139**, 240–242.

Roberts, S. D. and Resnick, M. I. (1986). Glycosaminoglycans content of stone matrix. *Journal of Urology* **135**, 1078–1083.

Robertson, W. G. Physical chemical aspects of calcium stone-formation in the urinary tract. In *Urolithiasis Research* (ed. H. Fleisch, W. G. Robertson, L. H. Smith, and W. Vahlensieck), pp. 25–39. New York: Plenum Press, 1976.

Robertson, W. G. (1999). Mild hyperoxaluria: a critical review and future outlook. In *Kidney Stones* (ed. L. Borghi, T. Meschi, A. Briganti, T. Schianchi, and A. Novarini), pp. 33–42. Cosenza, Italy: Editorial Bios, 1999.

Robertson, W. G. and Peacock, M. (1982). The pattern of urinary stone disease in Leeds and in the United Kingdom in relation to animal protein intake during the period 1960–1980. *Urologia Internationalis* **37**, 394–399.

Robertson, W. G., Peacock, M., and Nordin, B. E. C. (1968). Activity products in stone-forming and non-stone-forming urine. *Clinical Science* **34**, 579–594.

Robertson, W. G., Scurr, D. S., and Bridge, C. M. (1981). Factors influencing the crystallization of calcium oxalate in urine—critique. *Journal of Crystal Growth* **53**, 182–194.

Robertson, W. G. *et al.* (1978). Risk factors in calcium stone disease of the urinary tract. *British Journal of Urology* **50**, 449–454.

Robertson, W. G. *et al.* Possible causes of the changing pattern of the age of onset of urinary stone disease in the UK. In *Urolithiasis 2000* (ed. A. L. Rodgers, B. E. Hibbert, B. Hess, S. R. Khan, and G. M. Preminger), pp. 366–368. Cape Town, South Africa: University of Cape Town, 2000.

Rodman, J. S. and Mahler, R. J. (2000). Kidney stones as a manifestation of hypercalcemic disorders. Hyperparathyroidism and sarcoidosis. *Urological Clinics of North America* **27**, 275–285.

Romberg, R. W. *et al.* (1986). Inhibition of hydroxyapatite crystal growth by bone-specific and other calcium-binding proteins. *Biochemistry* **25**, 1176–1180.

Rose, G. A. and Sulaiman, S. (1982). Tamm–Horsfall mucoproteins promote calcium oxalate crystal formation in urine: quantitative studies. *Journal of Urology* **127**, 177–179.

Rossiter, B. J. and Caskey, C. T. Hypoxanthine-guanine phosphoribosyltransferase deficiency: Lesch Nyhan syndrome and gout. In *The Metabolic and Molecular Bases of Inherited Disease* (ed. C. R. Scriver, A. Beaudet, and W. S. Sly), p. 1679. New York: McGraw-Hill, 1995.

Ryall, R. L. (1996). Glycosaminoglycans, proteins and stone formation: adult themes and child's play. *Pediatric Nephrology* **10**, 656–666.

Ryall, R. L. (1997). Urinary inhibitors of calcium oxalate crystallization and their potential role in stone formation. *World Journal of Urology* **15**, 155–164.

Ryall, R. L. *et al.* (2000). The hole truth: intracrystalline proteins and calcium oxalate kidney stones. *Molecular Urology* **4**, 391–402.

Sarig, S. *et al.* (1982). A method for discrimination between calcium oxalate kidney stone formers and normals. *Journal of Urology* **128**, 645–649.

Scheid, C. R. *et al.* (1996). Ox toxicity in LLC-PK1 cells: role of free radicals. *Kidney International* **49**, 413–419.

Schwille, P. O. (1985). Urolithiasis research—where is it going? *Urological Research* **13**, 157–159.

Schwille, P. O. *et al.* (1988). Urinary pyrophosphate in patients with recurrent calcium urolithiasis and in healthy controls: a re-evaluation. *Journal of Urology* **140**, 239–245.

Schwille, P. O. *et al.* (2001). Calcium oxalate crystallization in undiluted postprandial urine of healthy male volunteers as influenced by citrate. *Arzneimittel Forschung, Drug Research* **51**, 848–857.

Scurr, D. C. and Robertson, W. G. (1986). Modifiers of calcium oxalate crystalliszation found in urine. III. Studies on the role of Tamm–Horsfall mucoprotein and of ion-stength. *Journal of Urology* **136**, 505–507.

Sharma, S. *et al.* (1992). Urinary excretion of inorganic pyrophosphate by normal subjects and patients with renal calculi in North-Western India and the effect of diclofenac sodium upon urinary excretion of pyrophosphate in stone formers. *Urologia Internationalis* **48**, 404–408.

Shiraga, H. *et al.* (1992). Inhibition of calcium oxalate crystal growth *in vitro* by uropontin: another member of the aspartic acid-rich protein superfamily. *Proceedings of the National Academy of Science* **89**, 426–430.

Siddiqiu, A. A. *et al.* (1999). Isolation of low molecular mass proteins from renal stones. *Bichemical Society Transactions* **18**, 1256–1257.

Sidhu, H. *et al.* Clinical significance of Oxalobacter formigenes: colonization studies in patients with cystic fibrosis, inflammatory bowel disease and calciumoxalate urolithiasis. In *Urolithiasis 2000* (ed. A. L. Rodgers, B. E. Hibbert, B. Hess, S. R. Khan, and G. M. Preminger), pp. 468–473. Cape Town, South Africa: University of Cape Town, 2000.

Silverberg, S. J. *et al.* (1990). Nephrolithiasis and bone involvement in primary hyperparathyroidism. *American Journal of Medicine* **89**, 327–334.

Smith, L. H. (1974). Medical evaluation of urolithiasis: etiologic aspects and diagnostic evaluation. *Urologic Clinics of North America* **1**, 241–260.

Smith, L. H. and Werness, P. G. (1983). Hydroxyapatite—the forgotten crystal in calcium urolithiasis. *Transactions of the American Clinical Association* **95**, 183–190.

Sorensen, S., Justesen, S. J., and Johnsen, A. H. (1995). Identification of a macromolecular crystal growth inhibitor in human urine as osteopontin. *Urological Research* **23**, 327–334.

Sorokina, E. A. and Kleinman, J. G. (1999). Cloning and preliminary characterization of a calcium-binding protein closelyrelated to nucleolin on the apical surface of inner medullary collecting duct cells. *Journal of Biological Chemistry* **274**, 27492–27496.

Sperling, O. Uric acid nephrolithiasis. In *Renal Tract Stone—Metabolic Basis and Clinical Practice* (ed. J. E. A. Wickham and A. C. Buck), pp. 349–365. Edinburgh: Churchill Livingstone, 1990.

Stapleton, A. M. F. *et al.* (1996). Further evidence linking urolithiasis and blood coagulation: urinary prothrombin fragment 1 is present in stone matrix. *Kidney International* **49**, 880–888.

Strohmaier, W. L. (2000). Course of calcium stone disease without treatment. What can we expect? *European Urology* **37**, 339–344.

Suzuki, M. *et al.* (2001). Excretion of bikunin and its fragments in the urine of patients with renal stones. *Journal of Urology* **166**, 268–274.

Thamilselvan, S. and Khan, S. R. (1998). Oxalate and calcium oxalate crystals are injurious to renal epithelial cells: results of *in vivo* and *in vitro* studies. *Journal of Nephrology* **11** (Suppl. I), 66–69.

Tiselius, H. G. (1981). The effect on pH on the urinary inhibition of calcium oxalate crystal growth. *British Journal of Urology* **53**, 470–474.

Tiselius, H. G. (1982). An improved method for the routine biochemical evaluation of patients with recurrent calcium oxalate stone disease. *Clinica Chimica Acta* **122**, 409–418.

Tiselius, H. G. (1984a). A simplified estimate of the ion-activity product of calcium phosphate in urine. *European Urology* **10**, 191–195.

Tiselius, H. G. (1984b). Effects of sodium urate and uric acid crystals on the crystallization of calcium oxalate. *Urological Research* **12**, 11–15.

Tiselius, H. G. Urinary pH and calcium oxalate crystallization. In *Pathogenese und Klinik der Harnsteine. Fortschritte der Urologie und Nephrologie* (ed. W. Vahlensieck and G. Gasser), pp. 184–187. Darmstadt: Steinkopff, 1984c.

Tiselius, H. G. (1989). Standardized estimate of the ion-activity product of calcium oxalate in urine from renal stone formers. *European Urology* **16**, 48–58.

Tiselius, H. G. Solution chemistry of supersaturation. In *Kidney Stones—Medical and Surgical Management* (ed. F. L. Coe, M. J. Flavus, C. Y. C. Pak, J. H. Parks, and G. M. Preminger), pp. 33–64. Philadelphia: Lippincott-Raven Publishers, 1996.

Tiselius, H. G. (1997a). Macromolecular substances—their role in urolithiasis. *Current Opinion in Urology* **7**, 234–239.

Tiselius, H. G. (1997b). Estimated levels of supersaturation with calcium phosphate and calcium oxalate in the distal tubule. *Urological Research* **25**, 153–159.

Tiselius, H. G. (1997c). Metabolic evaluation of patients with stone disease. *Urologia Internationalis* **59**, 131–141.

Tiselius, H. G. (1999). Factors influencing the course of calcium oxalate stone disease. *European Urology* **36**, 363–370.

Tiselius, H. G. (2000). Stone incidence and prevention. *Brazilian Journal of Urology* **26**, 452–462.

Tiselius, H. G. and members of the Advisory Board of Urolithiasis and the HCO Working Party of Lithiasis (2001). Possibilities for preventing recurrent calcium stone formation: principles for the metabolic evaluation of patients with calcium stone disease. *BJU International* **88**, 158–168.

Tiselius, H. G. *et al.* (1993). Effects of citrate on the different phases of calcium oxalate crystallisation. *Scanning Microscopy* **7**, 381–389.

Tiselius, H. G. *et al.* Is calcium phosphate the natural promoter of calcium oxalate crystallization. In *Urolithiasis 2000* (ed. C. Y. C. Pak, M. I. Resnick, and G. M. Preminger). Dallas: Millet the Printer Inc., 1996.

Tiselius, H. G. *et al.* (1999). Minimally invasive treatment of infection staghorn stones with shock wave lithotripsy and chemolysis. *Scandinavian Journal of Urology and Nephrology* **33**, 286–290.

Tiselius, H. G. *et al.* (2002). Stone disease: diagnosis and medical management. *European Urology* **76**, 1–9.

Traxer, O. *et al.* (2001). Risk of calcium oxalate stone formation with ascorbic acid ingestion. Abstract 1001. *Journal of Urology* **165**, 243.

Trinchieri, A. *et al.* (1991). The influence of diet on urinary risk factors in healthy subjects and idiopathic renal stone formers. *British Journal of Urology* **67**, 230–236.

Trinchieri, A. *et al.* (1998). Hyperoxaluria in patients with idiopathic calcium nephrolithiasis. *Journal of Nephrology* **11** (Suppl. 1), 70–72.

Umekawa, T. and Kurita, T. (1994). Calprotetin-like protein is related to soluble organic matrix in calcium oxalate urinary stone. *Biochemistry and Molecular Biology International* **34**, 309–313.

Umekawa, T., Kohri, K., Amasaki, N., Yamate, T., Yoshida, K., Yamamoto, K., Suzuki, Y., Sinohara, H., and Kurita, T. (1993). Sequencing of urinary stone protein identical to α1-antitrypsin. *Biochemical Biophysical Research Communications* **193**, 1049–1053.

von Unruh, G. E., Voss, S., and Hesse, A. Oxalate absorption, variability and modification. In *Urolithiasis 2000* (ed. A. L. Rodgers, B. E. Hibbert, B. Hess, S. R. Khan, and G. M. Preminger), pp. 461–463. Cape Town, South Africa: University of Cape Town, 2000.

Verkoelen, C. F. *et al.* (1995). Association of calcium oxalate monohydrate crystals with MDCK cells. *Kidney International* **48**, 129–138.

Verkoelen, C. F. *et al.* (1997). Cell cultures and nephrolithiasis. *World Journal of Urology* **157**, 376–383.

Wall, I. and Tiselius, H. G. (1990). Studies on the crystallisation of magnesium ammonium phosphate in urine. *Urological Research* **18**, 401–406.

Walton, R. C. *et al.* Chemical analysis and crystallisation properties of urine samples from stone formers and controls. In *Urolithiasis 2000* (ed. A. L. Rodgers, B. E. Hibbert, B. Hess, S. R. Khan, and G. M. Preminger), pp. 60–62. Cape Town, South Africa: University of Cape Town, 2000.

Werness, P. G. *et al.* (1985). EQUIL2: a basic computer program for the calculation of urinary saturation. *Journal of Urology* **134**, 1242–1244.

Whalley, N. A. *et al.* (1996). Long-term effects of potassium citrate therapy on the formation of new stones in groups of recurrent stone formers with hypocitraturia. *British Journal of Urology* **78**, 10–14.

Yoshioka, T. *et al.* (1989). Possible role of Tamm–Horsfall glycoprotein in calcium oxalate crystallization. *British Journal of Urology* **64**, 463–467.

Zanchetta, J. R. *et al.* (1996). Bone mineral density in patients with hypercalciuric nephrolithiasis. *Nephron* **73**, 557–560.

Zerwekh, J. E., Holt, K., and Pak, C. Y. C. (1983). Natural urinary macromolecular inhibitors: attenuation of inhibitory activity by urate salts. *Kidney International* **23**, 838–841.

Zoref, E., de Vries, A., and Sperling, O. (1997). Evidence for z-linkage of phosporibosylpyrophosphate synthetase in man: studies with cultured fibroblasts from a gouty family with mutant feedbackresistent enzyme. *Human Heredity* **27**, 73.

Appendices

Appendix 1 Principles of crystallization

In water as well as in urine, a salt AB is dissociated with release of the ions A^+ and B^-, whereby an equilibrium is established:

$$AB \leftrightharpoons A^+ + B^-$$

The ion-activity product of AB is defined as follows:

$$AP_{AB} = f_1 \cdot C_{A^+} \cdot f_1 \cdot C_{B^-}$$

where f_1 is the activity coefficient for monovalent ions and C_{A^+} and C_{B^-} the free ion concentrations of A^+ and B^-.

The activity coefficient f_z for any ion is determined by the charge of that ion (Z) and the ion strength (I):

$$f_z = \exp\left[-1.202Z^2\left(\frac{\sqrt{I}}{1+\sqrt{I}} - 0.285I\right)\right]$$

The ion strength in a solution is derived as follows, in which formula C_i is the concentration and Z_i the charge of the ion i:

$$I = 0.5\sum_{i=l}^{n} C_i Z_i^2$$

The activity coefficients for ions with charges of 1, 2, and 3, in urine with an average composition, are approximately 0.7, 0.3, and 0.06 respectively (Tiselius 1996).

The general expression of the ion-activity product of a salt A_nB_m with this equilibrium:

$$A_nB_m \leftrightharpoons nA^{x+} + mB^{y-}$$

takes the following form:

$$AP_{AB} = [f_x]^n \cdot [A^{x+}]^n \cdot [f_y]^m \cdot [B^{y-}]^m$$

The ion-activity product of calcium oxalate (AP_{CaOx}) accordingly is expressed as follows:

$$AP_{CaOx} = \lfloor C_{Ca^{2+}} \rfloor \cdot f_2 \cdot \lfloor C_{Ox^{2-}} \rfloor \cdot f_2$$

and that of HAP ($Ca_5(PO_4)_3OH$; AP_{HAP}):

$$AP_{HAP} = [C_{Ca^{2+}}]^5 \cdot [f_2]^5 \cdot [C_{OH^-}] \cdot f_1 \cdot \lfloor C_{PO_4^{3-}} \rfloor^3 \cdot [f_3]^3$$

As long as there is only one salt to consider in the solution it is fairly easy to calculate the ion-activity product. In solutions with a large number of ions, such as urine, numerous complexes are formed, the concentrations of which have to be known in order to derive the free-ion concentrations. Inasmuch as we lack methods to assess the free concentrations of most of the ions that are relevant for the stone forming process, computerized programs based on iterative approximation have been developed (Robertson *et al.* 1968; Werness *et al.* 1985). The total concentrations of each important ion provide the basis for computing the approximate concentrations of theoretically possible ion complexes. The concentration of an ion complex is determined by its stability constant ($K_{stability}$). For a complex AD^{2-} formed by a combination of the ions A^+ and D^{3-} the $K_{stability}$ is defined as follows:

$$K_{stability} = \frac{C_{AD^{2-}} \cdot f_2}{[C_{A^+} \cdot f_1] \cdot [C_{D^{3-}} \cdot f_3]}$$

For complexes that are electroneutral the activity coefficient is 1.0.

Appendix 2 Basic physical–chemical principles of crystallization

To precipitate any salt, the urine has to be sufficiently supersaturated. From a physical–chemical point of view it is the actual ion-activity product (AP) that determines the level of supersaturation with a salt.

For each salt a SP is defined as the ion-activity product below which the energy is too low to cause precipitation or growth of crystals. The solution is saturated with the solid phase. The level of supersaturation for the salt AB is expressed as the ratio between the actual AP_{AB} and SP_{AB}:

$$\text{Supersaturation} = \frac{AP_{AB}}{SP_{AB}}$$

For values greater than 1 there is a state of real supersaturation and less than 1, the urine (or the solution) is undersaturated.

The different levels of saturation relevant to urine is depicted in Fig. 10. At an AP below SP any salt should theoretically be dissolved. Although such a dissolution under physiological conditions might be very slow and usually insignificant for salts such as calcium oxalate, there is absolutely no chance for crystal formation (nucleation) in the under-saturated solution.

The formation product FP is defined as the ion-AP above which crystals can form. Crystallization thereby can be induced by facilitating factors (promoters) or occur spontaneously. In the first case we have a heterogeneous nucleation ($FP_{heterogeneous}$) and in the latter case

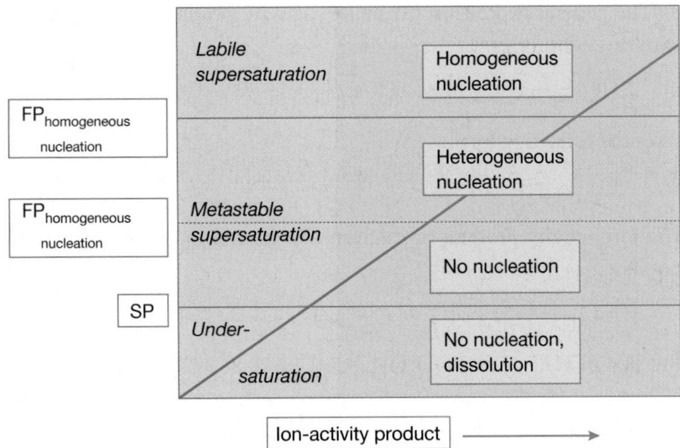

Fig. 10 Diagram showing the relationship between the ion-activity product and the different levels of saturation. Formation product (FP) and solubility product (SP).

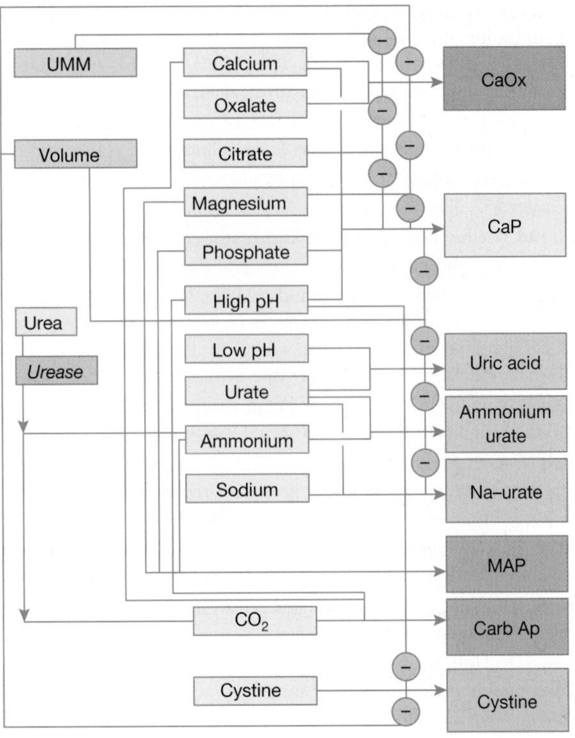

Fig. 11 Major determinants for the formation of various types of stone. Calcium oxalate (CaOx), calcium phosphate (CaP), sodium urate (Na–urate), magnesium ammonium phosphate (MAP), carbonate apatite (Carb Ap), and urinary macromolecules (UMM). The *minus* signs indicate inhibitory activity.

a homogenous nucleation ($FP_{homogeneous}$). Above $FP_{homogeneous}$ the urine has a labile state of supersaturation, which means that the energy is sufficient to create a new crystal. The interval between SP and $FP_{homogeneous}$ is termed the metastable range of supersaturation. Although promoters can bring about a heterogeneous nucleation within this range, the energy of the supersaturation is too low for spontaneous crystal formation. Any crystals that is present can, however, grow as long as AP exceeds SP. There are several inhibitors of crystallization that counteract crystal growth and crystal nucleation. Thus, the level of $FP_{heterogeneous}$ can be increased by inhibitors and decreased by promoters.

Important determinants of common stone constituents

As stated above, no salt will be precipitated unless the urine is sufficiently supersaturated with that salt. The most important determinants for the various types of stone are summarized in Fig. 11.

The prerequisites for precipitation of uric acid are fulfilled when the ion-activity product of the salt exceeds 5.0×10^{-9} $(mol/l)^2$, which is the formation product. This condition is met at a low pH in urine with or without a high concentration of urate (Sperling 1990). An estimate of the ion-activity product of uric acid (AP_{H_2U}) can be obtained with the formula below (Marshall and Robertson 1976; Tiselius 1996):

$$AP_{H_2U} = \frac{C_{Urate} \cdot 10^{-pH} \cdot 0.53}{(1 + 1.63 \cdot 10^5 \cdot 10^{-pH})}$$

At a pH in the range between 6 and 7 and in the presence of high concentrations of urate and NH_4, the preferred precipitate will be ammonium urate (Marshall and Robertson 1976; Tiselius 1996). The formation product of ammonium urate is 7.2×10^{-4} $(mol/l)^2$ and the ion-activity product of ammonium urate (AP_{NH_4HU}) can be calculated accordingly:

$$AP_{NH_4HU} = \frac{C_{Urate} \cdot C_{Ammonium} \cdot 0.53}{(1 + 1.63 \cdot 10^5 \cdot 10^{-pH})}$$

Stones composed of sodium urate are occasionally formed, but only when the concentrations of both sodium (Na) and urate are high (Marshall and Robertson 1976; Erwin and Nancollas 1981). The ion-activity product of sodium urate (AP_{NaHU}) is derived with this formula and the formation product has been estimated to be 1.3×10^{-3} $(mol/l)^2$:

$$AP_{NaHU} = \frac{C_{Urate} \cdot C_{Na} \cdot 0.53}{(1 + 1.63 \cdot 10^5 \cdot 10^{-pH})}$$

Infection stones are composed of MAP (struvite) and CarbAp, frequently also with some admixture of HAP (Griffith and Klein 1983; Wall and Tiselius 1990). The prerequisites for this kind of precipitation are high concentrations of NH_4 and carbonate ions as well as a high pH. These alterations in urine composition emerge as a result of infection with urease-producing microorganisms (see section on Infection stones). The ion-activity product of magnesium ammonium phosphate (AP_{MAP}) in a 24-h urine sample can approximately be estimated from the excretion of Mg, NH_4, PO_4, urine volume, and pH according to this formula, in which the volume is expressed in litres and the other urine constituents in mmol excreted during the collection period (Robertson *et al.* 1968; Wall and Tiselius 1990):

$$AP(MAP)\text{-index} = \frac{3.8 \cdot 10^{-4} \cdot Mg^{1.06} \cdot NH_4^{0.98} \cdot PO_4^{0.71} \cdot (pH - 4.5)^{6.3}}{Volume^{2.3}}$$

The formation product of MAP is approximately 2.5×10^{-13} $(mol/l)^3$ (Robertson *et al.* 1968).

Stones composed of cystine can only be produced in urine with an excessively high concentration of cystine. This prerequisite is encountered in patients with homozygous cystinuria. The formation product of cystine is 1.3×10^{-20} $(mol/l)^3$ and an estimate of the ion-activity product of cystine ($AP_{Cystine}$) can be obtained as follows:

$$AP_{Cystine} = \frac{(10^{-pH}) \cdot C_{Cystine} \cdot 0.155}{[1 + (0.39 \cdot 10^{10} \cdot 10^{-pH}) + ((10^{-pH})^2 \cdot 3.51 \cdot 10^{16})]}$$

Calcium phosphate occurs in stones in several different forms: OCP, HAP, Bru, whitlockite, and CarbAp. The first product that precipitates is an ACP, which subsequently is converted to the crystal phases OCP and HAP or occasionally Bru. Calculation of the ion-activity products of the various calcium phosphates can be made with computerized iterative approximation as described above, using all the important urine ions in order to estimate concentrations of the numerous complexes that might form (Werness *et al.* 1985). The ion-activity product of the calcium and the PO_4 ions thereby can be used to reflect indirectly the supersaturation with the various calcium phosphate crystal phases:

$$AP_{CaP} = \lfloor C_{Ca^{2+}} \rfloor \cdot f_2 \cdot \lfloor C_{PO_4{}^{3-}} \rfloor \cdot f_3$$

An extensive analysis of the urine composition is, however, required to calculate this parameter but a simplified estimate of the ion-activity product of calcium phosphate [AP(CaP)-index] can be obtained with an expression based only on the excretion of calcium, PO_4, citrate, the pH, and the urine volume (Tiselius 1984a). The formula below is valid for an AP(CaP)-index in a 24-h urine sample:

$$\text{AP(CaP)-index} = \frac{2.7 \cdot 10^{-3} \cdot \text{Calcium}^{1.07} \cdot \text{Phosphate}^{0.70} \cdot (\text{pH} - 4.5)^{6.8}}{\text{Citrate}^{0.20} \cdot \text{Volume}^{1.31}}$$

The two crystal phases in calcium oxalate stones are the monohydrate and the dihydrate. The crystal phase that first precipitates is calcium oxalate trihydrate (COT), but this salt is thermodynamically labile and therefore rapidly converts to COD. The formation product of calcium oxalate is so high that an ion-activity product at that level never can be expected physiologically. For calcium oxalate, we therefore have to consider a heterogeneous nucleation in the metastable range of supersaturation, that, is in the saturation range between SP and $FP_{homogeneous}$ (Fig. 10). Inasmuch as there are various promoters with the capacity to induce the precipitation of calcium oxalate, it is not possible to define an exact level of $FP_{heterogeneous}$, but it is assumed that the precipitation can occur at an ion-activity product between 1.5 and 2.8×10^{-8} $(mol/l)^2$ (Robertson *et al.* 1968; Höjgaard and Tiselius 1999).

Calculation of the ion-activity product of calcium oxalate is as complicated as that for calcium phosphate. It has been shown, however, that the most important determinants of this ion-activity product are the concentrations of oxalate, calcium, citrate, magnesium, and urine volume (Finlayson 1974; Robertson *et al.* 1981; Tiselius 1982). A simplified estimate of the ion-activity product of calcium oxalate [AP(CaOx)-index] based on all these variables is in good agreement with the ion-activity product obtained by computed iterative approximation (Werness *et al.* 1985; Tiselius 1996). The formula for AP(CaOx)-index in a 24-h urine sample is given below:

$$\text{AP(CaOx)-index} = \frac{1.9 \cdot \text{Calcium}^{0.84} \cdot \text{Oxalate}}{\text{Citrate}^{0.21} \cdot \text{Magnesium}^{0.12} \cdot \text{Volume}^{1.03}}$$

8.2 The medical management of stone disease

David S. Goldfarb and Fredric L. Coe

Introduction

The medical management of stone disease offers nephrologists and internists the opportunity to take care of a younger and healthier population than they might be used to seeing. It requires a broad knowledge of renal physiology, endocrinology, nutrition, and pharmacology. When successful, it will offer the gratifying experience of preventing much suffering, besides saving considerable expense and inconvenience. The amazing advances in the urological care of stone disease seen in the last 20 years have in no way reduced the pressing need for stone prevention among the sizeable proportion of the population that will have at least one stone or more in their lifetimes. Instead, a strategy of metabolic evaluation and treatment has been shown to be highly effective and leads to a significant cost savings (Parks and Coe 1996). Despite its efficacy, our impression is that stone prevention remains highly underutilized, with many patients never having appropriate consultations, and many nephrologists therefore remaining relatively inexperienced. We hope here to encourage the practice of stone prevention by reviewing what has and what has not been shown to be effective.

Evaluation of stone formers

Recommendations regarding the clinical evaluation of patients presenting with nephrolithiasis have evolved relatively little in the years between two sets of guidelines on this subject (National Institutes of Health Consensus Development Conference on Prevention and Treatment of Kidney Stones 1989; Tiselius *et al.* 2001). An appropriate history requires review of possible inciting factors. A family history of renal disease or stones might suggest polycystic kidney disease, renal tubular acidosis (RTA), medullary sponge kidney, or hyperparathyroidism associated with the multiple endocrine neoplasia syndromes. Extrarenal fluid losses reduce urine volume in patients who live or work in hot climates, who are physically active, and who have excessive gastrointestinal losses of water. A detailed medication list, including non-prescription drugs, vitamins, and herbal preparations, should be elicited. Higher rates of stone formation are associated with excessive ingestion of salt, animal protein, and oxalate-containing plant products, while diets higher in calcium content decrease stone risk. The physical examination rarely leads to diagnostic clues in stone disease and should be applied selectively.

Distinctions are often drawn between appropriate evaluations for patients presenting with their first stone, versus those whose stones have recurred. In all cases, laboratory testing should consist of the diagnostic tests listed in Table 1. The emphasis is on finding evidence of systemic diseases that may have long-term sequelae, such as renal tubular acidosis, hyperparathyroidism, sarcoidosis, or renal parenchymal disease. Stone analysis is always appropriate, even for recurrent stones, and should be performed only by labs specializing in determining stone composition either by X-ray crystallography or infrared spectroscopy, both of which are very reliable and inexpensive. Radio-opaque stones on plain radiography can be composed of calcium oxalate or phosphate, struvite, mixed uric acid and calcium oxalate; cystine stones are variably radio-opaque. Radiolucent stones visualized by computed tomography (CT) ultrasound, but not plain radiography, or seen as filling defects in studies using intravenous contrast, are most often composed of uric acid. Radiological imaging is performed to determine the presence of residual stones, to establish a baseline for surveillance, and to look for urological abnormalities. Helical or spiral CT is fast becoming the imaging modality of choice; it is quicker than intravenous pyelography and safer as it requires no radiocontrast. These features contribute to its declining cost.

The major difference between new stone formers and those with recurrent stones is the utility of the patient performing 24-h urine collections for analysis of urinary risk factors for stone formation. First-time stone formers, particularly young people, include many who will not have another stone for many years, and they may lack motivation to change habits of fluid intake and diet, or to take medications. Such patients should at least be informed of the relatively high mean rate of recurrence, estimated to be up to 30 per cent at 5 years, 50 per cent at 10 years, and 80 per cent at 20 years (Asplin and Chandhoke 1996). On the other hand, first-time stone formers also include patients whose stones did not simply pass spontaneously in the emergency department, but instead led to harrowing ordeals and urological interventions, whose motivations to prevent recurrence are strong. Other patients in whom initial evaluation might reasonably include 24-h urine collections include the elderly, whose risk of complications is increased while their tolerance declines, patients with a solitary kidney, with recurrent urinary tract infections or sepsis, those requiring urological intervention, and those with bowel disease, nephrocalcinosis, or RTA. For these patients, and for those with recurrent stones, current guidelines recommend diagnosis and treatment based on 24-h urine collections. Currently we recommend the patient provide two 'pretreatment' collections on their usual diet, and repeat this once after weeks of adhering to prescribed regimens, and then at yearly intervals. The standard measurements are of volume, pH, calcium, oxalate, citrate, sodium, creatinine, uric acid, potassium, magnesium, and phosphorus. Other urinary analytes sometimes reported are urea nitrogen and sulfate, both of which can be used to calculate the protein ingestion. All of these values can be used together calculate the relative supersaturation of the relevant stone-forming molecules.

Table 1 Diagnostic testing for nephrolithiasis

Test	Relevant conditions
Serum HCO_3 concentration	Low in distal RTA
Serum potassium concentration	Hypokalaemia seen in distal RTA; baseline for treatment with thiazides and potassium citrate
Serum Ca, ionized Ca concentrations	Hypercalcaemia suggests hyperparathyroidism, sarcoidosis
Serum PTH, intact	High values in parathyroidism
Serum creatinine concentration	High in renal parenchymal disease, more stones, more procedures, obstruction
Serum uric acid concentration	Hyperuricaemia seen in gout
Urine pH	$\leq$5.5 conducive to uric acid stones $\geq$6.5 suggestive of RTA $\geq$7.5 suggestive of infection, struvite stones
Urinalysis	Detect infection
Stone analysis	Correlates with pathophysiology
Cystine screen (if no stone analysis)	Cystinuria
24-h urine collections (usually reserved for recurrent or large stones)	To determine individual risk factors in selected patients

There are several advantages of having these values. They correlate well with stone composition and therefore appear to accurately reflect the underlying pathophysiology (Parks *et al.* 1997). They demonstrably improve with treatment and neatly summarize the net effects of changes in various urinary and stone constituents (Lingeman *et al.* 1998). Finally, the supersaturation is a simple number that can be used to educate and motivate the patient regarding the goals of therapy, much as contemporary patients are aware of their blood pressure, cholesterol, and prostate specific antigen values. Clinicians and patients waiting years to determine the efficacy of therapy can use the decline in supersaturation as a short-term surrogate.

The interpretation of urine testing is not entirely straightforward. Normal values vary among laboratories, and there is significant overlap seen between stone formers and non-stone-formers, so that they are not easily distinguished. Definitions of hypercalciuria and hypocitraturia, among others, are in flux and expressing results as absolute amounts, concentrations, and values normalized for body weight or creatinine excretion are competing strategies. Altering urinary variables that appear to be in the normal range in order to effect lower supersaturations is a sensible approach. Furthermore, many putative inhibitors and promoters of crystallization implicated in the clinical condition of nephrolithiasis have been studied, but their presence or absence is not routinely ascertained due to limitations of money, time, and a lack of ability to manipulate these factors in patients. We are limited in looking at and treating only the more easily measured and tested variables.

With these provisos in mind, further diagnostic considerations will arise and rational therapy can proceed from the results of serum testing and 24-h urine collections. An attempt to summarize some of what follows in the discussion of individual stone types is depicted in Fig. 1.

Calcium oxalate stones

The medical management of calcium stones continues to be controversial because of uncertainties regarding the aetiology of hypercalciuria, a common risk factor identified in patients with calcium stones. The attractive notion that identifying the source of the calcium in the urine (whether absorptive, resorptive, or due to failed renal reabsorption; see Chapter 8.1) would lead to specific therapies has not proved true. Both epidemiological studies and a randomized controlled trial confirm that restriction of calcium is ineffective for stone prevention, while thiazides are effective in the bulk of hypercalciuric patients, not solely those with renal leak hypercalciuria. Even patients with a component of absorptive hypercalciuria were, after therapy with low-calcium diets, in negative calcium balance, implying loss of bone mineral density. The understanding that has arisen in recent years then does not require specialized testing to determine the aetiology of hypercalciuria. This significantly simplifies the evaluation of calcium stone formers as detailed above, and reduces the therapeutic options to those best shown to be effective in the ultimate goal, that of stone prevention. We emphasize here, where available, the results of the relatively scarce randomized controlled trials in the field.

Fluids

Increasing urine volume for calcium stone prevention is a concept that patients intuitively understand. This therapy is critical not only to patients with hypercalciuria, but also to patients with other urinary risk factors, and to patients who are not classified. The decrease in supersaturation of calcium oxalate, calcium phosphate, and all other stone-forming salts that occurs with an increase in volume is continuous, but the steepest decrease occurs with volumes up to about 2–2.5 l, at which point further increases in volume will have progressively smaller effects and become less practical. Achieving this urine volume requires intake of about 2.5–3 l of fluid per day, to account for insensible losses. Fluid intake should occur around the clock, including before bedtime. For most recurrent stone formers fluid intake should lead to nocturia at least once and further intake of water should be taken upon awakening. Patients should understand that increasing fluid intake constitutes a serious medical therapy, and that it is safe, inexpensive, and effective.

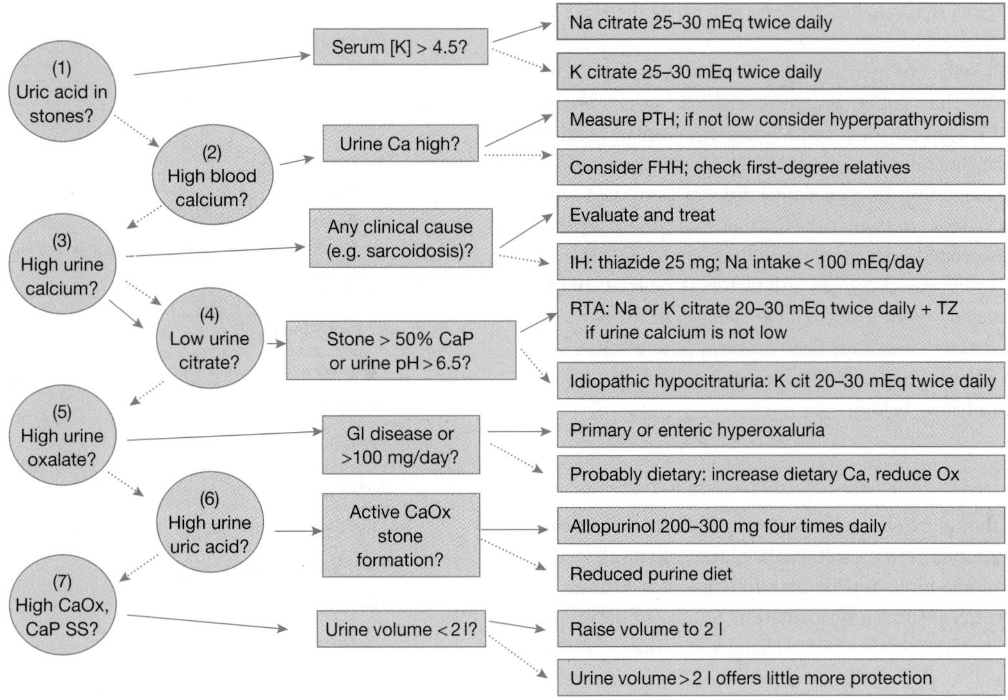

Fig. 1 Algorithm for management of nephrolithiasis. This algorithm depicts a simplified strategy for management of nephrolithiasis; patients may not all fit neatly into this schema, and more than one 'yes' answer may apply. Solid arrows signify a 'yes' answer to the questions, dashed arrows signify 'no'. FHH, familial hypocalciuric hypercalcaemia; IH, idiopathic hypercalciuria; RTA, renal tubular acidosis; CaOx, CaP SS, supersaturation of calcium oxalate or calcium phosphate; GI, gastrointestinal. Adapted with permission from Litholink Corp.

The effectiveness is in part demonstrated by the 'stone clinic effect', the term used to describe the decreased rate of stone recurrence in patients seen in specialty clinics devoted to stone care, not attributable to specific therapy. Simply giving patients advice regarding fluids leads to significant reduction in recurrence rates in those who comply with the recommendation. The effect of fluid is also suggested by a study that divided patients into quintiles of fluid intake based on dietary questionnaires and showed that the lower the fluid intake, the higher the risk of stone occurrence (Curhan *et al.* 1993).

One prospective randomized trial confirmed the hypothesis that fluid intake could effectively reduce stone disease (Borghi *et al.* 1996). In this study, patients with one previous episode of calcium stone disease (but not necessarily with hypercalciuria) were randomly assigned to a high intake of water without any dietary advice or to no recommendations regarding fluid intake. Patients were monitored for stone recurrence with radiological evaluations. Both men and women with stones in this study had lower urine volumes at entry as compared with non-stone-formers. Recurrences occurred during the 5 years of follow-up in 12 of 99 patients given advice about increased fluid intake (at an average time of 38.7 months) and in 27 of 100 patients (at an average time of 25.1 months) not given this advice ($p = 0.008$). Relative supersaturation of calcium oxalate, brushite and uric acid declined only in the former group. The urine volumes in the two groups were similar at baseline but quite different at yearly follow-up in years 1–5: range of 2.1–2.6 l in the high fluid intake group, versus 1.0–1.3 l in the control group. The efficacy of the regimen in patients with and without hypercalciuria was not reported. In short, an increase in fluid intake is a regimen that effectively reduces the incidence of stone recurrence when followed long-term.

The emphasis for patients should be properly placed on urine volume and not intake since under certain cirumstances intake will need to rise substantially to maintain moderate urine volumes. For example, hot climates increase insensible losses and intake requirements, and are associated with increased rates of stone formation. Certain occupations, such as those of athletes and life-guards, similar to physical exertion, have been associated with higher stone rates presumably related to increased water losses. Bowel disease may be associated with increased stool water content and contributes to the stone disease seen in patients with ileostomies and inflammatory bowel disease. However, some patients with bowel disease may have more stool output with increasing fluid intake rather than increased urine output.

One group of patients who may have difficulty with increasing fluid intake is that with urological disease, especially prostatic hypertrophy and incontinence of various aetiologies. These patients may have stones in part due to their voluntary limitation of fluid intake and resultant low urine volumes. Treatment of such stone formers may include medical therapy to address lower urinary tract obstruction, such as α-blockers for benign prostatic hypertrophy, or anticholinergic agents such as tolterodine to aid incontinence. Successful therapy may allow patients to increase fluid intake and increase urinary volume.

As to what fluids should constitute a stone former's intake, the simplest choice is tap water. Mineral water contains varying amounts of calcium and magnesium carbonates and phophates. Studies of stone incidence have not shown higher rates of stone formation with mineral water ingestion. In fact, short-term studies of its effect on urine composition show increased urinary citrate caused by the alkalinizing divalent ion salts, and decreases in urinary oxalate attributed to intestinal binding of oxalate by ingested calcium. Mineral water may therefore be of advantage for stone prevention.

Caffeine has a mild effect of increasing urine volume, and epidemiological studies show that coffee ingestion reduces stone disease (Curhan *et al.* 1998). Tea, on the other hand, is higher in oxalate content than coffee and is not generally recommended. In two large epidemiologic studies, regular ingestion of grapefruit juice was associated with atleast a 40 per cent increase in stone risk (Curhan *et al.* 1998). Orange juice has not been associated with more stone disease and its calcium-fortified form leads to improved urinary risk factors (Coe *et al.* 1992). Colas have been associated with unfavourable changes in urinary risk factors and increased rates of stones. Beer drinkers have consistently been shown to have a lower incidence of stones, and milk intake should be encouraged (see 'Calcium' below).

Diet

Diet has long been thought to be an important risk factor for stones. Excessive intake of animal protein, salt, oxalate, and calcium have all been implicated by epidemiological or pathophysiological studies as possible contributors to calcium stone formation. Studies of the effects of diet however tend to focus on short-term changes in urinary risk factors, rather than actual incidence of stone recurrence. There is a notable lack of prospective trials of dietary manipulation, and none showed benefit until very recently. More powerful epidemiological data have also confirmed that diminished, not increased, dietary calcium intake is associated with a higher rate of stone formation.

Calcium

The earlier focus on hyperabsorption of dietary calcium as one relatively common pathophysiological cause for idiopathic hypercalciuria made it seem reasonable to restrict dietary calcium intake, most of which is obtained from intake of dairy products. Epidemiological data demonstrated the reverse: higher dietary calcium was associated with fewer stones (Curhan *et al.* 1993, 1997). The putative mechanism of this effect is binding of dietary oxalate by dietary calcium in the intestinal lumen. The resultant poorly soluble complex is not absorbed by the bowel, leading to a decrease in urinary oxalate. This hypothesis was supported by a clinical series in which patients eating their *ad lib* diets had decreases in urinary oxalate excretion as dietary calcium increased, up to the range of about 800 mg/day, after which the effect lessened in magnitude (Lemann *et al.* 1996). While increases in dietary calcium intake lead to increased urinary calcium excretion, the net effect appears to be a decrease in supersaturation of calcium oxalate. In part this may be explained by the relative excess of urinary calcium as compared with oxalate; small changes in oxalate excretion lead to proportionately greater changes in the calcium–oxalate activity product than do changes in urinary calcium excretion.

One randomized trial confirmed the therapeutic importance of this effect by comparing low and high calcium intakes (10 and 30 mmol, respectively) in patients with hypercalciuria and recurrent calcium stones (Borghi *et al.* 2002). The composition of the diet is given in Table 2. Patients following the higher calcium intake had significantly fewer stone recurrences at 5 years. The design did not strictly test only the effects of changes in dietary calcium since although both groups followed restrictions in dietary oxalate intake, only the group with the higher calcium intake was also given restrictions in dietary sodium (50 mEq) and animal protein (52 g). Nonetheless, the results of 24-h urine collections suggested that the change in dietary calcium intake was the most important manoeuvre, since both groups had reductions in urinary calcium but urinary oxalate increased in the low-calcium group and declined in the high-calcium group.

Table 2 Composition of normal calcium diet for stone prevention in hypercalciuria (Borghi *et al.* 2002)

Calories (kcal)	2540
Total protein (g)	93
From meat or fish	21
From milk or milk products	31
From bread, pasta, and vegetables	41
Lipids (g)	93
Carbohydrates (g)	333
Fibre (g)	40
Sodium chloride (mmol)	50
Potassium (mmol)	120
Calcium (mmol)	30
Phosphorus (mmol)	49
Magnesium (mmol)	14.5
Oxalate (mmol)	2.2
Water in foods (ml)	1550

These data are strong enough that patients should be specifically told not to reduce calcium intake since the older recommendation to restrict it remains popular folklore and is still commonly prescribed by urologists. Calcium restriction will also lead to decreases in bone mineral demineralization and worsening of osteoporosis. Patients should be encouraged to ingest at least 800 mg of calcium per day (one 8-ounce glass of milk contains about 300 mg), particularly to accompany foods with relatively high oxalate content.

Protein

Many data link increased dietary animal protein intake to increased stone incidence (Goldfarb 1994). Data that support a causal relationship between these variables include epidemiological data showing more stones in people consuming more animal protein, demonstrations of greater protein intake in stone formers as compared with non-stone-forming controls, and studies of the effects of protein restriction on urinary composition. There are several ways that increased protein intake could increase urinary lithogenicity. Animal protein is a rich source of purines, the precursors to uric acid. Hyperuricosuria is itself a risk factor for calcium stone formation. Protein is also the major source in the 'Western' diet of protons, and it constitutes an acid load. This acid load in turn has two effects. First, it leads to decreased urinary citrate excretion since proximal tubular reabsorption of citrate, an endogenous inhibitor of calcium oxalate crystallization reabsorption, is pH sensitive. Second, the acid loads increases urinary calcium excretion, due both to a direct tubular effect to reduce calcium reabsorption and an effect to increase mobilization of calcium from bone. Finally, some data, but not all, demonstrate increases in urinary oxalate excretion following animal protein loads.

Despite these many persuasive data, there is little evidence of the therapeutic benefit of protein restriction. The study cited above, which demonstrated the benefit of increased calcium intake in patients with hypercalciuria also restricted animal protein; the relative effect of the protein restriction was not established (Borghi *et al.* 2002). One other randomized trial compared patients who either were or were not given recommendations on reducing dietary protein intake to 56–64 g/day (Hiatt *et al.* 1996). The study included patients with calcium oxalate stones but did not characterize them with respect to urinary risk factors. The low-protein group actually had an increase in stone recurrence. Whether a different result would have been obtained in patients with hypercalciuria is unknown.

Given the lack of convincing evidence, a reasonable course would be to more aggressively restrict animal protein intake only in patients who clearly have either high protein intake by history, or whose urine collections demonstrate sizeable protein catabolic rates, or elevated excretion of sulfate, a marker for animal protein ingestion. Patients should also be warned away from the 'Atkins diet', a ketogenic diet popular for weight loss, but associated with an increased rate of stone formation.

Sodium

Increases in urinary sodium excretion are accompanied by increases in urinary calcium excretion. The relationship appears stronger in patients with hypercalciuria than those with normal calcium excretion, with a steeper slope in the effect of increased sodium intake on urinary calcium (Wasserstein *et al.* 1987). In fact one limitation to the attempt to classify mechanisms of hypercalciuria is that urinary calcium excretion varies enough with sodium intake to blur the distinction between 'absorptive' and 'renal leak' hypercalciuria. Most patients with hypercalciuria will demonstrate a reduction in the degree of calciuria with sodium restriction. What remains unproven is whether excessive sodium intake is a primary cause of stones via hypercalciuria in patients who would otherwise remain stone-free. In women without stones, increased sodium intake appears to be associated with decreased bone mineral density, suggesting that sodium intake could be a direct and primary cause of calcium stone disease. However, most studies have not clearly delineated calcium stone-formers or hypercalciuric patients from control patients based on urinary sodium excretion. Epidemiological data have also not demonstrated that dietary sodium is a risk factor for a first episode of stone disease (Curhan *et al.* 1993).

There are no intervention trials of sodium restriction alone with stone recurrence as the primary end-point. The study by Borghi *et al.* (2002) included sodium restriction as a part of the experimental manoeuvre along with the high-calcium diet, and compared it with the low-calcium diet with unrestricted sodium intake. Both groups had similarly reduced urinary calcium restriction; in one group this was attributed to the reduction in calcium ingestion, while in the other, with the high-calcium diet, it was attributed to successful restriction of dietary sodium.

Sodium restriction is also important during thiazide therapy. Increases in urinary sodium excretion overcome the hypocalciuric effect of the drugs while urinary potassium excretion increases so that hypokalaemia and hypocitraturia ensue.

Despite the paucity of intervention data, the strength of the relationship makes restriction of dietary sodium a potentially important part of stone prevention in patients with hypercalciuria and those treated with thiazides. A serious limitation of this intervention is the inability of many people eating processed and canned foods to eliminate sodium readily from their diets. A goal of 100 mEq ingested per day is achievable only by significantly reducing these sources of salt and avoiding restaurants.

Oxalate

Given the above discussion suggesting that the benefits of increasing dietary calcium are mediated by the resultant decrease in intestinal oxalate absorption and urinary excretion, it might appear clear that oxalate restriction should also be an important manipulation. In fact, it remains untested in trials in which stone occurrence is the primary end-point.

There are many factors that continue to contribute to uncertainty about the contribution of dietary oxalate to stone disease (Holmes 2000; Holmes *et al.* 2001). There has been until recently debate about the proportion of urinary oxalate that derives from diet versus that produced by endogenous metabolism. While previous estimates had that proportion at approximately 20 per cent, recent estimates using more modern techniques of analysis place it as high as 80 per cent in some individuals. Some studies of oxalate excretion in response to dietary changes have failed to measure concomitant urinary excretion of citrate and organic anions, or measures of lithogenicity such as supersaturation or the upper limit of calcium oxalate metastability. Such studies neglect to measure the net effect of changes in urine composition. There is also evidence that oxalate absorption is influenced in part by genetic determinants so that selection of patients may lead to heterogenous study subjects (Holmes *et al.* 1998).

There have also been methodological issues interfering with the undisputed measurement of food content of oxalate, with some techniques suffering from a lack of specificity and interference by endogenous substances while more recent methodologies vary in accuracy, depending on whether the oxalate content is high or low (Holmes and Kennedy 2000). There are also questions about what proportion of oxalate in food is bioavailable, or absorbable by the intestine, since much of fruit and vegetable oxalate is potentially complexed with calcium or exists in other insoluble forms (Massey *et al.* 1993). Techniques of food preparation can also affect bioavailable or soluble oxalate content. The result of recent work is continued revision of tables of food oxalate content (Holmes and Kennedy 2000). Some of these results are shown in Table 3. A short list of some important foods to restrict would include dark, green, leafy vegetables such as spinach or chard; chocolate; tea; nuts; okra and rhubarb; green beans; beets; wheat bran; and soy products. There is a variable and inconsistent effect of ingested animal protein to increase urinary oxalate excretion as well.

A final practical problem with oxalate restriction is the confusion that patients express when they are told to reduce animal protein as well as some component of fruits and vegetables. Many middle-aged to older patients have already modified their diets to reduce their risk of cardiovascular disease and may find oxalate restrictions burdensome.

In the trial comparing low calcium intake with 'normal' calcium (the latter with restriction of salt and animal protein as well), both groups had oxalate intake restricted (Borghi *et al.* 2002). The difference in oxalate excretion was explained by the difference in calcium intake, suggesting that this variable appears to be as important or more so than oxalate intake in determining urinary oxalate excretion. Oxalate restriction is logical and probably useful in patients with calcium stones and hyperoxaluria, but at this point there is better evidence to support increasing dietary calcium intake to control urinary oxalate.

Table 3 Oxalate content of various foods (Assimos and Holmes 2000)

Food	Oxalate (mg/100 g)	Oxalate per serving (mg) (serving size, g)
Spinach	645	645 (100)
Fibre One cereal	142	43 (30)
Bran flakes	141	42 (30)
Green beans (steamed)	33	33 (100)
Potato (raw)	27.1	27.1 (100)
Snack bar (butterfinger)	53.5	24 (45)
Peanut butter	95.8	19.2 (20)
Tea (brewed)	7.5	18.8 (250)
Celery	61.2	18.4 (30)
Chocolate (American)	42.5	13 (30)
Ravioli	6.5	13 (200)
White bread	14.3	8.0 (56)
Carrots (raw)	5.7	5.7 (100)
Potato chips	9.4	3.0 (30)
White rice (steamed)	2.1	2.1 (100)
Broccoli (steamed)	1.8	1.8 (100)
Strawberry jelly	5.3	1.1 (20)
Corn flakes	1.9	0.6 (30)
Mustard	12.1	0.6 (5)
Apple (raw)	0.5	0.4 (100)
Peaches (canned)	0.3	0.3 (100)
Grape jelly	1.5	0.3 (20)

Ascorbate can be converted to oxalate, leading to concerns about high-dose vitamin C being a possible cause of hyperoxaluria. Studies of acute ingestion of such high doses are variable with respect to the resultant oxaluria. It is possible that non-enzymatic conversion of ascorbate to oxalate occurs not in the kidney but in the bladder where the reaction would have no implications for stone formation. There are also studies demonstrating either no increase in stone incidence in patients taking increased doses or a decrease (Gerster 1997). The potential harm of ascorbate conversion to oxalate may be more consequential for patients with renal failure.

Fibre

Increasing dietary fibre has been suggested to be a means of preventing stone recurrence in patients with hypercalciuria, but it has not been tested in randomized controlled trials. Increases in fibre intake in the form of rice bran were associated with reductions in hypercalciuria (Ebisuno *et al.* 1991) and stone formation in an uncontrolled study. This form of therapy was also associated with an increase in urinary oxalate excretion, so that selection of fibres with lower oxalate content might improve the efficacy of therapy. Increasing fibre intake via fruits and vegetables has a different effect, and may increase intestinal transit time, which is associated with a reduction in oxalate absorption and excretion.

The effects of fibre are not easily separated from the effects of phytic acid, also known as phytate or myo-inositol hexaphosphate. This molecule, derived from corn, soy products, and other cereal types has *in vitro* activity to inhibit crystallization of calcium oxalate and calcium phosphate. Epidemiological studies have suggested that patients with calcium oxalate stones consume less dietary phytate and have lower urinary phytate excretion (Grases *et al.* 2000). The efficacy of increasing dietary fibre to prevent stones remains untested, with the relative effects of increasing phytate and oxalate excretion unresolved.

Carbohydrate

Carbohydrate ingestion leads to increased urinary excretion of calcium and stone patients respond to glucose loads with more exaggerated calciuria than do non-stone-formers (Lemann *et al.* 1969). Epidemiological evidence has demonstrated that sucrose intake was correlated with a higher prevalence of stones in women, but not in men (Curhan *et al.* 1997). The therapeutic implications of these phenomena have not been explored, but it may be appropriate to reduce the ingestion of simple carbohydrates in patients with suggestive dietary histories.

Summary of dietary manipulations for calcium stone prevention

Though changes in several dietary components have the potential to affect risk factors for stone formation, only an increased fluid intake, and the normal calcium diet (with accompanying restriction of animal protein, salt, and oxalate), have demonstrated efficacy in randomized controlled trials. The most important component of these trials may have been the increased calcium intake in comparison with the control low calcium diet, since that manipulation was thought responsible for the reduction in urinary oxalate excretion that distinguished the successfully treated group from the control patients. Patients should be told to increase calcium intake via low-fat dairy products in order to not adversely affect serum lipid profiles. Lactose-free dairy products and calcium-fortified orange juice are available for those who are lactose-intolerant. The efficacy of this diet in calcium stone formers without hypercalciuria has not been established, but one would expect that calcium oxalate supersaturation would be favourably affected in a similar direction, if not with a similar magnitude. Also not tested is the concept of prescribing a diet to patients based specifically on their urinary risk factors. Such an approach would be difficult to test, but would have the appeal of directing patients to restrict specific nutrients, instead of a broad range of dietary components, possibly thereby enhancing compliance.

Pharmalogical therapy for specific risk factors

When stones recur, and dietary therapy is ineffective, because the magnitude of its effect is small, because the patient and physician are unable to identify culpable dietary constituents, or because the patient is relatively unable to make the requisite changes, pharmalogical therapy is indicated.

Hypercalciuria

Thiazides

Treatment with thiazide diuretics, or the non-thiazide drug indapamide, has been shown to be effective in three randomized controlled trails (Laerum and Larsen 1984; Ettinger *et al.* 1988; Borghi *et al.* 1993). These drugs have never been tested in comparison to diet, so that the relative efficacy of these techniques is unknown.

The term 'thiazides' will be used here to include commonly used thiazide diuretics, such as hydrochlorothiazide, bendroflumethiazide, trichlormethiazide, and two related drugs that are not strictly thiazides in structure, chlorthalidone and indapamide. The mechanism of the drugs' protective effect is the reduction in urinary calcium excretion. This hypocalciuric effect occurs as the result of thiazides' ability to inhibit electroneutral NaCl cotransport in the distal convoluted tubule, mediated by the protein called NCCT, for sodium chloride cotransporter. This inhibition, leading to less intracellular chloride, accompanied by basolateral chloride loss, may hyperpolarize the apical membrane of distal tubular epithelial cells. Hyperpolarization causes opening of voltage-gated calcium channels that then allow increased calcium entry and net absorption. That thiazides work in this manner is confirmed by the relatively rare Gitelman's syndrome, which, like the clinical effects of thiazides, is in part characterized by low urinary calcium excretion in patients with inactivating mutations of NCCT.

Some *in vitro* studies suggest that thiazide actions may be mediated by direct effects on bone mineralization. Though the clinical significance of such *in vitro* effects is not established, inhibition of osteoclast activity would be associated with positive calcium balance and a resultant reduction in urinary calcium excretion. Bone mineral density could also be affected by thiazides via their modest ability to inhibit activity of carbonic anhydrase, an enzyme whose activity is critical to mineral mobilization by osteoclasts. In addition, the thiazide-inhibitable NCCT is expressed in membranes of one osteoblast-like cell line, though an understanding of the transporter's integrated physiology and possible role in bone turnover has not yet been elucidated.

Regardless of the relative effects on bone mineralization and urinary calcium excretion, thiazides are associated with positive calcium balance and increased bone mineral density. This is a salutary effect that has been associated with a reduction in fracture rates in people with hypertension and osteoporosis treated with thiazides. This is a potentially important phenomenon in stone formers with hypercalciuria who demonstrate decreased bone density and increased fracture rates as compared with age and gender-matched non-stone-forming control patients (Lauderdale *et al.* 2001).

Finally, it is worth noting that a thiazide remains a first line agent for the treatment of hypertension. The class has had demonstrated efficacy in reducing stroke rate and cardiovascular morbidity in general, and in hypertensive subgroups including the elderly, those with diabetes mellitus, or with systolic hypertension. Thiazides are clearly the treatment of choice for calcium stone formers with concomitant hypertension.

There are three adequate randomized controlled trials demonstrating the stone-preventive properties of these drugs. The effect becomes statistically significant only after about 18 months. Studies in which patients were followed for less than 3 years have demonstrated inconsistent effects. A recent meta-analysis included such studies with inadequate duration of therapy, though still concluding that thiazides were effective (Pearle *et al.* 1999). We would suggest a longer duration of follow-up as a criterion for including trials in such an analysis. Some literature has suggested that the effect of thiazides to reduce calcium excretion is short-lived. Our own data in a large number of patients suggest that the effect is prolonged indefinitely (Coe and Parks 2000).

We briefly review the three randomized controlled trials. In the first study, 50 patients with recurrent calcium stones were randomly assigned to treatment with either 25 mg of hydrochlorothiazide twice daily with 0.6 g of potassium chloride or to placebo (Laerum and Larsen 1984). The majority of patients in both treatment arms did not have hypercalciuria and both groups were advised to restrict intake of calcium, salt, oxalate, and purines. During the period of follow-up, which averaged about 3 years, 48 per cent of patients in the placebo group had a new stone as compared with 22 per cent of the chlorthalidone group ($p = 0.05$). Among the patients with a new stone, the stone-free interval preceding it was 52 per cent longer in the treated group. The effect persisted among patients who were treated for an additional 12 months. The study was too small to conclude whether the effect was greater in patients with or without hypercalciuria. The results of urine collections for patients on therapy were not reported.

A second small study performed in patients with recurrent calcium stones assigned patients to three groups: placebo ($n = 31$) or 25 mg ($n = 19$) or 50 mg ($n = 23$) of chlorthalidone (Ettinger *et al.* 1988). Patients were advised to restrict dairy intake as well as salt, refined sugar, animal protein, and oxalate. Routine potassium supplementation was not specified. After 3 years, new calculous events, which included growth of pre-existing stones occurred in 45 per cent of patients taking placbo, 16 per cent of those taking 25 mg and 13 per cent of those taking 50 mg of chlorthalidone. Most patients did not have hypercalciuria and like the previously described study, the study lacked sufficient power to distinguish whether the benefit of the drug occurred in both those with and without hypercalciuria.

In a third randomized controlled trial, indapamide had a significant, similar benefit (Borghi *et al.* 1993). Similar to thiazides, indapamide has antihypertensive properties and works in the distal convoluted tubule. Only patients with hypercalciuria were included in this study and were assigned to three groups: advised regarding dietary restrictions and increased fluids; diet, fluids, and 2.5 mg of indapamide; or diet, fluids, indapamide, and 300 mg of allopurinol. After 3 years, the proportions of patients that remained stone-free were 57.2, 84.2, and 97.5 per cent in the three groups, respectively. Calcium excretion was reduced by 13, 48, and 50 per cent, respectively.

Treatment with all these drugs is often associated with some degree of potassium loss. Even in the absence of hypokalaemia, reduction of total body potassium can lead to shifts of protons into the cells of the proximal tubule, causing intracellular acidification. Proximal tubular sodium citrate cotransport is stimulated and hypocitraturia results. This may reduce the efficacy of thiazide's ability to inhibit stone formation in some patients. Potassium depletion can be prevented by supplementing most patients taking thiazides with potassium citrate (starting with 20–30 mEq/day), and adjusting doses based on urinary citrate excretion and serum potassium concentrations. In one study, supplementation of patients taking thiazides with potassium bicarbonate was associated with a greater reduction in urinary calcium excretion than treatment with thiazides alone, or thiazides with potassium chloride supplements (Frassetto *et al.* 2000). This effect was attributable to the effect of urinary alkalinization on calcium excretion. The effect of potassium bicarbonate and potassium citrate would be expected to have equivalent effects on urinary citrate and calcium excretion, though the citrate salt may be associated with less gastric production of carbon dioxide. Although not available commercially, a combination of both potassium and magnesium citrate may have better gastrointestinal tolerance while providing an equivalent amount of citrate (Ettinger *et al.* 1997).

Amiloride, a drug that blocks the epithelial sodium channel (ENaC), can also diminish potassium losses, and is available in combination with hydrochlorothiazide. Any effect of amiloride to stimulate calcium reabsorption by itself is small at best. Triamterene has the same potassium-sparing effect and also comes combined with thiazides but should be avoided as it is poorly soluble and itself a cause of stones.

Excessive sodium intake while taking thiazides leads to two important effects. Increased sodium excretion will reduce the hypocalciuric effect of the drug. Second, it will lead to greater potassium losses and more significant hypocitraturia. Patients on thiazide therapy therefore require advisement on reducing sodium intake, with a goal of ingesting no more than 100 mEq. Urine collections can be used to monitor success.

Other potential side-effects of thiazides are of minimal importance. Short-term effects on lipid profiles vanish within a year of starting therapy, and worsening glucose tolerance does not occur if hypokalaemia is prevented. Some patients, particularly young normotensives, may not tolerate the blood pressure lowering effect of the drugs. Occasionally at risk patients may have more frequent episodes of acute gout, and if necessary, allopurinol can be used to prevent these episodes.

Chlorthalidone may not only be the most potent in this class of drugs with respect to the hypocalciuric effect, and the longest acting, but may also be associated with the most potassium loss. Hydrochlorothiazide, bendroflumethiazide, and trichlormethiazide are also effective. Though indapamide was also associated with hypokalaemia, it did not cause hypocitraturia, though the decreased citrate excretion would be expected. No studies have examined the relative merits of these drugs in direct comparisons.

An unresolved question is the importance of using thiazides exclusively in patients with hypercalciuria, a strategy termed selective therapy. In part, this is truly a semantic issue since definitions of hypercalciuria vary. Since supersaturation varies with calcium excretion, lower calcium excretion is associated with fewer stones, regardless of the absolute amount, and whether the pretreatment amount meets some relatively arbitrary definition. One would expect proportionally more significant reductions in calciuria in patients with greater baseline calcium excretion, yet calcium oxalate supersaturation can be meaningfully reduced in patients with lower values of calcium excretion. Selective versus non-selective strategies have not been adequately compared for relative efficacy.

Citrate

Since citrate therapy has been shown to be useful in non-selected patients, those with or without hypocitraturia, supplementation of citrate may be effective in patients with hypercalciuria with normal citrate excretion. Citrate may reduce calcium excretion to a degree as well due to its alkalinizing effect, and usually is used along with thiazides as discussed above. The use of citrate is discussed further below in the section titled 'Hypocitraturia'.

Phosphates

Despite multiple mechanisms of potential benefit, and several different available preparations, no phosphate-containing preparations have been shown to be efficacious, safe, and practical in clinical use.

Cellulose phosphate serves as a calcium-binding resin, absorbing calcium in the intestinal lumen. It is not well tolerated, frequently causing diarrhoea and other gastrointestinal complaints. Its deleterious side-effects include negative calcium balance, negative magnesium balance, and potentially lower bone mineral density. There are no trials demonstrating its efficacy.

Oral administration of orthophosphate leads to increased urinary concentration of pyrophosphate, an *in vitro* inhibitor of calcium oxalate crystallization, but one of uncertain benefit *in vivo*. Urinary citrate also increases. Phosphate intake leads to reductions in calcitriol production. The result is diminished intestinal calcium absorption and urinary calcium excretion. Orthophosphate administration has not been shown to prevent stone in randomized trials, and likely causes negative calcium balance.

Preparations containing acid phosphate do not prevent stones. This form would be expected to inhibit renal calcium reabsorption, increase mobilization of bone calcium, and cause gastointestinal intolerance. Sodium phosphate would be expected to have less effectiveness in decreasing urinary calcium excretion due to the over-riding effect of the sodium load. These deleterious effects may be overcome by a newer preparation of neutral potassium phosphate, which increases urinary excretion of citrate and pyrophosphate. The preparation is not commercially available and has not been tested in randomized trials with stone prevention as an end-point. It appears to reduce urinary calcium excretion more than intestinal calcium absorption, causing positive calcium balance. In one randomized double-blind study, it reduced urinary calcium excretion at 3 months. In a 4-year study, it did not lead to a reduction in bone mineral density (Breslau *et al.* 1998).

Bisphosphonates

Given the evidence that mobilization of bone mineral may contribute to hypercalciuria, it follows that bisphosphonates might be useful in stone prevention. These drugs increase bone mineral density at least in part by decreasing osteoclast-mediated bone resorption. One study examined bisphosphonates in patients with recurrent calcium stones and hypercalciuria with low bone mineral density (Weisinger *et al.* 1997). A dose of 10 mg of alendronate was associated with decreased urinary calcium and increased bone mineral density at 1 year. The study was not designed to show an effect on stone prevention. Circulating, peripheral blood monocytes in the treated patients produced less interleukin 1 *in vitro*, a possible mediator of the drug's effect. There is also the possibility that these drugs, with a structural similarity to pyrophosphate, will also inhibit calcium salt crystallization in urine.

Measuring bone mineral density in patients with hypercalciuria, particularly older patients, may become routine. Currently it seems particularly sensible in postmenopausal women, a group in whom the discovery of osteoporosis has its own therapeutic implications. In women with stones and osteoporosis, both patients and internists are often uncertain regarding the advisability of taking calcium supplements. Treatment with bisphosphonates and calcium citrate supplements is a rational choice.

An epidemiological study suggested that women taking calcium supplements have an increased incidence of stones (Curhan *et al.* 1997). This study did not distinguish between use of carbonate and citrate forms of calcium or determine the timing of the supplements with respect to meals. Using the supplement within an hour of a meal allows it to serve as an oxalate binder. Calcium citrate has better gastrointestinal tolerance, has superior bioavailability even in the presence of achlorhydria, and unlike calcium carbonate, increases urinary citrate excretion. The net effect is no change in calcium oxalate supersaturation (Levine *et al.* 1994). While bisphosphonates and calcium citrate have not been shown to prevent stones, they do prevent osteoporosis, a disease with a significantly higher morbidity and even a higher mortality than stones.

Hypocitraturia

Low urinary citrate excretion is a common risk factor in patients with calcium stones. Definitions of the normal range of citrate excretion vary, and therefore the incidence of hypocitraturia varies considerably in different series. Different definitions are in use to define the low end of citrate excretion, but most studies consistently demonstrate that stone formers have somewhat lower citrate excretions than non-stone-formers. The significance of defining a lower limit of citrate excretion is diminished by the evidence that citrate supplementation is useful as a stone preventative even in patients who may not meet clinical criteria for hypocitraturia.

The importance of citrate arises from its ability to bind calcium and form a soluble complex. In this way, it can be thought of as competing with oxalate and phosphate to prevent their precipitation as insoluble calcium salts. In addition there is evidence that citrate inhibits the aggregation of calcium oxalate crystals, an important step in the growth of stones. The ability of citrate to inhibit calcium oxalate stone growth due to hyperuricosuria is uncertain; if heterogenous nucleation of calcium oxalate on uric acid crystals is responsible for this phenomenon, alkalinization would be expected to prevent uric acid crystal formation and inhibit it. If, on the other hand, 'salting out' of calcium oxalate by uric acid is the acting principle, changing uric acid supersaturation may be unimportant.

Several causes of low urinary citrate excretion have been elucidated, but the majority of individual patients with low citrate excretion and calcium stones have this risk factor on an idiopathic basis. Citrate, as a carboxylic anion, is a potential base, the metabolism of which in the liver leads to consumption of protons, the equivalent of generation of bicarbonate. Sodium citrate reabsorption in the proximal tubule is therefore stimulated by increased proton loads and metabolic acidosis. Increased ingestion of animal protein leads to an increase in net acid ingestion and excretion and lowers urinary citrate excretion. There are two causes of metabolic acidosis commonly associated with stone formation. Distal renal tubular acidosis (Type I RTA) causes hypocitraturia (as well as hypercalciuria). Gastrointestinal disease with bicarbonate loss, as seen in states of chronic diarrhoea, ileostomy, or inflammatory bowel disease, results commonly in hypocitraturia. Hypocitraturia could also be the result of decreased intestinal absorption of organic anions, or genetically determined changes in sodium citrate transport activity, but these mechanisms have not yet been shown to be operative. The difference in urine pH between patients with RTA and those with gastrointestinal losses highlights the contrasting pathophysiology: RTA is associated with an alkaline urine pH due to impaired acidification, while gastrointestinal losses are usually associated with an acid urine pH. These latter patients are therefore also at risk for uric acid stones, while patients with RTA are not. Most calcium oxalate stone formers with idiopathic hypocitraturia have a relatively normal urine pH, making their underlying pathophysiology less certain.

Increasing urinary citrate excretion can be accomplished with supplementation with either potassium or sodium citrate. The potassium salt is much preferred since increasing sodium excretion is accompanied by increased calcium excretion as well. The result is that while sodium citrate leads to an equivalent increase in urinary citrate, it leads to a much smaller change in calcium oxalate supersaturation than potassium citrate. Sodium citrate is reserved for patients who either cannot tolerate potassium supplementation due to gastrointestinal symptoms, or who have moderate hyperkalaemia. Potassium bicarbonate leads to an increase in urinary citrate excretion similar to that of potassium citrate, since systemic alkalinization leads to inhibition of sodium citrate reabsorption; the advantage of the citrate salt is that it is not titrated to carbon dioxide in the stomach and has better gastrointestinal tolerance. Most regimens consist of 30–60 mEq of potassium citrate divided into two doses. The relative benefit of using divided doses versus a single dose, assuming that both options lead to equivalent increases in 24-h citrate excretion has not been demonstrated. Urinary citrate can also be increased by ingestion of citrus fruit juices; lemon juice contains more citrate than other choices. Other juices have been associated with increased urinary oxalate excretion and therefore have no net effect on calcium oxalate supersaturation (Goldfarb and Coe 1999).

Two randomized controlled trials demonstrate the efficacy of citrate supplementation for prevention of calcium stones. In the first, 57 patients with recurrent stones, hypocitraturia, and no other metabolic abnormalities such as hypercalciuria were assigned to placebo or potassium citrate 30–60 mEq/day. At 3 years, 27.8 per cent of treated patients and 80 per cent of placebo-receiving patients had had a recurrence (Barcelo *et al.* 1993).

In a second study, a combination of magnesium and potassium citrate (one-third and two-thirds respectively, in milliequivalents provided) was used (Ettinger *et al.* 1997). It was compared with placebo in 64 patients with recurrent calcium stones who were not selected for urinary risk factors, and who were randomly assigned to the two treatment arms. At nearly 3 years of follow-up, 12.9 per cent of the patients receiving citrate had had a new calculous event, while 63.6 per cent of the placebo group had had one. The efficacy of magnesium supplementation to prevent stones has not been established. The potential importance of this preparation may be that decreasing potassium content could allow better gastrointestinal tolerance by sensitive patients as compared with potassium citrate alone, but this has yet to be demonstrated. In this study, however, there were higher rates of withdrawal and gastrointestinal symptoms in the citrate group, as is the case in trials of potassium citrate. This preparation is not currently commercially available. The relative benefit of giving potassium citrate to patients selected and not selected for hypocitraturia is not established, but the above studies demonstrated benefits for both groups.

Hyperoxaluria

Mild hyperoxaluria, usually defined as more than 40 mg (0.44 mmol) per day, is not uncommon. Its clinical significance is debatable in part because of the lack of controlled trials demonstrating that reductions in oxalate excretion can be maintained, and if maintained, can prevent stone recurrence. Variations in measurement methodology probably account for a wide range of estimates of prevalence. Patients with urinary oxalate levels greater than 60 mg (0.67 mmol) must be distinguished from those with the hereditary disease primary hyperoxaluria (PH) and those with enteric hyperoxaluria.

There is currently no proven medical therapy for hyperoxaluria in calcium stone formers who do not have the genetic disease PH. When increasing dietary calcium intake and restricting dietary oxalate content fail to lower oxalate excretion (see above), few other therapies are available, and literature supportive of long-term benefits are lacking. Ox-Absorb, studied in small numbers of patients with enteric hyperoxaluria (see below), has not been studied in patients with idiopathic hyperoxaluria.

Some patients with PH are sensitive to pyridoxine, a cofactor for activity of the critical enzyme alanine-glyoxalate aminotransferase (AGT). Whether any patients with hyperoxaluria who do not have the genetically determined defective enzyme also have a boost in hepatic metabolism of oxalate when given pyridoxine supplements has not been established. Some unusual patients may actually have a very mild form of PH induced by defective phosphorylation of pyridoxine to pyridoxal phosphate. Supplementation with 100 mg of pyridoxine may be associated with reductions in urinary oxalate excretion. In fact, epidemiological data support this possibility (Curhan *et al.* 1999). In this study of more than 85,000 women with no prior history of kidney stones, pyridoxine (Vitamin B_6) intake as both diet constituent and as contained in supplements was assessed. The relative risk of new stone formation for women in the highest category of pyridoxine intake (40 mg/day or more) compared with the lowest category (<3 mg/day) was 0.66 (95% confidence interval 0.44–0.98).

Several new therapies are currently being investigated but have no proven efficacy in stone prevention. The role of *Oxalobacter formigenes* in preventing stone disease could lead to new treatments for hyperoxaluria. This organism contains an oxalate-degrading decarboxylase to utilize oxalate as a substrate for production of ATP (Sidhu *et al.* 1999). The absence of the organism in patients treated with antibiotics could lead to diminished metabolism of oxalate in the intestine and result in increased urinary oxalate excretion. One therapeutic approach not yet investigated would be to recolonize patients lacking the organism as a part of their normal flora. However, the successful growth of the organism in a rat model of hyperoxaluria requires a high oxalate intake. The beneficial role of the organism where low dietary oxalate intake is prescribed is therefore uncertain. A strategy around this problem might be the administration of the oxalate-degrading enzyme.

In a recent study, a preparation of four lactic acid-producing organisms, including *Lactobacillus acidophilus*, was administered as a high-dose freeze-dried concentrate to six patients with mild hyperoxaluria (Campieri *et al.* 2001). All six patients experienced reductions in urinary oxalate excretion. These organisms lack the oxalase and the gene that codes for this protein product; the means by which they reduce urinary oxalate is not established.

Enteric hyperoxaluria

One specific aetiology of hyperoxaluria is attributable to intestinal malabsorption of fat, particularly in patients with inflammatory bowel disease, chronic pancreatitis, celiac sprue, and bowel resections. Luminal fatty acids bind calcium, leaving oxalate uncomplexed and free to be absorbed. Malabsorbed bile acids, especially with resection of the terminal ileum, increase colonic permeability, further facilitating oxalate absorption. Colonic resection with ileostomy reduces this oxalate absorption signficantly.

No therapy has been proven to be effective for this condition and series are small and not controlled, and report more often on changes in urinary composition than stone prevention. Reducing urinary oxalate in these patients is not easy. Restricting dietary oxalate is important and not always adequate. Increasing dietary calcium intake, or adding calcium supplements, leads to increased binding of luminal oxalate and prevents its absorption. Calcium citrate may be the preferred calcium salt, given that it also provides some of the calcium oxalate inhibitor citrate. It may dissociate to a greater degree than calcium carbonate and allow it to bind more oxalate. Reduction of dietary fat may lead to less steatorrhoea and reduced binding of calcium by fat instead of oxalate. Oral magnesium supplements could also bind intestinal oxalate while increasing urinary magnesium excretion. Frequently magnesium causes diarrhoea even in modest doses, and especially in patients with short bowels. Jejunal bypass is frequently associated with stones. While some of the above treatments may have some efficacy, recurrent stones may constitute a reason to reverse the surgery.

Ox-Absorb (made by Vitaline) is a calcium-charged organic colloid derived from seaweed that exchanges calcium for oxalate, which then passes out of the intestine in a non-absorbable form (Lindsjo *et al.* 1989). In small studies of patients with enteric hyperoxaluria due to the typical aetiologies, it reduced urinary oxalate excretion with a small, non-significant increase in urinary calcium excretion. The net effect was a reduction in the activity product index for calcium oxalate in eight of 10 patients. Seven of 10 patients with diarrhoea noted an improvement in the consistency of their stools. No studies of Ox-Absorb for stone prevention are available. Cholestyramine, more often used in the management of hyperlipidaemia, may bind both oxalate and bile acids.

Patients with this disorder often have other risk factors for stone disease. Patients with total colectomies may not have increased urinary oxalate excretion but may still be at risk due to these other features. Intestinal loss of bicarbonate leads to metabolic acidosis, which reduces urinary citrate excretion to very low levels. Urine pH falls, which predisposes to uric acid stones. Urine volume is often low, inversely related to intestinal losses. Magnesium is also malabsorbed and results in low urinary magnesium excretion, which may or may not also be important.

The treatment of such patients requires increasing urine volume, though some patients do not experience such an increase despite increased oral volume ingestion. Supplementation with potassium citrate to increase urinary citrate and urine pH is appropriate; sodium citrate should be used if urinary sodium excretion is low due to intestinal losses and calcium citrate may help lower urinary oxalate. Relatively large doses may be required. Fat intake should be limited.

Primary hyperoxaluria

Primary hyperoxaluria (PH1) is an autosomal recessive disease that causes excessive accumulation of oxalate (Leumann and Hoppe 2001). The defect is the mistargeting of the hepatic peroxisomal enzyme alanine : glyoxalate aminotransferase (AGT). The enzyme is functionally reduced in activity either as the result of its targeting to mitochondria instead of peroxisomes (the most common defect), or because the enzyme is defective or absent (Danpure 2000). This functional deficiency prevents normal metabolism of glyoxylate to glycine. The accumulated glyoxylate is oxidized to oxalate, and reduced to glycolate, both of which appear in the urine.

PH2 is considerably more rare, somewhat more mild, and attributable to a deficiency of an hepatic cytosolic enzyme with glyoxylate reductase, hydroxypyruvate, and glycerate dehydrogenase activity (Milliner *et al.* 2001). In these cases L-glyceric acid excretion is elevated. There are atypical cases, not fully characterized in sufficient numbers, that do not meet the diagnostic criteria for PH1 and PH2 that may merit a new designation of PH3.

For PH1, 50 per cent of patients have their first symptoms by age 5 and 50 per cent will have renal failure by age 25. The diagnosis is made in most cases in the first and second decades of life. These diagnoses should be considered in patients who present with calcium oxalate stones in childhood, young patients with stones and renal insufficiency, and patients of any age whose urinary oxalate excretion is unusually high (>1.2 mmol/1.73 m^2 for PH1, 1.0 mmol/1.73 m^2 for PH2). Occasionally patients with relatively more mild disease may present as young adults while a few others present with advanced renal insufficiency and no prior history of stones. Confirmation of the diagnosis can be accomplished by demonstrating increased urinary excretion of glycolate in PH1 and L-glycerate in PH2, as well as increased plasma oxalate concentrations, but both these tests may yield normal results in sizeable groups of affected patients. Definitive diagnosis requires liver biopsy and measurement of the activity of the relevant enzymes, a test performed by a limited number of laboratories throughout the world. As renal function worsens and plasma oxalate levels increase, deposition in all tissues can lead to disastrous effects including blindness, bone pain and fractures, and eventual renal failure and death.

The pace of stone formation and oxalate accumulation can be slowed to some extent by measures otherwise useful for prevention of calcium oxalate stones. No randomized trials have been performed. Maintaining high urine volumes is essential. Citrate supplementation is probably useful. Neutral orthophosphate, 30–40 mg of elemental phophorus per day in divided doses, for patients without advanced renal insufficiency may help forestall renal insufficiency in patients with both PH1 and PH2 (Milliner *et al.* 1994). Magnesium has not been proved to be effective. Pyridoxine is a cofactor for the AGT enzyme complex and up to one-third of patients, those with diminished, but not absent, activity, respond to high doses (5–10 mg/kg/day). It should be given for at least 3 months with repeated measures of urinary oxalate excretion to judge efficacy. Doses in the higher range may be associated with peripheral neuropathy, though the incidence is quite low. Dietary oxalate is a relatively small proportion of the oxalate excreted by the kidneys each day in affected patients, so that oxalate restriction of only the foods with the highest content should be stressed. Sodium chloride intake should be limited to reduce calciuria, while restrictions of calcium and protein intake are not important manipulations.

Treatment ultimately requires liver or kidney, or combined liver and kidney, transplantation, with the merits of these alternative strategies still being debated (Leumann and Hoppe 2001). Since liver donation is a more morbid procedure, and fewer livers are available, renal transplantation alone may significantly extend life expectancy with less risk, though without achieving a cure. Early liver transplantation, preempting renal failure, is attractive, but the timing is problematic since the progress of renal insufficiency is relatively unpredictable, and the procedure exposes the patient to the risk of surgery and immunosuppression. This procedure should be accomplished before significant renal failure has occurred, since declines of glomerular filtration rate to less than 20 ml/min are associated with progressive accumulation of oxalate in all tissues. Combined liver and kidney transplantation may be preferred when available. Neither haemodialysis nor peritoneal dialysis can maintain patients in negative oxalate balance so that tissue oxalate content increases dramatically despite more intensive dialysis. This accumulation then poses a risk to kidney function, whether native or transplanted, because metabolism of circulating oxalate causes mobilization of tissue oxalate stores into the circulation, threatening the kidneys with high urinary oxalate concentrations for months or even years. Patients treated with any of these transplant strategies require careful monitoring of plasma and urinary oxalate concentrations to forestall possible renal failure.

Hyperuricosuria

About 15–20 per cent of patients with calcium oxalate stones have isolated hyperuricosuria as their urinary risk factor. Hyperuricosuria has been demonstrated to be a risk factor for calcium stones via a single randomized controlled trial of allopurinol, a xanthine oxidase inhibitor, not known to affect any other urinary risk factor (Ettinger *et al.* 1986). This randomized, placebo-controlled trial selected 60 patients with recurrent calcium stones whose 24-h urinary uric acid excretion exceeded 800 mg in men, and 750 mg in women. Patients with hypercalciuria (>300 mg in men, 250 mg in women, or >4 mg/kg body weight in either gender) were excluded. The group treated with allopurinol 100 mg three times a day had a reduction in uric acid excretion from a mean of 1017 mg to less than 600 mg; the effect persisted at 24 months. New stone events, which included growth of pre-existing stones, occurred in 58 per cent of the placebo group and 31 per cent of the allopurinol group; the latter group had a longer time interval to recurrence.

The mechanism by which uric acid promotes calcium stone formation is probably due to salting out of calcium oxalate, a physicochemical reaction by which one ionic solute promotes precipitation of another.

Most often hyperuricosuria is the result of excessive ingestion of purine-containing animal protein. This dietary excess could be confirmed by measurement of urinary urea or sulfate or calculation of the protein catabolic rate. Dietary reduction of purine ingestion would be indicated, and if successful, would be expected to lead to reduced calcium excretion and increased citrate excretion. When diet is not successful, allopurinol would be appropriate prevention for the group with hyperuricosuria.

Studies of allopurinol in patients with hypercalciuria have failed to show benefit. Thiazides, on the other hand, are effective in patients with hyperuricosuria, probably in the absence of definite hypercalciuria. Their comparative efficacy has not been studied. Thiazides have a slight disadvantage in that their use requires monitoring of serum potassium and usually potassium citrate supplementation, while allopurinol has no such requirements. Allopurinol does have a small incidence of allergic reactions including the rare but serious Stevens–Johnson syndrome. Whether the efficacy of combining thiazides and allopurionol is superior to that of either alone has not been established but may increase the risk of allergic reactions.

Calcium phosphate stones

Although most calcium oxalate stones contain at least a minor component of calcium phosphate, stones that are greater than 50 per cent calcium phosphate are much less common, and stones composed almost entirely of calcium phosphate are even more rare. In one study looking at more than 11,000 renal and ureteral stones, calcium phosphate content exceeded calcium oxalate content in 16 per cent (Gault and Chafe 2000). Calcium phosphate stones are more frequent in women so that the male predominance among stone formers is lost when considering these stones. The crystalline form of calcium phosphate is most often hydroxyapatite, with brushite being uncommon, and tricalcium phosphate (whitlockite) and octocalcium phosphate quite unusual. Magnesium ammonium phosphate, or struvite, is considered below.

Though many calcium phosphate stones arise in patients with the same risk factors associated with calcium oxalate stones, two specific diagnoses should be considered where calcium phosphate comprises more than 50 per cent of a calcium stone: RTA and primary hyperparathyroidism. Prevention of calcium phosphate stones in patients lacking these two disorders should focus on increasing urine volume, and modifying other urinary risk factors as described above. No trials of therapy in patients with predominantly calcium phosphate stones have been performed.

Renal tubular acidosis

Distal RTA, also called Type I RTA, is caused by a defect in distal tubular acidification mechanisms. The disease may be hereditary, caused by mutations in the vacuolar H^+-ATPase and the anion exchanger AE-1 in the intercalated cells of the cortical collecting duct. It may be acquired particularly as the result of Sjögren syndrome and systemic lupus erythematosus. Hypercalciuria, particularly that of hereditary origin, may itself precede and cause RTA (Caruana and Buckalew 1988). The relative contribution of RTA to stone formation in syndromes also associated with hypercalciuria has not been determined.

Distal RTA is associated with calcium stone disease for several reasons (Buckalew 1989). Acidosis stimulates sodium citrate reabsorption in the proximal tubule and results in hypocitraturia. Hypokalaemia also may contribute to hypocitraturia. The relatively high characteristic urine pH, usually in the range of 6.2–6.5, increases supersaturation of calcium phosphate. The defect in distal tubular acidification causes metabolic acidosis, which in some patients inhibits calcium reabsorption and thereby promotes hypercalciuria. One series demonstrated that 32 per cent of patients with stones or nephrocalcinosis had hypercalciuria (Caruana and Buckalew 1988). Though calcium oxalate supersaturation may be high, the effect of pH is to specifically promote calcium phosphate crystallization; pure calcium phosphate stones are not unusual.

Patients with distal RTA frequently have osteoporosis. Young people with distal RTA have growth abnormalities attributed to metabolic acidosis, as do children with promixal, or Type II, RTA. But patients with distal RTA, and not those with proximal RTA, are in positive acid balance; part of their daily acid load is titrated by bone, causing dissolution of bone mineral, release of hydroxyapatite, and contributing to hypercalciuria. The absence of positive acid balance and negative calcium balance accounts for the lack of stone disease in proximal RTA, though these patients do have low urinary citrate excretion. Patients with Type IV RTA, most often caused by hyporenin-hypoaldosteronism, have also not been shown to have an increased rate of calcium stone disease.

The diagnosis is made in a patient with hyperchloraemic metabolic acidosis, an elevated urine pH, and the absence of diarrhoea. There is often a family history of stones and RTA. These patients also have a low urine cation gap, a surrogate for low urinary ammonium excretion. Nephrocalcinosis is also often present. Hypokalaemia of uncertain aetiology is often present; in a minority of patients this may be due to a defect in the H^+,K^+-ATPase in the medullary collecting duct. Chronic renal insufficiency is frequent and may progress to endstage renal disease.

The diagnosis of incomplete RTA is less straightforward since these patients have normal serum bicarbonate concentrations. Otherwise they have similar urinary abnormalities and an elicitable defect in urinary acidification. Some of these patients with incomplete RTA may progress to distal RTA with metabolic acidosis at a later time. An interesting finding is that they have hypocitraturia despite having a normal serum pH. One hypothesis is that these patients have a distinct disorder, suggested in part by their higher urinary ammonium excretion rates, and their lower urine pH after acidification (Donnelly *et al.* 1992). An inappropriately acidified proximal tubular cell would be expected to lead to hypocitraturia and elevated ammonium excretion, which perhaps is a cause of interstitial damage that eventually might cause distal RTA.

Giving ammonium chloride to test urinary acidification in order to distinguish patients with incomplete RTA from those with idiopathic calcium stone disease is not necessary from a clinical point of view. Though the distinction between distal RTA and incomplete RTA is of great interest, the recommended treatment is the same. Potassium citrate supplementation reduces stone recurrence, though it is associated with an increase in the already elevated urine pH. The potassium salt is preferred over the sodium salt since correction of hypokalaemia will aid in increasing citrate and avoiding the calciuria associated with natriuresis. No randomized controlled trials have been performed for stone prevention in distal RTA. The calculated supersaturation of calcium phosphate increases since the impact of citrate to lower supersaturation or lower calcium excretion is relatively smaller than the effect of pH to increase it. To a small degree, citrate might reduce urinary calcium excretion by systemic alkalinization. More recent data suggest that citrate has another, more potent effect of increasing the upper limit of metastability of calcium phosphate. The upper limit of metastability is the point at which addition of more solute to a supersaturated solution causes crystal formation.

Since many patients with distal RTA have hypercalciuria, a rational choice for stone prevention is to use thiazides as well as citrate. In this way, supersaturation of calcium phosphate can be lowered by reducing calciuria and countering the effect of citrate-induced urinary alkalinization. The incidence of osteoporosis in adults with distal RTA also warrants attention to measurement of bone mineral density and consideration of bisphosphonates for therapy of bone density and hypercalciuria.

Hyperparathyroidism

Primary hyperparathyroidism causes calcium phosphate stones, as well as calcium oxalate stones and mixtures of the two. Recent estimates of prevalence of stones among patients with hyperparathyroidism average less than 20 per cent, lower than previous estimates due to earlier diagnosis at an asymptomatic stage. Several pathophysiological mechanisms contribute to stone formation. Increases in parathyroid hormone (PTH) secretion lead to increased synthesis of the active 1,25-dihydroxy-vitamin D, leading to increased intestinal absorption of calcium and phosphorus. PTH stimulates resorption of bone, leading to dissolution and release of hydroxyapatite. The relative contributions of these two effects, intestinal absorption and bone resorption, varies among individuals. Some evidence suggests that younger patients have a greater activation of vitamin D, which in turn leads to some suppression of PTH secretion and more moderate PTH elevations (Patron *et al.* 1987). The greater activity of vitamin D might be attributable to better renal function. These patients have more intestinal absorption, hypercalciuria, and stones. Older patients tend to have less activation of vitamin D, less vitamin D-mediated suppression of PTH, higher PTH secretion, and more bone disease than stone formation.

PTH stimulates calcium reabsorption in the nephron and tends to reduce the hypercalciuria that results from the hypercalcaemia-induced increase in filtered load of calcium. As many as one-third of patients with hyperparathyroidism and stones will be normocalciuric. That patients have stones despite this mitigating effect suggests that other effects of hyperparathyroidism of promoting stone formation are also active, but evidence of associated hypocitraturia, hyperuricosuria, and changes that favour crystal growth and aggregation are either inconsistent or of uncertain significance. The contributions of mild RTA in some patients and an elevated urine pH in specifically promoting calcium phosphate stone formation in hyperparathyroidism are also not clear.

The diagnosis should be suspected in patients with calcium phosphate stones, in women, in patients with significant family histories of parathyroid disease or stones, and in patients with any degree of hypercalcaemia. As discussed above, primary hyperparathyroidism should be sought, with measurement of intact PTH, in patients with serum calcium concentrations in the high normal range. Ionized calcium concentration should also be measured and may reveal hypercalcaemia in some instances in which the total serum calcium concentration is normal. In cases with normocalcaemia, PTH secretion that is not suppressed is considered diagnostic of the disorder.

The therapy for primary hyperparathyroidism is surgical removal of the hyperplastic gland. The appropriateness of surgery increases in patients with more recurrent stones, diminished bone density, and more elevated serum calcium concentrations. Patients should be referred to an experienced surgeon who may proceed to exploration of the neck or perform imaging studies to localize abnormal glands preoperatively. Ultrasound, CT scanning, MRI, and nuclear imaging studies have all been used to identify the likely site of PTH secretion, but their role in reducing the time in the operating room or the morbidity of the procedure is not proven. Recurrent stone formation is prevented in most patients following parathyroidectomy.

Medical therapy of patients with hyperparathyroidism is limited to those with relative contraindications to surgery, though the safety of the procedure is high in experienced hands. Restriction of oral calcium intake is no longer recommended as it is expected to yield more negative calcium balance with mobilization from bone. Increased fluid intake and restriction of sodium intake are more appropriate. Thiazides can reduce hypercalciuria but at the risk of increasing serum calcium, which must be closely monitored. Bisphosphonates are also rational therapy with the potential to reduce urinary calcium excretion and increase bone density, but their use in stone prevention in this setting has not been investigated. Their long-term use in primary hyperparathyroidism may be accompanied by compensatory increases in PTH secretion. Ostrogen therapy in postmenopausal women may be useful. Calcimimetic agents that bind the calcium-sensing receptor and inhibit PTH secretion are effective in short-term studies but are not evaluated yet for the treatment of chronic primary hyperparathyroidism.

Urate stones

Uric acid

Uric acid stones are composed of crystals of diprotonated uric acid; a lesser component of monosodium urate may be present in patients with more sodium ingestion. Since the prime factor in determining the supersaturation of uric acid is urine pH, the prevention of uric acid stones begins with successful urinary alkalinization. The p*K* of uric acid in urine is approximately 5.3, so that in urine with pH values greater than 6.0, a proton will dissociate and solubilize the anionic urate. At pH values less than 5.3, little, if any, uric acid can remain soluble. The p*K* of the second proton is greater than 10 so that its dissociation is of no clinical significance. Since urine pH values greater than 6.0–6.5 are usually not difficult to achieve, uric acid stones can not only be prevented, but unlike calcium stones, they can also be dissolved.

The characteristic difference between uric acid stone formers and non-stone-formers is the former group's low urine pH in 24-h collections: 5.41 versus 6.06 (Asplin 1996). The uric acid stone formers also have such lower values for a greater proportion of the day. Fluctuations in urine pH are expected after meals, when gastric proton secretion is associated with a small increase in serum bicarbonate concentration. The resultant metabolic alkalosis causes a transient increase in urine pH known as the alkaline tide. This increase is sufficient to solubilize any uric acid crystals formed between meals during periods of more acid urine. The lack of this daily variation in urine pH is thought to be an important contributor to uric acid stones.

The pathophysiological basis for the low urine pH seen in most uric acid stone formers remains unresolved. A defect in ammoniagenesis, the basis for which remains only speculative, would account for the problem (Kamel *et al.* 2002). Such a defect, with diminished urinary excretion of NH_4^+, has been variably demonstrated in clinical studies of uric acid stone formers. Diminished availability of NH_3 to accept secreted protons would lead to a decrease in urine pH and an increase in urinary titratable acid, since urinary phosphate would be more fully titrated. Alternatively, an inappropriately alkaline proximal tubule cell would have inhibited ammoniagenesis and be accompanied by a lower urine pH; this mechanism has been postulated, but a basis for its occurrence has not been demonstrated (Kamel *et al.* 2002). It is instructive that another example of inhibited ammoniagenesis, Type IV RTA, is associated with metabolic acidosis, while uric acid stone formation is not. Patients with Type IV RTA have not been shown to have an increased rate of uric acid stones, further demonstrating the uncertainties regarding these disorders of acid–base handling.

Hyperuricosuria is a significantly less important cause of uric acid stones than low urine pH. Uric acid, excreted in amounts that constitute the normal or even low range, can easily become supersaturated at low urine pH values. Patients with bowel disease whose diarrhoea leads to a more acid urine pH can form uric acid stones regardless of the amount of uric acid excreted in a 24-h period. Hyperuricosuria may be the result of increased *de novo* synthesis as in gout, or due to an increase in ingestion of animal protein with the associated increase in ingestion of purines, the metabolic precursors of uric acid. The increase in animal protein intake would also be associated with increased dietary protons and the lowering of urine pH, particularly if NH_3 availability is limited. Low urine volume is also a cause of elevations in uric acid supersaturation, and contributes to stone formation in patients with bowel disease and intestinal fluid losses, and in hot climates where urine volume falls while insensible losses increase.

Gout is also a cause of uric acid stones, which occur in 10–20 per cent of patients with gout. A minority of patients with hyperuricaemia have overproduction of uric acid, and significant hyperuricosuria results. However, even in patients whose hyperuricaemia is caused by diminished rates of uric acid secretion, requiring higher levels of uricaemia to achieve uric acid balance, low urine pH is often seen. As is the case for idiopathic uric acid stone disease, the aetiology of low urine pH in gouty patients is attributed to defective ammoniagenesis, the basis for which has not been elucidated. Whether some patients with uric acid stones and no prior history of gouty arthritis actually have gout is not known. Patients with gout also have an increased incidence of calcium oxalate stones, in part as the result of hyperuricosuria.

There are several unusual causes of overproduction of uric acid that can result in hyperuricosuria and stone formation. Lesch–Nyhan syndrome is caused by a deficiency in hypoxanthine guanine phosphoribosyl transferase (HGPRT) leading to increased metabolism of hypoxanthine and guanine to uric acid. Increased activity of phosphoribosyl pyrophosphate aminotransferase (PRPP), and glycogen storage disease are also diseases associated with hyperuricaemia and high prevalence of uric acid stones. Myeloproliferative disease, with increased cell turnover, may also contribute to excessive purine degradation, and uric acid stones may result.

Uric acid stones are radiolucent unless mixed with calcium oxalate. Since calcium phosphate stones form only in an alkaline medium, uric acid stones do not occur mixed with calcium phosphate. Uric acid stones will not appear on plain radiography but are well visualized by CT scanning or ultrasound. They may appear as filling defects in the collecting system when radiocontrast is administered.

Prevention of uric acid stones requires treatment with potassium citrate or bicarbonate, with the goal of increasing urine pH to values greater than 6.0, and up to 7.0. The potassium salts are preferred over sodium citrate since the latter may be associated with increases in monosodium urate supersaturation despite increasing urinary pH, with increased uric acid clearance rates, and with hypokalaemia. Sodium citrate or sodium bicarbonate are reserved for cases where gastrointestinal side-effects are caused by potassium supplementation. All patients should be encouraged and instructed about maintaining urine volumes of at least 2 l. Acetazolamide can also increase urine pH but is not recommended since its use results in large potassium losses and metabolic acidosis.

Patients should be encouraged to measure urine pH regularly to demonstrate achievement of urine pH goals. This could be done once or twice a day at varying times over the course of several weeks. In patients in whom the goal is to dissolve pre-existing stones, alkalinization with urine pH values greater than 6.0, preferably 6.5, throughout the day is desirable. The success of stone dissolution can be followed by ultrasound at 3–4-month intervals. For prevention of new stones, it may be necessary to achieve higher urine pH values only once a day, or even every other day (Rodman 1991). Doses commonly used are 20–30 mEq of potassium or sodium citrate two or three times a day. Higher doses may be needed in patients with gastrointestinal disease such as ileostomies, where stool bicarbonate losses can be substantial. In some such patients, these higher doses may be futile as the potassium salts can exacerbate stool fluid losses and adversely affect urine volume. Patients with excessive dietary acid ingestion in the form of animal protein may also require higher doses. Citrate is also appropriate for patients with mixed uric acid and calcium oxalate stones as it will inhibit formation of the latter.

Allopurinol is reserved for patients with hyperuricosuria, particularly those with low urine pH who have not had a successful course of alkalinization. Reduction of uric acid excretion without correction of urine pH will not correct elevated uric acid supersaturations. Conversely, even very high rates of uric acid excretion can be treated successfully with citrate supplementation alone if alkalinization to a urine pH greater than 6.3 is achieved. Although allopurinol is quite well tolerated, it causes allergic manifestations, including rare instances of Stevens-Johnson syndrome, in about 1 per cent of patients. The usual dose is 300 mg/day, with reductions needed for reductions in glomerular filtration rate.

Ammonium acid urate

Ammonium acid urate is a relatively unusual component of stones in Western societies, but remains a frequent cause of stones in developing nations. In this molecule the anionic residue of uric acid binds NH_4^+ instead of H^+. This crystal is most often seen as a component of uric acid stones in the presence of inflammatory bowel disease, ileal resection, and laxative abuse. Ammonium acid urate may also be seen as a component of infectious stones resulting from urease-producing organisms and the associated increase in urinary ammonium content (Soble *et al.* 1999).

Diarrhoea with stool bicarbonate loss causes metabolic acidosis and stimulation of ammoniagenesis, leading to increased urinary ammonium excretion. Hypokalaemia is a further stimulus to ammoniagenesis. Low fluid volume in addition promotes urine formation with high content of uric acid and ammonium. The relative absence of sodium in the urine may permit ammonium to associate with urate; sodium depletion also impairs maximal distal acidification, causing a higher urine pH, and therefore less supersaturation of uric acid. Treatment should centre on potassium citrate for hypokalaemia and metabolic acidosis, and addressing causes of diarrhoea and urinary tract infection if present. The higher frequency of this crystal component in the developing world is attributed to diets deficient in protein and phosphate, and the high prevalence of infectious diarrhoea. In this setting, these stones have a particular proclivity for affecting children, more often boys, and for forming in the bladder.

2,8-Dihydroxyadenine

These rare stones occur in the setting of the autosomal recessive disorder of deficient production of adenine phophoribosyl transferase (APRT). The result of this enzyme deficiency is that adenine is not reused, but shifted towards production of the poorly soluble molecule 2,8-dihydroxyadenine. These stones can be mistaken for uric acid if chemical analysis is performed rather than infrared spectroscopy or X-ray crystallography. Renal failure due to interstitial deposition is a significant risk and can recur in renal transplants. Allopurinol is an important therapy with the potential to prevent progression of renal failure.

Struvite stones

Struvite stones, the most common composition of large staghorn calculi, form in the presence of infection with urease-producing organisms, most often *Proteus* species. Urea is metabolized to carbon dioxide and ammonia, a strong base, which increases urine pH by accepting a proton to form ammonium. The result of the high pH is precipitation of magnesium ammonium phosphate and carbonate apatite. The most critical step in the treatment and prevention of recurrence of these stones is elimination of the causative infection. Antibiotics sometimes suffice but their ability to penetrate and sterilize infected stones is poor, and recurrence rates are high. Medical therapy to inhibit urease activity is poorly tolerated.

The ultimate therapy of struvite stones is therefore surgical, with an emphasis on removing all infected stone material (Segura *et al.* 1994). There is no doubt that patients with stones left in place suffer high rates of urosepsis, renal failure, and death. Urological advances in recent years has led to a significant decrease in struvite stone recurrence and morbidity. Extracorporeal shock wave lithotripsy (ESWL) was associated with relatively high stone recurrence rates for all but the smallest struvite stones so that other options are now preferable. Flexible ureteroscopy with endoscopic lithotripsy of complex staghorn calculi is now highly successful, even in removing stones in the lower renal poles. Percutaneous nephostolithotomy has also improved and become more capable of rendering the infected collecting system stone-free with greater success rates and less morbidity than ESWL. The technological virtuousity needed to best put these techniques to use is not always available, so that the inferior option of ESWL is still frequently utilized by urologists with infrequent exposure to these complex stones.

Given the improvements in urological care, there is virtually no place for medical therapy of struvite stones today. Such therapies might be useful for patients where surgery is strongly contraindicated or where the requisite surgical expertise is lacking. Acetohydroxamic acid is an inhibitor of the enzyme urease, and it has been used to successfully prevent stone growth in several randomized controlled trials, all performed before the current era of endoscopic urology (Griffith *et al.* 1991). In each case, the drug was associated with less stone growth and increased rates of tremulousness, phelbitis, gastrointestinal intolerance, headache, and anxiety as compared with placebo, resulting in significant rates of patient withdrawal. The drug has not been shown to prevent stones after complete surgical removal, but might be useful in this setting where recurrent infection is likely. In renal insufficiency (serum creatinine >2.0 mg/dl) the drug is metabolized and fails to achieve adequate urinary concentration while producing a greater rate of side-effects.

Long-term therapy with culture-specific antibiotics may have the ability to reduce the magnitude of urinary tract infections and thereby the production of urease, with stabilization of stone growth even with the inevitable failure of sterilization. High rates of antibiotic resistance of the responsible organisms should be expected. Suppressive antibiotics such as nitrofurantoin, methenamine, or sulfamethoxazole are always given after urological interventions for struvite stone removal.

A significant proportion of patients with struvite stones, especially those whose stones include some component of calcium oxalate, are demonstrated to have metabolic abnormalities such as hypercalciuria and hyperoxaluria (Kristensen *et al.* 1987). Many such patients had typical episodes of stone passage preceding the discovery of their struvite stones, implying that typical calcium stone disease served to facilitate infection of their urinary tracts. The role of metabolic stone formation causing an inciting episode of calcium stone formation is much less in women, patients with pure struvite stones, and those with anatomical abnormalities such as spinal cord injury, duplicated collecting systems, or horseshoe kidneys. The role of treatment of specific metabolic risk factors has not been definitively established, but it is likely that modification of these factors would diminish stone recurrence in the population with mixed stones. Increased urine volume is clearly a rational therapy as it lowers supersaturation of the responsible stone constituents while preventing urinary stasis and reducing the rate of urinary tract infection.

It is of historical interest that phosphate depletion achieved with ingestion of low-phosphorus diets and aluminium-containing antacids has also been shown to reduce stone growth, but is poorly tolerated.

Cystine stones

Cystinuria results from a recessive mutation of the proximal tubule's cystine transporter (Goodyer *et al.* 2000). This poorly soluble amino acid is a dimer of the much more soluble amino acid cysteine. Although randomized controlled trials investigating cystine stone formation are lacking, the physiological principles that should lead to clinical benefit appear clear. The first goal in the prevention of cystine stone formation in cystinuria is to maintain the solubility of cystine. Increasing oral fluid intake to increase urine volume may suffice in some cases to lower cystine concentration and avoid stone formation (Barbey *et al.* 2000). A standard estimate of cystine solubility is that 250 mg (1 mmol) requires 1 l of urine to remain soluble. Cystine excretion can be measured in 24-h collections and oral fluid intake prescribed to maintain a concentration less than 250 mg/l. The most common phenotype, Type I cystinuria, is often caused by the genotype of homozygous mutations in the gene SLC3A1; such patients often have more than 1000 mg of cystine in their urine and may have difficulty maintaining urine volumes of 4 l or more. Even if these volumes are achieved, stone formation can continue unabated in some individuals. As in the case of calcium stones, the goal of fluid intake should be higher urine flow rates around the clock. Fluid intake at bedtime is recommended since increased urinary solute concentrations accompany sleep with its attendant decrease in fluid intake.

Another major determinant of cystine solubility is urine pH. Cystine solubility increases dramatically with urine pH values greater than 7.0 so that the goal of a programme of urinary alkalinization is values of 7.5–8.0. At pH 8.0, the solubility of cystine increases approximately fourfold, though the theoretical, and infrequent risk at this extreme is precipitation of calcium phosphate. Increased pH can be achieved through manipulation of diet and by oral supplementation with base. Dietary manipulation consists of restriction of animal protein, the major dietary source of protons. Reduction of ingestion of beef, poultry, pork, eggs, and fish can contribute to alkalinizing the urine. Reduction of protein intake is usually accompanied by reciprocal increases in ingestion of fruits and vegetables, which are relatively high in organic anions such as malate and citrate. These anions' carboxyl groups are metabolized by the liver, in the process of which protons are consumed, equivalent to generation of bicarbonate. Urine pH increases and cystine solubility improves.

Supplementation with oral base is often necessary for urinary alkalinization to the target range. The preferred supplement is potassium citrate, except in instances of decreased renal function when hyperkalaemia may occur. Citrate ingestion can come from dietary intake of citrus fruit and juices, particularly lemon juice, and pharmacological supplementation. Potassium citrate preparations are used in preference to sodium citrate since increases in urinary sodium excretion causes increases in urinary cystine excretion. For this reason, dietary restriction of sodium chloride is also recommended in prevention of cystine stones. Typical doses of potassium citrate are 20–30 mEq given two to four times per day, with one dose at bedtime to prevent nocturnal urinary acidification.

More difficult to achieve is a reduction in the absolute amount of cystine excreted. Reduced intake of methionine, the amino acid precursor of cystine, might be useful for patients who are willing to reduce animal protein intake, the major dietary source of methionine. However, even vegetarianism does not completely reduce cystine excretion, though individual patients and their physicians have claimed that the change made a difference. Unfortunately, such anecdotal reports are noteworthy due to the lack of any recent data demonstrating the benefit of reducing methionine intake. Literature examining the efficacy of diet as a preventive manipulation is scarce. Regardless of its utility to reduce cystine excretion, intake of animal protein serves also to alkalinize the urine and this effect may be the more persuasive indication for this recommendation.

If fluids, diet, and alkalinization fail to control cystine stone formation, the next modality available is the thiol drugs. Drugs containing thiol (sulfhydryl) groups can also reduce free cystine excretion. Such drugs reduce the cystine disulfide bridge, forming soluble drug–cysteine complexes. The most commonly used agents in this class are tiopronin (α-mercaptoproprionylglycine) and penicillamine. The rate of side-effects, particularly skin rashes and gastrointestinal intolerance, which limits use of thiols in as many as 40–50 per cent of patients, is somewhat less with tiopronin than with penicillamine so that it is now generally considered the first line thiol drug. Though never compared with each other in randomized trials, tiopronin may also be more effective than penicillamine.

The angiotensin-converting enzyme inhibitor captopril also contains a thiol and may have a modest effect on cystine excretion as well though the evidence is equivocal. Urine drug levels achieved with captopril are lower than with the other drugs, which may limit therapy (Coe *et al.* 2001). However, except for cough, it is well tolerated but should be avoided in women not using birth control. Hypertension in a patient with cystinuria would best be treated with captopril to take advantage of any effect it had on stone formation.

Doses of penicillamine and tiopronin often start at 500–1000 mg and are titrated upwards depending on urine volume and stone formation activity. Patients who cannot achieve target urine volumes need more thiol drugs to chelate more insoluble cystine. The dosing of these thiol drugs would be more straightforward if cystine assays were more reliable. One problem is the loss of precipitated cystine in urine that is not adequately alkalinized; such samples may yield falsely low values, corrected by alkalinizing the sample thoroughly before measuring cystine concentration (Nakagawa *et al.* 2000). Current assays may also not always clearly distinguish free cystine from drug–cysteine complexes, and may thereby obscure the effect of the drugs. Measurement of cystine supersaturation might be a more reliable method for assaying urine for cystine stone formation potential; such a technique is currently being developed (Nakagawa *et al.* 2000). Supersaturation is assayed by adding preformed cystine crystals to urine samples and measuring uptake or release of cystine by these crystals after a period of incubation. The ability of thiol drugs to affect supersaturation can then be measured directly. This technique, if validated, promises to change assessment of medical therapy of cystinuria.

Ascorbate (vitamin C), in a dose of 5 g/day, has been anecdotally reported to have efficacy in reducing the disulfide bridge of cystine and increasing cysteine excretion (Asper and Schmucki 1982). This effect is relatively small and unproven for long-term use in preventing stone formation. The argument has been made on physical chemistry grounds that the reaction actually cannot occur as ascorbate does not have sufficient reducing potential to drive the reaction (Ragone 2000).

Drugs and stones

Stones induced by or composed of drugs are relatively infrequent but several new drugs have led to new attention to this phenomenon. A careful drug history is an important consideration in evaluating patients with new onset of stones, or exacerbation of a previously recognized stone-forming syndrome. There are several mechanisms that account for drug-induced stones: insoluble drugs, drugs that alter urinary pH, drugs that cause hypercalciuria, hyperuricosuria, or hyperoxaluria, and drugs that lead to synthesis of other metabolites. The drugs are listed in Table 4.

Triamterene is often used as a potassium-sparing diuretic, as it blocks the ENaC. The drug is poorly soluble; its use can lead to triamterene stones, and probably causes calcium oxalate stones via heterogenous nucleation. Patients taking thiazides should be given amiloride or spironolactone for the treatment and prevention of hypokalaemia.

Most protease inhibitors are relatively insoluble, but indinavir also achieves relatively higher levels in the urine in patients with HIV infection. It is a frequent cause of stones as well as renal insufficiency associated with cast nephropathy. Although its pK is such that urinary acidification would boost its solubility, this is not a well-tolerated and entirely safe practice. Switching to another drug, such as nelfinavir, is preferred.

Sulfonamide precipitation with crystal formation or stones is less common today than in the past due to the use of more soluble preparations. It may still occur particularly in patients with HIV

Table 4 Drugs associated with stone formation listed by mechanism

Insoluble drugs
Triamterene
Sulfonamides
Felbamate
Ephedrine
Guafenisin
Aminophylline
Ciprofloxacin
Phenazopyridine
Acyclovir
Methyldopa
Nitrofurantoin
Calcium preparations
Vitamin D
Magnesium trisilicate
Effects on urine pH
Acetazolamide
Topiramate
Hypercalciuria
Calcium preparations
Vitamin D
Fursemide
Theophylline
Glucocorticoids
Hyperuricosuria
Probenecid
Hyperoxaluria
Ascorbate
Ethylene glycol
Piridoxilate
Other effects
Allopurinol

infection and toxoplasmosis treated with relatively high doses of sulfamethaxazole.

The best example of a drug that causes stones by altering urine pH is acetazolamide. This carbonic anhydrase inhibitor, most often used in the long term in the management of glaucoma, is active in the proximal and distal tubules, causing bicarbonaturia. Metabolic acidosis ensues, as does hypocitraturia; in the setting of a high urine pH, calcium phosphate stones occur as expected. Topiramate is a relatively new antiseizure medication, popular in management of paediatric epilepsy, associated with stone formation in as many as 1.5 per cent of treated patients. It has mild carbonic anhydrase activity, which might explain this association.

Allopurinol is the xanthine oxidase inhibitor often used in the management of gout and hyperuricosuria. Inhibition of uric acid synthesis allows the accumulation of xanthine. This intermediate metabolite, like uric acid, is poorly soluble in an acid medium; unlike uric acid, alkalinization does not help solubilize xanthine. Its accumulation is most likely to be of clinical significance in patients with lymphoproliferative disorders treated with allopurinol because of their risk of tumour lysis syndrome. Xanthine stones may also be seen in patients with Lesch–Nyhan syndrome treated with allopurinol.

References

Asper, R. and Schmucki, O. (1982). Cystinuria therapy by ascorbic acid. *Urology International* **37**, 91–109.

Asplin, J. R. (1996). Uric acid stones. *Seminars in Nephrology* **16**, 412–424.

Asplin, J. and Chandhoke, P. S. The stone-forming patient. In *Kidney Stones: Medical and Surgical Management* (ed. F. L. Coe *et al.*), pp. 337–352. Philadelphia: Lippincott-Raven, 1996.

Assimos, D. G. and Holmes, R. P. (2000). Role of diet in the therapy of urolithiasis. *Urologic Clinics of North America* **27**, 255–268.

Barbey, F. *et al.* (2000). Medical treatment of cystinuria: critical reappraisal of long-term results. *Journal of Urology* **163**, 1419–1423.

Barcelo, P. *et al.* (1993). Randomized double-blind study of potassium citrate in idiopathic hypocitraturic calcium nephrolithiasis. *Journal of Urology* **150**, 1761–1764.

Borghi, L. *et al.* (1993). Randomized prospective study of a nonthiazide diuretic, indapamide, in preventing calcium stone recurrences. *Journal of Cardiovascular Pharmacology* **22** (Suppl. 6), S78–S86.

Borghi, L. *et al.* (1996). Urinary volume, water and recurrences in idiopathic calcium nephrolithiasis: a 5-year randomized prospective study. *Journal of Urology* **155**, 839–843.

Borghi, L. *et al.* (2002). Comparison of two diets for the prevention of recurrent stones in idiopathic hypercalciuria. *New England Journal of Medicine* **346**, 77–84.

Breslau, N. A. *et al.* (1998). Physiological effects of slow release potassium phosphate for absorptive hypercalciuria: a randomized double-blind trial. *Journal of Urology* **160**, 664–668.

Buckalew, V. M. (1989). Nephrolithiasis in renal tubular acidosis. *Journal of Urology* **141**, 731–737.

Campieri, C. *et al.* (2001). Reduction of oxaluria after an oral course of lactic acid bacteria at high concentration. *Kidney International* **60**, 1097–1105.

Caruana, R. J. and Buckalew, V. M., Jr. (1988). The syndrome of distal (type 1) renal tubular acidosis. Clinical and laboratory findings in 58 cases. *Medicine (Baltimore)* **67**, 84–99.

Coe, F. L. and Parks, J. H. Pathogenesis and treatment of nephrolithiasis. In *The Kidney: Physiology and Pathophysiology* 3rd edn. (ed. D. W. Seldin and G. Giebisch), pp. 1841–1867. Philadelphia: Lippincott Williams & Wilkins, 2000.

Coe, F. L., Parks, J. H., and Webb, D. R. (1992). Stone-forming potential of milk or calcium-fortified orange juice in idiopathic hypercalciuric adults. *Kidney International* **41**, 139–142.

Coe, F. L. *et al.* (2001). Solid phase assay of urine cystine supersaturation in the presence of cystine binding drugs. *Journal of Urology* **166**, 688–693.

Curhan, G. C. *et al.* (1993). A prospective study of dietary calcium and other nutrients and the risk of symptomatic kidney stones. *New England Journal of Medicine* **328**, 833–838.

Curhan, G. C. *et al.* (1997). Comparison of dietary calcium with supplemental calcium and other nutrients as factors affecting the risk for kidney stones in women. *Annals of Internal Medicine* **126**, 497–504.

Curhan, G. C. *et al.* (1998). Beverage use and risk for kidney stones in women. *Annals of Internal Medicine* **128**, 534–540.

Curhan, G. C. *et al.* (1999). Intake of vitamins B6 and C and the risk of kidney stones in women. *Journal of the American Society of Nephrology* **10**, 840–845.

Danpure, C. J. (2000). Genetic disorders and urolithiasis. *Urologic Clinics of North America* **27**, 287–299, viii.

Donnelly, S. *et al.* (1992). Might distal renal tubular acidosis be a proximal tubular cell disorder? *American Journal of Kidney Diseases* **19**, 272–281.

Ebisuno, S. *et al.* (1991). Results of long-term rice bran treatment on stone recurrence in hypercalciuric patients. *British Journal of Urology* **67**, 237–240.

Ettinger, B. *et al.* (1986). Randomized trial of allopurinol in the prevention of calcium oxalate calculi. *New England Journal of Medicine* **315**, 1386–1389.

Ettinger, B. *et al.* (1988). Chlorthalidone reduces calcium oxalate calculous recurrence but magnesium hydroxide does not. *Journal of Urology* **139**, 679–684.

Ettinger, B. *et al.* (1997). Potassium–magnesium citrate is an effective prophylaxis against recurrent calcium oxalate nephrolithiasis. *Journal of Urology* **158**, 2069–2073.

Frassetto, L. A. *et al.* (2000). Comparative effects of potassium chloride and bicarbonate on thiazide-induced reduction in urinary calcium excretion. *Kidney International* **58**, 748–752.

Gault, M. H. and Chafe, L. (2000). Relationship of frequency, age, sex, stone weight and composition in 15,624 stones: comparison of results for 1980 to 1983 and 1995 to 1998. *Journal of Urology* **164**, 302–307.

Gerster, H. (1997). No contribution of ascorbic acid to renal calcium oxalate stones. *Annals of Nutrition and Metabolism* **41**, 269–282.

Goldfarb, D. S. and Coe, F. L. (1999). Beverages, diet, and prevention of kidney stones. *American Journal of Kidney Diseases* **33**, 398–400.

Goldfarb, S. (1994). Diet and nephrolithiasis. *Annual Reviews in Medicine* **45**, 235–243.

Goodyer, P., Boutros, M., and Rozen, R. (2000). The molecular basis of cystinuria: an update. *Experimental Nephrology* **8**, 123–127.

Grases, F. *et al.* (2000). Urinary phytate in calcium oxalate stone formers and healthy people—dietary effects on phytate excretion. *Scandinavian Journal of Urology and Nephrology* **34**, 162–164.

Griffith, D. P. *et al.* (1991). Randomized, double-blind trial of Lithostat (acetohydroxamic acid) in the palliative treatment of infection-induced urinary calculi. *European Urology* **20**, 243–247.

Hiatt, R. A. *et al.* (1996). Randomized controlled trial of a low animal protein, high fiber diet in the prevention of recurrent calcium oxalate kidney stones. *American Journal of Epidemiology* **144**, 25–33.

Holmes, R. P. (2000). Oxalate synthesis in humans: assumptions, problems, and unresolved issues. *Molecular Urology* **4**, 329–332.

Holmes, R. P. and Kennedy, M. (2000). Estimation of the oxalate content of foods and daily oxalate intake. *Kidney International* **57**, 1662–1667.

Holmes, R. P., Assimos, D. G., and Goodman, H. O. (1998). Genetic and dietary influences on urinary oxalate excretion. *Urological Research* **26**, 195–200.

Holmes, R. P., Goodman, H. O., and Assimos, D. G. (2001). Contribution of dietary oxalate to urinary oxalate excretion. *Kidney International* **59**, 270–276.

Kamel, K. S., Cheema-Dhadli, S., and Halperin, M. L. (2002). Studies on the pathophysiology of the low urine pH in patients with uric acid stones. *Kidney International* **61**, 988–994.

Kristensen, C. *et al.* (1987). Reduced glomerular filtration rate and hypercalciuria in primary struvite nephrolithiasis. *Kidney International* **32**, 749–753.

Laerum, E. and Larsen, S. (1984). Thiazide prophylaxis of urolithiasis. A double-blind study in general practice. *Acta Medica Scandinavica* **215**, 383–389.

Lauderdale, D. S. *et al.* (2001). Bone mineral density and fracture among prevalent kidney stone cases in the Third National Health and Nutrition Examination Survey. *Journal of Bone and Mineral Research* **15**, 1893–1898.

Lemann, J., Piering, W. F., and Lennon, E. J. (1969). Possible role of carbohydrate-induced calciuria in calcium oxalate kidney-stone formation. *New England Journal of Medicine* **280**, 232–237.

Lemann, J. *et al.* (1996). Urinary oxalate excretion increases with body size and decreases with increasing dietary calcium intake among healthy adults. *Kidney International* **49**, 200–208.

Leumann, E. and Hoppe, B. (2001). The primary hyperoxalurias. *Journal of the American Society of Nephrology* **12**, 1986–1993.

Levine, B. S. *et al.* (1994). Effect of calcium citrate supplementation on urinary calcium oxalate saturation in female stone formers: implications for prevention of osteoporosis. *American Journal of Clinical Nutrition* **60**, 592–596.

Lindsjo, M. *et al.* (1989). Treatment of enteric hyperoxaluria with calcium-containing organic marine hydrocolloid. *Lancet* **2**, 701–704.

Lingeman, J. *et al.* (1998). Medical reduction of stone risk in a network of treatment centers compared to a research clinic. *Journal of Urology* **160**, 1629–1634.

Massey, L. K., Roman-Smith, H., and Sutton, R. A. (1993). Effect of dietary oxalate and calcium on urinary oxalate and risk of formation of calcium oxalate kidney stones. *Journal of the American Dietetics Association* **93**, 901–906.

Milliner, D. S., Wilson, D. M., and Smith, L. H. (2001). Phenotypic expression of primary hyperoxaluria: comparative features of types I and II. *Kidney International* **59**, 31–36.

Milliner, D. S. *et al.* (1994). Results of long-term treatment with orthophosphate and pyridoxine in patients with primary hyperoxaluria. *New England Journal of Medicine* **331**, 1553–1558.

Nakagawa, Y. *et al.* (2000). Clinical use of cystine supersaturation measurements. *Journal of Urology* **164**, 1481–1485.

National Institutes of Health Consensus Development Conference on Prevention and Treatment of Kidney Stones (1989). *Journal of Urology* **141**, 705–808.

Parks, J. H. and Coe, F. L. (1996). The financial effects of kidney stone prevention. *Kidney International* **50**, 1706–1712.

Parks, J. H., Coward, M., and Coe, F. L. (1997). Correspondence between stone composition and urine supersaturation in nephrolithiasis. *Kidney International* **51**, 894–900.

Patron, P., Gardin, J. P., and Paillard, M. (1987). Renal mass and reserve of vitamin D: determinants in primary hyperparathyroidism. *Kidney International* **31**, 1174–1180.

Pearle, M. S., Roehrborn, C. G., and Pak, C. Y. (1999). Meta-analysis of randomized trials for medical prevention of calcium oxalate nephrolithiasis. *Journal of Endourology* **13**, 679–685.

Ragone, R. (2000). Medical treatment of cystinuria with vitamin C. *American Journal of Kidney Diseases* **35**, 1020.

Rodman, J. S. (1991). Prophylaxis of uric acid stones with alternate day doses of alkaline potassium salts. *Journal of Urology* **145**, 97–99.

Segura, J. W. *et al.* (1994). Nephrolithiasis Clinical Guidelines Panel summary report on the management of staghorn calculi. The American Urological Association Nephrolithiasis Clinical Guidelines Panel. *Journal of Urology* **151**, 1648–1651.

Sidhu, H. *et al.* (1999). Direct correlation between hyperoxaluria/oxalate stone disease and the absence of the gastrointestinal tract-dwelling bacterium *Oxalobacter formigenes*: possible prevention by gut recolonization or enzyme replacement therapy. *Journal of the American Society of Nephrology* **10** (Suppl. 14), S334–S340.

Soble, J. J., Hamilton, B. D., and Streem, S. B. (1999). Ammonium acid urate calculi: a reevaluation of risk factors. *Journal of Urology* **161**, 869–873.

Tiselius, H. G. *et al.* (2001). Guidelines on urolithiasis. *European Urology* **40**, 362–371.

Wasserstein, A. G. *et al.* (1987). Case–control study of risk factors for idiopathic calcium nephrolithiasis. *Mineral and Electrolyte Metabolism* **13**, 85–95.

Weisinger, J. R. *et al.* (1997). Role of bones in the physiopathology of idiopathic hypercalciuria: effect of amino-bisphosphonate alendronate. *Medicina (B Aires)* **57** (Suppl. 1), 45–48.

8.3 The surgical management of renal stones

Hugh Whitfield and Suresh K. Gupta

Introduction

During the last 15 years the surgical management of stones in the urinary tract has been radically altered. Advances in endoscopic instrument technology, the development of interventional uroradiological procedures, and the advent of extracorporeal shockwave lithotripters have combined to revolutionize the surgical approach to stone disease. The rate of change has been so rapid that even those close to the subject have had difficulty in keeping in touch with progress. Indications for the removal of stones have changed, since the newly introduced techniques are less invasive and minimize morbidity. Restraints that are present as a result of financial limitations in many parts of the world will be ignored in this chapter.

Percutaneous renal surgery

History and development

Credit for the first planned percutaneous nephrolithotomy (PCNL) must go to Fernström and Johannson (1976), whose report gave details of the first three procedures which they had performed a year earlier. Seldinger (1953) first reported the use of guide wires for angiography, and this technique is fundamental for the performance of all percutaneous renal surgeries. The first experience of antegrade renal radiology was reported by Wickbom (1954), and Goodwin *et al.* (1955) described the passage of a coaxial tube through a larger needle in order to drain the kidney. Fernström amalgamated and expanded these techniques, setting the scene for percutaneous renal surgery. His earliest cases involved the extraction of stones that were small enough to be removed intact through the tract. The first report of the planned disintegration of a large stone came from Rathbert *et al.* (1977), who used ultrasonic disintegration; Raney and Handler (1975) had used electrohydraulic disintegration of a retained stone, but with a track placed at open surgery.

The next significant landmark was the report by Thüroff and Hutschenriter (1980) from Mainz in Germany; a year later Alken *et al.* (1981) described 19 cases from the same centre and Wickham and Kellett (1981) reported the first five cases in the United Kingdom. Thereafter enormous enthusiasm for the technique developed worldwide.

Technique

There are two stages in performing a PCNL: first a track must be formed between the skin surface and the collecting system, and then the stone(s) must be removed endoscopically.

Forming a track

Applied anatomy

The usual puncture site lies between the subcostal margin and the iliac crest, lateral to the lateral border of the erector spinae. Although the right kidney lies at a lower level than the left, it is usual to find that only the lowest third of each kidney lies below the 12th rib; therefore the lower pole of the calyx is the most convenient point of access. Within each major calyceal group, minor calices are orientated in anterior, posterior, and lateral directions. A posterior or lateral calyx will give access to the rest of the collecting system, but with the patient lying prone or prone/oblique it is often impossible to gain access to the renal pelvis via a minor calyx disposed anteriorly (Fig. 1).

Although some of the superior calyceal groups can be explored through a lower calyceal track, the middle calyceal group may not be accessible. If the stone-bearing calyx is in the middle group, it may be necessary to dilate a track that lies above the 12th rib. The precise position of the pleural reflection varies, but it is usual to be able to avoid the pleura as long as the track is lateral to the midaxillary line, even if the puncture is above the 11th rib. If the pleural cavity is entered this

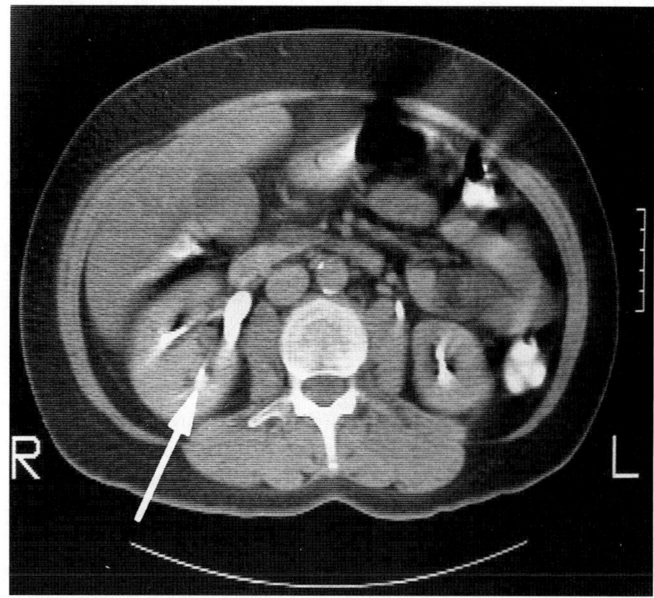

Fig. 1 A CT scan of a kidney. The arrow marks the line of approach to a posterior calyx.

is not an insuperable problem; a chest drain should be inserted at the end of the procedure, to drain any irrigating fluid that has entered the pleural cavity.

Track dilatation

In the very early days of PCNL the track was dilated under local anaesthetic over several days. PCNL is now commonly performed as a one-stage procedure under general anaesthetic.

The first step is to outline the collecting system, which is most conveniently done by passing a retrograde catheter up the ureter into the renal pelvis with the patient lying supine or in the lithotomy position. A small amount of methylene blue is mixed with the radiographic contrast so that it becomes easier to recognize when the puncture needle has entered the collecting system. With the catheter in position, the renal pelvis and calices may be gently distended to facilitate needle puncture. The catheter also helps to orient the operator during endoscopy and prevents stone fragments from passing into the ureter.

The patient is turned into the prone or prone/oblique position. Needle puncture is performed under either ultrasound or radiographic control. The usual puncture needle is of the Longdwell variety and has an outer Teflon sheath. The puncture must be made transparenchymally and as close to the convex border of the kidney as possible to ensure that there is minimal disturbance to the vascular supply of the kidney. During dilatation the parenchyma and the vessels which supply it are pushed aside; the track heals as a fine linear scar, with no detectable reduction of function (Webb and Fitzpatrick 1985). The theoretical risk of arteriovenous fistula formation has not been found to occur in practice, and this must be because there is minimal damage to vessels. Therefore, track dilatation is entirely different from the technique of renal biopsy, in which a core of tissue is removed. The transparenchymal approach is also essential for preventing the development of urinary fistula when the nephrostomy tube is finally removed.

When the needle tip lies within the collecting system the inner elements of the needle are removed and a guide wire is passed through the Teflon sheath. The tip of the guide wire should either pass down the ureter or curl up within the renal pelvis or in an upper pole calyx to provide anchorage during dilatation. Guide wires with flexible tips and stiffer shafts have the advantage of not kinking during dilatation (Fig. 2).

Three methods of dilatation have been described. A balloon dilator can be used, but these are expensive and cannot be reused. There is the advantage that dilatation of the track is quick and relatively straightforward. The balloon is backloaded with a 30 French guage Amplatz sheath. The balloon is passed over a stiff guide wire. The tip of the balloon must be within the selected calyx. The track is dilated by inflating the balloon with radio-opaque contrast to a pressure of 10–12 atm. If fibrosis of muscle layers and the perinephric tissues is present due to previous surgery, 'waisting' of the balloon may occur. Once the track is dilated the Amplatz sheath is placed over the inflated balloon to provide a conduit between the skin surface and the collecting system. The balloon is then deflated and removed. Graded Teflon dilators and metal telescopic bougies provide two alternative methods of dilating the track, and each has its advocates. Progress of the dilation is monitored radiologically to ensure that the tip of the dilator lies within, but not beyond, the collecting system.

Whatever the method of dilatation, the track must be kept patent by passing a sheath over the largest dilator, which is about 30 French gauge (a diameter of 9.5 mm). This sheath acts not only as a conduit between the skin surface and the collecting system for the passing of instruments during endoscopy but also tamponades the track and prevents bleeding.

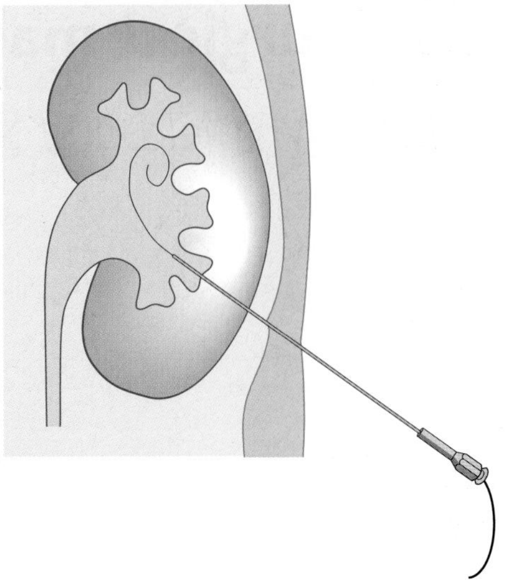

Fig. 2 Diagram showing the standard site of access for percutaneous renal surgery.

Stone removal

All the major urological instrument makers have now designed rigid endoscopes for percutaneous renal surgery, the majority of which incorporates an offset eye-piece so that a straight channel is available for instruments used in the removal and disintegration of stones.

Any stone which is accessible from the track and has the greatest diameter less than 9 mm can be grasped with an alligator or triradiate instrument and removed intact. Larger stones must first be disintegrated, and this can be done in different ways. If a flexible electrohydraulic probe is used, a high-tension spark is discharged at the end of the probe between a central core electrode and circumferential peripheral electrode. The frequency of the spark discharge can be altered from single shots to two to five passes with a frequency of up to 30 Hz; this is sufficient to fragment most stones, although those composed of calcium monohydrate, cystine, or uric acid can be very hard. Great care must be taken to ensure that the tip of the electrohydraulic probe is in contact with the stone; if it is not, serious damage to the collecting system can occur. The stone fragments which result are subsequently removed piecemeal.

Another method is to use ultrasonic energy, which is delivered at the end of a hollow probe to which suction is applied. This is particularly effective for dealing with infective triple-phosphate stones, when the 'hoovering' action of the probe can remove quite large amounts of calcified matrix material in a short time. No damage to the collecting system occurs if the probe is discharged when the tip is in contact with the mucosa. Calcium oxalate stones may also be disintegrated very satisfactorily; the hardest stones may take time, but can be fragmented with ultrasound and removed piecemeal rather than being suctioned out.

A third way of disintegrating stones, pneumatic lithotripsy, has been developed over the last 5 years. This is a safe and effective method of stone disintegration (Schulze *et al.* 1993). A suction device can be incorporated which enables small fragments that have been disintegrated to be removed during the process of disintegration. The latest modification incorporates the pneumatic disintegrator with an ultrasound probe so that simultaneous disintegration occurs with continuous suction of the very small stone fragments that are produced.

Whatever method of stone disintegration is used, on-table radiographs are taken to ensure that stones have been completely cleared. A large-size nephrostomy tube is left *in situ* for 24–48 h to tamponade the track and to provide drainage for any bleeding or clots that may occur. When the nephrostomy is removed the track usually closes within a few hours, although a urinary fistula occasionally persists for a day or two for no apparent reason. Most patients are fit to leave hospital on the second or third postoperative day. Some urologists advocate leaving no nephrostomy tube postoperatively. Punctures above the 11th or 12th rib are more painful postoperatively, and an intercostal block is an effective way of providing pain control.

Indications and contraindications

PCNL is usually reserved for stones that are larger than 2–2.5 cm in maximum diameter. Other factors that will influence the decision are stone composition. Very hard stones, such as cystine, are better treated with PCNL. The fate of fragments of non-opaque stones is difficult to follow, so again PCNL may be the preferred choice for stones less than 2 cm in diameter. Triple phosphate stones are relatively soft and respond poorly to extracorporeal shortwave lithotripsy (ESWL).

Renal pelvic stones

Stones which lie within the renal pelvis are the easiest to remove. Access through a lower-pole calyx is usually possible and good anchorage for the guide wire during dilatation should present no problem. The procedure becomes more difficult when a stone fills a small intrarenal pelvis. The ideal stone for percutaneous removal lies within a large extrarenal pelvis. Small stones can be removed intact, but larger stones need to be disintegrated.

Calyceal stones

It is always more difficult to remove stones from a calyx than from the renal pelvis; very often the track must be made directly on to the stone-bearing calyx, a procedure which demands a high degree of accuracy during track dilatation. Access to a lower-pole calyx is easier than access to middle- or upper-pole calyces, when the track has to be very oblique under the 12th rib or between the 11th and 12th ribs. When the stone-bearing calyx has a narrow infundibulum a direct puncture is essential. For the same reason, stones which have eroded the calyx in which they lie and stones within calyceal diverticula require a direct puncture.

It has often been suggested that stones in calyces cause few symptoms. Although many people live with a small stone that has not grown significantly over many years, calyceal colic is a very real entity. Whether chronic backache can be attributed to the presence of a stone can only be determined by removing the stone. Not infrequently the patient whose stone is removed will not only benefit from the absence of the pain but will also be aware of a significant improvement in his or her general well being.

Staghorn stones

The term 'staghorn' is used to describe different varieties of stone. A full staghorn occupies the renal pelvis and all the calyces, but stones which fill much but not all of the collecting system are also frequently, but incorrectly, termed staghorn. Moreover, the proportions of a staghorn stone which are calyceal and the proportions which are pelvic vary greatly depending on intrarenal anatomy.

Theoretically, and often in practice, there is no reason why staghorn stones should not be removed entirely by percutaneous surgery (Patterson *et al.* 1987). However, this may be time consuming and, where large calyceal fragments exist, multiple tracks will be required. Increasing operating time and/or operating sessions combined with the need for multiple tracks may sway the choice of procedure away from percutaneous surgery.

Ureteric stones

Stones which lie within the upper third of the ureter may be removed via an antegrade approach. In order to gain access to the ureter easily, the initial puncture should be placed in a middle or upper calyx. If the ureter above the stone is very dilated, an instrument of the calibre of a nephroscope may be accommodated. At other times a ureteroscope may be used. Stones may be removed intact or disintegrated *in situ* ultrasonically or electrohydraulically (Streem *et al.* 1988).

Contraindications

There are few absolute contraindications to percutaneous nephrostomy (Whitfield 1987). Although patients with a coagulopathy have often been mentioned as falling in this category, such a problem would also contraindicate other surgical methods of stone management. Gross spinal deformity may make a percutaneous approach impossible, but this is not necessarily so. A high kidney, an upper-pole stone, and a malrotated or horseshoe kidney may all cause difficulties, and success will depend on the expertise of the surgeon.

Complications

A catalogue of the possible complications related to percutaneous renal surgery would appear daunting but their incidence is very low (Whitfield 1983). The technique differs from open surgery in that the margin for error is much smaller. If bleeding occurs, if the track is lost, or if the collecting system is perforated, the operation has to be abandoned. However, if a large-size nephrostomy tube is left *in situ*, it is usually possible to complete the procedure 48–72 h later. The combined morbidity and the hospital stay of the two procedures remains less than that of open surgery.

Bleeding sufficiently severe to require transfusion or to necessitate abandoning the procedure occurs infrequently. Dilatation of the track can provoke severe bleeding if the initial puncture is placed too centrally. Veins around a calyceal neck can be damaged during dilatation of a narrow infundibulum or if an electrohydraulic probe is discharged in contact with the collecting system. Secondary haemorrhage has been described but is a problem which occurs very infrequently. Arteriovenous shunts have been demonstrated, but there are good reasons, already discussed, which make this more of a theoretical than a practical problem. If severe bleeding (primary or secondary) does occur, selective arterial embolization is the treatment of choice. Nephrectomy is the last resort which is needed very rarely.

Septicaemia is a potential hazard of any stone surgery, particularly when triple-phosphate stones which are infective in origin are being removed. It is not uncommon to find sterile urine in the presence of a stone from which organisms can be cultured. All patients undergoing PCNL should receive prophylactic parenteral antibiotics, but some may still develop septicaemia which must be treated appropriately.

If perforation of the collecting system goes unnoticed, large volumes of irrigating fluid may be extravasated in a very short time. Therefore, it is important to monitor the irrigant volumes being used and the amount recovered. Normal saline should always be the irrigant, not water or glycine, to lessen the potential for water overload. This is a recognized complication of lower urinary tract surgery but may also occur during PCNL. The irrigant should be warmed to body temperature and the patient should be placed on a warming mattress of some kind, since hypothermia can be encountered preoperatively (Miller and Whitfield 1985).

Hypertension probably occurs in patients with renal stone disease *per se*, particularly in those in whom infection and/or obstruction play a significant role, but there is no evidence that percutaneous surgery (or open surgery or lithotripsy) encourages the further development of hypertension.

Inadvertent transpleural puncture may go unrecognized and the patient will develop a pneumothorax or a haemo/hydropneumothorax. Removal of a high stone may need a supra-12 puncture, in which case a chest drain should be inserted as a planned manoeuvre.

There have been sporadic reports of perforation of the large bowel (Netto *et al.* 1988), the duodenum, the inferior vena cava, and the peritoneal cavity, but such untoward events are rare and can usually be avoided.

In the absence of any ureteric obstruction, leakage of urine from the kidney usually ceases within a few hours after the nephrostomy tube is removed since the parenchyma and soft tissues act as an effective sealing mechanism. Occasionally, a urinary fistula persists, but the insertion of a JJ stent usually resolves the problem quickly.

Results

Most centres in which percutaneous surgery is performed regularly would expect to achieve a success rate for one-stage PCNL of at least 95 per cent. There is learning curve (a euphemism for an early high failure rate) which has been encountered and endured by all urologists and by their patients (Whitfield and Mills 1985). The advent of ESWL has made the acquisition of percutaneous expertise more difficult, since stones that would be easy to remove percutaneously are almost always the most straightforward cases for ESWL. Improvement in performance depends upon acquiring expertise and experience in recognizing the potential difficulties of a case before deciding on the method of surgery.

Advantages and disadvantages

The advantages of percutaneous surgery compared with open surgery can be discussed separately from the relative merits of PCNL and endoscopic shockwave lithotripsy.

The morbidity attached to a percutaenous approach can be assessed in terms of the pain which occurs, the occurrence of postoperative ileus and its duration, the risks and rate of various complications, the length of hospital stay, and the time required for convalescence. By any of these criteria percutaneous surgery carries a morbidity which is an order of magnitude less than that of open surgery. A prospective comparative trial cannot be performed, since such a scientifically sound method could not be justified on ethical grounds (Preminger *et al.* 1985; Webb *et al.* 1985). The patient who has experienced both open and percutaneous surgery is in the best position to judge, and the surgeon who has been involved in the care of such patients after both types of surgery would also have no doubts.

There are no disadvantages for the patient who has a successful PCNL, but for the small percentage of failures a 'casualty syndrome' has been described, which at its worst results in open surgery following two or even more failed percutaneous procedures. However, there can be disadvantages for the surgeon. The techniques are difficult to learn, the learning curve is frustrating, and the potential hazards of irradiation exposure and auditory damage from ultrasonic disintegrators cannot be ignored (Bowsher *et al.* 1992).

Extracorporeal shockwave lithotripsy

History and development

The sudden explosion of ESWL on the medical scene in 1980 should not mask the painstaking development that had occurred in West Germany during the preceding years. A group of engineers in Munich were the first to recognize that focused shockwaves might be used to disintegrate renal stones. Collaboration between scientists and urologists led to the first clinical experience in Munich in 1980 (Chaussy *et al.* 1982). Although lithotripsy was initially used only for stones which were in the renal pelvis and which were considered to be metabolic rather than infective in origin, the indications were subsequently broadened. The second Dornier lithotripter to be installed was located in Stuttgart, where Eisenberger *et al.* (1985) exploited the potential of lithotripsy even further. This group was amongst the first to demonstrate the advantages of combining PCNL and ESWL. During 1983 and 1984 more lithotripters were installed throughout West Germany, and in December 1984 the first Dornier HM3 arrived in the United Kingdom. The following year the United States Food and Drugs Administration approved the machine for limited clinical trials and within a year large numbers of lithotripters began to appear all over the developed world. The Dornier HM3 became the gold standard against which all future lithotripters would be compared.

A general or epidural anaesthetic was required for lithotripsy using the Dornier HM3. The patient was secured on a frame so that the loin was exposed and was then lowered into a water bath. The water acted as a coupling medium between the shockwave and the patient, and prevented damage to the skin and soft tissue. The water was warmed to body temperature, degassed, and deionized. The shockwave was produced by a spark-gap mechanism (see below). The site of the shockwave focus was fixed and the stone had to be brought into the focus by moving the patient on the frame using two-dimensional radiographic control (Fig. 3). The number of shockwaves required for complete disintegration varied between 200 and 2000, depending on the size and composition of the stone. Progress was monitored by radiological screening. Since there was a risk that the shockwave might provoke cardiac dysrhythmias, the triggering was linked with an electrocardiogram (ECG) so that the shockwave was delivered during a refractory period of the cardiac cycle.

By the end of 1986 several 'second-generation' lithotripters were on the market, and by 1988 it was estimated that some 500,000 patients had received treatment worldwide. Upper and lower ureteric stones were also found to be within the scope of ESWL.

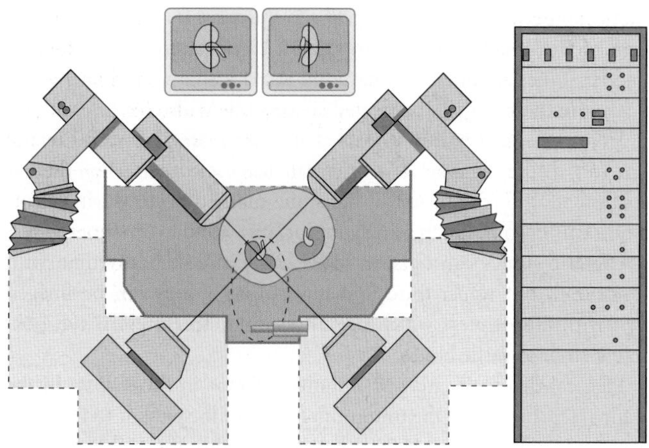

Fig. 3 The principle of a Domier HM3 lithotripter, showing biplanar X-ray tubes and a spark-gap electrode.

Principles of lithotripsy

All lithotripters require a mechanism producing a high-energy shockwave focus, a means of imaging the stone, and the ability to bring the shockwave focus and stone to coincidence. The lithotripters that are now available use different combinations of shockwave production and imaging. The ultimate goal to which the technique aspires is accurate imaging of a stone anywhere in the upper urinary tract followed by complete disintegration in all cases without the need for anaesthesia, analgesia, or sedation. At the present time, however, some compromise has to be reached between the power of the shockwave, the size of the energy focus, the pain produced, and the number of shockwaves required for complete stone disintegration.

Generating a shockwave

The three methods which are currently used for generating shockwaves are electrohydraulic, electromagnetic, and piezoelectric. The physical characteristics of the shockwaves produced by each method vary significantly, and it is these properties which not only dictate the way in which the stone disintegrates but also influence the clinical management during and after lithotripsy.

The five most important variables are the time taken for the shockwave to rise to peak pressure, the peak pressure itself, the extent to which the shockwave is biphasic, the angle of entry of the shockwave through the skin, and the surface area over which the shockwave enters the body on its way to the energy focus. The greater the peak pressure and the longer the time required to reach that pressure, the more acute the angle of entry, and the smaller the surface area through which the shockwave enters, the more painful the procedure.

Electrohydraulic

In many lithotripters the spark-gap principle is used for shockwave production. In the Dornier HM3 the life of the electrode was limited by the rapid rate of erosion of the opposing electrodes, and this contributed to its high running costs. Subsequent modifications in other lithotripters have helped to overcome this problem. A high-tension spark is discharged across two electrodes and the resulting shockwave produced at the first focus of a hemi-ellipsoid is brought to a second focus 1.5 cm × 0.7 cm × 0.5 cm by reflection from the sides of the hemi-ellipsoid. The diameter of the hemi-ellipsoid can be varied, altering the angle of entry of the shockwaves at the skin surface. The larger the diameter of the dish the less analgesia is required. General or epidural anaesthesia was necessary with both the Dornier HM3 and the original Technomed Lithostar, but subsequent modifications to both machines allow local anaesthesia and/or sedation to be used.

Piezoelectric

A mosaic of piezoelectric crystals covers the dish and each produces a shockwave which is brought to a small focus of dimensions 0.4 cm × 1.1 cm. Lithotripsy using these shockwaves can be performed without the need for analgesia, sedation, or anaesthesia, but the number of shockwaves required and the need for repeat treatments is greater than with other lithotripters.

Electromagnetic

A magnetic field, generated electrically, moves a flexible membrane to produce a pressure wave that is then focused. Some local, regional, or general anaesthesia and/or sedation is required.

Other methods

Laser-generated shockwaves have been tried in the United States, but so far without significant clinical success. A Japanese lithotripter using small explosive charges to generate shockwaves was designed, but the method was not adopted elsewhere.

Imaging

Radiological

Two-dimensional radiographic imaging was used in the Dornier HM3 and has been employed subsequently in many other lithotripters. The amount of radiation exposure during a treatment varies, largely depending on the experience of the operator, but it is not a hazard to the patient, being approximately equivalent to the exposure received during a barium enema. Radiological evidence of disintegration depends on seeing the density of the stone decrease and the size of the stone shadow increase. The resolution of radiographic screening may make it difficult to image stones which are not very radio-opaque, particularly in obese patients. Completely radiolucent stones can be treated by filling the collecting system with contrast, either after an intravenous injection or via a retrograde ureteric catheter, and then following the negative shadows.

Ultrasound

When ultrasound-guided lithotripters were introduced some radiologists doubted whether stones could be imaged accurately. There are several factors which combine to make this possible. First, the presence and position of a stone has been demonstrated radiologically and ultrasound has not been used to screen for stones. When the bright echo, characteristic of a stone, with a negative shadow behind it corresponds in position to a stone that has previously been demonstrated radiologically, the evidence becomes irrefutable. When the stone lies within a dilated part of the collecting system the echo is more distinct. In the upper ureter, a stone can be imaged if the ureter above the stone is dilated; in a non-dilated system stones in the upper ureter can be located with ultrasound using the lower pole of the kidney as an acoustic window. In the lower third of the ureter a stone can be seen through the full bladder which is used as an acoustic window. Imaging continues during lithotripsy, and the stone or stone particles can often be seen to bounce as the shockwaves occur. Tiny particles can sometimes be seen with ultrasound, but problems occur if there has been surgery previously because scarring within the kidney can produce confusing images.

Indications and contraindications

Lithotripsy is a two-stage process: the stone(s) must be disintegrated into fragments that are small enough to pass spontaneously, and then these fragments must be eliminated. The second phase requires adequate drainage of the entire upper and lower urinary tract. The presence of an impairment to ureteric urine flow, such as a ureterocele, or obstruction of the pelvi-ureteric junction, are obvious contraindications to lithotripsy. Intrarenal anatomy is also of vital importance: some stones seem to erode the calyx in which they lie, and drainage may be jeopardized. The size of the infundibulum is the crucial factor in deciding whether or not lithotripsy will be effective for calyceal stones. For the same reasons stones in a calyceal cyst or diverticulum are not suitable for lithotripsy.

The size of a stone may be a limiting factor. The disintegration of a large stone will produce a correspondingly large number of particles, which may exceed the capacity of the ureter to pass them spontaneously. The hardness of the stone and the type of lithotripter used are also related, since shockwaves generated by a spark discharge or electromagnetically fragment stones in a different way from piezoelectrically generated shockwaves: the first two methods split stones into halves, then quarters, then eighths, and so on, but piezoelectric shockwaves 'nibble' at the stones from the outside and the resulting particles are finer. As a general rule, any stone which has a maximum diameter greater than 2.5 cm can be treated by lithotripsy only in conjunction with the use of a ureteric stent, a nephrostomy tube, or a percutaneous procedure.

Cystine stones are extremely hard and may occasionally be totally resistant to disintegration by lithotripsy or break into large particles, making percutaneous surgery preferable.

Stones in horseshoe and malrotated kidneys can be treated with ESWL successfully provided that there is no obstruction to the urinary tract (Lampel *et al.* 1996), but pelvic kidneys are less suitable for this form of treatment. Stones in transplant kidneys can also be treated. Bladder stones are often very hard but those that are less than 2 cm in maximum diameter can be treated successfully with ESWL.

Stones that are tightly impacted in the ureter, the pelvi-ureteric junction, or the renal pelvis disintegrate less easily than when there is less potential for expansion of the stone mass to occur during treatment. This becomes increasingly important with harder stones.

Ureteric stones can be seen more easily radiologically than with ultrasound, but upper-third and lower-third stones can be imaged even with lithotripters which use ultrasound. Treatment is not possible if stones overlie bones.

Physical deformity may be a limiting factor in lithotripsy. In the original Dornier HM3 the minimum height of the patient to fit on the frame was said to be 135 cm, but adaptations for children much smaller than this were easily made. The upper weight limit of 135 kg was a bar to treatment in some cases. Most frequently, skeletal deformity made it impossible to secure the patient satisfactorily in the presence of a kyphoscoliosis, a fixed hip, or a fixed flexion deformity of the knees. Such problems do not arise to the same extent with second-generation machines.

Complications

The two complications that are encountered most commonly are obstruction and infection (Zink *et al.* 1988).

The aim of lithotripsy is to disintegrate the stone into particles of size 2 mm or less; larger fragments carry the risk of obstruction as they pass down the ureter. However, even small particles may cause obstruction if the sand mass exceeds the capacity of the ureter. Interlocked stone fragments accumulate on the principle of a dry stone wall and form a *stein strasse* (stone street) (Fig. 4). The degree to which this produces obstruction varies, but management must include prevention (Coptcoat *et al.* 1988). No stone with a maximum diameter of more than 2.5 cm should be treated by endoscopic shockwave lithotripsy without first introducing a JJ stent or performing a debulking PCNL.

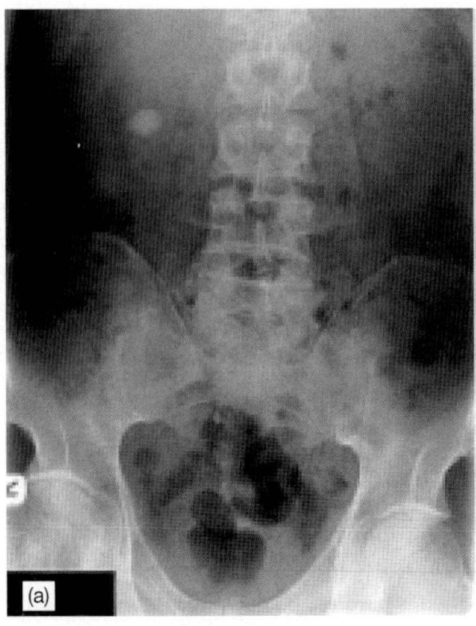

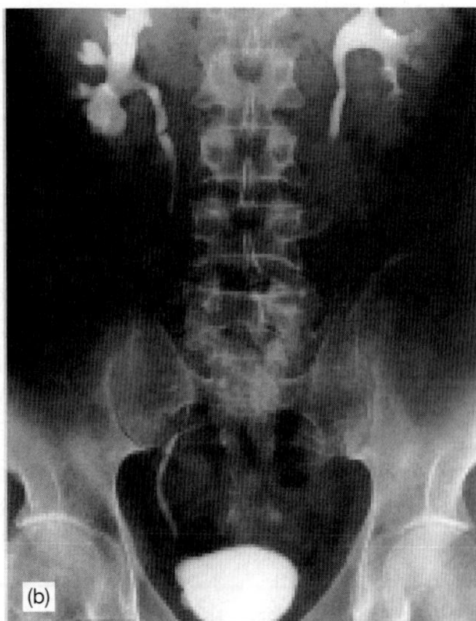

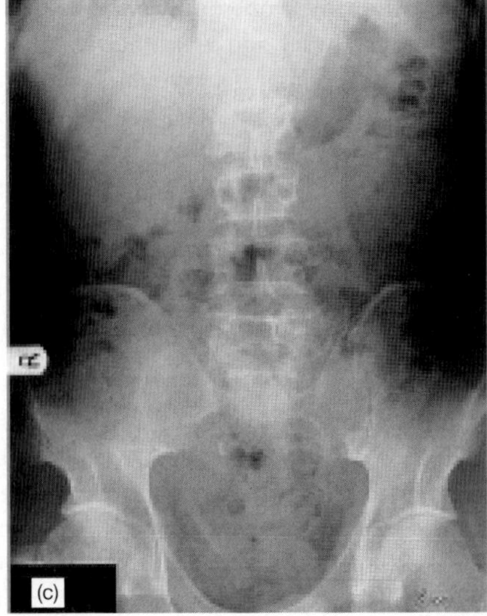

Fig. 4 (a) and (b) An intravenous urogram showing a 2-cm renal pelvic stone. (c) The *stein strasse* resulting from one treatment on the Wolf 2300 lithotripter.

If obstruction does occur after ESWL a percutaneous needle nephrostomy should be inserted under local anaesthesia to provide drainage. Peristalsis then returns to the previously dilated upper urinary tract and spontaneous passage of the *stein strasse* may occur. Ureteric endoscopic manoeuvres may be required or the *stein strasse* may be subjected to endoscopic shockwave lithotripsy. On rare occasions there is no alternative to performing open surgery (Sayed *et al.* 2001).

Infection may be provoked by endoscopic shockwave lithotripsy since stones may harbour organisms which are not exposed to prophylactic antibiotics. Although practice varies, many centres recommend oral antibiotic cover for all patients with metabolic stones. Parenteral antibiotic cover is indicated in patients with stones which are infective in origin. A combination of infection and obstruction demands urgent relief of the obstruction together with administration of a broad-spectrum parental antibiotic.

Subcapsular and perirenal haematomas occur; the vast majority are of no clinical significance and settle spontaneously (Krishnamurthi and Streem 1996), although there have been rare instances of very large haematomas which require drainage, usually percutaneously (Drach *et al.* 1986).

The suggestion that endoscopic shockwave lithotripsy provokes hypertension (Lingeman *et al.* 1988) is difficult to prove or disprove since a treatment effect is hard to distinguish from the natural history of the disease, particularly in the long term. Most subsequent prospective studies have either shown no increase in blood pressure (Montgommery and Shuttleworth 1989) or reported a minimal change, barely significant statistically or clinically (De Claro *et al.* 1993).

Patients almost always experience some haematuria during and for a short time after endoscopic shockwave lithotripsy owing to the abrasion of the mucosa by disintegrating stone fragments. The haematuria settles within a few hours and complications are rare (Chaussy and Fuchs 1989). The absence of haematuria may be evidence that the stone has not been imaged and hence has not been treated sufficiently.

High doses of shockwaves in experimental animals cause localized renal damage, but only slight transient changes in urinary enzyme excretion, creatinine excretion, and plasma renin concentration at clinical shockwave parameters. In one study of high-dose shockwave therapy for large stones ($>$2000 shocks from a Dornier HM3 lithotripter) renal biopsies were taken before and after the procedure; biopsies taken in the first 12 days showed minor histological changes including damage to small veins (Rigatti *et al.* 1989). Such slight and localized changes would not be expected to alter total renal function or morphology, and most clinical and experimental studies have failed to show any evidence of damage to the kidney following lithotripsy in which clinical levels of energy were used in adults (Boddy *et al.* 1987) or children (Goel *et al.* 1996).

Despite the timing of shockwaves to the cardiac cycle, an increase in extrasystoles and other minor arrhythmias has been shown in continuous ECG recordings during the procedure and even during treatment with a piezoelectric lithotripter, but clinically important arrhythmias are rare (Kataoka 1995).

Results

There has been much interest in and some controversy surrounding the value of lithotripsy. The ideal end result of any surgical stone management is a complete absence of stone, the elimination of infection, the restoration or preservation of renal function, and the resolution of symptoms. The extent to which the complete or partial absence of any of these criteria constitute failure is open to debate. Stone clearance rates will vary depending on the size, location, and composition of the stone and the intensity of the post-treatment investigations. Renal tomography and/or CT scanning reveal more stone fragments than a conventional plain radiograph, but what is not visible on a plain radiograph is unlikely to influence management.

Most centres have reported stone clearance rates in the region of 85 per cent 3 months after treatment (Drach *et al.* 1986; Bowsher *et al.* 1990). The term 'non-surgical fragment' has been coined to describe a residual stone of size 3 mm or less which causes no symptoms, provokes no infection, and does not produce an obstruction. It can and has been argued that the presence of residual 'non-surgical fragments' will promote stone recurrence and that the presence of even residual sand or dust particles, demonstrable only on CT scanning or tomography, will have the same effect. Clearly, long-term studies over at least 15 years will be required before a true comparison can be made between stone recurrence rates after open surgery, percutaneous surgery, and lithotripsy (Chaussy and Fuchs 1989), and most current conclusions are not based on randomized controlled trials.

Some comparisons between PCNL and lithotripsy for lower-pole calculi have shown a substantially greater stone recurrence rate in the first 2 years after lithotripsy (Lingeman *et al.* 1994; Carr *et al.* 1996); the presence of residual small calculi predicts clinical recurrence (Streem *et al.* 1996). The value of high fluid intake in preventing recurrence after lithotripsy has been confirmed in a controlled trial (Borghi *et al.* 1996). However, it is an irrefutable fact that stone recurrence does not carry the same threat to renal function or to the patient in general since the advent of methods of some management other than open surgery (Philp *et al.* 1988).

In about 10–15 per cent of cases lithotripsy needs to be combined with percutaenous surgery and/or endoscopic ureteric manoeuvres to achieve the best possible results (Das *et al.* 1988). Such additional intervention will usually be planned, but occasionally unforeseen developments after lithotripsy create the requirement for these secondary procedures.

Advantages and disadvantages

Advances in stone treatment occurred rapidly throughout the 1980s, and the indications for treatment changed as markedly as the methods used: in 1980 an incision of 18 cm was required to remove any renal stone, whereas in 1987 the same stone could be removed by painless lithotripsy on an out-patient basis. The difference in morbidity is self-evident, although not necessarily easy to quantify. Where prospective comparisons have been made, endoscopic shockwave lithotripsy has been shown to be superior in terms of conservation of renal function, general morbidity, and overall mortality (Whitfield 1988). Repeat treatment for recurrent or bilateral stones highlights these differences. The main disadvantages are that the resources in terms of medical manpower and finances are only available to the entire population in relatively few countries of the world.

Extracorporeal shockwave lithotripsy for ureteric stones

Many ureteric stones can be managed effectively with ESWL. Ultrasound imaging is possible in the upper third of the ureter using the lower pole of the kidney as an acoustic window. In the lower third of the ureter stones can be imaged using a full bladder as an acoustic window. In the absence of ureteric dilatation stones in the middle third of the ureter are difficult or impossible to image with ultrasound. As an alternative, radiological imaging can be used effectively and only where a stone overlies the sacro-iliac region is ESWL impossible (Birkens *et al.* 1998). Radiolucent calculi can be treated with ESWL if a contrast medium is injected to allow radiographic identification or by using ultrasound localization (Buchholz and Van Rossum 2001).

Second-generation lithotripters

At the time of writing there are more than a dozen different types of lithotripter in clinical use. Their price varies between $200,000 and 600,000. Although none of the available machines incorporates all features that could be described as ideal in every way, each functions very satisfactorily. The different combinations of imaging methods and shockwave production combine to provide a variety and a choice which may seem baffling. Radiological imaging is probably easier than ultrasound imaging, and more ureteric stones can be seen, and therefore treated, in machines which rely on radiological screening. However, lithotripters which use ultrasound imaging tend to be cheaper. Piezoelectric shockwaves are generally less powerful than those generated by a spark discharge or electromagnetically, resulting in virtually painless treatment but at the expense of an increased number of repeat treatments (Fig. 5). Very few centres can afford the luxury of two machines, one using ultrasound imaging with a relatively low-power shockwave focus energy and the other using radiological imaging and a more powerful shockwave delivery system. Therefore, the choice of a lithotripter can be very difficult and is further complicated by the certainty that newer machines are being produced all the time.

Endoscopic techniques

During the past 5 years ureteroscopy has become as much a routine for urologists as cystoscopy. The cost of instrumentation is only part of the capital outlay required; some form of radiographic screening must be available so that the position of guide wires and instruments within the ureter can be checked.

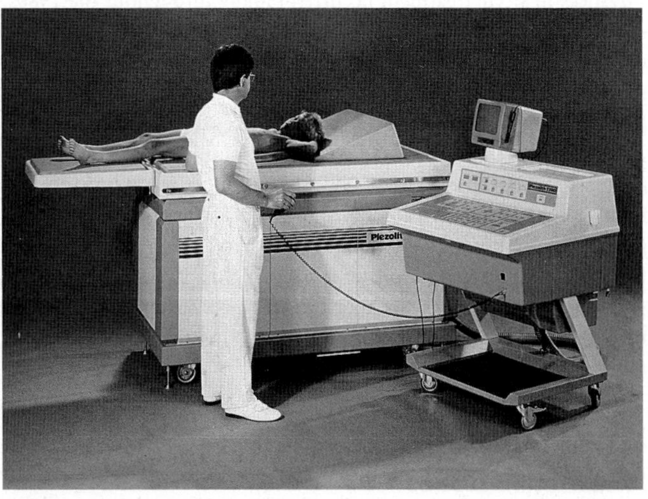

Fig. 5 A child undergoing treatment on a Wolf Piezolith 2300, requiring no analgesia or anaesthesia.

Instrumentation

Rigid ureteroscopes

Credit for the earliest ureteroscopy with a straight instrument belongs to Perez-Castro Ellendt and Martinez-Pinero (1980) who described how the normal ureter could be negotiated with a rigid endoscope, having first had the opportunity to ureteroscope a congenital mega-ureter using a standard cystoscope. All the major instrument manufacturers quickly developed purpose-built rod-lens instruments with which the entire length of the ureter could be visualized (Fig. 6). As with cystoscopy, vision is clarified by a flow of irrigant, which is inevitably slow because of the small calibre of both the instrument and the ureter. The channel through which irrigant flows can also accommodate a limited range of operating instruments. Shorter ureteroscopes are easier to use and are available in different circumferences and with offset eye-pieces. The smallest calibre of a rigid ureteroscope is 5.5 French gauge, that is a circumference of 5.5 mm, and the largest is 13.5 French gauge. The normal adult ureter has an external circumference of about 8 mm, and although the lumen is potential rather than actual the elasticity of the muscle wall may allow a rigid instrument to be passed without damage. However, it can be difficult or impossible to negotiate the ureteric orifice, the intramural ureter, or that part of the ureter which crosses the iliac vessels. Rigid ureteroscopy requires not only that the ureter has sufficient elasticity to accommodate the endoscope but also that the urinary tract can be straightened out between the external urethral meatus and the pelvi-ureteric junction. Therefore, the ureter must be raised from the posterior abdominal wall, which inevitably stretches, and sometimes overstretches, the blood supply of the ureter. Both this stretching of the blood supply and the distension from within the lumen have been implicated as causes of ureteric stricture formation (Boddy *et al.* 1988).

Flexible ureteroscopes

Fibre-optic technology has been applied to flexible ureteroscopes, which are available in sizes between 6 and 10 French. The theoretical advantages of flexible ureteroscopy are considerable (Bagley 1987): the calibre of the instruments is smaller, it is possible to manoeuvre the tip

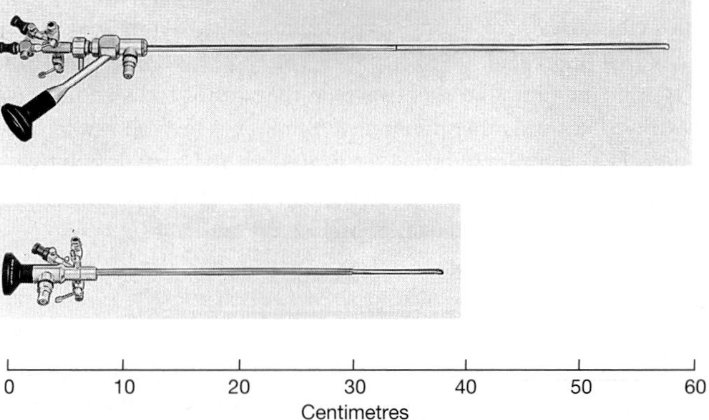

Fig. 6 A long and a short rigid ureteroscope.

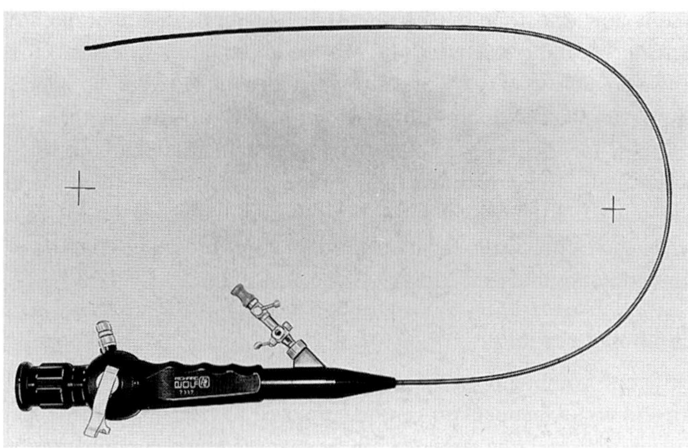

Fig. 7 A steerable flexible ureteroscope.

of the endoscope, and the instrument adapts to the course of the ureter. Technology has advanced so that the size of individual fibres is smaller and therefore the number of fibres that can be fitted into an instrument can be increased; the image quality is correspondingly improved. The graininess of the image is much less than before. However, fibres within the bundle can break (or be broken by careless use or maintenance of the scope) and the image quality is reduced. The irrigation/instrument channel is quite narrow, and the flow of irrigating fluid, which is always slow, is significantly reduced when an operating instrument is inserted. The flexibility of the instrument is restricted by both the ureter and any instrument within the operating channel. It is usually possible to have a view of the ureter, but operative manoeuvres are limited (Fig. 7).

Like most fibre-optic instruments, flexible ureteroscopes are expensive and have a limited lifespan, which can be extended if those involved in using and looking after the instrument treat it with care and respect.

Technique of ureteroscopy

For both dilatation and stone removal it is usual to have a guide wire in the ureter to minimize the risk of perforation to the ureteric wall by a dilator or instrument which has gone off course.

Ureteric dilatation

The ureteric orifice and the intramural ureter may have to be dilated before a ureteroscope can be passed (Rutner 1984). Graded Teflon or metal dilators may be passed over a guide wire under radiological control; alternatively, a balloon catheter or an appropriate length and calibre may be inflated. The ureter can also be dilated hydrostatically using either a pressurized infusion or a specially designed pump. With the smaller calibre instruments that are used currently, preliminary ureteric dilatation is required less often.

Stone removal

The technique of trapping ureteric stones within a wire basket passed up the ureter via a cystoscope has been in use for many decades (Dourmashkin 1945). The success of the procedure is greater and the technique is safer when the basket is manipulated under radiological control. Only stones in the lower third of the ureter were originally considered suitable for managing in this way and the stone needed to be small enough (5 mm) to be removed intact. The advent of ureteroscopy has made stone removal by this technique safer and more reliable, since the procedure can be monitored using a combination of radiological control and direct vision. Stones from anywhere within the ureter may be considered for treatment.

Radiological screening is important so that the basket can be controlled proximal to the stone when endoscopic vision is obscured by the stone itself. Direct viewing of the stone enables the operator to have a three-dimensional assessment of when the stone (or the ureter) is trapped by the basket. When the stone has been secured within the basket, it is pulled down onto the end of the ureteroscope and the two are withdrawn together, with the ureteroscope helping to dilate the ureter and to minimize trauma to the ureteric wall.

Stones that are too large to be removed intact can be disintegrated before they are removed (Marberger and Stackl 1983). Intracorporeal lithotripsy can be achieved using an electrohydraulic probe, electrokinetic probe, a pneumatic lithotripter, a laser fibre, or, very occasionally, an ultrasound probe. To avoid ureteric damage when using electrohydraulic disintegration particular care must be taken to discharge the probe only when its tip is in contact with the stone. The ultrasound probe is small and stone disintegration may be time consuming. A laser can be used to good effect within the ureter: the fibre size is very small, making the combination of laser disintegration through a flexible ureteroscope a practical proposition. The only disadvantage is the high cost of the laser. The pneumatic and electrokinetic mechanisms are very similar (Vorreuther *et al.* 1998; Menezes *et al.* 2000). The cost of the pneumatic disintegrator is of the order of $20,000, which is significantly lower than for a laser, which costs in the region of $75,000. The pneumatic probes are not disposable and this also adds to the cost-effectiveness of the treatment (Naqvi *et al.* 1994; Wadhwa *et al.* 1994).

When a stone of any size becomes impacted in the upper third of the ureter it is possible to dilate a percutaneous track to the kidney and then to perform antegrade ureteroscopy. The ureter above the stone is likely to be dilated, and if the renal access is placed through a middle or upper calyx negotiating the ureter becomes more straightforward. Disintegration can be performed or the stone can be removed intact, depending on size.

Indications

The majority of ureteric stones with which patients present acutely are small enough to pass spontaneously, and it is good clinical management to allow this to happen. Continuing pain, renographic evidence of impaired function, and failure of the stone to progress are sound indications for intervention. When the presence of a stone, which may cause further colic, leads to a restriction in employment activities, intervention may also be justified. The advent of endoscopic techniques has lowered the threshold for intervention in many of these circumstances.

The combination of proximal obstruction by the stone and infection is an absolute indication for immediate intervention, usually by inserting a percutaneous nephrostomy tube, since irreversible impairment of function will occur within hours. It is important that the clinical picture is recognized early.

Complications

The incidence of complications varies with the experience of the operator (Miller 1986). Every urologist will testify to the friability of the obstructed ureter, and perforation with a guide wire, a basket, or a ureteroscope is a potential hazard. The main concern then becomes the risk of extravasating large quantities of irrigating fluid. Normal saline at body temperature should always be used as an irrigant to minimize the possibility of water overload. If a perforation has occurred, a JJ ureteric stent should be left *in situ* at the end of the procedure (Ramsay *et al.* 1985). Some surgeons advocate the routine use of these stents after every ureteroscopy, but the author recommends a selective approach.

Infection may be provoked by any endoscopic surgery; since many stones contain an infective component in their make-up, routine antibiotic prophylaxis should be given.

Ureteric strictures are a late complication that can occur. The most probable cause is ischaemia due to overdistension of the ureter by an instrument which is too large. 'Bow-stringing' of the lower third of the ureter may also be a contributory factor, and there is experimental evidence that extravasation of infected urine or irrigant into the wall of the ureter may be implicated (Boddy *et al.* 1988). In most centres the incidence of strictures is less than 1 per cent, but when this complication does occur open surgery is usually necessary to correct it. Ureteric dilatation is almost inevitably followed by stricture recurrence.

Results

To achieve the highest possible success rate the urologist must have a range of ureteroscopes and their operating instruments, disintegrating devices, and radiological screening facilities available. Centres where this complete armamentarium is available will achieve successful endoscopic stone removal in over 95 per cent of cases. On occasions two endoscopic procedures will be necessary. For example, it can be an advantage to insert a JJ stent for a few days if access to a stone is impeded by a small-calibre ureter. The presence of even a small stent results in dilatation of the ureter. Nevertheless, the overall morbidity of the two endoscopic procedures and the length of hospital stay are almost always less than that which would be associated with open surgery, and certainly the ureter is at less risk. Endoscopic surgery has helped to avoid the surgical nightmare of repeated open operations on the ureter for recurrent stone formers. Another result of a minimally invasive surgical approach is that the indications for prolonged conservative management of stones have decreased, to the benefit of the patients and their renal function (Aronne *et al.* 1988).

Future developments

Continuing advances in fibre-optic technology may improve flexible ureteroscopy. The quality of the image improves as the number of fibres increases, and as the size of individual fibres becomes progressively smaller, the number of fibres within a bundle of a given size can be increased.

Integrated stone management

The importance of integrating stone management cannot be overemphasized (Das *et al.* 1988). Sometimes it is not possible to predict prior to surgery which method(s) of treatment will be necessary. For example, it is not always possible to know whether a renal stone will require a combination of percutaneous surgery to debulk the main stone mass and lithotripsy to disintegrate peripheral fragments. In the case of ureteric stones there is often even less certainty preoperatively about how the stone can be removed. It is very difficult to predict whether an upper ureteric stone will be impacted or whether it will prove possible to pass a JJ ureteric catheter past it. The best strategy is always to start with the simplest option and to proceed to more complex manoeuvres as necessary. The patient must be counselled accordingly. The aim of avoiding open surgery as far as possible is in the interest of the patient and for the good of the urinary tract, even when such a policy results in the need for two endoscopic episodes or for endoscopy and lithotripsy.

Combined techniques

Different combinations of lithotripsy, percutaneous surgery, and ureteroscopic manoeuvres can be employed to treat the same stone. For example, a large staghorn can be managed by a combination of lithotripsy with a JJ stent or by lithotripsy after percutaneous debulking. The underlying philosophy of both is that lithotripsy alone would produce a sand mass that would prove to be too large and which would almost inevitably result in ureteric obstruction. The combination of a percutaneous procedure to debulk a large stone with subsequent lithotripsy to disintegrate peripheral calyceal fragments has become a widely accepted *modus operandi* (Fig. 8). An alternative approach is to insert a JJ stent and to plan lithotripsy on a sessional basis, disintegrating only a limited part of the stone at any one time, and staging treatment in relation to the rate of disintegration and passage of stone particles.

Stones which are impacted in the upper third of the ureter may be pushed back into the renal pelvis using either a ureteric catheter or a long ureteroscope under radiological control. The stone may then be removed percutaneously, but if lithotripsy is planned for a later date a JJ stent will be inserted to reduce the chance of the stone's reimpacting.

JJ stents can be used for different purposes. When there has been any significant degree of trauma to the ureter during endoscopic procedures, the insertion of the JJ stent will prevent urinary extravasation and allow healing to occur with minimal risk of subsequent stricture formation. An indwelling ureteric stent causes the ureter to dilate within a few days, and this is beneficial if ureteroscopy has proved difficult or impossible because of a narrow ureter. Under such circumstances it is safer to insert a stent and then to repeat the ureteroscopic procedure 72 h or more later rather than risk causing ureteric damage. Ureteric dilatation around a JJ stent may also encourage the passage of stone particles when lithotripsy is performed on a large stone. The presence of a JJ stent may be associated with some adverse effects. Patients may experience discomfort from irritation of the trigone by the lower end of the stent. Pain in the kidney may occur during micturition as urine refluxes upwards. Encrustation of the stent can occur, particularly in stone formers, and large concretions may arise rapidly. Stent migration and fracture are other hazards. Unless the stent is inserted under radiological control the upper end can be pushed through the kidney or the ureter. It is essential that a stent register is maintained so that patients with stents are not lost to follow-up.

Open surgery

Less than 1 per cent of patients with urinary tract stones should require open surgery. In patients with staghorn calculi who have had no previous surgery and in whom the bulk of the stone is within narrow-necked calices; open surgery may be the most appropriate

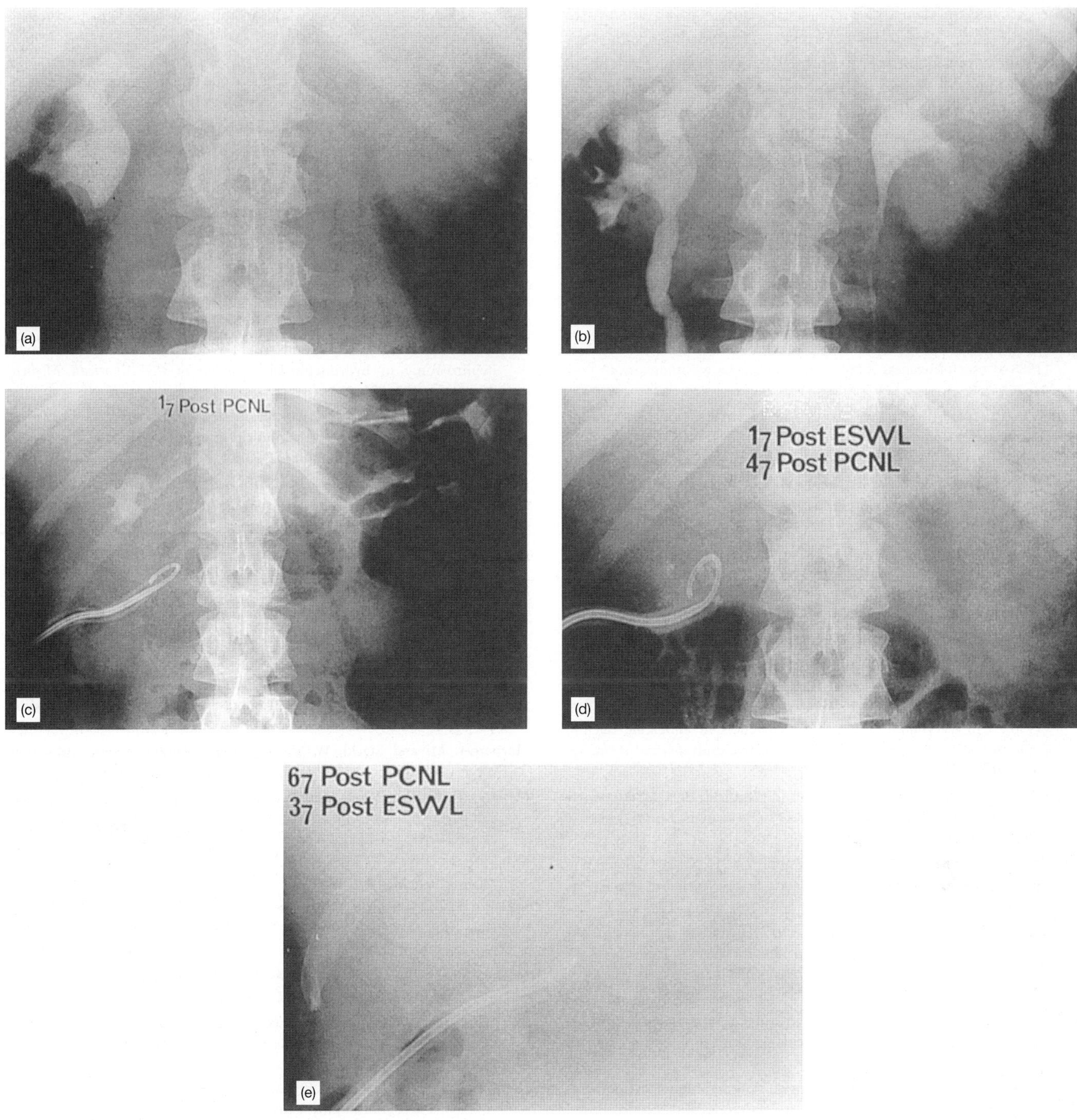

Fig. 8 (a) and (b) An intravenous urogram showing a staghorn calculus. (c) An upper calyceal fragment which remains following percutaneous debulking. (d) The fragmentation which occurred following lithotripsy. (e) Virtually complete stone clearance within 1 week of combined treatment.

treatment. Large stones which are impacted in the middle third of the ureter where it overlies the bony pelvis are not amenable to lithotripsy. A retrograde approach ureteroscopically may be less likely to succeed than an antegrade access, but both can be impossible if the ureter is very tortuous. However, the most frequent reason for resorting to open surgery is to correct a complication that has occurred following PCNL or ureteroscopy.

Medical treatment

Every patient who has had a urinary tract stone should be offered full metabolic screening. Analysis of stone fragments is useful, but retrieval of particles may not be possible, particularly after piezoelectric lithotripsy. Postlithotripsy urine analysis by scanning electron microscopy accurately identifies stone composition (Bowsher *et al.* 1990).

Most patients are keen to receive dietary advice in an attempt to reduce the chances of stone recurrence, and broad guidelines are worthwhile. Slavish pursuit of normocalciuria may be difficult to justify if anything other than moderate dietary restrictions are required, since, with the advent of minimally invasive techniques of stone management, such treatment may now be more irksome than the treatment of a recurrent stone.

References

Alken, P., Hutschenreiter, G., Gunther, R., and Marberger, M. (1981). Percutaneous stone manipulation. *Journal of Urology* **125**, 463–465.

Aronne, L. J., Brahma, R. L., Riehle, R., Vaughan, E. D., and Ruchlin, H. S. (1988). Cost effectiveness of extracorporeal shockwave lithotripsy. *Urology* **31**, 255–230.

Bagley, D. H. (1987). Ureteral endoscopy with passively deflectable irrigating flexible ureteroscopes. *Urology* **29**, 170–173.

Birkens, A. F. *et al.* (1998). Treatment of mid- and lower ureteric calculi; extracorporeal shock-wave lithotripsy vs laser ureteroscopy. A comparison of costs, morbidity and effectiveness. *British Journal of Urology* **81**, 31–35.

Boddy, S. A. M., Bomanji, J., Britton, K. E., Nimmon, C. C., and Whitfield, H. N. (1987). Radionuclide evaluation pre- and post-extracorporeal shockwave lithotripsy for renal calculi. *Journal of Nuclear Medicine* **28**, 1284–1289.

Boddy, S. A. M., Nimmon, C. C., Jones, S., Ramsay, J. W. A., Britton, K. E., Levison, D. A., Whitfield, H. N., and Wickham, J. E. A. (1988). Acute ureteric dilatation for ureteroscopy. An experimental study. *British Journal of Urology* **61**, 27–31.

Borghi, L., Meschi, T., Amato, F., Briganti, A., Novarini, A., and Giannini, A. (1996). Urinary volume, water and recurrences in idiopathic calcium nephrolithiasis: a 5 year randomised prospective study. *Journal of Urology* **155**, 839–843.

Bowsher, W., Crocker, P., Ramsay, J. W. A., and Whitfield, H. N. (1990). Single urine sample diagnosis: a new concept of stone analysis. *British Journal of Urology* **65**, 236–239.

Bowsher, W., Ramsay, J. W. A., Blott, P., and Whitfield, H. N. (1992). Radiation protection in percutaneous renal surgery. *British Journal of Urology* **69**, 231–233.

Buchholz, N.-P. N. and Van Rossum, M. (2001). The radiolucent ureteric calculus at the end of a contrast-medium column: where to focus the shock waves. *British Journal of Urology International* **88**, 325–328.

Carr, L. K., Honey, J. D.'A., Jewett, M. A. S., Ibanez, D., Ryan, M., and Bombardier, C. (1996). New stone formation: a comparison of extracorporeal shock wave lithotripsy and percutaneous nephrolithotomy. *Journal of Urology* **155**, 1565–1567.

Chaussy, C. G. and Fuchs, G. J. (1989). Current state and future developments of non-invasive treatment of human urinary stones with extracorporeal shockwave lithotripsy. *Journal of Urology* **141**, 782–789.

Chaussy, C. G., Schmiedt, E., Jochan, D., Brendel, W., Forssmann, B., and Walther, V. (1982). First clinical experience with extracorporeally induced destruction of kidney stones by shockwaves. *Journal of Urology* **127**, 417–420.

Coptcoat, M. J., Webb, D. R., Kellett, M. J., Whitfield, H. N., and Wickham, J. E. A. (1988). The Steinstrasse: a legacy of extracorporeal lithotripsy? *European Urology* **14**, 93–95.

Das, G. *et al.* (1988). 1500 cases of renal and ureteric calculi treated in an integrated stone centre. *British Journal of Urology* **62**, 301–305.

De Claro, J. A., Lima, M. L., Ferreira, U., and Netto, N. R., Jr. (1993). Blood pressure changes after extracorporeal shock wave lithotripsy in normotensive patients. *Journal of Urology* **150**, 1765–1767.

Dourmashkin, R. L. (1945). Cystoscopic treatment of stones in the ureter with special reference to large calculi: based on the study of 1550 cases. *Journal of Urology* **54**, 245–247.

Drach, G. W. *et al.* (1986). Report of the United States cooperative study of extracorporeal shockwave lithotripsy. *Journal of Urology* **135**, 1127–1133.

Eisenberger, F., Fuchs, G., Miller, K., Bub, P., and Rassweiler, J. (1985). Extracorporeal shockwave lithotripsy (ESWL) and endourology: an ideal combination for treatment of kidney stones. *World Journal of Urology* **3**, 41–47.

Fernström, I. and Johannson, B. (1976). Percutaneous pyelolithotomy. A new extraction technique. *Scandinavian Journal of Urology and Nephrology* **10**, 257–259.

Goel, M. C., Baserge, N. S., Babu, R. V. R., Sinha, S., and Kapoor, R. (1996). Pediatric kidney: functional outcome after extracorporeal shock wave lithotripsy. *Journal of Urology* **155**, 2044–2046.

Goodwin, W. E., Casey, W. C., and Woolf, W. (1955). Percutaneous needle nephrostomy in hydronephrosis. *Journal of the American Medical Association* **157**, 891–894.

Kataoka, H. (1995). Cardiac dysrhythmias related to extracorporeal shock wave lithotomy using a piezoelectric lithotriptor in patients with kidney stones. *Journal of Urology* **153**, 1390–1394.

Krishnamurthi, V. and Streem, S. B. (1996). Long-term radiographic and functional outcome of extracorporeal shock wave lithotripsy induced perineal hamatomas. *Journal of Urology* **154**, 1673–1675.

Lampel, A., Hohenfellner, M., Schult-Lampel, D., Lazica, M., Bohnen, K., and Thüroff, J. W. (1996). Urolithiasis in horseshoe kidneys: therapeutic management. *Urology* **47**, 182–186.

Lingeman, J. E., Evan, A. P., Wood, J. R., and Toth, P. D. (1988). The bioeffects of shockwaves and the risk of hypertension following ESWL. *Journal of Urology* **139**, 219a.

Lingeman, J. E., Siegel, Y. I., Stele, B., Nyhuis, A. W., and Wood, J. R. (1994). Management of lower pole nephrolithiasis: a critical analysis. *Journal of Urology* **151**, 663–667.

Marberger, M. and Stackl, W. (1983). New developments in endoscopic surgery for ureteric calculi. *British Journal of Urology* (Suppl.), 34–40.

Menezes, P., Kumar, P. V. S., and Timoney, A. G. (2000). A randomized trial comparing lithoclat with an electrokinetic lithotripter in the management of ureteric stones. *British Journal of Urology International* **85**, 22–25.

Miller, R. A. (1986). Endoscopic surgery of the upper urinary tract. *British Medical Bulletin* **42**, 274–279.

Miller, R. A. and Whitfield, H. N. (1985). Absorption of 1.5% glycine after percutaneous ultrasonic lithotripsy for renal stone disease. *British Medical Journal* **291**, 967.

Montgommery, B. S. I. and Shuttleworth, K. E. D. (1989). Does ESWL cause hypertension? *British Journal of Urology* **64**, 567–571.

Naqvi, S. A. A., Khaliq, M., Zafar, M. N., and Rizvi, S. A. H. (1994). Treatment of ureteric stones. Comparison of laser and pneumatic lithotripsy. *British Journal of Urology* **74**, 694–698.

Netto, N. R., Lemos, G. C., and Fruza, J. L. (1988). Perforation following percutaneous nephrolithotomy. *Urology* **32**, 223–224.

Patterson, D. E., Segura, J. W., and LeRoy, A. J. (1987). Long-term follow-up of patients treated by percutaneous ultrasonic lithotripsy for struvite staghorn calculi. *Journal of Endourology* **1**, 177–80.

Perez-Castro Ellendt, E. and Martinez Pinero, J. A. (1980). Transureteral ureteroscopy—a current urological procedure. *Archivos Espanöles de Urologia* **33**, 445–447.

Philp, T., Whitfield, H. N., Kellett, M. J., and Wickham, J. E. A. (1988). Painless lithotripsy: experience with 100 patients. *Lancet* **ii**, 41–43.

Preminger, G. N. *et al.* (1985). Percutaneous nephrostolithotomy vs open surgery for renal calculi. *Journal of the American Medical Association* **254**, 1054–1056.

Ramsay, J. W. A., Payne, S. R., Gosling, P. T., Whitfield, H. N., Wickham, J. E. A., and Levison, D. A. (1985). The effects of double J stenting on unobstructed ureters. *British Journal of Urology* **57**, 630–634.

Raney, A. M. and Handler, J. (1975). Electrohydraulic nephrolithotripsy. *Urology* **6**, 439–442.

Rathbert, P., Stumpf, V., Pohlmann, P., and Lutzeyer, W. (1977). Ultraschall Lithotripsie von Ureter and Niernsteinen Experimentelle und erste klinische Untersuchungen. Verhandlungs bericht Deutsches Gesellschaft. *Urologie* **16**, 365–367.

Rigatti, P., Colombo, R., Centemero, A., Francesca, F., Di Girolamo, V., Montorsi, F., and Trabucchi, E. (1989). Histological and ultrastructural evaluation of extracorporeal shock wave lithotripsy-induced acute renal lesions: preliminary report. *European Urology* **16**, 207–211.

Rutner, A. B. (1984). Ureteral balloon dilatation and stone basketing. *Urology* **23**, 44–53.

Sayed, M. A.-B., El-Taher, A. M., Aboul-Ella, and Shaker, S. E. (2001). Steinestrasse after extracorporeal shockwave lithotripsy: aetiology, prevention and management. *British Journal of Urology International* **88**, 675–678.

Seldinger, S. I. (1953). Catheter replacement of the needle in percutanous arteriography. *Acta Radiologica* **39**, 266–276.

Schulze, H., Hauptm, G., Pergiovanni, M., Wisard, M., Niderhausen, W., and Senge, T. (1993). The Swiss lithoclast: a new device for endoscopic stone disintegration. *Journal of Urology* **149**, 15–18.

Streem, S. B., Hall, P., Elch, M. G., Risius, N., and Geisinger, M. A. (1988). Endourologic management of upper and mid-ureteral calculi: percutaneous antegrade extraction vs transurethral ureteroscopy. *Urology* **31**, 34–37.

Streem, S. B., Yost, A., and Mascha, E. (1996). Clinical implications of clinical insignificant stone fragments after extracorporeal shock wave lithotripsy. *Journal of Urology* **155**, 1186–1190.

Thüroff, J. W. and Hutschenreiter, G. (1980). Fallbreicht: percutane Nephrostomie und instrumentelle Steinentfernung in Localanaesthesie. *Urologia Internationalis* **35**, 375–380.

Vorreuther, R. *et al.* (1998). Pneumatic versus electrokinetic lithotripsy in the treatment of ureteral stones. *Journal of Endourology* **12**, 233–236.

Wadhwa, S. N., Hemal, A. K., and Sharma, R. K. (1994). Intracorporeal lithotripsy with the Swiss lithoclast. *British Journal of Urology* **74**, 699–702.

Webb, D. R. and Fitzpatrick, J. M. (1985). Percutaneous nephrolithotripsy: a functional and morphological study. *Journal of Urology* **134**, 587–591.

Webb, D. R., McNicholas, T., Whitfield, H. N., and Wickham, J. E. A. (1985). Extracorporeal shockwave lithotripsy, endourology and open surgery. The management and follow-up of 200 patients with urinary calculi. *Annals of the Royal College of Surgeons of England* **67**, 337–340.

Whitfield, H. N. (1983). Percutaneous nephrolithotomy. *British Journal of Urology* **55**, 609–612.

Whitfield, H. N. Stone destruction and removal. In *Recent Advances in Urology/Andrology* Vol. 4 (ed. W. F. Hendry), pp. 41–60. Edinburgh: Churchill Livingstone, 1987.

Whitfield, H. N. (1988). New techniques for kidney stones. *The Practitioner* **232**, 338–341.

Whitfield, H. N. and Mills, V. A. (1985). Percutaneous nephrolithotomy: a report of 150 cases. *British Journal of Urology* **57**, 603–604.

Wickbom, L. (1954). Pyelography after direct puncture of the renal pelvis. *Acta Radiologica* **41**, 505–512.

Wickham, J. E. A. and Kellett, M. J. (1981). Percutaneous nephrolithotomy. *British Journal of Urology* **53**, 297–299.

Zink, R. A., Frohmueller, H. G., Eberhardt, J. U., and Kraemer, K. E. (1988). Urosepsis following ESWL. *Journal of Urology* **139**, 265a.

8.4 Nephrocalcinosis

Oliver Wrong

Definitions

The term 'nephrocalcinosis' means an increase in the calcium content of the kidneys and is usually reserved for generalized increases rather than localized increases such as those occurring in caseating renal tuberculosis or calcified renal infarcts. This increased calcium content takes three forms, representing increasing amounts of calcium and increasing degrees of renal damage:

(1) An increased concentration of calcium in renal cells, chiefly those of the tubular epithelium, can adversely affect renal structure and function and constitutes a *chemical nephrocalcinosis*. The underlying cause is usually hypercalcaemia, and in practice its features cannot be distinguished from *hypercalcaemic nephropathy*.

(2) Calcium may also precipitate in crystalline form, usually as phosphate or oxalate. The resultant mineral deposits may be too small to be seen except histologically, forming *microscopic nephrocalcinosis*, the form of nephrocalcinosis most studied in the laboratory rat.

(3) Larger areas of calcification can be seen by the naked eye or visualized by imaging techniques which do not require magnification, such as radiology or ultrasound, and constitute a *macroscopic nephrocalcinosis*.

In the last 10 years, dramatic advances in medical genetics and renal imaging have led to a great increase in knowledge of category 3 above, macroscopic nephrocalcinosis, the form of nephrocalcinosis of greatest relevance to clinical medicine. In contrast, there has been relatively little new knowledge in the field of category 1 above, so this section has been abbreviated to Table 1 in order to allow for expansion of the remaining sections, and for more detailed information the reader is referred to the 1998 2nd edition of this textbook.

Table 1 Hypercalcaemic nephropathy

Main causes
Autonomous hyperparathyroidism
Malignant disease: lytic bone lesions, or humoral effects of parathyroid-related peptide
Hypervitaminosis D, including hypercalcaemic sarcoidosis
Calcium excess ('milk/alkali' syndrome)
Rapidly progressive osteoporosis (e.g. immobilization, Cushing's)
Clinical features
Marked loss of renal salt and water reabsorbing capacity, with pre-renal uraemia which is largely reversible
Marked loss of renal concentrating ability, causing thirst and polyuria
Enhanced or impaired tubular hydrogen ion secretion, leading to mild alkalosis or even the full syndrome of renal tubular acidosis
Renal potassium-losing
Milder effects: increased renal magnesium and calcium loss, rarely renal glycosuria and aminoaciduria
Variable effect on urinary phosphate
Hypertension in 50% of patients, despite hypovolaemia, from direct effect of hypercalcaemia on systemic vasculature, and catecholamine release
Treatment
Parenteral resalination
Reduce plasma calcium (appropriate surgery, steroids, diphosphonates, calcitonin, calcium channel-blocking drugs)

Microscopic nephrocalcinosis

Man

At necropsy, the normal human kidney almost invariably contains microscopic deposits of calcium, usually in the renal medulla. Burry *et al.* (1976) described the patterns taken by this medullary calcification in over 2000 adult necropsies, and Shanks and MacDonald (1959) described histological nephrocalcinosis in 84 infants. The weakness of these studies is that they provided virtually no information on metabolic abnormalities or renal function during life.

Renal pathology texts contain little information about the microscopic appearances of the kidney affected by the various diseases causing nephrocalcinosis. The diagnosis of these conditions is made on biochemical grounds, not from renal histology. For example, practically no information is available on the early renal histology of the various forms of Bartter's syndrome, Fanconi syndrome, or distal renal tubular acidosis (dRTA). Kidneys from patients with endstage renal failure due to such metabolic renal diseases are also uninformative, being usually so severely distorted by fibrosis, atrophy, and round-cell infiltration that diagnosis of the primary disease is impossible; the best that the histopathologist can usually do is to diagnose 'chronic interstitial nephritis'. Calcium deposits can be visualized as amorphous von Kossa positive material, but the relationship of these deposits to the underlying renal structures is often obscured by chronic inflammatory changes, and this stain is for phosphate, rather than for calcium. Calcium oxalate deposits are best seen as doubly refractile crystals under polarized light.

In general, therefore, renal histology is of little value in the diagnosis of diseases associated with nephrocalcinosis, but there are a few exceptions to this rule. Thus in primary hyperoxaluria, gross renal failure may develop because of microscopic deposits of calcium oxalate throughout the kidneys which are often not shown by ultrasound or radiology (Cochran *et al.* 1968); an example is shown in Fig. 1. Occasional patients with long-standing hypercalcaemia, particularly from primary hyperparathyroidism or milk-alkali syndrome (Becker *et al.* 1952) have been shown to have microscopic nephrocalcinosis in the absence of macroscopic nephrocalcinosis. Acute oliguric renal failure caused by tubular obstruction with calcium phosphate casts has also occasionally followed episodes of hyperphosphataemia in man, usually as a complication of malignant disease (Carey *et al.* 1968; Kanfer *et al.* 1979). Histological nephrocalcinosis has also been shown in some children with the nephrotic syndrome, especially that due to minimal change glomerular change disease (Mocan *et al.* 2000), with small von Kossa-staining deposits lying in the lumen of cortical tubules; the suggestion has been made that the frusemide used as treatment of these patients has been responsible, in view of its role in other forms of nephrocalcinosis (see below).

Renal failure itself causes an increase in calcium in surviving renal tissue, both in man with various forms of primary renal disease (Kuzela *et al.* 1977; Giminez *et al.* 1987) and in the five-sixths nephrectomized uraemic rat (Ibels and Alfrey 1981); this may be an important factor leading to further progression of renal failure. In both species, this nephrocalcinosis has been mainly demonstrated by chemical analysis, but histological preparations show calcium deposits in the renal cortex, particularly in the tubular lumen and peritubular tissues (Kuzela *et al.* 1977; Ibels *et al.* 1981; Goligorsky *et al.* 1983, 1985). A raised plasma phosphate appears to be the most important factor leading to this renal calcification (Ibels and Alfrey 1981; Giminez *et al.* 1987); secondary hyperparathyroidism may also play a role through the effect of parathyroid hormone in increasing calcium entry into renal tubular cells (Borle and Uchikawa 1978; Goligorsky *et al.* 1986). The importance of hyperphosphataemia, which may operate both by increasing the plasma calcium × phosphate product and by leading to hyperparathyroidism, has been emphasized by the finding that the increased renal calcium content can be prevented by phosphate depletion (Ibels and Alfrey 1981), with improved preservation of residual renal function (Ibels *et al.* 1978).

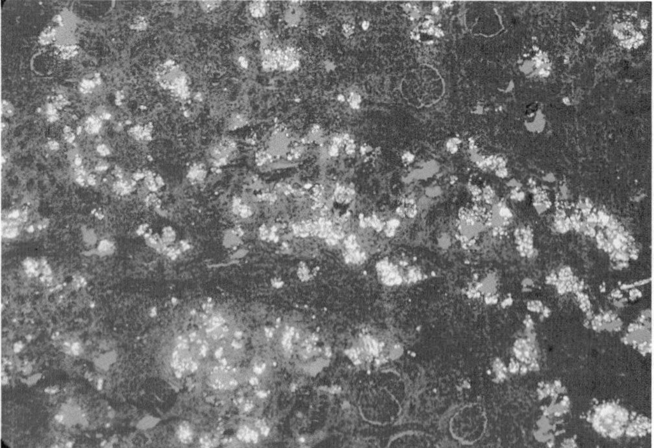

Fig. 1 Primary hyperoxaluria type I: low-power view of doubly refractile calcium oxalate crystals shown under partially polarized light in the renal cortex (note the presence of glomeruli) of a patient with medullary nephrocalcinosis and renal failure. This microscopic cortical nephrocalcinosis was not apparent in a plain film, which showed nephrocalcinosis only in the medulla.

Microscopic nephrocalcinosis has also been reported in a few metabolic diseases which have not yet been shown to progress to macroscopic nephrocalcinosis. One of these is the 'blue diaper syndrome', a rare familial metabolic disorder (only one family reported) which is probably inherited as an autosomal recessive trait, with defective intestinal absorption of tryptophan and mild hypercalcaemia (Drummond *et al.* 1964); the pathogenesis of the raised plasma calcium is not clear, but it is probably responsible for the microscopic nephrocalcinosis, predominantly medullary, in this condition. Microscopic nephrocalcinosis has also been described by Katz *et al.* (1988) in necropsy material from patients with cystic fibrosis; the deposits were within both tubular lumens and tubular epithelial cells, and appear to have been calcium phosphate. Urinary calcium was slightly raised in a similar group of surviving patients with cystic fibrosis, suggesting that hypercalciuria might have caused the microscopic nephrocalcinosis. The incidence of calcium oxalate renal calculi may be slightly increased in cystic fibrosis (Chidekel and Dolan 1996), but there appear to be no reports of macroscopic nephrocalcinosis in the condition.

Animal models

Microscopic nephrocalcinosis has been reported in the rabbit, hamster, mouse, gerbil, naked mole rat, horse, dog, squirrel monkey, chicken, and rainbow trout. However, it has been studied in detail only in the laboratory rat, partly because it develops very readily in this animal, but also because the rat is the principal animal used for chronic toxicity and carcinogenicity tests. Unfortunately, many of the records of these studies are contained in the confidential reports of industrial laboratories and private research organizations which have not been published. However, there can be little doubt that microscopic nephrocalcinosis has been more extensively investigated in the rat than in man. Several different patterns have been described.

Corticomedullary nephrocalcinosis in the rat

This takes the form of calcium phosphate deposits related to the basement membrane of tubules in medullary rays in the inner zone of the renal cortex and frequently extending into both cortex and medulla (Fig. 2), with some deposits within the tubular lumen, particularly in the straight segments of the proximal tubules. Electron microscopy shows that the initial stage is the appearance of intracellular crystals of apatite within tubular mitochondria and vacuoles (Caulfied and Schrag 1964; Battiflora *et al.* 1966). This type of nephrocalcinosis is so common in the rat that it has been described as 'invariable' once the weaning period has been passed (Cousins and Geary 1966). It increases with age and is more prominent in female rats (Geary and Cousins 1969), being partly oestrogen-dependent and affecting castrated females minimally, but becoming more marked even in male animals when they are given oestrogens.

The standard commercial pelleted feed for laboratory rats may play a role in the development of this nephrocalcinosis, for it contains added supplements designed to prevent mineral deficiencies, and nephrocalcinosis can be prevented by reducing the dietary content of calcium and phosphorus or increasing that of magnesium (Woodard 1971; Du Bruyn 1972; Phillips *et al.* 1986); conversely an increased calcium or phosphorus intake leads to an increased incidence of nephrocalcinosis (Fourman 1959; Al-Modhefer *et al.* 1986). Other precipitating factors include excess parathyroid hormone (Caulfield and Shrag 1964), vitamin D (Sanderson 1959), and acetazolamide (Harrison and Harrison 1955; Evans and MacPherson 1956; Heaton and Anderson 1965; Györy *et al.* 1970).

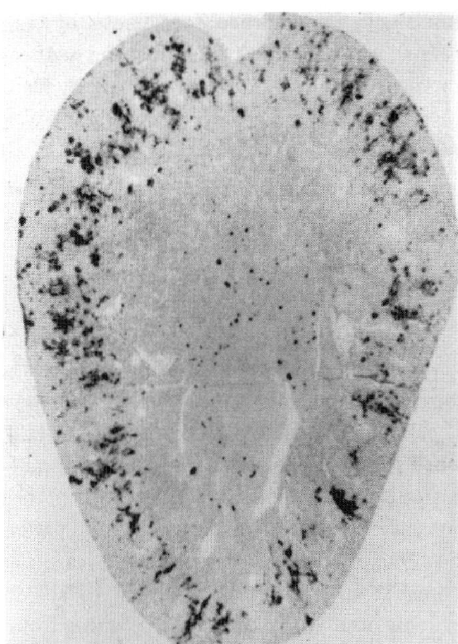

Fig. 2 Microscopic nephrocalcinosis in the rat kidney after parenteral phosphate. The nephrocalcinosis is maximal on the cortical side of the corticomedullary junction. Kernechtrot stain to show calcium. Magnification 3.5× (reproduced with permission from Fourman 1959).

Experimental magnesium depletion, which may be accompanied by hypercalcaemia, also leads to this type of nephrocalcinosis; a raised plasma calcium is not an essential prerequisite (Cramer 1932; MacIntyre and Davidson 1958; Heaton and Anderson 1965; Schneeberger and Morrison 1965; Battiflora *et al.* 1966). Thyroid hormone is protective against the nephrocalcinosis produced both by vitamin D (Newman 1973) and magnesium depletion (Reeves and Forbes 1972), whereas the hypothyroid state renders animals more sensitive to the development of nephrocalcinosis.

'Pelvic' nephrocalcinosis in the rat

This term has been applied to calcification affecting the renal papilla, either within the covering epithelium or just beneath it within the substance of the papilla, often attached to calcific material within the renal pelvis which may break free to form detached calyceal calculi. Calcium oxalate is the mineral responsible for this type of nephrocalcinosis when it follows hyperoxaluria caused by parenteral oxalate administration (Khan *et al.* 1982), or pyridoxine deficiency (Gershoff and Andrus 1961). Otherwise calcium phosphate, particularly apatite, is the usual material deposited, and this form of nephrocalcinosis can be induced by a diet high in calcium or low in magnesium content (Gershoff and Andrus 1961; Roginski and Mertz 1974; Roe 1989), as can the more common corticomedullary pattern of calcification. This 'pelvic' pattern of nephrocalcinosis is common in animals that are fed numerous carbohydrates, including the sugar alcohols sorbitol and xylitol (Bär 1985), the disaccharide lactose, and some chemically modified starches (De Groot *et al.* 1974) such as acetylated di-starch adipate, that are now widely used in the food industry because their physical properties, such as resistance to gelatinization on heating, are desirable in the manufacture of processed food. The underlying mechanism responsible for the nephrocalcinosis that arises in these circumstances appears to be the increased intestinal absorption of calcium which is promoted by many dietary carbohydrates, including starch and its derivatives (Hodgkinson *et al.* 1982; Wurzburg 1986; Roe 1989) and particularly by lactose (Lengemann and Comar 1961).

Other types of nephrocalcinosis in the rat

Small areas of calcification in the outer cortex have been found after acute hypercalcaemia caused by parenteral administration of calcium gluconate (Fourman 1959) associated with hypercalcaemia and hypercalciuria.

Medullary nephrocalcinosis has been reported in 'hyaline-droplet nephropathy'. In this condition, inhalation of volatile hydrocarbons leads to marked histological change and accumulation of low molecular weight α_{2u} globulins in the proximal tubules of male rats (female rats are practically unaffected), with secondary tubular cast information and nephrocalcinosis affecting the renal medulla (Busey and Cockrell 1984; Murty *et al.* 1988). This condition may turn out to be of interest as a rat model of human proximal tubular disease.

Functional studies in the rat

Disappointingly, there are few studies on the effects of nephrocalcinosis on renal function in the rat. Sanderson (1959), studying rats made hypercalcaemic by calciferol, found increased blood urea concentrations and reduced renal concentrating power, but these changes might have resulted from hypercalcaemic nephropathy rather than microscopic nephrocalcinosis. Al-Modhefer *et al.* (1986) found a marked prolongation of single nephron transit time, particularly in the distal tubule, in rats with diet-induced corticomedullary nephrocalcinosis, perhaps the result of calcium cast obstruction of distal tubules, but they made few observations on other renal functions. Occasionally, animals with 'pelvic' nephrocalcinosis have developed acute pyelonephritis or calculous ureteric obstruction with renal failure, as occurs in man with calculi arising in the renal pelvis. However, there appear to be no detailed studies of glomerular filtration or renal tubular function in these various models of nephrocalcinosis in the rat.

One must conclude that nephrocalcinosis in the rat is a poor model for the human condition because of the much greater ease with which it develops, its different distribution within the kidney, the paucity of observations on renal function, and the absence of a rat model for many of the diseases causing human nephrocalcinosis. It is true that there are some conditions, such as hypercalcaemia, hyperoxaluria, and exposure to acetazolamide, which cause nephrocalcinosis in both species, though this has a different distribution. 'Pelvic' nephrocalcinosis in the rat has a distribution which is similar to Randall's plaques, a human form of nephrocalcinosis which is discussed below. Comparison of nephrocalcinosis in the rat and in man is further complicated by the high incidence of spontaneous glomerulosclerosis in laboratory rats (Saxton and Kimball 1941; Greaves and Faccini 1984), often known as 'old rat nephropathy', which is common in animals of both sexes but almost invariable in male rats surviving beyond 2 years.

Macroscopic nephrocalcinosis in man

Imaging for nephrocalcinosis

Radiography

Conventional radiology as part of the KUB (kidneys, ureters, bladder) examination is the traditional technique, but has increasingly been supplemented by computed tomography (CT), of which good examples are shown in Fig. 3. A helical (spiral) CT scan is currently the gold standard, visualizing smaller calcium deposits than can be shown by other techniques, and giving precise information on the position of calcium deposits in the kidney, particularly the relationship to the collecting system. The use of contrast, especially with the CT scan, may distinguish stones in the minor calyces from deposits of nephrocalcinosis in the renal substance; it also assists the diagnosis of medullary sponge kidney (MSK) by showing ectatic tubules in parts of the renal medulla which are not affected by calcium deposition. The radiation exposure from a spiral CT scan is about 10 m-sieverts, or 10 times that of a single KUB film; this radiation dose must be placed in context, for many patients having a CT scan will require further renal radiographs in the course of their illness, and the risks of radiation exposure are proportional to the total dose of radiation.

Ultrasound (see also Chapter 1.6.1.i)

The non-invasive advantage of ultrasound has led to its wide adoption as the initial screen for renal calcification. The examination often picks up nephrocalcinosis at an earlier stage than a plain KUB film (Glazer *et al.* 1982; Alon *et al.* 1983; Jequier *et al.* 1986; see also Fig. 9), but is not as good as the CT scan in detecting very small calcium deposits, and requires greater experience than radiography, both in technique and in interpretation. The amateur may be deceived into diagnosing nephrocalcinosis by areas of increased echogenicity which do not represent calcium, especially papillary cysts or deposits of fat in the renal hilum. A particular problem arises with renal ultrasound in the full-term neonate, in whom increased renal medullary echogenicity has been recorded in about 50 per cent of cases (Starinsky *et al.* 1995; Howlett *et al.* 1997). Although the radiographic appearance of this echogenicity is not known, it is unlikely to be due to calcium deposition as it disappears within a few days of birth. This finding should not be confused with the true nephrocalcinosis of very premature babies (see below), which develops after birth and has been attributed mainly to excessive use of loop diuretics, particularly frusemide.

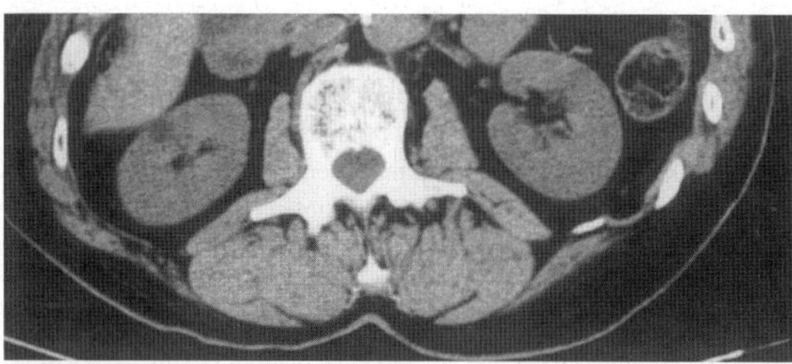

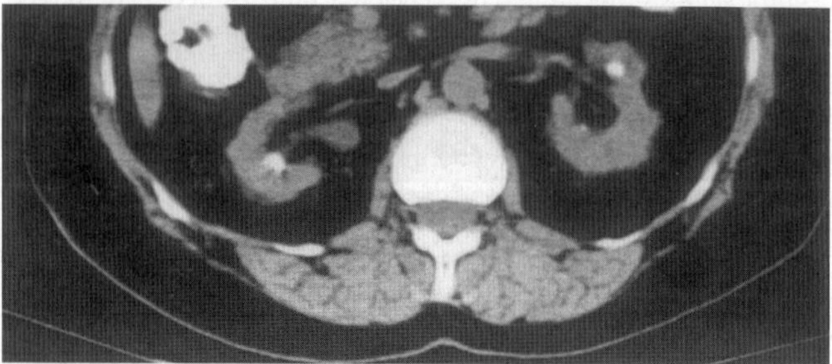

Fig. 3 Renal CT scans. Top—a healthy normal subject; bottom—a patient with chronic renal failure caused by analgesic nephropathy, showing irregular renal atrophy and the medullary nephrocalcinosis of calcified necrotic renal papillae. By courtesy of Dr Marc E. De Broe.

Magnetic resonance

This visualizes renal calcification poorly and so in general does not make a useful contribution to the detection of nephrocalcinosis.

Surveys of macroscopic nephrocalcinosis in man

The first analysis of a large number of cases was that of 91 patients described by Mortensen and Emmett 50 years ago (1954), 48 of them identified from a survey of the existing medical literature. A further report on 77 patients was made by Monserrat *et al.* (1979), but the largest published series is the personal one of Wrong and Feest (1976), now consisting of 375 patients, which was reviewed in the second edition of this book. This series consists mainly of adult patients seen over the years 1954–1995 in London, Manchester, Newcastle, and Dundee; a diagnostic breakdown of this series is shown in Table 2. Some case selection inevitably occurred in this series, resulting from the clinical

Table 2 Causes of macroscopic nephrocalcinosis in personal series of 375 patients

	Number of patients[a]	Percentage
Cortical	9	2.4
Chronic glomerulonephritis	3	0.8
Acute cortical necrosis (2 haemolytic–uraemic, 1 obstetric)	3	0.8
Chronic pyelonephritis	1	0.3
Benign nodular subcapsular	2	0.5
Medullary	366	97.6
Autonomous hyperparathyroidism	121.5	32.4
Milk alkali syndrome	12	3.2
Hypervitaminosis D	6	1.6
Sarcoidosis	6	1.6
Rapidly progressive osteoporosis	5.5	1.5
Idiopathic hypercalciuria	22	5.9
Amelogenesis imperfecta/ nephrocalcinosis syndrome	2	0.5
Oxalosis	12	4.3
Distal renal tubular acidosis	73	19.5
Acetazolamide	1.5	1.5
Dent's disease	16	4.2
Hypomagnesaemia–hypercalciuria syndrome	6	1.6
Medullary sponge kidney	42.5	11.3
Renal papillary necrosis	9	2.4
Others (Williams' and Bartter's syndrome, idiopathic Fanconi syndrome, hypothyroidism, glucocorticoid-suppressible aldosteronism, severe acute tubular necrosis)	6	1.6
Undiscovered cause	25	6.7
Total	375	

[a] 'Half' patients refer to one half of a double diagnosis.

interests of the authors, and in particular from the tracing of first-degree relatives of some patients with familial diseases. However, the frequency of the main clinical diagnosis corresponds well with those reported by Mortensen and Emmett. Many more disease entities are recorded in the more recent series, and the table is probably a fairly good indication of the incidence of the various causes of macroscopic nephrocalcinosis in adults in the United Kingdom over the last 50 years. Surveys of children have shown a greater proportion of congenital and familial disease, as well demonstrated in the series of 152 cases published by Rönnefarth and Misselwitz in 2000.

These surveys of large numbers of cases made clear that macroscopic nephrocalcinosis occurs in two main patterns, a rare cortical variety that is usually due to underlying destructive renal disease, particularly glomerulonephritis and cortical necrosis, and a much more common medullary pattern, which is usually the result of clear-cut metabolic diseases, most often diseases affecting calcium metabolism. Occasionally the distinction breaks down, nephrocalcinosis involving both cortex and medulla (as in primary hyperoxaluria), or the underlying renal disease obliterates the difference between renal cortex and medulla (e.g. polycystic disease), but in general the distinction is easily made and clinically useful.

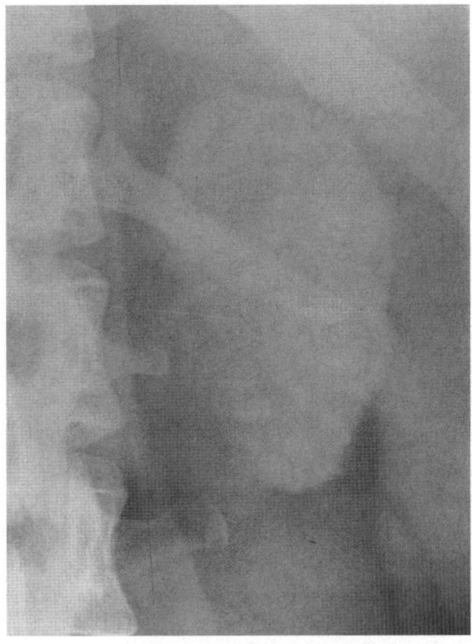

Fig. 4 Cortical nephrocalcinosis in a 38-year-old woman with chronic glomerulonephritis and endstage renal failure. The right kidney was similarly affected.

Cortical nephrocalcinosis in man

Nephrocalcinosis predominantly involving the renal cortex is usually the result of severe destructive cortical disease, many patients having endstage renal failure. Renal calcification may be either confluent or patchy, depending on the underlying renal disease; occasionally it extends to the renal medulla.

Chronic glomerulonephritis

The first five patients were reported by Sosman and his colleagues from the Peter Bent Brigham Hospital (Vaughan *et al.* 1947; Arons *et al.* 1955), and several reports of smaller numbers of cases have appeared since (Mortensen and Emmett 1954; Esposito 1967); the present series contains three such patients. Renal histology, available from three of the patients of Arons and one of our own, has shown in all a severe proliferative glomerulonephritis with crescent formation, and calcium deposits in periglomerular tissues but not in the glomeruli. Arons *et al.* noted that four of their five patients had consumed large amounts of milk, and one patient of ours (Fig. 4) had long standing post-thyroidectomy hypoparathyroidism for which she had been treated with calciferol; it is possible, therefore, that intermittent hypercalcaemia plays a part in the nephrocalcinosis of some patients. Cortical nephrocalcinosis has also been reported occasionally in other glomerular diseases, such as familial infantile nephrotic syndrome and Alport's syndrome (Page and Castleman 1961; Schepens *et al.* 2000). Calcification appears smooth or finely granular on radiographs, in keeping with the diffuse nature of the underlying glomerular disease.

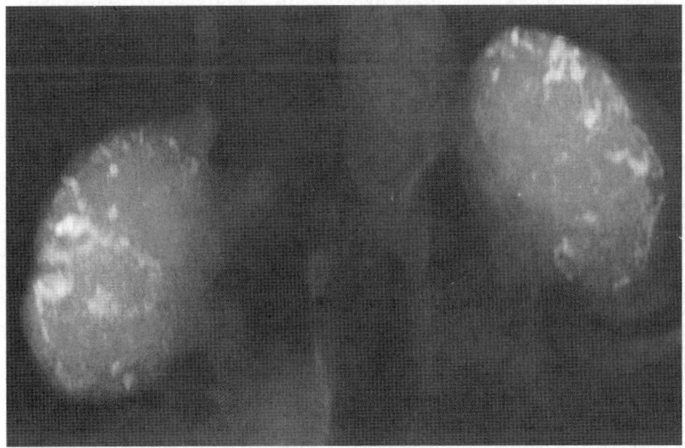

Fig. 5 Cortical nephrocalcinosis (necropsy specimen) in a 14-month-old male infant who developed haemolytic–uraemic syndrome at 6 months of age and was treated for 5 months by peritoneal dialysis (reproduced with permission from Wrong 1985).

Acute cortical necrosis (see also Chapter 10.2)

Patchy cortical nephrocalcinosis has been reported following the acute cortical necrosis of concealed accidental haemorrhage and toxaemia of pregnancy (Alwall *et al.* 1958; McAlister and Nedelman 1961; Cramer and Fuglestad 1965), snake bite (Oram *et al.* 1963), and haemolytic–uraemic syndrome (Moschos *et al.* 1972; Young 1979). Our own series included two infants with haemolytic–uraemic syndrome (Fig. 5) and a woman aged 24 years who developed cortical necrosis and a microangiopathic haemolytic anaemia 8 days after an apparently normal delivery at term. In most instances, nephrocalcinosis was discovered many weeks after the onset of acute renal failure, while the patient was kept alive by dialysis, and recovery of useful renal function was not observed, but Palmer (1970) described a patient whose renal function returned after an episode of acute renal failure associated with a toxaemic stillbirth, and in whom nephrocalcinosis was not discovered for a further 6 years. The term 'tram-line calcification' was applied by Lloyd-Thomas *et al.* (1962) to a pattern of nephrocalcinosis seen in an obstetric case of cortical necrosis, with a double line of calcification along the two sides of the necrotic zone in the cortex, but though the authors considered this finding characteristic of cortical necrosis it has not been described by others.

Chronic pyelonephritis

Ekengren (1973) described a linear pattern of cortical nephrocalcinosis in three children with chronic pyelonephritis and vesicoureteric reflux. Our series contains only one such patient (Fig. 6), in whom there was a marked difference in the extent of nephrocalcinosis on the two sides, in keeping with the focal nature of this disease.

Renal transplants (see also Chapter 13.3.3)

Cortical nephrocalcinosis was described as a late development in one patient following partial recovery from an acute transplant rejection episode (Harrison and Vaughan 1978). Renal transplants have also developed medullary nephrocalcinosis as a result of autonomous ('tertiary') hyperparathyroidism after successful transplantation (Walsh 1969; Leapman *et al.* 1976). Many transplanted kidneys develop the functional tubular abnormalities of dRTA (Better *et al.* 1969; Wilson and Siddiqui 1973), probably on an immune basis, and may therefore be at risk of the medullary nephrocalcinosis which is typical of this condition (Wrong *et al.* 1993), though this complication has not yet been recorded.

Oxalosis (see also Chapter 16.5.2)

Cortical nephrocalcinosis has been reported in both primary hyperoxaluria (Wilson *et al.* 1979; Luers *et al.* 1980) and the hyperoxaluria of methoxyflurane abuse (Brennan *et al.* 1988), though in our own hyperoxaluric patients radiography has shown a medullary pattern. The reported patients with primary hyperoxaluria who had a cortical distribution of nephrocalcinosis developed renal failure within the first year of life, suggesting that this findings indicates a particularly severe form of the disease.

Polycystic disease (see also Chapters 16.2.1 and 16.2.2)

Lucaya *et al.* (1993) have recently reported radiological nephrocalcinosis in seven of 11 children with the autosomal recessive disease who survived the immediate neonatal period. All patients had reduced glomerular filtration rates, but only in three were clearances less than 50 per cent of normal. The distorted renal architecture of this disease make it difficult to establish whether the renal calcifications are cortical or medullary in distribution. Anecdotal evidence suggests that the dominant adult form of polycystic disease may also lead to nephrocalcinosis; some of these areas of calcification may represent focal calcium infiltration of cysts affected by haemorrhage.

Benign nodular cortical nephrocalcinosis

Two patients with a nodular subcapsular form of cortical nephrocalcinosis and normal renal function were seen in our personal series, and have been described in detail by Hoffbrand *et al.* (1987). Nephrocalcinosis (Fig. 7) was discovered by chance in both patients, and there were no clinical, urinary, or biochemical indications of underlying renal disease. Renal biopsy in one patient showed a small nodule of calcium oxalate without any other cortical abnormality. The cause of this rare form of nephrocalcinosis remains a mystery.

Trauma

Bilateral cortical nephrocalcinosis has also been reported in a patient in whom lithotripsy for bilateral renal calculi was followed by permanent anuric renal failure (Calviño *et al.* 1999). This report quotes several other reports of patients with long-term reduction in renal function after this common form of treatment, but this is the first recorded complete and permanent loss of renal function due to cortical nephrocalcinosis following lithotripsy.

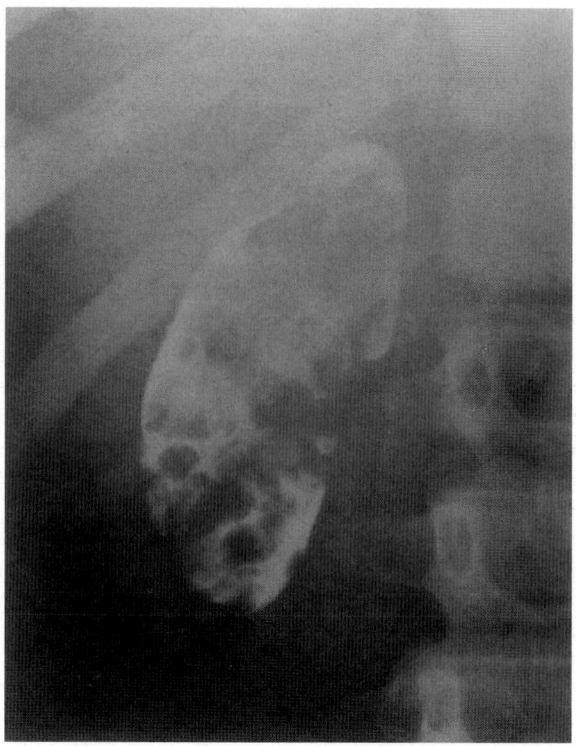

Fig. 6 Plain radiograph of right kidney of a 14-year-old boy with vesicoureteric reflux and chronic pyelonephritis. The left kidney was similarly but much less severely affected.

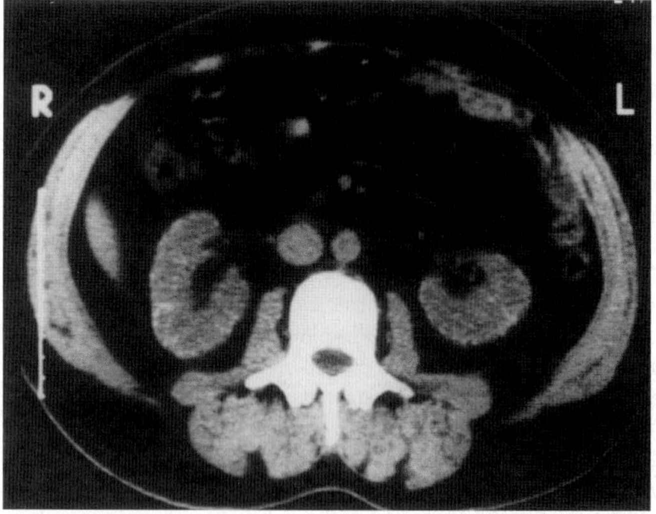

Fig. 7 CT scan of benign nodular cortical nephrocalcinosis in a 51-year-old man with normal renal function. Note the subcapsular distribution of renal calcification.

Medullary nephrocalcinosis in man

This is the usual pattern of macroscopic nephrocalcinosis, comprising over 97 per cent of our own patients and the vast majority of other reports. The nephrocalcinosis usually takes the form of small nodules of calcification clustered in each pyramid (Fig. 8), which gradually coalesce as the underlying disease progresses, producing a similar picture whatever the cause. Ultrasound of nephrocalcinosis induced by vitamin D therapy in patients with hereditary rickets (Patriquin and Robitaille 1986; Goodyer *et al.* 1987) showed that initial calcification was in the region of the corticomedullary junction, producing a 'ring' or 'doughnut' pattern. The appearances on imaging are seldom diagnostic of the underlying cause, except sometimes in papillary necrosis due to analgesic abuse where the whole papilla may be calcified, and in MSK, where the sharp definition of areas of calcification and their focal distribution may suggest the diagnosis. A common associated finding, best shown by CT, is the appearance of numerous small renal cysts, probably the result of tubular obstruction, throughout the renal substance; Igarashi *et al.* (1991) suggested that these are specific to distal renal tubular acidosis (dRTA), but they have been demonstrated also in Dent's disease (Wrong *et al.* 1994), in the nephrocalcinosis of the syndrome of apparent mineralocorticoid excess (Moudgil *et al.* 2000) and in one of the patients with the hypomagnesaemia/hypercalciuria syndrome reported here, so they appear to have no precise diagnostic value.

The renal pathology of some of the diseases causing nephrocalcinosis is well understood (e.g. oxalosis, analgesic nephropathy), but little is known about the histopathology of nephrocalcinosis formation. Because many of these diseases are characterized by hypercalcaemia or hypercalciuria, it is generally assumed that the first foci of calcification develop either in renal tubular cells or in the interstitium when hypercalcaemia is the important factor, or within the tubular lumen in conditions characterized by hypercalciuria. This question is not easily resolved by study of kidneys affected by nephrocalcinosis, since by the time they reach the pathologist, these have usually been so severely damaged by chronic inflammation, fibrosis, and nephron drop-out that it is difficult to define the primary site of mineral deposition.

Most recent studies of the local processes of stone formation in nephrolithiasis (concerned usually with enucleation and aggregation of calculous material) have been directed to urinary stone formation in general (see Chapter 8.1) and not specifically to nephrocalcinosis, but it is unlikely that the processes are different in the two situations. Two urinary factors which are likely to play a role in intrarenal calcium precipitation are hypercalciuria and hypocitraturia, of which one or other or both are present in most of the renal tubular syndromes causing nephrocalcinosis that are discussed below.

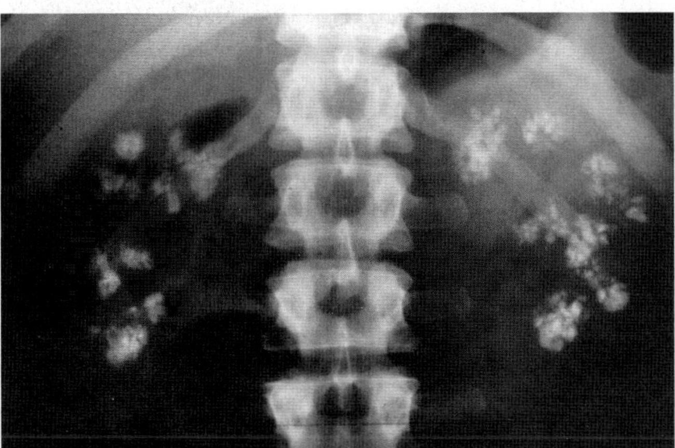

Fig. 8 Medullary nephrocalcinosis in a 25-year-old man with familial dRTA due to a Band 3^{WALTON} mutation (Toye *et al.* 2002). Note the pyramidal distribution of the clusters of nephrocalcinosis.

Individual diseases causing medullary nephrocalcinosis

Disturbances of calcium metabolism (see also Chapter 2.3)

Almost any condition causing a sustained or intermittent hypercalcaemia or hypercalciuria may cause nephrocalcinosis. Autonomous hyperparathyroidism (usually primary, but occasionally the result of previous nutritional vitamin-D deficiency or malabsorption) is the single most common cause in adults, accounting for 42 per cent of the series of Mortensen and Emmett and 32 per cent of our own, but is an unusual cause in children (Wenzl *et al.* 1968; Cremin *et al.* 1982; Rönnefarth and Misselwitz 2000). The incidence of nephrocalcinosis in this disease is not particularly high—22 per cent in a series of 138 patients studied by Lloyd (1968) and 16 per cent in a series of 700 consecutive patients coming to parathyroid surgery (A. G. A. Cowie and L. C. Watson, personal communication)—and the high frequency of parathyroid disease as a cause of nephrocalcinosis arises from the high prevalence of hyperparathyroidism in the general population.

Nephrocalcinosis is not usually marked (Kreel 1962) and its presence appears to be more closely related to the duration of hypercalcaemia than to its intensity; the mean plasma calcium in our own patients was 3.1 ± 0.3 mmol/l (12.5 ± 1.3 mg/100 ml) and urinary calcium varied from subnormal values in the presence of renal failure up to 27 mmol (1100 mg)/day. Nephrocalcinosis is not closely related to the degree of renal failure and chronic renal failure may complicate autonomous hyperparathyroidism even in the absence of demonstrable nephrocalcinosis.

Other conditions in which hypercalcaemia can lead to nephrocalcinosis are William's syndrome, or idiopathic infantile hypercalcaemia (Lightwood 1952; Shiers *et al.* 1957); and the so-called milk-alkali syndrome (Burnett *et al.* 1949; McMillan and Freeman 1965), which is really a form of chronic oral calcium poisoning resulting from consumption of large amounts of milk or calcium alkali for the relief of ulcer dyspepsia (in the United Kingdom, the latter is usually taken as Rennies Digestif tablets, each containing 680 mg of calcium carbonate). Milk-alkali syndrome in peptic ulcer disease has become much less common since the high milk intakes advocated by Sippy as treatment have been largely replaced by use of H2-receptor antagonists and proton pump inhibitors.

Ultrasound nephrocalcinosis has been reported in Down's syndrome infants in at least four centres (Proesmans *et al.* 1995; Filler *et al.* 2001). This may be a form of milk-alkali syndrome, as three of the infants were poor feeders who had been nourished with tube feeds based largely on milk, and their nephrocalcinosis and attendant hypercalciuria improved when a more normal dietary regime was established; however, Filler's patient was an intestinal calcium overabsorber who had received only recommended amounts of oral calcium and vitamin D, suggesting another basis for this syndrome.

Hypervitaminosis D

This is a well-recognized cause of hypercalcaemia with nephrocalcinosis which occasionally arisen by accident, or when overdoses are taken by normal subjects obsessed with self-administration of vitamins. Nephrocalcinosis has been reported in healthy children given prophylactic vitamin D in East Germany, to a total dose of 90 mg (3,600,000 IU) over 20 months (Rönnefarth and Misselwitz 2000). A report of a mass outbreak in Massachusetts, caused by gross over-fortification of a domestic milk supply, is reassuring in the small number of people who were clinically affected: the concentration of vitamin D_3 in the milk supplied to over 11,000 households over 6 years was 70–500 times greater than the recommended 400 IU/quart, but only 56 patients with symptoms of vitamin D excess were reported, usually with anorexia and weight loss, plasma calcium was only moderately increased to a maximum of 4.1 mmol/l, no patient died and only two patients were reported as showing nephrocalcinosis on renal ultrasound (Jacobus *et al.* 1992; Blank *et al.* 1995; Scanlon *et al.* 1995).

Iatrogenic hypervitaminosis D

Vitamin D preparations are widely used in the treatment of hypocalcaemia and various forms of metabolic bone disease, and nephrocalcinosis is being increasingly observed following this therapy, even in patients who have received recommended amounts and never shown to be hypercalcaemic. Hypoparathyroidism, both postsurgical and idiopathic, was probably the first condition where this problem arose, with marked hypercalciuria developing on treatment even when this was insufficient to raise plasma calcium to normal levels (Litvak *et al.* 1958); such patients have often developed nephrocalcinosis (Ferris *et al.* 1961). A similar situation has been observed in the rare form of familial hypocalcaemia/hypercalciuria which is due to a gain-of-function mutation of the calcium-sensing receptor (Pearce *et al.* 1996); patients with this autosomal dominant disease have sometimes been misdiagnosed as having familial hypoparathyroidism, and are likewise at risk of nephrocalcinosis when vitamin D preparations are used to treat their hypocalcaemia. Several centres have recently reported similar problems in the treatment of X-linked hypophosphataemic rickets; these patients have usually been given phosphate supplements in addition to vitamin D preparations, and though the latter is usually incriminated as the therapy responsible for nephrocalcinosis, there is some evidence suggesting that phosphate therapy contributes to this complication (Goodyer *et al.* 1987; Verge *et al.* 1991; Taylor *et al.* 1995; Seikaly *et al.* 1996). Other diseases where this problem has arisen include hypophosphatasia (Fraser 1957; Sumner *et al.* 1984), vitamin-D dependent rickets and hypophosphataemic 'non-rachitic' bone disease (Jequier *et al.* 1986; Patriquin and Robitaille 1986) and cystinotic Fanconi syndrome (Theodoropoulos *et al.* 1995). My own series includes five patients with iatrogenic nephrocalcinosis of this type: two with hypoparathyroidism and one each with bone disease caused by Lowe's syndrome, uraemic osteodystrophy and coeliac disease.

Sarcoidosis (see also Chapter 4.4)

This also frequently leads to hypercalcaemia, the result of increased conversion of 25-hydroxycholecalciferol to 1,25-dihydroxycholecalciferol within sarcoid granulomata (Mason *et al.* 1984), and nephrocalcinosis is a recognized result, though this is probably a less common problem now than it was 50 years ago when vitamin D was sometimes advocated as treatment for sarcoidosis (Curtis *et al.* 1947). In temperate climates, the hypercalcaemia of sarcoidosis is particularly liable to be episodic, as it may be apparent only with increased exposure to natural sunlight in the summer months, or when the patient is deliberately exposed to solar radiation in a winter vacation; hypercalcaemia then becomes more marked because the additional vitamin D synthesized by the irradiated skin contributes to the dietary vitamin D being 1-hydroxylated by sarcoid tissue. As in other patients with intermittent hypercalcaemia arising from hypervitaminosis D or excess calcium intake, the plasma calcium may be normal when nephrocalcinosis is first discovered, but previous episodes of hypercalcaemia can be suspected from the history and the finding of corneal calcification.

Rapidly progressive osteoporosis

This may also cause nephrocalcinosis. It may be of the postmenopausal or senile variety, or associated with prolonged immobilization, but is particularly a feature of Cushing's syndrome, both of endogenous origin and due to adrenocorticotrophic hormone (ACTH) or corticosteroid administration. The use of ACTH in treatment of infantile convulsions, usually continued for 6–18 weeks, has been particularly associated with this complication (Foley *et al.* 1982; Rausch *et al.* 1984). The standard explanation is that steroid-induced osteoporosis causes nephrocalcinosis by leading to hypercalcaemia and/or hypercalciuria, but other mechanisms have been suggested to explain renal calcification in infants receiving ACTH, including vitamin D excess and hyperparathyroidism (Riikonen *et al.* 1986).

Idiopathic hypercalciuria

Although this is one of the most common of the metabolic causes of renal stones, it is not a particularly common cause of nephrocalcinosis, comprising only 6 per cent of our present series. Idiopathic hypercalciuria, and nephrocalcinosis associated with the syndrome, both show a marked male predominance, and 18 of 22 patients in our own series were male (Fig. 9). The syndrome is heterogenous and probably contains several different diseases which are yet to be disentangled. Several published reports have shown a familial tendency (Fanconi 1963; Hamed *et al.* 1979; Aggarwal and Verrier Jones 1989) including a striking familial incidence of nephrocalcinosis (Eggert *et al.* 1998). In our own patients, nephrocalcinosis has usually been mild and has tended to diminish in severity when hypercalciuria has been successfully controlled by treatment. With hindsight, it appears likely that some of the reported cases might have had the hypomagnesaemia–hypercalciuria syndrome or Dent's disease (in keeping with their male predominance), rather than a truly idiopathic hypercalciuria, for a low plasma phosphate has often been found, and plasma magnesium and low-molecular-weight proteinuria have frequently not been examined.

Amelogenesis imperfecta/nephrocalcinosis/hypocalciuria syndrome

This bizarre association has been reported in four unrelated families from Australia, the United States and the Middle-East (MacGibbon 1972; Lubinsky *et al.* 1985; Phakey *et al.* 1995; Dellow *et al.* 1998). Each report was of a sibling pair, without involvement of other generations, and in one family, the parents were first-cousins, so the disease is likely to be an autosomal recessive though the identity of the gene defect is unknown. The dental condition is characterized by extremely thin and fragile enamel, affecting both primary and permanent dentitions, with delayed or absent eruption probably because the presence of enamel is essential for the normal eruption of teeth; the two patients in the writer's family still had some unerupted canines, premolars and molars of their permanent dentition when in their forties. The syndrome has been little studied with respect to renal tubular abnormalities, other than the finding of hypocalciuria under 1.0 mmol/day and normal urinary citrate, but Lubinsky reported normal urinary acidification. Nephrocalcinosis is of the usual medullary pattern, easily visualized in conventional radiographs, and glomerular filtration has been moderately reduced in several patients, in keeping with the degree of nephrocalcinosis. The author's two patients (Dellow *et al.* 1998) have

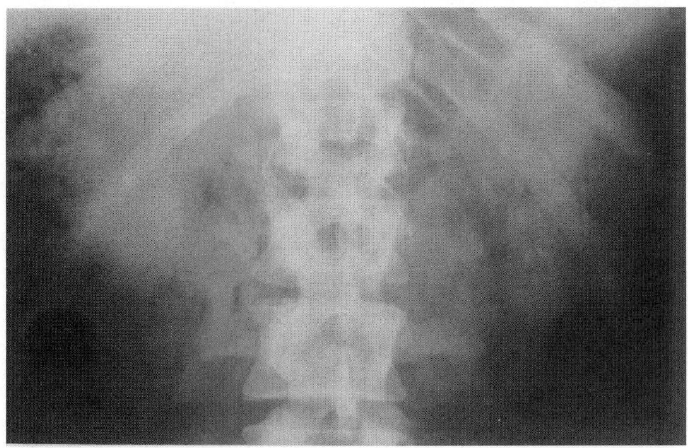

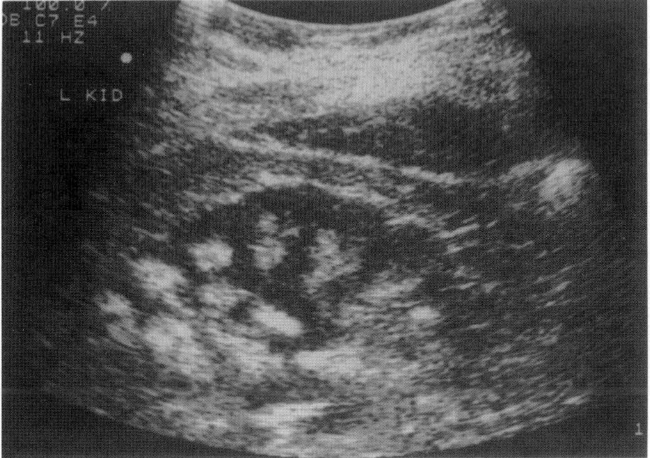

Fig. 9 Medullary nephrocalcinosis in a 42-year-old man with idiopathic hypercalciuria and a normal plasma creatinine. Top is KUB film, and bottom is ultrasonograph of left kidney. Note that ultrasound is better than KUB in showing nephrocalcinosis.

plasma creatinines of 71 and 137 μmol/l, but the original patients of MacGibbon both had end-stage renal failure by the time they were young adults. In one patient, plasma phosphate was reduced to 0.46–0.71 mmol/l. X-linked and autosomal dominant forms of amelogenesis imperfecta are also recognized, but unlike the recessive disease, these are not associated with nephrocalcinosis.

Other systemic metabolic diseases damaging the renal tubule

Oxalosis (see Chapter 16.5.2)

These syndromes are characterized by excess oxalate production in the body, so the usual descriptive term 'hyperoxaluria' is misleading, implying incorrectly the existence of a renal abnormality causing excess oxalate excretion. In so called 'primary' hyperoxaluria, increased urinary oxalate excretion is secondary to an increased synthesis of oxalate within the body, amounting to some 5–20 times normal, which causes deposition of calcium oxalate crystals in many organs, including a microscopic nephrocalcinosis (Fig. 1) which usually leads to renal failure in childhood or early adult life.

Nephrocalcinosis, when visible macroscopically, is usually of a medullary pattern, but a cortical distribution has also been described in very young children and represents a more fulminant form of the disease (Wilson *et al.* 1979; Luers *et al.* 1980). Both the more common type 1 (glycollic) hyperoxaluria (Scowen *et al.* 1959) and the much rarer type 2 (glyceric) hyperoxaluria (Williams and Smith 1968) can cause macroscopic nephrocalcinosis. In the present series of 12 patients with radiological nephrocalcinosis caused by oxalosis, nine had type 1, one had type 2, and two had enteric hyperoxaluria, caused by a jejunoileal bypass operation performed for extreme obesity in one patient, and an ileal resection for volvulus in a second. These last two patients are a reminder that nephrocalcinosis caused by hyperoxaluria is not confined to the familial hyperoxalurias, but can also occur from exogenous oxalate poisoning (Jeghers and Murphy 1945), increased intestinal oxalate absorption from primary intestinal disease (Chikos and McDonald 1976) or bypass surgery (Earnest 1979), or from ingestion of oxalate precursors such as ethylene glycol or methoxyflurane. However, the acute hyperoxaluria of oxalate and ethylene glycol poisoning is characterized by microscopic nephrocalcinosis and acute renal failure, which is often reversible (Jeghers and Murphy 1945; Friedman *et al.* 1962), whereas macroscopic nephrocalcinosis takes months or years to become visible and is therefore associated with more chronic hyperoxaluric states. In many cases, the enteric hyperoxaluria caused by intestinal bypass or disease is rather mild, passing unnoticed or leading to the passage of an occasional calcium oxalate stone, but in some patients it is very severe, running a course as devastating as primary hyperoxaluria and, if unchecked, leading to endstage renal failure within a few years (Gelbart *et al.* 1977).

Chronic hypokalaemic states (see also Chapter 2.2)

Nephrocalcinosis has been reported in several patients with longstanding hypokalaemia which was not known to be associated with primary renal disease, leading to the suggestion that persistent hypokalaemia may itself predispose to nephrocalcinosis. Case reports have included primary aldosteronism (Yang *et al.* 1994; Schmitt *et al.* 1995), Liddle's syndrome (Liddle *et al.* 1963), congenital 11β-hydroxysteroid dehydrogenase deficiency (Stewart *et al.* 1988), and the syndrome of apparent mineralocorticoid excess (White *et al.* 1997; Moudgil *et al.* 2000); my own series includes a patient with familial glucocorticoid-suppressible hyperaldosteronism. Chronic potassium deficiency is known to be associated with damage to the tubular epithelium (Relman and Schwartz 1958), and a low urinary citrate (Simpson 1983), both of which might predispose to precipitation of calcium salts. Persistent hypokalaemia is a feature of several other diseases dealt with in this chapter which lead to nephrocalcinosis (e.g. renal tubular acidosis, Bartter's syndrome and Dent's disease), where it may be a contributory factor to intrarenal calcium deposition.

Congenital hypothyroidism

This is a recognized cause of infantile nephrocalcinosis and our personal series contains one such patient whose mild nephrocalcinosis is stationary more than 60 years after her infantile cretinism was recognized and successfully treated. These infants have sometimes been hypercalcaemic (Naylor 1955), which might have explained their nephrocalcinosis, but in many the serum calcium has been normal (Tümay *et al.* 1962; Bateson and Chander 1965). Another more mysterious factor in their nephrocalcinosis might be the absence of some unexplained property of thyroid hormone which appears to protect against nephrocalcinosis, as demonstrated in several models of experimental nephrocalcinosis in the rat (Reeves and Forbes 1972; Newman 1973).

Other renal tubular diseases

Distal renal tubular acidosis (see also Chapter 5.4)

This is the second most common cause of macroscopic nephrocalcinosis after autonomous hyperparathyroidism, comprising 19 per cent of both the 1954 series of Mortensen and Emmett and of my own. Among diseases causing medullary nephrocalcinosis, it has one of the highest incidences of this complication, which was present in 77 per cent of the 44 adults and older children of Caruana and Buckalew (1988) with primary dRTA, and in 80 per cent of the 87 patients in my series. It also tends to produce a more gross nephrocalcinosis than occurs in other diseases, though of the usual medullary pattern (Figs 8, 10, and 11).

Most forms of primary dRTA have a high incidence of nephrocalcinosis: the transitory infantile form originally described over 65 years ago (Lightwood 1935; Butler *et al.* 1936); the familial disease, both dominant and recessive, caused by *AE1* gene mutations affecting the collecting duct bicarbonate/chloride band 3 exchanger (Wrong *et al.* 1996; Bruce *et al.* 1997, 2000); the recessive disease caused by mutations affecting subunits of the tubular H^+-ATPase (Karet *et al.* 1998; Smith *et al.* 2000); and the adult-onset female form of the disease that is associated with multiple autoimmune abnormalities (Wrong *et al.* 1993). Nephrocalcinosis has also been reported in the form of renal tubular acidosis associated with carbonic anhydrase II deficiency and osteopetrosis (Ismail *et al.* 1997), though here it is probably less common in keeping with the predominantly proximal, rather than distal, type of urinary acidification defect found in this syndrome. Because medullary nephrocalcinosis is itself a cause of secondary dRTA (Butler *et al.* 1936; Ferris *et al.* 1961), it is sometimes difficult to determine which came first, as in the nephrocalcinosis associated with analgesic nephropathy and MSK, two conditions which can cause both nephrocalcinosis and a urinary acidification defect, as discussed below. Apparent exceptions to the general rule that dRTA from any cause can lead to nephrocalcinosis are the renal transplant with an acquired urinary acidification defect (Better *et al.* 1969; Wilson and Siddiqui 1973), and the distal type of urinary acidification defect which complicates renal obstruction (Berlyne 1961) and has been used by physiologists as an experimental animal model of dRTA (Ribeiro and Suki 1986).

Most patients with dRTA have a hyperchloraemic acidosis, but a substantial proportion, 20–35 per cent in most series, are not acidotic (Buckalew *et al.* 1968; Feest and Wrong 1982; Caruana and Buckalew 1988; Wrong *et al.* 1993), mainly due to their preserved ability to excrete hydrogen ion as ammonium despite impairment of urinary acidifying power. These patients with 'incomplete' or non-acidotic dRTA usually come to notice because of unexplained nephrocalcinosis, renal stone formation or hypokalaemia, or are discovered during a search of relatives of patients with familial disease or of those with immune diseases often associated with dRTA, such as Sjögren's syndrome, systemic lupus erythematosus or autoimmune thyroid disease. Their reduced renal ability to lower urine pH can be revealed by an acidotic stress test (Wrong and Davies 1959; Elkinton *et al.* 1960), or the use of frusemide (furosemide) and fludrocortisone (Walter *et al.* 1999), methods which do not entail the fallacies inherent in the use of urinary $p\text{CO}_2$ as a measure of distal tubular H^+ secretion (Wrong 1991).

The mineral deposited in nephrocalcinosis of dRTA is probably some form of calcium phosphate. Carbonate–apatite has been the mineral form of calcium phosphate shown by X-ray diffraction of stones passed by dRTA patients under my care. Calcium phosphate is believed to precipitate from urine in the collecting ducts, though no unequivocal evidence exists that mineral deposition is primarily an intratubular event.

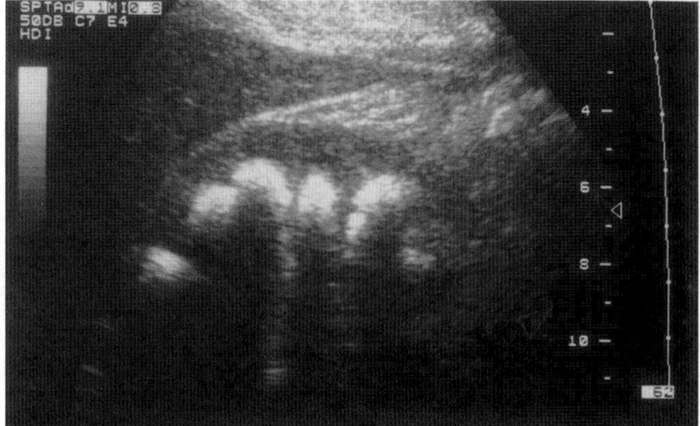

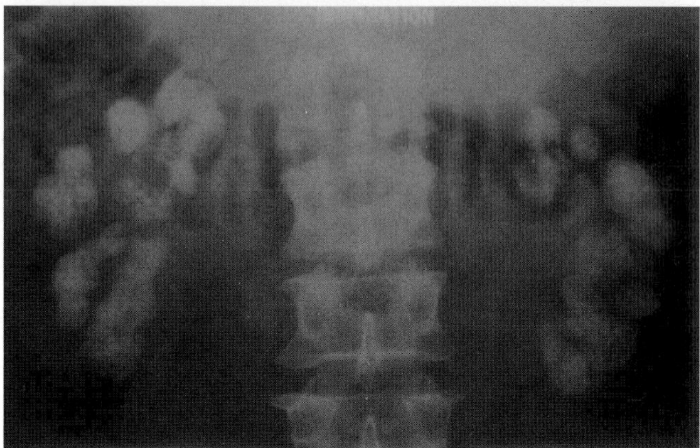

Fig 10 Medullary nephrocalcinosis in a 41-year-old man with dRTA caused by a band 3 Arg589Hist mutation (Bruce *et al.* 1997). Top shows ultrasonograph of right kidney; bottom shows KUB. Nephrocalcinosis appears to be better shown in KUB, because in the ultrasound picture acoustic shadowing caused by nephrocalcinosis in the outer medulla hides much of the inner medullary nephrocalcinosis.

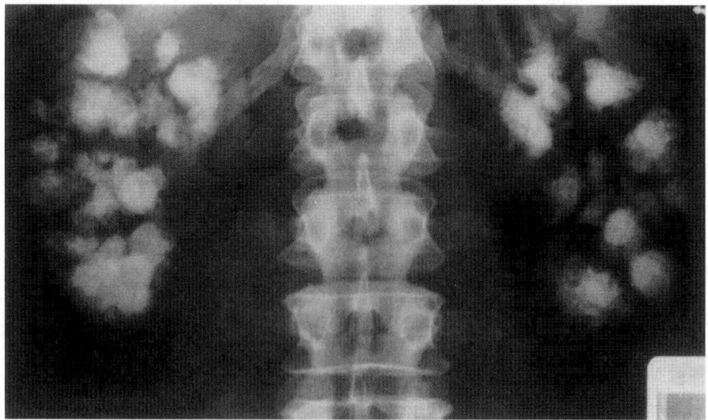

Fig. 11 Medullary nephrocalcinosis in a 56-year-old man with dRTA. This is the same patient shown in Fig. 8. Note the marked increase in nephrocalcinosis despite 31 years of continuous alkali (mainly sodium bicarbonate) treatment.

The likely local factors leading to renal deposition of this material in dRTA are (a) a low urinary citrate, (b) a relatively alkaline urine, usually in the pH range 6–7, and (c) hypercalciuria. The relatively high urine pH and low urinary citrate are cardinal features of the disease, but hypercalciuria is not, for it is the result of systemic acidosis and a well-recognized complication of acidosis from other causes. Hypercalciuria is usual in children with dRTA who are acidotic (Greenberg *et al.* 1966; McSherry and Morris 1978), but it is not a feature of the incomplete (non-acidotic) disease, or of patients whose acidosis has been corrected with alkalis, and it is absent in many adults with dRTA even in the presence of acidosis (Wrong and Feest 1980; Feest and Wrong 1982). The widespread but mistaken view that hypercalciuria is a cardinal feature of dRTA may have partly arisen because of early reports of hypercalciuria in patients who were incorrectly labelled as having dRTA, but subsequently shown to have another disease of which hypercalciuria is a basic feature. Thus early accounts of the hypomagnesaemia/hypercalciuria syndrome (Michelis *et al.* 1972), and Dent's disease (Buckalew *et al.* 1974; Kelleher *et al.* 1998), both of them inherited renal tubular disorders of which hypercalciuria is a cardinal feature, described both syndromes as familial forms of renal tubular acidosis, and these reports contributed to the erroneous concept that hypercalciuria is a cardinal feature in some dRTA families (Buckalew *et al.* 1974).

In normal subjects, urinary citrate increases as urine pH increases, and the concentration of citrate ion is sufficient to complex calcium in a soluble form and prevent its precipitation as calcium phosphate, which might otherwise be predicted from the insolubility of calcium phosphate in alkaline solution. Urinary citrate is invariably low in dRTA, despite the relatively alkaline urines (Dedmon and Wrong 1962; Brodwall *et al.* 1972; Norman *et al.* 1978). This low urinary citrate is generally attributed to an intracellular acidosis affecting renal tubular cells, a consequence both of systemic acidosis and frequently an associated potassium deficiency, for intracellular pH is known to markedly influence urinary citrate through its effect on proximal tubular reabsorption of filtered citrate (Simpson 1983). If this sequence were the whole explanation, treatment of distal renal tubular acidosis with alkali, particularly alkaline salts of potassium, should, by correcting intracellular acidosis, also correct the deficiency in urinary citrate. The author's experience has been that alkali therapy increases urinary citrate in most patients, but does not completely correct the urinary citrate/pH relationship, although it retards or even inhibits further development of nephrocalcinosis. In a few patients, urinary citrate is unresponsive to alkali, in either sodium or potassium form, in doses much greater than those required to correct acidosis or hypokalaemia; these are often the patients with the most relentlessly progressive nephrocalcinosis (Figs 8 and 11). The low urinary citrate of dRTA is, therefore, not fully explained, though an intracellular acidosis of proximal tubular epithelial cells may be a factor in many cases.

Despite the usual severity of the nephrocalcinosis in dRTA, renal function is fairly well maintained provided obstructive and infective episodes are properly treated. My own experience of 73 patients with nephrocalcinosis caused by primary dRTA (familial, sporadic, and immune-related), with a cumulative follow-up of over 1000 years since nephrocalcinosis was first noted, contains only three who have reached end-stage renal failure, and all three had suffered from episodes of bilateral calculous ureteric obstruction that had remained untreated for years, largely because they had failed to attend clinic.

Use of the carbonic anhydrase inhibitor acetazolamide has given rise to renal stones and nephrocalcinosis in both man and the rat (Parfitt 1969; Győry *et al.* 1970; Parikh and Nolan 1994), probably through its effect in increasing urine pH while reducing citrate excretion (Dedmon and Wrong 1962). My personal series includes two patients who developed nephrocalcinosis after many years of acetazolamide therapy for chronic glaucoma; one of these also took phenacetin for his associated headache, and probably both drugs contributed to his nephrocalcinosis. The acidosis caused by acetazolamide has features more of a proximal than of a dRTA (Leaf *et al.* 1954); as nephrocalcinosis is not usually regarded as a feature of *proximal* renal tubular acidosis, its occurrence after acetazolamide might seem surprising. The probable explanation for the apparent paradox is that most cases of spontaneous proximal renal tubular acidosis in man are associated with the multiple proximal tubular defects of the Fanconi syndrome, which include increased urinary losses of citrate (Milne *et al.* 1952; De Toni and Nordio 1959), amino acids and other organic anions which like citrate can form soluble complexes with calcium (Klement and Weber 1941), and that the excretion of these substances prevents development of nephrocalcinosis.

Fanconi syndrome (see also Chapter 5.3)

The common assumption that nephrocalcinosis is not a feature of Fanconi syndrome is incorrect, for it develops in the majority of males affected in the X-linked Dent's disease, discussed below, and even occurs rarely in women with this condition (Wrong *et al.* 1994). Nephrocalcinosis has also been reported in other forms of the Fanconi syndrome, including that due to Wilson's disease (Litin *et al.* 1959; Hoppe *et al.* 1993), Lowe's syndrome (Sliman *et al.* 1995), cystinosis (Saleem *et al.* 1995), tyrosinaemia (Russo and O'Regan 1990), and idiopathic Fanconi syndrome (Ruiz-Palomo *et al.* 1978; Wen *et al.* 1989). The Fanconi syndrome caused by type 1 glycogen storage disease also commonly leads to nephrocalcinosis (Fick and Beck 1992; Restaino *et al.* 1993) though here there are some features of distal RTA, including a low urinary citrate (Weinstein *et al.* 2001). My own series of nephrocalcinotic patients includes two with idiopathic Fanconi syndrome, in one of whom the disease is a Mendelian dominant and affects three generations of the family. Hypercalciuria has been demonstrated in most of the patients with Fanconi syndrome affected by nephrocalcinosis. As already noted, nephrocalcinosis has also developed in other patients with Fanconi syndrome who received vitamin D derivatives for metabolic bone disease.

Dent's disease (see also Chapter 5.3)

Dent's disease was first described in 1990 as a form of renal Fanconi syndrome which is characterized by low molecular weight proteinuria, hypercalciuria, medullary nephrocalcinosis, and a strong male preponderance (Wrong *et al.* 1990, 1994). A similar disease was shown to be X-linked in a very large kindred in upper New York state (Frymoyer *et al.* 1991), and described as 'X-linked recessive nephrolithiasis (XRN)'. Soon afterwards, low molecular weight proteinuria, often with nephrocalcinosis, was detected in some Japanese schoolboys ('Japanese variant of Dent's disease', Igarashi *et al.* 1995), picked up because of the national policy of examining schoolchildren's urine for low molecular weight protein. The three conditions are variants of the same disease, which was shown to be caused by mutations of the *CLCN5* gene which codes for an intracellular chloride channel in the proximal convoluted tubule (Lloyd *et al.* 1996). The disease is accompanied by other features of the Fanconi syndrome, particularly hypokalaemia, renal phosphate-losing, aminoaciduria, glycosuria, uricosuria, and a variable urinary acidification defect (Scheinman 1998). Rickets or osteomalacia occurs in about a quarter of cases; this bone disease is similar to that of other forms of Fanconi syndrome, in that excess renal phosphate loss is probably an important aetiological factor; unlike the bone disease of dRTA, systemic acidosis is not responsible. The disease though rare is widespread, with reports of families from the United Kingdom, United States, Canada, Italy, France, and Japan; some hundreds of patients have now been described, with more than 60 different mutations affecting all parts of the CLCN5 channel (Thakker 2000). In the past, the disease has been confused with other syndromes, particularly dRTA and absorptive hypercalciuria.

Nephrocalcinosis is found in the majority of males with Dent's disease, but rarely in affected females (Wrong *et al.* 1994). It can be very marked (Fig. 12) but its severity is not closely related to the degree of renal failure which can develop even in the absence of nephrocalcinosis. Figure 13 shows the progression of the renal atrophy and minimal nephrocalcinosis of a young man with the disease; his maternal uncle had Dent's disease with the same CLCN5 mutation, and had already reached renal failure and transplantation aged 51, but his native kidneys showed only the features of a severe chronic interstitial nephritis without calcification.

Familial magnesium-losing nephropathy

Rodriguez-Soriano *et al.* (1987) reviewed the several forms of this condition and emphasized that the hypomagnesaemia/hypercalciuria syndrome (Michelis *et al.* 1972; Manz *et al.* 1978) is the only one of which nephrocalcinosis is a part. The condition is transmitted as an autosomal recessive and results from mutations in the Paracellin-1 tight junction protein that determines the linked paracellular reabsorption of magnesium and calcium in the ascending limb of Henle's loop (Simon *et al.* 1999). Hypercalciuria is usually in the range of 0.1–0.25 mmol/kg/day, which is three to four times the normal value for children of this age, and is probably an important factor in nephrocalcinosis which is of typical medullary type. Urinary acidification may be slightly impaired, perhaps as a secondary effect of the nephrocalcinosis. Urinary citrate is low (Schärer and Manz 1985), in keeping with the effects of experimental magnesium depletion in the rat (Lifshitz *et al.* 1967). Clinically, the syndrome is characterized by tetany or convulsions of hypocalcaemic or hypomagnesaemic origin, occasional rickets and ocular abnormalities including myopia and horizontal nystagmus. Renal failure requiring renal replacement therapy in childhood or adolescence has been a common feature (Nicholson *et al.* 1995); in our personal series of six patients, currently aged 22–31 years, four are known to have reached endstage renal failure aged 9–22 years. The syndrome is quite distinct from familial dRTA, though frequently confused with it in the past when plasma magnesium was less easily measured.

Medullary sponge kidney (see Chapter 17.5)

MSK is a common cause of medullary calcification, though it can be argued that it is not a true nephrocalcinosis as the calcium lies in ectatic collecting ducts rather than in the renal substance. The appearances may closely mimic those of a metabolic nephrocalcinosis. The true diagnosis may be suspected because renal calcium deposits are uneven in distribution and often larger and more sharply defined than those of a metabolic disease. Hemihypertrophy of the body, often apparent in the bony proportions shown in a KUB film, should also suggest the diagnosis. Proof consists of demonstrating dilated collecting ducts in an excretory urogram which are not visualized in the plain film, but this may not be possible if every ectatic collecting duct is occupied by a stone.

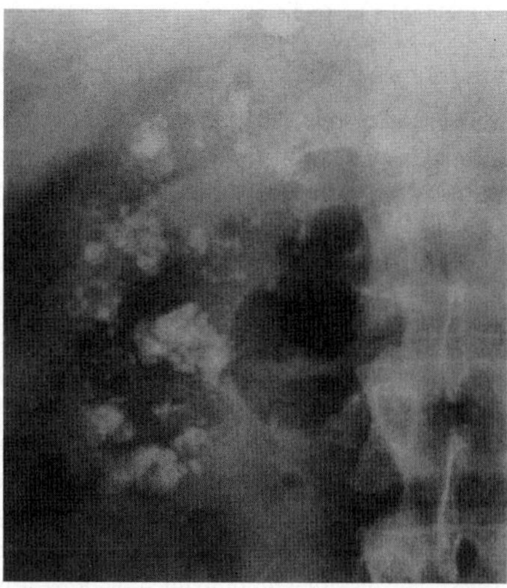

Fig. 12 Medullary nephrocalcinosis in 26-year-old man with Dent's disease due to a codon 200 missense mutation of chloride channel CLCN5 (Lloyd *et al.* 1996). The left kidney was similarly affected.

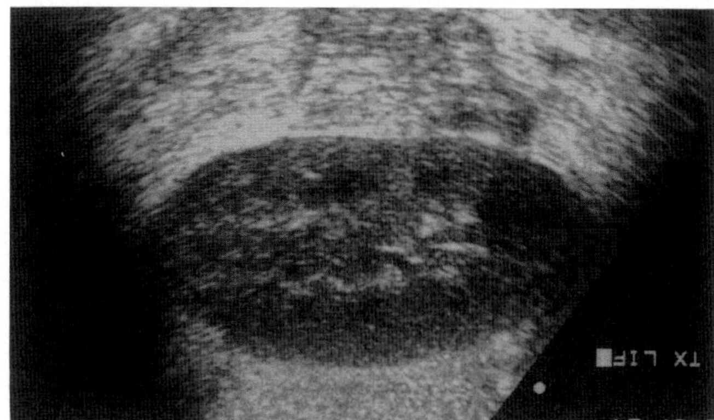

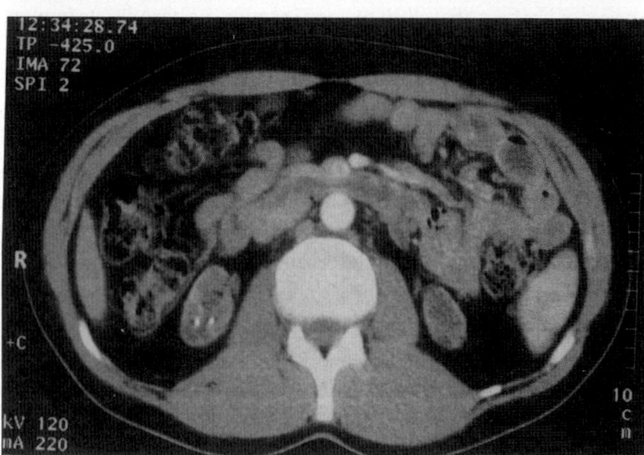

Fig. 13 Medullary nephrocalcinosis in a patient with endstage renal failure caused by Dent's disease from a CLCN5 intron 5 acceptor splice site mutation (Cox *et al.* 1999). Top (ultrasound) shows mild nephrocalcinosis in right kidney at the age of 26 years when patient still had residual renal function; bottom (CT) 3 years later shows further renal atrophy despite no worsening of nephrocalcinosis, patient already transplanted with native kidneys showing no excretion of contrast.

Sponge kidney is occasionally familial (Kuiper 1971). It is frequently associated with hypercalciuria: 88 per cent in the series of O'Neill *et al.* (1981), but only 25 per cent in our series. It is also associated with dRTA (Greenberg *et al.* 1971; Higashihara *et al.* 1984; Osther *et al.* 1994), the latter usually consisting of the incomplete syndrome with a distal type of acidification defect and a low urinary citrate but no acidosis. The finding of these functional tubular defects in patients with MSK has two important diagnostic implications: (a) the demonstration of idiopathic hypercalciuria or dRTA in a patient with nephrocalcinosis cannot be taken as proof that these conditions are the cause of the nephrocalcinosis, as the renal calcification may be secondary to an underlying MSK, and (b) some of the renal calcification in MSK might not lie in ectatic collecting ducts, but rather in the renal substance, for parenchymatous deposition of calcium is a feature of both dRTA and idiopathic hypercalciuria.

In my experience, MSK tends to be over-diagnosed in patients with nephrocalcinosis, usually because the renal calcification is first seen by a radiologist who does not have immediate access to the metabolic investigations which might uncover a different explanation for the nephrocalcinosis; the diagnosis of MSK, once made though often in error, tends to be accepted by other physicians who later see the patient. Because a correct diagnosis of a metabolic cause of nephrocalcinosis may have therapeutic and familial implications for the patient (e.g. in dRTA, Bartter's syndrome, and Dent's disease), MSK should not be diagnosed by exclusion, but by the positive identification at renal imaging of ectatic collecting ducts.

Bartter's syndrome (see Chapter 5.4)

The genetic basis of this group of recessive renal tubular diseases presenting with hypokalaemia, renal sodium-losing, hyperreninaemic hyperaldosteronism and juxtaglomerular hyperplasia has been well delineated over the last 10 years (Zelikovic 2001), and it is becoming more clear which forms are at most risk from nephrocalcinosis, though there is still insufficient information on the phenotypic differences between the various syndromes. Gitelman's variant of the syndrome, which is the most common and the least clinically severe, is associated with hypomagnesaemia and a low or normal urinary calcium, and is the result of mutations affecting the *SLC12A3* gene that codes for thiazide-sensitive NaCl cotransporter (NCCT) on the luminal membrane of the distal convoluted tubule (Simon *et al.* 1996a). Nephrocalcinosis is *not* a feature, in keeping with the absence of hypercalciuria.

The remaining patients have either a very severe form of Bartter's syndrome which presents antenatally with maternal polyhydramnios, infants being born prematurely with marked polyuria, hypercalciuria, renal sodium-losing, circulatory collapse and hypokalaemic alkalosis (also described as the 'hyperprostaglandin E syndrome', Seyberth *et al.* 1985), or a slightly milder disease in young children with the same features which has been designated 'true' Bartter's syndrome. The genetic basis for both these forms of the disease has been found to lie in mutations affecting four different ion transporters which together are responsible for the normal tubular reabsorption of sodium and chloride in the thick ascending limb: Bartter I is due to mutations of the *SLC12A1* gene that codes for the Na/K/2Cl (NKCC2) cotransporter in the thick ascending limb apical membrane (Simon *et al.* 1996b); Bartter II results from mutations affecting the *KCNJ1* gene that codes for the ROMK recycling potassium channel on the same membrane (Simon *et al.* 1996c); Bartter III syndrome is caused by mutations of the *CLCNKB* gene that codes for the chloride channel (ClCKb) on the baso-lateral membrane of this cell (Simon *et al.* 1997; Konrad *et al.* 2000); and Bartter IV syndrome is due to mutations of the *BSND* (Barttin) gene that codes for a renal protein which is probably an accessory subunit to this ClCKb chloride channel (Birkenhager *et al.* 2001; Estévez *et al.* 2001). Hypercalciuria is a feature of all four forms of the syndrome and nephrocalcinosis is almost a constant feature of Bartter I and II, but less common in Bartter III and IV. Bartter IV also features sensorineural deafness (Landau *et al.* 1995; Brennan *et al.* 1998) from the mutation affecting the *BSND* gene product in the inner ear, and some reports describe renal failure as a part of this particular syndrome, but there is clinical overlap between the various syndromes (Konrad *et al.* 2000) and it is not clear to what extent renal failure is usually a result of nephrocalcinosis and may complicate all varieties of the syndrome.

Other causes of medullary nephrocalcinosis

Total parental nutrition

Nephrocalcinosis has been reported quite frequently in this circumstance, usually in association with hypercalciuria. Patients are prone to metabolic bone disease, including rickets and osteomalacia, and because oral medication is impossible they have often been given parenteral calcium, phosphate, and vitamin D preparations. Hypercalciuria and medullary nephrocalcinosis have been noted despite the presence of bone disease and hypocalcaemia (Müller *et al.* 1998).

Neonatal nephrocalcinosis

In the last 25 years, many centres have reported medullary nephrocalcinosis in infants who have suffered the respiratory distress syndrome. This has been detected by ultrasound or radiography between 5 weeks and 2 years after birth, or at necropsy in infants who died of their lung disease (Hufnagle *et al.* 1982; Pearse *et al.* 1984). Affected infants have been very premature, with an average gestational age of 27 weeks and birth weight of 830 g in the patients of Ezzedeen *et al.* (1988); all were less than 1500 g in weight in the series of Jacinto *et al.* (1988). In keeping with their prematurity, these babies were extremely ill, requiring assisted ventilation, parenteral feeding, mineral and vitamin supplements, and various antibiotics and steroids, but the most important common factor leading to their nephrocalcinosis is now believed to be the loop-diuretic frusemide (furosemide), given as treatment for fluid retention caused by their pulmonary disease, often in large doses continued for many weeks. In comparison with infants who were not receiving frusemide, these infants have been markedly hypercalciuric, and some have shown features of skeletal demineralization; studies on other infants have shown that frusemide increases urinary calcium excretion (Atkinson *et al.* 1988) just as it does in adults. Some of these infants later develop renal stones, but in most cases, nephrocalcinosis improves and gradually disappears, though glomerular filtration rate may be moderately reduced up to at least 4 years of age (Downing *et al.* 1991). Although the evidence that frusemide is responsible for the nephrocalcinosis is fairly convincing, occasional patients have been reported in whom the diuretic was not used (Short and Cooke 1991; Karlowicz *et al.* 1993), and these very premature infants have numerous other metabolic abnormalities which may play a role (Campfield *et al.* 1994; Bérard *et al.* 1995).

Frusemide excess

Though the original discovery that long-term frusemide administration may cause nephrocalcinosis was made in very premature infants, it is now clear that this complication can arise after birth at term. Alon *et al.* (1994) found nephrocalcinosis in five children, born at 34–40 weeks gestation, who required large doses of the drug for heart failure caused by congenital heart disease; renal calcification appeared to improve in two of the children in whom it was possible to stop the diuretic. Nephrocalcinosis has been seen also in infants given long-term frusemide and acetazolamide for management of hydrocephalus (Stafstrom *et al.* 1992; Lamas *et al.* 2000), a combination of two drugs which can each cause nephrocalcinosis, so entailing a double risk of this complication.

Recently, Kim *et al.* (2001) found nephrocalcinosis in 18 Korean adults aged 21–59 years who had taken up to 2800 mg daily of the drug over a period of 3–25 years; patients were female in all but one case, and the drug had been taken to control weight or oedema. In view of the frequency with which diuretic abuse is encountered in the West, it is likely that many more adults with frusemide-induced nephrocalcinosis will be reported.

Frusemide-induced nephrocalcinosis can be regarded as a pharmacological model of Bartter I syndrome; in both conditions, hypercalciuria and renal sodium-losing result from lack of function of the normal frusemide-sensitive NKCC2 transporter in the thick ascending limb.

Renal papillary necrosis (see Chapter 6.2)

This often calcifies and presents as medullary nephrocalcinosis. This is not the acute papillary necrosis which complicates acute pyelonephritis, such as occurs in diabetes mellitus, but is a more slowly progressive papillary necrosis, and is particularly associated with phenacetin-induced analgesic nephropathy (Murphy 1968), in which an incidence of nephrocalcinosis of 47 per cent was recorded by Fellner and Tuttle (1969). The calcified papillae in this condition have even been known to ossify (Burry *et al.* 1966). Papillary necrosis can be associated with other drugs, especially non-steroidal anti-inflammatory drugs (Segasothy *et al.* 1994; Elseviers *et al.* 1995). Nephrocalcinosis from calcified necrotic papillae can arise from other causes, for it was described in the 1827 necropsy of Ludwig van Beethoven (Davies 1993), at least 60 years before any of these drugs were introduced.

The nephrocalcinosis of papillary necrosis can often be identified in radiographs as consisting of calcified papillae (Figs 3 and 14), rather than the speckled pattern of calcification seen in nephrocalcinosis of metabolic cause. Although such patients usually have some degree of renal failure, the finding of calcified papillae may paradoxically be a relatively favourable sign in comparison with patients whose necrotic papillae do not calcify, for the calcium that is deposited is probably derived from the urine, and urinary calcium usually becomes negligible in amount in advanced renal failure. Our own group of nine patients with nephrocalcinosis from analgesic nephropathy contained four with creatinine clearances greater than 45 ml/min, and during a 42-year total follow-up endstage renal failure developed in only two, including the patient shown in Fig. 14 in whom papillary calcification caused by excess calcium ingestion may have preceded the development of analgesic-induced papillary necrosis.

Randall's plaques

In the 1930s, Randall, a Philadelphia urologist, described calcium deposits lying immediately under the papillary epithelium which appeared to be 'the initiating lesions of renal calculus' (Randall 1936). These deposits consisted of plaques of carbonate apatite (Prien 1975) and, although up to 2 mm in diameter, and so of a size to render many of them visible radiographically, were usually demonstrated at surgery or necropsy.

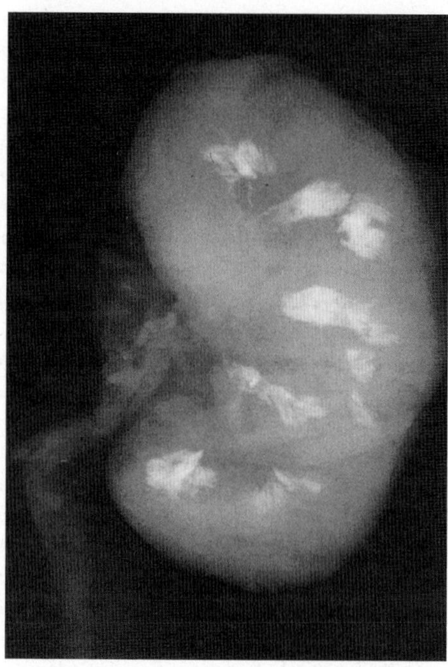

Fig. 14 Calcification of the renal papillae (necropsy specimen) in a 43-year-old woman, a pharmacy assistant who consumed large amounts of Rennies (calcium carbonate) and phenacetin during her work. The right kidney was similarly affected.

In a summary of his findings, Randall (1940) described deposits in 20 per cent of over 1000 necropsies; about one-fourth showed adherent urinary calculi lying in the calyceal system; plaques were twice as common in men as in women, and were most common in the age group 60–69 years. These observations were made before most of the renal tubular syndromes described in this chapter had been recognized. A more recent radiological study by Stoller *et al.* (1996) on 50 cadavers with a mean age of 56 years showed that 57 per cent had renal papillary calcific deposits of 0.3–4.0 mm in length, thus confirming the continued existence of Randall's plaques. La Mansa *et al.* (1998) has demonstrated similar deposits with renal ultrasound in 196 Neapolitan children, which they called 'calyceal microlithiasis'; patients had renal symptoms, usually renal pain or haematuria, many had a family history of renal stones, and a common metabolic finding was hypercalciuria. These recent reports indicate that the plaques described by Randall are still encountered, though the gist of this chapter is that it should usually be possible to make a metabolic diagnosis.

Other conditions

Nephrocalcinosis associated with hypercalciuria has recently been reported in several children with the familial sodium-losing renal tubular disease known as 'pseudohypoaldosteronism' (Shalev *et al.* 1994). It has also been reported in several patients with familial hypercholesterolaemia (Hill *et al.* 1991); no plausible pathogenetic mechanism was proposed. A particular interesting report is the description from Finland of nephrocalcinosis and hypercalciuria in five infants with congenital lactase deficiency (Saarela *et al.* 1995); hypercalciuria disappeared when the infants were given a lactose-free diet, suggesting that the presence of unhydrolyzed lactose in the intestine may have been responsible for excessive calcium absorption, as has been demonstrated in the rat (Lengemann and Comar 1961). Single instances of radiological nephrocalcinosis have also been described in fluorosis (Manigand *et al.* 1971) and alkaptonuria (Goldberg *et al.* 1976), which might be coincidence except that both diseases affect calcification and the latter is known to be associated with calcium phosphate lithiasis.

More remarkable are the diseases which are not associated with macroscopic nephrocalcinosis, including hyperthyroidism (despite the frequent occurrence of hypercalcaemia and hypercalciuria), familial benign (hypocalciuric) hypercalcaemia and the hypercalcaemia of malignant disease. A single case of medullary nephrocalcinosis has been reported in a male with hypercalcaemic thyrotoxicosis (Epstein *et al.* 1958), but the scarcity of this complication is surprising, and is further evidence of the protective action of thyroid hormone already mentioned. The author has not been able to trace any report of macroscopic nephrocalcinosis due to malignant hypercalcaemia, except that due to parathyroid carcinoma, although microscopic nephrocalcinosis and renal failure have been frequently reported; the important factor here is probably time, for patients with malignant disease seldom survive for long enough to develop macroscopic nephrocalcinosis.

In my personal series of patients with macroscopic nephrocalcinosis (Table 2), it was possible to place all but 7 per cent of patients in a firm diagnostic category. The rate of diagnostic success is even better than this figure suggests, for some important causes (e.g. Dent's disease, hypomagnesaemia/hypercalciuria, Bartter's syndrome) had not been described and so could not have been diagnosed when this series was started in 1954, and many of the patients in this small undiagnosed rump, all with *medullary* nephrocalcinosis, were either incompletely investigated for practical reasons, or had endstage renal failure which obliterates many diagnostic features. A similar proportion of patients with an undiagnosed cause (6 per cent of 152 cases) was found by Rönnefarth and Misselwitz (2000) in their survey of children with nephrocalcinosis.

Familial nephrocalcinosis

Table 3 contains a list of the many familial diseases which can be complicated by medullary nephrocalcinosis. It will be noted that the underlying diseases causing nephrocalcinosis vary from those which are invariably

Table 3 Familial diseases which may cause macroscopic medullary nephrocalcinosis

Disease	Inheritance	Remarks[a]
Multiple endocrine neoplasia, type 1, with hyperparathyroidism	Autosomal dominant	
Multiple endocrine neoplasia, type 2, with hyperparathyroidism	Autosomal dominant	
Distal renal tubular acidosis	Autosomal dominant or recessive	
Distal renal tubular acidosis with neurosensory deafness	Autosomal recessive	
Primary hyperoxaluria, type 1 (glycollic)	Autosomal recessive	
Primary hyperoxaluria, type 2 (glyceric)	Autosomal recessive	
Hypomagnesaemia–hypercalciuria syndrome	Autosomal recessive	
Amelogenesis imperfecta with nephrocalcinosis (MacGibbon–Lubinsky)	Autosomal recessive	
Idiopathic hypercalciuria	Usually autosomal dominant	Rarely familial
Dent's disease/X-linked recessive nephrolithiasis	X-linked	
Williams' disease	Uncertain	Rarely familial (Cortado *et al.* 1980)
Bartter's syndrome	Autosomal recessive	Caused by mutations of four different genes
Liddle's syndrome	Autosomal dominant	Chronic potassium depletion may be responsible for nephrocalcinosis (Liddle's syndrome; 11β-hydroxysteroid dehydrogenase deficiency; glucocorticoid-suppressible aldosteronism)
11β-Hydroxysteroid dehydrogenase deficiency	Uncertain	
Glucocorticoid-suppressible aldosteronism	Autosomal dominant	
Familial hypercholesterolaemia	Autosomal recessive	
Pseudohypoaldosteronism	Autosomal dominant and recessive forms	
Medullary sponge kidney	Probably autosomal dominant	Rarely familial (Kuiper 1971)
Alkaptonuria	Autosomal recessive	Only one case report
Wilson's disease	Autosomal recessive	Only one case report (Litin *et al.* 1959) with Fanconi syndrome
Hypophosphatasia	Various	Nephrocalcinosis usually iatrogenic but reported spontaneous by Sumner *et al.* (1984)
X-linked hypophosphataemic rickets	X-linked dominant	Nephrocalcinosis is iatrogenic, caused by vitamin D or derivatives, or oral phosphate supplements (X-linked hypophosphataemic rickets through Lowe's syndrome)
Vitamin-D-dependent rickets	Autosomal recessive	
Hypophosphataemic 'non-rachitic' bone disease	Autosomal dominant	
Nephropathic cystinosis	Autosomal recessive	
Lowe's syndrome	X-linked recessive	

[a] References in text except when well recognized or mentioned here.

familial (e.g. primary hyperoxaluria, Wilson's disease) to those that are rarely so (William's syndrome, medullary sponge kidney). The incidence of nephrocalcinosis in each disease also varies from the very common (autosomal dominant dRTA) to the very rare (alkaptonuria, Wilson's disease). The nephrocalcinosis in several familial forms of metabolic bone disease is iatrogenic in origin, associated with the use of vitamin D or its derivatives to cure the bone disease.

Clinical presentation of medullary nephrocalcinosis

Nodules of medullary nephrocalcinosis may erode through the papillary epithelium into the calyceal system to become urinary stones, so the usual presentation is with renal colic, passage of urinary stones, or haematuria. Urinary tract infections and formation of stag-horn calculi are common complications, particularly in women. Polyuria and thirst are also common presenting symptoms, caused by reduced renal concentrating power. Sometimes patients present with renal failure, or with some systemic feature of their underlying disease, and renal imaging then reveals the presence of nephrocalcinosis.

Hypertension is less common than in most forms of renal disease, probably because the juxtaglomerular apparatus is not initially involved, and the renal disease is often sodium-losing. Of my personal series of 375 patients, only 27 per cent had a casual resting blood pressure above 150/90, and the malignant phase of hypertension (hypertensive retinopathy Grade III or IV) was seen in only three.

Erythrocytosis with increased urinary erythropoietin has been reported in several cases of medullary nephrocalcinosis of various aetiologies (Feest *et al.* 1978; Agroyannis *et al.* 1992). The 16 patients I have seen with this complication had very marked nephrocalcinosis and included cases of primary hyperparathyroidism, dRTA, Dent's disease, type 1 primary hyperoxaluria, and MSK, suggesting that the nephrocalcinosis itself, rather than the underlying disease, is the cause. The possibility that their increased renal secretion of erythropoeitin is the result of hyperreninism (Gould *et al.* 1980), caused either by hypovolaemia consequent on renal sodium-losing, or by direct damage to small blood vessels and hence interference with perfusion of the juxtaglomerular apparatus, has not been explored, but provides obvious possibilities for treatment.

Urinary protein is not usually increased above normal values in medullary nephrocalcinosis, but in Dent's disease and other forms of Fanconi syndrome losses of low molecular weight proteins may exceed 2 g daily. Microscopic pyuria is almost invariable, even in the absence of urinary infection, and represents a chronic inflammatory response to the calcific deposits in the renal medulla; episodes of urinary tract infection are less common, and in the present series occurred in 50 per cent of women but in only 22 per cent of men.

Features of proximal tubular dysfunction are unusual, except for the tubular proteinuria and less frequent aminoaciduria of Dent's disease, but features of distal tubular dysfunction are common, in keeping with the medullary distribution of the nephrocalcinosis. Clinical states of sodium deficiency caused by excess renal losses are not common, but sometimes become apparent when sodium intake is impaired by intercurrent anorexia or vomiting, particularly in dRTA and milk-alkali syndrome.

Urinary acidification, as measured by urine pH during spontaneous acidosis or that induced by ammonium chloride, is frequently impaired, not just in primary dRTA where it is abnormal by definition, but in many patients with nephrocalcinosis caused by other diseases (Fig. 15). It is clear that medullary nephrocalcinosis of virtually any origin can cause secondary dRTA: for example, primary hyperparathyroidism (Butler *et al.* 1936), vitamin D intoxication (Ferris *et al.* 1961), excess treatment of X-linked hypophosphataemia (Seikaly *et al.* 1996). From this observation, it follows that, when nephrocalcinosis is present, primary dRTA should not be diagnosed from an acidification defect alone, but with the help of ancillary evidence such as familial incidence, gene defects known to be associated with dRTA, nerve deafness, or associated immune abnormalities.

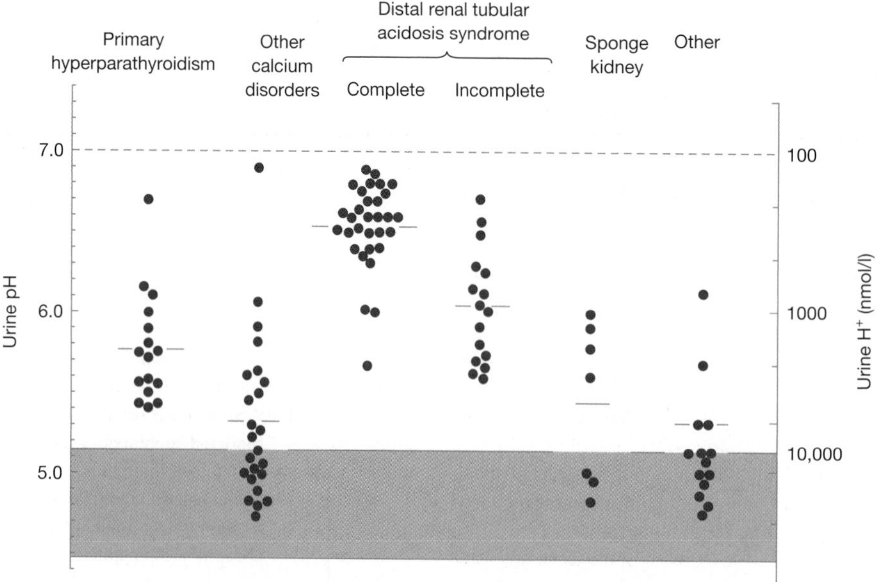

Fig. 15 Minimum urine pH during spontaneous acidosis or that induced by ammonium chloride in 108 patients with medullary nephrocalcinosis. The blue area shows the normal range (reproduced with permission from Wrong and Feest 1976).

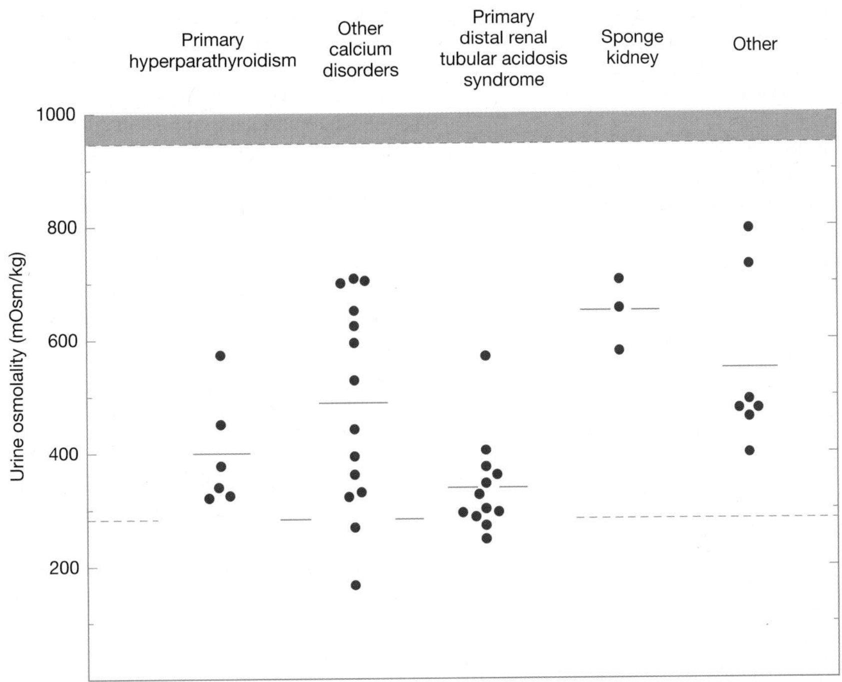

Fig. 16 Maximum urinary osmolality, stimulated by long-acting vasopressin, desmopressin or hydropenia in 42 patients with medullary nephrocalcinosis. The blue area shows the normal range (reproduced with permission from Wrong and Feest 1976).

Defects in urine concentrating power (Fig. 16) are almost invariable in medullary nephrocalcinosis of any cause. These are probably a non-specific effect of damage to the countercurrent multiplier caused by calcium deposition and chronic inflammatory change in the renal medulla, which distorts the normal intimate relationship between ascending and descending limbs of the loop of Henle, vasa recta and collecting ducts, on which the formation of a concentrated urine depends. This damage to the renal countercurrent multiplier, invariable in the presence of nephrocalcinosis, must also impair the normal function of the countercurrent multiplier in maintaining the high papillary carbon dioxide tension which is in equilibrium with the normal high $p\mathrm{CO}_2$ of alkaline urines (DuBose *et al.* 1982). In the diagnosis of dRTA, urinary $p\mathrm{CO}_2$ has been advocated as an indicator of collecting tubule proton secretion (Batlle 1986), but the use of this marker is probably invalid when urinary concentrating ability is impaired (Wrong 1991).

Treatment and natural history of medullary nephrocalcinosis

Once medullary nephrocalcinosis has become macroscopically visible, it usually persists for many years. The author has seen definite lessening of nephrocalcinosis in only two conditions—idiopathic absorptive hypercalciuria in which therapy has successfully reduced urinary calcium, and enteric hyperoxaluria after this has been corrected by bowel surgery—and even in these instances, study over several years was required to show convincing improvement. Slow lessening of nephrocalcinosis has also been reported in the childhood forms associated with use of frusemide or parenteral nutrition. In most other diseases, the renal lesion responsible for the nephrocalcinosis is to a great extent incurable (e.g. primary hyperoxaluria, dRTA, Dent's disease, papillary necrosis, magnesium-losing nephropathy) and the most that can usually be achieved by treatment is that the nephrocalcinosis should not become more marked. Such therapy includes treatment of type 1 primary hyperoxaluria with large doses of pyridoxine (which sometimes markedly lowers oxalate production), magnesium supplements in magnesium-losing nephropathy (increased urinary magnesium helps retain calcium in solution), and the use of alkalis, especially potassium alkali, in dRTA (which lower urinary calcium in acidotic cases and usually increase urinary citrate). But even in dRTA, where nephrocalcinosis tends to be more marked than in other diseases, the logical treatment with alkalis and potassium salts may fail to halt progression of nephrocalcinosis (Figs 8 and 11). Other general measures which might play a role in treatment include thiazide diuretics and dietary restriction of calcium or sodium (to lower urinary calcium), but so far no group of patients has been followed for long enough to see whether these extra measures are effective in halting progression of nephrocalcinosis.

The ulceration of nodules of medullary nephrocalcinosis into the calyceal system of the kidney to form separate stones, and the consequent hazards of urinary obstruction or infection, are ever-present risks in medullary nephrocalcinosis of any cause. Renal obstruction can develop without fresh symptoms, and a renal ultrasound examination every 2 or 3 years is a useful means of detecting change without recourse to radiation. Although these patients often pass renal calculi without experiencing urinary obstruction or infection, surgery is frequently required. Modern minimally invasive methods of stone removal (percutaneous nephrolithotomy, laser dissolution of stones, and shock-wave lithotripsy) have revolutionized the management of these problems. However, the prevailing current opinion is that no physical attempt should be made to try to remove nodules of nephrocalcinosis from within the renal substance, as this inevitably leads to further destruction of renal tissue.

Table 4 Macroscopic medullary nephrocalcinosis: prognosis for end-stage renal failure

Best	Idiopathic hypercalciuria
	Medullary sponge kidney
	Distal renal tubular acidosis
	Autonomous hyperparathyroidism and other reversible hypercalcaemias
	Papillary necrosis
	Dent's disease
	Hypomagnesaemia–hypercalciuria syndrome
Worst	Primary hyperoxaluria type 1

Renal failure is the major long-term hazard faced by patients with medullary nephrocalcinosis. Although this risk can be partly countered by close surveillance, especially with regard to episodes of urinary infection, calculous obstruction and management of hypertension, the problem is to a large extent a feature of the underlying renal disease and not simply a complication of nephrocalcinosis. Table 4 shows a league table of the major causes of medullary nephrocalcinosis, ranked according to the risk of renal failure, and based on combined personal experience and a survey of world literature. Patients with idiopathic absorptive hypercalciuria and MSK have the least risk of developing renal failure, which I have not seen in my personal series. At the opposite end of the table are those with type 1 primary hyperoxaluria, who usually already have renal failure when they first come to medical attention. Patients with the hypomagnesaemia/hypercalciuria syndrome and males with Dent's disease fare only slightly better, the majority developing end-stage renal failure between 20 and 50 years of age. The remaining diseases causing nephrocalcinosis lie between these extremes, or too few cases have been reported to allow generalizations about the development of renal failure.

Conclusions

The word 'nephrocalcinosis' has a beguiling simplicity which is misleading, for the term covers a wide variety of different pathological and clinical states. To avoid confusion, it is usually best to define what is meant by the word in respect of the species affected, the part of the kidney involved, and the degree of nephrocalcinosis, that is, whether chemical, microscopic, or macroscopic.

The usual form of human nephrocalcinosis seen by nephrologists is the macroscopic medullary type, visualized by radiography or ultrasound. There are many different metabolic causes of this condition, which in most cases can readily be identified. Endstage renal failure is a feature of some of these diseases, but others run a very benign renal course, so precise diagnosis of the cause is of great importance in clinical care.

References

Aggarwal, V. K. and Verrier Jones, K. (1989). Diffuse nephrocalcinosis and idiopathic renal hypercalciuria. *Archives of Disease in Childhood* **64**, 1055–1057.

Agroyannis, H. *et al.* (1992). Erythrocytosis in type 1 renal tubular acidosis with nephrocalcinosis. *Nephrology, Dialysis, Transplantation* **7**, 365–366.

Al-Modhefer, A. K. J. *et al.* (1986). Kidney function in rats with cortico-medullary nephrocalcinosis: effects of alterations in dietary calcium and magnesium. *Journal of Physiology* **380**, 405–414.

Alon, U., Brewer, W. H., and Chan, J. C. M. (1983). Nephrocalcinosis: detection by ultrasonography. *Pediatrics* **71**, 970–973.

Alon, U. S., Scagliotti, D., and Garola, R. E. (1994). Nephrocalcinosis and nephrolithiasis in infants with congestive heart failure treated with furosemide. *Journal of Pediatrics* **125**, 149–151.

Alwall, N. *et al.* (1958). Two cases of gross renal cortical necrosis in pregnancy with severe oliguria and anuria for 116 and 79 days respectively. *Acta Medica Scandinavica* **161**, 93–98.

Arons, W. L., Christensen, W. R., and Sosman, M. C. (1955). Nephrocalcinosis visible by X-ray associated with chronic glomerulonephritis. *Annals of Internal Medicine* **42**, 260–282.

Atkinson, S. A. *et al.* (1988). Mineral excretion in premature infants receiving various diuretic therapies. *Journal of Pediatrics* **113**, 540–545.

Bär, A. (1985). Urolithiasis and nephrocalcinosis in xylitol- and sorbitol-fed male rats of two different strains. *International Journal of Vitaminology and Nutrition Research* **28** (Suppl.), 69–89.

Bateson, E. M. and Chander, S. (1965). Nephrocalcinosis in cretinism. *British Journal of Radiology* **38**, 581–584.

Batlle, D. C. (1986). Segmental characterization of defects in collecting tubule acidification. *Kidney International* **30**, 546–554.

Battiflora, H. *et al.* (1966). The kidney in experimental magnesium deprivation. American *Journal of Pathology* **48**, 421–437.

Becker, D. L., Bagenstoss, A. H., and Weir, J. F. (1952). Parenchymal calcification of the kidneys in patients with duodenal ulcer. *American Journal of Clinical Pathology* **22**, 843–854.

Bérard, E. *et al.* (1995). Nephrocalcinosis and prematurity: importance of urate and oxalate excretion. *Nephron* **69**, 237–241.

Berlyne, G. M. (1961). Distal tubular function in chronic hydronephrosis. *Quarterly Journal of Medicine* **30**, 339–355.

Better, O. S. *et al.* (1969). Syndrome of incomplete renal tubular acidosis after cadaver kidney transplantation. *Annals of Internal Medicine* **71**, 39–45.

Birkenhager, R. *et al.* (2001). Mutation of *BSND* causes Bartter syndrome with sensorineural deafness and kidney failure. *Nature Genetics* **29**, 310–314.

Blank, S. *et al.* (1995). An outbreak of hypervitaminosis D associated with overfortification of milk from a home-delivery dairy. *American Journal of Public Health* **85**, 656–659.

Borle, A. B. and Uchikawa, T. (1978). Effects of parathyroid hormone on the distribution and transport of calcium in cultured kidney cells. *Endocrinology* **102**, 1725–1732.

Brennan, R. P., Pearlstein, A. E., and Miller, S. A. (1988). Computed tomography of the kidneys in a patient with methoxyflurane abuse. *Journal of Computer Asssisted Tomography* **12**, 155–156.

Brennan, T. M. H. *et al.* (1998). Linkage of infantile Bartter syndrome with sensorineural deafness to chromosome 1p. *American Journal of Human Genetics* **62**, 355–361.

Brodwall, E. K., Westlie, L., and Myhre, E. (1972). The renal excretion and tubular reabsorption of citric acid in renal tubular acidosis. *Acta Medica Scandinavica* **192**, 137–139.

Bruce, L. J. *et al.* (1997). Familial renal tubular acidosis is associated with mutations in the red cell anion exchanger (band 3, AE1) gene. *Journal of Clinical Investigation* **100**, 1693–1707.

Bruce, L. J. *et al.* (2000). Band 3 mutations, renal tubular acidosis and South-East Asian ovalocytosis in Malaysia and Papua New Guinea: loss of up to 95 per cent band 3 transport in red cells. *Biochemical Journal* **350**, 41–51.

Buckalew, V. M. *et al.* (1968). Incomplete renal tubular acidosis. *American Journal of Medicine* **45**, 32–42.

Buckalew, V. M. *et al.* (1974). Hereditary renal tubular acidosis. *Medicine* **53**, 229–254.

Burnett, C. H. *et al.* (1949). Hypercalcemia without hypercalciuria or hypophosphatemia, calcinosis and renal insufficiency. *New England Journal of Medicine* **240**, 787–794.

Burry, A. F., de Jersey, P., and Weedon, D. (1966). Phenacetin and renal papillary necrosis: results of a prospective autopsy investigation. *Medical Journal of Australia* **1**, 873–879.

Burry, A. F. *et al.* (1976). Calcification in the renal medulla. *Human Pathology* **7**, 43–49.

Busey, W. M. and Cockrell, B. Y. Non-neoplastic exposure-related renal lesions in rats following inhalation of unleaded gasoline vapors. In *Renal Effects of Petroleum Hydrocarbons. Advances in Modern Environmental Toxicology* Vol. VII (ed. H. A. Mehlman *et al.*), pp. 57–64. Princeton, NJ: Princeton Scientific Publishers, 1984.

Butler, A. M., Wilson, J. L., and Farber, S. (1936). Dehydration and acidosis with calcification at renal tubules. *Journal of Pediatrics* **8**, 489–499.

Calviño, J. *et al.* (1999). Cortical nephrocalcinosis induced by extracorporeal shock wave lithotripsy. *Nephron* **81**, 242–243.

Campfield, T. *et al.* (1994). Urinary oxalate excretion in premature infants: effect of human milk versus formula feeding. *Pediatrics* **84**, 674–679.

Carey, R. W. *et al.* (1968). Massive extraskeletal calcification during phosphate treatment of hypercalcaemia. *Archives of Internal Medicine* **122**, 150–155.

Caruana, R. J. and Buckalew, V. M. (1988). The syndrome of distal (Type 1) renal tubular acidosis. *Medicine* **67**, 84–99.

Caulfield, J. B. and Schrag, P. E. (1964). Electron microscopic study of renal calcification. *American Journal of Pathology* **44**, 365–381.

Chidekel, A. S. and Dolan, T. F. (1996). Cystic fibrosis and calcium oxalate nephrolithiasis. *Yale Journal of Biology and Medicine* **69**, 317–321.

Chikos, P. M. and McDonald, G. B. (1976). Regional enteritis complicated by nephrocalcinosis and nephrolithiasis. *Radiology* **121**, 75–76.

Cochran, M. *et al.* (1968). Hyperoxaluria in adults. *British Journal of Surgery* **55**, 121–128.

Cousins, F. B. and Geary, C. P. M. (1966). A sex-determined renal calcification in rats. *Nature* **211**, 980–981.

Cox, J. P. D. *et al.* (1999). Renal chloride channel, CLCN5, mutations in Dent's disease. *Journal of Bone and Mineral Research* **14**, 1536–1542.

Cramer, G. C. and Fuglestad, J. R. (1965). Cortical calcification in renal cortical necrosis. *American Journal of Roentgenology* **95**, 344–348.

Cramer, W. (1932). Experimental production of kidney lesions by diet. *Lancet* **2**, 174–175.

Cremin, B., Wiggelinkhuizen, J., and Bonnici, F. (1982). Nephrocalcinosis in children. *British Journal of Radiology* **55**, 413–418.

Curtis, A. C., Taylor, H. G., and Grekin, R. H. (1947). Sarcoidosis. I. Results of treatment with varying amounts of calciferol and dihydrotachysterol. *Journal of Investigative Dermatology* **9**, 131–150.

Davies, P. J. (1993). Beethoven's nephropathy and death; discussion paper. *Journal of the Royal Society of Medicine* **86**, 159–161.

Dedmon, R. E. and Wrong, O. (1962). The excretion of organic anion in renal tubular acidosis with particular reference to citrate. *Clinical Science* **22**, 19–32.

De Groot, A. P. *et al.* (1974). Two-year feeding and multigeneration studies in rats on five chemically modified starches. *Food and Cosmetics Toxicology* **12**, 651–663.

Dellow, E. L. *et al.* (1998). Amelogenesis imperfecta, nephrocalcinosis, and hypocalciuria syndrome in two siblings from a large family with consanguineous parents. *Nephrology, Dialysis, Transplantation* **13**, 3193–3196.

De Toni, E. and Nordio, S. (1959). The relationship between calcium–phosphorus metabolism, the 'Krebs cycle' and steroid metabolism. *Archives of Disease in Childhood* **34**, 371–382.

Downing, G. J. *et al.* (1991). Furosemide-related renal calcifications in the premature infant. A longitudinal ultrasonographic study. *Pediatric Radiology* **21**, 563–565.

Drummond, K. N. *et al.* (1964). The blue diaper syndrome: familial hypercalcemia with nephrocalcinosis and indicanuria. A new familial disease, with definition of the metabolic abnormality. *American Journal of Medicine* **37**, 928–948.

DuBose, T. D., Pucacco, L. R., and Green, J. M. (1982). Hydrogen ion secretion by the collecting duct as a determinant of the urine blood PCO_2 gradient in alkaline urine. *Journal of Clinical Investigation* **69**, 145–156.

Du Bruyn, D. B. (1972). Nephrocalcinosis in the white rat. Part II. The relationship between dietary magnesium, calcium and phosphorus content and kidney calcification and bone magnesium. *South African Medical Journal* **46**, 1588–1593.

Earnest, D. L. Enteric hyperoxaluria. In *Advances in Internal Medicine* Vol. 24 (ed. G. H. Stottermann), pp. 407–427. Chicago, IL: Year Book Medical Publishers, 1979.

Eggert, P., Müller, D., and Schröter, T. (1998). Nephrocalcinosis in three siblings with idiopathic hypercalciuria. *Pediatric Nephrology* **12**, 144–146.

Ekengren, K. (1973). Renal cortical calcification in pyelonephritis. *Annales de Radiologie* **16**, 223–226.

Elkinton, J. R. *et al.* (1960). The renal excretion of hydrogen ion in renal tubular acidosis. *American Journal of Medicine* **29**, 554–575.

Elseviers, M. M. *et al.* (1995). High diagnostic performance of CT scans for analgesic nephropathy with incipient to severe renal failure. *Kidney International* **48**, 1316–1323.

Epstein, F. H., Freedman, L. R., and Levitin, H. (1958). Hypercalcemia, nephrocalcinosis and reversible renal insufficiency associated with hyperthyroidism. *New England Journal of Medicine* **258**, 782–785.

Esposito, W. J. (1967). Specific nephrocalcinosis of chronic glomerulonephritis. *American Journal of Roentgenology* **101**, 688–691.

Estévez, R. *et al.* (2001). Barttin is a Cl channel β-subunit crucial for renal Cl^- reabsorption and inner ear K^+ secretion. *Nature* **414**, 558–561.

Evans, B. M. and MacPherson, C. R. (1956). Some observations on acetazolamide induced nephrocalcinosis in the rat. *British Journal of Experimental Pathology* **37**, 533–540.

Ezzedeen, F., Adelman, R. D., and Ahlfors, C. E. (1988). Renal calcification in preterm infants: pathophysiology and long-term sequelae. *Journal of Pediatrics* **113**, 532–539.

Fanconi, A. (1963). Idiopathische Hypercalciurie im Kindesalter. *Helvetica Paediatrica Acta* **18**, 306–322.

Feest, T. G. and Wrong, O. M. Renal tubular acidosis. In *Recent Advances in Renal Medicine* No. 2 (ed. N. F. Jones and D. K. Peters), pp. 243–271. Edinburgh: Churchill Livingstone, 1982.

Feest, T. G. *et al.* (1978). Nephrocalcinosis: another cause of renal erythrocytosis. *British Medical Journal* **2**, 605–606.

Fellner, S. K. and Tuttle, E. P. (1969). The clinical syndrome of analgesic abuse. *Archives of Internal Medicine* **124**, 379–382.

Ferris, T. *et al.* (1961). Renal tubular acidosis and renal potassium-wasting acquired as a result of hypercalcemic nephropathy. *New England Journal of Medicine* **265**, 924–928.

Fick, J. J. and Beck, F. J. (1992). Echogenic kidneys and medullary calcium deposition in a young child with glycogen storage disease. *Pediatric Nephrology* **22**, 72–73.

Filler, G., Kotecha, S., and Milanska, J. (2001). Trisomy 21 with hypercalcemia, hypercalciuria, medullary calcinosis and renal failure—a syndrome? *Pediatric Nephrology* **16**, 99–100.

Foley, L. C. *et al.* (1982). Nephrocalcinosis: sonographic detection in Cushing syndrome. *American Journal of Roentgenology* **139**, 610–612.

Fourman, J. (1959). Two distinct forms of experimental nephrocalcinosis in the rat. *British Journal of Experimental Pathology* **40**, 464–473.

Fraser, D. (1957). Hypophosphatasia. *American Journal of Medicine* **22**, 730–746.

Friedman, E. A. *et al.* (1962). Consequences of ethylene glycol poisoning. *American Journal of Medicine* **32**, 891–902.

Frymoyer, P. A. *et al.* (1991). X-linked recessive nephrolithiasis with renal failure. *New England Journal of Medicine* **325**, 681–686.

Geary, C. P. and Cousins, F. B. (1969). An oestrogen-linked nephrocalcinosis in rats. *British Journal of Experimental Pathology* **50**, 507–515.

Gelbart, D. R. *et al.* (1977). Oxalosis and chronic renal failure after intestinal bypass. *Archives of Internal Medicine* **137**, 239–243.

Gershoff, S. N. and Andrus, S. B. (1961). Dietary magnesium, calcium, and vitamin B_6 and experimental nephropathies in rats: calcium oxalate calculi, apatite nephrocalcinosis. *Journal of Nutrition* **73**, 308–316.

Giminez, L. F., Solez, K., and Walker, W. G. (1987). Relation between renal calcium content and renal impairment in 246 human renal biopsies. *Kidney International* **31**, 93–99.

Glazer, G. M., Callen, P. W., and Filly, R. A. (1982). Medullary nephrocalcinosis: sonographic evaluation. *American Journal of Roentgenology* **138**, 55–57.

Goldberg, B. H. *et al.* (1976). Alkaptonuria with nephrocalcinosis. *Journal of Pediatrics* **88**, 518–519.

Goligorsky, M. S. *et al.* (1983). X-ray microanalysis of uremic nephrocalcinosis. *Nephron* **35**, 89–93.

Goligorsky, M. S. *et al.* (1985). Calcium metabolism in uremic nephrocalcinosis: preventive effect of verapamil. *Kidney International* **27**, 774–779.

Goligorsky, M. S., Loftus, D. J., and Hruska, K. A. (1986). Cytoplasmic calcium in individual proximal tubular cells in culture. *American Journal of Physiology* **251**, F938–F944.

Goodyer, P. R. *et al.* (1987). Nephrocalcinosis and its relationship to treatment of hereditary rickets. *Journal of Pediatrics* **11**, 700–704.

Gould, A. B. *et al.* (1980). Interrelation of the renin system and erythropoietin in rats. *Journal of Laboratory and Clinical Medicine* **96**, 523–534.

Greaves, P. and Faccini, J. M. *Rat Histopathology*. Amsterdam: Elsevier, 1984.

Greenberg, A. J., McNamara, H., and McCrory, W. W. (1966). Metabolic balance studies in primary renal tubular acidosis: effects of acidosis on external calcium and phosphorus balances. *Journal of Pediatrics* **69**, 610–618.

Greenberg, P.-O., Lagergren, C., and Theve N. O. (1971). Renal function studies in medullary sponge kidney. *Scandinavian Journal of Urology and Nephrology* **5**, 177–180.

Györy, A. Z. *et al.* (1970). The relative importance of urinary pH and urinary content of citrate, magnesium and calcium in the production of nephrocalcinosis by diet and acetazolamide in the rat. *Clinical Science* **39**, 605–623.

Hamed, I. A. *et al.* (1979). Familial absorptive hypercalciuria and renal tubular acidosis. *American Journal of Medicine* **67**, 385–391.

Harrison, H. E. and Harrison, H. C. (1955). Inhibition of urine citrate excretion and the production of renal calcinosis in the rat by acetazolamide (Diamox) administration. *Journal of Clinical Investigation* **34**, 1662–1670.

Harrison, R. B. and Vaughan, E. D. (1978). Diffuse cortical calcification in rejected renal transplants. *Radiology* **126**, 635–636.

Heaton, F. W. and Anderson, C. K. (1965). The mechanism of renal calcification induced by magnesium deficiency in the rat. *Clinical Science* **28**, 99–106.

Higashihara, E. *et al.* (1984). Medullary sponge kidney and renal acidification defect. *Kidney International* **25**, 453–459.

Hill, S. C., Hoeg, J. M., and Avila, N. A. (1991). Nephrocalcinosis in homozygous familial hypercholesterolemia: ultrasound and CT findings. *Journal of Computer Assisted Tomography* **15**, 101–103.

Hodgkinson, A. *et al.* (1982). A comparison of the effects of lactose and of two chemically modified waxy maize starches on mineral metabolism in the rat. *Food and Chemical Toxicology* **20**, 371–382.

Hoffbrand, B. I. *et al.* (1987). Nodular cortical nephrocalcinosis: a benign and hitherto undescribed form of renal calcification. *Nephron* **46**, 370–372.

Hoppe, B. *et al.* (1993). Hypercalciuria and nephrocalcinosis, a feature of Wilson's disease. *Nephron* **63**, 460–462.

Howlett, D. C. *et al.* (1997). The incidence of transient renal medullary hyperechogenicity in neonatal ultrasound examinations. *British Journal of Radiology* **70**, 140–143.

Hufnagle, K. G. *et al.* (1982). Renal calcifications: a complication of long-term furosemide therapy in preterm infants. *Pediatrics* **70**, 360–363.

Ibels, L. S. and Alfrey, A. C. (1981). Effects of thyroparathyroidectomy, phosphate depletion and diphosphonate therapy on acute uraemic extraosseous calcification in the rat. *Clinical Science* **61**, 621–626.

Ibels, L. S. *et al.* (1978). Preservation of function in experimental renal disease by dietary restriction of phosphate. *New England Journal of Medicine* **298**, 122–126.

Ibels, L. S. *et al.* (1981). Calcification in end-stage kidneys. *American Journal of Medicine* **71**, 33–37.

Igarashi, T. *et al.* (1991). Renal cyst formation as a complication of primary renal tubular acidosis. *Nephron* **59**, 75–79.

Igarashi, T. *et al.* (1995). Hypercalciuria and nephrocalcinosis in patients with idiopathic low-molecular-weight proteinuria in Japan: is the disease identical to Dent's disease in United Kingdom? *Nephron* **69**, 242–247.

Ismail, E. A. R., Abul Saad, S., and Sabry, M. A. (1997). Nephrocalcinosis and urolithiasis in carbonic anhydrase II deficiency syndrome. *European Journal of Pediatrics* **156**, 957–962.

Jacinto, J. S. *et al.* (1988). Renal calcification incidence in very low birth weight infants. *Pediatrics* **81**, 31–35.

Jacobus, C. H. *et al.* (1992). Hypervitaminosis D associated with drinking milk. *New England Journal of Medicine* **326**, 1173–1177.

Jeghers, H. and Murphy, R. (1945). Practical aspects of oxalate metabolism. *New England Journal of Medicine* **233**, 208–215, 238–246.

Jequier, S. *et al.* (1986). Renal ultrasound in metabolic bone disease. *Pediatric Radiology* **16**, 135–139.

Kanfer, A. *et al.* (1979). Extreme hyperphosphataemia causing acute anuric nephrocalcinosis in lymphosarcoma. *British Medical Journal* **1**, 1320–1321.

Karet, F. E. *et al.* (1998). Mutations in the gene encoding B1 subunit of H^+-ATPase cause renal tubular acidosis with sensineural deafness. *Nature Genetics* **21**, 84–90.

Karlowicz, M. G., Katz, M. E., and Adelman, R. D. (1993). Nephrocalcinosis in very low birth weight neonates: family history and ethnicity as independent risk factors. *Journal of Pediatrics* **122**, 635–638.

Katz, S. M., Krueger, L. J., and Falkner, B. (1988). Microscopic nephrocalcinosis in cystic fibrosis. *New England Journal of Medicine* **319**, 263–266.

Kelleher, C. L. *et al.* (1998). CLCN5 mutation Ser 244 Leu is associated with X-linked renal failure without X-linked recessive hypophosphatemic rickets. *Kidney International* **53**, 31–37.

Khan, S. R., Finlayson, B., and Hackett, R. L. (1982). Experimental calcium oxalate nephrolithiasis in the rat. *American Journal of Pathology* **107**, 59–69.

Kim, K.-G. *et al.* (2001). Medullary nephrocalcinosis associated with long-term furosemide abuse in adults. *Nephrology, Dialysis, Transplantation* **16**, 2303–2309.

Klement, R. and Weber, R. (1941). Das Verhalten von Hydroxylapatit in Serum und ähnlichen Lösungen. *Biochemische Zeitschrift* **308**, 391–398.

Konrad, M. *et al.* (2000). Mutations in the chloride channel gene *CLCNKB* as a cause of classic Bartter syndrome. *Journal of the American Society of Nephrology* **11**, 1449–1459.

Kreel, L. (1962). Radiological aspects of nephrocalcinosis. *Clinical Radiology* **13**, 218–223.

Kuiper, J. J. (1971). Medullary sponge kidney in three generations. *New York State Journal of Medicine* **71**, 2665–2669.

Kuzela, D. C. *et al.* (1977). Soft tissue calcification in chronic dialysis patients. *American Journal of Pathology* **86**, 403–424.

Lamas, J. V. *et al.* (2000). Persistent nephrocalcinosis for acetazolamide and furosemide in a pediatric patient. *Nephron* **86**, 378–379.

La Mansa, A. *et al.* (1998). Calyceal microlithiasis in children: report of 196 cases. *Pediatric Nephrology* **12**, 214–217.

Landau, D. *et al.* (1995). Infantile variant of Bartter syndrome with sensorineural deafness: a new autosomal recessive disorder. *American Journal of Medical Genetics* **59**, 454–459.

Leaf, A., Schwartz, W. B., and Relman, A. S. (1954). Oral administration of a potent carbonic anhydrase inhibitor ('diamox'). *New England Journal of Medicine* **250**, 759–763.

Leapman, S. B. *et al.* (1976). Nephrolithiasis and nephrocalcinosis after renal transplantation: a case report and review of the literature. *Journal of Urology* **115**, 129–132.

Lengemann, F. W. and Comar, C. L. (1961). Distribution of absorbed strontium-85 and calcium-45 as influenced by lactose. *American Journal of Physiology* **200**, 1051–1054.

Liddle, G. W., Bledsoe, J., and Coppage, W. S. (1963). A familial disorder simulating primary aldosteronism but with negligible aldosterone secretion. *Transactions of the Association of American Physicians* **76**, 199–213.

Lifshitz, F. *et al.* (1967). Citrate metabolism and the mechanism of renal calcification induced by magnesium depletion. *Metabolism* **16**, 345–357.

Lightwood, R. (1935). Calcium infarction in the kidneys in infants. *Archives of Disease in Childhood* **10**, 205–206.

Lightwood, R. (1952). Idiopathic hypercalcaemia in infants with failure to thrive. *Archives of Disease in Childhood* **27**, 302–303.

Litin, R. B. *et al.* (1959). Hypercalciuria in hepatolenticular degeneration (Wilson's disease). *American Journal of the Medical Sciences* **238**, 614–620.

Litvak, J. *et al.* (1958). Hypercalcemic hypercalciuria during vitamin D and dihydrotachysterol therapy of hypoparathyroidism. *Journal of Clinical Endocrinology and Metabolism* **18**, 246–252.

Lloyd, H. M. (1968). Primary hyperparathyroidism: an analysis of the role of the parathyroid tumour. *Medicine* **47**, 53–71.

Lloyd, S. E. *et al.* (1996). A common molecular basis for three inherited kidney stone diseases. *Nature* **379**, 445–449.

Lloyd-Thomas, H. G., Balme, R. H., and Key, J. J. (1962). Tram-line calcification in renal cortical necrosis. *British Medical Journal* **1**, 909–911.

Lubinsky, M. *et al.* (1985). Syndrome of amelogenesis imperfecta, nephrocalcinosis, impaired renal concentration, and possible abnormality of calcium metabolism. *American Journal of Medical Genetics* **20**, 233–243.

Lucaya, J. *et al.* (1993). Renal calcifications in patients with autosomal recessive polycystic kidney disease: prevalence and cause. *American Journal of Roentgenology* **160**, 359–362.

Luers, P. R., Lester, P. D., and Siegler, R. L. (1980). CT demonstration of cortical nephrocalcinosis in congenital oxalosis. *Pediatric Radiology* **10**, 116–118.

MacGibbon, D. (1972). Generalized enamel hypoplasia and renal dysfunction. *Australian Dental Journal* **17**, 61–63.

MacIntyre, I. and Davidson, D. (1958). The production of potassium depletion, sodium retention, nephrocalcinosis and hypercalcaemia by magnesium deficiency. *Biochemical Journal* **70**, 456–462.

Manigand, G. *et al.* (1971). Fluorose osseuse associée à une néphropathie interstitielle chronique avec néphrocalcinose. *Annales de Médecine Interne* **122**, 191–198.

Manz, F. *et al.* (1978). Renal magnesium wasting, incomplete tubular acidosis, hypercalciuria and nephrocalcinosis in siblings. *European Journal of Pediatrics* **128**, 67–79.

Mason, R. S. *et al.* (1984). Vitamin D conversion by sarcoid lymph node homogenate. *Annals of Internal Medicine* **100**, 59–61.

McAlister, W. H. and Nedelman, S. H. (1961). The roentgen manifestations of bilateral renal cortical necrosis. *American Journal of Roentgenology* **86**, 129–135.

McMillan, D. E. and Freeman, R. B. (1965). The milk alkali syndrome: a study of the acute disorder with comments on the development of the chronic condition. *Medicine* **44**, 485–501.

McSherry, E. and Morris, R. C. (1978). Attainment and maintenance of normal stature with alkali therapy in infants and children with classic renal tubular acidosis. *Journal of Clinical Investigation* **61**, 509–527.

Michelis, M. F. *et al.* (1972). Decreased bicarbonate threshold and renal magnesium wasting in a sibship with distal renal tubular acidosis. *Metabolism* **21**, 905–920.

Milne, M. D., Stanbury, S. W., and Thomson, A. E. (1952). Observations on the Fanconi syndrome and renal hyperchloraemic acidosis in the adult. *Quarterly Journal of Medicine* **21**, 61–82.

Mocan, H. *et al.* (2000). Microscopic nephrocalcinosis and hypercalciuria in nephrotic syndrome. *Human Pathology* **31**, 1363–1367.

Monserrat, J. L. *et al.* (1979). La nefrocalcinosis como síndrome clínico (análisis de 77 casos). *Medicina Clinica (Barcelona)* **73**, 305–311.

Mortensen, J. D. and Emmett, J. L. (1954). Nephrocalcinosis: a collective and clinicopathologic study. *Journal of Urology* **71**, 398–406.

Moschos, A. *et al.* (1972). Renal cortical necrosis in an infant. *Archives of Disease in Childhood* **47**, 472–474.

Moudgil, A. *et al.* (2000). Nephrocalcinosis and renal cysts associated with apparent mineralocorticoid excess syndrome. *Pediatric Nephrology* **15**, 60–62.

Müller, D., Eggert, E., and Krawinkel, M. (1998). Hypercalciuria and nephrocalcinosis in a patient receiving long-term parenteral nutrition: the effect of intravenous chlorothiazide. *Journal of Pediatric Gastroenterology and Nutrition* **27**, 106–110.

Murphy, K. J. (1968). Calcification of the renal papillae as a sign of analgesic nephropathy. *Clinical Radiology* **19**, 394–399.

Murty, C. V. R. *et al.* (1988). Hydrocarbon-induced hyaline droplet nephropathy in male rats during senescence. *Toxicology and Applied Pharmacology* **96**, 380–392.

Naylor, J. M. (1955). A case of hypothyroidism with nephrocalcinosis. *Archives of Disease in Childhood* **30**, 165–168.

Newman, R. J. (1973). The effects of thyroid hormone on vitamin D-induced nephrocalcinosis. *Journal of Pathology* **111**, 13–21.

Nicholson, J. C. *et al.* (1995). Familial hypomagnesemia-hypercalciuria leading to end-stage renal failure. *Pediatric Nephrology* **9**, 74–76.

Norman, M. E. *et al.* (1978). Urinary citrate excretion in the diagnosis of distal renal tubular acidosis. *Journal of Pediatrics* **92**, 394–400.

O'Neill, M., Breslau, N. A., and Pak, C. Y. C. (1981). Metabolic evaluation of nephrolithiasis in patients with medullary sponge kidney. *Journal of the American Medical Association* **245**, 1233–1236.

Oram, S. *et al.* (1963). Renal cortical calcification after snake-bite. *British Medical Journal* **1**, 1647–1648.

Osther, P. J. *et al.* (1994). Urinary acidification and urinary excretion of calcium and citrate in women with bilateral medullary sponge kidney. *Urologia Internationalis* **52**, 126–130.

Page, L. B. and Castleman, B. (1961). Case records of the Massachusetts General Hospital. *New England Journal of Medicine* **264**, 930–936.

Palmer, F. J. (1970). Renal cortical calcification. *Clinical Radiology* **21**, 175–177.

Parfitt, M. (1969). Acetazolamide and sodium bicarbonate induced nephrocalcinosis and nephrolithiasis. *Archives of Internal Medicine* **124**, 736–740.

Parikh, J. R. and Nolan, R. I. (1994). Acetazolamide-induced nephrocalcinosis. *Abdominal Imaging* **19**, 466–467.

Patriquin, H. and Robitaille, P. (1986). Renal calcium deposition in children: sonographic demonstration of the Anderson–Carr progression. *American Journal of Roentgenology* **146**, 1253–1256.

Pearce, S. H. S. *et al.* (1996). A familial syndrome of hypocalcemia with hypercalciuria due to mutations in the calcium sensing receptor. *New England Journal of Medicine* **335**, 1115–1122.

Pearse, D. M. *et al.* (1984). Sonographic diagnosis of furosemide-induced nephrocalcinosis in premature infants. *Journal of Ultrasound Medicine* **3**, 553–556.

Phakey, P. *et al.* (1995). Ultrastructural study of tooth enamel with amelogenesis imperfecta in AI-nephrocalcinosis syndrome. *Connective Tissue Research* **32**, 253–256.

Phillips, J. C. *et al.* (1986). Studies on the mechanism of diet-induced nephrocalcinosis: calcium and phosphorus metabolism in the female rat. *Food and Chemical Toxicology* **24**, 283–288.

Prien, E. L. (1975). Riddle of Randall's plaques. *Journal of Urology* **114**, 500–507.

Proesmans, W., De Cock, P., and Eyskens, B. (1995). A toddler with Down syndrome, hypercalcaemia, hypercalciuria, medullary nephrocalcinosis and renal failure. *Pediatric Nephrology* **l9**, 112–114.

Randall, A. (1936). Initiating lesions of renal calculus. *Surgery, Gynecology and Obstetrics* **64**, 201–208.

Randall, A. (1940). Papillary pathology as a precursor of primary renal calculus. *Journal of Urology* **44**, 580–589.

Rausch, H. P., Hanefeld, F., and Kaufmann, H. J. (1984). Medullary nephrocalcinosis and pancreatic calcifications demonstrated by ultrasound and CT in infants after treatment with ACTH. *Radiology* **153**, 105–207.

Reeves, P. G. and Forbes, R. M. (1972). Prevention by thyroxine of nephrocalcinosis in early magnesium deficiency in the rat. *American Journal of Physiology* **222**, 220–224.

Relman A. S. and Schwartz, W. B. (1958). The kidney in potassium depletion. *American Journal of Medicine* **24**, 764–773.

Restaino, I. *et al.* (1993). Nephrocalcinosis, hypocitraturia, and a distal renal tubular acidification defect in Type 1 glycogen storage disease. *Journal of Pediatrics* **122**, 392–396.

Ribeiro, C. and Suki, W. N. (1986). Acidification in the medullary collecting duct following ureteral obstruction. *Kidney International* **29**, 1167–1171.

Riikonen, R. *et al.* (1986). Disturbed calcium and phosphate homeostasis during treatment with ACTH. *Archives of Disease in Childhood* **61**, 671–676.

Rodriguez-Soriano, J., Vallo, A., and Garcia-Fuentes, M. (1987). Hypomagnesaemia of hereditary renal origin. *Pediatric Nephrology* **1**, 465–472.

Roe, F. J. C. (1989). Relevance for man of the effects of lactose, polyols and other carbohydrates on calcium metabolism seen in rats: a review. *Human Toxicology* **8**, 87–98.

Roginski, E. E. and Mertz, W. (1974). Development and reversibility of urolithiasis in rats by mineral mixtures. *Journal of Nutrition* **104**, 599–604.

Rönnefarth, G. and Misselwitz, J. (2000). Nephrocalcinosis in children: a retrospective survey. *Pediatric Nephrology* **14**, 1016–1031.

Ruiz Palomo, F. *et al.* (1978). Sindrome de Fanconi y nefrocalcinosis: Una asociación exceptional. *Recista Clinica Española* **149**, 401–440.

Russo, F. and O'Regan, S. (1990). Visceral pathology in hereditary tyrosinemia type 1. *American Journal of Human Genetics* **47**, 317–324.

Saarela, T., Similä, S., and Kolvisto, M. (1995). Hypercalcemia and nephrocalcinosis in patients with congenital lactase deficiency. *Journal of Pediatrics* **127**, 920–923.

Saleem, M. A. *et al.* (1995). Hypercalciuria and ultrasound abnormalities in children with cystinosis. *Pediatric Nephrology* **9**, 45–47.

Sanderson, P. H. (1959). Functional aspects of renal calcification in rats. *Clinical Science* **18**, 67–79.

Saxton, J. A. and Kimball, G. C. (1941). Relation of nephrosis and other diseases of albino rats to age and to modifications of diet. *Archives of Pathology* **32**, 951–965.

Scanlon, K. S. *et al.* (1995). Subclinical health effects in a population exposed to excess vitamin D in milk. *American Journal of Public Health* **85**, 1418–1422.

Schärer, K. and Manz, F. (1985). Renal handling of citrate in children with various kidney disorders. *International Journal of Pediatric Nephrology* **6**, 79–88.

Scheinman, S. J. (1998). X-linked hypercalciuric nephrolithiasis: clinical syndromes and chloride channel mutations. *Kidney International* **53**, 3–17.

Schepens, D. *et al.* (2000). Renal cortical nephrocalcinosis. *Nephrology, Dialysis, Transplantation* **15**, 1080–1082.

Schmitt, K. *et al.* (1995). Aldosterone and testosterone producing adrenal adenoma in childhood. *Journal of Endocrinological Investigation* **18**, 69–73.

Schneeberger, E. E. and Morrison, A. B. (1965). The nephropathy of experimental magnesium deficiency. *Laboratory Investigation* **14**, 674–686.

Scowen, E. F., Stansfeld, A. G., and Watts, R. W. L. (1959). Oxalosis and primary hyperoxaluria. *Journal of Pathology and Bacteriology* **77**, 195–205.

Segasothy, M. *et al.* (1994). Chronic renal disease and papillary necrosis associated with the long-term use of non-steroidal anti-inflammatory drugs as the sole or predominant analgesic. *American Journal of Kidney Disease* **24**, 17–24.

Seikaly, M., Browne, R., and Baum, M. (1996). Nephrocalcinosis is associated with renal tubular acidosis in children with X-linked hypophosphatemia. *Pediatrics* **97**, 91–93.

Seyberth, H. W. *et al.* (1985). Congenital hypokalemia with hypercalciuria in preterm infants: a hyperprostaglandinuric tubular syndrome different from Bartter syndrome. *Journal of Pediatrics* **107**, 694–701.

Shalev, H. *et al.* (1994). Nephrocalcinosis in pseudohypoaldosteronism and the effect of indomethacin therapy. *Journal of Pediatrics* **125**, 246–248.

Shanks, R. A. and MacDonald, A. M. (1959). Nephrocalcinosis infantum. *Archives of Disease in Childhood* **35**, 115–119.

Shiers, J. A., Neuhauser, E. B. D., and Bowman, J. R. (1957). Idiopathic hypercalcemia. *AJR. American Journal of Roentgenology* **78**, 19–20.

Short, A. and Cooke, R. W. I. (1991). The incidence of renal calcification in preterm infants. *Archives of Disease in Childhood* **66**, 412–417.

Simon, D. B. *et al.* (1996a). Gitelman's variant of Bartter's syndrome, inherited hypokalaemic alkalosis, is caused by mutations in the thiazide-sensitive NaCl cotransporter. *Nature Genetics* **12**, 24–30.

Simon, D. B. *et al.* (1996b). Bartter's syndrome, hypokalaemic alkalosis with hypercalciuria, is caused by mutations in the Na–K–2Cl cotransporter *NKCC2*. *Nature Genetics* **13**, 183–186.

Simon, D. B. *et al.* (1996c). Genetic heterogeneity in Bartter's syndrome revealed by mutation in the K^+ channel, ROMK. *Nature Genetics* **14**, 152–156.

Simon, D. B. *et al.* (1997). Mutations in the chloride channel gene, *CLCKB*, cause Bartter's syndrome type III. *Nature Genetics* **17**, 171–178.

Simon, D. B. *et al.* (1999). Paracellin-1, a renal tight junction protein required for paracellular Mg^{2+} resorption. *Science* **285**, 103–106.

Simpson, D. P. (1983). Citrate excretion: a window on renal metabolism. *American Journal of Physiology* **244**, F223–F234.

Sliman, G. A. *et al.* (1995). Hypercalciuria and nephrocalcinosis in the oculocerebrorenal syndrome. *Journal of Urology* **153**, 1244–1246.

Smith, A. N. *et al.* (2000). Mutations in *ATP6N1B*, encoding a new kidney vacuolar proton pump 116-kD, cause recessive distal renal tubular acidosis with preserved hearing. *Nature Genetics* **26**, 71–75.

Stafstrom, C. E., Gillmore, H. E., and Kurtin, P. S. (1992). Nephrocalcinosis and urolithiasis complicating medical treatment of posthemorrhagic hydrocephalus. *Pediatric Neurology* **8**, 179–182.

Starinsky, R. *et al.* (1995). Increased renal medullary echogenicity in neonates. *Pediatric Nephrology* (Suppl. 1), S43–S545.

Stewart, P. M. *et al.* (1988). Syndrome of apparent mineralocorticoid excess. A defect in the cortisol–cortisone shuttle. *Journal of Clinical Investigation* **82**, 340–349.

Stoller, M. L. *et al.* (1996). High resolution radiography of cadaveric kidneys: unraveling the mystery of Randall's plaque formation. *Journal of Urology* **156**, 1263–1266.

Sumner, T. E. *et al.* (1984). Hypophosphatasia and nephrocalcinosis demonstrated by ultrasound and CT. *Clinical Nephrology* **22**, 317–319.

Taylor, A., Sherman, N. H., and Norman, M. E. (1995). Nephrocalcinosis in X-linked hypophosphatemia: effect of treatment versus disease. *Pediatric Nephrology* **9**, 173–175.

Thakker, R. V. (2000). Molecular pathology of renal chloride channels in Dent's disease and Bartter's syndrome. *Experimental Nephrology* **8**, 351–360.

Theodoropoulos, D. S. *et al.* (1995). Medullary nephrocalcinosis in nephropathic cystinosis. *Pediatric Nephrology* **9**, 412–418.

Toye, A. M. *et al.* (2002). Band 3 Walton, a C-terminal deletion associated with distal renal tubular acidosis, is expressed in the red cell membrane but retained internally in kidney cells. *Blood* **99**, 342–347.

Tümay, S. B., Bilger, M., and Hatemi, N. (1962). Skeletal changes and nephrocalcinosis in a case of athyreosis. *Archives of Disease in Childhood* **37**, 543–547.

Vaughan, J. H., Sosman, M. C., and Kinney, T. D. (1947). Nephrocalcinosis. *American Journal of Roentgenology* **58**, 33–45.

Verge, C. F. *et al.* (1991). Effects of therapy in X-linked hypophosphatemic rickets. *New England Journal of Medicine* **325**, 1843–1848.

Walsh, A. (1969). Néphrocalcinose sur rein greffé. *Journal d'Urologie et de Néphrologie* **75** (Suppl. 12), 244.

Walter, S. *et al.* (1999). Assessment of urinary acidification. *Kidney International* **55**, 2092.

Weinstein, D. A., Somers M. J. G., and Wolfsdorf, J. I. (2001). Decreased urinary citrate excretion in type Ia glycogen storage disease. *Journal of Pediatrics* **138**, 378–382.

Wen, S.-F., Friedman, A. L., and Oberley, T. D. (1989). Two case studies of a family with primary Fanconi syndrome. *American Journal of Kidney Disease* **13**, 240–246.

Wenzl, J. E. *et al.* (1968). Nephrolithiasis and nephrocalcinosis in children. *Pediatrics* **41**, 57–61.

White, P. C., Mune, T., and Agarwal, A. K. (1997). 11β-Hydroxysteroid dehydrogenase and the syndrome of apparent mineralocorticoid excess. *Endocrine Reviews* **18**, 135–156.

Williams, H. E. and Smith, L. H. (1968). L-Glyceric aciduria. *New England Journal of Medicine* **278**, 233–239.

Wilson, D. A., Wenzl, J. E., and Altshuler, G. P. (1979). Ultrasound demonstration of diffuse cortical nephrocalcinosis in a case of primary hyperoxaluria. *American Journal of Roentgenology* **132**, 659–661.

Wilson, D. R. and Siddiqui, A. A. (1973). Renal tubular acidosis after kidney transplantation. *Annals of Internal Medicine* **79**, 352–359.

Woodard, J. C. (1971). A morphologic and biochemical study of nutritional nephrocalcinosis in female rats fed semipurified diets. *American Journal of Pathology* **65**, 253–268.

Wrong, O. (1985). The significance of radiological nephrocalcinosis. *Hospital Update* **11**, 167–178.

Wrong, O. (1991). Distal renal tubular acidosis: the value of urinary pH, $p\text{CO}_2$ and NH_4 measurements. *Pediatric Nephrology* **5**, 249–255.

Wrong, O. and Davies, H. E. F. (1959). The excretion of acid in renal disease. *Quarterly Journal of Medicine* **28**, 259–313.

Wrong, O. M. and Feest, T. G. Nephrocalcinosis. In *Advanced Medidne* No. 12 (ed. D. K. Peters), pp. 394–406. London: Pitman Medical, 1976.

Wrong, O. M. and Feest, T. G. (1980). The natural history of distal renal tubular acidosis. *Contributions to Nephrology* **21**, 137–144.

Wrong, O. M., Norden, A. G. W., and Feest, T. G. (1990). Dent's disease: a familial renal tubular syndrome with hypercalciuria, tubular proteinuria, rickets, nephrocalcinosis and eventual renal failure. *Quarterly Journal of Medicine* **77**, 1086–1087.

Wrong, O. *et al.* (1996). Unravelling of the molecular mechanisms of kidney stones. *Lancet* **348**, 1561–1565.

Wrong, O. M., Feest, T. G., and MacIver, A. G. (1993). Immune-related potassium-losing interstitial nephritis: a comparison with distal renal tubular acidosis. *Quarterly Journal of Medicine* **86**, 513–534.

Wrong, O. M., Norden, A. G. W., and Feest, T. G. (1994). Dent's disease; a familial proximal renal tubular syndrome with low-molecular-weight proteinuria, hypercalciuria, nephrocalcinosis, metabolic bone disease, progressive renal failure and a marked male predominance. *Quarterly Journal of Medicine* **87**, 473–493.

Wurzburg, O. B. (1986). Nutritional aspects and safety of modified food starches. *Nutrition Reviews* **44**, 74–79.

Yang, C. W. *et al.* (1994). Nephrocalcinosis associated with primary aldosteronism. *Nephron* **68**, 507–508.

Young, L. W. (1979). Radiological case of the month. *American Journal of Diseases of Children* **133**, 203–204.

Zelikovic, I. (2001). Molecular pathophysiology of tubular transport disorders. *Pediatric Nephrology* **16**, 919–935.

8.5 Renal and urinary tract stone disease in children

William G. van't Hoff

Introduction

Urinary stone disease in children differs considerably from that in adults. The prevalence of paediatric urolithiasis is much less but certain groups of children (e.g. those born prematurely) are at increased risk. Throughout the world, the prevalence depends on geographical location with high rates in the endemic stone regions. Second, whereas the majority of adult patients are idiopathic, calcium oxalate stone formers, the likelihood of identifying a metabolic predisposition is much greater and is increasing in children. The frequency of a metabolic abnormality was only 16 per cent in a series of 120 paediatric patients with urolithiasis reported in 1977 (Barratt and Ghazali 1977), current data from the same institution suggests a frequency of nearly 50 per cent (Coward *et al.* 2003). Young children, in particular, have an increased risk of stones developing after urinary tract infection. A further important reason to study paediatric urolithiasis is that there is good evidence that both the incidence of stones, in all age groups, is increasing and the age of first stone formation is falling (Robertson *et al.* 1999). It is possible that changes in children's or adolescent's diet and/or lifestyles predispose them to early stone formation.

Presentation of stones

The clinical presentation of renal stones varies enormously in children. The classic picture of renal colic and haematuria is seen in older patients but young children cannot easily describe pain. Abdominal pain may be a presenting feature in only approximately 50 per cent children, indicating that in the other half, the parents had not perceived that the child might have pain or discomfort (Coward *et al.* 2003). In this age group, parents may report the passage of gravel or small stones into the nappy. Recurrent vomiting and poor appetite are commonly seen in children with a substantial stone burden and not infrequently, it is the subsequent investigation of the gastrointestinal tract that coincidentally reveals renal stones. Urinary tract infection is a common presenting feature. Infection with *Proteus mirabilis* is an especial risk for stone formation, more common in uncircumcised boys in whom it colonizes the foreskin. Persistent infection, resistant to antibiotic therapy, indicates the need to undertake imaging of the urinary tract to exclude the possibility of a stone. A significant number of renal stones in children are asymptomatic and are found during an incidental investigation (e.g. abdominal ultrasound). Not uncommonly the presentation is with spontaneous passage of stones into the nappy or toilet. When available these should always be sent for detailed analysis as the composition may readily identify an underlying disorder (e.g. cystinuria). Very rarely, analysis of such stones reveals artefacts (e.g. silicaceous material) indicating that the 'stone' was not formed in the urinary tract and that the illness is factitious (Munchausen by Proxy) (Senocak *et al.* 1995; Absolut de la Gastine *et al.* 1998). Acute renal failure may be the manifestation of rare metabolic defects of purine metabolism leading to acute crystal nephropathy (Simmonds *et al.* 1989).

Investigation

Imaging

The investigation of a child with stones is divided into two stages. First, detailed imaging is required to determine the optimal method of stone clearance and, second, a biochemical screen is undertaken to look for an underlying metabolic cause. Imaging for stones uses the same modalities as for adults, but ultrasonography is particularly helpful (and generally well tolerated) as most children are much slimmer than adults and, therefore, the quality of the image is much improved. Therefore, an ultrasound of the kidneys, ureters, and bladder is combined with a plain abdominal radiograph as the first-line investigations. An intravenous urogram is helpful in cases suspected of having ureteric calculi, but also provides very good information on calyceal anatomy. A dimercapto succinic acid (DMSA) radionuclide renal scan will demonstrate the differential function between both kidneys and focal defects in tracer uptake which may result from 'renal scarring' secondary to infection (Fig. 1). The surgical approach to a kidney with an extensive stone burden will vary considerably according to whether differential function is approximately equal on both sides or very poor (e.g. $<$10 per cent) for the affected kidney. It is feasible to combine the intravenous urogram and the DMSA scan in a single investigation, with injection of the radionuclide followed immediately and through the same needle by the contrast media.

Biochemical evaluation

The second stage of investigation is to determine whether the child has a metabolic abnormality, which may have predisposed to stone formation. The likelihood of finding an abnormality varies in different series, mainly dependent on the region under investigation. Epidemiological studies in developed countries show that approximately 50 per cent of children who have had renal stones have an underlying metabolic abnormality (Pietrow *et al.* 2002; Coward *et al.* 2003). In developing countries, metabolic abnormalities are less common, varying between 5 and 35 per cent in a number of series (Kamoun *et al.* 1999; Ece *et al.* 2000;

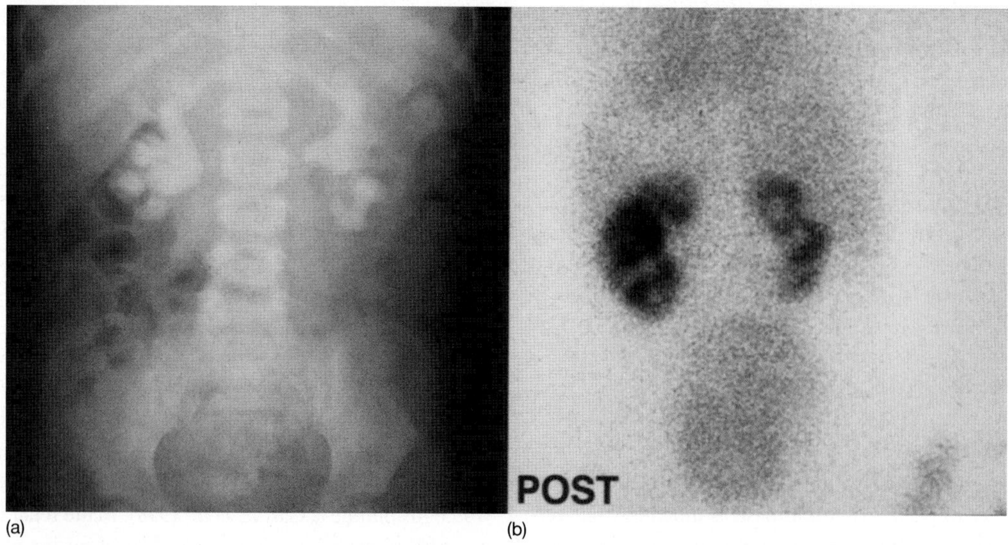

Fig. 1 Plain abdominal radiograph (a) and concurrent DMSA radionuclide scan (b) from a 5-year-old girl. The radiograph shows bilateral staghorn calculi, which were subsequently found to be composed of magnesium ammonium phosphate, occurring secondary to persistent urinary infection. The DMSA shows bilateral multiple focal defects and a high background count. These findings are due to bilateral renal scarring leading to severe renal damage (GFR 34 ml/min/1.73 m^2).

Sarkissian *et al.* 2001). Biochemical evaluation is important not only to determine the cause but also because metabolic abnormalities are associated with an increased number, with bilateral and with recurrent stone disease (Pietrow *et al.* 2002; Coward *et al.* 2003).

Analysis of the stone may reveal an underlying metabolic abnormality [e.g. cystine in cystinuria, 2,8-dihydroxyadenine in adenine phosphoribosyl transferase (APRT) deficiency]. This is even more important in paediatric practice as the incidence of metabolic abnormalities is greater yet the means to investigate children is more difficult. However, the finding of a triple phosphate stone, as is typically seen after urinary infection, should not prevent a full metabolic evaluation, as occasionally such stones can be the presenting episodes of an underlying metabolic disorder (Coward *et al.* 2003). Metabolic evaluation is based on a routine set of plasma biochemical tests (including bicarbonate, calcium, phosphate, magnesium, and urate) and analysis of the urine. Collection of 24 h urine samples is not feasible in very young children (generally under 3–4 years) and, in this age group, random, spot samples are all that can be tested. Normal ranges for urinary solute excretion in random samples in children are available although there is some variation, dependent on the sample group, timing of urines, relationship to diet or feeds, etc. (discussed under individual metabolic causes). Catherization is inappropriate other than in exceptional cases. The key urinary solutes to determine are calcium, oxalate, cystine, and urate. Measurement of urinary citrate may be helpful and abnormalities in any of the above should be confirmed on several samples, preferably with a 24 h collection. Further metabolic investigation may then be necessary (e.g. liver biopsy in hyperoxaluria, plasma, and urine clearance studies in purine disorders).

Causes of stones

Infective stones

Urinary tract infection was the predominant cause of nephrolithiasis in children until recent years (Ghazali *et al.* 1973). In current practice, infective stones still account for approximately one-fourth of paediatric cases. Such stones, typically composed of magnesium ammonium phosphate and calcium phosphate, can develop over a short timescale into extensive staghorn calculi. The classic infective organism is *Proteus mirabilis* but many other bacteria such as *Escherichia coli*, *Klebsiella*, and *Pseudomonas* species can split urea to form alkaline ammonium ions, favouring supersaturation of triple phosphate. Infective stones are more common in young children (<5 years), especially uncircumcised boys in whom *Proteus* colonizes the foreskin. They are often found incidentally during investigation of a child in whom a urinary tract infection has been diagnosed. In this age group, symptoms such as haematuria and renal colic are the exception and the most important diagnostic clue is persistent urinary infection. Occasionally, boys present with intermittent or complete urinary retention, due to a calculus causing urethral obstruction. Recurrence of infective calculi is uncommon *if* the child has a normal urinary tract, stone removal is complete, and infection is eradicated (Androulakakis *et al.* 1982).

Infective stones also occur in children with congenital renal anomalies or after urological surgery, including renal transplantation, but especially after bladder augmentation. Vesicoureteric reflux (VUR) is a common congenital urinary tract abnormality. Despite this, the incidence of stones in children with VUR is low at approximately 0.5 per cent (Roberts and Atwell 1989). Lesions such as pelvi-ureteric junction (PUJ) obstruction might predispose to stone formation either through their obstruction to urinary flow or following infection. In practice, calculi in PUJ kidneys are not as common as might be expected, sometimes occurring *following* surgery and may result from metabolic abnormalities such as increased urinary oxalate and calcium excretion (Tekin *et al.* 2001). Occasionally, stones are associated with a poorly functioning, xanthogranulomatous pyelonephritis, for which nephrectomy is the appropriate treatment (Quinn *et al.* 1999; Samuel *et al.* 2001). A review of 183 transplants in 146 children reported an incidence of stone formation of 2.7 per cent (Nuininga *et al.* 2001). This is a much higher figure than that determined in a recent retrospective series of adult renal transplants, where the incidence was 0.23 per cent (Rhee *et al.* 1999).

Children requiring clean intermittent catheterization (CIC) have an increased risk of calculi (Barroso *et al.* 2000). In a study of 403 children using CIC, the incidence of stone formation ranged between 5 and 10 per cent, with the higher rates in those catheterizing via a Mitrofanoff channel (Barroso *et al.* 2000). Most stones were asymptomatic and approximately one-third recurred. Approximately 10–15 per cent children with intestinal urinary reservoirs or augmented bladders develop calculi, the rate may vary according to which type of reservoir has been fashioned (Kronner *et al.* 1998; Mathoera *et al.* 2000; Woodhouse and Lennon 2001). In a series of 146 patients, all those with an augmented bladder drained by a suprapubic Mitrofanoff formed stones, whereas in those with a Kock pouch the incidence was 50 per cent and in those who catheterized urethrally it was 9 per cent. No patient who voided spontaneously formed stones, leading the authors to suggest that gravitational drainage of the bladder was a protective factor (Woodhouse and Lennon 2001). Matheora and colleagues emphasized that girls had a higher risk of stone formation and that children who had cloacal malformations, vaginal reconstructions, or anal atresia also had a higher incidence (Mathoera *et al.* 2000).

Hypercalciuria

Introduction

Hypercalciuria is the most common metabolic abnormality detected in children with calculi (Coward *et al.* 2003). Determination of urinary calcium in small children should be undertaken with a second morning urine since there is considerable diurnal variation; the upper limit of normal is then 0.74 mmol/mmol creatinine (0.25 mg/mg) (Ghazali and Barratt 1974). However, there is variation in reported normal ranges for urinary calcium/creatinine, depending on the timing of the samples (e.g. fasting/non-fasting), ethnic origin, geographic region, and, importantly, on age (So *et al.* 2001). Matos and colleagues undertook a cross-sectional study of solute excretion versus age and demonstrated much higher second morning urine calcium/creatinine values in infancy compared to older children (95th centile fell from 2.2 to 0.7 mmol/mmol between 1 month and 14 years) (Matos *et al.* 1997). In older children, a 24 h urine calcium greater than 0.1 mmol/kg/day (4 mg/kg/day) is considered abnormal (Ghazali and Barratt 1974). Urine calcium excretion is increased after surgery (due to immobilization) and may alter when stones are removed, so that metabolic evaluation should be undertaken after stone clearance (Ghazali and Barratt 1974). In view of the variability of calcium excretion, patients with excess calcium excretion should have several samples measured before the label of hypercalciuria is used.

In children, hypercalciuria is normally associated with a normal plasma calcium concentration. Indeed, hypercalcaemia as a cause of renal stones is rare in children (Coward *et al.* 2003). The most common cause of hypercalcaemia causing calculi is immobilization but other conditions such as hyperparathyroidism, hypothyroidism, hypophosphatasia, and vitamin D toxicity should be excluded.

Idiopathic hypercalciuria

The majority of children with hypercalciuria have no identifiable underlying tubulopathy or disorder and are thus described as idiopathic. Hypercalciuria is a common finding in children who were born premature and also in those treated with a ketogenic diet (see below). Children can present with haematuria, dysuria, polyuria, and polydipsia (in those with nephrocalcinosis and a secondary urinary concentration defect) or with symptoms of renal calculi (Kalia *et al.* 1981). Hypercalciuria can, however, be entirely asymptomatic. Studies of the outcome for children with hypercalciuria indicate a risk of forming stones of between 3 and 33 per cent (Alon and Berenbom 2000; Noe 2000; Polito *et al.* 2000). This variability is, in part, explained by differences in the study groups. Other factors may also be involved in stone formation in hypercalciuric children. In a Turkish study, hypocitraturia and hyperoxaluria were much more common in a group of 78 children with idiopathic calcium stones compared to controls whereas calcium excretion was no different (Tekin *et al.* 2000). Thus, it seems prudent to monitor children who have suffered from renal calculi and have ongoing hypercalciuria, as they require long-term follow-up and possible dietary or pharmacological therapy since the recurrence risk for further stones is significant.

Children treated with a ketogenic diet, usually for intractable epilepsy, frequently have hypercalciuria and stone formation is increased (Furth *et al.* 2000). In a series of 112 children, 40 per cent had hypercalciuria at initiation of the diet but 75 per cent had an elevated urinary calcium/creatinine ratio 6 months into the diet (Furth *et al.* 2000). Other urinary abnormalities included low urine pH (5.5–6) and low citrate excretion. Six (5 per cent) formed calculi (three uric acid and three mixed calcium/uric acid stones) (Furth *et al.* 2000).

Hypercalciuria and nephrolithiasis in renal tubulopathies

Routine biochemical investigations will reveal those with a more complex cause of hypercalciuria. The combination of nephrocalcinosis or stone formation, hypercalciuria, and proximal tubular dysfunction (aminoaciduria and low molecular weight proteinuria) in a boy raises the possibility of Dent's disease (Wrong *et al.* 1994). This is an X-linked disorder in which defective chloride channel function leads to this rare phenotype. Whilst nephrocalcinosis is commonly seen in affected boys, nephrolithiasis appears to be rarer in childhood. Hypercalciuria with early onset, severe nephrocalcinosis is a feature of distal renal tubular acidosis and the antenatal-onset form of Bartter's syndrome. However, calculi are rare in these disorders, especially in early childhood. Children with type 1 glycogen storage disease commonly have hypercalciuria associated with hypocitraturia, abnormalities which appear to worsen with age (Weinstein *et al.* 2001). These findings may reflect an incomplete distal renal tubular acidosis in this patient group (Restaino *et al.* 1993).

Hypomagnesaemia with hypercalciuria, nephrocalcinosis, and nephrolithiasis are all found in the Michaelis–Manz syndrome (Rodriguez-Soriano *et al.* 1987, for review; Praga *et al.* 1995). This is an autosomal recessive disorder with a phenotype seemingly similar to distal renal tubular acidosis, but the acidification defect is actually secondary to the nephrocalcinosis (Rodriguez-Soriano and Vallo 1994). Some patients also have ocular abnormalities. The condition arises as a result of mutations in a gene coding for a protein, paracellin-1 (Simon *et al.* 1999), which is expressed in the thick ascending limb of the loop of Henle (Simon *et al.* 1999). Paracellin-1 acts as a channel for magnesium and calcium across the cell tight junction, allowing paracellular flux. Mutations in the paracellin-1 gene lead to defective paracellular mineral flux and, hence, increased urinary calcium and magnesium losses.

Nephrolithiasis in ex-premature children

Children born prematurely (defined as birth at <37 weeks of gestation) have an increased incidence of nephrocalcinosis and nephrolithiasis. The more premature the birth, the greater the risk of stone formation: 17–21 per cent of babies born under 32 weeks gestation develop nephrocalcinosis and 5–9 per cent have calculi (Short and Cooke 1991; Monge *et al.* 1998). The risk of nephrocalcinosis is greater in babies with the lowest birth weights and in those who have required more intensive care. A number of other risk factors have been described including episodes of acute renal failure, hypophosphataemia, hypercalcaemia, bronchopulmonary dysplasia, and the use of frusemide, dexamethasone, theophylline, and thiazides (Ezzedeen *et al.* 1988; Short and Cooke 1991; Toffolo *et al.* 1997; Monge *et al.* 1998; Schell-Feith *et al.* 2000). Although the risk of calculi appears greatest in the sickest infants, a high incidence (9 per cent) has also been found in routine follow-up of school-age children who were born with very low birth weights and had *no* history of renal failure or frusemide therapy (Monge *et al.* 1998). In addition to the risk of stone formation, such children can have persistent hypercalciuria and hypocitraturia leading to reduced bone mineral density (Monge *et al.* 1998; Jones *et al.* 2001).

Infant nutrition may also affect the risk of stone formation in babies. The urinary oxalate/creatinine ratio is higher in preterm babies than in term babies and is higher in those fed formula milk compared to those breastfed (Hoppe *et al.* 1997a). The increased risk of stones in the sicker babies is compounded if they need total parenteral nutrition (TPN). Babies fed with TPN have a higher oxalate and calcium but lower citrate excretion, contributing to a higher calcium oxalate saturation (Hoppe *et al.* 1993). Furthermore, *in vitro* studies of crystal kinetics have shown that urine from preterm babies does not inhibit calcium oxalate crystal agglomeration as well as urine from babies born at term, predisposing them to nephrocalcinosis and stone formation (Schell-Feith *et al.* 2001).

Management of hypercalciuria

A major question in the management of hypercalciuria is whether any treatment is required. However, for children who have already developed a stone and are found to have ongoing hypercalciuria, there is a significant chance of recurrent stones and simple measures to try and reduce this risk are appropriate. It is not necessary and may be harmful to introduce dietary restrictions. Calcium restriction will tend to increase urinary oxalate excretion, which has even more potent lithogenic potential (Borghi *et al.* 2002). Protein restriction can be detrimental to children's growth. However, reducing the child's salt intake is worthwhile. Alon and Berenbom (2000) advised a subgroup of hypercalciuric children to take a low sodium, high potassium diet, which led to a 50 per cent decrease in urine calcium/creatinine ratio. Such a reduction may, however, be difficult to sustain in routine clinical practice. Potassium citrate administration may lower calcium crystallization. Thiazide diuretics act to reduce tubular calcium excretion, reduce hypercalciuria, and, indeed, improve bone mineral density (Reusz *et al.* 1998).

Cystinuria

Introduction

Cystinuria is an autosomal recessive disorder in which the proximal tubular transport of cystine and dibasic amino acids is defective. As a result, the urinary concentration of cystine is very high, exceeding its solubility and leading to nephrolithiasis, especially at low urine pH (Fig. 2). Historically, three different phenotypes were recognized according to the concentrations of urinary cystine in the heterozygous

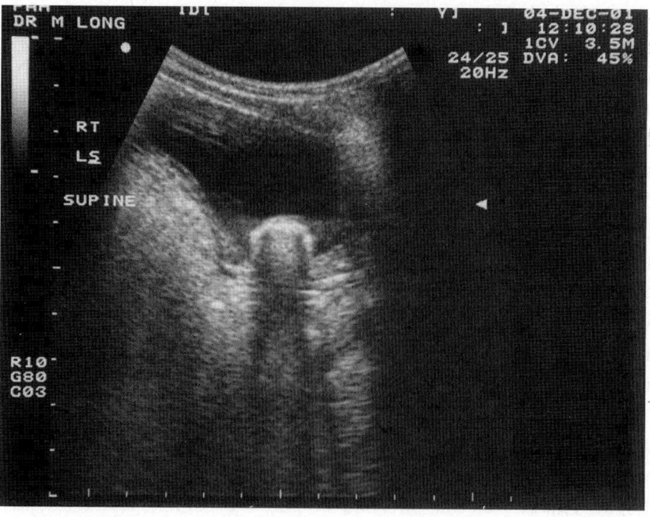

Fig. 2 Ultrasound of the bladder in a 2-year-old girl, showing large echobright stone with acoustic shadow. The stone was composed of cystine, confirming a diagnosis of cystinuria.

parents (Rosenberg *et al.* 1966). The heterozygous parents of type I cystinuria patients have normal urinary excretion of cystine and dibasic amino acids, whilst these levels are increased in heterozygotes of types II and III. Recent molecular genetic research has led to a fuller understanding and reclassification. Patients with type I cystinuria have mutations in the *SLC3A1* gene, which encodes a type II membrane glycoprotein rBAT (Calonge *et al.* 1994), leading to defective cystine transport and massively elevated urinary cystine levels. Patients with non-type I cystinuria have mutations in another gene (*SLC7A9*), localized on chromosome 19q, which encodes another transmembrane protein bo,+amino acid transporter, the light subunit of rBAT (Feliubadalo *et al.* 1999).

Severity in children

Patients with cystinuria in which both affected alleles have type I mutations are more severely affected than those with non-type I or compound heterozygotes forms of the disorder. Asymptomatic babies, identified through the Quebec Network of Genetic Medicine Screening programme as having urinary cystine excretion in the range for affected cystinuria patients, have been prospectively followed through childhood (Goodyer *et al.* 1993, 1998). Urinary cystine excretion is higher in type I/I homozygous children than in non-type I patients, often exceeding the limit of solubility (Goodyer *et al.* 1993). The risk of stone formation is greater and occurs at an earlier age in type I/I children than in others. Half the type I/I children (mean urinary cystine 4566 μmol cystine/g creatinine) formed stones within the first decade compared to none of the type I/II children (mean urinary cystine 1544 μmol cystine/g creatinine) (Goodyer *et al.* 1998). In the clinic, type I/I patients can be identified since their parents will have normal urinary cystine excretion. Given the worse severity, it appears logical to use more intensive measures to prevent stone formation in type I/I cystinuric children.

Management

The medical management of cystinuria is based on dietary modification, increased fluid intake, alkalinization of the urine, and treatment with sulfydryl chelating agents. In adults, dietary protein restriction has been shown to be associated with reduced cystine excretion (Rodman *et al.* 1984). However, this has not been demonstrated in children in whom protein restriction can have severe effects on growth and well being. Much more important is dietary sodium restriction which has clearly been shown to reduce cystine excretion (Norman and Manette 1990; Lindell *et al.* 1995a; Rodriguez *et al.* 1995). In children, marked dietary reduction of sodium intake from 6.0 to 1.5 mmol/kg/day was associated with a statistically significant reduction in urine cystine concentration from 328 to 14 mg/l, with no significant difference in urine volume between the two groups (Rodriguez *et al.* 1995). However, maintaining such a low sodium intake appears difficult for most UK children over the long term.

Increased fluid intake is the mainstay of medical management. The theoretical limit of solubility for cystine is approximately 1000 μmol/l, which is far lower than the usual urinary cystine concentration for type I/I patients (Goodyer *et al.* 1998). Fluid therapy is adjusted to bring the excreted urinary cystine to below the solubility limit of 1000 μmol/l. In practice, children will require a water intake of 1.5–2 l/m^2/day to achieve this. Measurement of urinary cystine concentrations at each clinic appointment can help to judge whether enough water is being administered. For small children, spot urine samples are all that can be collected. In older patients, a 24 h sample may provide a more representative value of daily urine cystine excretion (generally children over 3–4 years should be able to collect a 24 h sample). However, there is considerable diurnal variation in cystine excretion in adults (Lindell *et al.* 1995b) and it is likely to be equally evident in children (Goodyer *et al.* 1998). It is, therefore, important to give a large fluid volume just before the child's bedtime and, if they wake, more in the night.

Unfortunately, young children are rarely able to comply with such a large volume of fluid and additional therapeutic measures are necessary. The solubility of cystine is markedly increased at higher urine pH so that alkalinization is a useful adjunct to fluid therapy. Traditionally, treatment with sodium bicarbonate would achieve this, but the increased sodium load has the effect of increasing urinary cystine excretion (Lindell *et al.* 1995a; Rodriguez *et al.* 1995). Therefore, potassium citrate is the preferred alkalinization agent (except in patients with severe renal impairment) (Joly *et al.* 1999; Fjellstedt *et al.* 2001). The dose of citrate is titrated against urinary pH, aiming for values greater than 7.5. Monnens and colleagues emphasized the importance not only of extra fluid at bedtime, but also of trying to maintain alkalinization throughout the night by using an evening dose of acetozolamide (Monnens *et al.* 2000). Many children can be treated with a combination of extra fluids and potassium citrate. A minority, however, continue to form recurrent stones and require chelation therapy.

D-Penicillamine and tiopronine are sulfydryl compounds that undergo disulfide exchange with cystine, forming much more soluble mixed disulfides. These drugs are associated with a reduction in stone formation (Stephens 1989; Chow and Streem 1996; Barbey *et al.* 2000), but both are associated with significant side-effects including rashes, bone marrow suppression, proteinuria, and rarely membranous nephropathy (Stephens 1989). Although rash and mild proteinuria are common adverse effects, it is usually possible to continue therapy (Stephens 1989). Captopril (another sulfydryl compound) has also been used in the treatment of cystinuria although with conflicting results (reviewed in Joly *et al.* 1999).

In view of the recurrent stone formation in cystinuric patients, surgical therapy of cystine calculi utilizes minimally invasive techniques. Cystine stones are hard and may not be so amenable to disintegration with lithotripsy although more recent series report better success (reviewed in Joly *et al.* 1999). For larger (>15 mm) renal stones, percutaneous nephrolithotomy (PCNL) is the best approach (Chow and Streem 1998).

Hyperoxalurias

Introduction

Hyperoxaluria is a potent stimulus to stone formation and calcium oxalate stones are the most common type of calculi in children as well as in adults. In paediatric series, hyperoxaluria (defined as >0.5 mmol/24 h/1.73 m^2) is found in approximately 20 per cent children with stones and, of these children, approximately half have primary hyperoxaluria (Neuhaus *et al.* 2000). The remainder develop hyperoxaluria secondary to another disorder or have no clear cause (idiopathic). The absorption of oxalate is inversely proportional to that of calcium. Intestinal disorders such as malabsorption (steatorrhoea), inflammatory bowel disease, cystic fibrosis (CF), or surgical small bowel resection (e.g. for necrotizing enterocolitis) can lead to hyperoxaluria (Bohane *et al.* 1979; Neuhaus *et al.* 2000). Approximately 10 per cent of children with CF develop renal stones (Bohles *et al.* 2002). Metabolic evaluation has shown hyperoxaluria, demonstrated in 60 per cent CF children in ones serie (Turner *et al.* 2000), associated with hypocitraturia and hypercalciuria (Bohles *et al.* 2002; Perez-Brayfield *et al.* 2002). An additional factor is that CF children have a reduced rate of colonization of *Oxalobacter formigenes*, a commensal which degrades oxalate in the gut (Sidhu *et al.* 1998).

Primary hyperoxalurias

Biochemical basis

The primary hyperoxalurias (PH) are rare autosomal recessive disorders due to defects in oxalate metabolism with consequent overproduction and excessive urinary excretion of oxalate. Oxalate is metabolized in hepatic peroxisomes and a defect in alanine-glyoxalate transferase (AGT) is responsible for PH1. This enzyme requires pyridoxine as a cofactor and some cases are responsive to supraphysiological doses of this vitamin.

Mutations in the *AGTX* gene lead to failure of production of AGT or to its misdirection to mitochondria where it is non-functional (Danpure 1998). PH type 2 (PH2), which is less common and generally less severe, results from a deficiency of D-glycerate dehydrogenase/glyoxalate reductase. The biochemical sequelae of these defects are hyperoxaluria (often >1.0 mmol/day/1.73 m^2, normal children <0.5), glycolic aciduria (PH1), or L-glyceric aciduria (PH2). Oxalate is relatively insoluble in urine and readily precipitates forming crystals, leading to nephrocalcinosis and/or calculi. Severe nephrocalcinosis or recurrent stone disease can lead to progressive renal damage. Since oxalate is only excreted by the kidney, renal dysfunction leads ultimately to reduced oxalate clearance and then to systemic oxalate accumulation (oxalosis).

Clinical features and diagnosis

The clinical presentation of PH1 is extremely variable. The most common presentation is of a child with features of nephrolithiasis. Some children develop only nephrocalcinosis and indeed stones are very uncommon in the rare occurrence of PH1 manifesting in infants less than 1 year of age (Latta *et al.* 1990). These infants present with severe renal failure, nephrocalcinosis, and have evidence of advanced systemic oxalosis. By contrast, children with severe renal damage from recurrent oxalate calculi can have siblings, sharing the same genotype, but who are asymptomatic (Hoppe *et al.* 1997b). Some children develop only occasional calculi whilst others have recurrent stones and progressive renal damage. This variability inevitably affects strategies for treatment (see below). PH2 appears to be much more rare but may be under-diagnosed and confused with PH1. It generally causes less severe manifestations, usually with calculi presenting in older children (Fig. 3), and renal failure appears to be uncommon (Marangella *et al.* 1994; Milliner *et al.* 2001).

The diagnosis of PH1 is made on the basis of persistently elevated urinary oxalate usually with an elevated urinary glycollate. Urine should be acidified on collection to prevent ascorbate conversion to oxalate and plasma oxalate samples require careful handling (Kasidas 1995). Urine should also be sent for determination of L-glycerate, which is elevated in PH2. Confirmation of PH requires a liver biopsy and specialized determination of AGT and GR activities in hepatocytes (Rumsby *et al.* 1997; Giafi and Rumsby 1998). There are now recognized a small number of patients with significant hyperoxaluria with or without glycolic aciduria, who have normal AGT and glycerate reductase/human D-glycerate dehydrogenase (GR/HGD) activities (referred to as non-type 1, non-type 2 PH), probably resulting from as yet unrecognized disorders of oxalate metabolism (van Acker *et al.* 1996). The plasma oxalate concentration and plasma calcium-oxalate supersaturation (β-CaOx) are increased in children with PH1, even whilst renal function remains normal, increasing the risk of systemic oxalate deposition (Hoppe *et al.* 1998). β-CaOx increases as glomerular filtration rate (GFR) declines and the risk of significant systemic oxalate crystallization increases steeply once GFR is less than 30–40 ml/min/1.73 m^2 (Marangella *et al.* 1995; Hoppe *et al.* 1998). In children with PH, who are in endstage renal failure (ESRF) and maintained on haemodialysis, plasma oxalate, and β-CaOx are extremely elevated, even after aggressive haemodialysis. This indicates that systemic deposition of oxalate can continue unabated once a child is on dialysis (Hoppe *et al.* 1999). Systemic oxalosis occurs in many tissues, especially bone, retina, arteries, nerves, muscle, heart, and the testis. Hypothyroidism has also been described in severely affected infants (Frishberg *et al.* 2000).

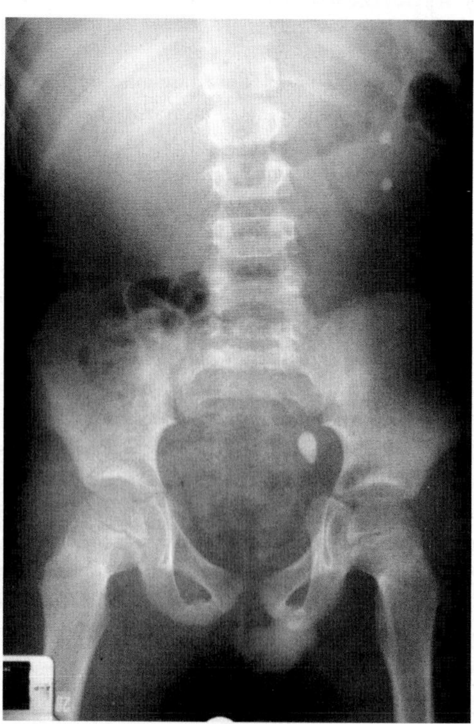

Fig. 3 Plain abdominal radiograph showing left renal and ureteric stones in a 9-year-old boy with primary hyperoxaluria type 2.

Medical management

The management of hyperoxaluria involves a high fluid intake ($>$1.5–2 l/m^2/day) and administration of inhibitors of crystallization, such as potassium citrate (Leumann *et al.* 1993). The dietary contribution of oxalate to the total oxalate pool is small and, thus, dietary restriction is not helpful. Supraphysiological doses of pyridoxine, the cofactor for AGT, can lead to a reduction in urinary oxalate, sometimes to within the normal range and can preserve renal function (see Fig. 4) (Milliner *et al.* 1994; Toussaint 1998). However, pyridoxine responsiveness only occurs in a proportion of patients and may not be maintained (Toussaint 1998). Serial monitoring of renal function is important in order to plan renal replacement therapy. This needs to be done at much higher levels of GFR than for non-PH patients, because systemic oxalosis can occur when the GFR is less than approximately 30–40 ml/min/1.73 m^2 (see above). In general, neither haemodialysis nor peritoneal dialysis lead to effective oxalate clearance so that further systemic deposition continues (Hoppe *et al.* 1996, 1999).

Transplantation in primary hyperoxaluria

Systemic oxalosis creates an additional hazard to a kidney transplant as rapid oxalate clearance occurs in the first few months after surgery. This contributes to the poor outcome for isolated kidney transplants performed for PH1 with graft survival rates in one large European paediatric series of 23 per cent for LD and 17 per cent for cadaveric kidneys at 3 years (Broyer *et al.* 1990). Isolated renal transplantation may, however, be a reasonable option for PH2 patients. In North America, isolated renal transplantation has remained a therapeutic option, requiring intensive perioperative dialysis and medical management, but in Europe most authorities opt for a combined liver–kidney transplant (Latta *et al.* 1995; Broyer *et al.* 1996; Cochat and Basmaison 2000). Liver transplantation provides a new source of AGT and hence can be considered as 'enzyme replacement therapy'. It has been combined with a kidney transplant in patients with renal failure and leads to an immediate reduction of endogenous oxalate production to normal. The inevitable systemic oxalate burden that such patients have prior to the transplant maintains an elevated plasma oxalate and significant hyperoxaluria for many months (Jamieson 1998). A recent review of 87 combined liver–kidney transplants in 80 patients (mean age 17 years) reported graft survival rates of 82, 78, and 62 per cent at 1, 2, and 5 years after surgery respectively. Survival was clearly better in those who received their grafts after short periods on dialysis compared to those with longer periods (e.g. $>$2 years), in whom systemic oxalate deposition was much greater (Jamieson *et al.* 1998). These successes have led some to consider pre-emptive liver transplantation in children

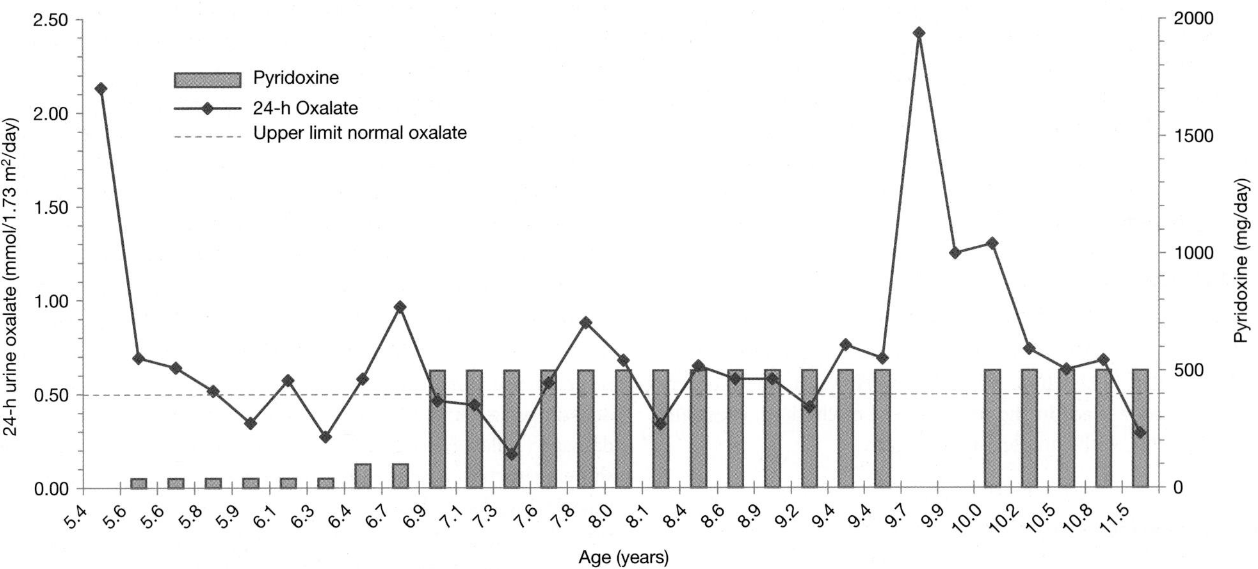

Fig. 4 Twenty-four hour urinary oxalate excretion in a child with biopsy-proven AGT deficiency (primary hyperoxaluria type 1), treated with AGT cofactor, pyridoxine. Subsequent withdrawal of the pyridoxine at 9.4 years led to increase in urinary oxalate, which returned towards the normal range (<0.5 mmol/1.73 m^2/day) when it was reintroduced.

not yet in ESRF. This strategy is controversial and patient selection is important because, even within one family, PH1 can have very variable manifestations (Hoppe *et al.* 1996). A reasonable strategy is to consider combined liver–kidney transplantation in PH patients with low GFR (<40 ml/min/1.73 m^2), in whom plasma oxalate and, hence, systemic oxalate deposition is increasing rapidly. In those with a better GFR, isolated liver transplantation may have a role (Cochat and Scharer 1993). Isolated liver transplantation has also been undertaken in the severely affected infants in whom combined transplantation is not feasible. Subsequent renal transplantation has then been performed when the child is in a better clinical condition (Latta *et al.* 1995; Ellis *et al.* 2001).

Purine disorders

Uric acid stones

Uric acid stones are more common in developing countries where hyperuricosuria is more prevalent and in these situations tend to be associated with urinary tract infection and tend to develop in the lower urinary tract, especially the bladder (Angwafo *et al.* 2000). Hyperuricosuria can lead to microscopic or macroscopic haematuria, even in the absence of stone formation and approximately 40 per cent patients may have coexistent hypercalciuria (La Manna *et al.* 2001). Conversely, hyperuricosuric children can develop microcalculi and loin pain without any evidence of haematuria (La Manna *et al.* 2001). It has been reported to occur in some children with CF consuming large doses of pancreatic enzyme supplements. Hyperuricosuria has also been associated with thin basement nephropathy (Praga *et al.* 1998). Hyperuricosuria can also occur as a result of drugs, such as some antibiotics. Hyperuricaemia and subsequent hyperuricosuria are major risk factors in the aetiology of tumour lysis syndrome in children with lymphomas and high cell count leukaemias (Vachvanichsanong *et al.* 1995). Patients with type 1 glycogen storage disease are also at risk of hyperuricaemia and hyperuricosuria, with consequent stone formation (Chen 1991), although coexistent hypercalciuria and hypocitraturia may be equally important factors (Restaino *et al.* 1993).

Adenine phosphoribosyl transferase deficiency

A deficiency of APRT leads to increased conversion of adenine (which it normally converted into AMP) to 2,8-dihydroxyadenine (2,8-DHA), which is much less soluble and, hence, forms stones (Cameron *et al.* 1993). Such stones need expert analysis as they may be confused for 'uric acid' stones. Children with APRT deficiency may be asymptomatic, may present with brown crystalluria, or with the more common manifestations of calculi. Occasionally, they may develop acute renal failure due to crystal nephropathy (Simmonds *et al.* 1989). Repeated stone episodes or long-standing crystal deposition can lead to chronic renal failure and recurrent deposition can occur after renal transplantation (Gagne *et al.* 1994). The plasma urate level is normal and confirmation of the diagnosis comes from stone analysis or detailed studies of the plasma and urine purine metabolite profiles. Treatment involves a high fluid intake and a low purine diet. Second, the diversion of adenine to 2,8-DHA requires xanthine oxidase (XO), which can be inhibited by administration of allopurinol, thereby preventing the potential long-term complications.

Xanthinuria

A deficiency of XO leads to an inability to metabolize xanthine and hypoxanthine to uric acid. As a consequence, the urinary xanthine concentration increases to levels in excess of the solubility, causing precipitation, crystal, and stone formation. Approximately 50 per cent of reported case have presented in childhood (Cameron *et al.* 1993). Children may suffer from an isolated defect of XO (classic, type I) or from a mutation in the molybdenum cofactor gene, which leads to not only XO deficiency, but also defective function of other dependent enzymes (aldehyde oxidase and sulfite oxidase). This latter form (type II) causes neonatal seizures and has a poor prognosis. The plasma uric acid concentration is normal in xanthinuria. Treatment with allopurinol is not effective.

Surgical treatment

Introduction

The majority of children with stones are treated with minimally invasive techniques, with rates of stone clearance matching those in adult series (Fraser *et al.* 1999; Choong *et al.* 2000). However, open surgery continues to have a place in the management of children, especially very young infants, with complex stone disease.

External shock wave lithotripsy

Children have now been treated with external shock wave lithotripsy (ESWL) for 20 years or more and it is the most frequent modality of stone removal employed. Young children (e.g. those aged <10 years) are usually treated under general anaesthesia. Practices such as placement of ureteric JJ stent prior to ESWL to enhance passage of fragments down the ureter and the use of prophylactic antibiotics vary from unit to unit. Recent UK paediatric series have demonstrated stone clearance rates of 88–91 per cent (Fraser *et al.* 1999; Choong *et al.* 2000), although these figures include a few children treated in more than one session or in combination with another technique. A comparison of ESWL stone clearance in adults and children treated in one centre indicated that children (aged 6 months–6 years) had better success rates than adults (Gofrit *et al.* 2001). In this study, stone clearance rates of 89–100 per cent were demonstrated for children and, interestingly, the improvement was most obvious in the subgroup of patients with larger (>20 mm) stones, although such stones often need more than one session. Brinkmann and colleagues reviewed 64 children (30 girls, mean age 5.6 years) with a total of 83 stones, treated by ESWL (Lithostar) (Brinkmann *et al.* 2001). The stone clearance rate was 83 per cent and the remaining fragments were deemed clinically insignificant.

There are some data suggesting that metabolic stones are harder to disintegrate. In a UK series of 43 children, three of the five cases who had residual stones after ESWL had metabolic calculi (Fraser *et al.* 1999). A particular difficulty to the paediatric urologist is the management of very small infants, often born prematurely, who have developed calculi. Their size and medical status (many have chronic lung disease as a sequel to ventilatory support in the newborn period) may make instrumentation (e.g. PCNL or endoscopy) difficult. ESWL has been applied very successfully to these infants. Shukla and colleagues reported a series of eight infants (mean age 13 months and weight 7.7 kg) treated with a Dornier HM3 lithotriptor, with adaptation of the gantry to accommodate the child (Shukla *et al.* 2001). At this size, the child requires foam pads to protect the lungs and viscera from the treatment. Each stone was successfully treated with a single ESWL session with no reported complications (Shukla *et al.* 2001). In a French series of 16 children aged 6 months to 2 years, Lottmann and colleagues reported a high success rate (87.5 per cent stone clearance) for ESWL in the treatment of staghorn calculi (Lottmann *et al.* 2001). However, the success of treatment in such specialized cases requires multidisciplinary input and obsessional care of fluid, electrolyte, and antibiotic therapy.

Concerns about the safety of ESWL are magnified in paediatric practice because of the theoretical effects that the shock wave might have on the developing kidney and because of the reduced calibre of the paediatric ureter. In practice, a number of series appear to show no clinically significant sequelae. Gofrit and colleagues demonstrated that the paediatric ureter is fully able to transport fragments after ESWL, when compared to adult series (Gofrit *et al.* 2001). Detailed studies have included imaging, plasma, and urine biochemistry. Villanyi and colleagues studied 16 children before and after ESWL, and found that there was a transient increase in urinary renal tubular enzymes and proteins (e.g. aspartate transaminase, alkaline phosphatase, lactate dehydrogenase, and β2-microglobulin), consistent with acute tubular damage (Villanyi *et al.* 2001). However, longitudinal measurements show a return to baseline values for these parameters within approximately 2 weeks (Villanyi *et al.* 2001). The same study found no structural changes on ultrasound imaging. Likewise, in Brinkmann's review of 64 children treated with ESWL, there was no difference in renal growth, assessed by ultrasound, between treated and untreated kidneys (Brinkmann *et al.* 2001). Lifshitz and colleagues monitored renal growth after ESWL in 29 children over a mean follow-up period of 9 years (Lifshitz *et al.* 1998). They found no significant difference in the sizes of the treated and untreated kidneys. Interestingly, at the time of ESWL, the stone-containing kidneys tended to be smaller than the mean size for age, whereas the normal kidneys were of appropriate length. When followed-up, the ESWL-treated kidneys had grown less compared to the untreated kidneys. Such reduced growth in the stone-containing kidney may be due to the presence of the stone (since the reduction is evident prior to treatment), but it remains possible that ESWL may have some effect (Lifshitz *et al.* 1998). In contrast to these findings, Lottmann and colleagues performed pre- and post-ESWL DMSA scans in 15 children (mean age 6.5 years) and found that ESWL-treated kidneys did not develop any new defect on the scan repeated 6 months after treatment (Lottmann *et al.* 1998).

Percutaneous nephrolithotomy

PCNL has been used in adults for some 25 years but paediatric experience is more limited, due mainly to technical constraints in the size of instruments available for children. In the last 15 years, however, PCNL has become a standard technique and recent, smaller equipment has improved its utility. Mor and colleagues reported a stone-free rate of 68 per cent after a single session of PCNL in a series of 25 children (Mor *et al.* 1997). Failure to completely clear the stone was more common with staghorn calculi and multiple stones. After an average follow-up period of 2 years, no complications were seen and in 10 cases, in whom repeat DMSA scans were performed, there were no significant changes in all but one child (Mor *et al.* 1997). Other groups have reported similar stone-clearance rates of between 70 and 90 per cent (Desai *et al.* 1999; Sahin *et al.* 2000). Jackman and colleagues reported their experience of a 11F 'peel-away' vascular sheath ('mini-perc') technique in a number of small children, averaging 3 years and 12 kg (Jackman *et al.* 1998). Stone clearance was obtained in 85 per cent of children with minimal morbidity. The main complications of PCNL are bleeding, infection, postoperative leakage, and incomplete stone removal.

Ureteroscopy

Ureteric stones in children have traditionally been managed by open surgery, but in recent years minimally invasive techniques such as ESWL, PCNL, and ureteroscopy have replaced ureterolithotomy in all but occasional situations. Ureteroscopy can be performed with rigid or flexible scopes, allowing baskets or lithotripsy probes to be inserted to clear the stone. There are now many reports of paediatric series of ureteroscopies. Al Busaidy and colleagues reviewed a large series of 50 ureteroscopic procedures in 43 children, using electrohydraulic lithotripsy as the main fragmentation technique and reported a stone-clearance rate of 93 per cent (Al Busaidy *et al.* 1997). Efficacy varied according to the position of the stone, with lesser success with upper ureteric calculi. Two children suffered ureteric perforation and follow-up cystograms demonstrated an incidence of VUR of 17 per cent, although this was felt to be of minor importance. Other techniques of ureteric stone disintegration include Holmium : YAG lithotripsy, which appears equally successful (Wollin *et al.* 1999). Schuster and colleagues reviewed 27 ureteroscopies performed in 25 children (mean age 9 years) and found that 92 per cent of the children were stone-free after one procedure and 100 per cent stone-free after two treatments. Approximately half the children required ureteric dilatation prior to treatment and stents were placed after the procedure in 70 per cent of the cases (Schuster *et al.* 2002). In a large series of 66 ureteroscopies, performed in 66 children (mean age 9 years), Bassiri reported a stone-clearance rate of 88 per cent using a variety of fragmentation techniques (Bassiri *et al.* 2002). Complications occurred in 23 per cent but were mostly limited to haematuria with one patient suffering colic and three developing pyelonephritis.

References

Absolut de la Gastine, G. *et al.* (1998). Urinary calculi and Munchausen syndrome. *Archives Pediatrie* **5**, 517–520.

Al Busaidy, S. S., Prem, A. R., and Medhat, M. (1997). Paediatric ureteroscopy for ureteric calculi: a 4-year experience. *British Journal of Urology* **80**, 797–801.

Alon, U. S. and Berenbom, A. (2000). Idiopathic hypercalciuria of childhood: 4- to 11-year outcome. *Pediatric Nephrology* **14**, 1011–1015.

Androulakakis, P. A. *et al.* (1982). Urinary calculi in children. A 5 to 15-year follow-up with particular reference to recurrent and residual stones. *British Journal of Urology* **54**, 176–180.

Angwafo, F. F. III *et al.* (2000). Pediatric urolithiasis in sub-Saharan Africa: a comparative study in two regions of Cameroon. *European Urology* **37**, 106–111.

Barbey, F. *et al.* (2000). Medical treatment of cystinuria: critical reappraisal of long-term results. *Journal of Urology* **163**, 1419–1423.

Barratt, T. M. and Ghazali, S. (1977). The aetiology of renal stones in children. *Postgraduate Medical Journal* **53** (Suppl 2), 35–40.

Barroso, U. *et al.* (2000). Bladder calculi in children who perform clean intermittent catheterization. *British Journal of Urology International* **85**, 879–884.

Bassiri, A. *et al.* (2002). Transureteral lithotripsy in pediatric practice. *Journal of Endourology* **16**, 257–260.

Bohane, T. D. *et al.* (1979). A clinical study of young infants after small intestinal resection. *Journal of Pediatrics* **94**, 552–558.

Bohles, H. *et al.* (2002). Antibiotic treatment-induced tubular dysfunction as a risk factor for renal stone formation in cystic fibrosis. *Journal of Pediatrics* **140**, 103–109.

Borghi, L. *et al.* (2002). Comparison of two diets for the prevention of recurrent stones in idiopathic hypercalciuria. *New England Journal of Medicine* **346**, 77–84.

Brinkmann, O. A. *et al.* (2001). Extracorporeal shock wave lithotripsy in children. Efficacy, complications and long-term follow-up. *European Urology* **39**, 591–597.

Broyer, M. *et al.* (1990). Kidney transplantation in primary oxalosis: data from the EDTA Registry. *Nephrology, Dialysis, Transplantation* **5**, 332–336.

Broyer, M. *et al.* (1996). Management of oxalosis. *Kidney International Supplement* **53**, S93–S98.

Calonge, M. J. *et al.* (1994). Cystinuria caused by mutations in rBAT, a gene involved in the transport of cystine. *Nature Genetics* **6**, 420–425.

Cameron, J. S., Moro, F., and Simmonds, H. A. (1993). Gout, uric acid and purine metabolism in paediatric nephrology. *Paediatric Nephrology* **7**, 105–118.

Chen, Y. T. (1991). Type I glycogen storage disease: kidney involvement, pathogenesis and its treatment. *Pediatric Nephrology* **5**, 71–76.

Choong, S. *et al.* (2000). The management of paediatric urolithiasis. *British Journal of Urology International* **86**, 857–860.

Chow, G. K. and Streem, S. B. (1996). Medical treatment of cystinuria: results of contemporary clinical practice. *Journal of Urology* **156**, 1576–1578.

Cochat, P. and Scharer, K. (1993). Should liver transplantation be performed before advanced renal insufficiency in primary hyperoxaluria type 1? *Pediatric Nephrology* **7**, 212–218.

Cochat, P. and Basmaison, O. (2000). Current approaches to the management of primary hyperoxaluria. *Archives of Diseases of Childhood* **82**, 470–473.

Coward, R. J. *et al.* (2003). Epidemiology of paediatric renal stone disease in the UK. *Archives of Diseases of Childhood* **88** (11), 962–965.

Danpure, C. J. (1998). The molecular basis of alanine : glyoxylate aminotransferase mistargeting: the most common single cause of primary hyperoxaluria type 1. *Journal of Nephrology* **11** (Suppl. 1), 8–12.

Desai, M. *et al.* (1999). Pediatric percutaneous nephrolithotomy: assessing impact of technical innovations on safety and efficacy. *Journal of Endourology* **13**, 359–364.

Ece, A. *et al.* (2000). Characteristics of pediatric urolithiasis in south-east Anatolia. *International Journal of Urology* **7**, 330–334.

Ellis, S. R. *et al.* (2001). Combined liver-kidney transplantation for primary hyperoxaluria type 1 in young children. *Nephrology, Dialysis, Transplantation* **16**, 348–354.

Ezzedeen, F., Adelman, R. D., and Ahlfors, C. E. (1988). Renal calcification in preterm infants: pathophysiology and long-term sequelae. *Journal of Pediatrics* **113**, 532–539.

Feliubadalo, L. *et al.* (1999). Non-type I cystinuria caused by mutations in SLC7A9, encoding a subunit (bo,+AT) of rBAT. International Cystinuria Consortium. *Nature Genetics* **23**, 52–57.

Fjellstedt, E. *et al.* (2001). A comparison of the effects of potassium citrate and sodium bicarbonate in the alkalinization of urine in homozygous cystinuria. *Urological Research* **29**, 295–302.

Fraser, M. *et al.* (1999). Minimally invasive treatment of urinary tract calculi in children. *British Journal of Urology International* **84**, 339–342.

Frishberg, Y. *et al.* (2000). Hypothyroidism in primary hyperoxaluria type 1. *Journal of Pediatrics* **136**, 255–257.

Furth, S. L. *et al.* (2000). Risk factors for urolithiasis in children on the ketogenic diet. *Pediatric Nephrology* **15**, 125–128.

Gagne, E. R. *et al.* (1994). Chronic renal failure secondary to 2,8-dihydroxyadenine deposition: the first report of recurrence in a kidney transplant. *American Journal of Kidney Diseases* **24**, 104–107.

Giafi, C. F. and Rumsby, G. (1998). Kinetic analysis and tissue distribution of human D-glycerate dehydrogenase/glyoxylate reductase and its relevance to the diagnosis of primary hyperoxaluria type 2. *Annals of Clinical Biochemistry* **35**, 104–109.

Ghazali, S. and Barratt, T. M. (1974). Urinary excretion of calcium and magnesium in children. *Archives of Diseases of Childhood* **49**, 97–101.

Ghazali, S., Barratt, T. M., and Williams, D. I. (1973). Childhood urolithiasis in Britain. *Archives of Diseases of Childhood* **48**, 291–295.

Gofrit, O. N. *et al.* (2001). Is the pediatric ureter as efficient as the adult ureter in transporting fragments following extracorporeal shock wave lithotripsy for renal calculi larger than 10 mm? *Journal of Urology* **166**, 1862–1864.

Goodyer, P. R. *et al.* (1993). Prospective analysis and classification of patients with cystinuria identified in a newborn screening program. *Journal of Pediatrics* **122**, 568–572.

Goodyer, P. *et al.* (1998). Cystinuria subtype and the risk of nephrolithiasis. *Kidney International* **54**, 56–56.

Hoppe, B. *et al.* (1993). Urinary saturation and nephrocalcinosis in preterm infants: effect of parenteral nutrition. *Archives of Diseases of Childhood* **69** (3), 299–303.

Hoppe, B. *et al.* (1996). Oxalate elimination via hemodialysis or peritoneal dialysis in children with chronic renal failure. *Pediatric Nephrology* **10**, 488–492.

Hoppe, B. *et al.* (1997a). Influence of nutrition on urinary oxalate and calcium in preterm and term infants. *Pediatric Nephrology* **11**, 687–690.

Hoppe, B. *et al.* (1997b). A vertical (pseudodominant) pattern of inheritance in the autosomal recessive disease primary hyperoxaluria type 1: lack of relationship between genotype, enzymic phenotype, and disease severity. *American Journal of Kidney Diseases* **29**, 36–44.

Hoppe, B. *et al.* (1998). Plasma calcium-oxalate saturation in children with renal insufficiency and in children with primary hyperoxaluria. *Kidney International* **54**, 921–925.

Hoppe, B. *et al.* (1999). Plasma calcium oxalate supersaturation in children with primary hyperoxaluria and end-stage renal failure. *Kidney International* **56**, 268–274.

Jackman, S. V. *et al.* (1998). Percutaneous nephrolithotomy in infants and preschool age children: experience with a new technique. *Urology* **52**, 697–701.

Jamieson, N. V. (1998). The results of combined liver/kidney transplantation for primary hyperoxaluria (PH1) 1984–1997. The European PH1 Transplant Registry report. European PH1 Transplantation Study Group. *Journal of Nephrology* **11** (Suppl. 1), 36–41.

Joly, D. *et al.* (1999). Treatment of cystinuria. *Pediatric Nephrology* **13**, 945–950.

Jones, C. A. *et al.* (2001). Hypercalciuria in ex-preterm children, aged 7–8 years. *Pediatric Nephrology* **16**, 665–671.

Kalia, A., Travis, L. B., and Brouhard, B. H. (1981). The association of idiopathic hypercalciuria and asymptomatic gross hematuria in children. *Journal of Pediatrics* **99**, 716–719.

Kamoun, A. *et al.* (1999). Urolithiasis in Tunisian children: a study of 120 cases based on stone composition. *Pediatric Nephrology* **13**, 920–925.

Kasidas, G. P. (1995). Plasma and urine measurements for monitoring of treatment in the primary hyperoxaluric patient. *Nephrology, Dialysis, Transplantation* **10** (Suppl. 8), 8–10.

Kronner, K. M. *et al.* (1998). Bladder calculi in the pediatric augmented bladder. *Journal of Urology* **160**, 1096–1098.

La Manna, A. *et al.* (2001). Hyperuricosuria in children: clinical presentation and natural history. *Pediatrics* **107**, 86–90.

Latta, K. and Brodehl, J. (1990). Primary hyperoxaluria type I. *European Journal of Pediatrics* **149**, 518–522.

Latta, K. *et al.* (1995). Selection of transplantation procedures and perioperative management in primary hyperoxaluria type 1. *Nephrology, Dialysis, Transplantation* **10** (Suppl. 8), 53–57.

Leumann, E., Hoppe, B., and Neuhaus, T. (1993). Management of primary hyperoxaluria: efficacy of oral citrate administration. *Pediatric Nephrology* **7**, 207–211.

Lifshitz, D. A. *et al.* (1998). Alterations in predicted growth rates of pediatric kidneys treated with extracorporeal shockwave lithotripsy. *Journal of Endourology* **12**, 469–475.

Lindell, A. *et al.* (1995a). The effect of sodium intake on cystinuria with and without tiopronin treatment. *Nephron* **71**, 407–415.

Lindell, A. *et al.* (1995b). Measurement of diurnal variations in urinary cystine saturation. *Urological Research* **23**, 215–220.

Lottmann, H. B. *et al.* (1998). 99mTechnetium-dimercapto-succinic acid renal scan in the evaluation of potential long-term renal parenchymal damage associated with extracorporeal shock wave lithotripsy in children. *Journal of Urology* **159**, 521–524.

Lottmann, H. B. *et al.* (2001). Monotherapy extracorporeal shock wave lithotripsy for the treatment of staghorn calculi in children. *Journal of Urology* **165**, 2324–2327.

Marangella, M., Petrarulo, M. and Cosseddu, D. (1994). End-stage renal failure in primary hyperoxaluria type 2. *New England Journal of Medicine* **330**, 1690.

Marangella, M. *et al.* (1995). The clinical significance of assessment of serum calcium oxalate saturation in the hyperoxaluria syndromes. *Nephrology, Dialysis, Transplantation* **10** (Suppl. 8), 11–13.

Mathoera, R. B., Kok, D. J., and Nijman, R. J. (2000). Bladder calculi in augmentation cystoplasty in children. *Urology* **56**, 482–487.

Matos, V. *et al.* (1997). Urinary phosphate/creatinine, calcium/creatinine, and magnesium/creatinine ratios in a healthy pediatric population. *Journal of Pediatrics* **131**, 252–257.

Milliner, D. S., Wilson, D. M., and Smith, L. H. (2001). Phenotypic expression of primary hyperoxaluria: comparative features of types I and II. *Kidney International* **59**, 31–36.

Milliner, D. S. *et al.* (1994). Results of long-term treatment with orthophosphate and pyridoxine in patients with primary hyperoxaluria. *New England Journal of Medicine* **8**, 1553–1558.

Monge, M. *et al.* (1998). Study of renal metabolic disturbances related to renal lithiasis at school age in very-low-birth-weight children. *Nephron* **79**, 269–273.

Monnens, L. A. H., Noordam, K., and Trijbels, F. (2000). Necessary treatment of cystinuria at night. *Pediatric Nephrology* **14**, 1148–1149.

Mor, Y. *et al.* (1997). The role of percutaneous nephrolithotomy in the management of pediatric renal calculi. *Journal of Urology* **158**, 1319–1321.

Neuhaus, T. J. *et al.* (2000). Urinary oxalate excretion in urolithiasis and nephrocalcinosis. *Archives of Diseases of Childhood* **82**, 322–326.

Noe, H. N. (2000). Hypercalciuria and pediatric stone recurrences with and without structural abnormalities. *Journal of Urology* **164**, 1094–1096.

Norman, R. W. and Manette, W. A. (1990). Dietary restriction of sodium as a means of reducing urinary cystine. *Journal of Urology* **143**, 1193–1195.

Nuininga, J. E. *et al.* (2001). Urological complications in pediatric renal transplantation. *European Urology* **39**, 598–602.

Perez-Brayfield, M. R. *et al.* (2000). Metabolic risk factors for stone formation in patients with cystic fibrosis. *Journal of Urology* **167**, 480–484.

Pietrow, P. K. *et al.* (2002). Clinical outcome of pediatric stone disease. *Journal of Urology* **167**, 670–673.

Polito, C. *et al.* (2000). Clinical presentation and natural course of idiopathic hypercalciuria in children. *Pediatric Nephrology* **15**, 211–214.

Praga, M. *et al.* (1995). Familial hypomagnesemia with hypercalciuria and nephrocalcinosis. *Kidney International* **47**, 1419–1425.

Praga, M. *et al.* (1998). Association of thin basement membrane nephropathy with hypercalciuria, hyperuricosuria and nephrolithiasis. *Kidney International* **54**, 915–920.

Quinn, F. M. *et al.* (1998). Xanthogranulomatous pyelonephritis in childhood. *Archives of Diseases of Childhood* **81**, 483–486.

Restaino, I. *et al.* (1993). Nephrolithiasis, hypocitraturia, and a distal renal tubular acidification defect in type 1 glycogen storage disease. *Journal of Pediatrics* **122**, 392–396.

Reusz, G. S. *et al.* (1998). Sodium transport and bone mineral density in hypercalciuria with thiazide treatment. *Pediatric Nephrology* **12**, 30–34.

Rhee, B. K., Bretan, P. N., Jr., and Stoller, M. L. (1999). Urolithiasis in renal and combined pancreas/renal transplant recipients. *Journal of Urology* **161**, 1458–1462.

Roberts, J. P. and Atwell, J. D. (1989). Vesicoureteric reflux and urinary calculi in children. *British Journal of Urology* **64**, 10–12.

Robertson, W. G. *et al.* The changing pattern of the age at onset of urinary stone disease in the UK. In *Kidney Stones* (ed. I. Borghi, T. Meschi, A. Briganti, T. Schiani, and A. Novarini), pp. 165–168. Editoriale Bios: Corenza, 1999.

Rodman, J. S. *et al.* (1984). The effect of dietary protein on cystine excretion in patients with cystinuria. *Clinical Nephrology* **22**, 273–278.

Rodriguez, L. M. *et al.* (1995). Effect of a low sodium diet on urinary elimination of cystine in cystinuric children. *Nephron* **71**, 416–418.

Rodriguez-Soriano, J. and Vallo, A. (1994). Pathophysiology of the renal acidification defect present in the syndrome of familial hypomagnesaemia–hypercalciuria. *Pediatric Nephrology* **8**, 431–435.

Rodriguez-Soriano, J., Vallo, A., and Garcia-Fuentes, M. (1987). Hypomagnesaemia of hereditary renal origin. *Pediatric Nephrology* **1** (3), 465–472.

Rosenberg, L. E. *et al.* (1966). Cystinuria: biochemical evidence for three genetically distinct diseases. *Journal of Clinical Investigation* **45**, 365–371.

Rumsby, G., Weir, T., and Samuell, C. T. (1997). A semiautomated alanine : glyoxylate aminotransferase assay for the tissue diagnosis of primary hyperoxaluria type 1. *Annals of Clinical Biochemistry* **34**, 400–404.

Sahin, A. *et al.* (2000). Percutaneous nephrolithotomy in older children. *Journal of Pediatric Surgery* **35**, 1336–1338.

Samuel, M. *et al.* (2001). Xanthogranulomatous pyelonephritis in childhood. *Journal of Pediatric Surgery* **36**, 598–601.

Sarkissian, A. *et al.* (2001). Pediatric urolithiasis in Armenia: a study of 198 patients observed from 1991 to 1999. *Pediatric Nephrology* **16**, 728–732.

Schell-Feith, E. A. *et al.* (2000). Etiology of nephrocalcinosis in preterm neonates: association of nutritional intake and urinary parameters. *Kidney International* **58**, 2102–2110.

Schell-Feith, E. A. *et al.* (2001). Modulation of calcium oxalate monohydrate crystallization kinetics by urine of preterm neonates. *American Journal of Kidney Diseases* **38**, 1229–1234.

Schuster, T. G. *et al.* (2002). Ureteroscopy for the treatment of urolithiasis in children. *Journal of Urology* **167**, 1813–1816.

Senocak, M. E., Turken, A., and Buyukpamukcu, N. (1995). Urinary obstruction caused by factitious urethral stones: an amazing manifestation of Munchausen syndrome by proxy. *Journal of Pediatric Surgery* **30**, 1732–1734.

Short, A. and Cooke, R. W. (1991). The incidence of renal calcification in preterm infants. *Archives of Diseases of Childhood* **66**, 412–417.

Shukla, A. R. *et al.* (2001). Urolithiasis in the low birth weight infant: the role and efficacy of extracorporeal shock wave lithotripsy. *Journal of Urology* **165**, 2320–2323.

Sidhu, H. *et al.* (1998). Absence of Oxalobacter formigenes in cystic fibrosis patients: a risk factor for hyperoxaluria. *Lancet* **352**, 1026–1029.

Simmonds, H. A. *et al.* (1989). Purine enzyme defects as a cause of acute renal failure in childhood. *Pediatric Nephrology* **3**, 433–437.

Simon, D. B. *et al.* (1999). Paracellin-1, a renal tight junction protein required for paracellular Mg^{2+} reabsorption. *Science* **285**, 103–106.

So, N. P. *et al.* (2001). Normal urinary calcium/creatinine ratios in African-American and Caucasian children. *Pediatric Nephrology* **16**, 133–139.

Stephens, A. D. (1989). Cystinuria and its treatment: 25 years experience at St. Bartholomew's Hospital. *Journal of Inherited Metabolic Disease* **12**, 197–209.

Tekin, A. *et al.* (2000). A study of the etiology of idiopathic calcium urolithiasis in children: hypocitruria is the most important risk factor. *Journal of Urology* **164**, 162–165.

Tekin, A. *et al.* (2001). Ureteropelvic junction obstruction and coexisting renal calculi in children: role of metabolic abnormalities. *Urology* **57**, 542–545.

Toffolo, A. *et al.* (1997). Non-furosemide-related renal calcifications in premature infants with bronchopulmonary dysplasia. *Acta Paediatrica Japanonica* **39**, 433–436.

Toussaint, C. (1998). Pyridoxine-responsive PH1: treatment. *Journal of Nephrology* **11** (Suppl. 1), 49–50.

Turner, M. A., Goldwater, D., and David, T. J. (2000). Oxalate and calcium excretion in cystic fibrosis. *Archives of Diseases of Childhood* **83**, 244–247.

Vachvanichsanong, P. *et al.* (1995). Severe hyperphosphatemia following acute tumor lysis syndrome. *Medical and Pediatric Oncology* **24**, 63–66.

van Acker, K. J. *et al.* (1996). Hyperoxaluria with hyperglycolic aciduria not due to alanine : glyoxalate transferase defect: a novel type of hyperoxaluria. *Kidney International* **50**, 1747–1752.

Villanyi, K. K. *et al.* (2001). Short-term changes in renal function after extracorporeal shock wave lithotripsy in children. *Journal of Urology* **166**, 222–224.

Weinstein, D. A., Somers, M. J., and Wolfsdorf, J. I. (2001). Decreased urinary citrate excretion in type 1a glycogen storage disease. *Journal of Pediatrics* **138**, 378–382.

Wollin, T. A. *et al.* (1999). Holmium : YAG lithotripsy in children. *Journal of Urology* **162**, 1717–1720.

Woodhouse, C. R. and Lennon, G. N. (2001). Management and aetiology of stones in intestinal urinary reservoirs in adolescents. *European Urology* **39**, 253–259.

Wrong, O. M., Norden, A. G. W., and Feest, T. G. (1994). Dent's disease: a familial proximal renal tubular syndrome with low-molecular weight proteinuria, hypercalciuria, nephrocalcinosis, metabolic bone disease, progressive renal failure and a marked male predominance. *Quarterly Journal of Medicine* **87**, 473–493.

9

The patient with renal hypertension

9.1 The structure and function of blood vessels in the kidney

Karlhans Endlich

Branching pattern and wall structure

The renal vasculature displays a high level of organization reflecting the close relationship between structure and function in the kidney (Lemley and Kriz 1994; Dworkin and Brenner 1996). The branching pattern (Fig. 1) and the ultrastructure of renal vessels are specialized with respect to:

- the glomerular capillary network and its supply, where a high capillary pressure drives glomerular filtration;
- the peritubular capillaries, where massive reabsorption takes place;
- the renal medulla, where urine concentration is controlled by the countercurrent system.

Last, but not the least, the renal vessels supply the metabolic needs of the kidney tissue. However, the high tissue perfusion of the kidney by far exceeds its metabolic demands. The vascular organization varies to a certain degree between species. The description presented in this chapter refers to the general pattern of the renal vasculature and includes pecularities of the human kidney.

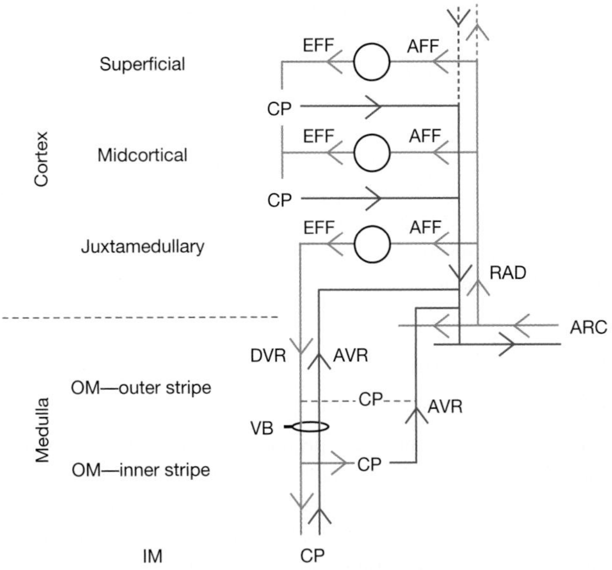

Fig. 1 Schematic drawing of the branching pattern of the renal vasculature. ARC, arcuate arteries or veins; RAD, cortical radial arteries or veins; AFF, afferent arterioles; EFF, efferent arterioles; CP, capillary plexus; DVR, descending vasa recta; AVR, ascending vasa recta; VB, vascular bundles; OM, outer medulla; IM, inner medulla.

Each kidney is supplied by one renal artery. The renal artery branches at the hilus giving rise to the interlobar arteries which enter the renal parenchyma at the cortico-medullary border. Each interlobar artery undergoes further divisions into the arcuate arteries. These vessels are called arcuate arteries because they run along the cortico-medullary border resulting in an arch-like pattern.

Cortex

The next level of branching after the arcuate arteries yields the cortical radial arteries ('interlobular arteries' in the old but still frequently used nomenclature). The cortical radial arteries ascend radially from the arcuate arteries within the cortex. During their course through the cortex, the cortical radial arteries undergo several divisions and give rise to the afferent arterioles. Occasionally, an aglomerular branch of the cortical radial artery reaches the renal capsule at the kidney surface. The afferent arterioles of midcortical and superficial glomeruli originate exclusively from the cortical radial arteries, while the afferent arterioles of the juxtamedullary glomeruli frequently branch off at the level of the arcuate arteries.

The feeding vessel of the glomerulus, the afferent arteriole, branches into several primary capillaries from which the interconnected capillary network of the glomerular tuft is established. A detailed description of the glomerular capillary network can be found in Chapter 3.1. The glomerular capillary network is drained by the efferent arteriole which already forms within the glomerulus. While the efferent arterioles of midcortical and superficial glomeruli divide into the capillaries of the peritubular network of the cortex, the wider efferent arterioles of juxtamedullary glomeruli become the vasa recta supplying the renal medulla.

The peritubular capillaries form a dense meshwork around the tubules of the cortex. In the cortical labyrinth, where the convoluted parts of the proximal and distal tubules are located, peritubular capillaries form a round-meshed network. In the medullary rays, containing the straight parts of the tubules, a long-meshed network of peritubular capillaries is observed. Both capillary meshworks are fed by midcortical and superficial efferent arterioles in such a way that different efferent arterioles participate in the supply of one nephron.

The blood of the cortical capillaries is collected by venules which drain into the cortical veins. The cortical veins accompany the cortical radial arteries in the cortical labyrinth and empty into the arcuate veins. A part of the cortical capillary network is directly connected to the arcuate veins. In contrast to the arcuate arteries, which are end-arteries, the arcuate veins form true anastomosing arches. In humans, a second type of cortical veins has been described. These veins collect the blood of the outer cortex, and traverse the cortex from the surface to the cortico-medullary border, where they empty into the arcuate veins.

Medulla

The renal medulla is supplied by the efferent arterioles of the juxtamedullary glomeruli. As the juxtamedullary efferent arterioles enter the outer stripe, they branch into the descending vasa recta. Branches of the juxtamedullary efferent arterioles/descending vasa recta that feed true capillaries are sparse in the outer stripe. In contrast, a large part of descending vasa recta terminates in the inner stripe, where they form a dense round-meshed capillary plexus. The remainder of descending vasa recta reaches the inner medulla. Here, the descending vasa recta successively terminate in a less dense long-meshed capillary plexus, which supplies the inner medulla.

The blood of the capillaries in the renal medulla is collected by venous vessels: the ascending vasa recta. The ascending vasa recta which drain the capillary plexus of the inner medulla successively join—as they emerge—the descending vasa recta forming the vascular bundles. The vascular bundles traverse the outer medulla as compact anatomical structures. Ascending and descending vasa recta are arranged in a checkerboard pattern in vascular bundles. This countercurrent arrangement facilitates diffusional exchange between ascending and descending vasa recta, thereby minimizing dissipation of solutes from the inner medulla.

The capillary plexus of the inner stripe is drained by a second type of ascending vasa recta. These ascending vasa recta do not join the vascular bundles. Instead, they ascend in the interbundle spaces and traverse the outer stripe constituting the main 'capillaries' in this region. This type of ascending vasa recta possesses a large contact area with the tubules in the outer stripe. The close arrangement of ascending vasa recta and tubules is supported by a very scarce interstitium, which contrasts with the well-developed interstitium of the inner medulla. Both types of ascending vasa recta finally empty into the arcuate veins and into the distal part of the cortical veins.

Structure

The intrarenal arterial vessels up to the proximal part of the afferent arteriole are similar to the arteries and arterioles of the same size in other regions of the body. In the distal part of the afferent arteriole, the smooth muscle cells are replaced by the renin-secreting juxtaglomerular cells. Since the number of renin-positive cells in the afferent arteriole can vary considerably under experimental conditions, smooth muscle cells of the afferent arteriole are likely to transdifferentiate into renin-secreting cells and vice versa. Endothelial cells are coupled by gap junctions in the cortical radial artery and in the proximal afferent arteriole, whereas the coupling of the smooth muscle cells in these vessels appears to be sparse. However, myoendothelial contacts containing gap junctions are frequently observed in the cortical radial arteries and in the whole afferent and efferent arterioles.

The glomerular capillaries are lined with fenestrated endothelium, the fenestrae of which do not possess diaphragms. The continuous basement membrane is covered by pericyte-like cells called visceral glomerular epithelial cells or podocytes. For a detailed description of the structure of the glomerular capillaries, the reader is referred to Chapter 3.1. The efferent arterioles of superficial and midcortical glomeruli usually possess one layer of smooth muscle cells, which becomes more and more loose in the distal portions.

The peritubular capillaries are made up by a fenestrated endothelium. The fenestrae, which are closed by diaphragms, comprise about 50 per cent of the capillary surface area. The proteinaceous nature of the diaphragms is responsible for the high permeability of the peritubular capillaries for water and small hydrophilic solutes. The cortical veins, which drain the peritubular capillaries, retain the fenestrated capillary wall structure implicating some reabsorptive function. It is not before the arcuate veins that smooth muscle cells emerge poviding the arcuate veins with a regular venous vessel wall.

The efferent arterioles of the juxtamedullary glomeruli differ clearly from their cortical counterparts in that they possess two to four layers of smooth muscle cells. The smooth muscle cell layers are progressively lost as the efferent arterioles of the juxtamedullary glomeruli branch into the descending vasa recta. The descending vasa recta are still lined by a continuous endothelium, but smooth muscle cells are replaced by contractile pericytes. The capillary plexus of the inner stripe and the inner medulla are made up of an endothelium with fenestrae closed by diaphragms—like the peritubular capillaries in the cortex. The ascending vasa recta keep the fenestrated capillary structure of the capillary plexus.

Vessel innervation

The intrarenal arteries, the afferent and efferent arterioles, and the descending vasa recta are innervated by postganglionic sympathetic nerves. These nerves regulate vascular tone via the release of transmitters with noradrenaline being the main transmitter. Neuropeptide Y has been identified as a frequent cotransmitter. Vasoactive intestinal peptide and substance P have also been described as cotransmitters (DiBona and Kopp 1997).

Function of the renal vasculature

The kidneys receive more than 20 per cent of cardiac output corresponding to a renal blood flow (RBF) of about 1.0–1.2 l/min resulting in a tissue blood perfusion of about 4 ml/min/g. One human kidney contains about one million glomeruli, from which a mean single glomerulus blood flow (GBF) of about 500 nl/min can be calculated. Considering this high blood perfusion of the renal tissue and the low oxygen extraction of 7 per cent, it becomes immediately clear that meeting metabolic demands is not the central task of the renal vasculature. Instead, the main functions of the renal vasculature are to enable and to regulate:

- glomerular filtration;
- peritubular reabsorption;
- medullary urine concentration.

To accomplish these functions, specific hydrostatic pressures have to be maintained in the different capillary networks of the kidney.

In the glomerular capillaries, the hydrostatic pressure ranges from 40 to 60 mmHg under physiological conditions as measured in various animal species. For filtration to occur, glomerular capillary pressure has to exceed the sum of the capillary oncotic pressure ($\approx$20 mmHg) and the hydrostatic pressure in Bowman's space ($\approx$12 mmHg), which is needed to push the filtrate and finally the urine through the tubular system into the renal pelvis. The unusual high hydrostatic pressure in the glomerular capillaries largely exceeds the sum of the two counteracting pressures (≈32 mmHg), preventing the filtration equilibrium being reached too early along the glomerular capillaries. In addition, the extremely high blood flow in the glomerular capillaries further ascertains that filtration proceeds practically along the whole length of the glomerular capillaries, without reaching filtration equilibrium too early, thereby maximizing the glomerular filtration rate (GFR).

The situation is completely opposite in the peritubular capillaries. Here, the capillaries should take up what is reabsorbed by the tubules (mainly water and sodium chloride). Accordingly, hydrostatic pressures in peritubular capillaries range between 10 and 15 mmHg—well below the oncotic pressure, which has considerably increased to about 35 mmHg at the beginning of the peritubular network due to glomerular filtration. Though difficult to measure, the hydrostatic pressure in the interstitium is thought to be close to 0 mmHg. As a result of extensive branching, flow velocity in peritubular capillaries is low, allowing the exploitation of the net inward filtration force until filtration equilibrium is reached.

Glomerular filtration

The regulation of glomerular filtration is the central task of the renal vasculature (Maddox and Brenner 1996). To understand the importance of the renal vessels for the regulation of GFR, one has to consider the determinants of GFR. Single nephron GFR (SNGFR) depends on the ultrafiltration coefficient (K_f) and on the mean effective filtration pressure ($\langle p_{eff} \rangle$)

$$\text{SNGFR} = K_f \cdot \langle p_{eff} \rangle$$

The ultrafiltration coefficient K_f is the product of the filtration surface area (S) and the hydraulic permeability (k): $K_f = S \cdot k$. The hydraulic permeability (k) of glomeruli (20–30 nl/min/mmHg/mm^2) is one to three orders in magnitude higher than the hydraulic permeability of continuous capillaries. By micropuncture of glomerular capillaries, it was demonstrated that the ultrafiltration coefficient K_f can change in response to physiologically relevant stimuli. However, it remains still unsettled whether changes in the ultrafiltration coefficient K_f are brought about by variation of the filtration surface area or by variation of hydraulic permeability or both. Mesangial contraction has been claimed to be able to reduce filtration area. On the other hand, changes in the molecular structure of the podocyte slit diaphragm may be able to alter hydraulic permeability. Recent progress in elucidating the molecular equipment of podocyte foot processes will shed light on the regulation of the ultrafiltration coefficient K_f (cf. Chapter 3.1).

On the other hand, the regulation of the mean effective filtration pressure $\langle p_{eff} \rangle$ is well understood. The mean effective filtration pressure $\langle p_{eff} \rangle$ is calculated by integrating the effective filtration pressure p_{eff} along the length coordinate of the capillaries. One obtains the effective filtration pressure by subtracting the capillary oncotic pressure and the hydrostatic pressure in Bowman's space from the capillary hydrostatic pressure. Because the capillary oncotic pressure increases along the capillaries due to filtration, which leaves the plasma proteins behind, effective filtration pressure decreases progressively. To obtain the mean effective filtration pressure $\langle p_{eff} \rangle$, the effective filtration pressure p_{eff} therefore has to be integrated over the length coordinate of the capillaries. As it has already been outlined above, both capillary hydrostatic pressure and blood flow affect the driving force for filtration directly, or indirectly by changing the rapidity with which filtration equilibrium is approached. Thus, the mean effective filtration pressure $\langle p_{eff} \rangle$ and consequently SNGFR are functions of glomerular capillary pressure and blood flow. Due to the variation of oncotic pressure along the capillaries necessitating the integration of the effective filtration pressure, SNGFR does not linearly depend on glomerular pressure and blood flow. However, it can be noted that elevating glomerular capillary pressure or glomerular capillary blood flow both increase SNGFR, with the former usually having the stronger impact on SNGFR.

Given the predominant dependence of GFR on glomerular capillary pressure and blood flow, the pivotal role of the renal vasculature in the regulation of GFR becomes obvious. The principal capacity to regulate glomerular haemodynamics resides in the pre- and postglomerular arterial and arteriolar vessels according to their wall structure. Most likely, the glomerular capillaries do not participate in the regulation of glomerular haemodynamics. This is because the glomerular capillaries form a branched and interconnected network, offering many parallel flow channels which considerably reduce haemodynamic resistance. Though it is almost impossible to measure the pressure drop along the glomerular capillaries—and this has never been done—pressure is believed to fall only by a few mmHg during the passage of blood through the glomerulus.

To facilitate the understanding of the regulation of glomerular haemodynamics by the renal vasculature, all resistances of the vessels from the renal artery down to the afferent arteriole can by lumped together in the preglomerular vascular resistance (R_{pre}). The postglomerular vascular resistance (R_{post}) mainly depends on the efferent arteriole. The peritubular capillaries and the venous vessels can be neglected in the regulation of glomerular haemodynamics, since their wall structure is not suited to actively regulate the lumen diameter to a substantial degree. Under conditions of stable systemic blood pressure, GBF depends on the total vascular resistance which is the sum of the pre- and postglomerular vascular resistances. On the other hand, the ratio between the postglomerular and total vascular resistances determines glomerular pressure (p_{glom}).

$$\text{GBF depends on: } R_{pre} + R_{post}$$
$$p_{glom} \text{ depends on: } R_{post}/(R_{pre} + R_{post})$$

Pre- and postglomerular vascular resistances can be adjusted independently from each other, which results in a spectrum of combinations to regulate GBF and p_{glom} under conditions of constant or varying systemic blood pressure. Special cases of changes in pre- and postglomerular vascular resistances are presented in Fig. 2, illustrating the regulation of glomerular haemodynamics by renal vessels. Pre- and postglomerular vascular resistances are controlled via the luminal diameter of the respective vessels. For example, a homogenous vasodilation of renal vessels by 10 per cent will increase GBF by 46 per cent, according to Hagen's and Poiseuille's law. Thus, small diameter changes are sufficient to powerfully regulate renal haemodynamics and GFR.

The postglomerular vascular resistance is controlled by the efferent arteriole, whereas the preglomerular vascular resistance is composed of resistances of several vessels. It is not evident a priori whether diameter changes in different vessels affect preglomerular vascular resistance to the same extent. Whether a given preglomerular vessel has the potential to importantly participate in the regulation of preglomerular vasclar resistance depends on its contribution to basal preglomerular vascular resistance. To illustrate this fact, let us assume that the

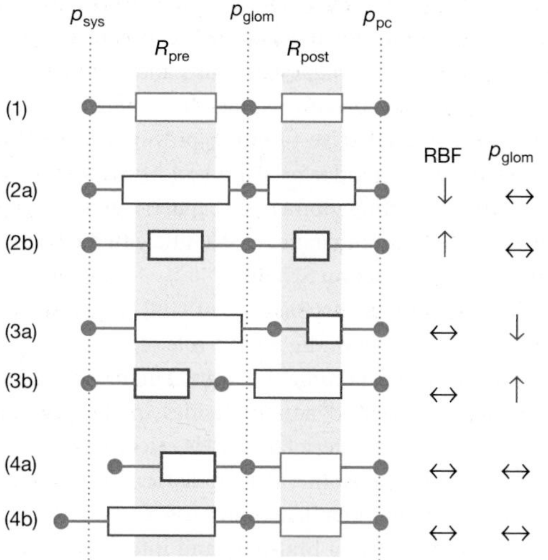

Fig. 2 Regulation of renal haemodynamics by pre- and postglomerular vascular resistances. The regulation of renal blood flow (RBF) and glomerular capillary pressure (p_{glom}) by preglomerular vascular resistance (R_{pre}) and by postglomerular vascular resistance (R_{post}) is illustrated. (1) Baseline condition. (2) Proportionally equal changes in pre- and postglomerular resistances affect RBF, while p_{glom} remains unchanged; (2a) vasoconstriction; (2b) vasodilation. (3) Shifting a part of resistance between pre- and postglomerular vessels without changing total vascular resistance selectively affects p_{glom}, while RBF remains constant; (3a) preglomerular vasoconstriction and postglomerular vasodilation; (3b) preglomerular vasodilation and postglomerular vasoconstriction. (4) If systemic blood pressure (p_{sys}) varies, RBF and p_{glom} will be maintained by appropriate changes in preglomerular resistance; (4a) fall in blood pressure and preglomerular vasodilation; (4b) rise in blood pressure and preglomerular vasoconstriction. Peritubular capillary pressure (p_{pc}) is assumed to be constant in all examples. ↑—increase; ↓—decrease; ↔—no change.

afferent arteriole would contribute 50 per cent to preglomerular vascular resistance under basal conditions. Isolated constriction of the afferent arteriole by 16 per cent would increase its resistance by 100 per cent, leading to an increase of preglomerular vascular resistance by 50 per cent (because we assumed that only half of the preglomerular vascular resistance were caused by the afferent arteriole). If the afferent arteriole contributed only 10 per cent to preglomerular vascular resistance, the same constriction by 16 per cent would increase preglomerular vascular resistance by 10 per cent only. Thus, it is essential to know the contribution of the different preglomerular vessels to preglomerular vascular resistance.

The pressure profile in the preglomerular vasculature provides information on how much each vessel contributes to preglomerular vascular resistance. Unfortunately, in the intact kidney, the preglomerular vessels are almost inaccessible to direct pressure measurements by micropuncture. Applying the stop flow technique, a few indirect measurements have been performed in rare branches of the cortical radial artery to the kidney surface and in superficial efferent arterioles in the rat. From these measurements, a pressure of 60–85 mmHg in the distal interlobular artery was inferred (Källskog *et al.* 1976; Boknam *et al.* 1981). Calculations based on data obtained in vascular casts indicate that a significant pressure drop may already occur in interlobar and arcuate arteries (Endlich *et al.* 1993). Thus, most likely all preglomerular vessels contribute to preglomerular vascular resistance. In particular, the contribution of the afferent arteriole to preglomerular vascular resistance may not exceed 50 per cent. A continuous fall in intravascular pressure along the precapillary vessels was observed in various organs, in which direct micropuncture measurements can be performed.

Peritubular reabsorption

At the beginning of this section where intravascular pressures have been considered, it has already been mentioned that several factors guarantee massive reabsorption in the peritublar capillaries: low hydrostatic pressure, high oncotic pressure, and low flow velocity due to extensive branching. The fenestrated endothelium in the peritubular capillaries further facilitates the reabsorption of water and solutes. Fenestrae in the endothelium are closed by diaphragms preventing leakage of plasma proteins into the interstitium, but also limiting the hydraulic permeability. Values of about 0.6 nl/min/mmHg/mm^2 for the hydraulic permeability (k) of peritubular capillaries were reported.

The reabsorption in the peritubular capillaries plays a crucial role for balancing glomerular filtration and reabsorption in the proximal tubule. A detailed balance between glomerular filtration and proximal tubular reabsorption helps to deliver a constant load to distal tubules, maintaining the optimal working range for water and salt regulatory processes in the distal tubule and collecting duct. Two mechanisms participate in the delivery of a constant load to distal tubules: the tubuloglomerular feedback (TGF), which does not involve peritubular capillaries, and the glomerular–tubular balance. The glomerular–tubular balance describes the phenomenon that an increase in GFR results in enhanced proximal tubular and peritubular capillary reabsorption. Fluid reabsorption is a two-step process, the first step being tubular transepithelial transport, and the second being transport from the interstitium into the peritubular capillary. Since an increase in GFR further augments protein concentration in peritubular capillaries, the increased capillary osmotic pressure enhances peritubular capillary reabsorption from the interstitium. However, the oncotic pressure of the peritubular blood also regulates a fraction of the fluid reabsorption across the epithelium—a mechanism that is not well understood. The means by which hormones and other mechanisms regulate the permeability of peritubular capillaries remains largely unknown.

Medulla

The renal medulla receives only 10–15 per cent of the total RBF. Notwithstanding, medullary blood flow plays a crucial role in the urinary concentrating mechanism due to the countercurrent arrangement of descending and ascending vasa recta in the vascular bundles. This anatomical arrangement of vasa recta prevents the loss of solutes from the medulla, helping to maintain osmotic gradients. At the same time, oxygen and nutrients are unable to enter the inner medulla in relevant amounts, because they rapidly diffuse from descending into ascending vasa recta. Thus, the special architecture of the medullary microcirculation accounts for the special metabolic situation and the high ischaemic vulnerability of the renal medulla. Changes in medullary blood flow alter osmotic gradients influencing the concentrating ability. An increase in medullary blood flow leads to wash-out of solutes from the interstitium, which in turn results in natriuresis. The homeostatic mechanism of 'pressure natriuresis' is thought to be mediated by generating natriuresis via proportional elevation of medullary blood flow as renal perfusion pressure increases.

Diameter changes of juxtamedullary efferent arterioles and of descending vasa recta control medullary blood independently from cortical blood flow. Many vasoactive hormones act on the vascular smooth muscle cells of juxtamedullary efferent arterioles and/or on the contractile pericytes of descending vasa recta. Especially the endocrine hormones arginine vasopressin and angiotensin II (ANGII) are potent constrictors of juxtamedullary efferent arterioles and descending vasa recta (Navar *et al.* 1996; Pallone and Silldorff 2001). In addition, medullary blood flow is regulated by many paracrine hormones (Navar *et al.* 1996; Pallone and Silldorff 2001), including adenosine, bradykinin, endothelin, and nitric oxide (NO). Renal medullary interstitial cells are a rich source of many paracrine vasoactive hormones.

Regulation of vasomotor tone

The renal vasculature plays a dominant role in the regulation of GFR, as described in the previous section. Changes of vasomotor tone in pre- and postglomerular vessels result in vasodilation or vasoconstriction, controlling glomerular pressure and flow (Maddox and Brenner 1996; Arendshorst and Navar 1997). Vasomotor tone of renal vessels is afffected by various mechanisms, some of which are kidney-specific:

- endocrine hormones;
- transmitter release from renal nerves;
- paracrine hormones generated mainly by endothelial and epithelial cells (including mediators of the TGF);
- autocrine hormones generated by vascular smooth muscle cells;
- haemodynamic forces (transmural pressure gradient and shear stress);
- signal transmission between cells in the vessel wall via gap junctions.

Our knowledge about the regulation of renal vasomotor tone stems mainly from animal experiments performed not only in rats, but also in dogs, rabbits, and increasingly in mice, because of the transgenic technology. While the renal vasculature had to be treated as a 'black box' in clearance, flowmeter, and micropuncture experiments, in the 1980s several models were developed allowing to directly access the renal vasculature (Navar *et al.* 1996; Steinhausen and Endlich 1996):

- isolated renal microvessels (cortical radial arteries, afferent, and efferent arterioles);
- the split hydronephrotic kidney, in which the whole renal vasculature can be visualized *in vivo* or *in vitro*;
- the *in vitro* perfused juxtamedullary nephron preparation.

In addtion, more recent progress in isolation and culture of vascular smooth muscle cells from preglomerular arterioles and small arteries further adds to our understanding of the cellular mechanisms regulating vasomotor tone and growth in the renal vasculature (Dussaule *et al.* 1989; Dubey *et al.* 1992; Endlich *et al.* 2000).

Cell–cell coupling in the renal vessel wall

It has already been described that endothelial and smooth muscle cells are coupled by gap junctions in pre- and postglomerular vessels (cf. 'Branching pattern and wall structure'). Gap junctions are formed by pairs of connexons, each connexon being a hexamer of connexins (Cx). Three connexins of the 13-member family are typically detected in vessels: Cx37, Cx40, and Cx43. While Cx43 localizes mainly to vascular smooth muscle cells, endothelial cells may express a combination of all three connexins. In the kidney, endothelial cells and predominantly smooth muscle cells in arteries and arterioles show immunoreactivity for Cx43 (Barajas *et al.* 1994; Hillis *et al.* 1997). Along the preglomerular vessels, Cx43 expression decreases in the afferent arterioles (Barajas *et al.* 1994). Cx40 is abundantly expressed in the endothelium of preglomerular vessels including the proximal portion of the afferent arteriole, but significantly less in the distal portion of the afferent arteriole (Hwan Seul and Beyer 2000). Interestingly, the renin-secreting cells in the juxtaglomerular portion of the afferent arteriole express Cx40, which is otherwise absent from smooth muscle cells in renal vessels. Finally, Cx37 has also been detected in the endothelium preferentially of larger preglomerular vessels (Arensbak *et al.* 2001). From these results, it appears that endothelial, smooth muscle, and renin-secreting cells are distinctly coupled, with a generally reduced coupling in the afferent arteriole. However, since the afferent arterioles possess only one layer of smooth muscle cells, signals may be as effectively transmitted in afferent arterioles as in larger preglomerular vessels.

Gap junctions permit small molecules, such as ions and second messengers, to diffuse from cell to cell. Thus, local changes in membrane potential or local changes in concentrations of second messengers may be propagated via gap junctions along renal vessels or within the renal vessel wall. Indeed, electrically induced vasomotor responses (constriction or dilation) are propagated in cortical radial arteries and in afferent arterioles, decaying exponentially with a length constant of around 150–400 μm (Steinhausen *et al.* 1997). Using microapplication of KCl to the distal afferent arteriole, upstream propagation of vasoconstriction with a length constant of 300 μm was observed (Wagner *et al.* 1997). The propagation of vasomotor responses in renal vessels may serve different functions:

- uniform vasoconstriction in response to focal release of transmitters from renal nerve varicosities;
- upstream propagation of the vasomotor response elicited by the TGF in the juxtaglomerular portion of the afferent arteriole;
- integration of spatially separated vasomotor changes in response to various nerval, humoral, and mechanical signals.

In addition, gap junctions functionally couple the endothelium and the smooth muscle layer in renal vessels. This allows signals originating in the endothelium to be transmitted to smooth muscle cells and vice versa. In this regard, gap junctions have been proposed to underly the vasodilation induced by the endothelium-derived hyperpolarizing 'factor' (EDHF). The renal acetycholine-induced vasodilation in the presence of inhibitors of NO and prostaglandin synthesis has recently been shown to be partially inhibited or to be abolished by disruption of gap junctions, utilizing small peptides homologous to the extracellular loop of Cx43 or Cx40, respectively (De Vriese *et al.* 2002). Moreover, gap junctions mediate a basal vasodilator tone in renal vessels, since intrarenal administration of gap-junction-disrupting peptides results in vasoconstriction (De Vriese *et al.* 2002).

Wall tension—myogenic response

Increases in renal perfusion pressure are not associated with proportional increases in RBF, as it would be expected for a rigid tube. In contrast, RBF remains quite constant despite changes in perfusion pressure within the range 80–180 mmHg. This phenomenon has been termed 'renal autoregulation'. To maintain constant RBF when perfusion pressure increases, renal vascular resistance must increase by the same proportion as perfusion pressure. Constriction of preglomerular vessels is responsible for the increase in renal vascular resistance (Steinhausen *et al.* 1990). Two mechanisms participate in the autoregulatory increase of preglomerular vascular resistance: a kidney-specific mechanism, the TGF (see below), and an intrinsic vascular mechanism, which is encountered in many vascular beds. In the case of the intrinsic vascular mechanism, called the 'myogenic response' or 'Bayliss effect', vasoconstriction is directly triggered by the increase in luminal pressure. The myogenic response of vessels is independent of an intact endothelium (Navar *et al.* 1996). Vascular smooth muscle cells sense the intraluminal pressure (or more precisely, the difference between intraluminal and interstitial hydrostatic pressure) through changes in wall tension. At the cellular level, mechano-sensitive proteins transduce the mechanical signal into a chemical or electrical one.

On the basis of several recent publications, the following signalling cascade of mechano-transduction in smooth muscle cells of preglomerular vessels has emerged (Fig. 3). Since Gd^{3+}, which is an inhibitor of stretch-activated cation channels, blocks the myogenic response in afferent arterioles and distal cortical radial arteries, a stretch-activated cation channel is most likely the sensor of wall tension (Takenaka *et al.* 1998a,b). In other organs, integrins, being the transmembranous link of extracellular matrix and the cytoskeleton, have been implicated in the myogenic response. However, RGD peptides, which mimic the binding sites of extracellular matrix proteins to integrins, induced constriction in isolated afferent arterioles, but did not interfere with myogenic vasoconstriction (Yip and Marsh 1997). In addition to stretch-activated cation channels, activation of phospholipase C (PLC) and release of Ca^{2+} from intracellular stores has been demonstrated to be involved in the pressure-induced contraction of afferent arterioles (Inscho *et al.* 1998). While stretch-activated channels may play a pivotal role in afferent arterioles and distal cortical radial arteries, activation of PLC appears to be crucially involved in mediating the myogenic response in preglomerular vessels upstream of the proximal cortical radial artery (Takenaka *et al.* 1998b). However, it remains unclear whether PLC is directly activated by mechanical force or whether PLC lies downstream of the actual mechanosensor.

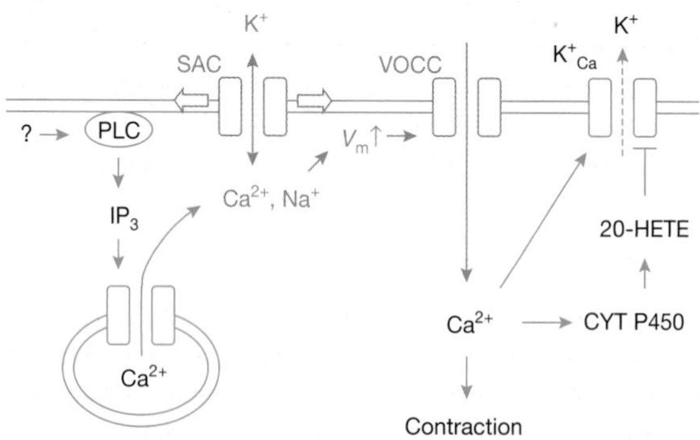

Fig. 3 Signalling pathway of myogenic vasoconstriction in preglomerular vascular smooth muscle. SAC, stretch-activated cation channel; VOCC, voltage-operated Ca^{2+} channel; K^+_{Ca}, Ca^{2+}-activated K^+ channel; PLC, phospholipase C; IP_3, inositoltrisphosphate; V_m, membrane potential; 20-HETE, 20-hydroxyeicosatetraenoic acid; CYT P450, cytochrome P450. The main pathway is shown in magenta. ⟶ release, formation, or activation; ⊣ inhibition.

Influx of Ca^{2+} and Na^+ through stretch-activated cation channels depolarizes smooth muscle cells opening L-type voltage-operated Ca^{2+} channels (Takenaka *et al.* 1998a). The depolarization of the membrane potential and the increase in intracellular Ca^{2+} in response to increased transmural pressure have been measured in isolated preglomerular vessels (Harder *et al.* 1987; Yip and Marsh 1996). Ca^{2+} influx through L-type voltage-operated Ca^{2+} channels is an obligate step in preglomerular myogenic constriction (Navar *et al.* 1996), indicating that Ca^{2+} influx through stretch-activated cation channels as well as Ca^{2+} release from intracellular stores is not sufficient to elicit vasoconstriction. The increase in intracellular Ca^{2+} concentration then activates the myosin light chain (MLC) kinase via calmodulin, resulting in enhanced vasomotor tone.

20-HETE (20-hydroxyeicosatetraenoic acid), an ω-hydroxylation product of arachidonic acid catalyzed by the cytochrome P450 enzyme family CYP 4A, plays an important role in the myogenic response (Roman 2002). Inhibitors of the formation of 20-HETE block the myogenic response of preglomerular vessels (Roman 2002). 20-HETE is endogenously produced by smooth muscle cells after an increase in intracellular Ca^{2+}. Once formed, 20-HETE increases smooth muscle tone by reducing the open-probability of Ca^{2+}-activated K^+ channels, which would otherwise limit depolarization-induced Ca^{2+} influx in a negative-feedback loop (Roman 2002).

Shear stress

Shear stress, which is exerted by the blood stream on the endothelial surface, regulates endothelial autacoid production and gene transcription. Augmentation of shear stress leads to vasodilation through the release of prostaglandins, NO, and an EDHF in many non-renal vascular preparations. That shear stress modulates renal vasomotor tone has been demonstrated in only a few studies. Increasing blood viscosity *in vivo* or perfusate viscosity *in vitro* does not decrease RBF, demonstrating vasodilation of the renal vasculature in response to elevated shear stress (Chen *et al.* 1989; Endlich *et al.* 1999). Shear stress-induced vasodilation in isolated perfused rat kidneys is mediated by NO and non-NO/non-prostanoid compound(s), suggesting shear stress-induced release of EDHF in renal vessels (Endlich *et al.* 1999). Furthermore, shear stress importantly modulates the myogenic response and the ANGII induced vasoconstriction in renal vessels via endothelium-derived NO (Juncos *et al.* 1995; Juncos *et al.* 1996; Endlich *et al.* 1999). The sensor(s) and signalling cascade(s) in the endothelium of renal vessel, which trigger the release of autocoids, are unknown.

Tubuloglomerular feedback

More than 30 years ago, Schnermann and coworkers presented the first direct evidence that the distal tubular NaCl load is able to regulate GFR. This coupling of tubular salt load and GFR was termed tubuloglomerular feedback. In the classical and still used approach to measure the response characteristics of TGF, tubular flow is interrupted at the level of the proximal tubule. The late proximal tubule is perfused with artificial solution allowing to vary the flow rate and the composition of tubular fluid that will reach the macula densa. Proximal to the interruption, SNGFR or tubular stop flow pressure, which reflects glomerular capillary pressure, are measured. With increasing late proximal flow rate, raising NaCl delivery to the macula densa, SNGFR gradually declines. The fall in SNGFR will reduce the filtered amount of NaCl, and would thus decrease the NaCl delivery to the distal tubule, if the proximal tubule were not interrupted. Thus, TGF constitutes a negative-feedback loop at the single-nephron level that aims to keep the NaCl load constant in the distal tubule in face of fluctuations in SNGFR. The TGF appears not to exert a tonic influence on SNGFR. Alterations in the sodium balance lead to changes in GFR, which are accompanied by a 'resetting' of the TGF, in such a way as to maintain maximal sensitivity of the TGF around the new set point of GFR. Thus, TGF most likely buffers SNGFR fluctuations that occur on a time scale of less than 1 hour (Schnermann *et al.* 1998).

The following concept as to how TGF works has evolved during the last decades of intense research (Navar *et al.* 1996; Schnermann and Briggs 2000) (Fig. 4). The macula densa cells sense the luminal NaCl load via a mechanism that depends on the Na^+–K^+–$2Cl^-$ cotransporter. Subsequent to the activation of the luminal sensing mechanism, an intracellular signalling cascade is thought to be activated, leading to the formation of a vasoactive substance. However, the intracellular signalling cascade is poorly defined, but could involve an increase in intracellular Ca^{2+} concentration. On the other hand, considerable evidence has been obtained in recent studies that adenosine is the diffusible mediator of the TGF (Thomson *et al.* 2000; Brown *et al.* 2001; Sun *et al.* 2001; Ren *et al.* 2002). Thus, increased NaCl transport in macula densa cells augments their metabolic activity leading to enhanced formation of adenosine, which diffuses to the afferent arteriole and

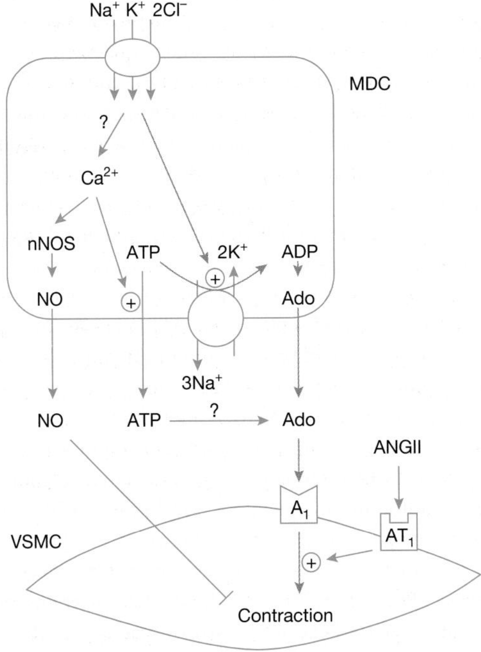

Fig. 4 Signalling pathway of tubuloglomerular feedback (TGF). Signal transduction starts at the luminal side of macula densa cells (MDC) with NaCl transport by the Na^+–K^+–$2Cl^-$cotransporter. Increasing concentrations of adenosine (Ado) in the basolateral compartment of MDC and diffusion to vascular smooth muscle cells (VSMC) of the afferent arteriole trigger vasoconstriction. nNOS, neuronal NO synthase; A_1, adenosine A_1 receptor; AT_1, ANGII AT_1 receptor. The main pathway is shown in magenta. ⟶ release, formation, or activation; ⊣ inhibition.

elicits vasoconstriction via adenosine A_1 receptors. In keeping with this hypothesis, TGF efficiency is significantly compromised, if adenosine A_1 receptors or 5′-nucleotidase are blocked (Thomson *et al.* 2000; Ren *et al.* 2002), or if adenosine activity is clamped by combining 5′-nucleotidase inhibition and A_1 receptor stimulation by a fixed amount of agonist (Thomson *et al.* 2000). Moreover, the TGF response is absent in adenosine A_1 receptor knock-out mice (Brown *et al.* 2001; Sun *et al.* 2001). ATP, which constricts the afferent arteriole through purinergic receptors, has also been suggested as a mediator of TGF (Navar 1998). However, the adenosine A_1 receptor knock-out mice clearly demonstrate that ATP cannot substitute for adenosine receptor deficiency.

There are several important modulators of the TGF response (Navar *et al.* 1996; Schnermann and Briggs 2000). Among these modulators, ANGII and NO play a dominant role. Adenosine needs the presence of ANGII in the juxtaglomerular portion of the afferent arteriole to induce A_1 receptor-mediated constriction. Consequently, the TGF response is absent in knock-out mice lacking the ANGII AT_1 receptor or the angiotensin I converting enzyme (Schnermann *et al.* 1997; Traynor *et al.* 1999). TGF in these knock-out mice can be restored by exogenous application of a constant amount of ANGII. However, the molecular mechanism underlying the interaction between adenosine and ANGII remains unclear. Because of the presence of renin in the juxtaglomerular portion of the afferent arteriole and the availability of all other components of the renin–angiotensin system in the kidney, ANGII is likely to be generated at the juxtaglomerular apparatus. Thus, during volume-depleted states the increased renin and ANGII activity will enhance the TGF response, whereas volume-expanded states will render TGF almost inactive. NO is generated in a Ca^{2+}-dependent manner by the neuronal NO synthase in macula densa cells. NO strongly attenuates the TGF response, and acute blockade of NO enhances the TGF response. Since NO production is increased by high salt intake, the attenuation of TGF by NO should facilitate sodium excretion. However, the TGF response remains unaltered if macula densa-derived NO is chronically absent in neuronal NO synthase knock-out mice (Vallon *et al.* 2001).

By securing a constant NaCl delivery to the distal tubule, the TGF response is a salt-conserving mechanism. However, the adenosine A_1 receptor knock-out mice, in which the TGF response is absent, exhibit neither any deviations in volume homeostasis nor changes in GFR. This finding indicates that TGF is dispensable for volume homeostasis under physiological conditions. However, it will be interesting to see if TGF is required to achieve maximum sodium reabsorption under conditions of restricted salt access.

Autoregulation of GBF and GFR

As it has already been described above (cf. 'Wall tension—myogenic response'), the renal autoregulation maintains RBF/GBF at a constant level in the face of fluctuations of renal perfusion pressure between 80 and 180 mmHg. Moreover, in the same pressure range, GFR/SNGFR are also kept constant by the same autoregulatory mechanisms. Given that the ultrafiltration coefficient (K_f) remains unchanged, SNGFR can be kept constant only if, besides GBF, glomerular capillary pressure (p_{glom}) is not altered by changes in renal perfusion pressure. Only preglomerular vascular resistance changes to adjust total renal vascular resistance in such a way as to keep RBF constant for a given renal perfusion pressure [cf. Fig. 2 (4a and b)]. As long as RBF remains constant, the pressure drop along the postglomerular vessels, which are not involved in the autoregulatory response, stays the same, and hence glomerular capillary pressure remains unchanged.

Both the myogenic response and TGF participate in renal autoregulation. The myogenic response in preglomerular vessels is triggered by changes in transmural pressure (cf. 'Wall tension—myogenic response'). The controlled variable of the TGF is the distal NaCl load (cf. 'Tubuloglomerular feedback'). However, before the autoregulatory mechanism is activated, an increase in renal perfusion pressure elevates GFR (via increasing GBF and glomerular capillary pressure), augmenting the delivery of NaCl to the distal tubule. Therefore, an increase in renal perfusion pressure activates the TGF, which in turn results in constriction of the afferent arteriole. Thus, the TGF is able to participate in renal autoregulation, though it does not directly sense any haemodynamic parameter.

There is a long-standing debate as to the individual contribution of the myogenic response and the TGF to renal autoregulation. It has become clear that both mechanisms are needed to account for the almost perfect autoregulation of RBF and GFR in the intact kidney (Navar *et al.* 1996). Using the juxtamedullary nephron preparation, in which both mechanisms are operative, an almost equal participation of both mechanisms could be demonstrated (Navar 1998). In contrast, in the hydronephrotic kidney, in which the tubular system has undergone complete degeneration, the myogenic response perfectly autoregulates GBF in the absence of TGF (Steinhausen *et al.* 1997). It will be interesting to study renal autoregulation in the adenosine A_1 receptor knock-out mice, which possess no TGF. An exact dissection of the two processes in the autoregulatory response is however difficult, because the two mechanisms interact. Constriction of the distal portion of the afferent arteriole by the TGF mechanism increases luminal pressure in the upstream vessels, evoking a myogenic response. Moreover, the myogenic and TGF responses are likely to be conducted along the preglomerular vessels (cf. 'Cell–cell coupling in the renal vessel wall'). Finally, the efficiency of the myogenic response and TGF appear to be pressure-dependent, with the myogenic response being more activated at higher pressures.

Typically, fluctuations in renal perfusion pressure occur over a broad range of time scales. Breathing and the heart beat produce the stongest variations in blood pressure with a time period of about 5 and 1 s, respectively. However, blood pressure fluctuates considerably also on longer time scales of minutes and hours. Because renal autoregulation rests on two different mechanisms, it becomes evident that the efficiency of renal autoregulation depends on the time scale under consideration. Contraction of vascular smooth muscle after activation in response to membrane stretch will only take several seconds. In contrast, to activate the TGF response, the pulse wave of increased GFR has to travel along the whole length of Henle's loop (this takes more than 20 s in rats), before it can be sensed at the macula densa. In response to a step decrease in renal perfusion pressure, a time-dependent recovery of RBF (autoregulation) has been observed consistent with the activation characteristics of the myogenic response and TGF (Walker *et al.* 2000; Just *et al.* 2001).

Pressure fluctuations arising from the heart beat can only be dampened by the passive wall properties of the vessels. Renal autoregulation starts to reduce the amplitude of pressure fluctuations that are slower than 10 s (Holstein-Rathlou and Marsh 1994). Due to the time which is necessary to activate the myogenic response or TGF, oscillations in renal perfusion pressure, occurring with a similar period as the activation time, result in amplified—instead of dampened—oscillations in RBF (pressure falls at the same time when the myogenic response or the TGF just respond with vasoconstriction to the prior activation by increased pressure). Resonance frequencies in the dynamic autoregulation of RBF around 0.2 Hz (~1/5 s) and 0.04 Hz (~1/25 s) have been measured, corresponding to the myogenic response and TGF, respectively (Holstein-Rathlou and Marsh 1994). Though pressure fluctuations arising from heart beat are too fast to be dampened by the myogenic response, recent results demonstrate that these pressure fluctuations, however, increase preglomerular vessel tone (Loutzenhiser *et al.* 2002), thereby reducing the transmission of peak pressures into glomerular capillaries.

Hormones

A wealth of hormones affects the tone of renal vessels. Renal vasoactive hormones have been the subject of several extensive reviews (Steinhausen *et al.* 1990; Navar *et al.* 1996; Steinhausen and Endlich 1996; Navar 1998), and will therefore only be briefly discussed in this section. By integrating the constrictory and/or dilatory actions on the different pre- and postglomerular vessel segments, one obtains the net effect of specific vasoactive hormones on RBF and GFR. It has to be kept in mind that, in the case of paracrine and autocrine hormones, the sites of hormonal action are largely determined by the fact where the hormone is produced or released, though sometimes receptors may be present in practically all vessel segments.

Endocrine, renally vasoactive hormones include adrenaline, ANGII, arginine vasopressin, atrial natriuretic peptide (ANP), and probably parathyroid hormone. ANP is unique in its capability to increase GFR through preglomerular vasodilation combined with efferent arteriolar constriction. Paracrine hormones are mainly released by three cell types: axon terminals of autonomic neurones, endothelial cells, and tubular epithelial cells. Excitation of renal nerves results mainly in the release of noradrenaline and NPY. The renal vascular endothelium is known to produce many potent vasoactive compounds including arachidonic acid metabolites (e.g. prostaglandins, thromboxane A_2), C-type natriuretic peptide, endothelin, EDHF, and NO. Because of the close anatomical relationship between vessels and tubules, tubular epithelial cells are a rich source of vasoactive hormones, comprising adenosine, arachidonic acid metabolites, ATP, bradykinin, dopamine, parathyroid hormone-related protein, and urodilatin—the renal natriuretic peptide. Since all elements of the renin–angiotensin system are expressed within the kidney, ANGII is thought to act as a paracrine renal hormone in addition to its endocrine mode of action. Vascular smooth muscle cells themselves generate vasoactive hormones which may act in an autocrine manner (e.g. arachidonic acid metabolites, parathyroid hormone-related protein). Besides the typical vasoactive hormones, growth factors may also exert important effects on renal vasomotor tone. Recently, it has been shown that the epidermal gowth factor modulates ANGII-induced vasoconstriction in the afferent arteriole (Carmines *et al.* 2001).

Signal transduction of hormone-induced vasoconstriction in renal vessels

Over the recent years, the intracellular signalling pathways that mediate renal constriction in response to vasoactive substances have been elucidated in increasing detail. Evidence has been accumulated that signal transduction mechanisms triggering agonist-induced vasomotor responses are fundamentally different between preglomerular vessels and efferent arterioles. While transduction of constriction in preglomerular vessels is similar to that observed in arteries and arterioles of other vascular beds, the transduction in the efferent arteriole is quite special. The importance of understanding the constrictory signalling cascades in renal vessels resides in the possibility to selectively block these pathways with pharmacological agents in the future. Instead of antagonizing the constriction induced by one hormone, blockade of intracellular signalling pathways offers the power to inhibit constriction in response to a whole class of hormones, which acts through a specific pathway. Ca^{2+} antagonists are a well-known example of a therapeutic agent which interferes with a specific signal transduction mechanism.

The main pathways transducing hormone binding into contraction are shown in Figs 5 and 6 for preglomerular vessels and for efferent arterioles, respectively. Already, the expression of myosin heavy chain isoforms differs between preglomerular vessels and efferent arterioles (Kimura *et al.* 1995); the functional role is however unknown. Contraction of smooth muscle is induced through phosphorylation of the regulatory MLC. The level of MLC phosphorylation and hence the degree of contraction is regulated by two enzymes, MLC kinase and MLC phosphatase (Pfitzer 2001). MLC kinase activity is stimulated by an increase of intracellular Ca^{2+}. Thus, the regulation of intracellular Ca^{2+} plays a crucial role for contraction. Regarding MLC phosphatase, considerable progress has been made in recent years in identifying pathways that induce contraction via the inhibition of MLC phosphatase activity (Pfitzer 2001).

The key difference in the constrictory signalling pathway between preglomerular vessels and efferent arterioles concerns the Ca^{2+} influx pathway. While Ca^{2+} enters preglomerular vascular smooth muscle cells (VSMC) through voltage-operated Ca^{2+} channels (VOCCs) of the L-, T-, and P-types (Hansen *et al.* 2000, 2001), in efferent arterioles Ca^{2+} passes through store-operated channels (SOCs) (Loutzenhiser and Loutzenhiser 2000). Thus, the regulation of the membrane potential plays a central role for Ca^{2+} influx in preglomerular vessels (Gordienko *et al.* 1994). Binding of vasoconstrictors to seven transmembrane receptors activates PLC (Takenaka *et al.* 1997), leads to production of inositoltrisphosphate (IP_3), and IP_3-mediated release of Ca^{2+} from intracellular stores. The Ca^{2+} released is of minor importance for prolonged contraction, but opens Cl^- channels which cause depolarization due to Cl^- efflux (Gordienko *et al.* 1994; Takenaka *et al.* 1996). VOCCs are gated by depolarization and Ca^{2+} enters the cell. Ca^{2+}-activated K^+ channels (K^+_{Ca}) limit Ca^{2+} influx via hyperpolarization, constituting a negative feedback loop (Gordienko *et al.* 1994). Furthermore, K^+_{Ca} channels can be directly activated by the EDHF, resulting in vasodilation. Since VOCCs are absent in efferent arterioles, EDHF-mediated vasodilation is only observed in preglomerular vessels (Wang and Loutzenhiser 2002). Besides vasoconstrictor hormones, the myogenic response, which is confined to preglomerular vessels, also elicits contraction via changes in membrane potential.

In efferent arterioles, the intracellular Ca^{2+} release leads to a depletion of intracellular stores, a process that triggers opening of SOCs. Depletion of intracellular stores blunts constriction of efferent arterioles demonstrating the relevance of this pathway (Imig *et al.* 2000). Furthermore, SOCs and possibly other non-selective cation channels, providing a route for Ca^{2+} entry in efferent arterioles, are known to be regulated by diacylglycerol and protein kinase C. Further studies are needed to clarify the role of the latter mechanisms in efferent arterioles.

Finally, binding of vasoconstrictors to seven transmembrane receptors can lead to activation of the small G protein RhoA. Activated

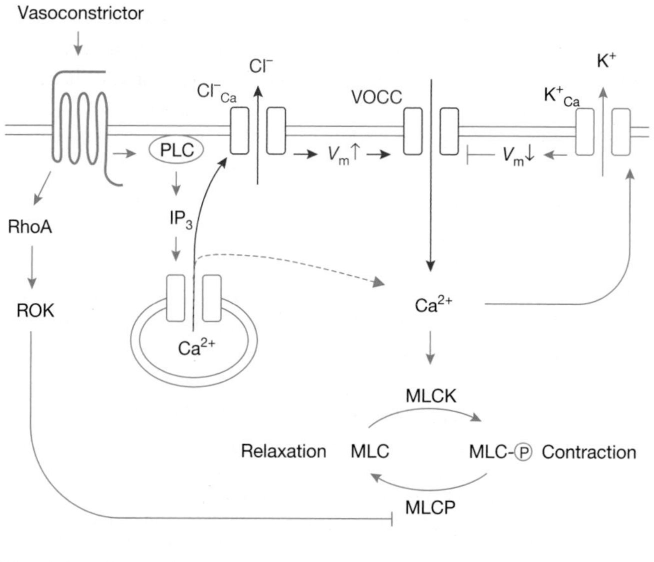

Fig. 5 Signalling pathway of vasoconstriction in preglomerular vessels. Signalling cascade of preglomerular vasoconstrictors that bind to G protein-coupled seven transmembrane receptors. Cl^-_{Ca}, Ca^{2+}-activated Cl^- channel; VOCC, voltage-operated Ca^{2+} channel; K^+_{Ca}, Ca^{2+}-activated K^+ channel; ROK, Rho kinase; PLC, phospholipase C; IP_3, inositoltrisphosphate; V_m, membrane potential; MLC, regulatory myosin light chain; MLCK, myosin light chain kinase; MLCP, myosin light chain phosphatase. The main pathway is shown in magenta. ⟶ release, formation, or activation; ⊣ inhibition.

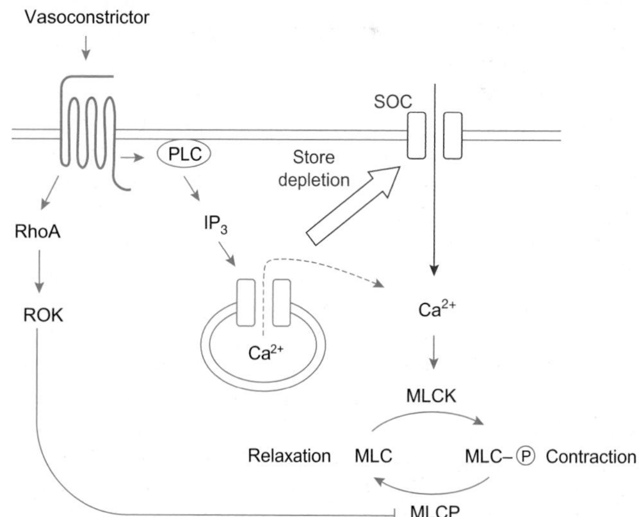

Fig. 6 Signalling pathway of vasoconstriction in efferent arterioles. Signalling cascade of efferent vasoconstrictors that bind to G protein-coupled seven transmembrane receptors. SOC, store-operated Ca^{2+} channel; ROK, Rho kinase; PLC, phospholipase C; IP_3, inositoltrisphosphate; MLC, regulatory myosin light chain; MLCK, myosin light chain kinase; MLCP, myosin light chain phosphatase. The main pathway is shown in magenta. ⟶ release, formation, or activation; ⊣ inhibition.

RhoA increases the activity of Rho kinase (ROK), which inactivates MLC phosphatase by phosphorylation (Pfitzer 2001). This pathway evokes contraction in the absence of changes in intracellular Ca^{2+}. ROK has been demonstrated to play an important role in the constriction of preglomerular vessels and efferent arterioles (Cavarape *et al.* 2003).

Renal vessels in kidney disease

The renal vasculature is involved in the development and progression of several forms of kidney disease. On the other hand, many pathological states of the kidney compromise renal vessel function perpetuating or aggravating renal malfunction. The following examples should illustrate the participation of renal vessels in pathological states.

Glomerular capillaries are exposed to rather high mechanical forces arising from glomerular flow and pressure. Glomerular hypertension is known to be an important determinant for the development of glomerular lesions and for the progression of glomerulosclerosis in humans (Bidani and Griffin 2002). The balance of vascular resistances between preglomerular vessels and efferent arterioles sets glomerular capillary pressure. Moreover, the myogenic constriction of preglomerular vessels prevents the undampened transmission of fluctuations of systemic blood pressure into the glomerulus. Accordingly, dysbalance of pre- and postglomerular vascular resistances and defects in the myogenic response have been demonstrated to precede the onset of glomerular damage in diabetic rats, in DOCA/salt hypertensive rats, and in fawn-hooded rats—a genetic model of focal segmental glomerulosclerosis (van Dokkum *et al.* 1999; Bidani and Griffin 2002; van Rodijnen *et al.* 2002). Thus, the renal vasculature may play a primary role in the pathogenesis of glomerulosclerosis.

Reduction of renal mass also results in an augmented haemodynamic load in glomerular capillaries (Bidani and Griffin 2002). The hypertrophied glomeruli of remnant kidneys are prone to glomerulosclerosis due to the altered haemodynamics. By mechanisms that are not well understood, glomerular blood flow and pressure increase, elevating SNGFR, in an effort to maintain total GFR despite the substantial loss of nephrons. Shear stress-induced vasodilation appears to be an indispensable mechanism in the adaptation of the kidney to acute ablation of renal mass, as demonstrated by lethality of 3/4 nephrectomy in vimentin knock-out mice which exhibit an impaired shear stress-dependent vasodilation in renal vessels (Terzi *et al.* 1997).

Renal vessels are the site where leucocytes and platelets adhere, releasing vasoactive substances and eventually transmigrating into the tissue. While leucocytes roll and adhere in glomerular and peritubular capillaries as well as in venules, platelets interact also with the arterial endothelium. Cell adhesion molecules represent a promising target for the treatment of various kidney diseases (Rosenkranz and Mayadas 1999). Mediators released in inflammation (e.g. serotonin, leukotrienes, thromboxane) induce constriction preferentially in larger preglomerular vessels, that is interlobar and arcuate arteries (Steinhausen and Endlich 1996). Constriction of large preglomerular vessels shuts down RBF in all regions of the kidney, eventually leading to acute renal failure. Understanding of signalling mechanisms which are specific to larger preglomerular vessels will allow to target large vessel constrictions in renal disease.

In addition to changes in vasomotor tone, growth processes of VSMC control vessel function by altering vascular geometry. Genetic disposition, exposure to specific growth factors, and changes in wall tension due to chronic dilation/constriction or changes in intravascular pressure result in remodelling of the vessel wall. VSMC proliferation is responsible for the progessive narrowing of large preglomerular vessels in chronic rejection of renal transplants (Shaikewitz and Chan 1994). Furthermore, arcuate arteries in spontaneously hypertensive rats exhibit an increase in wall thickness at a time when blood pressure is still normal (Smeda *et al.* 1988). In addition, afferent arteriolar narrowing is a predictor of the development of hypertension in the F2 generation of a cross of spontaneously hypertensive and normotensive rats (Mulvany 2002). Thus, dysregulation of VSMC growth in the renal vasculature could participate in the development of arterial hypertension. Interestingly, cultured VSMC of large preglomerular vessels possess different growth characteristics as compared to aortic VSMC (Endlich *et al.* 2000). Moreover, tubular epithelial cells produce a variety of growth factors that may link vessel structure to tubular function. Growth factor receptors may therefore represent an attractive target for the treatment of renal vascular dysfunction.

References

Arendshorst, W. J. and Navar, L. G. Renal circulation and glomerular hemodynamics. In *Diseases of the Kidney* 6th edn. (ed. R. W. Schrier and C. W. Gottschalk), pp. 59–106. Boston: Little Brown and Company, 1997.

Arensbak, B., Mikkelsen, H. B., Gustafsson, F., Christensen, T., and Holstein-Rathlou, N. H. (2001). Expression of connexin 37, 40, and 43 mRNA and protein in renal preglomerular arterioles. *Histochemistry and Cell Biology* **115**, 479–487.

Barajas, L., Liu, L., and Tucker, M. (1994). Localization of connexin43 in rat kidney. *Kidney International* **46**, 621–626.

Bidani, A. K. and Griffin, K. A. (2002). Long-term renal consequences of hypertension for normal and diseased kidneys. *Current Opinion in Nephrology and Hypertension* **11**, 73–80.

Boknam, L., Ericson, A. C., Aberg, B., and Ulfendahl, H. R. (1981). Flow resistance of the interlobular artery in the rat kidney. *Acta Physiologica Scandinavica* **111**, 159–163.

Brown, R., Ollerstam, A., Johansson, B., Skott, O., Gebre-Medhin, S., Fredholm, B., and Persson, A. E. (2001). Abolished tubuloglomerular feedback and increased plasma renin in adenosine A_1 receptor-deficient mice. *American Journal of Physiology Regulatory, Integrative and Comparitive Physiology* **281**, R1362–R1367.

Carmines, P. K., Fallet, R. W., Che, Q., and Fujiwara, K. (2001). Tyrosine kinase involvement in renal arteriolar constrictor responses to angiotensin II. *Hypertension* **37**, 569–573.

Cavarape, A., Endlich, N., Assaloni, R., Bartoli, E., Steinhausen, M., Parekh, N., and Endlich, K. (2003). Rho kinase inhibition blunts vasoconstriction mediated through distinct signaling pathways *in vivo*. *Journal of the American Society of Nephrology* **14**, 37–45.

Chen, R. Y., Carlin, R. D., Simchon, S., Jan, K. M., and Chien, S. (1989). Effects of dextran-induced hyperviscosity on regional blood flow and hemodynamics in dogs. *American Journal of Physiology* **256**, H898–H905.

De Vriese, A. S., Van de Voorde, J., and Lameire, N. H. (2002). Effects of connexin-mimetic peptides on nitric oxide synthase- and cyclooxygenase-independent renal vasodilation. *Kidney International* **61**, 177–185.

DiBona, G. F. and Kopp, U. C. (1997). Neural control of renal function. *Physiological Review* **77**, 75–197.

Dubey, R. K., Roy, A., and Overbeck, H. W. (1992). Culture of renal arteriolar smooth muscle cells. Mitogenic responses to angiotensin II. *Circulation Research* **71**, 1143–1152.

Dussaule, J. C., Bea, M. L., Baud, L., Ronco, P., Chansel, D., Helwig, J. J., and Ardaillou, R. (1989). Effects of bradykinin on prostaglandin synthesis and cytosolic calcium in rabbit subcultured renal cortical smooth muscle cells. *Biochimica et Biophysica Acta* **1005**, 34–44.

Dworkin, L. D. and Brenner, B. M. The renal circulations. In *The Kidney* 5th edn. (ed. B. M. Brenner), pp. 247–285. Philadelphia: W.B. Saunders Company, 1996.

Endlich, K., Kuhn, R., and Steinhausen, M. (1993). Visualization of serotonin effects on renal vessels of rats. *Kidney International* **43**, 314–323.

Endlich, K., Muller, C., Barthelmebs, M., and Helwig, J. J. (1999). Role of shear stress in nitric oxide-dependent modulation of renal angiotensin II vasoconstriction. *British Journal of Pharmacology* **127**, 1929–1935.

Endlich, N., Endlich, K., Taesch, N., and Helwig, J. J. (2000). Culture of vascular smooth muscle cells from small arteries of the rat kidney. *Kidney International* **57**, 2468–2475.

Gordienko, D. V., Clausen, C., and Goligorsky, M. S. (1994). Ionic currents and endothelin signaling in smooth muscle cells from rat renal resistance arteries. *American Journal of Physiology. Renal Physiology* **266**, F325–F341.

Hansen, P. B., Jensen, B. L., Andreasen, D., Friis, U. G., and Skott, O. (2000). Vascular smooth muscle cells express the α_{1A} subunit of a P-/Q-type voltage-dependent Ca^{2+} channel, and it is functionally important in renal afferent arterioles. *Circulation Research* **87**, 896–902.

Hansen, P. B., Jensen, B. L., Andreasen, D., and Skott, O. (2001). Differential expression of T- and L-type voltage-dependent calcium channels in renal resistance vessels. *Circulation Research* **89**, 630–638.

Harder, D. R., Gilbert, R., and Lombard, J. H. (1987). Vascular muscle cell depolarization and activation in renal arteries on elevation of transmural pressure. *American Journal of Physiology* **253**, F778–F781.

Hillis, G. S., Duthie, L. A., Mlynski, R., McKay, N. G., Mistry, S., MacLeod, A. M., Simpson, J. G., and Haites, N. E. (1997). The expression of connexin 43 in human kidney and cultured renal cells. *Nephron* **75**, 458–463.

Holstein-Rathlou, N. H. and Marsh, D. J. (1994). Renal blood flow regulation and arterial pressure fluctuations: a case study in nonlinear dynamics. *Physiological Review* **74**, 637–681.

Hwan Seul, K. and Beyer, E. C. (2000). Heterogeneous localization of connexin40 in the renal vasculature. *Microvascular Research* **59**, 140–148.

Imig, J. D., Cook, A. K., and Inscho, E. W. (2000). Postglomerular vasoconstriction to angiotensin II and norepinephrine depends on intracellular calcium release. *General Pharmacology* **34**, 409–415.

Inscho, E. W., Cook, A. K., Mui, V., and Imig, J. D. (1998). Calcium mobilization contributes to pressure-mediated afferent arteriolar vasoconstriction. *Hypertension* **31**, 421–428.

Juncos, L. A., Garvin, J., Carretero, O. A., and Ito, S. (1995). Flow modulates myogenic responses in isolated microperfused rabbit afferent arterioles via endothelium-derived nitric oxide. *The Journal of Clinical Investigation* **95**, 2741–2748.

Juncos, L. A., Ren, Y., Arima, S., Garvin, J., Carretero, O. A., and Ito, S. (1996). Angiotensin II action in isolated microperfused rabbit afferent arterioles is modulated by flow. *Kidney International* **49**, 374–381.

Just, A., Ehmke, H., Toktomambetova, L., and Kirchheim, H. R. (2001). Dynamic characteristics and underlying mechanisms of renal blood flow autoregulation in the conscious dog. *American Journal of Physiology. Renal Physiology* **280**, F1062–F1071.

Kallskog, O., Lindbrom, L. O., Ulfendahl, H. R., and Wolgast, M. (1976). Hydrostatic pressures within the vascular structures of the rat kidney. *Pflügers Archive: European Journal of Physiology* **363**, 205–210.

Kimura, K. *et al.* (1995). Diversity and variability of smooth muscle phenotypes of renal arterioles as revealed by myosin isoform expression. *Kidney International* **48**, 372–382.

Lemley, K. V. and Kriz, W. Structure and function of the renal vasculature. In *Renal Pathology with Clinical and Functional Correlations* 2nd edn. (ed. C. C. Tisher and B. M. Brenner), pp. 981–1026. Philadelphia: J.B. Lippincott Company, 1994.

Loutzenhiser, K. and Loutzenhiser, R. (2000). Angiotensin II-induced Ca^{2+} influx in renal afferent and efferent arterioles: differing roles of voltage-gated and store-operated Ca^{2+} entry. *Circulation Research* **87**, 551–557.

Loutzenhiser, R., Bidani, A., and Chilton, L. (2002). Renal myogenic response: kinetic attributes and physiological role. *Circulation Research* **90**, 1316–1324.

Maddox, D. A. and Brenner, B. M. Glomerular ultrafiltration. In *The Kidney* 5th edn. (ed. B. M. Brenner), pp. 286–333. Philadelphia: W.B. Saunders Company, 1996.

Mulvany, M. J. (2002). Small artey remodeling and significance in the development of hypertension. *News in Physiological Sciences* **17**, 105–109.

Navar, L. G. (1998). Integrating multiple paracrine regulators of renal microvascular dynamics. *American Journal of Physiology. Renal Physiology* **274**, F433–F444.

Navar, L. G., Inscho, E. W., Majid, S. A., Imig, J. D., Harrison-Bernard, L. M., and Mitchell, K. D. (1996). Paracrine regulation of the renal microcirculation. *Physiological Review* **76**, 425–536.

Pallone, T. L. and Silldorff, E. P. (2001). Pericyte regulation of renal medullary blood flow. *Experimental Nephrology* **9**, 165–170.

Pfitzer, G. (2001). Regulation of myosin phosphorylation in smooth muscle. *Journal of Applied Physiology* **91**, 497–503.

Ren, Y., Arima, S., Carretero, O. A., and Ito, S. (2002). Possible role of adenosine in macula densa control of glomerular hemodynamics. *Kidney International* **61**, 169–176.

Roman, R. J. (2002). P-450 metabolites of arachidonic acid in the control of cardiovascular function. *Physiological Review* **82**, 131–185.

Rosenkranz, A. R. and Mayadas, T. N. (1999). Leukocyte-endothelial cell interactions—lessons from knockout mice. *Experimental Nephrology* **7**, 125–136.

Schnermann, J. and Briggs, J. P. Function of the juxtaglomerular apparatus: control of glomerular hemodynamics and renin secretion. In *The Kidney: Physiology and Pathophysiology* 3rd edn. (ed. D. W. Seldin and G. Giebisch), pp. 945–980. Philadelphia: Lippincott Williams and Wilkins, 2000.

Schnermann, J. B., Traynor, T., Yang, T., Huang, Y. G., Oliverio, M. I., Coffman, T., and Briggs, J. P. (1997). Absence of tubuloglomerular feedback responses in AT_{1A} receptor-deficient mice. *American Journal of Physiology. Renal Physiology* **273**, F315–F320.

Schnermann, J., Traynor, T., Yang, T., Arend, L., Huang, Y. G., Smart, A., and Briggs, J. P. (1998). Tubuloglomerular feedback: new concepts and developments. *Kidney International* **67** (Suppl.), S40–S45.

Shaikewitz, S. T. and Chan, L. (1994). Chronic renal transplant rejection. *American Journal of Kidney Diseases* **23**, 884–893.

Smeda, J. S., Lee, R. M., and Forrest, J. B. (1988). Structural and reactivity alterations of the renal vasculature of spontaneously hypertensive rats prior to and during established hypertension. *Circulation Research* **63**, 518–533.

Steinhausen, M. and Endlich, K. (1996). Controversies on glomerular filtration from Ludwig to the present. *Pflügers Archive: European Journal of Physiology* **432** (Suppl.), R73–R81.

Steinhausen, M., Endlich, K., and Wiegman, D. L. (1990). Glomerular blood flow. *Kidney International* **38**, 769–784.

Steinhausen, M., Endlich, K., Nobiling, R., Parekh, N., and Schütt, F. (1997). Electrically induced vasomotor responses and their propagation in rat renal vessels *in vivo*. *The Journal of Physiology* **505**, 493–501.

Sun, D., Samuelson, L. C., Yang, T., Huang, Y., Paliege, A., Saunders, T., Briggs, J., and Schnermann, J. (2001). Mediation of tubuloglomerular feedback by adenosine: evidence from mice lacking adenosine 1 receptors. *Proceedings of the National Academy of Sciences USA* **98**, 9983–9988.

Takenaka, T., Kanno, Y., Kitamura, Y., Hayashi, K., Suzuki, H., and Saruta, T. (1996). Role of chloride channels in afferent arteriolar constriction. *Kidney International* **50**, 864–872.

Takenaka, T., Suzuki, H., Fujiwara, K., Kanno, Y., Ohno, Y., Hayashi, K., Nagahama, T., and Saruta, T. (1997). Cellular mechanisms mediating rat renal microvascular constriction by angiotensin II. *Journal of Clinical Investigation* **100**, 2107–2114.

Takenaka, T., Suzuki, H., Okada, H., Hayashi, K., Kanno, Y., and Saruta, T. (1998a). Mechanosensitive cation channels mediate afferent arteriolar myogenic constriction in the isolated rat kidney. *The Journal of Physiology* **511**, 245–253.

Takenaka, T., Suzuki, H., Okada, H., Hayashi, K., Ozawa, Y., and Saruta, T. (1998b). Biophysical signals underlying myogenic responses in rat interlobular artery. *Hypertension* **32**, 1060–1065.

Terzi, F., Henrion, D., Colucci-Guyon, E., Federici, P., Babinet, C., Levy, B. I., Briand, P., and Friedlander, G. (1997). Reduction of renal mass is lethal in mice lacking vimentin. Role of endothelin-nitric oxide imbalance. *Journal of Clinical Investigation* **100**, 1520–1528.

Thomson, S., Bao, D., Deng, A., and Vallon, V. (2000). Adenosine formed by 5′-nucleotidase mediates tubuloglomerular feedback. *Journal of Clinical Investigation* **106**, 289–298.

Traynor, T., Yang, T., Huang, Y. G., Krege, J. H., Briggs, J. P., Smithies, O., and Schnermann, J. (1999). Tubuloglomerular feedback in ACE-deficient mice. *American Journal of Physiology. Renal Physiology* **276**, F751–F757.

Vallon, V., Traynor, T., Barajas, L., Huang, Y. G., Briggs, J. P., and Schnermann, J. (2001). Feedback control of glomerular vascular tone in neuronal nitric oxide synthase knockout mice. *Journal of the American Society of Nephrology* **12**, 1599–1606.

van Dokkum, R. P., Sun, C. W., Provoost, A. P., Jacob, H. J., and Roman, R. J. (1999). Altered renal hemodynamics and impaired myogenic responses in the fawn-hooded rat. *American Journal of Physiology. Regulatory Integrative and Comparitive Physiology* **276**, R855–R863.

van Rodijnen, W. F., van Lambalgen, T. A., Tangelder, G. J., van Dokkum, R. P., Provoost, A. P., and ter Wee, P. M. (2002). Reduced reactivity of renal microvessels to pressure and angiotensin II in fawn-hooded rats. *Hypertension* **39**, 111–115.

Wagner, A. J., Holstein-Rathlou, N. H., and Marsh, D. J. (1997). Internephron coupling by conducted vasomotor responses in normotensive and spontaneously hypertensive rats. *American Journal of Physiology. Renal Physiology* **272**, F372–F379.

Walker, M., III, Harrison-Bernard, L. M., Cook, A. K., and Navar, L. G. (2000). Dynamic interaction between myogenic and TGF mechanisms in afferent arteriolar blood flow autoregulation. *American Journal of Physiology. Renal Physiology* **279**, F858–F865.

Wang, X. and Loutzenhiser, R. (2002). Determinants of renal microvascular response to ACh: afferent and efferent arteriolar actions of EDHF. *American Journal of Physiology. Renal Physiology* **282**, F124–F132.

Yip, K. P. and Marsh, D. J. (1996). $[Ca^{2+}]_i$ in rat afferent arteriole during constriction measured with confocal fluorescence microscopy. *American Journal of Physiology. Renal Physiology* **271**, F1004–F1011.

Yip, K. P. and Marsh, D. J. (1997). An Arg-Gly-Asp peptide stimulates constriction in rat afferent arteriole. *American Journal of Physiology. Renal Physiology* **273**, F768–F776.

9.2 Clinical approach to hypertension

Alison L. Brown and Robert Wilkinson

Definition of hypertension

Blood pressure (BP) in the general population has a Gaussian distribution skewed towards the higher end, making it difficult to choose one value to separate normotension from hypertension. However, for practical clinical purposes, it is necessary to agree to a BP level above which treatment should be commenced, with the aim of reducing morbidity and mortality. The threshold level of BP at which to start antihypertensive treatment, and the target BP level to aim for, will vary depending on coexistent risk factors. As new evidence on the benefits of treatment of various levels of BP has accumulated, the definition of 'normal' and 'high' BP has altered over recent years. The most recent British Hypertension Society (BHS) guidelines for the management of hypertension recommend that treatment should be considered for those with BP greater than 140/90 mmHg depending on coexistent risk factors (Ramsay *et al.* 1999). If systolic pressure is greater than or equal to 160 mmHg or diastolic pressure greater than or equal to 100 mmHg in those under the age of 65 years, greater than or equal to 90 mmHg in those aged over 60 years, then treatment is indicated regardless of other risk factors.

The BHS guidelines recommend that all adults should have their BP measured routinely at least every 5 years till the age of 80 years. Those with high–normal (135–139/85–89 mmHg) or high readings at any time should have annual BP checks. A minimum of two measurements at several visits, using a properly validated and maintained device and correctly fitted cuff, should be used.

The Sixth Report of the Joint National Committee (JNC VI 1997) also defines hypertension as a systolic blood pressure (SBP) of 140 mmHg or greater and a diastolic blood pressure (DBP) of 90 mmHg or greater. The JNC go on to define an optimal BP as less than 120/80 mmHg, normal BP as less than 130/85 mmHg, and high normal as less than 139/89 mmHg. Hypertension is divided into three stages: stage 1, less than 159/99 mmHg; stage 2, less than 179/109 mmHg; and stage 3, greater than or equal to 180/110 mmHg.

Twenty-four-hour ambulatory monitoring

Twenty-four-hour ambulatory blood pressure monitoring (24-h ABPM) is now widely available and allows half hourly or hourly documentation of BP during normal daily activity outside hospital or clinics. The 24-h ABPM also documents diurnal variation of BP, the normal pattern being a decline of around 10 per cent during sleep. There is evidence that 24-h ABPM may allow better prediction of risk, with better correlation with target organ damage such as left ventricular hypertrophy, than clinic BP (Verdecchia *et al.* 1995).

Mean daytime ABPM levels are lower than equivalent clinic BP so thresholds for treatment are also lower; normal daytime ABPM is less than 135/85 mmHg, and normal overnight resting BP below 120/75 mmHg (Staessen *et al.* 1996).

The 24-h ABPM remains expensive and is inconvenient for the patient. It may be best reserved for those with suspected 'white coat' hypertension where clinic BP recordings are consistently greater than readings at other times, those with apparent drug resistant hypertension, or those with hypotensive symptoms whilst taking antihypertensive medication.

In addition, abnormalities in the usual circadian rhythm of BP are common in renal hypertension. Many authors have reported an attenuation in the usual nocturnal decrease in BP ('dipping') to a decrease of less than 10 per cent ('non-dipping') (Ritz *et al.* 2001). The proportion of non-dippers increases as renal function worsens, and is particularly high in endstage renal failure (ESRF), irrespective of the type of dialysis. ABP values are highly predictive of coronary and cerebrovascular morbidity and mortality in patients with essential hypertension (Khattar *et al.* 1999); as there is some evidence to suggest a relationship between nocturnal BP and renal disease progression as well as survival (Ritz *et al.* 2001), 24-h ABPM may be particularly useful in guiding therapy in patients with renal disease.

Prevalence of hypertension

Hypertension is common in all industrialized countries and tends to increase with age.

Using the JNC V criteria, 24 per cent, or an estimated 43 million, of the adult population of the United States had hypertension in the third National Health and Nutrition Examination Survey between 1988 and 1991 (Burt *et al.* 1995). The prevalence of hypertension increased from 4 per cent of those aged 18–34 years to 58.5 per cent of those aged 65–74 years (NHANES III; Joffres *et al.* 2001).

In 1990, a Scottish population survey showed that the 'rule of halves', first described some 20 years earlier, still applied. Half the men with BP greater than or equal to 160/95 mmHg had not previously been detected as hypertensive; half of those whose hypertension had been previously detected were untreated; and in half of those receiving treatment, BP was not controlled (Smith *et al.* 1990).

A more recent French study of a working population with a mean age of 39 years showed a prevalence of hypertension of 16 per cent in men and 9 per cent in women. In this survey, for 50 per cent of men with

BP greater than 140/90 mmHg, their hypertension was undetected; only one-fourth of those with detected hypertension were untreated, but only one-third of those on treatment had BP controlled by treatment. Figures were better for women, with three-fourths being aware of their hypertension, almost 9 out of 10 under treatment, but still only one out of two controlled by treatment (Lang *et al.* 2001). This compares to 25 per cent of American hypertensives treated and controlled (NHANES III) and 13 per cent in a Canadian survey (CHHS) (Joffres *et al.* 2001).

The Health Survey for England 1996 reported that mean SBP among 13,131 adults was 136 mmHg, mean DBP 75 mmHg. A total of 23 per cent of all adults in this survey had BP greater than 160 SBP, greater than 95 DBP, or were on antihypertensive treatment.

Among those with high BP, more than half (59 per cent) were receiving antihypertensive medication. Of those on treatment, 64 per cent had SBP less than 160 and DBP less than 95 mmHg.

The 1998 Health Survey, using the *new* definition of high BP of SBP greater than or equal to 140 and DBP greater than or equal to 90, or on medication, found the prevalence of high BP to be 40.8 per cent for men and 32.9 per cent for women (Health Survey for England 1998).

Renal disease and hypertension

Only a small proportion of all hypertensives have primary renal parenchymal disease, perhaps around 4 per cent (Berglund *et al.* 1976).

However, loss of functioning nephrons from whatever cause leads inevitably to salt and water retention and progressive hypertension, which accelerates the rate of decline of renal function. Good BP control is essential to slow this process and prevent an inexorable decline towards ESRF.

There is no doubt that malignant hypertension is a definite cause of endstage renal disease, but controversy continues as to whether uncomplicated hypertension can lead to ESRF. In 2000, 27 per cent of patients with new endstage renal disease in the United States were judged to have hypertension as the cause of their ESRF, second only to diabetes mellitus at 45 per cent (USRDS 2001). However, the diagnosis of 'hypertensive nephrosclerosis' may be based on clinical grounds with no biopsy confirmation, and may be inaccurate. A prospective study of 56 Caucasian patients clinically diagnosed as having hypertensive nephrosclerosis found that on renal biopsy only 48 per cent had histological confirmation of the diagnosis, while 35 per cent had atheromatous vascular disease (Zuccelli and Zuccala 1996).

In 1990 the, incidence of ESRF was assessed in the 332,544 men screened between 1973 and 1975 for entry to the Multiple Risk factor Intervention Trial (MRFIT), who were followed up for an average of 16 years. Both SBP and DBP were shown to be strong independent predictors of endstage renal disease. The relative risk of ESRF for those with a BP of greater than or equal to 210 mmHg systolic or greater than or equal to 120 mmHg diastolic, compared with those with BP less than 120 mmHg systolic and less than 80 mmHg diastolic, was 22.1 (Klag *et al.* 1996).

Treatment of hypertension in renal disease

Nephrologists have long realized that the final common pathway of progressive renal damage from whatever cause is loss of functioning nephrons leading to salt retention and/or increased renin secretion leading to hypertension. This systemic hypertension is probably associated with glomerular hypertension and proteinuria, possibly mediated by angiotensin II, which accompanies the necessary hyperfiltration by residual nephrons and leads to further nephron loss and a progressive decline in glomerular filtration rate (GFR). Aggressive BP control, usually requiring multiple drugs, has been the main aim. Recent evidence suggests that reduction of glomerular protein leakage by angiotensin converting enzyme (ACE) inhibition seems to provide additional renoprotection.

Optimal management for maximum renoprotection is not yet clearly established, but several strategies are available (Herbert *et al.* 2001).

Non-diabetic renal disease

The Modification of Diet in Renal Disease (MDRD) Study assessed rate of progression of renal disease and proteinuria in 840 patients with a variety of different chronic renal diseases, mostly with proteinuria of less than 1 g/24 h—insulin treated diabetics were excluded (Peterson *et al.* 1995).

Patients with higher baseline proteinuria had faster decline in GFR and greater benefits from BP control to a mean arterial pressure of 92 mmHg or less (equivalent to a BP of 125/75 mmHg or less). Achieving the low BP goal was associated with a significant reduction in proteinuria and a slower subsequent decline in GFR.

The AIPRI (ACE Inhibition in Progressive Renal Insufficiency) trial was a multicentre European trial of the effectiveness of the ACE inhibitor (ACEI) benazepril in protecting residual renal function (Maschio *et al.* 1999). Five hundred and thirty-eight patients with non-diabetic renal disease and mild (creatinine clearance 46–60 ml/min) to moderate (creatinine clearance 30–55 ml/min) renal failure were randomized to receive benazepril or placebo plus other antihypertensive agents, with a target DBP of less than 90 mmHg. The benazepril group had a 53 per cent relative risk reduction of reaching end points of doubling of serum creatinine or starting renal replacement therapy at 3 years. Benazepril was effective in slowing the rate of progression of renal disease in those with chronic glomerular disease and proteinuria greater than 1 g/24 h. No difference between the benazepril and placebo groups was seen in those with hypertensive glomerulosclerosis or interstitial nephritis or polycystic kidney disease. The protective effect of benazepril was associated with a reduction in BP (3.5–4 mmHg lower in the benazepril group) and proteinuria (proteinuria decreased by 29 per cent in the benazepril group and increased by 9 per cent in the placebo group). The protective effect of benazepril was greater in patients with proteinuria of more than 3 g/24 h than in those with proteinuria of 1–3 g/24 h at randomization.

The REIN (Ramipril Efficacy in Nephropathy) study (GISEN group 1997) randomized 352 patients with chronic non-diabetic nephropathy to ramipril or placebo plus conventional antihypertensive therapy targeted at achieving a DBP less than 90 mmHg. The patients were stratified according to baseline proteinuria; 1–3 g/24 h or greater than or equal to 3 g/24 h. Those with baseline proteinuria of greater than or equal to 3 g/24 h had a faster decline in GFR than those with baseline proteinuria of less than 3 g/24 h (0.67 versus 0.25 ml/min/month). In the group with proteinuria greater than or equal to 3 g/24 h, the ramipril treated group had a significantly lower decline in GFR per month than the placebo group (0.53 versus 0.88 ml/min) and the risk of doubling of serum creatinine or reaching ESRF was halved. In the ramipril group, the percentage reduction in proteinuria was inversely correlated with decline in GFR and predicted the reduction in risk of doubling of baseline creatinine or ESRF (18 ramipril versus 40 placebo). The benefits seemed to exceed the reduction expected for the slightly lower BP in the ramipril treated group, and the study investigators felt the effect was probably due at least in part to the effect of ACE on glomerular protein trafficking.

A total of 186 REIN study patients with between 1 and 3 g/24 h proteinuria were followed-up for a median of 31 months after randomization and a similar reduction in the risk of ESRF was found in the ramipril treated group (relative risk in the non-ramipril group 2.72), particularly among those with a GFR of less than 45 ml/min at baseline (Ruggenenti *et al.* 1999).

A meta-analysis of 11 randomized controlled trials of ACEI therapy in non-diabetic renal disease confirmed reduction in proteinuria, which is more marked in those with greatest proteinuria, and slowing of rate of progression (Jafar *et al.* 2001).

Furthermore, the Heart Outcomes Prevention Evaluation Study (HOPE) showed that ramipril reduced the risk of cardiovascular death, myocardial infarction (MI), and strokes in high-risk patients, again with only a modest decrease in BP (about 3 mm SBP and 2 mm DBP), which seemed too small to account for the significant benefits (The Heart Outcomes Prevention Evaluation Study Investigators 2000a,b). Since cardiovascular disease is the single largest cause of morbidity and mortality in patients with chronic renal disease, the HOPE Study data provide evidence for the use of ACEIs wherever possible in renal patients.

Not everyone seems to benefit equally from ACE inhibition; those with greater proteinuria and faster progression seem to benefit more, and those with DD genotype for the ACE gene seem to benefit least (Parving *et al.* 1996). The underlying renal diagnosis is also relevant; loss of renal function is not slowed by ACE inhibition in patients with polycystic disease (Maschio *et al.* 1999). There are also differences in ACEI effect in different ethnic groups; for example, ACE monotherapy is less effective in African-Americans than Caucasians, though ACEI should still be used when indicated (JNC VI 1997).

Diabetic renal disease and hypertension

Type 1 diabetes

There is evidence of a genetic predisposition to hypertension in the 30 per cent of type 1 diabetics who develop nephropathy.

The earliest sign of diabetic nephropathy in both type 1 and type 2 diabetics is the development of urinary albumin excretion rates above normal; this is called microalbuminuria, and defined as albumin excretion rates 20–200 μg/min or 30–300 mg/day. Several factors, including a high degree of hyperglycaemia and high arterial BP, have been shown to be risk factors for the progression of microalbuminuria to macroalbuminuria (>300 mg/day) and overt nephropathy.

Early studies demonstrated the value of aggressive BP control using a variety of different antihypertensive agents in slowing progression to macroalbuminuria and progressive decline in GFR (Mogenson 1982). Later studies confirmed that ACEIs have a beneficial effect on albumin excretion rate and on the rate of progression of renal impairment in established nephropathy in type 1 diabetes (Lewis *et al.* 1993); benefit was also demonstrated for normotensive type 1 diabetics (Parving *et al.* 1989).

A meta analysis of several trials showed that in microalbuminuric type 1 patients, progression to macroalbuminuria decreases by about one-third and regression to normoalbuminuria increases threefold (ACE Inhibitors in Diabetic Nephropathy Trialist Group 2001).

BHS guidelines currently recommend a threshold for treatment of BP in type 1 diabetics without evidence of nephropathy of 140/90 mmHg, and an optimal BP target of less than 140/80 mmHg. The target is lowered to 130/80 mmHg in type 1 diabetics with nephropathy and less than 125/75 mmHg when there is proteinuria of greater than 1 g/24 h (Ramsay *et al.* 1999).

More stringent guidelines for BP targets for diabetics are recommended by the International Society of Hypertension (ISH), which suggest optimal or normal BP, below 130/85 mmHg; the National Kidney Foundation (NKF), which suggest a target BP of 130/80 mmHg; and the American Diabetes Association (ADA), which suggest a target of less than 130/80 mmHg (WHO–ISH Guidelines 1999; Bakris *et al.* for the NKF Hypertension and Diabetes Executive Committees Working Group 2000; American Diabetes Association 2002).

Type 2 diabetes

Diabetic nephropathy develops in about 40 per cent of type 2 diabetics and is now the commonest cause of ESRF in the United States and Europe.

The UKPDS study showed that an achieved BP of 144/82 mmHg compared with 154/87 mmHg over a median 8.4 years of follow-up substantially reduced the risk of microvascular disease (retinopathy, vitreous haemorrhage, and renal failure) as well as stroke (though not MI) (Adler *et al.* 2000). BP control in this trial was obtained using a beta blocker or ACEI and then adding in a loop diuretic, calcium channel blocker, or vasodilator.

The effect of ramipril on diabetic nephropathy was evaluated in the MICRO-HOPE substudy of the Heart Outcomes Prevention Evaluation study (HOPE Study Investigators 2000). The majority of the 3577 diabetics included were type 2 diabetics; ramipril lowered the risk of overt nephropathy in those with and without baseline microalbuminuria.

More recently, the angiotensin II receptor blockers (ARBs) losartan and irbesartan have been shown in large-scale trials to reduce incidence of doubling of serum creatinine and ESRF in type 2 diabetics with nephropathy by about 25–30 per cent in comparison with an antihypertensive regime which did not include an ARB or ACEI (Brenner *et al.* 2001; Lewis *et al.* 2001).

This additional protection against progression of type 2 nephropathy by ARBs could not be explained by differences in achieved BP in the two treatment groups.

Furthermore, treatment with irbesartan was shown to reduce significantly the rate of progression from microalbuminuria to clinical albuminuria in hypertensive type 2 diabetics over a 2-year follow-up, independent of the effect on BP (Parving *et al.* 2001). These trials are discussed in more detail below.

Renal transplant recipients

Cardiovascular disease is the major cause of mortality in renal transplant recipients. In addition to strenuous efforts to control BP, other risk factors such as smoking and lipids must be tackled. In the past, ACEIs and ARBs have been used rather sparingly in these patients because of the fear of underlying renal artery stenosis, which occurs in about 5 per cent of patients, and of hyperkalaemia. In view of the high cardiovascular risk in these patients, and of the established benefits of

ACEIs and more recently ARBs (Dahlof *et al.* 2002) in cardiovascular prevention, it seems likely that the use of these drugs in renal transplant recipients will increase in the future.

Furthermore, in chronic graft dysfunction, proteinuria has been shown to correlate with worse transplant function and long-term survival (Hohage *et al.* 1997); reduction of proteinuria by ACE inhibition would be expected to slow progression of renal impairment as in primary renal disease.

Renal artery stenosis

Fibromuscular dysplasia

This is a collection of vascular diseases that predominantly affects females between the ages of 15 and 50 years, but accounts for less than 10 per cent of all cases of renal artery stenosis. The cause is unknown. Fibromuscular dysplasia (FMD), most commonly of the media, causes multiple narrowings usually of the distal two-thirds of the renal artery (Safian and Textor 2001); dilated segments in between give the characteristic appearance of a string of beads or string of sausages on arteriography. In addition, single stenoses may occur and differentiation from atheroma depends on the absence of other evidence of atheroma on angiography. Tissue for histology is rarely available.

Unlike atherosclerotic renovascular disease (ARVD), FMD rarely progresses to occlusion of the renal artery. It is important to diagnose since the results of intervention with angioplasty are very good with 'cure' rates for hypertension of about 50 per cent (Ramsay and Waller 1990); a further 40 per cent are improved by intervention.

Atherosclerotic renovascular disease

This is the cause of 90 per cent of cases of renal artery stenosis and usually involves the ostium and proximal third of the renal artery and perirenal aorta, usually as part of generalized atheromatous disease, especially aortoiliac disease (Safian and Textor 2001). It is more common in the elderly. It may present with renin-dependent hypertension, progressive renal impairment, or as part of generalized athero-embolic disease. More rarely, ARVD presents as recurrent pulmonary oedema out of proportion to underlying left ventricular dysfunction, known as 'flash' pulmonary oedema (Pickering *et al.* 1988). The mechanism is thought to be greatly increased proximal tubular absorption of sodium and water caused by a combination of a direct effect of angiotensin II on the sodium hydrogen pump in the proximal renal tubule and the effects of angiotensin-induced efferent arteriolar constriction causing increased oncotic pressure and reduced hydrostatic pressure in the peritubular capillaries.

ARVD is a common and progressive disease; previous reports suggest progressive stenosis in 51 per cent of renal arteries 5 years after diagnosis, and development of renal atrophy in 21 per cent of those with renal artery stenosis of more than 60 per cent (Safian and Textor 2001).

However, although percutaneous transluminal renal angioplasty with or without stenting is successful in correcting renal artery stenosis, results of intervention on hypertension or renal impairment have been disappointing (Isles *et al.* 1999). It seems likely that the underlying intrinsic renal damage established before intervention may progress despite improved perfusion. Furthermore, the increased mortality in patients with renovascular compared to essential hypertension is due largely to an increase in MI and stroke rather than to renal failure (Krumme and Mann 2001).

Table 1 Features suggestive of renal artery stenosis

Onset of hypertension before the age of 30 years, especially without a family history (fibromuscular dysplasia)
Sudden onset of significant hypertension after the age of 50 years (atheromatous RAS)
Sudden worsening of previously stable hypertension
Severe or resistant hypertension (uncontrolled despite three or more drugs)
Abdominal bruit
Evidence of other vascular disease, e.g. absent pulses, bruits
Smoker
'Flash' pulmonary oedema
Acute deterioration in renal function with ACEI or ARB therapy
Unexplained renal impairment, especially with normal urine dipstix

Three randomized controlled trials comparing intervention, usually by angioplasty, and medical treatment, have shown little difference in the outcome between the two approaches (Plouin *et al.* 1998; Webster *et al.* 1998; van Jaarsveld *et al.* 2000). However, these trials included rather small numbers of patients followed for a short period of time and treatment generally did not include stenting. Furthermore, these trials defined renal artery stenosis as a decrease in luminal diameter of 50 per cent or more, which may not be haemodynamically relevant; it is possible that intervention only for tighter stenoses may result in more favourable outcomes.

Therefore, the benefits of intervention, by aggressive medical management including the use of ACEIs or ARBs, in comparison to angioplasty with or without stenting, on progression of renal impairment or BP control, remain unclear. Several prospective randomized trials of drug therapy versus stenting are currently underway.

Features suggestive of an underlying diagnosis of renal artery stenosis are listed in Table 1.

Detection and assessment of renal hypertension

The major challenge is to identify the small number with underlying renal disease from the huge majority of essential hypertensives. This is important because specific therapy may be available for the underlying renal problem and drug choice may be different.

Clinical history

A full medical history, including detailed family history, diet, exercise, smoking, alcohol intake, and drug treatment (including over-the-counter medicines such as non-steroidal anti-inflammatory drugs, NSAIDs) should be taken. Generally, reliable clues to underlying disease do not arise in the history but certain features (Tables 1 and 2) may be useful in selecting patients for further investigation.

The combined oral contraceptive pill is responsible for the development of hypertension in some women. The mechanism of this

Table 2 Clinical assessment in renal hypertension: features indicating the need for further investigation

Past or family history of renal disease
Symptoms of renal dysfunction, e.g. nocturia
Proteinuria or haematuria
Prospect of future pregnancies
Features suggestive of renal artery stenosis as listed in Table 1

hypertension is not known but the oestrogen component seems the most important since hypertension has been observed less frequently once the oestrogen component is reduced, though it does still occur. When hypertension does occur with the low-dose oestrogen pill, the possibility of underlying renal disease should be considered. Hypertension induced by the oral contraceptive pill may take up to 3 months to settle after withdrawal of the treatment and may fail to settle in some women.

NSAIDs may also lead to an increase in BP in normotensive individuals as well as those with pre-existing hypertension and renal impairment. NSAIDs may also attenuate the antihypertensive effects of diuretics, beta blockers, vasodilators, and ACEIs, probably by the suppression of renal and extrarenal cyclo-oxygenase with inhibition of prostaglandin synthesis. It seems sensible to assess the response to withdrawal of these drugs if possible before embarking on extensive investigation.

Physical examination

A general physical examination is essential, with particular attention to the heart, peripheral pulses, and fundi to assess the extent of end organ damage from the hypertension. The diagnosis of renal disease can rarely be made at the bedside but clinical clues can be found in some patients (Table 3). In patients with neurofibromatosis and hypertension, renal artery stenosis should be considered as well as the more classically associated phaeochromocytoma. An epigastric bruit in a young female may suggest fibromuscular renal artery stenosis; widespread vascular bruits and diminished peripheral pulses would raise the suspicion of atheromatous renal artery stenosis in an older arteriopath.

Investigation

Clinical history and physical examination thus fail to pick out the majority of patients with renal disease from the population with hypertension, and further investigation is necessary to detect most cases. A suggested plan of investigation is outlined in Table 4.

Laboratory investigation

Urinalysis and measurement of the plasma creatinine and electrolytes are obligatory in all patients with hypertension in order to identify those with renal damage as a consequence of hypertension as well as those few with primary renal disease. However, since only 40 per cent of those with chronic pyelonephritis have proteinuria (Arze *et al.* 1982) and patients with renovascular disease may have anything from absent to nephrotic range proteinuria, urinalysis may fail to identify patients with mild renal disease. The majority of patients with glomerulonephritis will have haematuria and proteinuria on dipstix testing but in some cases, for example IgA nephropathy, these abnormalities may be episodic. Proteinuria may occur as a consequence of essential hypertension rather than as a result of primary renal disease but is then obviously an important indicator of end organ damage and also a marker of increased cardiovascular risk (Agewall *et al.* 1997).

Table 3 Features on clinical examination suggesting renal hypertension

Bilateral palpable kidneys
  Polycystic kidney disease
  Tuberous sclerosis
  Von-Hippel–Lindau
(hydronephrotic kidneys often not palpable)

Systemic lupus erythematosis
Nerve deafness—Alport's syndrome
Partial lipodystrophy—mesangiocapillary glomerulonephritis
Adenoma sebaceum—tuberous sclerosis
Epigastric bruit—renal artery stenosis
Neurofibromatosis—renal artery stenosis or phaeochromocytoma

Note: Clinical clues are uncommon.

Table 4 Laboratory and radiological investigation to detect renal disease in hypertensives

Obligatory in all hypertensives
Urinalysis
  Glomerulonephritis—blood and/or protein in most cases. May be red cells or casts on microscopy
  'Chronic pyelonephritis' (reflux nephropathy)—may be blood/protein, may be normal. May be white cells on microscopy
  Polycystic disease: may be haematuria, perhaps frank, may be normal
  Renovascular disease: normal to nephrotic range proteinuria
Plasma creatinine—crude test of renal function
Plasma electrolytes—hypokalaemia without hypernatraemia clue to renovascular hypertension
Glucose, lipid levels to assess overall cardiovascular risk

When indicated
Renal ultrasonography
  Obstruction
  Polycystic kidneys
  Scarring in reflux nephropathy
  Small kidneys in chronic renal failure
  Asymmetry in renal artery stenosis
Renal duplex Doppler sonography
  Blood flow characteristics in renal vessels may suggest renal artery stenosis

Further imaging IVU—obstruction, stones, frank haematuria DTPA renogram to further investigate renal artery stenosis DMSA scan to confirm renal scarring, especially in children MR angiogram/CT scan to confirm renal artery stenosis Renal angiography for definitive diagnosis of renal artery stenosis and intervention—angioplasty, stent

Radiological, ultrasonographic, and isotope studies

Clinical examination is a relatively crude method for detecting end organ damage from hypertension. Left ventricular hypertrophy should be sought by performing an ECG; however, this will detect only 15 per cent of cases. Echocardiography is much more sensitive, though much more expensive. Accurate assessment of peripheral vasculature may require ultrasonography with colour Doppler assessment of flow. It is, however, not appropriate to subject the majority of patients with hypertension to further investigation since the yield is low and the cost plus possible complications of investigation would exceed any potential benefit. Essential hypertension is unusual before the age of 20 years and investigation is clearly worthwhile in the very young with hypertension, particularly in women of child-bearing age. The proportion of patients with secondary hypertension gradually decreases with increasing age and beyond the age of 40 years a routine search is seldom indicated. Investigation is indicated in those presenting with malignant hypertension, up to 30 per cent of whom may have renovascular disease (van Jaarsveld *et al.* 1994): when there is a clinical clue to underlying renal disease; or when hypertension is resistant to treatment with three or more drugs. A further indication is where drug treatment of hypertension has an implication for employment prospects.

Decisions for further investigation must be based on an overall assessment of each patient's particular circumstances. Some guidelines are listed in Table 4.

Imaging techniques (see also Table 4)

Ultrasound

This is a rapid, non-invasive, and relatively cheap method of assessing renal size and cortical thickness. It is the best method for the diagnosis of adult polycystic disease. Ultrasound will detect obstruction to outflow in the majority of cases, though an intravenous urogram or retrograde pyelogram will usually be required to identify the site of obstruction. However, very detailed scanning by an experienced ultrasonographer is required to identify abnormalities such as small differences in renal size due to renal artery stenosis, or cortical scarring due to reflux nephropathy, and this service may not be available on the routine ultrasound list. Increasing use of Doppler scanning to assess blood flow velocities in the renal vessels (duplex Doppler sonography) allows detection of renal artery stenosis by experienced operators. Sensitivity varies from 32 to 91 per cent and specificity from 94 to greater than 95 per cent, depending on the technique used (van Jaarsveld and Deinum 2001).

Finally, patient obesity and bowel gas may limit the use of this technique even in the best hands.

Intravenous urography

Rapid sequence intravenous urography (IVU) carries a risk of contrast medium allergy and also of nephrotoxicity; in addition, a significant dose of radiation is required. Unsatisfactory films will be obtained when there is significant renal impairment.

Although a unilateral renal artery stenosis may result in a small dense delayed pyelogram on IVU, there is an appreciable rate of false-positive and false-negative results even in unilateral disease, and the IVU is of little value in bilateral disease. Generally, initial investigation should be with non-invasive methods such as ultrasound where possible, and IVU reserved for specific indications such as locating the site of obstruction or a urothelial tumour. IVU is rarely indicated in the investigation of hypertension.

Renal isotope scans

Several different radiopharmaceuticals are in use. The most widely used is ^{99}Tc-diethylenetriaminepenta-acetic acid (DTPA). This is eliminated by glomerular filtration and so is a marker of GFR, giving good results when renal function is reasonable. ^{123}I-iodohippurate (OIH) and ^{99}Tc-mercaptoacetylglycylglycine (MAG3), which are excreted by glomerular filtration and tubular secretion, are markers of renal blood flow and are useful to assess renal perfusion when function is reduced. DMSA (^{99}Tc-dimercaptosuccinic acid) is a marker of tubular function (Pederson 1994) and DMSA static scanning is used to detect and monitor renal scarring in children with urinary tract infection. It is less reliable for this purpose in adults since other conditions, such as patchy renal infarction, may be indistinguishable from chronic pyelonephritis.

Isotope renography demonstrates altered excretion of the radioactive tracer in a poststenotic kidney, with delayed uptake, delayed time to peak, and delayed excretion compared to the contralateral kidney. The administration of an ACEI such as captopril 25 or 50 mg orally 1 h before the test increases the sensitivity of screening for RAS: so too does aspirin, which blocks prostaglandin-dependent vasodilatation in the poststenotic kidney. Single kidney GFR can be calculated using the disappearance of DTPA from the blood, and this technique can be helpful in bilateral renal artery stenosis. In some centres, isotope renography has to a large extent been superseded as a screening method by the newer imaging methods such as spiral computed tomography (CT) scanning or magnetic resonance angiography (MRA). However, isotope renography may be more readily available than other techniques in many hospitals and may precede the ultrasound; if the renogram is completely normal, no further investigation may be necessary. In addition, isotope renography is useful in monitoring patients following angioplasty or stenting.

Diagnosis of renal artery stenosis by CT and MR scanning

These are safer and less invasive procedures than the 'gold standard' intra-arterial angiography, though contrast which may affect renal function is still required in CT scanning. MRA is safe in patients with impaired renal function, though it requires the ability to hold the breath for 25–35 s to avoid respiratory artefacts; like CT scanning it is not suitable for those prone to claustrophobia. The median sensitivity of gadolinium-enhanced MRA is reported as 97 per cent (88–100 per cent) with a median specificity of 92 per cent (71–100 per cent) (Dong *et al.* 1999). MRA is only suitable for the detection of stenoses of the main renal artery; branch stenoses may be missed. It is therefore of value in older patients in whom atheromatous stenosis is likely but not in young patients since FMD often affects smaller vessels and may not be demonstrated.

Intra-arterial digital subtraction angiography

When indicated on the basis of clinical features and investigations, renal angiography with direct intra-arterial injection into the aorta and selectively into the renal arteries is necessary to directly visualize the lumen of the renal artery, and is still considered to be the gold standard for diagnosis of renal artery stenosis. Confirmation of renal artery stenosis can be followed immediately by intervention with percutaneous transluminal balloon angioplasty or stenting.

In the future, improved non-invasive screening such as MRA may allow identification of those patients who do not have a stenosis, allowing angiography to be reserved for those in whom angioplasty or stent placement is being considered.

Functional significance of renal artery stenosis

There is as yet no consensus on factors which predict response to intervention (van Jaarsveld and Deinum 2001). Recent reports of techniques such as resistance index measured by colour Doppler ultrasonography are promising (Radermacher *et al.* 2001). Renal vein renin studies have not proved to be useful.

Drug treatment

Target BP

Multiple drugs are usually necessary to achieve target BPs for optimal renal protection. Small doses of several agents may minimize side-effects and maximize efficiency, though compliance may become a problem due to the expense and inconvenience of taking large numbers of tablets on a daily basis, especially as hypertension and mild renal impairment are generally asymptomatic. It is essential to discuss the rationale and aims of treatment with patients to ensure understanding of and agreement with the treatment plan. Once daily dosages are also helpful for compliance.

It may also be helpful for patients to monitor BP themselves, using a reliable cuff device, and the correct cuff size (18 cm) in those with large upper arms (circumference > 32 cm). It is important for diabetics to measure BP, both sitting and standing, to detect orthostatic hypotension.

The JNC VI recommend a BP target of less than 135/85 mmHg in chronic renal disease, and less than 125/75 mmHg when there is a protein leak of 1 g or more.

Treatment of other cardiovascular risk factors

Cardiovascular risk is greatly increased in hypertensives with renal impairment, particularly diabetics. It is sensible to encourage general non-pharmacological measures such as weight loss, exercise, and stopping smoking, as well as a healthy low-salt, low-fat diet. Statin therapy should be considered depending on overall cardiovascular risk.

Alcohol intake above 21 units per week is associated with a rise in BP: alcohol consumption should be limited to no more than 20–30 g ethanol per day for men, and no more than 10–20 g ethanol per day for women.

Once BP is controlled, aspirin should be considered in patients over the age of 50 years in whom the risk of a vascular complication, calculated on the basis of BP, age, diabetic status and lipid profile, family history, and race, exceeds 20 per cent in 10 years. Aspirin should also be considered in patients who have already suffered a cardiovascular complication, including left ventricular hypertrophy, or have renal impairment or proteinuria (Ramsay *et al.* 1999).

Choice of Drugs

A list of drugs used and suggested strategy is shown in Table 5.

Table 5 Drug strategy in renal hypertension

ACEIs: use whenever possible for cardiovascular protection and renoprotection Monitor renal function and potassium Use with care in significant renal artery stenosis; consider angioplasty/stent to allow ACEI use if renal function worsens Use with care in hypovolaemia, congestive cardiac failure
ARBs: in those intolerant of ACEIs Monitor renal function and potassium Use with care in significant renal artery stenosis
Thiazide diuretic: if plasma creatinine < 200 μmol/l OR to amplify response to loop diuretics at higher serum creatinine concentrations
Loop diuretic: if plasma creatinine > 200 μmol/l OR resistant hypertension
β-Blockers: if coexisting angina, ischaemic heart disease, previous MI. Consider for cautious use in heart failure
Calcium channel blocker: use long acting preparation
α-Blocker: useful for prostatism
Methyldopa: still useful in resistant cases or pregnancy
Minoxidil: if all else fails (Note: fluid retention and hirsutism)
Aspirin, statins: to reduce cardiovascular risk, according to local guidelines

Angiotensin converting enzyme inhibitors

ACEIs block the renin–angiotensin system by inhibiting the enzymatic conversion of angiotensin I to angiotensin II via kininase II. This enzyme also inactivates bradykinin, so ACE inhibition also results in increased bradykinin levels which in turn stimulates endothelial nitric oxide release. It seems likely that this bradykinin-mediated effect contributes to reduction of BP, but the relative contribution of this additional vasodilator effect to reduced angiotensin II levels remains unclear. Inhibition of kininase II also increases the level of substance P in the lung which is believed to be important in causing the persistent dry cough which is a troublesome side-effect of ACEI therapy.

Many studies have demonstrated that ACEIs reduce morbidity and mortality due to heart failure: the Studies of Left Ventricular Dysfunction (SOLVD), the Survival and Ventricular Enlargement trial (SAVE), Acute Infarction Ramipril Efficacy (AIRE), the Trandolopril Cardiac Evaluation (TRACE) (Flather *et al.* 2000). The BHS and JNC VI guidelines list heart failure and left ventricular dysfunction as compelling indications for treatment with an ACEI. Type 1 diabetic nephropathy is also a compelling indication for ACEI.

More recently the HOPE study randomized 9297 high-risk older patients (with diabetes or vascular disease but not heart failure) to treatment with ramipril or placebo in addition to conventional therapy. There was a 22 per cent reduction in the combined primary end point of stroke, MI, and cardiovascular death from any cause in the ramipril group compared to the placebo group. This study provides further evidence for the use of ACEIs in high-risk patients, where possible. Whether the beneficial effects of ACEIs are a class effect or not is yet to be established.

Captopril is perhaps used less often today because of its short half-life. Ramipril, perindopril, lisinopril, enalapril, and quinapril are all widely used. The properties of commonly used ACEIs are shown in Table 6.

Caution is needed, however, in the use of ACEIs in renal impairment, and especially in renal artery stenosis (see below). In all patients there is a risk of first dose hypotension, but this is particularly likely in high renin states when large doses of diuretics are used. It is prudent

Table 6 Properties of ACEIs

ACEI	Active drug	Elimination half-life (h)	% renally excreted (active form)	Usual daily dose for hypertension (mg) (dose frequency)
Benazapril	Benazaprilat	11	18	10–80 (1–2×)
Captopril	Captopril	4–6	50	25–50 (2–3×)
Cilazapril	Cilazaprilat	9	53	2.5–5 (1×)
Enalapril	Enalaprilat	6	43	10–40 (1–2×)
Fosinopril	Fosinoprilat	12	75	10–40 (1×)
Lisinopril	Lisinopril	7	97	10–40 (1×)
Perindopril	Perindoprilat	3–10	22	2–8 (1×)
Quinapril	Quinaprilat	1.8	30	10–80 (1–2×)
Ramipril	Ramiprilat	13–17	70	2.5–10 (1–2×)
Trandolapril	Trandoprilat	10	14	1–4 (1×)

to omit diuretics for a day or two (if this can safely be done) prior to starting a low dose of ACEI to be taken just before retiring to bed. The ACEIs (and also ARBs which also reduce angiotensin II effect albeit by a different mechanism) may cause a substantial rise in creatinine and potassium in patients with renal parenchymal disease and may precipitate renal failure when there is bilateral significant renal artery stenosis or stenosis of an artery to a single functioning kidney. Renal failure during the administration of captopril to a renal transplant recipient was described shortly after the introduction of the drug (Farrow and Wilkinson 1979), and the possible mechanism subsequently suggested by Hricik *et al.* (1983). In haemodynamically significant renal artery stenosis, renal perfusion pressure is reduced distal to the stenosis and renin is produced in response to a reduction in pressure at the afferent arteriolar baroreceptor. This leads to the local production of angiotensin II, which acts preferentially on the efferent arteriole causing vasoconstriction and increased intraglomerular pressure. The GFR is thus maintained despite reduced glomerular plasma flow (Fig. 1a). ACEIs block the formation of angiotensin II and the resulting efferent vasodilatation leads to a reduction in GFR while renal plasma flow is maintained (Fig. 1b). In a patient with unilateral stenosis of a renal artery and a normal contralateral kidney there may be no discernable change in the plasma creatinine, although careful monitoring of renal function (e.g. single kidney GFR) may reveal some deterioration. However, in those with stenosis of the artery supplying a single functioning kidney, such as a transplant, or in patients with bilateral disease, severe renal failure may develop. This is usually reversible on withdrawal of the ACEI but there have been reports of renal artery occlusion leading to permanent loss of function of the affected kidney.

In patients with severe impairment of renal function but patent renal arteries, ACE inhibition causes only a slight reduction in the GFR (Heeg *et al.* 1987) even though it seems possible that angiotensin II induced efferent arteriolar constriction may contribute to the hyperfiltration by residual nephrons in chronic renal disease. In contrast to the effect in renal artery stenosis, when the renal artery is not stenosed the renal plasma flow can be maintained or increased (Grazi *et al.* 1989) during ACE inhibition, despite the reduction in systemic pressure because of reduced renal vascular resistance; although the

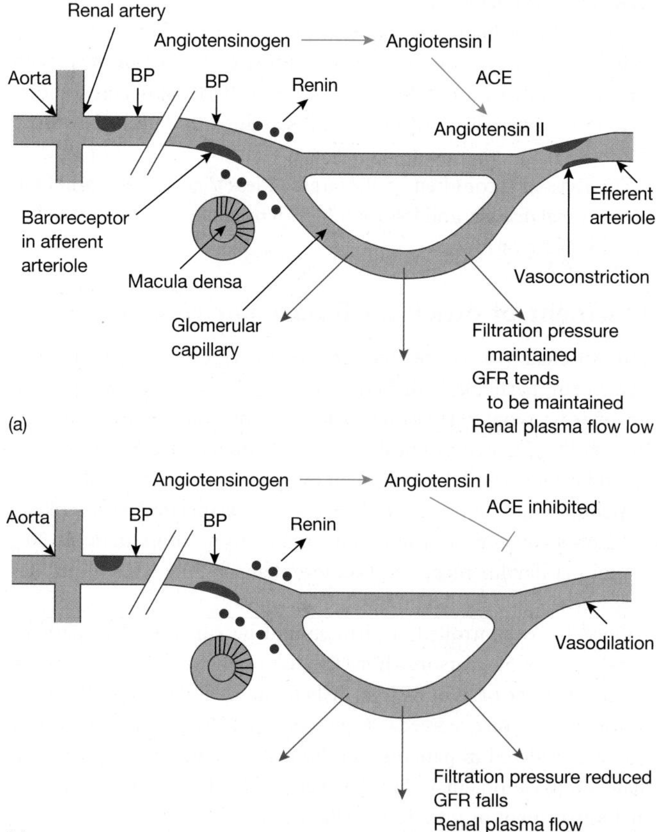

Fig. 1 Renal haemodynamic adaptation to reduced perfusion pressure in renal artery stenosis: (a) when the production of angiotensin II is intact and (b) in the presence of ACEIs.

filtration pressure is reduced by efferent vasodilatation, filtration tends to be maintained. Filtration is usually rapid from the first part of the glomerular capillary since hydrostatic pressure is at its highest and the osmotic pressure resisting filtration at its lowest. Along the capillary, hydrostatic pressure gradually declines and the osmotic pressure of plasma protein increases as a result of the filtration of water and crystalloids until a point of equilibrium is reached where filtration stops. If the perfusion pressure declines but plasma flow is maintained, then filtration is initially slower but continues further along the glomerular capillary before equilibrium is reached since the osmotic pressure increases less rapidly (Fig. 2). Thus, the GFR declines a little, but not to the extent seen in renal artery stenosis, and may even remain stable. However, reversible renal failure may occur in patients with renal parenchymal disease without renal artery stenosis treated with ACEIs, particularly in the presence of small vessel disease and with concomitant diuretic or non-steroidal anti-inflammatory treatment.

The other factor which may limit the use of ACEIs (and also ARBs) is their potential to cause hyperkalaemia. In renal failure, sodium balance continues to be governed at least in part by the renin–angiotensin system. When renin deficiency occurs for any reason, a state of hyporeninaemic hypoaldosteronism develops, with potentially dangerous hyperkalaemia. ACEIs (and ARBs) induce a state of hypoaldosteronism and serum potassium must be carefully monitored in patients with impaired renal function treated with ACEIs or ARBs. These drugs are often used inadvertently in patients with renovascular hypertension and the development of renal failure during treatment may be the first clue to the diagnosis. For this reason, plasma creatinine should be checked before and shortly after instituting therapy with ACEIs or ARBs in all patients, with particular care in older patients with evidence of vascular disease elsewhere. Careful monitoring should continue in those with renal impairment.

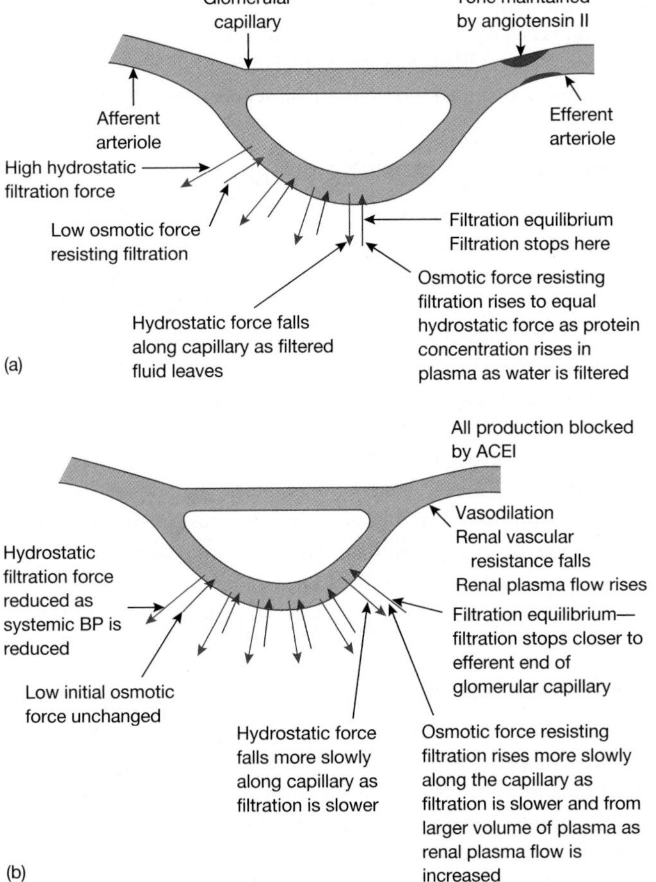

Fig. 2 A possible mechanism for the maintenance of GFR in patients with parenchymal renal disease during treatment with ACEIs: (a) showing filtration equilibrium reached early in the glomerular capillary in the presence of angiotensin II; (b) showing slower filtration continuing further along the capillary in the absence of angiotensin II during ACEI treatment.

One additional indication for the use of ACEIs is in the treatment of hypertension associated with scleroderma renal crisis, where their use has resulted in a dramatic improvement in survival (Steen *et al.* 1990).

Angiotensin II receptor antagonists (A2RAs, ARBs)

The final step of the renin–angiotensin cascade is binding of angiotensin II to receptors, resulting in their activation. Several angiotensin II receptor subtypes are now recognized, the clinically important receptors being AT1 and AT2. All known clinical effects of angiotensin II are mediated by the AT1 receptor which is found in kidney, heart, vascular smooth muscle cells, brain, adrenal gland, platelets, adipocytes, and the placenta (Burnier and Brunner 2000). These are the receptors that are blocked by the sartans or ARBs. The AT2 receptors are important during fetal development but are present only at low levels in adult tissues, mainly in uterus, adrenal, central nervous system, heart, and kidney. They are upregulated in experimental cardiac hypertrophy, MI, and vascular and wound healing, but their physiological role remains unclear.

Angiotensin receptor blockers provide more complete blockade of the renin–angiotensin system than ACEIs; long-term treatment with ACEIs results in a gradual return of circulating angiotensin II levels to pretreatment levels, thought to be due to conversion of angiotensin I to angiotensin II by alternative non-ACE enzymes such as chymase. The benefits of ACE inhibition persist with long-term treatment, however, raising the possibility that at least some of their effect is not due to renin–angiotensin system blockade. Thus, it seems likely that combination of such ACEI effect with more effective insurmountable renin-angiotensin blockade using ARBs will provide additional benefit.

The sartans (losartan, candesartan, eprosartan, irbestartan, telmisartan, and valsartan) are well tolerated, and in particular the frequency of cough is comparable to placebo. The properties of the ARBs are shown in Table 7.

The sartans have been shown to be effective antihypertensive agents but it is still unclear whether they are equivalent to or superior to ACEIs in heart failure and renoprotection. The benefits of using angiotensin II receptor blockade alone or in combination with ACEIs have yet to be fully established (Sleight 2002).

A recent study has shown that losartan-based treatment is superior to atenolol-based treatment in patients with hypertension and LVH with or without diabetes (Dahlof *et al.* 2002; Lindholm *et al.* 2002); cardiovascular morbidity and death were reduced to a greater degree in the losartan group despite similar reduction in BP.

Heart failure

The ELITE (Evaluation of Losartan in the Elderly) II trial, which compared captopril with losartan in patients with heart failure, did not demonstrate any significant difference between the two drugs on the

Table 7 Properties of the ARBs

Drug	Half-life (h)	Bioavailability (%)	Dose in renal impairment	Dose in mild/mod hepatic impairment	Usual dose (mg/day)
Candesartan	9	14	Half	Half	4–16 (32)
Eprosartan	5–9	13	Half	Half	400–800
Irbesartan	11–15	60–80	— No adjustment necessary —		150–300
Losartan	6–9	33	Reduce	Reduce	50–100
Telmisartan	>20	50	No adjustment necessary	<40 mg	40–80
Valsartan	9	23	Reduce	Hal	80–320

combined end point of mortality or hospitalization for a cardiovascular event (Pitt *et al.* 2000).

Diabetic nephropathy

There is now evidence from the Reduction of Endpoints in NIDDM with the Angiotensin II Antagonist Losartan (RENAAL) trial and the Irbesartan in type 2 diabetic nephropathy (IDNT) trial that ARBs are effective in delaying progression of renal impairment and delaying progression of microalbuminuria to proteinuria in type 2 diabetes (Lewis *et al.* 2001; Parving *et al.* 2001).

The RENAAL trial compared outcomes in 751 type 2 diabetics treated with losartan 50–100 mg daily plus conventional treatment excluding other ARBs and ACEIs, to 762 patients treated with placebo plus conventional antihypertensive therapy. Mean follow-up was 3.4 years. Losartan reduced the risk of doubling of serum creatine by 25 per cent and the risk of endstage renal disease by 28 per cent, but had no effect on the rate of death. Target BP was less than 140/90 mmHg; actual BP was 140/74 and 142/74 mmHg at the end of the study in the losartan and placebo groups, respectively. The study investigators felt the difference in BP between the losartan and placebo groups was too small to account for the risk reduction achieved.

The IDNT trial compared outcomes in 579 type 2 diabetics treated with irbesartan 300 mg daily, 567 treated with amlodipine 10 mg daily, and 569 allocated to placebo, all also treated with antihypertensive agents other than ARB, ACEI, or calcium channel blockers. Follow-up was for 2.6 years. Risk of doubling of serum creatinine was 33 per cent lower in the irbesartan group than the placebo group and 37 per cent lower in the irbesartan group than the amlodipine group. There were no significant differences in death rates or in the composite cardiovascular end point. Target BP was less than 135/85 mmHg, and subsequent mean BP in the irbesartan group 140/77 mmHg and in the amlodipine group 141/77 mmHg. The mean arterial BP was 3.3 mmHg lower in the irbesartan and in the amlodipine groups throughout the study. The study investigators felt that the differences in outcome were too large to be explained by the differences in BP achieved.

Combining ACEIs and ARBs

In theory, as discussed above, combining effective renin–angiotensin system blockade by using an ARB with the additional vasodilator effects of ACEIs might provide additional benefits.

Small short-term trials using a combination of ACEI and ARB have been reported. The CALM study (Candesartan and Lisinopril Microalbuminiuria study) showed a greater reduction in urinary albumin/creatinine ratio in microalbuminuric type 2 diabetics receiving candesartan 16 mg/day plus lisinopril 20 mg/day than in patients receiving either drug alone (Mogenson *et al.* 2000). However, this was a study of 199 patients for only 24 weeks, and DBP was also lower with combination therapy than with either candesartan or lisinopril alone.

A further study of eight normotensive patients with IgA nephropathy demonstrated a 73 per cent greater reduction in protenuria with losartan plus an ACEI than with either drug alone (Russo *et al.* 1999). However, these studies used submaximal doses of ACEIs and ARBs, so no conclusion on an additive effect is as yet possible.

α-Adrenoceptor blocking drugs

Prazosin, doxazosin, indoramin, and terazosin are selective post-synaptic α-adrenoreceptor blockers. They rarely cause tachycardia but may cause postural hypotension. They can be used with all other antihypertensives and have a favourable effect on dyslipidaemia, though the long-term benefits of this are unknown. They also have a beneficial effect on the symptoms of benign prostatic hypertrophy so should be considered for use in older men with this condition.

The ALLHAT study (Antihypertensive and Lipid lowering Treatment to Prevent Heart Attack Trial; ALLHAT Research Group 2000), comparing outcomes for chlorthalidone, amlodipine, lisinopril, and doxazosin, controversially stopped the doxazosin arm of the trial early because of an apparent increased risk of congestive cardiac failure. It seems reasonable at present to reserve doxazosin as a second-line treatment for hypertension, rather than as first-line monotherapy.

β-Adrenoreceptor blocking drugs

These drugs block the β-adrenoreceptors in the heart, peripheral vessels, bronchi, pancreas, and liver. The precise mechanism of action by which they lower BP is not known, but it may include reduction in cardiac output, suppression of renin (Buhler *et al.* 1972), and possibly a central effect. Some β-blockers are lipid soluble and some water soluble; generally, drugs with low lipid solubility are not taken up by the liver for metabolism and are filtered at the glomerulus but not reabsorbed from the tubule so that excretion depends on renal function. Atenolol, celiprolol, nadolol, and sotalol are the most water-soluble β-blockers; they tend to accumulate in renal failure as described above and a reduction in dosage may be required. Sotalol may induce torsade de pointes and should not be used in significant renal impairment.

Propranolol is lipid soluble and rapidly metabolized by the liver; only very small amounts are excreted unchanged in the urine, but because its metabolites are active and accumulate in uraemia the dose should be reduced slightly.

Labetalol, celiprolol, carvedilol, and nebivolol act by various mechanisms to cause vasodilatation in addition to β-adrenoreceptor blockade. Nebivolol alone stimulates the release of nitric oxide, though the long-term potential benefits on endothelial damage and atherosclerosis remain to be proven.

In addition to providing symptomatic benefit in ischaemic heart disease, some β-blockers reduce mortality post-MI. Bisoprolol, carvedilol, and modified release metoprolol have been shown to reduce mortality in some patients with heart failure. These coexisting conditions may provide compelling reasons to use β-blockade in these patients.

β-Blockers are often underused and wrongly withheld from many patients with ischaemic heart disease on dialysis or after transplantation, particularly diabetics, who would benefit from their use.

Calcium channel blockers

Calcium channel blockers interfere with the inward movement of calcium ions through the slow channels of active cell membranes. They influence myocardial cells, the conducting system of the heart, and vascular smooth muscle cells.

Dihydropridine calcium channel blockers (nifedipine, amlodipine, felodipine, isradipine, lacidipine, lercanidipine, and nisoldipine) undergo almost complete (95 per cent) hepatic oxidation to inactive metabolites that are excreted in the urine, and renal impairment does not significantly alter their pharmacokinetics. The drugs are not cleared to any significant extent by dialysis, probably because they are highly protein-bound and highly lipophilic. Thus, no adjustment of dose is required in renal failure or on dialysis.

Verapamil and diltiazem (non-dihydropyridine calcium channel blockers) can cause significant bradycardia, so in combination with β-blockers great caution is required.

Calcium channel blockers can be used with diuretics which, however, will not prevent the associated peripheral oedema which is a local effect.

Long-acting calcium channel blockers should be used and short-acting calcium channel blockers avoided. Calcium channel blockers are of proven benefit for the prevention of stroke in elderly patients.

The combination of an ACEI and a calcium channel blocker has been shown to be more renoprotective than ACEI monotherapy in diabetics (Bakris 2001).

Centrally acting drugs

Clonidine has the disadvantage that sudden withdrawal may cause a hypertensive crisis, but this is only a practical problem with high doses. A small dose of 50 μg three times daily has very few side-effects and is highly effective in renal patients, in whom sympathetic overactivity is believed to be an important cause of hypertension (Converse *et al.* 1992). Clonidine is occasionally useful when a patient has migraine in association with hypertension. Methyldopa is still widely used in pregnancy where its established safety record outweighs the disadvantage of side-effects such as tiredness. Side-effects are minimized if the daily dose is kept to less than 1 g. Although methyldopa undergoes some metabolism in the liver, there is also some renal excretion and so it may accumulate in renal failure. In practice this is rarely a problem since, as with all antihypertensive drugs, a low starting dose is used, building up gradually according to the patient's response.

Moxonidine is a more recently introduced centrally acting drug which is generally well tolerated though may cause bradycardia; the dose should be reduced in renal impairment.

Thiazide and loop diuretics

Thiazides are accepted first-line therapy for uncomplicated essential hypertension since many trials have shown a reduction in morbidity and mortality with these agents, and they are cheap. Thiazide diuretics become ineffective as monotherapy when plasma creatinine exceeds 200 μmol/l and should then be replaced by loop diuretics. All thiazide diuretics are equally effective at the appropriate dose. The dose–response curve is flat and thus low doses have virtually the same efficacy as higher doses but with much reduced metabolic side-effects of hypokalaemia, dyslipidaemia, hyperglycaemia, and hyperuricaemia.

Although thiazide diuretics in the doses usually used act predominantly on the distal part of the thick ascending limb of the loop of Henle and the first part of the distal convoluted tubule (the cortical diluting segment), at greater doses they also inhibit sodium chloride reabsorption in the proximal tubule, as do loop diuretics (Fernandez and Puschett 1973; Beyer 1982).

The proximal effect of thiazide diuretics is usually obscured by increased sodium absorption in the ascending limb of the loop of Henle, but if loop diuretics are given concomitantly, this increase is prevented and a sequential blockade of sodium reabsorption along the nephron by the combined effects of the two diuretics (covering the proximal convoluted tubule, the loop of Henle, and the cortical diluting segment) results in a synergistic diuretic action. The combination of a thiazide and a loop diuretic (e.g. metolazone and furosemide/frusemide) is therefore useful even in patients with renal impairment.

Loop diuretics are necessary when the plasma creatinine exceeds 200 μmol/l. They are almost always required to obtain control of hypertension as renal function deteriorates. Furosemide (frusemide) and bumetanide are very similar in action; both act within an hour of administration and diuresis is complete within 6 h. Torasemide has similar properties.

The dose-response curve with loop diuretics, unlike thiazides, is not flat and it is possible to obtain a useful diuresis even in patients with advanced renal failure, using doses up to 1 g of furosemide or 20 or 30 mg of bumetanide daily. In such large doses both drugs can cause deafness and bumetanide can cause myalgia.

As renal failure progresses, the fractional excretion of filtered sodium (FE_{Na}) increases even in the absence of diuretics so that by the time GFR has declined to 5 l/24 h, FE_{Na} has increased from the usual value of around 0.5 up to 20 per cent (Slatopolsky *et al.* 1968). This can be further increased by a loop diuretic so that fluid balance can be maintained down to a very low GFR. In advanced renal failure, hypertension is often resistant to multiple antihypertensives until sodium overload is corrected and very high doses of loop diuretic, plus dietary salt restriction, are often required to combat this. It is often preferable to use a combination of a thiazide diuretic with a more modest dose of loop diuretic to achieve sodium balance, as above. Such a combination may cause hypokalaemia even in renal failure, and

Table 8 Diuretics used in renal hypertension

Group	Drug	Dose	Comments
Thiazide	Bendrofluazide	2.5 mg daily	Flat dose response
	Metolazone	5–80 mg daily	Profound diuresis when used with frusemide
Loop	Furosemide (Frusemide)	40–2000 mg daily	Wide range of dose
	Bumetanide	1–50 mg daily	
	Torasemide	2.5–40 mg daily	
Potassium	Amiloride	5–20 mg daily	Monitor potassium
Conserving	Triamterene	50–200 mg daily	
	Spironolactone (aldosterone antagonist): avoid in moderate to severe renal impairment		

since oral potassium supplements may be ineffective or poorly tolerated, it may be necessary to add a potassium-sparing distal tubular diuretic. Potassium must then be very carefully monitored to avoid dangerous hyperkalaemia; amiloride (5–20 mg daily) or triamterene (50–200 mg daily) are preferred to spironolactone since they are less likely to cause hyperkalaemia and their extrarenal side-effects are less troublesome.

The plasma urea may increase markedly, and the plasma creatinine less markedly, during diuretic therapy. This may rarely be due to a drug-induced interstitial nephritis which will usually resolve on withdrawal of the diuretic. More commonly it is simply due to hypovolaemia and the stimulation of renin release resulting from the diuresis. In response to reduced renal perfusion, angiotensin II is formed locally in the juxtaglomerular apparatus and causes efferent arteriolar constriction; this maintains the filtration pressure but leads to reduced hydrostatic and increased osmotic pressure in the peritubular capillaries. As a result of this, and also in response to the direct action of angiotensin II, sodium and water reabsorption from the proximal tubule is increased and with it urea. Further reabsorption of urea occurs in the more distal parts of the tubule because of the reduced flow rate of tubular fluid.

Diuretics commonly used in renal hypertension are shown in Table 8.

Vasodilator antihypertensive drugs

Sodium nitroprusside may be given by intravenous infusion to control severe hypertensive crises, though it is very rare for parenteral treatment to be required. It may also be used to produce controlled hypotension when a short duration of action is necessary, for example, during surgery or to control hypertension during renal angioplasty when there may be a dramatic fall in BP immediately postprocedure.

Minoxidil is a very potent vasodilator that acts directly on the arterial wall blocking calcium uptake. Minoxidil and diazoxide are the most potent vasodilators available for oral use. Because of this property, both drugs cause fluid retention which may be massive, so concurrent diuretic therapy is required. Similar to the oedema that accompanies calcium antagonist therapy, this fluid retention is thought to be a local haemodynamic effect resulting from increased tissue capillary pressure that is a consequence of arteriolar dilatation. There may also be a hormonal element since the reduction in BP stimulates the release of renin by reflex sympathetic stimulation acting through the renal nerves and leading to secondary aldosteronism. There is no accumulation in renal failure and dose adjustment is not necessary.

Diazoxide can cause hyperglycaemia and is rarely used today. Minoxidil is used only for the most severe and resistant hypertensives since its side-effect of hypertrichosis is very problematic, especially for women. The vasodilatation is accompanied by increased cardiac output and tachycardia as well as fluid retention and a β-blocker should be prescribed as well as a diuretic.

References

ACE Inhibitors in Diabetic Nephropathy Trialist Group (2001). Should all patients with type 1 diabetes mellitus and microalbuminuria receive angiotensin-converting enzyme inhibitors?: a meta-analysis of individual patient data. *Annals of Internal Medicine* **134** (5), 370–379.

Adler, A. I. *et al.* (2000). Association of systolic blood pressure with macrovascular and microvascular complications of type 2 diabetes (UKPDS 36): prospective observational study. *British Medical Journal* **321**, 412–419.

Agewall, S. *et al.* (1997). Usefulness of microalbuminuria in predicting cardiovascular mortality in treated hypertensive men with and without diabetes mellitus. *American Journal of Cardiology* **80** (2), 164–169.

ALLHAT Collaberative Research Group (2000). Major cardiovascular events in hypertensive patients randomised to doxazosin vs chlorthalidone; the antihypertensive and lipid-lowering treatment to prevent heart attack trial (ALLHAT). *Journal of the American Medical Association* **283**, 1967–1975.

American Diabetes Association (2002). Standards of medical care for patients with diabetes mellitus. *Diabetes Care* **25**, S33–S49.

Arze, R. S. *et al.* (1982). The natural history of chronic pyelonephritis in the adult. *Quarterly Journal of Medicine* **51**, 396–401.

Bakris, G. L. (2001). A practical approach to achieving recommended blood pressure goals in diabetic patients. *Archives of Internal Medicine* **161** (22), 2661–2667.

Bakris, G. L. *et al.* for the National Kidney Foundation Hypertension and Diabetes Executive Committees Working Group (2000). *American Journal of Kidney Diseases* **36** (3), 646–661.

Berglund, G., Anderson, O., and Wilhelmson, L. (1976). Prevalence of primary and secondary hypertension: studies on a random population sample. *British Medical Journal* **2**, 554–556.

Beyer, K. H. (1982). Chlorothiazide. *British Journal of Clinical Pharmacology* **13**, 15.

Brenner, B. M. *et al.* (2001). Effects of losartan on renal and cardiovascular outcomes in patients with type 2 diabetes and nephropathy. *New England Journal of Medicine* **345**, 861–869.

Buhler, F. R. *et al.* (1972). Propranolol inhibition of renin secretion. *New England Journal of Medicine* **287**, 1209–1214.

Burnier, M. and Brunner, H. R. (2000). Angiotensin II receptor antagonists. *Lancet* **355**, 637–645.

Burt, V. L. *et al.* (1995). Prevalence of hypertension in the US adult population. Results from the Third National Health and Nutrition Examination Survey. *Hypertension* **25** (3), 305–313.

Converse, R. L., Jr. *et al.* (1992). Sympathetic overactivity in patients with chronic renal failure. *New England Journal of Medicine* **327**, 1912–1918.

Dahlof, B. *et al.* (2002). Cardiovascular morbidity and mortality in the Losartan Intervention for Endpoint Reduction in hypertension study (LIFE): a randomised trial against atenolol. *Lancet* **359**, 995–1004.

Dong, Q. *et al.* (1999). Diagnosis of renal vascular disease with MR angiography. *Radiographics* **19**, 1535–1554.

Farrow, P. R. and Wilkinson, R. (1979). Reversible renal failure during treatment with captopril. *British Medical Journal* **1**, 1680.

Fernandez, P. C. and Puschett, J. B. (1973). Proximal tubular actions of metolazone and chlorothiazide. *American Journal of Physiology* **225**, 954–961.

Flather, M. D. *et al.* (2000). Long-term ACE-inhibitor therapy in patients with heart failure or left ventricular dysfunction: a systematic overview of data from individual patients. ACE-inhibitor Myocardial Infarction Collaborative Group. *Lancet* **355**, 1575–1581.

Grazi, G. *et al.* (1989). Renal effects of enalapril in hypertensive patients with glomerulonephritis. *Nephrology, Dialysis, Transplantation* **4**, 396–398.

Gruppo Italiano di Studi Epidemiologici in Nefrologia (GISEN group) (1997). Randomised placebo-controlled trial of effect of ramipril on decline in glomerular filtration rate and risk of terminal renal failure in proteinuric, non-diabetic nephropathy. *Lancet* **349**, 1857–1863.

Health Survey for England. Cardiovascular disease. *Joint Health Surveys Unit.* London: The Stationery Office, 1998.

Heart Outcomes Prevention Evaluation (HOPE) Study Investigators (2000a). Effects of an angiotensin-converting enzyme inhibitor, ramipril, on death from cardiovascular causes, myocardial infarction and stroke in high risk patients. *New England Journal of Medicine* **342**, 145–153.

Heart Outcomes Prevention Evaluation (HOPE) Study Investigators (2000b). Effects of ramipril on cardiovascular and microvascular outcomes in people with diabetes: results of the HOPE study and MICRO-HOPE substudy. *Lancet* **355**, 253–259.

Heeg, J. E. *et al.* (1987). Reduction of proteinuria by angiotensin converting enzyme inhibition. *Kidney International* **32**, 78–83.

Herbert, L. A. *et al.* (2001). Renoprotection: one or many therapies? *Kidney International* **59**, 1211–1226.

Hohage, H. *et al.* (1997). Influence of proteinuria on long-term transplant survival in kidney transplant recipients. *Nephron* **75** (2), 160–165.

Hricik, D. E. *et al.* (1983). Captopril induced functional renal insufficiency in patients with bilateral renal artery stenosis or stenosis in a solitary kidney. *New England Journal of Medicine* **308**, 373–376.

Isles, C. G., Robertson, S., and Hill, D. (1999). Management of renovascular disease: a review of renal artery stenting in ten studies. *Quarterly Journal of Medicine* **92**, 159–167.

Jafar, T. Z. *et al.* (2001). Angiotensin-converting enzyme inhibitors and progression of nondiabetic renal disease: a meta-analysis of patient-level data. *Annals of Internal Medicine* **135** (2), 73–87.

Joffres, M. R. *et al.* (2001). Distribution of blood pressure and hypertension in Canada and the United States. *American Journal of Hypertension* **14**, 1099–1105.

JNC VI (1997). The Sixth Report of the Joint National Committee on Prevention, Detection, Evaluation and Treatment of High Blood Pressure. National Institutes of Health Publication, November.

Khattar, R. S. *et al.* (1999). Prediction of coronary and cerebrovascular morbidity and mortality by direct continuous ambulatory blood pressure monitoring in essential hypertension. *Circulation* **100**, 1071–1076.

Klag, M. J. *et al.* (1996). Blood pressure and end stage renal disease in men. *New England Journal of Medicine* **334**, 13–18.

Krumme, B. and Mann, F. E. (2001). Atherosclerotic renal artery stenosis in 2001—are we less confused than before? *Nephrology, Dialysis, Transplantation* **16**, 2124–2127.

Lang, T. *et al.* (2001). Prevalence and therapeutic control of hypertension in 30,000 subjects in the workplace. *Hypertension* **38**, 449–454.

Lewis, E. J. *et al.* (1993). The effect of angiotensin converting enzyme inhibition on diabetic nephropathy. *New England Journal of Medicine* **329** (20), 1456–1462.

Lewis, E. J. *et al.* (2001). Renoprotective effect of the angiotensin-receptor antagonist irbesartan in patients with nephropathy due to type 2 diabetes. *New England Journal of Medicine* **345**, 851–860.

Lindholm, L. H. *et al.* (2002). Cardiovascular morbidity and mortality in patients with diabetes in the Losartan Intervention for Endpoint reduction in hypertension study (LIFE): a randomised trial against atenolol. *Lancet* **359**, 1004–1011.

Maschio, G. *et al.* (1999). The ACE inhibition in progressive renal insufficiency (AIPRI) study group. *Journal of Cardiovascular Pharmacology* **33**, S16–S20.

Mogenson, C. E. (1982). Long-term antihypertensive treatment inhibiting progression of diabetic nephropathy. *British Medical Journal* **285**, 685–688.

Mogensen, C. E. *et al.* (2000). Randomised controlled trial of dual blockade of renin-angiotensin system in patients with hypertension, microalbuminuria and non-insulin dependent diabetes: the candesartan and lisinopril microalbumniuria (CALM) study. *British Medical Journal* **321**, 1440–1444.

Parving, H.-H. *et al.* (1989). Effect of captopril on blood pressure and kidney function in normotensive insulin dependent diabetics with nephropathy. *British Medical Journal* **299**, 533–536.

Parving, H.-H. *et al.* (1996). Effect of deletion polymorphism of the angiotensin converting enzyme gene on progression of diabetic nephropathy during inhibition of angiotensin converting enzyme: observational follow-up study. *British Medical Journal* **313**, 591–594.

Parving, H.-H. *et al.* (2001). The effect of irbesartan on the development of diabetic nephropathy in patients with type 2 diabetes. *New England Journal of Medicine* **345**, 870–879.

Pederson, E. B. (1994). Angiotensin converting enzyme inhibitor renography. Pathophysiological, diagnostic and therapeutic aspects in renal artery stenosis. *Nephrology, Dialysis, Transplantation* **9**, 482–492.

Peterson, J. C. *et al.* (1995). Blood pressure control, proteinuria and the progression of renal disease. The Modification of Diet in Renal Disease Study. *Annals of Internal Medicine* **123**, 754–762.

Pickering, T. G. *et al.* (1988). Recurrent pulmonary oedema in hypertension due to bilateral renal artery stenosis; treatment by angioplasty or surgical revascularisation. *Lancet* **II**, 551–552.

Pitt, B. *et al.* (2000). Effect of losartan compared with captopril on mortality in patients with symptomatic heart failure: randomised trial—the Losartan Heart Failure survival study ELITE II. *Lancet* **355**, 1582–1587.

Plouin, P. F. *et al.* (1998). Blood pressure outcome of angioplasty in atherosclerotic renal artery stenosis. *Hypertension* **31**, 823–829.

Radermacher, J. *et al.* (2001). Use of Doppler ultrasonography to predict the outcome of therapy for renal artery stenosis. *New England Journal of Medicine* **344** (6), 410–417.

Ramsay, L. E. and Waller, P. C. (1990). Blood pressure response to percutaneous transluminal angioplasty for renovascular hypertension; an overview of published series. *British Medical Journal* **300**, 569–572.

Ramsay, L. E. *et al.* (1999). Guidelines for management of hypertension: report of the third working party of the British Hypertension Society. *Journal of Human Hypertension* **13**, 569–592.

Ritz, E., Schwenger, V., Zeier, M., and Rychlik, I. (2001). Ambulatory blood pressure monitoring: fancy gadgetry or clinically useful exercise? *Nephrology, Dialysis, Transplantation* **16**, 1550–1554.

Ruggenenti, P. *et al.* (1999). Renoprotective properties of ACE-inhibition in non-diabetic nephropathies with non-nephrotic proteinuria. *Lancet* **354**, 359–364.

Russo, D. *et al.* (1999). Additive antiproteinuric effect of converting enzyme inhibitor and losartan in normotensive patients with IgA nephropathy. *American Journal of Kidney Disease* **33**, 851–856.

Safian, R. D., and Textor, S. C. (2001). Medical progress: renal artery stenosis. *New England Journal of Medicine* **344** (6), 431–442.

Smith, W. C., Lee, A. J., Crombie, I. K., and Tunstall-Pedoe, H. (1990). Control of blood pressure in Scotland: the rule of halves. *British Medical Journal* **300** (6730), 981–983.

Slatopolsky, E., Elkan, I. O., Weerts, C., and Bricker, N. S. (1968). Studies on the characteristics of the control system governing sodium excretion in uraemic man. *Journal of Clinical Investigations* **47**, 521–530.

Sleight, P. (2002). The renin–angiotensin system: a review of trials with angiotensin-converting enzyme inhibitors and angiotensin receptor blocking agents. *European Heart Journal Supplements* **4** (Suppl. A), A53–A57.

Staessen, J. A., Bieniaszewski, L., O'Brien, E. T., and Fagard, R. (1996). Special feature: what is a normal blood pressure in ambulatory monitoring? *Nephrology, Dialysis, Transplantation* **11**, 241–245.

Steen, V. D. *et al.* (1990). Outcome of renal crisis in systemic sclerosis: relation to availability of angiotensin converting enzyme (ACE) inhibitors. *Annals of Internal Medicine* **113** (5), 352–357.

USRDS (2001). US Renal Data System. Annual data report: Atlas of ESRD in the United States, National Institute of Health, National Institute of Diabetes and Digestive and Kidney Diseases, Bethesda, MD.

Van Jaarsveld, B. C. and Deinum, J. (2001). Evaluation and treatment of renal artery stenosis: impact on blood pressure and renal function. *Current Opinion in Nephrology and Hypertension* **10** (3), 399–404.

Van Jaarsveld, B. C. *et al.* (1994). Preliminary results of the Dutch Renal Artery Stenosis Intervention Cooperative (DRASTIC) study. *Netherlands Journal of Medicine* **44**, A65.

Van Jaarsveld, B. C. *et al.* (2000). The effect of balloon angioplasty on hypertension in atherosclerotic renal artery stenosis. *New England Journal of Medicine* **342** (14), 1007–1014.

Verdecchia, P. *et al.* (1995). Gender, day–night blood pressure changes and left ventricular mass in essential hypertension. Dippers and peakers. *American Journal of Hypertension* **8**, 193–196.

Webster, J. *et al.* (1998). Randomised comparison of percutaneous angioplasty vs continued medical therapy for hypertensive patients with atheromatous renal artery stenosis. *Journal of Human Hypertension* **12**, 329–335.

World Health Organisation–International Society of Hypertension Guidelines for the Management of Hypertension (1999). *Journal of Hypertension* **17**, 151–183.

Zucchelli, P., and Zuccala, A. (1996). Recent data on hypertension and progressive renal disease. *Journal of Human Hypertension* **10**, 679–682.

9.3 The kidney and control of blood pressure

Luis M. Ruilope

Introduction

The existence of a relation between arterial pressure and the kidney was first postulated by Bright (1836) even before it was possible to measure blood pressure. A simplified view of arterial hypertension considers it to be the consequence of the equilibrium among factors regulating volume and vasoconstriction. Mean arterial pressure (MAP) should be the final results of multiplying cardiac output (CO) by peripheral resistance (PR) (MAP = CO × PR). An elevation in arterial blood pressure can then be the consequence of a derangement in volume regulation or may arise as a consequence of an imbalance between factors enhancing or opposing vasoconstriction. Arterial hypertension can also be the consequence of a combined alteration of the two components, volume and vasomotion.

The kidney participates, through different mechanisms, in the regulation of both volume and vasoconstriction (see Table 1). It has been assumed that some defect in renal function must be present in any type of arterial hypertension. On the other hand, sustained elevation in systemic blood pressure irrespective of its cause may damage the kidney. This, in turn, will further contribute to the maintenance of elevated arterial pressure.

Disentangling cause and effect between kidney and arterial hypertension is particularly difficult in man, since patients are usually presented with established disease and the full sequence of changes can no longer be observed. Analysis of the relation is further complicated by the fact that once the renal regulation of volume or vasoactive substances has been altered, secondary mechanisms will be set in train, which may obscure the primary derangement. This chapter reviews first the renal mechanisms that participate in arterial pressure control. Subsequently, the role of the kidney in the initiation of arterial hypertension will be discussed in the different scenarios. Figure 1 (left panel), shows the scenario where the kidneys are at the origin (i.e. the primary cause) of human hypertension, either in the absence of a detectable renal defect, or in the presence of a renal defect, either primary or secondary. The right panel depicts the situation where the kidneys have suffered from the consequences of elevated arterial pressure. In both situations, the kidneys contribute to the elevation of arterial pressure. The signal that modifies the activity of the system and the effector pathways that result in the elevation of blood pressure will be analysed separately for each of these situations.

Table 1 Renal regulation of volume and vasoconstriction

Regulation of volume
Excretion of water and electrolytes (in particular sodium)
Regulation of vasoconstriction
Secretion of renin and other vasoconstrictive substances
Secretion of vasodepressor substances

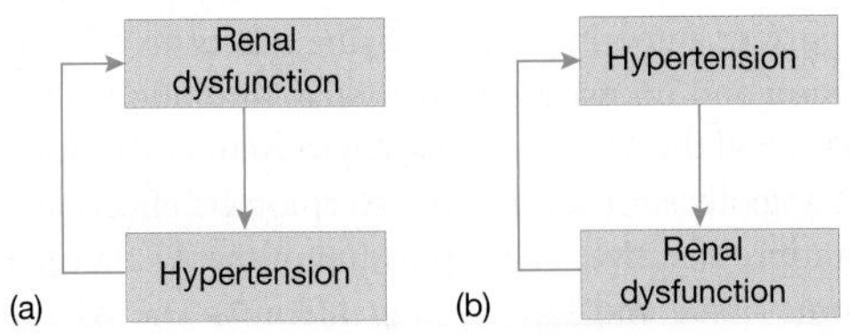

Fig. 1 Relationship between the kidneys and arterial pressure. Renal dysfunction can be the origin of arterial hypertension (b) or can be the consequence of the elevation in arterial pressure (a).

Renal mechanisms participating in the control of arterial pressure

Sodium and water excretion: the mechanism of pressure–natriuresis

It is well recognized that an elevation in renal perfusion pressure results in an increased excretion of sodium and water (pressure–natriuresis diuresis). According to the theory proposed by Guyton *et al.* (1972), whenever arterial blood pressure is elevated, activation of pressure–natriuresis promotes the excretion of sodium and water until blood volume is diminished sufficiently to return arterial blood pressure back to normal values. This theory predicts the existence of an infinite negative feedback gain for the long-term regulation of arterial pressure by adjusting blood volume and allowing the kidneys to serve as a servo-controller of arterial pressure. In other words, in the long run the kidneys will over-ride all other blood pressure control mechanisms.

Pressure–natriuresis is intrinsic to the kidney, because it can be demonstrated using an isolated perfused kidney preparation (Aperia *et al.* 1971). It is also independent of changes in glomerular filtration rate (GFR) and in renal blood flow (RBF), as depicted in Fig. 2. This figure represents the relationship between arterial pressure, natriuresis, GFR, and RBF. The latter parameters remain constant within the so-called limits of autoregulation, which operates in the range of perfusion pressure values between 80 and 200 mmHg. Variations in salt intake are followed by an exponential increase in natriuresis, but under normal circumstances they are accompanied only by very small changes in arterial pressure. Autoregulation of GFR and RBF is due to

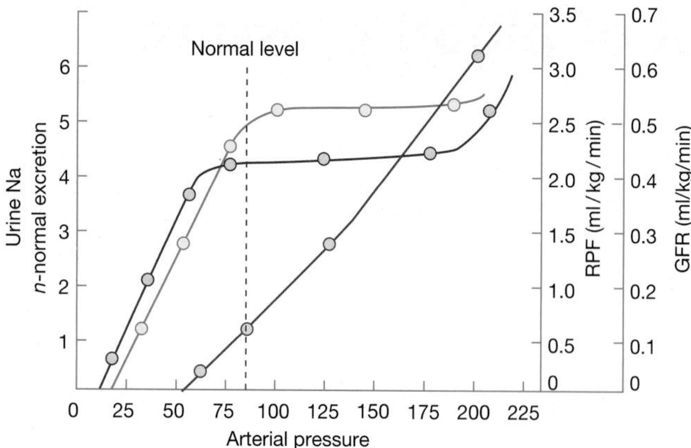

Fig. 2 Schematic representation of the pressure–natriuresis and autoregulation of renal haemodynamics for the long-term control of arterial pressure.

Table 2 Factors participating in the regulation and control of pressure–natriuresis

Renal nerves
Prostaglandins
Angiotensin II
Atrial natriuretic peptide
Nitric oxide
Kallikrein–kinin system
Vasopressin

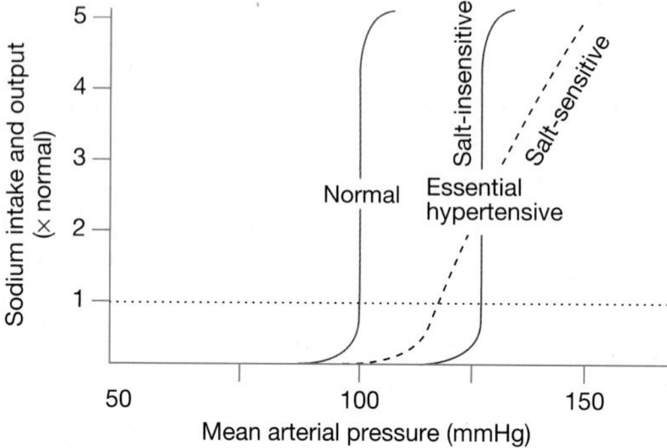

Fig. 3 Arterial pressure versus sodium intake and output curves for normal kidneys, and kidneys in salt-sensitive and -insensitive essential hypertensives.

preglomerular vasoconstriction that impedes the transmission of an elevated systemic arterial pressure to the glomeruli and peritubular capillaries of the kidney (Romero *et al.* 1988).

According to Cowley and Roman (1996), the mechanism underlying the relationship between an increase in arterial pressure and the subsequent increase in natriuresis, is the transmission of changes in systemic pressure into the renal interstitium via changes in renal medullary haemodynamics. Many factors, summarized in Table 2, are implicated in the endocrine and paracrine regulation of this phenomenon.

The pressure–natriuresis is at the origin of arterial hypertension, but it is in no way presumed that the abnormality leading to the elevation in arterial pressure is intrinsic to the kidney. It is equally possible that the changes of the pressure–natriuresis relationship results from the fact that the kidney reacts to extrarenal signals, for example, hormonal or neural in nature. In any case, the analysis of the pressure–natriuresis mechanism may provide a clue to understand the precise nature of the defect(s) responsible for altering kidney function in essential hypertension (Hall 1991). An example is the classification of the hypertensive population according to the response of arterial pressure to changes in salt intake. In response to changes in salt intake, patients segregate into those in whom arterial pressure is relatively insensitive to changes in the sodium content of the diet (salt-insensitive individuals) and those exhibiting relevant changes in arterial pressure with changes in salt intake (salt-sensitive individuals). Figure 3 depicts the pressure–natriuresis relationship in these two groups. Salt-insensitive hypertensives exhibit a shift of pressure–natriuresis curve to higher pressures in parallel with the normal curve. In contrast, salt-sensitive hypertensives in whom plasma renin activity is frequently low, the curve is also shifted to higher levels of arterial pressure, but the slope is flat. When salt content in the diet is low, blood pressure is normal, but it increases progressively, when the salt content in the diet is increased. Hall (1992) postulated that the presence of a flat slope indicates that additional abnormalities of renal function must be present besides a simple increase in glomerular resistance.

The renin–angiotensin system

The renin–angiotensin system serves as one of the most powerful regulators of arterial pressure and sodium balance. As can be seen in Fig. 4, in response to various stimuli that compromise blood volume, extracellular fluid volume, arterial pressure, stress, and trauma, three major mechanisms are activated, that is, the macula densa, baroreceptor reflex, and the sympathetic nervous system. All three mechanisms stimulate renin release by the cells of the juxtaglomerular apparatus. Renin hydrolyzes angiotensinogen that is synthesized in the liver to form angiotensin I. This decapeptide is rapidly converted to angiotensin II by the angiotensin-converting enzyme (ACE) present primarily in the lungs and endothelial cells. Angiotensin II, an octapeptide is the most active component of this system and is responsible for its most relevant actions. Angiotensin II plays a central role in regulating extracellular fluid volume as well as systemic vascular resistance. It is a unique hormone in that it regulates arterial pressure by acting on the circulating fluid volume, as well as on vascular resistance. Angiotensin II binds in humans to at least two receptors, that is, AT1 and AT2 receptors that have been cloned and pharmacologically characterized. Most of the known effects of angiotensin II are mediated through the AT1 receptor, for example, vasoconstriction, aldosterone and vasopressin release, salt and water retention through the kidney, and sympathetic activation, as well as important autocrine and paracrine effects on cell proliferation and migration and on extracellular matrix formation. The effects of the stimulation of the AT2 receptor seem to counteract the effect of the binding of angiotensin II to the AT1 receptor. Its effects are vasodilatory and antiproliferative. The expression of the AT2 receptor is high in embryonic tissue and low in adult lifetime. The AT2 receptor is re-expressed, however, in various pathological situations, suggesting that the AT2 receptor plays a role in pathophysiology (De Gasparo and Bullock 2000).

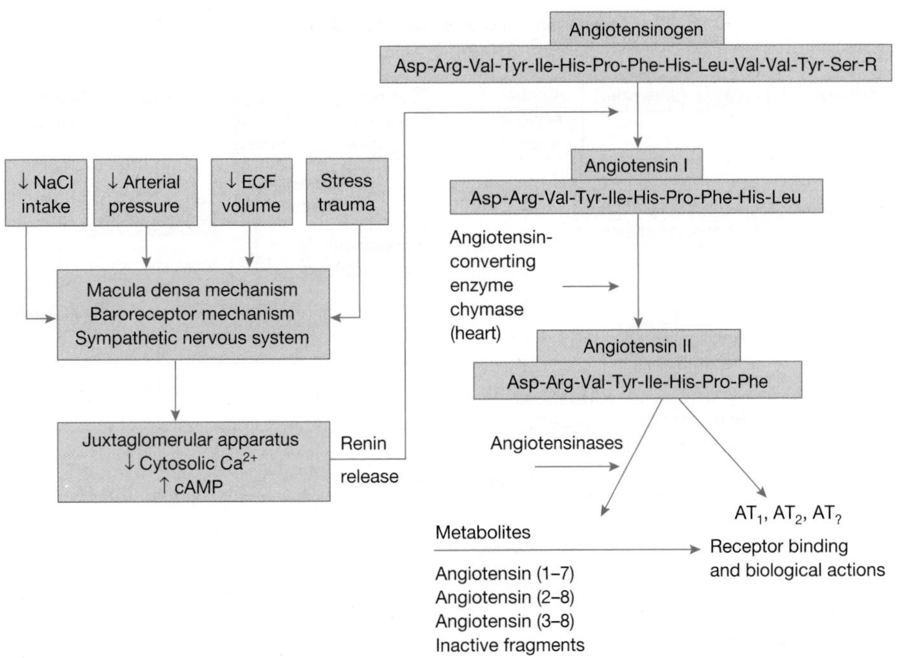

Fig. 4 Scheme of the renin–angiotensin system.

Recent studies have indicated that further angiotensin metabolites such as angiotensin (2–8), angiotensin (1–7), and angiotensin (3–8) also have biological actions, which may be mediated via alternative receptors.

Renin hypersecretion by the kidney is clearly responsible for hypertension in humans in two clinical situations. First, when renin is hypersecreted secondary to the existence of a renin-secreting tumour known as haemangiopericytoma (Mimran 1994). Second, when renin is secreted as a result of stenosing lesions in the renal vessels, causing renal ischaemia as in renovascular hypertension or in dialysis-resistant hypertension in patients with advanced renal disease (Wilkinson *et al.* 1970). The most clear-cut experimental example of the participation of this system in blood pressure elevation is the hypertension resulting from chronic infusion of angiotensin II. This model offers some insight into the complexity of mechanisms involved in the genesis of hypertension even when a single cause can be defined. Such multiple actions of angiotensin II and of further effectors of the system are depicted in Fig. 5. Obviously, angiotensin II has many actions that go far beyond its renal effects. Under physiological conditions the main task of angiotensin is to increase sodium reabsorption by the kidney in order to guarantee volume homeostasis, depicted in Fig. 6.

On the other hand, as previously stated, angiotensin II provokes vasoconstriction followed by an increase in arterial pressure. Direct vasoconstriction cannot be the only mechanism, however. When the correlation between plasma angiotensin II concentration and arterial pressure values is examined in patients with renin-secreting tumours, blood pressure values are much higher than those obtained by infusing angiotensin II to achieve similar plasma concentrations (Brown *et al.* 1979). In other words, chronic exposure to increased or even normal concentrations of angiotensin II in the presence of elevated arterial blood pressure amplifies the immediate pressure response. An analogous phenomenon has been demonstrated in rabbits and rats. Infusion of doses of angiotensin II that were insufficient to cause an acute increase in arterial pressure, when infused chronically over a period of days were capable of causing a gradual increase in arterial blood pressure (Dickinson and Lawrence 1963). This slow-pressor effect of angiotensin II can be attributed to several mechanisms. First, blood pressure becomes salt-sensitive because circulating angiotensin II is no longer suppressed in response to elevated blood pressure or because the balance between angiotensin II and nitric oxide in tissues is disturbed. Second, angiotensin II increases oxidative stress. Reactive oxidant species diminish the synthesis of nitric oxide, scavenge nitric oxide thus reducing its bioavailability, and cause lipid oxidation resulting in the formation of vasoconstrictor prostanoids. Third, angiotensin II causes vascular hypertrophy because of its known trophic effects (Dickingson 1981; Lever 1986; Elijovich *et al.* 1998). It was initially thought that high peripheral arterial resistance was maintained through structurally fixed luminal narrowing of resistance vessels. More recent studies in different forms of human hypertension have suggested, however, that the decrease in wall : lumen ratio of the resistance vessels is not the consequence of hypertrophy or hyperplasia, but is the consequence of rearrangement of the media around a reduced lumen (remodelling) (Mulvany 1994). Hypertrophy or remodelling of the resistance vessels, facilitated by the slow-pressor mechanism of angiotensin II or by other mechanism(s), increases resistance to flow even at maximal vasodilatation. It contributes to the maintenance of arterial hypertension since in elegant experiments scandinavian investigators showed that after remodelling of resistance vessels, the pressor dose–response curve was much steeper (Folkow 1982; Mulvany 1994).

Recent evidence suggests that the angiotensin receptors in different tissues are not only activated by circulating angiotensin II, but also by angiotensin II formed by local renin–angiotensin systems of different tissues (Deinum and Schalekamp 2000). The kidney secretes renin in to the circulation to be delivered to extrarenal tissues including heart, brain, and vessels to form both angiotensins I and II in these tissues. Furthermore, there is increasing evidence that in several tissues all components of the renin–angiotensin systems are available locally.

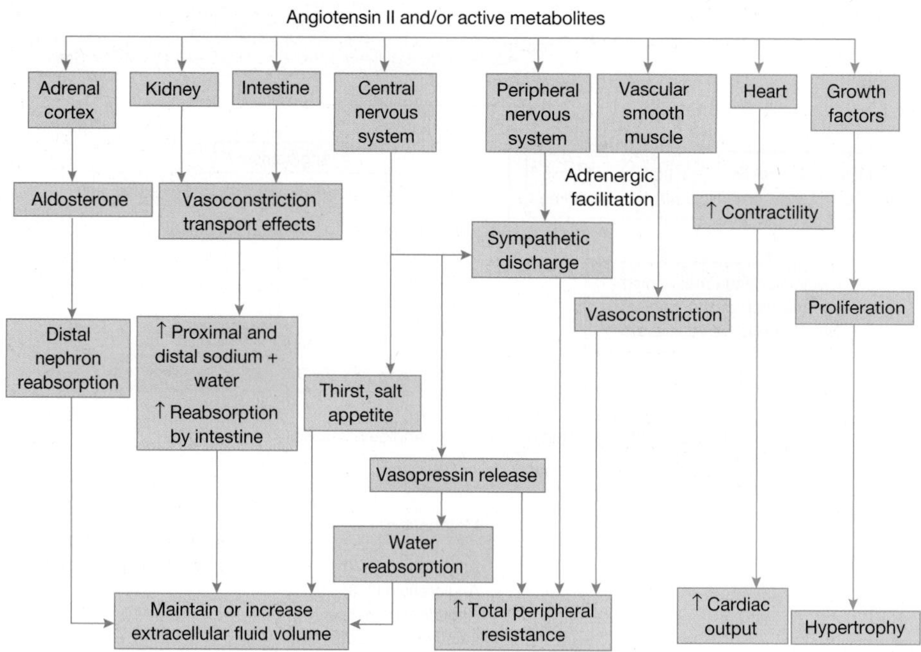

Fig. 5 Actions of angiotensin II and other active metabolites of the renin–angiotensin system.

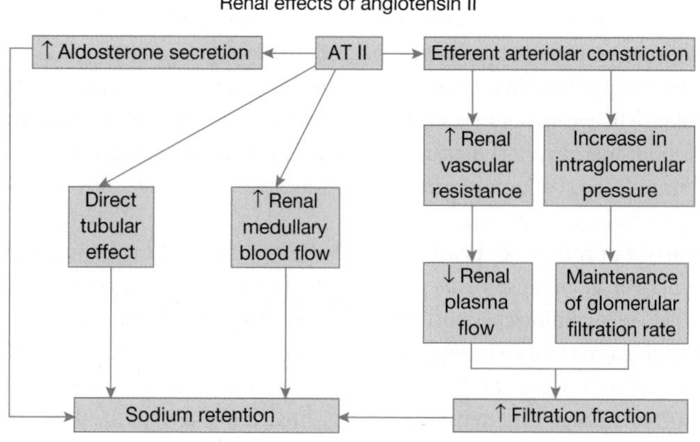

Fig. 6 Mechanisms by which angiotensin II facilitates sodium retention.

Formation of angiotensins I and II in intra- and extrarenal tissue compartments does not necessarily parallel the concentration of these peptides in plasma (Komine *et al.* 2002).

An example of this situation is diabetes mellitus where levels of circulating components of the system are low, but the intrarenal synthesis of angiotensin II is increased (Price *et al.* 1999). In this situation, angiotensin II acts as a paracrine and autocrine hormone. Tissue renin–angiotensin systems are of potential clinical relevance in light of the growing evidence that the beneficial effects of ACE inhibitors (ACEi) and angiotensin receptor blockers (ARBs) in heart failure, post-myocardial infarction, arterial hypertension, and renal disease do not depend solely on their actions on the circulating renin–angiotensin system.

Renal nerves

The sympathetic nervous system has been implicated in the pathogenesis of essential hypertension and in the spontaneously hypertensive rat (Folkow 1982). There is a good correlation between arterial pressure and renal nerve activity measured in crossbreeds of spontaneously hypertensive rats (Judy *et al.* 1976). Acute renal denervation shifts the relationship between sodium excretion and arterial pressure towards lower pressure values (Roman and Cowley 1985). On the other hand, reflex activation of the sympathetic tone markedly blunts the pressure–natriuresis in conscious dogs (Ehmke *et al.* 1990). These findings indicate that the renal nerves exert a tonic influence on the pressure–natriuresis relationship. In humans with mild arterial hypertension, when compared to normal individuals, sympathetic overactivity resulting from mental stress is accompanied, by a greater increase in arterial pressure and in GFR as well as a blunted natriuretic response (Schneider *et al.* 2001). The renal capacity to excrete sodium returned to normal after the administration of an ACEi. This indicates that angiotensin II is involved in blunting of the pressure–natriuresis, which is observed in individuals with mild hypertension during activation of the sympathetic nervous system.

On the other hand, renal afferent nerves can also increase the activity of the sympathetic nervous system in situations of renal ischaemia, such as renovascular hypertension or chronic renal failure of different origins (Johansson and Friberg 2000; Orth *et al.* 2001). The increase in sympathetic tone will contribute to maintain the elevation of arterial pressure by promoting further renal and systemic vasoconstriction and in the long run by facilitating the remodelling of resistance arterioles (Intengan and Schiffrin 2001). Interestingly, in the presence of chronic renal failure the participation of the sympathetic nervous system can also be counteracted by the administration of an ACEi (Ligtenberg *et al.* 1999).

Finally, a correlation is found between sodium balance and activity of the sympathetic nervous system. This observation could contribute to the resolution of one of the major problems of the pathogenesis of arterial hypertension: how does sodium and water retention give rise to elevated arterial pressure? Folkow and Ely (1987) demonstrated in normotensive and spontaneously hypertensive rats that a high sodium intake increases the amount of neurotransmitter released per nerve impulse at noradrenergic nerve endings. Salt restriction has the opposite effect, reducing the release of noradrenaline per nerve impulse. This effect was particularly pronounced in hypertensive rats. De Champlain *et al.* (1969) have shown an increased turnover of noradrenaline in deoxycorticosterone-salt hypertension, which is a well-known example of volume-mediated hypertension. Chemical sympathectomy has shown to prevent the development of hypertension in the same model (Okuno *et al.* 1985). Experiments conducted during the last two decades suggest that salt loading alters the activity of central alpha2-adrenergic receptors, resulting in a hypertensive hyperadrenergic state (Gavras and Gavras 2001).

Renal depressor mechanisms

Early experiments suggested that the positive sodium and water balance could not entirely explain the hypertension that follows bilateral nephrectomy. This hypothesis was upheld by further more complex studies. The existence of a renomedullary antihypertensive function was demonstrated in different animal models of arterial hypertension (Muirhead *et al.* 1971; Swales *et al.* 1987). The interstitial cells in the renal medulla contain two classes of antihypertensive lipid. One compound known as medullipin I is an inactive prohormone and requires conversion by the liver to the active compound medullipin II that is responsible for the arterial pressure lowering activity of the renal medulla (Muirhead 1994). Much more will have to be learnt regarding the physiology of this hormone and its involvement in the genesis of arterial hypertension. Its role in arterial blood pressure control seems to depend on its capacity to vasodilate, to inhibit sympathetic tone, and to promote natriuresis (Bergstrom *et al.* 1998). A deficit in renomedullary depressor substances does not seem to be causally involved in the genesis of all forms of hypertension. At least in one experimental model of hypertension, the spontaneously hypertensive rat, the droplet content of interstitial cells is increased and an appropriate increase is seen in response to a low salt intake (Kett *et al.* 2001).

Other systems or substances produced by the renal tissue and vessels that participate in the renal regulation of arterial pressure through haemodynamic or tubular effects are prostaglandins, the peptides of the kallikrein–kinin system, nitric oxide, and endothelin (Cowley and Roman 1996).

Situations where the kidney is involved in the genesis of human hypertension in the absence of an intrinsic renal defect

As previously mentioned, under normal conditions renal function in humans is characterized by the interaction of different systems that interact to maintain circulating blood volume and arterial blood pressure within normal limits. Despite an otherwise normal renal function, however, the kidney participates in the elevation of systemic arterial pressure by performing its physiological functions to an excessive degree. These forms of arterial hypertension can be cured when the faulty stimulus driving the kidney to overperform is corrected. I shall cite two examples resulting from inappropriate performance of an otherwise totally normal kidney, which responds to faulty extrinsic signals. One of these signals is renal ischaemia. This is perceived by the receptor of the juxtaglomerular apparatus as a low perfusion pressure, for example in the patient with renovascular hypertension. The other example is the patient with autonomous secretion of aldosterone, as a result of primary aldosteronism due to an adenoma. Aldosterone drives an otherwise normal kidney to increased reabsorption of sodium.

Arterial pressure normalizes after intervention on the renal artery by angioplasty or surgery, particularly in young women with renovascular hypertension due to unilateral fibromuscular dysplasia. In cases where atherosclerosis is the cause of the renal artery stenosis the success of intervention is less certain. The fact that arterial pressure returns to normal values and remains normal indicates that renal function in the affected kidney(s) is normal as well. At least when the duration of arterial hypertension has not been sufficiently long to bring about the above-mentioned vascular adaptations that perpetuate the elevation in arterial pressure.

Similarly, when an aldosterone secreting adrenal adenoma causing arterial hypertension is surgically removed, permanent normotension may be seen after the intervention. In this case, through increased sodium reabsorption and probably other mechanisms, the kidney facilitates the elevation of arterial pressure, but behaves absolutely normal once the stimulus of elevated aldosterone concentrations has disappeared.

These two situations exemplify how, in response to different signals (ischaemia or aldosterone), normally operating renal systems cause, or at least contribute to, increased arterial blood pressure.

Situations where a renal defect or disease is involved in the genesis of arterial hypertension

Evidence derived from transplantation experiments and from human renal transplantation

Over the last decades evidence has accumulated indicating that arterial hypertension can be transmitted to a normotensive recipient by the transplantation of the kidney of a hypertensive animal or hypertensive human donor. More precisely, cross-transplantation experiments have been performed between hypertensive strains of rats and their normotensive controls. To avoid confounding effects of the native kidneys of the recipients, bilateral nephrectomy had been performed before or during transplantation. The results of these experiments demonstrate that after transplantation, the blood pressure values of the recipient reach levels similar to those of the donor. Classical experiments of this kind were carried out by Dahl *et al.* (1972). Using inbreeding techniques, two strains of rats were obtained that were completely different with respect to the arterial pressure response to salt feeding. One of the strains developed high arterial pressure when fed a high-salt diet, while the other did not. Dahl transplanted the kidneys of hypertensive rats of the salt-sensitive strain to salt-resistant rats that were normotensive, while on a normal sodium intake. The result convincingly documented that the recipient animals developed hypertension (see Fig. 7). The transplantation experiments can be interpreted as the transplantation of a primary renal abnormality. From this perspective, hypertension is an epiphenomenon, not the primary transplanted abnormality. Results similar to those obtained in Dahl rats were seen when the kidneys from spontaneously hypertensive rats, stroke-prone spontaneously hypertensive rats, and Milan hypertensive rats were transplanted into the respective normotensive counterparts (Elijovich *et al.* 1998). Evidence for a primary role of the kidney in hypertension has also been provided by corresponding observations in human renal transplantation. In humans, a graft from a hypertensive donor, presumably genetically programmed for hypertension, kidney can transmit not only chronic hypertension, but also susceptibility to a greater rise in arterial pressure and more severe kidney impairment compared to recipients of grafts from normotensive donors (Guidi *et al.* 1998). On the other hand, kidneys from normotensive donors without a family history of arterial hypertension, when grafted into hypertensive recipients who had developed endstage renal disease due to nephrosclerosis, led to permanent normotension (Curtis *et al.* 1983).

What does the renal abnormality consist of?

There is a well-documented connection between hypertension and salt intake both in man and in different animals. The link between diet and arterial pressure could reside in the presence of a renal abnormality consisting in a restricted ability to excrete sodium (Woolfson and de Wardener 1996). In agreement is this hypothesis, the offspring of hypertensive parents experience a significant increase in arterial pressure in response to volume expansion with saline (Grim *et al.* 1979). This is accompanied by accelerated natriuresis (Wiggins *et al.* 1978), similar to what has been described in established hypertension. A positive correlation between urinary sodium excretion and systolic blood pressure is also found in the offspring of hypertensive parents (Hooft 1994).

Different theories have been proposed concerning the renal defect(s) accounting for the initiation of arterial hypertension. Hereditary hypertension is characterized, both in animals and in humans, by the presence of generalized membrane abnormalities (Aviv and Lasker 1990). It has been suggested that membrane transport functions could be markers of individual susceptibility to the pressor effects of salt. Membrane abnormalities present in blood cells could be paralleled by membrane alterations in the renal tubuli accounting for defective renal handling of dietary sodium. The existence of a primary renal defect in sodium handling could then lead to the elevation in arterial pressure, through extracellular volume expansion. It has also been proposed that volume expansion leads to increased concentrations of circulating ion transport inhibitors in an effort to counteract the renal abnormality. The increase in these factor(s) acting on both renal epithelial cells and vascular smooth muscle cells would restore natriuresis, but at the cost of increasing the intracellular content of calcium in smooth muscle cells facilitating vasoconstriction and elevating arterial pressure (Blaustein 1977).

A congenital reduction in the number of nephrons or in the filtration area per glomerulus (Brenner *et al.* 1988), or the presence of nephron population heterogeneity with a subpopulation of ischaemic nephrons hypersecreting renin chronically (Sealey *et al.* 1988), are other theories proposed to explain a primary renal origin of arterial hypertension.

Several years ago, we published a review on renal alterations and the origin of human arterial hypertension (Ruilope *et al.* 1994). We had concluded that, according to the data available in the literature, vasoconstriction was the most common finding in the kidneys of offspring of hypertensive patients as well as in borderline and established hypertension. The existence of preglomerular vasoconstriction would cause displacement of the relationship between arterial pressure and natriuresis to the right, as shown in Fig. 8. Higher renal perfusion pressure levels are needed to ensure balance between salt intake and salt excretion by the kidneys. Renal vasoconstriction is not an isolated phenomenon, but is seen in other vascular beds also, as the consequence of cardiovascular adaptation in primary hypertension (Folkow 1982). A lack of modulation of the renal vasculature in response to angiotensin II-increased sympathetic activity or withdrawal of dopaminergic activity could be the mechanism(s) underlying the apparent renal vasoconstriction. As can be seen in Fig. 9, renal vasoconstriction is functional in nature during the initial stages of the process and can be reversed preferentially by calcium channel blockers and ACEi. Later on, the maintenance of elevated arterial pressure leads to the appearance of nephrosclerosis causing further increase in renal vascular resistance. At this stage, renal vasoconstriction is no longer reversible.

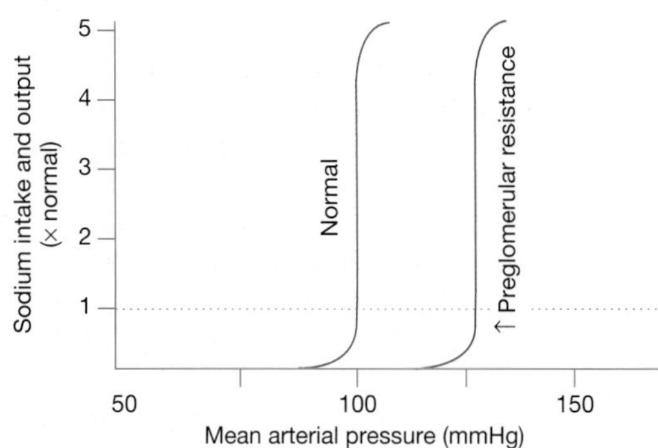

Fig. 7 Effect on arterial pressure of the transplantation of a kidney from a normotensive rat to a hypertensive rat and vice versa.

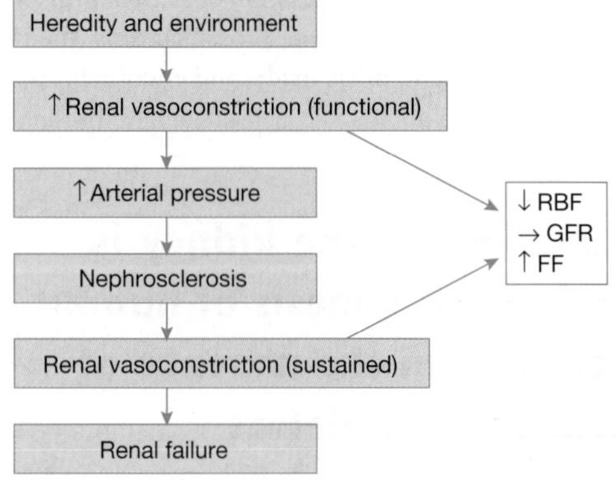

Fig. 8 Characteristic steady-state relationships between mean arterial pressure and an increase in preglomerular resistance.

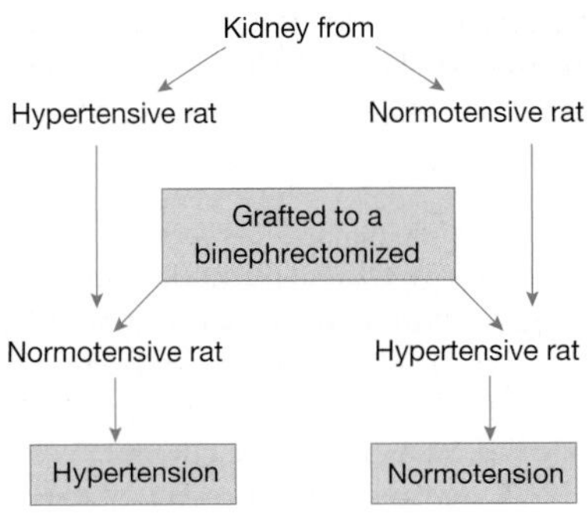

Fig. 9 Evolution of renal vasoconstriction during the development and maintenance of essential hypertension.

The issue of subtle acquired renal injury in the origin of arterial hypertension

Very recently, a unifying hypothesis has been proposed. Subtle abnormalities in renal function resulting from a primary insult causing sustained renal vasoconstriction should lead to the development of salt-sensitive hypertension (Johnson *et al.* 2002). As a consequence of persistent renal vasoconstriction, the resulting tubular ischaemia and preglomerular arteriolopathy should increase sodium reabsorption and decrease the filtered load of sodium, respectively. It was speculated that the ensuing elevation in arterial pressure should counteract the effects of tubular ischaemia and diminish single GFR. Renal sodium handling would then be normalized but at the price of persisting hypertension. Salt-sensitivity has been shown to be particularly prevalent in Black, in obese, and in elderly hypertensive patients. It is frequently associated with microalbuminuria, absence of the nocturnal decrease in arterial pressure and absence of modulation of renal blood flow in response to sodium loading. The above predisposing conditions are characterized by the frequent presence of a diminished renal function and by a significantly enhanced cardiovascular risk. Both renal and cardiovascular risk have been shown to run in parallel, and, in fact, mild alterations in renal function constitute the best predictors of an increased cardiovascular risk (Ruilope *et al.* 2001).

A look into the future

The mechanism(s) through which the kidneys participate in the development of arterial hypertension will certainly be better characterized in the future. Essential hypertension is recognized as a polygenic syndrome and most classifications of hypertension have been based on characterization of intermediate phenotypes. Some of these phenotypes are: salt-sensitivity, low or normal renin state, or an attenuated response of the adrenal and the renal vasculature to angiotensin II (Williams *et al.* 1992). The better characterization of the genetic basis of common phenotypic forms of hypertension will also facilitate the elucidation of the mechanisms through which the kidney mediates changes in arterial pressure. Although the products of many genes are involved in renal sodium handling, the possibility exists that a mutation in only one or a few of these genes may be sufficient to alter salt sensitivity in a given individual. An example is the recent description of how the homozygous expression of one single nucleotide polymorphism of the alpha adducin gene, the 460 Trp polymorphism, modifies sodium homeostasis and is associated with the intermediate phenotypes of salt-sensitivity and low-renin hypertension (Grant *et al.* 2002).

In summary, the kidneys can be at the root of the development of arterial hypertension or they can participate in the maintenance of hypertension and its sequels. Renal alterations interfering with the regulation of sodium homeostasis or facilitating the generation of vasoconstrictors particularly angiotensin II, are involved in the deregulation of arterial blood pressure that underlies the development of arterial hypertension. On the other hand, the kidney may suffer injury from a sustained elevation of arterial pressure that can end up in renal failure. Once the kidney has been damaged, it will contribute greatly to the increase of arterial pressure.

References

Aperia, A. C., Brobergen, C. G. O., and Sodenland, S. (1971). Relationship between renal artery perfusion pressure and tubular reabsorption. *American Journal of Physiology* **220**, 1205–1212.

Aviv, A. and Lasker, N. Proposed defects in membrane transport and intracellular ions as pathogenic factors in essential hypertension. In *Hypertension. Pathophysiology, Diagnosis and Management* (ed. J. H. Laragh and B. M. Brenner), pp. 923–937. New York, NY: Raven Press, 1990.

Bergstrom, G., Gothberg, G., Karlstrom, G., and Rudenstam, J. (1998). Renal medullary blood flow and renal medullary antihypertesive mechanisms. *Clinical and Experimental Hypertension* **20**, 1–26.

Blaustein, M. P. (1977). Sodium ions, calcium ions, blood pressure regulation, and hypertension: a reassessment and a hypothesis. *American Journal of Physiology* **232**, C165–C173.

Brenner, B. M., Garcia, D., and Anderson, S. (1988). Glomeruli and blood pressure. Less of one, more the other? *American Journal of Hypertension* **1**, 335–347.

Bright, R. (1836). Tabular view of the morbid appearances in 100 cases connected with albuminous urine. *Guy's Hospital Reports* **1**, 380–400.

Brown, J. J., Casals-Stedntzel, J., Cumming, A. M., Davies, D. L., Fraser, R., Lever, A. F., Morton, J. J., Semple, P. F., Tree, M., and Robertsson, J. I. S. (1979). Angiotensin II, aldosterone and arterial pressure: a quantitative approach. *Hypertension* **1**, 159–179.

Cowley, A. W. and Roman, R. J. (1996). The role of the kidney in hypertension. *Journal of the American Medical Association* **275**, 1581–1589.

Curtis, J. J., Luke, R. G., Dustan, H. P., Kashgarian, M., Whelchel, J. D., Jones, P., and Diethelm, A. G. (1983). Remission of essential hypertension after renal transplantation. *New England Journal of Medicine* **309**, 1009–1015.

Dahl, L. K., Heine, M., and Thompson, K. (1972). Genetic influence of renal homografts on the blood pressure of rats from different strains. *Proceedings of the Society for Experimental Biology and Medicine* **140**, 852–856.

De Champlain, J., Krakoff, L., and Oxelrod, J. (1969). Interrelationships of sodium intake, hypertension and norepinephrine storage in the rat. *Circulation Research* **24** (Suppl. I), 75–92.

De Gasparo, M. and Bullock, G. R. The AT1 and AT2 angiotensin receptors. In *Hypertension* (ed. S. Oparil and M. A. Weber), pp. 100–110. Philadelphia, PA: W.B. Saunders, 2000.

Deinum, J. and Schalekamp, M. A. D. H. Renin and prorenin. In *Hypertension* (ed. S. Oparil and M. A. Weber), pp. 70–76. Philadelphia, PA: W.B. Saunders, 2000.

Dickinson, C. J. (1981). Neurogenic hypertension revisited. *Clinical Science* **60**, 471–477.

Dickinson, C. J. and Lawrence, F. R. (1963). A slowly developing pressor response to small concentrations of angiotensin. *Lancet* **1**, 1354–1356.

Ehmke, H., Persson, P. B., Seyforth, M., and Kirchheim, H. R. (1990). Neurogenic control of pressure natriuresis in conscious dogs. *American Journal of Physiology* **259**, F466–F473.

Elijovich, F., Laffer, C. L., and Romero, J. C. (1998). Pathogenesis of essential hypertension: the kidney, slow pressor responses to angiotensin II and oxidative stress. *BioMedicina* **1**, 303–309.

Folkow, B. (1982). Physiological aspects of primary hypertension. *Physiological Reviews* **62**, 347–504.

Folkow, B. and Ely, D. L. (1987). Dietary sodium effects on cardiovascular and sympathetic neuroeffector function as studied in various rat models. *Journal of Hypertension* **5**, 383–395.

Gavras, I. and Gavras, H. (2001). Role of the alpha2-adrenergic receptors in hypertension. *American Journal of Hypertension* **14** (pt 2), 171S–177S.

Grant, F. D., Romero, J. R., Jeunemaitre, X., Hunt, S. C., Hopkins, P. N., Hollenberg, N. K., and Williams, G. H. (2002). Low-renin hypertension, altered sodium homeostasis, and alpha-adduci polymorphism. *Hypertension* **39**, 191–196.

Grim, C. E., Luft, F. C., Miller, J. Z., Brown, P. L., Gannon, M. A., and Weinberger, M. H. (1979). Effects of sodium loading and depletion in normotensive first-degree relatives of essential hypertensives. *Journal of Laboratory and Clinical Medicine* **94**, 764–771.

Guidi, E., Cozzi, M. G., Minetti, E., and Bianchi, G. (1998). Donor and recipient family histories of hypertension influence renal impairment and blood pressure during acute rejections. *Journal of the American Society of Nephrology* **9**, 2102–2107.

Guyton, A. C., Coleman, T. G., Cowley, A. W., Jr., Scheel, K. W., Manning, R. D., Jr., and Norman, R. A., Jr. (1972). Arterial pressure regulation: overriding dominance of the kidneys in long-term regulation and in hypertension. *American Journal of Medicine* **52**, 584–594.

Hall, J. E. (1991). Renal function in one-kidney, one-clip hypertension and low-renin essential hypertension. *American Journal of Hypertension* **4**, 523S–533S.

Hall, J. E., Mizelle, H. L., Brands, M. W., and Hildebrand, D. A. (1992). Pressure natriuresis and angiotensin II in reduced kidney mass, salt-induced hypertension. *American Journal of Physiology* **262**, R61–R71.

Hooft, I. M., ed. Renal sodium handling, intracellular sodium, sodium–potassium ATPase activity, and unsaturated fatty acids in offspring of hypertensive and normotensive parents. In *The Dutch Hypertension and Offspring Study* pp. 269–286. Den Haag: CIP-DATA Koninklijke Bibliotheek, 1994.

Intengan, H. D. and Schiffrin, E. J. (2001). Vascular remodeling in hypertension: role of apoptosis, inflammation, and fibrosis. *Hypertension* **38** (pt 2), 581–587.

Johansson, M. and Friberg, P. (2000). Role of the sympathetic nervous system in human renovascular hypertension. *Current Hypertension Reports* **2**, 319–326.

Johnson, R. J., Herrera-Acosta, J., Schreiner, G. F., and Rodriguez-Iturbe, B. (2002). Subtle acquired renal injury as a mechanism of salt sensitive hypertension. *New England Journal of Medicine* **346**, 913–923.

Judy, W. V., Watanabe, A. M., Henry, D. P., Besch, H. R., Murphy, W. R., and Hocket, G. M. (1976). Sympathetic nerve activity. Role in regulation of blood pressure in spontaneously hypertensive rats. *Circulation Research* **38** (Suppl. II), II-21–II-129.

Kett, M. M., Heideman, B. L., Bertram, J. F., and Anderson, W. P. (2001). Renomedullary interstitial cell lipid droplet content is increased in spontaneously hypertensive rats and by a low salt diet. *Journal of Hypertension* **19**, 1309–1313.

Komine, N., Khang, S., Wead, L. M., Blantz, R. C., and Gabbai, F. B. (2002). Effect of combining an ACE inhibitor and an angiotensin II receptor blocker on plasma and kidney tissue angiotensin II levels. *American Journal of Kidney Diseases* **39**, 159–164.

Lever, A. F. (1986). Slow-pressor mechanism in hypertension: a role for hypertrophy of resistance vessels. *Journal of Hypertension* **4**, 515–524.

Ligtenberg, G., Blankestijn, P. J., Oey, P. L., Klein, I. H., Dijkhorst-Oei, L. T., Boomsma, F., Wieneke, I., van Huffelen, A. C., and Koomans, H. A. (1999). Reduction of sympathetic hyperactivity by enalapril in patients with chronic renal failure. *New England Journal of Medicine* **340**, 1321–1328.

Mimran, A. Renin-secreting tumors. In *Textbook of Hypertension* (ed. J. D. Swales), pp. 858–864. Oxford: Blackwell Scientific, 1994.

Muirhead, E. E. Renomedullary vasodepressor lipid: medullipin. In *Textbook of Hypertension* (ed. J. D. Swales), pp 341–359. Oxford: Blackwell Science, 1994.

Muirhead, E. E., Rightsel, W. A., Leach, B. E., Byers, L. W., Pitcock, J. A., and Brooks, B. (1971). Reversal of hypertension by transplant of cultured renomedullary interstitial cells. *Laboratory Investigation* **36**, 162–172.

Mulvany, M. J. Resistance vessels in hypertension. In *Textbook of Hypertension* (ed. J. D. Swales), pp. 103–119. Oxford: Blackwell Scientific, 1994.

Okuno, T., Winternitz, S. R., Lindheimer, M. D., and Oparil, S. (1985). Central catecholamine depletion, vasopressin and blood pressure in the DOCA/NaCl rat. *American Journal of Physiology* **13**, H807–H811.

Orth, S. R., Amman, K., and Ritz, E. (2001). Sympathetic overactivity and arterial hypertension in renal failure. *Nephrology, Dialysis, Transplantation* **16** (Suppl. 1), 67–69.

Price, D. A., Porter, L. E., Gordon, M., De Oliveira, J. M., Laffel, L. M., Passan, D. R., Williams, G. H., and Hollenberg, N. K. (1999). The paradox of the low renin state in diabetic nephropathy. *Journal of the American Society of Nephrology* **10**, 2382–2391.

Roman, R. J. and Cowley, A. W., Jr. (1985). Characterization of a new model for the study of pressure–natriuresis in the rat. *American Journal of Physiology* **248**, F190–F198.

Romero, J. C., Ruilope, L. M., Bentley, M. D., Fiksen-Olsen, M. J., Lahera, V., and Vidal, M. J. (1988). Comparison of the effects of calcium antagonists and converting enzyme inhibitors on renal function under normal and hypertensive conditions. *American Journal of Cardiology* **62**, 59G–68G.

Ruilope, L. M., Lahera, V., Rodicio, J. L., and Romero, J. C. (1994). Are renal hemodynamics a key factor in the development and maintenance of arterial hypertension? *Hypertension* **23**, 3–9.

Ruilope, L. M., van Veldhuisen, D. J., Ritz, E., and Luscher, T. F. (2001). Renal function: the Cinderella of cardiovascular risk. *Journal of the American College of Cardiology* **38**, 1782–1787.

Schneider, M. P., Klingbeil, A. U., Schlaich, M. P., Langenfeld, M. R., Veelken, R., and Schmieder, R. E. (2001). Impaired sodium excretion during mental stress in mild essential hypertension. *Hypertension* **37**, 923–927.

Sealey, J. E., Blumenfeld, J. D., Bell, G. M., Pecker, M. S., Sommers, S. C., and Laragh, J. H. (1988). On the renal basis for essential hypertension: nephron heterogeneity with discordant renin secretion and sodium excretion causing a hypertensive vasoconstriction–volume relationship. *Journal of Hypertension* **23**, 3–9.

Swales, J. D., Bing, R. F., Edmunds, M. E., Russell, G. I., and Thurston, H. (1987). Reversal of renovascular hypertension: role of the renal medulla. *Canadian Journal of Physiology and Pharmacology* **65**, 1566–1571.

Wiggins, R. C., Basar, I., and Slater, J. D. H. (1978). Effect of arterial pressure and inheritance on the sodium excretory capacity of normal young men. *Clinical Science and Molecular Medicine* **54**, 639–647.

Wilkinson, R., Scott, D. F., Uldall, P. R., and Kerr, D. N. S. (1970). Plasma renin and exchangeable sodium in the hypertension of chronic renal failure. *Journal of Medicine* **39**, 377–394.

Williams, G. H., Dluhy, R. G., Lifton, R. P., Moore, T. J., Gleason, R., Williams, R., Hunt, S. C., Hopkins, P. N., and Hollenberg, N. K. (1992). Non-modulation as an intermediate phenotype in essential hypertension. *Hypertension* **20**, 788–796.

Woolfson, R. G. and de Wardener, H. E. (1996). Primary renal abnormalities in hereditary hypertension. *Kidney International* **50**, 717–731.

9.4 The effects of hypertension on renal vasculature and structure

Ulrich Wenzel and Udo Helmchen

Introduction

Mahomed was the first to suggest, in the late nineteenth century, that arterial hypertension might lead to renal scarring. The concept of a hypertensive nephrosclerosis was introduced by Volhard and Fahr in 1914 and has been extensively used in the literature since then (Wolf 2000). However, the very existence of a hypertensive nephrosclerosis is still far from consensus. While it is indisputable that malignant hypertension is a cause of endstage renal disease (ESRD), there remains a controversy as to whether the so-called benign nephrosclerosis can also lead to ESRD (Caetano *et al.* 1999; Luke 1999).

> Pressure, if it is great enough, will eventually disrupt any structure. Obviously, this is also true of blood pressure. It is therefore not surprising that an experimentally induced great increase in pressure disrupts the integrity of the blood-vessel wall.

This statement was made by Möhring (1977) as a criticism of the 'pressure hypothesis', which was regarded as the only explanation for the development of vascular disease in hypertensive individuals (Beilin and Goldby 1977). In fact, such vascular lesions may be caused or at least influenced by several factors: humoral factors such as angiotensin II, catecholamines, mineralocorticosteroids, prostaglandins, and vasopressin may increase vascular permeability, thereby damaging the vessel walls independently of, or superimposed upon, elevated blood pressure. Nephrosclerosis is literally defined as hardening of the kidney (Greek derivation: *nephros*, kidney; *sclerosis*, hardening). It refers to diseases with predominant pathological changes occurring in the preglomerular vasculature and secondary changes involving the glomeruli and interstitium. Therefore, it is appropriate to describe first those vascular lesions, which, at least under defined experimental conditions, are believed to be caused solely by the presence of hypertension.

Lessons from experimental models

The experimental models of chronic renal hypertension in dogs devised by Goldblatt provided the opportunity to study the structural effects of hypertension (Goldblatt 1938, 1964; Goldblatt *et al.* 1934, 1976). The experimental model of unilateral renal artery stenosis, referred to later as two-kidney one-clip hypertension, has one important advantage, that is, the clipped kidney is protected from the effects of hypertension. This provides a control organ with which vascular lesions occurring within the contralateral non-clipped kidney of the same animal can be compared. Extension of Goldblatt's model to rabbits and rats showed that arterial hypertension was the dominating factor causing vascular lesions within the non-clipped kidneys; vascular damage was not found in the clipped kidneys (Wilson and Pickering 1938; Wilson and Byrom 1939; Floyer 1955; Eng *et al.* 1994; Wenzel 2002b). These experiments documented the unique ability of the altered intrarenal vascular bed to initiate and sustain a vicious circle, that is, hypertension causes vascular lesions, which, in turn, further increase blood pressure (Wilson and Byrom 1941; Floyer 1955).

The morphological similarities between these experimentally produced vascular lesions and those seen in benign and malignant nephrosclerosis in human kidneys are striking (Page and McCubbin 1968). The following description of acute and chronic hypertensive lesions is derived from the rat models of two-kidney one-clip hypertension and desoxycorticosterone salt hypertension as well as from genetic models such as SHR and Dahl rats.

Three different types of preglomerular vascular change may develop in the non-clipped kidneys of animals with two-kidney one-clip hypertension. The first is characterized by medial thickening of the intrarenal arterial and arteriolar walls, leading to an increased wall-to-lumen ratio (Nordborg *et al.* 1983; Hampton *et al.* 1989; Vial and Boyd 1989) (Fig. 1). It is not clear if these changes in the kidney are also associated with an increased number of vascular cells and increased synthesis of vascular wall material, or whether they can be produced just by a remodelling of the vascular wall, that is, redistribution of existing cells and material (Lee 1987; Mulvany and Aalkjaer 1990). Recent data suggest that smooth muscle cell hypertrophy rather than hyperplasia is responsible for the medial thickening. Elevated DNA content of arteries in hypertension may be secondary to a marked increase in cells showing nuclear polyploidy and infiltration of blood-borne cells (Owens *et al.* 1981; Owens and Schwartz 1982; Chobanian *et al.* 1984; Ross 1993). Remodelling is usually an adaptive process that occurs in response to long-term changes in haemodynamic conditions, but it may subsequently contribute to the pathophysiology of hypertension and renal disease (Gibbons and Dzau 1994). The structural adaptation to the hypertensive state and the functional implications have been studied intensively by Folkow and coworkers (Folkow *et al.* 1958; Folkow 1971, 1990). Observations on altered resistance vessels in hypertension led them to suggest that vascular hypertrophy and arterial pressure are linked in a positive feedback relationship, in which minor but persistent overactivity of a pressor mechanism is amplified by hypertrophy. Blood pressure increases slowly and severe hypertension results (Lever 1986). These changes have also been shown to be valid for the renal vascular bed (Lundgren 1974; Berecek *et al.* 1980). Changes in the extracellular matrix in the aortic vascular wall caused by experimental hypertension have been described (Brecher *et al.* 1978; Khan 1987). It is likely that these changes also occur in the renal vasculature (Boffa *et al.* 1999).

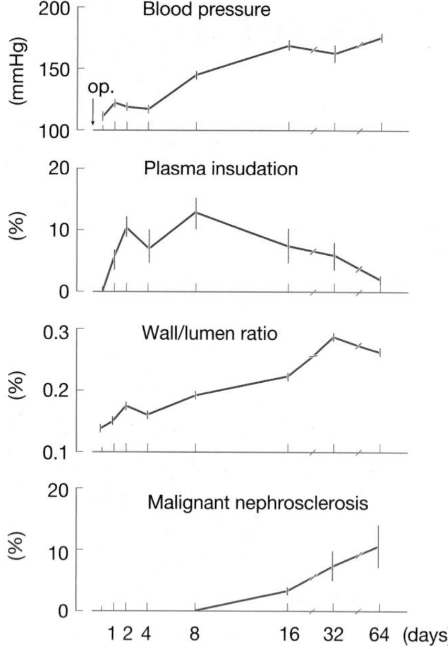

Fig. 1 Experimental two-kidney one-clip hypertension 1–64 days after unilateral renal artery constriction: systolic blood pressure, focal plasma insudation (hyalinosis, necrosis), wall-to-lumen ratio, and malignant nephrosclerosis in interlobular arteries of the pressure-exposed non-clipped kidneys (reproduced with permission from Helmchen *et al.* 1984a).

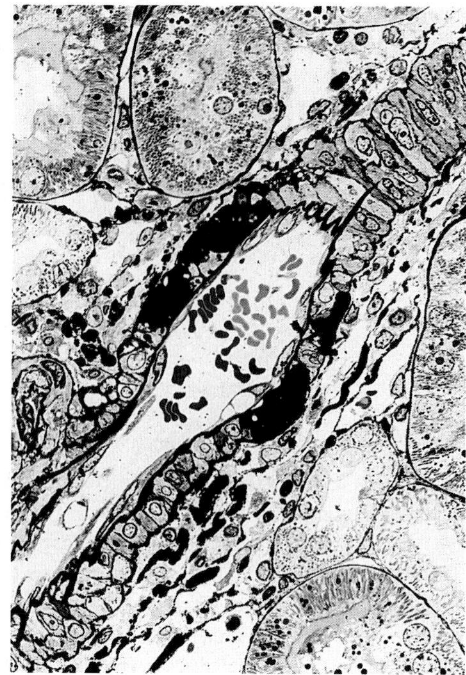

Fig. 2 Non-clipped kidney: focal medial necrosis (plasma insudation, hyalinosis) of an interlobular artery 24 h after unilateral renal artery constriction (immersion fixation, semithin section, silver impregnation; magnification 420×).

The second type of renal vascular alteration consists of segmental hyalinosis of the vessel wall, affecting mainly the interlobular arteries and afferent arterioles. This can be explained by the inability of local areas of these vessel segments to withstand the increased stress, resulting in a critical vascular dilatation. Broad gaps between the underlying endothelial cells may occur temporarily, followed by an intrusion of blood constituents into the vessel walls and by focal necrosis of medial smooth muscle cells (Figs 2 and 3). Indeed, segmental hyalinosis is more often associated with dilatation than with narrowing of the vessel lumen. These changes can also be produced if pressure is increased by other procedures, such as injection of angiotensin II, catecholamines, or vasopressin (Giese 1964a, 1973; Byrom 1976; Beilin and Goldby 1977; Wilson and Heptinstall 1984; Johnson *et al.* 1992; Wenzel *et al.* 2000, 2002a).

In vivo examination of cerebral, retinal, and mesenteric arterioles under different hypertensive conditions has shown that an increase in blood pressure is consistently followed by alternating patchy constrictions and dilatations of arterioles; injection of marker substances to which the vascular wall is normally impermeable, such as colloidal carbon, labelled dilated segments only (Giese 1964a,b; Byrom 1969; Goldby and Beilin 1972; Johansson 1976). After administration of angiotensin II the proportion of labelled arterioles correlated with arterial pressure, but not with the dose of the vasoconstricting agent; antihypertensive therapy with hydralazine prevented dilatation and carbon labelling of arterioles (Goldby and Beilin 1972). Wilson and Heptinstall (1984) obtained similar results under comparable conditions in interlobular arteries and afferent arterioles of rat kidneys. Since the hyaline vascular changes are considered to be potentially reversible, this type of arterial and arteriolar lesion might be assumed to be negligible. In practice, however, such lesions may reduce the autoregulatory potency

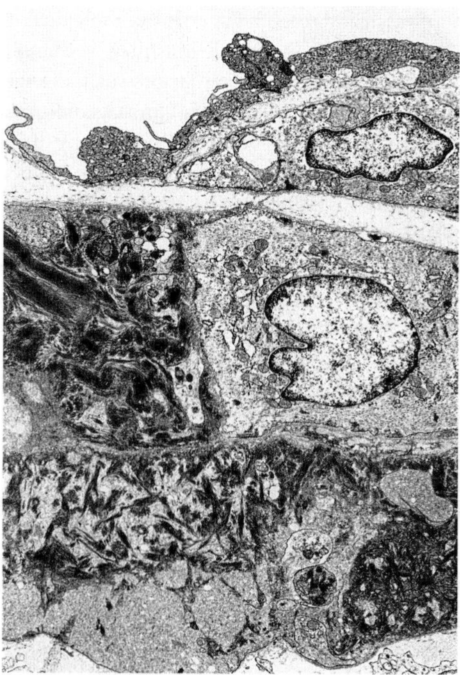

Fig. 3 Non-clipped kidney: electron microscopy findings in a hyaline segment of an interlobular artery 4 days after unilateral renal artery constriction. Plasmic constituents including fibrin precipitate within the partially necrotic media (immersion fixation, transmission electron microscopy; magnification 9000×).

of preglomerular vessels, favouring a transient exposure of the glomerular capillaries to abnormally increased filling pressures with the consequent development of hypertension-induced structural glomerular lesions (Ploth *et al.* 1981; Bidani *et al.* 1987). It seems that an increased preglomerular resistance is protective of glomeruli, whereas decreased resistance with increased flow/pressure is injurious (Olson *et al.* 1986). Similarly, the stenosed kidney is protected from immunological injury (Wenzel *et al.* 2002b). Therefore, antihypertensive drugs which adversely affect autoregulation and pressure transmission may not provide protection against hypertensive glomerular injuries (Wenzel *et al.* 1992, 1994; Griffin *et al.* 1995). In the early stages, these consist of focal and segmental destruction of the glomerular tufts, affecting endothelial, mesangial, and visceral epithelial cells. Capillary aneurysms may complicate these early glomerular lesions, finally resulting in focal and segmental glomerulosclerosis (Fig. 4). The loss of glomeruli will be followed by patchy tubular atrophy and interstitial fibrosis (Fig. 5). Thus, despite its potential reversibility, in the long-term preglomerular focal hyalinosis may contribute to a gradual loss of nephrons, and hence to the hypertensive state itself, by progressively reducing the renal excretory capacity.

The third and most severe type of hypertensive renal vascular lesion is closely related to 'malignant nephrosclerosis' (Fahr 1925; Klemperer and Otani 1931), a condition which really marks the final stage of a sequence of structural changes that develop mainly within the interlobular arteries. Initially, there is usually a widening of the intimal space which is entered by plasmic and corpuscular blood constituents that separate the endothelial cells from the internal elastic membrane (Fig. 6). Later, the intima becomes organized by collagen synthesizing cells, resulting in the typical onion-like appearance of

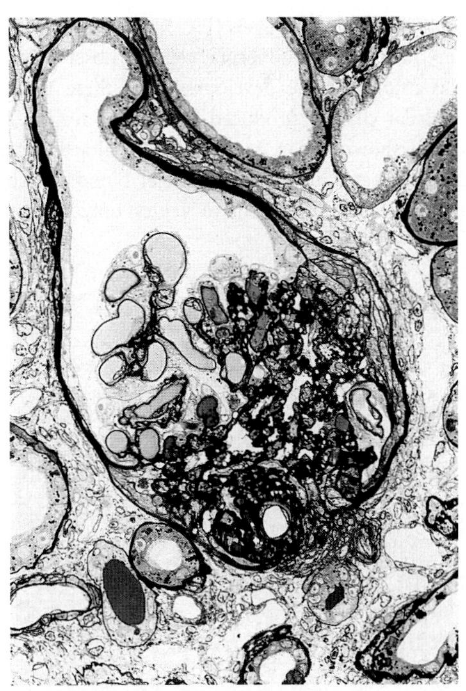

Fig. 5 Non-clipped kidney: glomerulosclerosis, tubular atrophy, and interstitial fibrosis 2 months after unilateral renal artery constriction (pressure-adjusted perfusion fixation, semithin section, silver impregnation; magnification 360×).

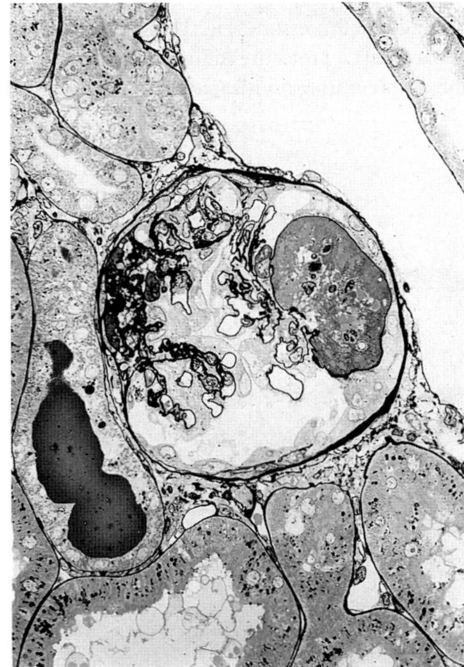

Fig. 4 Non-clipped kidney: capillary aneurysm and segmental sclerosis within a glomerulus 8 days after unilateral renal artery constriction (pressure-adjusted perfusion fixation, semithin section, silver impregnation; magnification 360×).

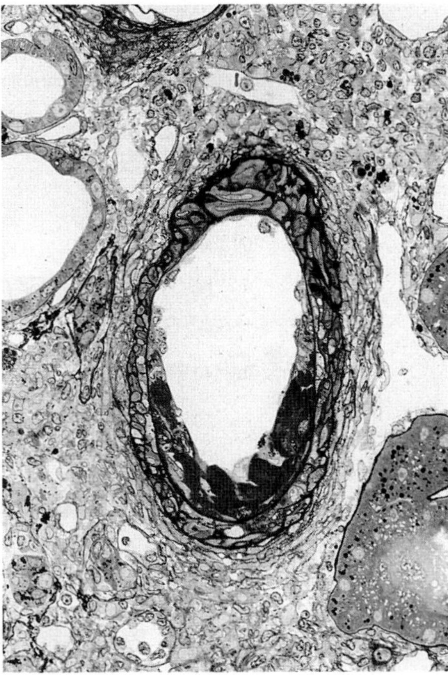

Fig. 6 Non-clipped kidney: early stages of malignant nephrosclerosis with widening of the intimal space containing plasmic material in an interlobular artery 2 months after unilateral renal artery constriction (pressure-adjusted perfusion fixation, semithin section, silver impregnation; magnification 360×).

these substantially narrowed vessels (Fig. 7). Frequently, an increased number of epithelioid juxtaglomerular cells are observed.

Sequential studies of the development of these three types of intrarenal vascular changes produced unexpected results (Helmchen *et al.* 1984a). As shown in Fig. 1, unilateral renal artery constriction induced the anticipated increase in arterial blood pressure which, however, reached stable hypertensive values only after 8 days. In contrast, segmental hyalinosis, reflecting both plasma insudation and focal medial necrosis of intrarenal arteries and arterioles, developed as early as 24 h after surgery. Since segmental vascular damage only occurred in the non-clipped kidneys, haemodynamic rather than humoral influences had to be regarded as causative factors; however, blood pressure was almost normal for the first 4 days. Continuous recording of blood pressure in conscious rats during the first 24 h after renal artery constriction showed the earliest stage of hypertension: short-lived intermittent hypertensive episodes with peaks of more than 200 mmHg occurred during the first 12 h of the experiment (Fig. 8). Such intermittent blood pressure peaks, which were not detected by the usual intermittent measurements, were sufficient to override the vascular resistance of interlobular arteries and afferent arterioles, thereby causing widespread segmental hyalinosis. Comparable intrarenal vascular lesions were observed after short-lived acute hypertensive periods produced by removal of the renal artery clip in the chronically hypertensive rat, thereby suddenly exposing the renal vasculature to high blood pressure (Byrom 1969; Helmchen *et al.* 1976), and after increasing the intravascular filling pressure by rapid intracarotid injections of saline (Byrom and Dodson 1948; Wolfgarten and Magarey 1959). The importance of blood pressure fluctuation for glomerular injury was also demonstrated by Bidani and colleagues: continuous radiotelemetric monitoring of conscious rats showed an exceedingly close correlation of glomerulosclerosis in individual animals with the number of blood pressure fluctuations (Bidani *et al.* 1993; Griffin *et al.* 1994, 2004).

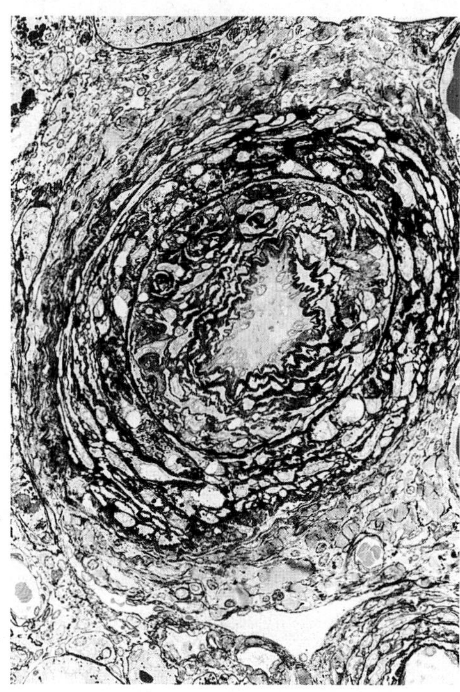

Fig. 7 Non-clipped kidney: late stage of malignant nephrosclerosis with concentric highly narrowing intimal fibrosis in an interlobular artery 4 months after unilateral renal artery constriction (pressure-adjusted perfusion fixation, semithin section, silver impregnation; magnification 420×).

Two weeks after one renal artery has been constricted, the wall-to-lumen ratio of intralobular arteries in the non-clipped kidney is significantly increased; this increase continues for at least 1 month (Fig. 1), mainly due to a widening of the media (Helmchen *et al.* 1984b). By this time, segmental arterial necrosis within interlobular arteries of non-clipped kidneys becomes significantly less common despite increasing blood pressure (Fig. 1). This suggests that medial hypertrophy may exert a protective influence during the hypertensive state, probably by preventing overdistension of the vessel walls. To test

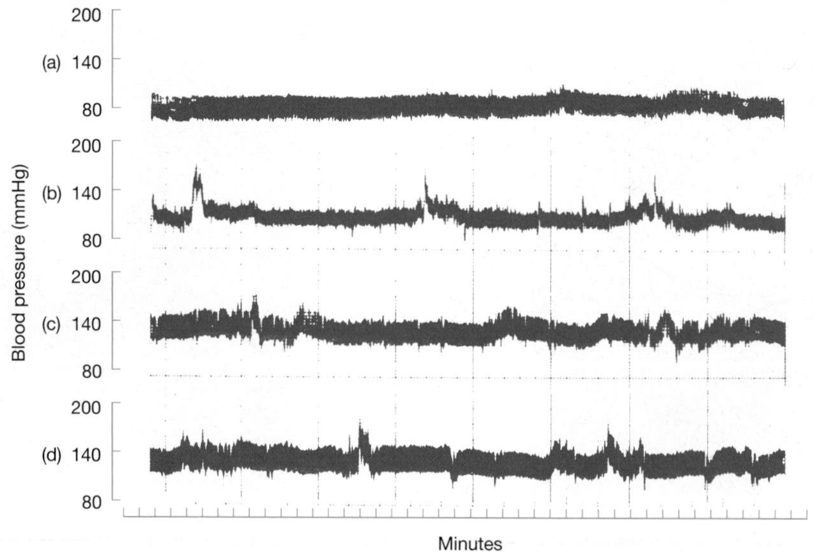

Fig. 8 Continuous blood pressure recording in conscious rats under resting conditions: (a) part of the blood pressure curve of a normotensive control rat; (b)–(d) blood pressure curves of three different rats obtained during the first 24 h after unilateral renal artery constriction (reproduced with permission from Helmchen *et al.* 1984a).

this hypothesis the unilateral renal artery clip was carefully removed from rats which had been hypertensive for 6–8 weeks; 24 h later severe hypertension was induced in these animals by three infusions of angiotensin II, each of 10 min duration (Helmchen *et al.* 1984b). Intravenous colloidal carbon was given just before the first angiotensin II infusion. After 24 h, focal carbon deposits were found predominantly in the kidney, which had previously been protected from the high blood pressure by the renal artery clip. Macroscopically, some of these kidneys appeared almost black. Microscopically, these organs showed carbon particles within foci of medial necrosis in interlobular arteries and afferent arterioles, in the glomerular mesangium, in glomerular aneurysms, and in tubular cells, as well as in the peritubular interstitium (Fig. 9). All these lesions were significantly less pronounced in the previously non-clipped kidneys in which the vessels could undergo structural adaptation. Therefore, it can be assumed that structural adaptation of the vessels may be protective even during extreme hypertension. Interestingly, in the previously non-adapted kidney, severe segmental lesions of interlobular arteries were exclusively confined to the media and were not accompanied by a widening of the intimal space. Only a few interlobular arteries of previously non-clipped pressure-adapted kidneys showed carbon particles within a subendothelial intimal oedema (Helmchen *et al.* 1984b).

Although very short-term increases in blood pressure constantly lead to segmental vascular hyalinosis, an experimental equivalent of benign nephrosclerosis, the earliest stage of malignant nephrosclerosis cannot be induced in intact interlobular arteries by this method. Since malignant nephrosclerosis only becomes apparent after vascular structural adaptation has occurred, it is suggested that medial hypertrophy and/or increased collagen content in the arterial wall might be prerequisites for the development of this severe complication of hypertension. If this is the case, hypertension-induced structural adaptation of the arterial wall may potentially reduce the risk of benign nephrosclerosis, but increase that of malignant nephrosclerosis. This is supported by data from Bidani *et al.* showing that renal ablation acutely transforms 'benign' renal changes to 'malignant' nephrosclerosis in spontaneously hypertensive rats (Bidani *et al.* 1994).

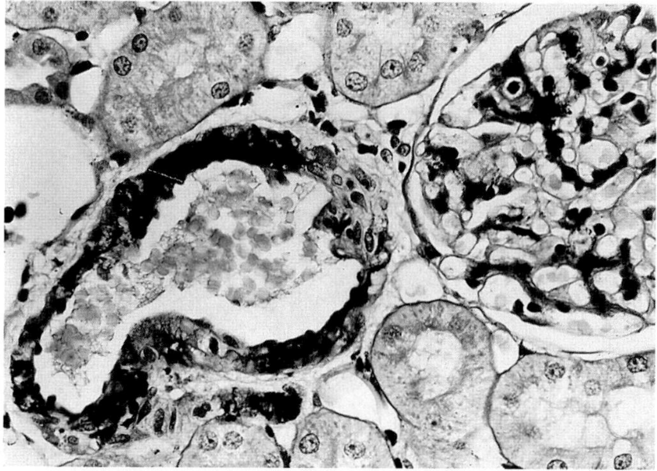

Fig. 9 Previously clipped non-adapted kidney 24 h after inducing hypertension by angiotensin II infusion and intravenous application of colloidal carbon. Marked carbon deposits can be seen within hyaline areas of an interlobular artery and in the glomerular mesangium (immersion fixation, periodic acid–Schiff reagent; magnification 336×).

The essential part played by intrarenal vascular lesions in the maintenance of hypertension, even after its primary cause has been removed, can be demonstrated by the following experiment in two-kidney one-clip hypertensive rats (Fig. 10): removal of the renal artery clip after maintenance of the hypertensive state for 1 year causes the blood pressure to decrease. However, this is temporary and hypertensive levels are regained within 1 week. This 'post-Goldblatt hypertension' may be a result of general atherosclerosis which may have developed during the preceding hypertensive period. Removal of the previously non-clipped kidney allows normotension to be maintained, indicating the pathogenic role of renal vascular disease including adaptive and destructive structural changes, such as severely obliterating lesions of interlobular arteries and afferent arterioles accompanied by focal glomerular sclerosis, tubular atrophy, and interstitial fibrosis. In contrast, at the end of the experiment the previously clipped kidneys of the same animals showed only minor focal vascular, glomerular, and tubular interstitial lesions that were obviously not sufficient to reinduce hypertension. Rettig *et al.* (1990) have also demonstrated that the non-clipped kidney can not only sustain but also induce hypertension: transplantation of non-clipped kidneys from two-kidney one-clip hypertensive rats induced sustained hypertension in the normotensive recipients. The lesions described above may also play a role in patients with 'pseudo renal artery stenosis syndrome'. In response to converting enzyme inhibitor therapy these patients have clinical signs suggestive of renal artery stenosis despite patent renal arteries. It is believed that long-standing hypertension has caused sufficient intrarenal arteriolar hypertrophy and sclerosis to interfere with renal blood flow and to induce the functional pattern of renal artery stenosis (Pettinger *et al.* 1989b; Toto *et al.* 1991).

Increased glomerular perfusion and the elevation of glomerular capillary pressure are important mechanisms underlying the subsequent structural damage within the glomerulus (Brenner 1985; Klahr *et al.* 1988). A close link between glomerular hypertrophy and sclerosis has been demonstrated (Fogo and Ichikawa 1989, 1991; Miller *et al.* 1991); however, this concept is not supported by all studies (Lafferty and Brenner 1990; Wenzel *et al.* 2002b). Analysis of individual glomeruli showed a biphasic pattern of these two parameters. Early development of glomerular sclerosis takes place together with hypertrophy of the glomerulus, and further advancement of sclerosis occurs with shrinkage

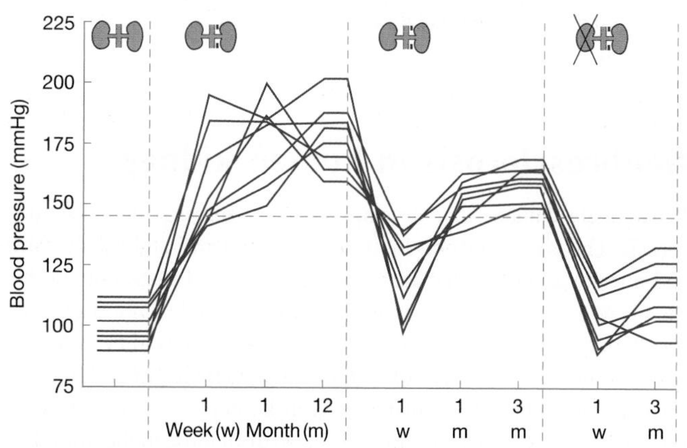

Fig. 10 Two-kidney one-clip hypertension of 12-month duration: post-Goldblatt hypertension after removal of the renal artery clip; sustained normotension after removing the previously non-clipped kidney (reproduced with permission from Helmchen *et al.* 1984b).

in glomerular size (Fogo and Ichikawa 1989, 1991). This finding was first described in the renal ablation model (Yoshida *et al.* 1989), but has also been demonstrated in the non-clipped kidney of rats with renovascular hypertension (Wenzel *et al.* 1992). Harvey *et al.* (1992) examined renal biopsies and found that glomeruli from hypertensive patients were larger than those from normotensive patients. The enlargement of glomeruli was probably a consequence of the loss of functioning glomeruli due to global sclerosis, which is, in turn, due to ischaemia. A reduced number of glomeruli with an increased volume was also found recently in patients with essential hypertension (Keller 2003).

The glomeruli have been a focal point of interest, particularly in view of the hyperfiltration hypothesis involving the degradation and sclerosis of remaining nephrons. However, the notion that tubulointerstitial fibrosis may be the cause rather than the result of decreased glomerular function has recently received strong support (Ong and Fine 1994; Luft and Haller 1995). Luft and coworkers have recently reported that an early expansion of the interstitial volume precedes hypertensive vascular changes and glomerular injury in the non-clipped kidney of renovascular hypertensive rats (Mai *et al.* 1993; Luft and Haller 1995). Increased matrix deposition was primarily found within the interstitium. Similar findings were reported by Eng *et al.* (1994). Moreover, both groups also described tubulointerstitial proliferation and dense focal interstitial monocyte/macrophage influx in the non-clipped kidney. These changes could be caused by mechanical damage of the renal microvasculature including obstruction of the postglomerular interstitial capillary network. Thus, both the tubules and the interstitium are actively involved and may be important initial sites of injury in hypertension. Short periods of hypertension can induce tubulointerstitial damage and rarefication of peritubular capillaries. Bohle *et al.* (1996) have reported that focal peritubular capillary loss is present in renal biopsies of patients with essential hypertension. To determine whether these changes were sufficient to induce salt-sensitive hypertension, angiotensin II was infused into normal rats for 2 weeks. During the infusion, blood pressure was elevated, and renal biopsy confirmed the development of microvascular and tubulointerstitial injury. After the angiotensin II infusion had been discontinued, the blood pressure returned to normal, and it remained normal when the rats were given a low-salt diet. In contrast, hypertension recurred in rats that were given a high-salt diet. These observations led to the hypothesis that in many persons in whom hypertension develops, the kidneys may initially be normal, but that some event leads to the development of subtle renal injury that alters the ability to excrete salt (Johnson *et al.* 2002).

Nephrosclerosis in human kidneys

Renal tissue damage that develops in hypertensive patients is non-specific. This is valid not only for the glomerulosclerosis, tubular atrophy, and interstitial fibrosis that are seen in the advanced stage, but also for the preglomerular lesions that are characteristic of, but not diagnostic for, hypertensive disease. These lesions do not allow differentiation between the different causes of high blood pressure. Light and electron microscopy studies of vascular lesions in kidneys from patients with essential hypertension are indistinguishable from those in the contralateral or unprotected kidney of individuals with renovascular hypertension (Fisher *et al.* 1966). The traditional use of the term 'nephrosclerosis' (Volhard and Fahr 1914; Fahr 1919, 1924, 1925), comprising the benign or malignant variety, encompasses a wide range of morphological findings, including primary injuries of the vessel walls and early and late tissue reactions.

Light microscopy shows that the component of benign nephrosclerosis found most regularly is segmental hyalinization of interlobular arteries and afferent arterioles (Fig. 11). It preferentially affects the media which then shows a diminished number of smooth muscle cell nuclei (Fahr 1925); the lumen of the hyalinized segments is not necessarily narrowed. Immunofluorescence and electron microscopy techniques have made possible the demonstration of several plasma constituents, such as immunoglobulins (IgM) and complement components (Clq, C3) within the hyalinized areas (Valenzuela *et al.* 1980) (Fig. 12). Thus arterial and arteriolar hyalinosis in humans, as in animal models, can be regarded as the structural result of an insudation of plasma constituents into the vessel walls during a period of increased permeability (Fisher *et al.* 1966). If vascular hyalinization is present in biopsies from younger non-diabetic patients, arterial hypertension can be suspected as its cause (Kimmelstiel and Wilson 1936) although it may be intermittent and only revealed by continuous blood pressure monitoring. The vascular hyalinization of benign nephrosclerosis is one of the most frequent findings on light microscopy of kidney biopsies. Many kidney biopsies taken from patients with minor mono- or oligosymptomatic renal disease show benign nephrosclerosis as the only pathological change (Katafuchi and Takebayashi 1987; Harvey *et al.* 1992) (Table 1). This may have clinical implications, since nephrosclerosis is frequently the only morphological diagnosis in patients with chronic renal disease at the start of dialysis (Malangone *et al.* 1989). The evidence for a relationship between mild to moderate hypertension and either nephrosclerosis or ESRD remains circumstantial. The Framingham population studies, which identified risk factors for

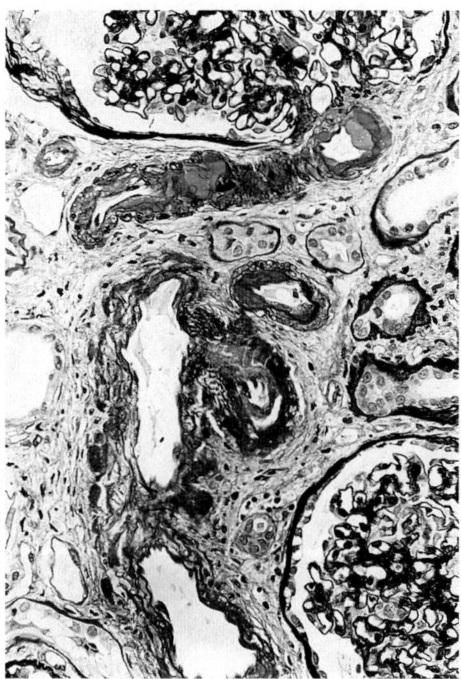

Fig. 11 Benign nephrosclerosis: segmental hyalinization of interlobular arteries and afferent arterioles; focal tubular atrophy and interstitial fibrosis. Renal biopsy of a hypertensive man, aged 36 years, with IgA nephropathy (periodic acid–Schiff reagent; magnification 360×).

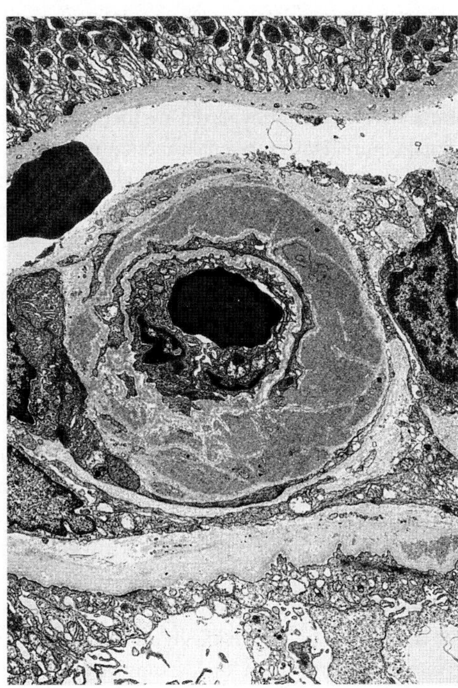

Fig. 12 Benign nephrosclerosis: plasmic material within the partially destroyed media of a peripheral interlobular artery. Renal biopsy of the same patient as in Fig. 11 (transmission electron microscopy; magnification 4800×).

Table 1 The most frequent diagnoses from the renal biopsies (all examined by light microscopy, immunohistology, and electron microscopy) of 560 oligosymptomatic patients

Morphological diagnosis	*n*	Percentage
IgA nephropathy	209	37.3
Benign nephrosclerosis	156	27.9
Focal tubular atrophy/interstitial fibrosis	44	7.7
Alport's syndrome	29	5.2
Thin basement membrane glomerulopathy	23	4.8

cardiovascular morbidity and mortality, did not evaluate the impact of hypertension on renal failure because of the low incidence of renal failure in that population (Kannel 1983). Patients with essential hypertension do not routinely undergo diagnostic renal biopsy. The frequency of hypertension as a reported cause of ESRD has increased in the past few years. This is seemingly paradoxical since effective pharmacological control of blood pressure in the past two decades has led to a decrease in the prevalence of malignant hypertension as well as cardiovascular morbidity related to hypertension. It should be noted, however, that the very protective effect of antihypertensive therapy against cardiovascular disease, by improving life expectancy, may prolong the time available for hypertensive renal disease to progress, thus increasing in the long run the number of patients suffering from terminal renal disease (Caetano *et al.* 1999). As a consequence, previously most hypertensive patients likely died from cardiovascular events before advanced nephrosclerosis became manifest. Hypertensive nephrosclerosis started to stand out as a presumed cause of ESRD only in the early 1980s, coinciding with a steady increase in the mean age of new dialysis patients. Nephrosclerosis is characterized by a very slow rate of progression. For this reason, very long follow-up, longer than the usual duration of trials looking at cardiovascular morbidity and mortality in arterial hypertension are required to investigate hypertensive nephrosclerosis. Increased serum creatinine at baseline, proteinuria and age are independent predictors for the development of a renal event in patients having the presumed diagnosis of nephrosclerosis (Segura *et al.* 2001). Our knowledge of the role of hypertension as a cause of chronic renal failure and our understanding of the human pathology is limited.

Nephrologists identify hypertension as the aetiology of nephrosclerosis in 25 per cent of patients initiating renal replacement therapy in United States (Weisstuch and Dworkin 1992). The percentage appears to be less in Europe and Australia. In a study performed in Leicester, England, which followed 176 patients with essential hypertension with suboptimal blood pressure control for 14 years, no patient reached ESRD (Tomson *et al.* 1991). Kincaid-Smith (1982, 1999) wrote: 'Benign hypertension does not cause clinically significant renal damage. The kidney in benign hypertension remains normal in both size and function'. However, Kincaid-Smith data pertain to a period that started in the 1960s. As mentioned above, at these times patients suffering from arterial hypertension died from cardiovascular events before reaching ESRD due to hypertensive nephrosclerosis. Certainly, the sequence of hypertension occurring for years before renal insufficiency or proteinuria develops, in the absence of any other primary renal disease is supportive of a diagnosis of hypertensive nephrosclerosis. The risk of hypertensive ESRD is believed to be greater in the Black population (Rostand *et al.* 1982). However, nephrologists are twice as likely to label an African-American patient as having hypertensive nephrosclerosis as a White patient, when presented with identical clinical history (Freedman *et al.* 1995). In contrast, a close agreement between clinical and histological diagnosis of hypertensive nephrosclerosis could be demonstrated in African-Americans as shown by Fogo and coworkers. In nearly 85 per cent of these patients, renal histological examination was consistent with the clinical diagnosis by revealing the presence of exclusively vascular lesions (Fogo *et al.* 1997). It has been demonstrated recently that strict blood pressure control can stabilize renal function in black patients thought to have hypertensive nephrosclerosis (Toto *et al.* 1995). Obviously, the estimates of the likelihood of essential hypertension causing ESRD vary among countries and between renal units depending upon the enthusiasm with which a primary diagnosis is pursued (Brown and Whitworth 1992). It also seems that renovascular disease, ischaemic nephropathy and cholesterol microembolization may either cause or accelerate renal insufficiency in a larger portion of the atherosclerotic population with hypertension and renal insufficiency than previously recognized (Jacobson 1988; Jacobson *et al.* 1994; Alcazar and Rodicio 2000; Saran *et al.* 2001). Familial clustering of ESRD attributed to hypertension and recent molecular genetic developments in hypertensive populations support the concept that inherited factors may predispose to renal failure (Zarif *et al.* 2000). A correlation between polymorphisms and ESRD due to nephrosclerosis is not available yet. It is of interest that mice lacking a functional angiotensinogen or angiotensin-converting enzyme gene have abnormal kidneys with renal vascular changes consisting of thickened walls (Krege *et al.* 1995; Smithies and Maeda 1995). The identification of factors and genes that predispose to nephrosclerosis is immensely important and would probably lead to an improved understanding of the factors producing renal disease (Schmieder *et al.* 1994).

Hypertension-induced benign nephrosclerosis may also accompany and aggravate other renal disorders. In a series of biopsies from patients with glomerulonephritis, the incidence of benign nephrosclerosis was 31 per cent (Table 2). In another study (Katafuchi *et al.* 1988), the same type of preglomerular vascular change was closely related to high blood pressure in patients with IgA glomerulonephritis. Other clinical and pathological studies have also indicated that the progression of IgA glomerulonephritis and the development of chronic renal failure may be enhanced by hypertension-induced intrarenal vascular lesions (Feiner *et al.* 1982; Alamartine *et al.* 1990). Segmental hyalinosis of interlobular arteries and efferent arterioles is frequently observed at a time when the glomerular and tubular interstitial structures are still completely preserved, and this probably reflects the earliest hypertension-induced intrarenal lesion. Arterial fibroplasia is a better correlate of high blood pressure than is parenchymal fibrosis, suggesting that blood pressure relates less to the renoprival state of nephron loss than it does to renal ischaemia in patients with nephrosclerosis (Tracy 1992; Tracy and Ishii 2000). Theoretically, it may undergo remission (McCormack *et al.* 1958; Tracy and Toca 1974), although it may also be followed by focal and segmental glomerular damage (Jones 1953, 1974, 1976). Focal glomerular sclerosis may also be found in biopsy specimens from patients with benign essential hypertension (Katz *et al.* 1979); although the laboratory findings were suggestive of glomerulonephritis, the morphological changes were indicative of benign nephrosclerosis. In fact, these glomerular lesions resemble focal and segmental glomerulonephritis, and the term 'alterative glomerulonephritis' (Kimmelstiel and Wilson 1936) is understandable. In the early stages of the glomerular injury, the capillary loops adjacent to the vascular pole characteristically show a widening of the mesangium, swelling of endothelial cells, and sometimes an occlusion of the lumina filled with condensed material derived from the plasma. Thereafter, formation of an irregular basement membrane and segmental extracapillary cell proliferations may lead to capsular adhesions, finally resulting in focal and segmental glomerulosclerosis (Fig. 13).

Data from the Hypertension Detection and Follow-Up Program and other studies show that antihypertensive therapy can prevent progression of renal failure. However, renal function was found to decline in some patients despite treatment (Brazy *et al.* 1989; Pettinger *et al.* 1989a; Weisstuch and Dworkin 1992; Toto 1995). Several studies have been performed in hypertensive patients with chronic renal failure in whom control of hypertension with various drugs and drug combinations demonstrated preservation or improvement in renal function (Maki *et al.* 1995; Toto 1995). No data are available on repeated measurement of renal function during prolonged treatment of mild hypertension in subjects with normal or near-normal renal function.

A second type of glomerular lesion is characterized by the ischaemic collapse of the glomerular tuft. This is more frequently seen in kidneys with pronounced narrowing of the preglomerular vessels, as is commonly observed in malignant nephrosclerosis (Fig. 14). Ischaemic wrinkling collapse of the glomerular tuft is seen much more commonly in hypertensive nephrosclerosis than is focal glomerulosclerosis, which is the characteristic lesion of the adapted hyperperfused nephron. The occurrence of irreversible hypertension-related glomerular injury marks the transition to 'decompensated benign nephrosclerosis' (Fahr 1925), which carries an increased risk of steadily advancing tubular atrophy and interstitial fibrosis (Bohle and Ratschek 1982). Progression to chronic renal insufficiency may be inevitable. Kannel (1977) stated that there is nothing benign in any kind of hypertension. From the morphological point of view, one may add that there is nothing benign in nephrosclerosis.

The principal difference between the two forms of nephrosclerosis is that the structural changes of the so-called benign variety are mainly

Table 2 Frequency of benign nephrosclerosis in the renal biopsies of 209 patients with IgA nephropathy

IgA nephropathy	*n*	Percentage
Women	62	30
Men	147	70
Hypertension	68	33
Age (years)		
1–20	60	29
21–45	106	51
46–70	43	20
Benign nephrosclerosis	64	31
Focal glomerulosclerosis	66	32
Focal tubular atrophy/interstitial fibrosis	162	78

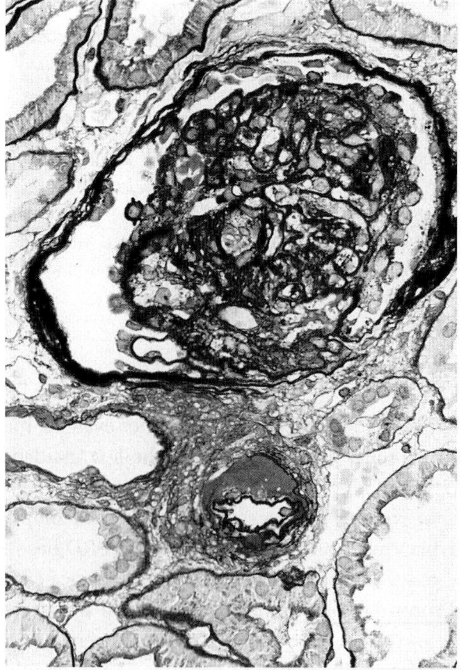

Fig. 13 Focal glomerulosclerosis in benign nephrosclerosis. Renal biopsy of a hypertensive man aged 41 years (periodic acid–Schiff reagent; magnification 360×).

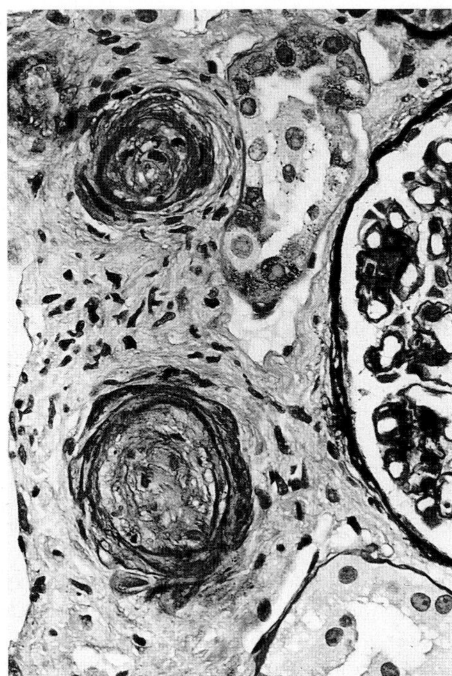

Fig. 14 Malignant nephrosclerosis: interlobular arteries with obliterating proliferative 'endarteritis Fahr'. Ischaemic collapse of capillary loops of an adjacent glomerulus. Renal biopsy of a man aged 32 years with accelerated hypertension (periodic acid–Schiff reagent; magnification 360×).

confined to the media, particularly during the early stages, whereas even the early lesions of malignant nephrosclerosis predominantly affect the intimal space. It is this subendothelial compartment of the vascular wall that becomes widened, initially containing plasma and corpuscular blood constituents, but during the later stages also containing numerous myointimal cells as well as collagen fibres. Although medial fibrinoid necrosis may also occur, the intimal process is the first phenomenon and remains dominating, potentially leading to an extreme narrowing of the vascular lumen. The term 'malignant nephrosclerosis' actually covers quite different morphological findings; at different stages a subendothelial oedema, an intimal cell proliferation ('endarteritis'; Fahr 1925), or the onion-like appearance of intimal scarring may predominate. The initial intimal oedema is assumed to be reversible following effective lowering of blood pressure (Olsen 1969; Pickering 1971; Helmchen and Kneissler 1976; Helmchen *et al.* 1976). This may be important, and suggests that even this type of nephrosclerosis may not necessarily be 'malignant'. Rigorous antihypertensive therapy should be encouraged, particularly when initial stages of malignant nephrosclerosis are detected (Kincaid-Smith 1991).

As in experimental animals, malignant nephrosclerosis in the human kidney also develops predominantly in the interlobular arteries and afferent arterioles. Secondary to a progressive narrowing of these vessels, hyperplasia of the juxtaglomerular epithelioid cells, ischaemic collapse of the glomerular tufts, tubular atrophy, and interstitial fibrosis may follow (Fahr 1919, 1925; Ellis 1942; Heptinstall 1953; Sommers *et al.* 1958; Zollinger 1966) (Fig. 14).

These morphological findings reflect the two basic mechanisms of the vicious circle of hypertension: the activation of the renin–angiotensin system and the impairment of the excretory renal capacity. Functionally, the situation resulting when hundreds of intrarenal arteries are significantly narrowed is comparable to severe stenosis of the main renal artery (Goldblatt 1964). In the presence of renal artery stenosis or malignant nephrosclerosis, pharmacological blockade of the renin–angiotensin system may be regarded as an effective antihypertensive therapy. However, this may cause a further undesired reduction in the residual glomerular filtration rate and may also accelerate tubular atrophy owing to reduction of the angiotensin-II-dependent tone of the efferent arterioles (Collste *et al.* 1979; Farrow and Wilkinson 1979; Helmchen *et al.* 1982; Hricik *et al.* 1983; Hollenberg 1984; Groene and Helmchen 1986).

It remains to be determined whether high blood pressure alone is sufficient to cause malignant nephrosclerosis in humans. Although the evidence seems to be conclusive in patients with renal hypertension, experimental results show that even under well-defined conditions additional factors might be required to initiate the crucial intimal thickening. If high blood pressure alone is the cause of malignant hypertension, the widespread use of antihypertensive medication and the increasing frequency of diagnosis of mild to moderate hypertension should have the effect that malignant hypertension becomes less common. However, there is only limited evidence for this (Kincaid-Smith 1985, 1991), and the incidence of malignant hypertension in the United Kingdom has failed to decline (Lip *et al.* 1994). In advanced malignant nephrosclerosis, autopsy and biopsy material do not indicate whether hypertension is the cause or the result of the vascular disorder, and there is no doubt that malignant nephrosclerosis can develop in previously normotensive patients suffering from haemolytic–uraemic syndrome or from postpartum acute renal failure (Gasser *et al.* 1955; Habib *et al.* 1967, 1969; Ponticelli *et al.* 1972; Bohle *et al.* 1973, 1976; Thoenes and John 1980).

Schürmann and MacMahon (1933) initially suggested that an alteration in the selective permeability of the endothelial barrier induced by chemical or biological agents, including bacterial toxins and humoral factors acting directly on the endothelium, allowed numerous components of blood to seep into the intimal space and to excite a proliferative reaction. Consequently, primary malignant nephrosclerosis precedes arterial hypertension in these cases (Bohle *et al.* 1973; Byrom 1976).

MacMahon (1966) suggested that most cases of malignant nephrosclerosis were hypertensive in origin. However, this is not certain, and the alternative possibility of a preponderance of primary malignant nephrosclerosis with secondary hypertension, as postulated by Fahr (1924, 1925), still deserves consideration. It is probable that humoral factors and pressure both play a role in the process of malignant nephrosclerosis. In any case, strict antihypertensive therapy should be encouraged, particularly when initial stages of malignant nephrosclerosis are detected (Kincaid-Smith 1991). The relationship between 'benign hypertension' and either nephrosclerosis or ESRD remains circumstantial. Nevertheless, strict blood pressure control is also crucial in patients with mild or moderate hypertension (Toto 1995; Wenzel 2001).

References

Alamartine, E., Sabatier, J. C., and Berthoux, F. C. (1990). Comparison of pathological lesions on repeated renal biopsies in 73 patients with primary IgA-glomerulonephritis: value of quantitative scoring and approach to final prognosis. *Clinical Nephrology* **34**, 45–51.

Alcazar, J. M. and Rodicio, J. L. (2000). Ischemic nephropathy: clinical characteristics and treatment. *American Journal of Kidney Diseases* **36**, 883–893.

Beilin, L. J. and Goldby, F. S. (1977). High arterial pressure versus humoral factors in the pathogenesis of the vascular lesions of malignant hypertension. The case for pressure alone. *Clinical Science* **52**, 111–113.

Berecek, K. H., Stocker, M., and Gross, F. (1980). Changes in renal vascular reactivity at various stages of deoxycorticosterone hypertension in rats. *Circulation Research* **46**, 619–624.

Bidani, A. K., Schwartz, M. M., and Lewis, E. J. (1987). Renal autoregulation and vulnerability to hypertensive injury in remnant kidney. *American Journal of Physiology* **252**, F1003–F1010.

Bidani, A. K., Griffin, K. A., Picken, M., and Lansky, D. M. (1993). Continuous telemetric blood pressure monitoring and glomerular injury in the rat remnant kidney mode. *American Journal of Physiology* **265**, F391–F398.

Bidani, A. K., Griffin, K. A., Plott, W., and Schwartz, M. M. (1994). Renal ablation acutely transforms 'benign' hypertension to 'malignant nephrosclerosis' in hypertensive rats. *Hypertension* **24**, 309–316.

Bohle, A. and Ratschek, M. (1982). The compensated and the decompensated form of benign nephrosclerosis. *Pathology, Research and Practice* **174**, 357–367.

Bohle, A., Grund, K. E., Helmchen, U., and Meyer, D. (1976). Primary malignant nephrosclerosis. *Clinical Science* **51**, 23s–25s.

Bohle, A. *et al.* (1973). Über die primäre und sekundäre maligne Nephrosklerose. *Klinische Wochenschrift* **51**, 841–847.

Bohle, A. *et al.* (1996). Pathogenesis of chronic renal failure in the primary glomerulopathies, renal vasculopathies, and chronic interstitial nephritides. *Kidney International* **49**, S2–S9.

Boffa, J. J., Tharaux, P. L., Placier, S., Ardaillou, R., Dussaule, J. C., and Chatziantoniou, C. (1999). Angiotensin II activates collagen type I gene in the renal vasculature of transgenic mice during inhibition of nitric oxide synthesis: evidence for an endothelin-mediated mechanism. *Circulation* **100**, 1901–1908.

Brazy, P. C., Stead, W. W., and Fitzwilliam, J. F. (1989). Progression of renal insufficiency: role of blood pressure. *Kidney International* **35**, 670–674.

Brecher, P., Chan, C. T., Franzblau, C., Faris, B., and Chobanian, A. V. (1978). Effects of hypertension and its reversal on aortic metabolism in the rat. *Circulation Research* **43**, 561–569.

Brenner, B. M. (1985). Nephron adaptation to renal injury or ablation. *American Journal of Physiology* **249**, F324–F337.

Brown, M. A. and Whitworth, J. A. (1992). Hypertension in human renal disease. *Journal of Hypertension* **10**, 701–712.

Byrom, F. B. *The Hypertensive Vascular Crisis. An Experimental Study*. London: Heinemann, 1969.

Byrom, F. B. (1976). Tension and artery: the experimental elucidation of pseudouraemia and malignant nephrosclerosis. *Clinical Science* **51**, 3s–11s.

Byrom, F. B. and Dodson, L. F. (1948). The causation of acute arterial necrosis in hypertensive disease. *Journal of Pathology and Bacteriology* **60**, 357–368.

Caetano, E. P., Zatz, R., and Praxedes, J. N. (1999). The clinical diagnosis of hypertensive nephrosclerosis—how reliable is it? *Nephrology, Dialysis, Transplantation* **14**, 288–290.

Chobanian, A. V., Prescott, M. F., and Haudenschild, Ch. C. (1984). Recent advances in molecular pathology. The effects of hypertension on the arterial wall. *Experimental and Molecular Pathology* **41**, 153–169.

Collste, P., Haglund, K., Lundgren, G., Magnusson, G., and Ostman, J. (1979). Reversible renal failure during treatment with captopril. *British Medical Journal* **ii**, 612–617.

Ellis, A. W. M. (1942). The natural history of Bright's disease. *Lancet* **i**, 1–6, 34–38, 72–76.

Eng, E. *et al.* (1994). Renal proliferative and phenotypic changes in rats with two-kidney, one-clip Goldblatt hypertension. *American Journal of Hypertension* **7**, 177–185.

Fahr, T. (1919). Über Nephrosklerose. *Virchows Archiv für Pathologische Anatomie* **226**, 119–178.

Fahr, T. (1924). Über atypische Befunde aus den Kapiteln des M. Brightii nebst anhangsweisen Bemerkungen zur Hypertoniefrage. *Virchows Archiv für Pathologische Anatomie* **248**, 323–336.

Fahr, T. Pathologische Anatomie des M. Brightii. In *Handbuch der Speziellen Anatomie und Histologie* (ed. F. Henke and O. Lubarsch), pp. 374–472. Berlin: Springer, 1925.

Farrow, P. R. and Wilkinson, R. (1979). Reversible renal failure during treatment with captopril. *British Medical Journal* **i**, 1680–1684.

Feiner, H. D., Calibi, S., Baldwin, D. S., Schacht, R. G., and Gallo, G. R. (1982). Intrarenal vascular sclerosis in IgA nephropathy. *Clinical Nephrology* **18**, 183–192.

Fisher, E. R., Perez-Stable, E., and Pardo, V. (1966). Ultrastructural studies in hypertension. I. Comparison of renal vascular and juxtaglomerular cell alterations in essential and renal hypertension in man. *Laboratory Investigation* **15**, 1409–1433.

Floyer, M. A. (1955). Further studies in the mechanisms of experimental hypertension in the rat. *Clinical Science* **14**, 163–181.

Fogo, A. and Ichikawa, I. (1989). Evidence for the central role of glomerular growth promoters in the development of sclerosis. *Seminars in Nephrology* **9**, 329–342.

Fogo, A. and Ichikawa, I. (1991). Evidence for a pathogenic linkage between glomerular hypertrophy and sclerosis. *American Journal of Kidney Diseases* **17**, 666–669.

Fogo, A. *et al.* (1997). Accuracy of the diagnosis of hypertensive nephrosclerosis in African Americans: a report from the African American Study of Kidney Disease (AASK) Trial. AASK Pilot Study Investigators. *Kidney International* **51**, 244–252.

Folkow, B. (1971). The haemodynamic consequences of adaptive structural changes of the resistance vessels in hypertension. *Clinical Science* **41**, 1–12.

Folkow, B. (1990). 'Structural factor' in primary and secondary hypertension. *Hypertension* **16**, 89–101.

Folkow, B., Grimby, G., and Thulesius, O. (1958). Adaptive structural changes of the vascular walls in hypertension and their relation to the control of peripheral resistance. *Acta Physiologica Scandinavica* **44**, 255–272.

Freedman, B. I., Iskandar, S. S., and Appel, R. G. (1995). The link between hypertension and nephrosclerosis. *American Journal of Kidney Diseases* **25**, 207–221.

Gasser, C., Gautier, E., Steck., A., Siebenmann, H. E., and Oechslin, R. (1955). Hämolytisch urämische Syndrome. Bilaterale Nebennierenrindennekrosen bei akuten erworbenen hämolytischen Anämien. *Schweizerische Medizinische Wochenschrift* **85**, 905–909.

Gibbons, G. H. and Dzau, V. J. (1994). The emerging concept of vascular remodeling. *New England Journal of Medicine* **330**, 1431–1438.

Giese, J. (1964a). Acute hypertensive vascular disease. 1. Relation between blood pressure changes and vascular lesions in different forms of acute hypertension. *Acta Pathologica Microbiologia Scandinavica* **62**, 481–496.

Giese, J. (1964b). Acute hypertensive arterial disease. II. Studies on the vascular reaction pattern and permeability changes by means of vital microscopy and colloidal tracer techniques. *Acta Pathologica Microbiologia Scandinavica* **62**, 497–515.

Giese, J. (1973). Renin, angiotensin and hypertensive vascular damage. *American Journal of Medicine* **55**, 315–332.

Goldblatt, H. (1938). Studies on experimental hypertension. VII. The production of the malignant phase of hypertension. *Journal of Experimental Medicine* **67**, 809–826.

Goldblatt, H. (1964). Hypertension of renal origin. Historical and experimental background. *American Journal of Surgery* **107**, 21–25.

Goldblatt, H., Lynch, J., Hanzal, R. F., and Summerville, W. W. (1934). Persistent elevation of systolic blood pressure by means of renal ischemia. *Journal of Experimental Medicine* **59**, 347–379.

Goldblatt, H., Haas, E., Klick, R. L., and Lewis, L. (1976). The effect of main artery occlusion of one kidney on blood pressure of dogs. *Proceedings of the National Academy of Sciences of the United States of America* **73**, 1722–1724.

Goldby, F. S. and Beilin, L. J. (1972). How an acute rise in arterial pressure damages arterioles. Electron microscopic changes following angiotensin infusion. *Cardiovascular Research* **6**, 569–584.

Goldby, F. S. and Beilin, L. J. (1974). The evolution and healing of arteriolar damage in renal clip-hypertension in the rat. An electron microscope study. *Journal of Pathology* **114**, 139–148.

Griffin, K. A., Picken, M. M., and Bidani A. K. (1994). Radiotelemetric BP monitoring, antihypertensives and glomeruloprotection in remnant kidney model. *Kidney International* **46**, 1010–1018.

Griffin, K. A., Picken, M. M., and Bidani, A. K. (1995). Deleterious effects of calcium channel blockade on pressure transmission and glomerular injury in rat remnant kidneys. *Journal of Clinical Investigation* **96**, 793–800.

Griffin, K. A., Picken, M. M., and Bidani, A. K. (2004). Blood pressure liability and glomerulosclerosis after normotensive 5/6 renal mass reduction in the rat. *Kidney International* **65**, 209–218.

Groene, H. J. and Helmchen, U. (1986). Impairment and recovery of the clipped kidney in two kidney, one clip hypertensive rats during and after antihypertensive therapy. *Laboratory Investigation* **54**, 645–655.

Habib, R., Mathieu, H., and Royer, P. (1967). Le syndrome hemolytique et urémique de l'enfant. *Nephron* **4**, 139–172.

Habib, R., Courtecuisse, V., Leclerc, F., Mathieu, H., and Royer, P. (1969). Etude anatomo-pathologique de 35 observations de syndrome hemolytique et urémique de l'enfant. *Archives Françaises de Pédiatrie* **26**, 391–416.

Hampton, J. A., Bernardo, D. A., Khan, N. A., Lacher, D. A., Rapp, J. P., Gohara, A. F., and Goldblatt, P. J. (1989). Morphometric evaluation of the renal arterial system of Dahl salt-sensitive and salt-resistant rats on a high salt diet. II. Interlobular arteries and intralobular arterioles. *Laboratory Investigation* **60**, 839–846.

Harvey, J. M., Howie, A. J., Lee, S. J., Newbold, K. M., Adu, D., Michael, J., and Beevers, D. G. (1992). Renal biopsy findings in hypertensive patients with proteinuria. *Lancet* **340**, 1435–1436.

Helmchen, U. and Kneissler, U. (1976). Role of the renin–angiotensin system in renal hypertension. An experimental approach. *Current Topics in Pathology* **61**, 203–238.

Helmchen, U., Khosla, M. C., Se, S., Khairallah, P. A., and Bumpus, F. M. (1976). Therapeutischer Effekt eines Angiotensin II-antagonisten bei experimenteller Nephrosklerose. *Verhandlungen Deutsche Gesellschaft für Pathologie* **60**, 308–309.

Helmchen, U., Grone, H. J., Kirchertz, E. J., Bader, H., Bohle, R. M., Kneissler, U., and Khosla, M. C. (1982). Contrasting renal effects of different antihypertensive agents in hypertensive rats with bilaterally constricted renal arteries. *Kidney International* **22** (Suppl. 12), 198–205.

Helmchen, U., Bohle, R. M., Kneissler, U., and Groene, H. J. (1984a). Intrarenal arteries in rats with early two-kidney, one clip hypertension. *Hypertension* **6**, III87–92.

Helmchen, U., Kneissler, U., Bohle, R. M., Reher, A., and Groene, H. J. (1984b). Adaptation and decompensation of intrarenal small arteries in experimental hypertension. *Journal of Cardiovascular Pharmacology* **6**, S696–S705.

Heptinstall, R. H. (1953). Malignant hypertension: a study of fifty-one cases. *Journal of Pathology and Bacteriology* **65**, 423–439.

Hollenberg, N. K. (1984). Renal hemodynamics in essential and renovascular hypertension: influence of captopril. *American Journal of Medicine* **76**, 22–32.

Hricik, D. E., Browning, P. J., Kopelman, R., Goorno, W. E., Madias, N. E., and Dzau, V. J. (1983). Captopril-induced functional renal insufficiency in patients with bilateral renal artery stenosis or renal-artery stenosis in a solitary kidney. *New England Journal of Medicine* **308**, 373–379.

Jacobson, H. (1988). Ischemic renal disease: an overlooked clinical entity? *Kidney International* **34**, 729–743.

Jacobson, H. R., Dean, R., Madias, N. E., Novick, A., Menon, M., and Schaeffer, A. J. (1994). Proceedings of the Symposium on Ischemic Renal Disease. *American Journal of Kidney Diseases* **24**, 614.

Johansson, B. B. (1976). Some factors influencing the damaging effect of acute arterial hypertension on cerebral vessels in rats. *Clinical Science* **51**, 415–435.

Johnson, R. J., Alpers, C. E., Yoshimura, A., Lombardi, D., Pritzl, P., Floege, J., and Schwartz, S. M. (1992). Renal injury from angiotensin II mediated hypertension. *Hypertension* **19**, 464–474.

Johnson, R. J. *et al.* (2002). Subtle acquired renal injury as a mechanism of salt-sensitive hypertension. *New England Journal of Medicine* **346**, 913–923.

Jones, D. B. (1953). Nephrosclerosis and the glomerulus. *American Journal of Pathology* **24**, 619–631.

Jones, D. B. (1974). Arterial and glomerular lesions associated with severe hypertension. Light and electron microscopic studies. *Laboratory Investigation* **3**, 303–313.

Jones, D. B. (1976). The renal vascular lesions of severe and malignant hypertension: a light-immunofluorescent microscopy, transmission and scanning electron-microscopy study. *Clinical Science* **51**, 27–29.

Kannel, W. B. Importance of hypertension as a major risk factor in cardiovascular disease. In *Hypertension, Physiology, and Treatment* (ed. J. Koiw, E. Genest, and O. Kuchel), p. 908. New York: McGraw-Hill, 1977.

Kannel, W. B. An overview of the risk factors for cardiovascular disease. In *Prevention of Coronary Heart Disease* (ed. N. M. Kaplan and J. Stamler), pp. 1–19. Philadelphia: W.B. Saunders, 1983.

Katafuchi, R. and Takebayashi, S. (1987). Morphometrical and functional correlations in benign nephrosclerosis. *Clinical Nephrology* **28**, 238–243.

Katafuchi, R., Takebayashi, S., and Taguchi, I. (1988). Hypertension-related aggravation of IgA-nephropathy: a statistical approach. *Clinical Nephrology* **30**, 261–269.

Katz, S. M., Lavin, L., and Swartz, C. (1979). Glomerular lesions in benign essential hypertension. *Archives of Pathology and Laboratory Medicine* **103**, 199–203.

Keller, G., Zimmer, G., Mall, G., Ritz, E., and Amann, K. (2003). Nephron number in patients with primary hypertension. *New England Journal of Medicine* **348**, 101–108.

Khan, N. A., Hampton, J. A., Lacer, D. A., Rapp, J. P., Gohara, A. F., and Goldblatt, P. J. (1987). Morphometric evaluation of the renal arterial system of Dahl salt-sensitive and salt-resistant rats on a high salt diet. I. Interlobar and arcuate arteries. *Laboratory Investigation* **57**, 714–723.

Kimmelstiel, P. and Wilson, C. (1936). Benign and malignant hypertension and nephrosclerosis: a clinical and pathologic study. *American Journal of Pathology* **12**, 45–81.

Kincaid-Smith, P. S. Renal hypertension. In *Hypertension—Mechanisms and Management* (ed. P. S. Kincaid-Smith and J. A. Whitworth), pp. 94–101. New York: ADIS Health Science Press, 1982.

Kincaid-Smith, P. S. What has happened to malignant hypertension? In *Handbook of Hypertension Epidemiology of Hypertension* Vol. 6 (ed. C. J. Bulpitt), pp. 255–265. Amsterdam: Elsevier, 1985.

Kincaid-Smith, P. S. (1991). Malignant hypertension. *Journal of Hypertension* **9**, 893–899.

Kincaid-Smith, P. S. (1999). Clinical diagnosis of hypertensive nephrosclerosis. *Nephrology, Dialysis, Transplantation* **14**, 2255–2256.

Klahr, S., Schreiner, G., and Ichikawa, I. (1988). The progression of renal disease. *New England Journal of Medicine* **318**, 1657–1666.

Klemperer, P. and Otani, S. (1931). Malignant nephrosclerosis (Fahr). *Archives of Pathology* **11**, 60–117.

Krege, J. H. *et al.* (1995). Male–female differences in fertility and blood pressure in ACE-deficient mice. *Nature, London* **375**, 146–148.

Lafferty, H. M. and Brenner, B. M. (1990). Are glomerular hypertension and 'hypertrophy' independent risk factors for progression of renal disease? *Seminars in Nephrology* **10**, 294–304.

Lee, R. M. K. W. (1987). Structural alterations of blood vessels in hypertensive rats. *Canadian Journal of Physiology and Pharmacology* **65**, 1528–1538.

Lever, A. F. (1986). Slow pressor mechanisms in hypertension: a role for hypertrophy of resistance vessels? *Journal of Hypertension* **4**, 515–524.

Lip, G. Y. H., Beevers, M., and Beevers, G. (1994). The failure of malignant hypertension to decline: a survey of 24 years' experience in a multiracial population in England. *Journal of Hypertension* **12**, 1297–1305.

Luft, F. C. and Haller, H. (1995). Hypertension-induced renal injury: is mechanically mediated interstitial inflammation involved? *Nephrology, Dialysis, Transplantation* **10**, 9–11.

Luke, R. G. (1999). Hypertensive nephrosclerosis pathogenesis and prevalence. Essential hypertension is an important cause of endstage renal disease. *Nephrology, Dialysis, Transplantation* **14**, 2271–2278.

Lundgren, Y. (1974). Adaptive changes of cardiovascular design in spontaneous and renal hypertension. Hemodynamic studies in rats. *Acta Physiologica Scandinavica* **408** (Suppl.), 5–62.

McCormack, L. J., Beland, J. E., Schneckloth, R. E., and Corcoran, A. C. (1958). Effects of hypertensive treatment on the evolution of the renal lesions in malignant nephrosclerosis. *American Journal of Pathology* **34**, 1011.

MacMahon, H. E. (1966). Malignant nephrosclerosis, 50 years later. *Journal of Historical Medicine* **21**, 125–146.

Mai, M., Geiger, H., Hilgers, K. F., Veelken, R., Mann, J. F. E., Dämmrich, J., and Luft, F. C. (1993). Early interstital changes in hypertension-induced renal injury. *Hypertension* **22**, 754–765.

Maki, D. D., Ma, J. Z., Louis, T. A., and Kasiske, B. L. (1995). Long-term effects of antihypertensive agents on proteinuria and renal function. *Archives of Internal Medicine* **155**, 1073–1080.

Malangone, J., Abuelo, J. G., Pezzullo, J. C., Lund, K., and McGloin, C. A. (1989). Clinical and laboratory features of patients with chronic renal disease at the start of dialysis. *Clinical Nephrology* **31**, 77–87.

Miller, P. L., Rennke, H. G., and Meyer, T. W. (1991). Glomerular hypertrophy accelerates hypertensive glomerular injury in rats. *American Journal of Physiology* **261**, F459–F465.

Möhring, J. (1977). High arterial pressure versus humoral factors in the pathogenesis of the vascular lesions of malignant hypertension. The case for humoral factors as well as pressure. *Clinical Science* **52**, 113–116.

Mulvany, M. J. and Aalkjaer, C. (1990). Structure and function of small arteries. *Physiological Reviews* **70**, 921–961.

Nordborg, C., Ivarsson, H., Johansson, B. B., and Stage, L. (1983). Morphometric study of mesenteric and renal arteries in spontaneously hypertensive rats. *Journal of Hypertension* **1**, 333–338.

Olsen, F. A. (1969). Rate and ways of resolution of hypertensive vascular disease. *Acta Pathologica Scandinavica* **77**, 39–48.

Olson, J. L., Wilson, S. K., and Heptinstall, R. H. (1986). Relation of glomerular injury to preglomerular resistance in experimental hypertension. *Kidney International* **29**, 849–857.

Ong, A. C. M. and Fine, L. G. (1994). Loss of glomerular function and tubulointerstitial fibrosis: cause or effect? *Kidney International* **45**, 345–351.

Owens, G. K. and Schwartz, S. M. (1982). Alterations in vascular smooth muscle mass in the spontaneously hypertensive rat. Role of cellular hypertrophy, hyperploidy, and hyperplasia. *Circulation Research* **51**, 280–289.

Owens, G. K., Rabinovitch, P. S., and Schwartz, S. M. (1981). Smooth muscle cell hypertrophy versus hyperplasia in hypertension. *Proceedings of the National Academy of Sciences of the United States of America* **78**, 7759–7763.

Page, I. H. and McCubbin, J. *Renal Hypertension*. Chicago, IL: Year Book, 1968.

Pettinger, W. A., Lee, H. C., Reisch, J., and Mitchell, H. C. (1989a). Long-term improvement in renal function after short-term 'strict' blood pressure control in hypertensive nephrosclerosis. *Hypertension* **13**, 766–772.

Pettinger, W. A., Mitchell, H. C., Lee, H.-C., and Redman, H. C. (1989b). Pseudo renal artery stenosis (PRAS) syndrome. *American Journal of Hypertension* **2**, 349–351.

Pickering, G. (1971). Reversibility of malignant hypertension. *Lancet* **i**, 413–418.

Ploth, D. W., Roy, R. N., Huang, E. C., and Navar, L. G. (1981). Impaired renal blood flow and cortical pressure autoregulation in contralateral kidneys of Goldblatt hypertensive rats. *Hypertension* **3**, 67–74.

Ponticelli, C., Imbasciati, E., Tarantino, G., Graziani, G., and Radpaelli, B. (1972). Post partum renal failure with microangiopathic haemolytic anaemia. Long-term survival after anticoagulant therapy. *Nephron* **9**, 227–241.

Rettig, R., Folberth, C. G., Stauss, H., Kopf, D., Waldherr, R., Baldauf, G., and Unger, T. (1990). Hypertension in rats induced by renal grafts from renovascular hypertensive donors. *Hypertension* **15**, 429–435.

Ross, R. (1993). The pathogenesis of atherosclerosis: a perspective for the 1990s. *Nature, London* **362**, 801–809.

Rostand, S. G., Kirk, K. A., Rutsky, E., and Pate, B. A. (1982). Racial differences in the incidence of treatment for end-stage renal disease. *New England Journal of Medicine* **306**, 1276–1279.

Saran, R. D. and Textor, S. C. (2001). Renal-artery stenosis. *New England Journal of Medicine* **6**, 431–442.

Schmieder, R. E., Veelken, R., Gatzka, C. D., Rüddel, H., and Schächinger, H. (1994). Predictors for hypertensive nephropathy: results of a 6-year follow-up study in essential hypertension. *Journal of Hypertension* **13**, 357–365.

Schürmann, P. and MacMahon, H. E. (1933). Die maligne Nephrosklerose, zugleich ein Beitrag zur Frage der Bedeutung der Blutgewebsschranke. *Virchows Archiv* **291**, 47–218.

Segura, J. *et al.* (2001). ACE inhibitors and appearance of renal events in hypertensive nephrosclerosis. *Hypertension* **38**, 645–649.

Smithies, O. and Maeda, N. (1995). Gene targeting approaches to complex genetic diseases: atherosclerosis and essential hypertension. *Proceedings of the National Academy of Sciences of the United States of America* **92**, 5266–5272.

Sommers, S. C., Relman, A. S., and Smithwick, R. H. (1958). Histologic studies of kidney biopsy specimens from patients with hypertension. *American Journal of Pathology* **34**, 685–715.

Spector, S., Ooshima, A., Iwatsuki, K., Fuller, G., Cardinale, G., and Udenfriend, S. (1978). Increased vascular collagen biosynthesis by hypertension and reversal by antihypertensive drugs. *Blood Vessels* **15**, 176–182.

Thoenes, W. and John, H. D. (1980). Endotheliotropic (hemolytic) nephroangiopathy and its various manifestation forms (thrombotic microangiopathy, primary malignant nephrosclerosis, hemolytic–uremic syndrome). *Klinische Wochenschrift* **58**, 173–184.

Tomson, C. R. V., Petersen, K., and Heagerty, A. M. (1991). Does treated essential hypertension result in renal impairment? A cohort study. *Journal of Human Hypertension* **5**, 189–192.

Toto, R. D., Mitchell, H. C., Lee, H.-C., Milam, C., and Pettinger, W. A. (1991). Reversible renal insufficiency due to angiotensin converting enzyme inhibitors in hypertensive nephrosclerosis. *Annals of Internal Medicine* **115**, 513–519.

Toto, R. D., Mitchell, H. C., Smith, R. D., Lee, H. C., McIntire, D., and Pettinger, W. A. (1995). 'Strict' blood pressure control and progression of renal disease in hypertensive nephrosclerosis. *Kidney International* **48**, 851–859.

Tracy, R. E. (1992). Blood pressure related separately to parenchymal fibrosis and vasculopathy of the kidney. *American Journal of Kidney Diseases* **20**, 124–131.

Tracy, R. E. and Ishii, T. (2000). What is 'nephrosclerosis'? Lessons from the US, Japan, and Mexico. *Nephrology, Dialysis, Transplantation* **15**, 1357–1366.

Tracy, R. E. and Toca, V. T. (1974). Nephrosclerosis and blood pressure. *Laboratory Investigation* **30**, 30–34.

Valenzuela, R., Gogate, P. A., Deodhar, S. O., and Gifford, R. W. (1980). Hyaline arteriolar nephrosclerosis. Immunofluorescence findings in the vascular lesions. *Laboratory Investigation* **43**, 530–534.

Vial, J. H. and Boyd, G. W. (1989). Histometric assessment of renal arterioles during DOCA and post-DOCA hypertension and hydralazine treatment in rats. *Journal of Hypertension* **7**, 203–209.

Volhard, F. and Fahr, T. *Die Brightsche Nierenkrankheit. Klinik, Pathologie und Atlas*. Berlin: Springer, 1914.

Weisstuch, J. M. and Dworkin, L. D. (1992). Does essential hypertension cause end-stage renal disease? *Kidney International* **41** (Suppl. 36), S33–S37.

Wenzel, U. O. (2001). Angiotensin-converting enzyme inhibitors and progression of renal disease: evidence from clinical studies. *Contribution Nephrology* **135**, 200–211.

Wenzel, U. O., Troschau, G., Schoeppe, W., Helmchen, U., and Schwietzer, G. (1992). Adverse effect of the calcium channel blocker Nitrendipine on nephrosclerosis in rats with renovascular hypertension. *Hypertension* **20**, 233–241.

Wenzel, U. O., Helmchen, U., Schoeppe, W., and Schwietzer, G. (1994). Combination treatment of enalapril with nitrendipine in rats with renovascular hypertension. *Hypertension* **23**, 114–122.

Wenzel, U. O. *et al.* (2000). Renovascular hypertension does not influence repair of the glomerular lesions induced by the anti-thymocyte glomerulonephritis. *Kidney International* **58**, 1135–1147.

Wenzel, U. O. *et al.* (2002a). Angiotensin II infusion ameliorates the early phase of a mesangioproliferative glomerulonephritis. *Kidney International* **61**, 1020–1029.

Wenzel, U. O. *et al.* (2002b). Repetitive application of anti Thy-1 antibody aggravates damage in the nonclipped but not in the clipped kidney of rats with Goldblatt hypertension. *Kidney International* **61**, 2119–2131.

Wilson, C. and Byrom, F. B. (1939). Renal changes in malignant hypertension. Experimental evidence. *Lancet* **i**, 136–139.

Wilson, C. and Byrom, F. B. (1941). The vicious circle in chronic Bright's disease. Experimental evidence from the hypertensive rat. *Quarterly Journal of Medicine* **10**, 65–93.

Wilson, C. and Pickering, G. W. (1938). Acute arterial lesions in rabbits with experimental renal hypertension. *Clinical Science* **3**, 343–356.

Wilson, S. K. and Heptinstall, R. H. (1984). Effects of acute, angiotensin-induced hypertension on intrarenal arteries in the rat. *Kidney International* **25**, 492–501.

Wolf, G. (2000). Franz Volhard and his students' tortuous road to renovascular hypertension. *Kidney International* **57**, 2156–2166.

Wolfgarten, M. and Magarey, F. R. (1959). Vascular fibrinoid necrosis in hypertension. *Journal of Pathology and Bacteriology* **60**, 357–368.

Yoshida, Y., Fogo, A., and Ichikawa, I. (1989). Glomerular hemodynamic changes versus hypertrophy in experimental glomerulosclerosis. *Kidney International* **35**, 654–660.

Zarif, L. *et al.* (2000). Inaccuracy of clinical phenotyping parameters for hypertensive nephrosclerosis. *Nephrology, Dialysis, Transplantation* **15**, 1801–1807.

Zollinger, H. U. *Niere und Ableitende Harnwege*. Berlin: Springer, 1966.

9.5 Ischaemic nephropathy

Paramit Chowdhury and John E. Scoble

Introduction

The relationship between renal artery narrowing and renal function is complex. There are features common to all causes of renal artery disease but also significant differences between the different causes. The most common cause of renal artery stenosis (RAS) in Europe is atherosclerosis but this is not the case for other parts of the world. The issues related to hypertension are dealt with in Chapter 10.6.5. There are a number of clinical problems associated with acute renal artery occlusion or atheroembolic disease and these are dealt with in Chapter 10.6.5.

The effect of renal artery narrowing on renal blood flow

The much-quoted paper of May *et al.* (1963) on canine femoral arteries showed that for a 50 per cent reduction of diameter (75 per cent reduction in luminal surface) there was a reduction in blood flow. Before this level there was no effect on blood flow, but after this constriction there was a major and progressively catastrophic reduction in blood flow. It has been interpreted widely that there is no significance to a degree of stenosis less than 50 per cent. This is true for blood flow in an experimental setting. However, in the clinical setting atherosclerotic disease is often asymmetrical. The routinely used gold standard test has been the intra-arterial angiogram but this can only view the lesion only in two dimensions. More complex procedures such as intra-vascular ultrasound are possible. Schoenberg *et al.* (2002) have repeated the earlier data recently for renal artery blood flow. These data showed effects similar to those originally observed but added that it is only above a 50 per cent reduction in diameter that there is a reduction in renal blood flow. This suggests that for any renal artery narrowing reduction in flow is a relatively late occurrence in RAS.

Textor *et al.* (1985) looked at the relationship of renal blood flow and renal function. In 16 patients with atherosclerotic renal artery narrowing, a reduction in blood pressure was induced with nitroprusside. In eight patients with bilateral disease there was a reversible reduction in renal plasma flow and glomerular filtration rate suggesting that even with a reduction in blood pressure this may not cause a reduction in renal function. Nahman *et al.* (1994) investigated the renal artery pressure gradient at angioplasty and demonstrated a dramatic reduction in pressure gradient from 109 to 12 mmHg. However, this reduction did not correlate with functional outcome.

From all these data it is clear that the presence of renal artery narrowing does not have a predictable effect on renal function. However, in the data derived from single kidney glomerular filtration rate it is clear that once renal artery occlusion occurs there is a dramatic reduction in renal function (Fig. 1a and b). The point at which the renal function is affected short of occlusion remains an area with little clarity.

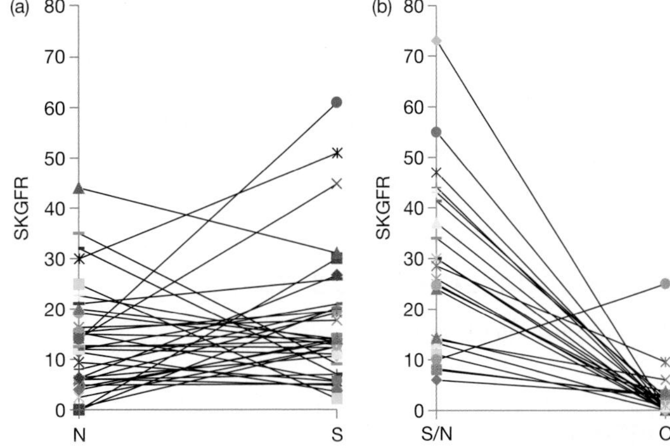

Fig. 1 (a and b) The relationship in atherosclerotic RAS of unilateral RAS and unilateral renal artery occlusion on renal function. Single kidney glomerular filtration rate in paired kidneys.

Experimental data on renal artery narrowing and renal dysfunction

The original observations by Goldblatt *et al.* (1934) were performed in a canine model with renal artery constriction. The histology showed that there was a pattern of changes in the kidney with imposed narrowing. These included marked interstitial fibrosis. Truong *et al.* (1992) showed that there was a process resembling the one seen in acute allograft rejection with the increased expression of histocompatibility antigens and an infiltrate of B-lymphocytes, T-helper lymphocytes, and macrophages in this rat model that was not possible to differentiate from other causes of interstitial nephritis. Subsequent investigators have shown that the reversal of the changes seen in the kidney with experimental renal artery narrowing can be reversed not only by removal of the renal artery clip causing narrowing of the renal artery but also by contralateral nephrectomy. Gobe *et al.* (1990) showed that in response to removal of the contralateral kidney there was renal hyperplasia and an increase in apoptosis within the remaining kidney with renal artery narrowing. Grone *et al.* (1996) showed that a number of processes initiated by experimental renal artery narrowing such as the Na,K-ATPase could be easily reversed by removal of the renal artery narrowing or removal of the contralateral kidney. It is counter-intuitive if the renal arteries narrowing remains but atrophic changes are reversed. Marcussen (1991) reported a series of 12 kidneys with RAS that were removed due to hypertension and three kidneys where there was RAS but no hypertension. He compared this with nephrectomies without renal artery narrowing. The study showed that the proximal tubular volume decreased and the interstitial fibrosis rose in consequence. He found a normal number of glomeruli but a large number of these were not connected to normal proximal tubules.

This suggests that the relationship between renal artery narrowing and renal function is complex. This is also due to the fact that there are effects separate from renal artery narrowing caused by the conditions that cause the renal artery narrowing. There are features common to all causes of renal artery disease but also significant differences between the different causes. Renal artery narrowing induces changes in the kidney downstream but these experimental data suggest that this effect can be reversed by other factors independent of renal artery narrowing.

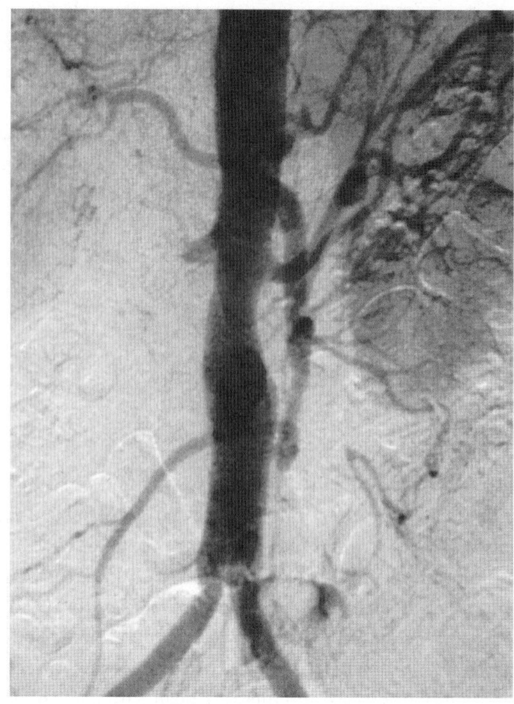

Fig. 2 Takayasu's arteritis. The abdominal angiogram of a young woman who previously had aortic occlusion and a thoracic aneurysm with aorto-bifemoral grafting who subsequently presented with right renal artery occlusion.

Renal collateral blood flow

This is discussed in Chapter 10.6.5.

Diseases causing RAS

Takayasu's arteritis

Takayasu's arteritis is a chronic inflammatory condition with a predilection for the aorta and its major branches. Figure 2 illustrates this condition. The first formal description of a case is ascribed to Mikito Takayasu, after whom the condition is now named (Numano and Tsunekazu 1996). However, the first description of a case was probably by Rokushu Yamamoto in 1830 in a document entitled *Kitsuo idan*, meaning 'Medical records of my private hospital with the big orange tree'. In it he described a 45-year-old man who, following high fever, who presented with absence of a pulse in one arm and a weak pulse in the other (Numano and Tsunekazu 1996).

It was not until after the Second World War that it was established with a systemic pathological survey of a young woman that these changes resulted from occlusion of the carotid arteries. The survey also revealed a panarteritis affecting the aorta and its main branches. Its characteristic clinical features led to coining the phrase 'pulseless disease' in 1948 (Numano *et al.* 2000). Due to its higher prevalence in Japan, the Ministry of Health and Welfare set up a research committee to study it and gave it its present day name.

Takayasu's disease is more commonly seen in South East Asia, South America, and the Mediterranean basin. It is rare in Caucasian populations, with an estimated incidence of 2.6 cases per million population in the United States (Toma 1995). In Israel, a study revealed that none of the 22 cases described were in Ashkenazi Jews who are of European descent, despite them making up 50 per cent of the Israeli population (Deutsch *et al.* 1974).

It is traditionally a disease of young women, who account for 90 per cent of cases in Japan (Koide 1992). It is interesting to note that surveys carried out in Japan demonstrate that the peak in the age distribution has shifted over the last three decades to older age groups (Kimura *et al.* 1996). Furthermore, it shows geographical variation, with the female to male ratio decreasing as one moves to the west (Sharma and Jain 1998).

The exact aetiology remains unclear. Autoimmune mechanisms have been postulated. Familial cases and three cases of monozygotic twins have been described and have led to genetic studies (Numano *et al.* 2000). HLA analysis has shown association with B52, B39.2, and DR2 in Japanese patients (Kimura *et al.* 1996), but has not been shown to hold true in Western populations, where a link with DR4 has been described (Volkman *et al.* 1982). A long-standing link with tuberculosis has been noted, with 70 per cent of Japanese patients demonstrating a positive tuberculin test.

Macroscopically, there is thickening of vessel walls with stenotic and dilated areas, often in alternating fashion. Normal areas forming a 'skipped' pattern separate the affected areas. It has been classified, according to extent of disease, as Type 1 (cranial branches), Type 2 (aortic arch), Type 3 (abdominal aorta), and Type 4 (diffuse extensive disease). Renal lesions are usually ostial at the origin of the main renal arteries. Other forms of renal involvement can occur, including mesangial proliferative, membrano-proliferative, and crescentic glomerulonephritis.

Microscopically, in the acute phase there is granulomatous inflammation with infiltrates of lymphocytes, plasma cells and occasional giant cells around the vasa vasorum. This gives way to chronic fibrotic changes with thickening of intimal and adventitial layers and destruction of the medial layer.

Classically, the condition has two phases. The first involves a systemic inflammatory phase with non-specific symptoms. These include fever, malaise, night sweats and arthralgia, making it difficult to distinguish from a number of more common inflammatory conditions. This is reflected in the laboratory findings, which include a raised erythrocyte sedimentation rate (ESR), C reactive protein (CRP), raised immunoglobulin levels, a leucocytosis, and normochromic anaemia. No specific markers have been isolated, and the ESR is used to monitor disease activity and response to treatment. However, in many cases this phase goes unrecognized.

The diagnosis is more commonly made in the late pulseless phase. Here presentation is related to symptoms of ischaemia secondary to arterial occlusion. Cardiovascular involvement leads to angina due to stenoses of coronary arteries and dyspnoea occurs due to congestive cardiac failure and aortic regurgitation. Although aortic involvement is usual, it should be a differential diagnosis in any young female with arterial disease, as isolated involvement of pulmonary and coronary vessels has been described.

Hypertension occurs in the late stage due to narrowing of the aorta at the origin of the renal arteries. Although a common finding, it shows interesting geographical variation related to distribution of disease. Japanese patients mainly show involvement of the aortic arch and its branches (Types 1 and 2), where as in patients from India and China, the abdominal aorta is predominantly affected (Types 3 and 4) (Zheng *et al.* 1992; Moriwaki *et al.* 1997). As a result, virtually all patients from the Indian subcontinent have hypertension, where Takayasu's accounts for 60 per cent of all cases of renovascular disease (Jain *et al.* 1996). In comparison, about 50 per cent of Japanese patients have hypertension, which is related to cardiovascular involvement. This is in marked contrast to Western populations, where atherosclerosis and fibromuscular dysplasia (FMD) account for the majority of cases of renovascular disease.

In 1990, the American College of Rheumatologists proposed a set of criteria including: (a) age less than 40 years; (b) claudication of an extremity; (c) decreased brachial pulse; (d) a 10 mmHg or more difference in systolic blood pressure between arms; (e) bruit over subclavian or aorta; and (f) angiographic evidence of a lesion involving the aorta or its main branches (Arend *et al.* 1990). This excluded a number of cases in older age groups and also those with isolated abdominal aortic involvement. Sharma *et al.* (1998) have suggested a further modification version of Ishikawa's criteria. These include removal of any age restrictions, the characteristic signs and symptoms being made a single major criterion, deletion of the absence of any iliac involvement as a minor criterion, and the inclusion of coronary artery lesions in patients under 30 as a minor criterion. With these modifications they claim a sensitivity of 92.5 per cent and specificity of 95 per cent when applied to 106 patients.

Total aortography is the gold standard. Figure 2 shows the angiogram of a young woman who had previously had aortic occlusion and a thoracic aneurysm with aortobifemoral grafting who subsequently presented with right renal artery occlusion. Imaging of the aorta and its branches is essential to document the extent of disease and allow intervention to prevent complications. Apart from being invasive, conventional angiography has the further disadvantages of requiring vascular access, a challenge in many of these patients, and requiring large volumes of contrast. Furthermore, it is not suitable as a means of following disease progression. Advances in spiral computed tomography (CT) technology and the wider availability of magnetic resonance imaging (MRI) have provided useful alternatives. Both have been shown to be as sensitive as conventional angiography in detecting lesions. These newer modalities are also able to look at vessel wall thickness rather than just luminal changes, hence are able to detect lesions at an earlier stage (Park 1996; Yeon and Lee 1998). Decreased thickening of arterial walls has also been seen in patients following successful steroid therapy, suggesting these modalities as a useful means of following up patients (Tanigawa *et al.* 1992). Duplex ultrasonography is also a non-invasive and cheap way of screening vessels, and is of particular use in evaluating carotid and renal artery involvement.

Treatment involves both medical and surgical components. Glucocorticosteroids remain the mainstay of medical treatment, guided by the ESR. Notable, however, is the fact that in up to 50 per cent of patients there are no reliable clinical or laboratory parameters to monitor disease. Ishikawa (1991) recommends careful and gradual tapering of steroid. When the ESR is persistently below 10 mm/h for 3–6 months, small dose reductions in maintenance therapy are allowed. For patient's whose disease is resistant to steroids, second line agents including methotrexate, mycophenolate mofetil, and leflunoamide have been used (Tyagi *et al.* 1993; Sharam *et al.* 1998; Daina *et al.* 1999). Surgical intervention is required to prevent complications, particularly renovascular hypertension, aneurysmal rupture, and total vessel occlusion. Surgical intervention should only be carried out after active disease has been controlled with medical therapy, which should be continued postoperatively.

Percutaneous transluminal angioplasty for stenotic lesions has shown considerable success. In the case of renal vessels, a success rate of 89.3 per cent was reported with a 13.5 per cent restenosis rate (Tyagi *et al.* 1993). Reports of successful stent deployment following angioplasty in lesions affecting a variety of arterial vessels have been described (Sharam *et al.* 1998). Reconstructive surgery has also proved successful in repairing aortic arch vessels to prevent cerebrovascular events, in renal artery involvement to cure hypertension (Giordano 2000), and in repairing aneurysms.

The prognosis is related to the prevention of complications, hence the importance of early diagnosis. Major causes of death are stroke, heart disease, aneurysmal rupture, and renovascular hypertension. It is felt to have a favourable prognosis with quoted mortality rates of around 3 per cent in the United States and Japanese studies (Ishikawa 1981; Kerr *et al.* 1994). However, studies have suggested significant morbidity. A better understanding of aetiology and availability of reliable disease markers are required to accurately document and improve outcome. In addition, improved awareness will lead to earlier and possibly increased diagnosis of this condition.

Fibromuscular dysplasia

Fibromuscular dysplasia is a non-inflammatory, non-atherosclerotic condition affecting medium to large arteries. Figure 3 shows the angiogram of a patient who presented with an intracranial bleed and hypertension and who was found to have fibromuscular disease of the carotid artery. Subsequent angiography revealed renal FMD. The condition was first described in 1933 affecting renal vessels (Stanley 1995). The renal arteries are the most commonly affected, accounting for 60–75 per cent of cases (Stanley 1995). The right renal artery is more commonly involved than the left. Other arteries affected include the carotid, vertebral, mesenteric, coeliac, hepatic, iliac and coronary vessels (Palubinskas and Ripley 1964).

FMD is the second most common cause of renovascular disease in the Western world, accounting for 25 per cent of cases. It is uncommon in Black and Asian populations. In its most common forms, it predominantly affects young to middle aged women, with a peak in the fourth decade of life (Kincaid *et al.* 1968). Autopsy studies have shown an incidence of 1–2 per cent in the general population (Heffelfinger *et al.* 1970).

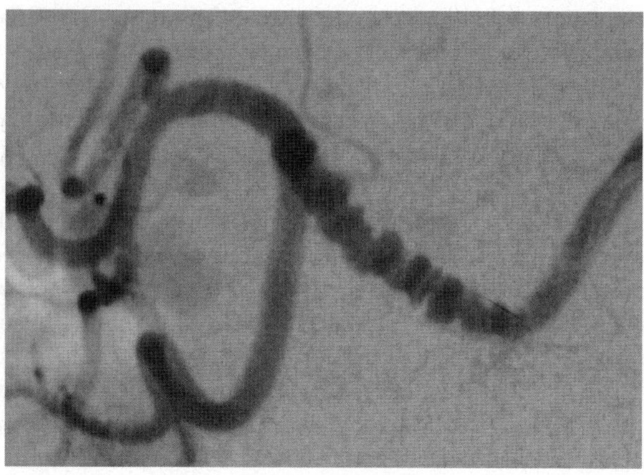

Fig. 3 Fibromuscular dysplasia. The figure shows the angiogram of a patient who presented with an intracranial bleed and hypertension and who was found to have fibromuscular disease of the carotid artery. Subsequent angiography revealed renal FMD.

The exact aetiology of FMD remains unknown. A familial version has been described, with an autosomal dominant pattern of inheritance suggested (Rushton 1980). Familial cases have been shown to be usually multifocal, bilateral, and diffuse (Panier-Moreau *et al.* 1997). Given the striking female preponderance, hormonal effects on vascular smooth muscle have been proposed, but remain unsubstantiated (Stanley 1995). Preferential involvement of the right renal artery has led to suggestions that mechanical stresses due to ptosis of the kidney are involved, ptosis more commonly affecting the right side (Stanley 1995). Other proposed mechanisms relate to mural ischaemia due to vasoconstriction of vasa vasorum. In keeping with this ischaemic aetiology, cigarette smoking has been shown to be a risk factor in predisposed individuals and associated with increased severity of disease (Sang *et al.* 1989; Bofinger *et al.* 1999). Studies have also described a link with α-1 antitrypsin deficiency (Schievink *et al.* 1998; Bofinger *et al.* 2000).

Three types have been identified, based on the dominant part of the vessel wall affected: intimal fibroplasia, medial fibroplasia, and periarterial (adventitial) fibroplasia. Medial fibroplasia is further divided into specific sub-types.

Intimal fibroplasia accounts for 5–10 per cent of cases. Children or young adults are more often affected. In contrast to other forms, there is no female preponderance. Radiologically, lesions take the form of smooth focal or tubular stenoses. Histologically, there is deposition circumferential of collagen without lipid in the intimal layer. The internal elastic lamina is always present, but may be fragmented or reduplicated. Multiple arteries can be involved, mimicking a systemic disease.

Medial fibroplasia accounts for the vast majority of cases (75–80 per cent). It typically affects women in the forth decade of life. Pathologically, there are areas of intimal and medial thinning with loss of the internal elastic lamina, leading to formation of aneurysms. These alternate with areas of medial thickening due to collagen deposition, leading to the classical 'string of beads' appearance seen on arteriography. The aneurysms are characteristically wider in diameter than the proximal unaffected portion of the artery. In contrast to atherosclerotic disease, the proximal one-third of the renal artery is spared. Disease may also extend into the primary branches and is bilateral in around 40 per cent of cases.

A less common variant of medial FMD, perimedial (or sub-adventitial) fibroplasia, is seen in around 10 per cent of cases. It predominantly affects young adults. Here fibrous tissue replaces the outer smooth muscle layer of the media, with sparing of the inner portion. It is a severely stenosing lesion predominantly affecting the right renal artery. The stenosing lesions can vary in severity, with alternating severe and milder stenoses giving a 'beaded' appearance. Unlike true medial hypoplasia, these do not represent aneurysms, and their diameter is less than that of the lumen of unaffected portions of the vessel. In some cases, medial and perimedial changes coexist, giving rise to a more diffuse picture.

A final rare variant of medial FMD is termed medial hyperplasia. Here, in contrast to other forms, there is true muscle hyperplasia as well as fibrosis, giving rise to long smooth stenoses as seen with intimal fibroplasia.

Adventitial fibroplasia is rarely seen, accounting for less than 1 per cent of cases. Collagen deposition can extend into surrounding tissues giving a similar picture to that seen in retroperitoneal fibrosis.

The presentation of FMD is usually with hypertension from renovascular involvement. Carotid involvement leads to a variety of neurological symptoms including dissection and an association with intracranial berry aneurysms (Cloft *et al.* 1998). Abdominal angina occurs when mesenteric vessels are involved. Iliac disease can give rise to symptoms of claudication.

In the diagnosis of FMD, arteriography remains the gold standard. A study of 20 patients suggested a role for helical CT angiography. MRA has the disadvantage of missing disease in branch vessels (Andreoni *et al.* 2002). Both modalities have the disadvantage that intraluminal pressures cannot be determined. Their roles as yet remain undetermined. In cases of diffuse involvement, when multiple vessels are affected, FMD can be difficult to distinguish from vasculitis.

In its common form of medial fibroplasia, FMD was thought to be non-progressive, however, more recent studies suggest this is not the case. Of 30 normotensive patients found to have FMD during screening for suitability as live renal donors, 26.6 per cent developed hypertension, compared with 6.1 per cent of healthy controls (Cragg *et al.* 1989). The rate of progression appears variable; one study of 42 proven cases showed progression in all sub-types (Goncharenko *et al.* 1981).

Medical control of hypertension should follow usual guidelines. For hypertension due to lesions of the main renal arteries, percutaneous transluminal renal angioplasty (PTRA) is the treatment of choice, with 70–90 per cent of patients showing improved blood pressure control at 1 year (Tegtmayer *et al.* 1995; Birrer *et al.* 2002). Restenosis rates vary from 8 to 23 per cent (Tegtmayer *et al.* 1995; Birrer *et al.* 2002). Complications include perforation of the renal artery and thrombosis with infarction but the incidence remains low.

For patients in whom PTRA is unsuccessful or not possible, reconstructive surgery remains an option. The operation is technically successful in 90 per cent of patients, with a mortality of around 2 per cent. Hypertension is cured in 36 per cent, and improved in 31 per cent. Five-year patency rates are reported at 74 per cent (Reiher *et al.* 2000). FMD is a very rare cause of endstage renal failure.

Middle aortic syndrome

Middle aortic syndrome (MAS) is a rare condition referring to isolated narrowing of the proximal portion of the abdominal aorta. Figure 4 shows an angiogram of a 17-year-old girl who presented with claudication at 100 m (Masterson *et al.* 2000). The first clinical descriptions of this condition date back to 1847, but the term 'middle aortic syndrome' was coined by Sen and his colleagues in 1963 (Sen *et al.* 1963).

A great deal of confusion exists with regard to terminology of lesions affecting the abdominal aorta. MAS is often confused with congenital lesions such as coarctation and hypoplasia. Some also consider it to be a specific variant of Takayasu's arteritis, but this wrongly infers an inflammatory aetiology. An association with neurofibromatosis has been described, but many consider the mesenchymal disease in this condition to represent a separate entity (Sumboonnanonda *et al.* 1992). The term 'middle aortic syndrome' should be considered a clinico-anatomical description without reference to aetiology. It should be reserved for cases demonstrating the characteristic focal, smooth, tubular narrowing of the proximal aorta in the absence of inflammation or other stigmata.

The aetiology remains unknown and the situation is further confused by the lack of clarity in its classification. Given its presentation in younger age groups, it has been suggested it is the result of a developmental abnormality. Its association with neurofibromatosis, William's syndrome, and other congenital conditions suggests a genetic component. Histological analysis of tissue in three cases showed fibrotic changes indistinguishable from FMD (Schwartz and White 1964).

MAS most commonly affects children and young adults. It presents with hypertension of upper limbs associated with weak femoral pulses and an abdominal bruit. Claudication secondary to ischaemia is not commonly encountered, in part due to large collateral formation. The hypertension can also be of renovascular origin, with RAS present in 90 per cent of cases. Multiple renal arteries are also frequently seen. There is also stenosis of the coeliac and superior mesenteric vessels but interestingly the inferior mesenteric artery is always spared. Lesions are typically ostial lesions at their origins, but mid vessel lesions have been described (Deal *et al.* 1992).

The treatment can often prove challenging due to the relatively young age of patients. Medical treatment consists of control of hypertension to prevent end organ damage. Without treatment death occurs before the fourth decade (Panayiotopoulos *et al.* 1996). Angioplasty of visceral branch lesions is increasingly successful option if technically feasible. However, balloon dilation of aortic lesions has a significant risk. Complications include aneurysm formation, rupture, and restenosis. These can be partly reduced by the use of stents, but this too poses problems in a patient whose is still growing.

In those patients with uncontrolled hypertension, declining renal function and/or ischaemic symptoms, surgery needs to be considered. Timing of these complex procedures in growing children requires considerable expertise. Aortic bypass surgery together with re-implantation of the renal arteries is the procedure most used. Renal autotransplantation may be required. If the coeliac axis is not involved, splenorenal or hepatorenal bypass may be an option. Repeat surgery is not uncommonly required as the patient grows. It is recommended in one series that surgery be withheld if at all possible in patients under 6 years of age (Panayiotopoulos *et al.* 1996).

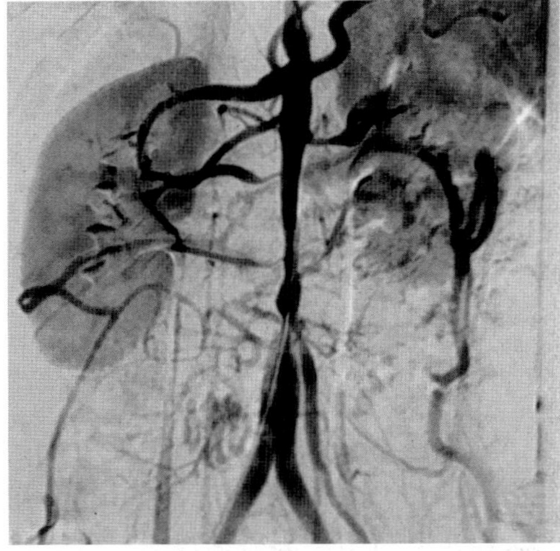

Fig. 4 Middle aortic syndrome. The figure shows an angiogram of a 17-year-old girl who presented with claudication at 100 m (Masterson *et al.* 2000).

Transplant renal artery stenosis

This tends to present more acutely both as occlusion and rapidly worsening renal function. It is dealt with in Chapter 10.6.5.

Atherosclerotic renal artery stenosis

Atherosclerotic disease of the renal arteries has been recognized for many years. The first clear evidence of the frequency of this problem was the Australian post mortem study of Schwartz and White (1964). The applicability of their exact estimates of the frequency of this problem may be open to dispute as this study was of individuals who had died in a hospital setting. Post mortem direct analysis of renal artery narrowing may be more accurate than has been achieved by subsequent imaging procedures as it measures directly artery and its narrowing. In spite of the limitation of the cohort examined the authors made two important points. The first is that whatever the exact incidence of atherosclerotic RAS (ARAS) the incidence increases with age. The second important point is that in none of the patients was RAS suspected ante mortem. Both of these points have been reinforced by all subsequent studies; Table 1.

These studies suggest that ARAS is a condition of the elderly population. However, the PDAY study (1993) showed that in individuals under the age of 35 years fatty streak deposition in the aorta is predominantly in the caudal half of the major abdominal aortic vessels; Fig. 5. ARAS is not a disease of the renal artery as in FMD but is a disease of the aorta. Harding *et al.* (1992) found a very low incidence of

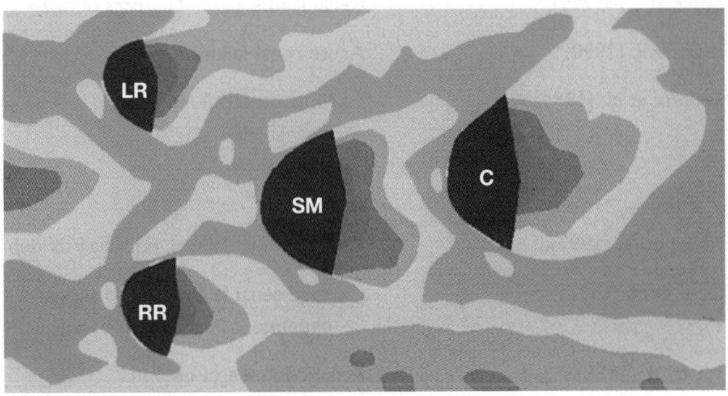

Fig. 5 Distribution of fatty streak in post mortems of individuals dying of a sudden or traumatic death (PDAY study 1993).

Table 1 Incidence of RAS in associated conditions

Author(s)	Association with RAS	% (total number)
Schwartz and White (1964)	Post mortem unselected	24 (154)
Holley *et al.* (1964)	Post mortem in hypertension	22 (295)
Sawicki *et al.* (1991)	Post mortem	
	All	4.3 (5194)
	Diabetes	8.3
Uzu *et al.* (1997)	Post mortem in myocardial infarction	12 (1788)
Kuroda *et al.* (2000)	Post mortem in stroke	10.4 (2167)
Maxwell *et al.* (1972)	Hypertension	36 (2442)
Ying *et al.* (1984)	Hypertension	37 (106)
	Hypertension + renal impairment	48 (21)
Carmichael *et al.* (1986)	Hypertension	36 (235)
Ramirez *et al.* (1987)	Coronary angiography	14 (102)
Harding *et al.* (1992)	Coronary angiography	30 (1235)
Jean *et al.* (1994)	Coronary angiography	18 (196)
Hnas and Zeskind (1995)	Carotid angiography	7 (401)
Rackson *et al.* (1990)	Aortic dissection	16 (63)
Olin *et al.* (1990)	Abdominal aortic aneurysm	38 (109)
Olin *et al.* (1990)	Aorto-occlusive disease	33 (21)
Valentine *et al.* (1993)	Aneurysmal or occlusive vascular disease	28 (346)
Dustan *et al.* (1964)	Peripheral vascular disease	37 (149)
Olin *et al.* (1990)	Peripheral occlusive vascular disease	39 (189)
Wilms and Marchal (1990)	Peripheral vascular disease	22 (100)
Choudhri *et al.* (1990)	Peripheral vascular disease	59 (100)
Swartbol *et al.* (1992)	Peripheral vascular disease	49 (450)
Missouris *et al.* (1994)	Peripheral vascular disease	45 (127)
Wachtell *et al.* (1996)	Peripheral vascular disease	31 (100)
		14 (100)
Metcalfe *et al.* (1999)	Peripheral vascular disease	36 (218)
Meyrier *et al.* (1988)	Renal failure	
	Retrospective	0.3 (5891)
	Prospective	1.4 (1087)
Scoble *et al.* (1989)	Renal failure (over 50 years of age)	14 (71)
Kalra *et al.* (1990)	Acute renal failure	16 (600)
Mailloux *et al.* (1994a)	Chronic renal failure	
	Age 15–40	1 (175)
	Age 41–61	5 (237)
	Age 61+	25 (271)
O'Neil *et al.* (1992)	Chronic renal failure, non-dialysis dependent	14 (21)
Appel *et al.* (1995)	Chronic renal failure, non-dialysis dependent in older patients	22 (45)
Vidt *et al.* (1988)	Renal cholesterol emboli	79 (24)
Neymark *et al.* (2000)	Potential renal donors, ARAS, and FMD	10.9 (716)

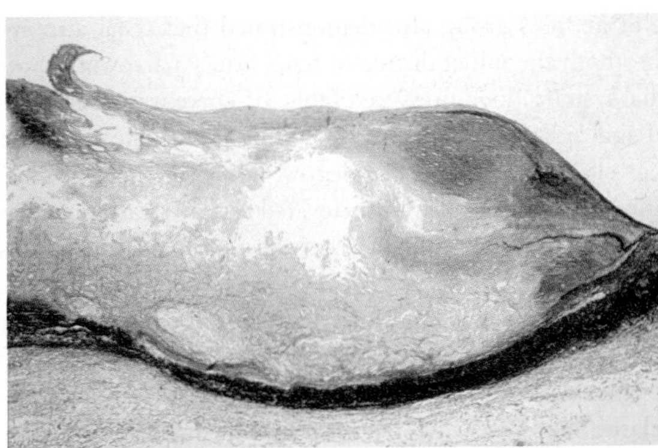

Fig. 6 A cross-section of a renal artery with atherosclerotic RAS. There is severe aortic atheroma but normal arterial architecture after the ostium.

Table 2 Associations of known ARAS

Authors	Association in known RAS	% (total number)
Louie *et al.* (1994)	% with severe carotid disease	46 (60)
Louie *et al.* (1994)	% with severe peripheral vascular disease	73 (60)
Zierler *et al.* (1998)	% with severe carotid disease	19 (149)
Zierler *et al.* (1998)	% with severe peripheral vascular disease	21 (149)
Missouris *et al.* (1998)	% with severe carotid disease	18 (38)

renal artery narrowing in patients with ARAS after the first centimetre of the renal artery. This is illustrated in Fig. 6, which shows that there is relatively little disease after the ostium. It seems likely that all ARAS is 'ostial' and that those lesions that are non-ostial are the result of dilatation of the aorta at this point. It would appear that ARAS is a programmed feature of longevity in many societies.

The role of ARAS in renal dysfunction was suggested by an early report that suggested that 14 per cent of patients with endstage renal failure not attributable to a known cause had ARAS; Table 1. Mailloux *et al.* (1995) have enlarged this early observation and suggested that 25 per cent of patients over the age of 60 years entering a renal replacement programme may have ARAS as the cause. The overall incidence of ARAS is unclear. Table 1 shows the associations previously reported and Table 2 shows the high incidence of associated vascular disease in those patients identified as having ARAS. The association of peripheral vascular disease with ARAS is stronger than any link with cardiac or cerebrovascular disease. There are significant associations with cardiac death and aortic aneurysmal disease as shown in Table 1. The study by Harding *et al.* (1992) illustrates these features very clearly; Table 3. The association of ARAS in patients undergoing coronary angiography was strongest with peripheral vascular disease and not with a number of other features that would be expected. As will be discussed later another association not apparent at the initial observation was of an enormously increased mortality in the ARAS group; Table 4.

Table 3 Predictors of ARAS in patients undergoing coronary angiography (Harding *et al.* 1992)

Feature	*P* value
Age	0.001
Peripheral vascular disease	0.001
Congestive heart failure	0.0001
Creatinine > 106 μmol/l	0.0019
Smoking	0.0081
Female	0.0156
Hypertension	0.0622
Diabetes mellitus	0.1207
History of CAD	0.4429
Hyperlipidaemia	0.7293

Table 4 Survival in atherosclerotic renovascular disease

Study and length of follow-up	Survival (%)
Mailloux *et al.* (1988)	
5-year survival endstage renal failure with RAS	12
Criqui *et al.* (1992)	
5-year severe peripheral vascular disease	69
Scoble *et al.* (1993)	
2-year survival RAS with intervention	80
2-year survival RAS without intervention	63
Connolly *et al.* (1994)	
2-year survival unilateral RAS	96
2-year survival bilateral RAS	74
2-year survival unilateral RAS and occlusion	47
Mailloux *et al.* (1994b)	
2-year survival endstage renal failure with RAS	55
5-year survival endstage renal failure with RAS	16
10-year survival endstage renal failure with RAS	5
15-year survival endstage renal failure with RAS	0
Khan *et al.* (1995)	
90 days with acute renal failure and RAS	7
Baboolal *et al.* (1998)	
5-year survival with bilateral RAS	55
Conlon *et al.* (1998)	
4-year survival of coronary angiography without RAS	86
4-year survival of coronary angiography with RAS	65
Cheung *et al.* (2002)	
5-year survival in unilateral renal artery occlusion	31

Atheroembolic disease

The clinical problem of acute atheroembolic disease is dealt with in depth in Chapter 10.6.5.

Progression in atherosclerotic RAS

The progression in renovascular disease is both that of the lesion and that of the underlying nephropathy; Table 5. In other vascular territories such as the coronary vessels progression with atherosclerotic disease would appear to be acute and catastrophic in atherosclerotic disease. However, in renal artery disease this is much less common. The first attempt at description of progression was by Meaney *et al.* in 1968 for the Cleveland Clinic. They observed that in 39 patients with atherosclerotic disease the lesion progressed in 10 cases and proceeded to occlusion in four but only occurred in two of the 40 patients with medial fibroplasia (Meaney *et al.* 1968). Two latter papers have suggested that the rate of occlusion was related to the initial degree of RAS (Schreiber *et al.* 1984; Tollefson and Ernst 1991). The study of Weibull *et al.* (1990) made the important observation that in 24 renal arteries that occluded between sequential angiograms there were no symptoms even with retrospective enquiry of the patients. In the Dutch DRASTIC study (van Jaarsveld *et al.* 1998) of angioplasty for the treatment of hypertension sequential angiograms were performed. This study showed that in the 25 patients with drug therapy alone 20 per cent had an increase in stenosis, 16 per cent regression and occlusion in 9 per cent of patients. This is the only prospective angiographic study of renal artery narrowing and progression. These observations were with angiography. The group of Strandness in Seattle have published a number of studies using sequential Doppler estimations of renal artery narrowing; Table 5. In these studies the individual renal arteries are assigned to either normal, less than 60 per cent stenosis, greater than 60 per cent stenosis, and occlusion. Renal atrophy was defined as a greater than 1 cm loss of bipolar length compared to the initial examination. Table 5 shows the relationship of the initial degree of stenosis both to progression of the lesion as well as atrophy in the kidney. In these studies it has been demonstrated that as in the angiographic papers the incidence of occlusion is related to the initial renal artery narrowing. Occlusion occurred in nine of the 295 renal arteries. Two were initially assessed at less than 60 per cent stenosis and seven in the greater than 60 per cent stenosis group. However, all were observed to have greater than 60 per cent stenosis prior to occlusion. The factors that predicted progression of the lesion were systolic blood pressure, diabetes mellitus and high-grade stenosis in either the ipselateral or contralateral renal artery.

Table 5 Progression in atherosclerotic renovascular disease

	Overall	Normal	<60% stenosis	>60% stenosis
% 2-year risk of atrophy (Caps et *al.* 1998a)		5.5	11.7	20.8
% 3-year risk of progression (Caps et *al.* 1998b)		18	28	49
% 1-year (van Jaarsveld et *al.* 1998) in known stenosis > 50%				
Progression	20			
Progression to occlusion	9			
% 2.6-year risk of progression (Crowley et *al.* 1998)	11.1%			

The Strandness group also demonstrated that renal atrophy was related to both the initial degree of renal artery narrowing as well as the initial systolic blood pressure (Table 5). There was a correlation of cortical end diastolic velocity and atrophy as well. The lower the end diastolic velocity, the higher the degree of atrophy. There was also a correlation of renal atrophy with elevated serum creatinine measurements. The progression of real atrophy also correlated with a decline in renal function.

The effect of effective lipid lowering therapy on ARAS is unclear. Data from such trials in cardiology such as AVERT (Pitt *et al.* 1999) suggest that effective lipid lowering therapy may be more useful than revascularization. One case report has shown regression of ARAS (Khong *et al.* 2001). This case report and the observations in DRASTIC may represent the increased use of powerful lipid lowering agents in recent years in these patients.

Progression of renal dysfunction with ARAS is a difficult area. The studies recently performed have included patient wall of whom have had intervention. Baboolal *et al.* (1998) reported a retrospective series of 51 patients without intervention. These patients had bilateral RAS and none had survival or radiological intervention. These authors found that the rate of loss of renal function was 4 ml/min/year with six patients progressing to renal failure. The mortality rate was high at 45 per cent at 5 years with and reduced the final number progressing to endstage renal failure. The predictor of progression to endstage renal failure was initial renal function. The mean glomerular filtration rate of those progressing to renal failure was 25 ml/min. This is not surprising as these patients had the lowest reserve at the start of then observation. Cheung *et al.* (2002) found that in patients with unilateral renal artery occlusion there was a loss of renal function 4.1 ml/min/year.

Mortality in ARAS

Atherosclerotic renovascular disease is not an isolated clinical problem. It is not unreasonable to expect the non-renal vascular disease to play an important part in the outcome of these patients. This has been born out by outcome data; Table 4. Mailloux *et al.* (1988) showed that in patients entering a dialysis programme those who suffered from atherosclerotic renovascular disease have the worst outcome for all diagnoses. Connolly *et al.* (1994) showed that the severity of the lesions predicted outcome with the worst in severe bilateral disease. Cheung *et al.* (2002) in unilateral RAS showed that the predicator of mortality or endstage renal failure was initial low baseline glomerular filtration rate. Harding *et al.* (1992) showed that in patients with demonstrable renovascular disease at the time of angiography for coronary artery disease there was a reduction. All these patients had unilateral renal artery occlusion in 4-year survival from 86 to 64 per cent. None of the patients died from renal impairment. Khan *et al.* (1995) have shown that in Aberdeen there was a 93 per cent mortality rate in those representing with ARAS by 90 days after initiation of dialysis treatment. Missouris *et al.* (1993) investigated a similar series of patients identified as having renovascular disease at the time of angiography for peripheral vascular disease. These patients on subsequent surgery for peripheral vascular disease had a mortality rate of 32 per cent for those with RAS and 0 per cent for those without in the early postoperative period. The series of 1058 patients with 4-year follow-up data and successful Palmaz stent insertion showed that the mortality rate was related to initial renal function (Dorros *et al.* 1998). In those with normal renal function the survival was 85 per cent, whereas in those with poor renal function it was 49 per cent.

In a group of 142 patients with established renovascular disease Fatica *et al.* (2001), while analysing the data from the US Renal Data System database, found that the mortality of patients with ESRF due to atherosclerotic renovascular disease was high. However, once the figures were adjusted for comorbidity, the survival was the same as patients without RAS but the same comorbidity.

The management of patients with atherosclerotic disease must take into account the high mortality rate when deciding on interventions to improve renal function. It is also clear that given the expected mortality rate any intervention may not need to be as durable as in other conditions.

Flash pulmonary oedema

Pickering *et al.* (1988) described a condition of recurrent pulmonary oedema associated with RAS. It appears to be associated with ARAS. The important feature that this report described was the cure of this condition by revascularization. Neither blood pressure nor renal function was a good predictor of the pulmonary oedema. These patients often have long-standing hypertension. Since the original report it has become recognized as a distinct clinical entity and the usual title of 'flash pulmonary oedema' is now commonly used. These patients have reasonable cardiac function but present with acute, and often, severe pulmonary oedema. In one series it was found that the average number of admissions was 2.3 prior to the diagnosis being made (Weatherford *et al.* 1997). In some of these cases this included ventilation for the pulmonary oedema. Figure 7 shows the renal angiogram of such a case. The patient had had an aortic graft, right nephrectomy and left saphenous vein graft from the aorta to the renal artery. She presented 24 years later with a modest impairment of renal function but severe pulmonary oedema (Farmer *et al.* 1999a). After angioplasty of the lesion there were no further admissions with pulmonary oedema. The exact physiology of the condition is unclear but one observation is that most cases present at night. It may be that in tight renal artery narrowing any diurnal variation in blood pressure may provoke a surge of angiotensin II. Kwan *et al.* (1997) described a case with diastolic left ventricular dysfunction that was cured by renal revascularization for bilateral RAS. Fascinatingly, 'flash pulmonary oedema' has been described following unilateral renal angioplasty in a patient with bilateral RAS (Harker *et al.* 1995). The Cornell group has more recently updated its original observation and found that the condition is more likely to occur in patients with bilateral stenosis or unilateral stenosis and occlusion (Bloch *et al.* 1999). In 41 per cent of patients with bilateral, RAS presenting for intervention a history of 'flash pulmonary oedema' could be obtained but in only 12 per cent of those with unilateral disease. In addition, those with unilateral disease were less likely to obtain benefit from revascularization that in this series was an endovascular stent placement. This condition appears to be usually seen in atherosclerotic disease although it has been described in FMD. There are case reports of this condition in a transplant RAS (Lye *et al.* 1996; Mansy *et al.* 1996).

The condition of 'flash pulmonary oedema' must be differentiated from the chronic congestive cardiac failure. Missouris *et al.* (1993) have described initially two patients but subsequently a series of nine patients who had congestive heart failure where there was a dramatic improvement in blood pressure and natriuresis following revascularization. It is not clear how common this condition is, although there have been other similar case reports (Ducloux *et al.* 1997). One report of patient presenting to a general medical clinic for congestive failure with a plasma creatinine of below 300 μmol/l showed that RAS was present in one-third of patients (McDowall *et al.* 1998). These patients did not all undergo revascularization and so any casual effect cannot be ascertained.

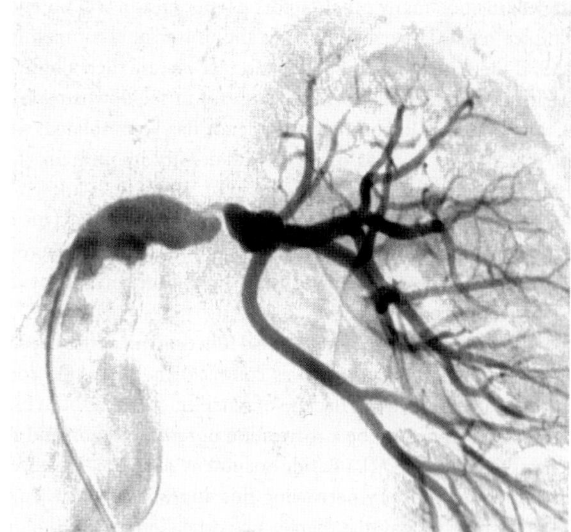

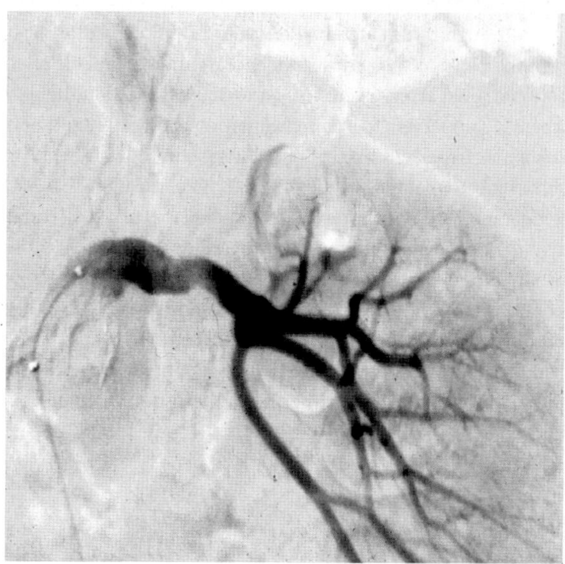

Fig. 7 Angiograms of a patient presenting 23 years after saphenous vein bypass graft to left kidney and right nephrectomy. The patient presented with pulmonary oedema and modestly elevated plasma creatinine (Farmer *et al.* 1999a).

Non-ischaemic damage—atherosclerotic nephropathy

The effects of renal artery narrowing may modulate the function of the downstream kidney. However, the milieu in which these kidneys will operate will include many other factors. Hypertension will independently induce renal damage and this is the universal accompaniment of ARAS. If there is significant aortic vascular disease then all the data show that there will be atheroembolic disease in the downstream kidneys, Chapter 10.6.5. Experimental evidence has accumulated, which suggest that factors such as oxidized low density lipoprotein (LDL) may influence renal function (Rahman *et al.* 1999). It is known that the atherosclerotic plaque is a potent site of LDL oxidation. This does illustrate one of the many potential agents produced by an atherosclerotic plaque that may affect downstream renal function independent of renal artery narrowing.

Renal artery narrowing may alter renal function but as has been previously discussed this relationship is complex. In ARAS, the role of renal artery narrowing in the decline of renal function has been examined. There does appear to be a correlation of renal function and renal artery narrowing in FMD (La Batide-Alanore *et al.* 2001). However, in atherosclerotic renal artery narrowing this appears less clear. Farmer *et al.* (1999b) have shown that there is no correlation in paired kidneys of function and the presence of unilateral RAS. This is shown in Fig. 1(a) and (b). Although in unilateral ARAS there is no correlation of function with the presence of stenosis, there is an understandable relationship between renal artery occlusion and renal dysfunction. In all these cases, there is comparison to a paired kidney obviating any effect of other factors such as hypertension or lipid abnormality. Suresh *et al.* (2000) reported a series 71 patients where there was no correlation between creatinine clearance and renal artery patency. Iglesias *et al.* (2000) reported a study of patients who underwent aortography for aorto-iliac disease. Of 201 patients, 49 per cent had some degree of renal artery narrowing. With long-term follow-up these patients did not have a greater decline in renal function than those with no renal artery narrowing. This suggests that in atherosclerotic disease there is a complex process causing renal dysfunction. This has been termed 'atherosclerotic nephropathy' (Scoble 1999).

Intervention in ARAS to improve renal function

Anecdotal reports over 20 years suggested that in individual patients renal failure could be averted by revascularization. Surgery has always been a modality for altering renal artery narrowing. Renal artery surgery for hypertension is dealt with in Chapter 10.6.5. A number of authors have shown that surgery in endstage renal failure can produce successful dialysis free survival (Kaylor *et al.* 1989; Hansen *et al.* 1995). The work of Lawrie *et al.* (1989) suggested that revascularization of a kidney in patients with a younger age and FMD had a better outcome. Only one study has compared surgery with angioplasty and no difference was found between the two (Weibull *et al.* 1993). There is considerable literature of surgery to stabilize renal function. Paty *et al.* (2001) have suggested that renal artery reconstruction with a prosthetic renal artery is successful. At the present time, considering the relative morbidity of surgery in most cases, intervention will be by angioplasty with or without stent insertion.

The paper of Ying *et al.* (1984) with angioplasty suggested that this was an important area for therapy and intervention in renal disease. These reports suggest that an improvement in renal function could be expected in one-third of patients with ARAS and stabilization in one-third, and worsening in one-third (Pattison *et al.* 1992; Dejani *et al.* 2000; Lederman *et al.* 2001). One series suggested reduced medication but continued hypertension after angioplasty in these patients (Kvist and Mulvany 2001). The differentiation between technically successful angioplasty and one with improvement in renal function was not often identified (Burket *et al.* 2000; Bush *et al.* 2001). The results published on improvement in hypertension are dealt with in Chapter 10.6.5 but none of these reports demonstrated an improvement in renal function (Plouin *et al.* 1998; van Jaarsveld *et al.* 1998; Webster *et al.* 1998).

It is important to try and identify the possible groups who may benefit from revascularization. One of the early series suggested an improvement in the renal function in those patients with an acute deterioration prior to angioplasty (Pattison *et al.* 1992). Two recent series have independently supported the concept that improvement in renal function is predicted by the pre-angioplasty rate of decline of renal function. Muray *et al.* (2002) reported a series of 73 patients with at least three plasma creatinine measurements prior to angioplasty. The steeper the decline in renal function prior to angioplasty, the better the response post angioplasty. In this series the renal size, pre-intervention plasma creatinine, and the degree of proteinuria did not correlate with the favourable outcome after angioplasty. The group of Beutler *et al.* (2001) examined a group of 63 patients with ostial ARAS. This study showed that in the 26 patients with stable renal function there was no improvement with angioplasty. However, in the 30 patients with deteriorating renal function there was stabilization of renal function. It is important to note that seven of the original group either died or reached endstage renal failure and were excluded from the study.

Other studies have used a decline pre-angioplasty renal function in order to identify patients for intervention and not stratify them. Harden *et al.* (1997) reported a series of 32 patients who had severe atherosclerotic renovascular disease and renal impairment with a range of creatinine of 197–391 μmol/l. Three patients were dialysis dependent. These patients had deteriorating renal function prior to angioplasty. Ten patients had bilateral RAS, 14 had unilateral RAS with contralateral renal artery occlusion, seven had unilateral stenosis, and one patient had bilateral occlusion. These patients had both renal insufficiency and also significant renal artery narrowing this represents severe renal artery diseases and this was associated with severe renal impairment. Three patients were dialysis dependent and the means age was 67 years. This study has been followed by a number of similar observations wherein severe renal impairment and severe atherosclerotic renal artery disease improvement can be documented. Watson *et al.* (2000) have shown that in a group of patients, with what they describe as global renovascular disease, the reciprocal plot was benefited by intervention. This study used renal artery stent placement in series of 33 patients. The use of a stent after angioplasty has been a major issue. In cardiac angioplasty it is now routine practice to perform stenting. The study of Blum *et al.* (1997) showed that renal artery stent placement was more effective in preventing restenosis that angioplasty alone in ostial RAS. This is the most common form of atherosclerotic renal artery involvement and it has been a criticism of earlier studies of intervention that have only used angioplasty without stent insertion (van Jaarsveld *et al.* 1998). However, this study included patients with good renal function and found no difference in renal function between the two groups in spite of a higher restenosis rate in the angioplasty group alone.

The major problem with a number of these series is that unilateral intervention might produce an improvement in overall renal function although the kidney undergoing intervention might not improve renal function. There are a number of series that have reported analysis of individual kidney function pre- and post-angioplasty. The first of these was from Jensen *et al.* (1995). This group looked at 137 patients undergoing angioplasty for hypertension. This also included patients with FMD. These patients as a group had good overall renal function with glomerular filtration rates of 78 and 48 ml/min/1.73 m^2 for the FMD and atherosclerotic groups, respectively. In the atherosclerotic group there was bilateral disease in 74 of the 107 patients. There is no mention of occlusion. The group suggested an improvement in blood pressure in both groups and an improvement in single kidney renal function from 29 to 32 ml/min. Overall there was a better response in term of function in those kidneys with FMD than atherosclerotic disease. However, in the atherosclerotic group with an overall glomerular filtration rate of 30 ml/min there were more individuals with a decline in renal function than an improvement. Another smaller series of ARAS pre- and post-single kidney glomerular filtration estimations there was no overall improvement in renal function (Farmer *et al.* 1998). In a smaller group of patients with single function kidneys it was observed that even after an initial good response to angioplasty progressive renal dysfunction could occur in the absence of restenosis (Mikhail *et al.* 1997). La Batide-Alanore *et al.* (2001) examined individual kidney function in a group with unilateral RAS including both atherosclerotic and FMD patients. These patients had relatively good renal function overall with a plasma creatinine of 96 μmol/l in the atherosclerotic group. They found an improvement in the kidney with RAS after angioplasty in both groups. Interestingly there was a mild decrement in renal function in the kidneys with normal renal arteries. However, in a series of 16 patients with angioplasty for renal dysfunction there was no overall improvement in individual kidney function. The pattern of response did not differ between those kidneys that had angioplasty or normal renal arteries. The difficulties in interpreting these data are that improvement in renal function is not important in those patients with good renal function. The Baboolal *et al.* (1998) data showed that the risk of renal impairment therapy was in those patients with relatively poor renal function.

Radermacher *et al.* (2001) have shown that the response to angioplasty can be predicted by the resistive index as measured by Doppler ultrasound in the cortex. Those patients with kidneys with a high resistive index had a higher rate of dialysis treatment and lower rate of improvement in renal function. The best predictor of improvement in renal function was the resistive index. However, in this series the best improvement in renal function was in those patients with the best renal function and thus those with the lowest possibility of renal replacement therapy.

All of these studies are hampered by the fact that there is no established relationship between renal artery narrowing and renal function in either the experimental or clinical setting. Unless renal artery occlusion has occurred the effect of RAS on renal function is unclear. At present trials are underway to assess the efficacy of intervention in ARAS.

Proteinuria, RAS, and intervention

Proteinuria has been regarded as a marker of glomerular disease whether this is an intrinsic glomerulonephritis or secondary to a systemic illness such as diabetes mellitus. There are a number of case reports where either treatment of RAS or nephrectomy of a kidney with renal artery narrowing has produced a cure for the nephrotic syndrome; Table 6. Bhowick *et al.* (1998) have reported case where the patient had unilateral renal artery obstruction but biopsy of the contralateral kidney had focal segmental glomerulosclerosis. Martinez Vea *et al.* (1987) reported as case of unilateral disease where ACEI resulted in a reduction in proteinuria from 16.2 g/day. This was followed by a reduction to only 1.9 g/day after nephrectomy. Montoliu *et al.* (1979) reported a patient whose 31 g/day proteinuria was reduced to less than 0.1 g/day after nephrectomy of the left kidney that had renal artery occlusion. Holman *et al.* (1990) have shown that ACEI can bring resolution of the proteinuria associated with left renal artery occlusion. More recently, Thadani *et al.* (1996) have suggested that in focal–segmental glomerulosclerosis over the age of 55 years, one-third of patients will have renovascular disease as the cause. One analysis has suggested that below a Cockroft and Gault calculated glomerular filtration rate of 25 ml/min proteinuria of greater than 0.5 per 24 h is universal (Makanjuola *et al.* 1999). The degree of proteinuria does not correlate with the proteinuria. The situation has now changed to one where proteinuria is expected in renovascular disease rather than a cause to seek another diagnosis. This is an important concept in maturity onset diabetes mellitus as proteinuria might be expected as a consequence of the diabetes but also there is a significant incidence of renovascular disease. It is also important, given the desire to reduce proteinuria with ACEI in these patients.

Drug therapy

There are no data on drug therapy in atherosclerotic renovascular disease. Many of the trials of ACEI in renal disease have specifically excluded either ARAS or significant renal impairment. In some series, there have been strict criteria for recruitment in terms of renal function. In others, although the terms of recruitment were liberal, the actual patients recruited had relatively good renal function. It seems logical that good blood pressure control as in other presentations of atherosclerotic disease is important in long-term outcome. ACEI or AII would appear to be useful agents in the treatment of renin driven hypertension and proteinuria. However, earlier reports have indicated the importance of ACEI in acute renal insufficiency in patients with atherosclerotic renovascular disease (Hricik *et al.* 1983). This study showed that in atherosclerotic renovascular disease with severe renal artery narrowing the introduction of an ACEI resulted in worsening of renal function. It is thought that this effect is reversible but some animal experimental data has cast doubt on this. In a small number of cases ACEI with other factors has been associated with renal artery thrombosis (Pontremoli *et al.* 1990). These cases appear to involve the additional use of diuretics. Some experimental models have suggested that ACEI plus renal artery narrowing can lead to progressive renal atrophy (Jackson *et al.* 1990). However, these results have not been universal.

A more novel approach has been suggested. Given the proven beneficial effects of ACEI angioplasty could be considered as a method of facilitating the introduction of ACEI or AII blockers (Goldsmith *et al.* 2000). The paradox to address in patients with ARAS is that without this condition ACEI would give a beneficial effect on long-term mortality but in the presence of ARAS it may give a short-term worsening of renal function that may not be reversible.

The role of statins as the most powerful of lipid lowering agents is unclear. In atheroembolic disease anecdotal reports have been given of their efficacy (Cabili *et al.* 1993; Woolfson *et al.* 1998). This is discussed

Table 6 Proteinuria and RAS

Author(s)	Number of patients	Comments	Nephrotic range (>3 g/24 h)	Mean proteinuria (g/24 h)
RAS				
Montoliu *et al.* (1979)	1	Normal renal biopsy in unaffected kidney, cured by nephrectomy	1	13–31
Kumar and Shapiro (1980)	3	Proteinuria cured by nephrectomy 2, aorto-renal graft 1	2	1.4–12.5
Takeda *et al.* (1980)	1	Improved with captopril	1	
Eiser *et al.* (1982)	1	Nephrectomy cured hypertension and proteinuria	1	3.4–3.6
Adams *et al.* (1984)	83	'Abnormal urinalysis' in 36% with worse response to intervention		
Martinez Vea *et al.* (1987)	1	Cured by nephrectomy, reduced by captopril	1	16.2
Sato *et al.* (1989)	1	Normal biopsy in unaffected kidney, cured by vein bypass to one kidney	1	4–7
Holman *et al.* (1990)	1	Left renal artery occlusion, proteinuria cured by enalapril	1	6.9
Docci *et al.* (1992)	1	Proteinuria cured by enalapril	1	4.5
Chen *et al.* (1995)	1	Proteinuria cured by nephrectomy	1	11.6
Thadhani *et al.* (1996)	8	Associated with FSGS, 24 hour protein in only 7/8 patients	6	4.4
Alkhunaizi and Chapman (1997)	1	FSGS in contralateral kidney but normal glomeruli in stenosed kidney. Cured by aortorenal bypass	1	11
Mikhail *et al.* (1997)	3	Patients with progressive dysfunction after angioplasty	0	0.7
Harden *et al.* (1997)	32	RAS prior to stent insertion	0	0.95
Makanjuola *et al.* (1999)	94	Proven RAS		
		GFR < 10 ml/min		1.95
		GFR 10–25 ml/min		1.4
		GFR 25–50 ml/min		0.6
		GFR > 50 ml/min		0.4
Bhowick *et al.* (1998)	1	Unilateral RAS with contralateral FSGS	1	6
Johnston and Alkhunaizi (1999)	1	Unilateral RAS with contralateral FSGS	1	11
Atheroembolic disease				
Greendyke and Akamatsu (1960)	3	1–3 plus protein in the patients		
Snyder and Shapiro (1961)	1	2–3 plus protein on Dipstix testing		
Moldveen-Geronimus and Merriam (1967)	2	1–3 plus protein		
Harrington *et al.* (1968)	2	1–3 plus protein		
Dalakos *et al.* (1974)	1	0.9 gm/l, no total given		
Regester (1979)	1			1.8
Varanasi *et al.* (1979)	1			0.3
Smith *et al.* (1981)	4	1 plus protein in 2/4		
Cosio *et al.* (1985)	7	1–2 plus protein in 4/7		
Hannedouche *et al.* (1986)	1	Necrotizing glomerulonephritis		2
Schwartz and McDonald (1987)	2	2 plus protein in 1/2		
Hyman *et al.* (1987)	1	2 plus protein		
Fine *et al.* (1987)	63	54% (34) had >1 plus proteinuria (review)	3	
Aujla *et al.* (1989)	1	Renal transplant proteinuria		2
Mannesse *et al.* (1991)	4		2	3.95
Case Records New England Journal of Medicine (1991)	1		1	3.5

Table 6 Continued

Author(s)	Number of patients	Comments	Nephrotic range (>3 g/24 h)	Mean proteinuria (g/24 h)
Wilson *et al.* (1991)	9	1–3 plus in 7/9		
Bendixen *et al.* (1992)	1	2 plus protein		
Sheehan *et al.* (1993)	1	2 plus protein		
Blakely *et al.* (1994)	1	Nephritic urinary sediment		1.1
Thadhani *et al.* (1995)	52	63% had >1 plus urine protein	2	
Haqqie *et al.* (1996)	4		4	8.3
Case Records New England Journal of Medicine (1996)	1		1	3.1
Greenberg *et al.* (1997)	24	FSGS in 15 patients	9	

in greater detail in Chapter 10.6.5. The AVERT study (Pitt *et al.* 1999) has suggested, in a similar vascular situation of stable artery narrowing but in a cardiac context, that aggressive lipid lowering was more effective than angioplasty and conventional lipid lowering. A trial of the effects of lipid lowering in ARAS has not been performed and it is unlikely to be done. Most patients with ARAS have a host of indications for lipid lowering including the enormous mortality rate already described. It is interesting that in patients with proven RAS the significant difference was a low value for high density lipoprotein rather than total cholesterol (Scoble *et al.* 1999). It is important to note that many of the early studies on progression of renal dysfunction and renal artery narrowing were performed in an era without major statin use. Recent results with single kidney glomerular filtration estimations in kidneys with RAS do not have a worse rate of decline than those kidneys without renal artery narrowing.

Aspirin use would appear beneficial although there are no data to confirm this in this group of patients.

Conclusion

RAS does have an effect on renal blood flow. The effect on renal function, however, seems to relate both to the renal artery narrowing and the cause of the renal artery narrowing. In terms of improvement in renal function it is at present unclear whether intervention will produce a beneficial effect. This is not to omit the obvious benefit to hypertension of intervention in FMD. In specific diseases causing RAS such as Takayasu's arteritis and atherosclerosis, treatment of the underlying disease is vitally important. However, it is also very clear that a very large proportion of the elderly population undergoing dialysis treatment have renal dysfunction as a result of atherosclerotic vascular disease.

References

Adams, M. B., Harris, S. S., Kauffman, H. M., and Towne, J. B. (1984). Effect of primary renal disease in patients with renovascular insufficiency. *Journal of Vascular Surgery* **1**, 482–486.

Alkhunaizi, A. M. and Chapman, A. (1997). Renal artery stenosis and unilateral focal and segmental glomerulosclerosis. *American Journal of Kidney Diseases* **29**, 936–941.

Andreoni, K. A. *et al.* (2002). Incidence of donor renal fibromuscular dysplasia: does it justify routine angiography? *Transplantation* **73**, 1112–1116.

Appel, R. G., Bleyer, A. J., Reavis, S., and Hansen, K. J. (1995). Renovascular disease in older patients beginning renal replacement therapy. *Kidney International* **48**, 171–176.

Arend, W. P. *et al.* (1990). The American College of Rheumatology 1990 criteria for the classification of Takayasu arteritis. *Arthritis and Rheumatism* **33**, 1129–1134.

Aujla, N. D., Greenberg, A., Banner, B. F., Johnston, J. R., and Tzakis, A. G. (1989). Atheroembolic involvement of renal allografts. *American Journal of Kidney Diseases* **13**, 329–332.

Baboolal, K., Evans, C., and Moore, R. H. (1998). Incidence of end-stage renal disease in medically treated patients with severe bilateral atherosclerotic renovascular disease. *American Journal of Kidney Diseases* **31**, 971–977.

Bendixen, B. H. *et al.* (1992). Cholesterol emboli neuropathy. *Neurology* **42**, 428–430.

Beutler, J. J. *et al.* (2001). Long-term effects of arterial stenting on kidney function for patients with ostial atherosclerotic renal artery stenosis and renal insufficiency. *Journal of the American Society of Nephrology* **12**, 1475–1481.

Bhowick, D., Dash, S. C., Jain, D., Agatwal, S. K., Tiwari, S. C., and Dinda, A. K. (1998). Renal artery stenosis and focal segmental glomerulosclerosis in the contralateral kidney. *Nephrology, Dialysis, Transplantation* **13**, 1562–1564.

Birrer, M., Do, D. D., Mahler, F., Triller, J., and Baumgartner, I. (2002). Treatment of renal artery fibromuscular dysplasia with balloon angioplasty: a prospective follow-up study. *European Journal of Vascular and Endovascular Surgery* **23**, 146–152.

Blakely, P., Cosby, R. L., and McDonald, B. R. (1994). Nephritic urinary sediment in embolic renal disease. *Clinical Nephrology* **42**, 401–403.

Bloch, M. J., Trost, D. W., Pickering, T. G., Sos, T. A., and August, P. (1999). Prevention of recurrent pulmonary edema in patients with bilateral renovascular disease through renal artery stent placement. *American Journal of Hypertension* **12**, 1–7.

Blum, U. *et al.* (1997). Treatment of ostial renal-artery stenoses with vascular endoprotheses after unsuccessful balloon angioplasty. *New England Journal of Medicine* **336**, 459–465.

Bofinger, A., Fawley, C., Daunt, N., Stowasser, M., and Gordon, R. (2000). Alpha-1-antitrypsin phenotypes in patients with renal arterial fibromuscular dysplasia. *Journal of Human Hypertension* **14**, 91–94.

Bofinger, A. M., Hawley, C. M., Fisher, P. M., Daunt, N., Stowasser, M., and Gordon, R. D. (1999). Increased severity of multifocal renal arterial fibromuscular dysplasia in smokers. *Journal of Human Hypertension* **13**, 517–520.

Burket, M. W. *et al.* (2000). Renal artery angioplasty and stent placement: predictors of a favourable outcome. *American Heart Journal* **139**, 64–71.

Bush, R. L. *et al.* (2001). Endovascular revascularization of renal artery stenosis: technical and clinical results. *Journal of Vascular Surgery* **33**, 1041–1049.

Cabili, S., Hochman, I., and Goor, Y. (1993). Reversal of gangrenous lesions in the blue toe syndrome with lovastatin. *Angiology* **44**, 821–825.

Caps, M. T. *et al.* (1998a). Risk of atrophy in kidneys with atherosclerotic renal artery stenosis. *Kidney International* **53**, 735–742.

Caps, M. D. *et al.* (1998b). Prospective study of atherosclerotic disease progression in the renal artery. *Circulation* **98**, 2866–2872.

Carmichael, D. J. S., Mathias, C. J., Snell, M. E., and Peart, S. (1986). Detection and investigation of renal artery stenosis. *Lancet* **1**, 667–670.

Case Records Case 2-1991 (1991). *New England Journal of Medicine* **324**, 113–120.

Case Records Case 11-1996 (1996). *New England Journal of Medicine* **334**, 973–979.

Chen, R., Novick, A. C., and Pohl, M. (1995). Reversible renin mediated massive proteinuria successfully treated by nephrectomy. *Journal of Urology* **153**, 133–134.

Cheung, C. M. *et al.* (2002). Epidemiology and renal dysfunction and patient outcome in atherosclerotic renal artery occlusion. *Journal of the American Society of Nephrology* **13**, 149–157.

Choudhri, A. H., Cleland, J. G. F., Rowlands, P. C., Tran, T. L., McCarthy, M., and Al-Kutoubi, M. A. (1990). Unsuspected renal artery stenosis in peripheral vascular disease. *British Medical Journal* **301**, 1197–1198.

Cloft, H. J., Kallmes, D. F., Kallmes, M. H., Goldstein, J. H., Jensen, M. E., and Dion, J. E. (1998). Prevalence of cerebral aneurysms in patients with fibromuscular dysplasia: a reassessment. *Journal of Neurosurgery* **88**, 436–440.

Conlon, P. J. *et al.* (1998). Survival in renal vascular disease. *Journal of the American Society of Nephrology* **9**, 252–256.

Connolly, J. O. *et al.* (1994). Presentation, clinical features and outcome in different patterns of atherosclerotic renovascular disease. *Quarterly Journal of Medicine* **87**, 413–421.

Cosio, F. G., Zager, R. A., and Sharma, H. M. (1985). Atheroembolic disease causes hypocomplementaemia. *Lancet* **2**, 118–121.

Cragg, A. H. *et al.* (1989). Incidental fibromuscular dysplasia in potential renal donors: long term follow-up. *Radiology* **172**, 145–147.

Criqui, M. H. *et al.* (1992). Mortality over a period of 10 years in patients with peripheral arterial disease. *New England Journal of Medicine* **326**, 381–386.

Crowley, J. J. *et al.* (1998). Progression of renal artery stenosis in patients undergoing cardiac catheterization. *American Heart Journal* **136**, 913–918.

Daina, E., Shieppati, A., and Remuzzi, G. (1999). Mycophenolate mofetil for the treament of Takayasu arteritis: report of three cases. *Annals of Internal Medicine* **130**, 422–426.

Dalakos, T. G., Streeten, D. H. P., Jones, D., and Obeid, A. (1974). 'Malignant' hypertension resulting from atheromatous embolization predominantly of one kidney. *American Journal of Medicine* **57**, 135–138.

Deal, J. E., Snell, T. M., Barratt, T. M., and Dillon, M. J. (1992). Renovascular disease in childhood. *Journal of Pediatrics* **121**, 378–384.

Dejani, H., Eisen, T. D., and Finkelstein, F. O. (2000). Revascularization of renal artery stenosis in patients with renal insufficiency. *American Journal of Kidney Diseases* **36**, 752–758.

Deutsch, V., Wexler, L., and Deutsch, H. (1974). Takayasu's arteritis: an angiographic study with remarks on ethnic distribution in Israel. *American Journal of Roentgenology* **122**, 13–28.

Docci, D., Moscatelli, G., Capponcini, C., Baldrati, L., and Feletti, C. (1992). Nephrotic-range proteinuria in a patient with high renin hypertension: effect of treatment with an ACE-inhibitor. *American Journal of Nephrology* **12**, 387–389.

Dorros, G. *et al.* (1998). Four-year follow-up of Palmaz–Schatz stent revascularization as treatment for atherosclerotic renal artery stenosis. *Circulation* **98**, 642–647.

Ducloux, D., Jamali, M., and Chapolin, J. M. (1997). Chronic congestive heart failure associated with bilateral renal artery stenosis. *Clinical Nephrology* **48**, 54–55.

Dustan, H. P., Humphries, A. W., De Wolf, V. G., and Page, I. H. (1964). Normal arterial pressure in patients with renal arterial stenosis. *Journal of American Medical Association* **187**, 1028–1029.

Eiser, A. R., Katz, S. M., and Swartz, C. (1982). Reversible nephrotic range proteinuria with renal artery stenosis: a clinical example of renin-associated proteinuria. *Nephron* **30**, 374–377.

Farmer, C. K. T., Cook, G. J. R., Blake, G. M., Reidy, J., and Scoble, J. E. (1999b). Individual kidney function in atherosclerotic nephropathy is not related to the presence of renal artery stenosis. *Nephrology, Dialysis, Transplantation* **14**, 2880–2884.

Farmer, C. K. T., Reidy, J., Kalra, P. A., Cook, G. J. R., and Scoble, J. (1998). Individual kidney function before and after renal angioplasty. *Lancet* **352**, 288–289.

Farmer, C. K. T., Reidy, J., and Scoble, J. E. (1999a). Flash pulmonary oedema in a patient 24 years after aorto-renal vein graft. *Nephrology, Dialysis, Transplantation* **14**, 1310–1312.

Fatica, R. A., Port, F. K., and Young, E. W. (2001). Incidence trends and mortality in end-stage renal disease attributed to renovascular disease in the United States. *American Journal of Kidney Diseases* **37**, 1184–1190.

Fine, M., Kapoor, W., and Falanga, V. (1987). Cholesterol crystal embolization: a review of 221 cases in the English literature. *Angiology* **38**, 769–784.

Giordano, J. M. (2000). Surgical treatment of Takayasu's arteritis. *International Journal of Cardiology* **75**, S123–S128.

Gobe, G. C., Axelsen, R. A., and Searle, J. W. (1990). Cellular events in experimental unilateral ischemic renal atrophy and in regeneration after contralateral nephrectomy. *Laboratory Investigation* **63**, 770–779.

Goldblatt, H., Lynch, J., Hanzal, R. F., and Summerville, W. W. (1934). The production of persistent elevation of systolic blood pressure by means of renal ischemia. *Journal of Experimental Medicine* **59**, 347–378.

Goldsmith, D., Reidy, J., and Scoble, J. (2000). Renal arterial intervention and angiotensin blockade in atherosclerotic nephropathy. *American Journal of Kidney Diseases* **36**, 837–843.

Goncharenko, V., Gerlock, A. J., Shaff, M. I., and Hollifield, J. W. (1981). Progression of renal artery fibromuscular dysplasia in 42 patients as seen on angiography. *Radiology* **139**, 45–51.

Greenberg, A., Bastacky, S. I., Iqbal, A., Borochovitz, D., and Johnson, J. P. (1997). Focal segmental glomerulosclerosis associated with nephrotic syndrome in cholesterol atheroembolism: clinicopathological correlations. *American Journal of Kidney Diseases* **29**, 334–344.

Greendyke, R. M. and Akamatsu, Y. (1960). Atheromatous embolism as a cause of renal failure. *Journal of Urology* **83**, 231–237.

Grone, H. J., Warnecke, E., and Olbricht, C. J. (1996). Characteristics of renal tubular atrophy in experimental renovascular hypertension: a model of kidney hibernation. *Nephron* **72**, 243–252.

Hannedouche, T. *et al.* (1986). Necrotizing glomerulonephritis and renal cholesterol embolization. *Nephron* **42**, 271–272.

Hansen, K. J. *et al.* (1995). Surgical management of dialysis-dependent ischemic nephropathy. *Journal of Vascular Surgery* **21**, 197–211.

Haqqie, S. S., Urizar, R. E., and Singh, J. (1996). Nephrotic-range proteinuria in renal atheroembolic disease: report of four cases. *American Journal of Kidney Diseases* **4**, 493–501.

Harden, P. N. *et al.* (1997). Effect of renal-artery stenting on progression of renovascular renal failure. *Lancet* **349**, 1133–1136.

Harding, M. B. *et al.* (1992). Renal artery stenosis: prevalence and associated risks factors in patients undergoing routine cardiac catheterization. *Journal of the American Society of Nephrology* **2**, 1608–1616.

Harker, C. P., Steed, M., Althaus, S. J., and Coldwell, D. (1995). Flash pulmonary edema; an acute and unusual complication of renal angioplasty. *Journal of Vascular and Interventional Radiology* **6**, 130–132.

Harrington, J. T., Sommers, S. C., and Kassirer, J. P. (1968). Atheromatous emboli with progressive renal failure. *Annals of Internal Medicine* **68**, 152–160.

Heffelfinger, M. J., Holley, K. E., Harrison, E. G., and Hunt, J. C. (1970). Arterial fibromuscular dysplasia studied at autopsy. *American Journal of Clinical Pathology* **54**, 274.

Hnas, S. S. and Zeskind, H. J. (1995). Routine use of limited abdominal aortography subtraction carotid and cerebral angiography. *Stroke* **26**, 1221–1224.

Holley, K. E., Hunt, J. C., Brown, A. L., Kincaid, O. W., and Sheps, S. G. (1964). Renal artery stenosis: a clinical–pathological study in normotensive and hypertensive patients. *American Journal of Medicine* **37**, 14–22.

Holman, N. D., Donker, A. J. M., and van der Meer, J. (1990). Disappearance of renin-induced proteinuria by an ACEI-inhibitor. *Clinical Nephrology* **34**, 70–71.

Hricik, D. E., Browning, P. J., Kopelman, R., Goorno, W. E., Madias, N. E., and Dzau, V. J. (1983). Captopril-induced functional renal insufficiency in patients with bilateral renal-artery stenoses or renal-artery stenosis in a solitary kidney. *New England Journal of Medicine* **308**, 373–376.

Hyman, B. T., Landas, S. K., Ashman, R. F., Schelper, R. L., and Robinson, R. A. (1987). Warfarin-related purple toes syndrome and cholesterol microembolization. *American Journal of Medicine* **82**, 1233–1237.

Iglesias, J. I., Hamburger, R. J., Feldamn, L., and Kaufman, J. S. (2000). The natural history of incidental renal artery stenosis in patients with aortoiliac vascular disease. *American Journal of Medicine* **109**, 642–647.

Ishikawa, K. (1981). Survival and morbidity after diagnosis of occlusive thromboaortopathy (Takayasu' disease). *American Journal of Cardiology* **47**, 1026–1032.

Ishikawa, K. (1991). Effects of Prednisolone therapy on arterial angiographic features in Takayasu's disease. *American Journal of Cardiology* **68**, 410–413.

Jackson, B., Franze, L., Sumithran, E., and Johnston, C. I. (1990). Pharmacological nephrectomy with chronic angiotensin converting enzyme inhibitor treatment in renovascular hypertension in the rat. *Journal of Laboratory and Clinical Medicine* **115**, 21–27.

Jain, S., Kumari, S., Ganguly, N. K., and Sharma, B. K. (1996). Current status of Takayasu arteritis in India. *International Journal of Cardiology* **54**, S95–S100.

Jean, W. J., Al-Bitar, I., Zwicke, D. L., Port, S. C., Schmidt, D. H., and Bajwa, T. K. (1994). High incidence of renal artery stenosis in patients with coronary artery disease. *Catheterization and Cardiovascular Diagnosis* **32**, 8–10.

Jensen, G., Zachrisson, B. F., Delin, K., Volkmann, R., and Aurell, M. (1995). Treatment of renovascular hypertension: one year results of renal angioplasty. *Kidney International* **48**, 1936–1945.

Johnston, R. J. and Alkhunaizi, A. M. (1999). Unilateral focal segmental glomerulosclerosis with contralateral sparing on the side of renal artery stenosis. *American Journal of Roentgenology* **172**, 35–37.

Kalra, P. S., Mamtora, H., Holmes, A. M., and Waldek, S. (1990). Renovascular disease and renal complications of angiotensin-converting enzyme inhibitor therapy. *Quarterly Journal of Medicine* **282**, 1013.

Kaylor, W. M., Novick, A. C., Ziegelbaum, M., and Vidt, D. G. (1989). Reversal of end stage renal failure with surgical revascularization in patients with atherosclerotic renal artery occlusion. *Journal of Urology* **141**, 486–488.

Kerr, G. S. *et al.* (1994). Takayasu arteritis. *Annals of Internal Medicine* **120**, 919–929.

Khan, I. H., Catto, G. R. D., Edward, N., and MacLoed, A. M. (1995). Death during the first 90 days of dialysis: a case control study. *American Journal of Kidney Diseases* **25**, 276–280.

Khong, T. K., Missouris, C. G., Belli, A. M., and MacGregor, G. A. (2001). Regression of atherosclerotic renal artery stenosis with aggressive lipid lowering therapy. *Journal of Human Hypertension* **15**, 431–433.

Kimura, A., Kitamura, H., Date, Y., and Numano, F. (1996). Comprehensive analysis of HLA genes in Takayasu arteritis in Japan. *International Journal of Cardiology* **54**, S65–S73.

Kincaid, O. W., Davis, G. D., Hallerman, F. J., and Hunt, J. C. (1968). Fibromuscular dysplasia of the renal arteries. *American Journal of Roentgenology* **104**, 271–282.

Koide, K. (1992). Takayasu arteritis in Japan. *Heart Vessels* **7**, S48–S54.

Kumar, A. and Shapiro, A. P. (1980). Proteinuria and nephrotic syndrome induced by renin in patients with renal artery stenosis. *Archives of Internal Medicine* **140**, 1631–1634.

Kuroda, S. *et al.* (2000). Prevalence of renal artery stenosis in autopsy patients with stroke. *Stroke* **31**, 61–65.

Kvist, S. and Mulvany, M. J. (2001). Reduced medication and normalization of vascular structure, but continued hypertension in renovascular patients after revascularization. *Cardiovascular Research* **52**, 136–142.

Kwan, T., Feit, A., Alam, M., Mandawat, M. K., and Clark, L. T. (1997). Pulsus alternans in diastolic left ventricular dysfunction. *Angiology* **48**, 1079–1085.

La Batide-Alanore, A., Azizi, M., Froissart, M., Raynaud, A., and Plouin, P. F. (2001). Split renal function outcome after renal angioplasty in patients with unilateral renal artery stenosis. *Journal of the American Society of Nephrology* **12**, 1235–1241.

Lawrie, G. M., Morris, G. C., Glaeser, D. H., and de Bakey, M. E. (1989). Renovascular reconstruction; factors affecting long term prognosis in 919 patients followed up to 31 years. *American Journal of Cardiology* **63**, 1085–1092.

Lederman, R. J., Mendelsohn, F. O., Santos, R., Phillips, H. R., Stack, R. S., and Crowley, J. J. (2001). Primary renal artery stenting: characteristics and outcomes after 363 procedures. *American Heart Journal* **142**, 314–323.

Louie, J., Isaacson, J. A., Zierler, R. G., Bergelin, R. O., and Strandness, D. E. (1994). Prevalence of carotid and lower extremity arterial disease in patients with renal artery stenosis. *American Journal of Hypertension* **7**, 436–439.

Lye, W. C., Leong, S. O., and Lee, E. J. C. (1996). Transplant renal artery stenosis presenting with recurrent acute pulmonary oedema. *Nephron* **72**, 302–304.

MacDowall, P., Kalra, P. A., O'Donoghue, D. J., Waldeck, S., Mamotora, H., and Brown, K. (1998). Risk of morbidity from renovascular disease in elderly patients with congestive cardiac failure. *Lancet* **352**, 13–16.

Mailloux, L. U., Napolitano, B., Belluci, A. G., Vernace, M., Wilkes, B. M., and Mossey, R. T. (1994a). Renal vascular disease causing end-stage renal disease, incidence, clinical correlates and outcomes: a 20-year clinical experience. *American Journal of Kidney Diseases* **24**, 622–629.

Mailloux, L. U., Belluci, A. G., Napolitano, B., Mossey, T., Wilkes, B. M., and Bluestone, P. A. (1994b). Survival estimates for 683 patients starting dialysis from 1970 through 1989: identification of risk factors for survival. *Clinical Nephrology* **42**, 127–135.

Mailloux, L. U., Napolitano, B., Bellucci, A. G., Mossey, R. T., Vernace, M. A., and Wilkes, B. M. Renal vascular end-stage disease. In *Renal Vascular Disease* (ed. A. Novick, J. Scoble, and G. Hamilton), pp. 315–321. London: W.B. Saunders, 1995.

Mailloux, L. U. *et al.* (1988). Predictors of survival in patients undergoing dialysis. *American Journal of Medicine* **84**, 855–862.

Makanjuola, A. D., Suresh, M., Laboi, P., Kalra, P. A., and Scoble, J. E. (1999). Proteinuria in atherosclerotic renovascular disease. *Quarterly Journal of Medicine* **92**, 515–518.

Mannesse, C. K., Blankestijn, P. J., Veld, A. J. M., and Schalekamp, M. A. D. H. (1991). Renal failure and cholesterol crystal embolization. *Clinical Nephrology* **36**, 240–245.

Mansy, H., Al-Harbi, A., El-Sherif, M., Al-Shareef, Z., and Shlash, S. (1996). Recurrent acute pulmonary edema as a presentation of renal artery stenosis in a renal transplant patient. *Clinical Nephrology* **46**, 216–217.

Marcussen, N. (1991). Atubular glomeruli in renal artery stenosis. *Laboratory Investigation* **65**, 558–565.

Martinez Vea, A., Garcia Ruiz, C., Carrera, M., Oliver, J. A., and Ricjart, C. (1987). Effect of Captopril in nephrotic-range proteinuria due to renovascular hypertension. *Nephron* **45**, 162–163.

Masterson, R., Scoble, J., Taylor, P., and Cook, G. (2000). Recovery of renal function following prolonged ischaemia in a patient with mid-aortic syndrome. *Nephrology, Dialysis, Transplantation* **15**, 1461–1463.

Maxwell, M. H., Bleifer, K. H., Franklin, S. S., and Varady, P. D. (1972). Cooperative study of renovascular hypertension: demographic analysis of study. *Journal of American Medical Association* **220**, 1195–1204.

May, A. G., De Weese, J. A., and Rob, C. G. (1963). Hemodynamic effects of arterial stenosis. *Surgery* **53**, 513–524.

Meaney, T. F., Dustan, H. P., and McCormack, L. J. (1968). Natural history of renal arterial disease. *Radiology* **91**, 881–887.

Metcalfe, W., Reid, A., and Geddes, C. G. (1999). Prevalence of angiographic atherosclerotic renal artery disease and its relationship to the anatomical extent of peripheral vascular disease. *Nephrology, Dialysis, Transplantation* **14**, 105–108.

Meyrier, A., Buchet, P., Simon, P., Fernet, M., Rainfray, M., and Callard, P. (1988). Atheromatous renal disease. *American Journal of Medicine* **85**, 139–146.

Mikhail, A., Cook, G. J. R., Reidy, J., and Scoble, J. E. (1997). Progressive renal dysfunction despite successful renal artery angioplasty in a single kidney. *Lancet* **349**, 926.

Missouris, C. G., Buckenham, T., Cappucio, F. P., and MacGregor, G. A. (1994). Renal artery stenosis: a common and important problem in patients with peripheral vascular disease. *American Journal of Medicine* **96**, 10–14.

Missouris, C. G., Buckenham, T., Vallance, P. J. T., and MacGregor, G. A. (1993). Renal artery stenosis masquerading as congestive heart failure. *Lancet* **341**, 1521–1522.

Missouris, C. G. *et al.* (1998). High prevalence of carotid artery disease in patients with atheromatous renal artery stenosis. *Nephrology, Dialysis, Transplantation* **13**, 945–948.

Moldveen-Geronimus, M. and Merriam, J. C. (1967). Cholesterol embolization. *Circulation* **35**, 946–953.

Montoliu, J., Botey, A., Torras, A., Darnell, A., and Revert, L. (1979). Renin-induced massive proteinuria in man. *Clinical Nephrology* **11**, 267–271.

Moriwaki, R., Node, M., Yajima, M., Sharma, B. K., and Numano, F. (1997). Clinical manifestations of Takayasu arteritis in India and Japan—new classification of angiographic findings. *Angiology* **48**, 369–379.

Muray, S. *et al.* (2002). Rapid decline in renal function reflects reversibility and predicts the outcome after angioplasty in renal artery stenosis. *American Journal of Kidney Diseases* **39**, 2002.

Nahman, N. S. *et al.* (1994). Renal artery pressure gradients in patients with angiographic evidence of atherosclerotic renal artery stenosis. *American Journal of Kidney Diseases* **24**, 695–699.

Neymark, E. *et al.* (2000). Arteriographic detection of renovascular disease in potential donors: incidence and effect on donor surgery. *Radiology* **214**, 755–760.

Numano, F. and Tsunekazu, K. (1996). Takayasu arteritis—five doctors in the history of Takayasu arteritis. *International Journal of Cardiology* **54**, S1–S10.

Numano, F., Okawara, M., Inomata, H., and Kobayashi, Y. (2000). Takayasu's arteritis. *Lancet* **356**, 1023–1025.

Olin, J. W., Melia, M., Young, J. R., Graor, R. A., and Risius, B. (1990). Prevalence of atherosclerotic renal artery stenosis in patients with atherosclerosis elsewhere. *American Journal of Medicine* **88**, 1-46N–1-51N.

O'Neil, E. A., Hansen, K. J., Canzanello, V. J., Pennell, T. C., and Dean, R. H. (1992). Prevalence of ischemic nephropathy in patients with renal insufficiency. *The American Surgeon* **58**, 485–490.

Palubinskas, A. J. and Ripley, H. R. (1964). Fibromuscular dysplasia in extrarenal arteries. *Radiology* **82**, 451–455.

Panayiotopoulos, Y. P., Tyrell, M. R., Koffman, G., Reidy, J. F., Haycock, G. B., and Taylor, P. R. (1996). Mid-aortic syndrome presenting in childhood. *British Journal of Surgery* **83**, 235–240.

Panier-Moreau, I. *et al.* (1997). Possible familial origin of multifocal renal artery fibromuscular dysplasia. *Journal of Hypertension* **15**, 1797–1801.

Park, J. H. (1996). Conventional and CT angiographic diagnosis of Takayasu arteritis. *International Journal of Cardiology* **54**, S135–S141.

Pattison, J. M. *et al.* (1992). Percutaneous transluminal renal angioplasty in patients with renal failure. *Quarterly Journal of Medicine* **85**, 883–888.

Paty, P. S. K. *et al.* (2001). Is prosthetic renal artery reconstruction a durable procedure? An analysis of 489 grafts. *Journal of Vascular Surgery* **34**, 127–132.

PDAY study (1993). Natural history of aortic and coronary atherosclerotic lesions in youth. *Arteriosclerosis and Thrombosis* **13**, 1291–1298.

Pickering, T. G. *et al.* (1988). Recurrent pulmonary oedema in hypertension due to bilateral renal artery stenosis: treatment by angioplasty or surgical intervention. *Lancet* **2**, 551–552.

Pitt, B. *et al.* (1999). Aggressive lipid-lowering therapy compared with angioplasty in stable coronary artery disease. *New England Journal of Medicine* **341**, 70–76.

Plouin, P. F., Chatellier, G., Darne, B., and Raynaud, A. (1998). Blood pressure outcome of angioplasty in atherosclerotic renal artery stenosis. *Hypertension* **31**, 823–829.

Pontremoli, R., Rampoldi, V., Morbidelli, A., Fiorini, F., Ranise, A., and Garibotto, G. (1990). Acute renal failure due to acute bilateral renal artery thrombosis: successful surgical revascularization after prolonged anuria. *Nephron* **56**, 322–324.

Rackson, M. E., Lossef, S. V., and Sos, T. A. (1990). Renal artery stenosis in patients with aortic dissection: increased prevalence. *Radiology* **177**, 555–558.

Radermacher, J. *et al.* (2001). Use of Doppler ultrasonography to predict the outcome of therapy for renal artery stenosis. *New England Journal of Medicine* **344**, 410–417.

Rahman, M. M., Varghese, Z., Fuller, B. J., and Moorhead, J. F. (1999). Scavengers of reactive oxygen species and L-arginine inhibit renal vasoconstriction induced by oxidized LDL. *Clinical Nephrology* **51**, 98–107.

Ramirez, G., Bugni, W., Farber, S. M., and Curry, A. J. (1987). Incidence of renal artery stenosis in a population having cardiac catheterization. *Southern Medical Journal* **80**, 734–737.

Regester, R. F. (1979). Renal failure secondary to spontaneous atheromatous microembolism. *Journal of the Tennessee Medical Association* 328–330.

Reiher, L., Pfeiffer, T., and Sandmann, W. (2000). Long-term after surgical reconstruction for renal artery fibromuscular dysplasia. *European Journal of Vascular and Endovascular Surgery* **20**, 556–559.

Rushton, A. R. (1980). The genetics of fibromuscular dysplasia. *Archives of Internal Medicine* **140**, 233–236.

Sang, C. N. *et al.* (1989). Etiological factors in renovascular fibromuscular dysplasia, a case–control study. *Hypertension* **14**, 472–479.

Sato, H., Saito, T., Kasai, Y., Abe, K., and Yoshinaga, K. (1989). Massive proteinuria due to renal artery stenosis. *Nephron* **51**, 136–137.

Sawicki, P. T., Kaiser, S., Heinemann, L., Frenzel, H., and Berger, M. (1991). Prevalence of renal artery stenosis in diabetes mellitus—an autopsy study. *Journal of Internal Medicine* **229**, 489–492.

Schievink, W. I., Meyer, F. B., Parisi, J. E., and Wijdicks, E. F. M. (1998). Fibromuscular dysplasia of the internal carotid artery associated with a1-antitrypsin deficiency. *Neurosurgery* **43**, 229–234.

Schoenberg, S. O. *et al.* (2002). Morphological and functional resonance imaging of renal artery stenosis: a multireader tricenter study. *Journal of the American Society of Nephrology* **13**, 158–169.

Schreiber, M. J., Pohl, M. A., and Novick, A. C. (1984). The natural history of atherosclerotic and fibrous renal artery disease. *Urological Clinics of North America* **11**, 383–392.

Schwartz, C. J. and White, T. A. (1964). Stenosis of renal artery: an unselected necropsy study. *British Medical Journal* **2**, 1415–1421.

Schwartz, M. W. and McDonald, G. B. (1987). Cholesterol embolization syndrome. *Journal of American Medical Association* **258**, 1934–1935.

Scoble, J. E. (1999). Atherosclerotic nephropathy. *Kidney International* **56**, S106–S109.

Scoble, J. E., Maher, E. R., Hamilton, G., Dick, R., Sweny, P., and Moorhead, J. F. (1989). Atherosclerotic renovascular disease causing renal impairment—a case for treatment. *Clinical Nephrology* **31**, 119–122.

Scoble, J. E., Sweny, P., Stansby, G., and Hamilton, G. (1993). Patients with atherosclerotic renovascular disease presenting to a renal unit: an audit of outcome. *Postgraduate Medical Journal* **69**, 461–465.

Scoble, J. E. *et al.* (1999). Lipid profiles in patients with atherosclerotic renal artery stenosis. *Nephron* **83**, 117–121.

Sen, P. K., Kinare, S. D., Engineer, S. D., and Parulkar, G. B. (1963). The middle aortic syndrome. *British Heart Journal* **25**, 610–618.

Sharam, S. *et al.* (1998). Results of renal angioplasty in non-specific aorto-arteritis (Takayasu disease). *Journal of Vascular and Interventional Radiology* **9**, 429–435.

Sharma, B. K. and Jain, S. (1998). A possible role of sex in determining distribution of lesions in Takayasu's arteritis. *International Journal of Cardiology* **66**, S81–S84.

Sharma, B. K., Jain, S., and Radotra, B. D. (1998). An autopsy study of Takayasu arteritis in India. *International Journal of Cardiology* **66**, S85–S90.

Sheehan, M. G., Condemi, J. J., and Rosenfeld, S. I. (1993). Position dependent livedo reticularis in cholesterol emboli syndrome. *Journal of Rheumatology* **20**, 1973–1974.

Smith, M. C., Ghose, M. K., and Henry, A. R. (1981). The clinical spectrum of renal cholesterol embolization. *American Journal of Medicine* **71**, 174–189.

Snyder, H. E. and Shapiro, J. L. (1961). A correlative study of atheromatous embolism in human beings and experimental animals. *Surgery* **49**, 195–204.

Stanley, J. C. Renal artery fibrodysplasia. In *Renal Vascular Disease* (ed. A. Novick, J. Scoble, and G. Hamilton), pp. 21–33. London: W.B. Saunders, 1995.

Sumboonnanonda, A., Robinson, B. L., Gedroyc, W. M., Saxton, H. M., Reidy, J. F., and Haycock, G. B. (1992). Middle aortic syndrome: clinical and radiological findings. *Archives of Diseases of Childhood* **67**, 501–505.

Suresh, M., Laboi, P., Mamtora, H., and Kalra, P. A. (2000). Relationship of renal dysfunction to proximal arterial disease severity in atherosclerotic renovascular disease. *Nephrology, Dialysis, Transplantation* **15**, 631–636.

Swartbol, P. (1992). Renal artery stenosis in patients with peripheral vascular disease and its correlation to hypertension. A retrospective study. *International Angiology* **11**, 195–199.

Takeda, R., Morimoto, S., Uchida, K., Kigoshi, T., Sumitani, T., and Matsubara, F. (1980). Effects of Captopril on both hypertension and proteinuria. *Archives of Internal Medicine* **140**, 1531–1533.

Tanigawa, K. *et al.* (1992). Magnetic resonance imaging detection of aortic and pulmonary artery wall thickening in the acute stage of Takayasu arteritis. Improvement of clinical and radiological findings after steroid therapy. *Arthritis and Rheumatism* **35**, 476–480.

Tegtmeyer, C. J., Matsumoto, A. H., and Angle, J. F. (1995). Percutaneous transluminal angioplasty in fibrous dysplasia and children. In *Renal Vascular Disease* (ed. A. Novick, J. Scoble, and G. Hamilton), pp. 363–383. London: W.B. Saunders, 1995.

Textor, S. C., Novick, A. C., Tazari, R. C., Klimas, V., Vidt, D. G., and Pohl, M. (1985). Critical perfusion pressure for renal function in patients with bilateral atherosclerotic renal vascular disease. *Annals of Internal Medicine* **102**, 308–312.

Thadhani, R., Pascual, M., Nickeleit, V., Tolkoff-Rubin, N., and Colvin, R. (1996). Preliminary description of focal segmental glomerulosclerosis in patients with renovascular disease. *Lancet* **347**, 231–233.

Thadhani, R. I., Camargo, C. A., Xavier, R. J., Fang, L. S. T., and Bazari, H. (1995). Atheroembolic renal failure after invasive procedures. *Medicine* **74**, 350–358.

Tollefson, D. F. J. and Ernst, C. B. (1991). Natural history of atherosclerotic renal artery stenosis associated with aortic disease. *Journal of Vascular Surgery* **14**, 327–331.

Toma, H. Takayasu's arteritis. In *Renal Vascular Disease* (ed. A. Novick, J. Scoble, and G. Hamilton), pp. 47–62. London: W.B. Saunders, 1995.

Truong, L. D., Farhood, A., Tasby, J., and Gillum, D. (1992). Experimental chronic renal ischemia: morphologic and immunologic studies. *Kidney International* **41**, 1676–1689.

Tyagi, S., Singh, B., Kaul, U. A., Seth, K. K., Arora, R., and Khalilullah, M. (1993). Balloon angioplasty for renovascular hypertension in Takayasu's arteritis. *American Heart Journal* **125**, 1386–1393.

Uzu, T. *et al.* (1997). Prevalence and predictors of renal artery stenosis in patients with myocardial infarction. *American Journal of Kidney Diseases* **29**, 733–738.

Valentine, R. J., Clagett, G. P., Miller, G. L., Myers, S. I., Martin, J. D., and Chervu, A. (1993). The coronary risk of unsuspected renal artery stenosis. *Journal of Vascular Surgery* **18**, 433–439.

van Jaarsveld, B. *et al.* (1998). The Dutch Renal Artery Stenosis Intervention Cooperative (DRASTIC) study: rationale, design and inclusion data. *Journal of Hypertension* **16**, S21–S27.

Varanasi, U. R., Moorthy, A. V., and Beirne, G. J. (1979). Spontaneous atheroembolic disease as a cause of renal failure in the elderly. *Journal of the American Geriatrics Society* **27**, 407–409.

Vidt, D. G., Eisele, G., Gephardt, G. N., Tubbs, R., and Novick, A. C. (1989). Atheroembolic renal disease: association with renal artery stenosis. *Cleveland Clinic Journal of Medicine* **56**, 407–413.

Volkman, D. J., Mann, D. L., and Fauci, A. S. (1982). Association between Takayasu's arteritis and B-cell alloantigen in North Americans. *New England Journal of Medicine* **306**, 464–465.

Wachtell, K., Ibsen, H., Olsen, M. H., Christoffersen, J. K., Norgaard, H., and Mantoni, M. (1996). Prevalence of renal artery stenosis in patients with peripheral vascular disease and hypertension. *Journal of Human Hypertension* **10**, 83–85.

Watson, P. S., Hadjipetrou, P., Cox, S. V., Piemonte, T. C., and Eisenhauer, A. C. (2000). Effect of renal artery stenting on renal function and size in patients with atherosclerotic renovascular disease. *Circulation* **102**, 1671–1677.

Weatherford, D. A., Freeman, M. A., Regester, R. F., Serrell, P. F., Stevens, S. L., and Goldman, M. H. (1997). Surgical management of flash pulmonary edema secondary to renovascular hypertension. *American Journal of Surgery* **174**, 160–163.

Webster, J. *et al.* (1998). Randomised comparison of percutaneous angioplasty vs continued medical therapy for hypertensive patients with renal artery stenosis. *Journal of Human Hypertension* **12**, 329–335.

Weibull, H., Bergqvist, D., Andersson, I., Choi, D. L., Jonsson, K., and Bergentz, S. E. (1990). Symptoms and signs of thrombotic occlusion of atherosclerotic renal artery stenosis. *European Journal of Vascular Surgery* **15**, 161–165.

Weibull, H., Bergqvist, D., Bergentz, S. E., Jonsson, K., Hulthen, L., and Manhem, P. (1993). Percutaneous transluminal renal angioplasty versus surgical reconstruction of atherosclerotic renal artery stenosis: a prospective randomized study. *Journal of Vascular Surgery* **18**, 841–852.

Wilms, G. and Marchal, G. (1990). The angiographic incidence of renal artery stenosis in the atherosclerotic population. *European Journal of Radiology* **10**, 195–197.

Wilson, D. M., Salazer, T. L., and Farkouh, M. E. (1991). Eosinophiluria in atheroembolic renal disease. *American Journal of Medicine* **91**, 186–189.

Woolfson, R. G. and Lachmann, H. (1998). Improvement in renal cholesterol emboli syndrome after simvastatin. *Lancet* **351**, 1331–1332.

Yeon, H. C. and Lee, W. R. (1998). Magnetic resonance imaging diagnosis of Takayasu arteritis. *International Journal of Cardiology* **66**, S175–S179.

Ying, C. Y., Tifft, C. P., Garvas, H., and Chobanian, A. V. (1984). Renal revascularisation in the azotemic hypertensive patient resistant to therapy. *New England Journal of Medicine* **311**, 1070–1075.

Zheng, D., Fan, D., and Lieu, L. (1992). Takayasu arteritis in China. A report of 530 cases. *Heart Vessels* **7**, S32–S36.

Zierler, R. *et al.* (1998). Carotid and lower extremity arterial disease in patients with renal artery atherosclerosis. *Archives of Internal Medicine* **158**, 761–767.

9.6 Hypertension and unilateral renal parenchymal disease

Michael Schömig and Ralf Dikow

Unilateral renoparenchymatous disease is a relatively rare cause of elevated blood pressure and is found in about 1–2 per cent of all patients with hypertension. In children and young adults, non-vascular unilateral renal disease, mostly the result of reflux nephropathy, is a prominent cause of hypertension. In principle, a great variety of renal parenchymal diseases may be associated with hypertension (Table 1).

Potential procedures to establish the diagnosis of unilateral renoparenchymal hypertension are shown in Table 2. The diagnostic strategies are further outlined in Chapter 9.1.

In the past, determination of peripheral plasma renin activity (PRA) and selective renal vein catherization to compare PRA of the diseased and non-diseased kidney had been very popular. A renin ratio greater than 1.5, that is, 50 per cent higher in the venous blood draining the affected kidney, was thought to prove hyper-reninism, indicating a high probability that the diseased kidney contributed to hypertension. But PRA and renin ratios are often confounded by variables such as blood pressure, sodium balance, antihypertensive treatment, and pulsatile renin secretion. As a result, they have only limited predictive value and have therefore been largely abandoned. A case in point is the 2-year follow-up study on normotensive patients with reflux nephropathy by Goonasekra *et al.* (1996) in which elevated PRA failed to predict the development of hypertension.

Table 1 Potential causes of hypertension resulting from unilateral renal parenchymal disease

Unilaterally small kidney
Segmental hypoplasia ('Ask-Upmark kidney')
Reflux nephropathy
Hypoplastic kidney
Radiation nephritis
Congenital abnormalities
Unilateral renal agenesis
Ectopic and ptotic kidney
Urinary tract malformation
Hydronephrosis
Simple renal cyst and unilateral multicystic kidney disease
Tuberculosis
Trauma
Tumour
Haemangiopericytoma (reninoma)
Wilms' tumour
Renal cell carcinoma
Unilateral nephrectomy (including donation of kidney)
Hypertension following renal transplantation

The unilaterally small kidney

Segmental hypoplasia ('Ask-Upmark kidney')

In 1929, Ask-Upmark described six patients with malignant hypertension, five of whom had a distinct renal anomaly that he considered to be a form of congenital segmental hypoplasia. By histology, the kidneys showed small areas with normal architecture separated by atrophic cortical grooves overlying dilated calyces without pyramids. In such patients, the parenchyma in these segments was reminiscent of thyroid tissue and did not contain glomeruli. The angiogram typically showed a normal renal artery; intravenous pyelography revealed a small kidney with irregular outlines, calyceal dilatation, and a thin cortical parenchyma. Scintigraphy or computed tomography (CT) also document the presence of segmental scarring or hypoplasia.

In most cases, segmental hypoplasia is strictly unilateral, but bilaterally symmetrical and asymmetrical renal disease have also been reported. Adults and even children with this condition may show variable degrees of renal failure. Most children and 60 per cent of adult patients are also hypertensive. There is a female predominance of 2 : 1.

Table 2 Diagnosis of unilateral renal parenchymal disease

Diagnosis of renal disease
History, physical examination
Proteinuria, leucocyturia, bacteriuria, acid fast bacteria, haematuria, casts
Ultrasound of the kidney
Duplex scan of renal vessels
Intravenous urography
Computed tomography or magnetic resonance tomography
Radionuclide renography with [^{131}J]Hippuran, MAG3, or [^{99}Tc^{m}]DTPA, with and without captopril and split renal function
Static renal imaging with radionuclides such as Tc-DMSA or gallium (^{67}Ga)
MRT angiography or selective renal arteriography
Renal biopsy

DMSA, dimercaptosuccinic acid; DTPA, diethylene triamine pentaacetic acid; MAG3, mercaptoacetyltriglycine.

Recent investigations cast doubt on the congenital nature of the Ask-Upmark kidney. The alternative hypothesis of an acquired atrophy secondary to vesicoureteral reflux (VUR) and infection has meanwhile been widely accepted (Laberke 1987) (Fig. 1). The role of renin in the pathogenesis of hypertension associated with this disease is uncertain: PRA is frequently elevated, particularly in the main or segmental renal veins, but normal or even low PRA has also been reported. The latter may be due to the loss of glomeruli in the hypoplastic areas, but immunohistochemical studies have demonstrated renin granules in sclerotic glomeruli, arterioles, and interstitial cells within atrophic areas devoid of glomeruli.

If the disease is strictly unilateral, segmental resection or nephrectomy may result in sustained lowering of blood pressure.

Vesicoureteral reflux, reflux nephropathy, and hypoplastic kidneys

Vesicoureteral reflux, that is, retrograde flow of urine from the bladder into the ureter or even into renal parenchyma, is a relatively common condition. It is noted in 0.5–2 per cent of the general population (Stefanidis 2001) (Fig. 2). Normally, the ureter is obliquely inserted into a tunnel traversing the bladder wall. This arrangement is functioning as a jack valve, so to speak: during micturition the ureter is compressed by the musculature of the bladder wall, thus preventing upstream movement of bladder urine. VUR develops when this tunnel is in an abnormal position or shortened. During embryonic development, the ureteric bud sprouts from the cloaca. It is responsible for the development of the ureter, and by interaction with the nephrogenic blastema, for the development of the ipsilateral kidney. It is thought that abnormal localization or delayed organization of the bud causes lateral displacement and abnormal development of the ureteric bud. When children grow up the bladder wall matures and thickens and particularly at the time of puberty the VUR often disappears. As a result, in the adult persisting renal scarring may be found and even a history of VUR may be obtained, but VUR may no longer be demonstrable. Since VUR is related to abnormal organogenesis of the urinary tract and the kidney, it is readily understood that the more lateral the site of insertion of the ureter and the more pronounced the VUR, the greater the risk of renal scarring. It is still controversial whether the reduction in renal parenchyma is secondary to reflux with or without infection or whether it reflects primarily faulty renal development. This may vary from case to case.

The clinical distinction between diffuse rarefication of renal parenchyma, as putative evidence of congenital reflux nephropathy, and segmental rarification of renal parenchyma, as putative evidence of acquired scarring from reflux nephropathy, is based on the pattern of tracer uptake by the renal parenchyma. Polito *et al.* (2000) performed DMSA (dimercaptosuccinic acid) scintigraphy. A diffuse reduction or abrogation of radiotracer uptake was interpreted as evidence of congenital reflux nephropathy. In contrast, segmentally reduced uptake, usually in the cranial and caudal segments of the kidney, was interpreted as evidence of postnatally acquired renal scarring. The more prominent involvement of cranial and caudal segments has been related to a more perpendicular course of collecting ducts in these segments, compared to the more oblique course in the middle renal segments. The perpendicular course is thought to permit easier propagation of elevated pressure from the pelvis into the renal parenchyma.

The VUR has a strong hereditary component. In most families it follows a pattern of autosomal dominant transmission. Recent studies showed that a locus on chromosome 1 cosegregates with the development of VUR (Feather *et al.* 2000). The family history is therefore of great importance when examining individuals with suspected VUR.

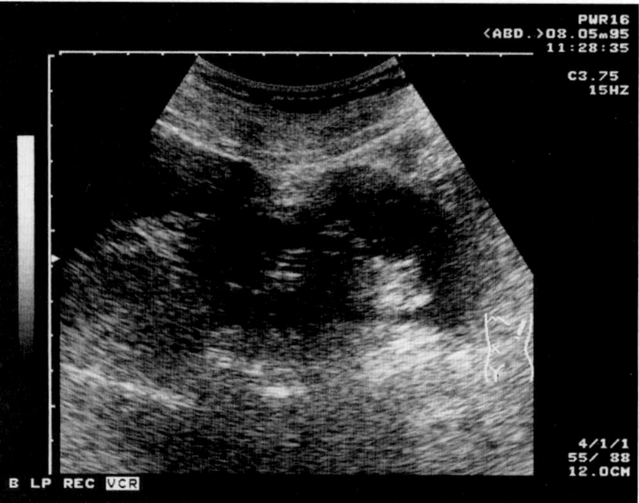

Fig. 1 Ultrasound of a kidney with segmental hypoplasia (Ask-Upmark kidney). Ultrasound view of the left kidney of a 50-year-old hypertensive female patient. It shows a major defect of renal mass caused by a deep scar. The lower pole of the kidney exhibits increased parenchymal width as a result of compensatory hypertrophy.

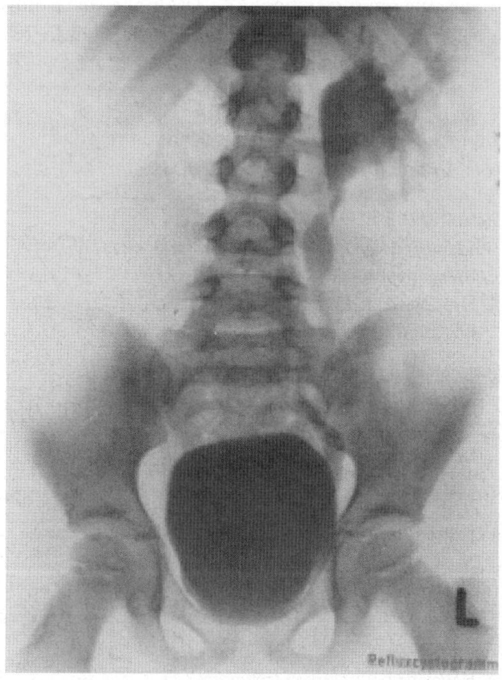

Fig. 2 Retrograde cystoureterogram of a patient with reflux nephropathy. The bladder of a female 40-year-old patient is filled with contrast agent. Note reflux of radiocontrast material from the bladder via the dilated ureter into the left pelvis. The ultrasound shows numerous parenchymal scars. On the right side there is no evidence of vesicoureteral reflux.

In one analysis, it could be shown that 50 per cent of siblings and offspring of patients had VUR. There is, however, some genetic heterogeneity and more than one locus is apparently involved. The causative genes have not been identified. Studies on some candidate genes on a priori grounds yielded negative results, for example, PAX-2, fibroblast growth factor receptor type 2, or glial cell line-derived neurotrophic factor receptor genes. The deletion allele (D/D) of the angiotensin converting enzyme (ACE) gene is more frequent in patients with renal scar formation (Ozen *et al.* 1999).

In individuals with acquired renal scarring, the issue arises whether scarring is the result of mechanical damage to renal parenchyma (water-hammer effect) or whether it results from recurrent upper urinary tract infections (pyelonephritis) (Fig. 3). Based on several studies (Berg and Johansson 1983; Smellie *et al.* 1985), the major pathogenic factor appears to be recurrent infections. This has led to the recommendation to provide prophylactic antibiotic treatment instead of antireflux surgery. Indeed, large studies comparing the results of conservative management including antibiotic prophylaxis with surgical correction of VUR did not show convincingly different outcomes between the two strategies in children with severe bilateral VUR and bilateral nephropathy when renal insufficiency was chosen as an endpoint (Smellie *et al.* 2001). Similarly, no difference of renal growth was seen (Olbing *et al.* 2000). Recommended antibiotics for long-term prophylaxis of recurrent infections are low-dose trimethoprim or (if renal function is normal) nitrofurantoin for up to 2 years, but there is no controlled study that confirmed that this form of treatment is superior to early detection and treatment of intercurrent infection (Jones 1993). Fluorchinolone antibiotics are contraindicated in children, but are an alternative in adults.

The major long-term sequelae of reflux nephropathy are hypertension and renal failure. Recent epidemiological observations suggest that the frequency of endstage renal disease caused by reflux nephropathy has decreased during the last few decades (Wennerstrom *et al.* 2000). This observation was made in Sweden where awareness of urinary tract infection and its consequences in VUR has been high. In contrast, the Australian and New Zealand dialysis and transplant registry found little evidence for a downward trend of endstage renal disease from reflux nephropathy (Craig *et al.* 2000). Although there is little controlled evidence, the majority of paediatricians are currently convinced that treatment of recurrent urinary tract infection, but not necessarily surgical correction of VUR, are the mainstay in the prevention of hypertension and endstage renal disease in individuals with reflux nephropathy. Our local policy is to restrict surgical correction to patients in whom recurrent breakthrough infections have occurred despite antibiotic prophylaxis.

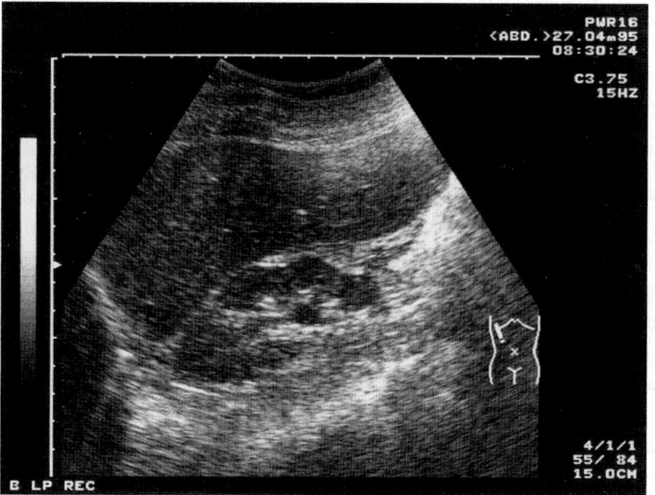

Fig. 3 Ultrasound of a kidney with reflux nephropathy. Ultrasound view of the right kidney of a 58-year-old female patient. The kidney is small (82 mm) with irregular contours caused by multiple scars.

The relation of VUR and specifically of reflux nephropathy to blood pressure is not well defined. In the short term, severe hypertension is relatively rare in children and adolescents with VUR. In a prospective cohort study of a cohort of children with reflux nephropathy, five of 55 patients developed systolic and two diastolic hypertension (Goonasekera *et al.* 1996). The PRA rose progressively above the values found in the control population, but PRA values were not individually predictive of the development of hypertension. There is immunohistochemical evidence for increased expression of renin, particularly in the border zones between scar tissue and functional renal parenchyma. Renin positive cells have been described in segmental renal hypoplasia by Menard *et al.* (1983). Clearly, therefore, the blood pressure in reflux nephropathy is renin-dependent and this pathomechanism is also suggested by the beneficial effects of pharmacological blockade of the RAS (Becker and Kincaid-Smith 1993; Lama *et al.* 1997).

When should nephrectomy be considered in the patient with unilateral reflux nephropathy or Ask-Upmark kidneys?

Unilateral nephrectomy may be considered when the affected kidney contributes less than 20 per cent to the total renal function, as evaluated by scintigraphic techniques. But nephrectomy should only be performed if the morphology and function of the contralateral kidney is completely normal and if proteinuria is absent. Otherwise prolonged treatment with antihypertensive medication including particularly ACE inhibitors or angiotensin receptor blockers is the preferred option.

Radiation nephritis (see Chapter 6.6)

Today, chronic radiation nephritis has become a very rare cause of hypertension. It may develop (often abruptly) months or years after irradiation of one or both kidneys. Because it may develop after radiation treatment of the spleen, the left kidney is more often affected than the right. Patients with radiation nephritis have usually been treated for Wilms' tumour, ovarian or testicular carcinoma, retroperitoneal lymphoma, osteogenic sarcoma, neuroblastoma, or intra-abdominal metastases. Renal damage occurs in most cases when a total dose of 20 Gy (2000 rads) or more has been administered. But late effects of radiation therapy have been seen in children even with a lower dose. In a study by Paulino *et al.* (2000), three of 55 children developed hypertension without decrease of renal function. This observation is in agreement with the findings of Maher (1989) that there is no tight relation between development of hypertension and loss of renal function.

Renin concentrations are increased in the vein draining the affected kidney, but PRA is not always increased. Histological examination shows intimal proliferation and fibrinoid lesions resembling malignant hypertension. Fibrinoid deposits may persist in the irradiated kidney for years. These findings led several authors to ascribe the development of hypertension to renal ischaemia as a result of vascular damage following irradiation (Shapiro *et al.* 1977; Lüscher *et al.* 1981a,b). In experimental radiation nephritis of rats, ACE inhibitors preserved renal function and structure, whilst a similar reduction in blood pressure by diuretics failed to do so (Juncos *et al.* 1993). If conservative treatment including ACE-inhibitor administration fails to improve hypertension, nephrectomy should be considered in cases of unilateral radiation nephritis.

Congenital abnormalities

Unilateral renal agenesis

Unilateral agenesis of the kidney, frequently associated with proteinuria and focal glomerulosclerosis of the single kidney (Kiprow *et al.* 1982), is usually discovered accidentally in adults. It may also be found, however, in various inherited familial disorders (Arfeen *et al.* 1993), including trisomy 8, lisencephaly syndrome, Kallmann syndrome, and VATER syndrome (see Chapter 17.4). It occurs in about 4.5 per cent of the first-degree relatives of patients with unilateral renal agenesis, compared to 0.3 per cent in a control population. Ultrasonographic screening of parents and siblings is therefore advised (Roodhoft *et al.* 1984).

There are conflicting reports on the incidence of hypertension, ranging from very low to about 90 per cent (Maschio *et al.* 1987). It has been suggested that complicating focal and segmental glomerulosclerosis is the result of long-standing hyperperfusion of the hypertrophied single kidney but a causal role of an intrinsic abnormality of the single kidney cannot be excluded. Renal disease was the cause of death in 35 of 232 patients who were born with solitary kidneys (Ashley and Mostofi 1960). Interestingly, the prevalence of VUR is increased in children with unilateral renal agenesis (Song *et al.* 1995).

Ptotic kidney

A number of symptoms, such as colic, lumbar pain, urinary tract infection, proteinuria, and others have been ascribed to renal ptosis (Boccardo *et al.* 1994). The conclusion was based on poorly controlled studies. In our experience ptotic kidneys are typical for underweight young females who as a rule lose this usually harmless finding when they gain weight. Surgical correction (nephropexy) is only indicated if one can consistently document lumbar pain in the upright position which rapidly disappears in a supine position or after micturition.

Urinary tract abnormalities: ureteral valves

Certain malformations such as ureteral valves lead to urinary tract obstruction. The diagnosis is made by intravenous and, if necessary, retrograde pyelography, which shows transverse defects of the obstructed ureter. The literature reports a few patients in whom this lesion was combined with hypertension. Whiting *et al.* (1983) described that hypertension resolved after surgical relief of ureteral obstruction (see Chapters 17.3 and 17.4).

Simple renal cyst and unilateral multicystic kidney

The prevalence of simple renal cysts is increasing with advancing age. In a study of 16,102 children, 37 cysts were detected by ultrasound in 35 patients, yielding a prevalence of 0.22 per cent (McHugh *et al.* 1991). The cysts measured from 0.3 to 7 cm in maximum diameter. In adults, the prevalence of single renal cysts is 10 per cent at the age of 70 (Pedersen *et al.* 1993). Fifty per cent of solitary cysts are found at the lower pole of the kidney, 30 per cent at the upper pole, and about 20 per cent are located centrally. While their diameter ranges from less than 1 cm to more than 7 cm, the majority of cysts are around 2 cm in diameter (Tada *et al.* 1983).

Hypertension due to a solitary renal cyst was first described by Farrell and Young (1942). Since then several cases have been reported. This constellation is usually seen in patients with large cysts in central localization, where they may impinge on hilar structures (Mast *et al.* 1985) compressing renal vessels and thus causing segmental ischaemia and increased renin production. The renin activity in the cyst fluid is not increased (Churchill *et al.* 1975; Lüscher *et al.* 1986). Improvement or cure of hypertension was seen after percutaneous needle decompression or surgical removal of the cyst. But even repeated puncture is often unsuccessful because cysts often refill rapidly. In such cases surgical correction should be considered if cysts are very large and increase in size.

Unilateral multicystic renal dysplasia is a rare cause of hypertension. It has been reported in a few newborn babies and children. Hypertension is renin-dependent (Chen *et al.* 1985). Additional urological and other anomalies (cardiac, intestinal) are responsible for the high mortality of these patients (Stockamp *et al.* 1974). Removal of the affected kidney may resolve hypertension. Nephrectomy is indicated if the function of the multicystic kidney is severely impaired and the function of the contralateral kidney is normal (Chen *et al.* 1985). It is advisable to search for accompanying extrarenal abnormalities (Stockamp *et al.* 1974).

Tuberculosis (see Chapter 7.3)

Mycobacterium tuberculosis bacteraemia initially affects both kidneys, but clinically manifest renal tuberculosis is usually unilateral (Corigliano and Leedom 1983). Approximately 4–8 per cent of patients with pulmonary tuberculosis will develop destructive lesions of the genitourinary tract after a latency from several months to more than 30 years. The diagnosis is made on the basis of history, cultures of a 24-h urine specimen or repeated morning urine specimens, and renal imaging. Polymerase chain reaction of the urine seems to be a promising new diagnostic tool. In late stages of renal tuberculosis with hypertension urine cultures are often negative. X-rays may reveal calcification of a deformed kidney.

Hypertension is an exceptional complication: its prevalence ranges from 2.5 to 4.5 per cent in patients with unilateral renal tuberculosis (Mast *et al.* 1985), and is less than 10 per cent in patients undergoing surgery for renal tuberculosis (Studer and Weidmann 1984). Hypertension develops only in patients with severe destruction of renal parenchyma, probably due to an obliterative arteritis of the larger intrarenal blood vessels (Corigliano and Leedom 1983). Renin may be elevated if measured in the segmental renal vein draining the tuberculous part of the kidney (Studer and Weidmann 1984). There is no evidence for an important role of the adrenergic system in this form of renal hypertension: noradrenaline and adrenaline in plasma and urine are normal (Studer and Weidmann 1984).

Conservative tuberculostatic treatment of renal tuberculosis may cure or reverse hypertension (Mast *et al.* 1985). If blood pressure is difficult to control, investigation for renal vein renin activity can be performed to identify those patients who may benefit from surgical intervention. Preoperative renal scintigraphy of the region of interest may be helpful. Resection of the affected part of the kidney is preferred to uninephrectomy. The antihypertensive effect of uninephrectomy is variable. In a series of 49 reported patients hypertension was improved or cured in 67 per cent (Beretta-Piccoli *et al.* 1982).

Hydronephrosis

In rat experiments, prolonged unilateral ureteral obstruction is followed by a substantial increase in blood pressure, associated with upregulation of the renin–angiotensin–aldosterone system and downregulation of tissue kallikrein mRNA in the involved kidney (El Dahr *et al.* 1993). Blockade of angiotensin II receptors with losartan prevents the increase in blood pressure after unilateral ureteral obstruction and lowers the blood pressure in chronically hypertensive rats with unilateral ureteral obstruction.

Hypertension is also common in patients with unilateral hydronephrosis which may be caused, for instance, by stenosis of the ureteropelvic junction, urolithiasis, ureterocele, aberrant segmental renal artery, external compression, internal occlusion, congenital malformation, and iatrogenic lesions.

Altered renal blood flow is a major pathogenetic factor in the genesis of hypertension due to hydronephrosis. Local renin formation is stimulated similar to that seen in renovascular hypertension. Microvascular disease of the ipsilateral, and later on of the contralateral, kidney produces a vicious circle: hydronephrosis leads to hypertension and hypertension in turn damages the renal vessels and thus aggravates hypertension.

When hypertension is of recent onset, there is little doubt that the process is renin mediated. Peripheral or renal vein renin may be elevated preoperatively and returns to normal after surgical relief of obstruction. Renin expression in the resected kidney may be increased and preferentially localized along the afferent arterioles of the juxtaglomerular apparatus at some distance from the glomeruli (Mizuiri *et al.* 1992).

When hydronephrosis and hypertension are chronic, peripheral renin activity is generally not elevated. In addition to angiotensin II, other vasoactive substances produced by the hydronephrotic kidney may play a modulating role: there may be an increased production of pressor prostaglandins, such as thromboxane A_2 and prostaglandin $F_{2\alpha}$, or an insufficient production of renomedullary depressor substances such as 'antihypertensive neutral renomedullary lipid'. This concept is fascinating, since the papilla is the portion of the renal parenchyma which disappears first in the hydronephrotic kidney thereby predisposing to hypertension; but clinical data to document this hypothesis are still lacking. There may also be reflex activation of the sympathetic nervous system, related to an increased pressure in the ureter or to the affected kidney with a consequent increase of vascular smooth muscle tone. A potential role for reduced sodium excretion with an increased intravascular volume has also been postulated.

The overall incidence of mild to moderate hypertension in patients with unilateral hydronephrosis was 20 per cent in the study of Wanner *et al.* (1987); other authors found hypertension in 50 per cent of patients with acute as compared to 10 per cent of patients with chronic unilateral hydronephrosis (Beretta-Piccoli *et al.* 1982).

Because of the risk of progressive organ damage, surgery is indicated in any case, even if hypertension is not present. Surgical restoration of urine flow or nephrectomy was reported to cure hypertension in 62 per cent and to improve blood pressure in an additional 19 per cent of the patients (Wanner *et al.* 1987). In another study blood pressure returned to normal in 70 per cent of the patients (Beretta-Piccoli *et al.* 1982).

Renal trauma

Renal trauma may induce transient or persistent hypertension, developing after days or even years. An initial traction injury, as may occur during deceleration trauma, may result in a tear of the intima of the renal artery with subsequent thrombosis or stenosis. Penetrating injuries may damage intra- or extrarenal blood vessels with subsequent haemorrhage. Renal biopsy may be complicated by an arteriovenous fistula, haematoma, or ureteral occlusion. Parenchymal kidney lesions are often associated with a compressive subcapsular or perirenal haematoma. In the absence of a haematoma, renal injury may be followed by renal scar formation. This can be documented by reduced radionuclide uptake (DMSA scintigraphy). On the other hand, however, no relation between renal scars and hypertension could be shown in the study of Surana *et al.* (1995). Figure 4 shows the classification of blunt renal injuries (Mendez 1977; Frohmüller 1983): contusions (grade I), lacerations of the renal parenchyma and/or the pelviureteral system (grade II), severe fractures (grade III), and pedicle injuries (grade IV).

Hypertension due to perirenal haematoma is explained by a mechanism first described by Page (1939) in dogs. One kidney was wrapped with cellophane and this was followed by perinephritic fibrosis and parenchymal compression. Today, the term 'Page kidney' is used to describe the rare syndrome of hyper-reninemic hypertension caused by unilateral compressive perinephritis. Blood or fluid that accumulates in the perinephric subcapsular space and forms a pseudocapsule compresses the renal parenchyma leading to ischaemia. Hypertension develops after a time interval of days, months, or several years

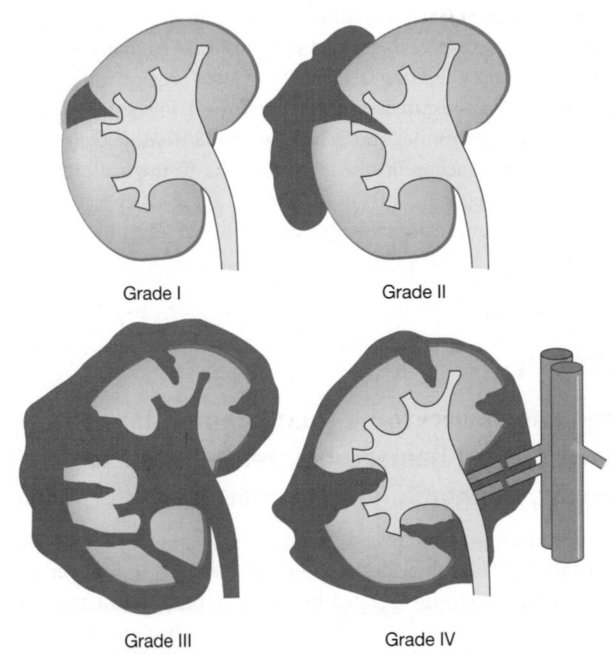

Fig. 4 Classification of blunt renal injury.

(Mast *et al.* 1985). Not only blunt renal injuries are responsible for a Page kidney, but also spontaneous subcapsular haematoma in patients with necrotizing vascular inflammation due to polyarteriitis nodosa (Pintar and Zimmerman 1998). Removal of the renal capsule and pseudocapsule can be curative in such cases (Moriarty *et al.* 1997).

The pathogenesis of hypertension following vascular lesions is similar to that described by Goldblatt *et al.* (1934) after experimental renal artery stenosis. After trauma, dull flank aching, headache, and haematuria may also be present. The intravenous pyelogram may show alterations of the renal outline, but a normal intravenous pyelogram does not exclude a severe lesion. On the other hand, it may reveal a completely non-functioning kidney.

Grading of the renal injury is performed by initial CT. Renal angiography will show lesions of the renal artery and its branches as well as cortical scarring (Meyrier *et al.* 1988). Today, lesions of the renal arteries could also be excluded using magnetic resonance angiography. A compressive haematoma located either in the subcapsular space or in the perirenal space between Gerota's fascia and the renal capsule induces renal ischaemia and renin secretion (Lüscher *et al.* 1985). Increased renin may also be the consequence of renal infarction. Peripheral plasma renin is often transiently elevated, but may decline after 1 or 2 years. Even normal PRA values may be found when renin secretion by the contralateral kidney is suppressed (Grim *et al.* 1975). Many authors have described an enhanced renal vein renin activity of the injured side (Grim *et al.* 1975; Spark and Berg 1976; Mast *et al.* 1985).

Complications including urinoma, sepsis, hydronephrosis, and persistent hypertension were particularly observed in grades III and IV (Abdalati *et al.* 1994). However, hypertension may also develop in less severe grades of kidney damage (grades I and II injuries) (Mast *et al.* 1985) (Fig. 4).

Major renal lacerations and vascular pedicle injuries often result in a loss of renal function and should be followed up closely because of the risk of delayed complications. For a patient with persistent hypertension and reduced size of the injured kidney, indicating renal ischaemia, unilateral nephrectomy may be considered (Maling *et al.* 1975). It can be effective in curing hypertension even many years after the trauma (von Knorring *et al.* 1981). After surgical intervention hypertension may be cured, or at least improved, in about 80 per cent of these patients (Wanner and Schollmeyer 1988). More conservative approaches are evacuation of the haematoma in the acute phase or removal of perinephritic scars in the chronic phase. After reabsorption of the haematoma, spontaneous restoration of normotension has been reported (Lüscher *et al.* 1985).

Tumour

Haemangiopericytoma (juxtaglomerular cell tumour, renal hamartoma, renin-producing tumour, reninoma, juxtaglomerular hyperplasia)

Renin-producing tumours are rare causes of potentially reversible hypertension. The initial description was made by Robertson *et al.* (1967). Renin is chiefly secreted by capillary pericytes of the juxtaglomerular apparatus. These cells may form a benign or very low grade malignant (Wesson 1982) tumour. In most cases the tumour is diagnosed in the second to fourth decades of life.

Symptoms include hypertension which is often severe and therapy resistant, increased PRA, secondary hyperaldosteronism, and hypokalaemia. Plasma renin secretion is not entirely autonomous: it may increase in response to upright posture, but not in response to sodium depletion.

Haemangiopericytomas are usually encapsulated and small (<1–4 cm in diameter); renal angiography may therefore fail to show a cortical filling defect. Magnification methods enhance the diagnostic yield. The value of CT for an exact localization must be documented in the future. Surgical local excision or nephrectomy result in a prompt reduction of plasma renin, angiotensin II, and aldosterone, with a parallel decline of blood pressure.

Surgically removed tumour tissue contains cells with a high renin content (Hirose *et al.* 1974). Ultrastructural studies documented the presence of characteristic secretory granules in tumour cells (Wesson 1982). Ectopic renin-producing tumours may also be encountered. Yokoyama *et al.* (1979) reported a 15-year-old girl with a tumour of the orbit which—although encapsulated—invaded the frontal lobe, sinuses, and pituitary. On light microscopy it resembled a juxtaglomerular cell tumour (Wesson 1982). Various other types of extrarenal tumours which occasionally secrete renin include hamartoma of the liver, carcinoma of lung and pancreas, and ovarian cancer (Menard *et al.* 1983).

Occasionally, the symptoms of a reninoma may be mimicked by unilateral juxtaglomerular hyperplasia with hypertension (or normotension), hypokalaemia, and lateralization of renin secretion. Angiography is usually negative (Küchel *et al.* 1993). Upon removal of the kidney blood pressure, PRA, and plasma electrolytes return to normal.

Wilms' tumour (nephroblastoma, embryoma)

Moderate hypertension is a common feature of Wilms' tumour, but severe elevation of blood pressure is unusual (Ganguly *et al.* 1973). About 1 per cent of hypertensive children suffer from this type of tumour (Wanner and Schollmeyer 1988).

Hypertension may be induced by renal ischaemia due to infiltration or compression of adjacent normal tissue with consecutive elevation of PRA (Ganguly *et al.* 1973; Wesson 1982); further abnormalities may contribute to the development of hypertension such as decreased afferent arteriolar blood flow caused by arteriovenous shunts and increased synthesis and secretion of renin by tumour tissue, particularly if it contains structures that resemble glomeruli (Mast *et al.* 1985).

Recurrence of hypertension after nephrectomy has been described in patients with metastases; blood pressure returned to normal after irradiation of the secondaries (Bradley and Pincoff 1938). This observation indicates that tumour tissue may produce a renin like substance (Brosman 1989) (for further discussion of Wilms' tumour see Chapter 18.2).

Renal cell carcinoma (hypernephroma, renal adenocarcinoma) (see also Chapter 18.1)

The prevalence of hypertension in patients with hypernephroma ranges from 10 to 50 per cent (Wesson 1982; Lüscher *et al.* 1985; Steffens *et al.* 1992): in a consecutive historical series of 56 patients with hypernephroma, hypertension was found in 12.5 per cent (Pillary *et al.* 1975). Symptoms of advanced tumours are flank and back pain, haematuria, and weight loss, but today this has become rare, because these tumours are usually detected at an earlier stage by ultrasonography. The age distribution ranges from 20 to 70 years (Melman *et al.* 1977) with a peak in patients older than 50 years.

Studies on the possible renin dependence of hypertension in patients with renal carcinomas yielded controversial results (Wesson 1982): peripheral renin may be elevated without increased blood pressure, and normal renin concentrations are seen in hypertensive patients who respond to nephrectomy. Hypertension is reversed after nephrectomy in about 50 per cent of patients (Morlock and Horton 1936; Horton 1940). In the study of Steffens *et al.* (1992), the pathogenetic relationship between tumour and hypertension was investigated in 129 patients with renal cell carcinoma. Of these patients, 41 (31.8 per cent) were hypertensive, six were found to have primary reninism (14.5 per cent), and in three of them autonomous renin production was demonstrated in cell culture. In five of six patients blood pressure returned to normal following nephrectomy. Renal cell carcinoma may also produce a variety of other ectopic hormones including erythropoietin (Hewlett *et al.* 1956; Brosman 1989), insulin, glucagon, parathyroid hormone (Greenberg *et al.* 1973), and norepinephrine (Koh *et al.* 2001). Erythropoietin and norepinephrine producing tumours may also cause hypertension.

In addition to primary reninism, coexistence of renal cell carcinoma and renal artery stenosis may occur. Furthermore, arteriovenous shunting in large tumours may be another cause of hyper-reninism and hypertension (Brosman 1989).

Unilateral nephrectomy (including donation of a kidney)

In experimental animals, ablation of renal mass leads to hypertension, progressive glomerulosclerosis, and renal failure. The susceptibility to these complications is different in various rat strains. In particular, the fawn-hooded rat is extremely vulnerable to the adverse effects of unilateral nephrectomy, suggesting the decisive role of genetic factors (Simons *et al.* 1993). Brown *et al.* (1996) could confirm this hypothesis experimentally by showing that in the fawn-hooded rat the susceptibility to develop chronic renal failure is under genetic control which is at least partially independent from the susceptibility to develop hypertension. Two genes Rf-1 and Rf-2 were responsible for about half of the genetic variance in key indices of renal impairment, but Rf-1 had no significant effect on blood pressure.

The effect of uninephrectomy on blood pressure and renal function in human is somewhat controversial. On the one hand, observations in healthy individuals losing one kidney because of trauma or organ donation showed a moderate increase in albumin excretion rate and occasionally also hypertension. As a consequence, today uninephrectomy of related or unrelated kidney donors is an accepted modality of treatment. The situation is somewhat different when nephrectomy is performed in individuals with known renal abnormalities. In children with an acquired solitary kidney the risk to develop hypertension, proteinuria, and renal insufficiency is higher. In a 25-year follow-up study, 138 children who underwent unilateral nephrectomy and had a normal contralateral kidney were examined. Survival of these Wilms's tumour patients was similar to that of an age-matched control group. However, in 30 patients an increased prevalence of proteinuria (27 per cent), renal insufficiency (30 per cent), and hypertension (10 per cent) was found (Argueso *et al.* 1992). Different results were reported by Robitaille *et al.* (1985). They studied 27 patients who had undergone unilateral nephrectomy in childhood at a mean age of 2.1 years. After a follow-up of 23.3 years the proportion of individuals with hypertension and evidence of glomerular damage was low. Thus, the concept that renal ablation at an early age predisposes to hypertension and progressive renal damage is not definitely proven.

In a meta-analysis of 313 adult patients, who had undergone unilateral nephrectomy for renal tuberculosis and were re-examined after a period ranging from 13.5 to 591 months, hypertension was found in 30.2 per cent, while serum creatinine levels averaged about 1.28 ± 0.53 mg/dl (Buccianti *et al.* 1993). Microalbuminuria was found in 51 per cent of the patients. According to these results the number of patients with progressive renal functional impairment after nephrectomy is low. Microalbuminuria did not appear to lead to progression of renal disease.

In follow-up studies of kidney donors, the reported frequency of hypertension was variable. Maschio *et al.* (1987) found a prevalence of about 10 per cent (60 out of 624 kidney donors). Talseth *et al.* (1986), who examined 86 kidney donors 9–15 years after uninephrectomy, found a slight, but significant, increase in blood pressure: 15 per cent (10 donors) were hypertensive at follow-up. Of these 10 hypertensives only three had been normotensive preoperatively, however, and a control group had not been examined.

Podjarny *et al.* (1986) reported an increased frequency of hypertension (75 per cent) after uninephrectomy when patients were aged more than 55 years. In men younger than 55 years the frequency of hypertension was the same as in the normal age-matched Israeli population (21.4 per cent). All of these 26 patients had been normotensive before uninephrectomy. Warnick *et al.* (1988) followed the clinical course of 29 persons for 9–18 years after kidney donation. The frequency of hypertension was 62 per cent as compared to 42 per cent in the control group. Proteinuria was seen in 14 per cent versus 6 per cent in the control group. Also, Hakim *et al.* (1984) reported a greater frequency of hypertension and proteinuria in male donors compared with age-matched controls 10–15 years after uninephrectomy. Different results were reported by Najarian *et al.* (1992) in 57 donors who had undergone unilateral nephrectomy 21–29 years earlier. Compared with age-matched siblings, renal donors had identical values for blood pressure, creatinine clearance, and protein excretion.

Hypertension following renal transplantation

Hypertension is very frequent after renal transplantation. The reader is referred to Section 13.

Management of the hypertensive patient with unilateral renal disease

In principle, the patient with hypertension resulting from unilateral renal disease should be managed as the patient with common forms of hypertension. If hypertension is mild to moderate, non-pharmacological treatment comprising restriction of dietary sodium intake, decreased alcohol consumption (very difficult in some European countries), reduction of body weight particularly in obese patients, and physical exercise should be recommended. This should be complemented by appropriate risk factor management, particularly cessation of smoking. If hypertension persists or hypertension is severe and cardiovascular risk factors or target organ damage are present, antihypertensive medication should be given. In view of the underlying pathomechanisms discussed above, there is a strong rationale for the use of ACE inhibitors or angiotensin receptor blockers.

Corrective interventions are indicated in the rare patients with perirenal haematoma, perirenal capsule formation, giant renal cysts, and hydronephrosis in whom surgical correction is possible. Apart from this nephrectomy is the only option in patients with advanced reflux nephropathy or other destructive diseases, for example, tuberculosis. This option should be considered only if the disease is strictly unilateral; failure of the contralateral kidney to undergo hypertrophy may indicate that this kidney is already damaged. Serum creatinine must be in the normal range, and the contribution of the diseased kidney to overall renal function should be less than 10–20 per cent. Increased renin secretion of the affected side with contralateral suppression indicates a greater probability of cure, but false-negative (12 per cent in unilateral renoparenchymal disease and 18 per cent in renovascular hypertension; Beretta-Piccoli *et al.* 1982) as well as false-positive tests limit its predictive reliability (Wanner *et al.* 1987). Complicating renovascular disease in the presumed healthy kidney should be excluded by angiography.

The success of surgical intervention in reversing hypertension varies in the different unilateral renoparenchymal diseases. Beretta-Piccoli *et al.* (1982) found a cure rate of 66 per cent. If the renal vein renin test was positive, the rate of improvement rose to 89 per cent; but false-negative tests did occur.

References

Abdalati, H. *et al.* (1994). Blunt renal trauma in children: healing of renal injuries and recommendations for imaging follow up. *Pediatric Radiology* **24** (8), 573–576.

Arfeen, S., Rosborough, D., Luger, A. M., and Nolph, K. D. (1993). Familial unilateral renal agenesis and focal and segmental glomerulosclerosis. *American Journal of Kidney Diseases* **21** (6), 663–668.

Argueso, L. R., Ritchey, M. L., Boyle, E. T., Jr., Milliner, D. S., Bergstralh, E. J., and Kramer, S. A. (1992). Prognosis of children with solitary kidney after unilateral nephrectomy. *Journal of Urology* **148** (2, Pt 2), 747–751.

Ashley, D. J. B. and Mostofi, F. K. (1960). Renal agenesis and dysgenesis. *Journal of Urology* **83**, 211–230.

Becker, G. J. and Kincaid-Smith, P. (1993). Reflux nephropathy: the glomerular lesion and progression of renal failure. *Pediatric Nephrology* **7**, 365–369.

Beretta-Piccoli, C., Weidmann, P., Boehringer, K., and Zingg, E. (1982). Hypertonie bei einseitigen Nierenparenchymkrankheiten: Ätiologie, Renin und chirurgischer Behandlungserfolg. *Aktuelle Urologie* **13**, 173–185.

Berg, U. B. and Johansson, S. B. (1983). Age as a main determinant of renal functional damage in urinary tract infection. *Archives of Diseases in Childhood* **58**, 963–969.

Boccardo, G., Ettari, G., De Prisco, O., Donato, G., and Maurino, D. (1994). Renal ptosis: nephrologic consequences of an organ malposition. *Minerva Urologia e Nefrologia* **46** (4), 195–204.

Bradley, J. E. and Pincoff, M. C. (1938). The association of adenomyosarcoma of the kidney (Wilm's tumor) with arterial hypertension. *Annals of Internal Medicine* **11**, 1613–1628.

Brosman, S. A. Tumours of the kidney and urinary tract. In *Textbook of Nephrology* Vol. 2, 2nd edn. (ed. S. G. Massey and R. J. Glassock), pp. 942–961. Baltimore: Williams and Wilkins, 1989.

Brown, D. M., Provoost, A. P., Daly, M. J., Lander, E. S., and Jacob, H. J. (1996). Renal disease susceptibility and hypertension are under independent genetic control in the fawn-hooded rat. *Nature Genetics* **11**, 44–51.

Buccianti, G. *et al.* (1993). Unilateral nephrectomy and progression of renal failure. *Renal Failure* **15** (3), 415–420.

Chen, Y. H., Stapleton, F. B., Roy, S., and Noe, H. N. (1985). Neonatal hypertension from a unilateral multicystic dysplastic kidney. *Journal of Urology* **133**, 664–665.

Churchill, D., Kimoff, R., Pinski, M., and Gault, M. H. (1975). Solitary intrarenal cyst: correctable cause of hypertension. *Urology* **6**, 485–489.

Corigliano, B. E. and Leedom, J. M. Renal tuberculosis. In *Textbook of Nephrology* Vol. 2, 2nd edn. (ed. S. G. Massey and R. J. Glassock), pp. 687–691. Baltimore: Williams and Wilkins, 1983.

Craig, J. C., Irwig, L. M., Knight, J. F., and Roy, L. P. (2000). Does treatment of vesicoureteric reflux in childhood prevent end-stage renal disease attributable to reflux nephropathy? *Pediatrics* **105**, 1236–1241.

El Dahr, S. S., Gee, J., Dipp, S., Hanss, B. G., Vari, R. C., and Chao, J. (1993). Upregulation of renin–angiotensin system and downregulation of kallikrein in obstructive nephropathy. *American Journal of Physiology* **64** (5, Pt 2), F874–F881.

Farrell, J. I. and Young, R. H. (1942). Hypertension caused by unilateral renal compression. *Journal of the American Medical Association* **118**, 711–712.

Feather, S. A., Malcolm, S., Woolf A. S., Wright, V., Blaydon, D., Reid, C. J., Flinter, F. A., Proesmans, W., Devriendt, K., Carter, J., Warwicker, P., Goodship, T. H., and Goodship, J. A. (2000). Primary, nonsyndromic vesicoureteric reflux and its nephropathy is genetically heterogeneous, with a locus on chromosome 1. *American Journal of Human Genetics* **66**, 1420–1425.

Frohmüller, H. (1983). Erfahrungsbericht über die Therapie des stumpfen Nierentraumas. *Unfallchirurgie* **9**, 268–273.

Ganguly, A., Gribble, J., Tune, B., Kempson, R. L., and Luetscher, J. A. (1973). Renin-secreting Wilms' tumour with severe hypertension. *Annals of Internal Medicine* **79**, 835–857.

Goldblatt, H., Lynch, J., Hanzal, R. F., and Summerville, W. W. (1934). Persistent elevation of systolic blood pressure by means of renal ischemia. *Journal of Experimental Medicine* **59**, 347–379.

Goonasekera, C. D., Shah V., Wade, A. M., Barratt, T. M., and Dillon, M. J. (1996). 15-year follow-up of renin and blood pressure in reflux nephropathy. *Lancet* **347**, 640–643.

Greenberg, P. B., Martin, T. J., and Sutcliffe, H. J. (1973). Synthesis and release of parathyroid hormone by a renal carcinoma in cell culture. *Clinical Science and Molecular Medicine* **45**, 183–191.

Grim, C. E., Mullins, M. F., Nilson, J. P., and Ross, G., Jr. (1975). Unilateral 'Page Kidney' hypertension in man: studies of the renin–angiotensin–aldosterone system before and after nephrectomy. *Journal of the American Medical Association* **231**, 42–45.

Hakim, R. M., Goldszer, R. C., and Brenner, B. M. (1984). Hypertension and proteinuria: long-term sequelae of uninephrectomy in humans. *Kidney International* **25**, 930–936.

Hewlett, J. S., Hoffman, G. C., Senhauser, D. A., and Battle, J. D., Jr. (1956). Hypernephroma with erythrocythemia. Report of a case and assay of the tumour of an erythropoietic-stimulating substance. *New England Journal of Medicine* **262**, 1058–1062.

Hirose, M. *et al.* (1974). Primary reninism with renal hamartomatous alteration. *Journal of the American Medical Association* **230**, 1288–1292.

Horton, B. T. (1940). The relationship of hypertension to renal neoplasm. *Proceedings of the Staff Meetings of the Mayo Clinic* **15**, 472–474.

Jones, K.V. (1993). What is the current recommendation in the management of covert (significant) bacteriuria in infants and preschool children? *Pediatric Nephrology* **7**, 146.

Juncos, L. I., Carrasco-Duenas, S., Cornejo, J. C., Broglia, C. A., and Cejas, H. (1993). Long-term enalapril and hydrochlorothiazide in radiation nephritis. *Nephron* **64** (2), 249–255.

Kiprov, D. D., Colvin, R. B., and McCluskey, R. T. (1982). Focal and segmental glomerulosclerosis and proteinuria associated with unilateral renal agenesis. *Laboratory Investigation* **46**, 275–281.

Koh, C. J., Bochner, B. H., Stein, J.P., Fedenko, A. N., Dequattro, V., and Skinner, D. G. (2001). Norepinephrine producing renal cell carcinoma. *Journal of Urology* **166**, 603.

Küchel, O., Horky, K., Cantin, M., and Roy, P. (1993). Unilateral juxtaglomerular hyperplasia, hyperreninism and hypokalaemia. *Journal of Human Hypertension* **7** (1), 71–78.

Laberke, H.-G. *Reflux Nephropathy*. Stuttgart: Gustav Fischer Verlag, 1987.

Lama, G., Salsano, M. E., Pedulla', M., Grassia, C., and Ruocco, G. (1997). Angiotensin converting enzyme inhibitors and reflux nephropathy: 2-year follow-up. *Pediatric Nephrology* **11**, 714–718.

Lüscher, T. F., Wanner, C., Hauri, D., Siegenthaler, W., and Vetter, W. (1985). Curable renal parenchymatous hypertension: current diagnosis and management. *Cardiology* **72** (Suppl. 1), 33–45.

Lüscher, T. F., Wanner, C., Siegenthaler, W., and Vetter, W. (1986). Simple renal cyst and hypertension: cause or coincidence? *Clinical Nephrology* **26**, 91–95.

Lüscher, T. *et al.* (1981a). Rare forms of renal hypertension. *Klinische Wochenschrift* **59**, 35–45.

Lüscher, T. *et al.* (1981b). Renal venous renin activity in various forms of curable renal hypertension. *Clinical Nephrology* **15**, 314–320.

Maher, J. F. Radiation nephropathy. In *Textbook of Nephrology* Vol. 1, 2nd edn. (ed. S. G. Massey and R. J. Glassock), pp. 860–863. Baltimore: Williams and Wilkins, 1989.

Maling, T. J. B., Little, P. I., Maling, T. K. J., Gunesekera, A., and Bailey, R. R. (1975). Renal trauma and persitent hypertension. *Nephron* **16**, 173–180.

Maschio, G., Rugiu, C., Oldrizzi, L., and Lupo, A. (1987). Proteinuria, hypertension and renal failure in a patient with unilateral renal agenesis (clinical conference). *American Journal of Nephrology* **7**, 243–249.

Mast, G. J., Braedel, H. U., and Ziegler, M. Fakultativ einseitige Nierenerkrankungen—Renale Hypertonie aus urologischer Sicht. In *Lehrbuch der Hypertonie* (ed. D. Ganten and E. Ritz), pp. 548–566. Stuttgart: Schattauer, 1985.

McHugh, K., Stringer, D. A., Hebert, D., and Babiak, C. A. (1991). Simple renal cysts in children: diagnosis and follow-up with US. *Radiology* **178**, 383–385.

Melman, A., Grim, E. C., and Weinberger, M. H. (1977). Increased incidence of renal cell carcinoma with hypertension. *Journal of Urology* **118**, 531–532.

Menard, J., Soubrier, F., Bariety, J., Camilleri, J.-P., and Corvol, P. Primary reninism. In *Hypertension* 2nd edn. (ed. J. Genest, O. Kuchel, P. Hamet, and M. Cantin), pp. 1034–1039. New York: McGraw-Hill, 1983.

Mendez, R. (1977). Renal trauma. *Journal of Urology* **118**, 698–703.

Meyrier, A., Rainfray, M., and Lacombe, M. (1988). Delayed hypertension after blunt renal trauma. *American Journal of Nephrology* **8**, 108–111.

Mizuiri, S. *et al.* (1992). Hypertension in unilateral atrophic kidney secondary to ureteropelvic junction obstruction. *Nephron* **61**, 217–219.

Moriarty, K. P., Lipkowitz, G. S., and Germain, M. J. (1997). Capsulectomy: a cure for the Page kidney. *Journal of Pediatric Surgery* **32**, 831–833.

Morlock, C. G. and Horton, B. T. (1936). Variations in systolic blood pressure in renal tumours. A study of 491 cases. *American Journal of the Medical Sciences* **191**, 647–658.

Najarian, J. S., Chavers, B. M., McHugh, L. E., and Matas, A. J. (1992). 20 years or more of follow-up of living kidney donors. *Lancet* **2**, 807–810.

Olbing, H., Hirche, H., Koskimies, O., Lax, H., Seppanen, U., Smellie, J. M., Tamminen-Mobius, T., and Wikstad, I. (2000). Renal growth in children with severe vesicoureteral reflux: 10-year prospective study of medical and surgical treatment: the International Reflux Study in Children (European branch). *Radiology* **216**, 731–737.

Ozen, S., Alikasifoglu, M., Saatci, U., Bakkaloglu, A., Besbas, N., Kara, N., Kocak, H., Erbas, B., Unsal, I., and Tuncbilek, E. (1999). Implications of certain genetic polymorphisms in scarring in vesicoureteric reflux: importance of ACE polymorphism. *American Journal of Kidney Diseases* **34**, 140–145.

Page, I. H. (1939). The production of persistent arterial hypertension by cellophane perinephritis. *Journal of the American Medical Association* **113**, 2046–2048.

Paulino, A. C., Wen, B. C., Brown, C. K., Tannous, R., Mayr, N. A., Zhen, W. K., Weidner, G. J., and Hussey, D. H. (2000). Late effects in children treated with radiation therapy for Wilms' tumor. *Interactional Journal of Radiation, Oncology, Biology, Physics* **46**, 1239–1246.

Pedersen, J. F., Emamian, S. A., and Nielsen, M. B. (1993). Simple renal cyst: relations to age and arterial blood pressure. *British Journal of Radiology* **66**, 581–584.

Pillary, G., Folco, J. D., and Lee, W. J. (1975). Hypernephroma and hypertension. *New York State Journal of Medicine* **79**, 865–867.

Pintar, T. J. and Zimmerman, S. (1998). Hyperreninemic hypertension secondary to a subcapsular perinephric hematoma in a patient with polyarteritis nodosa. *American Journal of Kidney Diseases* **32**, 503–507.

Podjarny, E., Richter, S., Magen, H., Bachar, L., and Bernheim, J. (1986). High incidence of hypertension in older patients after unilateral nephrectomy. A retrospective study. *Israel Journal of Medical Sciences* **22**, 861–864.

Polito, C., La Manna, A., Rambaldi, P. F., Nappi, B., Mansi, L., and Di Toro, R. (2000). High incidence of a generally small kidney and primary vesicoureteral reflux. *Journal of Urology* **164**, 479–482.

Robertson, P. W., Klidjian, A., Harding, L. K., Walters, G., Lee, M. R., and Robb-Smith, A. H. T. (1967). Hypertension due to a renin-secreting renal tumor. *American Journal of Medicine* **43**, 963–967.

Robitaille, P., Lortie, L., Mongeau, J. G., and Sinnassamy, P. (1985). Long-term follow-up of patients who underwent unilateral nephrectomy in childhood. *Lancet* **1**, 1297–1299.

Roodhoft, A. M., Birnholz, J. C., and Holmes, L. B. (1984). Familial nature of congential absence and severe dysgenesis of both kidneys. *New England Journal of Medicine* **310**, 1341–1345.

Shapiro, A., Cavallo, T., Cooper, W., Lapenas, D., Bron., K., and Berg, G. (1977). Hypertension in radiation nephritis. *Archives of Internal Medicine* **137**, 848–851.

Simons, J. L., Provoost, A. P., De Keijzer, M. H., Anderson, S., Rennke, H. G., and Brenner, B. M. (1993). Pathogenesis of glomerular injury in the fawn-hooded rat: effect of unilateral nephrectomy. *Journal of the American Society of Nephrology* **4** (6), 1362–1370.

Smellie, J. M., Barratt, T. M., Chantler, C., Gordon, I., Prescod, N. P., Ransley, P. G., and Woolf, A. S. (2001). Medical versus surgical treatment in children with severe bilateral vesicoureteric reflux and bilateral nephropathy: a randomised trial. *Lancet* **357**, 1329–1333.

Smellie, J. M., Ransley, P. G., Normand, I. C., Prescod, N., and Edwards, D. (1985). Development of new renal scars: a collaborative study. *British Medical Journal (Clinical Research Edition)* **290**, 1957–1960.

Song, J. T., Ritchey, M. L., Zerin, J. M., and Bloom, D. A. (1995). Incidence of vesicoureteral reflux in children with unilateral renal agenesis. *Journal of Urology* **153** (4), 1249–1251.

Spark, R. F. and Berg, S. (1976). Renal trauma and hypertension. *Archives of Internal Medicine* **136**, 1097–1100.

Stefanidis, C. J. (2001). Reflux nephropathy in children. *Nephrology, Dialysis, Transplantation* **16** (Suppl. 6), 117–119.

Steffens, J., Bock, R., Braeder, H. U., Isenberg, E., Bührle, C. P., and Ziegler, M. (1992). Renin-producing renal cell carcinomas—clinical and experimental investigations on a special form of renal hypertension. *Urological Research* **20** (2), 111–115.

Stockamp, K., Wulff, H. D., Skoluda, D., Greinacher, I., and Schäfer, A. (1974). Die multizystische Nierendysplasie im Kindes- und Erwachsenenalter. *Deutsche Medizinische Wochenschrift* **15**, 734–738.

Studer, U. E. and Weidmann, P. (1984). Pathogenesis and treatment of hypertension in renal tuberculosis. *European Urology* **10**, 164–169.

Surana, R., Khan, A., and Fitzgerald, R. J. (1995). Scarring following renal trauma in children. *British Journal of Urology* **75**, 663–665.

Tada, S., Yamagishi, J., Kobayashi, H., Hata, Y., and Kobari, T. (1983). The incidence of simple renal cyst by computed tomography. *Clinical Radiology* **34**, 437–439.

Talseth, T. *et al.* (1986). Long-term blood pressure and renal function in kidney donors. *Kidney International* **29**, 1072–1076.

Von Knorring, J., Fyhrquist, F., and Ahonen, J. (1981). Varying course of hypertension following renal trauma. *Journal of Urology* **126**, 798–801.

Wanner, C. and Schollmeyer, P. Einseitige (heilbare) renalparenchymatöse Hypertonie. In *Aktuelle Nephrologie* 21 Jahrgang (ed. Fresenius-Stiftung), pp. 503–526. Bad Hamburg: Wissenschaftliche Informationen, 1988.

Wanner, C., Lüscher, T. F., Schollmeyer, P., and Vetter, W. (1987). Unilateral hydronephrosis and hypertension: cause or coincidence? *Nephron* **45**, 236–241.

Warnick, T. J., Jenkins, R. R., Rackoff, P., Baumgarten, A., and Bia, M. J. (1988). Microalbumin and hypertension in long-term renal donors. *Transplantation* **45**, 59–65.

Wennerstrom, M., Hansson, S., Jodal, U., and Stokland, E. (2000). Primary and acquired renal scarring in boys and girls with urinary tract infection. *Journal of Pediatrics* **136**, 30–34.

Wesson, L. W. (1982). Unilateral renal disease and hypertension. *Nephron* **32**, 1–7.

Whiting, J. C., Stanisic, T. H., and Drach, G. W. (1983). Congenital ureteral valves: report of 2 patients, including one with a solitary kidney and associated hypertension. *Journal of Urology* **129**, 1222–1224.

Yokoyama, H., Yamane, Y., Takahara, J., Yoshinouchi, T., and Ofuji, T. (1979). A case of ectopic renin-secreting orbital hemangiopericytoma associated with juvenile hypertension and hypokalemia. *Acta Medica, Okayama* **33**, 315–322.

9.7 Renovascular hypertension

B. Krumme, J.-R. Allenberg, I. Dulau-Florea, and J.F.E. Mann

Definition

Renovascular disease is the narrowing of the main renal artery or of one of its branches by atherosclerotic, fibromuscular, or by inflammatory lesions. It may cause renovascular hypertension as well as potentially reversible renal failure, also called ischaemic nephropathy. Renal artery disease may occur asymptomatic, in association with hypertension, renal insufficiency or both. Renovascular hypertension is chronically raised blood pressure due to a significant renal artery stenosis, which improves after correction of the stenosis. Ischaemic nephropathy refers to the loss of renal function or parenchyma on the basis of atherosclerotic renal artery stenosis. In this chapter we will focus on renovascular hypertension rather than on ischaemic nephropathy; however, several diagnostic and therapeutic procedures are similar in both entities.

Unfortunately, renovascular hypertension so defined inexorably links the apparent accuracy of the diagnostic tests to the adequacy of treatment. Its invasive treatment may have no effect on blood pressure because renovascular disease is also associated with essential hypertension. In addition, narrowing of the renal artery may initiate high blood pressure that is then perpetuated by other mechanisms. Perpetuating events may include muscular hypertrophy of resistance vessels and contralateral nephrosclerosis, which are independent of the triggering stenosis.

Epidemiology

The prevalence of renovascular disease in the *unselected*, hypertensive population is not precisely known; estimates vary widely between well below 1 and 4 per cent (Table 1). It is reasonable to suggest that in referral centres 2–5 per cent of hypertensive patients might have renovascular hypertension, which is not complementary to renovascular disease. In a study involving more than 5000 hypertensive patients, renal artery stenosis was identified in 4 per cent, however, not all these patients had arteriography; only 67 (1.3 per cent of the total) underwent surgery (Gifford 1969). In another study of similar size, 0.18 per cent of hypertensives had an operable stenosis (Tucker and Labarthe 1977). Sinclair *et al.* (1987) investigated 3783 patients attending the Glasgow Blood Pressure Clinic, and found that 0.7 per cent of the hypertensives had renovascular disease. With the use of the saralasin test, Anderson *et al.* (1988) found 3 per cent renovascular hypertension among 3520 unselected hypertensive patients.

Table 1 Prevalence of renovascular disease among hypertensive populations

Reference	*n*	Prevalence (%)
Gifford (1969)	5000	4
Tucker and Labarthe (1977)	5000	0.18[a]
Berglund *et al.* (1976)	700	0.6
Atkinson (1974)	985	0[b]
Sinclair *et al.* (1987)	3783	0.7

[a] Percentage of patients referred to invasive treatment.

[b] Urography in all cases.

In non-selected autopsies, the prevalence of severe renal artery stenosis in patients who had died at less than 64 years was 5 per cent (Schwartz and White 1964). Among those who had died aged 64–74 years, the prevalence was 18 per cent, and the prevalence increased to 42 per cent for those who had died aged 75 years and more. In another large series of 5194 consecutive autopsies renal artery stenosis greater than 50 per cent was found in 4.3 per cent of all cases (Sawicki *et al.* 1991). Over 30 years ago, Holley *et al.* (1964) reported a 27 per cent overall prevalence of renal artery stenosis among 295 autopsies during a 10-month period. In a recent series of 2167 consecutive autopsies, 346 patients with clinical evidence of stroke were investigated and high grade renal artery stenosis was found in 10 per cent of cases (Kuroda *et al.* 2000).

The above data refer to adults, as does the remainder of this chapter. For renovascular disease in children, the reader is referred to Chapter 9.9 of this volume and to an extensive review of Ingelfinger (1993).

In certain subsets of the hypertensive population, renovascular disease is apparently much more frequent. Such populations include patients with grade III or IV retinopathy (Davies *et al.* 1979), in which the prevalence of renal artery stenosis was 43 per cent in Whites and 7 per cent in Blacks (total, 123 patients). Ying *et al.* (1984) detected stenosis of the renal artery in a quarter of more than 100 consecutive cases with hypertension that was 'difficult to control'. In this population, 21 patients had azotaemia; among these, 10 suffered from stenosis of the renal artery.

Atherosclerotic renal artery stenosis often coexists with peripheral vascular and aortic disease regardless of the presence of hypertension. In a prospective study of 395 aortic angiograms, done for the evaluation of peripheral vascular disease, Olin *et al.* (1990) found renal artery stenosis greater than 50 per cent in 38 per cent of the patients with abdominal aneurysms, in 33 per cent with aorto-occlusive disease and in 39 per cent with peripheral vascular disease. Similar results with 346 angiograms were reported by Valentine *et al.* (1993): renal artery stenosis greater than 50 per cent was present in 21 (29 per cent) patients with abdominal aneurysm, in 34 (26 per cent) patients with aorto-occlusive disease and in 43 (30 per cent) patients with peripheral vascular disease.

Likewise, patients with suspected coronary heart disease have a high prevalence of renal artery stenosis. In a consecutive series of 1235 patients referred for coronary angiography, renal artery stenosis greater than 50 per cent on aortography was detected in 188 (15 per cent). Hypertension only occurred in 100 (53 per cent) of these patients and failed to be a predictor for renal artery stenosis in this population (Harding *et al.* 1992). In a review collecting data from 11 angiographic studies among 3698 patients with peripheral or coronary atherosclerosis, the prevalence of unsuspected renal artery stenosis was 23 per cent (Greco and Breyer 1996).

When patients with one of several citeria (see Table 4) of renovascular disease were selected for clinical work-up, Fommei *et al.* (1991), Setaro *et al.* (1991), and Svetkey *et al.* (1989) detected 51, 54, and 22 per cent renovascular hypertension among 113, 424, and 140 patients, respectively, with clinical signs suggestive of the disease. The prevalence of renovascular hypertension is generally assumed to be lower in black Americans than in whites (Davies *et al.* 1979; Keith 1982). This assumption may be erroneous and may reflect the zeal with which the diagnosis is pursued in Black hypertensives.

In summary, renovascular disease is much more frequent than expected; however, renovascular hypertension is rare. This paradox is the dilemma of screening procedures (Salvetti *et al.* 1996) and of the stratification of different therapies (Plouin *et al.* 2001).

Aetiology

Renal artery stenosis may be due to one of several causes (Table 2). More than 90 per cent of cases are related to either atherosclerosis or fibromuscular dysplasia. In a study of 884 patients with renovascular hypertension (US Cooperative Study of renovascular hypertension; Bookstein *et al.* 1972a,b), one-third had fibromuscular dysplasia and two-thirds had atherosclerotic stenosis; this proportion is similar to that found in other studies (e.g. Sos *et al.* 1983; Kuhlmann *et al.* 1985). In our own (unpublished) series of more than 300 cases, fibromuscular disease was only found in 15 per cent. The exact prevalence depends on patient selection and referral population.

Other causes of renovascular disease (Table 2) are uncommon (Stair *et al.* 1990). These include thrombosis or embolism of a renal artery, intimal flaps after abdominal trauma, dissection of the renal artery (Fig. 1), coarctation of the aorta, inflammatory stenosis as with Takayashu's disease as well as aneurysms (Fig. 2) and tumours (including phaeochromocytomas). In children, fibromuscular dysplasia and coarctation of the aorta are more common than in adults. Further, in countries with a high prevalence of Takayashu's or Kawasaki's arteritis, these are a more frequent cause.

Table 2 Aetiology of renovascular hypertension

Atherosclerosis (*ca.* 75% of cases)
Fibromuscular dysplasia (*ca.* 15% of cases)
Dissecting aneurysms of the aorta
Dissecting aneurysms of the renal artery
Arteritis (e.g. Takayashu's arteritis)
Coarctation of the aorta
Renal thrombosis and embolism
Abdominal trauma with intimal tears
Arteriovenous fistulas
External compression by tumours
After renal transplantation
After radiation therapy
von Recklinghausen's disease
Angiomas

Pathological and radiological aspects

Atherosclerotic stenosis

Stenosis is usually located in the proximal 2–3 cm of the renal artery. Frequently aortic plaques are protruding into the ostial lumen of the renal artery. For example, ostial involvement was reported in three-fourths of 109 patients by Wollenweber *et al.* (1968), in 50 out of 125 by Canzanello *et al.* (1989), and in one-third of cases by Sos *et al.* (1983). The lesions are commonly bilateral: bilateral disease proved to be present in two-thirds of 109 cases reported by Wollenweber *et al.* (1968), in one-third of 884 cases in the US Cooperative Study (Bookstein *et al.* 1972a,b), and in about one-third of 100 cases investigated by Canzanello *et al.* (1989), where 30 per cent of cases also had only one functioning kidney. There is no agreement as to whether atherosclerotic lesions predominantly occur on the left or on the right (Wollenweber *et al.* 1968; Bookstein *et al.* 1972a,b). Segmental lesions were carefully looked

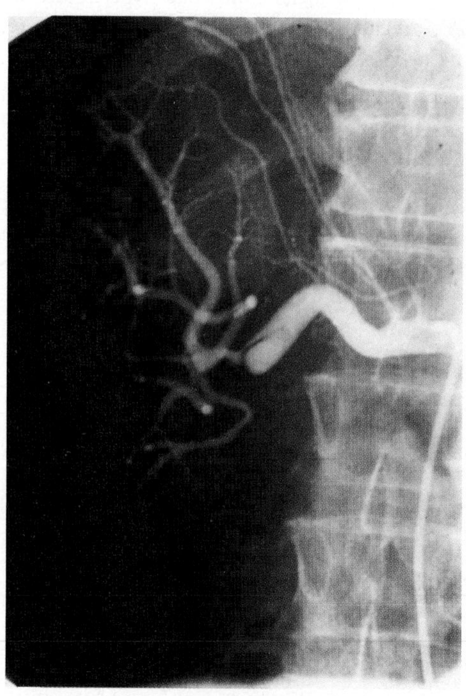

Fig. 1 Angiogram of the right renal artery showing a dissection in the distal part of the main artery. Intrarenal blood flow is almost absent.

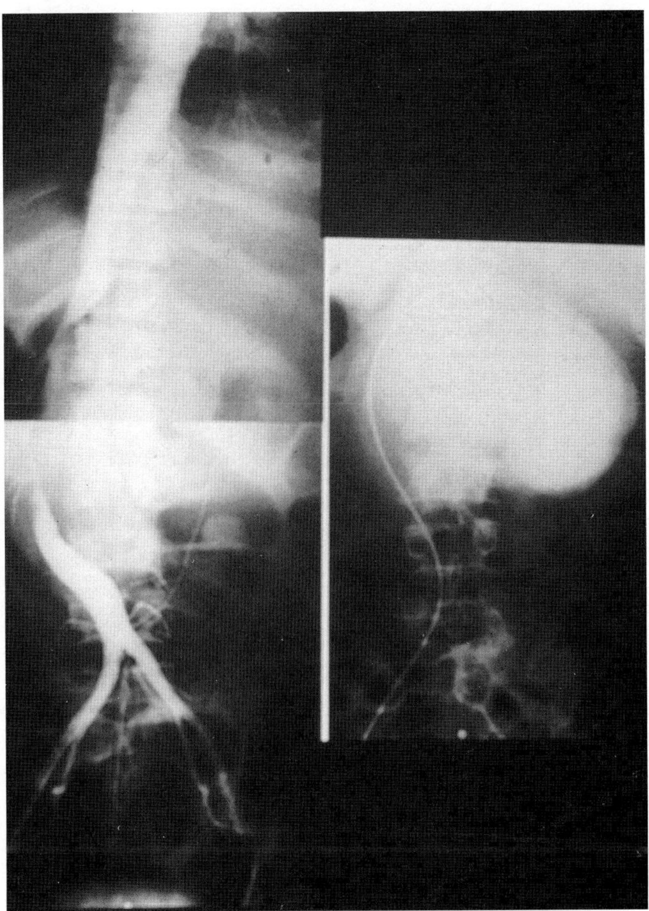

Fig. 2 Large aneurysm of the left renal artery leading to displacement and obstruction of the aorta. The diagnosis was confirmed at operation.

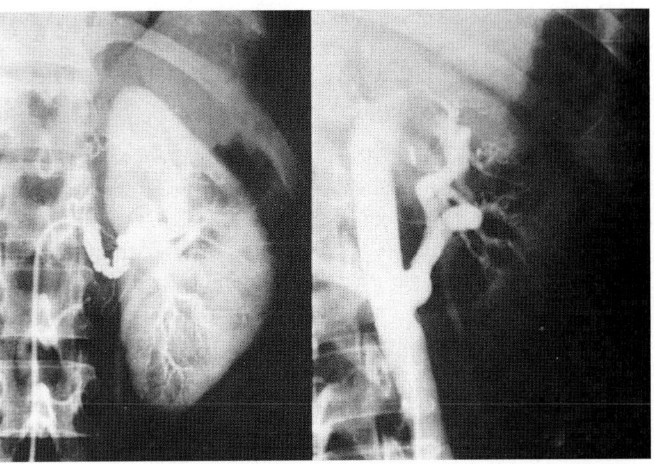

Fig. 3 Typical angiographic aspect of fibromuscular dysplasia. An angiogram recorded 2 years after operation is shown on the right-hand side. A double saphenous vein bypass to both segmental arteries was implanted.

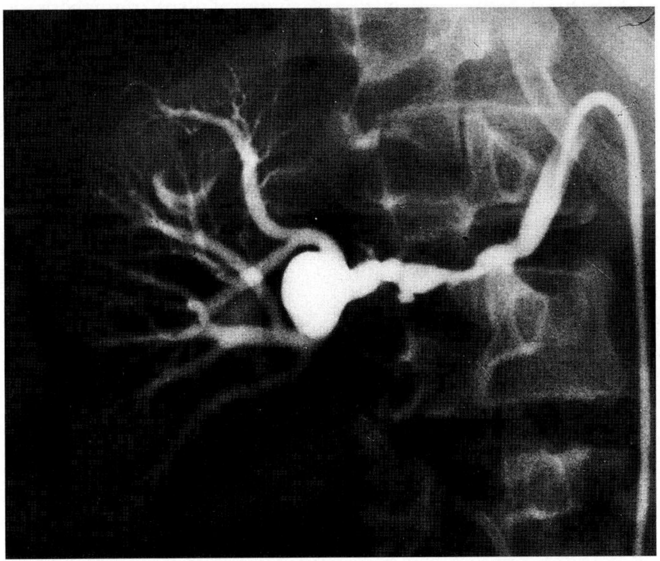

Fig. 4 Renal artery aneurysm combined with fibromuscular disease.

for in at least one large study and found in 10 per cent of patients (Bookstein *et al.* 1972a,b).

With increasing severity of stenosis, post-stenotic dilation and collateral circulation develop in the majority of patients (Bookstein *et al.* 1972a,b). However, it must be appreciated that the degree of stenosis seen by angiography is only a rough estimate of the reduction in vessel diameter. Recently, three independent studies evaluated interobserver variability between different radiologists for the grading of renal artery stenosis with intra-arterial renal angiography (Paul *et al.* 1999; Schreij *et al.* 1999; van Jaarsveld *et al.* 1999). Interobserver agreement in defining the severity of renal artery stenosis was poor. Kappa-values below 0.40 were reported. Especially excentric stenoses can be misleading. Therefore, the future diagnostic gold standard may be three-dimensional (3D) imaging and haemodynamic information from magnetic resonance imaging (MRI) studies.

Fibromuscular dysplasia

This is usually classified according to the criteria of Harrison and McCormack (1971). Lesions within the medial muscular layer are the major cause of this disease in adults (Fig. 3) and may also occur concomitantly in other arterial beds. In medial fibroplasia (60 per cent of fibromuscular dysplasias), there are areas of medial thickening and fibrosis alternating with aneurysmal dilation; this pattern leads to the typical beaded appearance on angiograms (Fig. 4). The diameter of the aneurysmal dilation may exceed that of the normal vessel (Harrison and McCormack 1971). In perimedial fibroplasia, the outer half of the media is involved, with proliferation of fibrous tissue and moderate, poststenotic aneurysmal dilation. However, in this form of fibromuscular hyperplasia, aneurysms are less common than in medial fibroplasia. The other types of fibromuscular dysplasia are rare. It is not clear whether histological subtypes of dysplasia can be differentiated angiographically. In a study by Scott *et al.* (1983), which involved six experienced radiologists, only 62 per cent of medial fibroplasias and 46 per cent of perimedial fibroplasias were correctly diagnosed from the angiogram alone (postoperative histology as 'gold standard').

In the US Cooperative Study (Bookstein *et al.* 1972a,b), fibromuscular dysplasia was predominantly found on the right side (two-thirds of cases). In 60 per cent of cases, involvement included the middle and distal third of the vessel; in 30 per cent the proximal third or the orifice of the main renal artery was involved; in less than 10 per cent segmental renal arteries were involved. About one-fourth of the fibromuscular lesions were bilateral.

Differential diagnosis

For purposes of differential diagnosis, the presence of aortic atherosclerosis is an excellent means of distinguishing between atherosclerotic and fibromuscular stenosis of the renal artery. Thus, Scott *et al.* (1983) found that stenosis in the absence of atherosclerosis of the abdominal aorta is almost always associated with fibromuscular disease. On the other hand, 90 per cent of atherosclerotic lesions in the renal artery are accompanied by aortic atherosclerosis. In Scott's study, all specimens of the renal artery were investigated histologically. A few cases of fibromuscular disease may be accompanied by some concomitant aortic atherosclerosis.

Occlusion of a renal artery by thrombosis or embolism

Thrombotic or embolic occlusion of the renal artery may cause hypertension; this is an uncommon finding but has been documented in a substantial number of unselected autopsies. Renal thrombosis or embolism may follow abdominal trauma, renal angiography, or angioplasty. It may also be associated with aneurysms or dissections of the aorta or of the renal arteries, and may be a consequence of other diseases such as vasculitis (including Takayashu's arteritis), atrial fibrillation, and neurofibromatosis. As outlined below, acute occlusion of the renal artery with flank pain is a medical emergency, which nonetheless is frequently overlooked or misdiagnosed as nephrolithiasis.

Aneurysms

Aneurysms of the renal artery have been described in both normotensives and hypertensives. High blood pressure may be a consequence of, or may contribute to, the development of such aneurysms. If hypertension is a consequence, stenosis of the adjacent vascular bed or microembolism of the kidney may be responsible for it. The aneurysms may be accompanied by vascular stenoses (Fig. 4), may increase in size, and may subsequently be mistaken for tumours or cysts. There is a definite risk of rupture for aneurysms that are greater than 2–3 cm in diameter. Pregnant women are especially at risk for this complication. As shown in Fig. 5, spontaneous involution of such aneurysms may also occur.

Other conditions

With the exception of Takayashu's disease, arteritis is rarely associated with stenosis of the renal artery and subsequent hypertension. Radiation therapy may lead to a atherosclerotic stenosis of vessels within the radiation field (Plouin *et al.* 2001). Stenosis of the renal artery after renal transplantation is discussed separately in this volume.

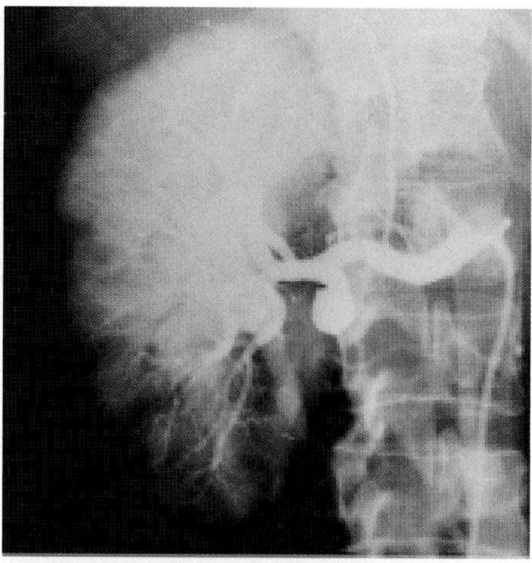

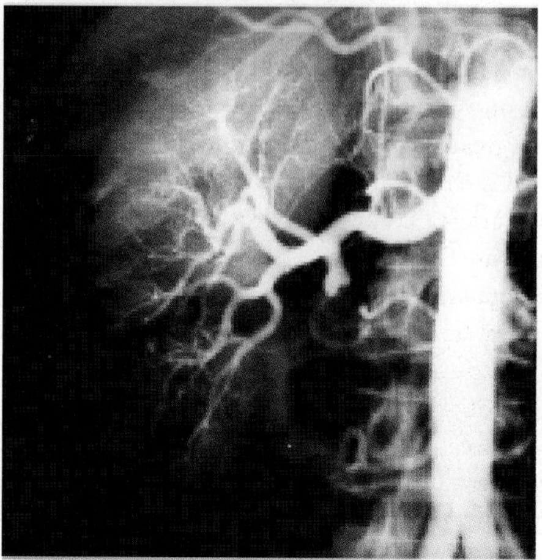

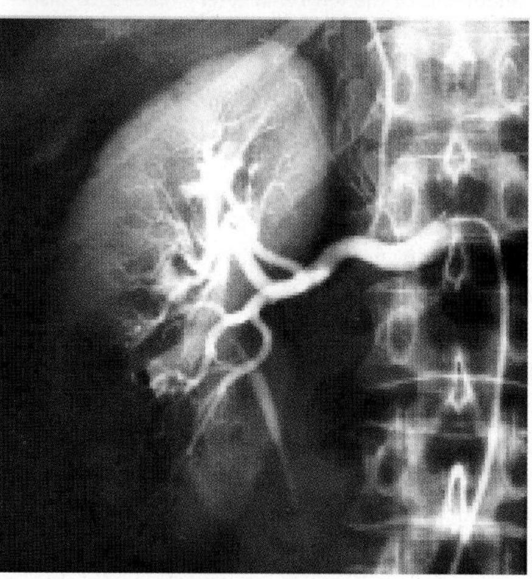

Fig. 5 Aneurysm of a right renal artery showing spontaneous regression from 1979 (top), to 1982 (middle), to 1985 (bottom).

Natural history

Atherosclerotic renovascular disease

The natural history of this condition is one of more or less relentless progression. Schreiber *et al.* (1984) retrospectively identified and followed up 85 patients with atherosclerotic, renovascular disease at the Cleveland Clinic. These patients had had two or more renal angiograms between 1960 and 1979 (Table 3). After a mean follow-up of 2 years, 39 per cent of those with 75–99 per cent stenosis progressed to complete occlusion. In those with 50–75 per cent stenosis, progression was found in almost half, with total occlusion in 10 per cent. In those with stenosis of less than 50 per cent, progression was observed in one-third. Schreiber also found that control of the blood pressure did not correlate with angiographically demonstrated progression. These data

Table 3 Progression of atherosclerotic renovascular stenosis

Original luminal narrowing (%)	*n*	No progression (%)	Progression without total occlusion (%)	Progression to occlusion (%)
75–99	18	61	—	39
50–75	30	53	37	10
<50	78	69	26	5

Adapted from Schreiber *et al.* (1984) who reviewed original and repeat renal angiograms after a mean follow-up of 2 years in 85 patients.

are in agreement with newer observations using noninvasive Duplex sonography for follow-up (Caps *et al.* 1998a). In 170 patients, the 3-year cumulative incidence of progression of renal artery stenosis initially classified as normal, below 60 per cent and greater than 60 per cent was 18, 28, and 49 per cent, respectively. Baseline factors such as renal artery stenosis greater than 60 per cent, diabetes mellitus, systolic blood pressure greater than 160 mmHg, as well as contralateral disease were associated with disease progression. However, in this population only nine renal artery occlusions occurred, exclusively in patients with high grad stenosis (Caps *et al.* 1998a).

Dean (1986) randomly allocated 48 patients with renovascular hypertension to medical treatment without surgical intervention. After a mean follow-up of 3 years, they found a decrease in the functioning renal mass in 18 of the 48 patients. In 17 patients there was a loss of renal length; another had a doubling of the serum creatinine. In a further observational study of 122 patients with renal artery stenosis the appearance of renal atrophy clearly correlated with elevations of serum creatinine concentrations (Caps *et al.* 1998b). Several studies confirmed the agressive nature of atherosclerotic renal artery stenosis in many but not all patients (Tollefson and Ernst 1991; Guzman *et al.* 1994; Zierler *et al.* 1994; Hupp and Allenberg 1995). These findings suggest that even optimal medical treatment does not prevent the progression to occlusion.

Anatomic progression of renovascular stenosis, however, is not necessarily associated with a high rate of endstage renal failure. Leertouwer *et al.* (2001) retrospectively studied 386 consecutive patients who underwent digital substraction angiography because of peripheral vascular disease, in whom incidental renal artery stenosis was detected in 126 people. None of the patients with or without renal artery stenosis, which was left untreated, developed endstage renal disease over a 8–10 year follow-up period. This finding is explained by the high rate of cardiovascular death in patients with atherosclerotic renal artery stenosis before reaching endstage renal disease, by the formation of collaterals of the renal artery and by the fact that the extent of renal insufficiency is primarily determined by intrarenal nephrosclerosis, not by the stenosis of the main renal artery.

Cholesterol embolism may have a major impact on the long-term prognosis of renal function in patients with atherosclerotic renal artery stenosis. The release of cholesterol plaques can occur spontaneously or more often after intravascular trauma with angiographic catheters or after the use of anticoagulants and thrombolytic agents. In the extensive review of Modi and Rao (2001), the incidence of atheroembolic renal disease ranges between 1.1 and 30 per cent after angiography, depending on the study population and on the diagnostic procedures of the various studies. Eosinophilia, hypocomplementaemia as well as increased levels of C-reactive protein may be present, however, these signs lack specificity and sensitivity. Meyrier *et al.* (1988) observed 30 patients with renal insufficiency who had atherosclerotic stenosis of the renal artery. Eight of these patients had biopsy-proven cholesterol embolism. There were two additional cases with such embolism but without a stenosis; both patients had heavily diseased aortas. Only five of the 10 patients with cholesterol embolism exhibited eosinophilia, and two of eight hypocomplementaemia.

The presence of atheroembolic renal disease also influences the patient survival after surgical revascularization of renal artery stenosis. In a group of 44 patients in whom concomitant intraoperative renal biopsy was performed, the 16 patients (36 per cent) with atheroembolic renal disease had significantly decreased 5-year survival of 54 versus 85 per cent in patients without atheroembolic renal disease (Krishnamurthi *et al.* 1999).

Atherosclerotic renovascular disease is an independent predictor for mortality in patients with endstage renal disease (Mailloux *et al.* 1994) and in patients undergoing coronary angiography (Conlon *et al.* 2001). In a population of 683 dialysis patients, the 83 patients with renovascular disease had the worst survival estimates, with a 25-month median survival and 5- and 10-year survival rates of 18 and 5 per cent, respectively (Mailloux *et al.* 1994). In a large cohort of 3987 patients with routinely performed abdominal aortography after coronary angiography, the presence and severity of renal artery stenosis was an independent predictor of all-cause mortality (Conlon *et al.* 2001). Significant renal artery stenosis, defined as greater than 75 per cent in this study was associated with a 4-year survival rate of 57 per cent. In contrast to previous studies (Harding *et al.* 1992), hypertension was strongly related to the presence of stenosis with more than 75 per cent luminal narrowing (Conlon *et al.* 2001). The nature of the link between atherosclerotic renal artery stenosis and mortality may be explained by several reasons. Renal artery stenosis may reflect more widespread atherosclerosis, severe hypertension and an increased activity of the renin–angiotensin system which is known to be associated with accelerated atherogenesis and left ventricular hypertrophy.

Older studies did also report a reduced survival rate of patients with atherosclerotic renal artery stenosis. Wollenweber *et al.* (1968) reported a significantly reduced 5-year survival of 66 per cent in their 109 patients as opposed to an expected actuarial rate of 92 per cent in a normal population. The rate was improved with better control of blood pressure, irrespective of the mode of treatment (surgical or medical). However, patients treated by surgery had lower blood pressure.

Fibromuscular dysplasia

The natural history of this dysplasia of the renal arteries is not well delineated since most patients are invasively treated. In one study of 42 patients, all had progressive disease during a follow-up period ranging from 1 month to 11 years. Almost 50 per cent of the patients were male and the lesions were bilateral in 79 per cent. A decrease in the size of the kidney of more than 0.5 cm occurred in 62 per cent; total occlusion was seen in one-fourth. Histological proof of fibromuscular dysplasia was subsequently obtained in 16 of these 42 patients (Goncharenko *et al.* 1981). Contrary to previous assumptions (Meaney *et al.* 1968), Goncharenko also found that all types of fibromuscular dysplasia may progress, independent of age, and may lead to total occlusion of the affected vessel. Pohl and Novick (1985) also described progression of fibromuscular renal artery disease in one-third of their patients but no occlusion.

Pathophysiology

Concepts of the pathophysiology and pathogenesis of renovascular hypertension are largely derived from animal experiments and stem from the pioneering work of Goldblatt *et al.* (1934). However, it is not clear which animal models are equivalent to the human state and to what extent findings in animals are applicable to man. Renal artery stenosis in animals is induced acutely whereas in man the lesions develop gradually. There are species-specific differences in the arterial blood supply of the kidney in mammals. In addition, the renovascular hypertension involving one of two kidneys, the one clip (2K1C)-type, is easily induced in rats but not sustainable in primates (Hofbauer and Wood 1988). The following models of renovascular hypertension are commonly used: two kidney–one clip (2K1C), two kidney–two clip (2K2C), one kidney–one clip (1K1C), and coarctation of the aorta between or above the renal arteries.

Renin–angiotensin involvement

Experimental models

There is firm evidence that the renin–angiotensin system plays a primary role in the initial phase of all types of renovascular hypertension. Several days or weeks after acute stenosis of the renal artery, the involvement of the renin system becomes less obvious. In the 1K1C model, blood pressure is only initially dependent on release of renin. Thereafter, retention of sodium and volume supervene and contribute to the high blood pressure. Depending on the extent of volume retention, and of blood pressure, release of renin diminishes and is then less involved in the maintenance of hypertension (Dargie *et al.* 1977). Other investigators have suggested that the activity of the renal nerves is increased in models of renovascular hypertension. Renal denervation has been shown to lower blood pressure (Katholi *et al.* 1982). In the chronic phase of the 2K1C model, renin levels tend to decline if the stenosis is of moderate degree but remain elevated with a higher grade of stenosis. The contribution of renin to the maintenance of hypertension in this phase may only be appreciated by prolonged administration of angiotensin II-receptor antagonists (Riegger *et al.* 1977). This observation indicates a 'slow pressor effect' of angiotensin II, which is not easily appreciated in acute studies. This effect may also be due to actions of angiotensin II on the central nervous system (Mann *et al.* 1978; Luft *et al.* 1989).

In the 2K1C model, the unclipped kidney is exposed to high pressure and excretes more sodium than the clipped kidney. In the rat, sodium losses may be so large that they must be replaced orally by a 2 per cent NaCl solution (Gross *et al.* 1975). Davies *et al.* (1983) made the interesting observation that the higher the blood pressure in humans with unilateral renovascular hypertension, the lower the total body sodium. In this situation, loss of sodium may further stimulate release of renin, which in turn contributes to even higher blood pressure and enhances further loss of sodium, so forming a vicious circle. Administration of sodium may be beneficial in this particular malignant hypertension (Gross *et al.* 1975). Vasopressin may also play a role in a malignant phase of 2K1C hypertension (Möhring *et al.* 1978), although the involvement of vasopressin has not been a universal finding (Rabito *et al.* 1981). As in the 1K1C model, there is evidence that the sympathetic nervous system and the renal nerves are involved in 2K1C renovascular hypertension in the rat (Dargie *et al.* 1977; Katholi *et al.* 1982). The role of afferent and efferent renal nerves, as well as involvement by the central nervous system, are discussed elsewhere (DiBona 1982; Faber and Brody 1985).

In 2K1C rats acute renal artery stenosis caused ipsilaterally acute upregulation and contralaterally downregulation of juxtaglomerular cyclooxygenase-2 (COX-2) expression. However, COX-2 blocker celecoxib did not change renin mRNA either in the clipped or in the contralateral intact kidney, indicating that COX-2-derived prostaglandins do not control renin expression during renal hypoperfusion (Mann *et al.* 2001).

With the 2K2C model some cases are similar to 1K1C renovascular hypertension, while others are more like the 2K1C model, depending on the extent of each stenosis (Mann *et al.* 1978).

Human disease

In humans the pathogenesis of renovascular hypertension is not fully elucidated. It must be appreciated that many patients with submaximal stenosis of the renal arteries do not develop hypertension (Van Velzer *et al.* 1961; Eyler *et al.* 1962; Holley *et al.* 1964). It is not obvious what differentiates patients developing hypertension from those who do not despite occlusive disease of the renal artery. The plasma renin is raised in the majority of patients with renovascular hypertension but clearly not in all of them (Breslin *et al.* 1982; Vaughan 1985; Müller *et al.* 1986). The response of the blood pressure to the inhibition of angiotensin II by converting enzyme inhibitors is not consistently enhanced in human renovascular hypertension (see Müller *et al.* 1986). It has been reasoned that whenever plasma renin is normal or low in renovascular hypertension, blood pressure is volume dependent (Brunner *et al.* 1971; Pickering *et al.* 1988a). However, it is not clear whether or not the volume–renin relationship, an accepted mechanism of physiological regulation, is altered in renovascular hypertension to the effect that renin levels are inappropriately raised for a given sodium–volume relationship. In addition, the regulation of blood pressure in renovascular hypertension is certainly more complex than can be appreciated from renin and volume status alone.

Other factors

The role of hormonal factors other than renin (e.g. endothelin, catecholamines) in human renovascular hypertension is poorly understood. There is some evidence that catecholamines are at least not suppressed and do contribute to maintenance of the blood pressure (Maslowski *et al.* 1983; Mathias *et al.* 1983). The role of vasodilatory substances (e.g. ANF, NO, kinins, prostaglandins) remains to be determined.

An association between nephroptosis and renovascular hypertension of the fibromuscular type has often been described (Kaufmann 1979). This association is discussed in detail by Pickering *et al.* (1988b). It is questionable whether this clinical association is more than a coincidence, because only half of the patients with fibromuscular dysplasia have enhanced mobility of the kidney. Moreover, most patients with enhanced mobility are not hypertensive.

There is some evidence that those with renovascular hypertension have more left ventricular dilatation and more cardiac hypertrophy than those with essential hypertension at similar degrees of blood pressure (Textor *et al.* 1983). This effect may be due to specific cardiotrophic effects of the renin system (Karam *et al.* 1989), or to the sympathetic nervous system, or to the fact that despite the similar blood pressures at any one measurement, pressure 'load' over 24 h is greater in secondary than in primary hypertension. An altered pattern of diurnal blood pressure elevation was shown by repetitive blood pressure measurements (Vetter *et al.* 1990).

There is also some evidence that angiotensin-converting enzyme (ACE) polymorphisms are related to the occurrence of atherosclerotic renal artery stenosis. Fifty-eight patients with angiographically documented renal artery stenosis had a significantly higher D allele frequency of the ACE gene than did the control population of 102 normotensive subjects without any evidence of atherosclerosis. A total of 48.3 per cent of patients were homozygous for the D-genotype suggesting a predisposing role for this ACE genetic polymorphism in the development and progression of atherosclerotic renal artery stenosis (Olivieri *et al.* 1999).

Diagnosis

Clinical characteristics

There are clinical characteristics that suggest the presence of renovascular disease (Working Group on Renovascular Hypertension 1987; Table 4). Unfortunately, none of these features is particularly specific. About half of the patients with atherosclerotic renal artery stenosis have abdominal or flank bruits; however, these are also found in 7 per cent of those with essential hypertension (Breslin *et al.* 1982). These bruits are characteristically heard only during systole and may be rather soft. The presence of a diastolic component greatly increases the likelihood of renal artery stenosis. The test is not sensitive but is moderately specific (Grim *et al.* 1979; England *et al.* 1988).

The blood pressure level may be a further indicator for the presence of renal artery stenosis in hypertensive patients. In 355 patients selected for renal arteriography clinical and biochemical criteria were tested to predict renal artery stenosis. Systolic and diastolic blood pressure on automatic recording above 160 and 100 mmHg, respectively, despite antihypertensive therapy was associated with a 30 per cent prevalence of renal artery stenosis (Bijlstra *et al.* 1996). The number of antihypertensive drugs needed to control hypertension is another simple but useful criterion to identify patients with renal artery stenosis. In a prospective study of 217 patients selected for arteriography the criterion of drug resistant hypertension (diastolic blood pressure > 95 mmHg with more than two antihypertensive drugs) revealed a 19 per cent prevalence of patients with renal artery stenosis greater than 50 per cent (Derkx *et al.* 1996).

Table 4 Clinical clues for renovascular hypertension

Accelerated, treatment-refractory, or malignant hypertension
Hypertension with peripheral vascular occlusive disease, with coronary artery disease, or with other signs of generalized arteriosclerosis
Moderate to severe hypertension beginning before the age of 30 or after the age of 50
Sudden worsening of hypertension or renal function
Decrease of glomerular filtration rate with inhibition of the renin system
Hypertension with unexplained renal failure
Unilaterally small kidney
Abdominal bruits

Age and the duration of hypertension may also have diagnostic significance. Simon *et al.* (1972) compared patients with essential hypertension and those with renovascular disease (see Table 2). They found that those with renovascular hypertension tended to have disease of more recent onset, were more likely to develop disease after the age of 50 years, slightly less commonly had a family history of hypertension, and had a more severe retinopathy than those with essential hypertension. Proteinuria, which may reach nephrotic range, was also more prevalent in renovascular than in essential hypertension. In a series of 34 patients with atherosclerotic renal artery stenosis (Meyrier *et al.* 1988), proteinuria from greater than 1 to 4 g/day was found in 13, of less than 1 g/day in 15, and no proteinuria (<250 mg/day) in four patients. We have seen a 37-year-old female patient with unilateral fibromuscular disease and proteinuria of 4.5–6 g/day; this abated completely after successful transluminal renal angioplasty.

An increased urinary *N*-acetyl-glucosaminidase excretion has been advocated as a useful marker for the presence of renovascular hypertension. However, the observation could not be reproduced in an animal model (Luft *et al.* 1979).

In the US Cooperative Study, patients with fibromuscular disease had a mean age of 35 years (Simon *et al.* 1972); most were female, as was also reported in a Swiss study of 96 patients (Lüscher *et al.* 1985). In another series of 42 somewhat older patients (mean age 49 years), there was only a slight predominance of females (Goncharenko *et al.* 1981).

Patients with atherosclerotic renal disease are usually older than those with fibromuscular disease. A mean age of 50 years was found in the co-operative study (Simon *et al.* 1972), of 58 years by Canzanello *et al.* (1989), and of 53 years by Wollenweber *et al.* (1968). Recent studies, in accordance with our own experience report a higher mean age (>60 years) of patients presenting with atherosclerotic renal artery stenosis (van Jaarsveld *et al.* 2000; Radermacher *et al.* 2001a).

Atherosclerotic renal disease is somewhat more common in males than in females (Wollenweber *et al.* 1968; Simon *et al.* 1972; Canzanello *et al.* 1989). Patients with renovascular hypertension tend to be less obese than matched patients with essential hypertension, and the vast majority are smokers (Nicholson *et al.* 1983).

As mentioned earlier, those with atherosclerotic renovascular hypertension typically have signs and symptoms of atherosclerosis in other vascular beds. We undertook renal angiography in 100 consecutive patients with hypertension and angina pectoris who underwent coronary angiography. Sixty-six of them were found to have coronary heart disease; six also had renovascular hypertension (Mann *et al.*, unpublished). Even higher prevalence of renovascular disease with coronary arteriosclerosis (Vetrovec *et al.* 1984; Jean *et al.* 1994)—and vice versa (Louie *et al.* 1994)—was described. The prevalence of renovascular hypertension is also increased in patients with intermittent claudication, mesenteric arterial obstruction, and occlusive disease of the carotid arteries (Carlsson *et al.* 1963; Hardin 1965; Schwartz 1965; Kuhlmann *et al.* 1983; Priollet *et al.* 1990; Missouris *et al.* 1994).

In fibromuscular hyperplasia, other vascular beds may also be involved. Such involvement includes predominantly the carotid arteries, but also the subclavian, coronary, mesenteric, and iliacofemoral arteries (Lüscher *et al.* 1985).

Several clinical indicators may suggest the presence of renovascular hypertension (Table 4). The occurrence of renovascular disease in patients presenting with congestive heart failure is particularly noteworthy because the treatment of such patients often includes inhibitors of angiotensin I-converting enzyme (ACE). These agents may not be tolerated in this clinical setting, particularly if the stenosis of the renal artery is bilateral. Meissner *et al.* (1988) found that six of 89 consecutive patients with congestive heart failure had renal artery stenosis; only three of the six had high blood pressure. We found a similar patient who did not tolerate reduction of afterload with ACE inhibitors but did so after successful transluminal angioplasty of his stenotic renal artery. Consequently, we advise concomitant angiography of the renal arteries in patients with congestive heart failure who undergo diagnostic coronary angiography.

It is increasingly being appreciated that decreased renal function may be a presenting symptom of atherosclerotic stenosis of the renal artery, and may also be an indication for invasive treatment (Mann *et al.* 1985; Grützmacher and Bussmann 1986; Grützmacher *et al.* 1988; Jacobson 1988; Canzanello *et al.* 1989). In a study of 100 consecutive patients with atherosclerotic, renovascular disease, 66 presented with a serum creatinine of greater than 1.5 mg/100 ml (Canzanello *et al.* 1989). Wollenweber *et al.* (1968) found that 15 per cent of their patients with renovascular hypertension had a serum creatinine of greater than 2.0 mg/100 ml. Underlying atheromatous disease of the kidney is responsible for an increasing number of patients with otherwise occult, endstage renal failure (Meyrier *et al.* 1988; Scoble *et al.* 1989).

Whether patients with diabetes mellitus (especially those with type 2 disease) have a lower than expected prevalence of renovascular hypertension (Tierney *et al.* 1989), or a higher prevalence (Sawicki *et al.* 1991), has not been studied in sufficient detail. In our series of more than 100 patients with atherosclerotic renovascular disease who had been treated by transluminal angioplasty, one-third had underlying type 2 diabetes mellitus.

A retrospective analysis developed a complex predictive index for renal artery stenosis from a cohort of 477 patients selected for renal arteriography because of drug-resistant hypertension or of an increase in serum creatinine during therapy with ACE inhibitors. The clinical clues age, sex, atherosclerotic vascular disease, recent onset of hypertension, smoking history, body mass index, abdominal bruit, serum creatinine, and cholesterol level were used to calculate a clinical score. With the calculation of a sum score the corresponding probability of a stenosis can be read from a graph. Receiver operator characteristics with sensitivity of 68 per cent and specificity of 87 per cent showed a predicted probability for renal artery stenosis of 30 per cent in these patients. The diagnostic accuracy of this clinical score was similar to that of renal scintigraphy in the same study (Krijnen *et al.* 1998). It is unknown how this score would perform in non-selected hypertensive patients.

Of considerable clinical interest are patients with mural thrombi and embolism of the renal artery. These have flank pain as a presenting symptom and are most often referred to urologists for suspected nephrolithiasis. Normal findings on sonography and a non-excretory urogram on the affected side are usually reported and should be followed by immediate renal angiography. Similar symptoms are found with spontaneous dissections of the renal artery (see Fig. 1) which may occur when the renal arteries are involved in dissecting aneurysms of the aorta or with a rare type of fibromuscular dysplasia. This unusual situation, described in detail by Beroniade *et al.* (1987), is amenable to surgery (Reilly *et al.* 1991).

Recurrent sudden or 'flash' pulmonary oedema may also be a presenting symptom in patients with renovascular hypertension; most also have impaired renal function (Missouris *et al.* 1993). This complication was retrospectively found in nearly one-quarter of 55 consecutive patients with renovascular hypertension, the vast majority of whom had bilateral disease (Pickering *et al.* 1988b).

Diagnostic techniques

Despite of considerable progress of the non-invasive renal imaging techniques there is no universal test available which reliably predicts the benefit of intervention in patients with renal artery stenosis. There are diagnostic tests which exclusively image renovascular anatomy (angiography, CT angiography), give additional haemodynamic information of renal blood flow (Doppler sonography, MRT angiography), or exclusively rely on functional renin-dependent tests (saralasin test, captopril test, and captopril renography).

Therefore, there is a definite need for sensitive and selective screening tests. Screening is particularly important because of the low prevalence of renovascular hypertension within the general population of patients with high blood pressure. The risk and expense of the tests must also be considered. A list of diagnostic procedures, including our own preferences, appears in Table 5.

Renal arteriography

Intra-arterial angiography is still considered to be the 'gold standard' for diagnosis of renal artery stenosis, although significant interobserver variability of the grading of stenoses has been reported (Paul *et al.* 1999; Schreij *et al.* 1999; van Jaarsveld *et al.* 1999). Frontal views are frequently not adequate for seeing both renal ostia; therefore, left anterior oblique and right anterior oblique projections may be necessary. Selective catheterization is valuable for clearly delineating segmental lesions, which can be obscured by overlying vessels. Even conventional angiography is not completely adequate for all radiological aspects in approximately 20 per cent of cases. In 6 per cent it may be inadequate for complete analysis of the main renal artery (US Cooperative Study; Bookstein *et al.* 1972a,b). These observations emphasize the fact that renal arteriography should only be stopped when adequate films of the ostia, the main renal arteries, and segmental arteries have been obtained. Multiple renal arteries may be present in as many as one-quarter of patients (Pick and Anson 1940; Bookstein *et al.* 1972a,b).

Digital recording of images is now standard with less need of contrast material. Current protocols obtain images using 20 ml of 150–300 mg/ml

Table 5 Diagnostic techniques for renovascular hypertension

Conventional or digital subtraction angiography
Radio-isotope renography (with captopril, with aspirin, during exercise)
Colour-coded duplex sonography
Spiral CT-angiography
Magnetic resonance angiography
Positron emission tomography
Plasma renin: captopril test, renal vein renins
Rapid-sequence intravenous pyelography
Saralasin test

contrast at a rate of 10 ml/s. As a result catheters of smaller size (4-French gauge) can be used leading to less traumatic procedures (Textor and Canzanello 1996). Intravenous digital subtraction angiography (see Havey *et al.* 1985, for review) was largely abandoned in recent years because of motion artifacts, incomplete imaging and the high load of contrast media.

The measurement of the trans-stenotic gradient was introduced to gather haemodynamic information of renal artery stenosis. Except for cases with subtotal stenoses, where the pass of the catheter through the very narrow lumen may be impossible, this technique may actually be the gold standard of stenotic grading. However, the trans-stenotic gradient did not predict the change of blood pressure or of renal function after angioplasty in a study of 231 patients with atherosclerotic renal artery stenosis (Nahman *et al.* 1994).

There is a risk associated with catheterization of a major artery. The incidence of complications is definitely greater for the axillary and for the translumbar approaches than for the femoral. With the femoral technique, complications occur in about 0.5–2 per cent of patients, depending on the experience of the investigator, the extent of the atherosclerosis, and the blood pressure and coagulation status. Most complications are due to bleeding and haematoma formation at the puncture site. However, thrombosis, embolism, false aneurysms, arteriovenous fistulae, arterial dissections, vascular spasm, vessel perforation, and even death may occur (in 0.02–0.05 per cent of patients). In the presence of generalized atherosclerosis the risk of cholesterol embolism with potentially lethal consequences is especially important (Gaines *et al.* 1988).

There is certainly an additional risk of contrast media-associated acute renal failure; however, the significance of this complication—which unfortunately is rarely differentiated from cholesterol embolism—has been overestimated in the past (Brezis and Epstein 1989; Parfrey *et al.* 1989; Fleischmann *et al.* 1993). This risk is definitely less than 5 per cent, and only approximately 10 per cent in patients with diabetes mellitus and pre-existing mild renal insufficiency (Parfrey *et al.* 1989). Non-ionic contrast agents have only limited advantages over ionic as far as nephrotoxicity is concerned (Schwab *et al.* 1989). A schema of contrast dosing in patients with renal insufficiency was found to be effective in a prospective study by Cigarroa *et al.* (1989).

Most of the above complications of arteriography are found in patients with widespread atherosclerosis and/or renal insufficiency with diabetes. It is in these patients that the risk of the procedure must be weighed against the possible benefit (e.g. invasive treatment of renal artery stenosis instead of dialysis).

Currently, our own approach is to use intra-arterial digital subtraction angiography of the renal arteries only in those patients who are selected for revascularization by patient's history, clinical clues and non-invasive techniques. Interventional treatment either by angioplasty or by additional stent placement can be performed in the same session to avoid a second invasive procedure associated with the above mentioned risks.

Spiral computed tomography angiography

Computed tomographic angiography (CTA) has become an established technique for minimally invasive imaging of renal artery stenosis. This method is based on the rapid volume acquisition capabilities of spiral CT, especially with the new multi-slice machines, and uses a properly timed intravenous contrast bolus to obtain a 3D data set from the renal vasculature. The data set, consisting of overlapping transaxial CT images, can be reviewed using arbitrary cut planes or it can be transformed into angiographic displays using maximum intensity projections or 3D shaded surface displays. Complete data acquisition is possible in a single breath-hold-phase to avoid respiratory artefacts. Although there is an absolute limit to spatial resolution with spiral CT angiography of diagnostic assessment of vessels less than 1 mm in diameter, main and accessory renal arteries can be reliably be visualized (Krumme and Blum 1998). Axial images and multiplanar reformats remain the most important display mode for CTA data and serve as the basis for diagnosis, whereas maximum intensity projections and 3D shaded surface display images provide a good overview of the anatomic situation.

In an animal model of renal artery stenosis, electron beam computed tomography (EBCT) allowed to study renal perfusion and tubular dynamics by the detection of contrast concentration. The change in cortical blood flow correlated with the degree of stenosis (Lerman *et al.* 1999).

With the combination of different CTA techniques excellent diagnostic accuracy with sensitivity of 88–99 per cent and specificity of 93–98 per cent was found in several angiographically controlled studies (Pedersen 2000). The variability of the grading of renal artery stenosis was very low (κ-value 0.9) between two observers in a study of 71 consecutive patients with suspected renal artery stenosis (Kaatee *et al.* 1997).

The arterial lumen is exactly visualized by spiral CTA. Thus the sectional area of a stenosis can be calculated more precisely than by conventional two-dimensional angiography. Further advantages of CT include visualization of the arterial wall, with localization and quantification of calcified plaques (Gayard *et al.* 2000), concomitant depiction of renal parenchyma and lack of arterial catheterization. However, the nephrotoxicity of contrast medium (100–150 ml i.v.) is the major drawback of this technique.

Magnetic resonance imaging

Magnetic resonance angiography (MRA) has evolved considerably over the past years as a valuable tool for the assessment of renovascular disease. It combines morphological and functional imaging by the use of different techniques. The two main techniques for imaging flowing blood in vessels are time-of-flight and phase-contrast sequences. The time-of-flight technique has shorter scanning time, however with less background suppression. Using the time-of-flight technique, Yucel *et al.* (1993) observed a sensitivity and specificity of 100 and 93 per cent, respectively, in the diagnosis of renovascular disease, at least of the main renal artery. Contrast-enhanced 3D gadolinum MRA rapidly images the aorta and its branches to overcome flow artefacts and saturation problems that limit the utility of MRA. This new technique is performed in a single breathhold with better resolution of the small arteries (Prince *et al.* 1997). With optimized techniques based on fast data acquisition, sensitivity and specificity values exceeding 95 per cent have been consistently reported in several studies (Pedersen 2000). Based on these data 3D MRA is being increasingly used as diagnostic modality for the assessment of renovascular disease. Recently, a new technique was introduced for the haemodynamic grading of renal artery stenosis (Schoenberg *et al.* 1997). Cardiac-gated MR cine phase-contrast flow measurements with high temporal resolution provide time-resolved velocity profiles of the renal artery. Gradual haemodynamic changes secondary to a stenosis can be detected by means of characteristic changes of the velocity curve profile. The changes of the flow pattern are similar to those which are well known from Doppler flow profiles of stenotic renal arteries as 'parvus and tardus flow' (Stavros *et al.* 1992).

In a multireader analysis with seven radiologists the diagnostic value of 3D gadolinum MRA in combination with cine phase-contrast flow measurements was tested in terms of interobserver and intermodality variability for the grading of renal artery stenosis (Schoenberg *et al.* 2002). Eighty-three patients were evaluated with both techniques including intraarterial digital subtraction angiography. The combined approach of 3D-Gd-MRA and cine phase-contrast flow measurements revealed the best interobserver variability (*K*-value 0.75) and almost perfect intermodality agreement with Doppler sonographic angiography (97 per cent of cases) (Schoenberg *et al.* 2002). Three-dimensional Gd-MRA with cine phase-contrast flow measurement may be the gold standard in the near future.

Radioisotope renogram and captopril renal scintigraphy

The simple radioisotope renogram was used in several studies in the 1960s and the 1970s for the detection of renovascular hypertension. It was found to have a sensitivity and specificity in the range of 75 per cent (see Havey *et al.* 1985, for review). Sequential scintigrams of the kidneys with simultaneous measurements of renal perfusion showed a somewhat higher sensitivity of 85 per cent (Arlart *et al.* 1979; Chiarini *et al.* 1982).

'Captopril scintigraphy' has been found to be much superior to conventional scintigraphy for the diagnosis of renovascular hypertension (Fommei *et al.* 1987; Geyskes *et al.* 1987a,b; Maher *et al.* 1988; Sfakianakis *et al.* 1988; Erbslöh-Möller *et al.* 1991; Mann *et al.* 1991; Davidson and Wilcox 1992; Dondi *et al.* 1992). The data on captopril renography have been comprehensively reviewed by Prigent (1993) and by Pedersen (1994). A consensus report provides guidelines for the performance and interpretation of captopril renography including a grading of the renographic curves (Taylor *et al.* 1996).

This technique involves sequential scintigrams (one frame/20 s) with ^{99}Tc-m-labelled diethylene-triaminepenta-acetic acid (DTPA), a marker of glomerular filtration (Fommei *et al.* 1987; Maher *et al.* 1988), or with ^{131}I-hippurate, a marker of renal blood flow (Geyskes *et al.* 1987a,b; Sfakianakis *et al.* 1988), or with ^{99}Tc-MAG, another marker of renal blood flow. These tracers are injected twice: with and without prior (1 h) administration of 25–50 mg (p.o.) captopril. I.V. enalapril (50 μg/kg) may also be given. Patients must stop taking diuretics and inhibitors of the renin system for about 3–5 days before the studies. Each of the four cited studies with 40–60 patients of whom roughly one-third had renovascular disease agreed that captopril definitely enhances the usefulness of scintigraphy in screening for renovascular hypertension. In one study, seven of 14 kidneys with 60–95 per cent arterial obstruction had normal, baseline DTPA and hippurate scintigrams; both types of renograms became abnormal after captopril in all cases. In the other seven kidneys, baseline DTPA and hippurate renograms were abnormal but not characteristic of renovascular disease; after captopril, the hippurate renogram became positive in all cases, but in only four of those seven for the DTPA study. A further four kidneys with more than 95 per cent arterial occlusion had abnormal baseline appearances, which did not change after captopril (Sfakianakis *et al.* 1988). Geyskes *et al.* (1987a,b) found a sensitivity of 80 per cent and a specificity of 100 per cent for combined analysis of DTPA- and hippurate-captopril renograms. They also found a good agreement between the captopril renogram and the success of invasive treatment, as also found by Fommei *et al.* (1987).

The published results of captopril renography must be interpreted with caution because the protocols are often complex and diagnostic criteria are not standardized. The endpoint or reference standard of captopril renography studies should be the response to revascularization rather than the angiographic evidence of renal artery stenosis (Taylor *et al.* 2000). A Dutch group published their 15-year experience with renography, retrospectively evaluated in 505 consecutive patients (van Jaarsveld *et al.* 1997). With various tracers, and with and without captopril they found sensitivity values of 65 and 68 per cent, respectively, with corresponding specificity of 90 per cent. The presence of renal artery stenosis greater than 50 per cent on angiography was the gold standard in this study. However, a stenosis of merely 50–70 per cent may not be haemodynamically effective in many patients. Therefore a negative result of captopril renography may have been correct despite of the presence of 50 per cent renal artery stenosis. Some authors recommend to start with captopril renography and only add a further renography without captopril if the former test is abnormal. This procedure reduces costs and examination time (Pedersen 2000).

Of particular interest to nephrologists is the observation of Maher *et al.* (1988), who found a positive captopril-DTPA scintigram not only in all patients with unilateral stenosis of the renal artery, but also in others with asymmetrical size and function of the kidneys. Renoparenchymal disease rather than renovascular disease was responsible for the abnormal scintigrams in that series. One would therefore expect the specificity of this test to be reduced in unilateral renoparenchymal disease. It is apparent that renography will give no useful information if perfusion of the respective kidney is much reduced (Datseris *et al.* 1994).

Exercise may accentuate the results of renography. Clorius *et al.* (1987) found an acceptable predictive value for exercise renography in the preoperative evaluation of hypertension in 18 patients with renovascular disease who were treated surgically. Nine of 10 patients with an abnormal exercise scintigram continued to be hypertensive after surgery; seven of eight with a normal exercise scintigram were cured. The preliminary encouraging results of Imanishi *et al.* (1994) with aspirin renography for the diagnosis of unilateral renovascular disease could not be confirmed in a larger group of patients (van de Ven *et al.* 2000). In 75 consecutive patients suspected of having renal artery stenosis, aspirin renography (20 mg/kg orally) and captopril renography (25 mg orally) were prospectively compared using 99m Tc-MAG as tracer. The sensitivities for unilateral renal artery stenosis or bilateral stenosis were, respectively, 88 and 88 per cent for captopril renography and 82 and 94 per cent for aspirin renography. The overall specificity was 75 per cent for captopril renography and 83 per cent for aspirin renography, which was not significantly different (van de Ven *et al.* 2000).

Colour coded duplex sonography

Since the first introduction of Doppler sonography for assessment of renovascular disease (Avasthi *et al.* 1984) there was a rapid technical progress resulting in high-end duplex machines with excellent colour coded imaging of the renal and abdominal vessels. Blood flow velocity of extra- and intrarenal vessels during cardiac cycle are monitored and several haemodynamic parameters can be calculated from the flow pattern. In principle, duplex scanning can be performed in two different ways to screen for renal artery stenosis (Krumme and Rump 1996). The first is the direct approach to the main renal artery obtaining the maximum velocity or the ratio of the renal and aortic maximum velocities, which are increased in case of stenosis (Hoffmann *et al.* 1991; Olin *et al.* 1995). However, in about 20 per cent of patients bowel motility or obesity hinder complete imaging of the main or accessory renal arteries. This disadvantage can be overcome by the second approach namely duplex scanning of intrarenal arteries with the calculation of indirect indices, such as resistive index (RI) or pulsatility index (PI) (Schwerk *et al.* 1994; Krumme *et al.* 1996; Riehl *et al.* 1997; Johansson *et al.* 2000; Radermacher *et al.* 2001a). Significant renal artery stenosis leads to a change of the poststenotic flow pattern of the affected kidney, which can be compared with the flow pattern of the contralateral kidney. Intrarenal Doppler signals can be obtained in almost every patient, however, diagnostic accuracy of this intrarenal approach is reduced in patients with bilateral disease (Krumme *et al.* 1996). Therefore the combined scanning of intra- and extrarenal arteries is the procedure of choice for the duplex sonographic screening of renal artery stenosis (Krumme *et al.* 1996; Malatino *et al.* 1998; Radermacher *et al.* 2001a).

The use of contrast enhancement does not improve diagnostic accuracy of colour coded duplexsonography. In a multicentre study with 198 patients and a crossover randomized design (Claudon *et al.* 2000), visualization of the renal arteries was improved by contrast medium, but not sensitivity and specificity for the diagnosis of renal artery stenosis as compared to duplexsonography without contrast. Some authors found improved diagnostic accuracy of intrarenal Doppler scanning after application of captopril (Rene *et al.* 1995; Veglio *et al.* 1995; Oliva *et al.* 1998). In 71 angiographically controlled patients sensitivity improved from 81 to 100 per cent and specificity from 98 to 100 per cent, respectively, after application of captopril when intrarenal RI was compared (Oliva *et al.* 1998).

Recently, Radermacher *et al.* (2001a) have shown that intrarenal RI was of value to predict the clinical outcome of technically successful transluminal angioplasty in 131 patients with renal artery stenosis greater than 50 per cent. In 34 of 35 patients with RI above 80, blood pressure did not improve and renal function declined in 80 per cent of these patients. In contrast, in 90 of 96 patients with intrarenal RI below 80, blood pressure improved and renal function worsened in only three of these patients (Radermacher *et al.* 2001a). If further studies confirm this outstanding predictive value of intrarenal RI, possibly indicating the extent of arterio-arteriolosclerosis, Doppler scanning may become a valuable tool to select patients for further invasive procedure.

Measurements of plasma renin activity

Müller *et al.* (1986) retrospectively analysed the validity of the so-called captopril test in 266 patients who were not receiving diuretics and who had a urinary sodium excretion of more than 50 mmol/day. No antihypertensive treatment was given in 171 of the patients. Blood was obtained in the seated position after 30 min rest, 50 mg captopril were then given orally, and blood was again obtained 1 h later for measurement of plasma renin activity. Fifty-six patients had angiographically defined, unilateral or bilateral stenosis of the renal artery of greater than 75 per cent. In addition, 14 of 56 patients had impaired renal function. Not surprisingly, the baseline plasma renin activity did not discriminate between renovascular and essential hypertension. However, plasma renin values after captopril, and the change in these values from baseline did discriminate. Müller *et al.* found a sensitivity of 100 per cent and a specificity of 95 per cent for unilateral and bilateral stenosis, respectively. The test was definitely less accurate in patients with pre-existing impairment of the kidney because of false-positive and possibly also false-negative findings.

Derkx *et al.* (1987) investigated the captopril test in 89 patients with essential hypertension, and in 62 with unilateral, and 28 with bilateral, renal artery stenosis. All had severe hypertension with a diastolic blood pressure above 120 mmHg, or above 100 mmHg while receiving combination treatment with at least three different antihypertensives. Antihypertensives were discontinued at least 2 weeks before the study and all patients underwent angiography. A sensitivity of 93 per cent and specificity of 84 per cent was found for the detection of renovascular hypertension with the captopril test. However, these values were clearly lower in patients with bilateral stenosis of the renal artery. Renal function was not reported. Salvetti *et al.* (1987) obtained considerably poorer results as did Postma *et al.* (1990) in 149 patients, reporting a sensitivity of only 39 per cent and a specificity of 96 per cent. Again, Frederickson *et al.* (1990) found a sensitivity of 100 per cent in 129 patients, 29 of which had renovascular hypertension. The latter authors used only the postcaptopril renin levels as test criterion.

Kutkuhn *et al.* (1988) investigated 67 patients of whom 43 had unilateral and nine bilateral, renal artery stenosis. Twenty-one of these patients had a negative captopril test, and vascular surgery was without effect in all 10 patients so treated. The other 31 patients had a positive captopril test; 19 of these successfully underwent surgery. The investigators also found that three patients with fibromuscular dysplasia, who were later successfully operated, had low, normal baseline for plasma renin activity. The increase in this activity after captopril was only 100–160 per cent, a value less than that considered diagnostic by Müller *et al.* (1986).

Svetkey *et al.* (1989), reviewing the available data, have suggested that measuring captopril-stimulated, peripheral renin activity may be the most useful and efficient, but less than perfect, procedure for identification of patients with renovascular hypertension. We do not share that view because blood sampling for and measurement of plasma renin is subject to many errors. Standard criteria for a positive test vary. If not done routinely, as it will be in most settings, such errors and the lack of standardization invalidate the test. Furthermore, the sensitivity of the captopril test is reduced in renal insufficiency and with bilateral disease (Davidson and Wilcox 1992).

Renal vein renin

Measurement of renal vein renin has been used for many years in the diagnosis of renovascular hypertension and also for predicting the response to invasive treatment. Despite this, there is no agreement on its usefulness, as was emphasized by the reviews of Grim and Weinberger (1984), Rudnick and Maxwell (1984), Sellars *et al.* (1985), and Weinberger *et al.* (1986). The technique involves catheterization of the abdominal vena cava with selective blood sampling from each renal vein, and from the vena cava above and below the origin of these veins. The ratio of plasma renin activity between the ischaemic and non-ischaemic kidney can be calculated; for greater diagnostic accuracy, a renin secretion index may also be calculated. In typical cases the secretion index not only predicts the extent of renin secretion by the ischaemic kidney, but also indicates renin extraction by the contralateral kidney (Fig. 6). If the contralateral kidney secretes more renin than the stenosed one, severe hypertensive lesions of the arterioles are present and invasive treatment of the stenosis will fail.

Studies of renal vein renin present various technical problems. Sodium deprivation before the measurement, and sampling while the patient is tilted improve sensitivity and specificity (Grim and Weinberger 1984) as does the acute administration of captopril (Re *et al.* 1978; Thibonnier *et al.* 1984). Malpositioning of the catheter (e.g. leading to admixture of blood from gonadal veins) must be prevented, and

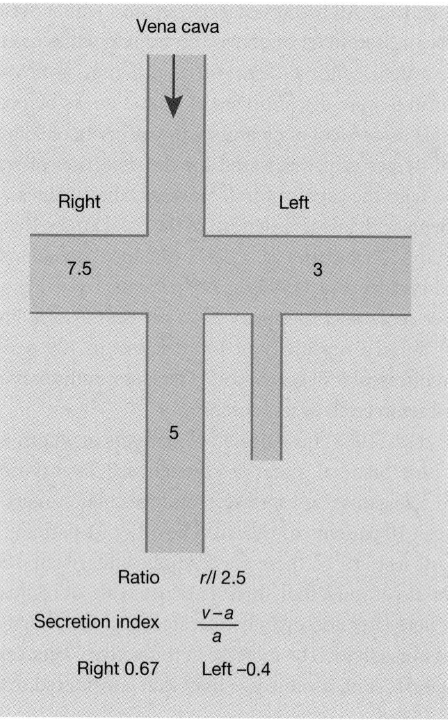

Fig. 6 A typical example of studies of renal vein renin in renovascular hypertension. The ratio of plasma renin activity is positive for the right side (>1.5). In addition, the secretion index indicates release of renin from the affected side and extraction of renin by the contralateral side, $v = 2$, $a = 2$.

the presence of multiple renal veins must be recognized. Because of the discontinuous release of renin, blood sampling should be done as quickly as possible. Some advocate the use of multiple catheters for simultaneous sampling both from renal veins and from the vena cava. If there is segmental stenosis of the renal artery, the respective subsegments of the renal veins should be catheterized.

With the above technical precautions, 90–95 per cent of patients with stenosis of the renal artery and a 'positive' renal vein renin (a renin ratio ischaemic/contralateral side > 1.5, or a positive secretion index of the ischaemic side) benefit from corrective intervention. However, 30–60 per cent of patients with 'negative' renal vein renin also benefit from invasive treatment (Grim and Weinberger 1984).

Saralasin test

Saralasin (Sar 1-Ala 8-angiotensin II), the angiotensin II-peptide receptor antagonist, was used in the late 1970s for the diagnosis of renovascular hypertension (Grim *et al.* 1979; Horne *et al.* 1979). The peptide was infused at a dose of 10 μg/kg/min for 30 min after pretreatment with diuretics. Lowering of blood pressure was regarded as a positive response. The test identified about 85 per cent of patients with renovascular hypertension but was also positive in about 10 per cent with essential hypertension. This is not surprising because blood pressure may become angiotensin II-dependent after administration of diuretics. Pressor responses with this peptide may also occur because saralasin is a partial agonist. The test is therefore considered to be of limited use (Vaughan 1985), and it is only rarely made in clinical practice today.

Baseline plasma renin activity

As outlined above, this is not a useful test for differentiating between patients with renal vascular hypertension and those with essential hypertension (Grim *et al.* 1979).

Diagnostic approaches

There is no uniform approach to the diagnosis of renovascular hypertension, even in departments with extensive experience. Our own approach is primarily based on clinical assessment of the patient. If there are signs or symptoms as outlined in Table 4, we proceed colour coded duplex sonography performing direct and indirect scanning as outlined above (Krumme *et al.* 1996). If colour coded duplex sonography is not available, captopril renography may be appropriate as initial screening tool (Mann 1995). This approach is cost effective and reduces the number of angiographies (Blaufox *et al.* 1996; Radermacher and Brunkhorst 1998). If one of these screening tests, in experienced hands, does not give a clear result, that is, Doppler sonographic angiography is only performed, if radiological or surgical intervention would be indicated due to resistant hypertension or rising of serum creatinine. It is a matter of debate, whether MRA should be performed as a new non-invasive gold standard including imaging of the vessels and haemodynamic profiles (Schoenberg *et al.* 2002). In our own experience, the rate of false positive results of MRA with present day machines is still too high.

The clinical signs that most commonly draw renovascular hypertension to our attention are summarized in Table 4. If the prevalence of renovascular hypertension is in the 5 per cent range, the positive predictive value of the above screening tests will be in the 30–40 per cent range, with a prevalence of 20 per cent in the 60–70 per cent range.

We also do not recommend routine studies of renal vein renin before invasive treatment because, even with negative results invasive treatment may benefit substantial number of patients (see above). However, the renal vein renin is useful in the demonstration of increased release of renin by the 'non-involved' kidney. It may also be helpful in the evaluation of unilateral parenchymal disease of the kidney. Smith (1956) contributed a classic clinical paper in which he demonstrated the futility of routinely removing such kidneys in the management of hypertension. We measure renal vein renins, before considering nephrectomy, in the few patients with hypertension and a unilateral small kidney. If the contralateral kidney is producing renin, we do not recommend surgery. Apart from personal experience, we are not aware of data supporting—or not—our approach.

In the decision for revascularization of renal artery stenosis the preservation of renal function has to be considered as well as the prevention of clinical events and last but not least the effect on blood pressure (Jacobson 1988; Kremer Hovinga *et al.* 1990; Allenberg and Hupp 1995). We will focus on renovascular hypertension rather than on the effect on renal function, which is extensively discussed in Chapter 9.5 of this textbook.

Treatment of renovascular hypertension

There is no universally accepted treatment in patients with renovascular hypertension. The choice of treatment may depend on age, actual and previous control of blood pressure, underlying renal function, concomitant diseases, estimated operative risk, the type, extent and site of stenosis, renal vein renin tests, local surgical or angiological experience, and last but certainly not least, the preference of the patient and the physician. It is not unusual for a patient with renovascular disease to be advised to take antihypertensive agents by one physician, to be treated by percutaneous transluminal renal angioplasty (PTRA) by another, and eventually to undergo vascular surgery by yet another. In recent times, there is a trend towards conservative treatment, supported by the fact that three randomized studies comparing PTRA with antihypertensive treatment in patients with renal artery stenosis showed no significant difference in blood pressure outcome (Plouin *et al.* 1998; Webster *et al.* 1998; van Jaarsveld *et al.* 2000). In addition, long-term follow-up of patients with atherosclerotic renal artery stenosis indicated, somewhat surprisingly, that the development of terminal renal failure is rare (Leertouwer *et al.* 2001).

However, one has to distinguish between fibromuscular and atherosclerotic renovascular disease in terms of blood pressure outcome as well as in terms of long-term renal function after revascularization. In 23 patients with fibromuscular renovascular disease, a younger age and a shorter duration of hypertension predicted a higher probability of blood pressure response after PTRA (Davidson *et al.* 1996).

In the following paragraphs we shall discuss aspects of medical treatment, PTRA, and surgery focusing on the more frequent atherosclerotic type of renal artery stenosis.

Medical treatment

Medical care for the patients with atherosclerotic renovascular disease has to consider the high cardiovascular mortality of these patients. Statins and antiplatelet agents as well as antihypertensive drugs should be provided, and smoking discouraged. None of the studies dealing with medical treatment of renovascular hypertension evaluated the effect of statins and antiplatelet drugs on the progression of renal artery stenosis, as has been successfully been done in patients with coronary heart disease. Some clinical and pathophysiological aspects of renovascular disease must be taken into account.

With unilateral disease, blood pressure is negatively correlated with sodium balance (Davies *et al.* 1983). Diuretics should therefore be used with care, a recommendation that does not apply to bilateral disease or to single kidneys. Inhibitors of the renin–angiotensin system are not the first choice, however they should be used, with caution, when blood pressure is not normalized because they are very effective antihypertensive agents with renovascular hypertension (Franklin and Smith 1985). Angiotensin II commonly contributes to the maintenance of glomerular filtration in an ischaemic kidney behind a stenosis, through its constrictive effects on the efferent glomerular arteriole. Inhibitors of the formation of angiotensin II (converting enzyme and renin inhibitors) or of its action (receptor blockers) may therefore not be the antihypertensive drug of first choice. Van de Ven *et al.* (1998) studied the effects of controlled exposure to ACE inhibitors on plasma creatinine in 108 patients at high risk for renovascular disease. In 69 patients, ACE inhibition caused at least a 20 per cent increase in plasma creatinine, in 26 cases after 4 days, in 31 after 2 weeks, and in 12 only after further blood pressure control by the addition of diuretics. The increase in serum creatinine during ACE inhibition was correlated with the degree of renovascular disease. However, no case of acute renal failure occurred with careful monitoring of renal function (Van de Ven *et al.* 1998). In a controlled trial 85 people with renal artery stenosis were randomized to either classical antihypertensive drugs or to ACE inhibitors. Serum creatinine increased somewhat more on ACE inhibitors during the 6-month follow-up, but blood pressure was much better controlled and no case of acute renal failure or anuria was noted (Franklin and Smith 1985). There are findings from animal experiments that prolonged inhibition of the formation of angiotensin II not only impairs filtration but also leads to loss of renal mass. In humans with renovascular disease, such a reduction in renal mass due to ACE inhibitors, or angiotensin blockers for that matter, has not been shown. In fact, roughly 20 per cent of patients with renal artery stenosis show a decline of GFR in the affected kidney with the administration of ACE inhibitors with wide interindividual variability.

Patients with renovascular hypertension frequently do not to show a nocturnal decrease in pressure. Therefore, long-acting antihypertensive agents must be given in order to ensure blood pressure control during the night-time hours.

Even with good control of blood pressure, a substantial number of patients will exhibit a decrease of renal mass with medical therapy (Dean *et al.* 1991; Guzman *et al.* 1994; Zierler *et al.* 1994). A sonographically controlled prospective study in 122 patients with renovascular disease showed that the 2-year cumulative incidence of renal atrophy was 5.5, 11.7, and 20.8 per cent in kidneys with a baseline renal artery disease classification of normal, less than 60 per cent stenosis, and more than or equal to 60 per cent stenosis, respectively (Caps *et al.* 1998a,b). In contrast, another retrospective angiographically controlled study recently showed that severity of renovascular disease of a single functioning kidney in 142 patients with contralateral renal artery occlusion was not predictive of baseline-GFR, calculated by the Cockcroft and Gault formula (Cheung *et al.* 2002). This surprising result emphasizes the importance of intrarenal parenchymal damage, rather than the haemodynamic effects of a given stenosis, in the pathogenesis of renal dysfunction in patients with atherosclerotic renovascular disease. In this context, medical treatment may be preferred even in patients with high-grade renal artery stenosis (Tullis *et al.* 1999).

Invasive treatment

Invasive treatment of renovascular hypertension has the potential disadvantage of immediate major complications which are rare but may be life-threatening. However, the potential advantages are substantial and apply to the majority of patients. They include cure, or improved control of high blood pressure; and improvement or preservation of renal function.

Percutaneous transluminal renal angioplasty

PTRA became a common invasive therapy for renovascular hypertension in the early 1980s. This technical progress was due to the pioneering work of Dotter and Indkins (1964) and Grüntzig *et al.* (1978). PTRA was initially advocated for the treatment of patients who had complications or were unlikely to survive surgery (Weinberger *et al.* 1979). When compared with surgery, which was the standard invasive treatment, PTRA offers the following advantages: (a) brief hospitalization; (b) lower cost; (c) can be used in those with poor operative risk; (d) low mortality and relatively low morbidity associated with the technique; (e) ready availability in hospitals with departments of angiography.

Obviously, the risks of PTA are considerable, particularly in inexperienced hands or in angiographic departments that infrequently undertake interventional procedures. In a compilation of findings from over 800 patients, major complications, even in experienced departments, occurred in 2–10 per cent of PTRAs; the death rate ranged from 0 to 3 per cent (mean < 1 per cent) (Mahler *et al.* 1986). The major complications are listed in Table 6, and may be divided into those related directly to manipulation of the renal artery, those caused by angiographic techniques, and to associated consequences such as changes in blood pressure, effects of contrast media, and coagulation complications.

The list of complications is indeed impressive. However, it must be weighed against the possible complications of alternative treatments (medical and surgical), and of hypertension itself. Mahler *et al.* (1986) have pointed out that the definition of a complication also varies widely.

Technique

We will only summarize here some general aspects of PTRA techniques (for reviews, see Castaneda-Zuniga 1983; Sos *et al.* 1986). The femoral artery serves as the common route of access. With extensive arteriosclerosis of the aorta and iliac artery an axillary approach may be necessary, with substantial additional risk to the patient.

The stenosis may be visualized by use of a selective angiographic catheter, which is directed into the lesion. A guide wire is advanced through the catheter across the stenosis. Thereafter, the catheter is exchanged for a balloon-tipped one with or without a stent. This technique is probably most common because angiographic catheters with a wide variety of configurations can be used, which are versatile and relatively easy to handle. However, there are some problems in crossing a 'tight' stenosis; vascular spasm and vessel damage by the wire are not uncommon.

Another technique uses a coaxial, Grüntzig-type, large-bore guiding catheter. After entering the renal artery, a balloon catheter is advanced through the guiding catheter into the stenosis. Steerable, soft-tipped wires may be advanced through the balloon catheter for the management of an eccentric, peripheral, or very tight stenosis. In addition, balloon catheters developed for coronary angiography can be used with the coaxial system. Some advocate 'overdilatation', that is, using balloons that are larger than the artery (Pickering *et al.* 1988a). It has been reported that overdilatation is associated with a lower recurrence of hypertension (Klinge *et al.* 1989). Angioplasty leads to intimal splitting and endothelial desquamation. The narrowing plaque is forced into the vessel wall, causing stretching and rupture of the media and stretching of the adventitia (Fig. 7).

Although rupture of the artery is an exceedingly rare event, dissections are frequently seen and the denuded endothelium is susceptible to thrombosis and spasm. Small dissections usually resolve spontaneously as do irregularities of the vessel wall. In other words, remodelling of the vessel wall is a common finding, especially with fibromuscular dysplasia.

Table 6 Reported major complications of percutaneous transluminal renal angioplasty

Occlusion of renal artery
Cholesterol embolism (to renal or peripheral arteries)
Puncture-site haemorrhage and aneurysm
Dissection of renal or angiographic access artery or of aorta
Spasm of renal artery with possible partial infarction (apparently a problem of guide-wire techniques)
Renal artery perforation
Cerebral or myocardial infarction
Arterial embolism
Haemorrhagic shock
Infections
Thyrotoxicosis (resulting from exposure to iodine)
Death

Results of PTA

Ideally, angioplasty will lead to normalization of blood pressure (or at least improvement of hypertension), to improvement of GFR, and to widening of the stenosis. PTRA is technically successful in roughly 80–90 per cent of those cases selected (non-randomly in all published series) for this procedure. In 10–20 per cent of patients, the stenosis either cannot be crossed with the guide wire or with the balloon, or it resists the pressure of the balloon. These difficulties may be an indication for stent-placement, which is discussed below. In fibromuscular disease, higher rates of technical success were reported (Lüscher *et al.* 1985; Klinge *et al.* 1989), even up to 100 per cent (Tegtmeyer *et al.* 1991). Technical success is difficult to evaluate with eccentric stenosis. We therefore look at the stenosis in at least two different projections.

Clinical success is easily assessed for renal function but the criteria for a satisfactory response in blood pressure are somewhat ambiguous. Specifically, many patients will show 'improved' control of hypertension, which is defined either as normotension with smaller amounts of antihypertensive medication, or as lower blood pressure with similar medication than before the angioplasty. However, the quantitative contribution of PTRA, and of more intense conservative management after PTRA, remain to be established. Observer bias and placebo effects must also be considered (Brawn and Ramsey 1987).

In patients with fibromuscular dysplasia, the clinical outcome of PTRA is similar to that of surgery (Table 7). More than half of this population are cured of their hypertension. In patients with atherosclerotic lesions, the clinical outcome is considerably worse. There are a number of reasons for this difference. First, atherosclerosis of the renal

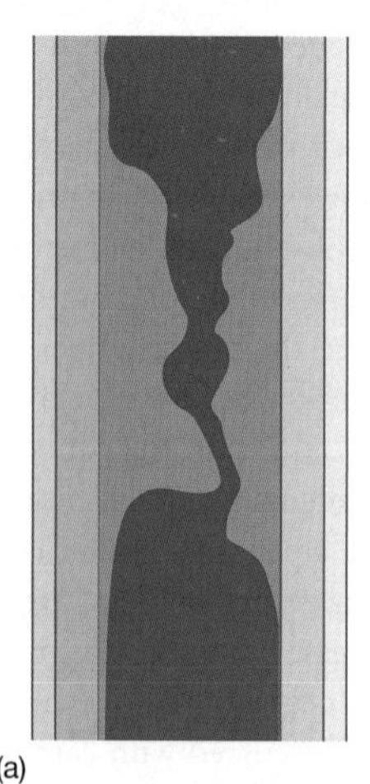

(a)

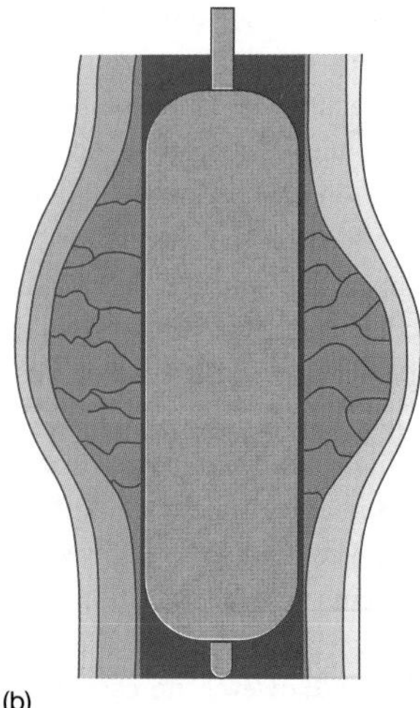

(b)

Fig. 7 Schematic diagram of transluminal angioplasty. The plaque is forced into the vessel wall with stretching and rupture of the media and adventitia.

Table 7 Effect of PTA on renal artery stenosis

Author(s), year	No. of patients	No. of stenoses	Ostial (%)	Bilateral (%)	Follow-up period (years)	Technical success (%)	Cured (%)	Improved (%)	Failed (%)	ΔBP (mmHg)	Re-stenoses (%)	Complications (%)	30-day mortality (%)
Colapinto *et al.* 1982 (ATS)	68				0.2–3	88	16	57	26				
Ingrisch, 1988 (ATS)	200				3	85–93		75	25		22		
Canzanello, 1989 (ATS)	100				2.4	73		43	57		NG		
Klinge *et al.* 1989					0.5–8								
ATS	134					78	13	90	12		12		
FMD	52					91	38	55	7		6		
Jeunemaitre *et al.* 1990 (ATS)	52				0.7	92	13	66	21		8		
Tegtmeyer *et al.* 1991 (FMD)	66				3	100	39	59	2		8		
Eldrup-Jorgensen *et al.* 1995	52	60		15.4	5 retro			67.3	8.33			3.8	1.19
Yutan *et al.* 2001 PTA + stent	76	88		94.7	10 retro	88	68	68			5	37	
Van Jaaresveld *et al.* 2000					1 prospect	92.9							
PTA	56			23.2			7.1	67.8	8.9	19–11	47.9	10.7	
Drugs	50			22			0	37.5	33.3	17–7	37.2	48	
Bonelli *et al.* 1995	320	396		23.75	14 retro								
ATS							8.4	61.6	30				2.2
FMD							22	41	27				
Von Knorring *et al.* 1996				24	4 prospect						8	12	4
ATS	38		9				11.1	74.1	14.8				
FMD	12		—				45.45	54.54	0				

Table 7 Continued

Author(s), year	No. of patients	No. of stenoses	Ostial (%)	Bilateral (%)	Follow-up period (years)	Technical success (%)	Cured (%)	Improved (%)	Failed (%)	ΔBP (mmHg)	Re-stenoses (%)	Complications (%)	30-day mortality (%)
Baumgartner *et al.* 1997		59	40.5	9	1 prospect					37–18	38	23.7	
ATS	37						8.6-sec.10.8	45.7-sec.59.5	45.7-sec.29.7				
FMD	13						8.3-sec.30.8	58.3-sec.53.8	33.4-sec.15.4				
Klow *et al.* 1998		552		134	12 retro		8	58	34			7.6	0.5
ATS	295										35		
FMD	49										31		
TX	74										30		
Plouin *et al.* (EMMA), 1998					0.5 prospect	100							0
PTA	23	23		0			6			11–10	3	6	
Drugs	26	26		0			0			8–5	0	2	
Webster *et al.* 1998					0.25–4.5 prospect								
PTA													
unilat	14										9–5		
bilat	16										19–4		
Drugs													
unilat	13										8–6		
bilat	12										2–2		
Paulsen *et al.* 1999	135	227		49.6	12 retro	93	6	36	47	70/24 22/14	45	9	1.5

ATS = atherosclerosis, FMD = fibromuscular dysplasia, TX = renal transplantation, retro = retrospective, prospect = prospective.

artery may not cause additional elevation of blood pressure but may be associated with essential hypertension. Second, the duration of the hypertension is usually much longer for atherosclerotic than for fibromuscular stenosis. In both instances, the duration of the hypertension is a strong predictor of a negative outcome. Third, atherosclerotic lesions commonly involve the ostium, and are caused by plaques in the aorta rather than in the renal artery. These stenoses are rarely amenable to PTRA and should be treated by stents (see below).

The rate of re-stenosis is higher with atherosclerotic (15–35 per cent) than with fibromuscular stenosis (5–20 per cent). Most of these re-stenoses occur during the first 3 months after PTRA (Grützmacher and Bussmann 1984, 1986; Plouin *et al.* 1993). In one study (Plouin *et al.* 1993) with re-angiography 9 months after PTRA in about 100 patients, re-stenosis was found in 16 per cent. Truncal stenoses were less prone to re-stenosis than branch or ostial lesions (12 versus 35 per cent). It is likely that aspirin may reduce the incidence of re-stenosis, as has been shown for PTA of the coronary arteries. The benefit or risk of adding clopidogrel to aspirin, especially after stent placement (Schomig *et al.* 1996), has not been explored in randomized studies with renal artery stenosis.

Renal artery stent placement

The introduction of stents for revascularization of PTA-refractory, mainly ostial, renal artery stenoses was another milestone in the treatment of renovascular disease. The primary failure of PTRA can be relieved by stents, as well as complications of PTA such as intimal dissection with obstructive intimal flaps or thombosis. Spontaneous dissecting aneurysms of the renal artery can also be covered by stents (Baert *et al.* 1994). Several types of stents such as the self-expandable Wallstent, the Strecker stent, the Nitinol stent and the Palmaz stent were tested for the use in the renal arteries. The Palmaz stent was used in most studies; is a slotted tube of stainless steel that becomes a wire mesh upon balloon expansion. The balloon size for stent delivery is chosen to be 1 mm greater than the renal artery lumen; such 'over-sizing' helps to ensure success of the procedure and reduces re-stenosis rates. For ostial lesions, the stent should be positioned 1–2 mm into the aorta in order to resist recoil of the aortic plaque and to prevent restenosis (Blum *et al.* 1997; Tuttle and Raabe 1998). Intravenous heparin should be given during the procedure and aspirin afterwards in a dosage of 100–300 mg/day. Some centres give clopidogrel for a period of 4 weeks after stent placement in accordance with stent studies in coronary artery disease (Schomig *et al.* 1996). However, prospective studies investigating different anticoagulation regimes during and after renal artery stenting are not available at present. The clinical outcome of stent placement is shown in Table 8.

A randomized prospective trial compared PTA with PTA plus stent placement in 85 patients with ostial atherosclerotic renal artery stenosis. At 6 months, the primary patency rate was 29 per cent for PTA (42 patients) and 75 per cent for PTRA with stent placement (43 patients). Re-stenosis after a successful procedure occurred in 48 per cent of patients for PTA and 14 per cent of patients for stenting. However the clinical results (plasma creatinine, blood pressure, medication) at 6 months did not differ in both groups (Van de Ven *et al.* 1999).

Harden *et al.* (1997) found in 32 patients with atherosclerotic renal artery stenosis that renal stent placement slows the progression of renovascular renal failure and may delay the need for renal replacement therapy.

In our own experience with 68 angiographically controlled patients treated with Palmaz stents for renal artery stenosis greater than 50 per cent, the re-stenosis-rate was 25 per cent. The secondary patency rate was 92 per cent during a mean follow-up of 27 months (Blum *et al.* 1997). Our initial results were confirmed by several studies listed in Table 8. Therefore, renal artery stenting can be recommended as initial treatment of ostial renal artery stenosis, if radiological intervention is warranted.

Surgical treatment

Because of the advent of PTRA including stenting and the increasing awareness of ischaemic disease of the kidney, indications for renovascular surgery have changed. In our department, hypertension was the major reason for renal artery reconstruction in 83 per cent of cases in the period from 1960 to 1979. Since 1980, this percentage has decreased to 37 per cent, and preservation or restoration of renal function has become the leading indication for renovascular surgery (Allenberg and Hupp 1995; Hansen *et al.* 2000). This situation is also related to the fact that we frequently correct stenosis of the renal artery in patients who are primarily operated upon for atherosclerotic aortoiliac disease (Fig. 8). The major indications for surgical treatment of renovascular occlusive disease are listed in Table 9. Depending upon the extent and site of the arterial lesion, different principles of reconstruction are applied.

Nephrectomy

Nephrectomy is only indicated in those hypertensives in whom the non-functioning kidney is known to be responsible for the hypertension. As indicated by Smith (1956), this state of affairs is seldom found. Sampling of renal vein renin may be helpful in this instance. Functional loss of a kidney can be expected if the longitudinal diameter is less than 7 cm in adults, and if scintigraphy shows severely compromised or absent function. Intrarenal stenosis or segmental occlusion of the artery may lead to indications for partial resection of a kidney. Nephrectomy must also be considered if vascular reconstruction is technically impossible or if its attempts fail.

Reconstruction

A variety of reconstructive techniques may be used, depending on the extent and site of the vascular lesions. Thromboendarterectomy consists of removal of the obstructive lesion in an intramural dissection plane. It can either be done by arteriotomy of the renal artery itself, or by a transaortic approach. If there is bilateral ostial stenosis of the renal artery, transaortic obliteration is preferred (Crinnion and Gough 1996). Thromboendarterectomy is also frequently combined with venous or prosthetic roof angioplasty (Fig. 9).

The aortorenal bypass is now the most frequently used and preferred method for stenoses in the middle or distal third of the renal artery, and for longer stenoses involving several centimetres of the renal artery. Saphenous vein or hypogastric artery may be used to form the bypass. In the presence of bilateral stenoses of the renal artery, revascularization may be performed by means of a vein bridge angioplasty. An aortic, side-to-side anastomosis and bilateral end-to-end anastomoses of the renal arteries are constructed. In selected cases the stenosis may be bypassed using synthetic material. This procedure, which is accompanied by a greater number of complications must be selected if no suitable vein or artery is available and if other time-consuming arterial reconstructions in the aortoiliac region must be made (Fig. 10).

Table 8 Effect of stent placement on renal artery stenosis

Authors, year	No. of patients	No. of stenoses	Ostial (%)	Bilateral (%)	Follow-up period (years)	Cured (%)	Improved (%)	Failed (%)	ΔBP mmHg	Complications (%)	30-day mortality (%)	Re-stenosis (%)	Initial technical success	Renal function improved-stabilized
Blum *et al.* 1997	68	74	—	8.8	2 prospect	16.2	61.8	22	20–25	4.4	—	10.8		
White *et al.* 1997	100	133		33	1 prospect				26			67		
Van de Ven *et al.* 1999	42 PTA 42 PTAS	50 52		19 24	6 mo prospect	4.8 14.3	42.8 40.5	50 40.5	15 20	38.1 42.8	—	48 14		
Rodriquez-Lopez *et al.* 1999	108	125	65.6		36 mo	13	55.5	32.4		8.3	3.7	15		
Leertouwer *et al.* 2000	678 PTAS 644 PTA	799 778			0.5–4 prospect	20 10	49 53	31 37			1	17 26	98 77	30 38
Baumgartner *et al.* 2000	123 PTA 64 S	200		22.7	4		43	11.7	12–4	3.1 8.6	1.6		34–83 80–66	32.7 5
Bush *et al.* 2001	73	85		16.4	6.5 retro					12		13.7	89	
Beutler *et al.* 2001	63				2						2.7	19		44.4 44.4
Isles *et al.* 1999	379	416	80	31		9				13	1.6	16	96–100	26 48

Mo, months; prospect, prospective; retro, retrospective.

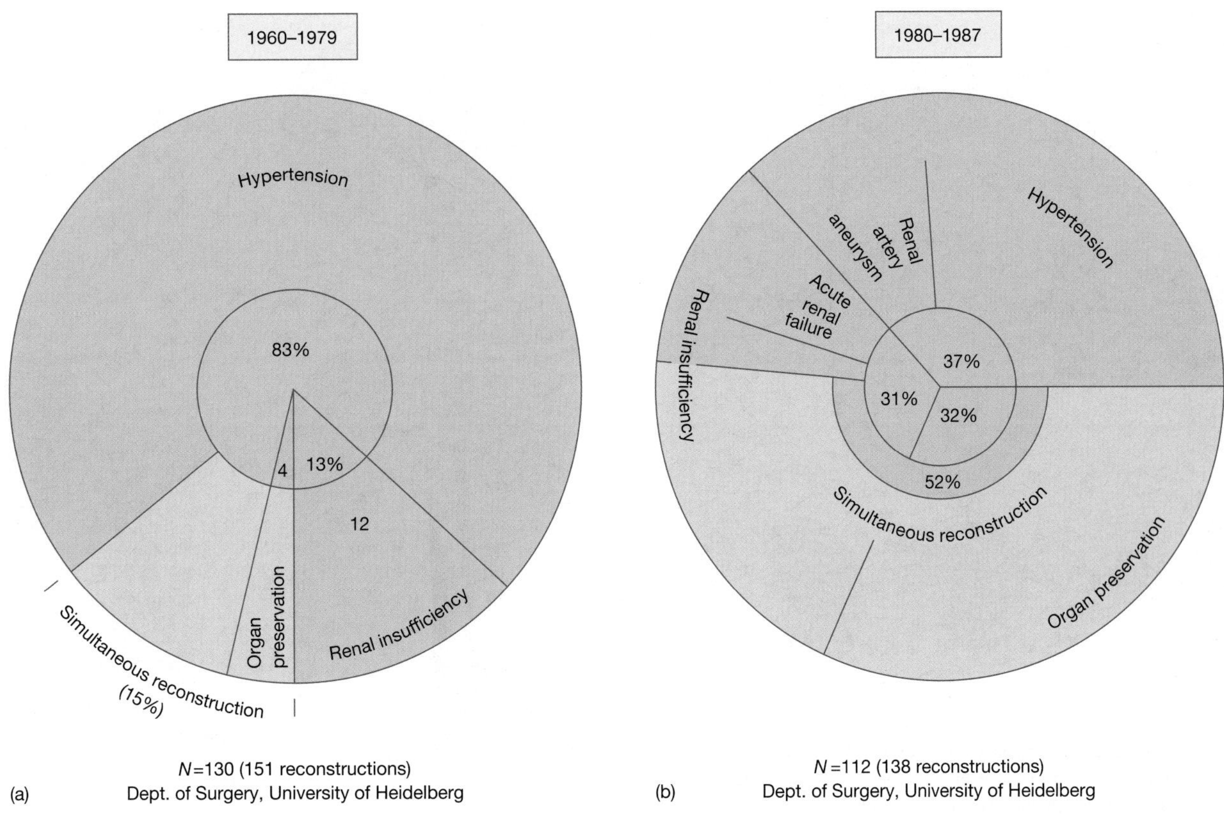

Fig. 8 (a) Indications for renal artery reconstruction in the period from 1960 to 1979: hypertension was the leading indication (83 per cent), organ preservation and renal insufficiency were indications in only 17 per cent, and simultaneous operations in the aortoiliac region were performed in 15 per cent. (b) Indications for renal artery reconstructions changed considerably in the period from 1980 to 1987: hypertension as the sole indication was present in only 37 per cent of cases, organ preservation in 32 per cent, and renal insufficiency in 31 per cent; simultaneous reconstructions in the aortoiliac region were made in 52 per cent of cases.

Table 9 Indications for the operative management of renal artery occlusive disease

Ostial stenosis of the renal artery
Simultaneous reconstruction of the aortoiliac vasculature
Severe contrast-media hypersensitivity
Renal artery aneurysm
Renal artery aneurysm combined with stenosis
Renal artery occlusion
Renal artery rupture
Re-stenosis after PTRA or unsuccessful PTRA
Renal artery stenosis secondary to kinking
Small non-functioning kidney (nephrectomy)
Peripheral multifocal stenosis

PTRA, percutaneous transluminal renal angioplasty.

Reinsertion of the renal artery must be considered if the stenosis involves its ostium or the proximal third and if it is kinked. Poststenotic dilatation facilities reinsertion in this case. In rare instances, such as kinking of the renal artery or stenosis in the middle third, segmental resection and an end-to-end anastomosis must be done.

Extra-anatomical bypass procedures must be considered in cases of stenosis recurring after surgery in the aortic or renal area. These procedures include the splenorenal bypass with preservation of the spleen (left side), the hepatorenal venous or prosthetic bypass (right side) (Fig. 11), or bypasses that originate from the celiac or mesenteric branches (Safian and Textor 2001). During reconstructive surgery, the renal ischaemia should not exceed 30–40 min. However, stenoses that have developed gradually over a long time allow longer periods of ischaemia because of abundant, collateral blood supply. If reconstruction of a renal artery is only possible with prolonged ischaemia cold perfusion *in situ* with modified Ringer's solution may help.

Due to technical problems, it may be impossible to reconstruct the renal vessels *in situ*. In these cases, two methods for extracorporal repair are currently in use: (a) the kidney may be removed and placed in front of the abdominal wall without dissection of the ureter; (b) the ureter may also be dissected free and the kidney may be repaired *ex vivo* on a work bench. The organ may then be reimplanted, either orthoptically or in the inguinal fossa, after the vascular repair. Perfusion with cold Ringer's solution again preserves the integrity of the kidney during these procedures.

Results of surgical treatment

The results of treatment described in representative studies are listed in Table 10. It is difficult to compare the various studies because the criteria for success, the selection of patients, and the surgical techniques vary

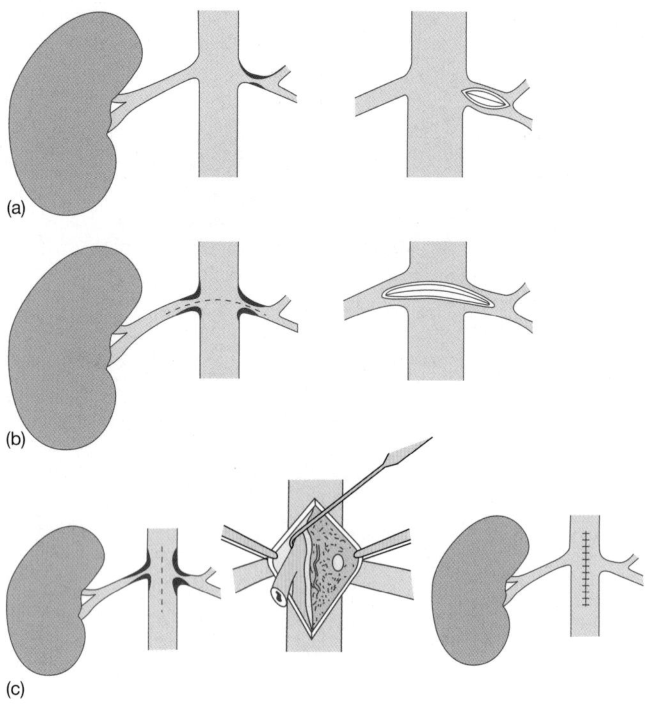

Fig. 9 Surgical approaches to renal artery stenosis: (a) direct thromboendarterectomy with vein or prosthetic roof patch angioplasty, (b) bilateral transaortic patch angioplasty, and (c) bilateral transaortic thromboendarterectomy.

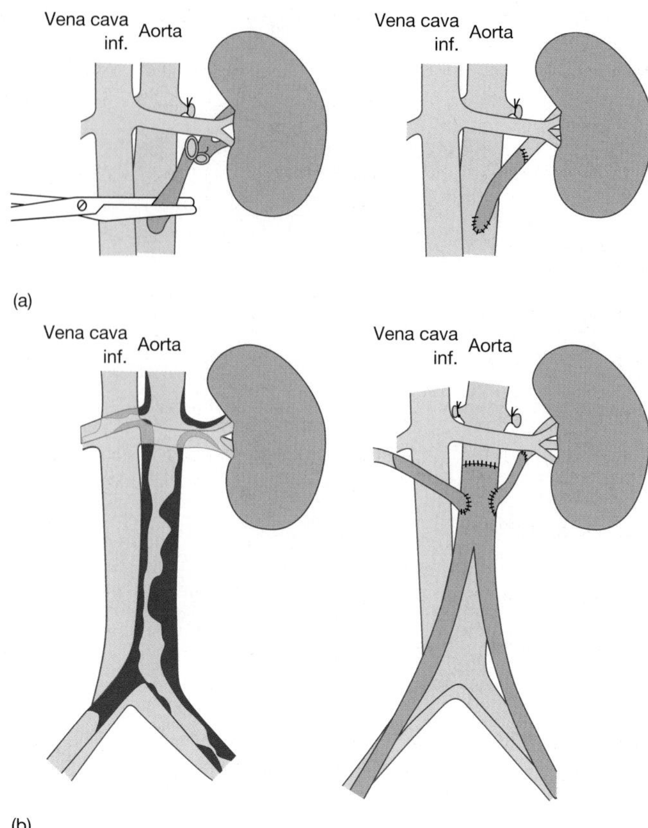

Fig. 10 (a) An aortorenal prosthetic bypass is used if a suitable vein is not available and (b) this bypass material can also be used if simultaneous time-consuming aortoiliac reconstructions are necessary.

significantly. Generally, cure of hypertension can be expected in nearly half, and improved control of blood pressure in a further 20–30 per cent of the patients treated surgically including fibromuscular and atherosclerotic stenosis. Hypertension due to fibromuscular stenosis of the renal artery is cured in 80–90 per cent of cases (Reiher *et al.* 2000). With atherosclerotic stenoses, the systemic blood pressure is normalized in only 30–50 per cent and improved in 15–20 per cent of patients (Steinbach *et al.* 1997).

Death at operation ranges from 0 to 10 per cent. Factors that increase perioperative mortality include the need for aortic reconstruction, the presence of severe perioperative azotemia, the need for bilateral renal bypass, and the use of an aortic graft as the source of aortorenal bypass. Independent predictors of an increased likelihood of death in the perioperative period include early graft failure, the presence of coronary artery disease, the presence of uncontrolled hypertension, and the need for abdominal aortic-aneurysm repair (Safian and Textor 2001).

In our own series with 261 patients and 338 revascularizations (62 per cent arteriosclerosis, 8 per cent fibromuscular, 12 per cent aneurysm), operative mortality was 2.3 per cent, patency rate of the stenoses 97 per cent, re-stenosis rate 3.5 per cent, and late occlusion was found in 1.2 per cent (Allenberg and Hupp 1995). Others provided similar results. For example, Novick (1991) operated 361 patients (arteriosclerosis in 241, fibrous disease in 104). Operative mortality was 2.1 per cent (restricted to arteriosclerotic disease), postoperative stenosis or thrombosis of the operated vessel 4.5 per cent. Hypertension was improved or cured in more than 90 per cent independent of the aetiology and renal function was stable or improved in 89 per cent.

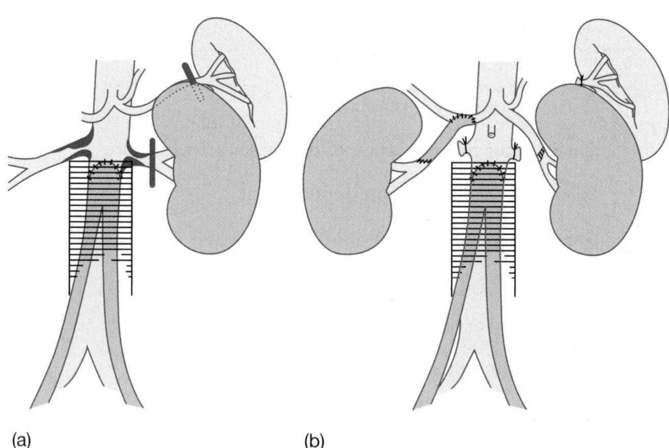

Fig. 11 Extra-anatomical bypass procedures can be performed with re-stenosis of the renal artery or with previous aortoiliac reconstructions. A splenorenal bypass and a hepatorenal bypass are shown.

Surgical correction of ischaemic nephropathy can retrieve renal function in selected patients dependent on dialysis characterized by a rapid decline in preoperative glomerular filtration rate in combination with global renal ischaemia treated by complete or bilateral renal vascularization. After renal artery repair, discontinuation of dialysis

Table 10 Results of surgical reconstruction on RAS in patients with renovascular hypertension

Reference	*n*	Systemic blood pressure at the end of the observation period			Minimum observation time (months)	Perioperative mortality (%)
		Normal	Improved	Unchanged		
Grim *et al.* (1982)	25 ATS	4 (16%)	20 (80%)	1 (4%)	24	—
	32 FMD	22 (69%)	10 (31%)	0	24	
Von Dongen *et al.* (1972)	200	132 (66%)	36 (18%)	32 (16%)	Preliminary	—
DeBakey *et al.* (1964)	115	80%	8%	6%	1–48	6
DeBakey *et al.* (1964)	225 ATS (83%) FMD (17%)	81%	8%	6%	24–60	5.80
Vollmar *et al.* (1971)	39 ATS	46%	23%	31%		—
	16 FMD	88%	6%	6%		
Breslin *et al.* (1982)	225 ATS	66%	30%	4%	12	2.1
	FMD	86%	14%	0		
Hansen *et al.* (1996)	54 ATS	72%		28%	96 retrospectively	7.4

ATS, atherosclerosis; FMD, fibromuscular dysplasia.

may be associated with improved survival rates when compared with continued dialysis dependence (Hansen *et al.* 1995).

Postoperative complications

Early thrombosis and stenosis are the main postoperative complications. Thrombotic occlusion after patch angioplasty is usually detected too late to save the kidney. Therefore, an intraoperative angiogram to assess the quality of the repair is recommended. In the early postoperative period, continuous monitoring of blood pressure, urinary output, and renal function are obligatory. Late complications include re-stenosis, occlusion, and the formation of aneurysms, especially with vein grafts, and rarely rupture—one single report in the literature (Travis *et al.* 2000). The rate of re-stenosis is estimated to be 5–20 per cent, and the survival rate is 65–81 per cent at 5 years. Independent predictors of increased late mortality include an age of more than 70 years at the time of the bypass, the presence of coronary artery disease, and preoperative uncontrolled hypertension (Safian and Textor 2001).

Postoperative use of anticoagulants

At the present time, prophylaxis of thrombosis with aspirin (about 200 mg/day) for at least 3 months is recommended in all patients after PTRA and surgical thromboendarterectomy. After aortorenal bypass, life-long treatment with warfarin may be useful.

Special problems of invasive treatment

Acute renal artery embolism and thrombosis

Information on embolism of the renal artery is confined to anecdotal reports because this unfortunate incident is rare in clinical practice. However, autopsy studies show a higher incidence of such embolism in up to 1 per cent of autopsies (Roberts *et al.* 1959). If the diagnosis is suspected, the patient should immediately undergo angiography to confirm the presence of embolism or thrombosis and to institute fibrinolysis, or to refer the patient for surgery. However, if thrombosis of the renal artery is a consequence of PTRA, fibrinolysis may lead to severe retroperitoneal bleeding through the previously damaged or dissected vessel. In this case, the patient should be referred to the vascular surgeon immediately.

Chronic occlusion of the renal artery

A kidney distal to a chronically occluded renal artery may be sufficiently perfused by collateral vessels to prevent its necrosis. These collateral vessels originate from gonadal, lumbar, ureteral, and suprarenal arteries. Because of these collaterals, renal salvage is often achieved by recanalization of the renal artery. PTRA has been successfully used for recanalization in half of obstructed arteries. There is little variability in the findings from various clinics (Gutierrez *et al.* 1981; Sniderman and Sos 1982; Mann and Allenberg 1985). In this instance the results of surgery are by far better than those of PTRA. As outlined above, recanalization should only be attempted if the results of diagnostic ultrasonography and scintigraphy suggest that the kidney will be viable.

Acute occlusion of a renal artery

This acute complex of symptoms is frequently misdiagnosed as urolithiasis (Table 11); patients with a functional, solitary kidney present with oliguria. For correct diagnosis and immediate treatment, a high level of suspicion is required.

Treatment with PTRA is possible (Fig. 12); however, such attempts should not delay surgery. As outlined above for chronic occlusion, PTRA and other catheter-conducted techniques are successful in only half of cases. Therefore, management must include surgical treatment; the administration of fibrinolytics should be avoided.

Figure 13 shows the operative course of a young patient who presented with acute oliguria of more than 10-h duration and flank pain for 5 days. He had only one functioning kidney. Spontaneous dissection of the renal artery was found (his angiogram is shown in Fig. 1). The intrarenal arteries were completely occluded by thrombi. After

Table 11 Symptoms, primary diagnosis, and management of nine patients with acute occlusion of a renal artery supplying a functional solitary kidney

Symptoms	
Oliguria	9/9
Flank pain	7/9
Haematuria	1/9
Primary diagnosis	
Urolithiasis	6/9
Pyelonephritis	1/9
Renal artery embolism	2/9
Assessment/management	
Initial serum creatinine	3–11 mg/100 ml
Dialysis required	4/9
Final serum creatinine (follow-up at least 6 months)	1–3 mg/100 ml

extracorporeal reconstruction, the patient required dialysis for 2 weeks. Thereafter, he regained normal renal function over a period of seven months. His creatinine decreased to 1.6 mg/100 ml. Figure 14 depicts the follow-up scintigrams. This case demonstrates that renal salvage is possible even after prolonged periods of ischaemia; there are other such instructive examples (Smith *et al.* 1974). Recent data of Reilly *et al.* (1991) support the salutary role of surgery in spontaneous renal artery dissection.

Medical treatment, percutaneous angioplasty or surgery for renal artery stenosis?

The results of four randomized trials are available which prospectively compared interventional with medical treatment of atherosclerotic renal artery stenosis (Plouin *et al.* 1998; Webster *et al.* 1998; Xue *et al.* 1999; van Jaarsveld *et al.* 2000). There was no benefit of angioplasty over medical treatment in terms of blood pressure control and of preservation of renal function. However, a closer look into the designs and the results of the above mentioned studies offers more detailed information. The DRASTIC-study of van Jaarsveld *et al.* (2000) randomized a total of 106 patients with renal artery stenosis greater than 50 per cent; 50 patients were assigned to drug therapy. Twenty-two of these 50 patients underwent angioplasty after 3 months because of drug-resistant hypertension. Three months after randomization mean blood pressure of these 22 patients was significantly higher and creatinine clearance was lower than the corresponding values of the 28 patients who were treated exclusively with antihypertensive drugs. However, in an intention-to-treat-analysis after 12 months blood pressure and creatinine clearance of the 50 patients originally assigned to medical treatment in total did not differ from the corresponding values of the 56 patients assigned to angioplasty though the latter needed less antihypertensive drugs. It is further of note that in the group assigned to medical treatment, renal artery occlusion occurred in eight patients but in none of the patients treated with angioplasty (van Jaarsveld *et al.* 2000). In a Scottish study less than half of 135 eligible patients ($N = 55$) with at least 50 per cent renal artery stenosis were randomized and subgroups of patients with unilateral and bilateral disease were analysed (Webster *et al.* 1998). In this small trial only patients with bilateral disease showed a significant decrease in systolic blood pressure after angioplasty as compared to drug treatment. In patients with unilateral disease, blood pressure did not significantly differ between both treatment arms and creatinine clearance was not different after 6 months (Webster *et al.* 1998).

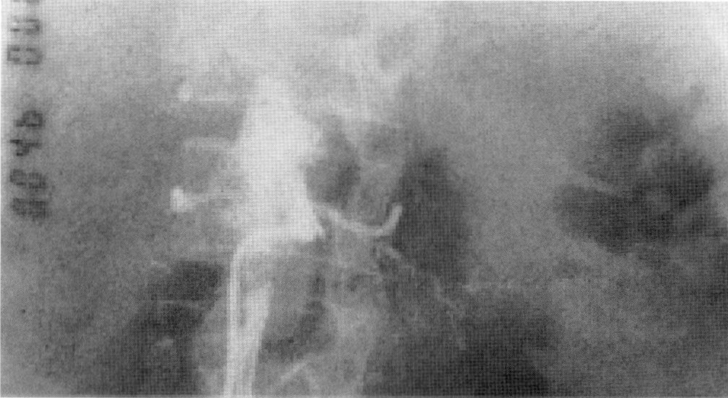
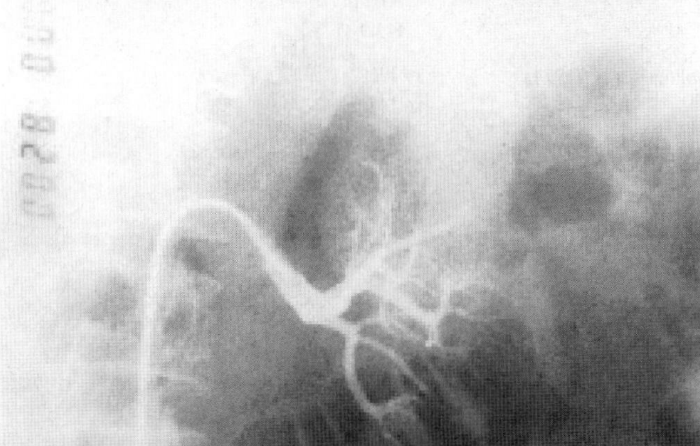
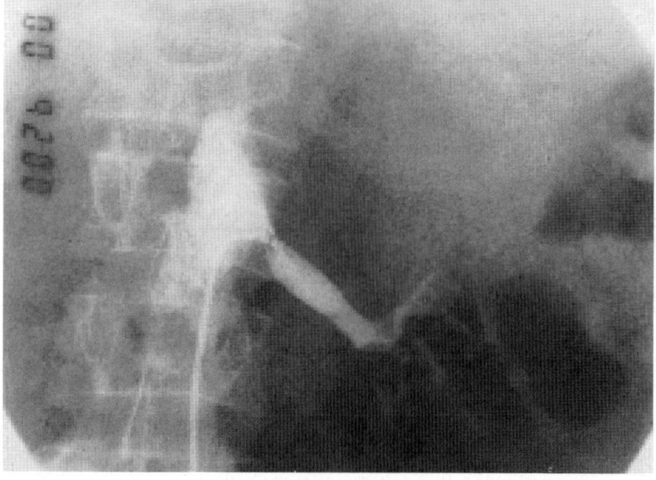

Fig. 12 Frames of a cineangiogram for a patient with known occlusion of the right renal artery who presented with acute anuria. The angiogram showed acute occlusion of the left renal artery. The stump of the left renal artery can be seen in the top frame. The middle frame shows a coronary percutaneous transluminal angioplasty guiding catheter (left) acutely traversing the thrombus of the renal artery. Several attempts with other guiding catheters and wires were unsuccessful. The bottom frame shows the remaining high-grade stenosis of the left renal artery. This could be successfully dilated. The patient died 3 years later of myocardial infarction, but had a stable serum creatinine.

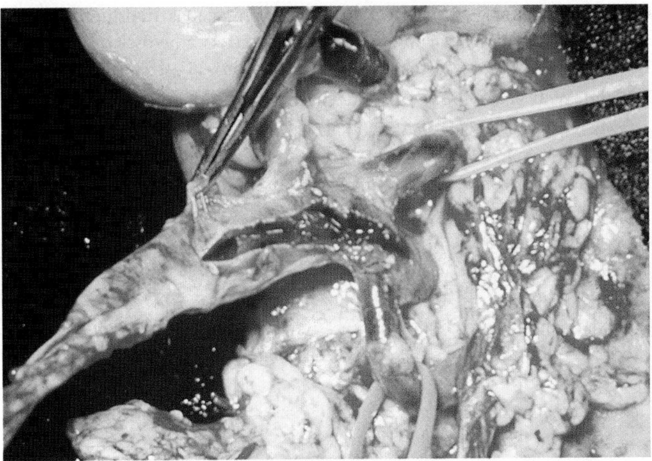

Fig. 13 Acute renal artery dissection with thrombosis of all segmental renal arteries. The angiogram and the hippurate renograms are shown in Figs 1 and 14, respectively.

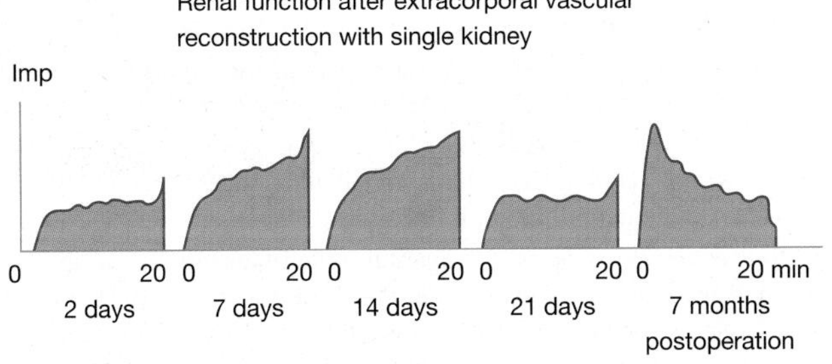

Fig. 14 ^{131}I-hippurate renograms after surgical reconstruction in the patient whose operative findings are shown in Fig. 13. The ordinate indicates the impulses, and the abscissa depicts the renograms 2 days, 7 days, 14 days, 21 days, and 7 months after operation.

In a prospective French study, 49 patients with renal artery stenosis greater than 50 per cent were randomized and 26 of them were assigned to medical treatment. Seven of these 26 patients required angioplasty due to drug-resistant hypertension during the follow-up of 6 months. The number of patients who needed more than two antihypertensives for blood pressure control was significantly higher in the medication group (Plouin *et al.* 1998).

These trials support the clinical practice to treat people with renovascular hypertension first by drugs. If blood pressure remains too high for more than 3 months, patients should be referred to PTA. This conservative approach is consistent with recent uncontrolled data from long-term follow-up of people with renal artery stenosis (Leertouwer *et al.* 2001). Surprisingly few of the participants of this retrospective analysis reached endstage renal disease and many died prematurely of cardiovascular diseases.

The initial cost for bypass grafting was found substantially higher than that for PTRA or stent placement by Xue *et al.* (1999). The choice of treatment in individual patients is often not as straightforward as the last paragraph of this chapter may suggest. The personal preferences of a patient, for example, opting for less drug-related side-effects after PTA, play a considerable role as does his potential life expectancy, etc. A high intrarenal vascular resistance strongly argues against invasive treatment because of extensive nephrosclerosis (Radermacher *et al.* 2001b).

References

Allenberg, J. R. and Hupp, T. (1995). Endovascular and open reconstructive surgery of renal artery lesions. *Chirurg* **66**, 101–111.

Anderson, G. H., Blakeman, N., and Streeten, D. H. P. (1988). Prediction of renovascular hypertension. Comparison of clinical diagnostic indices. *American Journal of Hypertension* **1**, 301–304.

Arlart, L. *et al.* (1979). Predictive value of radionuclide methods in the diagnosis of unilateral renovascular hypertension. *Cardiovascular Radiology* **1**, 115–125.

Avasthi, P. S., Voyles, W. F., and Greene, E. R. (1984). Noninvasive diagnosis of renal artery stenosis by echo-Doppler velocimetry. *Kidney International* **25**, 824–829.

Baert, A. L. (1994). Renal artery stent placement. *Radiology* **191**, 713–719.

Baumgartner, I., Triller, J., and Mahler, F. (1997). Patency of percutaneous transluminal renal angioplasty: a prospective sonographic study. *Kidney International* **51** (3), 798–803.

Baumgartner, I. *et al.* (2000). Stent placement in ostial and nonostial atherosclerotic renal arterial stenoses: a prospective follow-up study. *Radiology* **216** (2), 498–505.

Berglund, G., Andersson, O., and Wilhelmsen, L. (1976). Prevalence of primary and secondary hypertension: studies in random population samples. *British Medical Journal* **2**, 554–556.

Beroniade, V. *et al.* (1987). Primary renal artery dissection. *American Journal of Nephrology* **7**, 382–389.

Beutler, J. J. *et al.* (2001). Long-term effects of arterial stenting on kidney function for patients with ostial atherosclerotic renal artery stenosis and renal insufficiency. *Journal of the American Society of Nephrology* **12** (7), 1475–1481.

Bijlstra, P. J. *et al.* (1996). Clinical and biochemical criteria in the detection of renal artery stenosis. *Journal of Hypertension* **14**, 1033–1040.

Blaufox, M. D. *et al.* (1996). Cost efficacy of the diagnosis and therapy of renovascular hypertension. *Journal of Nuclear Medicine* **37**, 171–177.

Blum, U. *et al.* (1997). Treatment of ostial renal-artery stenoses with vascular endoprostheses after unsuccessful balloon angioplasty. *New England Journal of Medicine* **336**, 459–465.

Bonelli, F. S. *et al.* (1995). Renal artery angioplasty: technical results and clinical outcome in 320 patients. *Mayo Clinics Proceedings* **70** (11), 1041–1052.

Bookstein, J. J. *et al.* (1972a). Radiologic aspects of renovascular hypertension: I. Aims and methods of the radiology study group. *Journal of the American Medical Association* **220**, 1218–1224.

Bookstein, J. J. *et al.* (1972b). Radiologic aspects of renovascular hypertension: II. The role of urography in unilateral renovascular disease. *Journal of the American Medical Association* **220**, 1225–1230.

Brawn, L. A. and Ramsey, L. E. (1987). Is 'improvement' real with percutaneous transluminal angioplasty in the management of renovascular hypertension. *Lancet* **i**, 1313–1314.

Breslin, D. J. *et al. Renovascular Hypertension.* Baltimore: Williams & Wilkins, 1982.

Brezis, M. and Epstein, F. H. (1989). A closer look at radiocontrast-induced nephropathy. *New England Journal of Medicine* **320**, 179–180.

Brunner, H. R. *et al.* (1971). Hypertension of renal origin: evidence for two different mechanisms. *Science* **174**, 1344–1347.

Bush, R. L. *et al.* (2001). Endovascular revascularization of renal artery stenosis: technical and clinical results. *Journal of Vascular Surgery* **33** (5), 1041–1049.

Canzanello, V. J. *et al.* (1989). Percutaneous transluminal renal angioplasty in the management of atherosclerotic renovascular hypertension: results in 100 patients. *Hypertension* **13**, 163–172.

Caps, M. T. *et al.* (1998a). Prospective study of atherosclerotic disease progression in the renal artery. *Circulation* **98**, 2866–2872.

Caps, M. T. *et al.* (1998b). Risk of atrophy in kidneys with atherosclerotic renal artery stenosis. *Kidney International* **53**, 735–742.

Carlsson, E. *et al.* (1963). Renal arteriostenosis in cases of intermittent claudication and hypertension. *Journal of Cardiovascular Surgery* **4**, 393–400.

Castaneda-Zuniga, W. *Transluminal Angioplasty*. Stuttgart: Thieme, 1983.

Cheung, C. M. *et al.* (2002). Epidemiology of renal dysfunction and patient outcome in atherosclerotic renal artery occlusion. *Journal of the American Society of Nephrology* **13**, 149–157.

Chiarini, C. *et al.* (1982). Renal scintigraphy versus renal vein renin activity for identifying and treatment of renovascular hypertension. *Nephron* **32**, 8–13.

Cigarroa, R. G. *et al.* (1989). Dosing of contrast material to prevent contrast nephropathy in patients with renal disease. *American Journal of Medicine* **86**, 649–652.

Claudon, M. *et al.* (2000). Renal arteries in patients at risk of renal arterial stenosis: multicenter evaluation of the echo-enhancer SH U 508A at color and spectral Doppler US. Levovist Renal Artery Stenosis Study Group. *Radiology* **214**, 739–746.

Clorius, J. H. *et al.* (1987). Predictive value of exercise renography for presurgical evaluation of nephrogenic hypertension. *Hypertension* **10**, 280–286.

Colapinto, R. F. *et al.* (1982). Percutaneous transluminal dilatation of the renal artery. *American Journal of Roentgenology* **130**, 727–732.

Conlon, P. J. *et al.* (2001). Severity of renal vascular disease predicts mortality in patients undergoing coronary angiography. *Kidney International* **60**, 1490–1497.

Crinnion, J. N. and Gough, M. J. (1996). Bilateral renal artery atherosclerosis—the results of surgical treatment. *European Journal of Vascular and Endovascular Surgery* **11**, 353–358.

Dargie, J. H., Franklin, S. S., and Reid, J. L. (1977). Plasma noradrenaline concentrations in experimental renovascular hypertension in the rat. *Clinical Science and Molecular Medicine* **52**, 477.

Datseris, I. E. *et al.* (1994). Captopril renal scintigraphy in patients with hypertension and chronic renal failure. *Journal of Nuclear Medicine* **35**, 251–256.

Davidson, R. A. and Wilcox, C. S. (1992). Newer tests for the diagnosis of renovascular disease. *Journal of the American Medical Association* **268**, 3353.

Davidson, R. A., Barri, Y., and Wilcox, C. S. (1996). Predictors of cure of hypertension in fibromuscular renovascular disease. *American Journal of Kidney Diseases* **28**, 334–338.

Davies, B. A. *et al.* (1979). Prevalence of renovascular hypertension in patients with Grade III or IV hypertensive retinopathy. *New England Journal of Medicine* **301**, 1273.

Davies, D. L. *et al.* (1983). Body sodium and blood pressure: abnormal and different correlations in Conn's syndrome, renal artery stenosis and essential hypertension. *Proceedings of the European Dialysis and Transplant Association* **20**, 44–55.

Dean, R. H. (1986). Comparison of medical and surgical treatment of renovascular hypertension. *Nephron* **44** (Suppl. 1), 1012–1014.

Dean, R. H. *et al.* (1991). Evolution of renal insufficiency in ischemic nephropathy. *Annals of Surgery* **213**, 446–456.

DeBakey, M. E. *et al.* (1964). Lesions of the renal artery: urological technique and results. *American Journal of Surgery* **107**, 84–96.

Derkx, F. H. *et al.* (1996). Renal artery stenosis towards the year 2000. *Journal of Hypertension* **14**, S167–S172.

Derkx, F. M. H. *et al.* Captopril test for diagnosis of renal artery stenosis. In *Renovascular Hypertension* (ed. N. Glorioso *et al.*). New York: Raven Press, 1987.

DiBona, G. F. (1982). The functions of the renal nerves. *Reviews of Physiology Biochemistry and Pharmacology* **94**, 75–81.

Dondi, M. *et al.* (1992). Prognostic value of captopril renal scintigraphy in renovascular hypertension. *Journal of Nuclear Medicine* **33**, 2040–2044.

Dotter, C. T. and Indkins, M. P. (1964). Transluminal treatment of arteriosclerotic obstruction. Description of a new technique and a preliminary report of its application. *Circulation* **30**, 654–659.

Eldrup-Jorgensen, J. *et al.* (1995). Should percutaneous transluminal renal artery angioplasty be applied to ostial renal artery atherosclerosis? *Journal of Vascular Surgery* **21** (6), 909–914 (discussion 914–915).

England, W. L. *et al.* (1988). Cost-effectiveness in the detection of renal artery stenosis. *Journal of General Internal Medicine* **3**, 344–350.

Erbslöh-Möller, B. *et al.* (1991). Furosemide-^{131}I-hippuran renography after angiotensin-converting enzyme inhibition of the diagnosis of renovascular hypertension. *American Journal of Medicine* **90**, 23–29.

Eyler, W. R. *et al.* (1962). Angiography of the renal areas including a comparative study of renal arterial stenoses in patients with and without hypertension. *Radiology* **78**, 379–383.

Faber, J. E. and Brody, M. J. (1985). Afferent renal nerve-dependent hypertension following acute renal artery stenosis in the conscious rat. *Circulation Research* **57**, 676–688.

Fleischmann, E., Luft, F. C., and Mann, J. (1993). Die Kontrastmittelnephropathie. *Nieren- und Hochdruckkrankheiten* **22**, 177–186.

Fommei, E. *et al.* (1987). Renal scintigraphic captopril test in the diagnosis of renovascular hypertension. *Hypertension* **10**, 212–220.

Fommei, E., Mezzasalma, L., and Ghione, S. (1991). European captopril radionuclide test multicenter study. Preliminary results. Inspective renographic analysis. The European captopril radionuclide test multicenter study group. *American Journal of Hypertension* **4**, 716–720.

Franklin, S. S. and Smith, R. D. (1985). Comparison of effects of enalapril plus hydrochlorothiazide versus standard triple therapy on renal function in renovascular hypertension. *American Journal of Medicine* **79**, 14–23.

Frederickson, E. D. *et al.* (1990). A prospective evaluation of a simplified captopril test for the detection of renovascular hypertension. *Archives of Internal Medicine* **150**, 569–572.

Gaines, P. A. *et al.* (1988). Cholesterol embolisation: a lethal complication of vascular catherisation. *Lancet* **ii**, 168–171.

Gayard, P. *et al.* (2000). Spiral CT quantification of aorto-renal calcification and its use in the detection of atheromatous renal artery stenosis: a study in 42 patients. *Cardiovascular and Interventional Radiology* **23**, 17–24.

Geyskes, G. *et al.* (1987a). Renovascular hypertension identified by captopril-induced changes in the renogram. *Hypertension* **9**, 451–458.

Geyskes, G. *et al.* Unilateral renal failure after captopril in patients with renovascular hypertension. In *Renovascular Hypertension* (ed. N. Glorioso *et al.*), pp. 120–124. New York: Raven Press, 1987b.

Gifford, R. W. (1969). Evaluation of the hypertensive patient with emphasis on detecting curable causes. *Millbank Memorial Fund Quarterly* **47**, 170–186.

Goldblatt, H. *et al.* (1934). Studies on experimental hypertension. I. The production of persistent evaluation of systolic blood pressure by means of renal ischemia. *Journal of Experimental Medicine* **59**, 347–353.

Goncharenko, V. *et al.* (1981). Progression of renal artery fibromuscular dysplasia in 42 patients as seen on angiography. *Radiology* **139**, 45–51.

Greco, B. A. and Breyer, J. A. (1996). The natural history of renal artery stenosis: who should be evaluated for ischemic nephropathy? *Seminars in Nephrology* **16**, 2–11.

Grim, C. E. and Weinberger, M. H. The case for renin assays. In *Controversies in Nephrology and Hypertension* (ed. R. G. Narins), pp. 111–122. New York: Churchill Livingstone, 1984.

Grim, C. E. *et al.* (1979). Sensitivity and specificity of screening tests for renovascular hypertension. *Annals of Internal Medicine* **91**, 617–622.

Grim, C. E. *et al.* (1982). Unilateral renal vascular hypertension: surgery vs. dilatation. *Hypertension* **4**, 367–368.

Gross, F. *et al.* (1975). Salt loss as a possible mechanism eliciting an acute malignant phase in renal hypertensive rats. *Clinical and Experimental Pharmacology and Physiology* **2**, 323–330.

Grüntzig, A. *et al.* (1978). Treatment of renovascular hypertension with percutaneous transluminal dilatation of a renal artery stenosis. *Lancet* **i**, 801–803.

Grützmacher, P. and Bussmann, W. D. (1984). Behandlung der renovaskulären Hypertonie mittels Ballonkatheter. *Innere Medizin* **11**, 219–226.

Grützmacher, P. and Bussmann, W. D. (1986). Transluminale Dilatation und andere nichtoperative Kathetertechniken in der Behandlung der renovaskulären Hypertonie. *Klinische Wochenschrift* **64**, 884–896.

Grützmacher, P. *et al.* (1988). Non-operative revascularisation of renal artery occlusion by transluminal angioplasty. *Nephrology, Dialysis, Transplantation* **2**, 130–137.

Gutierrez, O. H., Izzo, J. L., Jr., and Burgener, F. A. (1981). Transluminal recanalization of an occluded renal artery: reversal of anuria in a patient with a solitary kidney. *American Journal of Radiology* **137**, 1254–1257.

Guzman, R. P. *et al.* (1994). Renal atrophy and arterial stenosis: a prospective study with duplex ultrasound. *Hypertension* **23**, 346–350.

Hansen, K. J. *et al.* (1995). Surgical management of dialysis-dependent ischemic nephropathy. *Journal of Vascular Surgery* **21** (2), 197–209 (discussion 209–211).

Hansen, K. J. *et al.* (1996). Is renal revascularization in diabetic patients worthwhile? *Journal of Vascular Surgery* **24** (3), 383–392 (discussion 392–393).

Hansen, K. J. *et al.* (2000). Management of ischemic nephropathy: dialysis-free survival after surgical repair. *Journal of Vascular Surgery* **32** (3), 472–481 (discussion 481–482).

Harden, P. N. *et al.* (1997). Effect of renal-artery stenting on progression of renovascular renal failure. *Lancet* **349** (9059), 1133–1136.

Hardin, C. A. (1965). The surgical importance of combined renal artery hypertension with cervical cephalic arterial occlusive disease. *Angiology* **16**, 754.

Harding, B. M. *et al.* (1992). Renal artery stenosis: prevalence and associated risk factors in patients undergoing routine cardiac catheterization. *Journal of the American Society of Nephrology* **2**, 1608–1616.

Harrison, E. G., Jr. and McCormack, L. J. (1971). Pathologic classification of renal arterial diseases in renovascular hypertension. *Mayo Clinic Proceedings* **46**, 161–167.

Havey, R. J. *et al.* (1985). Screening for renovascular hypertension. Is renal digital subtraction angiography the preferred non-invasive test? *Journal of the American Medical Association* **254**, 388–393.

Hofbauer, K. G. and Wood, J. M. (1988). Renin inhibitors as possible antihypertensive agents. *Klinische Wochenschrift* **66**, 906–913.

Hoffmann, U. *et al.* (1991). Role of duplex scanning for the detection of atherosclerotic renal artery disease. *Kidney International* **39**, 1232–1239.

Holley, K. E. *et al.* (1964). Renal artery stenosis. A clinical–pathological study in normotensive and hypertensive patients. *American Journal of Medicine* **37**, 14–22.

Horne, M. L. *et al.* (1979). Angiotensin II profiling with saralasin: summary of Eaton collaborative study. *Kidney International* **15**, 115–122.

Hupp, Th. and Allenberg, J. R. (1985). Akutes Nierenversagen durch Nierenarterienverschluss, ein chirurgisches Krankheitsbild. *Der Chirurg* **56**, 322–326.

Imanishi, M. *et al.* (1994). Aspirin renography to detect unilateral renovascular hypertension. *Kidney International* **45**, 1170–1176.

Ingelfinger, J. R. (1993). Renovascular disease in children. *Kidney International* **43**, 493–505.

Ingrisch, H. (1988). Perkutane Rekanalisation der Nierenarterie. In *Interventionelle Radiologie* (ed. R. W. Guenther and M. Thelan), pp. 44–57. Georg. Thieme Verlag Stuttgart.

Isles, C. G., Robertson, S., and Hill, D. (1999). Management of renovascular disease: a review of renal artery stenting in ten studies. *QJM: Monthly Journal of the Association of Physicians* **92** (3), 159–167.

Jacobson, H. R. (1988). Ischemic renal disease: an overlooked clinical entity? *Kidney International* **34**, 729–743.

Jean, W. J. *et al.* (1994). High incidence of renal artery stenosis in patients with coronary artery disease. *Catheterization and Cardiovascular Diagnosis* **32**, 8–10.

Jeunemaitre, X. *et al.* (1990). Intraluminal angioplasty in renovascular arterial hypertension—104 cases. *Presse Med.* **19**, 205–209.

Johansson, M. *et al.* (2000). Evaluation of duplex ultrasound and captopril renography for detection of renovascular hypertension. *Kidney International* **58**, 774–782.

Kaatee, R. *et al.* (1997). Renal artery stenosis: detection and quantification with spiral CT angiography versus optimized digital subtraction angiography. *Radiology* **205**, 121–127.

Karam, R., Lever, H. M., and Healy, B. P. (1989). Hypertensive hypertrophic cardiomyopathy or hypertrophic cardiomyopathy with hypertension? A study of 78 patients. *Journal of the American College of Cardiology* **13**, 580–584.

Katholi, R. E., Winternitz, S. R., and Oparil, S. (1982). Decrease in peripheral sympathetic nervous system activity following renal denervation or unclipping in the one-kidney one-clip Goldblatt hypertensive rat. *Journal of Clinical Investigation* **69**, 55–59.

Kaufmann, J. J. (1979). Renovascular hypertension: the UCLA experience. *Journal of Urology* **121**, 139–144.

Keith, T. A. (1982). Renovascular hypertension in black patients. *Hypertension* **4**, 438.

Klinge, J. *et al.* (1989). Percutaneous transluminal renal angioplasty: initial and long-term results. *Radiology* **171**, 501–506.

Klow, N. E. *et al.* (1998). Percutaneous transluminal renal artery angioplasty using the coaxial technique. Ten years of experience from 591 procedures in 419 patients. *Acta Radiologica* **39** (6), 594–603.

Kremer Hovinga, T. K. *et al.* (1990). Relief of renal artery stenosis: a tool to improve or preserve renal function in renovascular disease? *Nephrology, Dialysis, Transplantation* **5**, 481–488.

Krijnen, P. *et al.* (1998). A clinical prediction rule for renal artery stenosis. *Annals of Internal Medicine* **129**, 705–711.

Krishnamurthi, V., Novick, A. C., and Myles, J. L. (1999). Atheroembolic renal disease: effect on morbidity and survival after revascularization for atherosclerotic renal artery stenosis. *Journal of Urology* **161**, 1093–1096.

Krumme, B. and Blum, U. (1998). Imaging of renal artery stenosis. *Current Opinion in Urology* **8**, 77–82.

Krumme, B. and Rump, L. C. (1996). Colour Doppler sonography to screen for renal artery stenosis—technical points to consider. *Nephrology, Dialysis, Transplantation* **12**, 2385–2389.

Krumme, B. *et al.* (1996). Diagnosis of renovascular disease by intra- and extrarenal Doppler sonography. *Kidney International* **50**, 1288–1292.

Kuhlmann, U. *et al.* (1983). Häufigkeit und Bedeutung von Nierenarterienstenosen bei Patienten mit peripherer arterieller Verschlusskrankheit. *Klinische Wochenschrift* **61**, 339–342.

Kuhlmann, U. *et al.* (1985). Long-term experience in percutaneous transluminal dilatation of renal artery stenosis. *American Journal of Medicine* **79**, 692–698.

Kuroda, S. *et al.* (2000). Prevalence of renal artery stenosis in autopsy patients with stroke. *Stroke* **31**, 61–65.

Kutkuhn, B. *et al.* (1988). Captopril-stimulierte Plasma-Renina-Aktivität in der Diagnostik der renovaskulären Hypertonie. *Deutsche Medizinische Wochenschrift* **113**, 73–78.

Leertouwer, T. C. *et al.* (2000). Stent placement for renal arterial stenosis: where do we stand? A meta-analysis. *Radiology* **216** (1), 78–85.

Leertouwer, T. C., Pattynama, P. M. T., and Van Den Berg-Huysmans, A. (2001). Incidental renal artery stenosis in peripheral vascular disease: a case for treatment? *Kidney International* **59**, 1480–1483.

Lerman, L. O. *et al.* (1999). Noninvasive evaluation of a novel swine model of renal artery stenosis. *Journal of the American Society of Nephrology* **7**, 1455–1465.

Louie, J. *et al.* (1994). Prevalence of carotid and lower extremity arterial disease in patients with renal artery stenosis. *American Journal of Hypertension* **7**, 436–439.

Luft, F. C., Rankin, L. I., and Swain, R. R. (1979). Urinary *n*-acetylglucosaminidase excretion in rats with renovascular hypertension. *Proceedings of the Society for Experimental Biology and Medicine* **160**, 168–169.

Luft, F. C. *et al.* (1989). Angiotensin-induced hypertension in the rat: sympathetic nerve activity and the excretion of prostaglandins. *Hypertension* **14**, 396–403.

Lüscher, T. F. *et al.* (1985). Fibromuskuläre renovaskuläre Hypertonie: Vergleich von Operation, transluminaler Dilatation und medikamentöser Therapie. *Schweizer Medizinische Wochenschrift* **115**, 146–153.

Maher, E. R. *et al.* (1988). Captopril-enhanced 99m TcDTPA scintigraphy in the detection of renal-artery stenosis. *Nephrology, Dialysis, Transplantation* **3**, 608–611.

Mahler, F. *et al.* (1986). Complications in percutaneous transluminal dilatation of renal arteries. *Nephron* **44** (Suppl. 1), 60–63.

Mailloux, L. U. *et al.* (1994). Renal vascular disease causing end-stage renal disease, incidence, clinical correlates, and outcomes: a 20-year clinical experience. *American Journal of Kidney Diseases* **24**, 622–629.

Malatino, L. S. *et al.* (1998). Diagnosis of renovascular disease by extra- and intrarenal Doppler parameters. *Angiology* **49**, 707–721.

Mann, J. F. E. (1995). The diagnosis of renovascular hypertension: state of the art 1995. *Nephrology, Dialysis, Transplantation* **10** (8), 1285–1286.

Mann, J. F. E. and Allenberg, J. Renovaskuläre Hypertonie. In *Lehrbuch der Hypertonie* (ed. D. Ganten and E. Ritz), pp. 503–539. Stuttgart: Schattauer, 1985.

Mann, B. *et al.* (2001). Acute upregulation of COX-2 by renal artery stenosis. *American Journal of Physiology. Renal Physiology* **280**, F119–F125.

Mann, J. F. E. *et al.* (1978). Effects of central and peripheral angiotensin blockade in hypertensive rats. *American Journal of Physiology* **234**, H269–H637.

Mann, J. F. E. *et al.* (1985). Dilatation to avoid dialysis: angioplasty of an occluded renal artery with a coronary guiding catheter. *Lancet* **i**, 579–582.

Mann, S. J. *et al.* (1991). Captopril renography in the diagnosis of renal artery stenosis: accuracy and limitations. *American Journal of Medicine* **90**, 30–40.

Maslowski, A. H. *et al.* (1983). Mechanisms in human renovascular hypertension. *Hypertension* **5**, 597–603.

Mathias, C. J. *et al.* (1983). Clonidine lowers blood pressure independently of renin suppression in patients with unilateral renal artery stenosis. *Chest* **83** (Suppl.), 357s–361s.

Meaney, T. F., Dustan, H. P., and McCorman, L. J. (1968). Natural history of renal arterial disease. *Radiology* **91**, 881–887.

Meissner, M. D., Wilson, Ar., and Jessup, M. (1988). Renal artery stenosis in heart failure. *American Journal of Cardiology* **62**, 1307–1308.

Meyrier, A. *et al.* (1988). Atheromatous renal disease. *American Journal of Medicine* **85**, 139–146.

Missouris, C. G. *et al.* (1993). Renal artery stenosis masquerading as congestive heart failure. *Lancet* **341**, 1521–1523.

Missouris, C. G. *et al.* (1994). Renal artery stenosis: a common and important problem in patients with peripheral vascular disease. *American Journal of Medicine* **96**, 10–14.

Modi, K. S., and Rao, V. K. (2001). Atheroembolic renal disease. *Journal of the American Society of Nephrology* **12**, 1781–1787.

Möhring, J. *et al.* (1978). Plasma vasopressin concentrations and effects of vasopressin antiserum on blood pressure in rats with malignant two-kidney Goldblatt hypertension. *Circulation Research* **42**, 17–25.

Müller, F. B. *et al.* (1986). The captopril test for identifying unsuspected renovascular disease in hypertensive patients. *American Journal of Medicine* **80**, 633–644.

Nahman, N. S. *et al.* (1994). Renal artery pressure gradients in patients with angiographic evidence of atherosclerotic renal artery stenosis. *American Journal of Kidney Diseases* **24**, 695–699.

Nicholson, J. P. *et al.* (1983). Cigarette smoking and renovascular hypertension. *Lancet* **i**, 765–766.

Novick, A. C. (1991). Management of renovascular disease, a surgical perspective. *Circulation* **83**, 167–171.

Olin, J. W. *et al.* (1990). Prevalence of atherosclerotic renal artery stenosis in patients with atherosclerosis elsewhere. *American Journal of Medicine* **88**, 46–51.

Olin, J. W. *et al.* (1995). The utility of duplex ultrasound scanning of the renal arteries for diagnosing significant renal artery stenosis. *Annals of Internal Medicine* **122**, 833–838.

Oliva, V. L. *et al.* (1998). Detection of renal artery stenosis with Doppler sonography before and after administration of captopril: value of early systolic rise. *American Journal of Roentgenology* **170**, 169–175.

Olivieri, O. *et al.* (1999). Genetic polymorphisms of the renin–angiotensin system and atheromatous renal artery stenosis. *Hypertension* **34**, 1097–1100.

Parfrey, P. S. *et al.* (1989). Contrast material-induced renal failure in patients with diabetes mellitus, renal insufficiency or both. A prospective controlled study. *New England Journal of Medicine* **320**, 143–149.

Paul, J. F. *et al.* (1999). Interobserver variability in the interpretation of renal digital subtraction angiography. *American Journal of Roentgenology* **173**, 1285–1288.

Paulsen, D. *et al.* (1999). Preservation of renal function by percutaneous transluminal angioplasty in ischaemic renal disease. *Nephrology, Dialysis, Transplantation* **14** (6), 1454–1461.

Pedersen, E. B. (1994). Angiotensin-converting enzyme inhibitor renography. Pathophysiological, diagnostic and therapeutic aspects in renal artery stenosis. *Nephrology, Dialysis, Transplantation* **9**, 482–492.

Pedersen, E. B. (2000). New tools in diagnosing renal artery stenosis. *Kidney International* **57**, 2657–2677.

Pick, J. W. and Anson, E. J. (1940). The renovascular pedicle: anatomical study of 430 body-halves. *Journal of Urology* **44**, 411.

Pickering, T. G., Laragh, J. H., and Sos, T. H. Renovascular hypertension. In *Diseases of the Kidney* (ed. R. W. Schrier and C. W. Gottschalk), pp. 1597–1622. Boston: Little Brown, 1988a.

Pickering, T. G. *et al.* (1988b). Recurrent pulmonary oedema in hypertension due to bilateral renal artery stenosis: treatment by angioplasty or surgical revascularization. *Lancet* **i**, 551.

Plouin, P. F., Rossignol, P., and Bobrie, G. (2001). Atherosclerotic renal artery stenosis: to treat conservatively, to dilate, to stent, or to operate? *Journal of the American Society of Nephrology* **12**, 2190–2196.

Plouin, P. F. *et al.* (1993). Restenosis after a first percutaneous transluminal renal angioplasty. *Hypertension* **21**, 89–96.

Plouin, P. F. *et al.* (1995). Transluminal vascular stents for ostial atherosclerotic renal artery stenosis. *Lancet* **346** (8982), 1109.

Plouin, P. F. *et al.* (1998). Blood pressure outcome of angioplasty in atherosclerotic renal artery stenosis: a randomized trial. Essai Multicentrique Medicaments vs Angioplastie (EMMA) Study Group. *Hypertension* **31**, 823–829.

Pohl, M. A. and Novick, A. C. (1985). Natural history of atherosclerotic and fibrous renal artery disease: clinical implications. *American Journal of Kidney Diseases* **5**, A120–A130.

Postma, C. T. *et al.* (1990). The captopril test in the detection of renovascular disease in hypertensive patients. *Archives of Internal Medicine* **150**, 625–628.

Prigent, A. (1993). The diagnosis of renovascular hypertension: the role of captopril renal scintigraphy and related issues. *European Journal of Nuclear Medicine* **20**, 625–644.

Prince, M. R. *et al.* (1997). Hemodynamically significant atherosclerotic renal artery stenosis: MR angiographic features. *Radiology* **205**, 128–136.

Priollet, P. *et al.* (1990). Renal artery stenosis and peripheral vascular disease. *Lancet* **336**, 879 (letter).

Rabito, S. F., Carretero, O. A., and Scicli, A. G. (1981). Evidence against a role of vasopressin in the maintenance of high blood pressure mineralocorticoid and renovascular hypertension. *Hypertension* **3**, 34.

Radermacher, J. and Brunkhorst, R. (1998). Diagnosis and treatment of renovascular stenosis—a cost–benefit analysis. *Nephrology, Dialysis, Transplantation* **13**, 2761–2767.

Radermacher, J. *et al.* (2001a). Use of Doppler ultrasonography to predict the outcome of therapy for renal-artery stenosis. *New England Journal of Medicine* **344**, 410–417.

Radermacher, J., Weinkove, R., and Haller, H. (2001b). Techniques for predicting a favourable response to renal angioplasty in patients with renovascular disease. *Current Opinion in Nephrology and Hypertension* **10**, 799–805.

Re, R. *et al.* (1978). Inhibition of angiotensin converting-enzyme for diagnosis of renal artery stenosis. *New England Journal of Medicine* **298**, 582–586.

Reiher, L., Pfeiffer, T., and Sandmann, W. (2000). Long-term results after surgical reconstruction for renal artery fibromuscular dysplasia. *European Journal of Vascular and Endovascular Surgery* **20**, 556–559.

Reilly, L. M. *et al.* (1991). The role of arterial reconstruction in spontaneous renal artery dissection. *Journal of Vascular Surgery* **14**, 468–479.

Rene, P. C. *et al.* (1995). Renal artery stenosis: evaluation of Doppler US after inhibition of angiotensin-converting enzyme with captopril. *Radiology* **196**, 675–679.

Riegger, A. J. G. *et al.* (1977). Correction of renal hypertension in the rat by prolonged infusion of angiotensin inhibitors. *Lancet* **ii**, 1317–1319.

Riehl, J. *et al.* (1997). Renal artery stenosis: evaluation with colour duplex ultrasonography. *Nephrology, Dialysis, Transplantation* **12**, 1608–1614.

Roberts J. C., Jr., Wilkins, R. H., and Moses, C. (1959). Autopsy studies in atherosclerosis. Distribution and severity of atherosclerosis in patients dying without morphologic evidence of atherosclerotic catastrophy. *Circulation* **20**, 520.

Rodriquez-Lopez, J. A. *et al.* (1999). Renal artery stenosis treated with stent deployment: indications, technique, and outcome for 108 patients. *Journal of Vascular Surgery* **29** (4), 617–624.

Rudnick, M. R. and Maxwell, M. H. Limitations of renin assays. In *Controversies in Nephrology and Hypertension* (ed. R. G. Narins), pp. 123–160. New York: Churchill Livingstone, 1984.

Rudnick, M. R. ***et al.*** **for the Iohexol Cooperative Study** (1995). Nephrotoxicity of ionic and nonionic contrast media in 1194 patients: a randomized trial. *Kidney International* **47**, 254–261.

Safian, R. D. and Textor, S. C. (2001). Renal-artery stenosis. *New England Journal of Medicine* **344** (6), 431–442.

Salvetti, A. *et al.* Does humoral and hemodynamic response to acute ACE-inhibition identify true renovascular hypertension? In *Renovascular Hypertension* (ed. N. Glorioso *et al.*), pp. 305–317. New York: Raven Press, 1987.

Salvetti, A. *et al.* (1996). Renal artery stenosis in the nineties: screening dilemmas. *Contributions to Nephrology* **119**, 45–53.

Sawicki, P. T. *et al.* (1991). Prevalence of renal artery stenosis in diabetes mellitus—an autopsy study. *Journal of Internal Medicine* **229**, 489.

Schoenberg, S. O. *et al.* (2002). Morphologic and functional magnetic resonance imaging of renal artery stenosis: a multireader tricenter study. *Journal of the American Society of Nephrology* **13**, 158–169.

Schomig, A. *et al.* (1996). A randomized comparison of antiplatelet and anticoagulant therapy after placement of coronary stent. *New England Journal of Medicine* **334**, 1084–1089.

Schreiber, M. J., Pohl, M. A., and Novick, A. C. (1984). The natural history of atherosclerotic and fibrous renal artery disease. *Urological Clinics of North America* **11**, 383–392.

Schreij, G. *et al.* (1999). Interpretation of renal angiography by radiologists. *Journal of Hypertension* **17**, 1737–1741.

Schwab, S. J. *et al.* (1989). Contrast nephrotoxicity: a randomized controlled trial of non-ionic and an ionic radiographic contrast agent. *New England Journal of Medicine* **320**, 149–153.

Schwartz, D. T. (1965). Relation of superior-mesenteric-artery obstruction to renal hypertension: a review of 56 cases. *New England Journal of Medicine* **272**, 1318–1322.

Schwartz, C. J. and White, T. A. (1964). Stenosis of renal artery: an unselected necropsy study. *British Medical Journal* **2**, 1415–1419.

Schwerk, W. B. *et al.* (1994). Renal artery stenosis: grading with image-directed Doppler US evaluation renal resistive index. *Radiology* **190**, 785–790.

Scoble, J. E. *et al.* (1989). Atherosclerotic renovascular disease causing renal impairment—a case for treatment. *Clinical Nephrology* **31**, 119–122.

Scott, J. A. *et al.* (1983). Angiographic assessment of renal artery. Pathology: how reliable? *American Journal of Radiology* **141**, 1299–1303.

Sellars, L., Shore, A. C., and Wilkinson, R. (1985). Renal vein renin studies in renovascular hypertension: do they really help? *Journal of Hypertension* **3**, 177–181.

Setaro, J. F. *et al.* (1991). Simplified captopril renography in diagnosis and treatment of renal artery stenosis. *Hypertension* **18**, 289–298.

Sfakianakis, G. N., Jaffe, D. J., and Bourgoigie, J. J. (1988). Captopril scintigraphy in the diagnosis of renovascular hypertension. *Kidney International* **34** (Suppl. 25), 142–144.

Simon, N. *et al.* (1972). Clinical characteristics of renovascular hypertension. *Journal of the American Medical Association* **220**, 118–120.

Sinclair, A. M. *et al.* (1987). Secondary hypertension in a blood pressure clinic. *Archives of Internal Medicine* **147**, 1289–1293.

Smith, H. W. (1956). Unilateral nephrectomy in hyperstensive disease. *Journal of Urology* **76**, 685–701.

Smith, S. P. *et al.* (1974). Occlusion of the artery to a solitary kidney. *Journal of the American Medical Association* **230**, 1306–1307.

Sniderman, K. W. and Sos, T. A. (1982). Percutaneous transluminal recanalization and dilatation of totally occluded renal arteries. *Radiology* **142**, 607–610.

Sos, T. A. *et al.* (1983). Percutaneous transluminal renal angioplasty in renovascular hypertension due to atheroma or fibromuscular dysplasia. *New England Journal of Medicine* **309**, 274–279.

Sos, T. A. *et al.* (1986). Technical aspects of percutaneous renal angioplasty. *Nephron* **44** (Suppl. 1), 45–50.

Stair, D. C., Rios, W. A., and Black, H. R. (1990). Atypical causes of curable renovascular hypertension: a review. *Progress in Cardiovascular Diseases* **3**, 185–210.

Stavros, A. T. *et al.* (1992). Segmental stenosis of the renal artery: pattern recognition of tardus and parvus abnormalities with duplex sonography. *Radiology* **184**, 487–492.

Steinbach, F. *et al.* (1997). Long-term survival after surgical revascularization for atherosclerotic renal artery disease. *The Journal of Urology* **158**, 38–41.

Svetkey, L. P. *et al.* (1989). Prospective analysis of strategies for diagnosing renovascular hypertension. *Hypertension* **14**, 247–257.

Taylor, A. *et al.* (1996). Consensus report on ACE inhibitor renography for detecting renovascular hypertension. *Journal of Nuclear Medicine* **37**, 1876–1882.

Taylor, A. *et al.* (2000). Functional testing: ACEI renography. *Seminars in Nephrology* **20**, 437–444.

Tegtmeyer, C. J. *et al.* (1991). Results and complications of angioplasty in fibromuscular disease. *Circulation* **83**, 155–161.

Textor, S. C. and Canzanello, V. J. (1996). Radiographic evaluation of the renal vasculature. *Current Opinion in Nephrology and Hypertension* **5**, 541–551.

Textor, S. C., Novick, A. C., Steinmuller, D. R., and Streem, S. B. (1983). Renal failure limiting antihypertensive therapy as an indication for renal revascularization. *Archives of Internal Medicine* **143**, 2208–2211.

Thibonnier, M. *et al.* (1984). Improved diagnosis of unilateral renal artery lesions after captopril administration. *Journal of the American Medical Association* **251**, 56–60.

Tierney, W. M., McDonald, C. J., and Luft, F. C. (1989). Renal disease in hypertensive adults: effect of race and type II diabetes mellitus. *American Journal of Kidney Diseases* **12**, 485–493.

Tollefson, D. F. J. and Ernst, C. B. (1991). Natural history of atherosclerotic renal artery stenosis associated with aortic disease. *Journal of Vascular Surgery* **14**, 327.

Travis, J. A. (2000). Aneurysmal degeneration and late rupture of an aortorenal vein graft: case report, review of the literature, and implications for conduit selection. *Journal of Vascular Surgery* **32** (3), 612–615.

Tucker, R. M. and Labarthe, D. R. (1977). Frequency of surgical treatment for hypertension in adults at the Mayo Clinic from 1973 through 1975. *Mayo Clinic Proceedings* **52**, 549–555.

Tullis, M. J. *et al.* (1999). Blood pressure, antihypertensive medication, and atherosclerotic renal artery stenosis. *American Journal of Kidney Diseases* **33**, 675–681.

Tuttle, K. R. and Raabe, R. D. (1998). Endovascular stents for renal artery revascularization. *Current Opinion in Nephrology and Hypertension* **7**, 695–701.

Valentine, R. J. *et al.* (1993). Detection of unsuspected renal artery stenosis in patients with abdominal aortic aneurysms: refined indications for preoperative aortography. *Annals of Vascular Surgery* **7**, 220–224.

van de Ven, P. J. *et al.* (1998). Angiotensin converting enzyme inhibitor-induced renal dysfunction in atherosclerotic renovascular disease. *Kidney International* **53**, 986–993.

van de Ven, P. J. *et al.* (1999). Arterial stenting and balloon angioplasty in ostial atherosclerotic renovascular disease: a randomised trial. *Lancet* **353**, 282–286.

van de Ven, P. J. *et al.* (2000). Aspirin renography and captopril renography in the diagnosis of renal artery stenosis. *Journal of Nuclear Medicine* **41**, 1337–1342.

van Jaarsveld, B. C. *et al.* (1997). The place of renal scintigraphy in the diagnosis of renal artery stenosis. Fifteen years of clinical experience. *Archives of Internal Medicine* **157**, 1226–1234.

van Jaarsveld, B. C. *et al.* (1999). Inter-observer variability in the angiographic assessment of renal artery stenosis. DRASTIC study group. *Journal of Hypertension* **17**, 1731–1736.

van Jaarsveld, B. C. *et al.* (2000). The effect of balloon angioplasty on hypertension in atherosclerotic renal-artery stenosis. *New England Journal of Medicine* **342**, 1007–1014.

Van Velzer, Da., Burge, C. H., and Morris, G. C. (1961). Arteriosclerotic narrowing of renal arteries associated with hypertension. *American Journal of Roentgenology* **86**, 807.

Vaughan, D. E., Jr. (1985). Renovascular hypertension. *Kidney International* **27**, 811–827.

Veglio, F. *et al.* (1995). Assessment of renal resistance index after captopril test by Doppler in essential and renovascular hypertension. *Kidney International* **48**, 1611–1616.

Vetrovec, G. W. *et al.* (1984). High prevalence of renal artery stenosis in hypertensive patients with coronary artery disease. *Journal of American College of Cardiology* **3**, 518 (abstract).

Vetter, W. *et al.* Diagnostische und therapeutische Aspekte der 24-h-Blutdruckmessung. In *Indirekte 24-Stunden Blutdruckmessung* (ed. W. Meyer-Sabellek and R. Gotyen), pp. 135–140. Muenchen: Medikon Verlan, 1990.

Vollmar, J., Helmstadter, D., and Hallwachs, O. (1971). Complete occlusion of the renal artery: nephrectomy or revascularization? *Journal of Cardiovascular Surgery* **12**, 441–446.

Von Knorring, J., Edgren, J., and Lepantalo, M. (1996). Long-term results of percutaneous transluminal angioplasty in renovascular hypertension. *Acta Radiological* **37** (1), 36–40.

Webster, J. *et al.* (1998). Randomised comparison of percutaneous angioplasty vs continued medical therapy for hypertensive patients with atheromatous renal artery stenosis. Scottish and Newcastle Renal Artery Stenosis Collaborative Group. *Journal of Human Hypertension* **12**, 329–335.

Weinberger, M. H. *et al.* (1979). Percutaneous transluminal angioplasty for renal artery stenosis in a solitary functioning kidney: an alternative to surgery in the high-risk patient. *Annals of Internal Medicine* **91**, 684–688.

Weinberger, M. H. *et al.* (1986). Percutaneous transluminal angioplasty in complicated renal vascular hypertension. *Nephron* **44** (Suppl. 1), 51–53.

White, C. J. *et al.* (1997). Renal artery stent placement: utility in lesions difficult to treat with balloon angioplasty. *Journal of the American College of Cardiology* **30** (6), 1445–1450.

Wollenweber, J., Sheps, S. G., and Davis, G. D. (1968). Clinical course of atherosclerotic renovascular disease. *American Journal of Cardiology* **21**, 60–71.

Working Group on Renovascular Hypertension (1987). Detection, evaluation, and treatment of renovascular hypertension. *Archives of Internal Medicine* **147**, 820–829.

Xue, F. *et al.* (1999). Outcome and cost comparison of percutaneous transluminal renal angioplasty, renal arterial stent placement, and renal arterial bypass grafting. *Radiology* **212** (2), 378–384.

Ying, C. Y. *et al.* (1984). Renal revascularization in the azotemic hypertensive patient resistant to therapy. *New England Journal of Medicine* **231**, 1070–1075.

Yucel, E. K. *et al.* (1993). Time of flight renal MR angiography: utility in patients with renal insufficiency. *Magnetic Resonance Imaging* **11**, 925–930.

Yutan, E. *et al.* (2001). Percutaneous transluminal revascularization for renal artery stenosis: veterans affairs puget sound health care system experience. *Journal of Vascular Surgery* **34** (4), 685–693.

Zierler, R. E. *et al.* (1994). Natural history of atherosclerotic renal artery stenosis: a prospective study with duplex ultrasonography. *Journal of Vascular Surgery* **19**, 250–258.

9.8 Malignant hypertension

Ralf Dikow and Eberhard Ritz

Introduction

Renal function and blood pressure are intimately linked: on the one hand, hypertension adversely affects renal function in patients with renal impairment; on the other hand, renal dysfunction is a potent promotor of elevated blood pressure. Malignant hypertension represents the extreme of this spectrum. It is characterized by rapidly increasing blood pressure and declining renal function and confronts the clinician with a medical emergency. Early recognition and prompt management are crucial for the survival of the patient and for ensuring minimal damage to target organs, in particular, renal vascular lesions, which may lead to irreversible renal damage requiring long-term renal replacement therapy.

Major advances in the management of malignant hypertension have occurred in the past 40 years. The development and availability of potent blood pressure lowering agents and of renal dialysis allow to interrupt the vicious cycle and to substantially improve the previously dire prognosis of this condition. Nevertheless, many questions remain: which patients with essential hypertension or hypertension secondary to renal disease are at particular risk of developing malignant hypertension? What is the long-term prognosis of malignant hypertension? Which pathomechanisms underly the transformation of benign hypertension into the malignant form of hypertension? What is the optimal treatment?

The term 'accelerated hypertension' has traditionally been used to define patients with grade III hypertensive retinopathy, with retinal haemorrhages and exudates in association with high blood pressure (Keith *et al.* 1939), while the term 'malignant hypertension' was used in patients with papilloedema, or grade IV retinopathy. However, the prognosis of accelerated and malignant hypertension is similar. Fibrinoid necrosis of arterioles occurs in both conditions; since no sharp distinction can be drawn, the term 'malignant hypertension' is preferred. Although both the degree and rapidity of the increase in blood pressure are important in determining the development of malignant hypertension, it cannot be defined by an arbitrary cut-off of blood pressure. Malignant hypertension, that is, fibrinoid necrosis of arterioles, may develop with pressures as low as 150/100 mmHg and conversely, many patients have much higher blood pressure values for long periods without developing malignant hypertension.

Definition of malignant hypertension

Malignant hypertension should be distinguished from the hypertensive emergency. An acute increase in blood pressure may cause serious clinical problems, for instance, pulmonary oedema, cerebral haemorrhage, aortic dissection, and require active antihypertensive intervention. Funduscopy may show hypertensive retinopathy III or IV, that is, cotton wool exudates, flame-shaped haemorrhages, and papilloedema. If one were to obtain biopsies, fibrinoid necrosis of the arterioles would be absent.

In contrast, in patients with malignant hypertension one does not necessarily permanently find extremely elevated blood pressure values, although the diastolic pressure is usually above 115 mmHg. The funduscopic examination (retinopathy III or IV) is diagnostic and there is clinical evidence of target organ damage induced by fibrinoid necrosis of arterioles. Depending upon the balance between high perfusion pressure and narrowing of the vessels, one will find evidence of ischaemia and/or hyperperfusion, causing deteriorating renal function, left ventricular failure, hypertensive encephalopathy, etc.

Because in untreated patients 1-year mortality used to be 90 per cent as found in many malignancies, Volhard and Fahr (1914) adopted the term 'malignant' hypertension. This variety of hypertension is characterized by fibrinoid necrosis of the arteries and was distinguished from the usual form of hypertension which carried a much better prognosis and was therefore called 'benign' hypertension. Of course, today it is well known that life expectency is shortened in any form of hypertension so that the term 'benign' is clearly inappropriate. By histology, this variant of hypertension is characterized by elastic hyperplastic remodelling of arterioles.

Incidence and prognosis of malignant hypertension

Many patients presenting with malignant hypertension have a history of hypertension, although sometimes previously normotensive individuals can develop malignant hypertension as well, for instance, patients with pre-eclampsia or acute glomerulonephritis. In a retrospective study of 100 patients with severe hypertension, no less than 93 had a history of chronic hypertension (Bennett and Shea 1988). Although hypertension is very common in the general population, malignant hypertension has become rare according to most, but not all (Lip *et al.* 1994), recent reports. In early series, the frequency of malignant hypertension varied from 1 per cent (Kincaid-Smith *et al.* 1958) to 7 per cent (Perera 1955) in hypertensive patients. In the past two decades, obviously increasing recognition and prompt treatment of moderate to severe primary (or essential) hypertension led to a reduction in the number of patients developing malignant hypertension. Nevertheless,

Lip *et al.* (1994) reported that this complication is still found in 1–2 per cent of the hypertensive population and that the incidence in the general population is 1–2/100,000/year. In our experience, the incidence is lower by a factor of 5–10. Malignant hypertension occurs more frequently in males, and Blacks are at particular risk.

Pre-eclampsia and eclampsia can be considered variants of malignant hypertension. The frequency is approximately 4 per cent in primi-parae; it is considerably higher in patients with underlying renal disease and is excessive, in the range of 70 per cent, in patients with molar pregnancies (Sibai 1990). Hypertensive emergencies are frequent in primi-parae because in such patients a sudden major rise of blood pressure impacts on an unprepared vascular bed.

Although little is known about the relationship between pre-existing blood pressure level and development of malignant hypertension, some conclusions may be drawn from randomized placebo-controlled trials on treatment of patients with hypertension. In the Veterans Administration Cooperative Study (Veterans Administration Cooperative Study Group on Antihypertensive Agents 1967), a double-blind trial in 143 men with diastolic blood pressures in the range 115–129 mmHg, seven of 70 subjects (10 per cent) receiving placebo developed fundal changes of malignant hypertension over a mean period of 21 months. No patient receiving active treatment developed these changes. In contrast, in the Australian national blood pressure study (Reader *et al.* 1980), a trial of treatment in 3427 men and women aged 30–69 years with mild to moderate hypertension (diastolic blood pressure at entry 95–109 mmHg), severe retinopathy developed in only five of 1706 placebo-treated patients (0.29 per cent). The European Working Party on high blood pressure in the elderly trial (Amery *et al.* 1985) studied patients aged over 60 with initial diastolic blood pressures of 90–119 mmHg. Five of 424 subjects receiving placebo (1.2 per cent) developed papilloedema, retinal haemorrhages, or exudates over a 4.6 year follow-up, compared with none of 416 actively treated patients. Taken together, these observations suggest that the risk of developing malignant hypertension is very low in patients with mild and moderate essential hypertension, but—not surprisingly—is higher if hypertension is more severe.

A family history of malignant hypertension is an important predictor for hypertension in the offspring. Lopes *et al.* (2001) studied 42 offspring of parents with a history of malignant hypertension compared to 35 offspring of parents with normotension. In the offspring of hypertensive parents, body mass index (BMI), heart rate, and median blood pressure were significantly higher. Ambulatory blood pressure measurement showed inappropriately high night blood pressure and lower heart rate variability during daytime. Offspring also had lower HDL cholesterol, higher plasma insulin and norepinephrine concentrations, and higher insulin-to-glucose ratios than the offspring of normotensive patients.

The abysmal prognosis of malignant hypertension before the availability of effective antihypertensive therapy and renal replacement therapy is illustrated by the observation of Keith *et al.* (1939), that untreated patients of malignant hypertension had a 1-year mortality of 80 per cent, and a 5-year mortality of 100 per cent. In that classic study, 12-month survival was 65 and 20 per cent in patients with grades III and IV retinopathy, respectively; the corresponding survival rates at 24 months were 36 and 11 per cent. Similarly, 12-month survival was only 10 per cent in 197 patients with malignant hypertension and papilloedema studied by Kincaid-Smith in 1958.

In the past, several authors found that the prognosis was different in patients with grades III and IV retinopathy (Breckenridge *et al.* 1970): 5-year survival was 25 per cent for patients with grade IV retinopathy treated between 1952 and 1959 and 43 per cent for such patients treated between 1960 and 1967. For patients with grade III retinopathy, the corresponding survival rates were 70 and 71 per cent, respectively. More recent series have failed, however, to document a difference in survival between patients with grade III or grade IV hypertensive retinopathy, possibly as a result of antihypertensive treatment (Isles *et al.* 1985; Ahmed *et al.* 1986; Bing *et al.* 1986; McGregor *et al.* 1986). For example, as shown in Fig. 1, very similar survival rates were noted in a series of 139 consecutive patients with grade III or grade IV retinopathy. In 1994 Lip *et al.* reported 1-year survival rates of 76 per cent.

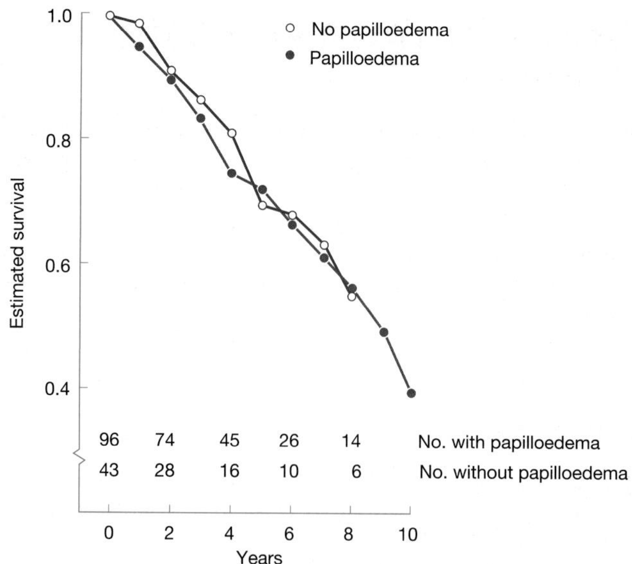

Fig. 1 Relationship between presence or absence of papilloedema and survival in 139 hypertensive patients with bilateral retinal haemorrhages and exudates, after controlling for age, gender, smoking, aetiology of hypertension, initial serum creatinine concentration, and initial and achieved blood pressure (reproduced from McGregor *et al.* 1986, with permission).

Renal function and survival

In addition to the beneficial effect of antihypertensive treatment on outcome, the prognosis has further been improved by the availability of renal replacement therapy. In the past, uraemia was the predominant cause of death (Keith *et al.* 1939; Heptinstall 1953). It accounted for 68 per cent of deaths in the Hammersmith series (Kincaid-Smith *et al.* 1958). Although the impact of the initial level of renal dysfunction on survival is no longer as dramatic as it was in the predialysis era, even today it remains an important prognostic factor.

Isles *et al.* (1985) compared 139 patients with malignant hypertension with controls matched for age, gender, and blood pressure: the only independent factors relating to patient survival were initial serum creatinine and the blood pressure achieved during treatment.

In patients presenting with malignant hypertension between 1974 and 1983, 10-year survival was 51 per cent in patients with impaired renal function compared to 81 per cent in those with normal renal function (Bing *et al.* 1986). Late cardiovascular events, particularly mesenteric ischaemia (Erdberg *et al.* 1992) are relatively common in patients with a history of malignant hypertension surviving on dialysis.

Outcome in relation to aetiology of malignant hypertension

Observations made before the availability of renal replacement therapy indicated that renal damage progressed more rapidly in patients with malignant hypertension without pre-existing renal disease than in patients with pre-existing renal disease. In contrast, when antihypertensive agents had become available, Harrington *et al.* (1959) no longer found a difference of survival in patients with malignant hypertension when patients with a history of essential hypertension were compared to those with primary renal disease. When renal impairment was found at presentation (blood urea > 60 mg/dl), patient survival and renal survival was higher in patients with pre-existing primary renal disease than in those with a history of essential hypertension. In the former, elevated creatinine was presumably the result of chronic renal disease, whilst in the latter it reflected renal damage induced by malignant hypertension.

Yu *et al.* (1986) noted no deaths in 17 patients with malignant hypertension and pre-existing essential hypertension who had been followed for up to 6 years, but nine deaths in 65 patients with a variety of renal and renovascular causes of malignant hypertension. More recent studies have not confirmed a consistent relationship between aetiology and outcome, however. Kawazoe *et al.* (1988) observed 100 per cent 5-year survival in 26 patients with a history of chronic glomerulonephritis, compared with 79 per cent 5-year survival in 33 patients with malignant hypertension and a history of pre-existing essential hypertension. In an analysis of factors determining survival in 139 patients with malignant hypertension (Isles *et al.* 1985), only initial serum creatinine and blood pressure achieved during antihypertensive treatment were independently related to outcome.

Development of renal impairment in essential hypertension

Hypertension is very common in patients with chronic renal failure, and nearly all patients with endstage renal failure are hypertensive, whatever the primary cause of renal failure (Curtis *et al.* 1969). Unless the specific lesions of malignant hypertension are present, hypertension is a relatively rare cause of renal failure: essential hypertension was documented as the primary disease in only 6.1 per cent of patients with endstage renal failure in the data of the European Dialysis and Transplant Association Registry (1986). A similar pattern existed also in the United States where the Dialysis Registry showed hypertensive nephrosclerosis was the aetiology of renal failure in 4.5 per cent of patients (Blythe 1985). These registry data must be taken with a grain of salt in the absence of biopsy confirmation of the diagnosis. In a clinicopathological study, Kincaid-Smith (1975) demonstrated that elevation of serum creatinine concentration as well as presence of nephrosclerosis at postmortem were similarly frequent in patients with essential hypertension and normotensive age-matched controls, again casting doubt on (primary) nephrosclerosis as a frequent cause of renal failure. Nevertheless, in a prospective study covering 300,000 individuals in the general population, Klag *et al.* (1996) noted that high blood pressure was correlated with the late development of endstage renal disease.

For reasons that remain unclear, primary hypertension is a much more frequent cause of progressive renal failure in Afro-American patients than in Caucasians. Rostand *et al.* (1982) reported that hypertension was the cause of 29 per cent of cases of endstage renal disease in Afro-American patients in Alabama, and estimated that hypertensive nephrosclerosis was nearly 18 times more common in Afro-Americans than in Caucasians. It is not known whether this large difference is merely the result of suboptimal detection and treatment of hypertension in the Afro-American population, or whether this group is inherently at greater risk because of unknown, possibly genetic, factors. A recent study suggests that the latter is the case: despite equal and adequate blood pressure control, renal function declined significantly in 25 per cent of Afro-American patients and only in 12 per cent of Caucasian patients during 12–174 months of follow-up (Rostand *et al.* 1989). Thus, at least in a subset of Afro-Americans, a given level of blood pressure causes disproportionately greater end-organ damage, which becomes manifest as nephrosclerosis and ventricular hypertrophy (Klahr 1989). The risk of malignant hypertension is also greater in Afro-American patients, further increasing the likelihood of renal failure. Perera (1958) observed that 46 per cent of a group of patients with malignant hypertension were Afro-American, although Afro-Americans accounted for only 31 per cent of the overall hypertensive population. Munro-Faure *et al.* (1979) compared hypertensive patients of African and Caucasian origin attending referral clinics in the United Kingdom with Caucasians matched for age and gender. He found grade III or grade IV retinopathy in 4.4 per cent of patients of African origin, but only in 0.74 per cent of Caucasian patients.

Renal function and renal survival in malignant hypertension

Primary hypertension has little effect on renal function, at least in the short term, although not necessarily in the long term (Klag *et al.* 1996); in contrast, rapid development of renal impairment is common when malignant hypertension develops.

Renal survival in patients with malignant hypertension is related to the level of renal function at presentation. In a group of 65 patients with malignant hypertension and a history of either primary hypertension or pre-existing renal disease overall 1-year renal survival was 66 per cent and 5-year renal survival was 51 per cent (Yu *et al.* 1986). In the 33 patients with an initial serum creatinine less than 300 μmol/l, glomerular filtration rate (GFR) remained stable or improved in 28 patients. Only three patients progressed to endstage renal failure. In contrast, 29 of the 32 patients with an initial serum creatinine greater than 300 μmol/l showed progressive deterioration in renal function, and 21 (67 per cent) required renal replacement therapy. In a survey of 69 patients, Kawazoe *et al.* (1987) observed an overall 5-year renal survival rate of 37 per cent; 5-year renal survival was 60 per cent in patients with underlying essential hypertension and 4 per cent in patients with chronic glomerulonephritis.

A more recent study showed a trend that end-organ damage becomes less severe in patients with malignant hypertension. Ohta *et al.* (2001) compared two series of patients with malignant hypertension (37 patients observed in the period from 1984 to 1999 versus 59 patients observed in the period from 1971 to 1983). Particularly the frequency of renal death 1-year after admission was significantly lower in the more recent series (30 versus 42 per cent). In addition, left ventricular hypertrophy was less frequent in the recent cases as well.

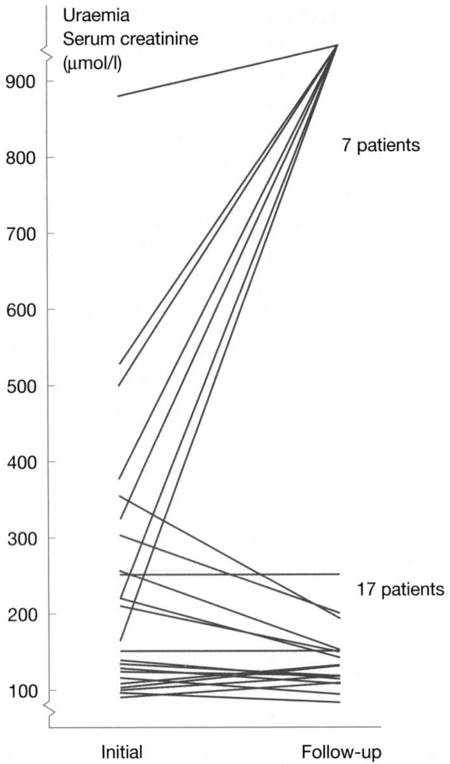

Fig. 2 Eventual renal function and serum creatinine concentration at presentation in 24 patients with malignant hypertension (reproduced from Herlitz *et al.* 1982, with permission).

Renal failure may be expected to progress in patients with underlying renal disease. Nevertheless, a significant proportion of patients with primary hypertension who develop malignant hypertension and uraemia will recover renal function when effective antihypertensive treatment is provided. Recovery of sufficient renal function so that dialysis can be stopped may take months (Yacoob *et al.* 1991). Intense and prolonged renal vasoconstriction, as shown by renal angiography, has been documented by Meyrier *et al.* (1990); reversal of renal failure may therefore be due, amongst others, to reversal of intense angiotensin II (AT II)-dependent vasoconstriction. Several studies have concluded that deterioration despite antihypertensive treatment is likely in patients with a serum creatinine of 300 μmol/l or more at presentation (Isles *et al.* 1984a,b). Seven of 24 patients with malignant hypertension and a history of primary hypertension had markedly elevated serum creatinine at diagnosis (Herlitz *et al.* 1982). The 17 patients with normal serum creatinine at presentation maintained renal function; GFR at presentation was 51 ml/min and at mean 6-year follow-up it was 62 ml/min. Considerable overlap of outcome was present in patients who presented with an initial serum creatinine in the range 170–350 μmol/l (Fig. 2). Hence, in this subgroup, particular attention must be paid to careful control of blood pressure, in order to minimize the risk of progressive renal failure.

Primary renal diseases—risk and evolution of malignant hypertension

Blood pressure starts to rise very early in the evolution of renal disease. Initially blood pressure increases within the range of normotensive values, but subsequently frank hypertension develops. Stefanski *et al.* (1996) compared blood pressure values in patients with IgA glomerulonephritis and normal inulin clearance with blood pressure values in controls matched for age, gender, and BMI. Although most values were still within the normotensive range they were significantly higher than the matched controls. If patients are in terminal renal failure, virtually all individuals are hypertensive with the exception of the rare patient with renal salt wasting. The risk to develop hypertension as well as the severity of hypertension are loosely related to the underlying renal disease. Hypertension is notoriously, frequent and severe in patients with focal glomerulosclerosis, IgA glomerulonephritis, reflux nephropathy, diabetic nephropathy, and systemic sclerosis. An infrequent but clinically important complication in patients with primary renal disease is the superimposition of atherosclerotic renal artery stenosis.

The above renal diseases are also the ones in which malignant hypertension is most frequently seen. What renal diseases are found in patients with malignant hypertension? In a series of 44 patients in whom postmortem confirmation of the diagnosis was available, 57 per cent had underlying 'chronic pyelonephritis' (Kincaid-Smith *et al.* 1958). These two groups of patients and those with essential hypertension could not be differentiated by degree of albuminuria or of renal impairment at presentation. In a study including renal biopsy, Rambausek *et al.* (1984) reported a notable frequency of malignant hypertension in IgA glomerulonephritis. This was confirmed by others (Nicholls *et al.* 1984; Rodicio 1984; Yu *et al.* 1986) and malignant hypertension may even be the presenting feature of IgA nephropathy. In a retrospective analysis of 66 patients with biopsy-proven IgA nephropathy, 24 patients were hypertensive at presentation and 10 were in the malignant phase of hypertension (Subias *et al.* 1987). In the series of Yu *et al.* (1986) of 83 patients with maligant hypertension, 25 had primary glomerular disease, the most common of which was IgA nephropathy (14 cases); focal segmental (non-IgA) glomerulonephritis was seen in four patients. Four of the 19 patients with renal disease as a result of systemic disease had systemic sclerosis and four had systemic lupus erythematosus (SLE). In contrast to previous opinion, malignant hypertension is not a common feature of vasculitis (except polyarteritis). In the study of Yu *et al.* necrotizing vasculitis, including Wegener's granulomatosis, was present in only three patients, whilst three patients had diabetic nephropathy. Thirteen patients had tubulointerstitial disease, the most common of which was reflux nephropathy (six cases), whilst polycystic kidney disease was seen in only one patient. Blood pressure values at the time when patients presented with malignant hypertension was similar irrespective of underlying primary renal disease.

Other conditions predisposing to malignant hypertension

A number of conditions other than primary renal disease may be associated with malignant hypertension. An important condition is renovascular disease, which is increasingly recognized as a cause of malignant hypertension. In the study of Kincaid-Smith *et al.* (1958) 3.2 per cent of patients had renovascular disease, compared to 15 per cent in a more recent series (Yu *et al.* 1986); others have claimed a considerably greater frequency of underlying renovascular disease in malignant hypertension. In a retrospective analysis of patients presenting with grade III or grade IV hypertensive retinopathy, renal arteriography had been performed in 93 per cent and renovascular hypertension was diagnosed in 30 per cent of patients (Davis *et al.* 1979). The criteria for the diagnosis were very liberal, however: even 20 per cent arterial narrowing was diagnosed as stenosis and no evidence of the functional relevance of the stenosis was provided. A particular note of caution is appropriate in patients with renal transplantation. A sudden rise in blood pressure should always alert the clinician to consider the possibility of a renal transplant artery stenosis. Duplex sonography should be performed in every case to exclude ischaemia of the transplant and if the clinical suspicion is strong, magnetic resonance (MR) angiography should be performed.

Malignant hypertension may also be the presenting feature of phaeochromocytoma or scleroderma crisis. Of particular interest is the occurrence of malignant hypertension in diseases in which primary damage to endothelial cells plays an important pathogenetic role, for example in the antiphospholipid syndrome (Julkunen *et al.* 1991; Cacoub *et al.* 1993) or familial homocysteinuria (Pousse *et al.* 1990).

Substance abuse and hypertension

Malignant hypertension is a known complication of illegal drug use, particularly ecstasy and cocaine, but also LSD, amphetamine, and metamphetamine (Swallwell and Davis 1999).

The problem is illustrated by the report of Woodrow *et al.* (1995) who described a 37-year-old man who took ecstasy (3,4-methylenedioxymethamphetamine) at a 'rave' party. He developed malignant hypertension with generalized headache, abdominal pain, vomiting, and acute renal failure. Blood pressure increased to 220/140 mmHg. Renal biopsy showed occlusion of arteries due to thrombi and fibrinoid changes. An increase of blood pressure and tachycardia are very common in healthy volunteers after consumption of 'ecstasy' (Downing 1986). In view of the widespread use of 'ecstasy' as a recreational drug in the 'techno scene', a detailed drug history should be obtained in adolescent patients with malignant hypertension Cocaine is a powerful vasoconstrictor (Ferdinand 2000) which is known to cause hypertensive crises and malignant hypertension, myocardial infarction, stroke, and sudden death. Cocaine should also be considered as a cause of endstage renal disease in patients without a clear cause of renal failure (Norris *et al.* 2001).

Renal pathology in malignant hypertension

Despite the diverse conditions leading to malignant hypertension, its clinical features and pathology are very homogenous and are readily identified. Characteristic lesions are found in the kidneys and other vascular beds. They are often superimposed on abnormalities due to preceding hypertension or underlying primary renal disease, respectively. The pathognomonic lesions of malignant hypertension in the kidney comprise proliferative endarteritis of the interlobular arteries, fibrinoid necrosis of the afferent arterioles and glomerular capillary tuft, and an associated necrotizing glomerulitis. Tubulointerstitial damage is also common. Although recognition of these features poses few problems, there is less agreement on which of these lesions correlates best with the severity of renal dysfunction.

Interlobular arteries

The larger renal arteries, including the arcuate arteries, do not show specific changes in malignant hypertension, although a characteristic proliferative end-arteritis of the interlobular arteries is seen. This may vary from minor intimal proliferation to almost total occlusion of the arterial lumen, the so-called onion-skin lesion (Fig. 3), in advanced malignant hypertension. The thickening of the intima is related to an increase in acid mucopolysaccharides (chondroitin sulfate and hyaluronic acid) as well as deposition of concentric pseudoelastic fibres consisting of a layer of elongated myointimal cells and fine connective tissue fibrils. In malignant hypertension of rapid onset the underlying media is not hypertrophied and is stretched around the thickened intima. Marked luminal narrowing may develop within interlobular arteries due to cellular intimal proliferation and oedema (Fig. 4). This lesion may appear within days after onset of malignant hypertension.

Afferent arteries

The hallmark of malignant hypertension is fibrinoid necrosis of the afferent arterioles. Fibrinoid necrosis (Fig. 5) is characterized by deposition of an acellular eosinophilic material within the media and intima. The deposits appear bright pink with haemotoxylin and eosin and deep red with trichrome staining; they stain positive for fibrin with immunofluorescence. This is associated with loss of cell nuclei and occasionally with inflammatory cells infiltrating the arteriole. Although considered pathognomonic of malignant hypertension, fibrinoid necrosis in afferent arterioles is a patchy process which affects only circumscribed segments of a minority of vessels (Kincaid-Smith *et al.* 1958). Loss of arteriolar endothelial integrity may also occur without evident fibrinoid necrosis, but may cause extravasation of blood cells into the arteriolar wall (Fig. 6).

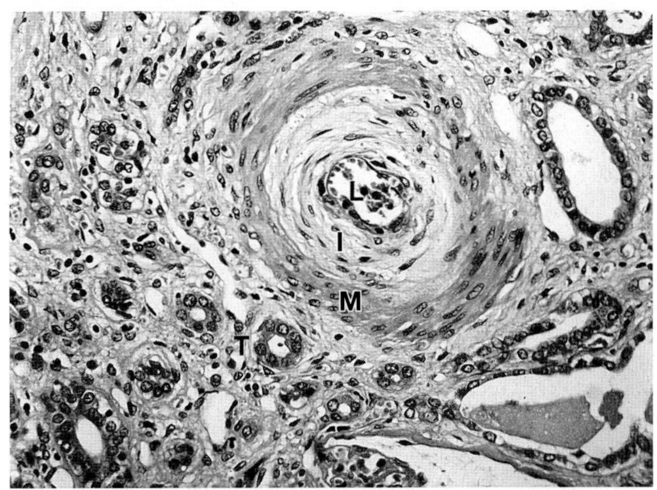

Fig. 3 Proliferative endarteritis of an interlobular artery in a patient with malignant hypertension. I, arterial intima showing gross proliferative change and 'onion-skin' appearance; L, severely narrowed arterial lumen; M, arterial media; T, tubular atrophy and interstitial fibrosis (by courtesy of Dr A.J. d'Ardenne).

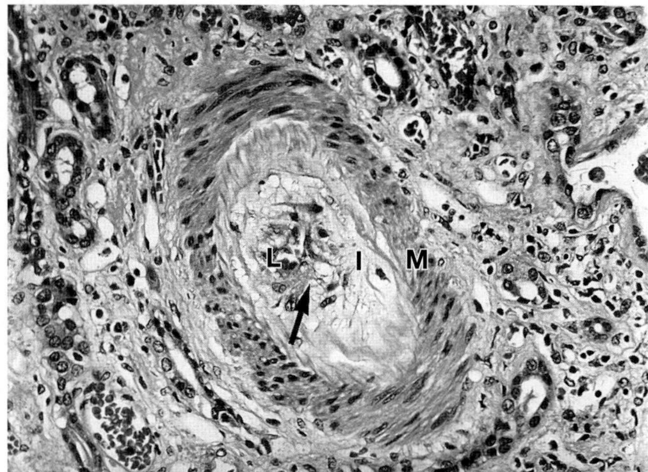

Fig. 4 Interlobular artery in malignant hypertension. Note hypertrophied arterial media (M), profound thickening of the intima (I), grossly narrowed arterial lumen (L), and circumscribed oedema of the intima (arrow) (by courtesy of Dr A.J. d'Ardenne).

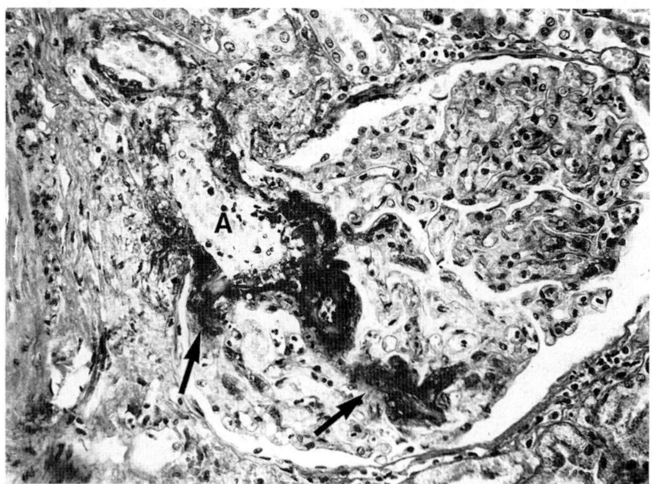

Fig. 5 Fibrinoid necrosis of an afferent arteriole extending into the glomerular tuft in a patient with malignant hypertension. A, afferent arteriole. Arrows show areas of fibrinoid necrosis (by courtesy of Dr A.J. d'Ardenne).

Glomeruli

Fibrinoid necrosis in the afferent arteriole often extends into the capillaries of the correspondening glomerular tuft (Fig. 5). In the glomerular capillaries necrosis is typically focal and segmental, with associated segmental proliferative changes and occasionally formation of glomerular crescents. In injured areas fibrin is deposed within the lumina of necrotic glomerular capillaries, which may also rupture, leading to haemorrhage into the capillary lumen or tubular lumen. If vessels are less severely damaged one usually notes thickening and wrinkling of the glomerular capillary walls with reduplication of the basement membrane.

In malignant hypertension the proportion of glomeruli affected may be quite small and variable. In Heptinstall's series of 51 cases, some even with terminal uraemia, the proportion of glomeruli with typical glomerulitis was only 5–30 per cent (Heptinstall 1953); the majority of glomeruli were normal or exhibited only slight thickening of the capillary wall. In late stages of the glomerulitis, when glomerular fibrinoid change are no longer present, the lesions may mimic those of chronic glomerulonephritis. The distinction then rests on the observation that the changes are focal rather than diffuse and global, and on the association of glomerular lesions with afferent arteriolar fibrinoid necrosis.

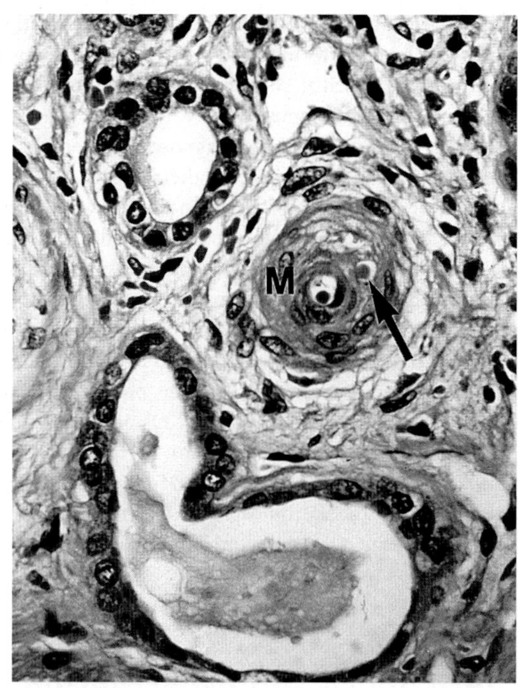

Fig. 6 Medial hypertrophy (M) of an arteriole in a patient with malignant hypertension. Note extravasation of erythrocyte into arteriolar wall (arrow) (by courtesy of Dr A.J. d'Ardenne).

Tubules and interstitium

When renal disease is severe in patients with malignant hypertension, tubular atrophy develops, partly due to ischaemia caused by severe narrowing of interlobular arteries and afferent arterioles. The interstitium in these areas is usually fibrosed and contains chronic inflammatory cells. Renal biopsies from patients with renal impairment complicating the accelerated phase may also show the changes of acute tubular necrosis (Isles *et al.* 1984a,b) and in such cases, the outlook for recovery of renal function is reasonably good.

Relationship between pathological changes and renal dysfunction

The vascular and parenchymal lesions of the kidney which characterize malignant nephrosclerosis occur late in the disease. In the Hammersmith series (Kincaid-Smith *et al.* 1958), renal lesions were minimal or even absent in some patients with clinical evidence of malignant hypertension who had died from non-renal causes and had no significant renal impairment. There is, moreover, considerable evidence that there is no tight relationship between arteriolar and glomerular fibrinoid necrosis and renal impairment. Remarkably fibrinoid necrosis was not found in patients of African origin in whom malignant hypertension is a common cause of renal failure (Pitcock *et al.* 1976). Rather hyalinization of arterioles and marked intimal hyperplasia of the interlobular arteries and larger arterioles was noted.

These findings are consistent with the view that the widening of the intima and narrowing of the lumina of interlobular arteries correlate most closely with the impairment of renal function in accelerated and malignant hypertension (Kincaid-Smith 1976). The relationship between renal impairment and arteriolar fibrinoid necrosis is quite variable. These conclusions are supported by more recent clinicopathological studies (Mittal and Almeida 1987). The dominant role of impaired perfusion and renal ischaemia in determining renal impairment may also explain the correlation which has been observed between renal dysfunction and tubular atrophy (Pitcock *et al.* 1976), since the latter is, amongst others, a marker of ischaemia.

The development of fibrinoid necrosis of renal arterioles is not limited to patients with grade IV retinal changes. Brown *et al.* (1966) described arteriolar fibrinoid necrosis in eight of 19 patients who had retinal haemorrhages and exudates, but no papilloedema. It remains uncertain whether proliferative endarteritis is as common in patients with grade III fundal changes as those with papilloedema.

Renal pathology and secondary malignant hypertension

The development of proliferative endarteritis and fibrinoid necrosis of arterioles is most common in untreated malignant essential hypertension: both abnormalities were present in 85 per cent of such patients, compared with 65 per cent of patients with chronic pyelonephritis and 45 per cent of patients with glomerulonephritis (Kincaid-Smith *et al.* 1958). In these latter conditions, histological examination of renal tissue usually shows the features of the underlying condition, for example, diffuse changes of chronic glomerulonephritis, or the patchy cortical scarring of 'chronic pyelonephritis'.

The histological changes of necrotizing vasculitis, especially microscopic polyarteritis, may include proliferative endarteritis and arteriolar fibrinoid necrosis, and these closely resemble those of malignant hypertension. However, an active cellular infiltrate in areas of necrosis is more common in polyarteritis. The distinction is aided by the presence of arteritic changes in larger vessels, including the arcuate arteries. In polyarteritis, elevation of blood pressure is usually mild to moderate and this disease is not a frequent cause of malignant hypertension. In contrast, the renal lesions in systemic sclerosis may be indistinguishable from those of malignant hypertension in patients with essential hypertension. The lesions comprise extensive arteriolar and glomerular fibrinoid necrosis and marked cellular intimal hyperplasia of the interlobular arteries in systemic sclerosis. The interlobular arteries may also exhibit fibrinoid necrosis, but this is rare in malignant hypertension. The recognition of systemic sclerosis as the underlying diagnosis is usually based on extrarenal manifestations such as sclerodactyly or oesophageal and pulmonary involvement.

In patients with the malignant phase of renovascular hypertension due to unilateral renal artery stenosis, the stenotic kidney may be histologically normal or show only ischaemic lesions, whilst the contralateral kidney exhibits the histological hallmarks of accelerated hypertension. Clinical observations such as these are in keeping with the experimental demonstration by Wilson and Byrom (1939) that lesions of malignant hypertension do not develop distal to a renal artery clamp. The fact that the lesions develop only in kidneys exposed to high blood pressure, highlights the primary importance of elevated blood pressure in the genesis of the specific histological lesions of malignant hypertension.

In a study of IgA nephropathy by Subias *et al.* (1987), 14 patients had benign hypertension and 10 malignant hypertension. There was no major difference in the proportion of patients in each group with mesangial, focal, or diffuse proliferative glomerulonephritis, interstitial fibrosis or infiltrates, or tubular atrophy. There was a higher proportion of glomeruli with crescents and segmental sclerosis in the patients with malignant hypertension associated with IgA nephropathy, three of whom had fibrinoid necrosis and proliferative endarteritis. However, the rate of progression to endstage renal disease was similar in all patients with malignant hypertension, whether or not these typical vascular changes were present. Thus in patients with underlying glomerulonephritis the correlation between impaired renal function and presence of proliferative endarteritis may not be as strong as it is when malignant hypertension develops in patients with primary hypertension.

Effects of antihypertensive treatment

The histological changes of malignant hypertension are rapidly reversed by effective antihypertensive treatment. Fibrinoid necrosis disappears within days, and fibrin in the walls of afferent arterioles and glomeruli is replaced by hyaline material (Harington *et al.* 1959). In contrast, the intimal proliferation and subsequent narrowing interlobular arteries do not disappear. Intimal proliferations are transformed into deposits of fibrous and elastic material, so that luminal narrowing and renal ischaemia persist. Obsolescence of those glomeruli is observed, which are fed by the lesioned upstream arteries. Obsolescence starts with wrinkling of the capillary basement membrane, and subsequently the capillary tuft shrinks. Kincaid-Smith (1976) suggested that in patients with malignant hypertension improvement of renal function after control of blood pressure is the result of hypertrophy of remaining nephrons that are fed by interlobular arteries which had remained intact. There is little reversibility in areas of profound ischaemic damage.

Pathology in other organs

The characteristic vascular changes of malignant hypertension are not only found in the kidney: similar changes occur in other organs, including pancreas, adrenals, liver, gastrointestinal tract, brain, retina, and skeletal and myocardial muscle. As in the kidney, narrowing of the arterial lumen leads to ischaemic changes in the area of supply of affected arteries. Proliferative endarteritis with associated focal necrosis within the pancreas is a relatively common finding at autopsy (Hranilovich and Baggenstoss 1953) and acute pancreatitis may complicate malignant hypertension, especially in uraemic subjects (Barcenas *et al.* 1978). Fibrinoid necrosis is also frequently present in the adrenal gland, which is usually hyperplastic as a result of secondary hyperaldosteronism because of the activation of the renin–angiotensin system. When 20 Afro-Americans with malignant hypertension were examined, cerebrovascular arteriolar fibrinoid necrosis was present in 65 per cent and fibrinoid necrosis of retinal vessels in 47 per cent (Chester *et al.* 1978).

Clinical presentation

The clinical presentation of malignant hypertension is explained as the result of three pathomechanisms:

(1) the effects of the acute increase in blood pressure;

(2) ischaemic organ dysfunction secondary to proliferative endarteritis;

(3) the result of pre-existing hypertension before malignant hypertension developed.

A general overview of the clinical manifestations is given in Table 1.

Blood pressure

There is no threshold of blood pressure above which malignant hypertension develops obligatory, though it is relatively uncommon when the diastolic pressure is below 115 mmHg in adults. Diastolic blood pressure in one recent series ranged from 100 to 180 mmHg, and systolic blood pressure from 150 to 290 mmHg (Yu *et al.* 1986). Similarly, the duration of hypertension prior to the development of malignant hypertension may range from days or weeks to 30 years (Perera 1955; Milliez *et al.* 1960).

Neurological symptoms

Headache is a common, but non-specific symptom: Clarke and Murphy (1956) documented headache in 77 per cent of 73 patients with malignant hypertension. The type of headache is usually headache in the morning affecting the back of the head. This is ascribed to elevated cerebrospinal fluid pressure induced during the phases of rapid eye movement (REM) sleep. Recently, thunderclap headache was also reported as a symptom of a reversible posterior leucoencephalopathy due to malignant hypertension (Tang-Wai *et al.* 2001). In such a case, clinical evaluation should exclude potential subarachnoid haemorrhage. Headache may develop months to years before the onset of malignant hypertension and is more common in younger patients. Impairment of vision, usually related to macular retinal vasculopathy, occurs in 60–90 per cent of patients (Schottstaedt and Sokolow 1953; Kincaid-Smith *et al.* 1958). More serious neurological complications may occur, ranging from focal cerebral ischaemia (18 per cent) and cerebral haemorrhage (16 per cent) to cranial nerve palsies (4 per cent) and subarachnoid haemorrhage (2 per cent) (Clarke and Murphy 1956).

Reversible focal neurological deficits, generalized convulsions, and coma may occur in association with acute blood pressure elevation. Such more serious central nervous system (CNS) symptoms suggest the presence of hypertensive encephalopathy, that is, cerebral hyperperfusion which is discussed in more detail below.

Optic fundus

Visual disturbance with or without headaches was the most common presenting feature (36 per cent) in the study of Lip *et al.* (1994). Grades I and II retinal changes after Keith *et al.* (1939) are manifestations of vascular remodelling. They occur with age and are not specific for hypertension and have little prognostic importance (Dollery 1983).

In contrast, neuroretinal grades III and IV changes are the specific consequence of malignant hypertension. They may appear with great rapidity in a previously normal fundus, or may be superimposed upon long-standing changes of retinal arteries. Animal studies have demonstrated that development of haemorrhage and exudates is preceded by loss of vascular autoregulation with development of areas of narrowing and dilatation in retinal vessels (Byrom 1963). Loss of endothelial integrity occurs in the dilated segments (Goldby and Beilin 1972), followed by leakage of plasma constituents and fibrin deposition in these segments of the vessel wall. Loss of endothelium may lead to haemorrhage, commonly from the radial peripapillary capillaries, in which intravascular pressure is higher than in more periphered vessels. Soft exudates (cotton wool spots) are due to ischaemic infarction of nerve fibres, and occur in relation to arteriolar endothelial breakdown (Hodge and Dollery 1964) subsequent wall swelling and luminal obstruction.

Table 1 Signs and symptoms at presentation

Involved organ	Pathology	Signs and symptoms	Diagnostic procedure
Heart	Myocardial ischaemia	Chest pain, dyspnoea, arrhythmia, and health failure	ECG, chest X-ray, and echocardiography
Vessels	Aortic dissection	Chest pain, back pain, and pulse difference (???)	Chest X-ray, sonography, and CT
CNS	Encephalopathy	Occipital morning headache, thunderclap headache, vomiting, seizures, occipital blindness, paresthesia, psychomotorical deficit, altered consciousness, decreased arousal, vertigo, convulsion, and coma	Neurological examination, CT, and MRI
	Neuroretinal lesions (striated haemorrhages, cotton wool exudates)		
Eyes	Papilloedema	Loss of vision	Funduscopy
Pancreas	Pancreatitis	Abdominal pain	Sonography, CT
Bowel	Mesenteric infarction	Abdominal pain, ileus, and GI bleeding	Angiography of mesenteric vessels
Kidney	Acute renal failure	Proteinuria, haematuria, casts, and oligoanuria	Urinary analysis, sonography (duplex)

The result is loss of transferency of the nerve layer as a result of blocked axonal transport. Hard exudates are caused by deposition of plasma constituents within intercellular spaces. Papilloedema denotes swelling of the optic disc with obliteration of the cup, and loss of the disc margins. Its cause is uncertain, but the most likely explanation is ischaemia. Papilloedema is not related to elevated cerebrospinal fluid pressure, which may be in the normal range (Kincaid-Smith *et al.* 1958). Optic atrophy may result from ischaemia in patients with malignant hypertension, especially in children. It is often provoked by abrupt lowering of blood pressure what results in tissue underperfusion because of loss of vascular autoregulation (Browning *et al.* 2001). It is therefore absolutely necessary to recognize malignant hypertension in children early and to treat it effectively but cautiously to avoid visual damage.

Heart

The effects of malignant hypertension and of so-called 'benign' hypertension on the heart differ to some extent. The so-called 'benign' hypertension is associated with concentric left ventricular hypertrophy and increased frequency of coronary heart disease. In contrast, the sudden onset of malignant hypertension often causes acute left heart failure presenting as pulmonary oedema (Milliez *et al.* 1960) as a result of the acute left ventricle (LV) pressure overload. More recent echocardiographic studies have shown that ventricular hypertrophy is often absent (Shapiro *et al.* 1981). In the era when antihypertensive treatment was not yet available, 13 per cent of deaths from malignant hypertension were due to heart failure and 1 per cent due to myocardial infarction (Kincaid-Smith *et al.* 1958). In contrast, after antihypertensive treatment had become available the prognosis in the same centre was considerably different: 5 per cent of the patients died from heart failure, but 27 per cent from myocardial infarction. The changing pattern presumably reflects increased survival permitting development of coronary atherosclerosis.

Hypertensive encephalopathy

Encephalopathy is a rare complication of malignant hypertension: in the series of Clarke and Murphy (1956) only one of 190 patients with malignant hypertension had reversible seizures unrelated to established cerebrovascular pathology. Most clinical (Healton *et al.* 1982) and pathological studies (Chester *et al.* 1978) of hypertensive encephalopathy have included only patients presenting with the fundal changes of malignant hypertension. Despite the presence of hypertensive encephalopathy, the optic fundi may appear completely normal (Jellinek *et al.* 1964), implying that abnormalities of the cerebral microcirculation induced by an acute rise in blood pressure are not necessarily associated with the retinal lesions of malignant hypertension. Consequently, hypertensive encephalopathy may occur in patients with malignant hypertension, but it is not specific, because it may also be seen after an acute rise in blood pressure in patients with hypertensive emergencies but without malignant hypertension.

Hypertensive encephalopathy was once believed to be due to cerebral vasospasm. Byrom (1954) demonstrated clearly that upon clipping of the renal artery in rats, a rapid increase in blood pressure was followed by seizures. Areas of cerebrovascular spasm were juxtaposed with areas of cerebrovascular dilatation. Areas of vasodilatation showed disruption of blood–brain barrier (Tamaki *et al.* 1984), exudation of plasma, initially increased cerebral blood flow, and cerebral oedema followed by a secondary decrease in cerebral blood flow (Byrom 1974). Using magnetic resonance imaging (MRI) technology evidence for hyperperfusion with exudation of plasma in the genesis of hypertensive encephalopathy has recently been provided in humans as well (Vaughan and Delanty 2000).

There is agreement that the precipitating event in encephalopathy is a loss of cerebral autoregulation resulting from an excessive increase in blood pressure, causing hyperperfusion with the consecutive breakdown of the blood–brain barrier (Lassen and Agnoli 1972). Strandgaard *et al.* (1973) documented that the autoregulatory curve for cerebral blood flow is shifted to the right in hypertensive patients. Intrinsic autoregulation will be overwhelmed, however, by an excessive increase of blood pressure. The absence of a shift of the autoregulatory curve in patients without a history of hypertension explains the observation that hypertensive encephalopathy is more common and occurs at lower blood pressure values in patients who had been normotensive before the hypertensive episodes.

In both experimental studies (Byrom 1954) and human observations (Jellinek *et al.* 1964), impairment of renal function prediposes to the development of hypertensive encephalopathy, possibly because of an underlying increase in blood–brain barrier permeability and the associated risk of autoregulation breakthrough. The blood–brain barrier disruption during a rapid blood pressure rise was less in spontaneously hypertensive rats, compared with normotensive animals (Mueller and Heistad 1980), but was even greater in renal hypertensive rats than in controls (Mueller and Luft 1982).

One iatrogenic cause of hypertensive encephalopathy is administration of erythropoietin (EPO). Winearls *et al.* (1986) reported on a rapid increase in blood pressure, culminating in seizures, in some patients started on EPO. The clinical findings in these patients—normal optic fundi, normal cerebrospinal fluid findings, and normal CT scans—are indistinguishable from those of acute hypertensive encephalopathy. This complication has virtually disappeared with more judicious administration of EPO and better management of the (avoidable) hypertension.

Laboratory investigations

Renin–aldosterone system

In malignant hypertension plasma renin and aldosterone are elevated (secondary hyperaldosteronism). As a result hypokalaemic metabolic alkalosis develops (Beevers *et al.* 1975). There is hyperplasia of both the juxtaglomerular apparatus and adrenal cortex. The stimulation of the juxtaglomerular apparatus may reflect injury to and stenosis of preglomerular vessels so that the baroreceptor senses spuriously low perfusion pressures, but in some patients renin hypersecretion is further aggravated by volume depletion. This pathogenetic sequence has been well documented in animal experiments (Möhring *et al.* 1976). Severe hypovolaemia causes non-osmotic release of arginine vasopressin (AVP), retention of osmotically free water and hyponatraemia, giving rise to the so-called 'hyponatraemic hypertensive syndrome'. The cause of hypovolaemia is pressure natriuresis. The risk of hyponatraemia is aggravated by AT II-dependent stimulation of thirst. Orth *et al.* (1976)

pointed to the importance of frusemide in triggering the hyponatraemic hypertensive syndrome. The pivotal role of AT II in the genesis of this syndrome is emphasized by its dramatic response to converting enzyme inhibition with captopril (Atkinson *et al.* 1979). Urinary kallikrein excretion is low (Hilme *et al.* 1992).

Urine

Proteinuria is a constant feature of malignant hypertension, but its degree varies widely. It is more pronounced (up to 20.5 g/24 h) in malignant hypertension of patients with primary renal disease compared to patients with a history of primary hypertension (up to 12 g/24 h), but there is considerable overlap. Signs and symptoms of overt nephrotic syndrome are rare, however (Kincaid-Smith *et al.* 1958). The urinary sediment usually shows granular casts, red cells (often dysmorphic) and white cells, and occasionally red cell casts; gross haematuria occurs in a minority of cases.

Haematology

The erythrocyte sedimentation rate is usually increased, occasionally to more than 100 mm/h. Several groups have drawn attention to the occurrence of microangiopathic haemolytic anaemia characterized by progressive anaemia, elevation of LDH and appearance of schistocytes in the blood smear (Linton *et al.* 1969; Gavras *et al.* 1975). It has been suggested that intrarenal intravascular coagulation might contribute to renal fibrin deposition, and hence to the pathogenesis of malignant hypertension. Isles *et al.* (1984a) have clarified this issue by demonstrating that similar blood abnormalities occur in patients without malignant hypertension but advanced renal impairment, indicating that they are primarily related to the presence of uraemia.

Pathogenesis of malignant hypertension

Malignant hypertension is a response to marked elevation of blood pressure, and its clinical and pathological features are similar whether the underlying hypertension is primary, renal, or endocrine in origin. This implies that the unique necessary condition for development of malignant hypertension is a severe and usually rapid increase in blood pressure whatever its origins. When the rate of rise is particularly rapid, especially in patients without previous hypertension and the associated vascular structural remodelling, malignant hypertension may occur at diastolic pressures as low as 105–110 mmHg. This may be seen in patients with acute glomerulonephritis or female patients with pre-eclampsia. Children after renal transplantation should also be mentioned, in whom a sudden rise of systolic blood pressure to only 150 mmHg can lead to cerebral symptoms.

The most parsimonious explanation for the development of arteriolar fibrinoid necrosis is that the very rapid increase in pressure leads to loss of autoregulation, development of areas of arteriolar dilatation with consequent endothelial breakdown from increased wall stress and extravasation of plasma constituents into the vessel walls, leading to fibrin deposition and necrosis of vascular smooth muscle cells. This results in ischaemia and infarction of tissue supplied by such vessels (Byrom 1974). Pre-existing chronic hypertension may lower the risk of malignant hypertension because adaptive vascular changes are protective.

Although there is considerable support from experimental and clinical observations for such a sequence of events (Dollery 1983), further questions arise. Why is development of malignant hypertension not related strictly to blood pressure level? Are there additional factors involved in the breakdown of the endothelial barrier and the increase in permeability? Which molecules induce the proliferation of myointimal cells which leads to luminal narrowing and ischaemia?

The role of the endothelium

The endothelial cells participate in the regulation of blood pressure via secretion of vasodilating substances such as nitric oxide (NO) or prostacyclin. The release of NO is controlled by endothelial agonists such as acetylcholine, bradykinin, or substance P (Furchgott *et al.* 1980). There are good arguments that release of vasodilating NO and/or bioavailability of NO are diminished in malignant hypertension.

On the other hand, an excess production of catecholamines and other vasopressors such as AT II, vasopressin (ADH), thromboxane, and endothelin-1 has been documented. These agents cause vasoconstriction and increase vascular resistance. Early studies of Byrom (1954) with *in vivo* observation of dural vessels showed that in the same vessel segments of intense vasodilatation (and even microaneurysm formation) alternate with segments of intense vasoconstriction. The latter is thought to be an autoregulatory response to increased perfusion and perfusion pressure, amplified by the systemic or local release of vasoconstrictors and inadequate availability of vasodilators. When perfusion pressure becomes excessive and/or the contractility of the vasculature is exhausted, vessels will be passively dilated.

The role of blood pressure

The key role of increased blood pressure in the pathogenesis of malignant hypertension is supported by experimental studies. The development of fibrinoid necrosis in renal clip hypertension of the rabbit is strictly correlated with the increase in blood pressure. Vessels which are not exposed to high blood pressure, such as those distal to a renal artery stenosis, do not develop fibrinoid necrosis. Conversely, in pure pulmonary hypertension with normal systemic blood pressure, development of fibrinoid necrosis of arterioles is confined to the pulmonary vasculature.

There are strong arguments, however, against the increase in blood pressure as the only explanation for the development of malignant hypertension. The level of blood pressure at which malignant hypertension develops is highly variable between patients. The risk of malignant hypertension is particularly pronounced in high-renin states and in renal failure. Malignant hypertension is infrequent, but does occur in low-renin states, however, for example, in DOCA-salt hypertension of the rat, the one-kidney–one-clip renal hypertension (Dietz *et al.* 1976), or in patients with primary hyperaldosteronism (Ideishi *et al.* 1990; Sunman *et al.* 1992). The latter observations document that excessive activation of the renin–angiotensin system is not a necessary condition for the development of malignant hypertension.

The role of the renin–angiotensin system

The most convincing argument for a pathogenetic role of this system was provided by Mullins *et al.* (1990) who found that transgenic rats expressing the additional mouse renin gene Ren-2 rapidly develop malignant hypertension in contrast to the genetic background population. The finding of elevated plasma renin activity is almost universal if malignant hypertension occurs secondary to renoparenchymal disease (Brown *et al.* 1966). A pathogenetic role on the renin system is further likely in view of experimental observations that administration of renin causes fibrinoid necrosis in nephrectomized rats (Giese 1963). Furthermore, in the rat model of aortic ligation it was plasma renin activity and not blood pressure, which correlated with the severity of arteriolar lesions (Chusilp *et al.* 1976). Not only the circulating but also the local renin systems play a role. Increased local generation of AT II has been documented in stroke-prone spontaneously hypertensive rat (SHRSP) (Kim *et al.* 1991; Fleming 2000). Finally, the role of AT II is also supported by *in vitro* studies documenting the proinflammatory action of AT II in vascular smooth muscle cells, as exemplified by induction of interleukin 6 expression (Funakoshi *et al.* 1999), accompanied by transcription of NF-$\kappa\beta$ (Funakoshi *et al.* 1999; Muller *et al.* 2000) and generation of reactive oxygen species (Mervaala *et al.* 1999). The latter is important because reactive oxygen species inactivate vasodilating NO. Increased endothelial expression of adhesion molecules including ICAM-1 and V-CAM-1 was shown in the transgenic rat model. This observation is important because it provides the molecular machinery for invasion of the vessel wall by inflammatory cells.

The role of AT II is illustrated by intervention studies. Ito *et al.* (2001) administered an AT1 receptor blocker to 10-week-old SHRSP. Hypertensive cerebral injury such as fibrinogen expression around micro-vessels or reduced expression of adhesion molecule-1 (ICAM-1) was abrogated. A benficial effect was also seen after administration of angiotensin-converting enzyme (ACE) inhibitors (Montgomery *et al.* 1998).

The role of genetic factors

When transgenic rats expressing the mouse renin gene Ren-2 were crossed with Edinburgh Sprague–Dawley rats, 73 per cent of the animals developed malignant hypertension. In contrast, when they were crossed with Hanover Sprague–Dawley rats, only 1 per cent developed malignant hypertension, illustrating the importance of genetic background (Whitworth *et al.* 1995). In humans marked ethnic predisposition to malignant hypertension and clustering of malignant hypertension in families would also be compatible with an important role of genetic factors. During that transition to malignant hypertension, there is a marked increase in the production of local endogenous rat renin in the juxtaglomerular apparatus underlining the importance of the local renin system (Whitworth *et al.* 1994). The factor triggering that transition still remains unclear.

The role of vasopressin

The vasopressin system is also involved: animal studies have demonstrated threefold elevation in plasma vasopressin in malignant compared with non-malignant DOCA-salt hypertension (Möhring *et al.* 1977). In patients with malignant hypertension vasopressin concentrations were increased twofold, but there was no correlation with blood pressure (Padfield *et al.* 1981) presumably because the concentrations observed were below the pressor range.

Increased non-osmotic vasopressin release, possibly secondary to volume depletion, may nevertheless aggravate malignant hypertension. It plays an important role in the hyponatraemic hypertensive syndrome (Orth *et al.* 1976; Atkinson *et al.* 1979). As discussed above this constellation occurs when an acute blood pressure increase is imposed upon a kidney which had been under near normotensive conditions and had not reset the pressure–natriuresis relationship. Excessive natriuresis and volume depletion will then not only activate the renin–angiotensin system and sympathetic nerve system, but also cause non-osmotic release of vasopressin. As a result the kidney retains water in excess of salt. The endresult is hyponatraemia. Because hypovolaemia also increase the pressor hormones AT II and AVP, a further increase in blood pressure occurs so that a vicious cycle is initiated. This explains the paradoxical observation that in the one-clip–two-kidney hypertension model administration of saline reverses the malignant phase of hypertension (Möhring *et al.* 1976). The hyponatraemic hypertension syndrome is seen in patients with malignant hypertension, particularly when natriuresis had been promoted by administration of frusemide. In the early phase of malignant hypertension body weight usually decreases as a result of pressure natriuresis (Barraclough 1966). Furthermore, before ACE inhibitors became available, volume repletion facilitated reversal of the malignant hypertension (Orth *et al.* 1976; Nanra *et al.* 1978). Today this intervention has been superseded by administration of ACE inhibitors or angiotensin receptor blockers, which interrupt the vicious cycle.

The role of other vasoactive systems

Elevated endothelin concentrations were shown in a rat model of genetically determined malignant hypertension, but administration of endothelin antagonists failed to reduce blood pressure (Whitworth *et al.* 1995).

Elevated concentrations of adrenomedullin and brain natriuretic peptide (BNP) were noted in a case with severe hypertension (270/160 mmHg initial blood pressure) (Nishikimi *et al.* 1996) and in a model of DOCA-salt spontane hypertensive rats (D-SHR) (Nishikimi 2001). Adrenomedullin appearantly plays a role in the vasodilatory defense, because a further increase in blood pressure was seen after infusion of the adrenomedullin antagonist calcitonin gene related peptide (CGRP).

Both in animal experiments and in patients with malignant hypertension intense sympathetic stimulation occurs. In some cases this may be triggered by hypovolaemia. In others it may the result of hypertensive encephalopathy. The importance of sympathetic stimulation is illustrated by the clinical obseration that pharmacological blockade of the system lowers blood pressure in patients with malignant hypertension.

Management

Prevention

It is obvious that malignant hypertension can be avoided by appropriate antihypertensive treatment, if hypertension is diagnosed and treated in time. It has been claimed that excess use of coffee and cigarette smoking play a role (Freestone *et al.* 1995), but further evidence for this relationship is needed.

General principles

The patient with malignant hypertension must be treated as an in-patient. The most important elements in the diagnosis are excessive blood pressure elevation (diastolic BP > 115 mmHg) plus retinopathy grade III or IV. If there is evidence of important target organ damage, particularly amaurosis, cardiac decompensation, renal failure, or encephalopathy (see Table 2), the patient should be treated in the intensive care unit. An indwelling arterial line may be placed for accurate monitoring of blood pressure, but this is not obligatory.

Before blood pressure is treated the following questions should be answered?

(1) How far should blood pressure be lowered?

(2) How fast should target blood pressure be reached?

(3) Which drugs are suitable for use in the hypertensive emergency?

(4) Are some drugs superior to others?

How far should blood pressure be lowered?

On the one hand, it is necessary to reduce the symptoms of hypertension induced end-organ damage such as left ventricular failure or seizures. On the other hand, blood pressure should not be decreased below the limit of cerebral autoregulation, because of the risk of iatrogenic ischaemia of the brain and the optic nerve. To avoid such fatal complications one should first check for signs of impending stroke (hemiparesis, amaurosis, aphasia, or motor deficits). If possible, stenotic lesions of the carotides should be excluded by carotid duplex ultrasonography. Unless there are emergencies (pulmonary oedema, aortic dissection), blood pressure should initially not be lowered to values less than 160–170/100–110 mmHg. This is also important because rapid lowering of blood pressure may cause acute renal failure superimposed upon pre-existing renal malfunction from malignant hypertension.

How fast should blood pressure be lowered?

In general, the recommended rate of blood pressure lowering must consider

(1) How long had excessive blood pressure values existed?

(2) Which organs show evidence of target-organ damage?

In established benign hypertension, the autoregulation curve for blood flow to the brain, kidneys, heart, and other organs is shifted rightward. This has repercussions on the rate at which blood pressure can acutely be reduced safely. The longer severe hypertension had been present the slower one should lower blood pressure. The generally recommended treatment targets are reduction of mean arterial blood pressure by no more than 20 per cent within 1–2 h (Calhoun and Oparil 1990). The physician should carefully look for signs of ischaemic target-organ damage (brain, eye, kidney), unless there is an absolute need for rapid blood pressure lowering imposed by aortic dissection, myocardial ischaemia, or left ventricular failure.

Which drugs can be used?

No class of antihypertensive agents is specific for the management of malignant hypertension. Several classes of drugs have been recommended in official guidelines and the most important ones are described below. Drugs recommended for intravenous use in the management of malignant hypertension are summarized in Table 2.

Sodium nitroprusside is suitable for administration in hypertensive emergencies. It has to be given intravenously and the bottle containing the drug should be shielded because sodium nitroprusside solution is light sensitive. Blood pressure lowering is immediate but short-lasting. The rate of infusion can therefore be titrated according to blood pressure values. In case of complications, the hypotensive effect is rapidly reversible after the infusion has been discontinued. Continous monitoring is required, if necessary with an indwelling arterial line. Nitroprusside is a direct vascular smooth muscle relaxant which dilates both arterial and venous vessels, thus reducing both cardiac preload and afterload. In the patient with malignant hypertension and angina pectoris or left ventricular failure, it is therefore the preferred drug because of its antianginal properties. It has been claimed that cerebral blood flow is preserved during nitroprusside administration even when blood pressure has been greatly reduced, although this is disputed (Henriksen and Paulson 1982). Prolonged administration causes accumulation of thiocyanate, resulting in fatigue, anorexia, blurred vision, and disorientation. Cyanide accumulation is a very rare complication.

Table 2 Management of hypertensive emergencies by intravenous medication

Drug	Dose	Onset	Duration	Clinical disadvantages
Sodium nitroprusside	0.25–10 μg kg^{-1} min^{-1}	Immediate	1–2 min	Nausea, vomiting, photodegradation, thiocyanate toxicity
Fenoldopam	0.1–1.6 μg kg^{-1} min^{-1}	15–30 min	15–30 min	Long-term tolerance, reflex tachycardia, headache, contraindicated in patients with glaucoma
Esmolol	Bolus 1 mg kg^{-1} over 30 s, then 150–300 μg kg^{-1} min^{-1} (infusion rate)	2 min	15–30 min	Bronchospasm in patients with history of asthma, bradycardia, decrease of peripheral blood flow
Labetalol	Bolus 20–80 mg (every 10 min), infusion: 2 mg min^{-1}	5–10 min	2–6 h	Bronchospasm in patients with history of asthma, bradycardia
Nicardipine	5–15 mg h^{-1} until target blood pressure received, then 3–5 mg h^{-1}	45–90 min	30–60 min	Reflex tachycardia, flushing
Enalaprilate	1.25 mg over 5 min every 6 h, titrated up to a maximum of 5 mg every 6 h	15 min	4–6 h	Hypotension, renal failure

Fenoldopam is a benzazepine derivative and the first selective dopamine-1-receptor agonist in clinical use (Wood 2001). It is a more potent DA-1-receptor agonist than dopamine but does not act as an agonist at DA-2-receptors or α- and β-adrenergic receptors (Hahn *et al.* 1982). It acts predominantly as a vasodilatator in peripheral arteries and as a diuretic in the kidney. It causes renal vasodilation, natriuresis, and increased renin release. It does not penetrate the blood–brain barrier.

A clinical trial by Panacek *et al.* (1995) showed that there is no significant difference in blood pressure lowering potency between nitroprusside and fenoldopam. Both drugs were equally well tolerated. One interesting difference was the significant increase in urinary output in the fenoldopam group. Tumlin *et al.* (2000) showed that fenoldopam could be used in hypertensive emergencies with signs of target-organ damage. The substance is given intravenously because of its poor bioavailability. The patients electrocardiogram (ECG) should be monitored carefully because T-wave inversion has been reported. The duration of action is longer than that of nitroprusside. Treatment should not be continued for more than 48 h and oral treatment with another drug should be started as soon as blood pressure has been stabilized.

Esmolol is a cardioselective β-adrenergic blocker with a very short duration of action; blood pressure is lowered within 1–2 min and wears off rapidly, 50 per cent of the blood pressure lowering effect is lost within 10–20 min. The agent can be used as a bolus or as a continuous infusion. It is safe in patients with acute myocardial infarction, even in patients who have relative contraindications against β-blockers (Mooss *et al.* 1994). Asthma and high-grade heart block are relative contraindications.

Labetolol has both α- and β-blocking activities. One advantage compared to a pure β-blocker is the maintenance of cardiac output, so that it can be safely administered even in patients with myocardial infarction (Pearce and Wallin 1994). One major disadvantage is the relatively long duration of action which is problematic in cases with drug-induced hypotension. Furthermore, life-threatening hyperkalaemia has been seen after intravenous labetolol injection for hypertensive emergencies in patients with endstage renal disease (Hamad *et al.* 2001). Labetolol is not approved in some European countries and is not the β-blocker of first choice in patients on haemodialysis.

Nicardipine is a dihydropyridine-type calcium channel blocker which is available as a solution for intravenous application. Halpern *et al.* (1990) showed that it potently decreases blood pressure in patients with severe hypertension. Its potency is comparable to that of nitroprusside. Because of its strong vasodilating action it reduces cardiac and cerebral ischaemia despite decreasing blood pressure (Schillinger 1987). Oral or sublingual preparations of the calcium channel blocker *nifedipine* had been very popular in the management of hypertensive emergencies, but it can no longer be recommended for patients with malignant hypertension because it lowers blood pressure abruptly and causes intense sympathetic counter-regulation. This explains why cerebral, renal, and myocardial ischaemic events have been reported following administration of nifedipine (Grossmann *et al.* 1996), especially in elderly patients. Because it can be administered only orally or sublingually, titration to reach target blood pressure is not possible.

Enalaprilate is an intravenous form of an ACE inhibitor with a duration of action of 6–12 h. Because AT II plays a role in the pathogenesis of malignant hypertension intravenous administration of enalaprilate has become popular in some therapy settings (Hirschl *et al.* 1997). The degree of blood pressure reduction with intravenous enalaprilate is correlated to the pretreatment concentration of AT II and plasma renin activity. In patients who are hypovolaemic or in those with underlying renal-artery stenosis intravenous administration of an ACE inhibitor can lead to a precipitous fall in blood pressure and increase in serum creatinine concentration. It should also be mentioned that enalaprilate is contraindicated in pregnancy.

Clonidine can be used both orally or as subcutaneous injection. Sympathetic activation plays an important role in malignant hypertension. The onset of action of clonidine is seen after 30 min and blood pressure is lowered gradually. Consequently it is a good choice for patients in whom rapid control of blood pressure is not required. Sedation is a well-known and, in some settings useful side-effect.

Diazoxide relaxes the arteriolar smooth muscle directly. If given intravenously, the onset of action is within 1 min. Because of significant side-effects diazoxide is not easy to handle. Side-effects include rapid lowering of blood pressure, compensatory reflex sympathetic activation (tachycardia, angina pectoris), compensatory salt and water retention, hyperglycaemia from impaired insulin secretion and others.

Today *Dihydralazine* is rarely used in the management of malignant hypertension because of the prolonged and unpredictable antihypertensive effects. This drug is a vasodilator acting directly on vascular smooth muscle cells (Ludden *et al.* 1980).

Antihypertensive emergencies in specific settings

Pre-eclampsia

Parenteral magnesium is the treatment of choice to prevent eclampsia. Hydralazine has been the antihypertensive treatment of choice in the past. Today labetalol is preferred in the acute critical care management in countries where the drug is licensed. An alternative is treatment with cardioselective β-blockers and possibly calcium channel blockers (although these drugs are not licensed for use in pregnancy). ACE inhibitors and angiotensin receptor blockers are strictly contraindicated because the babies may develop acute renal failure. Diuretics are not advisable in these hypovolaemic patients unless there is left ventricular failure. In refractory cases, termination of the pregnancy is the best option.

Acute aortic dissection

Aortic dissection is the most dramatic and most rapidly fatal complication of hypertensive emergencies. Blood pressure should be lowered rapidly to 100–110 mmHg systolic blood pressure. Treatment should be started as soon as there is evidence that aortic dissection may be present. A combination of β-blockers and intravenous vasodilators such as nitroprusside or fenoldopam is recommended. The β-blockers should be given first to prevent reflex tachycardia. The management must be decided upon in consultation with a cardiovascular surgeon.

Acute stroke

There is evidence of a better outcome in patients with acute stroke who have higher blood pressure in the phase immediately after event (but not thereafter). One reason is that autoregulation is disturbed so that perfusion in the ischaemic penumbra becomes pressure dependent. The common practise of 'normalizing' blood pressure should be avoided in the acute phase. Although there is no definite controlled evidence, most experts agree that antihypertensive therapy should be reserved for patients with a diastolic blood pressure greater than 120 mmHg in whom blood pressure should be reduced with great care. There is no preference of any class of antihypertensive drugs (Ringleb *et al.* 1998).

References

Ahmed, M. E. K., Walker, J. M., Beevers, D. G., and Beevers, M. (1986). Lack of difference between malignant and accelerated hypertension. *British Medical Journal* **292**, 235–237.

Amery, A. *et al.* (1985). Mortality and morbidity results from the European Working Party on high blood pressure in the elderly trial. *Lancet* **i**, 1349–1354.

Atkinson, A. B. *et al.* (1979). Hyponatraemic hypertensive syndrome with renal artery occlusion corrected by captopril. *Lancet* **ii**, 606–609.

Barcenas, C. G., Gonzales-Molina, M., and Hall, A. R. (1978). Association between acute pancreatitis and malignant hypertension with renal failure. *Archives of Internal Medicine* **138**, 1254–1256.

Barraclough, M. A. (1966). Sodium and water depletion with acute malignant hypertension. *American Journal of Medicine* **40**, 265–272.

Beevers, D. G. *et al.* (1975). The clinical value of renin and angiotensin estimations. *Kidney International* **8** (Suppl.), S181–S201.

Bennett, N. M. and Shea, S. (1988). Hypertensive emergency: case criteria, sociodemographic profile, and previous care of 100 cases. *American Journal of Public Health* **78**, 636–640.

Bing, R. F., Heagerty, A. M., Russell, G. I., Swales, J. D., and Thurston, H. (1986). Prognosis in malignant hypertension. *Journal of Hypertension* **4**, S42–S44.

Blythe, W. B. (1985). Natural history of hypertension in renal parenchymal disease. *American Journal of Kidney Diseases* **4**, A50–A56.

Breckenridge, A., Dollery, C. T., and Parry, E. H. O. (1970). Prognosis of treated hypertension: changes in life expectancy and causes of death between 1952 and 1967. *Quarterly Journal of Medicine* **39**, 411–429.

Brown, J. J., Davies, D. I., Lever, A. F., and Robertson, J. I. S. (1966). Plasma renin concentration in human hypertension III: renin in relation to complications of hypertension. *British Medical Journal* **i**, 505–508.

Browning, A. C., Mengher, L. S., Gregson, R. M., and Amoaku, W. M. (2001). Visual outcome of malignant hypertension in young people. *Archives of Disease in Childhood* **85**, 401–403.

Byrom, F. B. (1954). The pathogenesis of hypertensive encephalopathy and its relation to malignant phase of hypertension. Experimental evidence from the hypertensive rat. *Lancet* **ii**, 201–211.

Byrom, F. B. (1963). The nature of malignancy in hypertensive disease. Evidence from the retina of the rat. *Lancet* **i**, 516–520.

Byrom, F. B. (1974). The evolution of acute hypertensive arterial disease. *Progress in Cardiovascular Disease* **17**, 31–37.

Cacoub, P. *et al.* (1993). Malignant hypertension in antiphospholipid syndrome without overt lupus nephritis. *Clinical and Experimental Rheumatology* **11** (5), 479–485.

Calhoun, D. A. and Oparil, S. (1990). Treatment of hypertensive crisis. *New England Journal of Medicine* **323**, 1177–1183.

Chester, E. M. *et al.* (1978). Hypertensive encephalopathy: a clinicopathologic study of 20 cases. *Neurology* **28**, 928–939.

Chusilp, S., Hua, A. S., and Kincaid-Smith, P. (1976). Accelerated hypertension in the rat: relation between renin, renal vascular lesions, salt intake and blood pressure. *Clinical Science and Molecular Medicine* **51** (Suppl. 3), 69S–71S.

Clarke, E. and Murphy, E. A. (1956). Neurological manifestation of malignant hypertension. *British Medical Journal* **2**, 1319–1326.

Curtis, J. R. *et al.* (1969). Maintenance haemodialysis. *Quarterly Journal of Medicine* **38**, 49–89.

Davis, B. A. *et al.* (1979). Prevalence of renovascular hypertension in patients with grade III or grade IV hypertensive retinopathy. *New England Journal of Medicine* **301**, 1273–1276.

Dietz, R. *et al.* (1976). Does the renin–angiotensin system contribute to vascular lesions in renal hypertensive rats? *Clinical Science and Molecular Medicine* **51**, 33S–35S.

Dollery, C. T. Hypertensive retinopathy. In *Hypertension* 2nd edn. (ed. J. Genest, O. Kuchel, P. Hamet, and M. Cantin), pp. 723–731. New York, NY: McGraw-Hill, 1983.

Downing, J. (1986). The psychological and physiological effects of MDMA on normal volunteers. *Journal of Psychoactive Drugs* **18**, 335–340.

Erdberg, A., Korzets, Z., Neufeld, D., Rathaus, M., Cordoba, M., and Bernheim, J. (1992). Malignant hypertension; a possible precursor to the future development of mesenteric ischaemia in chronically haemodialysed patients. *Nephrology, Dialysis, Transplantation* **7** (6), 541–544.

European Dialysis and Transport Association Registry (1986). Demography of dialysis and transplantation in Europe, 1984. *Nephrology, Dialysis, Transplantation* **1**, 1–8.

Ferdinand, K. C. (2000). Substance abuse and hypertension. *Journal of Clinical Hypertension* **2**, 37–40.

Fleming, S. (2000). Malignant hypertension—the role of the paracrine renin–angiotensin system. *Journal of Pathology* **192**, 135–139.

Freestone, S., Yeo, W. W., and Ramsay, L. E. (1995). Effect of coffee and cigarette smoking on the blood pressure of patients with accelerated (malignant) hypertension. *Journal of Human Hypertension* **9**, 89–91.

Fukanoshi, Y., Ichiki, T., Ito, K., and Takeshita, A. (1999). Induction of interleukin-6-expression by angiotensin II in rat vascular smooth muscle cells. *Hypertension* **34**, 118–125.

Furchgott, R. F. and Zawadzky, J. V. (1980). The obligatory role of endothelial cells in the relaxation of arterial smooth muscle by acetylcholine. *Nature* **288**, 373–376.

Gavras, H. *et al.* (1975). Abnormalities of coagulation and the development of malignant phase hypertension. *Kidney International* **8**, 252–261.

Giese, J. (1963). Pathogenesis of vascular diseases caused by acute renal ischaemia. *Acta Pathologica Microbiologica Scandinavica* **59**, 417–427.

Goldby, F. S. and Beilin, L. J. (1972). How an acute rise in arterial pressure damages arterioles. Electron microscopic changes during angiotensin infusion. *Cardiovascular Research* **6**, 569–584.

Grossmann, E. *et al.* (1996). Should a moratorium be placed on sublingual nifedipine capsules given for hypertensive emergencies and pseudoemergencies? *Journal of the American Medical Association* **276**, 1328–1331.

Hahn, R. A., Wardell, J. R., Sarau H. M., and Ridley, P. T. (1982). Characterization of the peripheral and central effects of SK&F 82526, a novel dopamine receptor agonist. *The Journal of Pharmacology and Experimental Therapeutics* **223**, 305–313.

Halpern, N. A. *et al.* (1990). Postoperative hypertension. A prospective, placebo-controlled, randomized, double-blind trial, with intravenous nicardipine hydrochloride. *Angiology* **41**, 992–1004.

Hamad, A., Salameh, M., Zihlif, M., Feinfeld, D. A., and Carvounis, C. P. (2001). Life-threatening hyperkalemia after intravenous labetolol injection for hypertensive emergency in a hemodialysis patient. *American Journal of Nephrology* **21**, 241–244.

Harington, M., Kincaid-Smith, P., and McMichael, J. (1959). Results of treatment in malignant hypertension. A seven year experience in 94 cases. *British Medical Journal* **2**, 969–980.

Healton, E. B. *et al.* (1982). Hypertensive encephalopathy and the neurologic manifestations of malignant hypertension. *Neurology* **32**, 127–132.

Henriksen, L. and Paulson, O. B. (1982). The effect of sodium nitroprusside on cerebral blood flow and cerebral venous blood gases. Observations in awake man during successive blood pressure reduction. *European Journal of Clinical Investigation* **12**, 389–393.

Heptinstall, R. H. (1953). Malignant hypertension: a study of fifty-one cases. *Journal of Pathology and Bacteriology* **65**, 423–439.

Herlitz, H., Gudbrandsson, T., and Hansson, L. (1982). Renal function as an indicator of prognosis in malignant essential hypertension. *Scandinavian Journal of Urology and Nephrology* **16**, 51–55.

Hilme, E., Herlitz, H., Gyzander, E., and Hansson, L. (1992). Urinary kallikrien excretion is low in malignant essential hypertension. *Journal of Hypertension* **10** (8), 869–874.

Hirschl, M. M. *et al.* (1997). Impact of the renin–angiotensin–aldosterone system on blood pressure response to intravenous enalaprilat in patients with hypertensive crises. *Journal of Human Hypertension* **11**, 177–183.

Hodge, J. V. and Dollery, C. T. (1964). Retinal soft exudates. *Quarterly Journal of Medicine* **33**, 117–131.

Hranilovich, G. T. and Baggenstoss, A. H. (1953). Lesions of pancreas in malignant hypertension. *Archives of Pathology* **55**, 443–456.

Ideishi, M. *et al.* (1990). High renin malignant hypertension secondary to an aldosterone-producing adenoma. *Nephron* **54** (3), 259–263.

Isles, C. *et al.* (1984a). Abnormal haemostasis and blood viscosity in malignant hypertension. *Thrombosis and Haemostasis* **52**, 253–255.

Isles, C. G., McLay, A., and Boulton-Jones, J. M. (1984b). Recovery in malignant hypertension presenting as acute renal failure. *Quarterly Journal of Medicine* **53**, 439–452.

Isles, C. G. *et al.* (1985). Factors influencing mortality in malignant hypertension. *Journal of Hypertension* **3**, S405–S407.

Ito, H, Takemori, K., Kawai, J., and Suzuki, T. (2001). AT1 receptor antagonist prevents brain edema without lowering blood pressure. *Acta Neurochirurgica* **76** (Suppl.), 141–145.

Jellinek, E. H. *et al.* (1964). Hypertensive encephalopathy with cortical disorders of vision. *Quarterly Journal of Medicine* **33**, 239–256.

Julkunen, H., Kaaja, R., Jouhikainen, T., Teppo, A. M., and Friman, C. (1991). Malignant hypertension and antiphospholipid antibodies as presenting features of SLE in a young women using oral contraceptives. *British Journal of Rheumatology* **30** (6), 471–472.

Kawazoe, N. *et al.* (1987). Pathophysiology in malignant hypertension: with special reference to the renin-angiotensin system. *Clinical Cardiology* **10**, 513–518.

Kawazoe, N. *et al.* (1988). Long-term prognosis of malignant hypertension; difference between underlying diseases such as essential hypertension and chronic glomerulonephritis. *Clinical Nephrology* **29**, 53–57.

Keith, N. M., Wagener, H. P., and Barker, N. W. (1939). Some different types of essential hypertension: their cause and prognosis. *American Journal of Medical Sciences* **197**, 332–343.

Kim, S., Hosoi, M., Shimamoto, K., Takada, T., and Yamamota, K. (1991). Increased production of angiotensin II in the adrenal gland of stroke prone spontaneously hypertensive rats with malignant hypertension. *Biochemical and Biophysical Research Communications* **178** (1), 151–157.

Kincaid-Smith, P. *The Kidney: A Clinico-pathological Study*, p. 212. Oxford: Blackwell Scientific Publications, 1975.

Kincaid-Smith, P., Hua, A. S., Myers, J. B., MacDonald, I., and Fang, P. (1976). Prazosin and hydrallazine in the treatment of hypertension. *Clinical Science and Molecular Medicine* **3** (Suppl.), 617–619.

Kincaid-Smith, P., McMichael, J., and Murphy, E. A. (1958). Clinical course and pathology of hypertension with papilloedema. *Quarterly Journal of Medicine* **37**, 117–153.

Klag, M. J. *et al.* (1996). Blood pressure and endstage renal disease in men. *New England Journal of Medicine* **334**, 13–18.

Klahr, S. (1989). The kidney in hypertension—villain and victim. *New England Journal of Medicine* **320**, 731–733.

Lassen, N. A. and Agnoli, A. (1972). The upper limit of autoregulation of cerebral blood flow; on the pathogenesis of hypertensive encephalopathy. *Scandinavian Journal of Clinical and Laboratory Investigation* **30**, 113–116.

Lip, G. Y., Beevers, M., and Beevers, G. (1994). The failure of malignant hypertension to decline: a survey of 24 years' experience in a multiracial population in England. *Journal of Hypertension* **12** (11), 1297–1305.

Linton, A. L. *et al.* (1969). Microangiopathic haemolytic anaemia and the pathogenesis of malignant hypertension. *Lancet* **i**, 1277–1282.

Lopes, H. F., Bortolotto, L. A., Szlejf, C., Kamitsuji, C. S., and Krieger, E. M. (2001). Hemodynamic and metabolic profile in offspring of malignant hypertensive parents. *Hypertension* **38**, 616–620.

Ludden, T. M. *et al.* (1980). Hydralazine kinetics in hypertensive patients after intravenous administration. *Clinical Pharmacology and Therapeutics* **28**, 736–742.

McGregor, E., Isles, C. G., Jay, J. L., Lever, A. F., and Murray, G. D. (1986). Retinal changes in malignant hypertension. *British Medical Journal* **292**, 233–234.

Mervaala, E. M. *et al.* (1999). Monocyte infiltration and adhesion molecules in a rat model of high human renin hypertension. *Hypertension* **33**, 389–395.

Meyrier, A., Becquemont, L., Simon, P., and Laaban, J. P. (1990). Protracted anuria due to active vasoconstriction in primary or secondary malignant hypertension. *Nephrology, Dialysis, Transplantation* **5** (3), 174–178.

Milliez, P., Tcherdakoff, P., Smarcq, P., and Rey, L. P. The natural course of malignant hypertension. In *Essential Hypertension: An International Symposium* (ed. K. D. Bock and P. T. Coltier), pp. 60–78. Berlin: Springer, 1960.

Mittal, B. V. and Almeida, A. F. (1987). Malignant hypertension. *Journal of Postgraduate Medicine* **33**, 49–54.

Mohring, J. *et al.* (1976). Effects of saline drinking on malignant course of renal hypertension in rats. *American Journal of Physiology* **230**, 849–857.

Möhring, J. *et al.* (1977). Vasopressor role of ADH in the pathogenesis of malignant DOC hypertension. *American Journal of Physiology* **232**, F260–F269.

Montgomery, H. E. *et al.* (1998). Inhibition of tissue angiotensin converting enzyme acitvity prevents malignant hypertension in TGR(mREN2)27. *Journal of Hypertension* **16**, 635–643.

Mooss, A. N. *et al.* (1994). Safety of esmolol in patients with acute myocardial infarction treated with thrombolytic therapy who had relative contraindications to beta-blocker therapy. *The Annals of Pharmacotherapy* **28**, 701–703.

Mueller, S. M. and Heistad, D. D. (1980). Effect of chronic hypertension on the blood–brain barrier. *Hypertension* **2**, 809–812.

Mueller, S. M. and Luft, F. C. (1982). The blood–brain barrier in renovascular hypertension. *Stroke* **13**, 229–234.

Muller, D. N. *et al.* (2000). NF-κB inhibition ameliorates angiotensin-II-induced inflammatory damage in rats. *Hypertension* **35**, 193–201.

Mullins, J. J., Peters, J., and Ganten, D. (1990). Fulminant hypertension in transgenic rats harbouring the mouse Ren-2 gene. *Nature* **344**, 541–544.

Munro-Faure, A. D. *et al.* (1979). Comparison of black and white patients attending hypertension clinics in England. *British Medical Journal* **1**, 1044–1047.

Nanra, R. S. *et al.* (1978). Analgesic nephropathy: etiology, clinical syndrome and clinicopathologic correlations in Australia. *Kidney International* **13**, 79–92.

Nicholls, K. M., Fairley, K. F., Dowling, J. P., and Kincaid-Smith, P. (1984). The clinical course of mesangial IgA associated nephropathy in adults. *Quarterly Journal of Medicine* **210**, 227–250.

Nishikimi, T., Matsuoka, H., Ishikawa, K., Yoshihara, F., Kawano, Y., Kitamura, K., Saito, Y., Kangawa, K., Matsuo, H., and Omae, T. (1996). Antihypertensive therapy reduces increased plasma levels of adrenomedullin and brain natriuretic peptide concomitant with regression of left ventricular hypertrophy in a patient with malignant hypertension. *Hypertension Research* **19**, 97–101.

Nishikimi, T., Yoshihara, F., Kanazawa, A., Okano, I., Horio, T., Nagaya, N., Yutani, C., Matsuo, H., Matsuoka, H., and Kangawa, K. (2001). Role of increased circulating and renal adrenomedullin in rats with malignant hypertension. *American Journal Physiology. Regulatory, Integrative and Comparative Physiology* **281**, R2079–R2087.

Norris, K. C., Thornhill-Joynes, M., Robinson, C., Strickland, T., Alperson, B. L., Witana, S. C., and Ward, H. J. (2001). Cocaine use, hypertension, and end-stage renal disease. *American Journal of Kidney Diseases* **38**, 523–528.

Ohta, Y., Tsuchihashi, T, Ohya, Y., Fujii, K., Hirakata, H., Abe, I., and Fujishima, M. (2001). Trends in the pathophysiological characteristics of malignant hypertension. *Hypertension Research* **24**, 489–492.

Orth, H., Möhring, J., and Ritz, E. (1976). Maligne Hypertonie—Bedeutung der Hypovämie [Malignant hypertension—importance of hypovolemia]. *Deutsche Medizinische Wochenschrift* **101**, 1655–1659.

Padfield, P. L. *et al.* (1981). Blood pressure in acute and chronic vasopressin excess. Studies of malignant hypertension and the syndrome of inappropriate antidiuretic hormone secretion. *New England Journal of Medicine* **304**, 1067–1070.

Panacek, E. A., Bednarczyk, E. M., Dunbar, L. M., Foulke, G. E., and Holcslaw, T. L. (1995). Randomized, prospective trial of fenoldopam vs sodium nitroprusside in the treatment of acute severe hypertension. *Academic Emergency Medicine* **2**, 959–965.

Pearce, C. J. and Wallin, J. D. (1994). Labetalol and other agents that block both alpha- and beta-adrenergic receptors. *Cleveland Clinical Journal of Medicine* **61**, 59–69.

Perera, G. A. (1955). Hypertensive vascular disease; description and natural history. *Journal of Chronic Diseases* **1**, 33–42.

Perera, G. A. (1958). The accelerated form of hypertension—a unique entity. *Transactions of the Association of American Physicians* **71**, 62–69.

Pitcock, J. A. *et al.* (1976). Malignant hypertension in blacks. Malignant intrarenal arterial disease as observed by light and electron microscopy. *Human Pathology* **7**, 333–346.

Pousse, H., Ayachi, R., Essoussis, A. S., el May, A., and el Amri, H. (1990). Two familial cases of homocystinuria one of which was revealed by fatal hypertensive encephalopathy. *Annales de Pédiatrie* **37** (3), 189–192.

Rambausek, M., Waldherr, R., Andrassy, K., and Ritz, E. (1984). Hypertension in mesangial IgA glomerulonephritis. *Proceedings of EDTA-ERA* **21**, 693–697.

Reader, R. *et al.* (1980). The Australian therapeutic trial in mild hypertension: report by the management committee. *Lancet* **i**, 1261–1267.

Ringleb, P. A., Bertram, M., Keller, E., and Hacke, W. (1998). Hypertension in patients with cerebrovascular accident. To treat or not to treat? *Nephrology, Dialysis, Transplantation* **13**, 2179–2181.

Rodicio, J. L. (1984). Idiopathic IgA nephropathy. *Kidney International* **25**, 717–729.

Rostand, S. G. *et al.* (1982). Racial differences in the incidence of treatment for end-stage renal disease. *New England Journal of Medicine* **306**, 1276–1279.

Rostand, S. G. *et al.* (1989). Renal insufficiency in treated essential hypertension. *New England Journal of Medicine* **320**, 684–688.

Schillinger, D. (1987). Nifedipine in hypertensive emergencies: a prospective study. *The Journal of Emergency Medicine* **5**, 463–473.

Schottstaedt, M. F. and Sokolow, M. (1953). The natural history and course of hypertension with papilloedema (malignant hypertension). *American Heart Journal* **45**, 331–362.

Shapiro, L. M., Mackman, J., and Beevers, D. G. (1981). Echocardiographic features of malignant hypertension. *British Heart Journal* **46**, 374–379.

Sibai, B. M. (1990). Preeclampsia–eclampsia. *Current Problems in Obstetrics, Gynecology and Infertility* **13**, 3–45.

Stefanski, A., Schmidt, K. G., Waldherr, R., and Ritz, E. (1996). Early increase in blood pressure and diastolic left ventricular malfunction in patients with glomerulonephritis. *Kidney International* **50**, 1321–1326.

Strandgaard, S. *et al.* (1973). Autoregulation of brain circulation in severe arterial hypertension. *British Medical Journal* **1**, 507–510.

Subias, R., Botey, A., Darnell, A., Montoliu, J., and Revert, L. (1987). Malignant or accelerated hypertension in IgA nephropathy. *Clinical Nephrology* **27**, 1–7.

Sunman, W., Rothwell, M., and Sever, P. S. (1992). Conn's syndrome can cause malignant hypertension. *Journal of Human Hypertension* **6** (1), 75–76.

Swallwell, C. I. and Davis, G. G. (1999). Methamphetamine as a risk factor for acute aortic dissection. *Journal of Forensic Sciences* **44**, 23–26.

Tamaki, K. *et al.* (1984). Evidence that disruption of the blood–brain barrier precedes reduction in cerebral blood flow in hypertensive encephalopathy. *Hypertension* **6**, I-75–I-81.

Tang-Wai, D. F., Phan, T. G., and Wijdicks, E. F. M. (2001). Hypertensive encephalopathy presenting with thunderclap headache. *Headache* **41**, 198–200.

Tumlin, J. A. *et al.* (2000). Fenoldopam, a dopamine agonist, for hypertensive emergency: a multicenter randomized trial. *Academic Emergency Medicine* **7**, 653–662.

Vaughan, C. J. and Delanty, N. (2000). Hypertensive emergencies. *Lancet* **356**, 411–417.

Veterans Administration Cooperative Study Group on Antihypertensive Agents (1967). Effects of treatment on morbidity in hypertension. I. Results in patients with diastolic blood pressures averaging 115 through 129 mmHg. *Journal of the American Medical Association* **202**, 116–122.

Volhard, F. and Fahr, Th. *Die Brightsche Nierenkrankheit.* Berlin: Verlag Justus von Springer, 1914.

Whitworth, C. E. *et al.* (1994). Spontaneous development of malignant phase hypertension in transgenic Ren2-rats. *Kidney International* **46**, 1528–1532.

Whitworth, C. E. *et al.* (1995). A genetic model of malignant phase hypertension in rats. *Kidney International* **47**, 529–535.

Wilson, C. and Byrom, F. B. (1939). Renal changes in malignant hypertension; experimental evidence. *Lancet* **i**, 136–139.

Winearls, C. G. *et al.* (1986). Effect of human erythropoietin derived from recombinant DNA on the anaemia of patients maintained by chronic haemodialysis. *Lancet* **ii**, 1175–1178.

Wood, J. J. (2001). Fenoldopam—a selective peripheral dopamine-receptor agonist for the treatment of severe hypertension. *New England Journal of Medicine* **345**, 1548–1557.

Woodrow, G., Harnden, P., and Turney, J. H. (1995). Acute renal failure due to accelerated hypertension following ingestion of 3,4-methylenedioxymethamphetamine (ecstasy). *Nephrology, Dialysis, Transplantation* **10**, 399–400.

Yacoob, M., McClelland, P., and Ahmad, R. (1991). Delayed recovery of renal function in patients with acute renal failure due to accelerated hypertension. *Postgraduate Medical Journal* **67** (791), 829–832.

Yu, S.-H., Whitworth, J. A., and Kincaid-Smith, P. S. (1986). Malignant hypertension: aetiology and outcome in 83 patients. *Clinical and Experimental Hypertension. Part A, Theory and Practice* **A8**, 1211–1230.

9.9 The hypertensive child

Wolfgang Rascher

Arterial hypertension is a well-recognized manifestation of various forms of renal disease both in adults and children. Recently, standards for normal blood pressure have been satisfactorily defined in the paediatric age group.

Techniques for measuring blood pressure in children

Direct methods using catheters inserted into the umbilical artery have been used to establish normal blood pressure in neonates (Kitterman *et al.* 1969) and in preterm infants (Versmold *et al.* 1981). Direct arterial blood pressure recording is used only at neonatal care and paediatric intensive-care units when blood pressure monitoring is essential (e.g. during surfactant application in preterm neonates with respiratory distress syndrome, following cardiac surgery). Otherwise, indirect non-invasive techniques such as sphygmomanometry, oscillometry, or Doppler ultrasonography are used. Reliable measurement of blood pressure in infants and children requires procedures different from those used in adults. Detection of the pulse by auscultation, as in conventional sphygmomanometry, is often difficult in infants and children less than 3 years of age. This may be because the blood vessels do not transmit sufficient energy for the Korotkoff sounds to be audible with an ordinary stethoscope: the mistake of applying excessive pressure with the stethoscope on the cubital artery is common.

The width of the cuff bladder is crucial to achieving correct readings of blood pressure (Gómez-Marín *et al.* 1992). If very small cuffs are used, inappropriately high pressures are often recorded; with very large cuffs the recorded pressures are relatively low. The largest cuff that can be comfortably applied should be used, and its inflatable part (the bladder) should cover at least two-thirds of the circumference of the upper arm. A bladder 8 cm wide should be used for small children instead of the standard adult cuff with a bladder of 12–14 cm. The lower edge of the cuff should not touch the stethoscope when this covers the cubital artery. If necessary, an even smaller cuff of 5–6 cm width can be used. The child should be sitting relaxed and comfortable. There is a general agreement that the appearance of the first Korotkoff sound should be used as a criterion for measurement of the systolic blood pressure. However, there was some discrepancy in recommendations as to whether complete disappearance (phase 5) or muffling (phase 4) should be used as an indication of diastolic pressure. Whereas the Report of the Second Task Force on Blood Pressure Control in Children (1987) recommends phase 4 in children and phase 5 in adolescents older than 13, the Recommendations for Management of Hypertension in Children and Adolescents (1986) and the revised 1996 update of the recommendations of the Task force (Update on the 1987 Task force report on high blood pressure in children and adolescents, 1996) states that, in general, phase 5 should be used to indicate diastolic blood pressure in children and adolescents. If the value of phase 5 is close to 0, the measurement should be repeated: if the second measurement gives a similar value, phase 4 should be used.

Measurement of arterial blood pressure with Doppler ultrasound or oscillometric devices is particularly valuable for the detection of arterial hypertension in neonates and small infants. Doppler ultrasound devices only measure systolic pressure reliably (McLaughlin *et al.* 1971; Whyte *et al.* 1975), whereas oscillometry measures mean arterial blood pressure with a good approximation of both systolic and diastolic pressure.

Early reports demonstrated a fairly good correlation between intra-aortic pressures and systolic, diastolic, and mean arterial pressures measured by oscillometry (Friesen and Lichtor 1981; Colan *et al.* 1983); however, Doppler ultrasound was considerably more accurate than oscillometry for systolic arterial pressure in preterm and full-term neonates; the oscillometric method with the standard cuff was reasonably accurate for systolic and mean arterial pressure when several consecutive measurements were made, but diastolic blood pressure was not measured accurately (Pellegrini-Caliumi *et al.* 1982; Emery and Greenough 1992). Further studies in very low birthweight neonates have shown that larger cuffs are more appropriate (Sonesson and Broberger 1987), but hypotension cannot adequately be detected in these infants (Diprose *et al.* 1986). Normative oscillometrically derived blood pressures have been reported in very low birthweight infants (Tan 1988) and during the first 5 years of life (Park and Menard 1989).

Recent technological advances have enabled non-invasive, repetitive measurement of blood pressure over 24 h in individuals performing their normal activities. This newly introduced technique of ambulatory blood pressure monitoring is useful for the evaluation of arterial hypertension in adults as well as in children and adolescents (Loirat *et al.* 1991; Bald *et al.* 1994; Portman and Yetman 1994; Sorof and Portman 2001; Lurbe and Redon 2002). In the paediatric age group, oscillometric ambulatory blood pressure monitors are being used almost exclusively. Whereas blood pressure can be measured accurately in mildly active or inactive children, no reliable measurements are obtained during exercise and vigorous physical activity (Jacoby *et al.* 1993). As in adults, ambulatory monitoring is able to identify a considerable proportion of the children who have high blood pressure in the clinic but a normal mean ambulatory blood pressure elsewhere ('white-coat hypertension') (Hornsby *et al.* 1991; Sorof and Portman 2000). Systolic and diastolic blood pressure follow a typical circadian rhythm, values being 15–25 per cent less at night than during the day. Therefore, mean blood pressure should be calculated separately for the day and the night. Ambulatory blood pressure monitoring has the advantage when evaluating nocturnal blood pressure, which is particularly increased in renal hypertensive patients (Middeke and Schrader 1994; Lingens *et al.* 1995; Sorof and Portman 2001).

Blood pressure standards

A number of epidemiological studies have established normal blood pressures in different populations. Labarthe (1986) reviewed 88 epidemiological reports on blood pressure in children from 30 countries: a consistent increase in both systolic and diastolic blood pressure with age was observed in almost all surveys. A marked increase in average blood pressure with age in childhood and adolescence may be one aspect of normal growth and development. The patterns of blood pressure changes with age differ between populations: marked differences are probably related to methodological rather than population effects since only slight differences between population groups were noted when these were studied by the same investigators under comparable conditions (Voors *et al.* 1976; Kotchen and Kotchen 1978). Distribution and percentiles of general populations provide references for blood pressure in growing children: there is a progressive increase in random blood pressure of approximately 1.5 mmHg systolic and 0.7 mmHg diastolic per year of age. Serial observations can be used to predict subsequent values, especially when resting levels are obtained.

Combined data from several studies as references for random (casual) blood pressure have been published from studies in the United States (Report of the Second Task Force on Blood Pressure Control in Children 1987) and in Europe (De Man *et al.* 1991). The United States data included one European study, the Brompton study of more than 7000 children aged from 4 days to 5 years (De Swiet *et al.* 1976). Although the Task Force stresses the importance of making several recordings in any individual child before drawing conclusions about the blood pressure, only the first readings made in the 70,000 participants were used to prepare its standards, because in one of the nine studies just one measurement per individual was available. In an attempt to incorporate the important contribution of body size into the analysis, the Task Force has added the 90th percentile of height and weight for normal children at the bottom of the charts. The European percentile charts have related random blood pressure to height rather than to age (Fig. 1). Recently, tables for blood pressure in children were published taken into account both age and height (Rosner *et al.* 1993). However, these tables are rather difficult to use in daily practice.

Recently, reference values for ambulatory blood pressure monitoring of children and adolescents have been reported in a large cohort of 1141 children and adolescents that allowed the calculation of percentiles was studied in Germany to provide normal reference values (Soergel *et al.* 1997). Compared to reference values obtained from random (casual) measurements (Report of the Second Task Force on Blood Pressure Control in Children 1987; De Man *et al.* 1991), mean systolic daytime ambulatory blood pressure increased only moderately with height, from 110 to 118 mmHg (body height 120–170 cm), and mean diastolic daytime blood pressure was 72–74 mmHg, irrespective of height or gender (Fig. 2). In small children the mean systolic as well as diastolic daytime ambulatory blood pressure was significantly greater than the normal random blood pressure at rest, whereas this effect was less pronounced in taller adolescents.

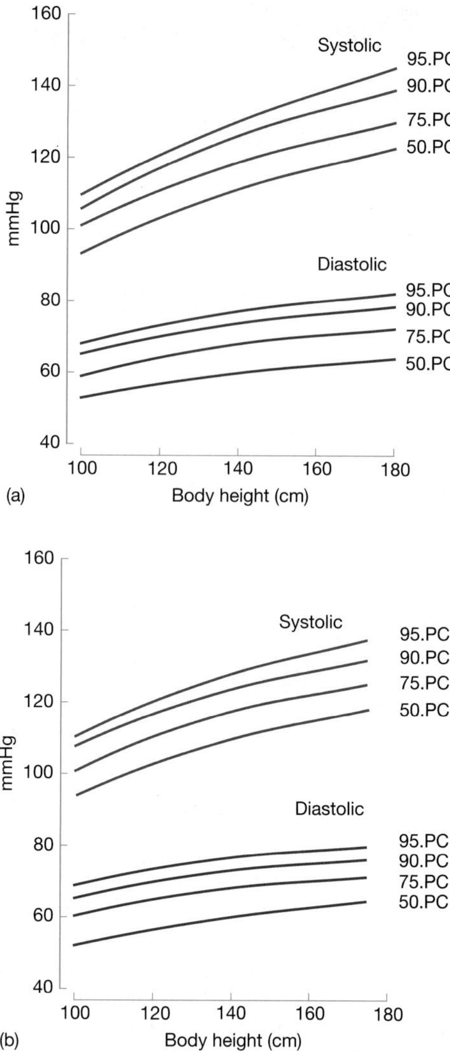

Fig. 1 Percentiles of blood pressure for children by height (combined European studies); Korotkoff phase V is given as diastolic pressure: (a) values for boys; (b) values for girls (according to De Man *et al.* 1991).

The reason for these discrepancies cannot be explained on a biological basis (e.g. higher level of physical activity throughout the day in younger children). Particularly lack of rise in diastolic blood pressure during maturation and lack of a gender difference in diastolic blood pressure do not correspond to casual measurements as verified in a variety of epidemiological studies (Report of the Second Task Force on Blood Pressure Control in Children 1987; De Man *et al.* 1991) (Fig. 3). Methodological differences (e.g. algorithm constructed for adults) might explain this phenomenon. The blood pressure recorder using the auscultatory method definitely show lower diastolic blood pressures as documented by Lambrechtsen *et al.* (1998) in a group of young adults. To resolve the problem with algorithms inadaequate for children companies should explain their algorithms or construct separate algorithms for devices used in children. Although we are using biologically inappropriate diastolic ambulatory blood pressures in children multiple readings during normal physical activity and during night time may improve diagnosis and treatment in children with renal hypertension.

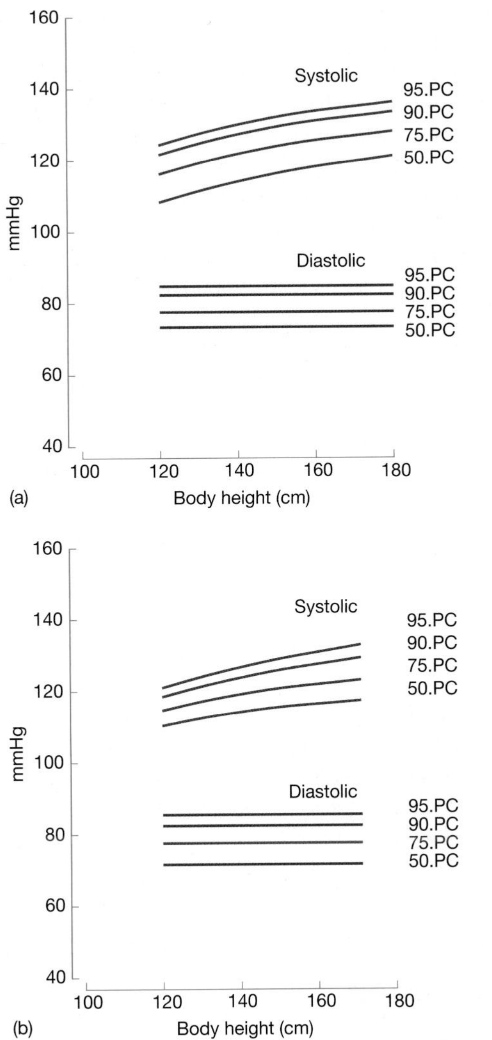

Fig. 2 Percentiles of daytime ambulatory blood pressure for 1141 children by height: (a) values for boys; (b) values for girls (Soergel *et al.* 1997).

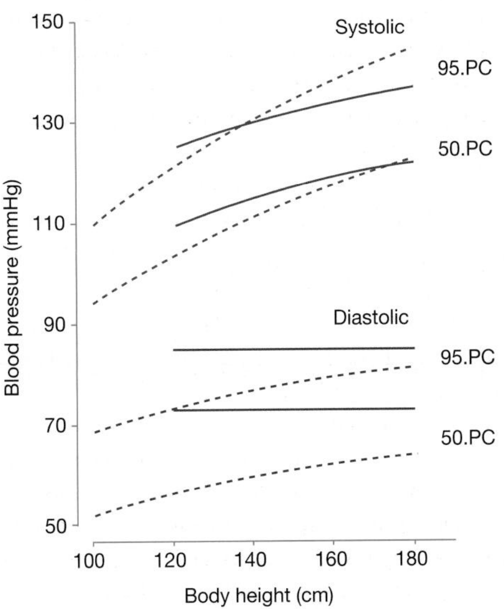

Fig. 3 Percentiles (dotted line) of blood pressure for children by height (combined European studies); Korotkoff phase V is given as diastolic pressure for boys (according to De Man *et al.* 1991) matched with the percentiles of daytime ambulatory blood pressure (solid line) for children by height for boys (Soergel *et al.* 1997).

There was a large decrease of blood pressure during the night, by more than 20 per cent of daytime pressure.

Determinants of blood pressure

The initial blood pressure measured has long been recognized to be the most powerful known predictor of primary hypertension (Cresenta and Burke 1986; Szklo 1986). The tendency of blood pressure to 'track', that is, to remain within a given age-related percentile over long periods of time, is less pronounced in children than in adults. But tracking of systolic blood pressure has been clearly demonstrated in a 15-year follow up population-based family study in Finland (Fuentes *et al.* 2002). Other determinants of blood pressure in children include heart rate, gender, race, degree of biological maturation, social class, environmental changes, and genetic factors (Szklo 1986).

Although the correlation coefficients are low, there are statistically significant relations between blood pressure and body size at all ages studied (Labarthe 1986; Szklo 1986). In the Bogalusa Heart Study of children aged 5–14 years, Voors *et al.* (1977) demonstrated that the relation between age and blood pressure disappeared when an adjustment was made for height, suggesting that among children the relation is explained by a correlate of height, which represents biological maturation. It is therefore better to relate blood pressure to height or some other measure of body size rather than to age (Voors *et al.* 1977; Lauer *et al.* 1986).

The increase in childhood obesity during the last 10–12 years is clearly associated with an elevation of blood pressure in children, the prevalence of obesity related hypertension and early cardiovascular risk (Luepker *et al.* 1996; Sinaiko *et al.* 1999).

Familial aggregation of blood pressure has been recognized in adults and some studies have shown significant correlations between systolic and diastolic pressures in mothers and infants (Hennekens *et al.* 1976; Lee *et al.* 1976). It is not clear to what extent these correlations are related to environmental or genetic factors; in the Montreal adoption study, correlations between the blood pressures of natural relatives were all significant, whereas correlations between blood pressures of adopted children and their new families were not (Biron and Mongeau 1978; Mongeau 1987). In the Minneapolis Children's Blood Pressure Study, mean systolic blood pressure was greater at the first screening in children with a family history of hypertension than in children without a history; this difference persisted at each of nine successive occasions over 8 years (Munger *et al.* 1988). These and other data point to the importance of family history in identifying children at risk for hypertension. In children whose parents are hypertensive, ambulatory monitoring detects an early increase of blood pressure when casual measurements are still indicating normotension (Ravogli *et al.* 1990).

Molecular genetic techniques with candidate gene and linkage analysis have been introduced to elucidate the genetic basis of hereditary hypertension. Recently, three monogenetic forms of hereditary hypertension have been identified. Liddle's syndrome is caused by constitutive activation of the renal epithelial sodium channel due to mutation in the β subunit (Skimkets *et al.* 1994) or by a mutation truncating the carboxy terminus of the gamma subunit of this channel (Hansson *et al.* 1995). Patients with glucocorticoid-remediable aldosteronism (GRA) possess chimeric gene duplications arising from unequal crossing-over, fusing regulatory sequences of steroid 11 β-hydroxylase to coding sequences of aldosterone synthase. These chimaeric genes are specific for GRA and explain the biochemistry, physiology, and genetics of this form of hypertension (Lifton *et al.* 1992; Dluhy *et al.* 2001).

Definition of hypertension in children

Criteria for the diagnosis of hypertension in adults are not applicable to children. A value of 140/90 mmHg for random (casual) blood pressure and 135/85 mmHg for daytime ambulatory blood pressure has been generally accepted as the upper limit of normal in adults, and this might also be true for adolescents. However, recent recommendations based on epidemiological and clinical studies define normal blood pressure of less than 130/85 mmHg as normal and values in the range 130–139/85–89 mmHg as high normal (World Health Organization—International Society of Hypertension Guidelines for the Management of Hypertension 1999). These figures should also be used for adolescents.

Since a linear relation exists between height and blood pressure and between log weight and blood pressure, a major determinant of blood pressure in childhood is body size (Voors *et al.* 1978). Therefore, it has been recommended that in the growing child blood pressure should be related to height (Cresenta and Burke 1986).

The range of 'normal' blood pressure is uncertain, and there is no agreement on the exact definition of hypertension at different ages. The most helpful criterion for definition of hypertension in children is the persistence of blood pressure above the 95th percentile.

Hypertension is only arbitrarily defined in terms of blood pressure or of standard deviation from the mean or percentile. For clinical purposes, values less than the 95th percentile should be considered as normal ('high normal' is between the 90th and the 95th percentiles); values above this, if confirmed by two further examinations, are compatible with the diagnosis of hypertension (Recommendations for Management of Hypertension in Children and Adolescents 1986; Report of the Second Task Force on Blood Pressure Control in Children 1987; Update on the 1987 Task force report on high blood pressure in children and adolescents 1996). For practical purposes (e.g. diagnostic investigation, treatment), mild forms of persistent hypertension should be separated from moderate to severe forms (>10–20 mmHg above the 95th percentile).

When ambulatory blood pressures taken with oscillometric devices are the basis for diagnosing arterial hypertension, separate reference values should be used (Soergel *et al.* 1997). Details are given in Tables 1 and 2 as well as in Figs 1 and 2.

Table 1 Paediatric reference values for casual blood pressure values

Body height (cm)	Boys		Girls	
	50.PC	95.PC	50.PC	95.PC
100	96/53	113/70	96/53	113/70
110	100/56	118/72	99/56	115/72
120	102/58	120/73	102/57	118/74
130	105/59	121/74	105/58	122/75
140	107/60	124/75	107/60	126/76
150	111/61	130/77	111/62	130/77
160	116/62	137/79	115/64	134/78
170	122/64	146/81	117/65	138/80
180	126/66	151/83		

PC, percentile.

Prevalence of primary and secondary hypertension

Although the definition of hypertension is necessarily somewhat arbitrary, the prevalence of hypertension in childhood is estimated at between 1 and 2 per cent, probably closer to 1 per cent (Leumann 1979; Cresenta and Burke 1986; Adrogue and Sinaiko 2001). The majority of these children have only a mild increase in blood pressure and belong to the category of primary (essential) hypertension; however, there is a small group of children with much increased blood pressures, most of

Table 2 Paediatric reference values for ambulatory blood pressure monitoring (ABPM)

Body height (cm)	Boys				Girls			
	Day		Night		Day		Night	
	50.PC	95.PC	50.PC	95.PC	50.PC	95.PC	50.PC	95.PC
120	112/73	132/85	95/55	104/63	111/72	120/84	96/55	107/66
130	113/73	125/85	96/55	107/65	112/72	124/84	97/55	109/66
140	114/73	127/85	97/55	110/67	114/72	127/84	98/55	111/66
150	115/73	129/85	99/56	113/67	115/73	129/84	99/55	112/66
160	118/73	132/85	102/56	116/67	116/73	131/84	100/55	113/66
170	121/73	135/85	104/56	119/67	118/74	131/84	101/55	113/66
180	124/73	137/85	107/56	122/67	120/74	131/84	103/55	114/66

Table 3 Cause of secondary persistent hypertension in childhood

	Still and Cotton (1967) (*n* = 52)	**Gill *et al.* (1976) (*n* = 98)**	**Uhari and Koskimies (1979) (*n* = 135)**	**André *et al.* (1980) (*n* = 46)**	**Loirat *et al.* (1982) (*n* = 88)**	**Dillon (1987) (*n* = 135)**	**Wyszynska *et al.* (1992) (*n* = 351)**	**Arar *et al.* (1994) (*n* = 102)**
Renoparenchymal disease (%)	73	79	59	81	89	73	68	76
Renovascular disease (%)	10	6	5	17	10	10	10	13
Coarctation of the aorta (%)	11	15	29	0	0	9	2	3
Endocrine and other causes (%)	6	1	7	2	1	8	20	10

whom suffer from secondary hypertension. The prevalence of persistent secondary hypertension in children is about 0.1 per cent (Leumann 1979; Rames *et al.* 1979), and renal disease predominates in this group: more than 80 per cent will have underlying kidney disease (Table 3). The consequences of untreated hypertension depend upon the severity, duration, and cause. Mild elevation of blood pressure rarely causes adverse effects until adult life. In contrast, severe sustained hypertension in children carries an increased risk of illness and death.

Causes of blood pressure elevation in childhood

In general, two forms of hypertension in childhood can be distinguished: transient and chronic sustained hypertension.

Transient hypertension

Renal diseases predominate as a cause of transient acute hypertension: such children may suffer from acute glomerulonephritis, Henoch–Schönlein nephritis, haemolytic–uraemic syndrome, or acute renal failure of any cause. The increase in blood pressure under these circumstances is mainly caused by sodium and water retention; however, under certain conditions, such as renal ischaemia or arteriolar damage, vasoconstrictor mechanisms, including the renin–angiotensin and sympathetic nervous systems, also contribute. According to Broyer *et al.* (1981), hypertension occurs in 46 per cent of children in the early stage of acute postinfectious glomerulonephritis. Blood pressure is elevated before steroid treatment is begun in children with idiopathic nephrotic syndrome associated with minimal glomerular changes (International Study of Kidney Disease in Children 1981; Küster *et al.* 1990). A possible mechanism is intravascular volume depletion, which results in the release of a variety of vasoconstrictors, including renin, vasopressin, and noradrenaline (Rascher and Tulassay 1987). The massive activation of these pressor mechanisms causes peripheral vasoconstriction to such an extent that, even in the presence of diminished intravascular volume, blood pressure increases. The treatment consists, paradoxically, of intravascular volume repletion using plasma, which lowers vasoconstrictor activity and, therefore, blood pressure.

Transient hypertension sometimes develops after urological surgery: this may be due to the release of renin in response to disturbance of the renal pedicle or kidney. In addition, in various forms of acute renal failure and after renal transplantation, transient hypertension may be observed and may require treatment.

Hypertension is also observed in the presence of increased intracranial pressure and in association with convulsions. Kaiser and Whitelaw (1988) have described a significant positive correlation between mean arterial pressure and intracranial pressure in infants. Hypertension was reported in various acute neurological diseases of childhood (Eden *et al.* 1977) and meningitis may present as hypertensive encephalopathy (Waters and Gills 1987). Possible hypertensinogenic mechanisms include disturbances of the medullary vasomotor centre, with subsequent increase in sympathetic nervous activity and activation of other vasoactive hormonal systems. Iatrogenic hypertension may develop during therapy with steroids (e.g. dexamethasone in preterm infants) (Greenough *et al.* 1992). Hypertension associated with skeletal traction in children has recently been reported (Heij *et al.* 1992).

Chronic sustained hypertension

The main causes of chronic hypertension in childhood are summarized in Table 4. Whereas in neonates and young infants coarctation of the aorta and renovascular disease (thrombosis after catheterization of the umbilical artery) predominate, renal disease is very likely in older infants, children and adolescents. Since coarctation of the aorta at the isthmus is nowadays surgically corrected within the neonatal period and the frequency and duration of umbilical artery catheters have been reduced, these causes of arterial hypertension are decreasing. Four different renal causes of persistent renal hypertension can be distinguished: diseases of the renal parenchyma; diseases of renal vessels (renovascular hypertension); chronic renal failure; and post-transplant hypertension.

Diseases of renal parenchyma

Chronic glomerulonephritis is one of the most frequent causes of hypertension in children as in adults (Table 5). Reduced capacity to excrete sodium and water, as well as reduced renal perfusion with subsequent activation of the pressor system, contribute to the pressure elevation. Failure to suppress vasoconstrictor hormones despite volume expansion has been implicated as a hypertensive mechanism, particularly in patients with glomerular diseases.

One of the most common causes of renal hypertension in childhood was pyelonephritic scarring (Table 5), which results from vesicoureteric reflux combined with urinary-tract infection in early life (Smellie and Normand 1975). It is also known as Ask-Upmark kidney

Table 4 Causes of chronic hypertension in childhood

1. Renal
   - Diseases of the renal parenchyma
     - Chronic glomerulonephritis
     - Reflux nephropathy (segmental renal scars)
     - Obstructive uropathy
     - Renal dysplasia
     - Polycystic kidney disease
     - Haemolytic–uraemic syndrome
     - Chronic renal failure
   - Renovascular disease
     - Renal artery stenosis (fibromuscular dysplasia, neurofibromatosis)
     - Anomalies of the renal artery (aneurysma, thrombosis, arteriovenous fistula)
     - Arteritis
   - Renal tumours
     - Wilms' tumour
     - Haemangioperiocytoma
     - Hamartoma
2. Coarctation of aorta
   - Thoracic
   - Abdominal
3. Endocrine
   - Catecholamine excess
     - Phaeochromocytoma
     - Neuroblastoma
   - Corticoid excess
     - Congenital adrenal hyperplasia
     - Conn's syndrome
     - Cushing's syndrome
   - Low renin states
     - Apparent mineralocorticoid excess (AME)
     - Glucocorticoid remediable aldosteronism (GRA)
4. Primary hypertension

(Ask-Upmark 1929), chronic pyelonephritis (Holland *et al.* 1975), asymmetrical renal parenchymal defect (Andersen *et al.* 1973), reflux nephropathy (Siegler 1976), and primary interstitial nephritis (Stickler *et al.* 1971). The lesions, characterized by segmental shrinking of the renal parenchyma containing hyalinized glomeruli, dilated tubules, thickened arterioles, and interstitial fibrosis, have been called 'segmental hypoplasia' in the French literature (Habib *et al.* 1965; Royer *et al.* 1971). Ask-Upmark kidney is sometimes listed under renovascular hypertension, since a primary vascular insult may be involved in the pathogenesis. Some authors use the misleading term 'neonatal reflux nephropathy'. In most cases, even with precise histological examination of the scarred, shrunken renal tissue, it is impossible to decide whether this is a consequence of a congenital disorder of renal development or segmental renal scar formation due to urinary tract infections and reflux in early life. The latter appears to be the most important cause and is preventable by early detection and treatment of acute pyelonephritis in infants. Reflux nephropathy is most common in girls. The occurrence of hypertension is closely related to the degree of scar formation in the kidney, but is a late stage of renal scarring, rarely developing in the first years of life. Approximately 10 per cent of children with renal scarring develop hypertension (Holland *et al.* 1975; Wallace *et al.* 1978). Plasma renin activity is usually elevated in children with hypertension and reflux nephropathy, and this is the major factor causing hypertension (Godard *et al.* 1973; Siegler 1976; Savage *et al.* 1978; Dillon and Smellie 1984). Renin release probably originates in ischaemic areas between scarred and normal renal parenchyma (Leumann 1979). In a considerable number of urinary-tract malformations, most of which are accompanied by chronic pyelonephritis, hypertension occurs before significant renal failure. With improved diagnosis and early treatment of acute pyelonephritis in infants and children the number of children with significant renal scarring and subsequent arterial hypertension appears to be decreasing substantially (Jansen and Scholtmeijer 1990).

In haemolytic–uraemic syndrome, the occurrence of hypertension is related to the type of histological lesion. Severe hypertension is present if microangiopathy has affected medium-sized branches of the renal arteries. This vascular form of haemolytic–uraemic syndrome occurs most frequently in older children; the glomerular form of microangiopathy mainly affects infants, in whom hypertension is rare

Table 5 Percentage frequency distribution of primary disease causing persistent renal hypertension

	Gill *et al.* (1976) (*n* = 83)	Uhari and Koskimies (1979) (*n* = 47)	André *et al.* (1980) (*n* = 45)	Broyer *et al.* (1981) (*n* = 238)	Loirat (1982) (*n* = 87)	Dillon (1987) (*n* = 260)	Wyszynska *et al.* (1992) (*n* = 272)	Arar *et al.* (1994) (*n* = 89)
Glomerular disease (glomerulonephritis)	42	26	22	29	38	29	26	42
Chronic pyelonephritis (including reflux nephropathy)	17	19	29	32	22	23	36	29
Obstructive uropathy	7	15	—	8	—	21	11	3
Polycystic kidney disease	5	11	—	1	8	7	9	11
Haemolytic–uraemic syndrome	7	2	9	6	16	5	6	—
Renovascular disease	7	8	18	20	10	16	12	15
Other nephropathies	14	19	23	3	6	3	1	—

and seldom severe. Hypertension appears to be a considerable long-term problem, that has been addressed recently (Tönshoff *et al.* 1994; Bald *et al.* 1996; Krmar *et al.* 2001).

Polycystic kidneys, an important cause of severe hypertension, are seen mainly in infants with the autosomal-recessive form of polycystic kidney disease. Insufficient control of blood pressure rather than renal failure was often associated with illness and death. Hypertension is often more severe in the first years of life than later, and may spontaneously return to normal. Ambulatory blood pressure is greater in asymptomatic children and adolescents with autosomal-dominant polycystic kidney disease than in normal controls (Zeier *et al.* 1993). Polycystic kidney disease may be associated with other congenital anomalies, such as tuberous sclerosis (Stapleton *et al.* 1980).

Renal tumours are only rarely the cause of hypertension in children: it has been reported in some patients with nephroblastoma (Wilms' tumour) (Ganguly *et al.* 1973; Sheth *et al.* 1978), juxtaglomerular-cell tumour/haemangiopericytoma (Warshaw *et al.* 1979; McVicar *et al.* 1993) and renal hamartoma. Renin secretion is the cause of hypertension in these tumours. In Wilms' tumour, renin is secreted as a consequence of arterial compression and subsequent ischaemia, or of excessive production by the tumour itself (Ganguly *et al.* 1973).

Renovascular hypertension

Diseases of the renal vessels resulting from lesions that cause unilateral or bilateral impairment of blood flow to kidneys are far rarer than diseases of the renal parenchyma (Table 5), accounting for about 10 per cent of cases of secondary hypertension in children, and tending to present more commonly in younger children (Leumann 1979). After coarctation of the aorta, usually at the isthmus and rarely of the abdominal aorta (Fig. 4), renal artery stenosis is the second most important surgically curable form of hypertension in children. Studies on the pathogenesis of hypertension and successful revascularization procedures have devoted particular attention to this form of hypertension in childhood. Renovascular disorders can generally be distinguished as those which are localized at the renal hilum and those occurring within the smaller vessels of the kidney (intrarenal) (Table 6).

Renal arterial stenosis is the most common cause of renovascular hypertension: approximately one-third to half of children have fibromuscular dysplasia (Deal *et al.* 1992b; Estepa *et al.* 2001), the cause of which is unknown.

Stenosis of the renal artery, associated with neurofibromatosis, is usually caused by intimal proliferation, which closely resembles fibromuscular dysplasia histologically. It is, therefore, essential to exclude neurofibromatosis in every child patient with renal artery stenosis. Although only the main renal artery is affected, lesions may subsequently develop in the contralateral artery (Müller-Wiefel 1978; Leumann 1979; Fossali *et al.* 2000). In 1978, 56 cases of renal arterial stenosis in neurofibromatosis were reviewed by Müller-Wiefel (1978). Most patients were young; 70 per cent were less than 16 years old. Radiography in 45 patients with vascular neurofibromatosis showed isolated abdominal coarctation in three and coarctation with renal artery stenosis in 10. The remainder of the patients had renal artery stenosis without coarctation. An example of stenosis with aneurysm in a 14-year-old boy with neurofibromatosis is shown in Fig. 5.

The renal artery may be compressed by a tumour, fibrous bands, haematoma, or surgical intervention. The observation that phaeochromocytomas may lead to renovascular hypertension by compression of the renal artery is of particular interest (Alvestrand *et al.* 1977). A similar aetiology has been suggested as cause of hypertension in a 5-year-old boy (Menschik *et al.* 2002).

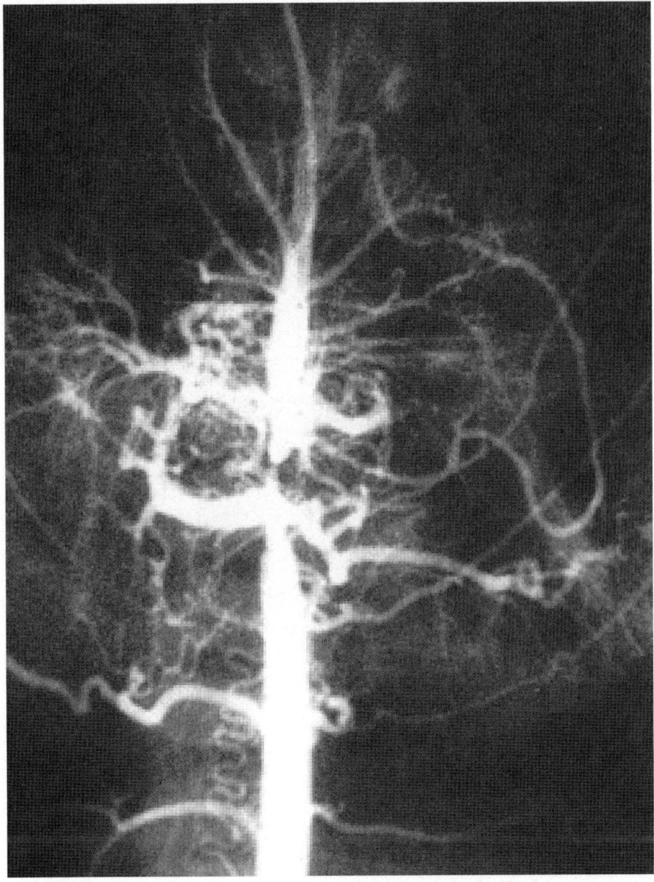

Fig. 4 Flush aortography in a 4-month-old girl with coarctation of the abdominal aorta, demonstrating extensive narrowing of that vessel.

Table 6 Renovascular causes of hypertension in childhood

Hilar compression by tumours of the kidney, adrenals, etc.
Stenosis of the renal artery and its main branches
Fibromuscular dysplasia, vascular neurofibromatosis, aneurysm, embolism, thrombosis (newborns), arteritis (Takayasu disease)
Coarctation of the abdominal aorta
Stenosis of the small arteries (intrarenal changes)[a]
Aneurysm (congenital, acquired, for example, after renal biopsy)
Irradiation nephritis, haemolytic–uraemic syndrome, general vascular disease: periarteritis nodosa, vasculitis, etc.
Vascular malformation (e.g. Klippel–Trenaunay syndrome)

[a] Some authors include 'segmental hypoplasia' (with reflux nephropathy in this category).

Takayasu's arteritis (aortic arch syndrome or pulseless disease) is an important cause of renovascular hypertension in non-White children (Wiggelinkhuizen and Cremin 1978); stenosis or occlusion on one or both renal arteries occurs in up to 75 per cent of cases. Other causes of renovascular hypertension in children include renal arterial aneurysm, arteriovenous fistula, renal arterial disruption, and arterial trauma.

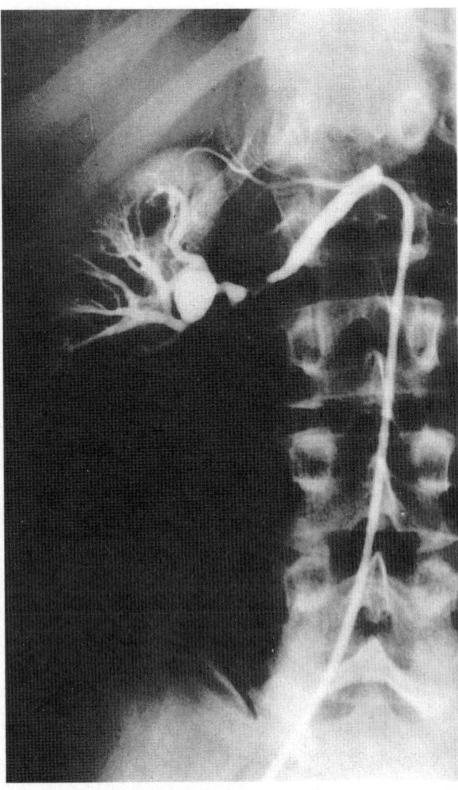

Fig. 5 Selective angiography of the right renal artery showing stenosis and poststenotic aneurysm in a 14-year-old boy with neurofibromatosis.

In neonates, the causes include renal arterial thrombosis associated with the use of umbilical arterial catheters, and renal arterial embolization from thrombosis of the ductus arteriosus (Adelman 1978). Renovascular hypertension in children has been reported in vascular malformation syndromes, such as the Klippel–Trenaunay syndrome (Proesmans 1982) or Moyamoya disease (Jansen *et al.* 1990). Marked stenosis of the renal vessel with hypertension is also found after radiation. Renin secretion following reduced renal perfusion into stenosed kidneys was also shown to be the cause of renal vascular hypertension in children (Dillon *et al.* 1978). Patients with Turner syndrome have vascular anomalies and are at risk for development of hypertension (Nathwani *et al.* 2000a,b).

Chronic renal failure and renal transplantation

Sustained hypertension frequently occurs in children with chronic renal failure, who are routinely treated by dialysis and renal transplantation. It must be stressed that, in almost all reports, patients with chronic renal failure have not been unequivocally differentiated from those with normal renal function, and it is often difficult to determine whether the hypertension was a direct consequence of the underlying renal disease or related to chronic renal failure. Between 1970 and 1978, 119 children and adolescents with persistently reduced renal function were analysed at the University Children's Hospital in Heidelberg (Table 7).

The frequency of hypertension in chronic renal failure varies considerably in relation to the stage of renal impairment, the primary disease and the treatment given. In the early stage of renal insufficiency, patients with glomerular diseases, segmental renal scars, and polycystic kidney disease usually have moderate to severe hypertension, whereas in the endstage only a few patients do not show elevation of blood pressure.

Table 7 Frequency of hypertension in 119 children with chronic renal failure before reaching endstage renal disease (glomerular filtration rate, GFR < 40 ml/min per 1.73 m^2)

	Number of patients		Mean serum creatinine at onset of hypertension (mg/dl)
	Total	Sustained hypertension	
Glomerular diseases	23	21	1.1
Chronic pyelonephritis (including urinary tract malformation)	40	33	2.2
Oligomeganephronic dysplasia	14	9	4.4
Nephronophthisis	18	12	4.0
Polycystic kidney disease	5	4	1.0
Other nephropathies	19	15	2.8

These patients suffer primarily from tubular or interstitial diseases or from renal hypoplasia (e.g. oligomeganephronic dysplasia), or have congenital malformations of the urinary tract.

After successful renal transplantation, hypertension occurs in 60–93 per cent of children and therefore appears to be more frequent than in adults (Tejani 1983; Ingelfinger 1984; Broyer *et al.* 1987; Baluarte *et al.* 1994). Pathogenetic mechanisms vary considerably. Up to 100 per cent of the children were hypertensive during the first post-transplant week, when volume expansion by plasma, colloid, or intravenous electrolytes commonly increases blood pressure. Acute rejection crises, treated with high-dose steroids, are also an important cause of transient increases in blood pressure. Patients with stable graft function have a lesser incidence of hypertension than those with chronic rejection. Broyer *et al.* (1987) studied 361 consecutive children given renal transplants over a period of 11 years, and found that 15 per cent never had hypertension, 12 per cent had hypertension within the first 6 months after transplantation, and 5 per cent exhibited transient hypertension when receiving high-dose steroid therapy. Sustained hypertension was present in 62 per cent, and 5 per cent were hypertensive until death or graft failure within the first 3 months. Chronic graft rejection was a major cause of sustained hypertension, as was renal arterial stenosis. Interestingly, the stenosis improved spontaneously in 15 out of 43 patients (Broyer *et al.* 1987). The main causes of sustained hypertension are given in Table 8. Others have reported a lower incidence of stenosis after transplantation: Malekzadeh *et al.* (1987) found 31 cases out of 400 cadaveric transplants performed at the Children's Hospital in Los Angeles. Renal arterial stenosis may result from insufficient suturing during the creation of the anastomosis, damage of the intima during removal or perfusion of the donor kidney, disproportion between the calibre of the transplanted renal artery and the recipient vessels, or from immunological reactions. From the clinical point of view, stenosis sometimes resembles acute rejection.

There is a close relation between the underlying primary renal disease and the occurrence of hypertension. Children whose primary disease is glomerulonephritis are more likely to develop severe hypertension after renal transplantation than those with other nephropathies.

Table 8 Main causes of sustained hypertension in 209 children after renal transplantation

	Per cent
Chronic rejection	59.0
Renal artery stenosis	20.5
Native kidney	4.5
Recurrence of primary renal disease	4.5
Non-viable kidney	1.5
No obvious cause	10.0

Clinical presentation

In children, even severe hypertension often occurs without any clinical symptoms. Physical signs are frequently minimal and often misinterpreted, unless blood pressure is recorded.

Presenting features differ with age. During infancy, congestive heart failure, respiratory distress, failure to thrive, vomiting, irritability, and convulsions are the most common features (Leumann 1979; Schärer *et al.* 1993). Headache, nausea, vomiting, polydipsia, polyuria, visual problems, irritability, tiredness, cardiac failure, facial palsy, epistaxis, and growth retardation are characteristic features in older children (Leumann 1979; Tirodker and Dabbagh 2001). The underlying disease accounts for many of the symptoms observed in the hypertensive child: nausea, tiredness, or polyuria might be related to underlying renal disease and not to specific hypertensive symptoms. In children suffering from phaeochromocytoma, palpitations, sweating, and pallor might be characteristic, but these symptoms sometimes occur with other causes of hypertension. Conditions suggesting increased risk of hypertension in infants are abdominal mass (polycystic kidney disease, neuroblastoma, Wilms' tumour), neurofibromatosis, failure to grow, indwelling umbilical arterial catheter, administration of glucocorticoids and/or ACTH, Turner's syndrome, Cushing's syndrome, Williams' syndrome, aortic coarctation, unexplained cardiac failure, and unexplained seizures.

Physical examination may reveal signs associated with the specific underlying cause of hypertension, for example, weak pulses or differences in blood pressure between the upper and lower limbs in coarctation of the aorta, *café-au-lait* skin patches or other features of neurofibromatosis with renal arterial disease, abdominal masses in polycystic kidney disease. Signs and symptoms of cardiomegaly, hypertensive retinopathy, or several neurological features are particularly important, since they indicate long-standing hypertension.

Diagnostic approach

The extent to which investigation of hypertension is justified depends on its severity and persistence, and the circumstances under which it is detected. The diagnostic strategy is clearly different for mild hypertension identified incidentally in an asymptomatic child and severe hypertension observed in a symptomatic patient. The investigation of the hypertensive child should reflect the relative frequencies of the diseases causing hypertension in children and should be as non-invasive as possible. In mild forms of persistent hypertension, the family history should be taken, together with a careful history on the use of drugs.

Table 9 Primary investigation of the child with moderate to severe forms of hypertension

Urinalysis (cells, protein)
Blood cell count
Serum chemistry (electrolytes, creatinine, urea, uric acid)
Plasma renin activity
Urinary catecholamine excretion (vanillylmandelic acid)
Abdominal ultrasound including Doppler sonography
^{99m}Tc-dimercaptosuccinic acid (static) scan of the kidney
Fundoscopy
Electrocardiography
Echocardiography (Chest radiography)

In moderate to severe forms of hypertension (>10–20 mmHg above the 95th percentile) the investigation should include urinalysis, blood-cell count, blood chemistry, abdominal ultrasonography, and some form of renal imaging (Table 9) (Recommendations for Management of Hypertension in Children and Adolescents 1986).

Apart from the routine biochemical profile, some measures of end-organ damage should be included. Two-dimensional echocardiography is more useful in identifying left ventricular hypertrophy and impaired left ventricular function than conventional radiographic examination of the heart. Bearing in mind the distribution frequency of secondary forms of hypertension (see Table 3), some form of renal imaging is mandatory and a combination of abdominal ultrasonography and [^{99m}Tc]dimercaptosuccinic acid static scanning is very useful. The latter method is a marker of renal parenchyma, the bound isotope reflecting the functioning proximal tubular mass, and is reportedly a very sensitive method for detecting segmental parenchymal scars (Merrick *et al.* 1980) and ischaemic areas due to renal vascular disease (Stringer *et al.* 1984). The [^{99m}Tc]dimercaptosuccinic acid scan also detects small or poorly functioning kidneys and provides information on differential renal function. The [^{99m}Tc]dimercaptosuccinic acid static scan is more sensitive than conventional intravenous urography, and requires less exposure to radiation (Fig. 6). The value of intravenous urography in the investigation of hypertension is limited in case of structural abnormalities. Voiding cystourethrography is only indicated if vesicoureteral reflux or obstructive uropathy are considered.

Abdominal ultrasonography detects tumours of the adrenal gland and the kidneys, and is also very valuable in the diagnosis of cystic renal diseases, renal calculi, dilatation of the collecting system, presence of a duplex system, ureterocele, and a thickened bladder wall. Since it does not show the degree of renal function it has to be combined with other forms of renal imaging. Colour-aided Doppler and duplex sonography have been occasionally used for vascular imaging in children with hypertension (Melter *et al.* 1992).

If any of the investigations mentioned above reveals an abnormality, or if hypertension is severe, further selected studies are indicated (Table 10). A dynamic scan of the kidney using [^{99}Tc^{m}]mercaptoacetyltriglycine ([^{99}Tc^{m}]MAG$_3$) scintigraphy gives information on renal function, glomerular filtration rate, renal transit time, and the collecting system. An additional scan following captopril administration (0.5–1.0 mg/kg orally) will show haemodynamically important

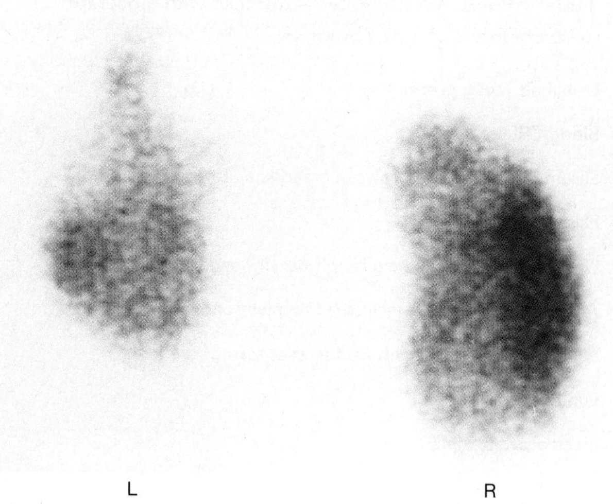

Fig. 6 [^{99m}Tc]dimercaptosuccinic acid static scan in a 10-year-old girl with vesicoureteric reflux demonstrating reduced isotope uptake in the upper pole of the left kidney indicating upper-pole scarring; a previous renal ultrasound examination looked normal.

Table 10 Supplementary investigation in the hypertensive child

In case of suspected renal aetiology
Glomerular filtration rate
Intravenous urography
Voiding cystourethrography
Colour-aided Doppler and duplex ultrasonography
[^{99}Tc^{m}]mercaptoacetyltriglycine (dynamic) scan of the kidney (under basic conditions and following captopril administration)
Renal angiography or digital substraction angiography
Renin sampling from renal veins and vena cava
Computed tomography (CT) scan
Renal biopsy
In case of suspected endocrine aetiology
Plasma catecholamines
If high:
^{123}I-m-iodobenzylguianidine (MIBG) scan
Vena cava sampling of catecholamines
Computed tomography (CT) scan
Angiography
Plasma aldosterone
If high:
Urine mineralocorticoids
Dexamethasone suppression
Adrenal scintigraphy
If low:
Urine mineralocorticoids
Other plasma mineralocorticoids
Cortisol response to ACTH or dexamethasone
In case of suspected cardiovascular aetiology
Echocardiography
Angiography or digital substraction angiography
Cardiac catheterization

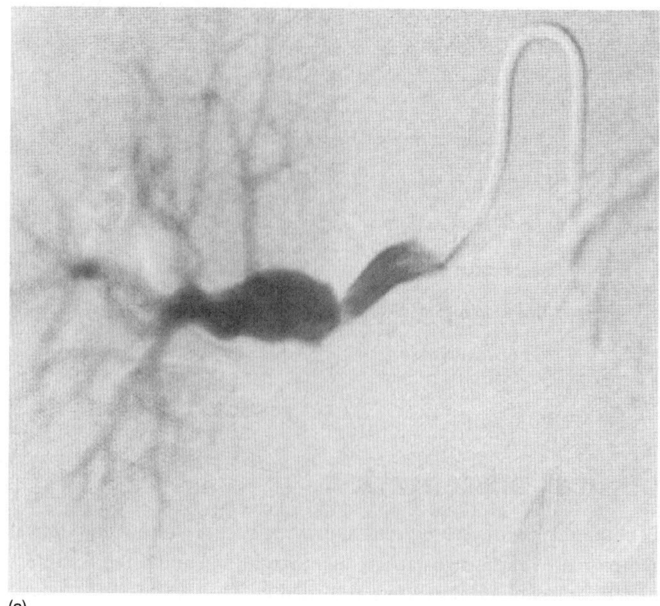

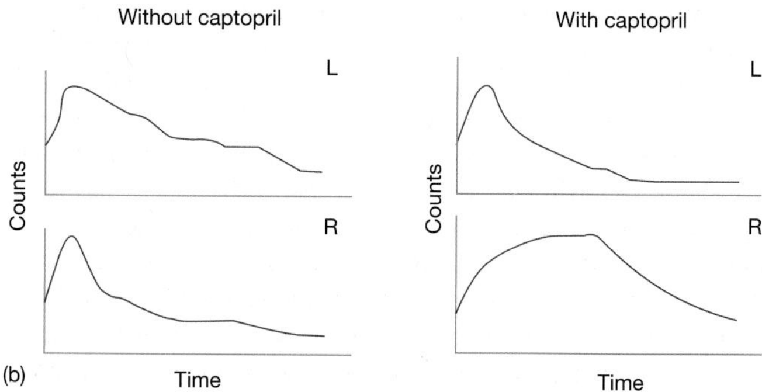

Fig. 7 (a) Selective digital-subtraction angiography in a 16-year-old boy who was successfully operated for renal arterial stenosis due to fibromuscular dysplasia 8 years ago. Hypertension developed again due to re-stenosis of the right renal artery. (b) Single-dose captopril scintigraphy (1 mg/kg 30 min before the second scan) revealed a haemodynamically significant stenosis of the renal artery as shown by the marked accumulation of the tracer ([^{123}I]hippuran) within the right kidney. Left : right ratio was 56 : 44 per cent before and 53 : 47 per cent afer captopril administration.

renovascular hypertension (Sfakianakis *et al.* 1987). Daman-Willems *et al.* (1989) have shown that the systolic and diastolic blood pressures after a single dose of captopril (0.7 mg/kg) were significantly correlated with initial plasma renin activity, and this might be a useful screening test for renin-dependent hypertension. In our hands, scintigraphy with captopril is most sensitive (Fig. 7).

Non-invasive studies (magnetic resonance angiography or three-dimensional computed tomography) are able to define the anatomy of the renal vasculature and may serve as screening method or will replace selective angiography for the diagnosis of renal artery stenosis in the future (Katayama *et al.* 2000; Leder and Nelson 2001).

Treatment of hypertension

The general management of hypertension in children includes non-pharmacological intervention, surgery, revascularization, and antihypertensive drugs. In primary hypertension, which is usually mild to moderate in adolescents, drug treatment should carefully be considered after non-pharmacological intervention has failed. Various interventions, such as reduction of dietary sodium chloride intake, reduction of body weight in obese children and adolescents, and dynamic exercises have been recommended (Recommendations for Management of Hypertension in Children and Adolescents 1986; Report of the Second Task Force on Blood Pressure Control in Children 1987; Rocchini *et al.* 1988, 1989; Beilin 1994). In adolescents, slightly increased blood pressure can be reduced by exercise and weight reduction, which are, therefore valuable therapeutic tools (Hagberg *et al.* 1984; Hofman *et al.* 1987). Although the therapeutic success of non-pharmacological intervention is so far not sufficiently established, this approach is recommended in mild forms of primary hypertension. Drug treatment is indicated if blood pressure continues to increase. Factors other than blood pressure that influence the decision to begin drug treatment include family history of early complications of hypertension (renal failure, stroke, heart disease), target-organ involvement (cardiac enlargement, left ventricular hypertrophy, retinal vascular changes), and the presence of other risk factors for coronary heart disease. There is no specific drug treatment for primary hypertension in children and adolescents: it follows the recommendations for secondary hypertension (see below).

Surgical treatment of coarctation of the aorta, tumours (e.g. phaeochromocytoma, neuroblastoma), and renovascular hypertension often lowers the blood pressure to normal. Revascularization procedures, such as percutaneous transluminal angioplasty for renovascular hypertension, have been successful in both children and adolescents (Chevalier *et al.* 1987). Various revascularization operations have been reported: direct reimplantation of the renal artery into the aorta, resection of the stenosed section of the renal artery with re-anastomosis of the remaining sections, aortorenal bypass, patch-extension angioplasty, and extracorporeal revascularization followed by autotransplantation of the kidney (Merguerian *et al.* 1990). Primary unilateral nephrectomy, formerly a routine procedure in renovascular hypertension of childhood, is rarely carried out today at specialized centres.

Surgical management is also possible in unilateral hydronephrosis, nephrolithiasis, and in rare cases of peripheral renal arterial stenosis or segmental renal scars where the blood pressure can occasionally be returned to normal by polar resection. Following surgery, it often takes weeks or months before the blood pressure becomes completely normal after discontinuation of antihypertensive therapy.

In the majority of children with renal hypertension, treatment is based on the long-term administration of antihypertensive drugs. As in adults, the number of pharmacological agents available for treating hypertension has been increased markedly within the last decade.

Antihypertensive agents in children

Pharmacological treatment of hypertension in children is based more on individual experience than on evidence based studies. Only few data on pharmacokinetics, dose finding, effectiveness, and safety of antihypertensive agents are available from prospective clinical trials in children and adolescents (Wells 1999). The primary reason for this is the lack of industry sponsored antihypertensive drugs trials in children. Since the prevalence of hypertension is low in that age group manufacturers had no incentive to do the trials. Furthermore, adequate dose recommendations based on careful dose finding studies are lacking as well as age-appropriate drug formulations. Some investigators initiated studies were performed as good examples with captopril and minoxidil more than 20 years ago (Sinaiko and Mirkin 1977; Mirkin and Newman 1985). Recent reports have reviewed the paediatric experience with various drugs (Sinaiko 1994; Wells 1999). Due to the FDA modernization act, an impetus was achieved to perform paediatric efficacy and safety data (Wells 1999). Dosages of antihypertensive agents in childhood based on personal and published experience (Table 11).

Diuretics

Paediatric experience has been reported with hydrochlorothiazide (Mirkin *et al.* 1977) and chlorthalidone (Bachmann 1984). Dosage for both drugs is 0.5–2 mg/kg per day. Chlorthalidone has a longer half-life and the dose interval is 24 or 48 h. Increasing the dose of thiazides affects blood pressure only marginally, but may be associated with increased incidence and severity of side-effects such as hypokalaemia, hyperuricaemia, impairment of glucose tolerance, and disturbances of lipid metabolism.

Loop diuretics such as frusemide are essential in children with advanced chronic renal failure; thiazides often are not effective. In contrast to the thiazide diuretics, frusemide induces calcium excretion and nephrocalcinosis has been reported with long-term treatment in preterm infants (Hufnagle *et al.* 1982).

Potassium-sparing diuretics (spironolactone, amiloride, triamterene) are only used occasionally to treat hypertension in children, always in combination with thiazides or frusemide to prevent hypokalaemia. They are strictly contraindicated in the presence of impaired renal function.

Table 11 Dosage of oral antihypertensive agents in childhood

	Dosage (mg/kg/day)	Interval (h)
Diuretics		
Hydrochlorothiazide	0.5–2	12–24
Chlorthalidone	0.5–2	24
Frusemide	1–5	8–12
Sympathetic inhibitors		
Propranolol	1–5	8–12
Atenolol[a]	1–3	24
Metoprolol	1–4	12
Clonidine	0.005–0.03	8–12
Methyldopa	10–40	8–12
Prazosin	0.02–0.5	8–12
Vasodilators		
Hydralazine	1–5	8–12
Minoxidil	0.01–0.5	12
Calcium antagonists		
Nifedipine	0.5–2	8–12[b]
Nitrendipine	0.5–1	12
Amlodipine	0.1–0.3	24
ACE inhibitors		
Captopril[a]	0.5–3	8–12
In newborns and small infants	0.1–0.5	8–12
Enalapril	0.1–0.4	24
Ramipril	1.5 mg/m^2	24

[a] Dose reduction in renal insufficiency.

[b] Retard preparation.

β-Adrenergic blockers

These are widely used to treat hypertension in children. Various studies have demonstrated that propranolol is effective and safe (Potter *et al.* 1977; Adelman 1978; Bachmann 1984). Doses up to 16 mg/kg per day are tolerated without significant side-effects. It is not clearly established whether an increase in dosage to more than 5 mg/kg per day has any further blood pressure-lowering effects, although this might be possible, since bioavailability varies between 20 and 50 per cent due to a high first-pass metabolism in the liver. The initial dose of propranolol is 1–2 mg/kg per day. Bradycardia and bronchoconstriction are side-effects reported in children.

Cardioselective β-adrenergic blockers have been recommended (Report of the Second Task Force on Blood Pressure Control in Children 1987). Atenolol is eliminated via the kidney and has a longer half-life than propranolol; a single morning dose is therefore sufficient (1–3 mg/kg per day). The dose has to be reduced in children with chronic renal failure. Metoprolol is metabolized within the liver and dose reduction during renal insufficiency is not required (1–4 mg/kg per day).

A fixed combination of the β-adrenergic blocker bisoprolol with the diuretic hydrochlorothiazide has recently been studied in a placebo controlled trial (Sorof *et al.* 2002). Blood pressure was reduced safely compared to placebo, but the large placebo effect and the failure of most subjects to reach the target blood pressure was not convincing.

Calcium antagonists

These are very useful in treating hypertensive emergencies in children. Over twenty-five years ago, Schärer *et al.* (1977) reported favourable effects of intravenous verapamil in children with renal hypertension. However, the cardiodepressive action of verapamil, particularly following intravenous application, had limited its use. Oral nifedipine has been shown to reduce blood pressure effectively and safely in paediatric hypertensive emergencies (Dilman *et al.* 1983; Rascher *et al.* 1986; Roth *et al.* 1986; Evans *et al.* 1988; Siegel and Brewer 1988; Blaszak *et al.* 2001). The dose used ranges between 0.3 and 0.5 mg/kg per day. Side-effects include headache, flush, and palpitations. Slow-release preparations of nifedipine are increasingly used as vasodilators to treat sustained renal hypertension in children in Germany, although this experience has not yet been reported in print. The dose used ranges between 0.5 and 2.0 mg/kg per day. Side-effects include gastrointestinal disturbances, constipation, oedema of the legs, and gingival hyperplasia, possibly due to an interaction with cyclosporin (Bökenkamp *et al.* 1994).

Recently, other long-acting calcium antagonists has been studied in children (Flynn and Pasko 2000). Oral nitrendipine was found to be effective and safe in children (Wells and Sinaiko 1991) as was shown for amlodipine (Pfammatter *et al.* 1998; Tallian *et al.* 1999; Flynn *et al.* 2000; Rogan *et al.* 2000).

Angiotensin converting enzyme inhibitors

The angiotensin-converting enzyme (ACE) inhibitor captopril was often used in children with severe renal hypertension (Friedman *et al.* 1980; Sinaiko *et al.* 1983; Mirkin and Newman 1985; Bouisson *et al.* 1986; Callis *et al.* 1986). It is of major interest that newborns and smaller infants require substantially lower doses per unit body surface than older infants and children for the control of hypertension (Sinaiko *et al.* 1986; O'Dea *et al.* 1988).

Cerebral and renal complications have been reported in newborns and small infants; these occur if the initial dose is too high (Tack and Perlman 1988; Perlman and Volpe 1989). In order to prevent a rapid decrease in blood pressure following the first dose of captopril, a low dose of 0.2 mg/kg (in newborns 0.05 mg/kg) should be given. If this dose is tolerated, the dose can be increased rapidly, to 1–2 mg/kg per day if necessary. Long-term treatment should not exceed 2–3 mg/kg per day, or 150 mg in adolescents, and the dose has to be reduced in children with renal insufficiency (Sinaiko *et al.* 1983).

Side-effects of captopril include skin rashes, taste disturbances, cough, and neutropenia. The last occurs between the third and twelfth week of treatment in patients with autoimmune disease and/or renal insufficiency, and regular blood counts should be done in these patients. Reported renal side-effects include proteinuria, membranous glomerulopathy, and haemodynamically mediated acute renal failure. The last occurs in patients with stenosis of both renal arteries or unilateral stenosis in a single kidney (e.g. after renal transplantation). This side-effect is reversible after discontinuation of the drug.

Enalapril is a pro-drug that must be metabolically converted to enalaprilat. Peak serum concentration occurred at 3–4 h after oral administration. The longer plasma half-life of 12 h might be an advantage to improve compliance in adolescents. Since enalapril is excreted by the kidneys, dosage should be reduced in patients with renal failure. As with captopril, approximately one-third of enalaprilat is cleared during haemodialysis. Experiences with the ACE inhibitor enalapril in children with renal hypertension have been reported (Miller *et al.* 1986) and recently pharmacokinetics of enalapril in children (Wells *et al.* 2001). Pharmocokinetics of enalapril in hypertensive infants aged 2 month up to adolescents aged 15 years was similar to values reported in healthy adults. Ramipril has also been used in children (Soergel *et al.* 2000).

Vasodilators

Hydralazine has frequently been used as a vasodilator. The recommended doses for children vary considerably: in adults 1–3 mg/kg per day are used; whilst in newborns, doses up to 9 mg/kg per day have been tolerated (Adelman 1978).

Minoxidil has been studied extensively in children (Makker 1975; Pennisi *et al.* 1977; Sinaiko and Mirkin 1977). It induces tachycardia and important salt and water retention, and side-effects, together with the hypertrichosis that may also occur, have limited its use.

Sympathetic blockers

Clonidine and α-methyldopa lower sympathetic outflow via central α_2-adrenergic stimulation. An important unwanted side-effect is centrally induced sedation. Clonidine and α-methyldopa are used if β-blockers are contraindicated.

This α_1-adrenergic blocker prazosin does not affect presynaptic α_1-receptors, as do phentolamine and phenoxybenzamine. Prazosin does not induce significant reflex tachycardia or renin release, but may have a profound first dose effect. It is used occasionally in children, but systematic studies are lacking.

Intravenous administered labetalol, an α_1- and β-adrenergic blocker, is able to control hypertension in hypertensive emergencies (Bunchman *et al.* 1992).

Approach to the treatment of children with antihypertensive agents

The management of children with chronically elevated blood pressure starts with low doses of a given drug and slowly reaching therapeutically effective levels. Treatment can be started with β-adrenergic-blocking drugs, with diuretic agents, with calcium antagonists or with ACE

Table 12 Drug treatment of hypertensive emergencies in childhood

Drug	Dose (mg/kg)	Application
Nifedipine	0.25–0.5	Oral
Nicardipine	0.3–3.0 (μg/kg/min)	Intravenous infusion
Clonidine	0.003–0.006	Subcutaneous Intramuscular, slowly IV
Labetalol	1–3	IV injection
Diazoxide	2.0–6.0	IV injection, start with low dose
Hydralazine	0.2–0.8	IV, intramuscular
Sodium nitroprusside	0.5–10.0 (μg/kg/min)	Intensive care unit

inhibitors. Very high-dose monotherapy should be avoided because of side-effects and a combination of two or more antihypertensive drugs should be used initially. The dosage of oral antihypertensive agents used in children is shown in Table 11. Hypertensive emergencies, particularly frequent in children with renal diseases, require immediate therapy (Deal *et al.* 1992a). In hypertensive emergencies (Table 12) with clinical signs of hypertensive encephalopathy or of pulmonary oedema, oral nifedipine at a dose of 0.3–0.5 mg/kg is the treatment of choice. If there is insufficient response within 15 min, the dose can be repeated. Lower doses of nifedipine are often sufficient if acute elevation of blood pressure occurs without clinical symptoms.

Alternatively, intravenous nicardipine has been studied in acute hypertensive emergencies and found to be effective and safe (Treluyer *et al.* 1993; Flynn *et al.* 2001). Doses range between 0.3 and 4 μg/kg per min with a mean dose of 1.8 μg/kg per min (Flynn *et al.* 2001).

Marked tachycardia may occur, which points to sympathetic stimulation, and therefore clonidine in a dose of 3–6 μg/kg is indicated, given either subcutaneously, intramuscularly, or slowly intravenously. The use of diazoxide (2–6 mg/kg) is established in childhood hypertension (Kohout *et al.* 1975), but no longer recommended as a first-line drug, since bolus injection may be associated with a precipitous reduction in blood pressure to hypotensive levels (Deal *et al.* 1992a). In states of fluid retention, frusemide (2–7 mg/kg IV) should be combined. If there is no satisfactory response to the drugs discussed above, sodium nitroprusside should be administered as a continuous infusion with the patient under constant surveillance (Gordillo-Paniagua *et al.* 1975). The infusion rate must be continuously adjusted to the changes in blood pressure. Thiocyanate levels should be monitored (Table 12).

References

Adelman, R. D. (1978). Neonatal hypertension. *Pediatric Clinics of North America* **25**, 99–110.

Adrogue, H. E. and Sinaiko, A. R. (2001). Prevalence of hypertension in junior high school-aged children: effect of new recommendations in the 1996 Updated Task Force Report. *American Journal of Hypertension* **14**, 412–414.

Alvestrand, A., Bergstroem, J., and Wehle, B. (1977). Pheochromocytoma and renovascular hypertension. A case report and review of the literature. *Acta Medica Scandinavica* **202**, 231–236.

Andersen, H. J., Jacobsson, B., Larsson, H., and Winberg, J. (1973). Hypertension, asymmetric renal parenchymal defect, sterile urine, and high *E. coli* antibody titre. *British Medical Journal* **2**, 14–18.

André, J. L., Fossati, A., Pierson, M., Neimann, N., Pernot, C., and Prévot, J. (1980). Nouveaux concepts sur l'etiologie de l'hypertensionartérielle de l'enfants. A propos de 68 observations recueilles en milieu hospitalier. *Médecine et Hygiène* **38**, 582–586.

Arar, M. Y., Hogg, R. J., Arant, B. S., and Seikaly, M. G. (1994). Etiology of sustained hypertension in children in the southwestern United States. *Pediatric Nephrology* **8**, 186–189.

Ask-Upmark, E. (1929). Über juvenile maligne Nephrosklerose und ihr Verhältnis zur Störung der Nierenentwicklung. *Acta Pathologica Microbiologica Scandinavica* **7**, 383–445.

Bachmann, H. (1984). Propranolol vs chlorthalidone—a prospective therapeutic trial in children with chronic hypertension. *Helvetia Paediatrica Acta* **39**, 55–61.

Bald, M., Kubel, S., and Rascher, W. (1994). Validity and reliability of 24 h blood pressure monitoring in children and adolescents using a portable, oscillometric device. *Journal of Human Hypertension* **8**, 363–366.

Bald, M., Lettgen, B., Wingen, A. M., and Bonzel, K. E. (1996). 24-Hour blood pressure monitoring in children and adolescents after recovery from hemolytic uremic syndrome. *Clinical Nephrology* **46**, 50–53.

Baluarte, H. J., Gruskin, A. B., Ingelfinger, J. R., Stablein, D., and Tejani, D. A. (1994). Analysis of hypertension in children post renal transplantation—a report of the North American Pediatric Renal Transplant Cooperative Study (NAPRTCS). *Pediatric Nephrology* **8**, 570–573.

Beilin, L. J. (1994). Non-pharmacological management of hypertension: optimal strategies for reducing cardiovascular risk. *Journal of Hypertension* **12** (Suppl. 10), S71–S81.

Biron, P. and Mongeau, J. G. (1978). Familial aggregation of blood pressure and its components. *Pediatric Clinics of North America* **25**, 29–33.

Blaszak, R. T., Savage, J. A., and Ellis, E. N. (2001). The use of short-acting nifedipine in pediatric patients with hypertension. *Journal of Pediatrics* **139**, 34–37.

Bökenkamp, A., Bohnhorst, B., Beier, C., Albers, N., Offner, G., and Brodehl, J. (1994). Nifedipine aggravates cyclosporine A-induced gingival hyperplasia. *Pediatric Nephrology* **8**, 181–185.

Bouisson, F., Meguira, B., Rostin, M., Fontaine, C., Charlet, J. P., and Barthe, P. H. (1986). Long-term treatment by captopril in children with renal hypertension. *Clinical and Experimental Hypertension* **A8**, 841–845.

Broyer, M., Bacri, J. L., and Royer, P. Renal forms of hypertension in children: report on 238 cases. In *Hypertension in Children and Adolescents* (ed. G. Giovannelli, M. I. New, and S. Gorini), pp. 201–208. New York: Raven, 1981.

Broyer, M., Guest, G., Gagnadoux, M. F., and Beurton, D. (1987). Hypertension following renal transplantation in children. *Pediatric Nephrology* **1**, 16–21.

Bunchman, T. E., Lynch, R. E., and Wood, E. G. (1992). Intravenously administered labetalol for treatment of hypertension in children. *Journal of Pediatrics* **120**, 140–144.

Callis, L., Vila, A., Catala, J., and Gras, X. (1986). Long-term treatment with captopril in pediatric patients with severe hypertension and chronic renal failure. *Clinical and Experimental Hypertension* **A8**, 847–851.

Chevalier, R. L., Tegtmeier, J., and Gomez, R. A., (1987). Percutaneous transluminal angioplasty for renovascular hypertension in children. *Pediatric Nephrology* **1**, 16–21.

Colan, S. D., Fujii, A., Borow, K. M., MacPherson, D., and Sanders, S. P. (1983). Noninvasive determination of systolic, diastolic and end-systolic blood pressure in neonates, infants and young children: comparison with central aortic pressure measurements. *American Journal of Cardiology* **52**, 867–870.

Cresenta, J. L. and Burke, G. L. Determinants of blood pressure levels in children and adolescents. In *Causation of Cardiovascular Risk Factors in Children* (ed. G. S. Berenson), pp. 157–189. New York: Raven, 1986.

Daman-Willems, C. E., Shah, V., Uchiyama, M., and Dillon, M. J. (1989). The captopril test: an aid to investigation of hypertension. *Archives of Disease in Childhood* **64**, 229–234.

Deal, J. E., Barratt, T. M., and Dillon, M. J. (1992a). Management of hypertensive emergencies. *Archives of Disease in Childhood* **67**, 1089–1092.

Deal, J. E., Snell, M. F., Barratt, T. M., and Dillon, M. J. (1992b). Renovascular disease in childhood. *Journal of Pediatrics* **121**, 378–384.

De Man, S. A. *et al.* (1991). Blood pressure in childhood: pooled findings of six European studies. *Journal of Hypertension* **9**, 109–114.

De Swiet, M., Fayers, P., and Shinebourne, E. A. (1976). Blood pressure survey in a population of newborn infants. *British Medical Journal* **ii**, 9–11.

Dillon, M. J. Clinical aspects of hypertension. In *Pediatric Nephrology* 2nd edn. (ed. M. A. Holliday, T. M. Barrat, and R. L. Vernier), pp. 743–757. Baltimore: Williams and Wilkins, 1987.

Dillon, M. J. and Smellie, J. M. Peripheral plasma renin activity, hypertension and renal scarring in children. In *Contribution to Nephrology, Reflux Nephropathy Update: 1983* (ed. C. J. Hodson, R. H. Heptinstall, and J. Winberg), pp. 68–80. Basel: Karger, 1984.

Dillon, M. J., Shah, V., and Barratt, T. M. (1978). Renal vein renin measurement in children with hypertension. *British Medical Journal* **ii**, 168–170.

Dilman, U., Caglar, M. K., Senses, D. A., and Kinik, E. (1983). Nifedipine in hypertensive emergencies of children. *American Journal of Diseases of Children* **137**, 1162–1165.

Diprose, G. K., Evans, D. H., Archer, L. N. J., and Levene, M. I. (1986). Dinamap fails to detect hypotension in very low birthweight infants. *Archives of Disease in Childhood* **61**, 771–773.

Dluhy, R. G., Anderson, B., Harlin, B., Ingelfinger, J., and Lifton, R. (2001). Glucocorticoid-remediable aldosteronism is associated with severe hypertension in early childhood. *Journal of Pediatrics* **138**, 715–720.

Eden, O. B., Sills, J. A., and Brown, J. K. (1977). Hypertension in acute neurological disease in childhood. *Developmental Medicine and Child Neurology* **19**, 437–445.

Emery, E. F. and Greenough, A. (1992). Non-invasive blood pressure monitoring in preterm infants receiving intensive care. *European Journal of Pediatrics* **151**, 136–139.

Estepa, R., Gallego, N., Orte, L., Puras, E., Aracil, E., and Ortuno, J. (2001). Renovascular hypertension in children. *Scandinavian Journal of Urology and Nephrology* **35**, 388–392.

Evans, J. H. C., Shaw, N. J., and Brocklebank, J. T. (1988). Sublingual nifedipine in acute severe hypertension. *Archives of Disease in Childhood* **63**, 975–977.

Flynn, J. T. and Pasko, D. A. (2000). Calcium channel blockers: pharmacology and place in therapy of pediatric hypertension. *Pediatric Nephrology* **15**, 302–316.

Flynn, J. T., Mottes, T. A., Brophy, P. D., Kershaw, D. B., Smoyer, W. E., and Bunchman, T. E. (2001). Intravenous nicardipine for treatment of severe hypertension in children. *Journal of Pediatrics* **139**, 38–43.

Flynn, J. T., Smoyer, W. E., and Bunchman, T. E. (2000). Treatment of hypertensive children with amlodipine. *American Journal of Hypertension* **13**, 1061–1066.

Fossali, E., Signorini, E., Intermite, R. C., Canalini, E., Lo varia, A., Maninetti, M. M., and Rossi, L. N. (2000). Renovascular disease and hypertension in children with neurofibromatosis. *Pediatric Nephrology* **14**, 804–810.

Friedman, A., Chesney, R., Ball, D., and Goodfriend, T. (1980). Effective use of captopril in severe childhood hypertension. *Journal of Pediatrics* **97**, 664–667.

Friesen, R. H. and Lichtor, J. L. (1981). Indirect measurement of blood pressure in neonates and infants utilizing an automatic noninvasive oscillometric monitor. *Anesthesia and Analgesia* **60**, 742–745.

Fuentes, R. M., Notkola, I.-L., Shemeikka, S., Tuomilehto, J., and Nissinen, A. (2002). Tracking of systolic blood pressure during childhood: a 15-year follow-up population based family study in eastern Finland. *Journal of Hypertension* **20**, 195–202.

Ganguly, A., Gribble, J., Tune, B., Kempson, R. L., and Luetscher, J. A. (1973). Renin-secreting Wilms' tumor with severe hypertension. Report of a case and brief review of renin-secreting tumors. *Annals of Internal Medicine* **79**, 835–837.

Gill, D. G., Mendes da Costa, B., Cameron, J. S., Joseph, M. C., Ogg, C. S., and Chantler, C. (1976). Analysis of 100 children with severe and persistent hypertension. *Archives of Disease in Childhood* **51**, 951–956.

Godard, C., Vallotton, M. B., and Broyer, M. (1973). Plasma renin activity in segmental hypoplasia of the kidneys with hypertension. *Nephron* **11**, 307–317.

Gómez-Marín, O., Prineas, R. J., and Rastam, L. (1992). Cuff bladder width and blood pressure in children and adolescents. *Journal of Hypertension* **10**, 1235–1241.

Gordillo-Paniagua, G., Velásquez-Jones, L., Martini, R., and Valdez-Bolanos, E. (1975). Sodium nitroprusside treatment of severe arterial hypertension in children. *Journal of Pediatrics* **87**, 799–802.

Greenough, A., Emery, E. F., and Gamsu, H. R. (1992). Dexamethasone and hypertension in preterm infants. *European Journal of Pediatrics* **151**, 134–135.

Habib, R., Courtecuisse, V., Ehrensperger, J., and Royer, P. (1965). Hypoplasie segmentaire du rein avec hypertension artérielle chez l'enfant. *Annales de Pédiatrie* **41**, 262–279.

Hagberg, J. M., Ehsani, A. A., Goldring, D., Hernandez, A., Sinacore, D. R., and Holloszy, J. O. (1984). Effect of weight training on blood pressure and haemodynamics in hypertensive adolescents. *Journal of Pediatrics* **104**, 147–151.

Hansson, J. H., Nelson-Williams, C., Suzuki, H., Schild, L., Shimkets, R., Lu, Y., Canessa, C., Iwasaki, T., Rossier, B., and Lifton, R. P. (1995). Hypertension caused by a truncated epithelial sodium channel gamma subunit: genetic heterogeneity of Liddle syndrome. *Nature Genetics* **11**, 76–82.

Heij, H. A., Ekkelkamp, S., and Vos, A. (1992). Hypertension associated with skeletal traction in children. *European Journal of Pediatrics* **151**, 543–545.

Hennekens, C. H., Jesse, M. J., Klein, B. E., Gourley, J. A., and Blumenthal, S. (1976). Aggregation of blood pressure in infants and their siblings. *American Journal of Epidemiology* **103**, 457–463.

Hofman, A., Walter, H. J., Connelly, P. A., and Vaughan, R. D. (1987). Blood pressure and physical fitness in children. *Hypertension* **9**, 188–191.

Holland, N. H., Kotchen, T., and Bhathena, D. (1975). Hypertension in children with chronic pyelonephritis. *Kidney International* **8** (Suppl. 5), 243–251.

Hornsby, J. L., Mongan, P. F., Taylor, T., and Treiber, F. A. (1991). *Journal of Family Practice* **33**, 617–623.

Hufnagle, K. G., Khan, S. N., Penn, D., Cacciarelli, A., and Williams, P. (1982). Renal calcifications: a complication of long-term furosemide therapy in preterm infants. *Pediatrics* **70**, 360–363.

Ingelfinger, J. R. Hypertension in children with ESRD. In *End Stage Renal Disease in Children* (ed. R. N. Fine and A. B. Gruskin), pp. 340–358. Philadelphia: Saunders, 1984.

International Study of Kidney Disease in Children (1981). Primary nephrotic syndrome in children: clinical significance of histopathologic variants of minimal change and of diffuse mesangial hypercellularity. *Kidney International* **20**, 765–771.

Jacoby, A. C., Fixler, D. E., and Torres, E. J. (1993). Limitations of an oscillometric ambulatory blood pressure monitor in physically active children. *Journal of Pediatrics* **122**, 321–326.

Jansen, H. and Scholtmeijer, R. J. (1990). Results of surgical treatment of severe vesicoureteric reflux grades 4 and 5. *British Journal of Urology* **65**, 413–417.

Jansen, J. N., Donker, A. J. M., Luth, W. J., and Smit, L. M. E. (1990). Moyamoya disease associated with renovascular hypertension. *Neuropediatrics* **21**, 44–47.

Kaiser, A. M. and Whitelaw, A. G. L. (1988). Hypertensive response to raised intracranial pressure in infancy. *Archives of Disease in Childhood* **63**, 1461–1465.

Katayama, H., Shimizu, T., Tanaka, Y., Narabayashi, I., and Tamai, H. (2000). Three-dimensional magnetic resonance angiography of vascular lesions in children. *Heart and Vessels* **15**, 1–6.

Kitterman, J. A., Phibbs, P. H., and Tooley, W. H. (1969). Aortic blood pressure in normal newborn infants during the first 12 h of life. *Pediatrics* **44**, 959–968.

Kohout, E. C., Wilson, C. J., and Leighton, L. (1975). Intravenous diazoxide in acute poststreptococcal glomerulonephritis. *Journal of Pediatrics* **87**, 795–798.

Kotchen, J. M. and Kotchen, T. A. (1978). Geographic effect of racial blood pressure differences in adolescents. *Journal of Chronic Diseases* **31**, 581–586.

Krmar, R. T., Ferraris, J. R., Ramirez, J. A., Ruiz, S., Salomon, A., Galvez, H. M., Janson, J. J., Galarza, C. R., and Waisman, G. (2001). Ambulatory blood pressure monitoring after recovery from hemolytic uremic syndrome. *Pediatric Nephrology* **16**, 812–816.

Küster, S., Mehls, O., Seidel, C., and Ritz, E. (1990). Blood pressure in minimal change and other types of nephrotic syndrome. *American Journal of Nephrology* **10** (Suppl. 1), 76–80.

Labarthe, D. R. (1986). Epidemiology of primary hypertension in the young. *Clinical and Experimental Hypertension* **A8**, 495–513.

Lambrechtsen, J., Rasmussen, F., Hansen, H. S., and Jacobsen, I. A. (1998). Ambulatory blood pressure in 570 Danes aged 19–21 years: the Odense Schoolchild Study. *Journal of Human Hypertension* 12, 755–760.

Lauer, M. R., Mohoney, L. T., and Clarke, W. R. (1986). Tracking of blood pressure during childhood: the Muscatine study. *Clinical and Experimental Hypertension* **A8**, 515–537.

Leder, R. A. and Nelson, R. C. (2001). Three-dimensional CT of the genitourinary tract. *Journal of Endourolology* **15**, 37–46.

Lee, Y., Rosner, B., and Gould, J. B. (1976). Familial aggregation of blood pressure of newborn infants and their mothers. *Pediatrics* **58**, 722–729.

Leumann, E. P. (1979). Blood pressure and hypertension in childhood and adolescence. *Ergebnisse Innere Medizin und Kinderheilkunde* **43**, 109–183.

Lifton, R. P. *et al.* (1992). Hereditary hypertension caused by chimaeric gene duplication and ectopic expression of aldosterone synthase. *Nature Genetics* **2**, 66–74.

Lingens, N., Soergel, M., Loirat, C., Busch, C., Lemmer, B., and Schärer, K. (1995). Ambulatory blood pressure monitoring in paediatric patients treated by regular hemodialysis and peritoneal dialysis. *Paediatric Nephrology* **9**, 167–172.

Loirat, C., Azancot-Benisty, A., Bossu, C., and Durant, I. (1991). Value of ambulatory blood pressure monitoring in borderline hypertension in the child. *Annales Pédiatrie (Paris)* **38**, 381–386.

Loirat, C., Pillion, G., and Blum, C. (1982). Hypertension in Children. *Advances in Nephrology* **11**, 65–98.

Luepker, R. V., Jacobs, D. R., Prineas, R. J., and Sinaiko, A. R. (1996). Secular trends of blood pressure and body size in a multi-ethnic adolescent population. *Journal of Pediatrics* **134**, 667–674.

Lurbe, E. and Redon, J. (2002). Reproducibility and validity of ambulatory blood pressure monitoring in children. *American Journal of Hypertension* **15**, 69S–73S.

McLaughlin, G. W., Kirby, R. R., Kemmerer, W. T., and deLemos, R. A. (1971). Indirect measurement of blood pressure in infants utilizing Doppler ultrasound. *Journal of Pediatrics* **79**, 300–303.

Makker, S. P. (1975). Minoxidil in refractory hypertension. *Journal of Pediatrics* **86**, 621–623.

Malekzadeh, M., Gruskin, C. M., Stanley, P., Brennan, L. P., Stiles, Q. R., and Lieberman, E. (1987). Renal artery stenosis in pediatric transplant recipients. *Pediatric Nephrology* **1**, 22–29.

McVicar, M., Carman, C., Chandra, M., Abbi, R. J., Teichberg, S., and Kahn, E. (1993). Hypertension secondary to a renin-secreting juxtaglomerular cell tumor: case report and review of 38 cases. *Pediatric Nephrology* **7**, 404–412.

Melter, M., Hoyer, P. F., Kotzerke, J., Schafer, C., and Brodehl, J. (1992). Unilaterale Nierenarterienstenose. Farbkodierte Doppler-Sonography und Captopril Szintigrapie bei einer 13-jährigen Patientin. *Monatsschrift Kinderheilkunde* **140**, 166–170.

Merguerian, P. A., McLorie, G. A., Balfe, J. W., Khoury, A. E., and Churchill, B. M. (1990). Renal autotransplantation in children: a successful treatment for renovascular hypertension. *Journal of Urology* **144**, 1443–1445.

Merrick, M. V., Uttley, W. S., and Wild, S. R. (1980). The detection of pyelonephritic scarring in children by radioisotope imaging. *British Journal of Radiology* **53**, 544–556.

Menschik, D., Lovvorn, H., Hill, A., Kelly, P., and Jones, D. P. (2002). An unusual etiology of hypertension in a 5-year-old boy. *Pediatric Nephrology* **17**, 524–526.

Middeke, M. and Schrader, J. (1994). Nocturnal blood pressure in normotensive subjects and those with white coat, primary and secondary hypertension. *British Medical Journal* **308**, 630–632.

Miller, K., Atkin, B., Rodel, P. V., and Walker, J. F. (1986). Enalapril: a well-tolerated and efficacious agent for the paediatric hypertensive patient. *Journal of Hypertension* **4** (Suppl. 5), 413–416.

Mirkin, B. L. and Newman, T. J. (1985). Efficacy and safety of captopril in the treatment of severe childhood hypertension. Report of the International Collaborative Study Group. *Pediatrics* **75**, 1091–1100.

Mirkin, B. L., Sinaiko, A. R., Cooper, M., and Anders, M. (1977). Hydrochlorothiazide therapy in hypertensive and renal insufficient children: elimination kinetics and metabolic effects. *Pediatric Research* **11**, 418.

Mongeau, J. G. (1987). Heredity and blood pressure in humans: an overview. *Pediatric Nephrology* **1**, 69–75.

Müller-Wiefel, D. E. (1978). Renovaskuläre Hypertension bei Neurofibromatose von Recklinghausen. *Monatsschrift Kinderheilkunde* **126**, 113–118.

Munger, R. G., Prineas, R. J., and Gomez-Marin, O. (1988). Persistent elevation of blood pressure among children with a family history of hypertension: the Minneapolis children's blood pressure study. *Journal of Hypertension* **6**, 647–653.

Nathwani, N. C., Unwin, R., Brook, C. G., and Hindmarsh, P. C. (2000a). The influence of renal and cardiovascular abnormalities on blood pressure in Turner syndrome. *Clinical Endocrinology* **52**, 371–377.

Nathwani, N. C., Unwin, R., Brook, C. G., and Hindmarsh, P. C. (2000b). Blood pressure and Turner syndrome. *Clinical Endocrinology* **52**, 363–370.

O'Dea, R. F., Mirkin, B. L., Alward, C. T., and Sinaiko, A. R. (1988). Treatment of neonatal hypertension with captopril. *Journal of Pediatrics* **113**, 403–406.

Park, M. K. and Menard, S. M. (1989). Normative blood pressure values in the first years in an office setting. *American Journal of Diseases of Children* **143**, 860–864.

Pelligrini-Caliumi, G., Agostino, R., Nodari, S., Maffei, G., Moretti, C., and Bucci, G. (1982). Evaluation of an automatic oscillometric method and of various cuffs for the measurement of arterial blood pressure in the neonates. *Acta Paediatrica Scandinavica* **71**, 791–797.

Pennisi, A. J. *et al.* (1977). Minoxidil therapy in children with severe hypertension. *Journal of Pediatrics* **90**, 813–819.

Perlman, J. M. and Volpe, J. J. (1989). Neurologic complications of captopril treatment of neonatal hypertension. *Pediatrics* **83**, 47–52.

Pfammatter, J. P., Clericetti-Affolter, C., Truttmann, A. C., Busch, K., Laux-End, R., and Bianchetti, M. G. (1998). Amlodipine once-daily in systemic hypertension. *European Journal of Pediatrics* **157**, 618–621.

Portman, R. J. and Yetman, R. J. (1994). Clinical use of ambulatory blood pressure monitoring. *Pediatric Nephrology* **8**, 367–376.

Potter, D. E., Schambelan, M., Salvatierra, O., Orloff, S., and Holliday, M. (1977). Treatment of high-renin hypertension with propranolol in children after renal transplantation. *Journal of Pediatrics* **90**, 307–311.

Proesmans, W. (1982). Syndrome de Klippel–Trenaunay avec hypertension artérielle et insuffisance rénale chronique. *Annales de Pédiatrie* **29**, 671–674.

Rames, L. K., Clarke, W. R., Connor, W. F., Reiter, M. A., and Lauer, R. M. (1979). Normal blood pressure and the evaluation of sustained blood pressure elevation in childhood. The Muscatine study. *Pediatrics* **61**, 245–251.

Rascher, W. and Tulassay, T. (1987). Hormonal water regulation in children with nephrotic syndrome. *Kidney International* **32** (Suppl. 21), 83–89.

Rascher, W., Bonzel, K.-E., Ruder, H., Müller-Wiefel, D. E., and Schärer, K. (1986). Blood pressure and hormonal responses to sublingual nifedipine in acute childhood hypertension. *Clinical and Experimental Hypertension* **A8**, 859–869.

Ravogli, A. *et al.* (1990). Early 24-hour blood pressure elevation in normotensive subjects with parental hypertension. *Hypertension* **16**, 491–497.

Recommendations for Management of Hypertension in Children and Adolescents (1986). *Clinical and Experimental Hypertension* **A8**, 901–918.

Report of the Second Task Force on Blood Pressure Control in Children (1987). *Pediatrics* **79**, 1–25.

Rocchini, A. P., Key, J., Bondie, D., Chico, R., Moorehead, C., Katch, V., and Martin, M. (1989). The effect of weight loss on the sensitivity of blood pressure to sodium in obese adolescents. *New England Journal of Medicine* **321**, 580–585.

Rocchini, A. P. *et al.* (1988). Blood pressure in obese adolescents: effect of weight loss. *Pediatrics* 82, 16–23.

Rogan, J. W., Lyszkiewicz, D. A., Blowey, D., Khattak, S., Arbus, G. S., and Koren, G. (2000). A randomized prospective crossover trial of amlodipine in pediatric hypertension. *Pediatric Nephrology* **14**, 1083–1087.

Rosner, B., Prineas, R. J., Loggie, J. M. H., and Daniels, S. R. (1993). Blood pressure nomograms for children and adolescents, by height, sex, and age. *Journal of Pediatrics* **123**, 871–886.

Roth, B., Herkenrath, P., Krebber, J., and Abu-Chaaban, M. (1986). Nifedipine in hypertensive crisis of infants and children. *Clinical and Experimental Hypertension* **A8**, 871–877.

Royer, P., Habib, R., Broyer, M., and Nouaille, Y. (1971). L'hypoplasie segmentaire du rein chez l'enfant. *Actualités Nephrologiques de l'Hopital Necker* **11**, 151–165.

Savage, J. M., Dillon, M. J., Shah, V., Barratt, T. M., and Williams, D. I. (1978). Renin and blood pressure in children with renal scarring and vesicoureteric reflux. *Lancet* **ii**, 441–444.

Schärer, K., Alatas, H., and Bein, G. (1977). Die Behandlung der renalen Hypertension mit Verapamil intramuscular Kindesalter. *Monatsschrift Kinderheilkunde* **125**, 706–712.

Schärer, K., Benninger, C., Heimann, A., and Rascher, W. (1993). Involvement of the central nervous system in renal hypertension. *European Journal of Pediatrics* **152**, 59–63.

Sfakianakis, G. N., Bourgoigne, J. J., Jaffee, D., Kyriakides, G., Perez-Stable, F., and Duncan, R. C. (1987). Single dose captopril scintigraphy in the diagnosis of renovascular hypertension. *Journal of Nuclear Medicine* **28**, 1383–1392.

Sheth, K. J., Tang, T. T., Blaedel, M. E., and Good, T. A. (1978). Polydipsia, polyuria, and hypertension associated with renin-secreting Wilms tumor. *Journal of Pediatrics* **92**, 921–924.

Siegel, R. L. and Brewer, E. D. (1988). Effect of sublingual or oral nifedipine in the treatment of hypertension. *Journal of Pediatrics* **112**, 811–813.

Siegler, R. L. (1976). Renin-dependent hypertension in children with reflux nephropathy. *Urology* **7**, 474–478.

Sinaiko, A. R. (1994). Treatment of hypertension in children. *Pediatric Nephrology* **8**, 603–609.

Sinaiko, A. R. and Mirkin, B. L. (1977). Management of severe childhood hypertension with minoxidil: a controlled clinical study. *Journal of Pediatrics* **91**, 138–142.

Sinaiko, A. R., Donahue, R. P., Jacobs, D. R., Jr., and Prineas, R. J. (1999). Relation of weight and rate of increase in weight during childhood and adolescence to body size, blood pressure, fasting insulin, and lipids in young adults: the Minneapolis children's blood pressure study. *Circulation* **99**, 1471–1476.

Sinaiko, A. R., Kashtan, C. E., and Mirkin, B. L. (1986). Antihypertensive drug therapy with captopril in children and adolescents. *Clinical and Experimental Hypertension* **A8**, 829–839.

Sinaiko, A. R., Mirkin, B. L., Hendrick, D. A., Green, T. P., and O'Dea, R. F. (1983). Antihypertensive effect and elimination kinetics of captopril in hypertensive children with renal disease. *Journal of Pediatrics* **103**, 799–805.

Skimkets, R. A. *et al.* (1994). Liddle's syndrome: heritable human hypertension caused by mutations in the beta subunit of the epithelial sodium channel. *Cell* **79**, 407–414.

Smellie, J. M. and Normand, I. C. S. (1975). Bacteriuria, reflux and renal scarring. *Archives of Disease in Childhood* **50**, 581–585.

Soergel, M., Kirschstein, M., Busch, C., Danne, T., Gellermann, J., Holl, R., Krull, F., Reichert, H., Reusz, G. S., and Rascher, W. (1997). Oscillometric twenty-four hour ambulatory blood pressure values in healthy children and adolescents: a multicenter trial including 1141 subjects. *Journal of Pediatrics* **130**, 178–184.

Soergel, M., Verho, M., Wühl, E., Gellermann, J., Teichert, L., and Schärer, K. (2000). Effect of ramipril on ambulatory blood pressure and albuminuria in renal hypertension. *Pediatric Nephrology* **15**, 113–118.

Sonesson, S. E. and Broberger, U. (1987). Arterial blood pressure in the very low birth weight neonate. *Acta Paediatrica Scandinavica* **76**, 338–341.

Sorof, J. M. and Portman, R. J. (2000). White coat hypertension in children with elevated blood pressure. *Journal of Pediatrics* **137**, 493–497.

Sorof, J. M. and Portman, R. J. (2001). Ambulatory blood pressure measurements. *Current Opinion in Pediatrics* **13**, 133–137.

Sorof, J. M., Cargo, P., Graepel, J., Humphrey, D., King, E., Rolf, C., and Cunningham, R. J. (2002). Beta-blocker/thiazide combination for treatment of hypertensive children: a randomized double-blind, placebo-controlled trial. *Pediatric Nephrology* **17**, 345–350.

Stapleton, F. B., Johnson, D., Kaplan, G. W., and Griswold, W. (1980). The cystic renal lesion in tuberous sclerosis. *Journal of Pediatrics* **97**, 574–579.

Stickler, G. B., Kelalis, P. P., Burke, E. C., and Segar, W. E. (1971). Primary interstitial nephritis with reflux. A cause of hypertension. *American Journal of Diseases of Children* **122**, 144–148.

Still, J. L. and Cotton, D. (1967). Severe hypertension in childhood. *Archives of Disease in Childhood* **42**, 34–39.

Stringer, D. A., de Bruyn, R., Dillon, M. J., and Gordon, I. (1984). Comparison of aortography, renal vein, renin sampling, radionuclide scans, ultrasound and the IVU in the investigation of childhood renovascular hypertension. *British Journal of Radiology* **57**, 111–121.

Szklo, M. (1986). Determinants of blood pressure in children. *Clinical and Experimental Hypertension* **A8**, 479–493.

Tack, E. D. and Perlman, J. M. (1988). Renal failure in sick hypertensive premature infants receiving captopril therapy. *Journal of Pediatrics* **112**, 805–810.

Tallian, K. B., Nahata, M. C., Turman, M. A., Mahan, J. D., Hayes, J. R., and Mentser, M. I. (1999). Efficacy of amlodipine in pediatric patients with hypertension. *Pediatric Nephrology* **13**, 304–310.

Tan, K. L. (1988). Blood pressure in very low birth weight infants in the first 70 days of life. *Journal of Pediatrics* **112**, 266–270.

Tejani, A. (1983). Post transplant hypertension and hypertensive encephalopathy in renal allograft recipients. *Nephron* **34**, 73–78.

Tirodker, U. H. and Dabbagh, F. (2001). Facial paralysis in childhood hypertension. *Journal of Paediatric Health* **37**, 193–194.

Tönshoff, B., Sammet, A., Sanden, I., Mehls, O., Waldherr, R., and Schärer, K. (1994). Outcome and prognostic determinants in the haemolytic uremic syndrome of children. *Nephron* **68**, 63–70.

Treluyer, J. M., Hubert, P., Jouvet, P., Couderc, S., and Cloup, M. (1993). Intravenous nicardipine in hypertensive children. *European Journal of Pediatrics* **152**, 712–714.

Uhari, M., and Koskimies, O. (1979). A survey of 164 Finnish children and adolescents with hypertension. *Acta Paediatrica Scandinavica* **68**, 193–198.

Update on the 1987 Task force report on high blood pressure in children and adolescents (1996). *Pediatrics* **98**, 649–658.

Versmold, H. T., Kitterman, J. A., Phibbs, R. H., Gregory, G. A., and Tooley, W. H. (1981). Aortic blood pressure in infants with birth weight 610 to 4220 grams. *Pediatrics* **67**, 607–613.

Voors, A. W., Foster, T. A., Frerichs, R. R., Webber, L. S., and Berenson, G. S. (1976). Studies of blood pressure in children, ages 5–14 years in a total biracial community. The Bogalusa Heart Study. *Circulation* **54**, 319–327.

Voors, A. W., Webber, L. S., and Berenson, G. S. (1978). Relationship of blood pressure levels to height and weight in children. *Journal of Cardiovascular Medicine* **3**, 911–918.

Voors, A. W., Webber, L. S., Frerichs, R. R., and Berenson, G. S. (1977). Body height and body mass as determinants of basal blood pressure in children—The Bogalusa Heart Study. *American Journal of Epidemiology* **116**, 276–286.

Wallace, D. M. H., Rothwell, D. L., and Williams, D. I. (1978). Longterm follow-up of surgical treated vesicoureteral reflux. *British Journal of Urology* **50**, 479–484.

Warshaw, B. L., Anand, S. K., Olson, D. L., Gruskin, C. M., Heuser, E. T., and Lieberman, E. (1979). Hypertension secondary to a renin-producing juxtaglomerular cell tumor. *Journal of Pediatrics* **94**, 247–250.

Waters, K. and Gills, J. (1987). Meningitis presenting as hypertension. *Archives of Disease in Childhood* **62**, 191–193.

Wells, T. G. (1999). Trials of antihypertensive therapies in children. *Blood Pressure Monitoring* **4**, 189–192.

Wells, T. G. and Sinaiko, A. R. (1991). Antihypertensive effect and pharmacokinetics of nitrendipine in children. *Journal of Pediatrics* **118**, 638–643.

Wells, T. G., Rippley, R., Hogg, R., Sakarcan, A., Blowey, D., Walson, P., Vogt, B., Delucchi, A., Lo, M. W., Hand, E., Panebianco, D., Shaw, W., and Shahinfar, S. (2001). The pharmacokinetics of enalapril in children and infants with hypertension. *Journal of Clinical Pharmacology* **41**, 1064–1074.

Whyte, R. K., Elseed, A. M., Frasier, C. B., Shinebourne, E. A., and deSwiet, M. (1975). Assessment of Doppler ultrasound to measure systolic blood pressure in infants and young children. *Archives of Disease in Childhood* **50**, 542–544.

Wiggelinkhuizen, J. and Cremin, B. J. (1978). Takayasu arteritis and renovascular hypertension in childhood. *Pediatrics* **62**, 209–217.

World Health Organization—International Society of Hypertension Guidelines for the Management of Hypertension (1999). *Journal of Hypertension* **17**, 151–183.

Wyszynska, T., Cichocka, E., Wieteska-Klimczak, A., Jobs, K., and Januszewicz, P. (1992). A single pediatric center experience with 1025 children with hypertension. *Acta Paediatrica* **81**, 244–246.

Zeier, M., Geberth, S., Schmidt, K. G., Mandelbaum, A., and Ritz, E. (1993). Elevated blood pressure profile and left ventricular mass in children and young adults with autosomal dominant polycystic kidney disease. *Journal of the American Society of Nephrology* **3**, 1451–1457.

10

Acute renal failure

10.1 Epidemiology of acute renal failure

Ciaran Doherty

Background

Acute renal failure (ARF) is a common clinical syndrome with a broad aetiological profile. It complicates about 5 per cent of hospital admissions and 30 per cent of admissions to intensive care units (ICU). It is associated with major morbidity and significant mortality due to the severity of the causative illness.

The true incidence of ARF is not easily discerned from published reports because of variation in methods of case ascertainment, definitions of ARF, and catchment populations. Most authors include patients with acute on chronic renal failure, some also include acute presentation of endstage renal disease (ESRD), while others exclude patients with ARF who remain dialysis dependent for over 90 days ('acute irreversible renal failure').

Most surveys of hospital populations cannot estimate true population incidence. Unselected hospital populations will include many patients never referred for nephrological opinion, for example, because ARF is in the context of untreatable terminal illness. Khan *et al.* (1997), in a study of 311 unselected hospital inpatients with ARF (serum creatinine = 300 μmol/l), observed that overall, only 22 per cent were referred to a nephrologist (34 per cent after excluding those with advanced cancer and age > 80 years) and that referral rates were significantly influenced by the age and co-morbidity of patients at presentation.

Hospital-based studies of ARF reflect selection bias as these populations are defined by the referral patterns to the site of care. (e.g. district general hospital, tertiary referral centre, general ICU, cardiothoracic ICU, etc.). Such populations will differ markedly; ICU patients will predominantly be those with acute tubular necrosis (ATN) in the setting of multiorgan failure, whereas general hospital admissions will reflect the wider spectrum of the disorder. Patients with isolated ARF compared to those with ARF in a multiorgan failure context, differ in age profile, aetiology, pathophysiology, site of care, and mortality rates (Liano *et al.* 1998). The age profile of the population studied must be taken into account because of the marked differences in age-specific incidence of ARF (see Fig. 1).

The setting in which ARF develops is another confounding variable. Kaufman (1991) in a study of 10,924 hospital admissions identified a 1 per cent incidence of community-acquired ARF of which 70 per cent were prerenal, 11 per cent renal, and 17 per cent obstructive ARF. The overall mortality was 15 per cent. Hou *et al.* (1983), in a prospective study of hospital-acquired ARF among 2216 consecutive admissions, found that ARF developed in 4.9 per cent, with iatrogenic factors (drugs and sepsis) accounting for 55 per cent of all episodes. The overall mortality was 25 per cent. In community-acquired ARF with mostly prerenal and postrenal causes, prognosis is, therefore, better than the 'nosocomial' disease developing during hospital admission.

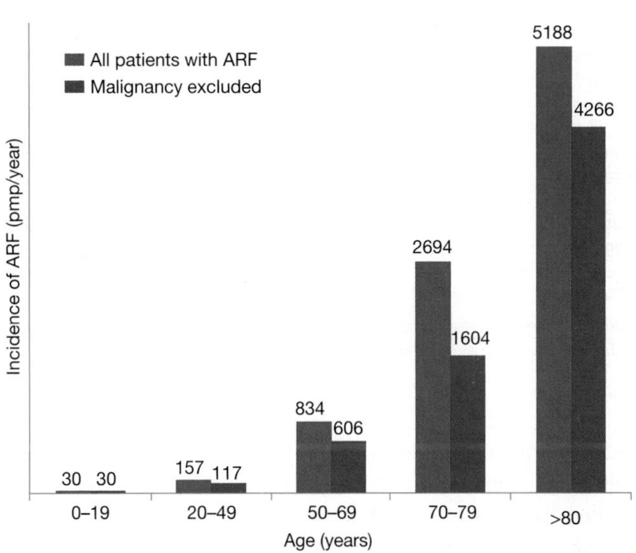

Fig. 1 The effect of age on the annual incidence of acute renal failure (ARF) in a predominantly Caucasian population of 506,100 in the Grampian region of Scotland. The overall incidence of ARF (serum creatinine > 300 μmol/l) was 620 per million population (pmp) and the age-related incidence ranged from 30 to 4266 pmp (Khan *et al.* 1997).

The use of arbitrary serum creatinine thresholds to define ARF is also unsatisfactory. Duncan *et al.* (2001) identified a substantial prevalence of significantly abnormal renal function among patients who have a serum creatinine within the laboratory normal range. Studies of ARF which include only patients with index serum creatinine values above a chosen elevated level, for example 300 μmol/l, will therefore, underestimate the true incidence of the disorder.

Incidence

Incidence in the general population

A limited number of studies have examined the true population incidence of ARF. They are listed in Table 1.

Based on these studies of adult populations in developed countries, the incidence of severe ARF (defined as serum creatinine > 500 μmol/l and including patients with acute on chronic renal failure) appears to

Table 1 Incidence and mortality of acute renal failure in the general population

Reference	Population studied	Definition of ARF	Incidence pmp/year	Mortality rate (%)
Hegarty *et al.* (2001)	South Wales (500,000)	Serum creatinine > 500 μmol/l Need for dialysis	736 138	46 (at discharge)
Stevens *et al.* (2001)	East Kent Health Authority (593,000)	Serum creatinine > 500 μmol/l Need for dialysis	486 83	44 (at discharge) 65 (at 1 year)
Metcalfe (2002)	Scotland (1,120,000)	Need for dialysis	203	73.5 (at 90 days)
Khan *et al.* (1997)	Scotland Grampian region (506,000)	Serum creatinine ≥ 300 μmol/l[a] Serum creatinine > 500 μmol/l Need for dialysis	620 102 50	At 2 years 20 (low risk) 58 (medium risk) 81 (high risk group)
Liano *et al.* (1996)	Madrid (4,227,837)	Sudden rise in serum creatinine > 177 μmol/l with prior normal renal function[b] Need for dialysis	209 85	45 (at discharge)
Doherty (1995)	Northern Ireland (1,660,000)	Tertiary referrals for ARF Need for dialysis	127 50	49 (at discharge)
Feest *et al.* (1993)	England (490,771)	Serum creatinine > 500 μmol/l Need for dialysis	172 22	46 (at 3 months) 66 (at 2 years)

[a] Prior chronic renal failure cases excluded.

[b] Excluded patients with prior chronic renal failure who had basal serum creatinine >3 mg/dl; included patients with basal chronic renal failure and serum creatinine <3 mg/dl who had a sudden rise in serum creatinine (50% or more).

exceed 500 pmp/year. This figure, however, includes the very elderly (>80 years), those with malignancy and terminal illness. Severe ARF needing dialysis is instead of the order of 200 pmp/year, and the incidence has increased over the past decade. This is probably due to more elderly patients undergoing operative interventions.

Incidence of acute renal failure in specific clinical settings

The incidence and mortality rates of ARF show wide variation according to the primary diagnosis (see Table 2), and different rates of survivor ESRD are observed (up to 15 per cent with survivors of abdominal aortic aneurysm surgery may require long-term dialysis). Particularly high-risk settings for ATN include postsurgical (abdominal aortic aneurysm, bowel resection, cardiothoracic surgery), multiple trauma, and multifactorial medical cases (poor cardiac output, sepsis, nephrotoxin). Patients in these latter high-risk groups often develop multiorgan failure, need intensive care, and have high mortality rates.

Many authors have used multivariate analysis to try and define factors which will identify those patients at high risk of ARF. Co-morbid factors which confer predisposition to ARF are advanced age, diabetes mellitus, arteriosclerosis, cancer, pre-existing chronic renal failure, fluid and electrolyte imbalance, and prescribing harm [non-steroidal anti-inflammatory drugs (NSAIDs), angiotensin-converting enzyme (ACE) inhibitors]. Some risk factors are more likely in certain situations, for example, the high incidence of occult renovascular disease in elderly patients with cardiac failure (MacDowall *et al.* 1998).

Behrend and Miller (1999) found that 106 (4 per cent) of 2392 admissions to a cardiac care unit during a 12-month period during 1996–1997 developed ARF, and 18 patients (17 per cent of those with ARF) needed dialysis. The aetiological factors in those with ARF were congestive heart failure (35 per cent), multifactorial (26 per cent), arrhythmia (13 per cent), contrast media (11 per cent), hypovolaemia (6 per cent), and sepsis (6 per cent). The overall mortality rate for those with ARF was 50 per cent but reached 70 per cent in those with an ejection fraction less than 25 per cent. The 50 per cent mortality rate in those who developed ARF contrasts with the 8 per cent figure in those who did not.

Cardiac surgeons and cardiologists may be reassured by the relatively low incidence of ARF following coronary artery bypass grafting (1.2 per cent) and percutaneous coronary interventions (0.73 per cent). (Fortescue *et al.* 2000; Gruberg *et al.* 2001). However, in those patients undergoing percutaneous coronary interventions who developed ARF (51 out of 7690 in Gruberg's series), the in-hospital mortality and 1-year survival was 27.5 and 54.5 per cent, compared to 1.0 and 6.4 per cent in those without ARF. Mahon and Desmond in a 10-year study of patients admitted to a Liverpool cardiothoracic ICU identified 58 patients with renal failure needing dialysis. These patients comprised three separate groups, the first with unexpected ARF (39 patients, mortality rate of 67 per cent), acute on chronic renal failure (eight patients, mortality rate 75 per cent), and patients already on renal replacement therapy for ESRD (10 patients, mortality rate 9 per cent).

Studies of ARF in the very elderly (>80 years) suggests that prognosis may be comparable to that found in the younger population and that acute dialysis should not be withheld solely on grounds of advanced age (Pascual *et al.* 1995; Andreucci *et al.* 1998; Baraldi *et al.* 1998).

Keller *et al.* (1995) studied 107 patients with decompensated liver disease and ARF, including 26 patients with hepatorenal syndrome. Of 43 patients assessed as having a favourable prognosis (defined by compensated renal failure, absence of malignancy, or selection for haemodialysis treatment), the 1 year survival rate was 38 per cent. They concluded that advanced liver disease including hepatorenal

Table 2 Incidence and mortality of acute renal failure in specific clinical settings

Setting (no. of patients)	Reference	ARF definition	Incidence (% of study group)	Mortality (%)
General ICU (26,669)	Ostermann *et al.* (2001)	Need for dialysis	27.6	56 (at hospital discharge)
Cardiothoracic ICU (58)	Mahon and Desmond (2000)	Need for dialysis	N/A	67 (ARF) 75 (acute on CRF) 9 (ESRD)
CCU (2392)	Behrend and Miller (1999)	Complex	4.0	50
Postcardiopulmonary bypass (47)	Ostermann *et al.* (2000)	Need for dialysis	2.0	53.8 (at ICU discharge)
CABG (9498)	Fortescue *et al.* (2000)	Need for dialysis	1.2	N/A
Percutaneous coronary interventions (7690)	Gruberg *et al.* (2001)	Need for dialysis	0.73	27.5 (at hospital discharge) 54.5 (at 1 year)
Pregnancy; Atlanta, USA (21)	Nzerue *et al.* (1998)	N/A	2 in 10,000 pregnancies	15.7
Severe alcoholic hepatitis; Birmingham (15)	Mutimer *et al.* (1993)	Serum creatinine >250 μmol/l	N/A	85.7
Earthquake crush syndrome; Turkey (635)	Erek *et al.* (2002)	Need for dialysis	74.6	15.2
Acute pancreatitis; Amsterdam (267)	Tran *et al.* (1993)	Serum creatinine >280 μmol/l or need for dialysis	16 13	81 (at hospital discharge) 100
Bone marrow transplant; Madrid (643)	Gruss *et al.* (1995)	Doubling of baseline serum creatinine and serum creatinine >177 μmol/l Need for dialysis	26 24	45.8 88

syndrome was not a contraindication to dialysis treatment (see also Chapter 10.6.4).

Aetiology

Overview

The classification of ARF reflects the pathophysiological concepts of prerenal (about 75 per cent of cases), intrinsic or parenchymal renal disease (25 per cent), and postrenal (5 per cent). Most intrinsic ARFs are induced by ischaemia and/or nephrotoxins and are associated with ATN.

Prerenal acute renal failure

Prerenal ARF is a physiological response to renal hypoperfusion in which a potentially reversible fall in glomerular filteration rate (GFR) is induced by four main mechanisms; true intravascular hypovolaemia, decreased 'effective' circulatory volume (e.g. cardiac failure), intrarenal vasoconstriction (radio contrast, cyclosporin, endotoxin), or borderline hypovolaemia in patients taking drugs that impair autoregulation of renal blood flow, for example, ACE inhibitors.

Intrinsic acute renal failure

Intrinsic ARF is categorized into diseases of large renal vessels (e.g. renal artery thrombosis), the renal microvasculature (e.g. vasculitis), the tubulointerstitium (e.g. allergic interstitial nephritis), and ATN due to ischaemia or toxins (see also Chapters 10.6.1 and 10.6.2).

Postrenal acute renal failure (see also Chapter 17.3)

Obstructive ARF is more more common in old age due to prostatic disease and pelvic cancer. Acute intratubular obstruction may occur when there is abrupt exposure of the kidneys to increased filtered loads of insoluble crystalline substances such as sodium biurate (following chemotherapy of leukaemia and lymphomas).

Historical variations in the aetiology of acute renal failure

Before 1975, approximately 60 per cent of ARF cases were related to surgery or trauma, 30 per cent occurred in a medical setting, and about 10 per cent were related to the complications of pregnancy. By the 1980s, in developed countries, obstetric cases had become rare (<3 per cent) and there was an increase in the incidence of ARF caused by 'medical' conditions (Beaman *et al.* 1987). This reflected improvements in obstetric care and the age of the population under treatment. By the 1990s, many medical cases of ARF included patients with profound medical problems and extremely poor prognosis independent of renal failure. In a longitudinal study of 1347 ARF patients seen over a 32-year period at Leeds General Infirmary Renal Unit, the median age was increased from 41 in the 1950s to 61 years in the 1980s (Turney *et al.* 1990). This trend has continued with a more recently reported series showing a mean age of 65 years (Hegarty *et al.* 2001). Other factors that contribute to change in the aetiological profile of ARF include the evolution of new causes of ARF, and development of new treatments for some causative disorders (Doherty 1993).

New causes of ARF identified in recent years are Chinese herbal medicine (Van Ypersele de Strihou and Van Herweghen 1995) (see Chapter 6.9), lithotripsy (Diaz-Tejeiro *et al.* 1993), human immunodeficiency virus infection (Rao 1998), abdominal compartment syndrome (Tan and Kua 1998), intravenous immunoglobulin therapy (Cantu *et al.* 1995), acyclovir (Perazella 1999), and medical misinformation on the Internet (Black and Hussain 2000).

New treatments which have altered the outcome of ARF include ACE inhibitors in scleroderma renal crisis (Steen *et al.* 1990) (see Chapter 4.8) and plasma infusions for haemolytic uraemic syndrome (Misiani *et al.* 1982). In a trial using activated protein C in patients with severe sepsis, the relative risk of death at 28 days was reduced by 20 per cent (Bernard *et al.* 2001). Clarke *et al.* (2000) and Pearson *et al.* (2000) have advocated protein C and early haemodiafiltration, respectively, as measures to reduce mortality in meningococcal septicaemia. Better understanding of the pathophysiology of acute pancreatitis has improved survival (Powell *et al.* 2000). The practice of nil by mouth in the management of acute pancreatitis is no longer recommended, as early enteral nutrition maintains gut barrier function and reduces septic complications. Computed tomography scan detection of infected pancreatic necrosis and early intravenous antibiotic therapy may also contribute to reduction in the number of deaths.

Authors of previous reports concluded that dialysis for ARF in the setting of hepatorenal syndrome was futile (Wilkinson *et al.* 1977). This view is challenged by recent experience of improved outcomes following treatment by albumin combined with the synthetic vasopressin analogue terlipressin, and also a modified dialysis method based on a molecular adsorbent recirculating system (MARS) which enables effective removal of albumin bound substances (Dagher and Moore 2001).

Recent case reports have documented recovery of renal function in cases of ARF due to cholesterol embolism after the use of statins (Woolfson and Lachman 1998) and oral corticosteroids (Nakahami and Sakaguchi 2001).

Geographical variations in the aetiology of acute renal failure (see Chapter 10.7.3)

The spectrum of causes of ARF is markedly different in developing and developed countries. Particular examples include copper sulfate ingestion (used widely in the agricultural and leather industries), a popular mode of suicidal poisoning. ARF occurs as a consequence of intravascular haemolysis and direct nephrotoxicity. Intravascular haemolysis in glucose 6-phosphate dehydrogenase deficiency provoked by malaria and analgesic drugs is common in India. In Asia, ARF following snake bites is a common problem. In the developed world, extensive trauma, abdominal and vascular catastrophies, and complicated open heart surgery are the leading causes of postsurgical ARF. Obstructive uropathy due to calculous disease is the most important surgical grouping in India (Chugh *et al.* 1989). Prakash *et al.* (1995), in a study of 426 patients in Eastern India, found that medical, surgical, and obstetric causes were responsible for 68.3, 17.8, and 14 per cent of cases, respectively. Diarrhoeal diseases (35.2 per cent), obstructive uropathy (13.3 per cent), and septic abortion (10.5 per cent) were the main causes for ARF in these groups (Table 3).

African studies of ARF have also found that medical causes were the dominant category, with herbal toxins and infections the most common aetiological factors in the medical subgroup (Seedat and Nattoo 1993). Tetanus, malaria, and typhoid featured among the infectious causes, and the most common nephrotoxin was a traditional herbal remedy, *Callilepsis laureola*, a tuberous plant that can cause liver and renal necrosis.

Age-related variations in the aetiology of acute renal failure (see Chapters 10.7.1 and 10.7.4)

The preponderance of elderly subjects in ARF practice is probably due to anatomical and physiological changes in the ageing kidney, the increased risk of ARF related to facilitating factors such as arteriosclerosis, diabetes, heart failure, and drug prescribing patterns in the elderly (ACE inhibitors, diuretics, NSAIDs), and the prevalence of obstructive uropathy (Pascual *et al.* 1995). In Liano and Pascual's multicentre study (1996), based on an adult population of 4.2 million in Madrid, 36 per cent of patients with ARF were aged over 70 years.

The aetiology of ARF in children differs from that in the adult population. Kaiser *et al.* (1994) in a study of 21,000 children admitted over a 3-year period to an American paediatric tertiary care centre identified only 105 children with ARF. The overall mortality was 40 and 10 per cent of survivors had ESRD. The causes included congenital renal disease, for example, posterior urethral valves and other obstructive lesions, a complication of surgery, sepsis, haemolytic uraemic syndrome, acute glomerulonephritis, and interstitial/tubular damage. Gallego *et al.* (1993) studied 138 cases of ARF in children admitted to Madrid hospitals. The median age was 26 months, the overall mortality was 48.3 per cent, and the aetiology was congenital heart disease 62 per cent, malignancy related 10 per cent, primary renal disease 11 per cent, and miscellaneous 17 per cent.

The past four decades have, therefore, seen changes in the pattern of disorders causing ARF both in developed and developing countries. These changes reflect an increase in the average age of the affected patients, the evolution of intensive care medicine, and of lowering of thresholds for surgical intervention.

Mortality

Trends in mortality rate

Fifty years ago, the mortality rate for ARF of the ATN-type in the clinical setting of war combat was over 90 per cent (Office of the Surgeon General, Department of the Army 1952). The mortality rate with the introduction of dialysis declined to 50 per cent (Kolff 1965) and has stubbornly remained around this figure since. Significant improvements in survival have occurred among patients with isolated ARF, but mortality rates from ARF in the setting of multiorgan failure have changed little over the past 30 years (Druml 1996). The likely explanation is that improvements in dialysis techniques, nutritional therapy, antibiotic therapy, and other supportive care have been counterbalanced by a trend towards increase in age, illness severity, prevalence of co-morbid illness, and the progressive shift to ARF occurring in the context of multiorgan failure rather than isolated organ failure.

Prognosis in individual patients

ARF is a syndrome with multiple aetiologies, each having its own individual prognosis. The overall mortality rates must be interpreted with

Table 3 Prevention of acute renal failure

Clinical setting	Therapeutic intervention	Comment	Reference
Contrast nephrotoxicity	Acetyl cysteine and saline infusion	Prevents contrast toxicity in patients with CRF	Tepel *et al.* (2000)
Ethyleneglycol poisoning	Fomepizole infusion	Superior to ethanol for treatment of acidosis. May reduce need for dialysis	Brent *et al.* (1999)
Septic shock	Hydroxyethyl starch avoidance	Avoid hydroxyethylstarch for volume replacement in patients at risk of ARF	Schertgen *et al.* (2001)
Acute renal failure postrenal transplant	Calcium blockers	Reduce incidence of ARF	Neumayer *et al.* (1992)
Rhabdomyolysis	Alkaline diuresis	Early treatment can prevent ARF	Better (1990)
Drug-induced ARF	Check renal function after starting ACE inhibitor, NSAID, warn patients about intercurrent vomiting and diarrhoea	Common cause of ARF of medical type in elderly patients	Kalpa *et al.* (1999), Jacobs *et al.* (2000)
Elderly patients postsurgery	Meticulous fluid and electrolyte balance	The most efficient general measure to prevent ATN	Lameire *et al.* (1995)
Rapidly progressive glomerulonephritis	Immunosuppression/plasma exchange	High index of suspicion needed for early detection	Cassidy *et al.* (1990)
Tumour lysis syndrome	Allopurinol and saline hydration	Established efficacy in ARF prevention	Lamiere (1994)
Cisplatinum therapy	Saline loading	Established efficacy	Ries (1986)
Critically ill patients on general wards	Early warning systems and medical emergency teams	As yet unproven but compelling logic	Subbe *et al.* (2001)
Scleroderma renal crisis	ACE inhibitor treatment	Reduces incidence of ARF	Steen *et al.* (1990)
Haemolytic uraemic syndrome	Plasma infusion	Improves survival and recovery of renal function	Misiani *et al.* (1982)
Atherosclerotic renal artery stenosis	Renal artery stenting/angioplasty	Controversial	Textor (1998)
Aminoglycoside toxicity	Computerized drug prescribing	Drug–drug and drug–patient interaction alerts may signal need to adjust dose for age and renal function	Bates *et al.* (1994)

caution if the study population includes patients with isolated ARF (low mortality rate) as well as cases of ARF in the setting of multiorgan failure (high mortality rate). Liano *et al.* (1996) have emphasized that crude mortality rate does not accurately reflect the contribution of ARF in the causation of death; while many patients die with ARF, the cause of death is most often the primary disorder or its subsequent complications, usually infective or cardiorespiratory. It may, therefore, be appropriate to exclude patients whose death was attributable to the primary disorder from analysis, and to give a 'corrected' or 'attributable' mortality rate. Druml (1995) in an extensive review of the prognosis of ARF over the period 1975–1995, also identified type and severity of the underlying disease and its complications as the strongest predictors of survival. He argued it was, therefore, more logical to speak of 'prognosis of the disease leading to ARF'.

Liano *et al.* (1996) reported mortality rates of 60 per cent for patients with ATN, 35 per cent for prerenal ARF, 35 per cent for acute on chronic renal failure, 27 per cent for obstructive ARF, and 26 per cent for renal disorders other than ATN. Mortality is highest in patients sufficiently ill to require admission to ICUs, with figures rising from 50 per cent for a combination of acute renal and respiratory failure towards 100 per cent with five system failure (Knaus *et al.* 1986).

Factors influencing the mortality rate

There is little consensus in the literature with regard to the predictive value of age, presence or absence of oliguria, and duration of renal dysfunction. Despite continued efforts to refine general prognostic models such as version II of the Acute Physiology and Chronic Health Evaluation (APACHE II), no model has been found to provide sufficient confidence for the prediction of outcome in individual patients (Fiaccadori *et al.* 2001). This reflects the inability of any prognostic tool to express the medical complexity of ARF adequately. The problems of validating and adapting prognostic models for ARF have been reviewed in detail recently (Lins *et al.* 2001). Probability models may, in the future, support clinical judgement, but will not replace it, and the final decision about initiation or withdrawal of dialysis will largely remain the responsibility of the individual clinician(s) involved.

Of the factors that do appear to influence the mortality rate, the most important are (i) the primary diagnosis or underlying cause of the ARF (Woodrow and Turney 1992; Jones *et al.* 1998) and (ii) the number of failing organ systems (Schwilk *et al.* 1997). In a prospective study carried out in South Wales hospitals, Sivalingam *et al.* (2001) described cases deemed to require high dependency care who were instead managed on general wards. There was a significant association between inappropriate site of care and mortality. The quality of early non-specialist management also appears to be important in the outcome of ARF (Stevens *et al.* 2001). The requirements are prompt recognition of renal dysfunction, early diagnosis of treatable disorders, appropriate adjustments to the drug prescription, and appropriate fluid and electrolyte administration. It is important not to miss pericardial tamponade and acute adrenal insufficiency as treatable causes of resistant shock (Korzets *et al.* 2001).

Co-morbid factors which influence mortality rate are chronic heart failure, myocardial infarction, respiratory failure, sepsis, and malignancy. The literature is conflicting with regard to the effect on ARF mortality of pneumonia, diabetes mellitus, and immune deficiencies (Chew *et al.* 1993) (Table 4).

The effect of treatment on outcome (see Chapter 10.4)

In many patients, ARF is not the ultimate cause of death, but a proxy for overall disease severity and complications of the primary diagnosis. The measures most likely to influence outcome are those directed at the underlying cause of ARF. This is exemplified in patients with ARF secondary to intra-abdominal sepsis.

Controversy persists over the effect of certain aspects of treatment on the mortality rate of established ARF. These include the choice of dialysis treatment (continuous renal replacement therapy or intermittent haemodialysis), the time of initiating dialysis treatment, the choice of membrane, and the dialysis prescription. Clinical trials in these areas are difficult to execute (Chertow *et al.* 2001) and the intrinsic heterogeneity of patients with ARF in respect of primary diagnosis, disease severity, and co-morbidity score. Other variations in care (e.g. inotropes, nutrition therapy) are further confounding variables.

Dialysis modality and intensity (dose) of dialysis (see also Chapter 10.4)

Randomized trials have not yet shown a survival advantage for continuous renal replacement therapy over intermittent haemodialysis (Mehta *et al.* 2001). Ronco *et al.* (2000) have reported that higher than standard doses of continuous venovenous haemofiltration may increase survival among patients with ARF while Schiffl *et al.* (2002) have argued that intensive daily haemodialysis reduces mortality.

Dialyser membrane and treatment outcome

The impact of dialyser membrane on mortality in ARF remains unresolved, due to the inherent limitations of reports published to date. Particular problems are the heterogeneity of populations studied and the overwhelming influence of illness severity on outcome in the context of multiorgan failure (Modi *et al.* 2001).

General measures (see also Chapter 10.2)

There is still no pharmacological intervention of proven efficacy for reversing or shortening established ATN. The results are awaited of clinical trials of endothelin receptor antagonists, atrial natriuretic peptide, nitric oxide synthase inhibitors, and other agents.

Upper gastrointestinal bleeding from stress ulceration is now a rare cause of death in critically ill patients, a benefit of improved nutrition, better dialysis, and ulcer prophylaxis using agents including H_2 receptor antagonists or sucralfate. Early enteral nutrition in critically ill patients reduces the risk of nosocomial infection and hospital stay (Marik and Zaloga 2001).

Treatment outcome in terms of recovery of renal function

The most frequent outcome measure used for ARF is hospital survival, with few series providing information on later survival or other outcomes such as length of admission and recovery of renal function (Chew *et al.* 1993). Bhandari and Turney (1996) studied 1095 patients with severe ARF between 1984 and 1995, and of these, 107 (16.2 per cent) remained dependent on long-term dialysis. They found that the frequency of ESRD in survivors varied between 3 and 41 per cent according to the cause of ARF, being highest in those with acute renal parenchymal disease and lowest in ARF due to obstetrics and trauma. These results suggest that ESRD resulting from ARF is more frequent than previously reported and may reflect the increasing age and co-morbidity profile of patients. Of cases classified clinically as having ATN, 10.5 per cent remained dialysis dependent. This latter figure contrasts with 20 years ago when there was a very low incidence (1 per cent) of non-recovery of renal function following ARF due to ATN (Kjellstrand *et al.* 1981).

Future directions

The incidence of ARF in adults in developed countries appears to be increasing both in the community and in hospitalized patients. The mean age of patients is increasing, duration for which dialysis support is required is increasing, and the dialysis prescriptions are being intensified. The overall effect of these changes is to increase workload and costs.

Table 4 Factors affecting the mortality of acute renal failure

Some evidence to support effect on mortality of ARF	No effect from evidence to date
Primary diagnosis (Woodrow and Turney 1992; Jones *et al.* 2001)	Type of dialysis modality (Mehta *et al.* 2001)
Co-morbidity (Chew *et al.* 1993; Khan *et al.* 1997)	Kidney membrane (Modi *et al.* 2001)
Quality of non-specialist management of ARF (Andreucci 1998; Stevens *et al.* 2001)	Low dose dopamine (Power *et al.* 1999)
Appropriate site of care (Sivalingham *et al.* 2001)	Frusemide (Kellum 1997)
Early referral to a nephrologist (Mehta *et al.* 1995)	Monoclonal antibody therapy to endotoxin (Hinds 1992)
Intensity of intermittent haemodialysis (Schiffl *et al.* 2002)	High-dose corticosteroid therapy (Bone *et al.* 1987)
Higher doses of CVVH (Ronco *et al.* 2000)	Decontamination of digestive tract (Sanderson 1989)

It is disappointing that despite previous recommendations (Liano 1994; Dubose *et al.* 1997; Renal Association 1997), reports still lack an agreed definition for ARF (covering inclusion/exclusion criteria) and treatment outcome measures (overall mortality, attributable mortality, length of stay, rate of survivor ESRD). Epidemiological studies and future clinical trials would be improved by agreement on these points. Better description of study populations to ensure equivalent demographics (especially age profile), aetiological profile, and inclusion criteria would allow meaningful comparison. Mortality should be reported in a common format, for example, a standardized mortality ratio and non-dialysis requiring ARF should be defined by a GFR threshold calculated from the Cockroft–Gault (1976) formula which takes account of age, gender, and body mass.

The continued high mortality rate and the fact that most patients are cared for by non-nephrologists underlines the need to improvement management of the early, potentially preventable phase of the disorder, and to minimize adverse renal-related events (Bates *et al.* 1994). Early detection protocols and outreach medical teams for critically ill ward patients should be encouraged. A group has recently been established, the Acute Dialysis Quality Initiative group to develop evidence-based practice guidelines for future management of ARF (Renal Research Institute: The Acute Dialysis Quality Initiative 2000). The increasing proportion of elderly patients who survive ARF only to remain dialysis dependent needs to be taken into account in planning ESRD programmes.

The staggering costs of treating patients with multi organ failure in the ICU will continue to attract attention. Korkeila *et al.* (2000) identified 62 of 3447 ICU admissions who required dialysis. The estimated cost per ARF 6-month survivor was US $80,000. Ostermann and colleagues (2001) studied 26,669 patients admitted to 21 ICUs in the United Kingdom during 1989–1996 and, excluding chronic renal failure patients, identified 2394 patients with ARF, of whom 660 (27.6 per cent) needed renal replacement. The hospital mortality of this group was 56 per cent (versus 25 per cent in those without ARF) and they consumed significantly more resource. The costs of treatment for patients with multiorgan failure in ICU increased from the 1960s through to the 1980s (Chew *et al.* 1993) but the more recent figures of Korkeila above suggest this trend may have reversed, as comparison with figures in the 1991 study by Gilbertson *et al.* (1991) showed a cost per life saved at that time in excess of US $90,000. It is often assumed that continuous renal replacement therapy is significantly more expensive than intermittent haemodialysis but Silvester (1998) disputes this.

Hamel *et al.* (1997) estimated the cost of dialysis and aggressive care of a critically ill patient with ARF at approximately US $128,000 per quality-adjusted life year saved. This compares to US $8300 for coronary artery bypass grafting for left main coronary disease or US $34,200 for the treatment of acute myocardial infarction with thrombolytic therapy. The accepted upper limit of cost-effective care is considered to be US $50,000. These data only serve to emphasize the need for continued research into prevention and improved treatment for ARF.

References

Andreucci, V. E., Fuiano, G., and Russo, D. (1998). Vasomotor nephropathy in the elderly. *Nephrology, Dialysis, Transplantation* **13** (Suppl. 7), 17–24.

Baraldi, A. *et al.* (1998). Acute renal failure of medical type in an elderly population. *Nephrology, Dialysis, Transplantation* **13** (Suppl. 7), S25–S29.

Bates, D. W. *et al.* (1994). Potential identifiability and preventability of adverse events using information systems. *Journal of the American Medical Informatics Association* **1**, 404–411.

Beaman, N. *et al.* (1987). Changing pattern of acute renal failure. *Quarterly Journal of Medicine* **62** (237), 15–23.

Behrend, T. and Miller, S. B. (1999). Acute renal failure in the cardiac care unit: aetiologies, outcomes and prognostic factors. *Kidney International* **56**, 238–243.

Bernard, G. R. *et al.* (2001). Efficacy and safety of recombinant human activated protein C for severe sepsis. *New England Journal of Medicine* **344**, 699–709.

Bhandari, S. and Turney, J. H. (1996). Survivors of acute renal failure who do not recover renal function. *Quarterly Journal of Medicine* **89**, 415–421.

Black, M. and Hussain, H. (2000). Fatal hepato-renal failure associated with hyrazine sulphate. *Annals of Internal Medicine* **133**, 877–880.

Bone, R. C. *et al.* (1987). A controlled clinical trial of high dose methylprednisolone in the treatment of severe sepsis and septic shock. *New England Journal of Medicine* **317**, 653–658.

Cantu, T. G. *et al.* (1995). Acute renal failure associated with immunoglobulin therapy. *American Journal of Kidney Diseases* **25** (2), 228–234.

Chertow, G. M. *et al.* (2001). Reasons for non-enrolment in a cohort study of acute renal failure in the critically ill: the PICARD experience and implications for a clinical trials network (abstract). *Journal of the American Society of Nephrology* **12**, A0862.

Chew, S. L. *et al.* (1993). Outcome in acute renal failure. *Nephrology, Dialysis, Transplantation* **8**, 101–107.

Chugh, K. S. *et al.* (1989). Changing trends in acute renal failure in third world countries—Chandigarh study. *Quarterly Journal of Medicine* **73** (272), 1117–1123.

Clarke, R. C., Johnston, J. R., and Mayne E. E. (2000). Meningococcal septicaemia treatment with protein C concentrate. *Intensive Care Medicine* **26** (4), 471–473.

Cockroft, D. W. and Gault, M. H. (1976). Prediction of creatinine clearance from serum creatinine. *Nephron* **16**, 31–41.

Dagher, L. and Moore, K. (2001). The hepatorenal syndrome. *Gut* **49**, 729–737.

Diaz-Tejeiro, R. *et al.* (1993). Irreversible acute renal failure after extracorporeal shock-wave lithotripsy. *Nephron* **63**, 242–243.

Doherty, C. C. (1993). Modern trends in acute renal failure. *Journal of Nephrology* **2**, 123–126.

Doherty, C. C. (1995). Acute renal failure in Northern Ireland. Personal communication in *DHSS Review of Renal Services in Northern Ireland*, 38.

Druml, W. (1996). Prognosis of acute renal failure 1975–1995. *Nephron* **73**, 8–15.

Dubose, T. D. *et al.* (1997). Acute renal failure in the 21st century: recommendations for management and outcomes assessment. *American Journal of Kidney Disease* **29**, 793–799.

Duncan, L. *et al.* (2001). Screening for renal disease using serum creatinine: who are we missing? *Nephrology, Dialysis, Transplantation* **16**, 1042–1046.

Erek, E. *et al.* (2002). An overview of morbidity and mortality in patients with acute renal failure due to Crush syndrome: the Marmara earthquake experience. *Nephrology, Dialysis, Transplantation* **17**, 33–40.

Feest, T. G., Round, A., and Hamad, S. (1993). Incidence of severe acute renal failure in adults: results of a community-based study. *British Medical Journal* **306**, 481–483.

Fiaccadori, E. *et al.* (2001). Incidence, risk factors and prognosis of gastrointestinal haemorrhage complicating acute renal failure. *Kidney International* **59** (4), 1510–1519.

Fortescue, E. B., Bates, D. W., and Chertow, G. M. (2000). Predicting acute renal failure after coronary bypass surgery: cross validation of two risk stratification algorithms. *Kidney International* **57**, 2594–2602.

Gallego, N. *et al.* (1993). Prognosis of children with acute renal failure: a study of 138 cases. *Nephron* **64**, 399–404.

Gilbertson, A. A., Smith, J. M., and Mostafa, S. M. (1991). The cost of an intensive care unit: a prospective study. *Intensive Care Medicine* **17** (4), 204–208.

Gruberg, L. *et al.* (2001). Acute renal failure requiring dialysis after percutaneous coronary interventions. *Catheterisation and Cardiovascular Interventions* **52** (4), 409–416.

Gruss, E. *et al.* (1995). Acute renal failure in patients following bone marrow transplantation: prevalence, risk factors and outcome. *American Journal of Nephrology* **15**, 473–479.

Hamel, M. B. *et al.* (1997). Outcomes and cost effectiveness of initiating dialysis and continuing aggressive care in seriously ill hospitalised adults. *Annals of Internal Medicine* **127**, 195–202.

Hegarty, J. *et al.* (2001). Clinical epidemiology of acute renal failure: a prospective population based study (abstract). *Journal of the American Society of Nephrology* **12**, 2001.

Hinds, C. J. (1992). Monoclonal antibodies in sepsis and septic shock. *British Medical Journal* **304**, 132–134.

Hou, S. H. *et al.* (1983). Hospital-acquired renal insufficiency: a prospective study. *American Journal of Medicine* **74**, 243.

Jones, C. H. *et al.* (1998). Continuous venovenous high-flux dialysis in multi-organ failure: a 5 year single centre experience. *American Journal of Kidney Diseases* **31** (2), 227–233.

Kaiser, B. A. *et al.* Acute renal failure in children. In *Paediatric Nephrology* Vol. 5 (ed. A. Drukaer and A. B. Gruskin), pp. 202–213. Basel: Karger, 1994.

Kaufman, J. *et al.* (1991). Community-acquired acute renal failure. *American Journal of Kidney Diseases* **XVII** (2), 191–198.

Keller, F. *et al.* (1995). Risk factors and outcome of 107 patients with decompensated liver disease and acute renal failure (including 26 patients with hepato-renal syndrome): the role of haemodialysis. *Renal Failure* **17** (2), 135–146.

Kellum, J. A. (1997). The use of diuretics and dopamine in acute renal failure: a systematic review of the evidence. *Critical Care (London)* **1** (2), 53–59.

Khan, I. H. *et al.* (1997). Acute renal failure: factors influencing nephrology referral and outcome. *Quarterly Journal of Medicine* **90**, 781–785.

Kjellstrand, C. N., Ebben, J., and Davin, T. (1981). Time of death, recovery of renal function, development of chronic renal failure and need for chronic haemodialysis in patients with acute renal failure. *Transactions of the American Society of Artificial Internal Organs* **28**, 45–50.

Knaus, W. A. *et al.* (1986). An evaluation of outcome from intensive care in major medical centres. *Annals of Internal Medicine* **104**, 410–418.

Kolff, W. J. (1965). First clinical experience with the artificial kidney. *Annals of Internal Medicine* **62**, 608–619.

Korkeila, M., Ruokonen, E., and Takala, J. (2000). Cost of care, long term prognosis and quality of life in patients requiring renal replacement therapy during intensive care. *Intensive Care Medicine* **26** (12), 1824–1831.

Korzets, A. *et al.* (2001). Resistant shock in a haemodialysed patient—why? *Nephrology, Dialysis, Transplantation* **16** (2), 418–419.

Liano, F. (1994). Severity of acute renal failure: the need of measurement. *Nephrology, Dialysis, Transplantation* **9** (Suppl. 4), 229–238.

Liano, F., Pascual, J., and the Madrid Acute Renal Failure Study Group (1996). Epidemiology of acute renal failure: a prospective, multi-centre, community-based study. *Kidney International* **50**, 811–818.

Liano, F. *et al.* (1998). The spectrum of acute renal failure in the intensive care unit compared with that seen in other settings. *Kidney International* **53** (Suppl. 66), S16–S24.

Lins, R. L., Elseviers, M., and Daelemans, R. (2001). Problems in the development, validation and adaptation of prognostic models for acute renal failure. *Nephrology, Dialysis, Transplantation* **16**, 1098–1101.

MacDowall, P. *et al.* (1998). Risk of morbidity from renovascular disease in elderly patients with congestive cardiac failure. *Lancet* **352** (9121), 13–16.

Mahon, S. V. and Desmond, M. J. (2000). Renal support in cardiothoracic intensive care. An analysis of a service based on veno-venous haemofiltration. *British Journal of Intensive Care* January/February, 6–10.

Marik, P. E. and Zaloga, G. P. (2001). Early enteral nutrition in acutely ill patients: a systematic review. *Critical Care Medicine* **29** (12), 2264–2270.

Mehta, R., Farkas, A., Pascual, M., and Fowler, W. (1995). Effect of delayed consultation on outcome from acute renal failure (ARF) in the ICU (abstract). *Journal of the American Society of Nephrology* **6**, 471.

Mehta, R. L. *et al.* (2001). A randomised clinical trial of continuous versus intermittent dialysis for acute renal failure. *Kidney International* **60**, 1154–1163.

Metcalfe, W. *et al.* (2002). Acute renal failure requiring renal replacement therapy: incidence and outcome. *Quarterly Journal of Medicine* **95**, 579–583.

Misiani, R. *et al.* (1982). Haemolytic uraemic syndrome: therapeutic effect of plasma infusion. *British Medical Journal* **285**, 1304–1306.

Modi, G. K., Pereira, B. J. G., and Jaber, B. L. (2001). Haemodialysis in acute renal failure: does the membrane matter? *Seminars in Dialysis* **14** (5), 318–321.

Mutimer, D. J. *et al.* (1993). Managing severe alcoholic hepatitis complicated by renal failure. *Quarterly Journal of Medicine* **86**, 649–656.

Nakahami, H. and Sakaguchi, K. (2001). Small dose oral corticosteroid treatment rapidly improved renal function in a patient with an acute aggravation of chronic renal failure due to cholesterol embolism. *Nephrology, Dialysis, Transplantation* **16**, 872–873.

Nzerue, C. M., Hewan-Lowe, K., and Nwawka, C. (1998). Acute renal failure in pregnancy: a review of clinical outcomes at an inner city hospital from 1986–1996. *Journal of the National Medical Association* **90** (8), 486–490.

Office of the Surgeon General, Department of the Army. *Clinical, Physiologic and Biochemical Correlation in Lower Nephron Nephrosis* Chapter 2, *Surgery in World War II*, p. 122. The Board for the Study of Severely Wounded, 1952.

Ostermann, M. E., Taube, D., and Morgan, C. J. (2000). Acute renal failure following cardiopulmonary bypass: a changing picture. *Intensive Care Medicine* **26** (5), 565–571.

Ostermann, M. E., Chang, R. W., and Nelson, S. R. (2001). Acute renal failure acquired in ICU and need for renal replacement therapy have a significant impact on outcome and resources. *Journal of the American Society of Nephrology* **12**.

Pascual, J., Liani, F., and Ortuno, J. (1995). The elderly patient with acute renal failure. *Journal of the American Society of Nephrology* **6**, 144–153.

Pearson G., Khandelwal P. C., and Naqvi, N. (2000). Early filtration and mortality in meningococcal septic shock? *Archives of Disease in Childhood* **83** (6), 508–509.

Perazella, M. A. (1999). Crystal-induced acute renal failure. *American Journal of Medicine* **106** (4), 459–465.

Powell, J. J., Fearon, K. C. H., and Siriwardena, A. K. (2000). Current concepts of the pathophysiology and treatment of severe acute pancreatitis. *British Journal of Intensive Care* March/April, 51–59.

Power, D. A., Duggan, J., and Brady, H. R. (1999). Renal dose (low dose) dopamine for the treatment of sepsis-related and other forms of acute renal failure: ineffective and probably dangerous. *Clinical and Experimental Pharmacology and Physiology Supplement* **26**, S23–S28.

Prakash, J. *et al.* (1995). Acute renal failure in Eastern India. *Nephrology, Dialysis, Transplantation* **10**, 2009–2012.

Rao, T. K. (1998). Acute renal failure in human immunodeficiency virus infection. *Seminars in Nephrology* **18** (4), 378–395.

Renal Research Institute: The Acute Dialysis Quality Initiative. In *Dialysis Times* Vol. 7 (ed. D. L. Leven, J. M. Lazarous, and S. Parnell). New York: Renal Research Institute, 2000.

Ronco, C. *et al.* (2000). Effects of different doses in continuous veno-venous haemofiltration on outcomes of acute renal failure: a prospective randomised trial. *Lancet* **356**, 26–30.

Sanderson, P. J. (1989). Selective decontamination of the digestive tract. *British Medical Journal* **299**, 1413–1414.

Schiffl, H., Lang, S. M., and Fischer, R. (2002). Daily haemodialysis and the outcome of acute renal failure. *New England Journal of Medicine* **346**, 305–310.

Schwilk, B. *et al.* (1997). Epidemiology of acute renal failure and outcome of haemofiltration in intensive care. *Intensive Care Medicine* **23** (12), 1204–1211.

Seedat, Y. K. and Nathoo, B. C. (1993). Acute renal failure in Blacks and Indians in South Africa—comparison after 10 years. *Nephron* **64**, 198–201.

Silvester, W. (1998). Outcome studies of continuous renal replacement therapy in the intensive care unit. *Kidney International* **53** (Suppl. 66), S138–S141.

Sivalingam, M. *et al.* (2001). Intensity of care and outcome in acute renal failure: a prospective population-based study. *Journal of the American Society of Nephrology* **12**.

Steen, V. *et al.* (1990). Outcome of renal crisis in systemic sclerosis: relation to availability of ACE inhibitors. *Annals of Internal Medicine* **113** (5), 352.

Stevens, P. E. *et al.* (2001). Non-specialist management of acute renal failure. *Quarterly Journal of Medicine* **94**, 533–540.

Tan, I. K. S. and Kua, J. S. W. (1998). Abdominal compartment syndrome and acute anuria. *Nephrology, Dialysis, Transplantation* **13**, 2651–2653.

The Renal Association's Standards Sub-Committee. *Treatment of Adult Patients with Renal Failure* 2nd edn., 1997, pp. 51–57.

Tran, D. D. *et al.* (1993). Acute renal failure in patients with acute pancreatitis: prevalence, risk factors, and outcome. *Nephrology, Dialysis, Transplantation* **8**, 1079–1084.

Turney, J. H. *et al.* (1990). The evolution of acute renal failure, 1956–1988. *Quarterly Journal of Medicine* **74** (273), 83–104.

van Ypersele de Strihou, C. and van Herweghem, J. L. (1995). The tragic pardigm of Chinese herbs nephropathy. *Nephrology, Dialysis, Transplantation* **10** (2), 157–160.

Wilkinson, S. P. *et al.* (1977). Dialysis in the treatment of renal failure in patients with liver disease. *Clinical Nephrology* **8**, 287–292.

Woodrow, G. and Turney, J. H. (1992). Cause of death in acute renal failure. *Nephrology, Dialysis, Transplantation* **7**, 230–234.

Woolfson, R. G. and Lachman, H. (1998). Improvement in renal cholesterol emboli syndrome after simvastatin. *Lancet* **351**, 1331–1332.

10.2 Acute renal failure: pathophysiology and prevention

Norbert Hendrik Lameire and Raymond Camille Vanholder

Introduction

Acute renal failure (ARF) is defined as a rapid (hours to weeks) deterioration of the glomerular filtration rate (GFR), associated with the accumulation of waste products such as urea and creatinine (azotaemia). Oliguria (urine output < 400 ml/day or <20 ml/h) is frequent (~50 per cent), but not invariable. It is a clinical syndrome that may be caused by many renal and extrarenal diseases. For purposes of differential diagnosis and management, ARF is conveniently subclassified into prerenal azotaemia, a physiological response to renal hypoperfusion in which the integrity of the renal tissue is preserved; intrinsic renal azotaemia in which ARF is caused by diseases of the renal parenchyma; and postrenal azotaemia due to acute obstruction of the urinary tract.

Prerenal factors contribute 30–60 per cent to all cases of ARF and is frequently community acquired, especially in the aged population (see Chapter 10.7.4).

Postrenal factors (e.g. intra- or extrarenal obstruction of urine flow) are much less frequently encountered (1–10 per cent of hospital-acquired ARF) and are almost always amenable to therapy.

The renal causes can be categorized according to the anatomic compartment predominantly involved in the injury. Although acute vascular, glomerular, and interstitial processes may cause ARF (~15 per cent of all cases of hospital-acquired ARF), the major cause of ARF is 'acute tubular necrosis' (ATN). ATN is caused by ischaemic or nephrotoxic injury to the kidney in 50 and 35 per cent of all causes of hospital-acquired ARF, respectively. However, in 50 per cent of the cases, the cause is multifactorial.

The term 'tubular necrosis' (commonly employed in clinical practice) is a misnomer because the alterations are not limited to the tubular structures and true cellular necrosis is often minimal. Neither the incidence nor the morbidity and mortality associated with ATN has declined despite improvements in supportive care and renal replacement therapy. One of the reasons for this lack of improvement is a change in the severity of the underlying diseases causing ARF.

Besides vascular derangements, tubular obstruction, and urinary backleak, newer concepts of the pathophysiology of ATN, including the role of inflammation, 'sublethal' cell injury, apoptosis, and cell repair after injury are emerging. The interplay of all these explain the acute decrease in GFR, which is the result of intrarenal vasoconstriction with a reduction in glomerular filtration pressure, vascular congestion in the outer medulla, activation of the tubuloglomerular feedback (TGF) as a result of enhanced delivery of solute to the macula densa ('the vascular component'), and tubular obstruction, transtubular backleak of the filtrate, and interstitial inflammation ('the tubular component') (Fig. 1).

Pathophysiology of prerenal failure

Prerenal azotaemia is the most common cause of both community- and hospital-acquired ARF and is an appropriate physiological response to

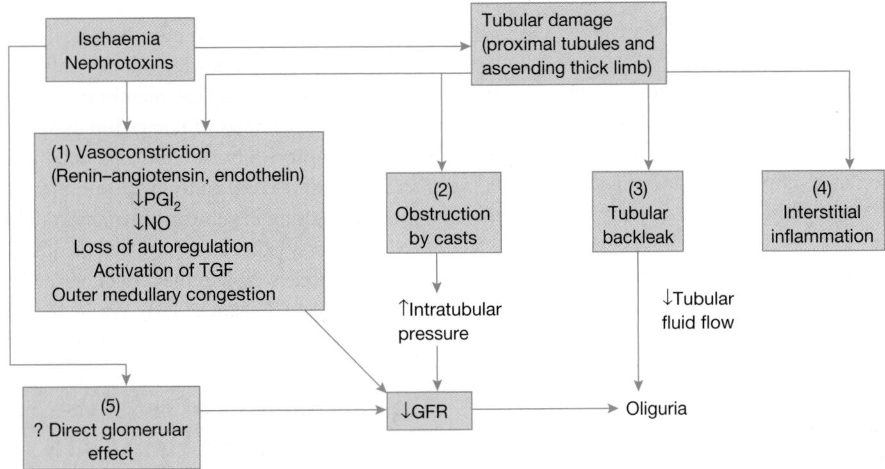

Fig. 1 Interplay of factors explaining the acute decrease in GFR. Adapted from Cotran, R., Kumar, V., and Robbins, S.L. (1994).

renal hypoperfusion (Blantz 1998). When not corrected, severe renal hypoperfusion will ultimately lead to ischaemic ATN and both prerenal azotaemia and ischaemic ATN are part of a continuum of manifestations of renal hypoperfusion. Prerenal disease can complicate any disease characterized by either 'true hypovolaemia' or a reduction in the 'effective circulating volume', such as low cardiac output, systemic vasodilatation, or intrarenal vasoconstriction. Hypovolaemia will lead to a reduction in systemic blood pressure, which, in turn, activates cardiovascular baroreceptors and initiates activation of the sympathetic nervous system, the renin–angiotensin–aldosterone system, and the release of vasopressin as well as other vasopressors, including endothelin. All these factors act in concert to maintain the blood pressure and preserve cardiac output and cerebral perfusion. Drugs interfering with the autoregulation of renal blood flow (RBF) and GFR may also provoke acute prerenal failure.

Protection of the renal perfusion in states of haemodynamic derangement

Autoregulation of RBF and GFR

The kidney responds to haemodynamic derangements by autoregulating RBF and GFR to a relatively constant level of renal perfusion pressure. When the blood pressure falls, a gradual vasodilatation of preglomerular arterioles, mediated primarily by an intrinsic myogenic mechanism, occurs. In the lower zone of autoregulation, concomitant vasoconstriction at the postglomerular arteriole, mainly under the influence of angiotensin II (A II), is necessary to maintain a constant glomerular capillary hydrostatic pressure. The autoregulation of RBF and GFR may be overcome under conditions of severe volume depletion or serious systemic circulatory derangement. In these situations, the decline in GFR is caused by a failure to increase the postglomerular vascular resistance because of the already high levels of A II.

The tubulo-glomerular feedback mechanism stabilizes both GFR and fluid delivery to the distal nephron. This is responsible for an inverse dependence of the single nephron GFR on late proximal flow and is mediated by complex communication between the macula densa and the glomerular microvasculature. In settings of acute volume depletion, associated with increased proximal reabsorption, tubulo-glomerular feedback mitigates the prerenal reduction in GFR, although this mitigation is partially countered by a resetting of the feedback (for review, see Blantz 1998).

Vasodilating substances

A variety of vasodilating substances are activated when systemic haemodynamics are compromised. Natriuretic peptides increase the GFR with a decrease in afferent arteriolar resistance and an increase in efferent arteriolar resistance; they inhibit renin and aldosterone secretion and interact with the sympathetic nerve system (Awazu and Ichikawa 1994).

A central part of the protective vasodilation is mediated by the secondary intrarenal generation of vasodilating products of arachidonic acid (AA) (i.e. PGI_2) (Dzau *et al.* 1984) and of nitric oxide (NO) (De Nicola *et al.* 1992).

Angiotensin stimulates synthesis of PGI_2 and PGE_2 within the kidney and the vasodilating prostaglandins act to preserve GFR in situations such as sodium depletion, surgical stress, and reduced cardiac output. Acute cyclo-oxygenase inhibition reduces the GFR and RBF in these conditions.

Nitric oxide

NO which mediates diverse functions including vasodilation (Wilcox 2000), is formed by a family of NO synthases (NOS) including the inducible isoform (iNOS) and the constitutively expressed isoforms neuronal (nNOS) and endothelial (eNOS) NOS. Although NO exerts similar tonic influences as an antagonist of A II, it also appears to stimulate the renin–angiotensin system such that chronic reduction in NO activity can result in reduced intrarenal A II generation (De Nicola *et al.* 1993).

Other important factors playing a role in the autoregulation process include serotonin, which is important for effective RBF autoregulation in ischaemic and nephrotoxic models of ARF.

Cytochrome P-450 metabolites of arachidonic acid (AA) (Maier and Roman 2001)

20-Hydroxyeicosatetraenoic acid (20-HETE) produced by renal vascular smooth muscle (VSM) cells is a potent vasoconstrictor. Inhibition of the formation of 20-HETE blocks the autoregulation of RBF and TGF responses *in vivo* and attenuates the renal vasoconstrictor response to A II, endothelin, norepinephrine, and vasopressin by approximately 50 per cent. Vasoconstrictor agonists stimulate the endogenous production of 20-HETE in renal VSM cells, and 20-HETE contributes to vasoconstrictor responses to these agonists. 20-HETE also plays an important role in the regulation of TGF responses in the kidney.

Prevention of prerenal acute renal failure

Prerenal azotaemia can be corrected if the extrarenal factors causing the renal hypoperfusion are reversed, for example, extracellular volume expansion, enhancement of cardiac output, correction of the causes of systemic vasodilatation, or stopping antihypertensive drugs.

The distinction between established ATN and prerenal failure is often difficult, especially in patients suffering from polyuric acute prerenal failure where the renal concentrating defect causes excessive water excretion with relative sodium chloride retention secondary to volume losses.

Acute tubular necrosis

Early studies on the pathophysiology of ATN were descriptive and an understanding of the mechanisms involved the development of experimental models. The morphological characteristics of ischaemia-induced ARF in animals include loss of the proximal tubular brush border, blebbing of apical membranes, cellular and mitochondrial swelling, and pyknosis of nuclei and apoptosis (Racusen 2001). With advanced injury, tubular epithelial cells detach from the basement membrane and contribute to intraluminal aggregation of cells and proteins resulting in tubular obstruction (Thadhani *et al.* 1996).

Controversy exists as to how well the histological findings observed in animal models explain the reduction in GFR that occurs in humans (Lieberthal and Nigam 2000). While the reported animal data are consistent, their relevance to human ischaemic ARF is debatable.

The mechanisms of renal vasoconstriction in experimental and human ATN (Fig. 2)

Renal vasoconstriction, the result of an increase in afferent and efferent arteriolar vascular resistance with a concomitant decrease in

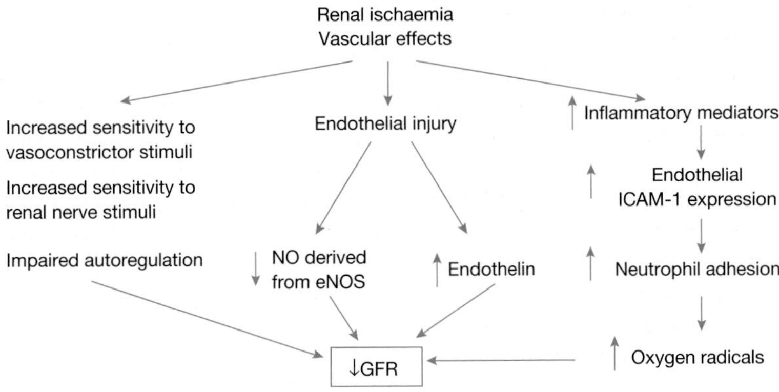

Fig. 2 Mechanisms of renal vasoconstriction. From Kribben *et al.* (1999).

glomerular plasma flow (~30–50 per cent decrease from normal values) and a resultant decrease in glomerular hydrostatic pressure, occurs both in the initiation phase and, to a lesser extent, in the maintenance phase of most ischaemic and toxic models of ARF (for review, see Conger 1998). Circulatory vasoconstrictors (e.g. catecholamines, A II, and endothelin) as well as renal sympathetic tone are frequently increased in the setting of ischaemic and nephrotoxic ATN (Lieberthal 1997). In addition, the renal vascular response to these vasoconstrictors is enhanced, in part due to the increase in cytosolic calcium concentration in the preglomerular arterioles (Yaqoob *et al.* 1997). However, the magnitude of the decline in RBF is, by itself, not sufficient to account for the almost complete cessation of the GFR. Moreover, following the initial insult, RBF may return to normal either spontaneously or in response to vasodilating pharmacological manoeuvres, yet GFR does not improve in parallel.

The role of the *renin–angiotensin* system in promoting renal vasoconstriction has attracted interest after the observations of increased juxtaglomerular cell granularity in kidneys of patients who died of ARF (Goormaghtigh 1945), together with the finding of increased activity of the renin–angiotensin system in early and sustained phases of experimental ATN (for review, see Conger 2001). However, no consistent evidence for a causative role of A II in the pathogenesis of ARF was found, in particular by maneuvers that suppress the renin–angiotensin system; including immunization against renin and treatment with angiotensin-converting enzyme (ACE) inhibitors.

Because both prior renal denervation and administration of phenoxybenzamine offers protection in some models of ARF, enhanced adrenergic activity and increased vascular sensitivity to renal nerve activity were considered as possible mediators of vasoconstriction. However, phenoxybenzamine failed to increase RBF in established ARF in humans, which argues against a significant adrenergic contribution (Conger and Schrier 1980).

Recent attention has focused on the importance of *sublethal ischaemic toxic endothelial cell injury*, causing an imbalance in the production of endothelin and endothelial NO (Lieberthal 1997). The vasoconstrictive and mitogenic actions of *endothelin* (ET-1) are mediated through two distinct subtypes of membrane receptors. Activation of the ET(A) receptor, which is abundant on VSM cells increases the intracellular calcium, leading to prolonged vasoconstriction. In contrast, activation of ET(B) receptors, localized on endothelial cells, induces the release of NO, leading to vasodilation (Rubanyi and Polokoff 1994). Increased circulating and kidney tissue ET-1 protein and ET(A) and ET(B) receptor gene expression have been demonstrated in ARF. It is possible that the sustained increase in ET-1 in ARF is caused, at least partly, by decreased neutral endopeptidase (NEP) expression in injured proximal tubular cells, leading to decreased ET-1 degradation (Ruschitzka *et al.* 1999). Endothelin receptor antagonists ameliorate the diminution of renal haemodynamics in experimental ARF (for recent summary see Lameire and Vanholder 2000).

Many of the actions of endothelin are counteracted by constitutively expressed, as well as endothelin-induced NO (Peters *et al.* 1999). The pivotal role of NO in endothelial dysfunction and its dual role in the pathophysiology of ARF have recently been summarized (Goligorsky *et al.* 2000). NO is vasodilatory and decreases endothelin expression and activity in the vascular endothelium, effects that should be protective against renal injury.

The response to endothelium-dependent vasodilators, such as acetylcholine and bradykinin, is reduced in experimental ARF, while the constrictor response to inhibition of NOS by N(G)-nitro-L-arginine-methyl ester (L-NAME) is increased. The eNOS activity is normal to increased, not decreased, in the renal vasculature. These findings suggest that NOS activity is operating at high intensity with maximal stimulation of the guanylate cyclase dilator pathway, such that NO agonists and donors have a reduced effect. It could be that this apparent increase in NOS activity acts as a protective counter-regulatory modulator of the response to an underlying vasoconstrictor stimulus produced by ischaemia. In contrast, a downregulation of eNO has been observed in other forms of ischaemic ARF (Whelton 2000), while in experimental sepsis, the NO secondary to iNOS downregulates eNOS (Schwartz and Blantz 1999).

Impaired autoregulation of RBF, observed in many models of ARF makes the kidney vulnerable to recurrent ischaemic injury (for review, see Conger 2001) because any decrease in mean arterial pressure results in a further decline in RBF and often in paradoxical vasoconstriction. This increased vulnerability is a possible reason for the finding of fresh tubular ischaemic lesions as much as 4 weeks after the initiation of human ARF (Solez *et al.* 1979). In some ARF models, changes in renal VSM cell calcium as well as changes in afferent arteriolar lumen diameter were observed. The calcium channel blocker, verapamil, dilated afferent arterioles and normalized the deteriorated autoregulation. The mechanisms underlying the loss of autoregulation are complex and involve injury to endothelial and VSM cells, causing an imbalance between vasodilator and vasoconstrictor systems (Conger 2001).

Other endothelial vasoconstrictors may also play a role, such as platelet activating factor (PAF), a vasoconstrictor metabolite of phospholipases (Kelly *et al.* 1996a), serotonin (Verbeke *et al.* 1998), and adenosine (Rudnick *et al.* 1996).

Adenosine has biphasic effects on RBF and renin release via intrarenal A_1 and A_2 adenosine receptor activation. Adenosine also reduces renal sympathetic activity, lowers the GFR, and controls the modulation of TGF mechanism via A_1 adenosine receptor activation. With A_2 adenosine receptor activation, it increases medullary blood flow. The role of A_3 adenosine receptor in the kidney is unknown at the present time.

Heterogeneity of renal blood flow

Heterogeneity of RBF plays an important role in the pathophysiology of ARF. The isolated rat kidney perfused with erythrocyte-free perfusate demonstrated a higher susceptibility for ischaemic damage in the inner stripe of the outer medulla where the tissue partial pressure of oxygen is lowest. This vulnerability has been attributed to the mismatch between the vigorous metabolic demand, and the inadequate oxygen delivery to the medullary thick ascending limb (mTAL) of Henle's loop (Brezis and Rosen 1995). The principal determinant of the medullary oxygen requirement is the rate of active sodium reabsorption along the mTAL, which is responsible for the generation of the medullary osmotic gradient. In view of the low ambient PO_2 in the medulla, the stage is set for tubular cell hypoxia and tubular dysfunction, should either oxygen delivery (e.g. RBF) fall or tubular cell oxygen demand increase. Dehydration, salt and volume depletion, and renal hypoperfusion are major stimuli of urine concentration and active sodium reabsorption, which may, therefore, exacerbate hypoxic tubular damage. Conversely, medullary hypoxia can be ameliorated by either increasing oxygen delivery (i.e. using vasodilators such as NO, PGE_2, and dopamine) (Chou *et al.* 1990) or reducing work. The latter can be achieved by proper hydration and salt loading, which obviate the need for urine concentration, or by inhibition of active transport by loop diuretics (e.g. frusemide) (Brezis and Rosen 1995). It is in this area that the TGF is thought to play an important role. The GFR in ARF may be decreased in part as a consequence of a reduced proximal tubular sodium reabsorption leading to an increased sodium chloride concentration and delivery to the macula densa. This enhanced delivery reduces the single nephron filtration rate as a consequence of an increase in Cl uptake through the $Na_2^-Cl^-K$ cotransporter at the macula densa which enhances the voltage in the macula densa cells. This causes increased TGF sensitivity and renin secretion (Schnermann and Briggs 2000), which in turn leads to a decrease in GFR, and to a decreased amount of sodium being presented to that tubule for reabsorption. This sequence of events leads to activation of TGF, manifested clinically as oliguria, which is an appropriate physiological response and has been called 'acute renal success' (Thurau and Boylan 1976).

The outer medullary ischaemia (Bankir *et al.* 1998) in ARF can at least in part be explained by enhanced leucocyte–endothelial interactions which physically impede blood flow in this segment due to a combination of endothelial injury together with leucocyte activation (Rabb and Postler 1998). Two molecules that have already been discussed, endothelin and NO, affect endothelial–leucocyte adhesion. ET-1 modulates neutrophil adhesion and enhances leucocyte rolling and adhesion, an effect abrogated by anti-P-selectin antibody (Sanz *et al.* 1999). After adherence and chemotaxis, infiltrating leucocytes release reactive oxygen species (ROS) and enzymes that damage the cells (Thadhani *et al.* 1996). Infusion of normal neutrophils accentuate severe ischaemia/reperfusion injury and decreases GFR during ischaemia, while oxygen radical deficient neutrophils did not influence the course of experimental ischaemic injury when infused in rats (Lauriat and Linas 1998). It is likely that both the release of potent vasoconstrictors including the prostaglandins, leukotrienes and thromboxanes, as well as direct endothelial injury, via release of endothelin and a decrease in NO are involved (Lieberthal 1997). The role of leucocyte infiltration into the renal interstitium is discussed in the section on tubular factors.

Besides affecting vascular tone and direct toxic effects on cells (see later), NO also modulates both neutrophil and epithelial cell adhesion. NO inhibits TNF-α-induced adhesion of neutrophils to endothelial cells, which should also be protective. It is possible that these leucocyte–endothelial interactions have a greater impact on outer medullary ischaemia than does vasoconstriction of preglomerular arterioles. Figure 3 summarizes the vascular and tubular effects of endothelin, NO, and leucocytes in the pathogenesis of ischaemic acute renal failure.

Clinical studies on renal haemodynamics in ARF

The severity and duration of ischaemia required to lead to ARF in humans are unknown. Following development of renal ischaemia, there is an interval that operationally defines the transition from functional prerenal to fixed postischaemic ARF. Restoration of RBF by volume expansion or vasodilators restores renal function during the functional stage but not after the establishment of fixed ARF. Whereas in some patients, severe and prolonged ischaemia may be inconsequential, susceptible patients may develop fixed ARF after only modest ischaemia of brief duration.

Clinical studies of fixed postischaemic ARF of variable duration have shown RBF ranging from 25 to 55 per cent of normal in the face of reductions in GFR to less that 5 per cent of normal (for review, see Conger 2001). Inert gas techniques have revealed a preferential cortical hypoperfusion (Hollenberg *et al.* 1968). It is now accepted that the cortical vasoconstriction is global in human ATN, but its pathogenetic role in maintaining the renal dysfunction in human ATN remains in doubt. Despite reversal of vasoconstriction by the intrarenal infusion of vasodilators, no improvement of renal function was noted (Conger 2001). It is likely that the persistent hypofiltration is attributable to other factors such as a decrease in glomerular permeability coefficient, K_f, or tubular factors such as tubular obstruction, or abnormal tubular leakiness (see later).

Careful investigations of the renal haemodynamics have been performed in renal transplant recipients with delayed graft function (DGF) (Corrigan *et al.* 1999).

Using both direct measurements and indirect estimates of GFR determinants, it was shown that renal plasma flow and the calculated net hydraulic driving force (ΔP) for primary glomerular filtration in recipients with DGF were low. The glomerular ultrafiltration coefficient was normal, and there was no evidence of tubular obstruction, pointing toward afferent arteriolar constriction (Alejandro *et al.* 1995a). Subsequently, using *p*-aminohippurate extraction, phase-contrast cine magnetic resonance imaging and intraoperative Doppler flowmeter, the same investigators found only small depressions in RBF despite

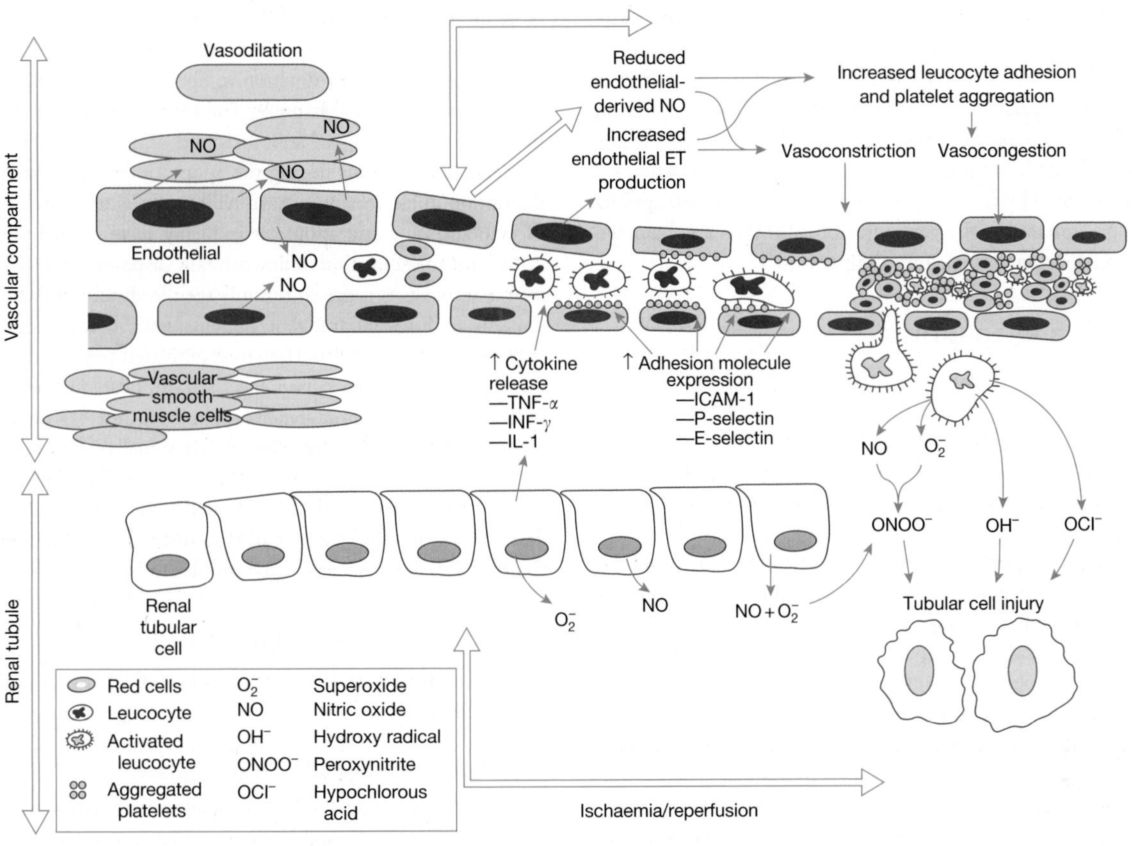

Fig. 3 Role of vascular and tubular effects of endothelin, NO, and leucocytes in the pathogenesis of ischaemic acute renal failure. From Lieberthal (1998).

profound reductions in GFR (Corrigan *et al.* 1999), suggesting that human postischaemic ARF occurs independent of a profound decrease in RBF (Ramaswamy *et al.* 2002).

On the other hand, other studies of the same group supported a higher role for tubular fluid backleak and possible increased sodium delivery from the proximal tubule to activate the tubulo-glomerular feedback system and reflex afferent arteriolar constriction (Kwon *et al.* 1999).

Despite the apparent contradictions in some of the data, it is believed that the reduced glomerular filtration pressure (ΔP) is more important than tubular obstruction. There is no information regarding changes in K_f, the glomerular ultrafiltration coefficient, in human postischaemic ARF.

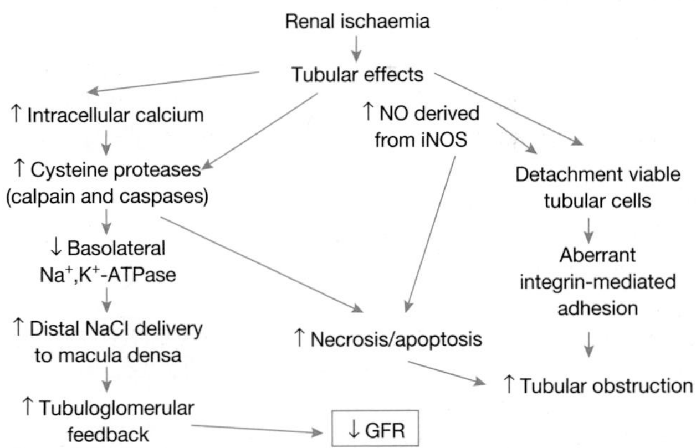

Fig. 4 Tubular factors in the pathophysiology of ATN. From Kribben *et al.* (1999).

Tubular factors in the pathophysiology of ATN (Fig. 4)

Morphological observations of luminal casts, tubule dilatation, and disruption in the integrity of tubular epithelium, although inconsistent, have been interpreted as indicative of tubule obstruction and backleak in human postischaemic ARF (Racusen 2001). Studies on the fractional urinary clearance of dextran molecules of graded size (clearance dextran/clearance inulin) in postischaemic, non-oliguric ARF following cardiac surgery have inferred that some 40–50 per cent of the filtrate was lost by tubular backleak (Myers *et al.* 1984). Observations on the kinetics of inulin excretion in patients with postischaemic, protracted ARF following cardiac surgery (beyond 14 days) have indicated the presence of sluggish tubular fluid flow, a finding consistent with, although not diagnostic of, severe and generalized intraluminal tubular obstruction.

Ischaemic or toxic injury to tissues triggers a complex series of metabolic disturbances, often culminating in cell death. Cell death may occur under two forms: necrosis or apoptosis. Furthermore, the importance of sublethal injury to tubular cells as it relates to the phenotype of cell death is increasingly appreciated (Lieberthal *et al.* 1998). Many intracellular mediators have been implicated in altering the balance between apoptosis and necrosis. Cellular necrosis results from the combined deleterious effects of a number of biochemical pathways precipitated by severe injury to the cell. In contrast, apoptosis although precipitated by the same injurious stimuli is an organized, genetically predetermined final common pathway.

Cell necrosis and apoptosis

The multiple biochemical pathways that are activated by severe cell injury and lead to cell necrosis include all of the following: severe depletion of cell energy stores [adenosine 5-triphosphate (ATP) depletion]; an increase in cytosolic free calcium; the generation of ROS; and the activation of multiple enzymes, including phospholipases, proteases, and endonucleases (Fig. 5).

Changes typical of apoptosis include condensation of the cell and of the nuclei, DNA fragmentation into nucleosomal units of 200-bp fragments, chromatin condensation, generation of evoluted membrane segments (zeiosis), formation of apoptotic bodies, cellular shrinkage, and disintegration of mitochondria. Unlike necrosis, apoptotic cell death is an active process that requires participation of the dying cell and changes in cellular biochemistry. Because apoptosis does not result in the release of intracellular material into the extracellular space, it does not result in an inflammatory response (Bonegio and Lieberthal 2002) (Fig. 6). In brief, almost all apoptotic stimuli induce the activation of some specific proteases, called caspases, which form a whole family of different cysteine-proteases cleaving target proteins at asparagine residues. An important function in apoptosis is also played by sphingomyelinases and ion channels. The mitochondrion is one of the key players in most forms of apoptosis and undergoes several typical and irreversible alterations during the apoptotic process, finally leading to disruption of electron transport, ATP production, as well as the release of cytochrome *c* and apoptosis-inducing factor, which are absolutely critical for the activation of downstream caspases and DNAses, respectively. Apoptosis is more commonly seen in distal tubular cells, both in animals and in allografts of patients with biopsy confirmed ATN (Oberbauer *et al.* 1999). The stress activated protein kinase (SAPK), p54 c-Jun *N*-terminal kinase, has been implicated in cell injury and is increased with ischaemia–reperfusion *in vivo* and ATP depletion *in vitro* (Pombo *et al.* 1994). The extracellular signal-related kinase (ERK) is activated in the distal cells but not in the proximal tubule cells (PTCs). c-Jun terminal kinase (JNK) is activated in both. This imbalance in ERK and p54 SAPK activity may partly account for the differential susceptibility of the proximal and distal tubules to injury.

Mechanisms of cellular damage

Figure 5 summarizes the most important biochemical pathways leading to cell necrosis.

Depletion of adenosine 5′-triphosphate

When cells are subjected to a severe deficiency of oxygen or to cytotoxic events, ATP depletion will be the proximate event; in cytotoxic injury,

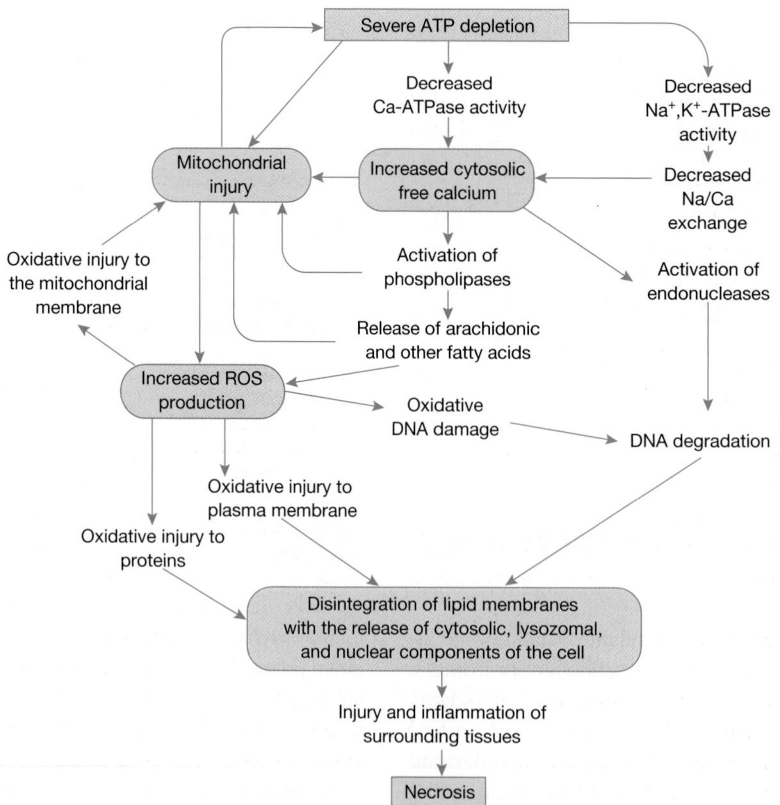

Fig. 5 Multiple biochemical pathways that lead to cell necrosis. From Levine and Lieberthal (2001).

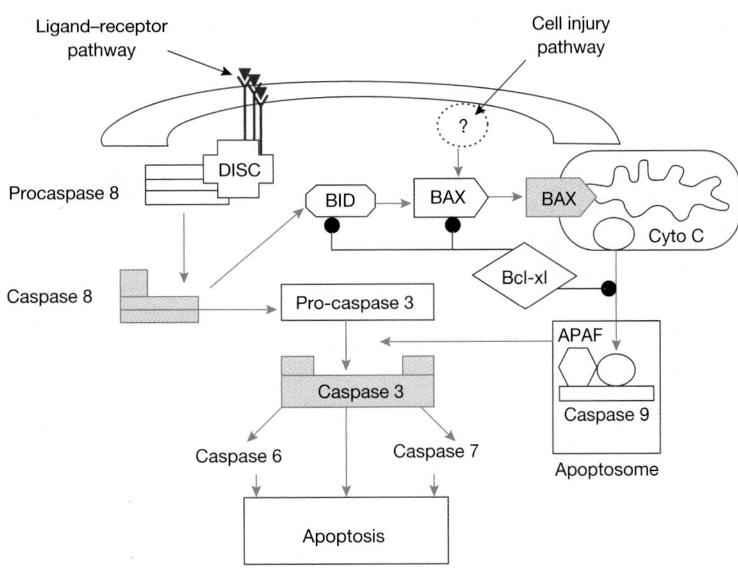

Fig. 6 Apoptotic stimuli that induce the activation of caspases. From Bonegio and Lieberthal (2002).

the initial damage may not be ATP depletion, but rather injury to cellular components such as cell membranes and proteins. However, these cytotoxic events will rapidly lead to mitochondrial injury, so that depletion of cell ATP stores ultimately occurs as a secondary event. For example, in ischaemic cell damage the rapid degradation of available ATP to adenosine 5′-diphosphate (ADP) and adenosine 5′-monophosphate (AMP) will, in case of prolonged hypoxia, lead to further metabolization of AMP to nucleosides (adenosine and inosine) and hypoxanthine.

These nucleosides are able to diffuse passively from the cell. As a result, metabolites that could serve as a reservoir for the rapid restoration of ATP during reperfusion become depleted. Eventual *de novo* synthesis of ATP from non-purine precursors, a process that itself requires a substantial amount of energy is not able to replace the ATP content.

Prolonged ischaemia ultimately leads to irreversible loss of mitochondrial function, further impairing rapid regeneration of ATP following reperfusion. Thus, the rate of recovery of cell ATP following reperfusion and the ability of the cell to survive ischaemia depend upon the duration of the ischaemic period (Lieberthal 1997).

The three most important factors that determine the sensitivity of individual renal tubular cells to ischaemic renal injury are the cell's energy requirements, its glycolytic capacity, and the severity of the hypoxia to which the cell is exposed. ATP can be generated via both glycolysis and oxidative phosphorylation. Cells that have a high glycolytic capacity are generally less sensitive to oxygen deprivation than cells that depend predominantly or exclusively on mitochondrial respiration. It is thus not surprising that the proximal tubule, which depends largely on mitochondrial respiration for its energy supply, is more susceptible to ATP depletion than more distal nephrons (Lieberthal and Nigam 1998).

Oxygen tensions vary widely within different regions in the kidney following ischaemia, with the medulla becoming far more hypoxic than the cortex. This probably explains the observation that the medullary straight portion of the proximal tubule (pars recta), which has more glycolytic capacity than the cortical segments of the proximal tubule, is more sensitive than cortical segments to ischaemic injury *in vivo* but more resistant than cortical segments to injury, when isolated tubular segments are subjected to hypoxia *in vitro* (Lieberthal and Nigam 1998).

Cytoskeleton

Cytoskeletal alterations occurring in PTCs during ischaemia play a major role in the structural, biochemical, and functional alterations that occur at both the cellular and the organ level (Atkinson and Molitoris 2001). The observed changes in ischaemia are secondary, in large part, to disruption of the cortical actin cytoskeleton, with distinctive disruption of apical brush border microvilli occurring rapidly and in a duration-dependent fashion. Microvillar membranes internalize into the cell's cytosol or are shed into the lumen as 'blebs'. These transformations result in a substantial loss of apical membrane surface area, thus reducing effective reabsorption and the blebs, shed into the lumen often aggregate, causing tubular obstruction. Actin and the actin-binding proteins, villin, and ezrin are concentrated in apical brush border microvilli. Changes in the distribution of these proteins manifest with the loss of cell polarity and consequently reduce the vectorial sodium transport. Alterations in the cortical actin cytoskeleton also mediate basolateral membrane changes, including untethering of surface membrane proteins and disruption of functional complexes. The normal localization of Na^+,K^+-ATPase to the basolateral membrane is regulated by direct interactions with the membrane-associated cytoskeletal proteins ankyrin, fodrin, and spectrin (Matlin and Caplan 2000).

In models of ischaemia using ATP depletion, the Na^+,K^+-ATPase relocates from its normal location on the basolateral plasma membrane to the apical membrane.

In humans, DGF is characterized by massive disruption of the cytoskeleton of the proximal tubular cells. Attenuation of the brush border of apical membranes and marked loss of basolateral membrane infoldings were evident in 50 per cent of the cells and approximately 50 per cent of Na^+,K^+-ATPase and the cytoskeletal proteins, ankyrin and fodrin, move from the basolateral membrane into the cytoplasm (Alejandro *et al.* 1995b).

Alterations in intracellular calcium

Hypoxia in isolated proximal rat tubules was associated with a significant increase in free intracellular calcium that preceded evidence of membrane damage. In the presence of glycine, an increase in free intracellular calcium was also observed during hypoxia in rat and in rabbit proximal tubules (Kribben *et al.* 1994). These results indicate that the observed increase in free intracellular calcium is not a consequence of lethal cell damage with disruption of the plasma membrane because prevention of lytic plasma membrane damage by glycine should have prevented the increase in free cytosolic calcium. Glycine is known to protect the cell against ischaemia-induced damage (Venkatachalam *et al.* 1996).

Low extracellular calcium also prevented the hypoxia-induced increase in free intracellular calcium, indicating that it is primarily due to net calcium entry (i.e. calcium influx > efflux) from the extracellular compartment into the cells. Reducing the free intracellular calcium using intracellular calcium chelators and by the extracellular calcium chelator EGTA to prevent net calcium entry into the cells resulted in marked cytoprotection against hypoxic proximal tubular injury (Kribben *et al.* 1994).

Activation of cysteine proteases

Calpain is a major Ca^{2+}-dependent cytosolic cysteine protease, which is ubiquitously present in most cell types. Activated calpain degrades cytoskeletal proteins involved in the interaction of the cell cytoskeleton with the plasma membrane. Calpain can also proteolyze substrate proteins after it is released into the cytosol. Calpain can also disassemble the anchoring of proteins in the plasma membrane, for example, the complex of Na^+,K^+-ATPase, ankyrin and spectrin, which will impair the anchoring of the Na^+,K^+-ATPase at the basolateral membrane.

Calpain is a mediator of hypoxic injury to rat proximal tubules (Edelstein 2000). Inhibition of the hypoxia-induced increase in calpain activity by chemically dissimilar cysteine protease inhibitors elicited cytoprotection against PTC membrane damage.

Other cysteine proteases include the caspases, which play, as explained above, a major role in apoptosis and in the activation of proinflammatory cytokines.

Phospholipase activation

The activation of several phospholipases is a characteristic feature of both ischaemic and nephrotoxic cellular damage. The substrate for cellular phospholipases are phospholipids in the membrane bilayer, which in turn are responsible for maintaining the integrity of the cell and the organelles. AA is an sn-2 fatty acid which is generated by action of phopholipase A2, and once liberated serves as the precursor for generation of vasoactive eicosnoids (e.g. prostaglandins). Besides direct hydrolysis of membrane phospholipids, additional mechanisms for cell damage following phospholipase A2 activation include direct toxicity of released fatty acids, vasoactive and chemoattractant properties of eicosanoids, direct toxicity of lysophospholipids and its PAF derivative, and the production of ROS, as a result of the metabolism of AA. Furthermore, AA directly compromises oxidative phosphorylation and it also impairs Na^+,K^+-ATPase activity (Levine and Lieberthal 2001).

Three major classes of phospholipase A2 have been recognized, based on their calcium dependence. In particular, cytosolic phospholipase A2 plays a major role in intracellular signal transduction, and is active at calcium concentrations that follow ATP depletion. Also the role of calcium-independent phospholipase A2 in tubule injury following ATP depletion has been well established. Specific inhibition of this enzyme was protective against tubule cell damage.

Nitric oxide (see also Fig. 3)

The role of NO in the haemodynamics of ARF has been described above, but NO is also an important mediator of hypoxia-induced PTC injury (Goligorsky *et al.* 2002). The prevention of iNOS induction by α-melanocyte-stimulating hormone (α-MSH) during ischaemia/reperfusion was associated with functional protection (Chiao *et al.* 1997); and *in vivo* targeting of iNOS with oligonucleotides specifically directed against iNOS–mRNA prevented both the induction of iNOS in whole kidney protein extracts and the increase in nitrite produced by isolated proximal tubules.

NO also plays a role in cell adhesion and locomotion and serves as a switch from stationary to a locomoting epithelial phenotype. In addition, NO, through the action of its metabolite peroxynitrite ($OONO^-$), impairs renal tubular epithelial cell–matrix attachment. This impairment of renal tubular epithelial cell–matrix adhesion may contribute to the tubular obstruction and delay recovery of the tubular epithelium during ARF.

Adhesion receptors and integrins and their role in tubular obstruction

Tubular obstruction has been described in sustained failure of GFR in animal models with an increase in proximal tubular pressure (de Rougemont *et al.* 1982). However, in general, tubular casts and dilated tubules are less frequently observed in human ARF than in animal models (Bohle *et al.* 1990).

Integrins are heterodimeric glycoproteins that recognize the most common universal tripeptide sequence, arginine–glycine–aspartic acid (RGD), which is present in a variety of matrix proteins (Goligorsky *et al.* 1993). These integrins can mediate cell–cell adhesion via an RGD inhibitable mechanism. In tubular cells exposed to oxidative stress, depletion of integrins expressed on the basal surface leads to the loss of anchorage to the basement membrane and cell desquamation. Detachment of viable tubular cells is caused by movement of integrins from a predominantly basolateral location to the apical membrane (Romanov *et al.* 1997). Desquamated cells and cellular conglomerates obstructing the tubular lumina were intensely stained with RGD peptides (Goligorsky *et al.* 1998). Expression of integrin receptors on the apical cell membrane may further lead to promiscuous interactions, for example, the adhesion of desquamated cells to the cells remaining *in situ*, thus initiating the process of tubular obstruction.

An additional potential mechanism of tubular obstruction is the binding of tubular cells to Tamm–Horsfall protein (THP). THP has a RGD sequence and neutrophil adhesion to THP is inhibited by synthetic RGD peptides (Toma *et al.* 1994). Therefore, a functionally significant specific RGD mediated binding between tubular cells and THP may promote tubule cast formation, distal tubular obstruction and decreased GFR.

These integrin-based interactions can be blocked by infusion of synthetic cyclic RGD peptides into the renal artery (Noiri *et al.* 1994). Components of integrin receptors are known substrates for calpain and NO. In cultured renal epithelial cells, both calpain and NOS inhibition prevent cell detachment from the extracellular matrix and it has been hypothesized that either NO, calpain or both cause decreased cell adhesion that results in proximal tubule detachment from the extracellular matrix (Edelstein *et al.* 1997).

Role of interstitial inflammation–leucocyte infiltration and adhesion molecules (Sheridan and Bonventre 2000)

Ischaemia–reperfusion injury involves an interstitial inflammatory response which results in leucocyte infiltration, oedema, and the compromise of microvascular blood flow. There are many mechanisms, recently reviewed (Heinzelmann *et al.* 1999), by which leucocytes potentiate renal injury, including the generation of ROS and the synthesis of phospholipase metabolites, which are important modulators of vascular tone.

Some controversy exists as to whether neutrophils or mononuclear cells infiltrate in ischaemia–reperfusion injury. The infiltration of macrophages and T lymphocytes may predominate over neutrophil infiltrate in the recovery phase of ARF. Although tissue injury is ameliorated by the prevention of neutrophil accumulation (for review, see Sheridan and Bonventre 2000), neutrophil depletion models may not adequately differentiate neutrophils from macrophages and T lymphocytes (De Greef *et al.* 1998).

The infiltration of leucocytes is dependent on the enhanced expression of adhesion molecules, including selectins and integrins. Integrins interact with immunoglobulin-like adhesion molecules such as interstitial cell adhesion molecules (ICAM-1) or vascular cell adhesion molecules (VCAM), which are expressed by endothelial cells and are upregulated after ischaemia in response to cytokines. ICAM-1 was implicated because the kidney was protected against ischaemia by using anti-ICAM-1 antibodies and ICAM-1 knockout mouse (Kelly *et al.* 1996b). Pretreatment with an ICAM-1 antisense oligodeoxyribonucleotide ameliorated the ischaemia-induced infiltration of granulocytes and macrophages and resulted in less cortical renal damage (Haller *et al.* 1996).

Chemokines, which recruit and activate leucocytes and selectins are upregulated by inflammatory cytokines, such as interleukin-1 (IL-1) and TNF-α. Local TNF-α-synthesis may be an early and pivotal event in renal ischaemic–reperfusion injury (Donnahoo *et al.* 1999). ROS may also upregulate chemokine expression. Transgenic mice that overproduce antioxidants are protected against ischaemic injury (Safirstein *et al.* 1991).

P-selectin, a molecule involved in adherence of circulating leucocytes to tissue in inflammatory states, is also involved in leucocyte infiltration during ischaemic injury (Rabb and Postler 1998).

Oxidant mechanisms in acute renal failure (for detailed review, see Ueda *et al.* 2001)

A large body of evidence indicates that partially reduced oxygen metabolites are important mediators of ischaemic, toxic, and immune-mediated tissue injury. Additionally, a new class of oxidants, NO-derived reactive nitrogen species, have emerged as important mediators of injury.

Central to the hypoxia response are a family of hypoxia-inducible transcription factors (HIF), which are activated when oxygen concentrations fall below a critical level. To date, three members of the family have been identified. Each is composed of a hypoxia-regulated α subunit (HIF-1α, -2α, and -3α) and an oxygen-insensitive β subunit (HIF-1β), which is also known as the arylhydrocarbon receptor nuclear translocator (ARNT). The HIF system regulates several target genes that have important functions in renal physiological and pathophysiological processes, including energy metabolism [glucose transporters (GLUT) and glycolytic enzymes], vasomotor regulation [NOS, haeme oxygenase-1 (HO-1), and endothelins], angiogenic growth [vascular endothelial growth factor and platelet-derived growth factor (PDGF)], matrix metabolism [collagens, collagen prolyl hydroxylases, matrix metalloproteinases, and transforming growth factor (TGF)-β isoforms], and apoptosis/cell survival decisions (NIP3 and Nix) (see Fine and Norman 2002).

Recently, the distribution of the hypoxia-inducible transcription factors HIF-1α and -2α in hypoxic and ischaemic kidneys has been outlined. This has advanced our understanding of how the kidney is able to 'take a deep breath' (at least from a cellular perspective) when it is deprived of oxygen (Rosenberger *et al.* 2002).

Reactive oxygen species (Fig. 7a)

The primary source of superoxide in reperfused tissues is the enzyme xanthine oxidase which exists in cells predominantly as the oxidized nicotinamide adenine dinucleotide (NAD$^+$)-dependent dehydrogenase (D-form). This form uses NAD^{2+} instead of O_2 as the electron acceptor during oxidation of purines and does not produce superoxide or hydrogen peroxide. Ischaemia, however, results in more of the

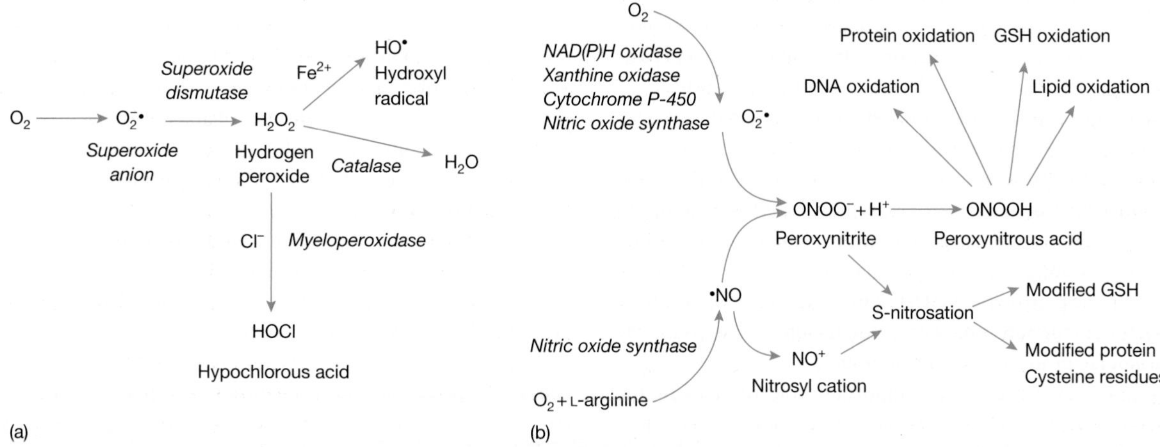

Fig. 7 (a) Reactive oxygen species, (b) reactive nitrogen species involved in the pathogenesis of renal ischaemia reperfusion. From Ueda *et al.* (2001).

radical-producing form of the enzyme (O-form). Conversion of xanthine dehydrogenase to xanthine oxidase (D to O conversion) occurs by a number of mechanisms, including limited proteolysis and chemical modification, or oxidation of sulfhydryl groups. During ischaemia, there is also a massive breakdown of the adenine nucleotide pool and adenosine is converted to inosine and then to hypoxanthine, resulting in its accumulation. Thus, after a period of ischaemia, there is an accumulation of xanthine oxidase (pre-existing and newly converted) and of its purine substrate, hypoxanthine. After reperfusion, the remaining substrate, molecular oxygen, re-enters the tissues and a burst of superoxide production ensues. The importance of this enzyme in kidney ischaemia–reperfusion is still unclear.

Mitochondria produce superoxide anions at two sites in the electron transport chain; the first site being the ubiquinone-to-cytochrome *b* region on the internal mitochondrial membrane; the second site is on the NADH-dehydrogenase that exists in the inner mitochondrial membrane. During ischaemia, the lack of molecular oxygen, and an inhibition of electron transfer lead to a high reduction of the components of the mitochondrial respiratory chain. Upon reperfusion, a burst of superoxide production occurs by the increased auto-oxidation of the major intramitochondrial sources of superoxide, ubisemiquinone, and NADH-dehydrogenase flavin semiquinone because of steady inhibition of electron transfer.

Microsomal and nuclear membranes also contain the electron transport systems cytochrome P-450 and cytochrome b5 that generate reactive oxygen metabolites; peroxisomes contain oxidases that generate hydrogen peroxide directly, without superoxide intermediate formation. The role of suborganelles as a source of reactive oxygen metabolites in the kidney is still unclear. AA metabolism via PGH synthase and lipo-oxygenase and the auto-oxidation of catecholamines or haem proteins such as myoglobin have also been shown to produce superoxide in the presence of NADH or NADPH.

Another potentially important source of reactive oxygen metabolites is leucocytes.

Iron has been shown to be important in various models of tissue injury. Iron chelators, such as desferrioxamine, which inhibit the generation of hydroxyl radical have been shown to be protective against ischaemia–reperfusion injury in several organs and in toxic, immune as well as in ischaemic injury to kidney (Paller and Neumann 1991). During reperfusion, a number of reactive and toxic aldehyde metabolites, such as malondialdehyde (MDA) and 4-hydroxynonenal (4-HNE), a product of lipid peroxidation, can be released. Inhibitors of lipid peroxidation, such as lazaroids (21-aminosteroid) and bioflavonoids, have been shown to reduce the formation of free radicals, lipid peroxidation, and kidney dysfunction in ischaemia–reperfusion injury.

The glutathione redox ratio-oxidized glutathione:reduced glutathione + oxidized glutathione [GSSG: (GSH + GSSG)] is considered a useful parameter for assessing oxidant stress and this ratio is decreased during ischaemia (McCoy *et al.* 1988). Ischaemia–reperfusion injury to the kidneys also affects the enzymatic antioxidant defence system, resulting in a significant decrease in superoxide dismutase (SOD), catalase, and glutathione peroxidase (GSH-Px) in the kidneys. The intrinsic cellular properties of the antioxidant enzymes in kidney tubule cells may be an important factor in susceptibility to injury.

There is much evidence for an important role of ROS in the pathogenesis of many forms of ARF, including ischaemia–reperfusion, lipopolysaccharide-induced renal injury, and gentamicin, glycerol, cisplatin, and cyclosporine A models of toxic ARF (for review, see Baliga *et al.* 1999). Of note, in glycerol-induced ARF, an animal model of rhabdomyolysis, there is enhanced generation of hydrogen peroxide, and scavengers of ROS and iron chelators provide protection. Although the dogma is that the myoglobin is the source of iron, recent studies suggest that cytochrome P450 may be an important source of iron in this model. In addition, there are marked alterations in antioxidant defenses, such as glutathione, as well as changes in haem oxygenase.

Reactive nitrogen species

As shown in Fig. 7(b), in an environment of oxidant stress, NO formation can lead to the generation of reactive nitrogen species. Oxidant stress may not only unmask the toxic potential of NO in the kidney but also augmented by the generation of NO and reactive nitrogen species. Proximal tubule NOS itself is capable of generating superoxide along with NO. When the expression of iNOS in the kidney was blocked using antisense oligonucleotides, both functional and morphologic indices of renal failure following ischaemia–reperfusion were greatly reduced. Furthermore, the evidence for the generation of peroxynitrite comes from immunohistochemical detection of nitrotyrosine–protein adducts in the kidney following ischaemia–reperfusion (Walker *et al.* 2000). The discovery that reactive nitrogen species can be generated in the kidney and participate in the development of ARF has uncovered a new therapeutic target. Over the past few years, selective iNOS inhibitors have been developed for treatment of a number of human diseases, in particular, septic shock. Non-selective NOS inhibitors that inhibit constitutive isoforms regulating vascular tone in addition to iNOS not only are ineffective but also can increase mortality (Petros *et al.* 1994). It may prove difficult to develop truly selective iNOS inhibitors. An alternative approach is to target reactive nitrogen species directly. The iron chelator desferrioxamine is one such drug and its ability to scavenge peroxynitrite, beyond its activity as an iron chelator may be responsible for many of its beneficial effects.

Heat shock proteins

During recovery from injury, the cell requires an efficient mechanism for restoring normal cell architecture and function by resurrecting disrupted proteins, shuttling misplaced proteins back to their correct location, and disposing of irreparably damaged proteins. All of these vital functions need to be accomplished in a confused cellular milieu. In addition, with an ischaemic injury, the essential mediators of protection and recovery would need to compete successfully for the residual pool of cellular ATP at a time when energy sources are depressed.

The heat shock proteins (HSPs) are ideally suited for this role (for review, see Van Why and Siegel 2001). Members of each HSP family assist intracellular protein trafficking and have been termed protein chaperones. Some of these stress proteins may prevent inappropriate peptide interactions in unfolding proteins, some can unfold protein substrates, and some can assist in the folding of polypeptides into their correct conformation.

The rapid induction of stress proteins in response to an insult occurs via activation of the preformed heat shock transcription factor (HSF). The activity of HSF appears to be modulated by constitutively expressed HSP-90 and HSP-70 proteins, which are themselves affected by levels of denatured proteins within the cell (Van Why and Siegel 2001). The principal trigger for the stress response in energy-depleted renal epithelium, both during ischaemia and nephrotoxicity is most probably the accumulation of disrupted, non-native, or denatured cellular proteins.

Following ischaemic injury in rat kidney, one of the inducible HSP-70 proteins, HSP-72 is rapidly detectable in the cortex and outer medulla, and is expressed most markedly in the cells that have sustained the most significant injury following ischaemia. Several other stress proteins, including the so-called small-stress proteins and endoplasmic reticulum chaperones, are induced by ischaemia. Because the small HSPs are involved in regulation of actin dynamics and because disorganization of the actin cytoskeleton is a prominent feature in ischaemic injury, it is relevant that increased levels of HSP-25 were detectable as early as 2 h of reflow after ischaemia and persisted for days. The particular pattern of HSP induction and elaboration of individual stress proteins has provided the initial insight into the role of stress proteins in cytoprotection and recovery from renal cell injury.

Whether stress proteins are instrumental in protecting the kidney against ischaemic injury is controversial issue (for review, see Van Why and Siegel 2001). When HSPs were examined in the intact rat kidney or in proximal tubules isolated from the injured kidney, minimal cytoprotection against ischaemia or hypoxia could be attributed to HSPs. Preconditioning ischaemia (Bonventre 2002) did protect proximal tubules from subsequent hypoxic injury, but the postischaemic HSP synthesis correlated poorly with the observed cytoresistance.

In conclusion, there is now compelling evidence that a series of stress proteins distributed throughout the cell in several compartments cooperate to prevent injury or promote recovery from a variety of insults to renal epithelia.

Repair of renal injury—role of growth factors (for in-depth review, see Ichimura and Bonventre 2001) (Fig. 8)

Proximal tubules are able to undergo repair, regeneration, and proliferation after ischaemic or nephrotoxic damage. In the outer cortex, the majority of cells are sublethally injured and undergo repair following adequate reperfusion. There are four major phases during this regeneration process. The first phase consists of the death and exfoliation of the proximal tubular cells. In this very early phase, stress response gene expression and the accumulation of mononuclear cells is observed. Growth factors may play a role in determining the fate of the epithelial cells and may contribute to the generation of signals that result in neutrophil and monocyte infiltration. The second phase of regeneration is the appearance of poorly differentiated epithelial cells. After both toxic or ischaemic injury, these cells have a flattened appearance with a poorly differentiated brush border. Cells express vimentin, an embryonic marker for multipotent kidney mesenchyme. This stage is, therefore, a 'de-differentiation' stage. The expression of vimentin and other proteins is similar to that expressed in the metanephric mesenchyme of the developing kidney and has led to the proposal that regeneration recapitulates aspects of development. The change from a differentiated phenotype to a less differentiated one might be important for remodeling of the proximal tubule architecture. Growth factors have been implicated in the control of cell differentiation. In the third phase, a marked increase in proliferation of the surviving PTCs is evident. These proliferating cells are derived from apparently mature PTCs, which have de-differentiated. Thus, differentiated PTCs retain the ability to de-differentiate and proliferate. Growth factors may also play an important role in this proliferative response. The last phase of the regeneration process is the stage of redifferentiation. In this late phase, the poorly differentiated regenerative tubular cells regain their differentiated character and produce a normal proximal tubule epithelium. These cells are already in a postmitotic stage when they differentiate. By the end of this phase, most damaged tubules have regained their essential functions.

Growth factors can have a number of beneficial effects on the kidney in the process of repair, from potentiation of adaptive responses to a reduction in functional mass and mediation of the proliferative processes after acute renal injury (Hammerman and Miller 1994). In addition, growth factors play important roles in angiogenesis and are also involved in epithelial cell differentiation (Hammerman 1998), an

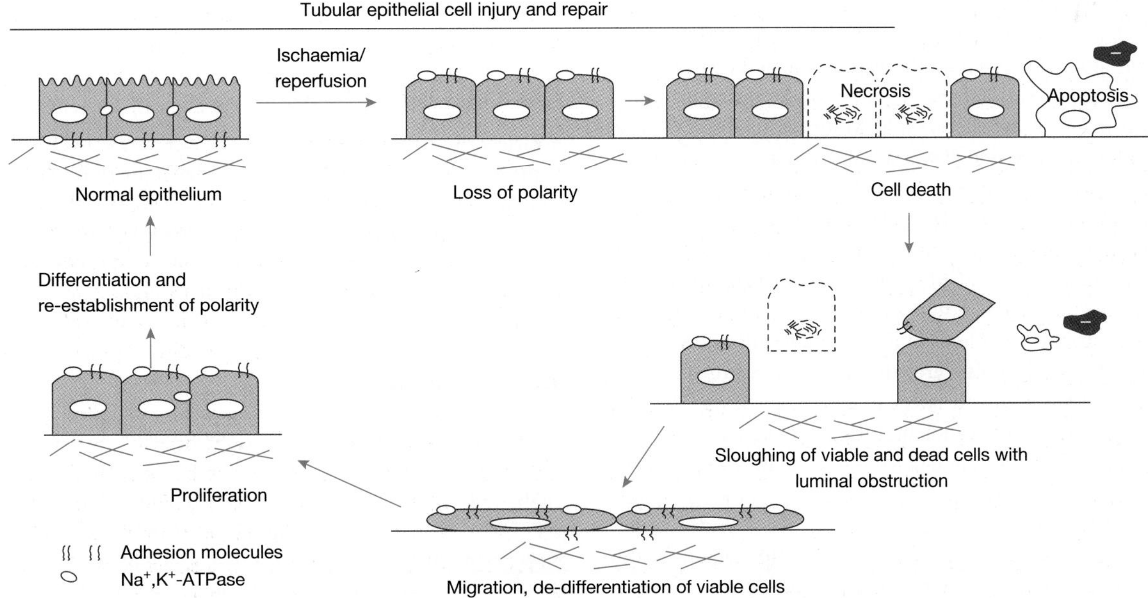

Fig. 8 Repair of renal injury. From Sheridan and Bonventre (2000).

important step in the restoration of function after injury. They can re-establish cell–ECM (ECM: extracellular matrix) and cell–cell interactions, functions that are very important for differentiation and functional integrity of the epithelium (Harris 1997).

Insulin-like growth factors

Collecting duct insulin-like growth factors (IGF-I) production is enhanced by growth hormone and epidermal growth factor (EGF), and is detectable in whole kidney and kidney cortex after damage, whether after challenge with folic acid, radiocontrast material or ischaemia. Administration of exogenous IGF-I can accelerate recovery of the postischaemic kidney in rats (Hammerman and Miller 1995). The mechanism of the enhanced recovery may be due to its ability to increase GFR, via altered haemodynamics, or to stimulate proximal tubule epithelial repair, regeneration, or proliferation. The effects of IGF-I may be direct or indirect, mediated by proteins whose expression is upregulated. As an example, osteopontin has been shown to be upregulated in ischaemic models of renal injury (Persy *et al.* 1999). This protein contains an RGD cell adhesion motif and has been implicated in tissue remodeling and repair. The clinical trials with IGF-I will be described later.

Epidermal growth factors and transforming growth factor-α

EGF is a mitogen for a broad spectrum of cells, including proximal tubule epithelial cells in culture (Ichimura and Bonventre 2001). EGF and TGF-α belong to the same gene family, and both act on the same EGF receptor. Both EGF and TGF-α precursors contain membrane-spanning regions that anchor them to the plasma membrane. Expression of EGF mRNA and protein decreases rapidly after ischaemic injury or gentamicin-induced renal injury; however, the binding capacity of EGF to the proximal tubules increases, presumably a reflection of an increased number of receptors. Exogenous EGF administration *in vivo* enhances proliferation and accelerates recovery of damaged proximal tubules after ischaemic or mercuric chloride-induced damage (Humes and Liu 1994).

Transforming growth factor-βs

These growth factors can either promote or inhibit cell proliferation or differentiation and also stimulate the expression of ECM proteins. These actions suggest that TGF-βs might be important regulators of tissue reconstruction. These effects on ECM formation, however, also contribute to the negative side of wound repair, that is, excessive fibrosis and sclerotic disease in the kidneys and other organs.

Renal TGF-β1 mRNA level is upregulated in regenerating proximal tubules in postischaemic kidney. Expression of several genes known to encode proteins that regulate ECM synthesis also increased in a TGF-β1-dependent manner. These results suggest involvement of TGF-β1 in the regulation of ECM synthesis in the postischaemic kidney.

The roles of PDGF, fibroblast growth factors, nerve growth factor, and vascular endothelial growth factor in experimental ARF are still not very well known and will not be further discussed. A detailed review of these factors can be found in Ichimura and Bonventre (2001).

Hepatocyte growth factor

Hepatocyte growth factor (HGF), known as scatter factor, is also involved in the adaptive response of the damaged kidney (Ichimura and Bonventre 2001). HGF and HGF activity are increased in chemically or ischaemia-damaged kidney. Serum HGF concentration increases in ARF patients compared with chronic renal failure patients (Libetta *et al.* 1998); this growth factor has been shown to protect the tubular epithelium from damage and to accelerate recovery from tubular injury in the postischaemic or nephrotoxic-damaged rat kidney (Miller *et al.* 1994).

Mitogen-activated protein kinase cascades and transcription responses in renal injury and repair

Growth factors exert their actions on cells via a number of different signalling mechanisms. One of the best studied pathways in ARF is the mitogen-activated protein (MAP) kinases pathways, the intracellular signaling events which ultimately lead to the transcription of genes whose encoded proteins mediate a response of proliferation, hypertrophy, differentiation, or apoptosis.

The best characterized of the three identified MAP kinase cascades in mammalian cells is the ERK. Numerous studies have demonstrated that the ERKs are critical to the mitogenic response, to cellular differentiation, and, in some cells, to the induction of hypertrophy (Bonventre and Force 1998). The ERKs are activated by cellular stress and by growth factors and many other agonists, including vasoactive peptides, via their receptors and associated molecules, including G-proteins. One of two other MAP kinase cascades is called the p54 MAP kinase, SAPKs, or JNK cascade.

Upon activation, ERK proteins translocate to the nucleus (Bonventre and Force 1998), where they phosphorylate and activate several members of the transcription factor family, including Elk-1, SAP1, Ets-1, and Ets-2.

SAPKs are not activated by ischaemia alone but are markedly activated by reperfusion of ischaemic kidney (Morooka *et al.* 1995), while others (DiMari *et al.* 1997) found that administration of A-acetylcysteine inhibited the ischaemia-induced increase in SAPK/JNK activity and partially protected the kidney against ischaemic injury. Whether the protection was related to the decrease in SAPK/JNK activity or to other antioxidant effects of *N*-acetylcysteine was not established.

Based on the intrarenal location of the activated ERK, it has been proposed that cell survival in the postischaemic kidney relies on ERK activation (di Mari *et al.* 1999).

Prevention of ARF

A variety of interventions and drugs have been tested for their ability to prevent or attenuate the injury, or hasten the recovery of ischaemic and toxic ATN. Some of these interventions are effective in altering the course of experimental models of ATN; however, only a few have consistently been shown to be of benefit in clinical ATN. The most important experimental and clinical drugs or interventions are summarized in Table 1.

Volume expansion

The preventive value of volume expansion alone is not always easy to estimate because fluids are often included as part of the overall management which will include the administration of diuretics and/or dopamine. As summarized by us (Lameire *et al.* 1995), hydration has been suggested to prevent contrast-, platinum-, amphotericin B-induced ATN and the intrarenal tubular precipitation of crystals after high doses of methotrexate, sulfonamides, and acyclovir. In the case of amphotericin-induced acute nephrotoxicity, the use of lipid formulations and changes

Table 1 Current and future drug therapy of clinical and experimental acute tubular necrosis

Pathogenetic mechanism	Current or future interventions in humans	Current interventions in animals
Renal vasoconstriction	Low-dose dopamine Calcium channel blockers Atrial natriuretic peptides Endothelin receptor antagonists Leukotriene receptor antagonists PAF antagonists	Low-dose dopamine Calcium channel blockers Atrial natriuretic peptides Endothelin receptor antagonists Leukotriene receptor antagonists PAF antagonists iNOS antisense oligonucleotides
Reperfusion injury	Anti-ICAM-1 mAB Anti-CD 18 m Ab Acetylcysteine	Anti-ICAM-1 mAB Anti-CD 18 m Ab Free radical scavengers Protease inhibitors α-MSH
Tubular obstruction	Diuretics	Diuretics RGD peptides iNOS antisense oligonucleotides
Tubular regeneration	Insulin-like growth factor Thyroxine	Insulin-like growth factor Epidermal growth factor Hepatocyte growth factor Thyroxine Osteopontin

iNOS, inducible nitric oxide synthase; PAF, platelet activating factor; RGD peptides, peptides containing the arginine–glycine–aspartic acid motif; mAB, monoclonal antibodies; ICAM-1, intercellular adhesion molecule-1; α-MSH, α-melanocyte-stimulating hormone.

in the rate of drug infusion may significantly affect renal dysfunction (Costa and Nucci 2001). In patients with chronic renal insufficiency undergoing cardiac angiography, hydration with 0.45 per cent saline provided better protection against acute decreases in renal function than did the same hydration protocol plus mannitol or frusemide (Solomon *et al.* 1994). Also patients about to receive chemotherapy or irradiation for cancer with rapid cell turnover should be pretreated with fluid loading to maintain a high urine output in combination with high doses of allopurinol, with or without sodium bicarbonate (Lameire 1994).

In crush syndrome, massive hydration with isotonic saline, together with a forced alkaline-mannitol diuresis can markedly reduce the renal toxicity. Such therapy should be initiated before the crush is relieved and the release of the haem pigments into the circulation (Better and Stein 1990).

Prevention with fluid therapy of postoperative ARF has been particularly well illustrated in aortic surgery, in surgery for obstructive jaundice, and after kidney transplantation (see review by Lameire and Vanholder 2000). This is difficult in patients with cardiac failure because fluid challenge may cause pulmonary oedema. Ultrafiltration or dialysis to 'rescue' such patients, should fluid be pushed too far, is essential in establishing confidence in avoiding volume depletion.

In sepsis, renal hypoperfusion may be a major factor in inducing renal failure, although other factors, such as endotoxins, release of cytokines may also play a role. The intriguing finding of a decreased renal sodium excretion in sepsis, even during prolonged oliguria, suggests an important influence of haemodynamic factors in this form of ARF. The therapeutic problem here is that even vigorous volume restitution under Swan–Ganz monitoring results in further fluid redistribution, with preferential sequestration to a 'third space' compartment.

Drug therapy with major impact on the vascular aspects of ARF (Verbeke *et al.* 1996; Dishart and Kellum 2000)

The classification of the drugs is based according to their principal action on the different pathophysiological mechanisms. This classification is to a large extent arbitrary, since many drugs act simultaneously in different ways.

Intrarenal vasoconstriction

Endothelin receptor blockers (Lameire and Vanholder 2000)

Several studies have shown a remarkable protection in experimental ischaemia–reperfusion animal models of ATN with either the non-peptide endothelin antagonist SB209670, BQ-123, a selective endothelin receptor antagonist or new, non-peptide, but selective ET receptor antagonists.

In the one multicentre study where the effect of intravenous SB209670, a mixed endothelin A and B receptor antagonist, in the prevention of radiocontrast-induced nephrotoxicity in patients with pre-existing chronic renal failure was investigated (Wang *et al.* 2000). An exacerbation of radiocontrast nephrotoxicity was observed, since the mean increase in serum creatinine 48 h after the angiography was higher in the patients receiving the experimental drug, compared to the placebo group.

Adenosine

Adenosine is a potent renal vasoconstrictor and has been thought to play a role in the initiation phase of ATN, mainly through its adenosine A1 receptor. However, this is in conflict with recent findings where both ischaemic preconditioning and adenosine pretreatment protected renal function and improved renal morphology in rats subjected to renal ischaemia (Lee and Emala 2000). In this study, an A_1 adenosine receptor agonist and A_3 adenosine receptor agonist protected and worsened renal function, respectively, after 45 min of renal ischaemia. An A_3 adenosine receptor antagonist protected renal function after ischaemic renal injury. Some studies administered *non-selective* adenosine-antagonists, either theophyllin (Erley 1999) or aminophylline (Abizaid *et al.* 1999) to patients with pre-existing chronic renal insufficiency, exposed to radiocontrast media. Both studies showed that the GFR is preserved by hydration alone without additional benefit of either drug. However, because non-selective adenosine receptor antagonist was used in their study, it is unclear which of the three adenosine receptors' antagonism protected renal function in these clinical situations.

Renal vasodilators

Low-dose dopamine

When infused in so-called 'renal doses' between 0.5 and 2 μg/kg/min, dopamine increases renal plasma flow, GFR, and sodium excretion. At higher doses, between 2 and 5 μg/kg/min, dopamine also binds to β-adrenergic receptors, and above 5 μg/kg/min, α-adrenergic receptors become activated. However, at each of these doses there is overlap in receptor activation as well as in intraindividual variation in binding activities. Although dopamine increased outer medullary blood flow in hypovolaemic rats, it failed to improve outer medullary oxygenation (Heyman *et al.* 1995). It is thus not easy to determine the extent to which a particular effect is purely dopaminergic in origin or is due to combined dopaminergic–adrenergic activation. A very large inter-individual variation in plasma clearances was found with a low dose 'renal' dopamine regimen in critically ill adult patients. Part of the renal improvement, if any, by dopamine can thus be explained by its inotropic effects, such as an increase in cardiac output and a rise in blood pressure.

Low doses of dopamine have been used and are still currently used to increase urine output in an attempt to prevent ATN in oliguric patients. However, according to several extensive reviews (Denton *et al.* 1996; Kellum and Decker 2001), the ability of dopamine to achieve these goals is poorly documented and largely anecdotal.

There is one study (Hall *et al.* 1992) reporting the protection of dopamine against radiocontrast nephrotoxicity in patients with pre-existing renal impairment, but few diabetic patients were included. In diabetic patients, a much higher frequency of contrast nephrotoxicity was previously found with dopamine (Weisberg *et al.* 1994). A prospective, randomized, controlled, single-blind trial was recently conducted where 98 participants were randomized to forced diuresis with intravenous crystalloid, frusemide, mannitol, and low-dose dopamine versus intravenous crystalloid and matching placebos (Stevens *et al.* 1999). This study suggests a modest benefit against contrast-induced nephropathy, provided a high urine flow rate can be achieved.

In a double-blind, randomized controlled trial (Lassnigg *et al.* 2000), a total of 126 patients with preoperative normal renal function undergoing elective cardiac surgery received a continuous infusion of either 'renal-dose' dopamine (2 μg/kg/min), frusemide (0.5 mg/kg/min), or isotonic sodium chloride as placebo, starting at the beginning of surgery and continuing for 48 h or until discharge from the intensive care unit. Acute renal injury (defined as an increase in serum creatinine >0.5 mg/dl) occurred more frequently in the patients treated with frusemide than in the two other groups. Also the creatinine clearance was lower in the patients treated with the loop diuretic. The continuous infusion of dopamine was ineffective for renal protection and was not superior to isotonic saline in preventing postoperative dysfunction after cardiac surgery. Another recent paper could also not demonstrate protection with low-dose dopamine in patients with mild renal insufficiency (Bellomo *et al.* 2000).

There are potential risks associated with low-dose dopamine regimens. These include the induction of tachycardia, cardiac arrhythmia, myocardial ischaemia, and possibly intestinal ischaemia (due to precapillary vasoconstriction), which might promote bacterial translocation from the intestinal lumen into the systemic circulation (Denton *et al.* 1996). Furthermore, in a series of elegant clinical investigations, the inhibitory effect of dopamine on the secretion of virtually all anterior-pituitary dependent hormones, in critically ill patients has been demonstrated (Van den Berghe and De Zegher 1996).

Atrial natriuretic peptide and urodilatin (Rushkoako 1992)

Atrial natriuretic peptide (ANP) appears to dilate the glomerular afferent arteriole but to constrict the efferent arteriole. Therefore, the increase in GFR is quite selective and may occur independently of an increase in RBF. Of further importance, ANP is reported to inhibit almost all tested vasoconstrictors that affect glomerular blood flow. Relevant for its potential action in ATN, ANP increases the tubular urinary flow rate and decreases the calcium influx into the cell. Several natriuretic peptides have been discovered, including urodilatin, likely to be produced by the kidney and with an equal or even greater natriuretic potency compared to human ANP. In most of the animal studies, where administration of ANP affords protection against ischaemic or toxic renal injury, the drug was administered either directly into the renal artery or intravenously in high doses; the latter often results in marked systemic hypotension (Conger 1996).

The first controlled clinical study (Rahman *et al.* 1994) in patients with established ATN showed that a combination of either intravenous or intrarenally infused human ANP together with frusemide or mannitol significantly increased the creatinine clearance by 8 h of ANP treatment. This effect persisted for 24 h after discontinuing ANP. Although there was a reduced need for dialysis in the ANP-treated group, the mortality rates between the treated and control groups were not significantly different. A larger and more rigidly controlled clinical trial with a 24-h infusion of ANP compared to placebo was then performed in patients with established ischaemic or nephrotoxic ATN (Allgren *et al.* 1997). Although ANP failed to show a beneficial effect in the general study population, a decrease in the incidence of dialysis and an increase in the dialysis-free survivorship was observed in the subgroup of oliguric ARF patients. In a follow-up study, patients with oliguric ARF were then enrolled into a multicentre, randomized, double-blind, placebo-controlled trial to assess prospectively the safety and efficacy of ANP compared with placebo (Lewis *et al.* 2000). Subjects were randomized to treatment with a 24-h infusion of ANP (anaritide, 0.2 μg/kg/min; synthetic form of human ANP) or placebo. Although a trend was present, there was no statistically significant beneficial effect of ANP in dialysis-free survival or reduction in dialysis in these subjects with oliguric ARF. In a more recent study (Sward *et al.* 2001) a long-term infusion (>48 h) of ANP improved RBF and GFR in patients with acute renal impairment after cardiac surgery. This renal vasodilatory effect was maintained during the infusion and seemed to be haemodynamically safe.

The efficacy of intravenous ANP to prevent radiocontrast-induced nephropathy (RCIN) was investigated in patients with stable chronic renal failure, with or without diabetes mellitus (Kurnik *et al.* 1998). There were no statistical differences in the incidence of RCIN.

Prostaglandin E1

Three different doses of prostaglandin E1 (10, 20, or 40 mg/kg/body weight per min) or placebo were administered to patients with renal impairment who underwent radiocontrast examinations. The mean elevation of the serum creatinine after the radiocontrast administration was markedly higher in the placebo group compared to the prostaglandin-infused patients (Koch *et al.* 2000). However, no clinically relevant changes regarding the creatinine clearance were observed in the four groups examined.

Role of infiltrating leucocytes

Anti-ICAM-1 antibodies, ICAM-1 antisense oligonucleotides, and IL-1 receptor blockers

As outlined above, the administration of monoclonal antibodies against ICAM-1 and an ICAM-1 antisense oligodeoxyribonucleotide (ODN) protected against ischaemic ARF in rats; similarly, ICAM-1 deficient mice were protected against renal ischaemia (Kelly *et al.* 1996b). The effect of a monoclonal anti-CD54 (anti-ICAM-1) antibody was also evaluated in a cisplatinum, nephrotoxic model of ARF. Striking protection of renal function but also of survival was observed in the animals that were treated with the antibody, compared to controls (Kelly *et al.* 1999).

IL-1 is a central component of many acute inflammatory processes and is believed to serve as one of the chemoattractants that can recruit leucocytes to areas of inflammation. IL-1 upregulates CD11/CD18 expression on leucocytes and increases ICAM-1 expression on endothelial cells (Springer 1990). Blocking IL-1 receptor (IL-1R) with IL-1R antagonist (IL-1Ra) or studying IL-1R knock-out mice has attenuated or ischaemia—reperfusion injury in the kidney, or at least significantly accelerated the recovery of renal function (Haq *et al.* 1998). This protection was associated with significantly less infiltration of polymorphonuclear leucocytes in postischaemic renal tissue.

α-Melanocyte-stimulating hormone

α-MSH is an anti-inflammatory cytokine that inhibits both neutrophil and NO pathways. α-MSH inhibits neutrophil migration and infiltration mediated by a number of mechanisms that have recently been summarized (Kohda *et al.* 1998). Administration of α-MSH inhibited renal injury even when started 6 h after injury in both mice and rats. However, this hormone also decreased renal injury when neutrophil effects were minimal or absent, as in ICAM-1 knock-out mice, indicating that α-MSH inhibits neutrophil-independent pathways of renal injury as well. α-MSH also inhibited cytokine-stimulated NO production in a cell line derived from proximal tubules.

Platelet-activating factor anatagonists

In animals treated with an oral PAF antagonist, (Ro-24-4736), prior to ischaemia, renal function was less impaired and histological abnormalities were less pronounced when compared to postischaemic kidneys from vehicle-treated animals (Kelly *et al.* 1996a). The coincident use of anti-ICAM-1 monoclonal antibody did not confer additional protection over that observed with the oral PAF antagonist alone. It is suggested that PAF has effects on leucocyte–endothelial interactions. A PAF antagonist seems also to protect against clinical post-transplant ARF (Grinyo *et al.* 1996) and against cyclosporin nephrotoxicity (Bagnis *et al.* 1996).

Drugs therapy with major impact on the tubular factors

Calcium entry blockers (Michael and Lee 1990)

A number of studies have shown that oral administration of a calcium entry blocker (calcium antagonist), protects against the fall in GFR that may occur after administration of hyperosmolar radiocontrast media. Many of the studies showing a protection contained a limited number of patients or showed other flaws in the experimental protocol. A number of investigators have demonstrated that the prophylactic administration of calcium channel blockers to recipients who receive renal grafts that are flushed with these drugs (e.g. diltiazem) protects the graft against post-transplant DGF (Alcaraz *et al.* 1991; Puig *et al.* 1991). When the recipient received the calcium antagonist immediately after the transplantation, but the graft was not perfused with diltiazem, the incidence of DGF was not significantly different from control. A criticism of these studies showing such a dramatic decrease in post-transplant ATN with calcium antagonists is that a similar low incidence of ATN can be obtained without calcium antagonists with an adequate hydration policy and the preoperative administration of a moderate dose of mannitol. An additional bias may be raised by the fact that diltiazem, verapamil, and nicardipine, but not nifedipine, interfere with the metabolism of cyclosporine through the P-450 cytochrome system (Wagner *et al.* 1988). Finally, a critical meta-analysis (Ladefoged and Andersen 1994) concluded that all studies showing a protective effect with these agents were uncontrolled, open studies while the studies where no effect could be demonstrated were the blinded, placebo-controlled investigations. These findings suggest at least that the issue of renal protection with calcium entry blockers in the prevention of post-transplant ATN is not settled.

Mannitol and loop diuretics

There are some theoretical arguments for the utilization of mannitol and/or loop diuretics in either the prevention or treatment of ATN. Both mannitol and loop diuretics can induce diuresis, potentially washing out obstructing cellular debris and casts. Mannitol may preserve mitochondrial function by osmotically minimizing the degree of postischaemic swelling, and by scavenging free radicals. Loop diuretics diminish active transport in the TAL, and the ensuing decrease in energy requirements may protect the cell in ischaemic conditions. In addition, loop diuretics may act as renal vasodilators in particular circumstances.

Mannitol

Prophylactic mannitol has been promoted in patients considered to be at high risk for ATN, such as those undergoing vascular aortic aneurysm surgery, cardiac surgery, renal transplantation, or patients developing obstructive jaundice or rhabdomyolysis. In any case, many of the studies, summarized in Kellum (1998), indicate that mannitol increases urine flow but does not reduce the incidence of ATN. In surgery for obstructive jaundice, the results are conflicting. Earlier studies found that mannitol reduced the incidence of ATN but a prospective evaluation (Sitges-Serra *et al.* 1992) found no additional beneficial effect of mannitol beyond adequate hydration. More convincing are the results obtained with the preventive administration of mannitol just before clamp release during renal transplantation surgery. In a randomized study comparing moderate hydration with or without mannitol, the incidence of post-transplant ATN was significantly lower in the mannitol group both in cyclosporin- and in azathioprine-treated patients (Van Valenberg *et al.* 1987). There are no formal studies on the prophylactic use of mannitol alone in patients with rhabdomyolysis. However, forced alkaline diuresis together with mannitol in severe crush injury is generally accepted as effective prevention of ATN.

Mannitol has been evaluated in the prevention of radiocontrast-induced acute nephropathy. In most of the recommended hydration protocols, mannitol (500 ml of 20 per cent), together with frusemide and hypotonic saline, is included. Some earlier studies have found that mannitol was successful in preventing deterioration of renal function in patients with mild to moderate chronic renal failure, undergoing intravenous pyelography. These studies employed historical controls, making the true contribution of mannitol difficult to assess. In contrast with current belief, another investigation (Weisberg *et al.* 1994) found that mannitol increased the incidence of acute contrast nephropathy in diabetic patients, but reduced the incidence in non-diabetic patients. Because similar results were obtained with two other renal vasodilators, dopamine, and ANP, this study suggests that the preventive administration of a renal vasodilator before a radiographic examination, cannot be recommended in diabetic patients. Moreover, a well-controlled study did not find additional benefit from mannitol beyond adequate hydration before and after radiocontrast administration to chronic renal failure patients (Solomon *et al.* 1994).

The potentially negative effects of mannitol include volume depletion and hypernatremia by too strong an osmotic diuretic effect. In contrast, volume expansion, hyponatremia, hyperkalaemia, and metabolic acidosis may develop when the hypertonic mannitol is retained. Excessively high plasma concentrations of mannitol ($>$1050 mg/dl) may actually cause ARF (Dorman *et al.* 1990).

Loop diuretics

Experience with loop diuretics, mainly frusemide, has closely parallelled that with mannitol. Frusemide has been advocated as part of prophylactic regimens for ATN, even though there is as yet no convincing evidence for its efficacy. In some studies, a favourable diuretic response was obtained when the diuretics, frusemide or ethacrynic acid, were given within the first 24 h after the onset of oliguria. All studies, except one (Anderson *et al.* 1977), have shown that loop diuretics do not lower the mortality in patients with ATN. Continuous infusion of frusemide may be more efficacious than bolus injections (Klinge 2001; van der Vorst *et al.* 2001).

A recent prospective, placebo-controlled, double-blind study examined the role of loop diuretics (frusemide and torasemide) in the treatment of oliguric ATN patients, all also treated by low-dose dopamine (Shilliday *et al.* 1997). No significant difference in any major outcome parameters (renal recovery, requirement for dialysis, or deaths) was observed. The use of loop diuretics in the setting of ATN is not without hazard. From an experimental point of view, frusemide may promote the aggregation of THP in the lumen of the tubules, a mechanism which is thought to cause intratubular obstruction (Sanders *et al.* 1990).

Large doses of frusemide or ethacrynic acid may cause deafness, which sometimes may become permanent. Coprescription of aminoglycosides increases the risk of ototoxicity. However, the incidence of permanent hearing loss is rather low and mostly reported when high doses were given in bolus injections. Finally, since frusemide may increase the risk of ATN due to aminoglycosides and cephalosporin antibiotics, it has no place in the prevention of these forms of ATN (Lieberthal and Levinsky 1990).

Drugs interfering with apoptosis

The finding that cells in postischaemic, regenerating nephrons undergo apoptosis suggests that regulators of apoptosis may be useful as therapeutic agents. However, before any strategies employing pro- or anti-apoptotic renal therapeutics can be designed and employed, it must be established whether a reduction or enhancement of apoptosis is beneficial or deleterious at a given time in a given clinical setting.

Therapeutic interventions that inhibit or promote apoptosis of tubular cells may either minimize the renal dysfunction or may accelerate the recovery after ATN (Ueda and Shah 2000; Levine and Lieberthal 2001). Administration of antiapoptotic agents such as IGF and a caspase inactivator (ZVAD-fmk) at the time of reperfusion after renal ischaemia in mice prevented the early onset of not only renal apoptosis, but also inflammation, tissue injury and kidney dysfunction (Daemen *et al.* 2000). All the available data have been obtained in experimental models of ARF and their clinical benefit has not yet been demonstrated.

Antioxidant therapy (Ueda *et al.* 2001)

Various scavengers of reactive oxygen metabolites, such as allopurinol, SOD, dimethylthiourea, catalase, reduced glutathione, *N*-acetylcysteine, or antioxidants such as vitamin E, have been reported to be protective against ischaemia–reperfusion injury, although conflicting results were obtained. In addition, feeding a selenium-deficient diet (which results in a marked reduction in GSH-Px, an enzyme that metabolizes hydrogen peroxide) and vitamin E, an antioxidant, has shown a marked susceptibility to ischaemia–reperfusion injury. In contrast, inhibition of catalase resulted in an exacerbation of injury following ischaemia–reperfusion.

Acetylcysteine

An important clinical trial (Tepel *et al.* 2000) was performed in 83 patients with chronic renal insufficiency (mean serum creatinine concentration 2.4 $\pm$ 1.3 mg/dl) and who were undergoing computed tomography with a non-ionic, low-osmolality contrast agent. The patients were pretreated with 0.45 per cent saline intravenously and either acetylcysteine or placebo. Only 2 per cent of the patients in the acetylcysteine group versus 21 per cent of the patients in the control group showed an increase in serum creatinine after the contrast study. In the acetylcysteine group, the mean serum creatinine concentration decreased, whereas in the control group the mean serum creatinine concentration increased (albeit insignificantly). These results need to be confirmed in a larger trial.

Drugs with main action on recovery, regeneration, and repair

Growth factors (reviewed by Hammerman 1998)

The expression and action of growth factor peptides during the recovery of functional and anatomic integrity of the nephron in ARF and the results of some experimental studies have led to clinical studies of growth factors in ARF patients. A double-blind, placebo-controlled multicenter study (Hirschberg *et al.* 1999) explored the effect of subcutaneous recombinant human IGF-I on the enhancement of the recovery of renal function in critically ill patients with ARF. Injections were started within 6 days of the onset of ARF. IGF-I did not accelerate the recovery of renal function in ARF patients with substantial comorbidity.

In another double-blind, placebo-controlled trial, it was shown that IGF-I administered postoperatively to patients undergoing surgery during which blood flow to the kidneys was interrupted, was well tolerated and prevented the fall in GFR that occurred in placebo-treated subjects (Franklin *et al.* 1997). However, the incidence of ARF was too low to allow conclusions of any protective action of IGF-I on the course of postoperative ARF.

Finally, although the administration of growth hormone can attenuate the catabolic response to injury, surgery, and sepsis, recent studies have shown that high doses of growth hormone administered to patients with critical illness are associated with increased morbidity and mortality (Takala *et al.* 1999).

Thyroxine

Thyroxine has been shown in experimental models to shorten the course of ARF (Michael *et al.* 1991). A prospective, randomized, placebo-controlled, double-blind trial of thyroxine had no effect on the course of clinical ARF and could even have had a negative effect on outcome through prolonged suppression of TSH. Critically ill euthyroid sick patients should not be given thyroid hormone.

The clinical treatment of patients with ARF is still largely supportive, but basic research has provided many, but still unproved, leads to future therapies (see Table 1). Additional experimental models that better reflect the multifactorial causes of clinical ARF are needed. Single drug therapy will probably never be effective and multiple agents may be needed to improve outcome in a disease in which different pathophysiological processes occur. In addition, drugs should be given as early as possible. Early detection of ARF, especially in the setting of the multiorgan failure syndrome, is crucial.

References

Abizaid, A. S., Clark, C. E., Mintz, G. S., Dosa, S., Popma, J. J., Pichard, A. D., Satler, L. F., Harvey, M., Kent, K. M., and Leon, M. B. (1999). Effects of dopamine and aminophylline on contrast-induced acute renal failure after coronary angioplasty in patients with preexisting renal insufficiency. *The American Journal of Cardiology* **83**, 260–263.

Alcaraz, A., Oppenheimer, F., Talbot-Wright, R., Fernandez-Cruz, L., Manalich, M., Garcia-Pages, E., Cetina, A., Vendrell, J. R., and Carretero, P. (1991). Effect of diltiazem in the prevention of acute tubular necrosis, acute rejection, and cyclosporine levels. *Transplantation Proceedings* **23**, 2383–2384.

Alejandro, V., Scandling, J. D., Jr., Sibley, R. K., Dafoe, D., Alfrey, E., Deen, W., and Myers, B. D. (1995a). Mechanisms of filtration failure during postischemic injury of the human kidney. A study of the reperfused renal allograft. *Journal of Clinical Investigations* **95** (2), 820–831.

Alejandro, V. S., Nelson, W. J., Huie, P., Sibley, R. K., Dafoe, D., Kuo, P., Scandling, J. D., Jr., and Myers, B. D. (1995b). Postischemic injury, delayed function and Na+/K+-ATPase distribution in the transplanted kidney. *Kidney International* **48** (4), 1308–1315.

Allgren, R. L., Marbury, T. C., Rahman, S. N., Weisberg, L. S., Fenves, A. Z., Lafayette, R. A., Sweet, R. M., Genter, F. C., Kurnik, B. R., Conger, J. D., and Sayegh, M. H. (1997). Anaritide in acute tubular necrosis. Auriculin Anaritide Acute Renal Failure Study Group (see comments). *New England Journal of Medicine* **336** (12), 828–834.

Anderson, R. J., Linas, S. L., and Berns, A. S. (1977). Non-oliguric acute renal failure. *New England Journal of Medicine* **296**, 1134–1138.

Atkinson, S. J. and Molitoris, B. A. Cytoskeletal alterations as a basis of cellular injury in acute renal failure. In *Acute Renal Failure—A Companion to Brenner & Rector's The Kidney* (ed. B. A. Molitoris and W. F. Finn), pp. 119–131. Philadelphia: W.B. Saunders, 2001.

Awazu, M. and Ichikawa, I. (1994). Alterations in renal function in experimental congestive heart failure. *Seminars in Nephrology* **14** (5), 401–411.

Bagnis, C., Deray, G., Dubois, M., Pirotzky, E., Jacquiaud, C., Baghos, W., Aupetit, B., Braquet, P., and Jacobs, C. (1996). Prevention of cyclosporine nephrotoxicity with a platelet-activating-factor antagonist. *Nephrology, Dialysis, Transplantation* **11**, 507–513.

Baliga, R., Ueda, N., Walker, P. D., and Shah, S. V. (1999). Oxidant mechanisms in toxic acute renal failure. *Drug Metabolism Reviews* **31** (4), 971–997.

Bankir, L., Kriz, W., Goligorsky, M., Nambi, P., Thomson, S., and Blantz, R. C. (1998). Vascular contributions to pathogenesis of acute renal failure. *Renal Failure* **20** (5), 663–677.

Better, O. S. and Stein, J. H. (1990). Early management of shock and prophylaxis of acute renal failure in traumatic rhabdomyolysis. *New England Journal of Medicine* **322** (12), 825–829.

Blantz, R. C. (1998). Pathophysiology of pre-renal azotemia. *Kidney International* **53** (2), 512–523.

Bohle, A., Christensen, J., Kokot, F., Osswald, H., Schubert, B., Kendziorra, H., Pressler, H., and Marcovic-Lipkovski, J. (1990). Acute renal failure in man: new aspects concerning pathogenesis. A morphometric study. *American Journal of Nephrology* **10** (5), 374–388.

Bonegio, R. and Lieberthal, W. (2002). Role of apoptosis in the pathogenesis of acute renal failure. *Current Opinion in Nephrology and Hypertension* **11** (3), 301–308.

Bonventre, J. V. (2002). Kidney ischemic preconditioning. *Current Opinion in Nephrology and Hypertension* **11** (1), 43–48.

Bonventre, J. V. and Force, T. (1998). Mitogen-activated protein kinases and transcriptional responses in renal injury and repair. *Current Opinion in Nephrology and Hypertension* **7** (4), 425–433.

Brezis, M. and Rosen, S. (1995). Hypoxia of the renal medulla—its implications for disease. *New England Journal of Medicine* **332** (10), 647–655.

Chiao, H., Kohda, Y., McLeroy, P., Craig, L., Housini, I., and Star, R. A. (1997). α-Melanocyte-stimulating hormone protects against renal injury after ischemia in mice and rats. *Journal of Clinical Investigation* **99**, 1165–1172.

Chou, S. Y., Porush, J. G., and Faubert, P. F. (1990). Renal medullary circulation: hormonal control. *Kidney International* **37** (1), 1–13.

Conger, J. (1998). Prophylaxis and treatment of acute renal failure by vasoactive agents: the fact and the myths. *Kidney International* **64** (Suppl.), S23–S26.

Conger, J. D. (1996). Effects of natriuretic peptides in acute renal failure. *Seminars in Dialysis* **9**, 460–463.

Conger, J. D. Vascular alterations in acute renal failure: roles in inititation and maintenance. In *Acute Renal Failure: A Companion to Brenner & Rector's The Kidney* (ed. B. A. Molitoris and W. F. Finn), pp. 13–29. Philadelphia: W.B. Saunders, 2001.

Conger, J. D. and Schrier, R. W. (1980). Renal hemodynamics in acute renal failure. *Annual Review of Physiology* **42**, 603–614.

Corrigan, G., Ramaswamy, D., Kwon, O., Sommer, F. G., Alfrey, E. J., Dafoe, D. C., Olshen, R. A., Scandling, J. D., and Myers, B. D. (1999). PAH extraction and estimation of plasma flow in human postischemic acute renal failure. *American Journal of Physiology* **277** (2 Pt 2), F312–F318.

Costa, S. and Nucci, M. (2001). Can we decrease amphotericin nephrotoxicity? *Current Opinion in Critical Care* **7**, 379–383.

Cotran, R. S., Kumar, V., and Robbins, S. L. The kidney. In *Pathologic Basis of Disease* (ed. R. S. Cotran, V. Kumar, and S. L. Robbins), pp 927–989. Philadelphia: W.B. Saunders Company, 1994.

Daemen, M. A. R. C., van t'Veer, C., Denecker, G., Heemskerk, V. H., Wolfs, T. G. A. M., Clauss, M., Vandenabeele, P., and Buurman, W. A. (2000). Inhibition of apoptosis induced by ischemia–reperfusion prevents inflammation. *Journal of Clinical Investigation* **104**, 541–549.

De Greef, K. E., Ysebaert, D. K., Ghielli, M., Vercauteren, S., Nouwen, E. J., Eyskens, E. J., and De Broe, M. E. (1998). Neutrophils and acute ischemia–reperfusion injury. *Journal of Nephrology* **11**, 110–122.

De Nicola, L., Blantz, R. C., and Gabbai, F. B. (1992). Nitric oxide and angiotensin II. Glomerular and tubular interaction in the rat. *Journal of Clinical Investigation* **89** (4), 1248–1256.

De Nicola, L., Thomson, S. C., Wead, L. M., Brown, M. R., and Gabbai, F. B. (1993). Arginine feeding modifies cyclosporine nephrotoxicity in rats. *Journal of Clinical Investigation* **92** (4), 1859–1865.

de Rougemont, D., Brunner, F. P., Torhorst, J., Wunderlich, P. F., and Thiel, G. (1982). Superficial nephron obstruction and medullary congestion after ischemic injury: effect of protective treatments. *Nephron* **31**, 310–320.

Denton, M. D., Chertow, G. M., and Brady, H. R. (1996). 'Renal-dose' dopamine for the treatment of acute renal failure: scientific rationale, experimental studies and clinical trials. *Kidney International* **50** (1), 4–14.

di Mari, J. F., Davis, R., and Safirstein, R. L. (1999). MAPK activation determines renal epithelial cell survival during oxidative injury. *American Journal of Physiology* **277**, F195–F203.

DiMari, J., Megyesi, J., Udvarhelyi, N., Price, P., Davis, R., and Safirstein, R. (1997). *N*-acetyl cysteine ameliorates ischemic renal failure. *American Journal of Physiology* **272** (3 Pt 2), F292–F298.

Dishart, M. K. and Kellum, J. A. (2000). An evaluation of pharmacological strategies for the prevention and treatment of acute renal failure. *Drugs* **59** (1), 79–91.

Donnahoo, K. K. *et al.* (1999). Early kidney TNF expression mediates neutrophil infiltration and injury after renal ischemia–reperfusion. *American Journal of Physiology* **277**, R922–R929.

Dorman, H. R., Sondheimer, J. H., and Chadnapaphomhai, P. (1990). Mannitol-induced acute renal failure. *Medicine* **69**, 153–159.

Dzau, V. J., Packer, M., Lilly, L. S., Swartz, S. L., Hollenberg, N. K., and Williams, G. H. (1984). Prostaglandins in severe congestive heart failure. Relation to activation of the renin–angiotensin system and hyponatremia. *New England Journal of Medicine* **310** (6), 347–352.

Edelstein, C. L. (2000). Calcium-mediated proximal tubular injury—what is the role of cysteine proteases? *Nephrology, Dialysis, Transplantation* **15** (2), 141–144.

Edelstein, C. L., Ling, H., and Schrier, R. W. (1997). The nature of renal cell injury. *Kidney International* **51** (5), 1341–1351.

Erley, C. M. (1999). Does hydration prevent radiocontrast-induced acute renal failure? (editorial). *Nephrology, Dialysis, Transplantation* **14**, 1064–1066.

Fine, L.G. and Norman, J. T. (2002). The breathing kidney. *Journal of the American Society of Nephrology* **13**, 1974–1976.

Franklin, S. C., Moulton, M., Sicard, G. A., Hammerman, M. R. and Miller, S. B. (1997). Insulin-like growth factor 1 preserves renal function postoperatively in patients at risk to develop acute renal failure. *American Journal of Physiology* **272**, F257–F259.

Goligorsky, M. S., Lieberthal, W., Racusen, L., and Simon, E. E. (1993). Integrin receptors in renal tubular epithelium: new insights into pathophysiology of acute renal failure. *American Journal of Physiology* **264** (1 Pt 2), F1–F8.

Goligorsky, M. S., Kessler, H., and Romanov, V. I., (1998). Molecular mimicry of integrin ligation: therapeutic potential of arginine–glycine–aspartic acid (RGD) peptides. *Nephrology, Dialysis, Transplantation* **13** (2), 254–263.

Goligorsky, M. S., Noiri, E., Tsukahara, H., Budzikowski, A. S., and Li, H. (2000). A pivotal role of nitric oxide in endothelial cell dysfunction. *Acta Physiologica Scandinavica* **168** (1), 33–40.

Goligorsky, M. S., Brodsky, S. V., and Noiri, E. (2002). Nitric oxide in acute renal failure: NOS versus NOS. *Kidney International* **61**, 855–861.

Goormaghtigh, N. (1945). Vascular and circulatory changes in renal cortex in anuric crush-syndrome. *Proceedings of the Society of Experimental Biology and Medicine* **59**, 303–305.

Grinyo, J. M., Torras, J., and Valles, J. (1996). The role of platelet-activating factor antagonists in the prophylaxis of posttransplant acute tubular necrosis. *Renal Failure* **18** (3), 445–451.

Hall, K. A., Wong, R. W., Gunter, G. C., Camazine, B. M., Rappaport, W. A., Smyth, S. H., Bull, D. A., McIntyre, K. E., Bernhard, V. M., and Misiorowski, R. L. (1992). Contrast-induced nephrotoxicity: the effects of vasodilator therapy. *Journal of Surgical Research* **53**, 317–320.

Haller, H., Dragun, D., Miethke, A., Park, J. K., Weis, A., Lippoldt, A., Gross, V., and Luft, F. C. (1996). Antisense oligonucleotides for ICAM-1 attenuate reperfusion injury and renal failure in the rat. *Kidney International* **50** (2), 473–480.

Hammerman, M. R. (1998). Growth factors and apoptosis in acute renal injury. *Current Opinion in Nephrology and Hypertension* **7** (4), 419–424.

Hammerman, M. R. and Miller, S. B. (1994). Therapeutic use of growth factors in renal failure (editorial). *Journal of the American Society of Nephrology* **5** (1), 1–11.

Hammerman, M. R. and Miller, S. B. (1995). Growth factor gene expression in tubular epithelial injury. *Current Opinion in Nephrology and Hypertension* **4** (3), 258–262.

Haq, M., Norman, J., Saba, S. R., Ramirez, G., and Rabb, H. (1998). Role of IL-1 in renal ischemic reperfusion injury. *Journal of the American Society of Nephrology* **9** (4), 614–619.

Harris, R. C. (1997). Growth factors and cytokines in acute renal failure. *Advances in Renal Replacement Therapy* **4** (2 Suppl. 1), 43–53.

Heinzelmann, M., Mercer-Jones, M. A., and Passmore, J. C. (1999). Neutrophils and renal failure. *American Journal of Kidney Diseases* **34**, 384–399.

Heyman, S. N., Kaminski, N., and Brezis, M. (1995). Dopamine increases renal medullary blood flow without improving regional hypoxia. *Experimental Nephrology* **3** (6), 331–337.

Hirschberg, R., Kopple, J., Lipsett, P., Benjamin, E., Minei, J., Albertson, T., Munger, M., Metzler, M., Zaloga, G., Murray, M., Lowry, S., Conger, J., McKeown, W., O'shea, M., Baughman, R., Wood, K., Haupt, M., Kaiser, R., Simms, H., Warnock, D., Summer, W., Hintz, R., Myers, B., Haenftling, K., and Capra, W. (1999). Multicenter clinical trial of recombinant human insulin-like growth factor I in patients with acute renal failure. *Kidney International* **55** (6), 2423–2432.

Hollenberg, N. K., Epstein, M., Rosen, S. M., Basch, R. I., Oken, D. E., and Merrill, J. P. (1968). Acute oliguric renal failure in man: evidence for preferential renal cortical ischemia. *Medicine (Baltimore)* **47** (6), 455–474.

Humes, H. D. and Liu, S. (1994). Cellular and molecular basis of renal repair in acute renal failure. *Journal of Laboratory and Clinical Medicine* **124** (6), 749–754.

Ichimura, T. and Bonventre, J. V. Growth factors, signaling, and renal injury and repair. In *Acute Renal Failure: A Companion to Brenner & Rector's The Kidney* (ed. B. A. Molitoris and W. F. Finn), pp. 101–118. Philadelphia: W.B. Saunders, 2001.

Kellum, J. A. (1998). Use of diuretics in the acute care setting. *Kidney International* **66** (Suppl.), S67–S70.

Kellum, J. A. and Decker, M. (2001). Use of dopamine in acute renal failure: a meta-analysis. *Critical Care in Medicine* **29**, 1526–1531.

Kelly, K. J., Tolkoff-Rubin, N. E., Rubin, R. H., Williams, W. W., Jr., Meehan, S. M., Meschter, C. L., Christenson, J. G., and Bonventre, J. V. (1996a). An oral platelet-activating factor antagonist, Ro-24-4736, protects the rat kidney from ischemic injury. *American Journal of Physiology* **271** (5 Pt 2), F1061–F1067.

Kelly, K. J., Williams, J. J., Colvin, R. B., Meehan, S. M., Springer, T. A., Guttierez-Ramos, J. C., and Bonventre, J. (1996b). Intracellular adhesion molecule-I deficient mice are protected against renal ischemia. *Journal of Clinical Investigation* **97**, 1056–1063.

Kelly, K. J., Meehan, S. M., Colvin, R. B., Williams, W. W., and Bonventre, J. V. (1999). Protection from toxicant-mediated renal injury in the rat with anti- CD54 antibody. *Kidney International* **56** (3), 922–931.

Klinge, J. (2001). Intermittent administration of furosemide or continuous infusion in critically ill infants and children: does it make a difference? *Intensive Care Medicine* **27** (4), 623–624.

Koch, J. A., Plum, J., Grabensee, B., and Modder, U. (2000). Prostaglandin E1: a new agent for the prevention of renal dysfunction in high risk patients caused by radiocontrast media? PGE1 Study Group. *Nephrology, Dialysis, Transplantation* **15** (1), 43–49.

Kohda, Y., Chiao, H., and Star, R. A. (1998). Alpha-melanocyte-stimulating hormone and acute renal failure. *Current Opinion in Nephrology and Hypertension* **7** (4), 413–417.

Kribben, A., Wieder, E. D., Wetzels, J. F. M., Yu, L., Gengaro, P. E., Burke, T. J., and Schrier, R. W. (1994). Evidence for role of cytosolic free calcium in hypoxia-induced proximal tubule injury. *Journal of Clinical Investigation* **93**, 1922–1929.

Kribben, A., Edelstein, C. L., and Schrier, R. W. (1999). Pathophysiology of acute renal failure. *Journal of Nephrology* **12** (Suppl. 2), S142–S151.

Kurnik, B. R., Allgren, R. L., Genter, F. C., Solomon, R. J., Bates, E. R., and Weisberg, L. S. (1998). Prospective study of atrial natriuretic peptide for the prevention of radiocontrast-induced nephropathy. *American Journal of Kidney Diseases* **31** (4), 674–680.

Kwon, O., Corrigan, G., Myers, B. D., Sibley, R., Scandling, J. D., Dafoe, D., Alfrey, E., and Nelson, W. J. (1999). Sodium reabsorption and distribution of Na^+/K^+-ATPase during postischemic injury to the renal allograft. *Kidney International* **55** (3), 963–975.

Ladefoged, S. D. and Andersen, C. B. (1994). Calcium channel blockers in kidney transplantation. *Clinical Transplantation* **8**, 128–133.

Lameire, N. (1994). Acute tumour lysis syndrome and the kidney (editorial; comment). *The Netherlands Journal of Medicine* **45** (5), 193–197.

Lameire, N. and Vanholder, R. (2000). Drug therapy of acute renal failure. *IDrugs* **3**, 1206–1216.

Lameire, N., Verbeke, M., and Vanholder, R. (1995). Prevention of clinical acute tubular necrosis with drug therapy. *Nephrology, Dialysis, Transplantation* **10** (11), 1992–2000.

Lassnigg, A., Donner, E., Grubhofer, G., Presterl, E., Druml, J., and Hiesmayr, M. (2000). Lack of renoprotective effects of dopamine and furosemide during cardiac surgery. *Journal of the American Society of Nephrology* **11**, 97–104.

Lauriat, S. and Linas, S. L. (1998). The role of neutrophils in acute renal failure. *Seminars in Nephrology* **18** (5), 498–504.

Lee, H. T. and Emala, C. W. (2000). Protective effects of renal ischemic preconditioning and adenosine pretreatment: role of A(1) and A(3) receptors. *American Journal of Physiology. Renal Physiology* **278**, F387.

Levine, J. S. and Lieberthal, W. Terminal pathways to cell death. In *Acute Renal Failure: A Companion to Brenner & Rector's The Kidney* (ed. B. A. Molitoris and W. F. Finn), pp. 30–59. Philadelphia: W.B. Saunders, 2001.

Lewis, J., Salem, M. M., Chertow, G. M., Weisberg, L. S., McGrew, F., Marbury, T. C., and Allgren, R. L. (2000). Atrial natriuretic factor in oliguric acute renal failure. Anaritide Acute Renal Failure Study Group. *American Journal of Kidney Diseases* **36** (4), 767–774.

Libetta, C., Rampino, T., Esposito, C., Fornoni, A., Semeraro, L., and Dal Canton, A. (1998). Stimulation of hepatocyte growth factor in human acute renal failure. *Nephron* **80** (1), 41–45.

Lieberthal, W. (1997). Biology of acute renal failure: therapeutic implications. *Kidney International* **52** (4), 1102–1115.

Lieberthal, W. (1998). Biology of ischemic and toxic renal tubular cell injury: role of nitric oxide and the inflammatory response. *Current Opinion in Nephrology and Hypertension* **7**, 289–295.

Lieberthal, W. and Levinsky, N. G. (1990). Treatment of acute tubular necrosis. *Seminars in Nephrology* **10**, 571–583.

Lieberthal, W. and Nigam, S. K. (1998). Acute renal failure. I. Relative importance of proximal vs. distal tubular injury. *American Journal of Physiology* **275**, F623–F631.

Lieberthal, W. and Nigam, S. K. (2000). Acute renal failure. II. Experimental models of acute renal failure: imperfect but indispensable. *American Journal of Physiology. Renal Physiology* **278** (1), F1–F12.

Lieberthal, W., Koh, J. S., and Levine, J. S. (1998). Necrosis and apoptosis in acute renal failure. *Seminars Nephrology* **18** (5), 505–518.

Maier, K. G. and Roman, R. J. (2001). Cytochrome P450 metabolites of arachidonic acid in the control of renal function. *Current Opinion in Nephrology and Hypertension* **10**, 81–87.

Matlin, K. S. and Caplan, M. J. Epithelial cell structure and polarity. In *The Kidney: Physiology and Pathophysiology* 3rd edn. (ed. D. W. Seldin and G. Giebisch), pp. 533–567. Philadelphia: Lippincott Williams & Wilkins, 2000.

McCoy, R. N., Hill, K. E., Ayon, M. A., Stein, J. H., and Burk, R. F. (1988). Oxidant stress following renal ischemia: changes in the glutathione redox ratio. *Kidney International* **33** (4), 812–817.

Michael, U. and Lee, S. M. The role of calcium antagonists in nephrotoxic models of renal failure. In *Calcium Antagonists and The Kidney* (ed. M. Epstein and R. Loutzenheimer), pp. 187–201. Philadelphia: Hanley, Belfus, 1990.

Michael, U., Logan, J. L., and Meeks, L. A. (1991). The beneficial effects of thyroxine on nephrotoxic acute renal failure in the rat. *Journal of the American Society of Nephrology* **1**, 1236–1240.

Miller, S. B., Martin, D. R., Kissane, J., and Hammerman, M. R. (1994). Hepatocyte growth factor accelerates recovery from acute ischemic renal injury in rats. *American Journal of Physiology* **266** (1 Pt 2), F129–F134.

Morooka, H., Bonventre, J. V., Pombo, C. M., Kyriakis, J. M., and Force, T. (1995). Ischemia and reperfusion enhance ATF-2 and c-Jun binding to cAMP response elements and to an AP-1 binding site from the c-jun promoter. *Journal of Biological Chemistry* **270** (50), 30084–30092.

Myers, B. D., Miller, D. C., Mehigan, J. T., Olcott, C. O., Golbetz, H., Robertson, C. R., Derby, G., Spencer, R., and Friedman, S. (1984). Nature of the renal injury following total renal ischemia in man. *Journal of Clinical Investigation* **73** (2), 329–341.

Noiri, E., Gailit, J., Sheth, D., Magazine, H., Gurrath, M., Muller, G., Kessler, H., and Goligorsky, M. S. (1994). Cyclic RGD peptides ameliorate ischemic acute renal failure in rats. *Kidney International* **46** (4), 1050–1058.

Oberbauer, R. *et al.* (1999). Apoptosis of tubular epithelial cells in donor kidney biopsies predicts early renal allograft function. *Journal of the American Society of Nephrology* **10**, 2006–2013.

Paller, M. S. and Neumann, T. V. (1991). Reactive oxygen species and rat renal epithelial cells during hypoxia and reoxygenation. *Kidney International* **40** (6), 1041–1049.

Persy, V. P., Verstrepen, W. A., Ysebaert, D. K., De Greef, K. E., and De Broe, M. E. (1999). Differences in osteopontin up-regulation between proximal and distal tubules after renal ischemia/reperfusion. *Kidney International* **56** (2), 601–611.

Peters, H., Border, W. A., and Noble, N. A. (1999). From rats to man: a perspective on dietary L-arginine supplementation in human renal disease. *Nephrology, Dialysis, Transplantation* **14** (7), 1640–1650.

Petros, A., Lamb, G., Leone, A., Moncada, S., Bennett, D., and Vallance, P. (1994). Effects of a nitric oxide synthase inhibitor in humans with septic shock. *Cardiovascular Research* **28** (1), 34–39.

Pombo, C. M. *et al.* (1994). The stress-activated protein kinases are major c-Jun amino-terminal kinases activated by ischemia and reperfusion. *Journal of Biological Chemistry* **269**, 26546–26551.

Puig, J. M., Lloveras, J., Oliveras, A., Costa, A., Aubia, J., and Masramon, J. (1991). Usefulness of diltiazem in reducing the incidence of acute tubular necrosis in Euro-Collins preserved cadaveric renal grafts. *Transplant Proceedings* **23**, 2368–2369.

Rabb, H. and Postler, G. (1998). Leucocyte adhesion molecules in ischaemic renal injury: kidney specific paradigms? *Clinical and Experimental Pharmacology and Physiology* **25** (3–4), 286–291.

Racusen, L. C. The morphologic basis of acute renal failure. In *Acute Renal Failure: A Companion to Brenner & Rector's The Kidney* (ed. B. A. Molitoris and W. F. Finn), pp. 1–12. Philadelphia: W.B. Saunders Company, 2001.

Rahman, S. N., Kim, G. E., Mathew, A. S., Goldberg, C. A., Allgren, R., Schrier, R. W. and Conger, J. D. (1994). Effects of atrial natriuretic peptide in clinical acute renal failure. *Kidney International* **45** (6), 1731–1738.

Ramaswamy, D., Corrigan, G., Polhemus, C., Boothroyd, D., Scandling, J., Sommer, F. G., Alfrey, E., Higgins, J., Deen, W. M., Olshen, R., and Myers, B. D. (2002). Maintenance and recovery stages of postischemic acute renal failure in humans. *American Journal of Physiology. Renal Physiology* **282** (2), F271–F280.

Romanov, V., Noiri, E., Czerwinski, G., Finsinger, D., Kessler, H., and Goligorsky, M. S. (1997). Two novel probes reveal tubular and vascular Arg-Gly-Asp (RGD) binding sites in the ischemic rat kidney. *Kidney International* **52** (1), 93–102.

Rosenberger, C., Mandriota, S., Jurgensen, J. S., Wiesener, M. S., Horstrup, J. H., Frei, U., Ratcliffe, P. J., Maxwell, P. H., Bachmann, S., and Eckardt, K. U. (2002). Expression of hypoxia-inducible factor-1alpha and -2alpha in hypoxic and ischemic rat kidneys. *Journal of the American Society of Nephrology* **13**, 1721–1732.

Rubanyi, G. M. and Polokoff, M. A. (1994). Endothelins: molecular biology, biochemistry, pharmacology, physiology, and pathophysiology. *Pharmacological Reviews* **46** (3), 325–415.

Rudnick, M. R., Berns, J. S., Cohen, R. M., and Goldfarb, S. (1996). Contrast media-associated nephrotoxicity. *Current Opinion in Nephrology and Hypertension* **5** (2), 127–133.

Ruschitzka, F., Shaw, S., Gygi, D., Noll, G., Barton, M., and Luscher, T. F. (1999). Endothelial dysfunction in acute renal failure: role of circulating and tissue endothelin-1. *Journal of the American Society of Nephrology* **10** (5), 953–962.

Rushkoako, H. (1992). Atrial natriuretic peptide: synthesis, release and metabolism. *Pharmacological Review* **44**, 479–602.

Safirstein, R. *et al.* (1991). Expression of cytokine-like genes JE and KC is increased during renal ischemia. *American Journal of Physiology* **261**, F1095–F1101.

Sanders, P. W., Booker, B. B., Bishop, J. B., and Cheung, H. C. (1990). Mechanisms of intranephronal proteinaceous cast formation by low molecular weight proteins. *Journal of Clinical Investigation* **85**, 570–578.

Sanz, M. J., Johnston, B., Issekutz, A., and Kubes, P. (1999). Endothelin-1 causes P-selectin-dependent leukocyte rolling and adhesion within rat mesenteric microvessels. *American Journal of Physiology* **277** (5 Pt 2), H1823–H1830.

Schnermann, J. and Briggs, J. P. Function of the juxtaglomerular apparatus: control of glomerular hemodynamics and renin secretion. In *The Kidney: Physiology and Pathophysiology* 3rd edn. (ed. D. W. Seldin and G. Giebisch), pp. 945–980. Philadelphia: Lippincott Williams & Wilkins, 2000.

Schwartz, D. and Blantz, R. C. (1999). Nitric oxide, sepsis, and the kidney. *Seminars in Nephrology* **19** (3), 272–276.

Sheridan, A. M. and Bonventre, J. V. (2000). Cell biology and molecular mechanisms of injury in ischemic acute renal failure. *Current Opinion in Nephrology and Hypertension* **9**, 427–434.

Shilliday, I. R., Quinn, K. J., and Allison, M. E. (1997). Loop diuretics in the management of acute renal failure: a prospective, double-blind, placebo-controlled, randomized study. *Nephrology, Dialysis, Transplantation* **12** (12), 2592–2596.

Sitges-Serra, A., Carulla, X., Piera, C., Martinez-Rodenas, F., Franch, G., Pereira, J., and Gubern, J. M. (1992). Body water compartments in patients with obstructive jaundice. *British Journal of Surgery* **79**, 533–536.

Solez, K., Morel-Maroger, L., and Sraer, J. D. (1979). The morphology of 'acute tubular necrosis' in man: analysis of 57 renal biopsies and a comparison with the glycerol model. *Medicine (Baltimore)* **58** (5), 362–376.

Solomon, R., Werner, C., Mann, D., D'Elia, J., and Silva, P. (1994). Effects of saline, mannitol and furosemide to prevent acute decreases in renal function by radiocontrast agents. *New England Journal of Medicine* **331**, 1414–1416.

Springer, T. A. (1990). Adhesion receptors of the immune system. *Nature (London)* **346**, 425–434.

Stevens, N. A., McCullough, P. A., Tobin, K. J., Speck, J. P., Westveer, D. C., Guido-Allen, D. A., Timmis, G. C., and O'Neill, W. W. (1999). A prospective randomized trial of prevention measures in patients at high risk for contrast nephropathy—results of the PRINCE study. *Journal of the American College of Cardiology* **33**, 403–411.

Sward, K., Valson, F., and Ricksten, S. E. (2001). Long-term infusion of atrial natriuretic peptide (ANP) improves renal blood flow and glomerular filtration rate in clinical acute renal failure. *Acta Anaesthesiologica Scandinavica* **45** (5), 536–542.

Takala, J., Ruokonen, E., Webster, N. R., Nielsen, N. S., Zandstra, D. F., Vundelinckx, G., and Hinds, C. J. (1999). Increased mortality associated with growth hormone treatment in critically ill patients. *New England Journal of Medicine* **341**, 785–792.

Tepel, M., van der Giet M., Schwarzfeld, C., Laufer, U., Liermann, D., and Zidek, W. (2000). Prevention of radiographic-contrast-agent-induced reductions in renal function by acetylcysteine. *New England Journal of Medicine* **343** (3), 180–184.

Thadhani, R., Pascual, M., and Bonventre, J. V. (1996). Acute renal failure. *New England Journal of Medicine* **334** (22), 1448–1460.

Thurau, K. and Boylan, J. W. (1976). Acute renal success. The unexpected logic of oliguria in acute renal failure. *American Journal of Medicine* **61** (3), 308–315.

Toma, G., Bates, J. M., Jr., and Kumar, S. (1994). Uromodulin (Tamm–Horsfall protein) is a leukocyte adhesion molecule. *Biochemical and Biophysical Research Communications* **200** (1), 275–282.

Ueda, N. and Shah, S. V. (2000). Tubular cell damage in acute renal failure—apoptosis, necrosis, or both. *Nephrology, Dialysis, Transplantation* **15** (3), 318–323.

Ueda, N., Mayeux, P. R., Baliga, R., and Shah, S. V. Oxidant mechanisms in acute renal failure. In *Acute Renal Failure: A Companion to Brenner & Rector's The Kidney* 1st edn. (ed. B. A. Molitoris and W. F. Finn), pp. 60–77. Philadelphia: W.B. Saunders Company, 2001.

Van den Berghe, G. and De Zegher, F. (1996). Anterior pituitary function during critical illness and dopamine treatment. *Critical Care in Medicine* **24** (9), 1580–1590.

van der Vorst, M. M., Ruys-Dudok, v. H., I, Kist-van Holthe, J. E., den Hartigh, J., Schoemaker, R. C., Cohen, A. F., and Burggraaf, J. (2001). Continuous intravenous furosemide in haemodynamically unstable children after cardiac surgery. *Intensive Care Medicine* **27** (4), 711–715.

Van Valenberg, P. L. J., Hoitsma, A., Tiggeler, R. W. G. L., Berden, J. H., van Lier, H. J., and Koene, R. A. (1987). Mannitol as an indispensable constituent of an intravenous hydration protocol for the prevention of acute renal failure after cadaveric renal transplantation. *Transplantation* **44**, 784–788.

Van Why, S. K. and Siegel, N. J. Heat shock proteins: role in prevention and recovery from acute renal failure. In *Acute Renal Failure: A Companion to Brenner & Rector's The Kidney* (ed. B. A. Molitoris and W. F. Finn), pp. 143–155. Philadelphia: W.B. Saunders, 2001.

Venkatachalam, M. A., Weinberg, J. M., Patel, Y., Saikumar, P., and Dong, Z. (1996). Cytoprotection of kidney epithelial cells by compounds that target amino acid gated chloride channels. *Kidney International* **49** (2), 449–460.

Verbeke, M., Van de Voorde, J., and Lameire, N. (1996). Prevention of experimental acute tubular necrosis: current clinical applications and perspectives. *Advances in Nephrology from the Necker Hospital* **25**, 177–216.

Verbeke, M., Van de Voorde, J., de Ridder, L., and Lameire, N. (1998). Influence of ketanserin on experimental loss of renal blood flow autoregulation. *Kidney International* **67** (Suppl.), S238–S241.

Wagner, K., Henkel, M., Heinemeyer, G., and Neumayer, H. H. (1988). Interaction of calciumblockers and cyclosporine. *Transplantation Proceedings* **20**, 561–568.

Walker, L. M., Walker, P. D., Imam, S. Z., Ali, S. F., and Mayeux, P. R. (2000). Evidence for peroxynitrite formation in renal ischemia–reperfusion injury: studies with the inducible nitric oxide synthase inhibitor L-*N*(6)-(one-iminoethyl)lysine. *Journal of Pharmacology and Experimental Therapeutics* **295** (1), 417–422.

Wang, A., Holcslaw, T., Bashore, T. M., Freed, M. I., Miller, D., Rudnick, M. R., Szerlip, H., Thames, M. D., Davidson, C. J., Shusterman, N., and Schwab, S. J. (2000). Exacerbation of radiocontrast nephrotoxicity by endothelin receptor antagonism. *Kidney International* **57** (4), 1675–1680.

Weisberg, L. S., Kurnik, P. B., and Kurnik, B. R. (1994). Risk of radio-contrast nephropathy in patients with and without diabetes mellitus. *Kidney International* **45**, 259–265.

Whelton, A. (2000). Renal and related cardiovascular effects of conventional and COX-2-specific NSAIDs and non-NSAID analgesics. *American Journal of Therapeutics* **7** (2), 63–74.

Wilcox, C. S. L-Arginine–nitric oxide pathway. In *The Kidney: Physiology and Pathophysiology* 3rd edn. (ed. D. W. Seldin and G. Giebisch), pp. 849–871. Philadelphia: Lippincott Williams & Wilkins, 2000.

Yaqoob, M. M., Alkhunaizi, A. A., Edelstein, C. L., Conger, J., and Schrier, R. W. ARF: pathogenesis, diagnosis, and management. In *Renal and Electrolyte Disorders* 5th edn. (ed. R. W. Schrier), pp. 449–506. New York: Lippincott-Raven, 1997.

10.3 The clinical approach to the patient with acute renal failure

J.D. Firth

Introduction

The diagnosis of renal failure is usually made when the plasma concentration of urea or creatinine is measured and found to be elevated; it cannot reliably be made on clinical grounds alone. Acute, as opposed to chronic, renal failure is diagnosed when the decline in renal excretory function and increase in plasma urea and creatinine concentrations occur over hours or days. The condition is frequently accompanied by oliguria [defined (arbitrarily) as a urinary volume of <400 ml/day] and sometimes by anuria (<100 ml/day). However, urinary volume can be maintained and hence the fact that a patient is passing a 'normal' volume of urine is no guarantee that they do not have acute renal failure.

Acute renal failure is a common clinical problem (see Chapter 10.1), for which there are a very large number of possible causes (Chapter 10.2). These can be usefully divided into prerenal, renal (intrinsic), and postrenal (obstructive) types (Table 1). However, in any given clinical context, few of these are likely to require consideration. Much of the most frequent scenario is of acute renal failure:

(1) occurring in the setting of circulatory disturbance caused by severe illness, trauma, or surgery—particularly if sepsis is involved, and in the presence of nephrotoxins or drugs with adverse effects on renal perfusion;

(2) in which the main renal pathology is thought to consist of tubular damage; and

(3) in which recovery of renal function is generally anticipated if the patient survives the precipitating insult and is given renal replacement therapy should they require it.

This clinical scenario, which accounts for 80–90 per cent of all cases of severe acute renal failure referred to renal units or managed in intensive care units, is known by a number of terms, including 'acute tubular necrosis' (the term used hereafter) and haemodynamically mediated acute renal failure.

This section describes a practical clinical approach to the patient with acute renal failure. Given the common and serious nature of the problem, this is something that all who have medical responsibility for acutely ill patients should be familiar with, but the nephrologist is frequently required to assist. The requirements are:

(1) to be able to deal effectively with life-threatening complications, in particular hyperkalaemia and pulmonary oedema;

(2) to be able to assess intravascular volume status correctly, recognize volume depletion, and resuscitate effectively if this is depleted;

(3) to be able to establish whether renal failure is indeed acute, rather than chronic;

(4) to be able to diagnose the cause of acute renal failure, or recognize the group of causes that are most likely in any particular case;

(5) to prescribe effective treatment, or refer appropriately to a specialist unit if this is required.

In cases where the cause of acute renal failure is not obvious, the importance of excluding urinary obstruction and intrinsic renal disease at an early stage is emphasized, since delay in making these diagnoses and initiating appropriate treatment can lead to the tragedy of avoidable permanent loss of renal function. Details of the specific treatment options for these conditions can be found as follows: urinary obstruction (see Chapter 17.3), nephritides (see Chapter 10.6.1), and vasculitides (see Chapter 10.6.1). Emphasis is given to the diagnosis, prevention, and treatment of acute tubular necrosis, also to those aspects of medical management common to all patients who have acute renal failure.

Table 1 Some causes of acute renal failure

Prerenal
Appropriate renal response to poor perfusion
Renal
Acute tubular necrosis/haemodynamically mediated acute renal failure
Following haemodynamic compromise, commonly with sepsis
Following exposure to nephrotoxins including drugs, chemicals, rhabdomyolysis, snake bite
Vascular causes
Acute cortical necrosis
Large-vessel obstruction
Small-vessel obstruction—accelerated-phase hypertension and systemic sclerosis
Glomerulonephritis and vasculitis
Interstitial nephritis
'Haematological' causes
Haemolytic–uraemic syndrome/thrombotic thrombocytopenic purpura
Myeloma
Hepatorenal syndrome
Postrenal
Urinary obstruction
Intrarenal—crystalluria
Postrenal—urinary stones, papillary necrosis, retroperitoneal fibrosis, bladder/prostate/cervical/rectal lesions, massive lymphadenopathy (lymphoproliferative conditions, secondary carcinoma)

Diagnosis of the presence of acute renal failure

A high index of clinical suspicion is required to diagnose acute renal failure at an early stage of its development. Very few patients know how much urine they pass, or what it looks like, and a reduction in urinary volume or change in colour—if commented upon—are invariably put down to the fact that they 'were not drinking'. Symptoms and signs attributable to the accumulation of urea and other toxins within the body are non-specific, and they are not evident until renal failure is far advanced. Inability to excrete salt and water can lead to the development of peripheral and/or pulmonary oedema, but these are also non-specific findings for which there are several more common causes than renal failure. Failure of renal acid excretion can lead to the development of systemic acidosis and induce a very characteristic sighing pattern of breathing (Kussmaul respiration). If the most common cause of this respiratory pattern, diabetic ketoacidosis, can be excluded, then its presence should strongly suggest the possibility of renal failure. In most cases, however, there are no features of the history or examination that enable the physician to make a confident declaration that acute renal failure is, or is not, present when a patient is first clinically assessed. If acute renal failure is present, then the clinical presentation is almost invariably dominated by that of the condition which precipitates it. Unsuspected hyperkalaemia is the greatest danger, since this rarely produces any recognized symptoms before inducing cardiac arrest.

On this background, all patients admitted to hospital with an acute illness should be considered to be at risk of having undiagnosed acute renal failure, and whilst they remain acutely ill to be at substantial risk of developing the condition. Those who have some pre-existing chronic impairment of renal function are particularly susceptible to acute exacerbations. This group includes all elderly patients, in whom a combination of low muscle mass and low dietary meat consumption may conspire to maintain an apparently 'normal' plasma creatinine, despite a reduction in glomerular filtration rate to as little as 25 per cent of that expected in a healthy young adult.

Given the lack of reliable clinical indicators, all patients admitted to hospital with an acute illness should have their plasma concentrations of creatinine and urea measured to establish whether or not they have impaired renal function, and routine measurement of electrolyte concentrations should allow detection of hyperkalaemia. Thereafter, one of the aims of basic medical and nursing care is to try to prevent the development of acute renal failure, or—failing that—to recognize its development at an early stage. This requires the careful monitoring of fluid input and output, daily weighing (where practicable), measurement of lying and standing (or sitting) blood pressure (at least once daily), and continued daily estimation of the plasma concentrations of creatinine, urea, and electrolytes whilst the patient remains acutely unwell. In conjunction with regular repeated clinical examination of the patient, the clinical and laboratory data must be appraised every day.

Nursing and clinical records

Recording of fluid input and output

The estimation of urinary output and of gastrointestinal losses is a simple matter in many patients, but can be impossible in some. Valid measurement of fluid output cannot be made in the incontinent patient, and is very difficult in those who vomit, or in those with fistulae. Aside from protecting the skin, the use of a urinary sheath or catheter in such cases has the advantage of enabling urinary output to be measured. Determination of fluid input can also be problematical, except in those who are only receiving fluids parenterally. Patients do not always drink all that they are given, and sometimes they help themselves to more. The most likely explanation for fluid-balance charts being difficult to interpret is that they are simply wrong.

Daily weighing

Daily weighing on accurate scales provides a more reliable picture of net overall fluid balance than do fluid charts. Patients who are acutely ill invariably lose flesh weight, commonly at a rate of up to a few hundred grams per day. If weight appears to fall faster than this, then negative fluid balance is almost certain. If the fluid balance charts do not suggest this, then record keeping may have been incorrect (or simply impossible), or the magnitude of 'insensible' losses through the skin and lungs may have been underestimated. This is particularly likely in those who are pyrexial, when insensible losses can amount to 1 l or more per day. If weight increases, then this must be due to positive fluid balance, whatever the input/output records suggest. It may not always be obvious from clinical examination where the fluid has gone, and the possibilities of sequestration in the peritoneal cavity or in the tissue interstitium, due to the development of a widespread 'capillary leak' in an acutely ill patient, should be recognized.

Postural measurement of blood pressure

The factor that precipitates the admission of many patients to hospital is the development of postural hypotension. When this develops, as a consequence of any illness, they are no longer able to get out of bed to go to the bathroom without feeling dizzy and light-headed, perhaps even collapsing in the attempt. Whilst postural hypotension may be caused by impairment of function of the autonomic nervous system, in those who are acutely ill the more common reason is intravascular volume depletion. Measurement of the blood pressure with the patient recumbent in bed can be falsely reassuring, a value of (say) 120/80 mmHg being taken as 'normal'. If a patient is fit enough to stand, the measurement should be repeated with them standing. If a patient is not well enough to stand, they should be helped to sit up and the blood pressure recorded in this position. If a significant reduction in blood pressure with postural change develops, then this should be taken as indicating intravascular volume depletion.

Diagnosis of the cause of acute renal failure

In the initial assessment by a nephrologist of a patient who appears to have acute renal failure four questions should be addressed.

Question 1: is the renal failure really acute?

The only secure basis for excluding the possibility of pre-existing chronic renal impairment is the knowledge of a previous normal measurement of renal function. A diligent search for such information can save much unnecessary work.

Some clinical features can help in deciding whether renal failure is acute or chronic: a history of vague ill health of some months duration, of nocturia, of pruritus; the findings of skin pigmentation, anaemia, evidence of long-standing hypertension or neuropathy, would all suggest chronicity (see Chapter 11.3.1). The fact that a patient may have been refused insurance at some time in the past, or had premiums loaded, or had a 'bit of protein in the urine' noted at a medical examination, or been told that they 'have a bit of a problem with their kidneys', are also likely to indicate long-standing renal disease. However, anaemia is not invariable in chronic renal failure (e.g. in polycystic kidney disease, the haemoglobin concentration is often normal) and anaemia can develop rapidly (over a few days) in acute renal failure, as may hypocalcaemia and hyperphosphataemia. Radiological evidence of renal osteodystrophy is only found in those with obviously long-standing chronic renal failure and rarely (if ever) aids the clinical distinction between acute and chronic renal failure.

An increase in the plasma concentration of urea leads to increased carbamylation of haemoglobin in circulating red cells. The level of such carbamylation has been measured in a research context: increased concentrations indicate long-standing elevation of the plasma urea concentration and chronic renal failure; low levels indicate that the biochemical derangement is of recent origin and that renal failure is acute (Davenport *et al.* 1993). However, this test has not become established in clinical practice since it is usually not difficult to distinguish between acute and chronic renal failure. Furthermore, when there is doubt, other methods in routine use, in particular ultrasound examination, enables the distinction of acute from chronic renal failure to be made in a satisfactory manner in most cases, and ultrasonography also provides other essential information.

Measurement of renal size

One of the first investigations will be imaging to determine renal size, and also to confirm that two kidneys are present. In most instances, chronic renal disease causes the kidneys to shrink, and it is the finding of 'two small kidneys' that most often indicates the presence of previously unsuspected chronic renal disease.

On a plain radiographic film of the abdomen, the outline of the kidneys can sometimes be traced, the normal length being 3.7 ± 0.4 times the height of the second lumbar vertebral body (Witten *et al.* 1977). Better definition of the renal outline can be obtained by intravenous urography, but this procedure is not recommended in patients with acute renal failure because high doses of contrast medium are necessary to obtain images in those with poor renal function, the images obtained in such circumstances tend to be of relatively poor quality, and there is concern that the contrast media used can be nephrotoxic. The standard imaging technique used to assess renal size is ultrasonography, which is non-invasive, has no known deleterious effects, and is also the first-line imaging technique to assess whether or not a patient has urinary obstruction. The normal kidney length measured by this method is 10–12 cm (Cook *et al.* 1977).

Radioisotopic methods ([^{131}I]iodohippurate, [^{99}Tc^{m}]DTPA, [^{99}Tc^{m}]DMSA) have been used to determine renal size in patients with renal failure, but they have not been found to be clinically helpful and are not routinely employed in this context. Computed tomography can also be used to measure the size of the kidneys, but is rarely required for this purpose alone.

Question 2: is urinary obstruction a possibility?

One of the merits of the traditional division of the causes of acute renal failure into prerenal, renal, and postrenal types is that it demands consideration of the possibility of urinary obstruction. This is a common cause of both acute and chronic renal impairments, with prostatic obstruction accounting for 25 per cent of cases of severe acute renal failure in the community-based study by Feest *et al.* (1993). It is obviously important that obstruction should not be missed because it is readily treatable and, if neglected, causes irreversible renal damage (Sacks *et al.* 1989).

A thorough urological history and examination is mandatory in those with acute renal failure in whom the cause is not obvious. Apart from asking the patient the obvious questions about whether they have ever had haematuria, passed urinary stones, had renal colic, had prostatic symptoms, had retroperitoneal or pelvic surgery, etc., it is worthwhile probing these aspects of the history in more detail. It is not uncommon to discover that a patient has, at some time in the past, had pain in the loin or back that lasted for a few days or weeks and then got better. At the time, this was plausibly attributed to a musculoskeletal problem, and when it went away it was forgotten. In retrospect, the interpretation has been that the episode represented unilateral renal obstruction, which was not recognized as such, not treated, and led to permanent loss of function of that kidney. The patient with a single functional kidney remaining then went on to develop acute renal failure as a consequence of its obstruction.

Palpation and percussion to see whether the bladder is distended are often neglected or done in a cursory manner during the 'routine' examination of the abdomen of a 'medical' patient. In any patient with renal failure, proper attention to this part of the physical examination should be given, also to examination of the genitalia, rectum, prostate, and the uterine cervix.

Even if there are no positive features in the history or examination to suggest obstruction, the diagnosis should still be considered where another positive diagnosis cannot be made. The presence of anuria or of alternating polyuria and oligoanuria are helpful clues. Although very uncommon, renal function may be significantly impaired due to obstruction despite the production of an apparently satisfactory 24-h urinary volume. The mechanisms responsible are poorly understood, but three factors present in obstruction tend to impair urinary concentrating ability and can thereby lead to preservation of urinary volume despite obstructive depression of the filtration rate. These factors are (a) structural damage to the inner medulla and papilla, (b) functional changes in the distal nephron resulting from increased intraluminal or interstitial pressure, and (c) loss of medullary hypertonicity at low filtration rates.

Renal imaging to detect obstruction

Ultrasonographic examination of the kidneys and bladder is the method of choice in most centres to investigate for the presence of obstruction (Fig. 1) (Green and Carroll 1986). However, ultrasound detects dilatation of the renal calyces and pelvis, not obstruction, and the diagnosis can be missed either because the calyces fail to dilate or do so minimally. In one series, such cases accounted for four of 80 patients presenting with acute obstructive anuria (Maillet *et al.* 1986). The most common cause of obstruction without dilatation is malignancy, which Spital *et al.* (1988) found to be the diagnosis in 17 out of 25 cases.

If, despite a 'negative' ultrasound report, obstruction is still a possible cause of acute renal failure, a number of options should be considered. Recognizing that obstruction without dilatation is possible, and also that the quality of image obtained by renal ultrasonography is variable—depending on the patient, the equipment, and on

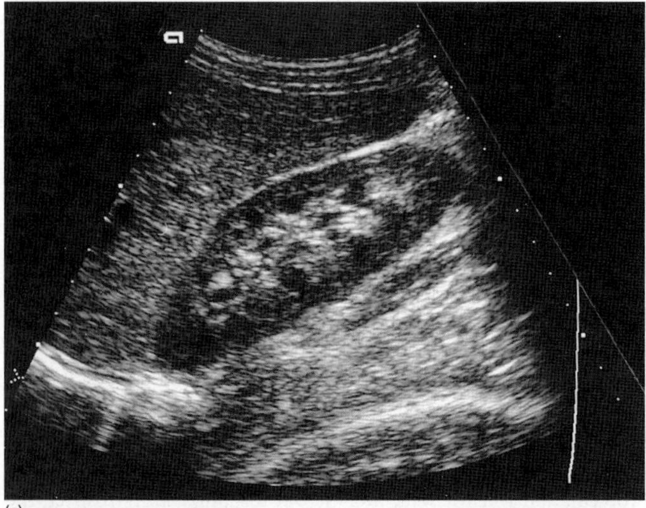

(a)

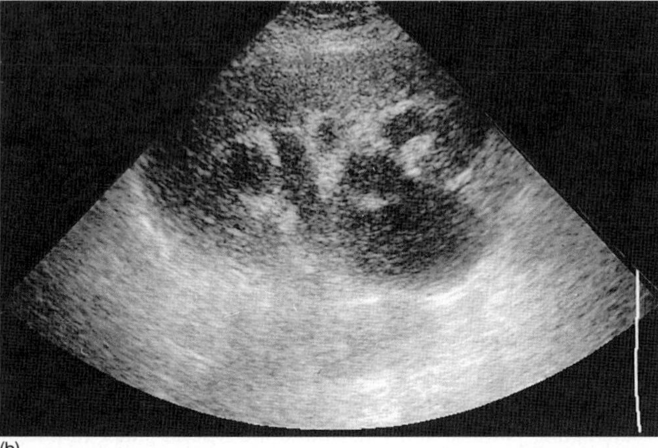

(b)

Fig. 1 Ultrasound appearances of (a) normal kidney and (b) an obstructed kidney, showing dilatation of the renal pelvis and calyces.

the operator—the case should be discussed with the person who made the original ultrasound examination and the scan repeated to see if appearances have changed. Further investigations then to be considered include computed tomography, cystoscopy with retrograde ureteropyelography, and (very rarely) antegrade nephrostomy. Radioisotope studies, such as DTPA renography with frusemide injection, can be useful in the diagnosis of urinary obstruction in those with normal or only slightly impaired renal function (see Chapter 1.6.1vii). However, since they depend on renal perfusion and glomerular filtration and/or tubular secretion to produce an image, they are rarely helpful in those with acute renal failure. In some cases, imaging alone may fail to resolve the problem unequivocally, and in these very rare instances it will be necessary to instigate a 'trial of urinary drainage'. This requires the renal pelvis(es) to be drained by either antegrade nephrostomy(ies) or retrograde stent(s) to see if this leads (over a few weeks) to functional improvement. Substantial recovery of renal function can occur after the relief of long-standing obstruction, up to 34 days of anuria in one series (Maillet *et al.* 1986).

Computed tomography, in common with ultrasound, demonstrates anatomy rather than function, but offers two major advantages. First, it produces 'hard copies' that can be shown to others whose opinion is valued. By contrast, ultrasound is a dynamic test, and the static images that are recorded often contain relatively little information: they provide reassuring visual confirmation for the clinician in obvious cases, but are of almost no value in those that are difficult. Second, computed tomography provides considerably better definition of retroperitoneal and pelvic anatomy: it is, therefore, much more likely than ultrasound to demonstrate a cause for obstruction, and to detect lesions that invade the retroperitoneal space causing obstruction without permitting dilatation. However, whilst some have reported that computed tomography scanning can reveal reliable secondary signs of acute obstruction, for example, obstructed kidney less dense than unobstructed on unenhanced scanning (Georgiades *et al.* 2001), others have emphasized that there is considerable interobserver variability in the assessment of scans and that computed tomography scanning is not good at differentiating between high grade (complete/near complete) or partial obstruction (Bird *et al.* 2002).

Magnetic resonance urography or 'virtual endoscopy' has also been used to examine the urinary tract in cases of obstruction. Very good images can be obtained in cases where the ureter is more than 5 mm in diameter, but it is not possible to obtain these in non-dilated systems because the technique depicts fluid in the urinary tract (Louca *et al.* 1999; Neri *et al.* 2000). However, magnetic resonance imaging can provide excellent anatomical images, is becoming more widely available, and is likely to be used increasingly in cases of possible urinary obstruction.

Cystoscopy with retrograde ureteropyelography, unlike ultrasound examination or computed tomography, is an invasive procedure which may require general anaesthesia, and trauma, haemorrhage and infection are recognized complications. It should not, however, be avoided in difficult cases, not least because the retrograde passage of ureteric stents can relieve any obstruction that is demonstrated.

Antegrade nephrostomy is usually done to obtain relief of obstruction after ultrasound (or computed tomographic) demonstration of pelvicalyceal dilatation. However, the procedure may also be warranted in the rare situation when there is genuine clinical suspicion that obstruction is present despite steadfastly 'equivocal' imaging results. Even though failure to observe dilatation of the renal pelvis and calyces makes the procedure technically more difficult and is a relative contraindication, the introduction of a fine needle into the pelvicalyceal system can usually be accomplished by a skilled operator. A small amount of contrast dye is introduced: obstruction is excluded if it passes freely down the ureter and into the bladder, an antegrade nephrostomy drainage tube (usually of the 'pig tail' variety) being inserted if it does not.

Relief of obstruction

If obstruction is diagnosed, then it should obviously be relieved by bladder catheterization, percutaneous (antegrade) nephrostomy, or cystoscopic retrograde insertion of ureteric stents, as a prelude to definitive treatment (where possible) of the underlying obstructive lesion. The most common causes of urinary obstruction causing acute renal failure are renal calculi, retroperitoneal fibrosis, malignant diseases of the uterine cervix, prostate, bladder, and rectum, benign prostatic hypertrophy, and conditions that cause massive retroperitoneal and pelvic lymphadenopathy (lymphoproliferative conditions and secondary carcinoma).

Renal obstruction needs to be relieved as soon as possible. If obstruction can be relieved by passage of a urethral or suprapubic catheter into the bladder, then this should be done immediately, since these are procedures that can be rapidly and safely performed in the general ward in the vast majority of cases. If, however, relief of obstruction requires antegrade nephrostomy, then considerations are somewhat different. There are no clinical data to determine whether a delay of (say) 24 h in relieving obstruction is significantly detrimental to long-term renal function, and the procedure carries risks, especially in the uncooperative patient. There is no justification for attempting antegrade nephrostomy in obviously suboptimal circumstances in order to try and avoid the need for dialysis. If the patient's clinical condition could be expected to improve with renal replacement therapy (see Chapter 10.4), then this should be given before nephrostomy is attempted. Furthermore, if the patient is not capable of cooperating, then some form of sedation will certainly be required, and one of the attending physicians should—if at all possible—accompany the patient to the ultrasound department to provide and supervise its administration.

If acute renal failure is caused by bilateral renal obstruction, then the obstruction to both kidneys should be relieved. This may require bilateral antegrade nephrostomies. In practice, however, it may not be possible to perform both procedures at the same sitting. If the first procedure is painful and traumatic for the patient, it may simply not be prudent to ask them to roll over and start on the other side. If the kidneys are asymmetrical, the one that appears to have the best-preserved cortex (and, by implication, the best potential for function) should be punctured first.

Question 3: are glomerulonephritis (Chapter 10.6.1), interstitial nephritis (Chapter 10.6.2), vasculitis, or other uncommon disorders possible?

The 'clues' to glomerulonephritis are sometimes very obvious, for example, the patient who is known to have systemic lupus erythematosus and says that their disease is active. However, it is important to explore all possible clinical leads in those in whom the cause of acute renal failure is not immediately apparent. The many extrarenal manifestations of multisystem disorders will not be listed here, but it is unwise to totally ignore any complaint or finding. Particular attention should be paid to a history or signs of a rash; to arthralgias or arthritis, to myalgias; and to eye, ear, or nose problems, which may be missed from the 'general medical assessment'. They provide the clues to multisystem disorder, vasculitic process, or rhabdomyolysis. Obtaining a complete drug history is essential: penicillins and non-steroidal anti-inflammatory agents, which in many countries are available without prescription, are the most common drugs that cause acute interstitial nephritis (see Chapter 10.6.2).

When referred a case of acute renal failure, it is important to ask 'What did the urine contain?' Although ward urinary microscopy may not be possible in some hospitals, urine dipsticks are widely available. It is to make the diagnosis of a renal inflammatory process, which although rare has vitally important management implications, that these tests are an absolute requirement. Urinary dipstick testing and—if this reveals the presence of blood and protein—microscopy of the urinary sediment are an essential part of the assessment of any patient with unexplained acute renal failure. These crucial investigations should not be delegated to those without a specific interest in the result. The technique for urinary microscopy should be as follows: 10–15 ml of urine should be spun at 1500 rpm for 5 min, all but 1 ml of the supernatant carefully discarded, and the pellet resuspended. Examination, looking primarily for red-cell casts (Fig. 2), should be made under high power, preferably after counterstaining. Their presence indicates renal inflammation caused by acute glomerulonephritis (of various types), renal vasculitis (of various types), accelerated-phase hypertension, or (rarely) interstitial nephritis. If they are present, then renal biopsy, together with other specialized blood tests (antiglomerular basement-membrane antibodies, antineutrophil cytoplasmic antibodies, antinuclear factor antibodies, etc.), will be required to establish a precise diagnosis.

Question 4: is an acute renal vascular event possible? (see Chapter 10.6.6)

The referral to renal units of increasing numbers of elderly patients with acute renal failure includes many who have widespread atheromatous vascular disease. Some of these will be dependent upon a single functioning kidney, the other having been lost as a result of occlusion of the renal artery at some time in the past. Imaging will demonstrate one kidney of normal size and one which is small, say less than 8 or 9 cm in length on ultrasound. Although acute renal failure may be due to acute tubular necrosis in these cases, there is clearly the possibility that it could be precipitated by acute occlusion, thrombotic or embolic, of the renal artery supplying the solitary functioning kidney. Risk factors include exposure to angiotensin-converting enzyme inhibitors, reduction in blood pressure secondary to antihypertensive agents or volume depletion, hypertension, radiological procedures requiring exposure to contrast media, and (sometimes) the instrumentation of the aorta (Roche *et al.* 1993).

The diagnosis of acute renal vascular occlusion is supported if the patient complains of flank pain, has macroscopic haematuria, if there is complete anuria, or—if the patient does pass some urine—by the finding of a urinary sodium concentration equal to that in plasma (Liano *et al.* 1994).

If renal artery occlusion is suspected, what is the best diagnostic technique and what is the most appropriate treatment? In most centres, the best test for detecting acute occlusion of the renal artery remains conventional arteriography, but the resolution of computed tomographic angiography and magnetic resonance angiography are improving (Kawashima *et al.* 2000; Urban *et al.* 2001; Vosshenrich and Fischer 2002). For detailed discussion of investigative techniques, see Chapter 10.6.6.

Decisions regarding treatment of renal artery occlusion are seldom straightforward. Occlusion caused by arterial thrombosis almost invariably arises on a background of long-standing atheromatous renal arterial disease, associated with the development of collateral blood supply from the suprarenal, lumbar, and ureteric vascular beds. In this situation, the kidney may remain viable after acute occlusion of its main arterial supply, even when the perfusion pressure from the collaterals is insufficient to support any glomerular filtration and the patient is totally anuric. Renal function can recover after revascularization even if this is delayed by weeks. Ramsay *et al.* (1983) reported a case in which bypass of an occluded renal artery produced recovery after 47 days of oliguric acute renal failure; Pontremoli *et al.* (1990) reported a case where bilateral revascularization after 42 days of anuria restored function. Fibrinolytic therapy can also be effective (Salam *et al.* 1993;

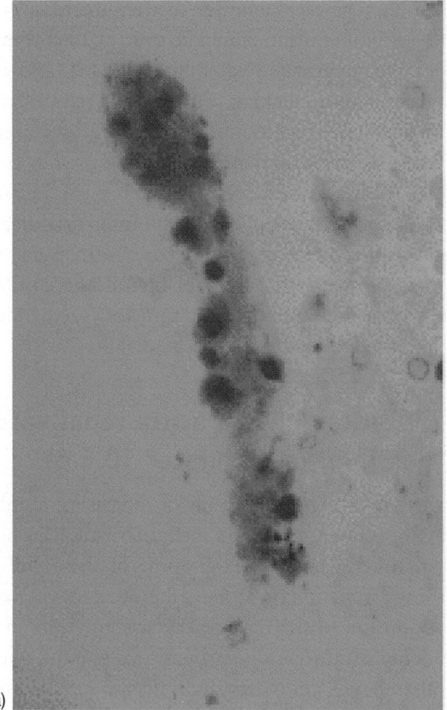

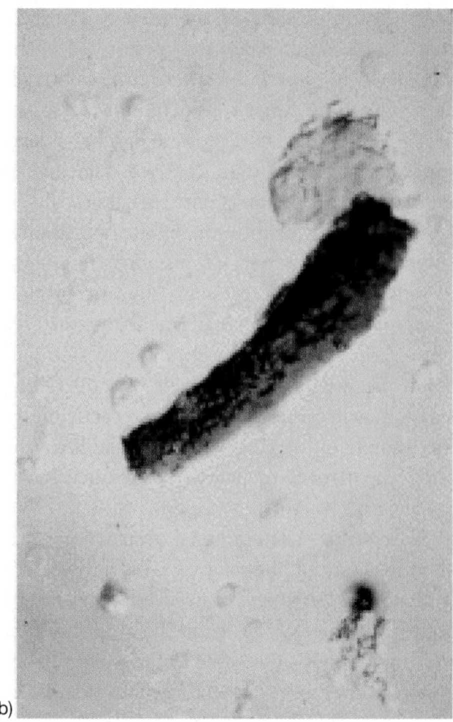

Fig. 2 A red cell cast seen in urine with (a) and without (b) counterstaining.

Takeda *et al.* 1993; Pilmore *et al.* 1995); however, the nephrologist will usually be faced with a frail, elderly, arteriopath who has been on dialysis for more than a week, posing the question, 'Should a substantial surgical procedure (renal revascularization, usually with a vein or prosthetic graft) that may result in some restoration of renal function, but with unknown chance of getting the patient off dialysis, be recommended when it undoubtedly carries a substantial risk of morbidity/mortality?' The decision will depend on the patient and the enthusiasm of the surgeon and/or radiologist, but there are little data to base that decision upon. By contrast, the prognosis is uniformly bad if the renal artery of a kidney that does not have a developed collateral supply is occluded. Blum *et al.* (1993) gave local thrombolytic therapy to 14 patients with acute unilateral embolic occlusion of a renal artery: in 13, the treatment was technically successful, but renal function did not recover in kidneys whose arteries had been completely occluded. They concluded that in this situation attempts to revascularize were 'not indicated once the ischaemic tolerance of the kidney (approximately 90 min) had been exceeded'.

Prerenal failure and acute tubular necrosis (see Chapter 10.2)

The vast majority of cases of acute renal failure will fall into the categories of prerenal failure or acute tubular necrosis. The term prerenal failure is used when renal dysfunction is entirely attributable to hypoperfusion and restoration of renal perfusion leads to rapid recovery. The term acute tubular necrosis is used, as indicated previously, to describe a particular clinical scenario: (a) it is seen in specific clinical contexts, frequently involving circulatory compromise, sepsis, and/or nephrotoxins; (b) urinary abnormalities (see later) usually suggest tubular dysfunction; and (c) essentially complete recovery of renal function is expected within days or weeks in most cases (if the patient survives the precipitating insult).

To use an obviously pathological expression, acute tubular necrosis, to describe what is almost invariably an entirely clinical diagnosis, is hard to justify. The term is eschewed by some because it implies that the pathological basis of the clinical syndrome is known. In its defence, it should be said that there is functional evidence that tubular integrity is breached in clinical cases of acute renal failure; studies of dextran clearance revealing that glomerular filtrate can leak back from the tubules into the circulation (Moran and Myers 1985). Furthermore, necrosis of tubular cells can usually be seen on renal biopsy (Solez *et al.* 1979), although the lesion may be inconspicuous. However, because of concerns about nomenclature, many other phrases have been devised to describe the syndrome in a more accurate and acceptable way. None have gained universal acceptance, but 'haemodynamically mediated acute renal failure' is one of the most frequently used alternatives (Myers and Moran 1986).

Acute renal failure of this type can be seen after virtually any episode of severe circulatory compromise, but not all causes of circulatory derangement are equally devastating to renal function. Primary impairment of cardiac performance, for example, following myocardial infarction, may cause plasma creatinine to increase somewhat, but rarely causes renal failure of sufficient severity to require renal replacement therapy. By contrast, haemodynamic upset caused by sepsis frequently does. Table 2 shows the causes of acute impairment of renal function (usually modest) in over 2000 consecutive medical and surgical admissions (Hou *et al.* 1983).

Many patients with haemodynamically mediated acute renal failure do not have a single cause for their renal failure: the kidney most typically fails when subjected to multiple insults. Rasmussen and Ibels (1982) defined and quantitatively assessed the risk factors and acute insults to which 143 patients with acute tubular necrosis had been exposed. Sixty-two per cent of patients had more than one acute insult, and 48 per cent more than one suspected risk factor. Statistical analysis suggested that hypotension, excessive exposure to aminoglycosides, pigmenturia, and dehydration were highly significant acute insults. Surprisingly, the study did not identify sepsis as a risk factor, probably because of the statistical method employed (sepsis not being significant after hypotension had been allowed for) and also due to a propensity of those caring for the patients to give aminoglycosides to those that they considered to be gravely ill. Most importantly, an additive interaction between insults was demonstrated, and the severity of acute renal failure was related to the number and magnitude of acute insults (Fig. 3).

Table 2 Causes of development of acute impairment of renal function in 2216 consecutive medical and surgical admissions

Acute tubular necrosis	
Hypovolaemia	22
Congestive cardiac failure	10
Sepsis	10
Nephrotoxins	25
Postsurgical	23
Other	12
Hepatorenal syndrome	5
Obstruction	3
Vasculitis	2
Other/multifactorial/unknown	17
Total	129 (4.9% of admissions)

Notes: (1) Acute impairment of renal function diagnosed when serum creatinine increased by predetermined amount (approximately one-third of baseline) during period of hospital admission; (2) during period of study 46 patients were excluded from analysis because they were either admitted specifically for treatment of acute renal failure or were recipients of long-term haemodialysis; (3) dialysis required in 10 cases. Modified from Hou *et al.* (1983).

Pathophysiology (see Chapter 10.2)

An understanding of the pathophysiology of any condition is a prerequisite for rational strategies for prevention or treatment. Although described in detail elsewhere, a summary is provided here to set the background for discussion of potential therapies.

In the case of acute tubular necrosis/haemodynamically mediated acute renal failure, our understanding is woefully incomplete. If the circulation is modestly compromised, compensatory mechanisms preserve the glomerular filtration rate by increasing the filtration fraction. This has repercussions on tubular function, which, along with other factors, leads to increased tubular reabsorption of sodium, water, and urea—a state rapidly reversed by the restoration of renal perfusion. However, following a more severe insult, renal function frequently deteriorates in a manner not immediately reversible when the circulation is restored. It is not obvious why this should be so. Under normal conditions, the kidney enjoys high blood flow, exceeded on a volume/weight basis only by the carotid body, and oxygen tension in the renal venous effluent is high, suggesting that oxygen supply greatly exceeds demand. Such a situation might be expected to confer protection from the effects of circulatory compromise, but no such benefit is observed. Indeed, the kidney appears more susceptible to damage than other organs. It is assumed that the mechanism is ischaemic, given (a) the clinical setting of profound haemodynamic disturbance in which acute renal failure is frequently seen, and (b) that acute renal failure resembling the clinical condition can be produced in animal models by manoeuvres that impair renal blood flow. Two main hypotheses, not necessarily mutually exclusive, have been proposed to explain why the kidney might be so prone to sustaining ischaemic damage. The first stresses that arteriovenous shunting of oxygen, resulting from the

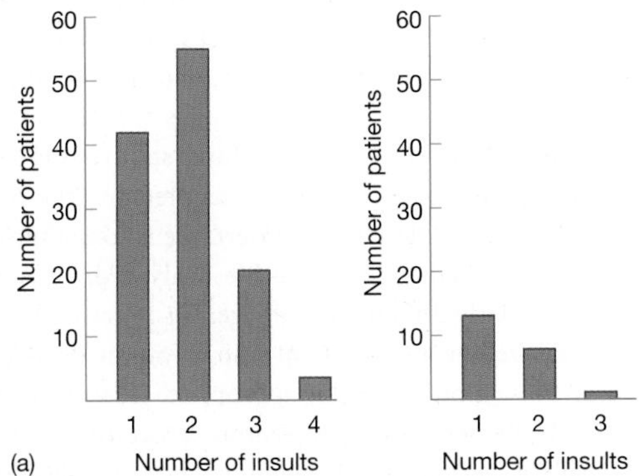

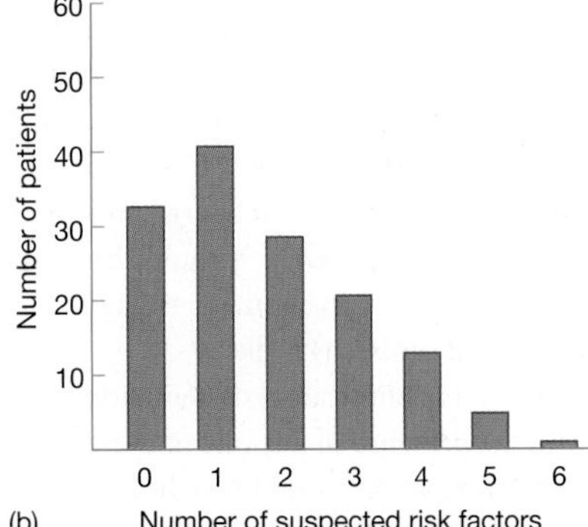

Fig. 3 Patients with acute tubular necrosis/haemodynamically mediated acute renal failure have frequently been subjected to more than one acute insult and have multiple suspected risk factors (from Rasmussen and Ibels 1982). (a) Distribution of the number of acute insults per patients in 121 patients without pre-existing renal disease and 22 patients with pre-existing renal disease. Acute insults considered were: hypotension, sepsis, excessive aminoglycoside exposure, parenteral administration of radiocontrast media, pigmenturia, severe liver disease, and dehydration. (b) Distribution of the number of suspected risk factors per patient in 143 patients. Factors considered were: an age of more than 59 years, hypertension, gout and/or hyperuricaemia, diabetes, pre-existing renal disease, and long-term diuretic medication.

specialized countercurrent arrangement of intrarenal arteries and veins, leads to the presence of areas of profound hypoxia within the normal kidney. These areas might, therefore, be operating on the verge of anoxia in the normal organ, and susceptible to ischaemic damage in response to modest compromise of whole-organ blood flow. The second hypothesis is based on clinical and experimental angiographic evidence of intense constriction of renal vessels during shock, and suggests that a very severe reduction in renal blood flow (perhaps only transient) may be responsible for the initiation of ischaemic damage.

Given the acknowledged imperfections in our understanding of the basic pathophysiology, the justification for many of the interventions proposed in the management of patients at risk of acute renal failure, or with established acute renal failure, is that they might preserve renal blood flow and/or reduce renal oxygen consumption, thus rendering the development of ischaemic injury less likely.

It seems plausible that the pathological basis for the distinction between the clinical syndromes of prerenal failure and established acute tubular necrosis/haemodynamically mediated acute renal failure is whether or not irreversible cellular damage has been sustained within the kidney. If it has not, then rapid recovery of renal function is possible. If it has, then restoration of function can only occur after the structure has been restored by cellular regeneration, and this process takes days or weeks rather than minutes or hours, although it may be possible to speed these processes up in the future.

Table 3 Evaluation of intravascular volume

Clinical signs of volume depletion
Jugular venous pressure low[a]
Hypotension, postural drop in blood pressure of >10 mmHg and rise in pulse rate of >10 beats/min (lying and sitting, if lying and standing not possible)
Collapsed peripheral veins and cool peripheries (nose, fingers, toes)
Fast, thready pulse
Clinical sings of volume overload
Jugular venous pressure high[a]
Gallop rhythm
Hypertension, peripheral oedema, liver congestion, pulmonary crepitations
Directly measurable indices of intravascular volume
Central venous pressure[a]
Pulmonary capillary-wedge pressure[a]
Therapeutic tests of volume depletion or excess
Trial of fluid infusion[b]
Trial of fluid removal [diuretic, haemofiltration/haemodialysis, venesection (exceptionally)]

[a] Absolute values deliberately not given: 'low' or 'high' relative to estimated optimal value for individual.

[b] Trials of fluid infusion should be undertaken with the patient under continuous medical observation and terminated immediately in the event of deterioration in the patient's condition.

Avoidance

One of the main aims of the basic management of all acutely ill patients is to minimize the chances of developing renal impairment. Regular measurement of the plasma creatinine concentration will permit early recognition of declining renal function, but is not of itself therapeutic. The cornerstones of good management are (a) the maintenance of optimal intravascular volume, and (b) the avoidance of, or reduction of exposure to, nephrotoxic agents.

Maintenance of optimal intravascular volume

The optimal intravascular volume is, from the nephrological point of view, the volume at which the kidneys are best perfused. However, there is no readily available method for measuring renal perfusion clinically: hourly measurement of urinary output is the closest we can get. In practical terms, the target is to improve and maintain the general state of the circulation as much as possible, whilst monitoring the urinary output. It is reasonable to assume that if the peripheries are well perfused, then there is a better chance that the kidneys will be too. In sepsis, this assumption is certainly flawed, but it is difficult to argue that the state of peripheral perfusion and arterial pressure should be completely ignored. If urinary output falls to less than about 0.5 ml/kg/h, then renal hypoperfusion (or another renal problem) is likely.

The features listed in Table 3 are indicators of depletion or excess of intravascular volume, and the presence of any one of these should lead to consideration of whether the patient would benefit from manoeuvres designed to increase or decrease that volume. Although a number of clinical signs are often stated to be of use in the diagnosis of volume depletion, for example, reduced skin turgor, reduced ocular tension, dry mouth, and tongue, these are very poor guides and may be seriously misleading, particularly in elderly people. The best indicators of intravascular volume depletion are (a) a low jugular venous pressure, and (b) postural hypotension; and of intravascular volume excess are (a) a raised jugular venous pressure, (b) a cardiac gallop rhythm, and (c) pulmonary crepitations.

Measurement of central venous pressure

It has become common practice in the management of acutely ill patients to use a central venous pressure line or pulmonary capillary-wedge pressure line to aid assessment of haemodynamic status. This deserves comment. A central venous pressure line certainly provides more precise measurement of right atrial pressure than can be gained from inspection of the jugular venous pulse, and the pulmonary capillary-wedge pressure line provides information on left-sided filling pressure that cannot be obtained clinically. However, the advantages of inserting these lines must be seen in perspective. There are some patients, particularly those with 'bull necks', in whom the jugular venous pulse cannot be seen at all. In such individuals a central venous pressure line is invaluable, but in most patients the jugular venous pulse can be seen, and the intravascular volume status easily assessed. In such cases, the benefits of a central venous pressure line may not outweigh the risks, and the decision to insert one is sometimes attributable to rigid protocols rather than sensible analysis of the clinical situation. It is particularly difficult and dangerous to try and insert a central venous pressure line into a patient who is volume depleted, and time spent on line insertion may delay appropriate treatment.

If the need is to gain venous access for resuscitation of the patient who is clearly hypovolaemic, a cannula should be inserted into a decent-sized peripheral vein—one in the forearm or antecubital fossa, but if these are constricted and cannot be cannulated, or if the patient is in extremis, then the femoral vein using the Seldinger technique is the best approach. The procedure is easiest if the patient can lie flat, but can be performed with the patient sitting if there is respiratory difficulty. The acronym NAVY (nerve artery vein Y-fronts) reminds the operator that the femoral vein lies medial to the artery. After cleaning the skin and giving local anaesthetic, the needle is inserted (with the bevel pointing forwards) just below the crease of the groin, one finger-breadth medial to the point of maximum pulsation of the femoral artery at an angle of about 60° to the skin and parallel to the long axis of the leg. Once the vein is punctured, the guidewire is passed into the vein and then the venous cannula is passed over it (after using dilators if inserting a large bore, e.g. dual lumen, cannula). The only significant complication of this procedure is inadvertent arterial puncture, the consequences of which are much less likely to be severe in the groin than in the neck or below the clavicle.

As regards cannulation of the internal jugular or subclavian veins, a study of over 5000 central venous access procedures conducted by Pittiruti *et al.* (2000) has provided useful information on the success and complication rates of various approaches. These are summarized in Table 4, the low lateral approach to the internal jugular vein being associated with the lowest incidence of accidental arterial puncture (1.2 per cent), catheter malposition (0.8 per cent), pneumothorax (none of 1767 cases), and a very low requirement for repeated attempts (3.3 per cent). The low lateral approach to the internal jugular vein is described in Fig. 4(a), the axial approach to the internal jugular vein is shown in Fig. 4(b), and the approaches to the subclavian vein in Fig. 5.

With the caveats stated in Table 3, in most patients, the central venous pressure—whether measured directly or estimated clinically from inspection of the jugular venous pulse—should be maintained at a level of 5–8 cm of water (measured from the mid-axillary line). However, it must be stressed that, even if the central venous pressure is measured directly, it is not uncommon to find that it is still difficult to decide whether intravascular volume is optimal in any particular patient. Three examples serve to illustrate this point. (1) After a large myocardial infarction there may be a fast, low volume pulse, hypotension, cool peripheries, a high jugular venous pressure, a gallop rhythm, and pulmonary crepitations—is the intravascular volume too high, too low, or optimal? (2) In someone with chronic right-sided cardiac dysfunction or pulmonary disease, the jugular venous pressure may be greatly in excess of that which would generally be regarded as normal, and ill-advised attempts to reduce the cardiac filling pressure could be catastrophic. (3) In many circumstances, the presence of peripheral or pulmonary oedema is associated, not with excess, but with contraction of intravascular volume. In some of these circumstances, the relation between left- and right-sided filling pressures may be abnormal and measurement of pulmonary capillary-wedge pressure can be very helpful. However, uncertainty as to whether intravascular volume is optimal may still persist, and the final strategy that can be employed is a trial of fluid infusion or removal (Table 3). If a decision to give a fluid challenge is made, then this should be done carefully, with the patient under continuous medical observation, accepting the possibility that pulmonary oedema might be induced. Two hundred and fifty millitres of colloid or 0.9 per cent saline should be administered rapidly, and the patient then observed closely for the next 5 min. If there is no perceptible deterioration, then the process can be repeated.

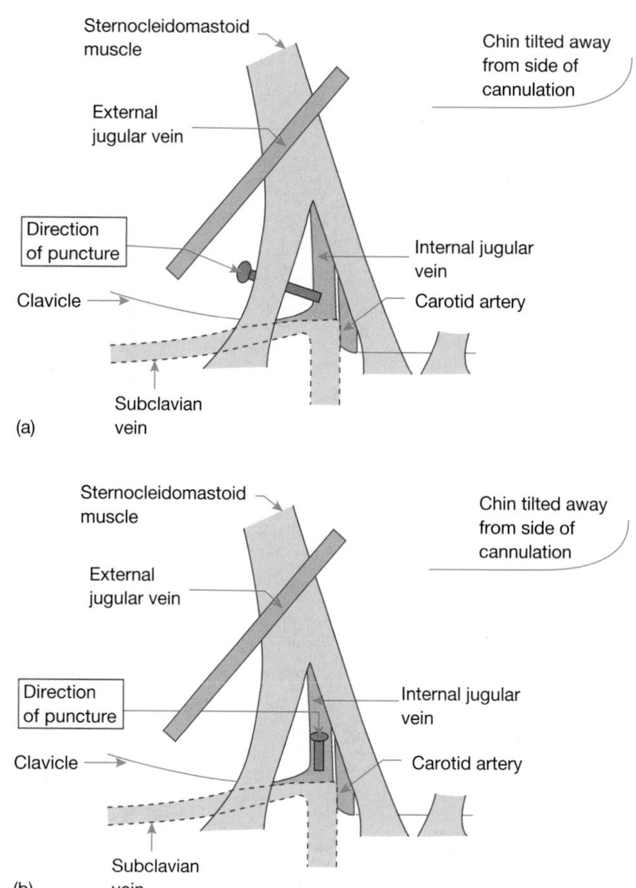

Fig. 4 The low lateral (b) and axial (b) approaches to the internal jugular vein. (a) The patient is supine with the head turned away from the side of the puncture. A towel may be placed under both shoulders to extend the neck. After preparation of the skin and drapes, and insertion of local anaesthetic, the bed is tilted to a 25° head down position. The needle is inserted lateral to the posterior border of the clavicular head of the sternocleidomastoid muscle, about one finger-breadth above the clavicle. It is then advanced parallel to the line of the clavicle and just behind the sternocleidomastoid muscle. The internal jugular vein, which lies superficially at this point, is cannulated close to its junction with the subclavian vein. As soon as the vein is entered the needle is angulated caudally to ease cannulation, the guidewire passing directly into the innominate vein. (b) The patient is positioned as described for the low lateral approach to the internal jugular vein. The needle is inserted in the centre of the triangle defined by the sternal and clavicular heads of the sternocleidomastoid muscle and the clavicle itself. It should be angulated caudally, at about 60° to the skin, and in a line pointing towards the ipsilateral anterior superior iliac spine.

Prescription of drugs and avoidance/reduction of exposure to nephrotoxins

Many drugs are excreted by the kidney and must be given in reduced dosage or at longer intervals than normal in patients with renal failure. Protein binding and extrarenal metabolism of drugs may also be altered in uraemia. All those prescribing for patients with acute renal failure should have access to information about the dose adjustments required. The changes in dosage recommended for those with impaired renal function should be regarded as a guide, and whenever possible plasma concentrations should be monitored to avoid the problems of underdosing on the one hand and toxicity on the other.

A large number of drugs have been reported to cause alteration of renal function and hence might be described as nephrotoxins. Indeed, as virtually all acutely ill patients are receiving drugs of one form or another, it is rarely possible to exclude the possibility that a drug may

Table 4 Complications during insertion of 5465 central vein catheters

Approach	Number of procedures	Complication					
		Pneumothorax (%)	Arterial puncture (%)	Repeated puncture, meaning two or more consecutive attempts to puncture a vein using the same approach (%)	Necessity to shift to another approach (%)	Failure to cannulate central vein, even after shifting to another approach (%)	Malposition of catheter (%)
Femoral vein	1014	Not relevant	9	5	4	0.1	0.1
High approach to internal jugular	460	0	7.7	9	22	0.5	4.5
Low lateral approach to internal jugular	1767	0	1.2	3.3	12	0.1	0.8
Axial approach to internal jugular	104	1	7	12	20	1	2
Infraclavicular approach to subclavian vein	1273	2.5	2.8	6.5	8.6	0.4	2.6
Supraclavicular approach to subclavian vein	847	1.1	3.6	4	8	0.2	1.4

Data from Pittiruti *et al.* (2000). *Journal of Vascular Access* **1**, 100–107.

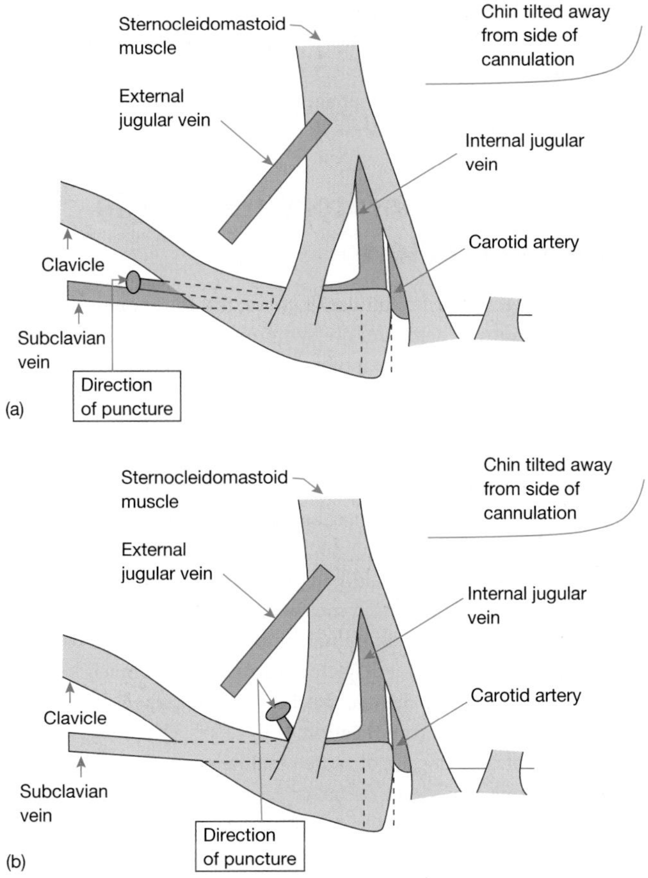

Fig. 5 The infraclavicular (a) and supraclavicular (b) approaches to the subclavian vein. (a) The patient is positioned as described for the low lateral approach to the internal jugular vein [Fig. 4(a)], excepting that instead of a towel being placed under both shoulders it should be positioned under the spine, allowing the shoulders to retract to reduce the risk of pneumothorax. The needle enters the skin below the mid-point of the lower border of the clavicle and is advanced under the clavicle towards the upper edge of the junction of the clavicle with the manubrium. (b) The patient is positioned as described for the infraclavicular approach to the subclavian vein. The needle is inserted into the angle between the superior border of the clavicle and the posterior border of the clavicular head of sternocleidomastoid and advanced caudally, medially, and ventrally.

be responsible for a case of acute renal failure, or be an exacerbating factor. However, for most drugs, the evidence of frequent significant nephrotoxicity is unconvincing and, if prescribed for the correct indication, the benefits of their prescription should far outweigh the risks. However, a few commonly used agents predictably induce detrimental changes to renal haemodynamics when the circulation is compromised or are directly injurious to renal tissue: these are listed in Table 5. For these drugs, the benefit/risk balance in the acutely ill patient is much more difficult to judge. They should be avoided unless they can reasonably be said to offer significant advantage over less noxious alternatives.

Non-steroidal anti-inflammatory agents, angiotensin-converting enzyme inhibitors, and angiotensin II receptor antagonists

An increasing number of patients take angiotensin-converting enzyme inhibitors or angiotensin II receptor antagonists, and many consume

Table 5 Common drugs to be used with caution in acutely ill patients or those with renal failure

Antimicrobials	
Aminoglycosides, e.g. gentamicin	See text
Amphotericin B	Incorporate into the pore structure of renal tubular cell membranes and cause damage related to cumulative dose (Porter and Bennett 1981; Kaloyanides 1994) Liposomal preparation less toxic, but extremely expensive
Tetracyclines (except doxycycline)	Retained in renal failure and exacerbate uraemia by catabolic effect (Ribush and Morgan 1972)
Cephaloridine, cephalothin (not other cephalosporins) (Rankin and Sutherland 1989)	Toxicity dependent follows cellular accumulation via organic anion transporter and lipid peroxidation (Kaloyanides 1994) Interaction with aminoglycoside to cause increased nephrotoxicity (Rankin and Sutherland 1989)
Non-steroidal anti-inflammatory agents and angiotensin-converting enzyme (ACE) inhibitors	
In the setting of circulatory compromise, renal blood flow and glomerular filtration are substantially supported by intrarenal generation of vasodilator prostaglandins and angiotensin II. Administration of non-steroidal anti-inflammatory agents (Clive and Stoff 1984) or ACE inhibitors (Suki 1989; Mason 1990) in such circumstances can lead to dramatic reduction in renal perfusion and induce acute renal failure	

non-steroidal anti-inflammatory agents. These agents can all cause renal dysfunction (Clive and Stoff 1984; Mason 1990; Lee and Kim 2001), and clinical experience suggests that they are particularly likely to do so when taken in combination. In one study, the notes of 1500 patients, greater than 75 years of age, were studied: 12 were taking both an angiotensin-converting enzyme inhibitor and a non-steroidal anti-inflammatory agent, two developed acute renal failure, and four showed deterioration of renal function (Adhiyaman *et al.* 2001). These drugs should usually be stopped in patients with acute renal failure.

Aminoglycosides

The drugs most commonly implicated as causing or exacerbating acute renal failure are the aminoglycoside antibiotics. However, aminoglycoside nephrotoxicity has become less of a clinical issue in recent years with the introduction of many alternative non-nephrotoxic antibiotics that are very effective in circumstances in which aminoglycosides (gentamicin in particular) previously used to be employed as first-line therapy, for example, Gram-negative septicaemia.

Aminoglycosides are cationic and those that are more strongly positively charged have greater nephrotoxic potential. The mechanism of this is partly understood as follows: aminoglycosides bind to negatively charged phospholipids on the surface of renal tubular cells, are delivered to megalin in coated pits, following which the complex is endocytosed and trafficked to the endosome. This has the effect of inhibiting endosome fusion, both *in vivo* and *in vitro*, but precisely how this leads to functional consequences for renal function is not known (Molitoris 1997).

In a review of 144 studies of aminoglycoside nephrotoxicity, Kahlmeter and Dahlager (1984) reported that 14 per cent of courses of treatment with gentamicin were associated with some evidence of this complication, with a slightly lower incidence following the use of tobramycin (12.9 per cent), amikacin (9.4 per cent), and netilmicin (8.7 per cent). There have been a number of randomized studies comparing the incidence of nephrotoxicity following the use of two or more of amikacin, gentamicin, netilmicin, sisomicin, and tobramicin. Taken individually, most have reported no significant difference between these agents, but a quantitative overview of the literature concluded that patients receiving gentamicin or sisomicin seemed to run a higher risk than those given amikacin; and the risk with tobramicin was lower than that for gentamicin but higher than that for netilmicin (Buring *et al.* 1988). In those who develop nephrotoxicity, the typical clinical picture is said to be of relatively mild, non-oliguric renal failure, with tubular proteinuria, and impairment of urinary concentrating ability. Proximal tubular damage involves the brush border, reflected by increased urinary excretion of γ-glutamyl transferase, alanine aminopeptidase, and of lysosomal enzymes (Humes 1988). Recovery may be slow, delayed or incomplete.

All patients receiving aminoglycosides are susceptible to nephrotoxicity, but those with longer duration of therapy, higher plasma concentrations, liver disease, advanced age, pre-existing renal impairment, and (possibly) females may be at increased risk (Smith *et al.* 1986). In an endeavour to prevent renal side-effects, and also because of the risk of ototoxicity, aminoglycosides should never be prescribed without the precaution of monitoring both renal function and the serum concentration of antibiotic. In the patient with normal renal function, a typical recommendation would be to start gentamicin (1.33 mg/kg) three times daily, aiming for a peak concentration of 5–10 mg/l 60 min after intravenous injection, and a trough value of less than 2.5 mg/l before the next dose. For once daily dosing (typically giving 7 mg/kg), a level of less than 1 mg/l at 24 h would be satisfactory, 1–2 mg/l borderline (reduce dose frequency to 36 hourly), and greater than 2 mg/l unsatisfactory (change to an alternative agent if possible). Despite the fact that such guidelines are widely known, audit studies reveal that monitoring is neglected in 15–20 per cent of courses of aminoglycoside therapy (Li *et al.* 1989; Shrimpton *et al.* 1993).

Radiographic contrast media

The incidence of acute renal failure associated with the use of radiographic contrast media has been reported to vary over a range from 0 to 50 per cent. This extraordinary variability reflects both differences in definition of acute renal failure and differences in the populations examined. Prospective studies in which careful attention has been paid to the maintenance of adequate hydration have shown a very low incidence of clinically significant renal impairment, even in groups reported to be at increased risk (diabetes, myeloma) (Parfrey *et al.* 1989). This applies to both ionic and non-ionic contrast media (Schwab *et al.* 1989). It seems probable that the high incidence of radiocontrast-induced nephrotoxicity reported in many of the earlier studies was due to the practice of restricting fluid intake before the radiological examinations.

Surgical procedures in those who are acutely ill or have acute renal failure

Elective surgical procedures should not be performed on those who are acutely ill, but there are occasions when surgery is essential for survival. This scenario is accompanied by a very high risk of acute renal failure (Hou *et al.* 1983; Turney *et al.* 1990), the chances of which can be minimized by the avoidance of hypovolaemia and unnecessary exposure to nephrotoxins. There is no evidence that giving frusemide, mannitol, dopamine, or any other agent confers additional protection.

Clinical and laboratory findings in acute renal failure

In the early stages of acute tubular necrosis, the commonest cause of acute renal failure, there are no symptoms attributable to renal dysfunction: unsuspected but potentially fatal hyperkalaemia is the greatest danger. The clinical picture is almost certain to be dominated by the primary condition of which acute tubular necrosis is a complication, and by the effects of intravascular volume depletion. As many as 50 per cent of cases in some series are not oliguric (Anderson *et al.* 1977). In the later stages, there may be manifestations of uraemia with anorexia, nausea, and vomiting (occasionally diarrhoea), muscular cramps, and signs of encephalopathy—including a 'metabolic' flapping tremor (asterixis), depressed consciousness, and *grand mal* convulsions (see Chapter 11.3.14). Skin bruising and gastrointestinal bleeding may occur. Uraemic haemorrhagic pericarditis occurs much less frequently in acute than in chronic renal failure, but when it does it is another potentially fatal complication.

If the patient does not die of acute renal failure, either because the degree of uraemia is modest or renal replacement therapy is provided, then renal recovery from acute tubular necrosis occurs in most of those who survive the precipitating insult. This may begin at any time from a few days to a few months (median 10–14 days) after the onset of acute renal failure, with progressive increase in urinary volume typically preceding improvement in plasma creatinine and urea. Restoration of the ability to concentrate the urine often lags behind recovery of other aspects of renal function, such that a period of polyuria is commonly seen, placing the patient temporarily at risk of sodium and water depletion. Indeed, although most patients with acute tubular necrosis can be expected to recover clinically normal renal function, testing reveals that the urinary concentration and acidification mechanisms are not completely restored in 50 per cent of cases (Briggs *et al.* 1967). Of greater consequence, however, is the fact that renal function does not always recover, particular in older patients with multiple co-morbidities (see later Discussion of prognosis).

Biochemical, haematological, and immunological findings

Biochemical findings

The clinical diagnosis of renal failure, acute or chronic, is made when plasma concentrations of urea and creatinine are elevated. Other important biochemical changes include the development of hyperkalaemia, metabolic acidosis, hypocalcaemia, and hyperphosphataemia. Hyperkalaemia is due not only to reduced urinary excretion, but also to potassium release from cells—either as a consequence of cell death or as a result of metabolic acidosis. Particularly rapid increases are to be expected when there is extensive tissue damage or hypercatabolism, as in rhabdomyolysis, burns, and sepsis. Transfusion of stored blood is sometimes said to cause dangerous hyperkalaemia in oliguric patients. It may, however, not be the transfused blood that is really to blame, but the circumstances that demand transfusion. Red-cell lysis and the absorption of a considerable potassium load follow loss of blood into the gastrointestinal tract or body tissues.

In acute renal failure, the renal systems for excreting acid fail, leading to the development of metabolic acidosis (see Chapter 2.6). This is usually modest in degree (plasma pH 7.2–7.35), but can on occasion be severe, manifesting as sighing Kussmaul respiration and/or with circulatory compromise. Acidosis is sometimes the metabolic abnormality most obviously necessitating urgent institution of renal replacement therapy, but overzealous administration of bicarbonate to all patients in which the plasma pH is less than normal should be avoided (see below).

Many patients with acute renal failure have hypocalcaemia and hyperphosphataemia, probably secondary to disordered vitamin D metabolism and failure of phosphate excretion, respectively. These abnormalities can develop within a few days, but they are usually asymptomatic, although tetany and fits can be provoked by over-rapid correction of acidosis causing a reduction in ionized calcium. If hypocalcaemia (say, corrected total calcium < 2.0 mmol/l) and hyperphosphataemia (say, phosphate > 2.5 mmol/l) are profound, then the diagnosis of rhabdomyolysis should always be considered. This can be confirmed by the presence of myoglobin in the urine (which looks brown, like 'cola', and tests positive for blood with reagent strips, but no red blood cells are seen on microscopy) and a greatly elevated concentration of blood creatine kinase (typically $>10{,}000$ IU/ml). Transient hypercalcaemia is common during the recovery phase of acute renal failure. This is also prominent after rhabdomyolysis, although the mechanism responsible is contentious, some arguing that hyperparathyroidism is important (Llach *et al.* 1981), others that it is not (Akmal *et al.* 1986). The hypercalcaemic phase may be prolonged and accompanied by widespread metastatic calcification in those who have sustained extensive muscle injury, a tendency that may be prolonged if calcium has been administered during the hypocalcaemic phase (Petit *et al.* 1992).

In acute renal failure, the plasma sodium concentration is usually normal, since deficits of sodium are usually matched by those of water: hence extracellular fluid volume may be reduced, but plasma sodium concentration remains unchanged. On occasion, however, intake of water—perhaps driven by hypovolaemia—may exceed the rate at which it can be excreted (which is depressed when the glomerular filtration rate is very low) and hyponatraemia results.

Retention of uric acid, sulfate, and magnesium occurs in acute renal failure, but these biochemical abnormalities are rarely clinically significant. Concentrations of uric acid can, however, be particularly high in rhabdomyolysis and tumour lysis, when they may warrant specific treatment.

Haematological findings

Anaemia develops within a few days of the onset of acute renal failure, the haemoglobin typically settling to approximately 8–9 g/dl. This is caused by impaired erythropoiesis, attributable both to erythropoietin deficiency and to 'toxic' effects of uraemia on the marrow, and to reduced survival of red blood cells or bleeding. The leucocyte count is often elevated—sometimes, but not always, indicating the presence of infection. Eosinophilia is rarely seen, but when present should lead to consideration of the diagnosis of acute interstitial nephritis or vasculitis (in particular the Churg–Strauss syndrome). The platelet count is often slightly reduced ($100–150 \times 10^9$/l) and defective platelet function contributes towards a tendency to bleed.

A number of distinctive haematological pictures need to be recognized in those with acute renal failure because they have diagnostic and therapeutic significance.

Disseminated intravascular coagulation

This typically presents with bleeding from multiple sites, most frequently the nose, mouth, gastrointestinal tract, and skin punctures, and most seriously into the brain or lungs. Laboratory tests show anaemia of greater severity than usual (frequently Hb < 8 g/dl), profound thrombocytopenia, and derangement of clotting tests (prolonged prothrombin, partial thromboplastin, and thrombin times; increased levels of fibrin degradation products and D-dimers). If a patient presenting with acute renal failure has this picture, the most likely diagnosis is septicaemia (Gram-positive or Gram-negative), but such a picture can also be found in those with burns, fat embolism, eclampsia, amniotic fluid embolism, missed abortion, severe heat stroke, liver failure, diabetic ketoacidosis, leukaemia, and neoplasia. Aside from treatment of the underlying condition, management involves giving platelets and clotting factors (cryoprecipitate, fresh-frozen plasma).

Haemolytic–uraemic syndrome (see Chapter 10.6.3)

This is recognized by the presence of profound anaemia and thrombocytopenia, together with a blood film showing gross morphological abnormality of the red blood cells (schistocytes).

Myeloma (see Chapter 4.3)

This diagnosis should be considered in any patient, particularly those over 50 years of age, if the cause of acute renal failure is not obvious. The first clues may be hypercalcaemia, the presence of rouleaux and clumping on the blood film, or the finding of a very high erythrocyte sedimentation rate.

Immunological findings

In the patient with acute renal failure due to acute tubular necrosis or urinary obstruction, it is not necessary to perform immunological tests. However, when the presence of proteinuria and/or haematuria suggest that a renal inflammatory condition is possible, it is essential to obtain immunological tests that—together with renal biopsy—are necessary to reach a precise diagnosis. The immunological tests that are required in this situation are listed in Table 6, further details being found in Chapter 10.6.1.

Urinary electrolytes

Prerenal failure and acute tubular necrosis almost invariably occur in the context of circulatory disturbance, that is, shock. If the patient is not in such a state, or has not recently been so, then it is unlikely that their acute renal failure is attributable to either of these conditions and it becomes particularly important to exclude obstructive or intrinsic renal causes. Circumstances predisposing to prerenal failure are almost invariably associated with increased plasma levels of antidiuretic hormone. This acts on the collecting duct to increase tubular reabsorption of both water and urea (see Chapter 2.1), hence plasma urea increases out of proportion to creatinine in prerenal failure. Plasma urea may also appear to be disproportionately increased with sepsis, corticosteroid use, tetracyclines (catabolic effect), and gastrointestinal haemorrhage (protein load).

Emphasis is often given to strategies designed to try and discern whether a patient is in prerenal failure or acute tubular necrosis based

Table 6 'Immunological' investigations in patients with acute renal failure suspected of having renal inflammation (cause unknown)

Test	Comment
Antiglomerular basement membrane antibodies*	Positive in Goodpasture's disease
Antineutrophil cytoplasmic antibodies (ANCA)* Antiproteinase 3 antibodies Antimyeloperoxidase antibodies	Positive in systemic vasculitis, but non-specific ANCA positivity (i.e. indirect immunofluorescence test positive, but with negative specific tests for antiproteinase 3 and antimyeloperoxidase antibodies) can be found in a variety of conditions, including infection. A negative ANCA indirect immunofluorescence test makes Wegener's granulomatosis or microscopic polyangiitis very unlikely unless there is strong clinical, radiological, or histological evidence to support the diagnosis
Antinuclear antibodies (ANA)*	Positive in systemic lupus erythematosus (SLE) and other autoimmune disorders, but many positive results are not clinically significant. If ANA positive, then screening for autoantibodies directed against a variety of autoantigens should be pursued as an aid to diagnosis. Anti ds-DNA autoantibodies have the highest specificity for the diagnosis of SLE
Serum immunoglobulins* Serum protein electrophoresis* Bence Jones proteinuria*	Presence of monoclonal band in serum or urine indicates myeloma if combined with suppression of other immunoglobulins Polyclonal increase in immunoglobulins is a non-specific finding seen in many inflammatory conditions
Cryoglobulins	Positive in cryoglobulinaemia, also sometimes in SLE and postinfectious disease
Complement activity* C3* C4*	Low serum complement activity (CH_{50}) is a feature of acute poststreptococcal glomerulonephritis (GN), type II membranoproliferative glomerulonephritis (MPGN), diffuse proliferative lupus nephritis, subacute bacterial endocarditis, 'shunt' nephritis, and essential cryoglobulinaemia Very low C3 with normal/mildly depressed C4 is a feature of poststreptococcal disease and MPGN type II Low C4 with relatively preserved C3 is a feature of type II cryoglobulinaemia and should alert the clinician to the possibility of this diagnosis Proportionate decrease in C3 and C4 is found in SLE and bacterial endocarditis
C-reactive protein (CRP)*	Entirely non-specific, but elevated in most renal inflammatory conditions excepting SLE
Antistreptolysin O Anti-DNAse B	Elevated titres suggest recent streptococcal infection and support the diagnosis of poststreptococcal GN in the appropriate clinical context

Note: The tests marked * should be performed in any patient presenting with unexplained acute renal failure that might be due to nephritis, that is, when there is proteinuria/haematuria/urinary red cell casts. The other tests listed may be indicated, depending on the clinical context (as may other tests not listed).

on urinary analysis, with the implication that this knowledge will be useful (Table 7). In the 'typical' case of prerenal failure, the urinary electrolytes are said to reflect the response of normal tubules to impaired renal perfusion. There is avid retention of sodium and water, leading to low urinary sodium and high urinary urea and creatinine concentrations, together with a high urinary osmolarity. Restoration of renal perfusion leads to rapid improvement in renal function. By contrast, in the 'typical' case of acute tubular necrosis, the urinary sodium concentration is elevated and the urinary urea and creatinine concentrations, and urinary osmolality are relatively low—features suggestive of tubular dysfunction. In such instances, whatever the treatment, renal function rarely improves rapidly.

Is urinary electrolyte analysis helpful in cases of acute renal failure? The measurements most frequently made are of sodium, urea, and creatinine concentrations in plasma and urine, together with urinary and plasma osmolality. The values obtained are used to derive a number of variables: the ratios of urine to plasma concentrations of urea, creatinine, and osmolality; fractional sodium excretion [FE_{Na} = (urinary sodium × plasma creatinine × 100)/(plasma sodium × urinary creatinine)]; and 'renal failure index' [(urinary sodium × plasma creatinine)/urinary creatinine]. The 'typical' findings expected are shown in Table 7. Of these, there is most information on the use of the FE_{Na} as a predictor of outcome. Espinel reported that patients with prerenal azotaemia had a FE_{Na} less than 1 per cent, whereas those with acute tubular necrosis had a value greater than 3 per cent, and concluded that the test was, therefore, of 'considerable clinical value' (Espinel 1976). In a subsequent publication, the same author found that using a FE_{Na} value of 1 per cent to divide those with prerenal failure and glomerulonephritis (<1 per cent) from those with acute tubular necrosis or obstruction (>1 per cent) resulted in the misclassification of only one patient out of 87 (Espinel and Gregory 1980). Myers *et al.* (1982) studied 30 cases of non-oliguric acute renal failure following open heart surgery. They measured the clearances of dextrans of various molecular weights and used the results to divide the patients into those with prerenal failure (no evidence of back-leak through the tubules) and those with acute tubular necrosis (evidence of back-leak present). The prerenal group, all of whom recovered renal function spontaneously, had an average FE_{Na} of 0.5 ± 1.0 per cent, whereas those with evidence of back-leak, 14 out of 16 of whom required dialysis, had an average FE_{Na} of 5.1 ± 1.5 per cent.

However, not all have found urinary tests to be so discriminating. Durakovic *et al.* (1989) were unable to separate those with a clinical

Table 7 Urinary biochemical indices in prerenal failure and acute tubular necrosis

Indices	'Typical' prerenal failure	'Typical' acute tubular necrosis
Urinary sodium (mmol/l)	<20	>40
Urine osmolarity (mOsm/l)	>500	<350
Urine/plasma urea	>8	<3
Urine/plasma creatinine	>40	<20
Urine/plasma osmolarity	>1.5	<1.1
Fractional sodium excretion (%)	<1	>2
Renal failure index	<1	>2

Notes: Fractional sodium excretion, FE_{Na} = (urinary sodium × plasma creatinine × 100)/(plasma sodium × urinary creatinine). Renal failure index = (urinary sodium × plasma creatinine)/urinary creatinine.

Reasons why urinary biochemical indices are of very limited clinical use:
(1) intermediate values common;
(2) 'typical' values do not reliably predict renal prognosis—it is increasingly recognized that cases which are otherwise indistinguishable from 'typical' acute tubular necrosis can have low urinary sodium (Brosius and Lau 1986);
(3) diuretics have frequently been given rendering urinary indices uninterpretable;
(4) in hepatorenal syndrome (see Chapter 10.6.4) indices are prerenal;
(5) treatment is not dictated by urinary indices.

diagnosis of prerenal failure from those with acute tubular necrosis on the basis of urinary measures. Brosius and Lau (1986) studied 41 patients who had a greater than twofold increase in their baseline plasma creatinine concentration that persisted for at least 7 days, those with volume depletion, obstruction, vasculitis, or glomerulonephritis having been excluded. Sixteen (40 per cent) were found to have a low FE_{Na} (<1 per cent). This was associated with milder insults (lower peak plasma creatinine concentration), earlier determinations (FE_{Na} measured sooner after the onset of acute renal failure), or significant hypotension at some time in the 3 days before the measurements were taken. Ten patients who were initially in this low-FE_{Na} group had measurements repeated at a later time; seven had converted to a high FE_{Na} value. The conclusion was reached that whilst 'a high FE_{Na} in the setting of acute renal failure is suggestive of intrinsic renal failure, a low FE_{Na} can be observed in similar patients with prolonged acute renal insufficiency'.

Most practising nephrologists would agree that measurement of urinary concentrations of sodium, urea, etc., and calculations based upon this information, have little merit in routine clinical practice. They do not reliably predict outcome in acute renal failure, and treatment is begun on exactly the same lines whether the diagnosis is of prerenal failure or of acute tubular necrosis. The response to initial treatment retrospectively defines the diagnosis and determines further management.

There are, however, two conditions in which measurement of urinary sodium concentration may be very helpful in the diagnosing the cause of acute renal failure. First, the hepatorenal syndrome (Chapter 10.6.5), in which the urinary sodium concentration is less than 10 mmol/l, and often as low as 2–5 mmol/l (Wong and Blendis 2001). Second, total acute renal artery occlusion. Liano *et al.* (1994) examined sodium excretion in the urine of three groups (10 patients in each) with acute renal failure: group 1 had total acute renal-artery occlusion; group 2 had unilateral acute renal-artery occlusion with a functioning contralateral kidney; and group 3 had acute tubular necrosis, without arterial thrombosis, following a major abdominal vascular procedure. In all of the group-1 and group-2 patients, and some of those in group 3, the status of the renal arteries was confirmed by arteriography. The mean urinary sodium concentration in group 1 was 133 ± 5 mmol/l (very similar to plasma); in group 2, 48 ± 10 mmol/l; and in group 3, 63 ± 8 mmol/l. The mean values of FE_{Na} were 91 ± 12 per cent (group 1), 6.5 ± 3.1 per cent (group 2), and 4.4 ± 1.0 per cent (group 3). It would, therefore, seem worthwhile to measure the urinary sodium concentration in the small volume of urine that can sometimes be obtained from patients with acute renal failure in whom acute renal arterial occlusion seems a possible diagnosis. When the urinary concentration of sodium (also urea and creatinine) is similar to that in plasma, then the presumptive diagnosis is acute bilateral occlusion of the renal arteries.

Medical management of acute renal failure

Many patients with acute renal failure are extremely ill, and the first priority in management is to treat any life-threatening problems. The nephrologist must remember not to concentrate on the kidneys to the exclusion of all else: if the patient is not breathing properly, then the first priority is to remedy this, if necessary by intubation and ventilation. The two life-threatening complications of renal failure are hyperkalaemia and pulmonary oedema, the specific management of which are discussed below. The next priority is the prompt diagnosis and treatment of hypovolaemia. Finally, the specific diagnosis and treatment of the underlying condition should be addressed.

Life-threatening complications

Hyperkalaemia

Hyperkalaemia is most dangerous in acute renal failure and is important because it can cause sudden cardiac arrest. Patients may occasionally suffer from muscular weakness or paralysis (Freeman and Fale 1993; Naumann *et al.* 1994), but these symptoms are rarely prominent, and if they do occur their significance is rarely appreciated (except in patients on long-term dialysis who have had them before).

As the plasma potassium concentration increases, there is a reduction in the transmembrane potassium concentration gradient and a reduction in the resting membrane potential. It also acts to shorten the duration of the cardiac action potential by increasing the velocity of cellular repolarization, possibly by altering membrane permeability to potassium. These changes correlate with 'tenting' of the T-waves and shortening of the QT interval on the surface electrocardiogram when the plasma potassium concentration increases to greater than about 5.5 mmol/l (Surawicz 1967; Ettinger *et al.* 1974). More severe hyperkalaemia lowers the resting membrane potential further, and also decreases the upstroke velocity of the action potential, causing slowing of intraventricular conduction, manifest by widening of the QRS complex. Because atrial muscle is more sensitive to these effects than the specialized fibres of the SA and AV nodes, the P-wave becomes smaller and the PR interval lengthens. Eventually, the P-wave disappears and the widened QRS complex becomes distorted (occasionally producing a pattern resembling infarction; Simon 1988), eventually assuming an irregular sinusoidal pattern. In one particularly dramatic case, inadvertent administration of a massive dose of potassium chloride to a patient undergoing open heart surgery was recognized when the surface electrocardiogram showed the characteristic sine-wave pattern and the heart was seen to beat in a 'serpentine' manner, with waves of contraction advancing slowly over the myocardium (Burket *et al.* 1992).

Not all patients are equally susceptible to the cardiac effects of hyperkalaemia, and in a series of patients, the plasma potassium concentration of each could not reliably be predicted from examination of their electrocardiogram (Wrenn *et al.* 1991). However, an individual's risk of hyperkalaemic cardiac arrest can be gauged from the appearance of their electrocardiogram, and for this reason all doctors who work with acutely ill patients should be able to recognize the characteristic electrocardiographic manifestations of hyperkalaemia (Fig. 6 and Table 8). Any change more pronounced than tenting of the T-waves demands treatment, and severe changes demand this immediately, as described in Table 8 (Anon 1989; Salem *et al.* 1991; Allon 1993).

Patients with severe hyperkalaemic cardiotoxicity should be given intravenous calcium: initially 10 ml of 10 per cent calcium gluconate over 60 s, repeated until the electrocardiogram shows clear signs of improvement (Fig. 6). It is not known why this treatment works: the plasma potassium concentration does not change at all, so that the effect on the heart is attributed to 'membrane stabilization'. There is some evidence for such action in the isolated, perfused heart preparation, where the conduction disturbances and tendency to ventricular fibrillation caused by hyperkalaemia can be reversed or lessened by increasing the extracellular concentration of calcium (Surawicz 1967). From a clinical viewpoint, it is important to recognize that the effect of calcium infusion is relatively transient. If the plasma potassium concentration is not reduced by other means, then any electrocardiographic improvement that has been obtained is likely to be lost over a period of 20–60 min.

After giving calcium to those with life-threatening hyperkalaemia, and in cases of moderately severe hyperkalaemia, the plasma potassium

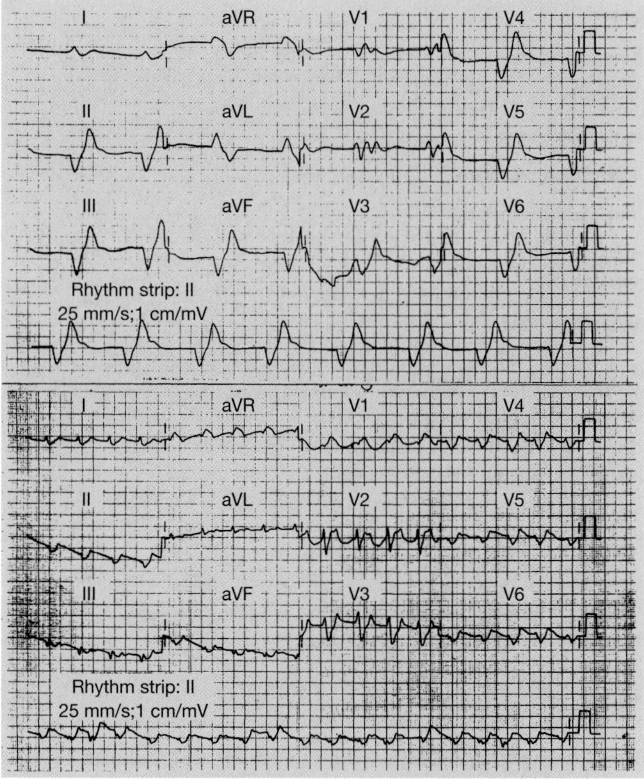

Fig. 6 The electrocardiogram of a patient with a plasma potassium concentration of 9.1 mmol/l, before (upper panel) and 2 min after (lower panel) the administration of intravenous calcium gluconate.

Table 8 Electrocardiographic manifestations and treatment of hyperkalaemia

Electrocardiographic changes

As serum potassium rises the following changes occur progressively

- 'Tenting' of the T-wave
- Reduction in size of P-waves, increase in PR interval, widening of QRS complex
- Disappearance of P-wave, further widening of QRS complex
- Irregular 'sinusoidal' waveform

Treatment

Method	Comment
1. Intravenous calcium (10 ml of 10% calcium gluconate, over 60 s, repeated until ECG improves)	Acts instantly to 'stabilize' cardiac membranes (mechanism unknown); does not alter serum potassium
2. Intravenous insulin and glucose (10 units rapidly acting insulin + 50 ml 50% glucose, over 10 min)	Insulin stimulates Na,K-ATPase in muscle and liver, thus driving potassium into cells; serum potassium falls by 1–2 mmol/l over 30–60 min
3. Salbutamol (10 mg via nebulizer)	Stimulation of β2-adrenergic receptors leads to activation of Na,K-ATPase, thus driving potassium into cells
4. Cation exchange resins, e.g. sodium or calcium polystyrene sulfonate (15 g by mouth 6-hourly or 15–30 g per rectum 6-hourly)	Exchange sodium or calcium for potassium in gut lumen and thus induce loss of potassium from body (unlike 1–3 above); take 4 h to produce effect; precautions required to prevent severe constipation
5. Haemodialysis/filtration	Except in those rare cases where renal function can rapidly be restored, e.g. relief of obstruction, it is likely that hyperkalaemia will recur and haemodialysis or high-volume haemofiltration will be required

concentration can be reduced by 1–2 mmol/l over 30–60 min by giving an intravenous infusion of glucose and insulin (50 ml of 50 per cent glucose with 10 units of rapidly acting insulin over 15 min) (Lens *et al.* 1989; Allon and Copkney 1990). The insulin acts by stimulating the Na,K-ATPase pump in skeletal and cardiac muscle, liver, and (possibly) in fat, thus driving potassium into cells (Moore 1983). The purpose of the glucose is to prevent hypoglycaemia.

Some physicians recommend intravenous sodium bicarbonate (50–100 ml of 4.2 per cent solution over 15 min) as an adjunct or alternative to glucose and insulin treatment. Its effect, typically a reduction of plasma potassium concentration of 1–2 mmol/l, has traditionally been ascribed to an increase in blood pH, thought to reduce the plasma potassium concentration by stimulating exchange of intracellular protons for extracellular potassium ions (Levinsky 1966). This may not be the correct explanation. In one study of 14 patients, it was found that the plasma potassium concentration declined by the same amount in those whose pH rose (mean change in pH, +0.12 units) as in those whose pH did not alter (mean change in pH, +0.01 units) (Fraley and Adler 1977). In another study, it was demonstrated that intravenous hypertonic saline (100–250 ml of 5 per cent solution), rather than bicarbonate, could cause a substantial reduction in plasma potassium concentration and reverse the electrocardiographic manifestations of severe hyperkalaemic cardiotoxicity (Garcia-Palmieri 1962). However, the routine use of intravenous sodium bicarbonate to treat hyperkalaemia cannot be recommended. Many patients with acute renal failure are already volume overloaded, and the treatment necessitates the administration of a considerable sodium load. Second, hypertonic solutions of sodium bicarbonate are extremely irritant, and their extravasation can cause chemical tissue burns so they must only be given via central veins. Third, in some patients the treatment can induce a dramatic reduction in the plasma ionized calcium, with the risk that this might precipitate tetany and epileptic seizures. Fourth, the treatment has no advantages over glucose and insulin. The one circumstance in which intravenous hypertonic sodium bicarbonate does seem appropriate is in the treatment of hyperkalaemia associated with profound acidosis, in particular when such acidosis is associated with (and may be causing) hypotension.

Stimulation of β_2-adrenergic receptors leads to activation of the Na,K-ATPase pump and the movement of potassium into cells. This property has been exploited to treat hyperkalaemia in patients with renal failure. Both intravenous salbutamol (0.5 mg over 15 min) and nebulized salbutamol (10 or 20 mg) can reduce plasma potassium concentration by a mean of about 1 mmol/l over 30–60 min (Montoliu *et al.* 1987; Allon *et al.* 1989; Lens *et al.* 1989). This treatment is now used regularly for the treatment of hyperkalaemia on some renal units, but agitation, tremor, and tachycardia are common side-effects such that most nephrologists prefer intravenous glucose/insulin, although there are circumstances, for example, when it is very difficult to obtain venous access or in children, where nebulized salbutamol can be extremely useful.

It must be emphasized that none of the treatments described above actually remove potassium from the body. They may be sufficient as treatment for hyperkalaemia on their own if rapid recovery of renal function can be anticipated, for example, following resuscitation of those with prerenal failure or relief of urinary obstruction. However, if rapid recovery cannot be expected, then hyperkalaemia will recur over a period of 2–4 h as potassium leaks back out of cells, with further doses of calcium, glucose, and insulin tending to have diminished efficacy. Here the period of temporary respite from dangerous hyperkalaemic cardiotoxicity must be used to initiate treatment that will remove potassium from the body. Cation-exchange resins may suffice in less severe cases (sodium or calcium polystyrene sulfonate, 15 g in water by mouth or 30 g in methylcellulose as a retention enema every 6 h, in both cases with precautions against the treatment inducing constipation). In most cases, some form of dialysis or haemofiltration will be required (see Chapter 10.4). Cases have been described in which hyperkalaemia has resulted in cardiac arrest, and conventional resuscitation manoeuvres have been unsuccessful until the patient was put on haemodialysis to remove potassium (Lin *et al.* 1994).

Avoidance of hyperkalaemia

Hyperkalaemia is most commonly a complication of acute, or acute on chronic, renal failure, but some types of chronic renal disease, in particular those causing hyporeninaemic hypoaldosteronism (see Chapter 2.2), are more likely than others to present with the condition. Drugs may also exacerbate the problem. The risks of hyperkalaemia in those taking potassium-sparing diuretics are well known, but recent studies demonstrating a survival advantage of patients with congestive cardiac failure taking spironolactone have led to this agent being given to many with impaired renal function. This can precipitate dangerous hyperkalaemia, one study reporting 25 such cases (Schepkens *et al.* 2001), so close monitoring is required. A number of other agents may also exacerbate problems in potassium homeostasis associated with renal failure. These include angiotensin-converting enzyme inhibitors (Ahuja *et al.* 2000) and heparin (Oster *et al.* 1995), which both induce hypoaldosteronism, and trimethoprim, which acts like amiloride to block the apical-membrane sodium channels in the distal nephron (Perazella 2000).

Pulmonary oedema

The most serious complication of salt and water overload in acute renal failure is the development of pulmonary oedema. Regrettably, many cases are iatrogenic. Patients admitted with severe illnesses are appropriately resuscitated, but the fact that they are in renal failure is not recognized, and two, three, or more litres per day of intravenous fluids are infused until the patient accrues a considerable positive balance and pulmonary oedema predictably ensues. This is commonly attributed to 'heart failure', although the heart is actually doing a very good job. Severe cases are dramatic. The patient is terrified, restless, and confused. Examination reveals cyanosis, tachypnoea, tachycardia, widespread wheeze or crepitations in the chest, and a gallop rhythm (if the heart sounds can be heard at all). Investigation demonstrates arterial hypoxaemia and widespread interstitial shadowing on the chest radiograph.

The immediate management of pulmonary oedema is to sit the patient up, which redistributes fluid from the pulmonary to systemic circulations and alters the pattern of perfusion within the lung in a manner favourable to gas exchange, and give oxygen by face mask and reservoir bag in as high a concentration as possible. Frusemide, or other diuretic agents, are of little benefit in producing diuresis in cases of pulmonary oedema associated with acute renal failure, although they have some vasodilator action that can be beneficial. Intravenous morphine in small doses (2.5 mg, repeated depending upon the response) is very helpful as both a vasodilator and an anxiolytic. Intravenous nitrate (e.g. isosorbide dinitrate 2–10 mg/h) can also be used to vasodilate and thereby reduce pulmonary capillary hydrostatic pressure. However, in renal failure definitive treatment requires the removal of excess fluid and pulmonary oedema is one of the indications for emergency haemodialysis or haemofiltration. In extremis, fluid can be removed by venesection, ideally with the blood returned to the patient later when their pulmonary oedema has resolved and they are comfortably established on haemodialysis or haemofiltration (if local blood transfusion practice will allow this).

Recognition and treatment of volume depletion

If features suggestive of intravascular volume depletion (listed in Table 3) are present, then the deficit should be corrected rapidly. Large-bore intravenous access should be established and fluid infused at maximum rate. If large veins in the forearms or antecubital fossae are not available, then access should be established through one of the femoral veins, as described previously. To emphasize the point made earlier, attempts to cannulate the central veins should not be made in those who are obviously hypovolaemic.

The fluid infused should be of a type that remains substantially within the intravascular compartment (blood, colloid, saline); it should mimic as closely as possible the nature of the fluid lost; and it should be given as rapidly as the tubing and vascular access will permit. The patient should be observed continuously and the infusion stopped when features of volume depletion have disappeared, but before volume overload has been induced.

There has been much debate about which type of replacement fluid is best for resuscitation. Methodologies and conclusions have been challenged, but Cochrane analyses have concluded that there is no evidence to support the use of colloids over crystalloids (Alderson *et al.* 2002a; Bunn *et al.* 2002a), no evidence that hypertonic crystalloid is better than isotonic (Bunn *et al.* 2002b), and that use of albumin is associated with higher mortality than other solutions (Alderson *et al.* 2002b). It would seem logical for the replacement fluids to include blood when blood has obviously been lost, or the haemoglobin concentration is less than 10 g/dl. Dextrose saline (containing 0.15 per cent saline) or 5 per cent dextrose infusions have no place in the correction of depleted intravascular volume, since these solutions partition throughout the total body water and only a small fraction remains within the vascular compartment. An all too common cause of gross oedema in patients referred with acute renal failure is inappropriate administration of dextrose-based solutions.

Other measures believed to improve renal function

In those whose acute renal failure is prerenal in origin, urine output and renal function will improve (by definition) when intravascular volume is restored. In many cases, however, this will not be the case, and urine output remains low (say 30 ml/h or less). In these instances, it is common practice to prescribe other measures in the hope of improving renal function. What is the evidence that any of these measures are helpful?

Loop diuretics

These agents, of which frusemide is the most commonly used, act primarily to inhibit function of the sodium/potassium/chloride cotransporter in the luminal membrane of the thick ascending limb of the loop of Henle. There are several theoretical reasons, some more fanciful than others, why they may be beneficial in cases of acute renal failure, or those at high risk of developing the condition (Shilliday and Allison 1994).

1. The countercurrent flow of blood in the vasa rectae (important for the mechanism of urinary concentration) creates a state in which the oxygen tension in the deeper parts of the cortex and the medulla of the normal kidney is very low. The medullary thick ascending limb may, therefore, be operating on the verge of anoxia, and be particularly susceptible to ischaemic/hypoxic damage if the circulation is perturbed, as described previously. By inhibiting sodium transport, loop diuretics reduce the metabolic work done by this segment of the renal tubule, and might thereby protect it against ischaemic/hypoxic damage.
2. By increasing the flow of urine down the tubules, loop diuretics may 'flush out' intratubular casts and reduce tubular obstruction.
3. Tubuloglomerular feedback is the process whereby an increased delivery of chloride to the macula densa of a nephron leads to a reduction in the filtration rate of that nephron. Loop diuretics inhibit this process, and may, therefore, preserve filtration rate in cases of acute renal failure. It should be noted, however, that such action may not necessarily be 'good' in this context. When a tubule is damaged, the tubuloglomerular feedback mechanism may serve an important protective function in preventing it from being inundated with fluid that it cannot reabsorb, which would cause an obligatory natriuresis and diuresis that could be detrimental (Thurau and Boylan 1976).
4. Renal blood flow is typically reduced in acute tubular necrosis. In normal individuals, loop diuretics reduce renal vascular resistance and increase renal blood flow, in part via effects on renal prostaglandin production. If they have the same actions in those with, or at risk of, acute renal failure (which is not proven), then they may be beneficial.

Treatment of acute renal failure

A very large number of publications report the effects of giving loop diuretics to patients with acute renal failure. Unfortunately, very few are helpful in determining whether the treatment is of any use. Cantarovich *et al.* (1973) divided 58 patients with acute renal failure who had not responded to fluid challenge or mannitol infusion into control ($n = 19$, no diuretics) and treatment groups ($n = 39$, 2 g of frusemide per day). The inequality of the numbers in the two groups arising from the fact that those who had received diuretic therapy before referral were not allowed to enter the control group, an obvious potential source of bias. Frusemide reduced the period of oliguria (urine output < 400 ml/day: 7 versus 14 days), reduced the time until the patients passed more than 2 l of urine/day (10 versus 20 days), and reduced the number of haemodialysis treatments given (five versus nine). It did not, however, speed up the recovery of renal function, as judged by the time until the serum creatinine fell to 1.5 mg/dl, or significantly reduce mortality (46 versus 58 per cent).

Kleinknecht *et al.* (1976) corrected intravascular volume depletion and then randomized 66 patients with oliguric renal failure to control ($n = 33$, no diuretics) and treatment groups ($n = 33$, frusemide 3 mg/kg per hour, then according to a sliding scale whereby less diuretic was given if urine output increased, and vice versa: maximum dose 1200 mg/day). This diuretic regimen did not appear to help: the period of oliguria was not significantly shortened, the time until plasma urea fell spontaneously was not altered, the number of haemodialyses required was unchanged, and there was no effect on mortality.

Brown *et al.* (1981) randomized 56 consecutive dialysis-requiring patients with acute renal failure to control ($n = 28$, frusemide 4 mg/kg per min for 4 h) and treatment groups ($n = 28$, frusemide as control, followed by 2 mg/kg per min continuously or 1 g orally three times per day). The group given the larger dose of diuretic had a shorter period of oliguria, but the time until the plasma creatinine concentration declined to less than or equal to 300 μmol/l was not altered, the number of dialyses required by survivors was unchanged, and mortality was the same in both groups. Transient or permanent deafness and/or tinnitus were noted as side-effects of high-dose frusemide.

The best study of the use of loop diuretics in acute renal failure was reported by Shilliday *et al.* (1997). Ninety-two patients whose renal function did not recover with appropriate volume expansion and who were presumed to have acute tubular necrosis were randomized into three groups, receiving (in a double blind manner) torasemide (3 mg/kg every 6 h, reducing if/when renal function improved), frusemide (also 3 mg/kg every 6 h, reducing if/when renal function improved), or placebo. All received dopamine and mannitol in the same way. Both diuretics increased urinary volume, but renal recovery, the need for dialysis and patient survival were no different in the three groups.

Prevention of acute renal failure (Chapter 10.2)

There has been one high-quality clinical study of the effect of frusemide and mannitol (separately) in a situation where the risk of developing acute renal failure was thought to be considerable. Solomon *et al.* (1994) randomized 78 patients with chronic renal impairment who were to undergo cardiac angiography into three groups: the first receiving 0.45 per cent saline (1 ml/kg/h) alone for 12 h before and 12 h after the procedure, the second receiving saline plus mannitol (25 g), and the third saline plus frusemide (80 mg). An acute radiocontrast-induced decrease in renal function was defined as an increase of at least 44 μmol/l over the baseline plasma creatinine concentration within 48 h. This happened in 11 per cent of the controls, 28 per cent of those given mannitol, and 40 per cent of those receiving frusemide. The investigators drew the obvious conclusion, namely that hydration with 0.45 per cent saline afforded better protection against renal dysfunction than did saline plus mannitol or frusemide.

Similar evidence that frusemide might actually be detrimental has come from a study in which 126 patients with preoperatively normal renal function undergoing elective cardiac surgery received a continuous infusion of either dopamine, frusemide (0.5 μg/kg/min), or isotonic sodium chloride (placebo) (Lassnigg *et al.* 2000). The postoperative increase in plasma creatinine was twice as high in the group given frusemide as in either of the other two groups, and acute renal injury [defined as a rise in creatinine over baseline >0.5 mg/dl (approximately 50 μmol/l)] occurred in 6/41 patients receiving frusemide, compared to 1/82 in the other two groups.

Mannitol

Intravenous mannitol is a potent osmotic diuretic, inducing large natriuresis and diuresis in those with normal renal function. As with loop diuretics, there are a number of theoretical reasons why its effects may be beneficial in cases of acute renal failure (Shilliday and Allison 1994).

1. An increase in flow rate through the tubules might flush out intratubular casts.
2. Mannitol may increase renal blood flow.
3. Damage to renal cells causes them to swell, causing vascular congestion and impairing blood flow. The osmotic effect of hypertonic mannitol may prevent this.
4. The same action that reduces cell swelling causes expansion of the intravascular volume and reduces the haematocrit, which may confer protection against ischaemic insult.
5. Mannitol may reduce the influx of calcium into mitochondria that occurs after ischaemia, and thereby preserve mitochondrial function in this situation.
6. Toxic free-radical species are generated during reperfusion of tissue after ischaemia. Mannitol can act as a free-radical scavenger.

The paucity of good-quality studies, lamented for the use of loop diuretics in the treatment of acute renal failure, is even more notable in the case of mannitol. Various computerized searches of the literature and perusal of many articles have failed to reveal a controlled trial of the use of mannitol in patients with established acute renal failure, although there are a number of case reports describing acute renal failure caused by mannitol (Docci *et al.* 1994; Lin *et al.* 1995). There are, however, a number of reports in the older literature describing the effects of mannitol in patients considered to be at high risk of developing acute renal failure in the context of surgical procedures. Many of these studies have not included a control population of any sort. The controlled studies that have been done have only included small numbers of patients, and in most if not all the conclusions reached are not relevant to modern surgical and anaesthetic practice, where the importance of prevention, detection, and treatment of hypovolaemia is widely recognized (Williams *et al.* 1960; Barry *et al.* 1961; Beall *et al.* 1963).

One particular circumstance in which mannitol infusion has been vigorously advocated is in the treatment of traumatic rhabdomyolysis. Better and colleagues (Ron *et al.* 1984; Better and Stein 1990) have reported that intravenous infusion at a rate of 12 l/day of a solution containing sodium (110 mmol/l), chloride (70 mmol/l), bicarbonate (40 mmol/l), glucose (5 per cent), and mannitol (1 per cent)—beginning as soon as possible (whilst the patient is being extricated from whatever has crushed them)—can prevent the development of renal failure. It is not, however, possible to say which particular aspects of this treatment regimen are important: it is entirely possible that adequate fluid replacement with saline alone would be sufficient. It would certainly be much simpler to administer.

Dopamine

Dopamine is an important modulator of renal function, playing a significant part in the regulation of sodium excretion. It is synthesized physiologically in proximal tubular cells from L-dopa taken up from the tubular lumen, and acts on a variety of renal dopamine receptors. The DA-1 receptor subtype is found in the vasculature and both the luminal and basolateral proximal tubular membranes; the DA-2 subtype in the sympathetic nerve terminals innervating the blood vessels. Activation of DA-1 receptors, which are more sensitive to dopamine than the DA-2 subtype, leads to renal vasodilatation and to inhibition of tubular sodium reabsorption. In normal individuals, an intravenous infusion of dopamine at a low dose (1–5 μg/kg per min) causes an increase in renal blood flow, glomerular filtration rate, and sodium excretion (Lokhandwala and Amenta 1991). It should be noted, however, that whilst such an infusion is frequently referred to as 'renal dose' dopamine, this is a misnomer, implying action exclusively on the kidney, whereas some of the effects on renal function are undoubtedly attributable to its inotropic action on the heart (Duke and Bersten 1992). Notwithstanding this quibble, the changes induced by the infusion of a low dose of dopamine in normal individuals might conceivably be beneficial (if they occur) in those with, or at risk of, acute renal failure, and are the rationale for the widespread use of the agent in this situation. However, as with the loop diuretics and mannitol, good studies are rare.

Treatment of acute renal failure

There have been no randomized trials of the use of dopamine in the treatment of patients with established acute renal failure.

Prevention of acute renal failure

Hans *et al.* (1990) studied 60 patients with pre-existing renal insufficiency who were to be given radiographic contrast media when they underwent arteriography. Those in the treated group received a low dose of dopamine for 12 h starting at the beginning of the procedure; those in the control group received a placebo infusion. In the control group, the plasma creatinine concentration rose significantly afterwards, in the dopamine group it did not. By contrast, in a similar study, Weisberg *et al.* (1993) reported that patients with chronic renal impairment who received an infusion of dopamine (2 μg/kg per min) for 2 h at the time of cardiac catheterization did not fare better than those who received an equivalent volume of saline: one-third of the patients in each group had a greater than 25 per cent rise in their plasma creatinine concentration 2 days after the procedure.

Baldwin *et al.* (1994) randomized 37 patients undergoing elective repair of an abdominal aortic aneurysm or aortobifemoral grafting into a group receiving dopamine (3 μg/kg per min) and a group receiving placebo. Plasma creatinine and urea concentrations, and creatinine clearance, were measured preoperatively and on the first and fifth postoperative days. No statistically or clinically significant differences were found between the outcomes in the two groups. Myles *et al.* (1993) randomized 52 patients undergoing elective coronary artery surgery into groups receiving dopamine (200 μg/min) or placebo for 24 h from induction of anaesthesia. The incidence of transient renal impairment was the same in both (dopamine, 36 per cent; placebo, 50 per cent). Similar findings were reported by Lassnigg *et al.* (2000).

Parks *et al.* (1994) randomized 23 patients undergoing surgical relief of obstructive jaundice into a control group ($n = 10$), receiving 3 l of 5 per cent dextrose intravenously during the 24 h before surgery and a bolus dose of intravenous frusemide (1 mg/kg) at induction, and an experimental group receiving an additional infusion of dopamine (3 μg/kg/min, started at induction and continued for 48 h). The outcome was the same in both groups. None of the patients developed clinically significant acute renal failure.

Marik and Iglesias (1999) randomized 395 patients with septic shock and oliguria into three groups: no dopamine, low-dose dopamine (2.5 μg/kg/min), and high-dose dopamine (16 μg/kg/min). There was no difference in the incidence of acute renal failure, need for dialysis, or 28-day mortality between the three groups. A similar conclusion came from the excellent multicentre study performed by the Australian and New Zealand Intensive Care Society (ANZICS) Clinical Trials Group (Bellomo *et al.* 2000): 328 patients (23 centres) with at least two criteria for the systemic inflammatory response syndrome and oliguria or an increase in serum creatinine concentration were randomized to receive a continuous infusion of dopamine (2 μg/kg/min) or placebo (double blind) whilst on the intensive care unit. There was no difference in the peak serum creatinine concentration during treatment in the two groups [245 (dopamine) versus 249 (placebo) μmol/l] or in any other parameter measured.

Some have argued that dopamine might be harmful, rather than simply being ineffective. Tang *et al.* (1999) reported that dopamine (2.5–4 μg/kg/min) increased the urinary excretion of retinol-binding protein (used as a marker of early tubular injury) after coronary artery surgery and, therefore, argued that it should not be given in this context because it exacerbated tubular injury.

By contrast with the studies described above, which paint a uniformly discouraging picture with regard to dopamine in acute renal failure, evidence that it may have some beneficial effect (albeit temporary) has come from a cross-over study in which eight critically ill patients with mild non-oliguric renal impairment (creatinine clearance 30–80 ml/min) received placebo for 4 h, dopamine 3 μg/kg/min for 48 h, then a final 4 h placebo period (Ichai *et al.* 2000). Urine flow, creatinine clearance, and fractional sodium excretion increased significantly 4 h after starting dopamine, reaching a maximum at 8 h (urine flow up 50 per cent, creatinine clearance up 37 per cent, fractional sodium excretion up 85 per cent) before dwindling to control (placebo) levels by 24 and 48 h.

A meta-analysis of 17 randomized clinical trials ($n = 854$ patients) of the use of dopamine in the prevention and/or treatment of renal dysfunction in patients with critical illness concluded that it did not prevent death, onset of acute renal failure, or need for dialysis and argued that it should be eliminated from routine clinical use (Kellum and Decker 2001).

Other agents

In a plethora of animal models, a wide variety of agents has been shown to ameliorate the development of acute renal failure, usually when given before, or at the same time as, the causative insult (see Chapter 10.2). These studies can be of use in elucidating the pathophysiological basis of renal failure in particular experimental situations, but they cannot be used to justify clinical practice; at best they may usefully indicate new avenues in which clinical trials should be conducted. The following treatments fall into this category: calcium-channel blockers; natriuretic peptides; ATP–$MgCl_2$; glycine and alanine; thyroxine; antioxidant defence strategies; RGD peptide inhibitors; manoeuvres designed to modulate the nitric oxide or endothelin systems, the action of lipid-derived mediators or cellular adhesion molecules; and growth factors (Fischereder *et al.* 1994; Lake and Humes 1994; Edelstein *et al.* 1997; Humes 1997; Lieberthal 1997).

As regards clinical studies, there is some evidence of effect of calcium-channel blockers (Lumlertgul *et al.* 1989, 1991; Neumayer *et al.* 1989), and one study has reported infusion of atrial natriuretic peptide to be beneficial (Rahman *et al.* 1994). Promising results have been reported in a small study using urodilatin (ularitide) (Meyer *et al.* 1997), but not confirmed in another (Herbert *et al.* 1999). One study of the use of thyroxine found it to be of no benefit (Acker *et al.* 2000).

Since recovery from acute tubular necrosis depends on cellular regeneration, there has been much interest in the possibility that administration of a growth factor might speed recovery, and this has been demonstrated in many experimental models (Coimbra *et al.* 1990; Ding *et al.* 1993). A multicentre clinical trial of recombinant human insulin-like growth factor-I (rhIGF-I) in patients with acute renal failure was reported in 1999 (Hirschberg *et al.* 1999). Those given rhIGF-I 100 μg/kg every 12 h for up to 14 days fared no better than those given placebo, but given the dramatic effects seen in clinical models of acute renal failure, and the efficacy of growth factors in other clinical situations (e.g. treatment of renal anaemia, restoration of white cell counts in haematological practice) this approach may eventually produce benefit.

None of the agents described above has yet found its way into routine clinical practice and none should be given except in the context of properly conducted research trials.

Practical recommendations on the use of other measures alleged to improve renal function

On the basis of the evidence described above, it is hard to disagree with the general conclusion reached by Cronin (1986), namely that in acute renal failure 'these pharmacological therapies increase the complexity and cost of care with little tangible evidence of benefit to the patient or the physician caring for the patient'. However, many nephrologists have had the experience of observing occasional patients in whom, after intravascular volume had been restored and treatment of any precipitating condition initiated, treatment with frusemide and dopamine appeared to initiate a diuresis and clinical improvement. It is, of course, impossible to say for certain whether or not the frusemide and/or dopamine caused the improvement (except in those cases where cessation led to deterioration and re-instigation led to re-improvement), but clinical practice is rarely as cut and dried as this. Thus, whilst the trials described above clearly indicate that the vast majority of patients with acute renal failure do not obtain substantial benefit from frusemide and dopamine, it remains clinical experience that a few do. For those physicians who wish to instigate a 'therapeutic trial' of treatment, Fig. 7 gives practical recommendations.

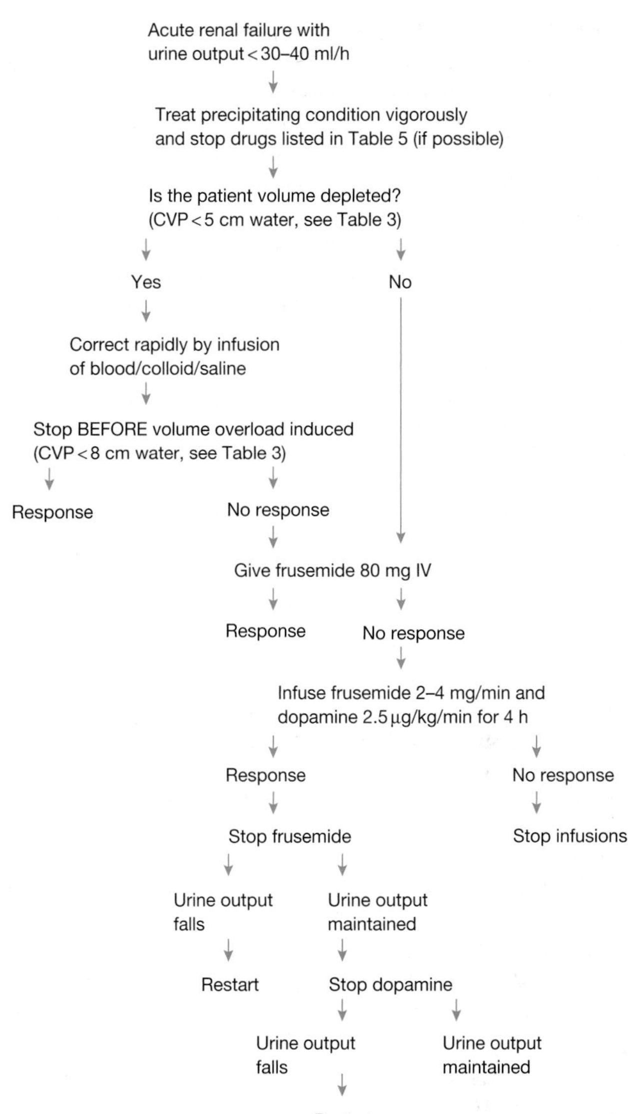

Notes:
(1) Total dose of frusemide not to exceed 1 g per day because of risk of ototoxicity.
(2) After restoration of intravascular volume fluid input (average sodium concentration 70–80 mmol/l) should equal measured output plus 0.5–1 l/day (insensible losses).

Fig. 7 Algorithm showing practical recommendations for the use of frusemide and dopamine in patients with acute tubular necrosis.

Fluid and electrolyte requirements in established acute renal failure

Most patients with acute renal failure will have intravascular volume depletion at the time of presentation. This must be corrected as quickly as possible by the rapid administration of appropriate fluid (see above). Once this has been accomplished—as evidenced by improvement in peripheral perfusion, fall in pulse rate, loss of postural drop in blood pressure, and rise in jugular venous pressure—the fluid requirements of the patient change considerably. If the kidneys are not working normally, care must be taken to ensure that the intake of fluids and electrolytes matches the sum of losses in the urine, from the gastrointestinal tract, and from other 'insensible' sources. Those with normal renal function are usually, but not always, able to cope with intravenous regimens—sometimes prescribed prospectively without clinical assessment of the patient—that infuse (say) 3 l per day of a variety of fluids. Those with acute renal failure cannot do this, yet a not uncommon indication for emergency haemodialysis/haemofiltration is pulmonary oedema caused by iatrogenic fluid overload.

As a working rule, fluid intake in those with acute renal failure should be limited to the volume of the previous day's urine output, plus the volume of other measurable fluid losses, plus 500 ml for insensible losses (an allocation that may need to be substantially increased in the presence of fever or in hot environments). However, as discussed previously, fluid-balance charts are frequently inaccurate: thus unthinking adherence to the 'output plus 500 ml' rule can lead to problems. There is no substitute for careful, twice-daily clinical examination for signs of intravascular volume depletion or excess, supplemented by accurate daily weighing to gauge overall net fluid balance, with a flexible response to the findings.

Sodium requirements in patients with acute renal failure are very variable. Those who are oliguric may lose, and therefore require, only 15–30 mmol/day. Those who are polyuric may excrete very considerable amounts of sodium (many hundred mmol/day), and run the danger of developing intravascular volume depletion if this is not replenished (with the risk of thereby exacerbating their acute renal failure). In the polyuric phase of acute tubular necrosis, the kidneys do not have the capacity to modulate sodium excretion in the normal manner, such that the urinary sodium concentration is typically in the range 50–70 mmol/l. Hence, if urine output is 3 l/day, over 200 mmol of sodium may be required to prevent negative balance. On occasion the urine output in polyuric acute renal failure can be extremely high (over 5 l/day is not uncommon). These cases can be difficult to manage: if the therapeutic response is to administer an even greater quantity of fluid (output plus insensible losses), then it is possible to contrive a vicious circle whereby ever-increasing urinary output is met by ever-increasing fluid infusion. Such a danger should be recognized in the polyuric patient, and a fluid-replacement strategy employed that avoids this by limiting input to a volume equal to the urinary output alone, and allowing other fluid losses to establish a mild overall negative balance. Regular clinical examination and weighing should alert the physician to the risk of development of significant intravascular volume depletion.

Because hyperkalaemia is one of the great dangers in those with acute renal failure, it is essential to check plasma potassium concentrations at least daily. In those with hypercatabolism or gastrointestinal bleeding, or who require surgery, more frequent estimations are advisable. In oliguric cases, high-potassium foods should be avoided. By contrast, in polyuric acute renal failure, very substantial urinary losses of potassium can occur (many hundred mmol/day), and avoidance of hypokalaemia can be difficult. In these circumstances, measurement of the urinary potassium concentration can be helpful in estimating how much is required. In the very rare patient that passes 500 ml of urine per hour or more, potassium may need it to be infused at a rate of up to 40 mmol/h, necessitating central venous access and very frequent measurement of the plasma potassium concentration.

Renal replacement therapy in acute renal failure (see Chapter 10.4)

When should renal replacement therapy be started?

Mandatory indications for the urgent instigation of life-saving renal replacement therapy are: (a) severe refractory hyperkalaemia; (b) intractable fluid overload causing pulmonary oedema; (c) overt uraemia manifesting as encephalopathy, pericarditis, or uraemic bleeding; and (d) acidosis producing circulatory compromise. It is more common, however, to see a state in which a patient's renal function gradually declines over a period of a few days whilst they are in hospital. In this circumstance, there is no hard and fast rule as to when renal replacement therapy should be initiated. Leaving patients until they are grossly uraemic is clearly to be avoided, but there is no threshold of nitrogenous waste at which the patient suddenly becomes susceptible to overt uraemic sequelae. It is clearly not sensible to wait until an obvious uraemic complication arises. Modern practice is to initiate renal replacement therapy sooner rather than later, for example, when the plasma urea concentration reaches 25–30 mmol/l and the plasma creatinine concentration 500–700 μmol/l, perhaps even earlier, unless there is clear evidence that renal function is about to recover. A plasma urea concentration of greater than 45 mmol/l usually requires urgent institution of treatment. There are, however, no controlled trials relevant to modern practice that can be used to justify the initiation of renal replacement therapy at one specific plasma urea or creatinine concentration rather than another.

What sort of renal replacement therapy, and how much?

There are a large number of different ways of giving renal replacement therapy, as described in Chapter 10.4.

Peritoneal dialysis

Peritoneal dialysis is technically the simplest form of renal replacement therapy and is still commonly used worldwide, although very little has been published about its use in acute renal failure (Ash 2001). The main differences from its use in chronic renal failure (see Chapter 12.4) are (a) that catheters are used that can be inserted percutaneously, without tunnelling, using a metal stylet (although some use the same type of catheter as that used for continuous ambulatory treatment), and (b) that smaller volume exchanges with shorter dwell-times are the norm. The technique obviously requires an intact peritoneum and is, therefore, precluded in the many patients whose renal failure follows abdominal surgery. Other problems include difficulty in maintaining dialysate flow, leakage, peritoneal infection, protein losses, and restricted ability to clear fluid and uraemic wastes. Peritoneal dialysis is rarely capable of providing good dialysis of the adult patient with acute renal failure as judged by contemporary standards, and is virtually never the first choice modality for renal replacement therapy in those centres that have a range of techniques at their disposal. Peritoneal dialysis is, however, the preferred treatment modality for acute renal failure in paediatric practice.

Haemodialysis, haemofiltration, and related techniques

Patients that are haemodynamically stable can be managed with intermittent techniques, requirements for the technical aspects of haemodialysis being the same as those for chronic haemodialysis (see Chapter 12.3). Patients who are haemodynamically unstable are best managed using continuous modalities, which allow for continuous fine-tuning of intravascular volume, but there is no reason to prefer one practical arrangement, for example, pumped veno-venous haemodiafiltration, over another, for example, pumped veno-venous haemofiltration. The only randomized head-to-head comparison of an intermittent and a continuous technique showed no clear benefit for one or other approach (Mehta *et al.* 2001). What is used in any particular centre typically depends on local skills and experience, but a few general comments are appropriate.

Pumpless arteriovenous haemofiltration should not be used, excepting where pumped veno-venous systems are not available. They provide inferior clearances and increased risk, in particular from haemorrhage with dislodgement of short (to reduce pressure decrement) cannulae in the femoral artery (Kierdorf and Sieberth 1995).

A number of recent studies have shown that patients with acute renal failure who receive renal replacement therapy that provides higher clearances of metabolic wastes seem to do better than those who receive treatment giving lower clearances. One randomized controlled trial found that continuous veno-venous haemofiltration at filtration rates of 35 or 45 ml/kg/h produced a better outcome than the lower rate of 20 ml/kg/h (Ronco *et al.* 2000). Another randomized study that assigned patients to receive daily or alternate-day intermittent haemodialysis showed that daily treatment resulted in better control of uraemia, fewer hypotensive episodes during dialysis, and more rapid resolution of acute renal failure (Schiffl *et al.* 2002). Given that many renal and intensive care units are stretched to the limit of their resources, these findings come as a significant challenge, both to the units themselves, and those who pay for the care they provide.

Many studies have looked at the effect of different dialysis membranes on the outcome of patients with acute renal failure: are more biocompatible membranes preferable to less biocompatible membranes? A number of randomized controlled trials have been performed (Hakim *et al.* 1994; Schiffl *et al.* 1994; Himmelfarb *et al.* 1998; Jorres *et al.* 1999): these have drawn conflicting conclusions, but taken overall there is a trend to show benefit of more biocompatible (strictly less bioincompatible) membranes (Vanholder *et al.* 2000).

Other issues in the management of patients with acute renal failure

Indications for renal biopsy

Most cases of acute renal failure are due to prerenal failure or to acute tubular necrosis (Turney *et al.* 1990). They occur in a recognized clinical context and can be expected to follow a predictable time course, with recovery of renal function anticipated over the course of a few weeks. Renal biopsy is not routinely performed in such instances because the risks of the procedure are not warranted, given that the information obtained is exceedingly unlikely to influence clinical management. There are, however, circumstances in which renal biopsy is essential to establish a correct diagnosis of the cause of acute renal failure, with important implications for both management and prognosis. Biopsy should be performed:

(1) when the history, examination, or laboratory tests suggest the possibility of a systemic disorder amenable to treatment that could cause acute renal failure and could be diagnosed by renal biopsy;

(2) when the urine sediment contains red-cell casts, indicating the presence of an inflammatory renal condition that may require treatment with immunosuppressive agents;

(3) when the case history is atypical, that is when there is no convincing documentation of circulatory disturbance to support a diagnosis of acute tubular necrosis.

Most nephrologists have advocated this conservative attitude towards renal biopsy in acute renal failure for many years. Solez and colleagues (Solez *et al.* 1994; Solez and Racusen 2001) have argued that it is not. They give an extensive list of potential new therapies for those with acute renal failure and argue that examination of renal tissue might enable a rational choice of one, rather than another, to be made at some time in the future.

Some nephrologists advocate that patients with acute renal failure should undergo renal biopsy if function has not recovered after about 6 weeks. The usual justification for this is the belief that it will give prognostic information by determining whether or not there is cortical necrosis: if this is present, recovery would not be expected, whereas if it is not, recovery remains a possibility. There is no strong evidence to support this approach, which seems fundamentally flawed. If the aim is to diagnose the presence of cortical necrosis, then renal biopsy is not the correct investigation because the condition is often patchy. Renal angiography and contrast-enhanced computed tomography scanning are preferable in that they provide information about perfusion of the cortices of the whole of both kidneys. In acute cortical necrosis, renal angiography reveals attenuation of interlobular arteries, an increase in the subcapsular vessels, and a negative outer cortical nephrogram: contrast-enhanced computed tomography scanning shows enhancement of the renal medulla, but no enhancement of the renal cortex and no excretion of contrast. It is not, however, known if these investigations can usefully be employed to predict renal outcome and it seems unlikely that they would alter management, which in this clinical context (acute renal failure which persists after 4–6 weeks) is to prepare the patient for long-term renal replacement therapy.

The main risk of renal biopsy is haemorrhage. In order to minimize this risk, it is important to (a) correct clotting abnormalities (see below); (b) use a well-recognized biopsy technique; and (c) avoid dialysis for 24 h afterwards (if possible).

Nutrition

Patients with acute renal failure are always catabolic, more so if they are also septic, and they can lose flesh weight very rapidly. Specific uraemic toxic effects, insulin resistance, hormonal derangements, metabolic acidosis, circulating proteases, inflammatory mediators, and dialysis-related losses of nutritional substrates all contribute to protein catabolism (Druml 1998). Those that are in the greatest negative caloric balance have the highest mortality (Mault *et al.* 1983), an observation which led naturally to the idea that improving nutrition might also improve outcome. It has become accepted wisdom that 'dietary manipulation and often vigorous nutritional intervention (i.e. parenteral nutrition) are a must for these patients' survival' (Varella and Utermohlen 1993). Others have said that 'despite the notorious difficulty to demonstrate clear-cut benefits of nutritional interventions and especially, of parenteral nutrition on prognosis in critically ill patients, there can be no doubt that nutritional therapy presents a cornerstone in the treatment of patients with ARF' (Druml 2001). However, it has not been proven in controlled trials of patients with acute renal failure that any form of nutritional support can either reliably generate positive nitrogen balance, improve nutritional status (Sponsel and Conger 1995), or alter mortality. This is not a justification for allowing patients with acute renal failure to starve.

Feeding should be by the enteral route whenever possible. If the gut is not working and parenteral feeding is required, the regimen used should not be unduly complex to make and to administer, and should not be unnecessarily costly. Since the amino acids are the most expensive ingredients, two small prospective trials performed on patients with acute renal failure by Feinstein and colleagues are of note (Feinstein *et al.* 1981, 1983). In the first study, 30 patients were randomized into three groups: each received the same total energy intake, but one was given this in the form of glucose alone, the second as glucose plus 21 g/day of essential amino acids, and the third as glucose plus 21 g/day of essential amino acids plus 21 g/day of non-essential amino acids. There were no differences between the groups in survival (although this would not be anticipated in such a small study), in rate of recovery of renal function, or in a number of biochemical measures of nutritional status. In the second study, 11 similar patients were randomized between two regimens: glucose plus 21 g/day essential amino acids, and glucose plus 76 g/day essential and non-essential amino acids. Nitrogen balance was negative and not significantly different in the two groups.

Suggested enteral and parenteral feeding regimens for patients with acute renal failure are shown in Table 9.

Bleeding

Some patients with acute renal failure bleed. The causes are multiple—defective platelet aggregation, decreased platelet adhesiveness, decreased availability of platelet factor III, all leading to prolongation of the bleeding time (Jubelirer 1985)—and they are frequently compounded by the effects of anaemia (Anand and Feffer 1994). The haemorrhagic tendency is usually mild, producing ecchymoses and purpura, but it can be severe and become the dominant clinical problem. A number of therapeutic options should then be considered (Table 10).

It would be useful to have a test capable of predicting which patients with acute renal failure were likely to have serious bleeding problems. Some have suggested that prolongation of the bleeding time can be used to define a subgroup at high risk (Steiner *et al.* 1979), but in a critical analysis of the literature, Rodgers and Levin (1990) concluded that in patients with acute renal failure it predicted significant bleeding no better than did knowledge of the platelet count or haematocrit.

Bleeding from the gastrointestinal tract used to be the second commonest cause of death in those with acute renal failure (after sepsis) (Kleinknecht *et al.* 1971). This is no longer the case, almost certainly because of the earlier institution of renal replacement therapy and the use of H2-blockers, which has become routine practice in the management of acute renal failure in many centres. There have been no randomized studies of the prevention of gastrointestinal haemorrhage in patients with uncomplicated acute renal failure, but many reports of the advantages of H2-receptor antagonists, antacids and/or sucralfate in preventing such bleeding in patients on intensive care units (Tryba 1991). However, sucralfate should be avoided in those with renal failure because toxic levels of aluminium can accumulate (Mulla *et al.* 2001), antacids are inconvenient because they have to be given very frequently (and some may cause toxicity in renal failure), hence H2-blockers are the agents usually given.

Table 9 Suggested enteral and parenteral feeding regimens for patients with acute renal failure

Recommended daily adult requirements (per kg body weight)

Total energy	35 kcal
Protein	1 g
Nitrogen	0.16 g

Patients with acute renal failure require this in a restricted fluid volume, with reduced amounts of sodium, potassium, and phosphate (if oliguric). For practical purposes it is sensible to have enteral and parenteral feeding fluids which satisfy these needs available routinely; since it is easier to add extra volume and electrolytes if these are required, rather than to take them away when they are not!

Enteral

Most enteral feeding preparations do not contain enough kcal/ml to be useful for patients with oliguria, and they also contain too much sodium, potassium, and phosphate. Commercial preparations designed for renal patients are available. For example, 'Nepro': 237 ml can provide 474 kcal (2 kcal/ml), 17 g protein, 9 mmol sodium, 6 mmol potassium, and 1.7 mmol phosphate. Feeding at 50 ml/h for 20 h per day provides 2000 kcal, 68 g protein, 36 mmol sodium, 24 mmol potassium, and 6.8 mmol phosphate, in 1000 ml total volume. Additional sodium, potassium, and phosphate can be given if required

Parenteral

Many hospital pharmacies make up their own bags of total parenteral nutrition (TPN) fluid. For renal patients a 'standard' regimen for an oliguric patient would involve giving each day:

- TPN fluid containing: dextrose 250 g; nitrogen 12–15 g; minimum electrolyte content (more may be added if required)—sodium 35 mmol, potassium 30 mmol, magnesium 2.5 mmol, phosphate 15 mmol, chloride 35 mmol; in a total volume of 1000 ml
- Lipid: 500 ml; various commercial preparations based on soya bean oil and other fats
- Vitamins and trace elements; various preparations

Note: These regimens are suggestions only! There is no good evidence to base strict stipulations regarding the optimal intake of calories and nitrogen/protein: some would advocate more of both in those that were hypercatabolic.

Infection

Many cases of acute renal failure are caused by infectious pathogens or are exacerbated and complicated by them (Wiecek *et al.* 1994). At one end of the spectrum are patients whose acute renal failure is caused by organisms that can be described as nephrotrophic in that the kidneys usually suffer the brunt of the clinical manifestations, for example, hantavirus infection (see Chapter 10.6.6), and leptospirosis (see Chapter 10.7.3). In the middle of the spectrum are cases in which acute tubular necrosis develops in the context of documented septicaemia, frequently in association with failure of other organ systems (Jochimsen *et al.* 1990).

Table 10 Practical strategies for the management of bleeding in acute renal failure

Exclude possibility of heparin effect
Increase haematocrit to >30% by blood transfusion (Livio *et al.* 1982; Anand and Feffer 1994)
Cryoprecipitate (10 bags): maximal effect between 1 and 12 h after administration; effect disappears at 24–36 h (Janson *et al.* 1980)
Desmopressin (0.3 μg/kg IV): acts by increasing factor VIII coagulant activity Shown in acute renal failure to shorten prolonged bleeding time (Mannucci *et al.* 1983) Many reports of clinical efficacy in those with severe haemorrhagic problems (Juhl and Jorgensen 1987) Lesser effect with repeated doses (Canavese *et al.* 1985) Can work after intranasal administration (Shapiro and Kelleher 1984) Cerebral thrombosis reported as a complication (Byrnes *et al.* 1988)
Conjugated oestrogen: 0.6 mg/kg/day IV for 5 days Shown to reduce bleeding time (effect beginning after 6 h and lasting 14 days) in patients with chronic renal impairment and haemorrhagic tendency (Liu *et al.* 1984; Livio *et al.* 1986; Vigano *et al.* 1988)

Septicaemic episodes are common in those who have acute renal failure for any reason, Frost *et al.* (1991) reporting that 50 (12 per cent) of 419 patients had positive blood cultures at some time during their admission. At the other end of the clinical spectrum are the many cases in which there is strong clinical suspicion, but no hard proof, that sepsis underlies the inexorable slide towards worsening renal and multiorgan failure of some patients who have been apparently successfully resuscitated from major trauma or surgery. Sepsis is an important predictor and cause of death in those with acute renal failure (Frost *et al.* 1991).

Aside from the provision of supportive measures, how should these patients be managed? In some instances, the answer is straightforward. Proven infection should be treated aggressively with appropriate antimicrobial agents, but these should not be used as an excuse to prevent localized sources of sepsis from being sought and dealt with vigorously. Occasionally, this may involve the drainage of abscesses, the aspiration of joints, the amputation of a limb, or many other procedures. If these are required, but not done, the patient will not recover. The oft-heard excuse that someone was 'too ill' for a particular procedure is always invalid unless a definite decision has been made to withdraw treatment: the more gravely ill, the more urgently remedy is required, and the only acceptable delay is a brief one to allow for resuscitation.

In cases where there is strong clinical suspicion of sepsis, but laboratory confirmation is not yet available, antimicrobial therapy should be initiated on a 'best guess' basis immediately after appropriate cultures have been obtained. The antimicrobials selected will be determined by the clinical context. In cases where the illness arises in the community the antimicrobials selected should provide broad-spectrum activity against both Gram-positive and Gram-negative organisms. When staphylococcal infection is thought to be likely, then a first-line antistaphylococcal agent should be included (if the cover would otherwise be weak in this respect); and when the chest is thought to be the primary focus of infection a drug such as erythromicin should be added to cover atypical organisms such as *Legionella*. In community-acquired sepsis, the organisms involved are relatively unlikely to be resistant to antimicrobials, but the best choice of regimen will be governed by what is known of antimicrobial resistance patterns in the local population, which vary enormously from place to place. When sepsis arises in hospital, particularly during a lengthy admission, the chances of a resistant organism being responsible are much greater, and it is vitally important to get the best information possible on the likelihood of this before selecting an antimicrobial combination. The possibility of fungal infection might also need to be considered in this group, and in those who are immunosuppressed a wider differential may need to be entertained.

Cases in which the diagnosis of sepsis is not secure, for example, the patient with a low-grade fever who simply seems to be deteriorating, present real difficulty. Unused intravenous lines and urinary catheters should be removed, and the patient examined regularly for signs of a septic focus. There should be a low threshold for repeated, thorough microbiological investigation, together with imaging (usually by ultrasound or computed tomography) to look for localized collections. In many instances, no firm evidence of sepsis is forthcoming despite these endeavours, and a 'trial of antimicrobial therapy' has to be considered. It is better that patients die after such a trial, rather than before it. There is, however, a danger of this argument being used to justify indiscriminate and prolonged use of powerful antimicrobials on renal and intensive care units. This is difficult to defend: trials of antimicrobial therapy should be exactly that—if no clear evidence of improvement has been produced within (say) 48 h, they should be stopped, and cultures and other appropriate tests repeated. Fevers can be caused by non-infection pathology, for example, serositis, drugs, and malignancy.

Is something wrong in the abdomen?

The patient with acute renal failure in the context of suspected or proven intra-abdominal mischief, for example, with a tender abdomen, or after surgery for perforated or ischaemic bowel, is a special case. This scenario is not uncommon, and the important clinical point is that imaging of the abdomen cannot exclude the presence of a surgically correctable condition with complete confidence. Although the wider availability and improvement of computed tomography scanning has helped physicians and surgeons enormously, laparotomy is often a necessary diagnostic manoeuvre. In 1978, Milligan reviewed 76 consecutive patients with acute renal failure and severe intra-abdominal infection: 50 after various types of abdominal surgery, 18 following trauma, seven cases of pancreatitis, and one primary pneumococcal peritonitis in a patient with the nephrotic syndrome (Milligan *et al.* 1978). Repeated surgical abdominal explorations were made on 70 occasions in 40 patients on the basis of physical findings, fever, and leucocytosis. Diagnostic procedures were not useful in predicting those who turned out to have correctable conditions, a group with lower mortality than those that did not. Surgeons should be encouraged to open the abdomen of a very ill patient even in the absence of what they recognize as a definite surgical indication such as peritonism, for such signs become less and less reliable as patients deteriorate. If a patient who has had a laparotomy for perforated or ischaemic bowel deteriorates inexplicably (e.g. they are looking less well with raised white cell count and increasing acidosis), then the explanation is likely to lie in the abdomen.

Prognosis (see Chapter 10.1)

Will the patient survive?

Acute renal failure is a potentially lethal condition: the mortality of all cases that required renal replacement therapy being about 40 per cent in the 1985–1988 cohort of the large series reported by Turney *et al.* (1990). However, it is clear that not all patients are at equivalent risk, and for many reasons it is important to know whether a particular patient or group of patients falls into a higher or lower category of risk. This information has many implications: most crucially for the counselling of individual patients and their relatives, and also for sensible interpretation of survival figures reported in the published literature.

The most important prognostic factor in those with acute renal failure is whether or not the kidneys are the only organ system that has failed. Many studies of patients requiring dialysis for acute renal failure have shown that the need for artificial ventilation has a massive effect on outcome. In Turney's series, 40 per cent of all patients needed mechanical ventilation, and in these the mortality rate was just over 60 per cent (Turney *et al.* 1990). In 250 consecutive cases of acute renal failure treated on an intensive care unit, 106 of 173 (61 per cent) of those that required ventilation died, in comparison with 12 of 77 (16 per cent) of those that did not (Barton *et al.* 1993). If patients with acute renal failure are classified into low, medium, and high risk groups on the basis of comorbidity and age, then one population-based study found survival of the three groups at 2 years to be 80, 42, and 19 per cent, respectively (Khan *et al.* 1997).

Will renal function recover?

The conventional belief is that renal function almost invariably recovers following acute tubular necrosis if the patient survives. This certainly used to be the case: in 1981, Kjellstrand *et al.* (1981) reported that only 4/432 cases of acute tubular necrosis needed chronic haemodialysis and that such patients were 'not very time-demanding on the capacity of dialysis units'. A recent study showed similar findings, with only 3/188 (1.6 per cent) of patients surviving acute renal failure on intensive care units in Scotland (UK) developing endstage renal failure (Noble *et al.* 2001), but the situation is no longer so clear-cut. Bhandari and Turney reported the outcome of 1095 cases of acute renal failure seen in Leeds (UK) between 1984 and 1995 (Bhandari and Turney 1996; Firth 1996). In 1984–1986, 166 patients were treated, 90 survived to 90 days (54 per cent), with five requiring long-term dialysis (6 per cent of survivors). By contrast, in 1993–1995, 411 patients were treated, 247 survived to 90 days (60 per cent), and 52 required long-term dialysis (21 per cent of survivors). One intensive care unit based study showed that three of 26 (12 per cent) of patients who required renal support for more than 4 weeks failed to recover renal function (Spurney *et al.* 1991). Middle aged and elderly patients receiving renal replacement therapy for presumed acute tubular necrosis should be told that, if they survive, there is a 10 per cent chance that their kidneys will not recover and they will need lifelong renal support, and the same should be explained to their relatives.

For many reasons, it would be helpful to know which patients will fail to recover renal function. Decisions regarding the strategy for long-term renal replacement could be made at an earlier stage, and in some cases, the knowledge that renal function was exceedingly unlikely to recover would appropriately lead to discussion about whether or not active treatment should be continued. No test in routine clinical use will provide the necessary information, although measurement of renal plasma flow shows promise. Holland *et al.* (1987) used a single-injection, single blood-sample technique to measure effective renal plasma flow rate in 33 haemodynamically stable patients receiving dialysis for presumed acute tubular necrosis. Eight patients died before their kidneys recovered, did not undergo autopsy, and were excluded from analysis. Of the remaining 25, six either remained on dialysis after 6 months or were considered to have 'irreversible renal disease at autopsy', and 19 became independent of dialysis. The effective renal plasma flow in the former group was 90 ± 11 ml/min and in the latter 204 ± 20 ml/min. Initial effective renal plasma flow was greater than 125 ml/min in 15 of the 19 who recovered, but in none of those who did not (false-positive rate 21 per cent, false-negative rate 0 per cent). Similar findings have been reported in 31 patients by Ilic *et al.* (2000). However, further prospective studies are needed before measurement of renal plasma flow could be advocated as a useful predictive test.

References

Acker, C. G. *et al.* (2000). A trial of thyroxine in acute renal failure. *Kidney International* **57** (1), 293–298.

Adhiyaman, V. *et al.* (2001). Nephrotoxicity in the elderly due to co-prescription of angiotensin converting enzyme inhibitors and nonsteroidal anti-inflammatory drugs. *Journal of the Royal Society of Medicine* **94** (10), 512–514.

Ahuja, T. S. *et al.* (2000). Predictors of the development of hyperkalemia in patients using angiotensin-converting enzyme inhibitors. *American Journal of Medicine* **20** (4), 268–272.

Akmal, M. *et al.* (1986). Hypocalcemia and hypercalcemia in patients with rhabdomyolysis with and without acute renal failure. *Journal of Clinical Endocrinology and Metabolism* **63** (1), 137–142.

Alderson, P. *et al.* (2002a). Colloids versus crystalloids for fluid resuscitation in critically ill patients (Cochrane Review). *The Cochrane Library*. Oxford: Update Software. Issue 2.

Alderson, P., Bunn, F., Lefebvre, C., Li Wan Po, A., Li, L., Roberts, I., and Schierhout, G. (2002b). Human albumin solution for resuscitation and volume expansion in critically ill patients (Cochrane Review). The Albumin Reviewers. *The Cochrane Library.* Oxford: Update Software. Issue 2.

Allon, M. (1993). Treatment and prevention of hyperkalemia in end-stage renal disease. *Kidney International* **43** (6), 1197–1209.

Allon, M. and Copkney, C. (1990). Albuterol and insulin for treatment of hyperkalemia in hemodialysis patients. *Kidney International* **38** (5), 869–872.

Allon, M. *et al.* (1989). Nebulized albuterol for acute hyperkalemia in patients on hemodialysis. *Annals of Internal Medicine* **110** (6), 426–429.

Anand, A. and Feffer, S. E. (1994). Hematocrit and bleeding time: an update. *Southern Medical Journal* **87** (3), 299–301.

Anderson, R. J. *et al.* (1977). Nonoliguric acute renal failure. *New England Journal of Medicine* **296** (20), 1134–1138.

Anon (1989). Hyperkalaemia—silent and deadly. *Lancet* **1** (8649), 1240.

Ash, S. R. (2001). Peritoneal dialysis in acute renal failure of adults: the safe, effective, and low-cost modality. *Contributions to Nephrology* **132**, 210–221.

Baldwin, L. *et al.* (1994). Effect of postoperative low-dose dopamine on renal function after elective major vascular surgery. *Annals of Internal Medicine* **120** (9), 744–747.

Barry, K. G. *et al.* (1961). Mannitol infusion II. The prevention of acute functional renal failure during resection of an aneurysm of the abdominal aorta. *New England Journal of Medicine* **264**, 967–971.

Barton, I. K. *et al.* (1993). Acute renal failure treated by haemofiltration: factors affecting outcome. *Quarterly Journal of Medicine* **86** (2), 81–90.

Beall, A. C. *et al.* (1963). Mannitol-induced osmotic diuresis during vascular surgery. *Archives of Surgery* **6**, 34–42.

Bellomo, R. *et al.* (2000). Low-dose dopamine in patients with early renal dysfunction: a placebo-controlled randomised trial. Australian and New Zealand Intensive Care Society (ANZICS) Clinical Trials Group. *Lancet* **356**, 2139–2143.

Better, O. S. and Stein, J. H. (1990). Early management of shock and prophylaxis of acute renal failure in traumatic rhabdomyolysis. *New England Journal of Medicine* **322** (12), 825–829.

Bhandari, S. and Turney, J. H. (1996). Survivors of acute renal failure who do not recover renal function. *Quarterly Journal of Medicine* **89** (6), 415–421.

Bird, V. G. *et al.* (2002). A comparison of unenhanced helical computerized tomography findings and renal obstruction determined by furosemide 99m technetium mercaptoacetyltriglycine diuretic scintirenography for patients with acute renal colic. *Journal of Urology* **167** (4), 1597–1603.

Blum, U. *et al.* (1993). Effect of local low-dose thrombolysis on clinical outcome in acute embolic renal artery occlusion. *Radiology* **189** (2), 549–554.

Briggs, J. D. *et al.* (1967). Renal function after acute tubular necrosis. *British Medical Journal* **3** (564), 513–516.

Brosius, F. C. and Lau, K. (1986). Low fractional excretion of sodium in acute renal failure: role of timing of the test and ischemia. *American Journal of Nephrology* **6** (6), 450–457.

Brown, C. B. *et al.* (1981). High dose frusemide in acute renal failure: a controlled trial. *Clinical Nephrology* **15** (2), 90–96.

Bunn, F. *et al.* (2002a). Colloid solutions for fluid resuscitation (Cochrane Review). *The Cochrane Library*. Oxford: Update Software. Issue 2.

Bunn, F. *et al.* (2002b). Hypertonic versus isotonic crystalloid for fluid resuscitation in critically ill patients (Cochrane Review). *The Cochrane Library*. Oxford: Update Software. Issue 2.

Buring, J. E. *et al.* (1988). Randomized trials of aminoglycoside antibiotics: quantitative overview. *Reviews of Infectious Diseases* **10** (5), 951–957.

Burket, M. W. *et al.* (1992). 'Serpentine heart'. Direct observation of the human heart during profound hyperkalemia. *International Journal of Cardiology* **36** (1), 109–110.

Byrnes, J. J. *et al.* (1988). Thrombosis following desmopressin for uremic bleeding. *American Journal of Hematology* **28** (1), 63–65.

Canavese, C. *et al.* (1985). Reduced response of uraemic bleeding time to repeated doses of desmopressin. *Lancet* **1** (8433), 867–868.

Cantarovich, F. *et al.* (1973). High dose frusemide in established acute renal failure. *British Medical Journal* **4** (5890), 449–450.

Clive, D. M. and Stoff, J. S. (1984). Renal syndromes associated with nonsteroidal antiinflammatory drugs. *New England Journal of Medicine* **310** (9), 563–572.

Coimbra, T. M. *et al.* (1990). Epidermal growth factor accelerates renal repair in mercuric chloride nephrotoxicity. *American Journal of Physiology* **259** (3 Pt 2), F438–F443.

Cook, J. H., III *et al.* (1977). Ultrasonic demonstration of intrarenal anatomy. *American Journal of Roentgenology* **129** (5), 831–835.

Cronin, R. E. (1986). Drug therapy in the management of acute renal failure. *American Journal of Medical Science* **292** (2), 112–119.

Davenport, A. *et al.* (1993). Differentiation of acute from chronic renal impairment by detection of carbamylated haemoglobin. *Lancet* **341** (8861), 1614–1617.

Ding, H. *et al.* (1993). Recombinant human insulin-like growth factor-I accelerates recovery and reduces catabolism in rats with ischemic acute renal failure. *Journal of Clinical Investigation* **91** (5), 2281–2287.

Docci, D. *et al.* (1994). Mannitol-induced acute renal failure. *Nephron* **68** (1), 141.

Druml, W. (1998). Protein metabolism in acute renal failure. *Mineral and Electrolyte Metabolism* **24** (1), 47–54.

Druml, W. (2001). Nutritional management of acute renal failure. *American Journal of Kidney Diseases* **37** (1 Suppl. 2), S89–S94.

Duke, G. J. and Bersten, A. D. (1992). Dopamine and renal salvage in the critically ill patient. *Anaesthesia and Intensive Care* **20** (3), 277–287.

Durakovic, Z. *et al.* (1989). The lack of clinical value of laboratory parameters in predicting outcome in acute renal failure. *Renal Failure* **11** (4), 213–219.

Edelstein, C. L. *et al.* (1997). Emerging therapies for acute renal failure. *American Journal of Kidney Diseases* **30** (5 Suppl. 4), S89–S95.

Espinel, C. H. (1976). The FENa test. Use in the differential diagnosis of acute renal failure. *The Journal of American Medical Association* **236** (6), 579–581.

Espinel, C. H. and Gregory, A. W. (1980). Differential diagnosis of acute renal failure. *Clinical Nephrology* **13** (2), 73–77.

Ettinger, P. O. *et al.* (1974). Hyperkalemia, cardiac conduction, and the electrocardiogram: a review. *American Heart Journal* **88** (3), 360–371.

Feest, T. G. *et al.* (1993). Incidence of severe acute renal failure in adults: results of a community based study. *British Medical Journal* **306**, 481–483.

Feinstein, E. I. *et al.* (1981). Clinical and metabolic responses to parenteral nutrition in acute renal failure. A controlled double-blind study. *Medicine (Baltimore)* **60** (2), 124–137.

Feinstein, E. I. *et al.* (1983). Total parenteral nutrition with high or low nitrogen intakes in patients with acute renal failure. *Kidney International* (Suppl.) **16**, S319–S323.

Firth, J. D. (1996). Acute irreversible renal failure. *Quarterly Journal of Medicine* **89** (6), 397–399.

Fischereder, M. *et al.* (1994). Therapeutic strategies in the prevention of acute renal failure. *Seminars in Nephrology* **14** (1), 41–52.

Fraley, D. S. and Adler, S. (1977). Correction of hyperkalemia by bicarbonate despite constant blood pH. *Kidney International* **12** (5), 354–360.

Freeman, S. J. and Fale, A. D. (1993). Muscular paralysis and ventilatory failure caused by hyperkalaemia. *British Journal of Anaesthesia* **70** (2), 226–227.

Frost, L. *et al.* (1991). Prognosis in septicemia complicated by acute renal failure requiring dialysis. *Scandinavian Journal of Urology and Nephrology* **25** (4), 307–310.

Garcia-Palmieri, M. R. (1962). Reversal of hyperkalemic cardiotoxicity with hypertonic saline. *American Heart Journal* **64**, 483–488.

Georgiades, C. S. *et al.* (2001). Differences of renal parenchymal attenuation for acutely obstructed and unobstructed kidneys on unenhanced helical CT: a useful secondary sign? *American Journal of Roentgenology* **176** (4), 965–968.

Green, D. and Carroll, B. Ultrasound of renal failure. In *Genitourinary Ultrasound* (ed. H. Hricak), pp. 55–88. Edinburgh: Churchill Livingstone, 1986.

Hakim, R. M. *et al.* (1994). Effect of the dialysis membrane in the treatment of patients with acute renal failure. *New England Journal of Medicine* **331** (20), 1338–1342.

Hans, B. *et al.* (1990). Renal functional response to dopamine during and after arteriography in patients with chronic renal insufficiency. *Radiology* **176** (3), 651–654.

Herbert, M. K. *et al.* (1999). Concomitant treatment with urodilatin (ularitide) does not improve renal function in patients with acute renal failure after major abdominal surgery—a randomized controlled trial. *Wiener Klinische Wochenschrift* **111** (4), 141–147.

Himmelfarb, J. *et al.* (1998). A multicenter comparison of dialysis membranes in the treatment of acute renal failure requiring dialysis. *Journal of the American Society of Nephrology* **9** (2), 257–266.

Hirschberg, R. *et al.* (1999). Multicenter clinical trial of recombinant human insulin-like growth factor I in patients with acute renal failure. *Kidney International* **55** (6), 2423–2432.

Holland, M. D. *et al.* (1987). Predictive value of bedside effective renal plasma flow for renal recovery in severe acute renal failure. *Renal Failure* **10** (2), 83–89.

Hou, S. H. *et al.* (1983). Hospital-acquired renal insufficiency: a prospective study. *American Journal of Medicine* **74** (2), 243–248.

Humes, H. D. (1988). Aminoglycoside nephrotoxicity. *Kidney International* **33** (4), 900–911.

Humes, H. D. (1997). Acute renal failure—the promise of new therapies. *New England Journal of Medicine* **336** (12), 870–871.

Ichai, C. *et al.* (2000). Prolonged low-dose dopamine infusion induces a transient improvement in renal function in hemodynamically stable, critically ill patients: a single-blind, prospective, controlled study. *Critical Care Medicine* **28** (5), 1329–1335.

Ilic, S. *et al.* (2000). The predictive value of 131I-hippurate clearance in the prognosis of acute renal failure. *Renal Failure* **22** (5), 581–589.

Janson, P. A. *et al.* (1980). Treatment of the bleeding tendency in uremia with cryoprecipitate. *New England Journal of Medicine* **303** (23), 1318–1322.

Jochimsen, F. *et al.* (1990). Impairment of renal function in medical intensive care: predictability of acute renal failure. *Critical Care Medicine* **18** (5), 480–485.

Jorres, A. *et al.* (1999). Haemodialysis-membrane biocompatibility and mortality of patients with dialysis-dependent acute renal failure: a prospective randomised multicentre trial. International Multicentre Study Group. *Lancet* **354** (9187), 1337–1341.

Jubelirer, S. J. (1985). Hemostatic abnormalities in renal disease. *American Journal of Kidney Diseases* **5** (5), 219–225.

Juhl, A. and Jorgensen, F. (1987). DDAVP and life-threatening diffuse gastric bleeding in uraemia. Case report. *Acta Chirurgica Scandinavica* **153** (1), 75–77.

Kahlmeter, G. and Dahlager, J. I. (1984). Aminoglycoside toxicity—a review of clinical studies published between 1975 and 1982. *The Journal of Antimicrobial Chemotherapy* **13** (Suppl. A), 9–22.

Kaloyanides, G. J. (1994). Antibiotic-related nephrotoxicity. *Nephrology, Dialysis, Transplantation* **9** (Suppl. 4), 130–134.

Kawashima, A. *et al.* (2000). CT evaluation of renovascular disease. *Radiographics* **20** (5), 1321–1340.

Kellum, J. A. and Decker, J. M. (2001). Use of dopamine in acute renal failure: a meta-analysis. *Critical Care Medicine* **29** (8), 1526–1531.

Khan, I. H. *et al.* (1997). Acute renal failure: factors influencing nephrology referral and outcome. *Quarterly Journal of Medicine* **90**, 781–785.

Kierdorf, H. and Sieberth, H. G. (1995). Continuous treatment modalities in acute renal failure. *Nephrology, Dialysis, Transplantation* **10** (11), 2001–2008.

Kjellstrand, C. M. *et al.* (1981). Time of death, recovery of renal function, development of chronic renal failure and need for chronic hemodialysis in patients with acute tubular necrosis. *Transactions—American Society for Artificial Internal Organs* **27**, 45–50.

Kleinknecht, D. *et al.* (1971). Factors influencing immediate prognosis in acute renal failure, with special reference to prophylactic hemodialysis. *Advances in Nephrology from the Necker Hospital* **1**, 207–230.

Kleinknecht, D. *et al.* (1976). Furosemide in acute oliguric renal failure. A controlled trial. *Nephron* **17** (1), 51–58.

Lake, E. W. and Humes, H. D. (1994). Acute renal failure: directed therapy to enhance renal tubular regeneration. *Seminars in Nephrology* **14** (1), 83–97.

Lassnigg, A. *et al.* (2000). Lack of renoprotective effects of dopamine and furosemide during cardiac surgery. *Journal of the American Society of Nephrology* **11** (1), 97–104.

Lee, H. Y. and Kim, C. H. (2001). Acute oliguric renal failure associated with angiotensin II receptor antagonists. *The American Journal of Medicine* **111** (2), 162–163.

Lens, X. M. *et al.* (1989). Treatment of hyperkalaemia in renal failure: salbutamol v. insulin. *Nephrology, Dialysis, Transplantation* **4** (3), 228–232.

Levinsky, N. G. (1966). Management of emergencies. VI. Hyperkalemia. *New England Journal of Medicine* **274** (19), 1076–1077.

Li, S. C. *et al.* (1989). Prospective audit of aminoglycoside usage in a general hospital with assessments of clinical processes and adverse clinical outcomes. *The Medical Journal of Australia* **151** (4), 224–232.

Liano, F. *et al.* (1994). Use of urinary parameters in the diagnosis of total acute renal artery occlusion. *Nephron* **66** (2), 170–175.

Lieberthal, W. (1997). Biology of acute renal failure: therapeutic implications. *Kidney International* **52** (4), 1102–1115.

Lin, J. L. *et al.* (1994). Outcomes of severe hyperkalemia in cardiopulmonary resuscitation with concomitant hemodialysis. *Intensive Care Medicine* **20** (4), 287–290.

Lin, S. L. *et al.* (1995). Mannitol-induced acute renal failure. *Nephrology, Dialysis, Transplantation* **10** (1), 120–122.

Liu, Y. K. *et al.* (1984). Treatment of uraemic bleeding with conjugated oestrogen. *Lancet* **2** (8408), 887–890.

Livio, M. *et al.* (1986). Conjugated estrogens for the management of bleeding associated with renal failure. *New England Journal of Medicine* **315** (12), 731–735.

Llach, F. *et al.* (1981). The pathophysiology of altered calcium metabolism in rhabdomyolysis-induced acute renal failure. Interactions of parathyroid hormone, 25-hydroxycholecalciferol, and 1,25-dihydroxycholecalciferol. *New England Journal of Medicine* **305** (3), 117–123.

Lokhandwala, M. F. and Amenta, F. (1991). Anatomical distribution and function of dopamine receptors in the kidney. *The FASEB Journal* **5** (15), 3023–3030.

Louca, G. *et al.* (1999). MR urography in the diagnosis of urinary tract obstruction. *European Urology* **35** (2), 102–108.

Lumlertgul, D. *et al.* (1989). Beneficial effect of intrarenal verapamil in human acute renal failure. *Renal Failure* **11** (4), 201–208.

Lumlertgul, D. *et al.* (1991). Intrarenal infusion of gallopamil in acute renal failure. A preliminary report. *Drugs* **42** (Suppl. 1), 44–50.

Maillet, P. J. *et al.* (1986). Nondilated obstructive acute renal failure: diagnostic procedures and therapeutic management. *Radiology* **160** (3), 659–662.

Mannucci, P. M. *et al.* (1983). Deamino-8-D-arginine vasopressin shortens the bleeding time in uremia. *New England Journal of Medicine* **308** (1), 8–12.

Marik, P. E. and Iglesias, J. (1999). Low-dose dopamine does not prevent acute renal failure in patients with septic shock and oliguria. NORASEPT II Study Investigators. *The American Journal of Medicine* **107** (4), 387–390.

Mason, N. A. (1990). Angiotensin-converting enzyme inhibitors and renal function. *DICP: The Annals of Pharmacotherapy* **24** (5), 496–505.

Mault, J. R. *et al.* (1983). Starvation: a major contribution to mortality in acute renal failure? *Transactions—American Society for Artificial Internal Organs* **29**, 390–395.

Mehta, R. L. *et al.* (2001). A randomized clinical trial of continuous versus intermittent dialysis for acute renal failure. *Kidney International* **60** (3), 1154–1163.

Meyer, M. *et al.* (1997). Urodilatin (INN : ularitide) as a new drug for the therapy of acute renal failure following cardiac surgery. *Clinical and Experimental Pharmacology and Physiology* **24** (5), 374–376.

Milligan, S. L. *et al.* (1978). Intra-abdominal infection and acute renal failure. *Archives of Surgery* **113** (4), 467–472.

Molitoris, B. A. (1997). Cell biology of aminoglycoside nephrotoxicity: newer aspects. *Current Opinion in Nephrology and Hypertension* **6** (4), 384–388.

Montoliu, J. *et al.* (1987). Potassium-lowering effect of albuterol for hyperkalemia in renal failure. *Archives of Internal Medicine* **147** (4), 713–717.

Moore, R. D. (1983). Effects of insulin upon ion transport. *Biochimical Biophysica Acta* **737** (1), 1–49.

Moran, S. M. and Myers, B. D. (1985). Pathophysiology of protracted acute renal failure in man. *The Journal of Clinical Investigation* **76** (4), 1440–1448.

Mulla, H. *et al.* (2001). Plasma aluminum levels during sucralfate prophylaxis for stress ulceration in critically ill patients on continuous venovenous hemofiltration: a randomized, controlled trial. *Critical Care Medicine* **29** (2), 267–271.

Myers, B. D. and Moran, S. M. (1986). Hemodynamically mediated acute renal failure. *New England Journal of Medicine* **314** (2), 97–105.

Myers, B. D. *et al.* (1982). Glomerular and tubular function in non-oliguric acute renal failure. *The American Journal of Medicine* **72** (4), 642–649.

Myles, P. S. *et al.* (1993). Effect of 'renal-dose' dopamine on renal function following cardiac surgery. *Anaesthesia and Intensive Care* **21** (1), 56–61.

Naumann, M. *et al.* (1994). Hyperkalaemia mimicking acute Guillain–Barre syndrome. *Journal of Neurology, Neurosurgery, and Psychiatry* **57** (11), 1436–1437.

Neri, E. *et al.* (2000). MR virtual endoscopy of the upper urinary tract. *American Journal of Roentgenology* **175** (6), 1697–1702.

Neumayer, H. H. *et al.* (1989). Prevention of radiocontrast-media-induced nephrotoxicity by the calcium channel blocker nitrendipine: a prospective randomised clinical trial. *Nephrology, Dialysis, Transplantation* **4** (12), 1030–1036.

Noble, J. S. *et al.* (2001). Renal and respiratory failure in Scottish ICUs. *Anaesthesia* **56** (2), 124–129.

Oster, J. R. *et al.* (1995). Heparin-induced aldosterone suppression and hyperkalemia. *The American Journal of Medicine* **98** (6), 575–586.

Parfrey, P. S. *et al.* (1989). Contrast material-induced renal failure in patients with diabetes mellitus, renal insufficiency, or both. A prospective controlled study. *New England Journal of Medicine* **320** (3), 143–149.

Parks, R. W. *et al.* (1994). Prospective study of postoperative renal function in obstructive jaundice and the effect of perioperative dopamine. *The British Journal of Surgery* **81** (3), 437–439.

Perazella, M. A. (2000). Trimethoprim-induced hyperkalaemia: clinical data, mechanism, prevention and management. *Drug Safety* **22** (3), 227–236.

Petit, P. *et al.* (1992). Computed tomographic detection of skeletal muscle calcifications in rhabdomyolysis. *Canadian Association of Radiologists Journal* **43** (6), 443–446.

Pilmore, H. L. *et al.* (1995). Acute bilateral renal artery occlusion: successful revascularization with streptokinase. *American Journal of Nephrology* **15** (1), 90–91.

Pittiruti, M. *et al.* (2000). Which is the easiest and safest technique for central venous access? A retrospective survey of more than 5400 cases. *The Journal of Vascular Access* **1**, 100–107.

Pontremoli, R. *et al.* (1990). Acute renal failure due to acute bilateral renal artery thrombosis: successful surgical revascularization after prolonged anuria. *Nephron* **56** (3), 322–324.

Porter, G. A. and Bennett, W. M. (1981). Nephrotoxic acute renal failure due to common drugs. *The American Journal of Physiology* **241** (1), F1–F8.

Rahman, S. N. *et al.* (1994). Effects of atrial natriuretic peptide in clinical acute renal failure. *Kidney International* **45** (6), 1731–1738.

Ramsay, A. G. *et al.* (1983). Renal functional recovery 47 days after renal artery occlusion. *American Journal of Nephrology* **3** (6), 325–328.

Rankin, G. O. and Sutherland, C. H. (1989). Nephrotoxicity of aminoglycosides and cephalosporins in combination. *Adverse Drug Reactions and Acute Poisoning Reviews* **8**, 73–88.

Rasmussen, H. H. and Ibels, L. S. (1982). Acute renal failure. Multivariate analysis of causes and risk factors. *The American Journal of Medicine* **73** (2), 211–218.

Ribush, N. and Morgan, T. (1972). Tetracyclines and renal failure. *Medical Journal of Australia* **1**, 53–55.

Roche, Z. *et al.* (1993). Reversible acute renal failure as an atypical presentation of ischemic nephropathy. *American Journal of Kidney Diseases* **22** (5), 662–667.

Rodgers, R. P. and Levin, J. (1990). A critical reappraisal of the bleeding time. *Seminars in Thrombosis and Hemostases* **16** (1), 1–20.

Ron, D. *et al.* (1984). Prevention of acute renal failure in traumatic rhabdomyolysis. *Archives of Internal Medicine* **144** (2), 277–280.

Ronco, C. *et al.* (2000). Effects of different doses in continuous veno-venous haemofiltration on outcomes of acute renal failure: a prospective randomised trial. *Lancet* **356** (9223), 26–30.

Sacks, S. H. *et al.* (1989). Late renal failure due to prostatic outflow obstruction: a preventable disease. *British Medical Journal* **298** (6667), 156–159.

Salam, T. A. *et al.* (1993). Local infusion of fibrinolytic agents for acute renal artery thromboembolism: report of ten cases. *Annals of Vascular Surgery* **7** (1), 21–26.

Salem, M. M. *et al.* (1991). Extrarenal potassium tolerance in chronic renal failure: implications for the treatment of acute hyperkalemia. *American Journal of Kidney Diseases* **18** (4), 421–440.

Schepkens, H. *et al.* (2001). Life-threatening hyperkalemia during combined therapy with angiotensin-converting enzyme inhibitors and spironolactone: an analysis of 25 cases. *American Journal of Medicine* **110** (6), 438–441.

Schiffl, H. *et al.* (1994). Biocompatible membranes in acute renal failure: prospective case-controlled study. *Lancet* **344** (8922), 570–572.

Schiffl, H. *et al.* (2002). Daily hemodialysis and the outcome of acute renal failure. *New England Journal of Medicine* **346** (5), 305–310.

Schwab, S. J. *et al.* (1989). Contrast nephrotoxicity: a randomized controlled trial of a nonionic and an ionic radiographic contrast agent. *New England Journal of Medicine* **320** (3), 149–153.

Shapiro, M. D. and Kelleher, S. P. (1984). Intranasal deamino-8-D-arginine vasopressin shortens the bleeding time in uremia. *The American Journal of Nephrology* **4** (4), 260–261.

Shilliday, I. and Allison, M. E. (1994). Diuretics in acute renal failure. *Renal Failure* **16** (1), 3–17.

Shilliday, I. R. *et al.* (1997). Loop diuretics in the management of acute renal failure: a prospective, double-blind, placebo-controlled, randomized study. *Nephrology, Dialysis, Transplantation* **12** (12), 2592–2596.

Shrimpton, S. B. *et al.* (1993). Audit of prescription and assay of aminoglycosides in a UK teaching hospital. *The Journal of Antimicrobial Chemotherapy* **31** (4), 599–606.

Simon, B. C. (1988). Pseudomyocardial infarction and hyperkalemia: a case report and subject review. *The Journal of Emergency Medicine* **6** (6), 511–515.

Smith, C. R. *et al.* (1986). Studies of risk factors for aminoglycoside nephrotoxicity. *American Journal of Kidney Diseases* **8** (5), 308–313.

Solez, K. and Racusen, L. C. (2001). Role of the renal biopsy in acute renal failure. *Contributions to Nephrology* **132**, 68–75.

Solez, K. *et al.* (1979). The morphology of 'acute tubular necrosis' in man: analysis of 57 renal biopsies and a comparison with the glycerol model. *Medicine (Baltimore)* **58** (5), 362–376.

Solez, K. *et al.* (1994). New approaches to renal biopsy assessment in acute renal failure: extrapolation from renal transplantation. *Kidney International Supplement* **44**, S65–S69.

Solomon, R. *et al.* (1994). Effects of saline, mannitol, and furosemide to prevent acute decreases in renal function induced by radiocontrast agents. *New England Journal of Medicine* **331** (21), 1416–1420.

Spital, A. *et al.* (1988). Nondilated obstructive uropathy. *Urology* **31** (6), 478–482.

Sponsel, H. and Conger, J. D. (1995). Is parenteral nutrition therapy of value in acute renal failure patients? *American Journal of Kidney Diseases* **25** (1), 96–102.

Spurney, R. F. *et al.* (1991). Acute renal failure in critically ill patients: prognosis for recovery of kidney function after prolonged dialysis support. *Critical Care Medicine* **19** (1), 8–11.

Steiner, R. W. *et al.* (1979). Bleeding time in uremia: a useful test to assess clinical bleeding. *American Journal of Hematology* **7** (2), 107–117.

Suki, W. N. (1989). Renal hemodynamic consequences of angiotensin-converting enzyme inhibition in congestive heart failure. *Archives of Internal Medicine* **149**, 669–673.

Surawicz, B. (1967). Relationship between electrocardiogram and electrolytes. *American Heart Journal* **73** (6), 814–834.

Takeda, M. *et al.* (1993). Successful fibrinolytic therapy using tissue plasminogen activator in acute renal failure due to acute thrombosis of bilateral renal arteries. *Urological Internationalis* **51** (3), 177–180.

Tang, A. T. *et al.* (1999). The effect of 'renal-dose' dopamine on renal tubular function following cardiac surgery: assessed by measuring retinol binding protein (RBP). *European Journal of Cardio-thoracic Surgery* **15** (5), 717–721; discussion 721–722.

Thurau, K. and Boylan, J. W. (1976). Acute renal success. The unexpected logic of oliguria in acute renal failure. *The American Journal of Medicine* **61** (3), 308–315.

Tryba, M. (1991). Prophylaxis of stress ulcer bleeding. A meta-analysis. *Journal of Clinical Gastroenterology* **13** (Suppl. 2), S44–S55.

Turney, J. H. *et al.* (1990). The evolution of acute renal failure, 1956–1988. *The Quarterly Journal of Medicine* **74** (273), 83–104.

Urban, B. A. *et al.* (2001). Three-dimensional volume-rendered CT angiography of the renal arteries and veins: normal anatomy, variants, and clinical applications. *Radiographics* **21** (2), 373–386; questionnaire 549–555.

Vanholder, R. *et al.* (2000). The role of dialyzer biocompatibility in acute renal failure. *Blood Purification* **18** (1), 1–12.

Varella, L. and Utermohlen, V. (1993). Nutritional support for the patient with renal failure. *Critical Care Nursing Clinics of North America* **5** (1), 79–96.

Vigano, G. *et al.* (1988). Dose–effect and pharmacokinetics of estrogens given to correct bleeding time in uremia. *Kidney International* **34** (6), 853–858.

Vosshenrich, R. and Fischer, U. (2002). Contrast-enhanced MR angiography of abdominal vessels: is there still a role for angiography? *European Radiology* **12** (1), 218–230.

Weisberg, L. S. *et al.* (1993). Dopamine and renal blood flow in radiocontrast-induced nephropathy in humans. *Renal Failure* **15** (1), 61–68.

Wiecek, A. *et al.* (1994). Role of infection in the genesis of acute renal failure. *Nephrology, Dialysis, Transplantation* **9** (Suppl. 4), 40–44.

Williams, R. D. *et al.* (1960). The effect of hypotension in obstructive jaundice. *Archives of Surgery* **81**, 335–340.

Witten, D. M. *et al. Emmetts Clinical Urography*. Philadelphia: Saunders, 1997.

Wong, F. and Blendis, L. (2001). New challenge of hepatorenal syndrome: prevention and treatment. *Hepatology* **34** (6), 1242–1251.

Wrenn, K. D. *et al.* (1991). The ability of physicians to predict hyperkalemia from the ECG. *Annals of Emergency Medicine* **20** (11), 1229–1232.

10.4 Renal replacement methods in acute renal failure

Vincenzo D'Intini, Rinaldo Bellomo, and Claudio Ronco

Acute renal failure—the changing pattern

There has been a significant change in the spectrum of severe acute renal failure (ARF) such that it is no longer mostly a single organ phenomenon but rather a complex multisystem clinical problem. Isolated severe ARF in Western hospitals is now less common, with 80 per cent of cases now associated with multiple organ failure (MOF). The significance of this epidemiological shift is that, despite great advances in renal replacement technique, mortality from ARF, when part of MOF, remains over 50 per cent (Brivet *et al.* 1996). The changing nature of ARF requires a new approach using the new advanced technology. Historically, management of ARF has been the responsibility of nephrologists, but the high incidence of ARF-MOF with its associated high mortality means that most patients require the combined expertise of intensive care and nephrology. Currently, a universal definition for ARF is yet to be agreed (Bellomo *et al.* 2001). Knochel in 1983 defined ARF as, 'a syndrome characterized by a sudden decrease in renal function'. Such a vague definition is inappropriate for clinical trials, so most researchers create their own, explaining the existence of over 30 definitions of ARF in the literature. Recently, an international task force has addressed this and other issues in ARF and its management. The Acute Dialysis Quality Initiative (ADQI) aims at establishing evidence based guidelines, set consensus recommendations for best practice, help standardize care, and identify questions for future research (Ronco *et al.* 2002).

Blood purification technologies have developed and improved rapidly over the last decades providing more options for the treatment of renal failure. Clinicians can provide therapies tailored to time constraints (intermittent, continuous, or extended intermittent), haemodynamic, and metabolic requirements and aimed at molecules of variable molecular weight. The renal replacement therapies (RRTs) available are listed in Table 1. The ideal RRT should mimic the functions and physiological mechanisms of the native organ, ensuring qualitative and quantitative blood purification, be free of complications, have good clinical tolerance and restore and maintain homeostasis, thus favouring organ recovery. Table 2 describes the technical and clinical requirements of an ideal RRT.

Initiation and indications for substitutive therapy

There is a wide variation in clinical practice in the timing for the commencement of RRT. At present, no consensus guidelines are available. A fixed rule for RRT initiation is inappropriate and potentially harmful to the patient. The complex nature of the severe ARF syndrome requires careful individual assessment with an individualized management plan. There are two levels of indications for starting RRT: they are divided into those that are urgent, which if not corrected immediately, carry a high risk of immediate death and those which are less urgent which may later, according to the clinical situation, become urgent. Bellomo *et al.* (1998) proposed a set of criteria for the initiation of RRT (Table 3).

The urgent indications include hyperkalaemia especially when associated with electrocardiographic abnormalities, diuretic resistant pulmonary oedema, severe metabolic acidosis, and encephalopathy.

Recent evidence supports the belief that commencing RRT early maybe prudent (Gettings *et al.* 1999; al-Khafaji *et al.* 2001). However, before initiating any RRT, one must consider the possibility that it may aggravate the situation and complicate other aspects of management.

Choice of replacement therapy

The Korean war provided the first large-scale clinical opportunity for artificial renal support to be applied and studied (Teschan *et al.* 1960). Since that time, extracorporeal therapies have undergone enormous technical improvement. There are now many available options divided into three groups:

(1) peritoneal dialysis (PD);

(2) intermittent therapies; and

(3) continuous therapies.

These groups differ in their clinical tolerability, method of delivery and efficiency. There is wide variability worldwide in the methods used for the treatment of ARF. The reasons for this variation include local practice (nephrologist or intensivist based management), the centre's experience of the various techniques, organization, and health resources. Because there is no consensus on the definition of ARF and no definitive treatment guidelines can be published due to lack of Level I evidence, variation in clinical practice will continue. Technical support and adequate training of personnel is essential for the performance of each substitutive treatment. Some techniques require less investment in terms of equipment and personnel and may therefore be preferred in spite of their limited efficacy. There are also certain clinical situations in which only a particular therapy is indicated, for example, continuous therapies in critically ill subjects with cardiovascular instability. Distinguishing whether ARF is a result of single organ dysfunction or part of MOF is a key factor. These two groups of

Table 1 Summary of renal replacement options available in ARF. Intermittent therapies can be utilized in various schedules depending on the clinical indications

Technique	Diffusion	Convection	Replacement fluid	Dialysis fluid	Back-filtration
Intermittent haemodialysis (IHD)	+++++	+	No	Yes	+
Daily haemodialysis (DHD)	+++++	+	No	Yes	+
Intermittent haemofiltration (HF)		+++++	Yes		
Intermittent haemodiafiltration (HDF)	+++	+++	Yes	Yes	+
Intermittent high flux dialysis (HFD)	++++	++	No	Yes	+++++
Sustained low efficiency dialysis (SLED)	+++	+	No	Yes	+
Continuous venovenous haemofiltration (CVVH)		+++++	Yes		
Continuous venovenous haemodialysis (CVVHD)	+++++	+	No	Yes	
Continuous venovenous haemodiafiltration (CVVHDF)	+++	+++	Yes	Yes	
Continuous venovenous high flux dialysis (CVVHFD)	++++	++	No	Yes	+++++
Intermittent ultrafiltration (UF)		+++++	No		
Slow continuous ultrafiltration (SCUF)		+++++	No		
Slow continuous ultrafiltration with dialysate (SCUF-D)	++	+++	No	Yes	
High volume haemofiltration (HVHF)		+++++	Yes ++++		
Coupled plasmafiltration-adsorption (CPFA)[a]	[a]	[a]	[a]	[a]	[a]

[a] This treatment can be performed in conjunction with CVVH, CVVHD, or CVVHDF.

Table 2 Technical and clinical requirements for an optimal renal replacement therapy in acute renal failure

Rapid and easy institution with simple treatment monitoring
Efficiency and efficacy which satisfies therapy prescription
Volume control without causing cardiovascular instability
Allows fluid administration/nutrition maintaining euvolaemia
Maintains stable acid–base balance
High biocompatibility with minimal interaction with blood
Clinical tolerance
No deleterious effects on renal function or duration of acute renal failure
Easy and predictable adjustment of drug dosing
Inexpensive

Table 3 Proposed indications for the initiation of renal replacement therapy

Anuria or oliguria (urine output < 200 ml/12 h)
Hyperkalaemia (K > 6.5 mmol/l)
Severe acidaemia (pH > 7.1)
Azotaemia (urea > 30 mmol/l)
Clinically significant organ oedema (particularly lung)
Uraemic encephalopathy
Uraemic pericarditis
Uraemic neuropathy/myopathy
Severe dysnatraemia ([Na] > 160 or < 115 mmol/l)
Hyperthermia
Drug overdose with a dialysable toxin

One criteria can be an indication for the initiation of RRT. Two or more criteria make RRT mandatory. Multiple criteria are a reason for early initiation of RRT.

subjects differ substantially and should be treated differently. ARF without MOF is less complex, can be managed outside the critical care unit and the same RRT techniques used for the treatment of chronic renal failure can be applied. On the other hand, ARF associated with MOF is a more complex condition and requires more flexible RRT.

Institution and monitoring

Any treatment should be easy to apply, rapid to institute, and simple to monitor. Both complex haemodialysis (HD) machines and various PD techniques require well-trained nurses. Similarly, continuous renal replacement therapy (CRRT) must be carried out by experienced personnel to guarantee its safety. The choice of the treatment will therefore depend on the clinical practice and resources of a given department than on precise clinical indication. A proficient and accountable team, experienced in various dialytic modalities with a quality assurance education program would be ideal. If this is not possible, the best combination of simple and easy treatment schedules, which are functional and efficient with no significant increases in personnel demand or labour intensity must suffice.

Efficiency and efficacy

ARF results in the accumulation of toxic substances. Pathogenetic molecules such as advanced glycation endproducts (AGEs), advanced lipid oxygenation compounds (ALEs), carbonyl and oxidative stress (which may produce malnutrition), β-2-microglobulin, and inflammatory mediators (C-reactive protein, CRP; cytokines; tumour necrosis factor, TNF) are now thought to be harmful. Despite the discovery of newer toxins, the original surrogate marker for blood purification efficiency used since the dawn of dialysis is still being used. RRT efficiency is measured by the quantitative removal of urea. While the amount of urea to be removed can be easily calculated from a daily urea nitrogen balance record (Borah *et al.* 1978), for other solutes (creatinine, uric acid, phosphate, chemically active mediators, β-2-microglobulin etc.) the 'adequate' amount to be removed has not yet been defined. Because of this gross deficiency, a treatment is considered adequate when it guarantees a daily urea clearance in litres greater or equal to the volume of total body water (TBW) and a daily clearance of vitamin B_{12} (chosen as a molecular marker for larger solutes) in litres more than or equal to 60 per cent of TBW. TBW can be calculated from anthropometric tables, or simply as 60 per cent of body weight. In practice:

$$\text{Efficiency} = \text{Urea } Kt/V \geq 1 \qquad \text{Efficacy} = \text{Vitamin B}_{12}\ Kt/V \geq 0.6$$

where K = clearance in ml/min, t = time of treatment in minutes, and V = volume in litres of TBW (Ronco *et al.* 1988; Gotch *et al.* 1989). These parameters guarantee a satisfactory blood purification for urea and other waste products in the majority of patients, even in presence of a severe catabolic state (Ronco *et al.* 1985a,b). While efficiency depends on the operational parameters of the treatment, efficacy is mostly related to the type of treatment and to the membrane utilized.

Maintenance of euvolaemia

Optimizing volume status provides many benefits to the clinical state of the patient by avoiding organ and tissue oedema. Defining the ideal volume status can, however, be difficult. Using both clinical assessment and invasive measurements, the maintenance of an ideal volume state, in combination with adequate perfusion, helps avoid respiratory and cardiovascular complications. This may also influence the outcome of the syndrome and recovery of renal function. Continuous therapies are generally superior at controlling volume status.

Clinical tolerance and haemodynamic response

The RRT modality and prescription should be well tolerated and not induce complications. This may be particularly difficult in critically ill subjects with MOF in which there is altered regulation of systemic vascular resistance and where vascular tone acts independent of intravascular volume. Continuous therapies are much better tolerated than intermittent treatments in regard to haemodynamics and volume control (Fig. 1). With PD, the intra-abdominal volume may interfere with ventilation by increasing intra-abdominal pressure.

Correction of electrolyte and acid–base disturbances

Continuous therapies achieve and maintain better control of electrolyte and acid–base balance compared to intermittent therapies as there is greater access to the various body pools (Uchino *et al.* 2001). For the correction of acid–base imbalance, bicarbonate is the most physiologic buffer but other buffers such as acetate or lactate can be used.

Biocompatibility

The treatment should cause the least interaction of the materials with blood. To improve the biocompatibility of the system, pyrogen-free dialysate and sterile replacement solutions are strongly recommended. The membrane for extracorporeal treatments may be important. Cellulosic membranes can stimulate monocyte activation with release

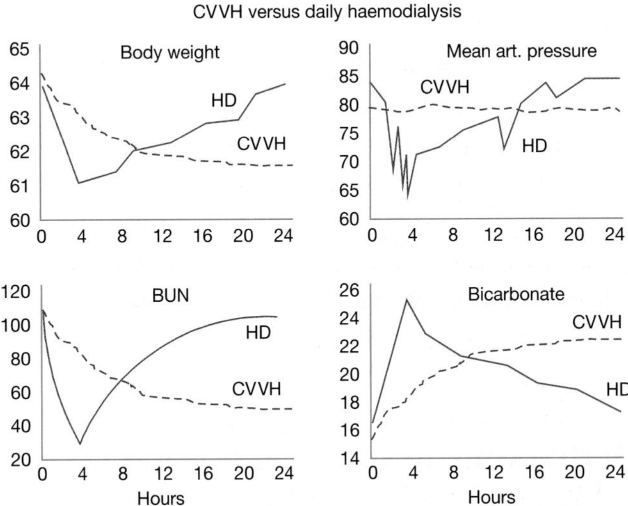

Fig. 1 Comparisons of MAP, body weight, blood urea nitrogen (BUN), and bicarbonate control with continuous and intermittent therapies demonstrating smoother and less varied control of all parameters with continuous treatment.

of cytokines and chemical mediators possibly causing a delay in the recovery from acute tubular injury (Hakim 1994). Synthetic membranes have the advantage of producing little or no inflammatory effects and may reduce the plasma concentration of several inflammatory mediators by filtration/adsorption (De Vriese *et al.* 1999).

Low rate of complications and cost effectiveness

The treatment must be safe and free of major technical and clinical complications. The costs should be appropriate to the results achieved and the treatment should not result in significantly greater workloads both for doctors and nursing staff.

Renal replacement therapies in acute renal failure

The term dialysis is derived from the Greek term 'δια−λυω', which when literally translated means to 'pass across'. The mechanisms involved in renal replacement therapies are founded upon the principle of water and solute transport whereby the composition of a solution is altered by exposing it to a second solution through a semipermeable membrane. Water and low molecular weight molecules can pass through the membrane pores while larger molecules are deterred depending on the membrane pore size.

There are a wide range of artificial membranes and techniques available for use for renal replacement therapy such that treatments can be tailored to individual patient needs. The general principles of different techniques are summarized in Fig. 2.

The membranes used can be divided into cellulose-based or synthetic (non-cellulose) types: cellulosic-hydrophilic (cuprophan, hemophan, cellulose acetate) and synthetic-hydrophobic (polysulfone, polyamide, polyacrylonitrile, AN69S). Cellulose-based membranes are generally considered low flux membranes, that is, membranes with a permeability coefficient to water, $K_m < 10$ (ml/h) × (mmHg/m^2). They are extremely thin (wall thickness of 5–15 μm), have a symmetric structure with uniform porosity, and are essentially hydrophilic. Synthetic membranes are high flux membranes with a $K_m > 30$ (ml/h) × (mmHg/m^2). Wall thickness ranges between 40 and 100 μm with an asymmetric structure composed of an inner skin layer and a surrounding sponge layer. They have larger pores and are hydrophobic. These membranes have high sieving coefficients for solutes of a wide range of molecular weights and are therefore more suitable for convective treatments. Because of these properties, high filtration rates are achieved mainly by convection.

In PD, the peritoneal mesothelium is used as a living membrane to separate the dialysis solution infused into the peritoneal cavity from the blood of the peritoneal microcirculation.

Mechanisms of solute and water transport across semipermeable membranes

Solutes that can pass through membrane pores are transported by two different mechanisms: diffusion and ultrafiltration (UF) (convection).

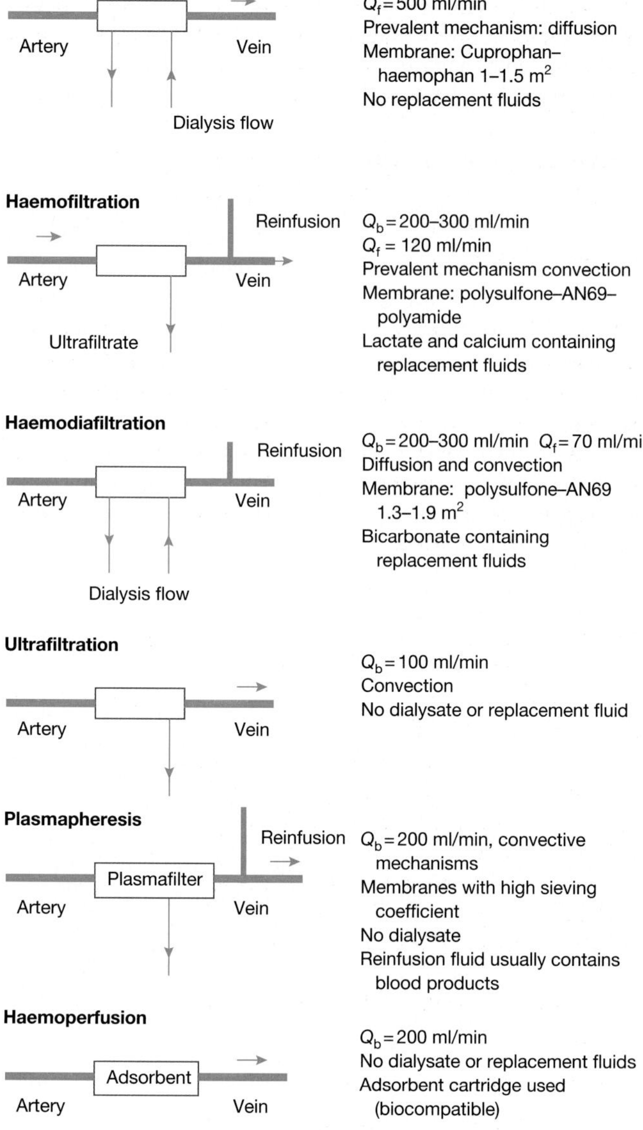

Fig. 2 Different techniques of intermittent extracorporeal therapies. Q_b, arterial blood flow; Q_f, dialysate blood flow.

Diffusion

This term defines the movement of solute with a statistical tendency to reach the same concentration of solute in the available distribution space on each side of the membrane. The practical result is a passage of molecules from the more concentrated compartment into the less concentrated compartment. Solute transport is governed by the following formula:

$$J_d = DTA(\delta c/\delta x)$$

where J is the solute flux, D the diffusion coefficient, T the temperature of the solution, A the surface area of the membrane, δc the concentration gradient between the two compartments, and δx the thickness of the membrane.

In dialysis, blood and dialysate are separated by a membrane. Bidirectional diffusive transport of molecules occurs in response to a concentration gradient. Clearances can be calculated in dialysis from the formulas

$$K = [(Q_{bi} \times C_{bi}) - (Q_{bo} \times C_{bo})]/C_{bi} \quad \text{or} \quad (Q_{do} \times C_{do})/C_{bi}$$

where Q_{bi} and Q_{bo} = inlet and outlet blood flows; C_{bi} and C_{bo} = inlet and outlet blood concentrations; Q_{do} = dialysate effluent flow; C_{do} = solute concentration in the effluent dialysate (leaving the dialyser or the peritoneal cavity).

Convection (ultrafiltration)

This occurs when water is driven either by a hydrostatic or osmotic force across a semipermeable membrane carrying solutes which can pass through uninhibited. This is also referred to as 'solvent drag'. The water pushed through the membrane is accompanied by solutes at similar concentrations to the original solution. Larger molecules are held back. Filtration occurs in response to a transmembrane pressure gradient according to the formula

$$Q_f = K_m \times \text{TMP} = K_m(P_b - P_{uf} - \pi)$$

where K_m is the permeability coefficient of the membrane, TMP the transmembrane pressure, P_b the hydrostatic pressure of blood, P_{uf} the hydrostatic pressure in the ultrafiltrate compartment, and π the oncotic pressure of blood.

Once UF occurs, solutes are carried on the other side of the membrane at various rates according to their membrane rejection coefficient (σ) with σ being close to 1 for albumin and near 0 for small solutes like urea. Assuming a relation of $S = 1 - \sigma$, we can derive that the sieving coefficient for a solute (S), will be inversely correlated with the membrane rejection coefficient. In clinical practice, the sieving coefficient is measured from the ratio between the concentration of solute in the ultrafiltrate and its concentration in plasma water. In convective treatments therefore, the transport (J_c) of solute x will be governed by the formula

$$J_c = \text{UF } [x]\text{UF}$$

where UF is the volume of ultrafiltrate and $[x]$UF is the concentration in the ultrafiltrate of the solute x. From this, we may derive that clearance in convective treatments is

$$K = Q_f[x]\text{UF}/[x]P_w$$

where Q_f is the UF rate and $[x]\text{UF}/[x]P_w$ is the ratio of the solute concentrations in the ultrafiltrate and plasma water or the sieving coefficient S. From this formula, we may observe that when the sieving coefficient is 1, clearance equals the UF rate.

Despite these distinctions, we should point out that diffusion and convection often act simultaneously and it is almost impossible to distinguish between these transport mechanisms. Thus, the term HD may not accurately describe a mode of treatment and a more suitable term would be 'haemodiafiltration' (HDF) (if replacement solution is needed) or 'high flux dialysis' (HFD) (if a filtration–back-filtration mechanism is present and no replacement fluid is required).

Osmosis

This mechanism operates in PD. Glucose is utilized as the osmotic agent in the PD solution. The low rate of glucose absorption from the peritoneal cavity enables the dialysis solution to have the osmotic effect to permit water transport. In this particular modality, water movement proportional to the osmotic power of the solution is achieved and the patient's hydration can be controlled. In PD however, the net fluid removal takes into account other processes such as transcapillary UF and lymphatic reabsorption.

Treatment nomenclature

The need to standardize definitions and procedures has spurred interest in a fixed nomenclature. This was created in 1996 (Bellomo *et al.* 1996) and subsequently endorsed by ADQI in 2000. The basic concepts are schematically shown in Fig. 1.

Haemodialysis

This term defines a mainly diffusive treatment in which blood and dialysate are circulated in counter-current mode, and a low permeable cellulose-based membrane is usually employed. UF rate is programmed approximately to the scheduled weight loss. This treatment can be performed intermittently (3–8 h three times per week), daily (2–4 h), or continuously. When the treatment is performed continuously, the circuit can be utilized both in arteriovenous or venovenous haemodialysis mode (CAVHD-CVVHD, respectively).

Haemofiltration

This term defines an exclusively convective treatment performed with highly permeable membranes. The ultrafiltrate produced is replaced completely or in part by a sterile solution. Any weight loss results from the difference between UF and reinfusion rates (no dialysis fluid is used). This treatment can be performed intermittently (30 l/session three times per week), daily, or continuously in venovenous mode (CVVH).

Haemodiafiltration

This is a combined treatment in which diffusion and convection are combined utilizing a highly permeable membrane. Blood and dialysate are circulated as in HD but typically a UF in excess of the scheduled weight loss is produced. To achieve fluid balance, sterile solution is reinfused to the patient at an appropriate rate. This treatment can be performed intermittently (3–5 h and 15 l exchanges/session three times per week), daily (3 h with 9 l exchanges), or continuously (CVVHDF).

High flux dialysis

This modality requires highly permeable membranes in conjunction with a UF control system. Blood and dialysate are circulated as in HD, but due to the high permeability coefficient of the membrane, excessive UF beyond the desired level patient weight loss would occur. Therefore, a positive pressure is applied to the dialysate compartment to reduce the amount of UF and to avoid the need of replacement solution. Due to the peculiar structure of hollow fibre dialysers, filtration takes place in the proximal part of the filter, while back filtration occurs in the distal part. Diffusion and convection therefore are still combined because the high filtration rate occurring in the proximal part of the dialyser is masked by a back filtration occurring in the distal part. Replacement is not required as it occurs within the filter by the mechanism of back filtration. It is essential therefore that the dialysate solution is sterile and pyrogen free.

Ultrafiltration

This term defines a treatment in which fluid removal is the main target of the therapy. Highly permeable filters are utilized and fluid is removed from the body without replacement. UF can be performed intermittently or daily with variable ultrafiltration rates applied depending on the haemodynamic stability of the subject. In clinical practice, UF has also been used in sequence with HD to improve cardiovascular tolerance. In critically ill patients, it can also be performed continuously at very low filtration rates (1–2 ml/min) with or without the addition of dialysate (slow continuous UF—SCUF or SCUF-D).

Plasmapheresis

This utilizes a particular membrane with a molecular weight cut-off much higher than that of a haemofilter. Whole plasma is filtered and blood is replaced by the infusion of plasma derivatives, fresh frozen plasma, albumin, or other fluids. The treatment is indicated for removing proteins or protein bound solutes that cannot be removed by simple HF.

Haemoperfusion

This term defines a form of treatment in which blood is circulated through a cartridge coated with activated charcoal or carbon to remove solutes by adsorption. Sorbent technology has been used for nearly a century. In the 1970s, they were used to increase the efficiency of dialysis but with only modest improvement. Earlier, sorbents were plagued with bioincompatibility (thrombocytopenia), but later technology utilizing better pore dimensions and biocompatible components has created new interest. The technique is specifically indicated in cases of toxic ARF, poisoning, or intoxication. Unlike HD, haemoperfusion (HP) has the ability to clear protein bound substances since charcoal can compete with plasma proteins for drugs. It is also very effective for lipid soluble substances.

Peritoneal dialysis

PD was once the main method used for the treatment of ARF especially in the paediatric population, but has been superseded by extracorporeal therapies. Plagued by a high incidence of complications and low efficiency, indications for its use are very limited today. PD offers little or no advantages over extracorporeal therapies.

It requires the use of pyrogen free solutions infused into the peritoneal cavity and drained in a series of cycles. Diffusive removal of solutes is achieved by a concentration gradient between blood flowing in the peritoneal capillary network and dialysate. Convective removal of water and solutes is obtained by increasing dialysate osmolality. This represents the major component of peritoneal transmembrane pressure. There are large individual variations in peritoneal membrane characteristics. Intermittent peritoneal dialysis (IPD) consists of a series of rapid exchanges with complete drainage of fluid at the end of each cycle. Continuous equilibration peritoneal dialysis (CPD) utilizes long intraperitoneal dwell times in order to achieve a dialysate/plasma equilibration with reduced fluid usage (Posen *et al.* 1979). Equilibration for urea occurs at about a 4 h dwell time. In tidal peritoneal dialysis (TPD), 1 l of solution is maintained in the peritoneal cavity while rapid one liter exchanges are continuously performed. This schedule reduces the time in which the peritoneal cavity is empty. While short exchanges are indicated for fast transporters to achieve less glucose reabsorption and higher UF rates, long dwell times are indicated in normal to low transporters. A new modality has recently emerged called continuous flow peritoneal dialysis (CFPD) where a double lumen catheter allows to circulate PD fluid continuously and to achieve the highest levels of clearance possible in PD. Such form is still under evaluation and clinical results in acute patients are awaited.

Efficiency

IPD regimes can achieve remarkable clearance and UF values, however, large amounts of fluid are required, so continuous monitoring is mandatory. CPD requires much less dialysis solution, but its efficiency is rather low. TPD offers a compromise although PD machinery is generally required for its performance. The final efficiency is obtained by the product (clearance × time) and it is expressed in litres of clearance per 24 h. In IPD, urea clearances up to 25 l/day can be achieved at an average dialysate flow rate of 5 l/h, while with other PD techniques lower clearances are generally achieved.

Despite its low efficiency in most uncomplicated patients, PD can effectively control urea concentration because of its continuous action guaranteeing stable biochemistry and significant solute extraction. Furthermore, the unique permeability of the peritoneal membrane allows for remarkable clearances of larger molecules other than urea and has the capacity for the removal of peptides of up to 50,000 Da (Scribner 1975).

Clinical indications

PD still provides a useful option in the management of uncomplicated ARF, however, in the critically ill adult patient with a high catabolic rate, adequate control of electrolytes, BUN and fluid cannot be achieved. Paediatric patients are ideal candidates for this therapy.

The obvious requirement of an intact abdomen limits its use since a proportion of patients who develop ARF have had abdominal surgery. Furthermore, critically ill patients often suffer from an ileus which may reduce even further the efficiency of PD. Some unique indications where PD may be considered include toxic ARF to remove the offending agent, in particular, iodinated contrast material. In one study, peritoneal clearance of iodide was reported as high as 12 ml/min and 56 per cent of iodide was removed over a period of 64 h of treatment (Brookes *et al.* 1973). Numerous reports concerning the removal of drugs and poisons with PD have also been published (Berman *et al.* 1964; Winchester *et al.* 1977).

Complications

Complications are numerous and potentially serious and include peritonitis, hyperglycaemia, substantial protein loss, disturbance of respiratory mechanics, and visceral perforation while inserting the catheter.

Intermittent extracorporeal therapies

These techniques require good vascular access and specially trained nurses to carry out the dialysis. A water treatment system including a water softener, which can de-ionize water, a reverse osmosis module and on line ultrafilters are needed to achieve a bacterial and pyrogen free dialysate. The dialysis machine must meet high standards of reliability and safety with an adequate blood module, a precise dialysate preparing module with adequate warming and de-aeration systems, and all parts must have active alarms to avoid accidents. Until recently, this combination was only available in renal units but modern intensive care units are becoming autonomous and able to initiate treatment without the need of nephrological input.

Haemodialysis

This treatment is carried out in a session of 3–5 h with a blood flow of 250–500 ml/min. A low-permeability membrane such as Cuprophan or Hemophan is utilized with an average surface area of 1–1.5 m^2. Dialysate flow is 500 ml/min and the rate of UF can be set as clinically indicated. In continuous modes (CVVHD), the dialysate flow rate is only 10–30 ml/min. HD relies on a mainly diffusive mechanisms and small molecular weight solutes are removed faster than medium- to large-sized molecules.

Haemofiltration

For this technique, treatment time is dependent on the rate of UF and the total amount of fluid to be exchanged. Blood flow is around 300 ml/min and no dialysate is present. A highly permeable membrane is used and solutes are removed by convection. Synthetic membranes like polysulfone provide a sieving capacity of approximately 1 for a wide spectrum of molecular weights. On the other hand, for cellulosic membranes, sieving coefficients significantly decrease even for moderate increases of molecular weight. For this reason, synthetic membranes are used in HF during which high amounts of ultrafiltrate are generated. The ultrafiltrate is completely or partially replaced with sterile substitution fluid and solute concentrations in plasma are essentially normalized. Net fluid balance is the difference between UF and reinfusion. High permeability membranes allow different sized molecules to be removed. The standard treatment duration for a 30 l exchange HF is 3–4 h.

Haemodiafiltration

HDF combines HD and HF techniques. Highly permeable membranes are used allowing clearance of a wide molecular weight range solutes. A total of 10–15 l of ultrafiltrate are produced in each session and substitution fluid is reinfused according to the patient's fluid requirement.

High flux dialysis

This system requires a highly permeable membrane and a precise UF control apparatus. A pressure rise in the dialysate compartment counterbalances the excessive filtration provided by the membrane and creates a typical mechanism of filtration–back-filtration in the dialyser. As a consequence, a certain degree of convection is still maintained in conjunction with diffusion. Replacement solution is not required since the back filtration in the distal part of the dialyser ensures a correct fluid balance. The use of a sterile or ultrapure dialysate is strongly recommended.

Vascular access

Vascular access is generally obtained by percutaneous cannulation of the femoral, subclavian, or jugular veins. Modern polyurethane catheters with a double lumen are used and connected with blood pump circuits. Complications related to these procedures are the same as those of any kind of central venous catheterization which include haemorrhage, thrombosis, pneumothorax, pulmonary embolism, and haematomas. Subclavian vein catheterization is associated with the highest complication rate. This particular catheterization is also associated with a high incidence of late subclavian vein stenosis of up to 50 per cent which can cause problems if an arteriovenous fistula is subsequently required (Bambauer *et al.* 1994). For subjects with a high risk of progression to endstage renal failure, subclavian vein use should be avoided. Femoral vein catheterization in neonates and young children is associated with high rates of thrombosis and should also be avoided.

Catheters may stay in place for days and even weeks but special care must be taken in avoiding exit site infection and bacteraemia. Much controversy exists in the literature over the site with the highest risk of infection and the length of time a catheter should remain *in situ* before removal.

Ultrasound guidance of central venous catheterization has been reported to reduce the insertion failure and complication rates.

One of the more frustrating problems with catheters is maintaining their patency for long-term use. Although new heparin bonded catheters are now commercially available, there are no prospective *in vivo* data in adult patients to show an advantage over standard catheters.

Anticoagulation

Bleeding complications have been reported in 5–26 per cent of treatments making anticoagulation one of the most important issues in RRT for ARF. Although no consensus guidelines exist for heparinization, circuit heparinization using unfractionated heparin (MW 5–50 kDa) is perhaps the most common anticoagulant regimen adopted when no contraindications exist. This is achieved using a continuous infusion of heparin at a rate of 500–1000 IU after an initial loading dose of 1000–5000 IU. This generally permits safe anticoagulation with minimal or no systemic effects. Therapeutic monitoring with regular activated partial prothrombin time (aPPT) levels is advisable. Complications associated with unfractionated heparin include bleeding, hypoaldosteronism, thrombocytopenia, osteoporosis, pruritus, itching, and hypersensitivity reactions.

Low molecular weight heparins (2–8 kDa) are becoming more popular because of their easier dosing (single dose). Efficacy can be monitored by anti-Xa levels as aPPT is unaffected. These heparins accumulate in renal failure and when dosing one should take renal function into account.

Although citrate and prostacyclin are alternatives to heparin, they are rarely used. However, in patients with a high risk of bleeding, dialysis can be carried out with lower doses or even without heparin (Ivanovich *et al.* 1983). Heparin free dialysis is performed with periodic saline flushes through the dialyser every 30–60 min. When a constant blood flow is provided by a well functioning access and a calibrated blood pump, clotting of the fibres rarely occurs.

Regional heparinization is an effective technique that prevents systemic anticoagulation. Heparin is infused in the arterial limb and neutralized by protamine infused in the venous line. This method is often used when systemic anticoagulation is contraindicated and some form of anticoagulation is needed to prevent circuit clotting. Caution must be taken with protamine as it can accumulate in ARF.

Efficiency and prescription

Table 4 contrasts the clearances of these techniques. All techniques achieve a Kt/V index greater than 1 in the single session while HF,

Table 4 Comparisons of clearances for various quantitative blood purification techniques. Intermittent treatment provides highly efficient clearances over a short period but the overall efficiency is greater in long lasting treatments even though their instantaneous clearances are smaller

Parameter	Daily short HD	SLED	CVVH
K (ml/min)	200	80	20
Urea$[C]_o$ (mg/dl)	110	110	70
Urea$[C]_c$ (mg/dl)	30	30	65
Tx time (min)	180	480	1440
Kt/v	1.12	1.24	0.8
Total clearance (l)	36	38.4	28.8
Urea removed (g)	18	27	30.6

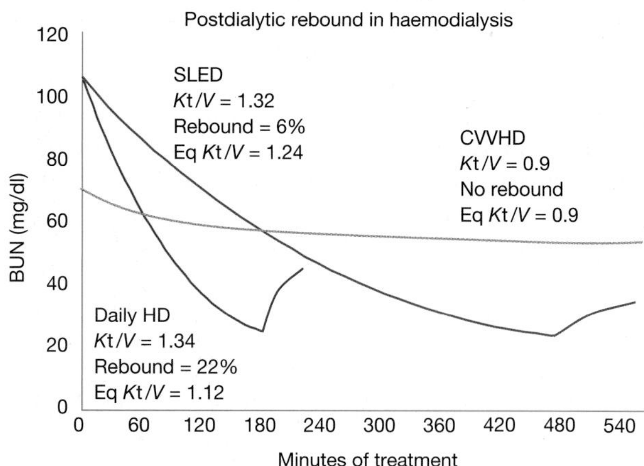

Fig. 3 Comparisons of urea rebound for various modalities.

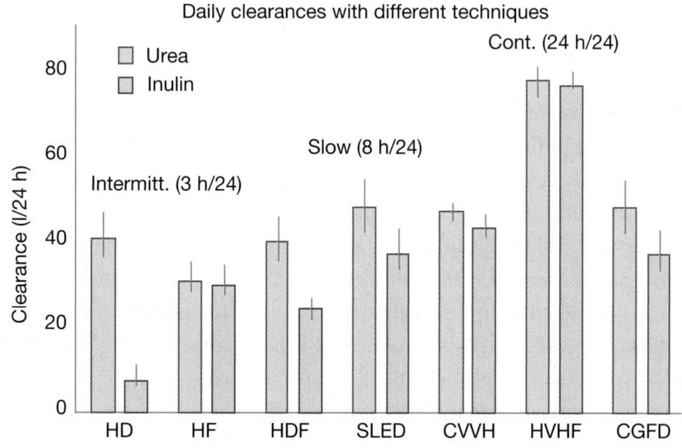

Fig. 4 Comparisons of clearances in intermittent, extended, and continuous therapies.

HDF, and HFD are significantly more efficient in removing molecules of higher molecular weight. The clinical significance and toxicity of such substances in ARF patients is still controversial. Intermittent techniques are characterized by a rapid decrease in solute plasma concentrations. Because of the brevity of the treatment, all blood pools are not well accessed and while clearance values remain fairly stable, the solute extraction tends to decrease and the final amount of solute removed from the body may be less in comparison with other, less efficient, but continuous therapies (Fabris *et al.* 1988). The smaller urea rebound seen in continuous therapies compared to intermittent therapies confirms this (Fig. 3). The speed of removal by dialysis is therefore faster than the capacity of equilibration between interstitial and vascular spaces and intracellular and extracellular compartments. This phenomenon, not only reduces the efficacy of the therapy, but also supports the theory of a 'non-physiological approach' of intermittent treatments (Fig. 4).

Dialysate composition

Replacement fluid and/or dialysate should contain a buffer and electrolytes in concentrations aiming for physiological levels and taking into account pre-existing deficits or excesses and all inputs and losses. Most commercially available solutions do not contain phosphate, which is not a problem with intermittent therapies but requires supplementation during prolonged CRRT. Frequent monitoring of serum electrolytes is imperative in critically ill patients. Supraphysiological glucose concentrations usually result in excessive glucose administration and hyperglycaemia and should be avoided (Monaghan *et al.* 1993).

Lactate and bicarbonate are the most common buffers available. Lactate buffered fluids can cause hyperlactataemia and, therefore, should not be used in patients with lactic acidosis. There is much controversy over the preferred buffer for RRT (Thomas *et al.* 1997). Irrespective of the buffer used, careful monitoring of acid–base status is recommended.

When replacement fluid or dialysate is directly administered to the patient's circulation it must be sterile, particularly in the case of high flux treatments where back diffusion occurs. Minimal blood/membrane interactions are guaranteed by the use of synthetic membranes (Hoenich *et al.* 1986; Hakim 1994). It should be noted, however, that highly permeable membranes may lead to a risk of back-filtration of non-sterile dialysate with a consequent back transport into the blood of endotoxin fragments able to stimulate complement and macrophage activation and IL-1 production.

Complications

Acute hypotension is the most common complication of intermittent dialysis treatment, especially in acutely ill patients (Korchik 1978). Achieving ideal fluid balance within a limited time can potentially cause cardiovascular instability. In chronic patients, it has been shown that the frequency of hypotensive episodes during dialysis is significantly correlated with the UF rate prescribed Fig. 5 (Ronco *et al.* 1988). Acute patients are generally less stable and potentially more sensitive to smaller UF rates. Several factors have been proposed in the pathogenesis of dialysis hypotension. The acute decrease in plasma osmolality may contribute to significant fluid shifts and hypotension (Kjellestrand *et al.* 1980). This phenomenon is partially avoided in HF where iso-osmotic UF takes place.

Bleeding episodes are uncommon if the coagulation status is carefully monitored. A low rate of heparinization and the possible use of protamine sulfate may result in a very low incidence of this complication.

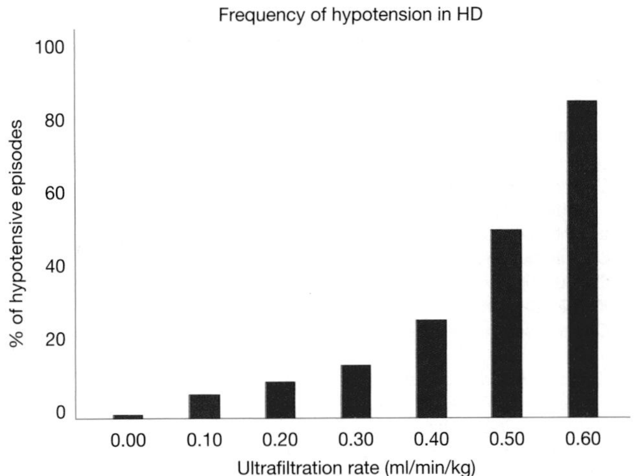

Fig. 5 Hypotensive episodes associated with the rate of ultrafiltration. The number of hypotensive episodes increases almost exponentially with the rate of ultrafiltration.

Technical complications related to the dialysis machine or equipment are seldom observed and the quality of modern machines guarantees safe and reliable dialytic procedure.

Sustained low-efficiency dialysis

Sustained low-efficiency dialysis (SLED) is a recently developed hybrid technique of RRT which applies a conventional HD machine with reduced blood flow and dialysate flow rates usually performed nocturnally for an extended period of time (10–12 h). The benefit of this form of treatment is that it provides a high dialysis dose, which can also be applied in unstable patients with the advantage of allowing unrestricted access to patients for daytime procedures (Marshall *et al.* 2001, 2002) (Table 4).

Continuous renal replacement therapies

CRRT is the closest modality that can achieve and maintain a physiological equilibrium. It has practical and theoretical advantages over intermittent therapies in haemodynamically unstable or severely catabolic patients with ARF.

The slow acceptance of CRRT in intensive care and renal units for the management of ARF is somewhat surprising. Using the previously established innovations of Henderson (1967) and Silverstein *et al.* (1974), who used UF as a treatment for fluid overload and azotemia, Kramer *et al.* in 1977 developed this technique by accidentally accessing the femoral artery instead of the vein creating an arteriovenous circuit which gave birth to the very primitive but innovative approach (Kramer *et al.* 1977). Problems with low flow and coagulation problems left this idea dormant until Lauer *et al.* (1983), described the unique operational characteristics of the system and the enormous potential for the treatment of ARF in intensive care departments. It was not until the application of blood pumps and the switch from arteriovenous to venovenous circuitry that current CRRT practice was born. Since then, the concept has remained unchanged but the technology has improved enormously.

The more common types of CRRT used include CVVH and CVVHDF (Fig. 6). CAVH is no longer used because of the multiple technical complications including low flow, poor efficiency, prolonged arterial cannulation, and the requirement of a satisfactory mean arterial pressure to drive the circuit. Arterial access itself can have grave complications such as haemorrhage, distal ischaemia, arterial thrombosis, traumatic fistula formation, and pseudoaneurysms. With the advent of compact and efficient peristaltic blood pumps, venous circuitry is the method of choice and arterial driven circuits have been superseded.

Despite the absence of consensus guidelines, CRRT is becoming the preferred extracorporeal treatment once ARF develops in critically ill patients with MOF (Mehta *et al.* 1999). Highly technologically advanced machines, which are continually improving are now available providing continuous, efficient, well tolerated, multifunction blood purification systems, which are simple and easy to use.

The principles

CRRT in diffusion mode (CVVHD) utilizes the same principles as in intermittent HD with solutes driven by their electrochemical gradient to move across the membrane into the sterile countercurrent flowing dialysate. However, during CRRT, dialysate flow is slow (10–30 ml/min) compared to intermittent HD (500 ml/min).

In CRRT using convection (CVVHF), solute movement across the membrane is driven by solvent drag. The solvent (plasma water) is pushed across the membrane by the filtrating pressure generated by blood flow through a process, which is identical to glomerular UF. Solvent takes all plasma water solutes with it. The ultrafiltrate is discarded and replaced with a sterile physiological solution. Diffusion and convection can be combined into a process appropriately named haemodiafiltration (CVVHDF). In this technique, the advantages of diffusion and convection are maximized for an improved clearance of small and larger molecules.

The membranes used for CRRT (especially polyacrylonitrile and polysulfone) have a significant adsorptive capacity particularly for several inflammatory mediators (De Vriese *et al.* 1999). CVVHF, because of its greater ability to remove middle molecules, its safety, and the ease of operation by nursing staff even at high exchange volumes, appears the technical approach of choice.

CRRT offers complete control of fluid balance. The amount of isotonic fluid removed over a given period of time can be easily regulated by setting the effluent pump and replacement fluid pump so that greater than 200 ml/h can be removed in excess of what is replaced. The rate of fluid removal and the total amount are set by the clinician according to clinical assessment and need for fluid administration. If the effluent rate is relatively high (i.e. 2 l/h) and the replacement fluid is administered after the filter (so-called postdilution), significant haemoconcentration will result from the removal of plasma water during transit of blood through the filter. Maintaining reasonable flows greater than 200 ml/min may offset the propensity for clotting. Administration of replacement fluid before the filter (so-called predilution) is preferred to prevent haemoconcentration.

HF replacement fluid contains supra-normal concentrations of buffer (typically either lactate or bicarbonate) tending to alkalinize blood, providing effective regulation of acid–base balance. Lactate can increase lactic acid levels in blood and therefore should not be used in

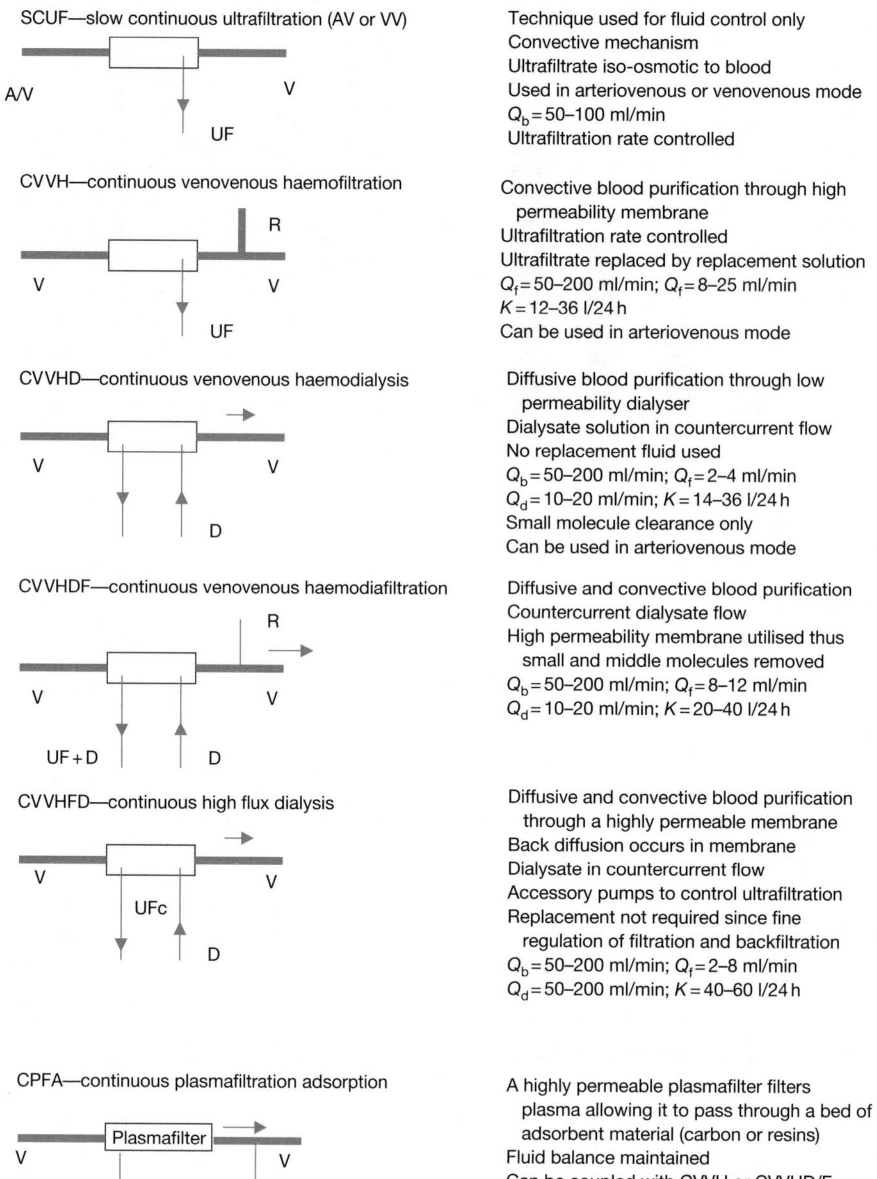

Fig. 6 Schematic representation and definitions of the different continuous renal replacement therapies according to standard nomenclature. A, artery; V, vein; D, dialysate; UF, ultrafiltrate; Ufc, ultrafiltrate control pump; Q_b, arterial flow; Q_f, ultrafiltration rate; Q_d, dialysate flow; P_f, plasmafiltration rate; K, clearance.

patients with lactic acidosis or liver failure. However much controversy exists over the preferred buffer (Thomas *et al.* 1997).

Technology

Nomenclature for these techniques is now established and illustrated in Fig. 6 (Bellomo *et al.* 1996). Adaptations to the standard technology include high-volume HF (Bellomo *et al.* 1998) and more complex circuit modifications aimed at increasing blood purification in septic shock or removing excess plasma water during cardiac surgery (Journois *et al.* 1998; Tetta *et al.* 1998b,c). The same circuit can be used to perform plasma exchange. Plasmafiltration and HP techniques (described earlier in this chapter) can also be used with CRRT technology.

Recently, CRRT machines have been designed specifically for ARF in intensive care patients (Table 5 and Fig. 7). These machines are equipped with integrated safety alarms, fluid balancing controls, and connected blood modules with the possibility to perform CVVH, CVVHD, and CVVHDF with increased levels of efficiency. Blood flows up to 500 ml/min and dialysate/replacement fluid flow rates in the same ranges can lead to urea clearances which may reach levels close to standard HD machines. The highly permeable membranes utilized in CRRT systems achieve improved clearances of the larger molecular weight solutes. Due to the higher blood and dialysate flow rates achievable in the system, higher surface areas can now be utilized and more efficient treatments can be carried out. The fluid control is achieved via gravimetric or volumetric control systems, which drive

Table 5 Specific data on the latest machines used in CRRT

	Company	Pumps	Q_b (ml/min)	Q_d (ml/min)	Fluid handed 1 (l)	Heater	Heparin pump	Reinfusion site	Pressure sensors	Printer/ RS-332 P	Scales	Available treatments
Acquarius	Ew L S Baxter	4	0–450	0–165	10	Yes	Yes	Pre Post Pre–post	4	No Yes	2	(IHD-IHFD)-IHF, PEX-PAP SCUF-CVVH-CVVHD-CVVHFD Pediatric Tx
BM 25	Ew L S Baxter	3	30–500	0–150	16	No	No	Pre Post	2	No Yes	2	SCUF-CVVH-CVVHD-PEX Pediatric Tx (Q_b = 5–150 ml/min)
Diapact	B.Braun	3	10–500	5–400	25	Yes	No	Pre Post	4	No Yes	1	IHD-IHFD-IHF, PEX-PAP SCUF-CVVH-CVVHD-CVVHFD
Equa-Smart	Medica	2[a]	5–400	0–150	10	Yes	Yes	Pre Post	3	Yes Yes	3	SCUF-CVVH-CVVHD-CVVHDF-PEX-Pediatric Tx
Multifiltrate	FMC	4[b]	0–500	0–70	24	Yes in-line	Yes	Pre Post Pre–post	4	No Yes	4	SCUF-CVVH-HV-HF CVVHD CVVHFD-CVVHDF-PEX
Multimat B	Bellco	2[c]	0–400	0–75	25	No	Yes	Pre Post	3	No No	1	SCUF-CVVH-CVVHD-CPFA
HF 400	Informed	4	0–450	0–200	12	Yes	Yes	Pre Post Pre–post	4	No Yes	2	IHD-IHFD-IHF, PEX, SCUF-CVVH-CVVHD-CVVHFD-CVVHDF- Pediatric Tx
Hygeia Plus	Kimal	4	0–500	0–65	4	Yes	Yes	Pre Post Pre–post	4	Yes Yes	Volumetric	SCUF-CVVH-CVVHD CVVHDF-PEX
Performer	Rand	4[d]	5–500	0–500	20	Yes	Yes	Pre Post	4	Yes Yes	1	IHD-IHFD-IHF, PEX-PAP-SCUF-CVVH-CVVHD-CVVHFD-CVVHDF
Prisma	Hospal	4	0–180	0–40	5	Blood warmer	Yes	Pre Post Pre–post	4	No Yes	3	SCUF-CVVH-CVVHD-CVVHFD-CVVHDF-PEX

[a] Two pumps plus two 'intelligent' clamps.

[b] The three pumps for dialysate and fluid are built in the hydraulic circuit of the machine.

[c] Each pump contains two line segments.

[d] The machine is equipped with several temperature probes.

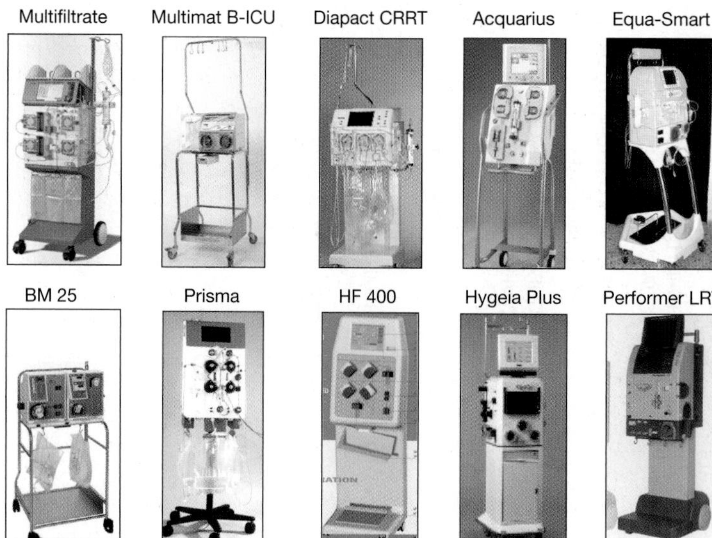

Fig. 7 The latest renal replacement therapy machines used in the treatment of acute renal failure.

Note:

The Multifiltrate from Fresenius Medical Care, Bad Homburg, Germany: This is the latest machine introduced into the market, specifically designed to perform all the CRRT techniques including plasma separation procedures (MPS). The system includes a high-resolution LCD colour screen, four roller pumps, four robust high precision scales, two individually bag heating systems, and heparin pump. The special construction of the scales enables the Multifiltrate to hold up to 24 l of haemofiltration solution to perform High Volume CVVH according to the increasing need of renal replacement therapies. The Multifiltrate disposables can easily be fitted through a cartridge which gives the user the possibility to select from a range of haemofilters, plasmafilters, and haemoperfusion columns. The user menu clearly displays all process and parameter sequences leading the user step by step. Pre, post, and simultaneous pre–post dilution modes are available.

The Multimat B-ICU from Bellco, Mirandola, Italy: The machine is basically derived from the Multimat system for HD with a modified software. The system presents two pumps, each of them containing two tubing sets. Ultrafiltration in CVVH is 15% of the blood flow while dialysate flow in CVVHD is 30% of the blood flow. The total fluid handling capacity is 25 l in a single scale. Warming of dialysate must be done externally while the heparin pump is included. In the configuration with one additional pump, the machine has been used to perform coupled plasmafiltration-adsorption (CPFA).

The Diapact CRRT from B.Braun, Melsungen, Germany: The machine is derived from a series of prototypes called ECU (emergency case units). The system presents three pumps with a wide range of blood flows (10–500 ml/min) and dialysate flows (5–400 ml/min). Fluid handling and ultrafiltration control is gravimetric with one scale. Dialysate is warmed and the heparin pump is included. Reinfusion can be performed either in pre or in post dilution mode during hemofiltration. The machine is particularly suited for continuous high flux dialysis with possibility of operating either in single pass or in recirculation mode.

The Acquarius from Edwards Life Sciences/Baxter: This is the latest machine for CRRT appeared on the market. The system includes four pumps and two scales with a possibility of performing all the CRRT techniques. The blood flow can be varied from 0 to 450 ml/min while the dialysate flow rate ranges between 0 and 165 ml/min. The system includes a pre-assembled tubing set and a wide colour screen with a friendly user interface. The priming procedure is automatic. Fluid heater and the heparin pump are included in the machine. Two independent scales allow for an accurate and continuous fluid balancing while four pressure sensors help to monitor the extracorporeal circuit function. Pre, post, and simultaneous pre–post dilution modes are available. A remarkable flexibility and versatility characterize the machine.

The Equa-Smart from Medica, Mirandola, Italy: The machine is derived from the original HP 300 and the Equaline fluid balancing system. It presents now an integrated fluid control with three load cells and one pump for fluid reinfusion. The two 'smart' clamps operate as a further system for fluid control. The system handles up to 10 l with the possibility of pre and post dilution modes. A built-in printer allows obtaining a complete treatment report with the possibility of tracing the previous treatments. The storing capacity is up to 99 days.

The BM 25 from Edwards Life Sciences/Baxter: The machine constitutes a 'classic' equipment for CRRT. Two different tubing sets are available for the paediatric and the adult treatments with variable blood and dialysate flow ranges. The system presents two scales and three pumps while the heater and the heparin pump are not included. The fluid handling capacity is up to 16 l.

The Prisma from Hospal-Gambro, Lyon, France: The Prisma machine has been the first integrated equipment specifically designed for CRRT. The machine features a pre-assembled cartridge including lines and the dialyser. Tubing loading is automatic as well as the priming procedure. The presence of four pumps and three independent scales allow performing all the CRRT techniques. Blood flows can vary from 0 to 180 ml/min while dialysate flow ranges between 0 and 40 ml/min. The fluid handling capacity is 5 l. Pre, post, and simultaneous pre–post dilution modes are available.

The HF 400 from Infomed, Geneva, Switzerland: The machine presents four pumps and a friendly user interface well suited to perform different CRRT techniques. Blood flows between 0 and 450 ml/min are available while dialysate flow ranges between 0 and 200 ml/min. Two scales permit an accurate ultrafiltration and fluid balance control. Fluid can be reinfused in pre, post, and pre–post dilution modes. Fluid warmer and heparin pump are included. The machine is equipped with a friendly user interface and a wide colour screen. Priming and rinsing procedures are automatic.

The Hygeia Plus from Kimal, London, UK: The machine is designed for use in a clinical environment where automated programs are required to control the extracorporeal and fluid circuits necessary to perform different continuous renal replacement therapies. The system incorporates the latest touch screen technology and colour graphic representation. This provides clear indications of essential treatment parameters as well as simplifying set-up and use. The machine features four pumps and a volumetric fluid control. Blood flows can vary from 0 to 500 ml/min while dialysate flow ranges between 0 and 65 ml/min. The fluid handling capacity is 20 l. Pre, post, and simultaneous pre–post dilution modes are available. The heater and the heparin pump are included.

The Performer LRT from RAND, Mirandola, Italy: The machine is one of the latest equipment appeared on the market. It is an integrated system able to support a variety of therapeutic applications in different medical fields (oncology, apheresis, and dialysis). The system includes: four peristaltic pumps, with adjustable flow rates (5–500 ml/min) according to the method in use; high performance heater, and syringe pump for heparin; haematocrit and oxygen saturation (SO_2) in-line measuring and monitoring; external independent monitoring of temperatures, by means of medical probes; graphic user-friendly operator interface, with 'touch screen' monitor; integrated in-line printer.

peristaltic pumps both for UF and reinfusion. The priming procedures are simplified because of the step-by-step on-line help and the self-loading preassembled tubing sets.

The new machines are also equipped with a user-friendly interface: this leads to increased confidence by nursing personnel supervising the treatment, while constant levels of efficiency can be obtained without major problems or complications. Table 5 and Fig. 7 show comparisons of various machines. Some of the new machines present operational conditions similar to those utilized for chronic HD. This provides the possibility of using the machine for different treatments and purposes.

The metabolic control of ARF generally requires at least 30 l of urea clearance per day. The combination of diffusion and convection has shown that satisfactory clearances of small and medium large molecules can generally be achieved. Furthermore, in the case of sepsis, patients may present increased levels of substances in the middle molecular weight range (500–5000 Da) such as chemical mediators of the humoral response to endotoxin. In this case, the treatment should control not only urea and other waste products, but also the circulating levels of these proinflammatory substances (Ronco *et al.* 1999). To achieve such a complex task, high convective rates may be required and can be obtained in CVVHF, CVVHDF, or in continuous high flux HD with continuous dialysate volume control. In HFD, substitution fluid is not required and the balance is obtained by a mechanism of internal back-filtration. If performed continuously, the treatments can provide weekly Kt/V in the range of 7–10, thus resulting in a treatment efficiency much higher than that achieved with other intermittent dialysis therapies.

The clinical application of CRRT

CRRT offers extraordinary physiological and practical advantages over intermittent HD or PD in the treatment of ARF. With CRRT, volume control is continuous and immediately adaptable to the rapidly changing clinical circumstances commonly seen in critically ill patients. Because of this adaptability, CRRT can immediately treat volume overload or prevent it without inducing acute volume depletion. The avoidance of intravascular volume depletion and hypotension is likely to prevent treatment-associated ischaemic renal injury, which has been reported during standard IHD (Manns *et al.* 1997).

Control of uraemia with CRRT is superior to that achieved with standard IHD (Clark *et al.* 1994) with a more consistent maintenance of lower urea and creatinine levels (Uchino *et al.* 2001). Recent data show that delivery of a greater 'dialysis dose' is associated with a better outcome in critically ill patients (Paganini *et al.* 1996; Ronco *et al.* 2000). Frequency of dialysis is another important determinant of treatment dose and intensity. The results of a randomized controlled trial, which compared daily to alternate day IHD in patients with ARF also show a statistically significant increase in survival in those patients treated with daily IHD (Schiffl *et al.* 2002). Dose can be increased in intermittent therapies, but cannot ever reach the levels obtained in CRRT.

CRRT offers more rapid improvement and control of metabolic acidosis and more rapid and reliable control of serum phosphate levels (Bellomo *et al.* 1995). A combination of high phosphate clearance and simultaneous initiation of feeding can lead to hypophosphataemia. Thus, phosphate levels should be monitored and phosphate replaced appropriately. CRRT allows better nutritional support. With standard IHD, adequate azotaemic control is difficult and a degree of protein restriction is often required to prevent uncontrolled uraemia, which can induce protein starvation and negative daily nitrogen balances (Bouffard *et al.* 1987). CRRT permits a protein rich nutritional policy with a neutral nitrogen balance preventing protein malnutrition (Bellomo *et al.* 1991; Frankenfield *et al.* 1995). Amino acid, trace element, and vitamin losses through the filter do occur and are not appreciably greater than those seen during a session of IHD or during PD, but should be replaced (Story *et al.* 1999). The benefits of achieving a near neutral nitrogen balance remain unknown.

CRRT is also indicated for patients at risk of or with increased intracranial pressure (neurosurgical patients, patients with encephalitis, meningo-encephalitis, or acute liver failure). CRRT prevents the surge in intracranial pressure associated with intermittent therapies (Davenport *et al.* 1989, 1993).

The clinical benefits of HF have also been reported for cardiac surgery patients (Caprioli *et al.* 1993). The possible mechanisms include decreased fluid overload, myocardial oedema, a decrease in left ventricular end diastolic pressure, optimization of the Starling relationship, increased myocardial performance, and the removal of circulating myocardial depressant factors (Blake *et al.* 1996).

Sepsis and the non-infectious systemic inflammatory response syndrome (SIRS) are a major cause of ARF (Silvester *et al.* 2001). CRRT appears to have beneficial effects on haemodynamics and inflammation in animal models of sepsis (Lee *et al.* 1998; Tetta *et al.* 1998b), thus providing a biologic rationale for using CRRT in septic shock and ARF in humans. Standard CRRT technology has been modified by either using a more permeable membrane, coupling continuous plasma filtration with continuous adsorption (Tetta *et al.* 1998c) or increasing the plasma water exchange rate. These modifications are aimed at moving CRRT from the simple treatment of ARF to the adjunctive treatment of sepsis, but whether they can yield clinically significant benefits remains unknown.

Initiating and terminating CRRT

There are also non-renal indications for CRRT (Table 6). Haemodynamic instability may not necessarily be a contraindication to the initiation of CRRT. Early initiation may increase survival (Gettings *et al.* 1999).

Table 6 Non-renal indications and functions of CRRT. With its multifunction potential, CRRT is the ideal modality as a multiple organ support therapy (MOST)

Blood purification and renal support
Temperature control
Acid–base control
Fluid balance control
Cardiac support
Protective lung support
Cerebral protection
Bone marrow protection
Blood detoxification and liver support
Septic therapy—immunomodulation and endothelial support

No guidelines exist on the timing and mode for the cessation of CRRT. If renal function is returning in the form of an increased urinary output (>1 l/day) associated with an improvement in the clinical condition, CRRT can be temporarily stopped. CRRT or another modality of RRT can be restarted if indications for further treatment are present. CRRT can be momentarily stopped and set in a recirculation mode using a heparinized saline bag as the site for connection of arterial and venous lines if urgent disconnection from the patient is required.

The controversies

Several controversies surround the use of CRRT and the most pressing question is that of whether CRRT offers an important survival advantage over IHD in the management of ARF. To answer this question, a randomized controlled trial of larger numbers of subjects and extremely strict criteria would be required (Bellomo and Boyce 1993). Such a trial would be extremely difficult to undertake and attempts to date have fallen short of providing a decisive result (Kellum *et al.* 2002).

To date, there are only three prospective randomized trials comparing CRRT to other forms of renal replacement with two published in abstract form (Simpson *et al.* 1993) and the other failing to achieve balanced randomization (Mehta *et al.* 2001). In addition, there are several observational studies. Most observational studies have reported improved survival with CRRT, even though CRRT patients were often sicker at baseline (Bartlett *et al.* 1986; Mauritz *et al.* 1986; Simpson *et al.* 1987; Bastien *et al.* 1991; Bosworth *et al.* 1991; McDonald *et al.* 1991; Kruczynski *et al.* 1993; Bellomo *et al.* 1995; Van Bommel *et al.* 1995). However, some have reported worse outcomes (Bosworth *et al.* 1991; Van Bommel *et al.* 1995). In the largest randomized controlled trial of 166 patients, there was no difference in outcome but there were significant baseline differences in severity of illness between groups, making comparison difficult (Mehta *et al.* 2001). A recent meta-analysis of all studies up to the end of 2000 showed a trend in favour of CRRT but this was not statistically significant (Kellum *et al.* 2002). One interesting finding from the largest randomized controlled study to date demonstrated that patients treated with CRRT who survived were more likely to have renal recovery than patients treated with IHD (92.3 versus 59.4 per cent; $p < 0.01$) (Mehta *et al.* 2001). These findings suggest that mortality may not be the only appropriate end point for future trials and that CRRT may increase recovery of renal function after ARF.

The need for continuous anticoagulation has been considered an important disadvantage of CRRT. This concern is not justified as CRRT can easily be conducted without any anticoagulation in patients at risk of bleeding without significantly compromising filter life (Favre *et al.* 1996).

Cost comparisons has been analysed by several authors and the general consensus is that the difference in cost between CRRT and IHD is minimal and depends more on the structure of ICU and nephrological care than on disposables (Hoyt *et al.* 1997).

Plasmafiltration and haemoperfusion

CRRT application can modified and supplemented with other modalities in order to achieve ultra high clearances. CRRT utilizing plasma membranes and HP devices (sorbents) are two such modalities currently being investigated.

Plasma filters differ from high flux membranes in that they have larger pores and sieving coefficients and can remove molecules with higher molecular weights including proteins and inflammatory mediators (Tetta *et al.* 1998a). There appears to be some advantages in clinical trials, however, it is too early to predict its benefits as further large scale trials are needed to confirm this (Reeves *et al.* 1999). At this time, both high costs from excessive plasma substitution fluids and unregulated losses of beneficial plasma constituents may limit this modality of treatment.

HP alone does not provide sufficient purification for the treatment of ARF but in combination with CVVH or CVVHDF is able to provide a broader purification removing molecules that are not removed by CVVH or HD alone. Coupled plasma filtration adsorption (CPFA) is a technique of blood purification in which plasma is separated from whole blood and circulated in a sorbent cartridge (HP). The plasma is then returned to the blood circuit which then undergoes standard HD or filtration. This modality has been shown to remove cytokines with high efficiency and most impressively has the ability to restore leucocyte responsiveness to endotoxin in *ex vivo* testing, suggesting an added immunomodulatory effect (Tetta *et al.* 1999; Ronco *et al.* 2002). The potential for CPFA in the treatment of MOF seems exciting but its role in the management of ARF has not been established and we await further clinical testing to appreciate its value is awaited.

Slow continuous ultrafiltration

This is a continuous therapy, which can achieve safe and effective management of fluid overload. It utilizes standard HD circuitry without dialysate or replacement fluid. Volumetric control of ultrafiltration may be required to maintain the UF rate at the desired value (Ronco *et al.* 2001). Fluid removed is similar to plasma water, therefore iso-osmotic.

Multiple organ support therapy

The extraordinary success achieved with the highly advanced renal replacement machines used in renal failure has brought about a novel concept recently named 'multiple organ support therapy' (MOST). In the setting of MOF, management is extended beyond simple renal support in the hope of achieving a global and optimal blood purification to assist and correct multiple organ dysfunction. CRRT has uses beyond renal support alone which can treat the complications seen in MOF (Table 6). Still, in the early phases of clinical evaluation, the potential of this therapy has been recognized and is currently being evaluated in clinical trials (Ronco and Bellomo 2002).

Conclusion

The future of RRTs is bright. Ultimately, the ideal machine will simulate normal kidney function. The technology available is rapidly approaching this goal. A change from intermittent to continuous therapy is certainly a step in the right direction. An understanding of the mechanisms that help in the recovery of renal function may be the next step in directing renal replacement planning and technology.

References

al-Khafaji, A. and Corwin, H. L. (2001). Acute renal failure and dialysis in the chronically critically ill patient. *Clinics in Chest Medicine* **22** (1), 165–174.

Bambauer, R., Inniger, R., Pirrung, K. J., Schiel, R., and Dahlem, R. (1994). Complications and side effects associated with large-bore catheters in the subclavian and internal jugular veins. *Artificial Organs* **18**, 318–321.

Bartlett, R. H., Mault, J. R., Dechert, R. E., Palmer, J., Swartz, R. D., and Port, F. K. (1986). Continuous arteriovenous hemofiltration: improved survival in surgical acute renal failure? *Surgery* **100**, 400–408.

Bastien, O., Saroul, C., Hercule, C., George, M., and Estanove, S. (1991). Continuous venovenous hemodialysis after cardiac surgery. *Contributions to Nephrology* **93**, 76–78.

Bellomo, R., and Boyce, N. (1993). Does continuous hemodiafiltration improve survival in patients with critical illness and associated acute renal failure? *Seminars in Dialysis* **6**, 16–19.

Bellomo, R., Martin, H., Parkin, G., Love, J., Kearly, Y., and Boyce, N. (1991). Continuous arteriovenous haemodiafiltration in the critically ill: influence on major nutrient balances. *Intensive Care Medicine* **17**, 399–402.

Bellomo, R., and Farmer, M., Parkin, G., Wright, C., and Boyce, N. (1995). Severe acute renal failure: a comparison of acute continuous hemodiafiltration and conventional dialytic therapy. *Nephron* **71**, 59–64.

Bellomo, R., Ronco, C., and Mehta, R. (1996). Nomenclature for continuous renal replacement therapies. *American Journal of Kidney Diseases* **28** (Suppl. 3), S2–S7.

Bellomo, R., Baldwin, I., Cole, L., and Ronco, C. (1998). Preliminary experience with high-volume hemofiltration in human septic shock. *Kidney International* **53** (Suppl. 66), S182–S185.

Bellomo, R., Kellum, J. A., and Ronco, C. (2001). Acute renal failure: time for consensus. *Intensive Care Medicine* **27**, 1685–1688.

Bergstrom, J. *et al.* (1978). Ultrafiltration without dialysis for the removal of fluid and solutes in uremia. *Clinical Nephrology* **9**, 156–161.

Berman, L. B. *et al.* (1964). Removal rates for barbiturates using two types of peritoneal dialysis. *New England Journal of Medicine* **270**, 77–80.

Blake, P., Hasegawa, Y., Khosla, M. C., Fouad-Tarazi, F., Sakura, N., and Paganini, E. (1996). Isolation of 'myocardial depressant factor(s) from the ultrafiltrate of heart failure patients with acute renal failure. *ASAIO Journal* **42**, M911–M915.

Borah, M. F. *et al.* (1978). Nitrogen balance during intermittent dialysis therapy of uremia. *Kidney International* **14**, 491–497.

Bosworth, C., Paganini, E. P., Cosentino, F., and Heyka, R. J. (1991). Long-term experience with continuous renal replacement therapy in intensive-care unit acute renal failure. *Contributions to Nephrology* **93**, 13–16.

Bouffard, Y., Viale, J. P., Annat, G., Delafosse, B., Guillame, C., and Motin, J. (1987). Energy expenditure in the acute renal failure patient mechanically ventilated. *Intensive Care Medicine* **13**, 401–404.

Brivet, F. G., Kleinknecht, D. J., Loirat, P., and Landais, P. J. (1996). Acute renal failure in intensive care units—causes, outcome, and prognostic factors of hospital mortality; a prospective, multicenter study. French Study Group on Acute Renal Failure. *Critical Care Medicine* **24** (2), 192–198.

Brookes, M. H. *et al.* (1973). Removal of iodinated material by peritoneal dialysis. *Nephron* **12**, 10–17.

Caprioli, R., Favilla, G., Palmarini, D., Comite, C., Gemignani, R., Rindi, P., and Cioni, L. (1993). Automatic continuous venovenous hemodiafiltration in cardiosurgical patients. *ASAIO Journal* **39**, M606–M608.

Clark, W. R. and Ronco, C. (1998). Renal replacement therapy in acute renal failure: solute removal, mechanisms and dose quantification. *Kidney International* **53** (Suppl. 66), S133–S137.

Clark, W. R., Alaka, K. J., Mueller, B. A., and Macias, W. L. (1994). A comparison of metabolic control by continuous and intermittent therapies in acute renal failure. *Journal of the American Society of Nephrology* **4**, 1413–1420.

Davenport, A., Finn, R., and Goldsmith, A. J. (1989). Management of patients with acute renal failure complicated by cerebral edema. *Blood Purification* **7**, 203–209.

Davenport, A., Will, E. J., and Davison, A. M. (1993). Effect of renal replacement therapy on patients with combined acute renal failure and fulminant hepatic failure. *Kidney International* **43** (Suppl. 41), S245–S251.

De Vriese, A. S., Colardyn, F. A., Philippe, J. J., Vanholder, R. C., De Sutter, J. H., and Lameire, N. H. (1999). Cytokine removal during continuous hemofiltration in septic patients. *Journal of the American Society of Nephrology* **10** (4), 846–853.

Fabris, A. *et al.* (1988). Total solute extraction versus clearance in the evaluation of standard and short haemodialysis. *ASAIO Transactions* **34**, 627–632.

Favre, H., Martin, P. Y., and Stoermann, C. (1996). Anticoagulation in continuous extracorporeal renal replacement therapy. *Seminars in Dialysis* **9**, 112–118.

Frankenfield, D. C. and Reynolds, H. N. (1995). Nutritional effect of continuous hemodiafiltration. *Nutrition* **11**, 388–393.

Gettings, L. G., Reynolds, H. N., and Scalea, T. (1999). Outcome in post-traumatic acute renal failure when continuous renal replacement therapy is applied early vs. late. *Intensive Care Medicine* **25**, 805–813.

Gotch, F. A. *et al.* (1989). A mechanistic analysis of the National Cooperative of Dialysis Study. *Kidney International* **28**, 526–533.

Groeneveld, A. B., Tran, D. D., van der Meulen, J., Nauta, J. J., and Thijs, L. G. (1991). Acute renal failure in the medical intensive care unit: predisposing, complicating factors and outcome. *Nephron* **59** (4), 602–610.

Hakim, R. M. (1994). Effect of the dialysis membrane in the treatment of patients with acute renal failure. *New England Journal of Medicine* **20**, 1338–1342.

Henderson, L. W. (1967). Blood purification by ultrafiltration and fluid replacement (diafittration). *ASAIO Transactions* **17**, 216–221.

Hoenich, N. A. *et al.* (1986). Biocompatibility of haemodialysis membranes. *Journal of Biomedical Engineering* **8**, 3–11.

Hoyt, D. B. (1997). CRRT in the area of cost containment: is it justified? *American Journal of Kidney Diseases* **30** (Suppl. 4), S102–S104.

Ivanovich, P. *et al.* (1983). Studies of coagulation and platelet functions I., heparin free haemodialysis. *Nephron* **33**, 116–122.

Journois, D. (1998). Hemofiltration during cardiopulmonary bypass. *Kidney International* **53** (Suppl. 66), S174–S177.

Kellum, J. *et al.* (2002). Continuous versus intermittent renal replacement therapy: a meta-analysis. *Intensive Care Medicine* **28**, 29–37.

Kjellestrand, C. M. *et al.* (1980). Hypotension during haemodialysis. Osmolality fall is an important pathogenic factor. *ASAIO Journal* **3**, 11–14.

Kolff, W. J. (1967). First clinical experience with the artificial kidney. *Annals of Internal Medicine* **62**, 608–612.

Korchik, W. P. (1978). Haemodialysis induced hypotension. *International Journal of Artificial Organs* **I**, 151–157.

Kramer, P. *et al.* (1977). Arteriovenous haemofiltration: a new and simple method for the treatment of overhydrated patients resistant to diuretics. *Klinische Wochenschrift* **55**, 1121–1128.

Kruczynski, K., Irvine-Bird, K., Toffelmire, E. B., and Morton, A. R. (1993). A comparison of continuous arteriovenous hemofiltration and intermittent hemodialysis in acute renal failure patients in the intensive care unit. *ASAIO Journal* **39**, M778–M781.

Lauer, A. *et al.* (1983). Continuous arteriovenous hemofiltration in the critically ill patient. *Annals of Internal Medicine* **99**, 455–460.

Lee, P., Weger, G. W., Pryor, R. W., and Matson, J. R. (1998). Effects of filter pore size on efficacy of continuous arteriovenous hemofiltration therapy for *Staphylococcus aureus*-induced septicemia in immature swine. *Critical Care Medicine* **26**, 730–737.

Manns, M., Siegler, M. H., and Teehan, B. P. (1997). Intradialytic renal hemodynamics—potential consequences for the management of the patient with acute renal failure. *Nephrology, Dialysis, Transplantation* **12**, 870–872.

Marshall, M. R., Golper, T. A., Shaver, M. J., Alam, M. G., and Chatoth, D. K. (2001). Sustained low-efficiency dialysis for critically ill patients requiring renal replacement therapy. *Kidney International* **60** (2), 777–785.

Marshall, M. R., Golper, T. A., Shaver, M. J., Alam, M. G., and Chatoth, D. K. (2002). Urea kinetics during sustained low-efficiency dialysis in critically ill patients requiring renal replacement therapy. *American Journal of Kidney Diseases* **39** (3), 556–570.

Mauritz, W., Sporn, P., Schindler, I., Zadrobilek, E., Roth, E., and Appel, W. (1986). Acute renal failure in abdominal infection. Comparison of hemodialysis and continuous arteriovenous hemofiltration. *Anasthestologie, Intensivtherapie, Notfallmedizin* **21**, 212–217.

McDonald, B. R. and Mehta, R. L. (1991). Decreased mortality in patients with acute renal failure undergoing continuous arteriovenous hemodialysis. *Contributions to Nephrology* **93**, 51–56.

Mehta, R. L. and Letteri, J. M. (1999). Current status of renal replacement therapy for acute renal failure. *American Journal of Nephrology* **19**, 377–382.

Mehta, R. *et al.* (2002). A randomized clinical trial of continuous versus intermittent dialysis for acute renal failure. *Kidney International* **60**, 1154–1163.

Monaghan, R., Watters, J. M., Clancey, S. M., Moulton, S. B., and Rabin, E. Z. (1993). Uptake of glucose during continuous arteriovenous hemofiltration. *Critical Care Medicine* **21**, 1159–1163.

Paganini, E. P., Tapolay, M., Goormastic, M., Halstenberg, W., Kozlowski, L., Leblanc, M., Lee, J. C., Moreno, L., and Sakai, K. (1996). Establishing a dialysis therapy/patient outcome link in intensive care unit acute dialysis for patients with acute renal failure. *American Journal of Kidney Diseases* **28** (Suppl. 3), S81–S89.

Posen, G. A. *et al.* (1979). Continuous equilibration peritoneal dialysis in the treatment of acute and chronic renal failure. *Proceedings of Clinical Dialysis Transplantation Forum* **9**, 50–63.

Reeves, J. H. *et al.* (1999). Continuous plasmafiltration in sepsis syndrome. Plasmafiltration in Sepsis Study Group. *Critical Care Medicine* **27** (10), 2096–2104.

Ronco, C. and Bellomo, R. (2002). Acute renal failure and multiple organ dysfunction in the ICU: from renal replacement therapy (RRT) to multiple organ support therapy (MOST). *The International Journal of Artificial Organs* **25** (8), 733–747. Review.

Ronco, C. *et al.* (1985a). Continuous arterio-venous haemofiltration. *Contributions to Nephrology* **48**, 70–78.

Ronco, C. *et al.* (1985b). Arteriovenous haemodiafiltration (AVHDF) combined with continuous aerteriovenous haemofiltration (CAVH). *ASIAIO Transactions* **31**, 349–355.

Ronco, C. *et al.* (1988). Comparison of four different short dialysis techniques. *International Journal of Artificial Organs* **3**, 169–174.

Ronco, C., Ghezzi, P., and Bellomo, R. (1999). New perspective in the treatment of acute renal failure. *Blood Purification* **17**, 166–172.

Ronco, C., Bellomo, R., Homel, P., Brendolan, A., Dan, M., Piccinni, P., and La Greca, G. (2000). Effects of different doses in continuous veno-venous haemofiltration on outcomes of acute renal failure: a prospective randomised trial. *The Lancet* **356**, 26–30.

Ronco, C., Bellomo, R., and Ricci, Z. (2001). Hemodynamic response to fluid withdrawal in overhydrated patients treated with intermittent ultrafiltration and slow continuous ultrafiltration: role of blood volume monitoring. *Cardiology* **96** (3–4), 196–201.

Schiffl, H., Lang, S., and Fisher, R. (2002). Daily hemodialysis and the outcome of acute renal failure. *New England Journal of Medicine* **346**, 305–310.

Scribner, B. H. (1975). Long term perintoneal dialysis. *EDTA Proceedings* **12**, 131–137.

Silverstein, M. E. *et al.* (1974). Treatment of severe fluid overload by ultrafiltration. *New England Journal of Medicine* **291**, 747–752.

Silvester, W., Bellomo, R., and Cole, L. (2001). Epidemiology, management, and outcome of severe acute renal failure of critical illness in Australia. *Critical Care Medicine* **29** (10), 1910–1915.

Simpson, K. and Allison, M. E. M. (1993). Dialysis and acute renal failure: can mortality be improved? *Nephrology, Dialysis, Transplantation* **8**, 946 (abstract).

Simpson, H. K., Allison, M. E., and Telfer, A. B. (1987). Improving the prognosis in acute renal and respiratory failure. *Renal Failure* **10**, 45–54.

Story, D. A., Ronco, C., and Bellomo, R. (1999). Trace element and vitamin concentrations and losses in critically ill patients treated with continuous venovenous hemofiltration. *Critical Care Medicine* **27** (1), 220–223.

Teschan, P. E. *et al.* (1960). Prophylactic hemodialysis in the treatment of acute renal failure. *Annals of Internal Medicine* **53**, 992–1016.

Tetta, C., Cavaillon, J. M., Camussi, G., Lonnemann, G., Brendolan, A., and Ronco, C. (1998a). Continuous plasma filtration coupled with absorbents. *Kidney International* **53** (Suppl. 66), S186–S189.

Tetta, C. *et al.* (1998b). Removal of cytokines and activated complement components in an experimental model of continuous plasma filtration coupled with sorbent adsorption. *Nephrology, Dialysis, Transplantation* **13**, 1458–1464.

Tetta, C., and Mariano, F., Ronco, C., and Bellomo, R. Removal and generation of inflammatory mediators during continuous renal replacement therapies. In *Critical Care Nephrology* (ed. C. Ronco and R. Bellomo), pp. 143–152. Dordrecht: Kluwer Academic Publishers, 1998c.

Tetta, C. *et al.* (1999). Use of adsorptive mechanisms in continuous renal replacement therapies in the critically ill. *Kidney International* **56** (Suppl. 72), S15–S19.

Thomas, A. N., Guy, J. M., Kishen, R., Geraghty, I. F., Bowles, B. J., and Vadgama, P. (1997). Comparison of lactate and bicarbonate buffered haemofiltration fluids: use in critically ill patients. *Nephrology, Dialysis, Transplantation* **12**, 1212–1217.

Uchino, S., Bellomo, R., and Ronco, C. (2001). Intermittent versus continuous renal replacement therapy in the ICU: impact on electrolyte and acid–base balance. *Intensive Care Medicine* **27** (6), 1037–1043.

Van Bommel, E. *et al.* (1995). Acute dialytic support for the critically ill: intermittent hemodialysis versus continuous arteriovenous hemodiafiltration. *American Journal of Nephrology* **15**, 192–200.

Winchester, J. F. *et al.* (1977). Dialysis and hemoperfusion of poisons and drugs—update. *ASAIO Transactions* **23**, 762–767.

10.5 Dialysis and haemoperfusion treatment of acute poisoning

Günter Seyffart

Introduction

For over 5000 years, mankind has used poisons for homicide, suicide, and chemical warfare, but only in the past 100 years has there been a search for treatment of poisonings. Prior to the era of dialysis, treatment of intoxications was, in general, symptomatic and supportive, although some specific measures of toxin removal such as gastric lavage and stimulation of endogenous pathways of elimination were used. Treatment of severe intoxications entered a new era with the availability of extracorporeal measures allowing the removal of exogenous substances, especially drugs in overdose and known toxins, directly from the blood compartment by haemodialysis and peritoneal dialysis, and later by haemoperfusion. The new techniques were usually implemented by nephrologists familiar with the handling of extracorporeal blood circuits.

History

The first report of an extracorporeal procedure for the removal of an exogenous poison in humans was published by Doolan *et al.* (1951), who showed that substantial quantities of salicylate could be removed by haemodialysis. The seminal paper by Schreiner (1958), listing 15 removable drugs was published one decade after the introduction of haemodialysis. It laid down the criteria for dialysis in poisonings, which are still applicable today, albeit with some minor modifications (see below). Reviews appeared then annually until 1977; the last review (Winchester *et al.* 1977) listed 142 dialysable agents with a corresponding 44 exogenous poisons removable by haemoperfusion, covering 80 pages and citing 953 references. The review was discontinued because the volume of information became too great and other sources became available (Seyffart 1977; Haddad and Winchester 1983).

There is a large body of published literature in the small field of treatment of poisoning by extracorporeal methods. Although most ascribe real value to the method involved, many are anecdotal and lack essential data such as the type of dialyser used, the body weight and haematocrit of the patient, or the method used to calculate clearances.

Epidemiology

The incidence of poisonings by both intended or accidential drug overdose was much greater during the period 1950–1970 than today. The most obvious reasons for that decline are:

1. Many sedatives and hypnotics, such as barbiturates, glutethimide, meprobamate, and methaqualone, and a variety of strong analgesics were developed and introduced during the 1950s and 1960s, and these were often the agents involved in accidental overdoses and suicide attempts. The use of barbiturates declined with the advent of newer sedatives, including benzodiazepines. Because the newer sedatives were less effective central nervous system (CNS) depressants, their use in suicide attempts declined. Classic analgesics such as acetylsalicylic acid and propoxyphene, sedatives and hypnotics such as carbromal, bromisoval, and glutethimide, were replaced by new generations of 'safer' drugs.
2. Non-steroidal anti-inflammatory drugs (NSAIDs), at present widely used as analgesics, have rarely been used in attempting suicide, and accidental overdose is also rare.
3. Since the 1970s, individuals with and without psychotic illnesses and those considering suicide have had greater access to psychiatric support, which may have prevented many suicide attempts.
4. Drug abuse and addiction entered the scene dramatically in the 1960s and it became evident that persons at risk of suicide were becoming drug abusers.
5. Increasing ecological awareness has led to a decrease in the use of pesticides and herbicides, which in the past had often caused severe intoxications by accident or suicides.

Extracorporeal techniques

The general treatment of intoxication includes: (a) limiting further exposure by skin decontamination, artificial emesis, gastric lavage, gastrointestinal instillation of adsorbents (usually activated charcoal), forced (osmotic) diuresis, administration of antidotes and chelating agents, plasma and blood exchange, and detoxification methods, and (b) supportive treatments like artificial ventilation and correction of metabolic derangement. Techniques include peritoneal dialysis, haemodialysis, haemodiafiltration, continuous haemodialysis and haemofiltration methods, haemoperfusion, combined haemoperfusion–haemodialysis, and plasmapheresis.

Peritoneal dialysis

In comparison to other techniques, peritoneal dialysis has low and slow mass transfer. No toxin is entirely removed by peritoneal dialysis. It has, therefore, only a limited place in the treatment of poisoning. It has been used successfully in (accidental) sodium chloride intoxication in children (Finberg *et al.* 1963), in whom haemodialysis is usually more difficult to perform. In adults, it has been successful in severe ethanol intoxication when the clinical situation precludes the use of other techniques.

Haemodialysis

Haemodialysis involves simple (passive) diffusion of substances from the blood to a dialysis solution across a semipermeable membrane. The dialysis membranes used today possess pores of such a wide range of sizes that the molecules of all toxins can pass the membrane without hindrance. All toxins are in the range of 100–2000 Da only and the cut-off of high-flux membranes is greater than 10,000 Da. The mass transfer is dependent on variables such as the blood flow rate, the active surface area, and the dialysate flow rate. The clearance (dialysance) for small molecules with a molecular weight of up to 200 Da usually equals the blood flow rate.

Several mathematical models for the description of kinetics during haemodialysis and the measurement of the dialysance have been described (Hoenich *et al.* 1989; Sargant and Gotch 1989).

The technique of haemodialysis is generally the same in intoxicated patients as it is in the patient with uraemia. The use of bicarbonate buffer in the dialysis solution is mandatory because it helps to correct the acidosis caused by many toxic substances without relying on hepatic conversion of lactate.

The removal of various substances is limited principally by physicochemical factors. Toxins eliminated by glomerular filtration are removed efficiently by dialysis. The efficiency of haemodialysis is further affected by the total body clearance, the distribution of the toxin in the body, and the rate of equilibration of the toxic agent from the peripheral tissues to blood.

Haemodialysis in the treatment of poisoning is not time-limited because the permeability of the membrane is usually not affected by duration of use and the dialysis solution is prepared continuously. In thallium intoxication, haemodialysis sessions of more than 100 h have been performed.

Differential indications for the use of haemodialysis in poisonings have recently been published (Seyffart 1997).

The removal of lipid-soluble toxins is very limited since the dialysis solution is in an aqueous phase. Also, any toxins bound to plasma proteins cannot cross the dialyser membrane.

Haemofiltration

In haemofiltration, an arteriovenous pressure difference generates convective transport of solutes through hollow fibre or flat sheet (disc) membranes. It allows a high flux of plasma water and molecules with a relative molecular mass of up to 40,000 Da. Because of the convective nature of the filtration process, the removal rate of a solute with a molecular mass less than the cut-off mass for the membrane is proportional to its concentration in the blood and independent of its size. Because of the high blood flow rate of more than 300 ml/min needed to derive the necessary transmembrane pressure, haemofiltration must be used with care in hypotensive patients. Since most toxins have a molecular weight of less than 1000 Da, they can be removed easily by haemodialysis, so the indication for haemofiltration in acute poisoning is limited.

Haemoperfusion

In haemoperfusion, blood circulates from the patient through a cartridge or column containing adsorbent material. Guenzet *et al.* (1985) have proposed a mathematical description of the theory of haemoperfusion for drugs obeying different one-compartment pharmacokinetic models. In practice, the clearance by haemoperfusion can be calculated with mathematical models used for haemodialysis. The rate-limiting factors in toxin removal during haemoperfusion are the affinity of the adsorbent for the toxin, the rate of blood-flow through the adsorbent, the total body clearance and the distribution of the toxin in the body, and the rate of equilibration of the toxic agent from the peripheral tissue to blood.

The process of haemoperfusion was introduced by Muirhead and Reid (1948) who used a mixture of charged cation- and anion-exchange resin for the removal of uraemic toxins. Their investigations, and later that of others using separate anion- and cation-exchange resins, revealed serious side-effects such as electrolyte disturbances, pyrogenic reactions, thrombocytopenia, and haemolysis. The use of charged resins was therefore not pursued.

Yatzidis (1964) and Yatzidis *et al.* (1965) introduced the first usable haemoperfusion device for removal of poisons and other solutes by using activated charcoal. Rosenbaum *et al.* (1970) introduced a non-ionic (electrically neutral) polystyrene exchange resin (Amberlite XAD) as an alternative adsorbent to activated charcoal in haemoperfusion. Both activated charcoal (uncoated and coated) and the uncoated exchange resin Amberlite XAD-4 have undergone further developments. Because of the dramatic decline in poisonings, to date, Amberlite XAD-4 and activated charcoal haemoperfusion devices are no longer available in all countries.

Differential indications for the use of haemoperfusion using activated charcoal and exchange resins in poisonings are described in detail by Seyffart (1997).

Activated charcoal

Active carbon is manufactured by the carbonization (pyrolytic decomposition of the starting material to derive pure carbon) followed by activation, almost exclusively of vegetable products (Smisek and Cerny 1970; Cooney 1995). During activation, carbon (charcoal) is treated with steam at 600–900°C to erode selectively the internal surface of the charcoal in order to develop a greater and finer network of pores, increasing the surface area available for adsorption. Prior to activation, charcoal has a specific surface area of several m^2/g, but after activation the surface area is in the range of 600–2000 m^2/g. The adsorption capacity of activated charcoal is due to van der Waals forces (electronic interactions) between pure carbon and the uncharged molecule of an agent.

Activated charcoal adsorbs unpolar (uncharged) agents on non-polar sites of molecules. It is held to be the universal antidote, but this is not the case. There is limited adsorption capacity for ionized agents such as electrolytes (sodium, potassium, calcium) and acids and bases in the stage of ionization (at a certain pK_a, see below).

Exchange resin

The procedure of adsorption by exchange resins is similar to that of activated charcoal, utilizing van der Waals forces at a large surface area provided by a polymer. Amberlite XAD-4 is an uncharged (electrically neutral) resin, consisting of small, highly porous globules that possess an apparent active surface area of 750 m^2/g and which come directly in contact with blood (uncoated). As with activated charcoal, predominantly unionized agents will be adsorbed. In contrast to activated charcoal, the binding is reversible so that the material may be regenerated.

Hydrophobic (lipophilic) substances may be adsorbed in relatively larger amounts by Amberlite XAD-4 than by activated charcoal. Exchange resins, unlike activated charcoal, are not the first choice adsorbents (antidotes). According to the manufacturer, the adsorptive property and capacity *per se* cannot be predicted for toxins; so present knowledge is based on *in vitro* experiments and the results from clinical detoxification.

Combined haemodialysis–haemoperfusion

De Broe *et al.* (1979) published the first results of the application of prolonged combined haemodialysis–haemoperfusion to cases of severe poisoning. The extracorporeal circuit consisted of haemoperfusion and haemodialysis placed in series whereby the cartridge is placed between blood pump and dialyser (predialysis) (Fig. 1). The combination utilizes two physicochemically different mechanisms, adsorption and diffusion. For many drugs the overall clearance is significantly greater than if only one method is used because both the free and the protein-bound agent are eliminated (Verpooten and de Broe 1984). The combination is very efficient for the removal of toxins with a small volume of distribution. Most agents will be removed within 4–6 h. For toxins having a larger volume of distribution (1–3 l/kg of body weight) treatment can be prolonged to 10 h or more, to be efficient, providing the advantage of removing the agent during redistribution (rebound phenomenon). This combination, by removing the greatest quantity of toxins within the shortest time, has obvious clinical advantages.

In clinical practice, haemodialysis is an important adjunctive treatment of various complications of toxin action, including metabolic acidosis, electrolyte disturbance, hypothermia and hyperthermia, fluid overload and pulmonary oedema, and acute renal failure.

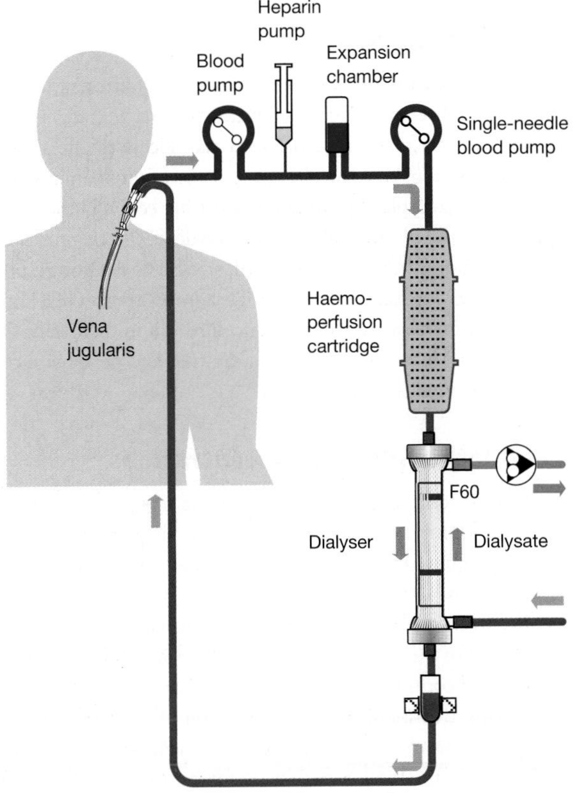

Fig. 1 Haemodialysis–haemoperfusion circuit (single-needle setting).

Continuous detoxification methods (see Chapter 10.4)

Combinations of different renal replacement measures have gained interest for the treatment of acute renal failure or diuretic-resistant fluid overload in critically ill patients with multiple organ failure, haemodynamic instability, electrolyte imbalance, or acid–base disturbances. In the continuous haemoperfusion system, a cartridge containing activated charcoal or exchange resins is used.

Drug removal

In addition to low-flow techniques of replacement of renal function, there is a significant removal of drugs and toxins during continuous treatment (Pond *et al.* 1987; Riegel 1995). In severe intoxication, conventional haemodialysis or haemoperfusion should be performed first and when the toxins redistribute (rebound phenomenon), continuous methods should be instituted thereafter. Continuous methods are useful for intoxicants such as paraquat, lithium, thallium, methotrexate, procainamide, and methanol. They are useful even if the treatment of an intoxication is initiated many hours or days after exposure.

Plasmapheresis

Plasmapheresis involves the removal of the patient's plasma by means of centrifugal or filtration devices, with substitution of fresh plasma or crystalloid solution. It involves exchange of 1–3 l of plasma per session; the maximal quantity of drug removed will be its concentration multiplied by the volume of plasma removed.

It has been used, albeit infrequently, in the treatment of poisoning. It is most useful for the removal of strongly protein-bound agents or complexes. Its efficacy in various poisonings has been reported anecdotally, but the role in treatment of poisonings is not clearly established (Seyffart 1982).

Factors determining, and indications for, extracorporeal removal of toxins

As a general guideline, any extracorporeal detoxification measure is clinically valuable only if the rate of removal of the toxins contributes a significant addition to the spontaneous rate of elimination either by biotransformation or renal, hepatic, and/or pulmonary excretion. This will depend on certain pharmacokinetic and toxicokinetic parameters (conditions). Some of these, such as plasma protein binding and volume of distribution, play a minor role in choosing the appropriate treatment of poisoning.

In drug overdose and toxic doses of poisons, toxicokinetics usually differ significantly from pharmacokinetics. They are unknown in extremely high doses and tend to become unpredictable if toxic lesions diminish or damage the function of certain organs or systems (hepatic failure, hypotension). They are difficult to predict in patients with underlying diseases, and there are differences between adults and children and the elderly. In clinical practice, the general indications for, and evaluation of application of, extracorporeal detoxification require knowledge of the following:

(1) toxic and 'lethal' dose;

(2) toxic and lethal plasma concentrations;

(3) plasma concentration;

(4) plasma protein binding;

(5) ionization and non-ionic diffusion;

(6) distribution in body compartments, including entering organs or cells, binding to receptors, and storage elsewhere;

(7) redistribution;

(8) (specific) toxic symptoms and the grade of their severity;

(9) the available capacity of the treatment modality.

Other pharmacokinetic parameters are less decisive. Neither the molecular weight of the intoxicant nor its water and lipid solubility in plasma is a limiting factor (see above). Biotransformation is a complex but not a determining factor; various metabolites are effectively removable, for example trichloroethanol and trichloroacetic acid in chloral hydrate poisoning. The rate of natural excretion is relevant only in so far as it competes with technical removal. In severe poisoning, auxiliary (aggressive) removal may be indicated to prevent life-threatening adverse effects, despite apparently sufficient natural removal.

Toxic dose

Determination

A toxic dose can be defined as the amount of toxin causing particular symptoms and signs in an otherwise healthy subject. When considering the indication for extracorporeal removal measures, the borderline of a toxic dose is difficult to define because doses presumed to be toxic do not necessarily cause distinct and comparable symptoms in different organisms or individuals. The amount of toxin administered is seldom precisely known, especially in attempted suicide. In practice, the dose of a toxin is crudely interpreted from the remaining content of bottles or drug boxes, or the description by the patient or poisoner. Vomiting before and after admission, gastric lavage (see below), and renal excretion may modify the amount of the toxin available. One should therefore be cautious in considering aggressive toxin removal, except for the most dangerous, and be guided by the severity of toxic symptoms (see below). In principle, an estimated toxic dose in the gram-range is potentially life-threatening with most drugs and almost all known toxins, and should be an indication to adopt active measures.

Influence by digestive absorption

The absorption, predominantly from the gastrointestinal tract, is an important factor when estimating the toxic dose. Digestive absorption varies, from one substance to another, between 2 and 95 per cent of the ingested dose. Absorption may be unimpeded and complete but is often delayed. Since the plasma concentration of an agent between the phase of absorption and distribution is the key to the efficacy of haemodialysis and haemoperfusion, knowledge of the toxin's fate in the gut is essential. When there are severe toxic symptoms it should be assumed that absorption is complete and toxic plasma concentrations are already at their peak or declining. However, if a large overdose of a toxin, known for its delayed absorption, has been ingested and toxic symptoms are actually not severe, the reverse is likely to be true. With increasing doses, absorption may decrease because of a limitation of the agent's liberation, saturation of active absorption processes, a dose-related decrease of blood circulation, or limitation of the velocity of the solution caused by paralysis of the intestine with decreased motility, for example in overdose of anticholinergic drugs. When there is delayed absorption, increasing toxicity is to be expected, and the need for aggressive treatment should be considered. If toxic symptoms increase with time, it implies that (continuous) extracorporeal toxin removal should have been applied earlier.

Influence of gastric decontamination

The apparent toxic dose is modified by the efficacy of toxin elimination by gastric lavage and instilled adsorbents prior to absorption. If the amount ingested is known, which is unfortunately often not the case, it would be ideal to calculate the remaining dose as well as plasma and total body concentration by estimating the portion being lavaged and adsorbed. During lavage, fragments of the toxic agent (tablets) can be harvested and the concentration of the intoxicant can be measured in the lavage solution. The adsorptive capacity of activated charcoal is known for many toxins. However, this procedure cannot be conducted in most cases. Gastric 'decontamination' is usually the first measure of intoxication treatment.

'Lethal' dose

In the past, the lethal dose of an intoxicant has been predicted from either animal experiments (LD_{50}) or human case reports. Human data have often been derived from dead patients or patients who died shortly after admission or during the clinical course. With the advent of dialysis and haemoperfusion, the value of existing data of lethal doses became less reliable because patients are now able to survive much higher than those receiving routine support only. Thus, for most toxic agents a 'classical lethal dose' cannot be assumed any longer. In any intoxicated patient, a high toxic dose is an absolute indication to employ appropriate extracorporeal detoxification measures.

Plasma concentration

Intoxicants enter the plasma by gastrointestinal, pulmonary, or skin absorption, or by direct intravenous administration.

Since any extracorporeal measure only has access to the systemic circulation, it is obvious that the plasma concentration of an intoxicant must be high. For example, digoxin, of which 1 per cent of a therapeutic dose is present in the blood, will, even in overdose, not be removed in an appreciable amount. On the other hand, acute intoxication resulting from a solitary overdose of a drug or a single administration of a known toxin will usually increase the plasma concentration immediately. Only later can an equilibrium between plasma, central, and peripheral compartments be assumed (see below).

Toxic and lethal plasma concentrations

In contrast to the toxic and 'lethal' dose, a toxic plasma concentration correlates more closely with toxic symptoms. Toxic plasma concentrations have been quoted to correlate with different stages and clinical severity (degrees) of actual toxicity. As with toxic doses, toxic and lethal plasma concentrations are usually derived from case reports (Winek 1976). The proof of the efficacy of haemodialysis and haemoperfusion in poisonings has commonly been documented either as a significant reduction during treatment or, as a significant clinical improvement following a reduction in the plasma concentration. For technical reasons, the part of the total dose of an intoxicant removed in dialysis solution or in the content of the cartridge has rarely been documented.

In most cases, the removal rate was in the range of 1–10 per cent of dose. The intoxicant is first removed from the plasma and later from the central compartment (see below). In general, a toxic plasma concentration that is associated with a risk of death (lethal plasma concentration) and that is associated with severe clinical symptoms is an absolute indication for an attempt at extracorporeal detoxification.

Plasma protein binding

A key factor influencing the actual distribution of a drug in the blood is its binding to plasma proteins. Drugs vary in their degree of protein binding and for a variety of intoxicants this is unknown. Examples of compounds for which there is virtually no protein binding are: alcohols, acids, aminoglycosides, atenolol, and lithium; examples of toxins with high protein binding are: arsenic, calcium-channel blockers, benzodiazepines, phenytoin, and tricyclic antidepressants. However, plasma protein binding is usually reversible, since an agent can be distributed only when released from plasma protein.

Plasma protein binding is a limiting factor in extracorporeal removal of intoxicants, by haemodialysis and haemofiltration (see above). Additionally, in drug overdose, following high drug concentration in plasma, the degree of binding will decrease in most cases because of saturation of the available protein. With regard to extracorporeal detoxification, plasma protein binding has two toxicological aspects. First, the capacity is unpredictable and may soon be exhausted, so that more free drug than expected (or estimated by experimental data) may be available for clearance. Second, if an agent is present in a state in which the bound portion is, for example, 80 per cent and the binding is reversible, early removal of the unbound agent by diffusion (haemodialysis and continuous methods) may lead to liberation of bound drug, and thus increase removal significantly.

Shortly after ingestion of an overdose with an intoxicant possessing high plasma protein binding, a high percentage of free substance is expected to be available because plasma protein binding may be incomplete or saturated. In this phase, haemodialysis may be worthwhile. Usually haemodialysis is not used for drugs that are highly protein-bound.

Ionization and non-ionic diffusion

On its way from the circulation to the target organ or cell, an intoxicant has to pass several membranes. Different physicochemical mechanisms are capable of carrying agents across a succession of membrane barriers. The mechanism of penetration through the capillary membrane is relevant to intoxication.

Most drugs, as well as various toxins, are either acids or bases. They are present in solution as both the non-ionized and ionized species. The non-ionized (non-polar) molecules are usually lipid soluble, the ionized are more water soluble. The major mechanism by which agents pass through membranes is penetration via the lipoprotein system. This system carries only non-ionized molecules (non-ionic diffusion). In contrast, ionized agents are unable to penetrate lipid membranes, they are distributed into the organism by diffusion through pores in membranes. In organic membranes, the number of pores is very limited, thus the disappearance of ionized agents from the circulation is slow.

The extent of ionization is expressed by the pK_a, for both acids and bases. The pK is that pH at which the electrolyte (drug or toxin) exists half in the ionized and half in the non-ionized form (Henderson–Hasselbalch equation). Since most substances exist as weak acids or bases, and the pH in most regions of the body is generally stable at about 7.4, pK_a is an important determinant of lipid solubility and, consequently, of the rate of membrane transport. For example, diazepam is a weak base with a pK_a of 3.31. It exists in blood mostly in non-ionized (lipid-soluble) form and is, thus, rapidly and almost completely distributed throughout the body. Thus, the more a toxic agent exists, or remains in plasma, in its ionized form, the more can be removed by haemodialysis.

Distribution, volume of distribution, and redistribution

In addition to toxic symptoms, the most important factor determining the indication for extracorporeal detoxification is the distribution of the intoxicant to body compartments and its removal. Distribution will depend on the route of administration, plasma and tissue protein binding, blood flow, diffusion rate, degree of ionization (pK_a), and partitioning to different tissues.

Apparent volume of distribution

The extent to which a substance distributes throughout the body is estimated by relating the plasma concentration after distribution to the amount of substance in the body, the volume of distribution. The volume of distribution is an imaginary space (apparent volume of distribution, l/kg of body weight). Thallium, for example, a non-polar compound, is supposed to possess an extremely large volume of distribution of 20 l/kg, that is in a patient of 70 kg of body weight it would be 1400 l. Commonly, only one volume of distribution is assumed, as demonstrated with thallium. This is inadequate for understanding the efficiency of intoxicant removal. The agent disappears initially (and mostly rapidly) from the blood compartment (volume 5.5 l, 8 per cent of body volume) to the central compartment, consisting of major organs such as the lungs, brain, heart, liver, kidneys, and intestine (volume about 7 l, 10 per cent of body volume, blood flow rate 1000–5700 ml/min), and is then slowly distributed to the peripheral compartment, which includes the muscles, adipose tissue, skin, and bones (volume about 57.5 l, 72 per cent of the body volume, blood flow rate 200–1200 ml/min) (Fig. 2). Assuming that an equilibrium exists after a certain period following intoxication, more than 70 per cent of a dose will be in the peripheral compartment.

However, the actual situation is more complicated because intoxicants are often concentrated in a specific tissue. Some may achieve greatest concentration at their site of toxic action, such as carbon monoxide in haemoglobin and paraquat in the lungs. Other agents concentrate at sites other than the site of toxic action. Lead, for example, is stored in the bone, while the toxic effects are due to lead in the soft tissue. The compartment where the intoxicant is concentrated can be thought of as a storage depot.

With regard to the apparent volume of distribution, consider the case of amitriptyline which is extremely high (20 l/kg). Because of its high plasma protein binding (almost 95 per cent), dialysis is ineffective, but it can be removed from plasma by haemoperfusion. A toxic dose of 1 g given to a 70-kg person will yield a plasma concentration of 0.0007 mg/ml. With maximal extraction by haemoperfusion at a blood flow rate of 200 ml/min, the clearance may reach 200 ml/min. Even with the almost total removal from the blood compartment,

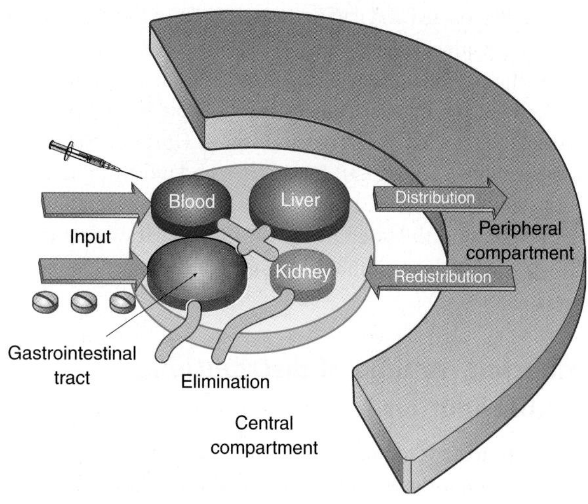

Fig. 2 Pharmacokinetic compartments.

the actual amount of drug removed by haemoperfusion will be 0.14 mg/min, or 33.6 mg in a session lasting 4 h. Thus, haemoperfusion is a highly efficient way of removing amitriptyline from the blood compartment, but is obviously relatively slow in effecting total elimination.

The relationship between the virtual volume of distribution and efficacy of extracorporeal detoxification

At any volume of distribution less than 0.5 l/kg, a significant amount of an intoxicant will be removed by haemoperfusion from both the plasma and the central compartment because of rapid redistribution to the 'empty' plasma space. This usually results in clinical improvement because the toxin has not yet been distributed to the peripheral compartment (high affinity to central organs, a target organ, or receptors). But if the volume of distribution greatly exceeds 0.5 l/kg and the equilibration is complete, the intoxicant will, as in the first case, be removed by haemoperfusion initially from the blood and then from the central compartment. However, the concentration in the central compartment will be much less because of the filling of the huge peripheral space. Since the redistribution from the peripheral compartment is greatly delayed, the low concentration of the central compartment will be decreased more rapidly, resulting in clinical improvement. When redistribution is slow, storage depots can be considered as protecting organs, preventing high concentrations of the intoxicant from being achieved at the site of its toxic action.

This toxicokinetic rule is often not taken into account. It emphasizes the usefulness of extracorporeal detoxification. In severe poisoning the outcome can usually not be predicted, but an attempt with intoxicant removal is always worthwhile in view of the complex toxicokinetics. Clearly, the earlier extracorporeal removal can be started, the less the toxin will be distributed. This is not usually possible in suicide cases.

For a variety of agents, such as paraquat, extracorporeal measures can remove the agent more rapidly from the plasma than it can be replaced from tissue stores by redistribution (rebound phenomenon). The treatment will become inefficient after a certain period and should therefore be discontinued and repeated later. Treatment of patients poisoned by agents with a significant redistribution requires continuous measures to stop the intoxicant from repeating its toxic effects. Fluctuating improvement and deterioration caused by the rebound phenomenon is well recognized in severe poisoning.

However, in cases of irreversible toxic damage to a target organ, for example by death-cap toxins, the value of eliminating intoxicants following redistribution is questionable.

Toxic symptoms

These can be divided into early and late symptoms, and those of actual organ injury. Early symptoms, such as nausea, vomiting, fatigue, disorientation, dizziness, confusion, and coma grades I and II (Reed *et al.* 1952), are not usually indications for extracorporeal detoxification. The exception is the perfidious toxin which leads initially to a 'silent' period or minor symptoms. If the late symptoms, such as coma grades III and IV (Reed *et al.* 1952), characterized by paralysis which leads to cardiac and respiratory disorders or arrest, hypothermia and hyperthermia, are present, haemodialysis and/or haemoperfusion are mandatory if toxin removal is possible by these methods. The exception is hypotension resistant to any therapy and cardiopulmonary arrest.

Extracorporeal measures are usually useless in (late) organ injury such as hepatic failure and disseminated intravascular coagulation. Paraquat is an exception. In the third stage, some days after exposure, lung injury supervenes and, surprisingly, haemoperfusion has been associated with unexpected improvement.

Drug concentrations and plasma half-life

In most intoxications, drug concentrations and plasma half-life do not predict or correlate with the state of toxicity in the patients. But the technical effectiveness of haemodialysis and haemoperfusion may be evaluated by measuring changes in the plasma half-life. Phenobarbital, for example, has a total body clearance of about 5 ml/min. Its plasma protein binding is small (about 20 per cent). During a haemodialysis treatment with a clearance of 65 ml/min, its removal accounts for 93 per cent of the total elimination so that the plasma half-life is diminished to 8 h (7 per cent of normal). A significant decrease in plasma half-life is of great clinical importance in massive overdose in view of threatening adverse effects such as coma and pneumonitis. However, the determination of actual plasma concentrations of many drugs and almost all toxic agents is time-consuming and not available in the majority of hospitals.

Clinical indications and choice of method of extracorporeal detoxification

Despite several decades of extensive experience, indications for extracorporeal detoxification are not clear-cut. With supportive treatment alone, spontaneous recovery usually occurs in 98 per cent of poisoned patients in intensive-care units (Bismuth 1990). Precise and critical indications and differential indications exist for a significant number of drugs in overdose and recognized toxins (Seyffart 1983, 1997; Haddad and Winchester 1990, 1997). Simple tools for the evaluation of indications are given in tables, in which agents are listed which have been removed either by haemodialysis or haemoperfusion not only in poisoning but also when used therapeutically (Gibson and Nelson 1977; Winchester *et al.* 1977; Takki *et al.* 1978; Pond *et al.* 1979; Rosenberg *et al.* 1981; Verpooten and de Broe 1984; Winchester 1986; Cutler *et al.* 1987; Schreiner 1987; Garella 1988; Vale 1993). Tables presenting a summary of the indications and differential indications for choice of modality for a large number of agents are available (Seyffart 1997; Schreiner 1987).

Indications regarding time-span of exposure to admission

Following accidental poisonings, patients are usually brought to hospital immediately; thus decisions for treatment modalities are guided by the immediate situation. In contrast, suicide or homicide patients are usually seen in hospitals after several hours or days. Most of the toxin will have been absorbed, entered the central and peripheral compartments, and may have caused serious and irreversible damage. Examples include paracetamol, amanitins, and phalloidins from death cap, paraquat, and arsenic. They are partly present in blood and tissues, and a significant amount can be removed by haemoperfusion. The toxic lesions are nevertheless irreversible despite significant removal, and extracorporeal removal is therefore pointless. This paradox may be difficult to explain to colleagues and relatives of the patient.

Differential indication regarding haemodialysis and haemoperfusion

The characteristics of the intoxicant point to the need for either haemodialysis or haemoperfusion. The differential indications have been worked out for the common and most important agents (Seyffart 1997), but there is still uncertainty for rarer toxins. The choice is influenced more by empirical and experimental experience rather than by results of research. Often the combined use of both techniques is warranted.

Differential indications regarding haemoperfusion with activated charcoal or exchange resin

Both adsorbents are effective in unpolar intoxicants. Since the principle of adsorption is the same in both adsorbents, there are no differential indications. The postulation that resins bind lipophilic agents to a greater extent than charcoal has little physicochemical justification. The adsorptive capacity of activated charcoal has been investigated systematically, mainly with regard to drugs dangerous in overdose and toxins, such as pesticides. However, clinical experience with resins is limited.

Contraindications

Established contraindications do not exist, relative contraindications are: hypotension resistant to any therapy and cardiovascular, pulmonary, and hepatic failure.

Amanita phalloides

The complexity of extracorporeal detoxification in severe poisoning is well illustrated by one of the most terrible and commonly fatal poisonings. It is caused by the toxins amanitin and phalloidin from the death cap (*Amanita phalloides*) (Fig. 3) (Seyffart 1997). The molecular weight of the toxins is less than 1000 Da, and following absorption none is bound to plasma proteins; thus, extracorporeal detoxification measures have frequently been used for their removal. Almost all have failed because of the particular actions of these toxins. The first toxic phase, within 6–40 h of ingestion, is characterized by gastrointestinal symptoms caused by the phalloidins. After a latent phase of 3–5 days, the illness enters the second, dramatic phase, characterized by severe hepatic damage, almost always fatal, caused by amanitins. Amanitins are rapidly absorbed, distributed, and enter hepatic cells during the first phase. They slowly begin to destroy the endoplasmic reticulum, leading to a chain reaction that triggers cleavage reactions which destroy almost all liver cells. This chain reaction is unstoppable, even when the toxin is no longer present. Because of this, even early attempts to remove the toxin fail. It should be remembered that in poisoning with a potentially lethal dose of death caps (consumption of more than one developed toadstool) a substantial amount of toxin reaches the liver and other organs quicker than it could be eliminated by any extracorporeal detoxification measure. The initial toxic symptoms usually show up 8–10 h after ingestion, after which all desperate attempts will be unsuccessful and death is inevitable.

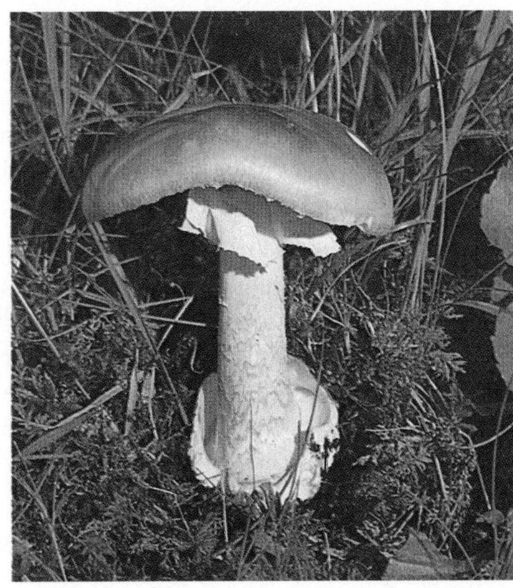

Fig. 3 Death cap (*Amanita phalloides*).

Summary

Despite the controversy with which haemodialysis, haemoperfusion, and related effective extracorporeal detoxification measures are surrounded, valuable general criteria for their use do exist.

The indications for *dialysis* have been clearly set out by Schreiner (1958).

1. The poison molecule should diffuse through a dialysis membrane such as cellulose from plasma water and should have a reasonable removal rate, or 'dialysance'.

2. The poison must be sufficiently well distributed in accessible body-fluid compartments. If substantial fractions of the absorbed poison are bound to protein, concentrated in inaccessible fluid compartments (e.g. cerebrospinal fluid), or attain a significant

intracellular concentration, then the effect of dialysis will be limited. The restriction is diminished, however, if the inaccessible portion rapidly equilibrates with the plasma.

3. There should be a relationship between the blood concentration, the duration of the body's exposure to the circulating poison, and toxicity.
4. The amount of poison dialysed must constitute a significant addition to the normal body mechanism for dealing with the particular poison under consideration. This should include metabolism, conjugation, and elimination of the substance by bowel and kidney.

With time the indications have been broadened and haemoperfusion has become available. These indications have been summarized by Rosenbaum *et al.* (1980), Winchester (1986), and Pond (1991), and are set out below.

1. Progressive clinical deterioration despite intensive supportive therapy and appropriate clinical management.
2. Severe intoxication with abnormal vital signs, including depression of mid-brain function leading to hypoventilation or apnoea, severe hypothermia and hypotension despite fluid replacement, and when vasoactive therapy is needed.
3. Prolonged coma grades III and IV, and prolonged assisted ventilation for more than 48 h.
4. Development of complications of coma, such as pneumonia or septicaemia, underlying conditions predisposing to such complications (e.g. obstructive lung disease), and peripheral neuropathy due to pressure ischaemia.
5. Acute renal failure caused by a (potentially) nephrotoxic intoxicant.
6. Impairment of metabolism and excretion of the intoxicant in the presence of hepatic, cardiac, or renal insufficiency.
7. Intoxication with agents with metabolic and/or delayed effects, such as methanol, ethylene glycol, and paraquat.
8. Intoxication with an extractable drug or poison, which can be removed at a rate exceeding endogenous elimination by liver or kidney.
9. Ingestion and probable absorption of a highly toxic (potentially lethal) dose (best determined after gastric decontamination). An estimated toxic dose in the gram-range is potentially life-threatening with most drugs and almost all genuine toxins.
10. A potentially fatal plasma concentration as assessed by previous experience of risk of death and severe clinical sequelae.

References

Bismuth, C. (1990). Biological valuation of extra-corporeal techniques in acute poisoning. *Acta Clinica Belgica* **45** (Suppl. 13), 20–28.

Cooney, D. O. *Activated Charcoal in Medical Applications.* New York, NY: Marcel Dekker, 1995.

Cutler, R. E., Forland, S. C., Hammond, P. G. S., and Evans, J. R. (1987). Extracorporeal removal of drugs and poisons by hemodialysis and hemoperfusion. *Annual Review of Pharmacology and Toxicology* **27**, 169–191.

De Broe, M. E., Verpooten, G. A., and van Haesebrouck, B. (1979). Recent experience with prolonged hemoperfusion–hemodialysis treatment. *Artificial Organs* **3**, 188–190.

Doolan, P. D., Walsh, W. P., Kyle, L. H., and Wishinsky, H. (1951). Acetylsalicylic acid intoxication: a proposed method of treatment. *Journal of the American Medical Association* **146**, 105–106.

Finberg, L., Kiley, J., and Luttrell, C. N. (1963). Mass accidental salt poisoning in infancy. A study of a hospital disaster. *Journal of the American Medical Association* **184**, 121–124.

Garella, S. (1988). Extracorporeal techniques in the treatment of exogenous intoxications. *Kidney International* **33**, 735–754.

Gibson, T. P. and Nelson, H. A. (1977). Drug kinetics and artificial kidneys. *Clinical Pharmacokinetics* **2**, 403–426.

Guenzet, J., Bourin, M., Laurent, D., and Aminou, T. (1985). Theoretical study of haemoperfusion: drugs obeying a one-compartment pharmacokinetic model. *Methods and Findings in Experimental Clinical Pharmacology* **7**, 259.

Haddad, L. M. and Winchester, J. F., ed. *Clinical Management of Poisoning and Drug Overdose* 1st edn. Philadelphia, PA: Saunders, 1983.

Haddad, L. M. and Winchester, J. F., ed. *Clinical Management of Poisoning and Drug Overdose* 2nd edn. Philadelphia, PA: Saunders, 1990.

Haddad, L. M., Shannon, M. W., and Winchester, J. F., ed. *Clinical Management of Poisoning and Drug Overdose* 3rd edn. Philadelphia, PA: Saunders, 1997.

Hoenich, N. A., Woffinden, C., and Ward, M. K. Dialysers. In *Replacement of Renal Function by Dialysis* 3rd edn. (ed. J. F. Maher), pp. 144–180. Dordrecht: Kluwer Academic Publishers, 1989.

Muirhead, E. E. and Reid, A. F. (1948). Resin artificial kidney. *Journal of Laboratory and Clinical Medicine* **33**, 841–844.

Pond, S. M. (1991). Extracorporeal techniques in the treatment of poisoned patients. *Medical Journal of Australia* **154**, 617–622.

Pond, S. M., Rosenberg, J., Benowitz, N. L., and Takki, S. (1979). Pharmacokinetics of haemoperfusion for drug overdose. *Clinical Pharmacokinetics* **4**, 329–354.

Pond, S. M. *et al.* (1987). Repeated hemoperfusion and continuous arteriovenous hemofiltration in a paraquat poisoned patient. *Journal of Toxicology. Clinical Toxicology* **25**, 305.

Reed, C., Driggs, M. F., and Foote, C. C. (1952). Acute barbiturate intoxication: a study of 300 cases based on a physiologic system of classification of the severity of the intoxication. *Annals of Internal Medicine* **37**, 290.

Riegel, W. (1995). Behandlung exogener Intoxikationen. *Anästhesiologie Intensivmedizin* **36**, 299.

Rosenbaum, J. L., Winsten, S., Kramer, M. S., Moros, J., and Raja, R. (1970). Resin hemoperfusion in the treatment of drug intoxication. *Transactions of the American Society of Artificial Internal Organs* **16**, 134.

Rosenbaum, J. L., Kramer, M. S., Raja, R. M., Krug, M. J., and Holiday, C. G. (1980). Current status of hemoperfusion in toxicology. *Clinical Toxicology* **17**, 493.

Rosenberg, J., Benowitz, N. L., and Pond, S. (1981). Pharmacokinetics of drug overdose. *Clinical Pharmacokinetics* **6**, 161–192.

Sargant, J. A. and Gotch, F. A. Principles and biophysics of dialysis. In *Replacement of Renal Function by Dialysis* 3rd edn. (ed. J. F. Maher), pp. 87–143. Dordrecht: Kluwer Academic Publishers, 1989.

Schreiner, G. E. (1958). The role of hemodialysis (artificial kidney) in acute poisoning. *Archives of Internal Medicine* **102**, 896–913.

Schreiner, G. E. (1987). Perspectives on the hemoperfusion of drugs and toxins. *Biomaterials, Artificial Cells, and Artificial Organs* **15**, 305–321.

Seyffart, G. *Poison Index. Dialysis and Haemoperfusion in Poisonings* 1st edn. Friedberg: Bindernagel, 1977.

Seyffart, G. (1982). Plasmapheresis in the treatment of acute intoxication. *Transactions of the American Society of Artificial Internal Organs* **28**, 673.

Seyffart, G. *Poison Index: Dialysis and Haemoperfusion in Poisonings* 3rd edn. Friedberg: Bindernagel, 1983.

Seyffart, G. *Poison Index. The Treatment of Acute Intoxication* 4th edn. Lengerich: Pabst Scientific Publishers, 1997.

Smisek, M. and Cerny, S. *Active Carbon. Manufacture, Properties and Applications*. Amsterdam: Elsevier, 1970.

Takki, S., Gambertoglio, J. G., Honda, D. H., and Tozer, T. N. (1978). Pharmacokinetic data. Pharmacokinetic evaluation of hemodialysis in acute drug overdose. *Journal of Pharmacokinetics and Biopharmaceutics* **6**, 427–442.

Vale, J. A. (1993). Reviews in medicine: clinical toxicology. *Postgraduate Medical Journal* **69**, 19–32.

Verpooten, G. A. and de Broe, M. E. (1984). Combined hemoperfusion–hemodialysis in severe poisoning: kinetics of drug extraction. *Resuscitation* **11**, 275–289.

Winchester, J. F. (1986). Evolution of artificial organs: extracorporeal removal of drugs. *Artificial Organs* **10**, 316–323.

Winchester, J. F., Gelfand, M. C., Knepshield, J. H., and Schreiner, G. E. (1977). Dialysis and hemoperfusion of poisons and drugs—update. *Transactions of the American Society of Artificial Internal Organs* **23**, 762–842.

Winek, C. L. (1976). Tabulation of therapeutic, toxic, and lethal concentrations of drugs and chemicals in blood. *Clinical Chemistry* **22**, 832–836.

Yatzidis, H. (1964). A convenient hemoperfusion micro-apparatus over charcoal for the treatment of exogenous and endogenous intoxications. Its use as an artificial kidney. *Proceedings of the European Dialysis and Transplant Association* **1**, 83.

Yatzidis, H., Oreopoulos, D., Triantaphylidis, D., Voudiclaris S., Tsaparas, N., and Gavras, H. (1965). Treatment of severe barbiturate poisoning. *Lancet* **2**, 216–217.

10.6 Special acute renal failure problems

10.6.1 Glomerulonephritis, vasculitis, and the nephrotic syndrome

Philip D. Mason

Introduction

About 10 per cent of cases of acute renal failure (Espinel and Gregory 1980; Turney *et al.* 1990) are caused by glomerulonephritis. Its incidence is similar outside Europe and North America (Chugh *et al.* 1989; Bamgboye 1993), and it may be relatively more common in children (McCrory 1970; Kandoth *et al.* 1994) and in the elderly (Hass *et al.* 2000). Early recognition is essential, since treatment may result in preservation or recovery of renal function. Acute renal failure with glomerulonephritis is common in small vessel vasculitis and systemic lupus erythematosus, and is uncommon, although well recognized, in many multisystem diseases. It is rare in association with 'primary' glomerular diseases. Some reports suggest that the prognosis is improving (Turney *et al.* 1990), but such retrospective reviews are difficult to interpret because of the change in case mix. A heterogeneous group of conditions are capable of causing rapidly progressive glomerulonephritis; all of these are fully discussed elsewhere (see also Chapter 3.10).

The term rapidly progressive glomerulonephritis is often used to describe the clinical syndrome of acute renal failure developing over a few months or weeks (but occasionally days) in patients found to have a proliferative, and often crescentic and necrotizing, glomerulonephritis. The term is not particularly useful, since an underlying glomerulonephritis will not be evident until a renal biopsy has been examined. Moreover, acute renal failure may develop in nephrotic patients with non-proliferative glomerulopathies (e.g. membranous, minimal change, and focal–segmental glomerulosclerosis) (see also Chapters 3.5 and 3.7), and may be caused by acute interstitial nephritis (see also Section 6), or may have a quite independent cause, for example acute tubular necrosis (see also Section 10).

The histological findings in acute renal failure caused by proliferative glomerulonephritis are of a focal necrotizing glomerulonephritis usually with crescents (Couser 1982; Neild *et al.* 1983; Glassock 1985) (see also Chapter 3.10). Caution is necessary in interpreting histological reports of 'crescents' because:

1. There is no universally accepted definition of a crescent; rather, there is a spectrum of abnormalities ranging from mild extracapillary proliferation (defined as more than two cells thick in Bowman's space) to extremely cellular circumferential proliferation with glomerular tuft compression and necrosis (Fig. 1). The appearances may also be confounded by the level of the glomerular section.
2. Crescents may be 'fresh' and cellular, representing acute active inflammation, or show a degree of organization and sclerosis (the descriptive terms cellular, fibrocellular, and fibrous crescents are often used) (Fig. 2). Relatively acellular and sclerotic crescents

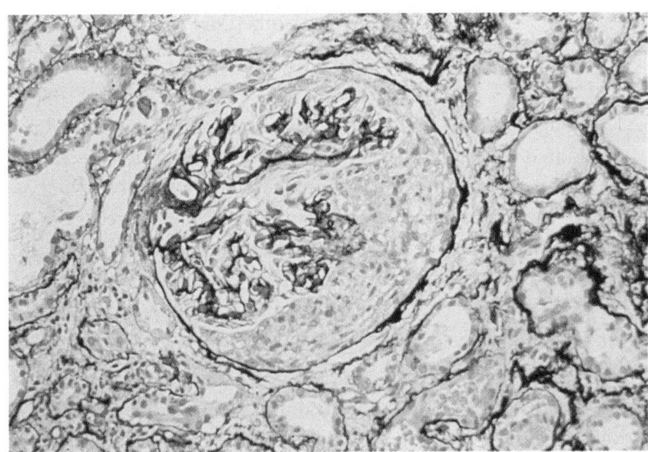

Fig. 1 Photomicrograph of a cellular crescent with necrosis and glomerular tuft compression from a patient with small vessel ANCA-positive vasculitis.

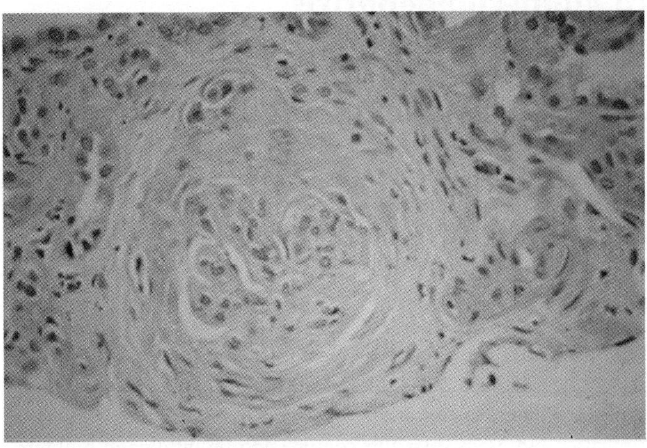

Fig. 2 Photomicrograph of a fibrous crescent.

alone suggest inactive disease, while the presence of fibrous and cellular crescents suggests an active disease process of some duration. This latter pattern is often seen in patients with antineutrophil antiplasmic antibody (ANCA) positive vasculitis but not in anti-glomerular basement membrane (anti-GBM) disease in which all glomeruli appear to be damaged synchronously.

3. Many of the conditions associated with crescentic nephritis are focal and, as a result of sampling error, the proportion of affected glomeruli may vary greatly in two tissue cores taken from the same kidney at the same time and may also change significantly over the course of a few days.

4. Crescents of some description affecting a minority of glomeruli are a relatively common finding, particularly in postinfectious nephritis (see Chapter 3.9), and represent a non-specific response to injury, probably the consequence of fibrin in the capsular space (Heptinstall 1992). There are experimental and clinical data to suggest that crescents may disappear with or without treatment (Faarup *et al.* 1978; Heptinstall 1992). They may be seen in conditions other than glomerulonephritis, for example, in accelerated phase hypertension and even in Alport's syndrome (Heptinstall 1992).

5. There are well-documented cases in which the initial renal biopsy revealed mild diffuse proliferative glomerulonephritis with few or absent crescents which developed, sometimes very rapidly, into a severe necrotizing glomerulonephritis with 100 per cent crescents (Teague *et al.* 1978; Briggs *et al.* 1979).

6. Although in some studies there is a correlation between the proportion of glomeruli (particularly if they are necrotic) affected by crescents and the prognosis for renal recovery (Whitworth *et al.* 1976; Morrin *et al.* 1978), the clinical outcome correlates most closely with the underlying cause of the glomerulonephritis and renal function at the time of treatment (Evans *et al.* 1986). This may be because crescent formation is a consequence of other more complex factors (Atkins *et al.* 1996).

Treatment should be decided mostly from the knowledge of the underlying disorder and the clinical context rather than by the pathological appearance of a kidney biopsy.

Table 1 Causes of acute renal failure associated with glomerular disease

Primary systemic vasculitis
Wegener's granulomatosis
Microscopic polyarteritis
'Idiopathic' or 'lone' nephritis
Churg–Strauss syndrome
Polyarteritis nodosa (uncommon)
Giant-cell arteritis (rare)
Takayasu's arteritis (rare)
Kawasaki's disease (very rare)
Other systemic conditions
Systemic lupus erythematosus
Mixed essential cryoglobulinaemia
Henoch–Schönlein purpura
Behçet's disease
Rheumatoid disease
Relapsing polychondritis
Systemic sclerosis
Infection-related glomerulonephritis
Postinfectious glomerulonephritis
Infective endocarditis
Ventricular shunt infection ('shunt nephritis')
Other infections (e.g. abscesses)
Goodpasture's disease (anti-GBM disease)
'Primary' glomerulonephritis
Mesangial IgA nephropathy
Mesangiocapillary glomerulonephritis
Membranous nephropathy
Minimal change nephropathy
Focal segmental glomerulosclerosis
Neoplasia associated
Carcinoma
Lymphoma
Leukaemia
Drug associated
Hydralazine
Penicillamine
Rifampicin

Causes of acute renal failure due to glomerulonephritis

Table 1 lists the causes of acute renal failure associated with glomerulonephritis and crescents. In Europe and North America small vessel vasculitis ('polyangiitis'), systemic lupus erythematosus, and anti-GBM disease are the usual causes, but infection-associated glomerulonephritis is probably the most common cause worldwide (see Chapter 3.12).

Table 2 Mechanisms of acute renal failure in glomerulonephritis

Glomerular capillary obliteration by inflammation
Vasculitis of larger vessels causing distal ischaemia
Vasomotor tone abnormalities
Endothelin release from damaged endothelium
Reduced nitric oxide production
Sequestration of nitric oxide (e.g. by haemoglobin)
Tubular toxicity
Haemoglobin, free iron

Pathogenesis

The precise mechanism of acute renal failure in glomerulonephritis is likely to be multifactorial (Table 2). The traditional explanation for the reduced glomerular filtration rate (GFR), namely obliteration of capillaries and glomerular tuft compression by influx and proliferation of cells, is undoubtedly true, particularly in fulminant cases of 'crescentic nephritis'. However, it is now evident that other more subtle mechanisms may also be important (Heyman and Brezis 1995), and these may explain the discrepancy between the pathology (including the proportion of glomeruli affected by crescents), the renal function at the time of biopsy, and the final outcome (Evans *et al.* 1986). Reduced GFR may result from vasculitis affecting vessels not represented in the biopsy or changes in vasomotor tone. For instance, endothelial cell damage results in the generation of endothelins and a reduction of nitric oxide production, both of which will reduce glomerular blood flow (Brezis *et al.* 1991). Haemoglobin binds nitric oxide strongly, and its presence in the blood-filled tubules has been suggested as causing vasoconstriction of medullary vessels, potentiating medullary hypoxia and leading to 'acute tubular necrosis' (Heyman and Brezis 1995). Yet another potential mechanism is a direct toxic effect on tubular cells of red blood cells or their contents (particularly the haem pigments or free iron).

Diagnosis

Acute glomerulonephritis with or without systemic vasculitis must always be considered in the differential diagnosis of acute renal failure. The history and examination often provide important clues to the underlying cause of renal failure, and a number of laboratory and radiological tests will add further diagnostic information. In the absence of a clear-cut cause of acute renal failure, a renal biopsy provides the most rapid route to the diagnosis. However, the wider availability of ANCA tests and solid phase enzyme-linked immunosorbent assay (ELISA) to detect anti-MPO and PR3 antibodies has resulted in earlier recognition of small vessel vasculitis, particularly in hospitals in which renal biopsy is not available.

Clinical features (see also Chapter 10.3)

The history and examination often provide vital clues to the diagnosis of acute renal failure due to glomerulonephritis, particularly when associated with systemic disorders. The history will often indicate other possible causes of renal failure, such as acute tubular necrosis due to sepsis, hypotension, or rhabdomyolysis. It is important to question patients about fever, possible preceding infections, travel, and their medication history. The thorough systemic review should include enquiries about myalgia, arthralgia/arthritis, skin rashes, mouth ulcers and ear, nose, throat, and eye problems, chest pain, haemoptysis, and symptoms of neuropathy.

Some symptoms and signs such as lethargy, nausea, oedema, and hypertension have little discriminatory value, while others may strongly indicate a single diagnosis or a small-number of differential diagnoses. For instance, the presence of a vasculitic rash with arthritis/arthralgia suggests the possibility of vasculitis either of the primary small-vessel type or secondary to lupus, cryoglobulinaemia, Henoch–Schönlein purpura, or endocarditis (Table 3). The common clinical features are listed in Table 3. Not all features will be present in every patient, and the presence of symptoms and signs other than those indicated does not automatically exclude the diagnosis. For instance, while hypertension is common in renal failure with fluid retention whatever the cause, severe hypertension (with 'accelerated phase') is well recognized in systemic

Table 3 Symptoms and signs in multisystem disease-associated acute renal failure

	GD	PV	SLE	CG	HSP	SS	BD	RD	RP	PIGN	IE
Fever		+	+	+	+		+	+			+
Severe HT			+			+				+	
Skin rash		+	+	+	+	a	b				+
Alopecia			+								
Mouth ulcers		+	+				+				
Arthralgia		+	+	+	+	+	+	+	+	+	+
Myalgia		+	+							+	+
ENT		+[c]							+		
Eyes		+	+				+	+	+		
Pleurisy		+	+								+
Haemoptysis	+	+	+								
Neuropathy		+	+	+				+	d		+
Abdominal pain		+	+		+	+					
Diarrhoea		(+)	+			+					
Murmur			+								+

[a] Skin is involved but not usually as a rash.

[b] Pustular lesions/erythema nodosum.

[c] ENT involvement suggests Wegener's granulomatosis.

[d] Usually by entrapment or amyloid in well-established cases.

GD, Goodpasture's disease; PV, primary vasculitis; SLE, systemic lupus erythematosus; CG, cryoglobulinaemia; HSP, Henoch–Schönlein purpura; SS, systemic sclerosis; BD, Behçet's disease; RD, rheumatoid disease; RP, relapsing polychondritis; PIGN, postinfectious glomerulonephritis; IE, infectious endocarditis; HT, hypertension; ENT, ear, nose, and throat.

Common or characteristic features are indicated. Many features need careful interpretation; for example, fever may have many causes, particularly infection, hypertension is a feature of established renal failure, particularly with fluid overload, arthritis may accompany arthralgia, and heart murmurs may be related to anaemia or fluid overload. Not all features are apparent in every patient. For some of the conditions, certain features listed occur only rarely, for example haemoptysis in Behçet's disease and sclerodema.

lupus and systemic sclerosis. Similarly, haemoptysis has been reported occasionally in patients with cryoglobulinaemia, systemic sclerosis, and rheumatoid disease, but commonly occurs in Goodpasture's disease, primary small vessel vasculitis, and lupus. It must also be remembered that more than one pathology may coexist, for example one of the conditions listed in Table 3 together with infection may result in pleurisy, abdominal pain, diarrhoea, fever and anaemia and fluid overload may result in functional heart murmurs.

Oliguria is usual in glomerulonephritis associated acute renal failure. Complete anuria is infrequent except in fulminant glomerulonephritis, particularly in anti-GBM disease. The presence of proteinuria is unhelpful unless it is very heavy, but urine microscopy is very useful (see Chapter 1.2). Haematuria is common in acute renal failure, particularly if a bladder catheter is in place. Microscopy (preferably positive phase contrast) of freshly voided urine may reveal a high proportion of dysmorphic erythrocytes, particularly acanthocytes, which are indicative of glomerular bleeding (Fairley and Birch 1982), and red-cell casts which are highly suggestive of 'crescentic' glomerulonephritis. However, they are occasionally seen in acute interstitial nephritis and rarely (in small numbers) in acute tubular necrosis. Leucocytes and abundant granular and cellular casts are also frequently found in the urine of patients with active glomerulonephritis.

A number of laboratory investigations (Table 4) are helpful. It is reasonable to expect to obtain reports of ANCA, anti-GBM, and anti-DNA binding antibodies, and complement abnormalities in patients in whom there is a strong presumptive evidence of glomerulonephritis within 24 h. Other investigations will help to exclude myeloma and rhabdomyolysis, which will be possibilities in oliguric patients with normal-sized kidneys. Apart from the 'specific' tests, the abnormal investigations listed in Table 4 have many alternative causes but a probable differential diagnosis often emerges from the combination of clinical features, laboratory investigations, imaging, and renal biopsy.

As in all cases of acute renal failure, renal ultrasound is essential to define the size (and number) of the kidneys and the cortical thickness, and to exclude obstruction. Most cases of glomerulonephritis-associated acute renal failure have normal-sized or slightly enlarged kidneys, often with increased cortical echogenicity indicating swelling and inflammation. Chest radiography is often informative. Diffuse alveolar air-space shadowing may suggest pulmonary oedema (particularly with fluid overload and/or heart failure), pulmonary haemorrhage, or infection. Haemorrhage and oedema may be difficult to differentiate, particularly in the absence of haemoptysis (Fig. 3). Computed tomography (CT) may help resolve the difference, but the carbon monoxide transfer coefficient (*K*co) is most useful. A high value or an increase of 30 per cent greater than the baseline is very suggestive of haemorrhage (Ewan *et al.* 1976). Round homogeneous lesions with or without cavities on the chest radiograph suggest a diagnosis of Wegener's granulomatosis, but are also a manifestation of infection, for example, Staphylococcal abscess. CT may help in such cases since it often demonstrates multiple small granulomatous lesions that are not apparent on the plain radiograph (Fig. 4). Sinus disease is found in Wegener's granulomatosis but is also common in the general population, although actual bone destruction strongly supports the diagnosis of Wegener's granulomatosis. Angiography may help in the diagnosis of vasculitis of medium-sized vessels (polyarteritis nodosa and sometimes Churg–Strauss syndrome) (Fig. 5). These conditions are not often associated with acute renal failure (see Section 10). Echocardiography (preferably transoesophageal because of its greater sensitivity and resolution) is an essential investigation in patients in whom infective endocarditis is a possibility.

Table 4 Laboratory investigations in rapidly progressive glomerulonephritis

Specific	
Anti-GBM antibodies	Anti-GBM disease
ANCA	Systemic vasculitis
Anti-ds DNA antibodies	SLE
Anti-Sm antibodies	SLE
C3 nephritic factor	MCGN type II (sometimes SLE)
ASOT	Poststreptococcal GN (titre may also increase with hyperglobulinaemia and SLE)
Anti-DNAse	
Non-specific	
Complement	
Low C4, normal C3	MEC, SLE
Low C4 and C3	SLE, MCGN type I, MEC
Low C3, normal C4	MCGN type II, postinfectious GN, sometimes SLE
Raised C3 and C4	Systemic vasculitis
Cryoglobulins	MEC (and others including SLE, postinfectious GN, usually at lower levels)
Immunoglobulins	
Raised IgG, IgM	SLE, systemic vasculitis, postinfectious GN
Raised IgE	Churg–Strauss syndrome
Raised IgA	IgA nephropathy/Henoch–Schönlein purpura
Paraprotein (usually IgM)	MEC, myeloma
Rh factor	
CRP	Most GN, particularly systemic vasculitis, but usually not SLE
Raised alkaline phosphatase	Systemic vasculitis
Haematology	
Neutrophilia, thrombocytosis	Systemic vasculitis
Eosinophilia	Churg–Strauss syndrome
Lymphopenia, thrombocytopenia	SLE
Positive bacteriological cultures	Infection-related disease, particularly endocarditis

SLE, systemic lupus erythematosus; ASOT, antistreptolysin titre; GN, glomerulonephritis; MCGN, mesangiocapillary glomerulonephritis; MEC, mixed essential cryoglobulinaemia; CRP, C-reactive protein.

Initial management of glomerulonephritis-associated acute renal failure (see also Chapters 3.10 and 3.11)

When indicated, general measures, including dialysis and ultrafiltration, antibiotics are indicated if there is evidence of infection—perhaps with a lower threshold if the patient is, or has been, immunosuppressed will be applied. The use of H_2 antagonists or proton-pump inhibitors has become standard practice as prophylaxis against stress ulcers in patients with acute renal failure and for those given high-dose steroids. The

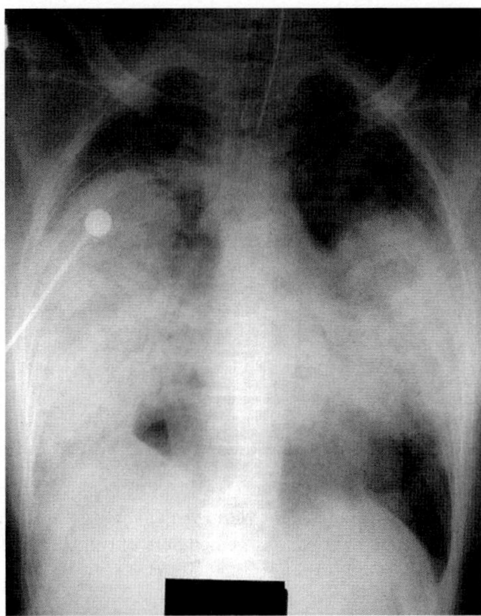

Fig. 3 Chest radiograph showing bilateral alveolar air-space shadowing due to pulmonary haemorrhage in a patient with small vessel vasculitis. The differential diagnosis includes pulmonary oedema and infection. An elevated *K*CO reliably suggests haemorrhage (see text).

prophylactic oral nystatin, amphotericin, or fluconazole for fungal infection, and cotrimoxazole for pneumocystis are logical treatments for those who are immunosuppressed. Although routine, this practice is not evidence-based in this setting. As for other causes of acute renal failure, the early introduction of enteral or parenteral nutrition for patients unable or unwilling to maintain an appropriate caloric and nitrogen intake is believed to be valuable.

Urgent disease directed treatment is essential for acute renal failure associated with anti-GBM disease, systemic vasculitis, isolated focal necrotizing crescentic glomerulonephritis, or systemic lupus erythematosus, particularly when the clinical course is one of rapid renal function deterioration. If the clinical context is strongly suggestive of such disease, and if serious infection is unlikely, there is little to be lost by starting treatment with corticosteroids, for example prednisolone 1 mg/kg/day and cyclophosphamide 2.5 mg/kg/day (2 mg/kg/day for patients aged over 60 years, but with dose reduction with severely impaired renal function) until the diagnosis can be confirmed. Others advocate the administration of methylprednisolone (e.g. 0.5 or 1 g intravenously). Further treatment can be decided once the diagnosis is established, and will include plasma exchange that seems to be superior to methylprednisolone (Gaskin *et al.* 2002). The white count of patients on cyclophosphamide should be monitored daily, and a steadily declining count should be met with a dose reduction or temporary withdrawal depending on the rate of decline (see also Chapter 3.10).

The renal failure of patients with an underlying 'immunological' disease needs particularly careful management. For instance, patients with Goodpasture's disease, primary small vessel vasculitis, and lupus are at particular risk of pulmonary haemorrhage which can be exacerbated or provoked by fluid overload and sepsis. They should therefore be kept as 'dry' as possible (assuming that they have established renal failure), and particular care must be taken to avoid line and other sepsis. The threshold for line removal/replacement should be especially low. The risk of infection is increased more by steroids than by cyclophosphamide or plasma exchange (Cohen *et al.* 1982), and so it is important to review the steroid dose regularly, taking account of the underlying disease and the patient's progress. Because of the risk of pulmonary haemorrhage, dialysis should be performed with minimal or no heparin cover. If plasma exchange is performed, care is needed to avoid transient fluid overload. Two to four units of fresh frozen plasma should be given at the end of each exchange if the patient is within 72 h of surgery or renal biopsy; or if there is a risk of pulmonary haemorrhage.

(a)

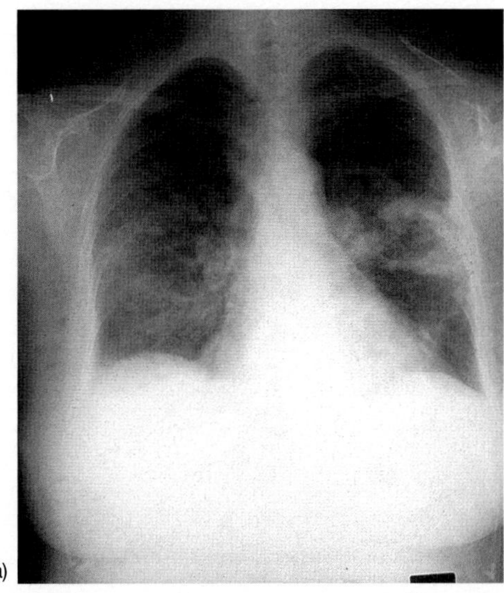

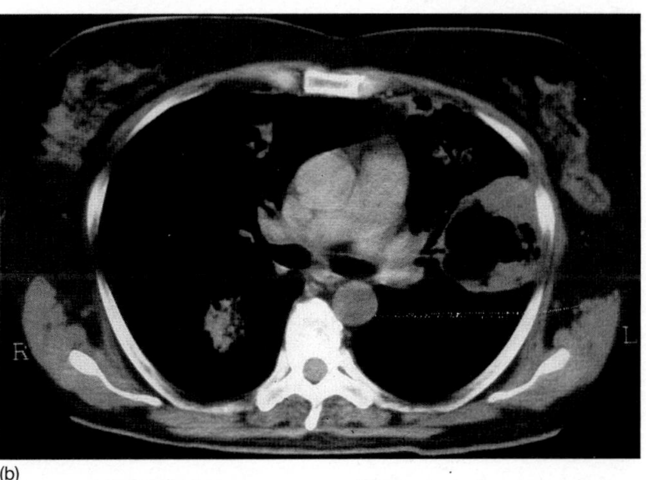

(b)

Fig. 4 (a) Chest radiograph showing rounded opacities in both lung fields; the lesion on the right appears to be cavitating. (b) A CT image of the same patient which reveals multiple cavitating lesions. The patient had Wegener's granulomatosis and positive c-ANCA.

Acute renal failure in patients with glomerulonephritis

The development of acute or acute-on-chronic renal failure in a patient already known to have an underlying glomerulonephritis needs careful assessment as the differential diagnosis is wide (Table 5).

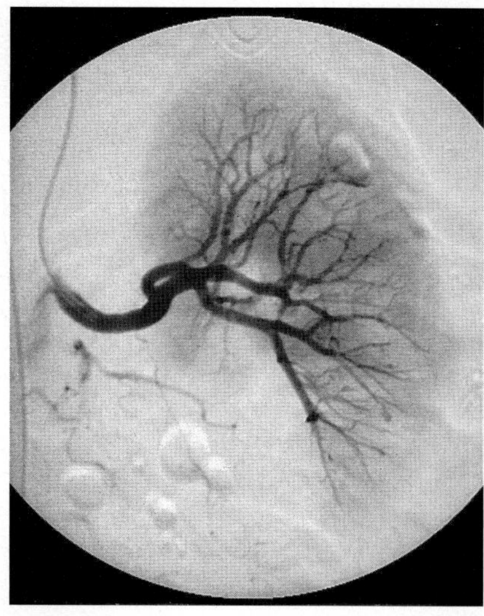

Fig. 5 A selective renal angiogram showing multiple aneurysms in a patient with polyarteritis nodosa.

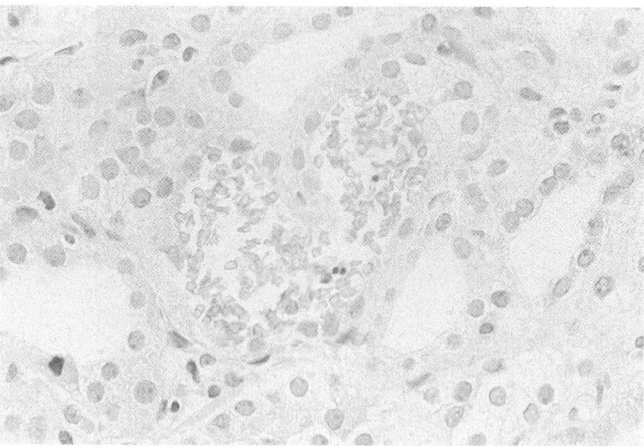

Fig. 6 A renal biopsy from a patient with IgA nephropathy and acute renal failure. Many of the tubules contain large numbers of red blood cells. (Courtesy of Dr D. Davies.)

Table 5 Differential diagnosis of acute renal failure in patients with pre-existing glomerulonephritis

Crescentic change	
Nephrotic associated renal failure Renal vein thrombosis	In nephrotic patients
Acute tubular necrosis: dehydration, sepsis, rhabdomyolysis, etc.	
Drug-induced acute interstitial nephritis	
Drug-induced—NSAIDs	
Other causes of acute renal failure (unrelated to glomerulonephritis)	
Accelerated phase hypertension	

NSAIDs, non-steroidal anti-inflammatory drugs; GN, glomerulonephritis.

Acute renal failure associated with crescents on the renal biopsy has been described in mesangial IgA nephropathy, mesangiocapillary glomerulonephritis, and membranous nephropathy. Acute renal failure with crescents is well recognized in mesangial IgA nephropathy (Nicholls *et al.* 1984a,b; Welch *et al.* 1988) (see Chapter 3.6), and may be the initial presentation, but acute renal failure may also occur in other circumstances (Schena 1990; Delclaux *et al.* 1993; Packham *et al.* 1994). Deterioration of renal function may be more common than generally realized, especially during prolonged episodes of macroscopic haematuria (Praga *et al.* 1985).

A variety of mechanisms for the development of acute renal failure without severe glomerular infiltration have been proposed. These include tubular obstruction by red blood cells but although macroscopic haematuria is commonly present in these circumstances (Fig. 6), there are data suggesting that obstruction is not the cause of the renal failure (Fogazzi *et al.* 1995). An alternative explanation is the toxic effect of the red cells or their contents (Packham *et al.* 1994; Heyman and Brezis 1995). In such cases, recovery of renal function is usually spontaneous. However, occasional or fibrous crescents are not uncommon in patients with IgA disease without acute renal failure. A variety of measures, including corticosteroids, immunosuppressive drugs, and plasma exchange, have been advocated for the treatment of patients with crescentic IgA nephropathy with acute renal failure (Lai *et al.* 1987; D'Amico *et al.* 2001), but there has been little convincing evidence of their efficacy. A multicentre trial of cyclophosphamide and corticosteroids in this group is being performed (see also Chapter 3.6).

Patients with mesangiocapillary glomerulonephritis who are nephrotic are likely to progress to endstage renal failure relatively quickly (see also Chapter 3.8). Rapid progression is sometimes associated with crescents on the renal biopsy (Kim *et al.* 1982; Korzets *et al.* 1987). Patients usually present with this clinical pattern, although transition to a crescentic form may develop after a period of less severe nephritis (McCoy *et al.* 1975). There is no convincing evidence that treatment is effective, although a variety of regimens, including steroids, immunosuppressive drugs, anticoagulants, and plasma exchange, have been tried.

Crescentic change in primary membranous nephropathy causing acute renal failure has also been described (Abreo *et al.* 1986) (see also Chapter 3.7) but is rare, and an underlying condition such as systemic lupus erythematosus or infection should be considered. These glomerular diseases are frequently associated with severe nephrotic syndrome which may itself result in acute renal failure (see below). Various drugs may cause acute interstitial nephritis in this group—non-steroidal anti-inflammatory drugs, antibiotics, diuretics, cimetidine, and allopurinol are the most common agents implicated (Cameron 1988) (see also Chapter 10.6.1). The diagnosis is suggested by the presence of fever, rash, arthralgia, eosinophilia, and eosinophiluria. These may be absent, particularly when non-steroidal anti-inflammatory drugs are the cause. A renal biopsy is necessary to confirm the diagnosis.

Renal disease is common in mixed 'essential' cryoglobulinaemia, with a mesangiocapillary glomerulonephritis being the most common glomerular lesion (see Chapter 3.8). Reversible clinical exacerbations are frequent and up to 25 per cent of patients present with an acute deterioration of renal function, but acute oliguric renal failure occurs in less than 5 per cent of cases (D'Amico *et al.* 1989). The diagnosis is suggested by the association of vasculitic skin rash, arthralgia, peripheral neuropathy, and Raynaud's phenomenon with glomerulonephritis. Complement components are characteristically low, and a rheumatoid factor and cryoglobulins are detected (Table 3). Patients with severe renal failure are usually treated aggressively (Ferri *et al.* 1986; D'Amico *et al.* 1989; Frankel *et al.* 1992) with plasma exchange to remove the cryoglobulin, usually with cyclophosphamide in an attempt to reduce or prevent resynthesis, and with corticosteroids to suppress glomerular inflammation. The response is unpredictable and there are potential serious side-effects in patients who are hepatitis C positive or have underlying lymphoma.

Although the acute nephritic syndrome is common in Henoch–Schönlein purpura, affecting up to half of the patients, it occurs less often in children under 5 years (see Chapter 4.5.2). These patients, like those with cryoglobulinaemia and lupus, present with glomerulonephritis, arthritis, and rash (Table 3), often with abdominal pain. Although infrequent, acute oliguric renal failure may also occur. Renal biopsy usually reveals a high proportion of crescents (Habib *et al.* 1993). Although steroids and cytotoxic drugs have not been proven to be of value, they are often given to patients with severe (crescentic) renal disease. Pulse methylprednisolone, plasma exchange, and intravenous immunoglobulin have also been applied but their effect on outcome is hard to judge.

Infection-related glomerulonephritis (see also Chapter 3.12)

Postinfectious glomerulonephritis exemplified by poststreptococcal disease is still a common entity in tropical and developing countries, and may occasionally result in acute renal failure. The incidence is low in Europe and North America, possibly more common in children (Stilmant *et al.* 1979). The proportion of patients with poststreptococcal nephritis who develop acute renal failure requiring dialysis is difficult to estimate because of the large numbers who have 'subclinical' disease, but it is likely to be considerably less than 5 per cent. Several series of patients with acute renal failure have been reported, and are reviewed by Salant *et al.* (1988). Most are oliguric and have a high proportion of crescents on renal biopsy. Overall, about 50 per cent (of 39 patients) recovered completely, but the prognosis was poor in older patients and those who had had a longer period of oliguria. A low C3 component of complement may be a clue to the diagnosis, although this depression is often transient (Table 4).

Asymptomatic nephritis (with microscopic haematuria and proteinuria) is almost invariable in patients with bacterial endocarditis, but acute renal failure is rare (Neugarten and Baldwin 1984). Recovery is usual provided the infection is controlled. Complement components (C3 and C4) may be low, but the concentrations do not correlate with clinical features. Cyroglobulins, rheumatoid factor, and hyperglobulinaemia are also commonly found.

Many other infections, for example, deep abscesses are associated with glomerulonephritis and, perhaps not surprisingly when acute renal failure develops, the biopsy usually shows severe lesions, including crescents (Salant *et al.* 1988; Montseny *et al.* 1995). Obviously, treatment to control or cure the infection is essential. However, steroids and cyclophosphamide have been given because of the intense glomerular inflammation seen in some patients, with apparent success in some reported cases (Montseny *et al.* 1995).

Acute renal failure complicating nephrotic syndrome

Acute renal failure complicates the nephrotic syndrome more often than is generally appreciated (see also Chapter 10.2). Renal failure may develop in the absence of glomerular inflammation, and may occur either around the time of presentation or much later. There are several possible causes, including hypovolaemia, drug-induced interstitial nephritis, renal vein thrombosis, and acute tubular necrosis secondary to sepsis. However, most are believed to be secondary to the abnormal renal haemodynamics associated with the nephrotic syndrome itself. The explanation of these changes remains uncertain, but several factors are probably involved (Table 6).

Clinical features

Most reported cases are in adults although children may also be affected (Steele *et al.* 1982; Springate *et al.* 1987; Sakarcan *et al.* 1994). Smith and Hayslett (1992) reviewed 79 episodes of acute renal failure in 75 patients reported in the English literature since 1966. The incidence of a significant fall in GFR is more common than dialysis-dependent renal failure, and may occur in up to 30 per cent of children (ISKD 1978) and adults (Nolasco *et al.* 1986). Older patients predominated (average 58 $\pm$ 2 years), two-thirds were male and proteinuria was usually heavy (11.6 $\pm$ 0.6 g/day) with low serum albumin concentrations (19 $\pm$ 1 g/l). Renal failure developed an average of 29 days after the onset of nephrotic syndrome and persisted for 7 weeks. The renal failure was, in some patients, irreversible and, although many such patients had underlying mesangiocapillary glomerulonephritis or focal segmental glomerulosclerosis, there are reports of patients in whom only minimal or minor glomerular lesions were demonstrated (Raij *et al.* 1975). Although hypovolaemia was alleged to be responsible for the acute renal failure in many of the cases, objective evidence of this was provided in only a few and blood pressures were normal or even elevated (Smith and Hayslett 1992).

Features consistent with acute tubular necrosis are the most common histopathological finding, being present in 60 per cent of patients (Smith and Hayslett 1992). However, there are contradictory reports in the literature. In some there was apparently little evidence of tubular damage (Cameron *et al.* 1974; Lowenstein *et al.* 1981), but in others,

Table 6 Possible causes of acute renal failure in nephrotic syndrome

Prerenal failure (hypovolaemia $\pm$ diuretics)
Acute tubular necrosis
Reduced glomerular filtration rate secondary to hypoproteinaemia (exacerbated by inhibition of prostaglandin synthesis)
Interstitial oedema
Rapid progression (focal segmental glomerulosclerosis)
Crescentic transformation (mesangiocapillary glomerulonephritis, membranous nephropathy)
Renal vein thrombosis/renal artery thrombosis
Interstitial nephritis

severe changes were reported (Esparza *et al.* 1981). Jennette and Falk (1990) found tubular damage in 71 per cent of adults with minimal change nephrotic syndrome and a creatinine more than 177 μmol/l compared with 0 per cent in those with a creatinine less than 133 μmol/l. They also found more atherosclerosis in those with renal impairment (but they were also older).

Mechanisms of acute renal failure in nephrotic syndrome

The mechanisms of acute renal failure are summarized in Table 6 (see also Chapter 10.2).

Hypovolaemia

Hypovolaemia resulting from a reduced plasma oncotic pressure is the obvious mechanism proposed to explain prerenal and established acute renal failure in severe nephrosis. However, the majority of patients with nephrotic syndrome do not have reduced plasma volumes (Dorhout Mees *et al.* 1984). This has been demonstrated in experimental animals, human volunteers rendered hypoproteinaemic, and in nephrotic patients. The reasons are uncertain but appear to be due, at least in part, to a reduction in the colloid osmotic pressure of interstitial fluid which compensates for the lower plasma oncotic pressure. The situation may be more complicated, since other data suggest that nephrotic patients have a greater than normal reduction in plasma volume on standing and that the cardiovascular system is less able to respond to extra stress (Geers *et al.* 1986). Under these circumstances hypovolaemia may be a contributory factor, particularly if induced by diuretics. Diuretic treatment of severely nephrotic patients should therefore be carefully monitored with daily measurement of weight (aiming for no more than a 3 kg loss per day), postural blood pressure, haematocrit, urea, and creatinine to reduce the risk of precipitating hypovolaemic acute renal failure. Similarly, other causes of hypovolaemia, such as diarrhoea and vomiting, haemorrhage, or surgery, may not be sufficiently compensated for and should be treated promptly.

Glomerular filtration rate in nephrotic syndrome

When the nephrotic syndrome is secondary to glomerular inflammation, this itself may be responsible for a reduced GFR. However, patients with minimal change nephrotic syndrome also have a mild to moderate decrease of GFR which increases on remission (Smith and Hayslett 1992). This is probably due to the basement membrane changes and the epithelial cell foot process fusion which occurs in nephrosis (Robson *et al.* 1974; Carrie *et al.* 1981). This reduction in GFR occurs despite the theoretical increase predicted to be a consequence of low plasma oncotic pressure which should increase the effective filtration pressure. In fact, a greater reduction in GFR may be prevented by prostaglandin-dependent afferent arteriolar vasodilatation. Renal plasma flow may be normal or even increased in these patients (Geers *et al.* 1986; Furuya *et al.* 1993). Nephrotics are as a result particularly susceptible to acute renal failure induced by non-steroidal anti-inflammatory drugs (Clive and Stoff 1984). Fortunately, recovery is usual after withdrawal of the drug (Arisz *et al.* 1976; Vriesendorp *et al.* 1986).

The filtration fraction is also low (Dorhout Mees *et al.* 1979; Lowenstein *et al.* 1981; Geers *et al.* 1984; Furuya *et al.* 1993). This has been attributed to increased intratubular or interstitial pressure secondary to interstitial oedema. Sometimes renal failure reverses with aggressive treatment of oedema with diuretics and recurs with reaccumulation of oedema (Stephens *et al.* 1979). Although it is unlikely that such changes in intratubular or interstitial pressure alone would be sufficiently large to cause acute renal failure, they may predispose to it by further reducing compensatory capacity. Another hypothesis is that intratubular obstruction occurs as a result of protein casts (Kuroda *et al.* 1979; Imbasciati *et al.* 1981), a hypothesis supported by the finding of prominent intratubular casts in such cases (Raij *et al.* 1975; Imbasciati *et al.* 1981).

Drug-induced acute renal failure

Non-steroidal anti-inflammatory drugs are able to induce acute renal failure in nephrotic patients because of their profound effect on GFR in situations in which prostaglandins maintain it. Their detrimental effect is potentiated by salt restriction and diuretics. They should be avoided altogether or used with extreme care. Interstitial nephritis can be the cause of acute renal failure. Drugs used in managing the nephrotic syndrome including antibiotics, diuretics, and cimetidine are occasional culprits. There are well-documented cases of interstitial nephritis in minimal change nephropathy (van Ypersele de Strihou 1979; Finkelstein *et al.* 1982), sometimes, but not always, associated with the characteristic allergic features (see Chapter 10.6.2).

Renal vein thrombosis

The hypercoagulable state, which accompanies the nephrotic syndrome predisposes to renal vein thrombosis (see also Chapter 3.4). Most patients suffering this complication do not have specific features, but the consequences of pulmonary emboli alert the physician to the possibility (Llach *et al.* 1980). It rarely presents acutely with acute renal failure (Duffy *et al.* 1973; Llach *et al.* 1980). In such cases, epigastric or loin pain with haematuria are suggestive. Although colour Doppler ultrasound may be diagnostic, confirmation or exclusion usually requires angiography or magnetic resonance venography.

Miscellaneous causes

Nephrotic patients are particularly susceptible to infections which may occasionally result in sepsis-associated acute tubular necrosis (Cameron 1988). Other nephrotoxins (e.g. radiographic contrast media) may occasionally be implicated, but there is no convincing evidence of any increased risk to nephrotic patients over and above that caused by dehydration.

Management

There are no specific management measures for incipient or established acute renal failure in nephrotic patients. A patient presenting with acute renal failure and nephrotic syndrome often needs a renal biopsy to establish whether the cause is the glomerular pathology or a superadded interstitial nephritis. If minimal change nephropathy or focal segmental glomerulosclerosis is found, corticosteroids should be administered. Whether they should be used in other conditions is debatable, although patients with florid nephrotic syndrome associated IgA deposits may respond to steroids as if they had minimal change nephropathy (Lai *et al.* 1986; Cheng *et al.* 1989).

Hypovolaemia should be corrected, and this is best done using central venous pressure monitoring. Volume expansion with 20 per cent albumin is logical, and it minimizes the additional sodium load. Infusion of 0.5–1 g/kg body weight albumin over 1–2 h has been recommended to increase the blood volume by 15–30 per cent. However, hypertension and pulmonary oedema may develop in some patients following overexpansion of the blood volume. This is a particular risk in children (Reid *et al.* 1996). Fluid removal by ultrafiltration or haemofiltration are alternative options, particularly in grossly oedematous or oliguric patients.

Aggressive treatment of oedema with diuretics with or without albumin, has been advocated to reduce intrarenal interstitial pressure, and this has been claimed to reverse renal failure (Stephens *et al.* 1979). Loop diuretics with thiazides are a particularly potent combination and are sometimes synchronized with albumin infusions. It should be remembered that marked hypokalaemia is a side-effect of such treatment. 'Renal-dose' dopamine is another commonly used 'treatment', but this is of doubtful value and may be detrimental (Thompson and Cockrill 1994).

Once established, acute renal failure should be managed along conventional lines. If it is secondary to acute tubular necrosis, the prognosis is good with recovery occurring within 6–7 weeks (Smith and Hayslett 1992).

References

Abreo, K., Abreo, F., Mitchell, B., and Schoemer, G. (1986). Idiopathic crescentic membranous glomerulonephritis. *American Journal of Kidney Diseases* **8**, 257–261.

Arisz, L., Donker, A. J. M., Brentjens, J. R. H., and van der Hem, G. K. (1976). The effect of indomethacin on proteinuria and kidney function in the nephrotic syndrome. *Acta Medica Scandinavica* **199**, 121–125.

Atkins, R. C., Nikolic-Paterson, D. J., Song, Q., and Lan, H. Y. (1996). Modulators of crescentic glomerulonephritis. *Journal of the American Society of Nephrology* **7** (11), 2271–2278.

Bamgboye, E. L., Mabayoje, M. O., Odutola, T. A., and Mabadeje, A. F. (1993). Acute renal failure at the Lagos University Teaching Hospital. *Renal Failure* **15**, 77–80.

Brezis, M., Heyman, S. N., Dinur, D., Epstein, F. H., and Rosen, S. (1991). Role of nitric oxide in renal medullary oxygen balance. Studies in isolated and intact rat kidneys. *Journal of Clinical Investigation* **88**, 390–395.

Briggs, W. A., Johnson, J. P., Teichman, S., Yeager, H. C., and Wilson, C. B. (1979). Antiglomerular basement membrane antibody-mediated glomerulonephritis and Goodpasture's syndrome. *Medicine* **58**, 348–361.

Cameron, J. S. (1988). Allergic interstitial nephritis: clinical features and pathogenesis. *Quarterly Journal of Medicine* **66**, 97–115.

Cameron, J. S., Turner, D. R., Ogg, C. S., Sharpstone, P., and Brown, C. B. (1974). The nephrotic syndrome in adults with 'minimal change' glomerular lesions. *Quarterly Journal of Medicine* **43**, 461–488.

Carrie, B. J, Salyer, W. R., and Myers, B. D. (1981). Minimal change nephropathy: an electrochemical disorder of the glomerular membrane. *American Journal of Medicine* **70**, 262–268.

Cheng, I. K., Chan, K. W., and Chan, M. K. (1989). Mesangial IgA nephropathy with steroid-responsive syndrome: disappearance of mesangial IgA deposits following steroid-induced remission. *American Journal of Kidney Diseases* **14**, 361–369.

Chugh, K. S., Sakhuja, V., Malhotra, H. S., and Pereira, B. J. G. (1989). Changing trends in acute renal failure in third-world countries—Chandigarh study. *Quarterly Journal of Medicine* **73**, 1117–1123.

Clive, D. M. and Stoff, J. S. (1984). Renal syndromes associated with non-steroidal anti-inflammatory drugs. *New England Journal of Medicine* **310**, 563–572.

Cohen, J., Pinching, A. J., Rees, A. J., and Peters, D. K. (1982). Infection and immunosuppression. A study of infective complications of 75 patients with immunologically-mediated disease. *Quarterly Journal of Medicine* **51**, 1–23.

Couser, W. G. (1982). Idiopathic rapidly progressive glomerulonephritis. *American Journal of Nephrology* **2**, 57–69.

D'Amico, G., Colasanti, G., Ferrario, F., and Sinico, R. A. (1989). Renal involvement in essential mixed cryoglobulinaemia. *Kidney International* **35**, 1004–1014.

D'Amico, G., Napodano, P., Ferrario, F., Rastaldi, M. P., and Arrigo, G. (2001). Idiopathic IgA nephropathy with segmental necrotizing lesions of the capillary wall. *Kidney International* **59**, 682–692.

Delclaux, C., Jacquot, C., Callerd, P., and Kleinknecht, D. (1993). Acute reversible renal failure with macroscopic haematuria in IgA nephropathy. *Nephrology, Dialysis, Transplantation* **8**, 195–199.

Dorhout Mees, E. J, Greers, A. B., and Koomans, H. A. (1984). Blood volume and sodium retention in the nephrotic syndrome: a controversial pathophysiological concept. *Nephron* **36**, 201–211.

Dorhout Mees, E. J., Roos, J. C., Boer, P., Oei, Y. H., and Simatupang, T. A. (1979). Observations on edema formation in the nephrotic syndrome. *American Journal of Medicine* **67**, 378–384.

Duffy, J. L., Letteri, J., Cinque, T., Hsu, P. P., Molho, L., and Churg, J. (1973). Renal vein thrombosis and the nephrotic syndrome. Report of two cases with successful treatment of one. *American Journal of Medicine* **54**, 663–672.

Esparza, A. R., Kahn, S. I., Garella, S., and Abuelo, J.G. (1981). Spectrum of acute renal failure in nephrotic syndrome with minimal (or minor) glomerular lesions; role of haemodynamic factors. *Laboratory Investigation* **45**, 510–521.

Espinel, C. H. and Gregory, A. W. (1980). Differential diagnosis of acute renal failure. *Nephrology* **13**, 73–77.

Evans, D. J., Savage, C. O. S., Winearls, C. G., Rees, A. J., Pusey, C. D., and Peters, D. K. (1986). Renal biopsy in prognosis of treated 'glomerulonephritis with crescents'. *Abstracts of the 10th International Congress of Nephrology*, 60.

Ewan, P. W., Jones, N. A., Rhodes, G. G., and Hughes, J. M. B. (1976). Detection of intrapulmonary haemorrhage with carbon monoxide uptake. Application in Goodpasture's syndrome. *New England Journal of Medicine* **328**, 1651–1657.

Faarup, P., Nørgaard, T., Elling, F., and Jensen, H. (1978). Structural changes in kidneys of patients with oliguric extracapillary glomerulonephritis during immunosuppressive therapy. *Acta Pathologica Microbiologica Scandinavica A* **86**, 409–414.

Fairley, K. F. and Birch, D. F. (1982). Hematuria: a simple method for identifying glomerular bleeding. *Kidney International* **21**, 105–108.

Ferri, C., Moriconi, L., Gremigani, G., Migliorini, P., Paleologo, G., Fosella, P. V., and Bombardieri, S. (1986). Treatment of the renal involvement in mixed cryoglobulinaemia with prolonged plasma exchange. *Nephron* **43**, 246–253.

Finkelstein, A., Fraley, D. S., Stachura, I., Feldman, H. A., Gandy, D. R., and Bourke, E. (1982). Fenoprofen nephropathy: lipoid nephrosis and interstitial nephritis. A possible T-lymphocyte disorder. *American Journal of Medicine* **72**, 81–87.

Fogazzi, G. B., Imbasciati, E., Moroni, G., Scalia, A., Mihatsch, M. J., and Ponticelli, C. (1995). Reversible acute renal failure from gross haematuria due to glomerulonephritis: not only in IgA nephropathy and not associated with intratubular obstruction. *Nephrology, Dialysis, Transplantation* **10**, 624–629.

Frankel, A. H., Singer, D. R. J., Winearls, C. G., Evans, D. J., Rees, A. J., and Pusey, C. D. (1992). Type II essential mixed cryoglobulinaemia: presentation, treatment and outcome in 13 patients. *Quarterly Journal of Medicine* **82**, 101–124.

Furuya, R., Kumagai, H., Ikegaya, N., Kobayashi, S., Kimura, M., Hishida, M., and Kaneko, E. (1993). Reversible acute renal failure in idiopathic nephrotic syndrome. *Internal Medicine* **32**, 31–35.

Gaskin, G., Jayne, D. R., and the European Vasculitis Study Group (2002). Adjunctive plasma exchange is superior to methylprednisolone in acute renal failure due to ANCA-associated glomerulonephritis. *Journal of the American Society of Nephrology* **13**, 2A–3A.

Geers, A. B., Koomans, H. A., Roos, J. C., Boer, P., and Dorhout Mees, E. J. (1984). Functional relationships in the nephrotic syndrome. *Kidney International* **26**, 324–330.

Geers, A. B., Koomans, H. A., and Dorhout Mees, E. J. (1986). Effect of changes in posture on circulatory homeostasis in patients with nephrotic syndrome. *Clinical Physiology* **6**, 63–75.

Glassock, R. J. (1985). Natural history and treatment of primary proliferative glomerulonephritis: a review. *Kidney International* **28** (Suppl. 17), 5136–5142.

Haas, M., Spargo, B. H., Wit, E. J., and Meehan, S. M. (2000). Etiologies and outcome of acute renal insufficiency in older adults: a renal biopsy study of 259 cases. *American Journal of Kidney Diseases* **35**, 433–437.

Habib, R., Niaudet, P., and Levy, M. Schönlein–Henoch purpura nephritis and IgA nephropathy. In *Renal Pathology with Clinical and Functional Correlations* (ed. C. C. Tisher and B. M. Brenner), pp. 472–523. Philadelphia, PA: Lippincott, 1993.

Heptinstall, R. H. Crescentic glomerulonephritis. In *Pathology of the Kidney* 4th edn. (ed. R. H. Heptinstall), p. 626. New York, NY: Churchill Livingstone, 1992.

Heyman, S. N. and Brezis, M. (1995). Acute renal failure in glomerular bleeding: a puzzling phenomenon. *Nephrology, Dialysis, Transplantation* **10**, 591–593.

Imbasciati, E., Ponticelli, C., Case, N., Altieri, P., Bolasco, F., Mihatsch, M. J., and Zollinger, H. U. (1981). Acute renal failure in idiopathic nephrotic syndrome. *Nephron* **28**, 186–191.

ISKD (1978). Nephrotic syndrome in children: prediction of histopathology from clinical and laboratory characteristics at time of diagnosis. A report of the International Study of Kidney Disease in Children. *Kidney International* **13**, 159–165.

Jennette, J. C. and Falk, R. J. (1990). Adult minimal change glomerulopathy with acute renal failure. *American Journal of Kidney Diseases* **16**, 432–437.

Kandoth, P. W., Agarwal, G. J., and Dharnidharka, V. R. (1994). Acute renal failure in children requiring dialysis therapy. *Indian Pediatrics* **31** (3), 305–309.

Kim, Y., Michael, A. F., and Fish, A. J. Idiopathic membranoproliferative glomerulonephritis. In *Nephrotic Syndrome* (ed. B. M. Brenner and J. Stein), p. 237. New York, NY: Churchill Livingstone, 1982.

Korzets, Z., Bernheim, J., and Bernheim, J. (1987). Rapidly progressive glomerulonephritis (crescentic glomerulonephritis) in the course of type I idiopathic membranoproliferative glomerulonephritis. *American Journal of Kidney Diseases* **10**, 56–61.

Kuroda, S., Aynedjian, H. S., and Bank, N. (1979). A micropuncture study of renal sodium retention in nephrotic syndrome in rats: evidence for increased resistance to tubular fluid flow. *Kidney International* **16**, 561–571.

Lai, K. N., Lai, F. M., Ho, C. P., and Chan, K. W. (1986). Corticosteroid therapy in IgA nephropathy with nephrotic syndrome: a long-term controlled trial. *Clinical Nephrology* **26**, 174–182.

Lai, K. N., Lai, F. M., Leung, A. C., Ho, C. P., and Vallance-Owen, J. (1987). Plasma exchange in patients with rapidly progressive idiopathic IgA nephropathy: a report of two cases and review of literature. *American Journal of Kidney Diseases* **10**, 66–70.

Llach, F., Papper, S., and Massry, S. G. (1980). The clinical spectrum of renal vein thrombosis: acute and chronic. *American Journal of Medicine* **69**, 819–827.

Lowenstein, J., Schacht, R. G., and Baldwin, D. S. (1981). Renal failure in minimal change nephrotic syndrome. *American Journal of Medicine* **70**, 227–233.

McCoy, R. C., Clapp, J., and Seigler, H. F. (1975). Membranoproliferative glomerulonephritis. Progression from pure form to a crescentic form with recurrence after transplantation. *American Journal of Medicine* **59**, 288–292.

McCrory, W. W. (1970). Glomerulonephritis: pediatric aspects. *Bulletin of the New York Academy of Medicine* **10**, 789–796.

Montseny, J.-J., Meyrier, A., Kleinknecht, D., and Callard, P. (1995). The current spectrum of infectious glomerulonephritis. Experience with 76 patients and review of the literature. *Medicine* **74**, 63–73.

Morrin, P. A. F. *et al.* (1978). Rapidly progressive glomerulonephritis. A clinical and pathologic study. *American Journal of Medicine* **65** (3), 446–460.

Neild, G. H. *et al.* (1983). Rapidly progressive glomerulonephritis with extensive glomerular crescent formation. *Quarterly Journal of Medicine* **52**, 395–416.

Neugarten, J. and Baldwin, D. S. (1984). Glomerulonephritis in bacterial endocarditis. *American Journal of Medicine* **77**, 297–304.

Nicholls, K., Fairley, K. F., Dowling, J., and Kincaid-Smith, P. (1984a). The clinical course of mesangial IgA nephropathy. *Quarterly Journal of Medicine* **53**, 227–250.

Nicholls, K., Walker, R. G., Kincaid-Smith, P., and Dowling, J. (1984b). Malignant IgA nephropathy. *American Journal of Kidney Diseases* **5**, 42–46.

Nolasco, F. Cameron, J. S., Heywood, E. F., Hicks, J., Ogg, C., and Williams, D. G. (1986). Adult-onset minimal change nephrotic syndrome: a long-term follow-up. *Kidney International* **29**, 1215–1223.

Packham, D. K., Hewitson, T. D., Yan, H. D., Elliott, C. E., Nicholls, K., and Becker, G. J. (1994). Acute renal failure in IgA nephropathy. *Clinical Nephrology* **42**, 349–353.

Praga, M. *et al.* (1985). Acute worsening of renal function during episodes of macroscopic hematuria in IgA nephropathy. *Kidney International* **28**, 69–74.

Raij, L, Kaene, W. F., Leonard, A., and Shapiro, F. L. (1975). Irreversible renal failure in idiopathic nephrotic syndrome. *American Journal of Medicine* **61**, 207–214.

Reid, C. J. D., Marsh, M. J., Murdoch, I. M., and Clark, G. (1996). Nephrotic syndrome in childhood complicated by life threatening pulmonary oedema. *British Medical Journal* **312**, 36–38.

Robson, A. M., Giangiacomo, J., Kienstra, R. A., Naqvis, T., and Inglefinger, J. R. (1974). Normal glomerular permeability and its modification by minimal change nephrotic syndrome. *Journal of Clinical Investigation* **54**, 1190–1199.

Sakarcan, A., Timmons, C., and Seikaly, M. G. (1994). Reversible idiopathic acute renal failure in children with primary nephrotic syndrome. *Journal of Pediatrics* **125**, 723–727.

Salant, D. J., Adler, S., Bernard, D. B., and Stilmant, M. M. Acute renal failure associated with renal vascular disease, vasculitis, glomerulonephritis, and nephrotic syndrome. In *Acute Renal Failure* 2nd edn. (ed. B. M. Brenner and J. M. Lazarus), pp. 371–490. New York, NY: Churchill Livingstone, 1988.

Schena, F. P. (1990). A retrospective analysis of the natural history of primary IgA nephropathy world-wide. *American Journal of Medicine* **89**, 209–215.

Smith, J. D. and Hayslett, J. P. (1992). Reversible renal failure in the nephrotic syndrome. *American Journal of Kidney Diseases* **19**, 201–213.

Springate, J. E., Coyne, J. F., Karp, M. P., and Feld, L. G. (1987). Acute renal failure in minimal change nephrotic syndrome. *Pediatrics* **80**, 946–948.

Steele, B. T., Bacheyie, G. S., Baumal, R., and Rance, C. Ph. (1982). Acute renal failure of short duration in minimal change nephrotic syndrome. *International Journal of Pediatric Nephrology* **3**, 59–62.

Stephens, V. J., Yates, A. P. B., Lechler, R. I., and Baker, L. R. I. (1979). Reversible uraemia in normotensive nephrotic syndrome. *British Medical Journal* **ii**, 705–706.

Stilmant, M., Bolton, W., Sturgill, B., Schmitt, G. W., and Couser, W. G. (1979). Crescentic glomerulonephritis without immune deposits: clinicopathologic features. *Kidney International* **15**, 184–195.

Teague, C. A., Doak, P. B., Simpson, I. J., Rainer, S. P., and Herdson, P. B. (1978). Goodpasture's syndrome: an analysis of 29 cases. *Kidney International* **13**, 492–504.

Thompson, B. T. and Cockrill, B. A. (1994). Renal-dose dopamine: a siren song? *Lancet* **344**, 7–8.

Turney, J. H., Marshall, D. H., Brownjohn, A. M., Ellis, C. M., and Parsons, F. M. (1990). The evolution of acute renal failure (1956–1988). *Quarterly Journal of Medicine* **74**, 83–104.

van Ypersele de Strihou, C. (1979). Acute oliguric interstitial nephritis (Nephrology Forum). *Kidney International* **16**, 751–765.

Vriesendorp, R., Donker, A. J. M., De Zeeuw, D., De Jong, P. E., and Van der Hem, G. K. (1986). Effects of non-steroidal anti-inflammatory drugs on proteinuria. *American Journal of Medicine* **81** (Suppl. 2B), 84–94.

Welch, T. R., McAdams, A. J., and Berry, A. (1988). Rapidly progressive IgA nephropathy. *American Journal of Diseases of Childhood* **41**, 789–793.

Whitworth, J. A., Morel-Maroger, L., Mignon, F., and Richet, G. (1976). The significance of extracapillary proliferation. Clinicopathological review of 60 patients. *Nephron* **16**, 1–19.

10.6.2 Acute tubulointerstitial nephritis

Alexandre Karras, Frank Martinez, and Dominique Droz

Acute tubulointerstitial nephritis (ATIN) has a clinical and a pathological definition—acute renal failure with predominantly interstitial inflammation (Cavallo 1998). The infiltrate is composed of lymphocytes and sometimes of granulocytes, and can include granulomas. It is usually associated with interstitial oedema and some degree of tubular damage. When the interstitial inflammatory reaction is moderate, it may be difficult to decide whether the patient has ATIN or acute tubular necrosis because there is overlap between these two entities (Zollinger and Mihatsch 1979). The term acute interstitial nephritis is sometimes used to designate this entity, but ATIN is now preferred to emphasize that tubular *and* interstitial changes are both present (Colvin and Fang 1994; Cavallo 1998).

General features of acute tubulointerstitial nephritis

Clinical features

The incidence of ATIN is difficult to estimate because the presenting symptoms are not specific and diagnosis requires biopsy or autopsy. Petterson *et al.* (1984) found a prevalence of 0.7 per 100,000 in young Finnish military recruits who had renal biopsies because of persistent haematuria or proteinuria. ATIN was found in only 1–3 per cent of the renal biopsies done in a renal unit (Laberke and Bohle 1980; Colvin and Fang 1994); 40–60 per cent of these cases were associated with prior drug treatment. The incidence of ATIN was 6.5–14 per cent in series of patients biopsied because of unexplained acute renal failure (Linton *et al.* 1980; Davison *et al.* 1998), and in most the diagnosis was not suspected before biopsy.

The main causes of ATIN are given in Table 1. Sometimes the history may suggest the possibility of acute interstitial nephritis if there is systemic infection, a typical drug reaction, sarcoidosis, Sjögren's syndrome, or uveitis. However, most of the clinical features are non-specific. The urinary output is variable and urinalysis usually reveals mild to moderate proteinuria with an increased number of red and white blood cells. Leucocyte and red-cell casts are frequently found. There may be gross haematuria. The fractional excretion of sodium is often high, but in some cases, particularly those with hypovolaemia, low fractional excretions have been found (Lins *et al.* 1986). Proteinuria in the nephrotic range is uncommon and almost always in the rare cases of drug-induced ATIN with an associated minimal-change glomerulonephropathy (Pirson and Van Ypersele de Strihou 1986).

Blood eosinophilia and eosinophiluria are inconstant findings but, when present, tend to support the diagnosis of allergic, drug-induced, ATIN. The reported frequency of eosinophiluria ranges from 40 to 100 per cent, varying according to the criteria used for definition (e.g. a proportion of the urinary leucocytes ranging from 1 to 33 per cent), and the technique used for staining the cells (Ten *et al.* 1988). The absence of eosinophiluria does not exclude the possibility of ATIN. On the other hand, eosinophiluria is not specific for this nephritis, as it may also be found in chronic interstitial nephritis of

Table 1 Main causes of acute tubulointerstitial nephritis (ATIN)

Drug-related ATIN (see Table 2)
Infection-related ATIN (see Table 5)
Immune-mediated and systemic diseases
Lupus erythematosus
Sarcoidosis
Sjögren's syndrome
TINU syndrome
With anti-TBM antibodies
Malignancy
Lymphoma
Myeloma cast nephropathy
Other
Idiopathic ATIN

various causes, in transplant rejection, and in eosinophilic cystitis (Nolan *et al.* 1986). Increased amounts of major basic protein (MBP), which is contained in eosinophil cytoplasmic granules, have been found in the urine of patients with biopsy-proven acute interstitial nephritis, but there is an overlap with findings in patients with other renal diseases (Ten *et al.* 1988). Eosinophiluria is not therefore an accurate test for diagnosing ATIN (Ruffing *et al.* 1994).

Imaging reveals kidneys that are normally sized or enlarged. Renal ultrasonography shows increased cortical echogenicity, which correlates with the extent of interstitial infiltration in the biopsy. Marked renal uptake of gallium has been found in ATIN, but is also seen in subacute or chronic cases of interstitial nephritis, and in some patients with rapidly progressive glomerulonephritis (Linton *et al.* 1985; Shibasaki *et al.* 1991). Gallium uptake is not, however, increased in acute tubular necrosis. This overlap emphasizes the value of renal biopsy for distinguishing between these different pathological processes.

Pathological features (Colvin and Fang 1994; Cavallo 1998)

The most striking histological finding is the presence of numerous cells, mainly mononuclear, in the renal interstitium. Tubular changes, characterized by areas of epithelial injury and interstitial oedema, or fibrosis and oedema, are usually seen, but with a variable distribution. As there is often a scarce interstitial cellular infiltration in primary acute tubular necrosis (see Section 5), the diagnosis of ATIN requires careful evaluation of the abundance of the cellular infiltrate versus the tubular changes. Glomerular changes are usually limited to a degree of ischaemia (collapsed glomerular tuft with splitting of the capillary walls). The absence of glomerular lesions and of significant glomerular deposits by immunofluorescence is required for differential diagnosis from primary glomerular disease, lupus glomerulonephritis, essential mixed cryoglobulinaemia, and vasculitis—all conditions in which prominent interstitial cell infiltrates may be present.

Interstitial infiltrates

By light microscopy, the interstitial infiltrates of mononuclear cells are of variable density (Fig. 1). When of low density they may predominate in the corticomedullary area; in contrast, when they are profuse the cortical interstitium looks like a 'cell carpet' in which glomeruli seem to stand out. Infiltration is usually less prominent in the medulla. The mononuclear cells are mainly lymphocytes but some mature plasma cells are also seen. There are also numerous monocytes/macrophages but these are difficult to recognize in standard preparations. Polymorphonuclear cells constitute only a minor part of the cell infiltrate as compared to lymphocytes, even in the early phases of the disease and in acute interstitial nephritis related to sepsis. When present, eosinophils form only a small proportion of the interstitial cells, even in drug-induced, ATIN.

Epithelioid and non-caseating giant-cell granulomas are found in some cases, especially in those in which ATIN is related to drugs (Magil 1983). Epithelioid and giant-cell interstitial granulomas, which are the morphological expression of delayed-type, cell-mediated hypersensitivity, must be differentiated from giant-cell reactions seen around basement membrane material when tubulorrhexis is present. Non-caseating granulomas are either perivascular or disseminated in the interstitium (Fig. 2). Usually they are in moderate number, three or four per biopsy, and several levels will need to be examined for their identification.

Monoclonal antibodies have been used to improve characterization of these interstitial infiltrates. The majority of the interstitial lymphocytes are of the T lineage, CD3-positive (Fig. 3). Except in Sjögren's syndrome, there are only a few B cells, usually less than 10 per cent of the cells. In the majority of cases, CD4+ cells and CD8+ T cells occur in roughly equal proportions. In those receiving β-lactam antibiotics (Boucher *et al.* 1986), the CD4+ population predominates, while in those receiving cimetidine or non-steroidal anti-inflammatory drugs (NSAIDs) (Bender *et al.* 1984; Boucher *et al.* 1986; Cheng *et al.* 1989), CD8+ outnumber the CD4+ cells. Activation markers of the infiltrating T cells have also been examined expression of HLA class II antigen on T lymphocytes has been observed (Husby *et al.* 1981) but CD25 expression (interleukin-2 receptor) was rarely found (Boucher *et al.* 1986). Natural killer or large granular lymphocytes constitute only a small proportion of the lymphocytes (Cheng *et al.* 1989).

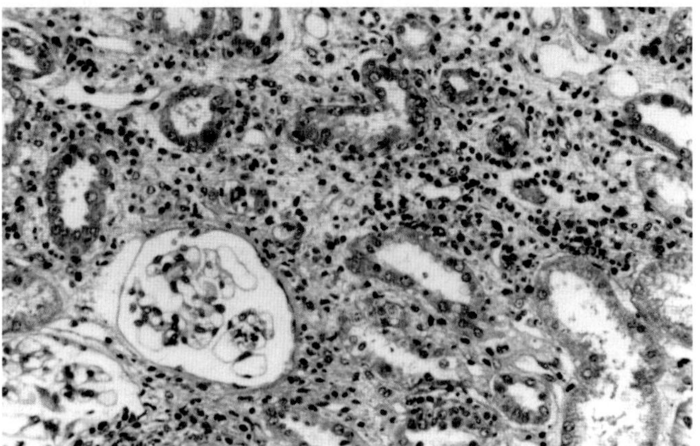

Fig. 1 Interstitial cell infiltration with oedema. Note the absence of glomerular change. Tubular cells are necrotic with appearance of 'tubulitis' (Masson's trichrome, 109×).

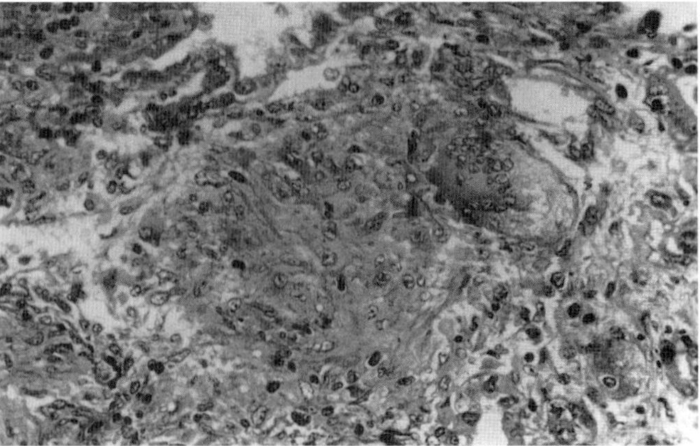

Fig. 2 Interstitial granuloma with epithelioid and giant cells in acute interstitial nephritis (Masson's trichrome, 170×).

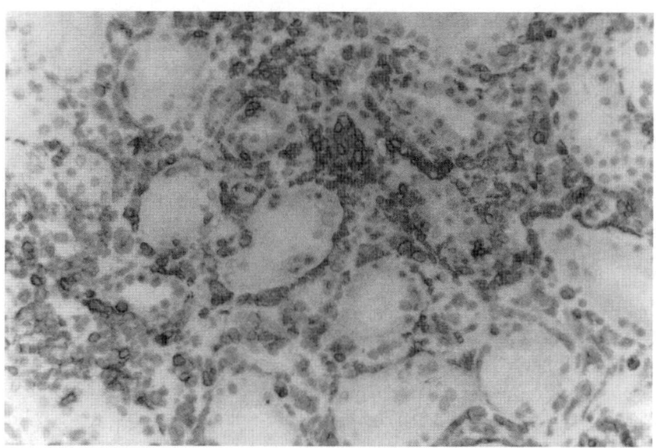

Fig. 3 CD3-positive lymphocytes in acute tubulointerstitial nephritis (immunoperoxidase, 109×).

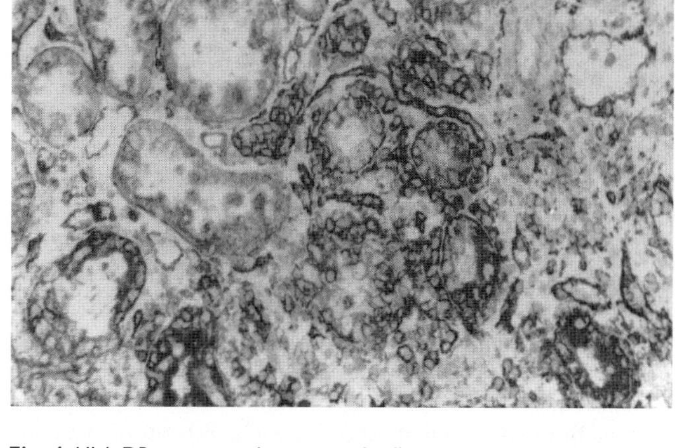

Fig. 4 HLA-DR expression by interstitial cells, capillary endothelium, and tubular cells in acute tubulointerstitial nephritis (immunoperoxidase, 109×).

The use of monoclonal antibodies has proved the importance of the monocytic/macrophage population in the renal infiltrates: up to 50 per cent of the infiltrating cells are CD14+ macrophages (Boucher *et al.* 1986; Cheng *et al.* 1989). When non-caseating granulomas are present, macrophages and CD4+ T lymphocytes predominate (Boucher *et al.* 1986). Overall, the phenotypic studies of interstitial cells in ATIN have not been helpful in identifying the cause, but have furthered understanding of the immunopathogenic mechanisms (see below).

Cell-adhesion molecules have a role in leucocyte recruitment, adherence to the endothelium, extravasation, and migration to sites of tissue injury. Two members of the integrin family, namely leucocyte function-associated antigen (LFA)-1 (CD11a/CD18) and very late antigen (VLA)-4 ($\alpha_4\beta_1$-integrin or CD49d/CD29), are independent leucocyte-adhesion molecules for attachment to the endothelium by interacting specifically with endothelial cell-surface molecules, intercellular adhesion molecule (ICAM)-1, ICAM-2, and vascular-cell adhesion molecule (VCAM)-1. Immunohistochemical studies have shown that a large proportion of interstitial infiltrating cells express LFA-1 and VLA-4 molecules (Mampaso *et al.* 1992). Mononuclear inflammatory cells in interstitial infiltration express the CCR5 molecule, which is the receptor for the C–C chemokine RANTES (Segerer *et al.* 1999).

Tubular lesions

There are almost always epithelial lesions of variable intensity. Swelling of the tubular cells with alteration of the tubular brush border, progressing to necrosis, are frequently seen. There may be a T lymphocyte infiltrate, mainly CD8+ cells, between the tubular cells, as in other pathological conditions such as acute transplant rejection. Such lesions are referred to as 'tubulitis' and mainly affect the distal part of the nephron (Racusen *et al.* 1999). Rupture of the tubular basement membranes, better seen in silver-stained sections, occurs in only the most severe cases. In these, there may be a giant-cell reaction close to the necrotic material.

Immunohistological studies have shown aberrant expression of HLA class II molecules, by tubular cells in ATIN (Boucher *et al.* 1986; Cheng *et al.* 1989) (Fig. 4), but no correlation between HLA-DR in tubular epithelium and the intensity or the phenotype of interstitial cell infiltrates (Cheng *et al.* 1989). This phenomenon is not restricted to any particular cause of ATIN and is also observed in other pathological conditions such as lupus nephritis, vasculitis, primary glomerular disease, and transplant rejection (Boucher *et al.* 1986). As antigen presentation takes place in a context of HLA class II molecules, DR+ tubular cells would be able to present antigen to helper T cells and thus initiate or amplify local immune reactions and tissue damage. As in other conditions such as allograft rejection or severe glomerulonephritis, *de novo* expression of ICAM-1 is observed in acute interstitial nephritis at the apical pole of proximal tubular cells, whereas VCAM-1 is detected at the basolateral part of some tubules (Mampaso *et al.* 1992). Interleukin-6 is expressed by damaged tubules in correlation with the DR expression (Fukatsu *et al.* 1993).

Glomeruli and vessels

The glomeruli show a variable degree of ischaemia, except in ATIN and the nephrotic syndrome induced by NSAIDs, where minimal-change glomerular lesions with fusion of epithelial foot processes are seen. In rare cases, evolution towards focal glomerular sclerosis has been described, but such lesions are more frequent in elderly patients and must be interpreted with caution. Exceptional cases of ATIN with membranous glomerulonephritis have been described (Champion de Crespigny *et al.* 1988).

Aside from the vascular lesions that relate to the patient's age or condition, vasculitis has rarely been found, mainly in drug-induced acute interstitial nephritis (Kleinknecht *et al.* 1983). Significant congestion of intertubular capillaries, often with interstitial haemorrhage in the outer medulla, is suggestive of hantavirus nephropathy (Van Ypersele de Strihou *et al.* 1986) or nephropathia epidemica (see Chapters 6.7 and 10.6.6).

ICAM-1, a counter-receptor of the leucocyte LFA-1 molecule, is strongly expressed on endothelial cells of vessels. In addition, *de novo* expression of VCAM-1 can be observed on some peritubular endothelia (Mampaso *et al.* 1992).

Immunofluorescence

In the great majority of cases, immunofluorescence shows scarce and non-specific deposition of immune reactants that can be found in many other conditions including renal ageing. When oedema is present, fibrin can be seen in the interstitium. There is often granular or pseudolinear fixation of C3 along some tubular and capsular basement membranes. Complement and IgM deposits in the arteriolar walls correspond to the arteriosclerotic lesions.

In a minority of cases, immunofluorescence provides positive information. Linear fixation of IgG and C3 along the tubular basement membrane indicates the presence of autoantibodies directed against membrane antigens. The demonstration of circulating antibodies to tubular basement membrane by indirect immunofluorescence is positive in some of these cases.

In another small group of patients, granular deposits of immunoglobulins and complement are found along the tubular basement membrane and in the interstitium, suggesting immune-complex deposition.

Evolution of the lesions

Little is known about long-term pathological sequelae of ATIN because most patients recover and follow-up biopsies have rarely been taken. There is no doubt that in severe cases, where there is significant tubular damage (especially disruption of basement membrane), the injury will lead to fibrous scars and irreversible damage. Fibrosis develops more often when there are granulomas (Colvin and Fang 1994). Complement components, including the membrane attack complex (MAC C5b–C9), are often found along the tubular basement membrane in a variety of renal diseases with chronic interstitial lesions (Falk *et al.* 1983). From experiments in the rat, it has also been proposed that increasing intrarenal ammonia through a reduction of renal mass may activate the alternate complement pathway and lead to non-immune-mediated C3 deposition, thus perpetuating the tubulointerstitial damage.

More recently, attention has been drawn to the molecular mechanism of renal fibrogenesis. Several cytokines released by infiltrating inflammatory cells may activate fibroblasts. Monocyte/macrophages produce a variety of mediators, such as interleukin-1, fibroblast growth factor, platelet-derived growth factor, and transforming growth factor-β, that promote fibroblast proliferation or enhance the synthesis of extracellular matrix components. Moreover, it seems that tubular epithelial cells are also capable of producing factors that influence the biological behaviour of fibroblasts (Müller *et al.* 1992).

Drug-related acute interstitial nephritis (see also Chapter 19.2)

Numerous drugs may cause ATIN (Table 2). The most commonly implicated are the β-lactam antibiotics and NSAIDs. Sulfonamides, rifampicin, phenindione, thiazide diuretics, triamterene, cimetidine, allopurinol, and more recently, antiviral drugs, have all been held responsible for some cases of acute interstitial nephritis. Most of the remaining descriptions are single case reports and many of these patients had received more than one drug. It is not always clear whether the related symptoms were due to ATIN or to the underlying disease.

Table 2 Drugs associated with acute tubulointerstitial nephritis

Antibiotics	Analgesics and salicylates	Others
β-Lactam antibiotics	***Analgesics and salicylates***	***Diuretics***
Amoxicillin	Aminopyrine	Chlorthalidone
Ampicillin[a,b]	Antrafenin	Frusemide[a,b]
Carbenicillin	Aspirin[a]	Indapamide
Cloxacillin	Indapamide	Thiazides[b]
Methicillin[a,b]	Floctafenin[b]	Tienilic acid[b]
Nafcillin	Mesalazine (5-ASA)	Triamterene[a,b]
Oxacillin	Glafenin[b]	***Anticonvulsive agents***
Penicillin G[b]	Paracetamol[b] (acetaminophen)	Carbamazepine
Piperacillin	Noramidopyrine	Diazepam
Cefaclor	Salicylazosulfapyridine	Diphenylhydantoin[a,b]
Cefotaxime	Sulfinpyrazone	Phenobarbitone
Cefotetan	***Non-steroidal anti-inflammatory drugs***	Phenytoin[a]
Cephalexin	Alclofenac	Valproic acid
Cephalothin	Clometacin[b]	Lamotrigine[b]
Cephradine	Diclofenac[b]	***Others***
Other antibiotics	Diflunisalb	Ajmaline
Erythromycin	Fenclofenac	Allopurinol[a,b]
Ethambutol	Fenoprofen[a,b]	α-Methyldopa
Gentamicin	Flurbiprofen	Amphetamine
Isoniazid	Ibuprofen[a,b]	Azathioprine
Lincomycin	Indomethacin[b]	Bethanidineb
Polymyxin sulfate[b]	Ketoprofen	Captopril[b]
Quinolones	Mefenamic acid[a]	Cimetidine[a,b]
Piromidic acid	Naproxen[a]	Clofibrate
Ciprofloxacin[a,b]	Niflumic acid	Contrast agents
Norfloxacin	Phenazone	D-Penicillamine
Rifampicin[a,b]	Phenylbutazone	Gold and bismuth salts
Spiramycin[b]	Piroxicam[a,b]	Herbal medicines (aristolochic acid)
Sulfonamides[a,b]	Pirprofen	Interferon-α
Co-trimoxazole[a,b]	Sulindac	Interleukin-2
Tetracyclines	Tolmetin	Nicergoline
Minocycline	Zomepirac	Omeprazole[a]
Teicoplanin	Rofecoxib	Phenindione[a,b]
Vancomycin[b]	Celecoxib	Ranitidine
Antiviral agents		Warfarin sodium
Acyclovir[b]		Clozapine
Adefovir		Propyl-thiouracil
Cidofovir		
Foscarnet		
Indinavir[a]		
Tenofovir		

[a] Most frequently reported drugs.

[b] With possible granuloma formation.

Clinical and pathological features

The clinical picture may be characteristic, as in ATIN from β-lactams antibiotics. The reaction develops in a small number of patients, several days or weeks after taking the drug, and is not dose-dependent except in some cases after penicillin G and allopurinol (Rossert 2001). The signs and symptoms are fever, skin rash, arthralgias, sometimes liver involvement, gross haematuria, blood eosinophilia, and a variable degree of acute renal failure. Mild proteinuria and microscopic haematuria are always present, with urinary white- and red-cell casts. Proteinuria within the nephrotic range is almost exclusively found in NSAIDs-related acute interstitial nephritis. The renal failure is often non-oliguric and dialysis is required in one-third of patients. Hyperchloraemic acidosis and impaired urinary concentration have been reported, and may persist for months after withdrawal of the drug (Table 3).

The value of symptoms and signs of systemic allergy in predicting ATIN has been evaluated in a collaborative study: the positive predictive value of fever, arthralgias, blood eosinophilia, and/or hepatocellular damage was only 0.60 because these symptoms were also found in 24 per cent of patients with drug-induced acute tubular necrosis (Landais *et al.* 1987). Because of this overlap, the diagnosis of ATIN can only be established by renal biopsy.

In early biopsies, interstitial infiltrates of mononuclear cells, mainly lymphocytes and monocytes/macrophages, are commonly found, together with some eosinophils (see above). Epithelioid granulomas within the interstitium are an important histological feature, particularly when the clinical picture is not characteristic or when there are no eosinophils within the interstitium (Vanhille *et al.* 1987). In two series, interstitial granulomas were found in 27 per cent (Vanhille *et al.* 1987) and 45 per cent (Kleinknecht *et al.* 1983) of patients with drug-related acute interstitial nephritis. Those with interstitial granulomas are more often oliguric and more likely to suffer permanent renal damage than those without. Granulomas are not pathognomonic of drug-induced acute interstitial nephritis, and are also found in ATIN related to infections or in cases of unknown aetiology. In late biopsies, interstitial fibrosis and tubular atrophy are obvious.

Many of the laboratory tests used for diagnosing a hypersensitivity reaction lack both sensitivity and specificity (Rossert 2001). Circulating antibodies to penicillin, rifampicin, or glafenin and their derivatives have been found in some cases of acute interstitial nephritis attributed to these drugs. Circulating antibodies against the tubular basement membrane have been described in some case reports of acute interstitial nephritis after the use of methicillin, cephalothin, and phenytoin.

Most patients recover fully, provided the responsible agent is discontinued. The recovery of renal function depends on how long renal failure was present before the discovery of acute interstitial nephritis (Laberke and Bohle 1980). A few patients die during the acute phase from an underlying disease or from non-renal causes. Persistent renal failure may occur, particularly in older patients, and in those with prolonged renal failure and with diffuse, rather than focal, infiltrates or with interstitial granulomas (Vanhille *et al.* 1987; Colvin and Fang 1994).

The benefit of treatment with steroids remain a matter of debate. The evidence for using steroids in drug-related acute interstitial nephritis comes from anecdotal reports (Pusey *et al.* 1983) and from small, uncontrolled, non-randomized studies (Galpin *et al.* 1978; Laberke and Bohle 1980). Patients treated with prednisone have an earlier and more complete return to baseline serum creatinine than those left untreated. The risk of this therapy must be weighed against its benefit in any given patient. Some authors believe that a limited course of high-dose prednisone is advisable for biopsy-proven, acute interstitial nephritis if renal failure has persisted for more than 1 week after removal of any inciting factor.

Table 3 Diagnostic features in drug-related, acute tubulointerstitial nephritis

Proteinuria, usually <1 g/24 h; rarely >1 g/24 h (NSAIDs)
FE_{Na}, usually >1
Increased urinary leucocytes without pyuria
Macroscopic haematuria
Fever, skin rash, arthralgias, and/or hepatocellular damage
Blood eosinophilia
Eosinophiluria
Thrombocytopenia, autoimmune, haemolysis
Gallium scanning—positive
Renal biopsy—characteristic (see text)

Antibiotics

β-Lactams

These agents give the most characteristic picture of drug-induced ATIN (Table 4) (Galpin *et al.* 1978).

Many cases of methicillin-induced ATIN were reported during the 1970s. The incidence of renal dysfunction ranged between 12 and 20 per cent of patients treated for staphylococcal infections, or receiving prophylactic treatment before cardiac surgery. This agent is no longer used and other antistaphylococcal antibiotics are now preferred. Signs and symptoms of 'ATIN' have appeared between 2 and 60 days after the start of treatment. Fever often occurred in a bimodal pattern, the first rise being due to the infection, and the recurrence to a hypersensitivity reaction. Macroscopic haematuria, skin rash, blood eosinophilia, and eosinophiluria were present in one-third of the

Table 4 Main clinical and pathological features observed in acute tubulointerstitial nephritis related to β-lactams and NSAIDs

	β-Lactams	**NSAIDs**
Age	Any	Older
Male : female	3 : 1	1 : 2
Time of development	2–60 days	Months
Fever, rash, blood eosinophilia, and/or eosinophiluria	Frequent	Rare
Non-oliguric, acute renal failure	Frequent	Frequent
Nephrotic syndrome	Very rare	Frequent
Requirement for dialysis	15–20%	30–40%
Cellular infiltrates in renal biopsy		
Lymphocytes	Common	Common
Eosinophils	Frequent	Sometimes
Epithelioid granulomas	Sometimes	Rare
Circulating anti-TBM[a] antibodies	Inconstant	Absent
Renal recovery	Usual	Frequent
Efficacy of steroid therapy	Unproven	Unproven

[a] TBM, tubular basement membrane.

patients. Half of the adults with ATIN had an increased blood urea; mild renal impairment seemed to be the rule in children. Recovery occurred in 90 per cent of cases. Sodium wasting, hyperkalaemia, and/or distal tubular acidosis were prominent features in some patients.

There are only a few reported cases of ATIN in association with other penicillin derivatives, including ampicillin, amoxicillin, penicillin G, and piperacillin (Pusey *et al.* 1983; Kleinknecht *et al.* 1986; Joh *et al.* 1989). An allergic reaction is thus much less frequent than in methicillin-related acute interstitial nephritis. Renal and extrarenal symptoms may recur if the patient is again challenged with the drug or with a chemically related one, and all β-lactam antibiotics are best avoided in anyone who developed acute interstitial nephritis during treatment with a penicillin compound or a cephalosporin. Cephalosporins are rarely responsible for ATIN. Cross-sensitization to a penicillin derivative has not been found consistently in these patients.

Methicillin- and penicillin-related acute interstitial nephritis is often cited as an example of a lesion induced by antibodies against tubular membrane because dimethoxyphenylpenicilloyl hapten, with linear IgG and C3 deposits, has been detected along that membrane and circulating antibodies of this type have also been found in some patients (Border *et al.* 1974).

Sulfonamides

About 40 cases of acute interstitial nephritis following the use of normal or high doses of co-trimoxazole (trimethoprim and sulfamethoxazole) have been reported to date (Kleinknecht *et al.* 1983; Pusey *et al.* 1983; Cryst and Hammer 1988). Some of these patients had previous chronic renal insufficiency, but the dosage of co-trimoxazole had not been reduced. Two patients with transplants developed renal failure while on prednisone. Signs of hypersensitivity were often absent. Severe interstitial infiltrates with eosinophils and granulomas were frequently found in renal biopsies, and full renal recovery was not the rule.

Others

A number of cases of ATIN after rifampicin have been reported (Kleinknecht *et al.* 1983; Muthukumar *et al.* 2002). The reason for giving this drug was always tuberculosis. The regimen was either intermittent or discontinuous, with a medication-free period before starting the treatment again, more often a result of non-compliance than design. A few hours or days after taking the drug, the patients developed chills, myalgia, fever, lumbar pain, nausea or vomiting, and dark but not haematuric urine. Skin rash, eosinophilia, thrombocytopenia, haemolysis, or even hepatitis were occasional but inconstant features. Most had oliguric acute renal failure requiring dialysis but tubular dysfunction with or without progressive renal failure has also been described (Quinn and Wall 1989).

In half of the cases, renal biopsies showed a typical acute interstitial nephritis with only focal tubular necrosis or atrophy. In the remainder, marked injury of proximal tubules and little interstitial infiltration was the rule. Interstitial granulomas were sometimes present and associated proliferative glomerulonephritis has also been described (Neugarten *et al.* 1983). With a few exceptions, immunofluorescence studies were negative. High titres of circulating, antirifampicin antibodies have occasionally been found during the acute phase. These observations argue against an immune-complex pathogenesis and suggest, at least in some cases, a direct toxic effect (Colvin and Fang 1994).

After stopping the drug, most patients recover normal renal function over several weeks, but a few are left with residual interstitial fibrosis and permanent damage. There is no evidence that steroids hasten recovery, and renal failure may progress despite continuous prednisone therapy. A further challenge with rifampicin in affected patients should obviously be avoided.

Acute interstitial nephritis has been documented in a handful of cases after simultaneous treatment with isoniazid and ethambutol. Rifampicin was sometimes prescribed at the same time, but did not prevent improvement of renal function (Garcia-Martin *et al.* 1991).

Vancomycin has been implicated in the development of ATIN in a small number of cases. Patients developed fever, skin rash, eosinophilia and/or eosinophiluria, and renal failure (Ratner 1988). These signs were reversed when vancomycin was stopped. In all reports, the nephritis was suspected clinically but renal biopsies were not performed.

This nephritis has also been associated with the use of other antibiotics such as erythromycin (Singer *et al.* 1988), minocyclin (Kiessling *et al.* 2001), and nitrofurantoin (Korzets *et al.* 1994), and quinolone derivatives such as norfloxacin (Boelart *et al.* 1986) and ciprofloxacin (Lien *et al.* 1993).

Antiviral agents

Several antiviral agents have been associated with ATIN. A granulomatous form of interstitial nephrits has been described with acyclovir, but several new drugs such as cidofovir, adefovir, and tenofovir, which are nucleotide analogues that share a same molecular structure, have been responsible for ATIN presenting as renal failure and Fanconi syndrome.

Indinavir is distinguishable from other HIV-protease inhibitors by its ability to induce crystalluria and urolithiasis. Crystals and kidney stones are composed of monohydrated indinavir. Three to 10 per cent of patients treated with indinavir develop renal colic and or nephrolithiasis (Martinez *et al.* 1998). Less frequently indinavir could induce ATIN, without urological symptoms. In these cases, renal biopsies showed crystals—composed of indinavir—in the lumen of some collecting ducts, and a mixed lymphocytic–histiocytic interstitial infiltrate with prominent fibrosis. Indinavir is soluble in acidic environment, however, there are several reports where the urine pH was 5.0–5.5 at the time of diagnosis of nephrolithiasis or nephropathy. Chronic renal dysfunction can persist several months after indinavir withdrawal. Ample hydration is recommended in order to prevent indinavir-associated crystalluria and urolithiasis.

Non-steroidal anti-inflammatory drugs (see also Chapter 6.3)

A number of functional disturbances of the kidney and examples of acute renal failure have been reported with the use of a large variety of NSAIDs (Clive and Stoff 1984; Kleinknecht 1995) (see Chapter 6.3 and Table 2). In some instances, the nephritis developed after taking various of these drugs in clinical use. Most of these patients were over 60 years of age, an age group in which these drugs are heavily consumed, often without medical prescription.

The clinical picture is somewhat different from that of acute nephritis related to β-lactams (Table 4). There may be no symptoms and signs of hypersensitivity, and renal insufficiency has a progressive onset, discovered several months or years after the start of treatment. Extrarenal signs are rare. Vasculitis has been reported in a few cases. Patients taking mefenamic acid often present with abdominal pain, diarrhoea, and vomiting.

More than 80 per cent of patients with acute interstitial nephritis related to NSAIDs develop a nephrotic syndrome; less than 1 per cent do so where it is related to β-lactams. In biopsies, the glomeruli show minimal changes in addition to the tubulointerstitial lesions already described. Epithelioid granulomas are sometimes associated features (Kleinknecht *et al.* 1986; Schwarz *et al.* 1988). Minimal-change nephrotic syndrome without acute interstitial nephritis has also been reported with many NSAIDs (Colvin and Fang 1994; Kleinknecht 1995) (for the pathogenesis of this particular type, see Chapter 6.3).

The place of steroid therapy remains controversial. In many cases, acute interstitial nephritis and the nephrotic syndrome remit within weeks or months of discontinuation of the drugs. There is some evidence that prednisone may hasten recovery in patients with epithelioid granulomas. Considering that chronic renal failure may develop (Kleinknecht 1986; Schwarz *et al.* 1988), it seems advisable to give prednisone to those patients before irreversible lesions have appeared.

Acute renal failure may or may not recur after resuming therapy with the same NSAIDs or with a different one (Kleinknecht 1995). ATIN has now been described with the newer NSAIDs, selective inhibitors of COX-2 enzyme, namely rofecoxib and celecoxib (Rocha *et al.* 2001; Henao *et al.* 2002).

Other drugs

Analgesics and salicylates (see also Chapter 6.2)

Some cases with definite ATIN have been described after the intake of glafenin, an analgesic formerly used in Europe and now withdrawn from the market.

Biopsy-proven ATIN has been found in a few patients receiving therapeutic doses of paracetamol (Kleinknecht *et al.* 1983; Pusey *et al.* 1983) but various other drugs were sometimes taken with this (Singer *et al.* 1988).

Salicylate derivatives may occasionally be responsible for some cases of tubulointerstitial nephritis, including 5-aminosalicylic acid, also called mesalazine, used as an adjunctive therapy for ulcerative colitis (Frandsen *et al.* 2002).

Diuretics

During the 1970s, there were some reports of patients with the idiopathic nephrotic syndrome who had received thiazides or frusemide, or a combination of both, and who developed rash, fever, or blood eosinophilia. Renal biopsy showsed numerous interstitial infiltrates of lymphocytes and eosinophils, associated with pre-existing glomerular lesions. Withdrawal of the diuretics and steroid therapy resulted in prompt recovery of renal function.

More recently, ATIN has been reported in patients without underlying renal disease who were taking a combination of hydrochlorothiazide (or another thiazide) and triamterene (Magil *et al.* 1980; Kleinknecht *et al.* 1983; Vanhille *et al.* 1987). Acute renal failure developed several weeks after the start of treatment, together with signs and symptoms of systemic allergy. On biopsy, most of these patients had interstitial infiltrates and epithelioid granulomas; immunofluorescence was negative. Withdrawal of the drug, with or without steroids, led to rapid recovery of renal function in all cases. It seems that triamterene potentiates the deleterious effect of thiazides, because some cases of acute interstitial nephritis have appeared after the use of triamterene alone or in combination with frusemide (Magil *et al.* 1980).

Miscellaneous

Severe hypersensitivity reactions to allopurinol, causing ATIN, have been described in several patients with pre-existing renal impairment and relative overdosing of the drug resulting from simultaneous treatment with diuretics (Grüssendorf *et al.* 1981; Cameron and Symmonds 1987). There was often widespread organ involvement, with renal, and sometimes hepatic, granulomas. A return to baseline renal function occurred after stopping allopurinol. The systemic reaction may have been favoured by increased serum concentrations of allopurinol, and of oxypurinol, a metabolite, because both renal insufficiency and diuretics decrease the urinary excretion of these compounds.

ATIN has been associated with the use of cimetidine, an H_2-receptor antagonist. The presentation is of fever, myalgia, and non-oliguric renal insufficiency several weeks after the start of treatment. Eosinophils were often found in serum, urine, and within the interstitium in biopsies. Most patients regained normal renal function after withdrawal of the drug, but residual renal damage was found in some cases (Kaye *et al.* 1983). There was some evidence that steroids hastened recovery in one case. Ranitidine, another selective H2-receptor blocker, was responsible for at least three cases of tubulointerstitial nephritis, including one with Fanconi syndrome and renal tubular acidosis (Gaughan *et al.* 1993; Neelakantappa *et al.* 1993). Even the use of proton-pump inhibitors such as omeprazole may be associated with interstitial nephritis (Ruffenach *et al.* 1992; Myers *et al.* 2001).

Captopril was reported to induce ATIN in a few patients, as did phenytoin. Interestingly, Hyman *et al.* (1978) demonstrated the presence of phenytoin along the tubular basement membrane, within the renal interstitium, and in the arteriolar walls, raising the possibility that the acute nephritis was associated with the formation of antibodies to the tubular membrane. Almost all other reports of acute interstitial nephritis are of single cases (see Table 2). Detailed references for these cases can be found in reviews (Colvin and Fang 1994; Rossert 2001) to which may be added anecdotal cases of ATIN associated with fenofibrate, D-penicillamine, warfarin, streptokinase as well as several anticonvulsant drugs such as valproate, phenobarbital, phenothiazines, and lamotrigine.

Two cases of tubulointerstitial nephritis following the use of recombinant interleukin-2 have been reported (Feinfeld *et al.* 1991; Vlasveld *et al.* 1993). The investigators suggested that renal damage could be the result of a cytotoxic, lymphocyte-mediated reaction induced by the cytokine therapy.

Interstitial nephritis rapidly progressing towards fibrosis has been observed in association with the use of certain Chinese herbal medicines (Vanherweghem *et al.* 1993). The herbs prescribed were taken as a slimming regimen by young women, mainly in Belgium, and contained aristolochic acid, a known nephrotoxin. Renal function continues to worsen after withdrawal of the offending agent, leading in most cases to irreversible renal failure and later, urothelial malignancies. This new type of nephropathy illustrates the need for a search for a toxic agent in any case of unexplained interstitial nephritis (see Chapter 6.8).

Acute tubulointerstitial nephritis and infection

Despite the introduction of antibiotics, and better recognition of the drug-induced variety, the most common forms of ATIN are related to infection. This is particularly so in children, in whom drug-related ATIN is rare (Ellis *et al.* 1981). In some cases, it should be difficult to assess whether the nephritis may should be attributed to the drug given to treat the infection or to the infection itself. ATIN may result from direct invasion of the renal parenchyma by the infective organism or from the reaction to the systemic infection (Table 5).

Septicaemia

Direct bacterial invasion of the renal parenchyma may complicate septicaemia due to various micro-organisms such as *Escherichia coli*, *Proteus*, Staphylococci, and *Candida albicans*. In many cases, the origin is an infection of the urinary tract itself, with or without obstruction. Predisposing factors are often present: old age, diabetes, or prolonged treatment with cytotoxic drugs, steroids, or NSAIDs.

The clinical picture is often that of a typical acute pyelonephritis (see also Section 7). Atypical cases are not exceptional, and presenting features may include fatigue, weight loss, gastrointestinal disturbances, or recurrent cystitis. Non-nephrotic proteinuria with progressive renal failure is common. Most patients are not oliguric. Renal biopsies show interstitial infiltration by polymorphonuclear leucocytes, forming microabscesses in some cases (Thomsen *et al.* 2002). A computed tography scan with contrast enhancement shows typically wedge-shaped or round, hypodense areas, diffuse hypodensity and/or abscesses, frequently accompanied by perirenal oedema (Meyrier *et al.* 1989). These lesions may not be obvious on intravenous pyelograms and by ultrasonography.

Prompt control of the acute infection is essential to rescue renal function and to prevent renal scarring (Meyrier *et al.* 1989). Uncontrolled infection results in extensive renal suppuration and a risk of death. Superimposed acute bacterial interstitial nephritis may exacerbate an existing chronic renal failure.

Table 5 Infections associated with acute tubulointerstitial nephritis

Bacteria
Streptococci, diphtheria, pneumococci, brucellosis[a], legionella, tuberculosis[a], typhoid fever[a], *Yersinia pseudotuberculosis*, enterobacteriaceae
Spirochaetes
Syphilis, leptospirosis
Rickettsia
Rocky Mountain and Mediterranean spotted fevers
Viruses
Human immunodeficiency virus, cytomegalovirus, Epstein–Barr virus[a], hantavirus, measles, echovirus, coxsackie virus, adenovirus, mumps, influenza, herpes simplex, hepatitis A and B, polyomavirus (BK type)
Others
Toxoplasma[a], mycoplasma, leishmania, chlamydia infections

[a] With possible granuloma formation.

Leptospirosis

Systemic infection by spirochaetes is rare in Europe and is mainly due to *Leptospira interrogans* serotype. During the second week of the disease, ATIN develops; the infiltrate contains lymphocytes, monocytes, plasma cells, and neutrophils, associated with various degrees of tubular necrosis (Yang *et al.* 2001). Leptospires can be demonstrated within the kidneys in two-thirds of cases (Colvin and Fang 1994). In the majority of cases, the renal lesions subside within a few weeks after resolution of the disease, although some interstitial infiltration may persist for several months in individual patients, generally those with persistent spirochaetes in the urine. There may be residual interstitial fibrosis and renal insufficiency.

Haemorrhagic fever with renal syndrome (see also Chapter 10.6.6)

Haemorrhagic fever due to hantaviruses is recognized in Europe with increasing frequency (Van Ypersele de Strihou *et al.* 1986). Biopsy shows tubular dilation or atrophy, interstitial oedema with mononuclear infiltrates, and often areas of medullary haemorrhage. Renal failure resolves rapidly leaving few late sequelae.

Polyomavirus (BK virus) infection

Recent studies have revealed that ATIN can be caused by a specific polyomavirus named BK virus (Ramos *et al.* 2002). This disease is mainly seen in renal transplant recipients who receive high-dose immunosuppressive regimens. The virus reactivation is reponsible for progressive renal graft dysfunction. Renal pathology shows extensive tubular necrosis, predominantly of distal medullary tubules and collecting ducts, associated with marked interstitial inflammation. This diagnosis is made by finding viral inclusions inside tubular cells, but also with indirect signs such as the presence of 'decoy' cells in the urine. A urine polymerase chain reaction test is now available.

Miscellaneous infections

ATIN may complicate infections in the absence of bacteraemia or acute renal parenchymal invasion. Before the antibiotic era, such nephritis was a relatively common complication of scarlet fever and diphtheria. The lesions occurred early in the course of the infection, usually within the first week or the first few days. Focal or diffuse interstitial infiltration by mononuclear cells was prominent. These lesions are quite different from those of pyelonephritis, because of their perivascular distribution, mostly in the corticomedullary region. Since the introduction of effective antibiotics, the incidence of such cases has declined (Ellis *et al.* 1981), but remains significant in some paediatric and adult series (Colvin and Fang 1994).

Many other infections may occasionally cause ATIN (Table 5). Of interest are occasional cases related to infectious mononucleosis (Ten *et al.* 1988; Verma *et al.* 2002), as renal interstitial fibrosis may persist after the acute episode. The Kawasaki disease virus has also been implicated in some instances of tubulointerstitial nephritis

(Colvin and Fang 1994). Some cases of ATIN related to *Yersinia pseudotuberculosis* infection have been reported in Japan (Okada *et al.* 1991). In the Mediterranean area, *Rickettsia prowazekii* and *R. conorii* (Almirall *et al.* 1995) may also be responsible.

Renal biopsy in patients infected by HIV-1 has revealed the relatively high frequency of ATIN (Nochy *et al.* 1993). The histopathological analysis showed large amounts of mononuclear cells (mainly CD8+ lymphocytes, macrophages, and plasma cells) in the interstitium. Such interstitial involvement can be associated with or without the glomerular lesions and is observed in both Black and in White patients. The frequency of hypergammaglobulinaemia, as well as the lymphocytic infiltration of other organs such as salivary glands and liver, suggests that acute lymphoplasmocytoid tubulointerstitial nephritis could be related to a virus-induced immune disorder.

Other types of acute interstitial nephritis

Systemic diseases

The renal lesions occurring during systemic diseases primarily affect the glomeruli, and tubulointerstitial involvement is secondary (see Section 4). However, prominent tubulointerstitial lesions with oliguric, acute renal failure have been observed in a handful of cases of systemic lupus erythematosus. Granular deposits of IgG and complement were found along the tubular basement membrane, and glomerular changes were mild, apparently not responsible for the renal failure. Primary tubulointerstitial lesions with limited glomerular involvement may also occur in transplanted kidneys.

Renal insufficiency from tubulointerstitial nephritis may develop in rare cases of primary Sjögren's syndrome (Rayadurg and Koch 1990 and reviewed by Bacon and Winearls 1996). On pathological examination, the interstitium is invaded by lymphocytes of the CD4 phenotype and by plasma cells. Immunoglobulin and complement deposits have been detected along the tubular basement membranes. A dramatic improvement in renal function may follow steroid therapy.

Sarcoidosis may present as isolated, acute renal failure (Brause *et al.* 2002). Multinucleated giant cells or interstitial granulomas are found in biopsies. The infiltrating lymphocytes are of the CD4 subset. In some patients, the renal interstitium may contain eosinophils but not granulomas, mimicking a drug-related acute interstitial nephritis (Colvin and Fang 1994). The renal failure responds promptly to prednisone, but persistent dysfunction is not uncommon if diagnosis is delayed (see also Chapter 4.4).

ATIN, associated or not with renal granulomas has been observed in polyglandular autoimmune syndrome and in common variable immunodeficiency (Hanningan 1996; Fakhouri 2001).

Malignancy

Massive invasion of the kidneys by malignant cells may occur in lymphoproliferative disorders and in plasma-cell dyscrasias (see Chapter 4.3). Other causes of renal failure should be excluded in these patients, such as ureteral obstruction or metabolic disorders (tumour lysis syndrome with hypercalcaemia, and hyperuricaemia). Irradiation of the kidneys or chemotherapy may rapidly improve renal function.

Idiopathic

Over the last years, there has been an increasing number of reports of ATIN associated with unilateral or bilateral uveitis or iritis (Ten *et al.* 1988; Gafter *et al.* 1993; Sessa *et al.* 2000). Uveitis may occur in many systemic disorders, but is rarely associated with ATIN. This association has therefore been called renal–ocular syndrome or tubulointerstitial nephritis and uveitis (TINU syndrome).

Initial symptoms occur mostly in adolescent girls or in adult females, and include fever, weight loss, myalgia, blood eosinophilia with eosinophiluria, mild renal failure, and hypergammaglobulinaemia. Proximal and/or distal tubular dysfunction may be associated features. Histologically there is ATIN, with or without eosinophils and tubular lesions. Steroids dramatically improve the renal and ocular lesions, but spontaneous improvement has also been observed. Topical steroids can be prescribed in cases with relapsing uveitis. Chronic renal failure requiring dialysis may develop in the absence of steroid therapy. TINU syndrome is a cell-mediated disease associated with suppressed peripheral T-helper cell function (Gafter *et al.* 1993).

ATIN of unknown cause has been described in the absence of uveitis. Clinical, biological, and histological features are identical to those found in the TINU syndrome, and this form also responds favourably to steroids. Associated systemic diseases, such as chronic active hepatitis, primary biliary cirrhosis, ulcerative colitis, light-chain disease, idiopathic cranial diabetes insipidus, Whipple's disease, or eosinophilic fasciitis have sometimes been present in individual cases.

Pathogenesis of acute tubulointerstitial nephritis: experimental models and their human counterparts (see reviews by Wilson 1989; Kelly *et al.* 1991; Michel and Kelly 1998)

Various experimental models, especially in rodents, have been devised to induce tubulointerstitial damage, but only a few really mimic human ATIN as defined above. The available models were once classified into two main groups: antibody mediated and cell mediated. However, these two largely overlap and a schematic division based on immunofluorescence findings appears more appropriate as it corresponds to what is observed in human disease. In fact, whatever the histological appearance on light microscopy (presence of interstitial cell infiltrates), the use of immunofluorescence allows greater discrimination: no significant immune deposits in the interstitium and along the tubular basement membrane (majority of the cases); the linear fixation of IgG along that membrane (antitubular basement membrane disease); granular deposits of immunoglobulins and complement fractions along the tubular membrane and in the interstitium.

Antitubular basement membrane disease (see also Chapter 3.11)

Although it is the least common of the conditions in man, antitubular basement membrane disease has been extensively studied in animals (see Wilson 1989). The first models were induced in the guinea pig in 1971 by immunization with a crude preparation of rabbit tubular basement membrane in Freund's adjuvant. The animals developed renal insufficiency related to tubular damage and interstitial infiltration by mononuclear and giant cells. Immunofluorescence showed linear IgG and C3 fixation along the tubular membrane and circulating antibodies to the membrane were found in the serum. Linear fixation along the glomerular basement membrane and circulating antibodies to that membrane were also present in half of the animals, but the glomeruli looked normal by light microscopy. There were strain differences in susceptibility, which segregated with the major histocompatibility complex (MHC) (Hyman *et al.* 1976). The disease was easily transferred with antibody but not with immune cells, suggesting a major role for antibodies against tubular basement membrane in the pathogenesis. Both IgG1 and IgG2 isotypes transferred the disease and generated autoimmune amplification. The injection of heterologous anti-idiotypic antibodies inhibited production of antibody to the tubular membrane, and decreased tubulointerstitial damage. The depletion of complement with cobra-venom factor also inhibited the tubular interstitial disease, implying a role of complement in this model. Guinea pig antibodies to the tubular membrane enhanced *in vitro* antibody-dependent cell-mediated cytotoxicity (Neilson and Phillips 1981).

An antitubular basement membrane disease model has been developed in Brown–Norway or Lewis × Brown–Norway F1 rats by immunization with Sprague-Dawley rat kidney homogenate or with bovine tubular basement membrane. Passive transfer of sensitized cells in naive rats resulted in mild tubulointerstitial nephritis. The characterization of renal inflammatory cells in Brown–Norway rats with the disease showed sequential accumulation of T cells with predominant T helper cells, then monocytes/macrophages after an initial polymorphonuclear leucocyte infiltration, coincident with the deposition of antitubular basement membrane antibodies and complement. Monocyte/macrophage interstitial infiltration increased after 2 weeks of the disease and then constituted 40 per cent of the total cells recovered from infiltrates when fibrosis and histological evidence of chronicity became apparent (Mampaso and Wilson 1983). When given early, and in high daily doses, cyclosphosphamide impaired the immune response and prevented tubulointerstitial nephritis. When given to animals with established disease it limited progression (Agus *et al.* 1986). Administration of cyclosporin A also impaired production of antibodies to tubular membrane and reduced tubulointerstitial damage (Gimenez *et al.* 1987).

By using monoclonal-antibody reactivity, several target antigens (which may share common epitopes) of antitubular basement membrane disease have been identified. The first one was a glycoprotein called 3M-1, with molecular mass of 48 kDa in man and 30 kDa in mice, secreted by proximal tubular cells and attached to the outer surface of the tubular basement membrane (Clayman *et al.* 1986). 3M-1 protein belongs to a family of intermediate filament-associated proteins. Although segments of this glycoprotein are preserved among different species, some polymorphism of expression occurs within a given species. This polymorphism may explain the development of anti-TBM antibodies after renal transplantation. Antibodies against 3M-1 can be found in different strains of mice, but nephrotoxicity appears only in selected strains such as SJL, SWR, or BALB/c (Neilson and Phillips 1982), which suggests that other factors, as susceptibility genes, are involved in this animal model.

A 58-kDa glycoprotein reacting with antitubular basement membrane antibodies has also been isolated (Butkowski *et al.* 1990). The full amino acid sequence of the 58-kDa target has been established, as well as its functional similarities to the cathepsin family of cysteine proteinases (Butkowski *et al.* 1994). This macromolecule, expressed essentially on proximal tubule cells (Chen *et al.* 1996), interacts with laminin and type IV collagen and seems to promote tubular epithelial cell adhesion (Kalfa *et al.* 1994). Anti-TBM antibodies in human have been shown to recognize this specific antigen in some cases (Ivanyi *et al.* 1998), but the pathogenic significance of these antibodies has not been proved.

Finally, antibodies that react to proximal tubule epithelial cells brush border have been observed in Heymann nephritis, a well-established animal model for membranous nephropathy. In this experimental model, interstitial infiltrates and injury are seen in addition to the classical and early glomerular lesions. One of the antigens involved has recently been identified as a membrane glycoprotein of the renal proximal tubule brush border named megalin, a multiligand receptor (Farqhar *et al.* 1995). However, autoantibodies against megalin have not been described in human tubulointerstitial nephritis.

The tolerance towards tubulointerstitial antigens can probably be broken by impairing normal surveillance systems with immunosuppressive drugs, by introducing a foreign antigen that cross-reacts with a self-structure, or by creating a neoantigen. This hapten–carrier conjugate responsible for the production of antibody to tubular membrane is a possible mechanism in some cases of human ATIN related to drugs, especially methicillin (Border *et al.* 1974), cephalotin, phenytoin, and possibly allopurinol (Grüssendorf *et al.* 1981). In one case of methicillin-associated ATIN with antibodies to tubular membrane, the dimethoxyphenylpenicilloyl breakdown products of methicillin were bound to that membrane together with IgG (Border *et al.* 1974). In a case of phenytoin-associated ATIN with these antibodies, phenytoin and IgG were present in a linear pattern along the tubular membrane.

However, in the great majority of human cases of ATIN, evidence for an antibody to tubular basement membrane is lacking. Moreover, no correlation has been found between titres of circulating antibodies to that membrane (when present) and disease activity. The passive transfer of human antitubular membrane antibodies fails to induce tubulointerstitial lesions in the rat although the antibodies bind to rat or guinea pig tubular basement membrane (Brentjens *et al.* 1989). Anti-TBM antibodies have been documented in a broad spectrum of renal disease such as antiglomerular membrane nephritis (Andres *et al.* 1978), membranous nephropathy (Ivanyi *et al.* 1998), lupus nephritis (Makker *et al.* 1980). Therefore, even when present, the pathogenic significance of such antibodies in acute interstitial nephritis remains uncertain. This is emphasized by findings in patients with renal transplants, who develop antibodies to tubular membrane that bind to the graft tubules but do not significantly impair renal function (Rotellar *et al.* 1986).

Immune-complex-mediated tubulointerstitial disease

Granular deposits of immunoglobulin and complement along the tubular basement membrane and in the interstitium characterize this group of tubulointerstitial diseases. Several experimental models have been developed. The process is triggered by either heterologous or autologous antigen. None results in ATIN but all produce interstitial infiltrates.

Chronic immunization of rabbits with large doses of bovine serum albumin leads, in addition to membranous glomerulonephritis, to granular deposits of the bovine albumin, IgG, and C3 along the tubular basement membrane and in peritubular areas. Tubulointerstitial lesions with IgG and C3 deposits along the tubular membrane can be produced in rabbits using various patterns of immunization (see Wilson 1989). Granular deposits along the tubular basement membrane together with tubulointerstitial lesions can also be found in late phases of Heymann nephritis (see Wilson 1989). A similar model of tubulointerstitial disease has been developed in rat by immunization with Tamm–Horsfall protein (Hoyer 1980). The rats developed autoantibodies to the protein; the immune deposits appear to be a consequence of *in situ* immune-complex formation. A similar experimental model in the rabbits, using endotoxin-free Tamm–Horsfall protein, results in chronic tubulointerstitial disease even in the absence of antibodies to the protein. Antibodies to that protein have been reported in humans with urinary tract infection, often in those with vesicoureteral reflux (Fasth *et al.* 1984). However, it has not been demonstrated that these antibodies are associated with renal deposits of the protein or that these deposits are related to interstitial inflammation (Chambers *et al.* 1986).

Certain strains of mice with autoimmune disease (NZB/W/F1, MRL/1) spontaneously develop granular deposits along the tubular basement membrane, and an interstitial cell infiltrate late in the course of the disease (see Wilson 1989). In lupus nephritis in man, granular deposits of IgG, C3, and C1q are frequently found along the tubular basement membrane, in the interstitium, and in the vessel walls, an observation that has a diagnostic value. However, in those rare patients with systemic lupus who present with acute renal failure, tubulointerstitial disease with abundant immune deposits is found in the absence of severe glomerular damage. Immunophenotyping of renal cell infiltrates has shown DR-positive T cells, with a predominance of either the CD4 or CD8 phenotype. In Sjögren's syndrome, immune-complex interstitial nephritis, more often of focal type, may occur. However, the role of immune complexes and/or that of cell-mediated immunity in this aspect of Sjögren's syndrome is not clear; the interstitial infiltrates contain mostly T cells with an increased proportion of CD4+ cells, but there are also nodules of B cells.

In a murine model, true ATIN was induced by challenge with specific antibody to the appropriate hapten–carrier antigen (Joh *et al.* 1989). In this model, humoral reactions with immune-complex formation appear to play a major part in inducing the renal lesions, and this could be relevant to some types of drug-induced ATIN in man.

Cell-mediated tubulointerstitial disease

This form of ATIN is characterized by the presence of mononuclear-cell infiltrates in the absence of significant deposits (either linear or granular) along the tubular basement membrane. Although incompletely understood, this pattern is the predominant form of human tubulointerstitial nephritis. Two main channels of injury are recognized: a delayed-type hypersensitivity reaction, involving mainly macrophages and CD4+ T lymphocytes, and direct T cell cytotoxicity involving mainly CD8+ T lymphocytes.

With regard to autologous or homologous antigens, several models of tubulointerstitial nephritis have been developed in Lewis rats by immunization with Lewis or Brown–Norway renal basement membranes (Sugisaki *et al.* 1980; Bannister *et al.* 1987). In Bannister's model, nodular tubulointerstitial nephritis with granuloma-like lesions are found in the cortex and the outer medulla. The disease is easily transferred to normal rats by cells from lymph nodes of immunized animals.

There has been wide interest in the spontaneous, chronic tubulointerstitial nephritis of *kdkd* mice. These mice develop, after 8 weeks of life, a fatal renal disease characterized by severe interstitial damage with tubular dilatation. Neither immunoglobulin deposits nor antibodies directed against tubulointerstitial determinants have been demonstrated (Neilson *et al.* 1984). The development of the renal lesions is markedly inhibited by thymectomy or by treatment with adoptively transferred T cells from CBA/Ca mice. The destructive renal lesions are mediated by tubular antigen-specific, H2-K-restricted, effector T cells of LyT-2+ phenotype, whose expression is facilitated by abnormal contrasupppression (Kelly and Neilson 1987). Both CD4+ and CD8+ T cells are involved in tubulointerstitial damage. Their cytotoxicity against tubular epithelial cells can be either direct, via expression of granzyme and perforine, or mediated by a delayed-type hypersensitivity reaction, leading to granuloma formation (Meyers *et al.* 1991, 1994; Heegers *et al.* 1994). The role of cell-adhesion molecules in the renal lesions has been demonstrated in that model; the injection of monoclonal antibody against murine ICAM-1 results in a significant reduction of tubulointerstitial lesions and proteinuria (Harning *et al.* 1992).

A human counterpart of cell-mediated ATIN is imprecisely recognized. However, the morphology of the lesions (granulomas and/or predominance of CD4+ T cells and macrophages in the interstitium) suggests that cell-mediated reactions of delayed-type hypersensitivity may occur in cases of drug-related ATIN (Magil 1983). In other forms of the nephritis (or in rapid deterioration of renal function), there is some evidence for a cell-mediated hypersensitivity reaction in sarcoidosis, and also in Wegener's granulomatosis. The association of ATIN with uveitis, where epithelioid and giant-cell granulomas also occur, could fit into this group of cell-mediated acute tubulointerstitial nephritides (Gafter *et al.* 1993).

In ATIN associated with NSAIDs and in the rare cases related to cimetidine, as well as those cases related to cytomegalovirus infection, the predominance of CD8+ T lymphocytes in the interstitium suggest the possibility of cell-mediated cytotoxicity (Bender *et al.* 1984; Boucher *et al.* 1986). However, in the majority of cases, CD4+ T lymphocytes were also found and sometimes were in the majority. Therefore, as phenotypic expression of T cells does not correlate with functional activity, and as the interstitial cell reaction is dynamic, reliable evidence for a predominantly cytotoxic reaction in human ATIN is lacking.

Direct hypersensitivity reactions

In direct, type I allergic reactions, the exposure to the sensitizing antigen leads to T cell activation, with maturation of specific B cells into plasma cells producing IgE antibodies against the antigen. The IgE antibodies bind to the mast cells and basophils, which, in turn, bind to the antigen, finally resulting in release of inflammatory mediators such as eosinophil chemotactic factors. Eosinophils as well as mast cells release proteases, leukotrienes, superoxides, peroxidases, and proteins, which have inflammatory effects.

Many patients with ATIN have signs of direct, type I hypersensitivity: fever, skin rashes, high serum concentrations of IgE, eosinophilia, eosinophiluria (Toto 1990), and the presence of eosinophils in the renal interstitial infiltrates. Such reactions mainly occur in drug-related ATIN: antibiotics, NSAIDs, phenobarbital (Kleinknecht *et al.* 1983).

Thus, it appears that several immune mechanisms may be implicated in the same case (humoral, cellular, IgE-mediated), either at the same time or sequentially, all resulting in the clinical disease and the histological appearances.

References

Agus, D. *et al.* (1986). The effects of daily cyclophosphamide administration on the development and extent of primary experimental interstitial nephritis in rats. *Kidney International* **29**, 635–640.

Almirall, J., Torremorell, D., Andreu, X., and Font, B. (1995). Acute renal failure as a complication of Mediterranean spotted fever. *Nephron* **69**, 338–339.

Andres, G., Brentjens, J., Kohli, R., Anthone, R., Baliah, T., Montes, M., Mookerjee, B. K., Prezyna, A., Sepulveda, M., Venuto, R., and Elwood, C. (1978). Histology of human tubulo-interstitial nephritis associated with antibodies to renal basement membranes. *Kidney International* **13**, 480–491.

Bacon, N. C. and Winearls, C. G. (1996). The patient with chronic renal failure of unknown origin—don't forget Sjögren's syndrome. *Nephrology, Dialysis, Transplantation* **11**, 1645–1648.

Bannister, K. M., Ulich, T. R., and Wilson, C. B. (1987). Induction, characterization and cell transfer of autoimmune tubulointerstitial nephritis in the Lewis rats. *Kidney International* **32**, 642–651.

Bender, W. L., Whelton, A., Beschorner, M. E., Darwish, M. O., Hall-Craggs, M., and Solez, K. (1984). Interstitial nephritis, proteinuria, and renal failure caused by nonsteroidal anti-inflammatory drugs. Immunologic characterization of the inflammatory infiltrate. *American Journal of Medicine* **76**, 1006–1012.

Boelart, J., de Jaegere, P. P., Daneels, R., Schurgers, M., Gordts, B., and Van Landurt, H. W. (1986). Case report of renal failure during norfloxacin therapy. *Clinical Nephrology* **25**, 272.

Border, W. A., Lehman, D. H., Egan, J. D., Stass, H. J., Glode, J. E., and Wilson, C. B. (1974). Antitubular basement-membrane antibodies in methicillin associated interstitial nephritis. *New England Journal of Medicine* **291**, 381–384.

Boucher, A., Droz, D., Adafer, E., and Noe, L. H. (1986). Characterization of mononuclear cell subsets in renal cellular interstitial infiltrates. *Kidney International* **29**, 1043–1049.

Brause, M., Magnusson, K., Degenhardt, S., Helmchen, U., and Grabensee, B. (2002). Renal involvement in sarcoidosis. *Clinical Nephrology* **57**, 142–148.

Brentjens, J. R. *et al.* (1989). Immunologic studies in two patients with antitubular basement membrane nephritis. *American Journal of Medicine* **86**, 603–608.

Butkowski, R. J., Langenveld, J. P. M., Wieslander, J., Brentjens, I. R., and Andres, G. A. (1990). Characterization of a tubular basement membrane component reactive with autoantibodies associated with tubulointerstitial nephritis. *Journal of Biology and Chemistry* **266**, 21091–21098.

Butkowski, R., Nelson, T., Klafa, T., and Charonis, A. S. (1994). Structure and function of tubulointerstitial nephritis antigen. *Journal of the American Society of Nephrology* **5**, 801.

Cameron, J. S. and Symmonds, H. A. (1987). Use and abuse of allopurinol. *British Medical Journal* **294**, 1504–1505.

Cavallo T. Interstitial nephritis. In *Heptinstall's Pathology of the Kidney* Vol. II, 5th edn. pp. 667–724. Boston: Little Brown, 1998.

Chambers, R., Groufsky, A., Hunta, J. S., Lyun, K. L., and McGiven, A. R. (1986). Relationship of abnormal Tamm–Horsfall glycoprotein localization to renal morphology and function. *Clinical Nephrology* **26**, 21–26.

Champion de Crespigny, P. J., Becker, G. J., Ihle, B. H., Walter, N. M. A., Wright, C. A., and Kincaid-Smith, P. (1988). Renal failure and nephrotic syndrome associated with sulindac. *Clinical Nephrology* **30**, 52–55.

Chen, Y., Krishnamurti, U., Wayner, E. A., Michael, A. F., and Charonis, A. S. (1996). Receptors in proximal epithelial cells for tubulointerstitial nephritis antigen. *Kidney International* **49**, 153–157.

Cheng, H. F., Nolasco, F., Cameron, J. S., Hildreth, G., Neild, G., and Hartley, B. (1989). HLA-DR display by renal tubular epithelium and phenotype of infiltrate in interstitial nephritis. *Nephrology, Dialysis, Transplantation* **4**, 205–215.

Clayman, M. D., Michaud, L., Brentjens, J., Andres, G. A., Kefalides, N. A., and Neilson, E. G. (1986). Isolation of the target antigen of human antitubular basement membrane antibody-associated interstitial nephritis. *Journal of Clinical Investigation* **72**, 1143–1147.

Clive, O. M. and Stoff, J. J. (1984). Renal syndromes associated with nonsteroidal anti-inflammatory drugs. *New England Journal of Medicine* **310**, 563–572.

Colvin, R. B. and Fang, L. S. T. Interstitial nephritis. In *Renal Pathology with Clinical and Functional Correlations* Vol. 1 (ed. C. C. Tisher and B. M. Brenner), pp. 723–768. Philadelphia: Lippincott, 1994.

Cryst, C. and Hammer, S. P. (1988). Acute granulomatous interstitial nephritis due to co-trimoxazole. *American Journal of Nephrology* **8**, 483–488.

Davison, A. M. and Jones, C. H. (1998). Acute interstitial nephritis in the elderly: a report from the UK MRC Glomerulonephritis Register and a review of the literature. *Nephrology, Dialysis, Transplantation* **13** (Suppl. 7), 12–16.

Ellis, D., Fried, W. A., Yunis, E. J., and Blan, E. B. (1981). Acute interstitial nephritis in children: a report of 13 cases and review of the literature. *Pediatrics* **67**, 862–870.

Falk, R. J. *et al.* (1983). Neoantigen of the polymerized ninth component of complement. Characterization of a monoclonal antibody and immunohistochemical localization in renal disease. *Journal of Clinical Investigation* **72**, 560–573.

Fakhouri, F., Robino, C., Lemaire, M., Droz, D., Noël, L. H., Knebelmann, B., and Lesavre, Ph. (2001). Granulomatous renal disease in a patient with common variable immunodeficiency. *American Journal of Kidney Diseases* **38**, E7.

Farqhar, M. G., Saito, A., and Kerjaschki, D. (1995). The Heymann nephritis antigenic complex: megalin (gp330) and RAP. *Journal of the American Society of Nephrology* **6**, 35–47.

Fasth, A., Bjure, J., Hjalmas, K., Jacobsson, B., and Jodal, U. (1984). Serum autoantibodies to Tamm–Horsfall protein and their relation to renal damage and glomerular filtration rate in children with urinary tract malformations. *Contributions to Nephrology* **39**, 285–295.

Feinfeld, D. A., D'Agati, V., Dutcher, J. P., Werfel, S. B., Lynn, R. I., and Wiernik, P. H. (1991). Interstitial nephritis in a patient receiving adoptive immunotherapy with recombinant interleukin-2 and lymphokine-activated killer cells. *American Journal of Nephrology* **11**, 489–492.

Frandsen, N. E., Saugmann, S., and Marcussen, N. (2002). Acute interstitial nephritis associated with the use of mesalazine in inflammatory bowel disease. *Nephron* **92**, 200–202.

Fukatsu, A., Matsuo, S., Yuzana, Y., Miyai, H., Futenma, A., and Kato, K. (1993). Expression of interleukin 6 and major histocompatibility complex molecules in tubular epithelial cells of diseased human kidneys. *Laboratory Investigation* **69**, 58–67.

Gafter, U. *et al.* (1993). Tubulointerstitial nephritis and uveitis: association with suppressed cellular immunity. *Nephrology, Dialysis, Transplantation* **8**, 821–826.

Galpin, J. E. *et al.* (1978). Acute interstitial nephritis due to methicillin. *American Journal of Medicine* **65**, 756–765.

Garcia-Martin, F., Mampaso, F., De Arriba, G., Moldenhauer, F., Martin-Escobar, E., and Saiz, F. (1991). Acute interstitial nephritis induced by ethambutol. *Nephron* **59**, 679–680.

Gaughan, W. J., Sheth, V. R., Francos, G. C., Michael, H. J., and Burke, J. F. (1993). Ranitidine-induced acute interstitial nephritis with epithelial cell foot process. *American Journal of Kidney Diseases* **22**, 337–340.

Gimenez, A., Leyva-Cobian, F., Fierro, C., Rio, M., Bricio, T., and Mampaso, F. (1987). Effect of cyclosporin A on autoimmune tubulointerstitial nephritis in the Brown–Norway rat. *Clinical and Experimental Immunology* **69**, 550–556.

Grüssendorf, M., Andrassy, K., Waldherr, R., and Ritz, E. (1981). Systemic hypersensitivity to allopurinol with acute interstitial nephritis. *American Journal of Nephrology* **1**, 105–109.

Hanningan, N. R., Jabs K., Perez-Atayde A. R., and Rosen S. (1996). Autoimmune interstitial nephritis and hepatitis in polyglandular autoimmune syndrome. *Pediatric Nephrology* **10**, 511–514.

Harning, R., Pelletier, J., Van, G., Takei, F., and Merluzzi, V. J. (1992). Monoclonal antibody to MALA-2 (ICAM1) reduces acute autoimmune nephritis in *kdkd* mice. *Clinical Immunology and Immunopathology* **64**, 129–134.

Heegers, P. S., Smoyer, W. E., Saad, T., Albert, S., Kelly, C. J., and Neilson, E. G. (1994). Molecular analysis of the helper T cell response in murine interstitial nephritis: T cells recognizing an immunodominant epitope use multiple TCR Vbeta genes with similarities across CDR3. *Journal of Clinical Investigation* **94**, 2084–2092.

Henao, J., Hisamuddin, I., Nzerue, C. M., Vasandani, G., and Hewan-Lowe, K. (2002). Celecoxib-induced acute interstitial nephritis. *American Journal of Kidney Diseases* **39**, 1313–1317.

Hoyer, J. R. (1980). Tubulointerstitial immune complex nephritis in rats immunized with Tamm–Horsfall protein. *Kidney International* **17**, 284–292.

Husby, G., Tung, K. S. K., and Williams, R. C. (1981). Characterization of renal tissue lymphocytes in patients with interstitial nephritis. *American Journal of Medicine* **70**, 31–38.

Hyman, L. R., Steinberg, A. D., Colvin, R. B., and Bernard, E. F. (1976). Immunopathogenesis of autoimmune interstitial nephritis. II. Role of an immune response gene linked to the major histocompatibility complex. *Journal of Immunology* **17**, 1894–1897.

Ivanyi, B., Haszon, I., Endreffy, E., Szenohradszky, P., Petri, I. B., Kalmar, T., Butkowski, R. J., Charonis, A. S., and Turi, S. (1998). Childhood membranous nephropathy, circulating antibodies to the 58-kd TIN antigen and anti-tubular basement membrane nephritis: an 11-year follow-up. *American Journal of Kidney Diseases* **32**, 1068–1074.

Joh, K. *et al.* (1989). Experimental drug-induced allergic nephritis mediated by antihapten antibody. *International Archives of Allergy and Applied Immunology* **88**, 337–344.

Kalfa, T. A., Thull, J. D., Butkowski, R. J., and Charonis, A. S. (1994). Tubulointerstitial nephritis antigen interacts with laminin and type IV collagene and promotes cell adhesion. *Journal of Biology and Chemistry* **269**, 1654–1659.

Kaye, W. A., Passero, M. A., Solomon, R. J., and Johnson, L. A. (1983). Cimetidine-induced interstitial nephritis with response to prednisone therapy. *Archives of Internal Medicine* **143**, 811–812.

Kelly, C. J. and Neilson E. G. (1987). Contrasuppression in autoimmunity. Abnormal contrasuppression facilitates expression of nephritogenic effector T cells and interstitial nephritis in *kdkd* mice. *Journal of Experimental Medicine* **165**, 107–123.

Kelly, C. J. Roth, D. A., and Meyers, C. M. (1991). Immune recognition and response to the renal interstitium. *Kidney International* **39**, 518–531.

Kiessling, S., Forrest, K., Moscow, J., Gewirtz, A., Jackson, E., Roszman, T., and Goebel, J. (2001). Interstitial nephritis, hepatic failure, and systemic eosinophilia after minocycline treatment. *American Journal of Kidney Diseases* **38**, E36.

Kleinknecht, D. (1995). Interstitial nephritis, the nephrotic syndrome, and chronic renal failure secondary to nonsteroidal anti-inflammatory drugs. *Seminars in Nephrology* **15**, 228–235.

Kleinknecht, D. *et al.* (1983). Acute interstitial nephritis due to drug hypersensitivity: an up-to-date review with a report of 19 cases. *Advances in Nephrology* **13**, 277–308.

Kleinknecht, D., Landais, P., and Goldfarb, B. (1986). Analgesic and nonsteroidal anti-inflammatory drug-associated acute renal failure: a prospective collaborative study. *Clinical Nephrology* **25**, 275–281.

Korzets, Z., Elis, A., Bernheim, J., and Bernheim, J. (1994). Acute granulomatous interstitial nephritis due to nitrofurantoin. *Nephrology, Dialysis, Transplantation* **9**, 713–715.

Laberke, H. G. and Bohle, A. (1980). Acute interstitial nephritis: correlations between clinical and morphological findings. *Clinical Nephrology* **14**, 263–273.

Landais, P., Goldfarb, B., and Kleinknecht, D. (1987). Eosinophiluria and drug-induced acute interstitial nephritis. *New England Journal of Medicine* **316**, 1664.

Lien, Y. H. *et al.* (1993). Ciprofloxacin-induced granulomatous interstitial nephritis and localized elastolysis. *American Journal of Kidney Diseases* **22**, 598–602.

Lins, R. L., Verpooten, G. A., De Clerck, D. S., and De Broe, M. (1986). Urinary indices in acute interstitial nephritis. *Clinical Nephrology* **26**, 131–133.

Linton, A. L., Richmond, J. M., Clark, W. F., Lindsay, R. M., Driedger, A. A., and Lamki, L. M. (1985). Gallium scintigraphy in the diagnosis of acute renal disease. *Clinical Nephrology* **24**, 84–87.

Magil, A. B. (1983). Drug-induced acute interstitial nephritis with granulomas. *Human Pathology* **13**, 36–41.

Magil, A. B., Ballon, H. S., Cameron, E. C., and Rae, A. (1980). Acute interstitial nephritis associated with thiazide diuretics: clinical and pathologic observation in three cases. *American Journal of Medicine* **69**, 939–943.

Makker, S. P. (1980). Tubular basement membrane antibody-induced interstitial nephritis in systemic lupus erythematosus. *American Journal of Medicine* **69**, 949–952.

Mampaso, F. M. and Wilson, C. B. (1983). Characterization of inflammatory cells in autoimmune tubulointerstitial nephritis in rats. *Kidney International* **23**, 448–457.

Mampaso, F., Sanchez-Madrid, F., Molina, A. Bricio, T., Liano, F., and Alvarez, V. (1992). Expression of adhesion receptor and counterreceptors from leukocyte-endothelial adhesion pathways LFA-1/ICAM-1 and VLA-4/ VCAM-1 on drug-induced tubulointersitial nephritis. *American Journal of Nephrology* **12**, 391–392.

Martinez, F., Mommeja-Marin, H., Estepa-Maurice, L., Beaufils, H., Bochet M., Daudon, M., Deray, G., and Katlama, C. (1998). *Nephrology, Dialysis, Transplantation* **13**, 750–753.

Meyers, C. M. and Kelly, C. J. (1991). Effector mechanisms in organ-specific auto-immunity. Characterization of a CD8+ T cell line that mediates murine interstitial nephritis. *Journal of Clinical Investigation* **88**, 408–416.

Meyers, C. M. and Kelly, C. J. (1994). Inhibition of murine nephritogenic effector T cells by a clone-specific suppressor factor. *Journal of Clinical Investigation* **94**, 2093–2104.

Meyrier, A. *et al.* (1989). Frequency of development of early cortical scarring in acute primary pyelonephritis. *Kidney International* **35**, 696–703.

Michel, M. M. and Kelly, C. J. (1998). Acute interstitial nephritis. *Journal of the American Society of Nephrology* **9**, 506–515.

Müller, G. A., Markovic-Lipkovksi, J., Frank, J., and Rodemann, H. P. (1992). The role of interstitial cells in the progression of renal diseases. *Journal of the American Society of Nephrology* **2**, S198–S205.

Muthukumar, T., Jayakumar, M., Fernando, E. M., and Muthusethupathi, M. A. (2002). Acute renal failure due to rifampicin: a study of 25 patients. *American Journal of Kidney Diseases* **40**, 690–696.

Myers, R. P., McLaughlin, K., and Hollomby, D. J. (2001). Acute interstitial nephritis due to omeprazole. *American Journal of Gastroenterology* **96**, 3428–3431.

Neelakantappa, K., Gallo, G. R., and Lowenstein, J. (1993). Ranitidine-associated interstitial nephritis and Fanconi syndrome. *American Journal of Kidney Diseases* **22**, 333–336.

Neilson, E. G. and Phillips, S. M. (1981). Cell-mediated immunity in interstitial nephritis. IV. Antitubular basement membrane antibodies can function in antibody-dependent cellular cytotoxicity reactions. Observation on a nephritogenic effector mechanism acting as an informational bridge between the humoral and cellular immune response. *Journal of Immunology* **126**, 1990–1993.

Neilson, E. G. and Phillips, S. M. (1982). Murine interstitial nephritis. I. Analysis of disease susceptibility and its relationship to pleimorphic gene products defining both immune-response genes and a restriction requirement for cytotoxic T cells at H-2 K. *Journal of Experimental Medicine* **155**, 1075–1085.

Neilson, E. G., McCafferty, E., Feldman, A., Clayman, M. D., Zakheim, B., and Korngold, R. (1984). Spontaneous interstitial nephritis in *kdkd* mice. I. An experimental model of autoimmune renal disease. *Journal of Immunology* **133**, 2560–2565.

Neugarten, J., Gallo, G. R., and Baldwin, D. S. (1983). Rifampicin-induced nephrotic syndrome and acute interstitial nephritis. *American Journal of Nephrology* **3**, 38–42.

Nochy, D. *et al.* (1993). Renal disease associated with HIV infection: a multicentric study of 60 patients from Paris hospitals. *Nephrology, Dialysis, Transplantation* **8**, 11–19.

Nolan, C. R., III, Anger, M. S., and Kelleher, S. P. (1986). Eosinophiluria—a new method of detection and definition of the clinical spectrum. *New England Journal of Medicine* **315**, 1516–1519.

Okada, K. *et al.* (1991). Acute tubulointerstitial nephritis associated with *Yersinia pseudotuberculosis*. *Clinical Nephrology* **35**, 105–109.

Pettersson, R., Von Bonsdorff, M., Tornroth, T., and Lindholm, H. (1984). Nephritis among young Finnish men. *Clinical Nephrology* **22**, 217–222.

Pirson, Y. and Van Ypersele de Strihou, C. (1986). Renal side effects of nonsteroidal anti-inflammatory drugs: clinical relevance. *American Journal of Kidney Diseases* **8**, 338–344.

Pusey, C. D., Saltissi, D., Bloodworth, L., Rainford, D. J., and Christie, J. L. (1983). Drug associated acute interstitial nephritis: clinical and pathological features and the response to high dose steroid therapy. *Quarterly Journal of Medicine* **52**, 194–211.

Quinn, B. P. and Wall, B. M. (1989). Nephrogenic diabetes insipidus and tubulointerstitial nephritis during continuous therapy with rifampicin. *American Journal of Kidney Diseases* **14**, 217–220.

Racusen L. C. *et al.* (1999). The Banff 97 working classification of renal allograft pathology. *Kidney International* **55**, 713–723.

Ramos, E., Drachenberg, C., Papadimitriou, J., Hamze, O., Fink, J., Klassen, D., Drachenberg, R., Wiland, A., Wali, R., Cangro, C., Schweitzer, E., Bartlett, S., and Weir, M. (2002). Clinical course of polyoma virus nephropathy in 67 renal transplant patients. *Journal of the American Society of Nephrology* **13**, 2145–2151.

Ratner, S. J. (1988). Vancomycin-induced interstitial nephritis. *American Journal of Medicine* **84**, 561–562.

Rayadurg, J. and Koch, A. E. (1990). Renal insufficiency from interstitial nephritis in primary Sjögren's syndrome. *Journal of Rheumatology* **17**, 1714–1718.

Rocha, J. and Fernandez-Alonso, J. (2001). Acute tubulointerstitial nephritis associated with the selective COX-2 enzyme inhibitor, rofecoxib. *Lancet* **357**, 1946–1947.

Rossert J. (2001). Drug-induced acute interstitial nephritis. *Kidney International* **60**, 804–817.

Rotellar, C., Noël, L. H., Droz, F., Kreis, H., and Berger, J. (1986). Role of antibodies directed against tubular basement membranes in human renal transplantation. *American Journal of Kidney Diseases* **7**, 157–161.

Ruffenach, J. R., Siskind, M. S., and Lien, Y. H. (1992). Acute interstitial nephritis due to omeprazole. *American Journal of Medicine* **93**, 472–473.

Ruffing, K. A., Hoppes, P., Blend, D., Cugino, A., Jarjonra, D., and Whittier, P. C. (1994). Eosinophils in urine revisited. *Clinical Nephrology* **41**, 163–166.

Schwarz, A., Krause, P. H., Keller, F., Offermann, G., and Mihatsch, M. J. (1988). Granulomatous interstitial nephritis after nonsteroidal anti-inflammatory drugs. *American Journal of Nephrology* **8**, 410–416.

Segerer, S., MacK, M., Regele, H., Kerjaschki, D., and Schlondorff, D. (1999). Expression of the C-C chemokine receptor 5 in human kidney diseases. *Kidney International* **56**, 347–348.

Sessa, A., Meroni, M., Battini, G., Vigano, G., Brambilla, P. L., and Paties, C. T. (2000). Acute renal failure due to idiopathic tubulo-intestinal nephritis and uveitis: 'TINU syndrome'. *Journal of Nephrology* **13**, 377–380.

Shibasaki, T., Ishimoto, F., Sakai, O., Joh, K., and Aizawa, S. (1991). Clinical characterization of drug-induced allergic nephritis. *American Journal of Nephrology* **11**, 174–180.

Singer, D. R. J., Simpson, J. G., Catto, G. R. D., and Johnston, A. W. (1988). Drug hypersentivity causing granulomatous interstitial nephritis. *American Journal of Kidney Diseases* **11**, 357–359.

Sugisaki, T., Yoshida, T., McCluskey, R. T., Andres, G. A., and Klassen, J. (1980). Autoimmune cell-mediated tubulointerstitial nephritis induced in Lewis rats by renal antigens. *Clinical Immunology and Immunopathology* **15**, 33–43.

Ten, R. M., Torres, V. E., Milliner, D. S., Schwab, T. R., Holley, K. E., and Gleich, G. J. (1988). Acute interstitial nephritis: immunologic and clinical aspects. *Mayo Clinic Proceedings* **63**, 921–930.

Thomsen O. F. and Ladefoged J. (2002). Pyelonephritis and interstitial nephritis—clinical-pathological correlations. *Clinical Nephrology* **58**, 275–281.

Toto, R. D. (1990). Review: acute tubulointerstitial nephritis. *American Journal of the Medical Sciences* **299**, 392–410.

Vanherweghem, J. L. *et al.* (1993). Rapidly progressive interstitial renal fibrosis in young women: association with slimming regimen including Chinese herbs. *Lancet* **341**, 387–391.

Vanhille, P. *et al.* (1987). Néphrites interstitielles granulomateuses d'origine médicamenteuse. *Néphrologie* **8**, 41–42.

Van Ypersele de Strihou, C., Van der Groen, G., and Desmyter, J. (1986). Hantavirus nephropathy in Western Europe: ubiquity of hemorrhagic fevers with renal syndrome. *Advances in Nephrology* **15**, 143–172.

Verma, N., Arunabh, S., Brady, T. M., and Charytan, C. (2002). Acute interstitial nephritis secondary to infectious mononucleosis. *Clinical Nephrology* **58**, 151–154.

Vlasveld, L. T. *et al.* (1993). Possible role for cytotoxic lymphocytes in the pathogenesis of acute interstitial nephritis after recombinant interleukin-2 treatment for renal cell cancer. *Cancer Immunology, Immunotherapy* **36**, 210–213.

Wilson, C. B. (1989). Study of the immunopathogenesis of tubulointerstitial nephritis using model systems. *Kidney International* **35**, 938–953.

Yang, C. W., Wu, M. S., and Pan, M. J. (2001). Leptospirosis renal disease. *Nephrology, Dialysis, Transplantation* **16** (Suppl. 5), 73–77.

Zollinger, H. V. and Mihatsch, M. J. (1979). Morphology of acute interstitial nephropathies. *Contributions to Nephrology* **10**, 118–125.

10.6.3 Acute renal failure associated with microangiopathy (haemolytic–uraemic syndrome and thrombotic thrombocytopenic purpura)

C. Mark Taylor and Guy H. Neild

Introduction

Definition

The syndromes known as haemolytic–uraemic syndrome (HUS) and thrombotic thrombocytopenic purpura (TTP) share similarities in their clinical presentation and pathology. Both are defined by Coomb's test negative haemolytic anaemia with fragmented red cells and thrombocytopenia [microangiopathic haemolytic anaemia (MAHA)].

The pathology is broadly described as thrombotic microangiopathy (TMA) in which mixed platelet–fibrin thrombi occur in capillaries, arterioles, and sometimes arteries in the absence of vascular inflammation.

Early descriptions

TTP was first described in the papers of Moschcowitz (1925), who described a teenage girl with fever, anaemia, and hyaline thromboses in the terminal arterioles and capillaries, and Baehr *et al.* (1936) who recognized the significance of thrombocytopenia. TTP was characterized by striking MAHA, usually with a history of malaise, fever, and fluctuating neurological abnormalities. Early reports were of adults, neurological involvement was emphasized, and renal failure was either not a significant feature or overlooked.

In 1955, Gasser *et al.* described five young children with the syndrome. Postmortem revealed extensive renal cortical necrosis in every case. In one, TMA was found in many organs including the heart and brain as well as the kidney. Emphasizing the importance of kidney involvement and the young age of his patients, Gasser coined the diagnostic term *Hämolytisch-urämische syndrome*. Medical texts did not apply this to adult patients until about 1970.

Gasser acknowledged the heterogeneous nature of the condition. Two of his cases had pneumonia, and one of these developed red cell polyagglutination, a subsequently recognized sub group. Another child had a dysenteric illness suggestive of verocytotoxin-producing *Escherichia coli* (VTEC) infection, now by far the most common cause of the syndrome.

Renal impairment is a required criterion for the diagnosis of HUS. However, the clinical features of HUS and TTP overlap. CNS disturbance can complicate HUS, just as moderate renal impairment occurs in 20 per cent of TTP cases so that the clinical features of the two form part of a spectrum. In general, nephrologists refer to the syndrome they see as HUS and haematologists call it TTP.

HUS associated with (D+) or without (D−) diarrhoea

Until the mid-1970s and the advent of specialized paediatric renal services, the mortality in children with HUS was high. Later, it became recognized that those presenting with diarrhoea had a better outcome than those without. This led to the clinically useful subdivision between D+ (diarrhoea associated) and D− forms of the syndrome (Levin and Barratt 1984); a distinction equally applicable in adults (Melnyk *et al.* 1995). In industrialized countries, and using routine laboratory techniques, it appears that at least three quarters of D+ HUS is caused by VTEC (Milford *et al.* 1990). D+ HUS would have a different connotation in parts of the Indian subcontinent or Africa where Shigella dysenteriae type 1 is a major cause of HUS (Bhimma *et al.* 1997).

Towards an aetiological classification of HUS, TTP, and related disorders

The D+ HUS/D− HUS terminology is simple to apply and clinically useful, but can mislead. For example, VTEC infection causes the majority of D+ HUS cases in the developed world, but not all. HUS has been described in patients with evidence of VTEC infection but no diarrhoeal component. Likewise, a diarrhoeal illness may precipitate HUS in patients with a different aetiology such as complement factor H deficiency. While some presentations are distinctive and suggest a likely aetiology, this is not the case in at least 10 per cent of children and the majority of adults.

The terms *epidemic*, *sporadic*, or *atypical HUS* should be avoided. Only a minority of cases of VTEC-induced HUS are part of an epidemic, most occur in isolation. Until a specific subgroup of HUS is properly defined, it is unhelpful to describe any case as *atypical*.

Recent advances in understanding the causal mechanisms of these disorders requires a revised classification based on aetiology and pathogenesis, rather than clinical description (Furlan and Lammle 2001). This is important, as it is likely that the syndrome comprises different disorders, each requiring specific management. A very thorough past and family history should be taken in all cases, enquiring into unexplained anaemia, complications of pregnancy, renal disease, and deaths in an attempt to identify the underlying mechanism. The chapter pursues this concept, and uses aetiological classifications wherever there is good evidence for them, and descriptive terms such as D+, D− where there is not. A proposed, but doubtless interim, classification is given in Table 1, and a checklist of diagnostic investigations in Table 2. Three important concepts of pathogenesis are addressed in detail: VTEC infection, complement factor H deficiency, and von Willebrand protease deficiency.

The clinical diagnosis of HUS and related disorders

Microangiopathic haemolytic anaemia

Central to the diagnosis of HUS, TTP, and related disorders is MAHA, a Coombs test negative haemolytic anaemia with characteristic red cell fragmentation seen on the blood film (Fig. 1). The mechanism is unknown. The hypothesis that fragmentation is the result of mechanical injury as red cells pass through intravascular fibrin strands seems unlikely as massive haemolysis may occur with relatively little microangiopathy and vice versa. Haemolysis is intravascular and the plasma concentration of lactate dehydrogenase (LDH), specifically the red

Table 1 A classification of HUS, TTP, and related disorders

Infection
Shiga toxin and verocytotoxin-/Shiga-like toxin producing organisms; i.e. *Shigella dysenteriae type 1* and enterohaemorrhagic *E. coli*
Neuraminidase producing organisms; red cell polyagglutination syndrome; i.e. *Streptococcus pneumoniae*
Human immunodeficiency virus
Drug and treatment induced
Mitomycin C
Cyclosporin A, tacrolimus
Quinine
Ticlopidine, clopidogrel
Genetic forms
Haemolytic complement abnormalities, e.g. Factor H
von Willebrand proteinase deficiency
Cobalamin metabolic disorders
Autosomal recessive not part of the above
Autosomal dominant not part of the above
Pregnancy associated
Pregnancy asssociated
Puerperium associated
HELLP syndrome
Acquired von Willebrand protease deficiency
Auto-antibody against vWF protease
Superimposed on existing disorder
Associated with malignancy
Associated with bone marrow transplantation
Associated with vasculitis
Associated with glomerulonephritis
Accelerated phase hypertension
Currently unknown, idiopathic

cell isoenzyme, is elevated, and haptoglobin is very low or absent. The latter is a valuable and very sensitive test of intravascular haemolysis and often the last abnormality to normalize in remission.

Thrombocytopenia occurs because of intravascular platelet activation and consumption. The majority of radio-labelled platelets end up in the liver and spleen (Katz 1973). The plasma concentrations of ADP and platelet factor 4 are increased (Appiani *et al.* 1982). Circulating platelets may be degranulated and show reduced aggregation *in vitro* (Sassetti *et al.* 1999).

Tests of coagulation are normal, and often the prothrombin (PT) and partial thromboplastin times (PTTs) are shortened and the plasma fibrinogen concentration is not reduced. This is distinctly different from the consumptive coagulopathy of disseminated intravascular coagulation (DIC) that accompanies sepsis or surgical shock in which PT and PTT are prolonged. Given this difference and the fact that the disorders that give rise to HUS and DIC are different, it is usual to draw a clear separation between the two. For example, in meningococcal sepsis there may be thrombocytopenia, anaemia, and microvascular damage leading to renal impairment, but there would be good evidence of DIC and little of red cell fragmentation. The terms HUS or TTP would not apply.

In HUS, thrombin–anti-thrombin III complexes and PT fragments are increased. There is an increase in D-dimers indicating local dissolution of thrombi although the overall fibrinolytic potential of the plasma, a balance between plasminogen activators and inhibitors, is reduced (Nevard *et al.* 1997; Chandler *et al.* 2002).

Acute renal failure

Abrupt onset of oligo-anuria is typical of some forms of HUS such as VTEC-induced disease. Polyuric renal failure can occur, and in some cases urine production is normal but plasma creatinine and urea rise or fluctuate. Insidious onset of renal impairment suggests a diagnosis other than VTEC infection. Microscopic haematuria is usual, but occasionally the urine appears red either from haemoglobinuria or haematuria. Proteinuria (1–2 g/day in adults) is to be expected, and rarely massive protein losses can produce a nephrotic syndrome either at presentation or during recovery.

Hypertension may occur at any stage. It is usually renin mediated, and angiotensin-converting enzyme inhibitors are the drugs of choice in its management. In D− HUS, hypertension is typically severe, and relapses of HUS are often associated with an increase in blood pressure. However in children with VTEC-induced HUS hypertension is usually mild and transient, often developing at the time that renal function starts to return.

Circulatory abnormalities

HUS may lead to vascular volume depletion. In severe cases, endothelial damage causes a capillary leak, which initially leads to loss of crystalloid, but can cause loss of colloid (albumin) into the extracellular fluid, further compromising the circulating blood volume. With D+ HUS, this may be established by the time patients present, and is made worse by diarrhoea and vomiting. Hypovolaemia increases the haematocrit, masking the severity of the anaemia.

Cardiac failure can have many causes including volume overload, hypertension, and uraemia. Microthrombi have been reported in coronary vessels in various forms of HUS and TTP at postmortem. Clinical manifestations of cardiomyopathy are rare. The latter may occur in post partum HUS and up to 3 months after an episode of diarrhoea associated HUS when recovery from the initial toxaemia and renal impairment is well under way (Poulton *et al.* 1987). Echocardiography shows dilatation and a reduced ejection fraction. Resolution generally occurs within a few weeks.

Pulmonary oedema is common in adults with VTEC (Dundas *et al.* 1999), but it has not been established as a primary complication of the condition. Patients are often elderly and are easily overloaded with fluid; nevertheless there could be a low-pressure pulmonary oedema as part of the capillary leak that occurs.

Neurological involvement

Patients with TTP or D− HUS of any aetiology may present with fluctuating neurological signs. In patients with TTP, there is often a history of malaise, nausea, headache, drowsiness, and weakness of recent onset. TMA has been found in the cerebral microcirculation of many cases at postmortem. Rarely, stroke-like events occur and there is evidence of large vessel occlusion or intracranial haemorrhage. Hypertensive encephalopathy may complicate any HUS presentation.

Table 2 Check list of investigation towards subgroup aetiology

Subgroup diagnosis	Investigation and comment
Verocytotoxin-producing *E. coli* infection (Shiga-like toxin-producing *E. coli* infection)	Rarely presents without diarrhoea. Culture stool for VTEC, test stool for cytotoxin neutralizable by specific antibody, probe for VT plasmid, test acute and convalescent serum for locally relevant O-serotype; e.g. O157 in UK and N. America
Complement regulation disorders	Persistently low C3 suggests defect of complement regulation, but normal C3 does not exclude Factor H deficiency. Genomic diagnosis required. Exclude systemic lupus erythematosis and mesangiocapillary glomerulonephritis. Screen family members. Measure Factor H in plasma
von Willebrand factor protease abnormality	Plasma SDS-1% agarose electrophoresis to reveal multimeric pattern of vWF. Ultra large multimers may be a transient feature suggesting fresh release of vWF from activated endothelium. Persistent large multimers suggest a causative defect in multimer processing, can be familial or acquired. Protease measurement required. Genomic diagnosis possible
Platelet binding autoantibodies	Various antibodies described, e.g. anti-CD36 platelet receptor GPIV, also a quinine-dependant antibody against GPIIb/IIIa, GPIb/IX
Erythrocyte polyagglutination, exposure of T-antigen	Usually discovered during attempts to cross match. The peanut lectin *hypogyea* identifies exposure of the Thomsen–Freidenreich crypt antigen where sialic acid has been cleaved from the cell surface by neuraminidase. Look for the causative infection, usually *S. pneumoniae*
Inborn error of Cobalamin	Very rare intra cellular defect of cobalamin-dependant conversion of homocysteine to methionine, and methylmalonyl-CoA to succinate Usually neonates, but older children described. Screen urine for methylmalonic acid and homocysteine
Pregnancy	Overlap with pre-eclampsia, and HELLP syndrome. Check pregnancy status in teenage girls. Check liver enzymes
Underlying primary glomerulopathy	HUS may complicate other primary glomerular diseases and vasculitis. Consider renal biopsy
Primary antiphospholipid syndrome	Measure anti cardiolipin antibodies and functional test for 'lupus anticoagulant'
Acquired immunodeficiency	May overlap other causes. HIV serology

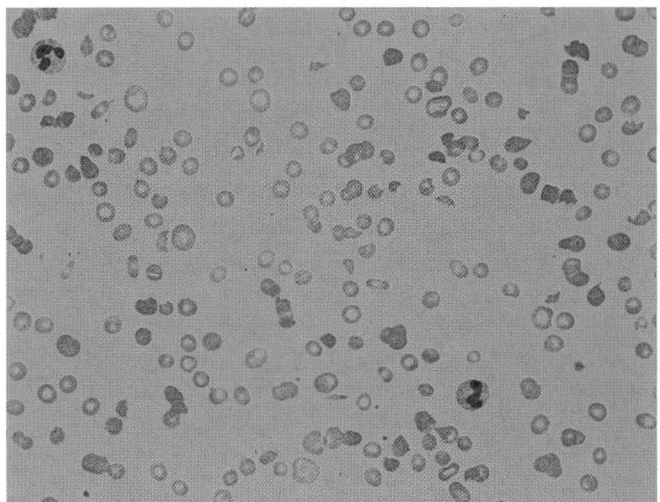

Fig. 1 Blood film showing microangiopathic haemolytic anaemia.

In children with VTEC-induced HUS, somnolence, irritability, hallucinations, cranial nerve palsies, seizure, or coma are seen in about a fifth of cases (Milford 1994). The commonest cause of death in the acute phase is a neurological catastrophe, often with a very rapid evolution. Much of this relates to cerebral oedema, which is most often caused by dilutional hyponatraemia in the uraemic state, compounded by a generalized capillary leak. VT is probably responsible for the latter, although it may also be directly toxic to neuronal tissue. In some cases of fatal brain stem herniation, no electrolyte or perfusion pressure abnormality precedes the acute brain swelling, and there may be no evidence of TMA in cerebral vessels.

Disease of other systems

Gastrointestinal involvement is largely related to the VTEC infection itself (see below).

TMA within the pancreas can cause insulin-dependent diabetes mellitus and exocrine pancreatic dysfunction. In VTEC-induced HUS, this complication tends to affect those with coexisting CNS disease. Pancreatic insufficiency may resolve in remission.

Petechiae and purpura are rare in most forms of HUS, but occur with profound thrombocytopenia ($<20 \times 10^9$ platelets/ml).

Early reports of TTP emphasized the frequency with which the adrenal glands were involved at autopsy (Amorosi and Ultmann 1966). This would suggest that although clinically relevant adrenal insufficiency does occur, it is not often recognized.

Pathology

In her adaptation of the term TMA to renal disease, Habib (1992) identified three broad sub groups: glomerular TMA, arterial TMA, and cortical necrosis with TMA.

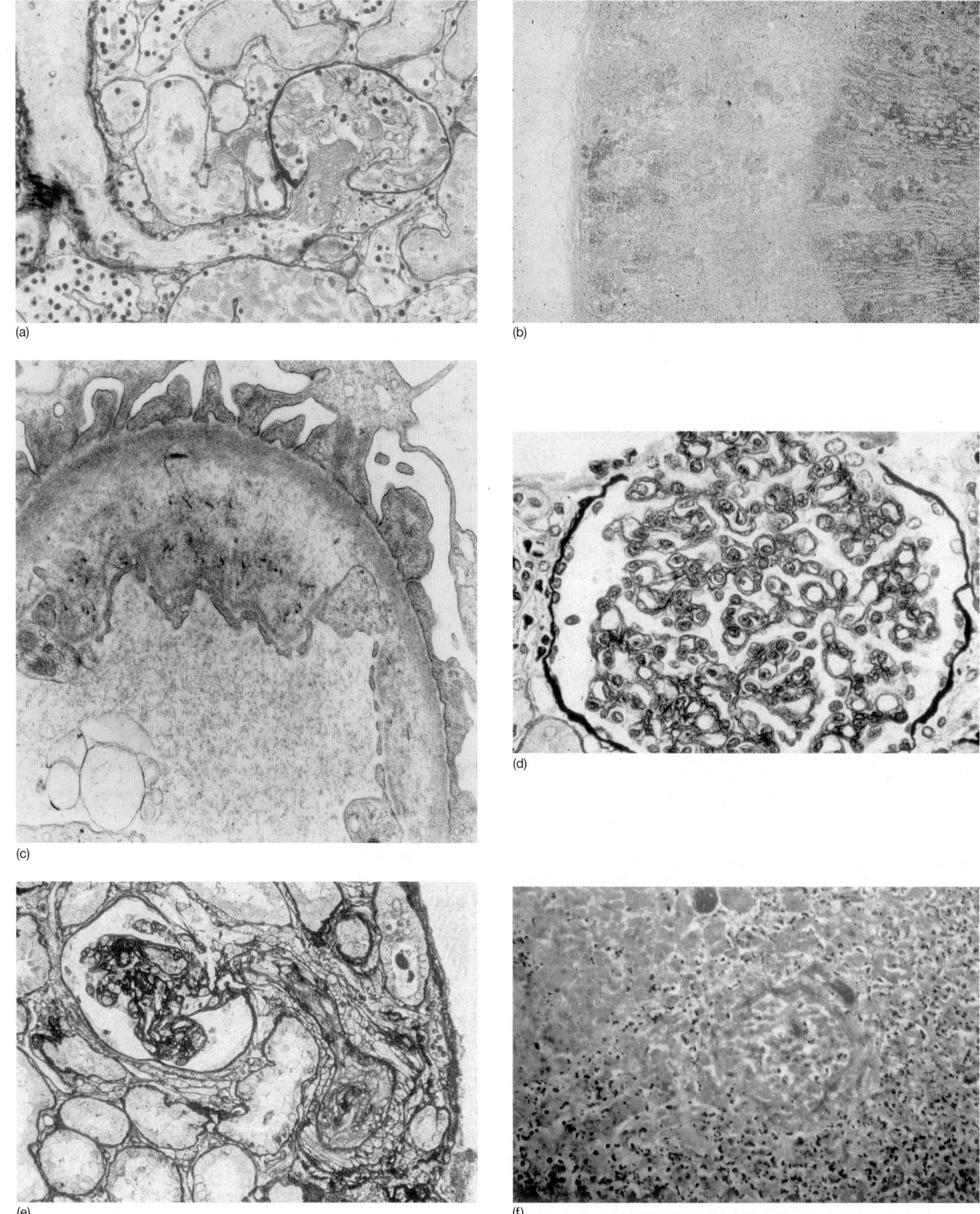

Fig. 2 Pathology of HUS. (a) Glomerular thrombotic microangiopathy in D+ HUS at postmortem showing a glomerulus distended with thrombus. (b) Low-power view showing extensive cortical necrosis in D+ HUS. (c) Electron micrograph showing endothelial detachment in a case of D+ HUS. (d) Thrombotic microangiopathy in a case of Factor H deficiency in which mesangial proliferation gives double contours to capillary walls (silver stain). (e) Arterial thrombotic microangiopathy in a teenager with an insidious onset D− HUS with fluctuating neurological signs. (f) Pancreas from the postmortem of a child with D+ HUS showing thrombosis in the peri-islet microvasculature.

Glomerular TMA describes a lesion of the glomerular capillary wall. By light microscopy the capillary wall appears thickened. In one pattern, the glomeruli are large with capillaries distended by red cells and platelet fibrin-thrombi that may extend proximally into the afferent arteriole (Fig. 2a). This appearance is typical of D+ HUS in children (Richardson *et al.* 1988; Inward *et al.* 1997). Ultrastructural appearances are characteristic, with endothelial swelling and separation from the glomerular basement membrane with subendothelial accumulation of electron lucent material and sometimes fibrin (Fig. 2c). A second pattern, more often seen in HUS caused by other aetiologies, includes mesangial cell swelling and in some cases mesangiolysis (Koitabashi *et al.* 1991). Later, mesangial interposition into the subendothelial space may be seen giving prominent double contours to the capillary loops (Fig. 2d). The afferent arterioles are involved with fibrinoid necrosis and scanty thrombosis.

Arterial TMA involves arterioles and interlobular, but not interlobar arteries. Acutely, fibrin may be found in the subendothelial space and the lumen. Later, one sees intimal proliferation with luminal stenosis, and the glomeruli show shrinkage and wrinkling of the basement membrane of the collapsed capillaries (Fig. 2e). Arterial TMA is more often seen in non-VTEC forms of HUS or TTP, and is typically associated with severe hypertension. The renal prognosis for severe arterial involvement is poor (Morel-Maroger *et al.* 1979; Thoenes and John 1980).

Patchy cortical necrosis of varying severity can be found in many cases of HUS, probably due to ischaemic damage following interruption of the local microcirculation. Rarely, massive cortical necrosis occurs that seems out of proportion to the TMA. Cortical necrosis with TMA is found in infants with HUS, and VTEC infection has been implicated in some cases (Fig. 2b). VT may cause direct damage to cortical epithelial cells (Karpman *et al.* 1998; Taguchi *et al.* 1998).

In paired acute and sequential biopsies, the proportion of glomeruli with TMA in the acute sample matched that with complete sclerosis a year later. From this it was deduced that TMA is often irreparable (Habib *et al.* 1982). Survivors of HUS may therefore have a reduced number of nephrons. Moghal *et al.* (1998) undertook biopsies in children who had proteinuria 5 years after D+ HUS. In these, the glomeruli had undergone considerable hypertrophy consistent with the hypothesis of compensatory glomerular hyperfiltration (Fig. 3).

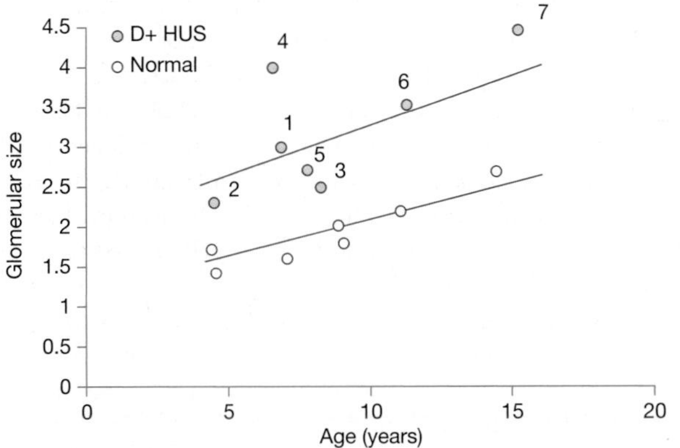

Fig. 3 Glomerular size in children with proteinuria 5 years after D+ HUS (Moghal *et al.* 1998).

An overview of clinical management

Standard supportive therapy

As with any case of acute renal failure, blood volume should be assessed clinically and hypovolaemia corrected. Volume depletion may be a consequence of diarrhoea and vomiting. In severe cases, endothelial damage causes a capillary leak, which initially leads to loss of crystalloid, but can cause loss of colloid (albumin) into the extracellular fluid, further compromising the circulating blood volume.

Anaemia may be profound, and if the haemoglobin falls below 8 g/dl, red cell transfusion will be necessary. Thrombocytopenia itself is not an indication to give platelets and may worsen the microcirculatory thrombosis. Platelet transfusion should be reserved for the rare patient with active bleeding or needing an operative procedure. Transfusion of blood products requires careful monitoring of vascular volume and serum potassium to prevent pulmonary oedema and hyperkalaemia.

When the patient is first seen, acute renal failure may not be established. Apart from hypovolaemia, there can be other causes of renal failure, such as haemoglobinuria, hyperbilirubinaemia, and urate crystal nephropathy. Vigorous therapy with crystalloids and intravenous frusemide (Rousseau *et al.* 1990) can induce a diuresis in some patients and either avoid the need for dialysis or at least make fluid balance management easier.

Hypertension can be severe, especially in non-diarrhoeal forms of HUS (Fitzpatrick *et al.* 1992a). It is usually renin-mediated, and therefore, angiotensin-converting enzyme or receptor inhibitors are the drugs of choice, once hypovolaemia and hyperkalaemia have been corrected. Rigorous control of blood pressure is essential in the management of relapsing HUS. Relapses are often associated with or triggered by a marked increase in blood pressure. The pressure may fall with plasma therapy (see below).

Specific strategies

Beyond the standard management of severe anaemia (with transfusions), renal failure (by dialysis if necessary), and withdrawal of causative drugs, certain specific strategies can be used to limit the vascular injury.

Plasma therapy

Fresh frozen plasma (FFP) has been used empirically in both adults and children with non-VTEC forms of HUS and TTP with considerable success (Misiani *et al.* 1982). When first described, untreated TTP used to have a 1-year mortality of 90 per cent, but with fresh plasma infusions and plasma exchange, the mortality is now around 10 per cent (Eknoyan and Riggs 1986; Bell *et al.* 1991). Similarly, the poor outcome for children with idiopathic HUS was improved by plasma exchange in some studies (Fitzpatrick *et al.* 1993; Renaud *et al.* 1995). However, a controlled trial of FFP in children with D+ HUS did not show a benefit, and there are no logical arguments for its use or PEX in this form of HUS (Loirat *et al.* 1988; Rizzoni *et al.* 1988).

FFP 10 ml/kg/day is sufficient to induce remission in patients with an inherited deficiency of von Willebrand protease. Remission can be maintained with repeated infusions at 2–3 week intervals. The plasma dosage for those with acquired protease depletion with an antiprotease antibody is less clear. There is anecdotal evidence that plasma therapy can induce remission in HUS associated with complement Factor H deficiency, probably by replacing missing Factor H, but the dose needed appears to be much larger and plasma exchange is needed to accommodate this volume, especially if renal function is compromised. A single volume plasma exchange is 50 ml/kg body weight.

The problem with a newly diagnosed patient is that the aetiology may not be known and an empirical initial approach is needed. A loading dose of FFP 30–40 ml/kg and then a daily dose of 15–20 ml/kg has been recommended (Misiani *et al.* 1982). This can be continued until the platelet count has returned to normal values and haemolysis has ceased. If this is unsuccessful, or if the volume load cannot be tolerated, plasmapheresis can be instituted using FFP as the replacement fluid. It is conceivable that in cases associated with a causative autoantibody, plasma exchange, perhaps with immunosuppression, may assist antibody clearance, but there is as yet no scientific confirmation of this approach.

Other therapies

'Anti-platelet' drugs, anticoagulants, and thrombolytics have not been shown to be of benefit. However, new evidence that increased thrombin generation and impaired thrombolysis precedes renal injury suggests that these treatments may have been given too late (Chandler *et al.* 2002). Recombinant tissue plasminogen activator therapy has not been applied in HUS.

Prostacyclin infusion may inhibit platelet–endothelial interactions and help promote a diuresis. Published anecdotal reports claim only limited success (Taylor and Milford 1997). However, these failures could represent late cases in which vascular injury was too advanced to allow recovery. No controlled study has been performed. It is usual to start with a dose of 2.5 ng/kg/min and gradually increase to 5 ng/kg, or higher if the drug is tolerated without troublesome hypotension or abdominal discomfort. In D+ HUS, prostacyclin can make the haemorrhagic colitis worse, and may potentiate cerebral oedema.

Severe cases, refractory to standard therapy, have remitted following splenectomy, corticosteroids, vincristine, or high-dose intravenous gammaglobulin (Thompson *et al.* 1992). Cases of coma with refractory HUS/TTP have remitted following bilateral nephrectomy. These are acts of therapeutic desperation with little rationale. The association of antibodies to von Willebrand factor (vWF)-cleaving protease in TTP gives some credence to the use of immunosuppression (Furlan *et al.* 1998).

Verocytotoxin-induced (Shiga-like toxin-induced) HUS

VTEC infection accounts for at least 80 per cent of all paediatric HUS in Western Europe, the Americas, and Australasia, and has become the commonest cause of community acquired acute renal failure in childhood.

Verocytotoxin-producing *Escherichia coli*

In 1977, it was discovered that a strain of *E. coli* secreted a powerful exotoxin to which vero cells were especially susceptible, hence the toxin's name (Konowalchuk *et al.* 1977). Homology with Shiga toxin was shown, leading to the alternative name *Shiga-like toxin*, the two terms being interchangeable (O'Brien and Laveck 1983). In 1982, VTEC were linked to haemorrhagic colitis and consequently acquired the title *enterohaemorrhagic E. coli* (EHEC). The report by Karmali *et al.* (1983) that positively associated VTEC with HUS in children followed a year later, radically altering the understanding of the syndrome.

VTEC infection is a zoonosis and HUS is the most extreme human manifestation. The strains of VTEC that are pathogenic in humans have additional virulence factors. One of these is the property, shared with *enteropathogenic E. coli* (EPEC), to bind to the brush border of enterocytes and form a characteristic attachment and effacing lesion (Kaper *et al.* 1998). The genes responsible for this reside in the locus for enterocyte effacement (LEE), a 35.6 kb pathogenicity island that is incorporated into the bacterial chromosome. This includes the genes for intimin and the translocated intimin receptor, *eaeA* and *tir*, respectively.

These *E. coli* have a mechanism for inserting their own bacterial receptor into the host enterocyte which then binds intimin expressed on the outer membrane of the bacterium. Binding between intimin and its translocated receptor locks the bacterium to the surface of the host (Fig. 4). The enterocyte responds with cytoskeletal changes that truncate the normal villous structure and replace it with the nest-like pedicle that typifies this form of adhesion (reviewed by Frankel *et al.* 1998). EHEC are, therefore, positioned to deliver exotoxin in the immediate vicinity of the enterocyte. Neither EPEC nor EHEC is enteroinvasive, unlike *Shigella dysenteriae type 1*.

The Shiga toxin family

Verocytotoxins (Shiga-like toxins) share varying degrees of sequence homology with Shiga toxin, the exotoxin of *Shigella dysenteriae type 1*. VT1, VT2, and VT2 variants are associated with human disease, while VT2e causes oedema disease in piglets, a disorder comprising diarrhoea, encephalopathy, and capillary leakage. VT1 and Shiga toxin are identical except for one amino acid in the A-sub unit and are serologically indistinct. There is approximately 55 per cent homology between VT1 and VT2. All Shiga family toxins are composed of an A-subunit linked to a pentamer of B-subunits. Whereas Shiga toxin is encoded in the chromosome of *Shigella dysenteriae type 1*, VT1 and VT2 are contained within plasmids. They can therefore be transferred to naive *E. coli* strains or other coliforms. For example, one outbreak of HUS was attributed to *Citrobacter freundii* bearing the VT2 plasmid (Schmidt *et al.* 1993). The operon structure and gene for the A-subunit is upstream from the B-subunit. Some of the factors that regulate toxin production are known. These include contact with intestinal mucus, the availability of iron and, interestingly, neutrophil derived superoxide (Wagner *et al.* 2001).

The B-subunit is essential for cell recognition and uptake. It binds the terminal carbohydrate moiety, galactose $\alpha 1$–4β galactose on globotriaosylceramide (Gb3) (CD77) (Stein *et al.* 1992). The distribution of receptors determines which cells and which species are susceptible to the toxin, and to some extent the pattern of disease. Gb3 is strongly expressed in primates, mostly on gut and renal tubular epithelial cells, as a differentiation marker in lymphocytes, and in a number of different cancers. Many species, such as domestic cattle, do not express Gb3 and are consequently unaffected by the toxin. On the other hand pigs express Gb4, and are vulnerable to VT2e, which preferentially binds Gb4 (Boyd *et al.* 1993).

Once engaged with the receptor, the holotoxin is endocytosed within a clathrin-coated pit by a calcium and energy dependant process. From the endosome it may be re-exported or fused with a lysosome for degrading. Alternatively, it may be routed to various intracellular destinations by retrograde transport through the Golgi apparatus to the endoplasmic reticulum (Sandvig and Van Deurs 1996). Binding and intracellular trafficking is influenced by the fatty acid component of the Gb3 glycolipid receptor. Shorter isoforms (C : 16, C : 18) track to the endoplasmic

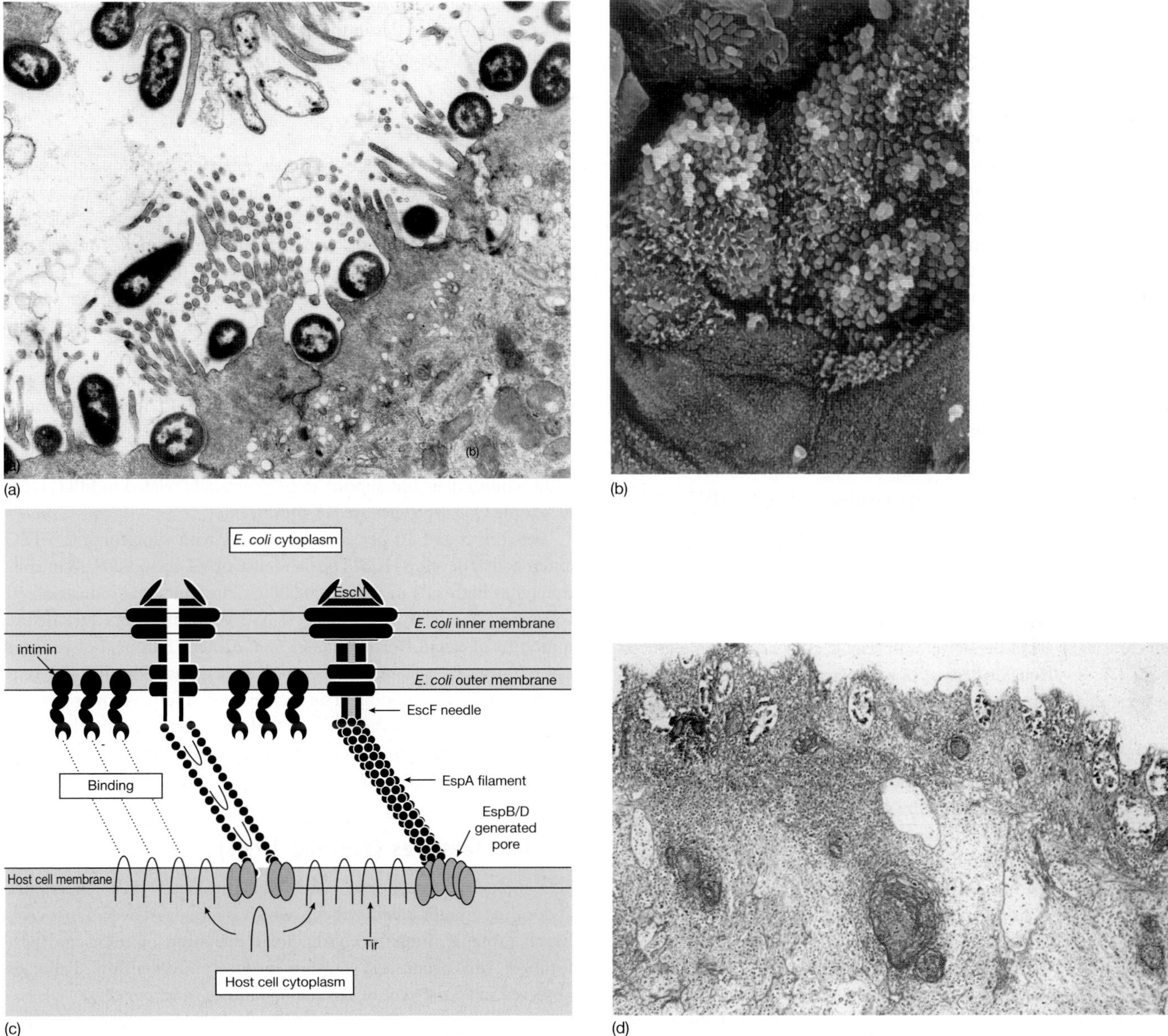

Fig. 4 VTEC-induced enteropathy. (a) Transmission electron micrograph showing enteropathogenic *E. coli* forming pedestal-like attachment and effacing lesions on enterocytes. (b) Scanning electron micrograph showing VTEC O157 attached to the apical surface of a human colonic epithelial cell with loss of the normal villous structure. (c) Cartoon of type III secretion by which *E. coli* inject translocated intimin receptor into host enterocytes to permit intimin binding and attachment. (d) Histological section of colon from a child with VTEC-induced HUS who required emergency bowel resection showing oedema, necrosis, and haemorrhage.

reticulum and the nuclear envelope, while longer ones (C : 22, C : 24) are transported to the trans-Golgi network (Arab and Lingwood 1998). Wide variations in cytotoxicity appear to be attributable to the different intracellular destinations of the toxin.

During intracellular trafficking, the holotoxin is cleaved by furin or calpain to release the A-subunit into the cytosol. Conserved regions of the A-subunit function enzymatically to depurinate a specific adenine residue near the 3′ end of the 28S ribosomal RNA at a point where aminoacyl transfer RNA is assembled within the 60S ribosome (Furutani *et al.* 1992). Only a very small amount of an intracellular ribotoxin is needed to prevent peptide assembly and arrest protein synthesis.

Toxicology

Cytotoxicity is dependent upon the cell type, expression of receptor, and the stage of the cell cycle (Pudymaitis and Lingwood 1992). While cytotoxicity is generally held to be the consequence of protein synthesis inhibition, the events leading to cell death are more complex as similar degrees of protein synthesis inhibition by other agents, such as cycloheximide, can have different effects.

VT kills cells through apoptosis or necrosis. Vero cells (Inward *et al.* 1995) and cultured foreskin microvascular endothelial cells (Pijpers *et al.* 2001), both of which bear the Gb3 receptor, die through apoptosis.

Primary cultures of human renal epithelial cells are exquisitely sensitive to VT1 (Hughes *et al.* 2000a) but appear to die through necrosis (Williams *et al.* 1999). Both human umbilical and glomerular endothelial cells are comparatively resistant to VT, but pretreatment with the inflammatory cytokines TNFα, IL-1β, or bacterial lipopolysaccharide makes them sensitive through the upregulation of Gb3 (van de Kar *et al.* 1992; Van Setten *et al.* 1997a). Human mesangial cells are resistant to VT (Van Setten *et al.* 1997b).

VT, like other protein synthesis inhibitors, induces the production of the IL-8 and other members of the C-X-C chemokine family from human enterocytes in culture, a phenomenon that involves the p38/mitogen activated protein kinase pathway, the primary response gene c-jun and NFκB (Thorpe 1999, 2001). Monocytes have also been shown to produce TNFα in the presence of VT. In animal models, there is an early and massive release of proinflammatory cytokines (Taylor *et al.* 1999a,b) and evidence that TNFα is produced in the kidney (Harel *et al.* 1993; Taylor *et al.* 1999b).

Pathogenesis of verocytotoxin-induced HUS

VTEC colonize the colonic epithelium and liberate free VT in the immediate vicinity of the mucosa. Toxin delivered to the sub mucosa by transcytosis is assumed to be responsible for the microvascular lesion of the colon. There is oedema, haemorrhage, and thrombosis affecting all layers of the bowel wall [Fig. 4(c)]. The overlying mucosa is shed, and various degrees of bowel infarction may be seen leading to toxic dilatation of the colon. VT induces the release of IL-8 from enterocytes explaining the high concentration in plasma IL-8 found in patients and the neutrophil infiltration of the colon.

There is good evidence that a procoagulant state during VTEC infection precedes the renal failure of HUS, and that the renal lesion is primarily one of intraglomerular thrombosis, microvascular obstruction and parenchymal ischaemia (Chandler *et al.* 2002). Also, neutrophilia occurs early in the disease in those who progress to HUS, and the magnitude of this response predicts outcome (Walters *et al.* 1989; Coad *et al.* 1991). Moreover, the plasma of HUS patients contains high concentrations of elastase which suggests that neutrophils are activated within the circulation (Fitzpatrick *et al.* 1992b).

A widely held view is that glomerular thrombosis follows endothelial cell toxicity, but it is not clear if or how this occurs. One possibility is that VT is delivered from the gut to endothelial sites that have a high affinity for the toxin. Human kidneys strongly express Gb3, but on tubular cells not the vasculature. The glomeruli have weak expression, except perhaps in young children (Lingwood 1994). However, endothelial Gb3 can be increased *in vitro* by TNFα and IL-1β, and there is evidence that TNFα is increased early in human HUS, supporting the hypothesis that the glomerular microcirculation might be preferentially targeted.

How the toxin is delivered is not known. VT has not been found in plasma. A novel finding that VT binds to the surface of neutrophils via a low affinity receptor raises the possibility that neutrophils might transfer VT to cytokine stimulated endothelium or other cells expressing Gb3 (Te Loo *et al.* 2000). Toxin induced endothelial injury, cell retraction, or detachment would expose procoagulant material in the subendothelial matrix and cause local thrombosis. In diarrhoea associated HUS, renal biopsies have shown detachment of glomerular endothelium and fibrin in a subendothelial location supporting this view. However, the acute inflammatory response that accompanies VTEC infection (King 2002) or sublethal effects of VT may also induce procoagulant properties in the endothelium and be important in the pathogenesis (Morigi *et al.* 1995, 2001).

Epidemiology

VTEC colonize a wide range of animals, often without inducing disease, and can persist outside their animal hosts in soil and surface water. Cattle are a major reservoir and several epidemics of human infection have been traced to beef, milk products, and water supplies or vegetable produce contaminated by farm slurry. However, the majority of cases of infection are sporadic and the source is never discovered. Secondary person-to-person spread is well recognized and careful sanitary intervention is needed to prevent it.

Many VTEC implicated in human disease share the same O-serotypes as EPEC, for example O26 and O111. However, the most important serotype in the Americas and much of Europe is O157 with or without the flagella type H7. O157 does not have an immediate EPEC counterpart but appears to be genetically related to EPEC O55, H7; some O55 serotypes are VT producers.

Between 5 and 10 per cent of patients with symptomatic VTEC enterocolitis develop HUS. The incidence of VT-induced HUS in children is as high as 3 or 4 per 100,000 children in some industrialized countries. The peak age of onset is 1–2 years. It is very rare before 6 months of age in North America and Western Europe, but younger age of onset is seen in South America, perhaps reflecting different practices of infant feeding. The incidence in adults is lower than in children. There is growing evidence that a proportion of healthy adults have IgG antibodies to VT2 suggesting subclinical exposure, and that antitoxin antibodies might be protective (Ludwig *et al.* 2001).

Clinical features (Milford 1994)

The majority of children with VTEC-induced HUS experience abdominal cramps and diarrhoea, which is bloody in over 70 per cent. Rectal prolapse, intussusception, toxic dilatation of colon and perforation can occur and require surgical intervention. Pallor is observed in 90 per cent of cases and jaundice in 35 per cent.

At the time of the diagnosis of HUS, about half of the cases appear to be normally hydrated, a quarter overloaded, and the remainder dehydrated. Low plasma sodium concentrations are common at diagnosis and tend to be lower in those with clinical hypovolaemia. Hypovolaemic shock occurs in about 2 per cent of children. Oligoanuria is recognized between 1 and 14 days after the onset of diarrhoea, usually between days 4 and 7, and is preceded by thrombocytopenia and anaemia. The anaemia is usually maximal about a day after the onset of oliguria. Hypertension occurs in one-third of patients.

The most common extrarenal manifestation is central nervous system disturbance affecting a fifth of all childhood cases. These are usually seizures, less often coma, or focal signs. This typically occurs within the first 48 hours of diagnosis, and is often accompanied by hyponatraemia. Cardiomyopathy and diabetes mellitus affect less than 5 per cent of patients.

Laboratory investigation for VTEC

Stool culture on sorbitol MacConkey agar is conventionally used where O157 is the prevalent VTEC serotype. Colonies can then be identified serologically. However, the yield is low partly because of the insensitivity of the test, and partly because VTEC excretion may be transient and missed. More sophisticated methods include the use of PCR to recognize toxin producing strains. This allows unexpected serotypes to be identified. Pulse field gel electrophoresis provides a molecular fingerprint of the plasmid and is important in tracing epidemics to their source. A rising antibody titre to a relevant VTEC O-serotype can be diagnostic in patients whose stools no longer contain the pathogen. However, all these tests together fail to identify infection in about 20 per cent of cases, even in thoroughly investigated epidemics.

Treatment

In the interval between the onset of diarrhoea and diagnosis of HUS, various treatments have been tried to prevent or reduce the severity of HUS. Although VTEC are sensitive to a wide range of antibiotics, their use in enterocolitis has been associated with an increased risk of HUS, and as a general rule, antibiotics should not be given (Pavia *et al.* 1990; Proulx *et al.* 1992). *In vitro*, certain antibiotics cause increased toxin release from VTEC (Zhang *et al.* 2000). However, in a Japanese report, the use of fosfomycin appeared protective (Ikeda *et al.* 1999). Antidiarrhoeal agents may also be harmful and should be avoided (Cimolai *et al.* 1994). Administration of Synsorb, a resin with high affinity and capacity for VT given orally to bind free toxin in the gut has not proved beneficial. Experimentally, passive immunization with antiverocytotoxin antibody can ameliorate disease models, and may become a therapy in humans.

Clinical management is supportive, and demands particular attention to detail (Taylor and Milford 1997). Vascular volume, electrolyte disturbance (hyperkalaemia, hyponatraemia, and acidosis), hypertension, and anaemia should be corrected. In a few oliguric patients, a high dose of frusemide will induce a diuresis allowing dialysis to be avoided. There is no evidence that dialysis itself has any effect on the course of the disease, and there is no evidence or rationale for the use of plasma therapy. Peritoneal dialysis is contraindicated if a surgical complication of the colitis is suspected, in which case haemodialysis should be instituted.

Seizures, confusional states, drowsiness, irritability and hallucination are ominous signs, and may be the first indication of raised intracranial pressure or an evolving neurological catastrophe. Management at this point should involve neurologists or intensivists. Seizures require immediate treatment with anticonvulsants, and EEG monitoring is helpful.

Outcome

The early mortality of HUS in children is less than 3 per cent, and largely due to CNS complications, particularly, acute cerebral oedema and hindbrain herniation. The severity and mortality of VTEC-induced HUS in the elderly and in epidemics is substantially higher (Dundas 1999).

Long-term outcome for survivors of VTEC-induced HUS is not yet established. This is because VTEC has only been recognized as a cause of HUS since the mid 1980s, and even after that time follow-up studies tended to include patients with different aetiologies. However, given that D+ HUS cases from this period are largely if not exclusively VTEC in origin, the outcome of D+ HUS is a reasonable guide. Less than 5 per cent of children progress straight from acute to endstage renal failure. Between 20 and 30 per cent of survivors experience adverse renal outcome consisting of proteinuria, hypertension, or renal impairment (Fitzpatrick 1992). An adverse outcome is more likely if the patient required more than 14 days of dialysis during the acute stage.

Because glomerular TMA is destructive of nephrons (see 'Pathology' section above), it is not advisable to discharge patients from long-term follow-up. Occasionally, individuals with normal creatinine, protein excretion, and blood pressure 5 or more years after onset will show proteinuria and reduced kidney function several years later. The burden of chronic renal failure in adults attributable to childhood HUS may not become apparent for another decade or more. Patients who are left with, or who develop, proteinuria are likely to benefit from the 'reno-protection' of angiotensin converting enzyme inhibitors. Although this has not been formally tested in this group there is a broad consensus that such treatment is appropriate.

There are no special precautions required in transplanting patients who reach endstage, and relapse of VTEC-induced HUS does not occur.

Shigella dysenteriae type 1-induced HUS

This is a rare condition in industrialized countries, and is usually imported by travellers returning from endemic areas such as the Indian subcontinent and Africa. Like VTEC infection, there is bloody diarrhoea before the onset of HUS, children are more often affected than adults, and Shiga toxin is implicated in the pathogenesis. However, *Shigella dysenteriae* is enteroinvasive and patients are febrile, have a massive leucocytosis, and may become bacteraemic (Koster *et al.* 1978). The mortality in undeveloped countries is high, partly because of disease severity but also because of delayed access to health care (Bhimma *et al.* 1997).

HUS associated with complement Factor H deficiency

Isolated reports of HUS with complement abnormalities have occurred over the last 25 years. Following the work of Warwicker *et al.* (1998), a form of HUS has now been linked to primary abnormalities of the complement regulator Factor H (Noris *et al.* 1999).

Pathogenesis

Factor H has a central role in the regulation of complement, both in the fluid phase and on the surface of cells (Fig. 5). Produced mainly in the liver as a single peptide glycoprotein, it circulates in plasma at a concentration of 500 mg/l, and binds to anionic sites on vascular endothelium. Its gene lies within a cluster of complement regulating genes on chromosome 1q32. The molecule consists of 20 folded, globular domains known as short consensus repeats (SCR). The tertiary structure of the molecule leaves the *C*-terminal SCR 20 exposed, suggesting an important role for this site (Caprioli *et al.* 2001; Perez-Caballero *et al.* 2001; Richards *et al.* 2001). Factor H contains three binding sites for heparin and other polyanions by which it can attach to cell surfaces. It has three binding regions for C3, each being specific for a different part of the C3 molecule. These appear in SCRs 1–4, the

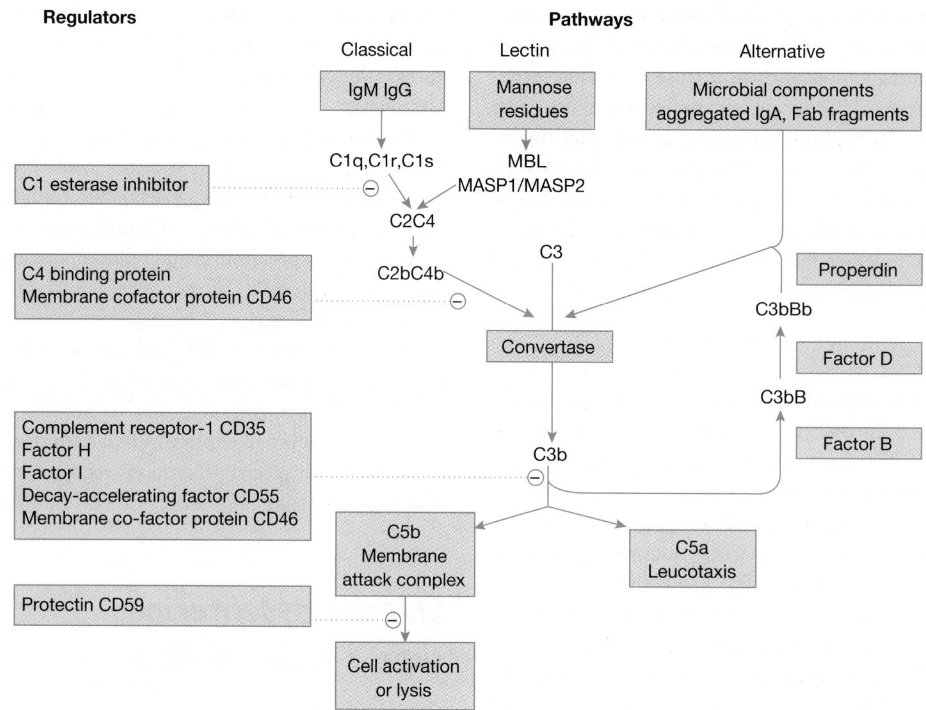

Fig. 5 The complement pathway and its regulation.

site responsible for C3b binding and Factor I cofactor activity, SCRs 6–10 and the terminal SCRs 16–20 (Zipfel 2001).

Strategically placed on host surfaces, Factor H downregulates complement activation and prevents bystander injury to host structures. It does so by competing with Factor B for freshly generated C3b and acts as a cofactor for Factor I in C3b degradation. This prevents both the amplification step of C3 convertase and the generation of downstream products, leucotactic C5a and the membrane attack complex C5b–C9. Complement is an essential participant in some models of glomerular thrombosis, for example, an accelerated immune model of glomerular TMA in rats that resembles HUS (Nangaku *et al.* 1998; Hughes *et al.* 2000b).

Various mutations predicted to cause loss of function of Factor H have been described, mostly in the terminal region SCR 16–20. However, the observation that Factor H deficient patients occasionally have long remissions from HUS or do not present until middle age, suggests that Factor H deficiency only predisposes patients to HUS and a 'second hit' is needed. Perhaps endothelial injuries that in normal circumstances would resolve, lead to complement activation, propagation of vascular injury, and full expression of the disease in vessels that are poorly defended by Factor H.

Clinical features, treatment, and outcome

These patients present either sporadically, or sometimes with a family history. Both autosomal dominant and recessive patterns of inheritance have been described. There is a wide range of age of onset from the neonatal period to adult life (reviewed by Ault 2000; Taylor 2001). There is an impression that homozygous patients with the lowest plasma concentrations of Factor H (<10 per cent of normal) present earlier, often in the first months of life, have persistently low plasma concentrations of complement C3 and evidence of consumption of alternative pathway factors. Heterozygotes are more difficult to detect, as hypocomplementaemia may not be evident. In these, Factor H protein is often present in plasma at about 50 per cent of expected range, but in some cases the factor is present in normal amounts but is non-functional. Genetic testing is required to identify these cases.

Some patients appear to have a prodromal infective illness such as an upper respiratory tract infection. The clinical course is notable for persistent severe hypertension, marked haemolysis, and a high rate of relapse. Structural damage to the kidney progresses with repeated relapses leading to a step-wise loss of kidney function. Once in end-stage renal failure, the haemolysis and thrombocytopenia tend to remit although low concentrations of plasma haptoglobin suggest mild ongoing intravascular haemolysis.

Renal biopsy usually shows mesangial proliferation, increased matrix, and mesangial cell interposition leading to the reduplication of the basement membrane. These features may indicate the chronic nature of the lesion. There may also be arterial changes. Complement deposition in glomeruli is often present within capillary loops but is not extensive.

There is anecdotal evidence that treatment with fresh frozen plasma, which contains Factor H, can induce remission. Little is known about the appropriate dose and it is usually administered with plasmapheresis to avoid vascular overload when renal function is compromised. In an unreported case, an exchange of twice the plasma volume was needed to improve the plasma concentration of C3 and normalize factor B. The effect lasted for about 5 days. There is concern that the benefit of plasma therapy seems to reduce with time.

There is an increased risk of relapse of HUS after transplantation (Loirat and Niaudet 2003). Although the actual risk is not known it appears to be approximately 30 per cent. Some clinicians try to avoid cyclosporin and tacrolimus but it is unclear whether these promote relapse in Factor H-deficient individuals. One should be very careful when considering live donation within the family, as potential donors might be similarly affected. Liver transplantation has been undertaken to correct the complement deficiency in two cases (Remuzzi *et al.* 2002).

von Willebrand protease deficiency

von Willebrand factor

von Willebrand factor is essential for normal platelet activation. It is constitutively secreted into plasma by endothelial cells, and stored in the alpha granules and Wiebel–Palade bodies of platelets and endothelial cells, respectively. vWF is synthesized as dimers which polymerize to form multimers of up to 40 dimeric subunits, giving a molecular mass of up to 20,000 kDa. However, it does not normally circulate in these very large multimeric forms. If endothelium is stimulated or damaged, vWF is released from storage sites as very large multimers that are then cleaved by a plasma protease at a specific site, Tyr-842-Met-843, giving rise to smaller forms (Dent *et al.* 1990). The proteolytic process is enhanced by shear stress, probably by unfolding the molecule to reveal cleavage sites (Tsai *et al.* 1994). The different patterns of multimeric size in plasma can be revealed by electrophoresis.

In addition to being the carrier protein for clotting factor VIII, and having binding sites for collagen and platelet glycoprotein IIb/IIIa, vWF has a high affinity for the platelet glycoprotein receptor complex Gp Ib-IX. It is this interaction that is capable of activating and aggregating platelets under flow conditions at high shear stress, such as might occur in the arterial circulation. Ultra-large vWF multimers, unfolded by shear stress, exhibit a 10-fold greater ability to activate platelets than multimers with lower molecular weight (Frederici *et al.* 1989).

vWF protease in HUS and TTP

Various abnormalities have been described in the plasma concentration of vWF and in the pattern of vWF multimers in patients with HUS and TTP (Moake *et al.* 1982; Galbusera *et al.* 1999). Since the development of a bioassay for the vWF metalloproteinase, and more recently, identification of its structure and gene, these findings have taken on a new perspective. The vWF protease has been partly purified and from its amino acid sequence shown to be a member of the ADAMTS family of metalloproteinases ('a disintegrin-like and metalloproteinase with thrombospondin motif') and designated ADAMTS13. The gene for this has been identified on chromosome 9, and the predicted full amino acid sequence published (Zheng *et al.* 2001). This allows two patient groups to be distinguished.

Constitutional vWF protease deficiency

The first is a rare group of patients with familial or congenital relapsing TTP in whom the protease is constitutionally absent or non-functioning (Furlan *et al.* 1998; Allford *et al.* 2000; Barbot 2001). In four pedigrees, mutations have been found in the ADAMTS13 gene (Levy *et al.* 2001). The disorder behaves as an autosomal recessive with unaffected heterozygotes having reduced protease activity, but not the near absence of activity (<5 per cent) that is required to express disease. The majority of these patients present in early infancy, although some have their first TTP episode in adult life. Having presented, they tend to relapse at intervals of about a month. The fact that some do not manifest the disease until later life suggests that abnormal vWF processing is necessary, but not in itself a sufficient reason for disease expression, and a second factor is required to trigger the disorder. The patients have ultra-large vWF multimers in their plasma in remission and respond to plasma infusions.

FFP contains the protease, so administration of sufficient plasma to bring the patient's plasma protease activity to above 10 per cent of normal will reverse the thrombocytopenia and haemolysis. Inhibitors of the protease have not been reported in this clinical group. The half-life of the infused protease is estimated to be between 2 and 4 days, and regular infusion of plasma at 2-weekly intervals appears to maintain remission (Furlan *et al.* 1999).

Acquired vWF protease deficiency

A second group consists of patients with non-familial TTP who have very low vWF protease activity due to an inhibitor. In two simultaneous publications describing 61 adult subjects, vWF protease was less than 5 per cent of expected in all but four during the acute episode of TTP (Furlan *et al.* 1998; Tsai *et al.* 1998). Mixing experiments showed that the plasma of these patients contained an inhibitory IgG autoantibody. The multimeric analysis of vWF in the acute presentation is variable and often there is loss of the large molecular weight multimers. Perhaps this is because they are precipitated in the arteriolar and capillary circulation with platelets aggregates. However, on entering remission the multimeric pattern normalizes, unlike patients with the constitutive protease deficiency in whom ultra large multimers persist. However, the multimeric analysis of vWF cannot be used as a reliable short cut to diagnose these forms of TTP or HUS, and the protease activity must be measured, and evidence of an inhibitor sought.

Treatment by plasma exchange rather than plasma infusion alone makes sense in that this will remove the autoantibody as well as replace the protease. The improvement in outcome for all cases of TTP from a historic mortality of about 90 per cent to less than 20 per cent has been attributed to plasma treatment. However, in some cases high titres of protease inhibitor make patients refractory to plasma exchange (Tsai 2000).

A similar autoantibody has been reported in cases of TTP associated with the platelet inhibitory drugs ticlopidine and clopidogrel, and increased binding of vWF to platelets has been demonstrated (Tsai *et al.* 2000; Sugio *et al.* 2001). TTP became apparent within 7 weeks of starting ticlopidine. Stopping the drug and daily plasma exchange for up to 10 exchanges led to sustained remission. Recently, in a case of TTP related to human immunodeficiency virus (HIV) infection a similar autoimmune inhibition of vWF proteinase was demonstrated (Sahud *et al.* 2002). This raises the possibility that other forms of thrombotic microangiopathy may share this pathogenesis. However, it is already clear that this mechanism does not participate in diarrhoea associated HUS, and probably not in the form of HUS/TTP that complicates bone marrow transplantation.

Other aetiologies and associations of HUS

HUS and TTP associated with pregnancy (see Chapter 10.7.2)

There are three separate conditions that appear to overlap, cause similar manifestations, and that need to be distinguished; pre-eclampsia,

HELLP (haemolysis, elevated liver enzymes, low platelet count) syndrome, and postpartum HUS.

Pre-eclampsia, characterized by hypertension, proteinuria, oedema, and at times abnormal coagulation, affects 5–10 per cent of women during pregnancy. Renal impairment occurs, but liver dysfunction, abnormal coagulation, and platelet consumption are relatively mild and fever is rare (Walker 2000).

Pre-eclampsia is associated with a contracted circulating volume, a low cardiac output and vasoconstriction. Patients require a vasodilator to control blood pressure. After a maximum dose of methyldopa (750 mg three times daily), nifedipine SR 20 mg twice a day can be tried. A small fetus suggests poor uteroplacental blood flow which would be made worse with beta-adrenergic blockade. Pregnancy-induced hypertension is a different condition and is associated with an expanded blood volume and high cardiac output. Blood pressure can be lowered by beta blocker.

HELLP syndrome is a very rare form of pre-eclampsia associated with severe liver dysfunction, thrombocytopenia, and a microangiopathic haemolytic anaemia. In both eclampsia and HELLP, immediate delivery of the baby is essential.

Postpartum HUS may develop during or immediately after delivery, during what is often an entirely uneventful pregnancy. Very rarely there is a family history of the syndrome, but the mechanism is unknown. Unfortunately, often due to the late re-presentation of patients who have already gone home, there is severe preglomerular vascular injury, irreversible renal failure, and severe hypertension. In early reports, a cardiomyopathy was a common feature. An important clinical issue is the distinction of HUS from the more common obstetric complications, pre-eclampsia and HELLP syndrome. Clinical suspicion of HUS requires urgent intervention with plasma treatment, while pre-eclampsia and HELLP syndrome typically resolve spontaneously following delivery (McMinn and George 2001).

Acute fatty liver is part of the differential diagnosis of peripartum obstetric medical emergencies. This is a rare but frequently fatal complication of late pregnancy that has many features in common with pre-eclampsia. It is diagnosed in about 1 : 10,000 pregnancies, but milder forms are now recognized. Patients present with severe abdominal pain and vomiting, and they become jaundiced rapidly and develop liver failure, hypoglycaemia, and disseminated intravascular coagulation. It is more common with multiple pregnancies and male fetuses. There is both a perinatal and maternal mortality of 70–80 per cent in severe cases, but milder cases are now recognized. In both this condition and in pre-eclampsia, the plasma urate concentration is increased disproportionately to the creatinine, although with pre-eclampsia the urate tends to increase in proportion to the blood pressure. Management consists of rapid termination of pregnancy and supportive therapy for renal and liver failure.

Neuraminidase and the red cell polyagglutination syndrome

HUS is associated with *S. pneumoniae* infection and red cell polyagglutination. Polyagglutination is the unexpected laboratory finding that patient's red cells are agglutinated *in vitro* by blood group ABO compatible serum. In this case, it is caused by naturally occurring IgM that recognizes the Thomsen–Friedenreich (T) antigen (Klein *et al.* 1977). On healthy cells the T epitope, galactose-β-1-3-galactose-*N*-acetyl-glucosamine, is masked by sialic acid. In cancers and in ageing red cells, the antigen becomes exposed. Neuraminidase, produced by *S. pneumoniae,* Clostridia species and influenza viruses, has the potential to cleave *N*-acetyl-neuraminic (sialic) acid from cell surfaces to reveal the T cryptantigen. The naturally occurring anti-T is an IgM cold antibody and unlikely to cause agglutination *in vivo.* Desialylation of red cells has been shown to remove the complement inhibitory effect of Factor H making them vulnerable to complement induced lysis (Fearon 1978). Given the association between HUS and Factor H deficiency, the pathogenesis of neuraminidase related HUS needs re-evaluation (Eder and Manno 2001).

Patients are usually infants and preschool age children. The onset of haemolysis, thrombocytopenia, and oliguria is abrupt and severe. The diagnosis should be suspected in any child with a microangiopathic haemolytic anaemia associated with sepsis but normal clotting. Often, it becomes clear when cross matching is undertaken. T-antigen exposure is confirmed by testing with the peanut lectin *Arachis hypogea*. It is traditional advice to minimize the administration of plasma products that contain the naturally occurring IgM. For example, if red cells or platelet transfusions are required the cells are washed to remove plasma. This advice presupposes that the naturally occurring IgM antibody is potentially pathogenic. Management is otherwise supportive for the acute renal failure and anaemia. The mortality has been regarded as high, but this may be historic (Brandt *et al.* 2002). Survivors usually regain renal function and there are no reports of relapse (Krysan and Flynn 2001).

Human immunodeficiency virus infection

In half of the cases reported, patients have had no previous symptoms of HIV-related disease. Some, however, have a preceding history of idiopathic immune thrombocytopenia (ITP). The presenting symptoms are similar to those of classic TTP and include fever in 75 per cent, and involvement of the central nervous system in 40 per cent, often with extremely low platelet counts (Thompson *et al.* 1992). Until proved otherwise, it must always be assumed that the patient has a complicating septicaemic illness.

In a single centre review of ARF occurring in the course of HIV infection, HUS was the commonest cause of ARF in 32 of the 92 patients (Peraldi *et al.* 1999). In another single centre review of 214 patients dying of AIDS, 7 per cent had evidence of TMA at the time of death and in half of those, their death was attributed to TMA (Gadallah *et al.* 1996). While patients who develop HUS but who do not have AIDS may recover, those with AIDS do not.

HUS and TTP associated with drugs

Oral contraceptives

HUS will sometimes first occur while taking oral contraceptives. The mechanism is unknown and other underlying causes of HUS should be sought. Survivors of the non-diarrhoeal form of the syndrome should be advised against the use of oral contraceptives.

Calcineurin inhibitors (cyclosporin, tacrolimus)

HUS with cyclosporin therapy was first reported as occurring after bone marrow transplantation (Shulman *et al.* 1981), and subsequently has been reported after both liver and renal transplantation. The syndrome has usually arisen within the first few weeks of transplantation, when the blood concentrations of the drug have been high. In renal allografts, platelet–fibrin thrombi in glomerular capillaries were also seen frequently in the first few weeks after transplantation (Neild *et al.* 1985), but these cases were invariably associated with very high concentrations of cyclosporin and are now rarely seen. Cyclosporin is not toxic to cultured endothelial cells in doses that inhibit prostacyclin synthesis (Brown and Neild 1987).

Although the renal vascular pathology described in *renal allografts* with chronic cyclosporin toxicity is non-specific with glomerular collapse and obsolescence, arteriolar hyalinosis, and tubular atrophy with interstitial fibrosis, the gross vascular pathology seen in *native kidneys* in heart transplant patients is indistinguishable from a chronic TMA (Griffiths *et al.* 1996). Despite this striking vascular pathology, it is exceptional for clinical features of HUS to be observed.

Chemotherapy

There are several cytotoxic drugs, including mitomycin-C (Giroux and Bettez 1985), 5-fluorouracil (Crocker and Jones 1983), bleomycin, epirubicin, and cisplatin (van der *et al.* 1998), and more recently the antimetabolite gemcitabine, whose use is associated with HUS.

There are several unusual features of the HUS that occurs with mitomycin C. Onset is acute but often some months after the last dose of mitomycin, and the condition can be precipitated by blood transfusion; the toxicity is related to the cumulative dose (>30 mg/m^2). The condition has a very poor prognosis, even when the tumour being treated appears to be in remission (Giroux and Bettez 1985; Verweij *et al.* 1987). Mitomycin is directly toxic to endothelial cells and when it was infused into the renal artery of a rat it caused a TMA in the ipsilateral kidney (Cattell 1985).

Quinine

Allergy to quinine may cause haemolytic anaemia, thrombocytopenia, TMA. In one series of 132 patients with HUS or TTP, who were asked specifically about current drug intake, 11 per cent had taken quinine and 6 per cent other drugs associated with this syndrome (Kojouri *et al.* 2001). Presensitized patients have developed quinine-dependent antibodies to erythrocytes, granulocytes, and the glycoprotein, Ib/IX and IIb/IIIa expressed on the platelet surface (Glynne *et al.* 1999). In most cases the renal involvement has not been conspicuous.

Ticlopidine, clopidogrel

These two closely related thienopyridines act by blocking an ADP-binding site on platelets which inhibits the expression of glycoprotein IIb/IIIa receptor that in turn binds fibrinogen and large multimers of vWF. The incidence of HUS with ticlopidine was estimated to be 1 case in 1600–5000 patients treated. The incidence with clopidogrel is not determined, but seems less common. With clopidogrel, the syndrome started within 2 weeks of starting treatment whereas with ticlopidine, the onset was later (2–12 weeks). It also appeared that patients with ticlopidine responded more promptly and with less likelihood of relapse compared with clopidogrel. In both groups, there is evidence of antibodies to vWF-cleaving protease (Bennett *et al.* 2000).

Other drugs

There is an increasing number of drugs associated with HUS, in addition to the above (Table 3). In some cases, a pathogenetic mechanism is known or has been proposed. Most commonly evidence of vWF-cleaving protease has been found (Bennett *et al.* 2000).

Table 3 Drugs associated with HUS

Oral contraceptives
Calcineurin inhibitors (cyclosporin, tacrolimus)
Cytotoxic therapy Mitomycin-C 5-Fluorouracil Gemcitabine Bleomycin Deoxycoformycin
Thienopyridines (ticlopidine, clopidogrel)
Quinine
Interferon-α (in treatment of chronic myeloid leukaemia)
'Crack' cocaine

HUS associated with malignancy

HUS occurring with untreated neoplastic disease is well described, but patients have more often received cytotoxic drugs such as mitomycin (see above). The tumour is usually a mucin-producing adenocarcinoma, most commonly a gastric adenocarcinoma followed by carcinoma of the breast, colon, and small cell lung carcinoma (Gordon and Kwaan 1999). Although there may be severe haemolysis and thrombocytopenia, renal involvement is often mild and fibrin thrombi rarely found at autopsy. In 1979 the median survival time was only 21 days (Antman *et al.* 1979).

There appears to be a particular association of interferon therapy inducing HUS when used to treat chronic myeloid leukaemia (Ravandi-Kashani *et al.* 1999).

Crow–Fukase disease or *POEMS* (polyneuropathy, organomegaly, endocrinopathy, monoclonal antibody, skin changes) syndrome is rarely reported outside of Japan. The renal lesion is a form of immune-complex negative membranoproliferative glomerulonephritis with striking endothelial injury similar to that seen in renal TMA. All features of HUS have been reported in this condition (Chazot *et al.* 1994).

Transplantation

Recurrence after transplantation

VTEC-related HUS does not recur following transplantation (Ferraris *et al.* 2002). However, non-diarrhoeal, idiopathic, or familial forms commonly recur. Of 63 children who received a total of 77 kidneys after D− HUS, 13 (21 per cent) had recurrence. Of the 17 known to have Factor H mutations, recurrence occurred in 35 per cent. There is no evidence that the likelihood of recurrence is related either to use of calcineurin-inhibitors or type of donor (Loirat *et al.* 1988).

In adults, the situation seems worse. In a single centre review from France of 16 patients transplanted in the period 1975–1995, 9 (56 per cent) developed definite evidence of recurrence, while four others had features of HUS which could not be differentiated with certainty from acute vascular rejection (Lahlou *et al.* 2000). One-year graft survival was 63 per cent. In the literature, to date 71 adult patients have received 90 kidneys with a 54 per cent rate of recurrence. The authors noted that in this combined experience the rate of recurrence appeared lower in those who had had a bilateral nephrectomy (Lahlou *et al.* 2000).

In autosomal recessive HUS, 11 patients received 14 kidneys with recurrence in 57 per cent of grafts (reviewed in Kaplan *et al.* 1997); in the dominant form 22 patients received 32 kidneys with recurrence in 65 per cent (Kaplan and Leonard 2000). In this group of patients bilateral nephrectomy did not appear to have a protective effect.

Renal allografts

The vascular injury of *acute* vascular rejection may be so severe that massive platelet consumption occurs in the kidney resulting in MAHA and HUS. The glomerular pathology is acute TMA. Thus, when idiopathic or familial HUS *recurs* shortly after transplantation it may be impossible to differentiate it with certainty from acute vascular rejection (Lahlou *et al.* 2000). Fortunately, the latter is now very rarely seen. Furthermore, *de novo* HUS can occur following renal transplantation. It has generally occurred in the presence of toxic blood concentrations of calcineurin inhibitors, both cyclosporin and tacrolimus (see above).

Other exotic causes of TMA in renal allografts are acute infection with parvovirus B19 (Murer *et al.* 2000); and a case report of disseminated BK-related polyoma virus (Petrogiannis-Haliotis *et al.* 2001). There are also increasingly frequent reports of *de novo* renal TMA occurring in recipients known to be hepatitis C positive, most of whom have anticardiolipin antibodies (Baid *et al.* 1999).

Bone marrow transplantation

Following bone marrow transplantation (BMT) there are a number of renal lesions, which are defined by the timing of their onset, into *early* and *late*. Acute renal failure associated with BMT is often the result of infection and its treatment with nephrotoxic drugs. Other causes of renal disease early after BMT include the tumour lysis syndrome, marrow infusion toxicity, cyclosporin toxicity and a hepatorenal-like syndrome (Zager 1994).

Cohen *et al.* use the term 'bone marrow transplant nephropathy' to describe a later-onset renal syndrome occurring more than three months after BMT (Cohen 2000). They identified a kidney lesion resembling radiation nephritis and HUS and reported an incidence of 20 per cent at 1-year post-BMT. They implicated pretransplant total body irradiation, because the clinical presentation was similar to radiation nephritis, and believed the lesion resulted from radiation injury to the endothelial cell of the kidney, similar to the pathogenesis of veno-occlusive disease after BMT (Rabinowe *et al.* 1991; Cruz *et al.* 1997).

Others, however, have reported BMT-nephropathy in patients not subjected to radiation and recognized a wide variation in the clinical features, severity, and response to therapy (Pettitt and Clark 1994). They suggest TMA as the underlying disorder. TMA is reported in up to 6 per cent of patients following BMT (Pettitt and Clark 1994) with a higher incidence among recipients of allografts (Zeigler *et al.* 1995).

In summary, several important factors are thought to be involved in the pathogenesis for TMA following BMT. These include, cyclosporin, graft-versus-host disease, irradiation, intensive conditioning chemotherapy, and infection. Nevertheless, the syndrome may occur after the use of autologous marrow when none of these factors apply (Zager 1994).

HUS associated with immunological diseases

Systemic lupus erythematosus

Rarely, patients with active systemic lupus erythematosus (SLE) may show features of HUS with the typical pathology of the syndrome superimposed upon the underlying lupus nephritis. These patients generally have arteriolar thrombi in multiple organs. Although this is rare, it is also likely to be missed when present, since the only feature of HUS that is not consistent with active systemic lupus is the microangiopathic haemolysis.

Much more commonly in SLE there is histological evidence of glomerular TMA with only individual clinical features of HUS, such as isolated thrombocytopenia, or fragmented red cells. In one single centre report from France, eight patients with TMA complicating active SLE were described of whom only one had MAHA, four thrombocytopenia, and five had a lupus anticoagulant. Five patients had severe hypertension (Bridoux *et al.* 1998).

Serum haptoglobin concentration should always be measured if this pathology is suspected. The correct differential diagnosis is important as treatment with FFP and plasma exchange may be more important then ever-increasing immunosuppression. The lupus should be treated in a conventional manner and the thrombotic microangiopathy with infusions of fresh frozen plasma (Gelfand *et al.* 1985). An association of this overlapping state with anticardiolipin antibodies or lupus anticoagulant is likely, but not yet clear.

Primary antiphospholipid syndrome

This is still a poorly characterized condition that manifests clinically in different and sometimes overlapping ways—from arterial and venous thrombosis and recurrent miscarriage to a catastrophic multi-system illness with a TMA involving the affected organs (Rennke 1999). The latter can be associated with all the features of HUS (Asherson *et al.* 2001).

The diagnosis is made by the presence of either the lupus anticoagulant or anticardiolipin antibodies (or antibodies to β2-glycoprotein I), or both. The lupus anticoagulant is found by measuring the activated PTT, and the dilute Russell's viper venom test. These laboratory abnormalities are found more commonly in patients with SLE and the clinical presentation can reflect both conditions (Levine *et al.* 2002).

Hepatitis C-induced cryoglobulinaemia

Mixed essential type II cryoglobulinaemia is a systemic vasculitis often associated with hepatitis C infection. Patients have undetectable complement 4 levels and an IgM *kappa* paraprotein rheumatoid factor. Typically, there is a palpable purpuric rash affecting the limbs, plus intermittent arthralgia, abdominal pains, severe hypertension, and a characteristic diffuse membranoproliferative glomerulonephritis. Full-blown and fatal HUS may complicate this condition and the TMA may have been underdiagnosed hitherto (Herzenberg *et al.* 1998). This pathology could partly explain the severe hypertension that is so common in this condition.

There are also increasing reports of recurrent TTP associated with chronic hepatitis C infection (Ramanan *et al.* 1999), and case reports of TTP occurring during interferon-α2b therapy (Iyoda *et al.* 1998).

Polymyositis and dermatomyositis

Full-blown and fatal HUS may complicate this condition (Miyaoka *et al.* 1997) and the TMA component may have hitherto been underdiagnosed. This complication should be suspected when such patients present with severe hypertension which is difficult to control (Anonymous 2001).

Scleroderma

Renal failure in this condition is usually associated with an acute onset and malignant hypertension. Either thrombocytopenia or a MAHA can occur, although neither is usually a prominent feature. The diagnosis of systemic sclerosis can occasionally be missed, particularly when patients have only a short history of Raynaud's disease. The increased blood pressure is probably secondary to the renal lesion, as acute renal failure occurs in up to 20 per cent of cases without hypertension (Cannon *et al.* 1974). Renal arteriolar thrombosis may be seen in acute scleroderma, even in patients without thrombocytopenia. Antibodies against Scl-70 or RNA polymerase support the diagnosis.

Glomerulonephritis

HUS complicating an underlying primary glomerulonephritis is unusual, but well documented. It has been reported with postinfectious glomerulonephritis, membranoproliferative glomerulonephritis, membranous glomerulonephritis, minimal-change disease, focal–segmental glomerulosclerosis, and with other unbiopsied cases of nephrotic syndrome (Siegler *et al.* 1989).

Malignant (accelerated) hypertension

Haematological features of HUS may occur with malignant hypertension (Linton *et al.* 1969). In patients under 50 years of age, it must always be assumed that the malignant phase of hypertension is secondary to an underlying renal disorder, whereas in older patients it is accepted that essential hypertension may enter a malignant phase.

The histological features of malignant hypertension are so similar to those of TMA that there may be uncertainty as to whether the patient has D− HUS (Bohle *et al.* 1977). Nevertheless, too often renal vascular pathology is blamed on the blood pressure when in fact the hypertension is probably secondary to or exacerbated by the renovascular pathology occurring as a primary event.

Idiopathic HUS

Previously, aetiological diagnoses were not found in the majority of adult cases of HUS. However, a recent review of 55 patients from a single centre in Paris (Tostivint *et al.* 2002) showed that only 10 were idiopathic. The others were related to HIV infection (18 cases), other nephropathies (10 cases), transplantation (seven cases), malignancy (five cases), VTEC (3 cases), pregnancy and the contraceptive pill (one case each). In childhood D− HUS about one-third can be allocated to one of the subgroups using the classification above, and two-thirds remain unexplained. In part, this is because developments in aetiology and pathogenesis are very recent, and routine laboratory investigations are often insufficient to reach a subgroup diagnosis. Support from active research groups is therefore helpful. It also suggests that there may be other aetiologies to discover. For example, not all patients with early onset relapsing or familial disease have disorders of Factor H or von Willebrand protease. It seems inevitable that other congenital and inheritable patterns of HUS exist.

It is difficult to define the prognosis in this contracting group of patients. In the past, there was often major preglomerular vascular pathology and irreversible renal failure both in children (Fitzpatrick 1992) and adults. However, data from the United Kingdom (Neild and Barratt 1998) suggest that the outcome in adults is better than was previously assumed with 62 per cent of 24 patients getting off dialysis. This is supported by an Italian registry, which showed that 59 per cent of 43 adults with primary or secondary forms of HUS were alive and independent of dialysis at 1 year of follow-up (Schieppati *et al.* 1992). A recommendation to manage idiopathic cases with plasma therapy and supportive measures as detailed seems justified.

Acknowledgements

The authors are grateful to Drs A.J. Howie and P. Ramani for providing Figs 2(a)–(e) and 4(d), to Dr Stuart Knutton for providing Figs 4(a)–(c), and to the late Dr L. Taitz for Figure 2(f).

References

Allford, S. L., Harrison, P., Lawrie, A. S., Liesner, R., Mackie, I. J., and Machin, S. J. (2000). von Willebrand factor-cleaving protease activity in congenital thrombotic thrombocytopenic purpura. *British Journal of Haematology* **111**, 1215–1222.

Amorosi, E. L. and Ultmann, J. E. (1966). Thrombotic thrombocytopenic purpura: a report of 16 cases and review of the literature. *Medicine (Baltimore)* **45**, 139–159.

Anonymous (2001). Case records of the Massachusetts General Hospital. Weekly clinicopathological exercises. Case 26-2001. Hypertensive encephalopathy with impaired renal function in a 67-year-old woman with polymyositis. *New England Journal of Medicine* **345** (8), 596–605.

Antman, K., Skarin, A., Mayer, R., Hargreaves, H., and Canellos, G. (1979). Microangiopathic hemolytic anemia and cancer: a review. *Medicine* **58** (5), 377.

Appiani, A. C., Edefonti, A., Bettinelli, A., Cossu, M. M., and Parachini, M. L. (1982). The relationship between plasma levels of the factor VIII complex and platelet release products (beta-thrombuglobulin and platelet factor 4) in children with the hemolytic–uremic syndrome. *Clinical Nephrology* **17**, 195–199.

Arab, S. and Lingwood, C. A. (1998). Intracellular targeting of the endoplasmic reticulum/nuclear envelope by retrograde transport may determine cell hypersensitivity to verotoxin via globotriaosyl ceramide fatty acid isoform traffic. *Journal of Cellular Physiology* **177**, 646–660.

Asherson, R. A. *et al.* (2001). Catastrophic antiphospholipid syndrome: clues to the pathogenesis from a series of 80 patients. *Medicine (Baltimore)* **80** (6), 355–377.

Ault, B. H. (2000). Factor H and the pathogenesis of renal diseases. *Pediatric Nephrology* **14**, 1045–1053.

Baehr, G., Klemperer, P., and Schifrin, A. (1936). An acute frbrile anaemia and thrombocytopenic purpura with diffuse platelet thromboses of capillaries and arterioles. *Transactions of the Association of American Physicians* **51**, 43–58.

Baid, S. *et al.* (1999). Renal thrombotic microangiopathy associated with anticardiolipin antibodies in hepatitis C-positive renal allograft recipients. *Journal of the American Society of Nephrology* **10** (1), 146–153.

Barbot, J., Costa, M., Barreirinho, M. S., Isvarlal, P., Robles, R., Gerritsen, H. E., Lammle, B., and Furlan, M. (2001). Ten years of prophylactic treatment with fresh-frozen plasma in a child with chronic relapsing thrombotic thrombocytopenic purpura as a result of a congenital deficiency of von Willebrand factor-cleaving protease. *British Journal of Haematology* **113**, 649–651.

Bell, W. R., Braine, H. G., Ness, P. M., and Kickler, T. S. (1991). Improved survival in thrombotic thrombocytopenic purpura/hemolytic uremic syndrome. *New England Journal of Medicine* **325**, 298–403.

Bennett, C. L. *et al.* (2000). Thrombotic thrombocytopenic purpura associated with clopidogrel. *New England Journal of Medicine* **342** (24), 1773–1777.

Bhimma, R., Rollins, N. C., Coovadia, H. M., and Adhikari, M. (1997). Postdysenteric haemolytic uremic syndrome in children during an epidemic of Shigella dysentery in Kwazulu/Natal. *Pediatric Nephrology* **11**, 560–564.

Bohle, A. *et al.* (1977). Malignant nephrosclerosis in patients with haemolytic uraemic syndrome. *Current Topics in Pathology* **65**, 81–113.

Boyd, B., Tyrrell, G., Maloney, M., Gyles, C., Brunton, J., and Lingwood, C. (1993). Alteration of the glycolipid binding specificity of the pig edema toxin from globotetraosyl to globotriaosyl ceramide alters *in vivo* tissue targetting and results in a verotoxin 1-like disease in pigs. *Journal of Experimental Medicine* **117**, 1745–1753.

Brandt, J., Wong, C., Mihm, S., Roberts, J., Smith, J., Brewer, E., Thiagarajan, R., and Warady, B. (2002). Invasive pneumococcal disease and hemolytic uremic syndrome. *Pediatrics* **110**, 371–376.

Bridoux, F. *et al.* (1998). Renal thrombotic microangiopathy in systemic lupus erythematosus: clinical correlations and long-term renal survival. *Nephrology, Dialysis, Transplantation* **13** (2), 298–304.

Brown, Z. and Neild, G. H. (1987). Cyclosporin inhibits prostacyclin production by cultured human endothelial cells. *Transplantation Proceedings* **19**, 1178–1180.

Cannon, P., Hassar, M., Case, D., Casarella, W., Sommers, S., and LeRoy, E. (1974). The relationship of hypertension and renal failure in scleroderma (progressive systemic sclerosis) to structural and functional abnormalities of the renal cortical circulation. *Medicine* **53**, 1–46.

Caprioli, J., Bettinaglio, P., Zipfel, P., Amadei, B., Daina, E., Gamba, S., Skera, C., Marziliano, N., Remuzzi, G., and Noris, M. (2001). The molecular basis of familial hemolytic uremic syndrome: mutation analysis of factor H gene reveals a hot spot in short consensus repeat 20. *Journal of the American Society of Nephrology* **12**, 297–307.

Cattell, V. (1985). Mitomycin-induced haemolytic uraemic syndrome (rat model). *American Journal of Pathology* **121**, 88–95.

Chandler, W. L., Jelacic, S., Boster, D. R., Ciol, M. A., Williams, G. D., Watkins, S. L., Igarashi, T., and Tarr, P. I. (2002). Prothrombotic coagulation abnormalities preceding the hemolytic uremic syndrome. *New England Journal of Medicine* **346**, 23–32.

Cimolai, N. *et al.* (1994). A continuing assessment of risk factors for the development of *Escherichia coli* O157:H7-associated haemolytic uremic syndrome. *Clinical Nephrology* **42**, 85–89.

Coad, N. A. G., Marshall, T., Rowe, B., and Taylor, C. M. (1991). Changes in the postenteropathic form of the haemolytic uremic syndrome in children. *Clinical Nephrology* **35**, 10–16.

Cohen, E. P. (2000). Radiation nephropathy after bone marrow transplantation. *Kidney International* **58** (2), 903–918.

Chazot, C. *et al.* (1994). Crow–Fukase disease/POEMS syndrome presenting with severe microangiopathic involvement of the kidney. *Nephrology, Dialysis, Transplantation* **9** (12), 1800–1802.

Crocker, J. and Jones, E. (1983). Haemolytic-uraemic syndrome complicating long-term mitomycin C and 5-fluorouracil therapy for gastric carcinoma. *Journal of Clinical Pathology* **36**, 24–29.

Cruz, D. N., Perazella, M. A., and Mahnensmith, R. L. (1997). Bone marrow transplant nephropathy: a case report and review of the literature. *Journal of the American Society of Nephrology* **8** (1), 166–173.

Dent, J. A., Berkowitz, S. D., Ware, J., Kasper, C. K., and Ruggeri, Z. M. (1990). Identification of a cleavage site directing the immunochemical detection of molecular abnormalities in the type IIA von Willebrand factor. *Proceedings of the National Academy of Sciences of the USA* **87**, 6306–6310.

Dundas, S., Murphy, J., Soutar, R. L., Jones, G. A., Hutchinson, S. J., and Todd, W. T. (1999). Effectiveness of therapeutic plasma exchange in the 1996 Lanarkshire *Escherichia coli* O157:H7 outbreak. *Lancet* **354**, 1327–1330.

Eder, A. F. and Manno, C. S. (2001). Does red-cell T activation matter? *British Journal of Haematology* **114**, 25–30.

Eknoyan, G. and Riggs, S. A. (1986). Renal involvement in patients with thrombotic thrombocytopenic purpura. *American Journal of Nephrology* **6**, 117–131.

Fearon, D. T. (1978). Regulation by membrane sialic acid of β1H-dependent decay-dissociation of amplification C3 convertase of the alternative complement pathway. *Proceedings of the National Academy of Sciences of the USA* **75**, 1971–1975.

Ferraris, J. R., Ramirez, J. A., Ruiz, S., Caletti, M. G., Vallejo, G., Piantanida, J. J., Araujo, J. L., and Sojo, E. T. (2002). Shiga toxin-associated hemolytic uremic syndrome: absence of recurrence after renal transplantation. *Pediatric Nephrology* **17**, 809–814.

Fitzpatrick, M. M. Long-term outcome of the hemolytic uremic syndrome in children. In *Hemolytic Uremic Syndrome and Thrombotic Thrombocytopenic Purpura* (ed. B. S. Kaplan, R. S. Trompeter, and J. L. Moake), pp. 441–451. New York: Marcel Dekker, 1992.

Fitzpatrick, M. M., Dillon, M. J., Barratt, T. M., and Trompeter, R. S. Atypical hemolytic uremic syndrome. In *Hemolytic Uremic Syndrome and Thrombotic Thrombocytopenic Purpura* (ed. B. S. Kaplan, R. S. Trompeter, and J. L. Moake), pp. 163–178. New York: Marcel Dekker, 1992a.

Fitzpatrick, M. M., Shah, V., Filler, G., Dillon, M. J., and Barratt, T. M. (1992b). Neutrophil activation in the haemolytic uraemic syndrome: free and complexed elastase in plasma. *Pediatric Nephrology* **6**, 50–53.

Fitzpatrick, M. M., Walters, M. D., Trompeter R. S., Dillon, M. J., and Barratt, T. M. (1993). A typical (non-diarrhea associated) hemolytic uremic syndrome in childhood. *Journal of Pediatrics* **122**, 532–537.

Frankel, G., Phillips, A. D., Rosenshine, I., Dougan, G., Kaper, J. B., and Knutton, S. (1998). Enteropathogenic and anterohaemorrhagic *Escherichia coli*: more subversive elements. *Molecular Microbiology* **30** (5), 911–921.

Frederici, A. B. *et al.* (1989). Binding of von Willebrand factor to glycoprotein Ib and IIb/IIIa complex: affinity is related to multimeric size. *British Journal of Haematology* **73**, 93–99.

Furlan, M. and Lammle, B. (2001). Aetiology and pathogenesis of thrombotic thrombocytopenic purpura and haemolytic uraemic syndrome: the role of von Willeband factor-cleaving protease. *Best Practice and Research Clinical Haematology* **14**, 437–454.

Furlan, M., Robles, R., Galbusera, M., Remuzzi, G., Kyrle, P. A., Brenner, B., Krause, M., Scharrer, I., Aumann, V., Mittler, U., Solentahaler, M., and Lammle, B. (1998). Von Willebrand factor-cleaving protease in thrombotic thrombocytopenic purpura and the haemolytic uremic syndrome. *New England Journal of Medicine* **339**, 1578–1584.

Furlan, M., Robles, R., Morelli, B., Sandoz, P., and Lammle, B. (1999). Recovery and half-life of von Willebrand factor-cleaving protease after plasma therapy in patients with thrombotic thrombocytopenic purpura. *Thrombosis and Haemostasis* **81**, 8–13.

Furutani, M., Kashiwagi, K., Ito, K., Endo, Y., and Igarashi, K. (1992). Comparison of the modes of action of a vero toxin (a shiga-like toxin) from *Escherichia coli*, of ricin, and of α-sarcin. *Archives of Biochemistry and Biophysics* **293**, 140–146.

Gadallah, M. F., el Shahawy, M. A., Campese, V. M., Todd, J. R., and King, J. W. (1996). Disparate prognosis of thrombotic microangiopathy in HIV-infected patients with and without AIDS. *American Journal of Nephrology* **16** (5), 446–450.

Galbusera, M., Benigni, A., Paris, S., Ruggenenti, P., Zoja, C., Rossi, C., and Remuzzi, G. (1999). Unrecognized pattern of von Willebrand factor abnormalities in haemolytic uremic syndrome and thrombotic thrombocytopenic purpura. *Journal of the American Society of Nephrology* **10**, 1234–1241.

Gasser, C., Gautier, E., Syeck, A., Siebermann, R. E., and Oechslin, R. (1955). Haemolytisch-uramische syndrome: bilaterale nierenrindennekrosen bei akuten erworbenen hamoytischen anamien. *Schweizische Medizinische Wochenschrift* **85**, 905–909.

Gelfand, J., Truong, L., Stern, L., Pirani, C., and Appel, G. (1985). Thrombotic thrombocytopenic purpura syndrome in systemic lupus erythematosus: treatment with plasma infusion. *American Journal of Kidney Diseases* **VI** (3), 154–160.

Giroux, L. and Bettez, P. (1985). Mitomycin-C nephrotoxicity: a clinicopathologic study of 17 cases. *American Journal of Kidney Diseases* **6**, 28–34.

Glynne, P., Salama, A., Chaudhry, A., Swirsky, D., and Lightstone, L. (1999). Quinine-induced immune thrombocytopenic purpura followed by hemolytic uremic syndrome. *American Journal of Kidney Diseases* **33** (1), 133–137.

Gordon, L. I. and Kwaan, H. C. (1999). Thrombotic microangiopathy manifesting as thrombotic thrombocytopenic purpura/hemolytic uremic syndrome in the cancer patient. *Seminars in Thrombosis and Hemostasis* **25** (2), 217–221.

Griffiths, M. H. *et al.* (1996). Cyclosporin nephrotoxicity in heart and lung transplant patients. *The Quarterly Journal of Medicine* **89**, 751–763.

Habib, R. Pathology of the haemolytic uremic syndrome. In *Hemolytic Uremic Syndrome and Thrombotic Thrombocytopenic Purpura* (ed. B. S. Kaplan, R. S. Trompeter, and J. L. Moake), pp. 315–353. New York: Marcel Dekker, 1992.

Habib, R., Levy, M., Gagnadoux, M. F., and Broyer, M. (1982). Prognosis of the haemolytic uremic syndrome in children. *Advances in Nephrology* **11**, 99–128.

Harel, Y. *et al.* (1993). A reporter tans gene indicates renal-specific induction of tumor necrosis factor (TNF) by Shiga-like toxin. Possible involvement of TNF in hemolytic uremic syndrome. *Journal of Clinical Investigation* **92**, 2110–2116.

Herzenberg, A. M., Telford, J. J., De Luca, L. G., Holden, J. K., and Magil, A. B. (1998). Thrombotic microangiopathy associated with cryoglobulinemic membranoproliferative glomerulonephritis and hepatitis C. *American Journal of Kidney Diseases* **31** (3), 521–526.

Hughes, A. K., Stricklett, P. K., Schmid, D., and Kohan, D. E. (2000a). Cytotoxic effect of shiga toxin-1 on human glomerular epithelial cells. *Kidney International* **57**, 2350–2359.

Hughes, J., Nangaku, M., Alpers, C. E., Shankland, S. J., Couser, W. G., and Johnson, R. J. (2000b). C5b-9 membrane attack complex mediates endothelial cell apoptosis in experimental glomerulonephritis. *American Journal of Physiology, Renal Physiology* **278**, F747–F757.

Ikeda, K., Ida, O., Kimoto, K., Yakatorige, T., Nakanishi, N., and Tarata, K. (1999). Effect of early fosfomycin treatment on prevention of hemolytic uremic syndrome accompanying *Escherichia coli* O157:H7 infection. *Clinical Nephrology* **52**, 357–362.

Inward, C. D., Howie, A. J., Fitzpatrick, M. M., Rafaat, F., Milford, D. V., and Taylor, C. M. (1997). Renal histology in fatal cases of diarrhoea-associated haemolytic uraemic syndrome. *Pediatric Nephrology* **11**, 556–559.

Inward, C. D., Williams, J., Chant, I., Crocker, J., Milford, D. V., Rose, P. E., and Taylor, C. M. (1995). Verocytotoxin-1 induces apoptosis in vero cells. *Journal of Infection* **30**, 213–218.

Iyoda, K. *et al.* (1998). Thrombotic thrombocytopenic purpura developed suddenly during interferon treatment for chronic hepatitis C. *Journal of Gastroenterology* **33** (4), 588–592.

Kaper, J. B., Elliot, S., Sperandio, V., Perna, N. T., Mayhew, G. F., and Blattner, F. R. Attaching and effacing intestinal histopathology and the locus of enterocyte effacement. In *Escherichia coli O157:H7 and Other Shiga Toxin Producing E. coli Strains* (ed. J. B. Kaper and A. D. O'Brien), pp. 163–182. Washington DC: American Society of Microbiology Press, 1998.

Kaplan, B. S. and Leonard, M. B. (2000). Autosomal dominant hemolytic uremic syndrome: variable phenotypes and transplant results. *Pediatric Nephrology* **14** (6), 464–468.

Kaplan, B. S., Papadimitriou, M., Brezin, J. H., Tomlanovich, S. J., and Zulkharnain (1997). Renal transplantation in adults with autosomal recessive inheritance of hemolytic uremic syndrome. *American Journal of Kidney Diseases* **30** (6), 760–765.

Karmali, M. A., Petric, M., Steele, B. T., and Lim, C. (1983). Sporadic cases of haemolytic uraemic syndrome associated with faecal cytotoxin and cytotoxin-producing *Escherichia coli* in stools. *Lancet* **i**, 619–620.

Karpman, D., Hakansson, A., Perez, M. T., Isaksson, C., Carlemalm, E., Caprioli, A., and Svanborg, C. (1998). Apoptosis of renal cortical cells in the hemolytic–uremic syndrome: *in vivo* and *in vitro* studies. *Infection and Immunity* **66**, 636–644.

Katz, J., Krawitz, S., Sacks, P. V., Levin, S. E., Thomson, P., Levin, J., and Metz, J. (1973). Platelet, erythrocyte, and fibrinogen kinetics in the hemolytic-uremic syndrome of infancy. *Journal of Pediatrics* **83**, 739–748.

King, A. J. (2002). Acute inflammmation in the pathogenesis of hemolytic–uremic syndrome. *Kidney International* **61**, 1553–1564.

Klein, P. J., Bulla, M., Newman, R. A., Muller, P., Uhlenbruck, G., Schaefer, H. E., Kruger, G., and Fisher, R. (1977). Thomsen–Friedenreich antigen in haemolytic–uraemic syndrome. *Lancet* **2** (8046), 1024–1025.

Koitabashi, Y., Rosenberg, B. F., Shapiro, H., and Bernstein, J. (1991). Mesangiolysis: an important glomerular lesion in thrombotic microangiopathy. *Modern Pathology* **4**, 161–166.

Kojouri, K., Vesely, S. K., and George, J. N. (2001). Quinine-associated thrombotic thrombocytopenic purpura-hemolytic uremic syndrome: frequency, clinical features, and long-term outcomes. *Annals of Internal Medicine* **135** (12), 1047–1051.

Konowalchuk, J., Speirs, J. I., and Stavric, S. (1977). Vero response to a cytotoxin of *Escherichia coli*. *Infection and Immunity* **18**, 775–779.

Koster, F., Levin, J., Walker, L., Tung, K. S. K., Gilman, R. H., Rahaman, M. M., Majid, M. A., Islam, S., and Williams, R. C. (1978). Hemolytic–uremic syndrome after Shigellosis. Relation to endotoxemia and circulating immune complexes. *New England Journal of Medicine* **298**, 927–933.

Krysan, D. J. and Flynn, J. T. (2001). Renal transplantation after *Streptococcus pneumoniae*-associated hemolytic uremic syndrome. *American Journal of Kidney Diseases* **37** (2), E15.

Lahlou, A. *et al.* (2000). Hemolytic uremic syndrome. Recurrence after renal transplantation. Groupe Cooperatif de l'Ile-de-France (GCIF). *Medicine (Baltimore)* **79** (2), 90–102.

Levin, M. and Barratt, T. M. (1984). Haemolytic uraemic syndrome. *Archives of Disease in Childhood* **59**, 397–400.

Levine, J. S., Branch, D. W., and Rauch, J. (2002). The antiphospholipid syndrome. *New England Journal of Medicine* **346** (10), 752–763.

Levy, G. G., Nichols, W. C., Lian, E. C., Foroud, T., McClintick, J. N., McGee, B. M., Yang, A. Y., Siemieniak, D. R., Stark, K. R., Gruppo, R., Sarode, R., Shurin, S. B., Chandrasekaran, V., Stabler, S. P., Sabio, H., Bouhassira, E. E., Upshaw, J. D., Ginsburg, D., and Tsai, H. M. (2001). Mutations in a member of the ADAMTS gene family cause thrombotic thrombocytopenic purpura. *Nature* **413**, 488–494.

Lingwood, C. A. (1994). Verotoxin-binding in human renal sections. *Nephron* **66**, 21–28.

Linton, A. L. *et al.* (1969). Microangiopathic haemolytic anaemia and the pathogenesis of malignant hypertension. *Lancet* **1**, 1277–1282.

Loirat, C. and Niaudet, P. (2003). The risk of recurrence of hemolytic uremic syndrome after renal transplantation in children. *Pediatric Nephrology* **18**, 1095–1101.

Loirat, C., Sonsino, E., Hinglais, N., Jais, J. P., Landais, P., and Fermanian, J. (1988). Treatment of childhood haemolytic uraemic syndrome with plasma. *Pediatric Nephrology* **2**, 279–285.

Ludwig, K., Karmali, M. A., Sarkim, V., Bobrowski, C., Petric, M., Karck, H., and Muller-Wiefel, D. (2001). Antibody response to Shiga toxins Stx2 and Stx1 in children with enterpathic haemolytic–uremic syndrome. *Journal of Clinical Microbiology* **39**, 2272–2279.

Melnyk, A. M. S., Solez, K., and Kjellstrand, C. M. (1995). Adult hemolytic–uremic syndrome. *Archives of Internal Medicine* **155**, 2077–2084.

McMinn, J. R. and George, J. N. (2001). Evaluation of women with clinically suspected thrombotic thrombocytopenic purpura–hemolytic uremic syndrome during pregnancy. *Journal of Clinical Apheresis* **16** (4), 202–209.

Milford, D. V. (1994). A National study of the epidemiology, clinical features and microbiology of the haemolytic uraemic syndromes. MD Thesis, University of Southampton.

Milford, D. V., and Taylor, C. M. (1990). New insights into the haemolytic uraemic syndromes. *Archives of Disease in Childhood* **65**, 713–715.

Milford, D. V., Taylor, C. M., Guttridge, B., Hall, S. M., Rowe, B., and Kleanthous, H. (1990). Haemolytic uraemic syndromes in the British Isles 1985–8: association with verocytotoxin producing *Escherichia coli*. Part 1: clinical and epidemiological aspects. *Archives of Disease in Childhood* **65**, 716–721.

Misiani, R., Appiani, A. C., Edefonti, A., Gotti, E., Bettinelli, A., Giani, M., Rossi, E., Remuzzi, G., and Mecca, G. (1982). Haemolytic uraemic syndrome: therapeutic effects of plasma infusion. *British Medical Journal* **285**, 1304–1306.

Miyaoka, Y. *et al.* (1997). A case of dermatomyositis complicated by thrombotic thrombocytopenic purpura. *Dermatology* **194** (1), 68–71.

Moake, J. L., Rudy, C. K., Troll, J. H., Weinstein, M. J., Colannino, N. M., Azocar, J., Seder, R. H., Hong, S. L., and Deykin, D. (1982). Unusually large plasma factor VIII: von Willebrand factor multimers in chronic relapsing thrombotic thrombocytopenic purpura. *New England Journal of Medicine* **307**, 1432–1435.

Moghal, N. E., Ferreira, M. A. S., Howie, A. J., Milford, D. V., Rafaat, F., and Taylor, C. M. (1998). The late histologic findings in diarrhea-associated hemolytic uremic syndrome. *Journal of Pediatrics* **133**, 220–223.

Morel-Maroger, L., Kanfer, A., Solez, K., Sraer, J. D., and Richet, G. (1979). Prognostic importance of vascular lesions in acute renal failure with microangiopathic hemolytic anaemia (hemolytic uremic syndrome) clinicopathologic study in 20 adults. *Kidney International* **15**, 548–558.

Morigi, M., Micheletti, G., Figliuzzi, M., Imberti, B., Karmali, M. A., Remuzzi, A., Remuzzi, G., and Zoja, C. (1995). Verotoxin-1 promotes leukocyte adhesion to cultured endothelial cells under physiologic flow conditions. *Blood* **86**, 4553–4558.

Morigi, M., Galbusera, M., Binda, E., Imberti, B., Gastoldi, S., Remuzzi, A., Zoja, C., and Remuzzi, G. (2001). Verotoxin-1 induced up-regulation of adhesive molecules renders microvascular endothelial cells thrombogenic at high shear stress. *Blood* **98**, 1828–1835.

Moschowitz, E. (1925). An acute febrile pleiochromic anaemia with hyaline thrombosis of the terminal arterioles and capillaries. An undescribed disease. *Archives of Internal Medicine* **36**, 89–93.

Murer, L. *et al.* (2000). Thrombotic microangiopathy associated with parvovirus B 19 infection after renal transplantation. *Journal of the American Society of Nephrology* **11** (6), 1132–1137.

Nangaku, M., Alpers, C. E., and Pippin, J. (1998). CD59 protects glomerular endothelial cells from immune-mediated thrombotic microangiopathy in rats. *Journal of the American Society of Nephrology* **9**, 590–597.

Neild, G. H. and Barratt, T. M. Acute renal failure associated with microangiopathy. In *Oxford Textbook of Clinical Nephrology* (ed. S. Cameron, A. M. Davison, J. Grunfeld, D. Kerr, and E. Ritz), pp. 1649–1666. Cambridge: Oxford University Press, 1998.

Neild, G. H., Reuben, R., Hartley, R. B., and Cameron, J. S. (1985). Glomerular thrombi in renal allografts associated with cyclosporin therapy. *Journal of Clinical Pathology* **38**, 253–258.

Nevard, C. H., Jurd, K. M., Lane, D. A., Philippou, H., Haycock, G. B., and Hunt, B. J. (1997). Activation of coagulation and fibrinolysis in childhood diarrhoea-associated haemolytic uraemic syndrome. *Thrombosis and Haemostasis* **78**, 1450–1455.

Noris, M., Ruggenenti, P., Perna, A., Orisio, S., Caprioli, J., Skerka, C., Vasile, B., Zipfel, P. F., and Remuzzi, G. (1999). Hypocomplementemia discloses genetic predisposition to hemolytic uremic syndrome and thrombotic thrombocytopenic purpura: role of factor H abnormalities. *Journal of the American Society of Nephrology* **10**, 281–293.

O'Brien, A. D. and Laveck, G. D. (1983). Purification and characterization of a *Shigella dysenteriae* 1-like toxin produced by *Escherichia coli*. *Infection and Immunity* **40**, 675–683.

Pavia, A. T. *et al.* (1990). Hemolytic uremic syndrome during an outbreak of *Escherichia coli* O157:H7 infection in intitutions for mentally retarded persons: clinical and epidemiological observations. *Journal of Pediatrics* **116**, 544–551.

Peraldi, M. N., Maslo, C., Akposso, K., Mougenot, B., Rondeau, E., and Sraer, J. D. (1999). Acute renal failure in the course of HIV infection: a single-institution retrospective study of ninety-two patients and sixty renal biopsies. *Nephrology, Dialysis, Transplantation* **14** (6), 1578–1585.

Perez-Caballero, D., Gonzalez-Rubio, C., Gallardo, M. E., Vera, M., Lopez-Trascasa, M., Rodrigues de Cordoba, S., and Sanches-Corral, P. (2001). Clustering of missense mutations in the *C*-terminal of factor H in atypical hemolytic uremic syndrome. *American Journal of Human Genetics* **68**, 478–484.

Petrogiannis-Haliotis, T. *et al.* (2001). BK-related polyomavirus vasculopathy in a renal-transplant recipient. *New England Journal of Medicine* **345** (17), 1250–1255.

Pettitt, A. R. and Clark, R. E. (1994). Thrombotic microangiopathy following bone marrow transplantation. *Bone Marrow Transplantation* **14** (4), 495–504.

Pijpers, A. H., van Setten, P. A., van den Heuvel, L. P., Assmann, K. J., Dijkman, H. B., Pennings, A. H., Monnens, L. A., and van Hinsberg, V. W. (2001). Verocytotoxin-induced apoptosis of human microvascular endothelial cells. *Journal of the American Society of Nephrology* **12**, 767–778.

Poulton, J., Taylor, C. M., and De Giovanni, J. V. (1987). Dilated cardiomyopathy associated with haemolytic uraemic syndrome. *British Heart Journal* **57**, 181–183.

Proulx, F., Turgeon, J. P., Delage, G., Lafleur, L., and Chicoine, L. (1992). Randomised, controlled trial of antibiotic therapy for *Escherichia coli* 0157:H7 enteritis. *Journal of Pediatrics* **121**, 299–303.

Pudymaitis, A. and Lingwood, C. A. (1992). Susceptibility to verotoxin as a function of the cell cycle. *Journal of Cell Physiology* **150**, 632–639.

Rabinowe, S. N. *et al.* (1991). Hemolytic–uremic syndrome following bone marrow transplantation in adults for hematologic malignancies. *Blood* **77** (8), 1837–1844.

Ramanan, A. S., Thirumala, S., and Chandrasekaran, V. (1999). Thrombotic thrombocytopenia purpura: a single institution experience. *Journal of Clinical Apheresis* **14** (1), 9–13.

Ravandi-Kashani, F., Cortes, J., Talpaz, M., and Kantarjian, H. M. (1999). Thrombotic microangiopathy associated with interferon therapy for patients with chronic myelogenous leukemia: coincidence or true side effect? *Cancer* **85** (12), 2583–2588.

Remuzzi, G., Ruggenenti, P., Codazzi, D., Noris, M., Caprioli, J., Locatelli, G., and Gridelli, B. (2002). Combined liver and kidney transplantation for familial haemolytic uraemic syndrome. *Lancet* **359**, 1671–1672.

Renaud, C., Niaudet, P., Gagnadoux, M. F., Broyer, M., and Habib, R. (1995). Haemolytic uraemic syndrome: prognostic features in children over 3 years of age. *Pediatric Nephrology* **9**, 24–29.

Rennke, H. G. (1999). Case records of the Massachusetts General Hospital. Weekly clinicopathological exercises. Case 18-1999. A 54-year-old woman with acute renal failure and thrombocytopenia. *New England Journal of Medicine* **340** (24), 1900–1908.

Rousseau, E., Blais, N., and O'Regan, S. (1990). Decreased necessity for dialysis with loop diuretic therapy in haemolytic uremic syndrome. *Clinical Nephrology* **34**, 22–25.

Richards, A., Buddles, M. R., Donne, R. L., Kaplan, B. S., Kirk, E., Venning, M. C., Tielemans, C. L., Goodship, J. A., and Goodship, T. H. (2001). Factor H mutations in haemolytic uraemic syndrome cluster in exons 18–20, a domain important for host cell recognition. *American Journal of Human Genetics* **68**, 485–490.

Richardson, S. E., Karmali, M. A., Becker, L. E., and Smith, C. R. (1988). The histopathology of the hemolytic uremic syndrome associated with verocytotoxin–producing *Escherichia coli* infections. *Human Pathology* **19**, 1102–1108.

Rizzoni, G. *et al.* (1988). Plasma infusion for hemolytic uremic syndrome in children: results of a multicentre controlled trial. *Journal of Pediatrics* **112**, 284–290.

Sabio, H., Bouhassira, E. E., Upshaw, J. D., Ginsburg, D., and Tsai, H.-M. (2001). Mutations in a member of the ADAMTS gene family cause thrombotic thrombocytopenic purpura. *Nature* **413**, 488–495.

Sahud, M. A., Claster, S., Liu, L., Ero, M., Harris, K., and Furlan, M. (2002). von Willebrand factor-cleaving protease inhibitor in a patient with human immunodeficiency syndrome-associated thrombotic thrombocytopenic purpura. *British Journal of Haematology* **116**, 909–911.

Sandvig K. and Van Deurs, B. (1996). Endocytosis, intracellular transport, and cytotoxic action of shiga toxin and ricin. *Physiological Reviews* **76**, 949–966.

Sassetti, B., Vizcarguenaga, M. I., Zanaro, N. L., Silva, M. V., Kordich, L., Florentini, L., Diaz, M., Vitacco, M., and Sanchez Avalos, J. C. (1999). Hemolytic uremic syndrome in children: platelet aggregation and membrane glycoproteins. *Journal of Pediatric Hematology and Oncology* **21**, 123–128.

Schieppati, A. *et al.* (1992). Renal function at hospital admission as a prognostic factor in adult haemolytic syndrome. *Journal of the American Society of Nephrology* **2**, 1640–1644.

Schmidt, H. *et al.* (1993). Shiga-like toxin II-related cytotoxins in *Citrobacter freundii* strains from human and beef samples. *Infection and Immunity* **61**, 534–543.

Shulman, H., Striker, G., Deeg, H. J., Kennedy, M., Storb, R., and Thomas, E. D. (1981). Nephrotoxicity of cyclosporin A after allogeneic marrow transplantation: glomerular thromboses and tubular injury. *New England Journal of Medicine* **305**, 1392–1395.

Siegler, R., Brewer, E., and Pysher, T. (1989). Hemolytic uraemic syndrome associated with glomerular disease. *American Journal of Kidney Diseases* **13** (2), 144–147.

Stein, P. E., Boodhoo, A., Tyrell, G. J., Brunton, J. L., and Read, R. J. (1992). Crystal structure of the cell-binding B oligomer of verotoxin-1 from *E. coli*. *Nature* **355**, 748–750.

Sugio, Y., Okamura, T., Shimoda, K., Matsumoto, M., Yagi, H., Ishizashi, H., Niho, Y., Inaba, S., and Fujimura, Y. (2001). Ticlopidine-associated thrombotic thrombcytopenic purpura with an IgG-type inhibitor to von Willebrand factor-cleaving protease activity. *International Journal of Hematology* **74**, 347–351.

Taguchi, T., Uchida, H., Kiyokawa, N., Mori, T., Sato, N., Horie, H., Takeda, T., and Fujimoto, J. (1998). Verotoxins induce apoptosis in human renal epithelium derived cells. *Kidney International* **53**, 1681–1688.

Taylor, C. M. (2001). Hemolytic–uremic syndrome and complement factor H deficiency: clinical aspects. *Seminars in Thrombosis and Hemostasis* **27**, 185–190.

Taylor, C. M. and Milford, D. V. Haemolytic uraemic syndrome in Baillière's Clinical Paediatrics Vol. 5, No. 4. In *Therapeutic Strategies in Renal Disease* (ed. W. Proesmans), pp. 557–593, 1997.

Taylor, C. M., Williams, J. M., Lote, C. J., Howie, A. J., Thewles, A., Wood, J. A., Milford, D. V., Rafaat, F., Chant, I., and Rose, P. E. (1999a). A laboratory model of toxin-induced hemolytic uremic syndrome. *Kidney International* **55**, 1367–1374.

Taylor, F. B., Tesh, V. L., DeBault, L., Li, A., Chang, A. C. K., Kosanke, S. D., Pysher, T. J., and Siegler, R. L. (1999b). Characterization of the baboon responses to Shiga-like toxin. *American Journal of Pathology* **154**, 1285–1299.

Te Loo, D. M. W. M., Monnens, L. A. H., van der Velden, T. J. A. M., Vermer, M. A., Preyers, F., Demacker, P. N. M., van den Heuvel, L. P. W. J., and van Hinsberg, V. W. M. (2000). Binding and transfer of verocytotoxin by polymorphonuclear leukocytes in hemolytic uremic syndrome. *Blood* **995**, 3396–3402.

Thoenes, W. and John, H. D. (1980). Endotheliotropic (haemolytic) nephroangiopathy and its various manifestation forms: thrombotic microangiopathy, primary malignant nephrosclerosis, hemolytic uremic syndrome. *Klinische Wochenschrift* **58**, 173–184.

Thompson, C. E., Damon, L. E., Ries, C. A., and Linker, C. A. (1992). Thrombotic Microangiopathies in the 1980s: clinical features, response to treatment, and the impact of the human immunodeficiency virus epidemic. *Blood* **80**, 1890–1895.

Thorpe, C. M., Hurley, B. P., Lincicome, L. L., Jacewicz, M. S., Keusch, G. T., and Acheson, D. W. (1999). Shiga toxins stimulate secretion of interleukin-8 from intestinal epithelial cells. *Infection and Immunity* **67**, 5985–5993.

Thorpe, C. M., Smith, W. E., Hurley, B. P., and Acheson, D. W. K. (2001). Shiga toxins induce, superinduce, and stabilize a variety of C-X-C chemokine mRNAs in intestinal epithelial cells resulting in increased chemokine expression. *Infection and Immunity* **69**, 6140–6147.

Tostivint, I., Mougenot, B., and Flahault, A. (2002). Adult haemolytic and uraemic syndrome: causes and prognostic factors in the last decade. *Nephrology, Dialysis, Transplantation* **17**, 1228–1234.

Tsai, H.-M. (2000). High titers of inhibitors of von Willebrand factor-cleaving metalloproteinase in a fatal case of acute thrombotic thrombocytopenic purpura. *American Journal of Hematology* **65**, 251–255.

Tsai, H.-M. and Lian, E. C.-Y. (1998). Antibodies to von Willebrand factor-cleaving protease in acute thrombotic thrombocytopenic purpura. *New England Journal of Medicine* **339**, 1585–1594.

Tsai, H.-M., Rice, L., Sarode, R., Chow, T. W., and Moake, J. L. (2000). Antibody inhibitors to von Willebrand factor metalloproteinase and increased binding of von Willebrand factor to platelets in ticlopidine-associated thrombotic thrombocytopenic purpura. *Annals of Internal Medicine* **132**, 794–799.

Tsai, H. M., Sussman, I. I., and Nagel, R. L. (1994). Sear stress enhances the proteolysis of von Willebrand factor in normal plasma. *Blood* **83**, 2171–2179.

van der Heijden, M., Ackland, S. P., and Deveridge, S. (1998). Haemolytic uraemic syndrome associated with bleomycin, epirubicin and cisplatin chemotherapy—a case report and review of the literature. *Acta Oncologica* **37** (1), 107–109.

Van de Kar, N. C., Monnens, L. A., Karmali, M. A., and van Hinsberg, V. W. (1992). Tumor necrosis factor and interleukin-1 induce expression of the verocytotoxin receptor globotriaosylceramide on human endothelial cells. *Blood* **80**, 2755–2764.

Van Setten, P. A., van Hinsberg, V. W., Van der Velden, T. J., van de Kar, N. C., Vermeer, M., Mahan, J. D., Assmann, K. J., van den Heuvel, L. P., and Monnens, L. A. (1997a). Effects of TNF alpha on vero cytotoxin cytotoxicity in purified human glomerular microvascular endothelial cells. *Kidney International* **51**, 1245–1256.

Van Setten, P. A., van Hinsberg, V. W., Vanden Heuvel, L. P., van der Velden, T. J., van de Kar, N. C., Krebbers, R. J., Karmali, M. A., and Monnens, L. A. (1997b). Verocytotoxin inhibits mitogenesis and protein synthesis in purified human glomerular mesangial cells without affecting cell viability: evidence for two distinct mechanisms. *Journal of the American Society of Nephrology* **8**, 1877–1888.

Verweij, J., van der Burg, M., and Pinedo, H. (1987). Mitomycin C-induced hemolytic uraemic syndrome. Six case reports and review of the literature on renal, pulmonary and cardiac side effects of the drug. *Radiotherapy and Oncology* **8**, 33–41.

Wagner, P. L., Acheson, D. W. K., and Waldor, M. K. (2001). Human neutrophils and their products induce shiga toxin production by enterohemorrhagic *Escherichia coli*. *Infection and Immunity* **69**, 1934–1937.

Walker, J. J. (2000). Pre-eclampsia. *Lancet* **356** (9237), 1260–1265.

Walters, M. D. S. *et al.* (1989). The polymorphonuclear leucocyte count in childhood haemolytic uraemic syndrome. *Pediatric Nephrology* **3**, 130–134.

Warwicker, P., Goodship, T. H. J., Donne, R. L., Pirson, Y., Nicholls, A., Ward, R. M., Turnpenny, P., and Goodship, J. A. (1998). Genetic studies into inherited and sporadic hemolytic uremic syndrome. *Kidney International* **53**, 836–844.

Williams, J. M., Boyd, B., Nutikka, A., Lingwood, C. A., Barnett Foster, D. E., Milford, D. V., and Taylor, C. M. (1999). A comparison of the effects of verocytotoxin-1 on primary human renal cell cultures. *Toxicology Letters* **105**, 47–57.

Zager, R. A. (1994). Acute renal failure in the setting of bone marrow transplantation. *Kidney International* **46**, 1443–1458.

Zeigler, Z. R., Shadduck, R. K., Nemunaitis, J., Andrews, D. F., and Rosenfeld, C. S. (1995). Bone marrow transplant-associated thrombotic microangiopathy: a case series. *Bone Marrow Transplant* **15** (2), 247–253.

Zhang, X., McDaniel, A. D., Wolf, L. E., Keusch, G. T., Waldor, N. K., and Acheson, D. W. (2000). Quinolone antibiotics induce shiga toxin-encoding bacteriophages, toxin production, and death in mice. *Journal of Infectious Diseases* **181**, 664–670.

Zheng, X., Chung, D., Takayama, T. K., Majerus, E. M., Sadler, J. E., and Fujikawa, K. (2001). Structure of von Willebrand factor cleaving protease (ADAMTS13), a metalloprotease involved in thrombotic thrombocytopenic purpura. *Journal of Biological Chemistry* **276**, 41059–41063.

Zipfel, P. F. (2001). Complement factor H: physiology and pathophysiology. *Seminars in Thrombosis and Hemostasis* **27**, 191–199.

10.6.4 Acute renal failure in liver disease

Vicente Arroyo Pérez, Andrés Cárdenas, José M. Campistol, and Pere Ginès

Introduction

Hepatorenal syndrome (HRS), a common form of renal failure in liver disease, may develop in patients with advanced cirrhosis or with acute liver failure. This type of renal failure is functional in nature and occurs due to a significant impairment in circulatory function which leads to renal hypoperfusion. Functional renal failure in HRS may progress to acute tubular necrosis particularly in cases of acute hepatic failure. Acute renal failure may be secondary to drug toxicity in patients with decompensated cirrhosis or with acute liver failure. Additionally, renal failure frequently complicates the postoperative course of patients with obstructive jaundice or those undergoing liver transplantation. Finally, acute renal failure in patients with liver disease and cirrhosis may be caused by glomerulonephritis secondary to IgA deposits or by cryoglobulinaemic glomerulonephritis as a consequence of hepatitis C virus infection.

Renal failure in cirrhosis

Hepatorenal syndrome

HRS is defined as renal failure developing in patients with advanced liver disease, liver failure, and portal hypertension in the absence of any identifiable renal pathology. Patients with HRS develop a severe disturbance in their systemic haemodynamics with resulting activation of endogenous vasoactive systems. In the kidney, intense renal vasoconstriction leads to a reduction in glomerular filtration rate (GFR), whereas in the extrarenal circulation there is predominant arterial vasodilation, which results in diminished systemic vascular resistance and, consequently, arterial hypotension. Although HRS occurs predominantly in advanced cirrhosis, it may also develop in other liver diseases associated with severe liver failure and portal hypertension, such as alcoholic hepatitis and acute liver failure (Arroyo *et al.* 1996). HRS is a major complication of cirrhosis, with a reported incidence of 8–10 per cent in hospitalized patients with ascites (Ginès *et al.* 1993). It develops in the late phases of decompensated cirrhosis and is an important determinant of survival.

Functional renal abnormalities in cirrhosis

Sodium retention, impaired free water excretion and renal vasoconstriction with decreased renal perfusion, and GFR are the main renal functional abnormalities. The onset of each of these abnormalities differs in time and, consequently, the course of cirrhosis can be divided into phases according to renal function. Renal dysfunction in cirrhosis usually follows a progressive course, so, in the final phase of the disease, when HRS develops, all the three abnormalities are present.

Sodium retention without activation of the traditional sodium-retaining systems

Sodium retention is the earliest manifestation of renal impairment in cirrhosis. Patients with compensated cirrhosis (i.e. without a history of ascites—the pre-ascitic phase) have subtle abnormalities in renal sodium handling. Patients may not be able to escape the effect of mineralocorticoids and develop continuous sodium retention and ascites (LaVilla *et al.* 1992). They may also be unable to excrete a sodium overload, as occurs in patients with cirrhosis who consume a large amount of salt in their diet or receive saline infusions. Arterial vasodilation, already present in compensated cirrhosis with portal hypertension probably plays an important role (Bosch *et al.* 1980).

As the disease progresses, the renal ability to excrete sodium diminishes and a critical point is reached when sodium excretion is less than sodium intake. The patient then develops sodium and water retention that accumulates as ascites. During this phase, renal perfusion, GFR, the renal ability to excrete free water, plasma renin activity (PRA) and the plasma concentrations of aldosterone and norepinephrine are normal (Saló *et al.* 1995). Sodium retention, therefore, cannot be attributed to the effect of the renin–angiotensin–aldosterone system (RAAS) and the sympathetic nervous system (SNS), the two most important sodium-retaining systems so far identified. Moreover, since plasma natriuretic peptides are also markedly increased in cirrhosis (Ginès *et al.* 1988), sodium retention cannot be attributed to reduced production of such endogenous natriuretic substances. Renal function at this stage is not dependent on renal prostaglandins, so that non-steroidal anti-inflammatory agents (NSAIDs) do not reduce renal perfusion and GFR at this stage (Arroyo *et al.* 1986). It has been suggested that arterial vasodilation in this phase of the disease is not intense enough to stimulate the RAAS and SNS, but it may enhance an unknown and extremely sensitive sodium-retaining mechanism (renal or extrarenal) (Arroyo and Jiménez 2000). An alternative proposal is that sodium retention is unrelated to circulatory function. An increased renal sensitivity to aldosterone, a decreased hepatic synthesis of a natriuretic factor, or a 'hepatorenal reflex' promoting sodium retention are possible mechanisms suggested by others (Bernardi *et al.* 1999). However, no substantial data support this mechanism. Sodium retention in the absence of a circulatory dysfunction would increase arterial pressure, a feature not observed at this stage of the disease.

Stimulation of RAAS, SNS, and antidiuretic hormone with preserved renal perfusion and GFR

With the exception of alcoholic cirrhosis in which hepatic, circulatory, and renal function may improve after alcohol withdrawal, the degree of sodium retention increases with the progression of disease. Patients with intense sodium retention have increased PRA, aldosterone, and norepinephrine (Arroyo 2002). The plasma volume, cardiac output,

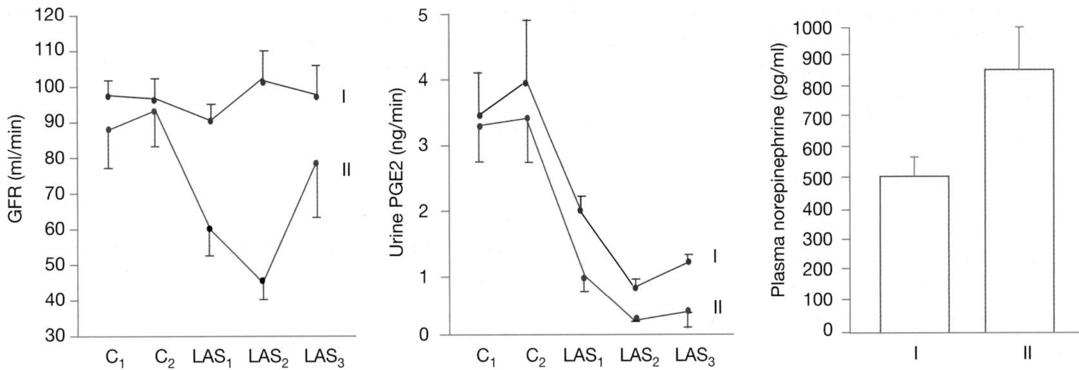

Fig. 1 Glomerular filtration rate and urinary excretion of prostaglandin E2 (mean ± SEM) before and after the intravenous injection of 450 mg of lysine acetylsalicylate (LAS) in 19 patients with cirrhosis and ascites. Patients were divided into two groups according to whether they developed renal insufficiency (II; 11 patients) or not (I; eight patients) after the administration of the drug. C_1 and C_2 represent two 30-min periods before the administration of LAS. LAS_1, LAS_2, and LAS_3 represent three 30-min periods after the administration of LAS. Values of plasma noradrenaline correspond to those of samples obtained before LAS injection (from Arroyo *et al.* 1983 with permission).

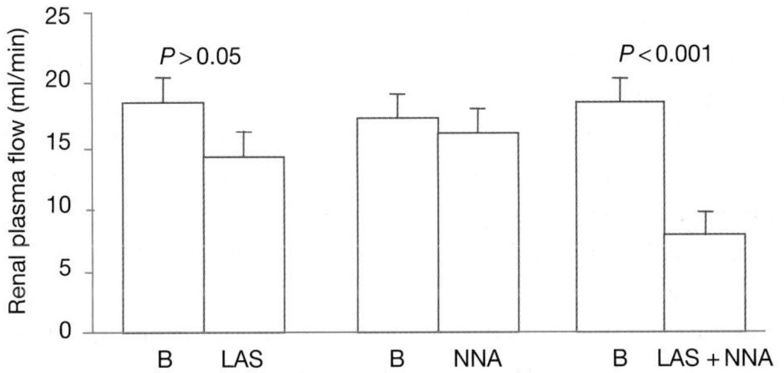

Fig. 2 Renal plasma flow in baseline conditions (B), following prostaglandin inhibition with LAS, following nitric oxide inhibition with L-nitro-arginine (NNA), and following the administration of both inhibitors in rats with cirrhosis and ascites (from Ros *et al.* 1995 with permission).

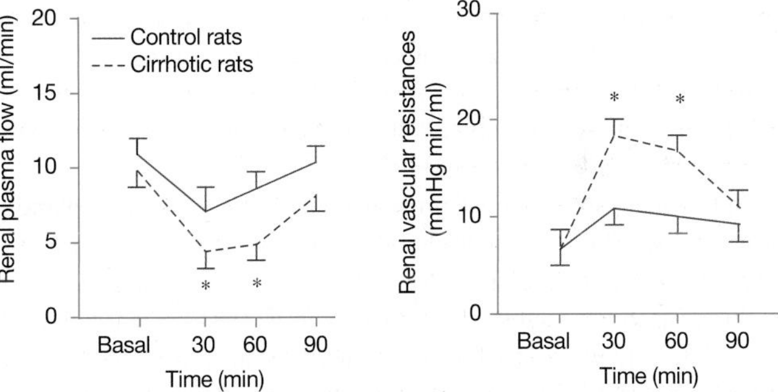

Fig. 3 Renal blood flow and renal vascular resistance in control (solid line) and cirrhotic rats with ascites (dotted line) under baseline conditions and at 30, 60, and 90 min after administration of a specific antagonist of endogenous natriuretic peptide receptors. Significance denoted in the figure are versus baseline values. $^*p < 0.05$ (from Angeli *et al.* 1994 with permission).

and peripheral vascular resistance do not differ from the previous phase (Bosch *et al.* 1980). Circulatory dysfunction, however, is greater at this stage of the disease since increased activity of the SNS and RAAS are required to maintain arterial pressure within normal limits.

Renal perfusion and GFR are normal or moderately decreased at this phase of intense sodium retention but are nonetheless critically dependent on an increased renal production of prostaglandins (Arroyo *et al.* 1986). These are vasodilators that antagonize the vasoconstrictor effect of angiotensin-II and norepinephrine. A syndrome indistinguishable from HRS can be produced in patients with cirrhosis, ascites and increased PRA following prostaglandin inhibition with NSAIDs (Fig. 1) (Boyer *et al.* 1979). The renal kallikrein–kinin system is also stimulated in decompensated cirrhosis (Pérez-Ayuso *et al.* 1984a,b) and seems to have an important role in the maintenance of renal haemodynamics.

Another factor that appears to be important in the maintenance of renal perfusion at this stage of the disease is nitric oxide (NO), a potent vasodilator (Angeli *et al.* 1994; Ros *et al.* 1995). While prostaglandin inhibition with NSAIDs in rats with ascites induces a moderate decrease in renal perfusion; NO inhibition does not affect renal haemodynamics and increases the renal production of prostacyclin. In contrast, simultaneous inhibition of both substances produces a profound decrease in renal blood blow (Fig. 2). Therefore, both prostacyclin and NO participate in the maintenance of renal perfusion in cirrhosis. Inhibition of one substance is partially or totally compensated for by the other and renal blood flow is maintained. Additionally, blockade of the vascular effect of natriuretic peptides reduces renal perfusion in normal rats and in rats with cirrhosis and ascites, but the impairment in renal haemodynamics is far more intense in the latter group (Fig. 3). Therefore, renal perfusion in advanced cirrhosis with ascites is maintained within normal or near normal limits by increased renal production of several vasodilator substances that antagonize the vasoconstrictor effect of RAAS and SNS, including prostaglandins, NO, and natriuretic peptides.

The renal ability to excrete free water is also impaired in patients with advanced cirrhosis (Arroyo *et al.* 1981; Arroyo and Jimenez 2000). Nonetheless, only a few show significant hyponatraemia (serum sodium concentration < 130 mEq/l). Water retention and dilutional hyponatraemia develop when renal water metabolism is severely impaired (free water clearance after water load < 1 ml/min; normal 6–12 ml/min). Impairment in free water clearance in cirrhosis is related to a non-osmotic hypersecretion of antidiuretic hormone (ADH) (Gines *et al.* 1998).

An increase in synthesis of prostaglandin E2 by the collecting tubules antagonizes the tubular effect of ADH and this explains why the renal ability to excrete free water is relatively preserved at this phase of the disease despite high plasma levels of this hormone.

Development of hepatorenal syndrome

This is the final phase of the disease. HRS is characterized by low arterial pressure, marked increase in plasma renin, norepinephrine, aldosterone, and ADH, and a low GFR (<40 ml/min) (Arroyo *et al.* 1996; Cardenas *et al.* 2000). Impairment in GFR in HRS is secondary to a dramatic reduction in renal perfusion secondary to renal vasoconstriction. Renal histology is normal. Since renal vascular resistance correlates closely with RAAS and SNS, HRS is likely to be related to extreme stimulation of these vasoconstrictor systems.

The plasma concentration of endothelin, a vasoconstrictor peptide of endothelial origin, is also increased in cirrhosis with ascites. Endothelin has also been proposed as a factor participating in the regulation of arterial pressure and a mechanism of HRS (Moore *et al.* 1992). However, several features in HRS do not support this contention: (a) arterial pressure in cirrhosis with ascites does not decrease following the administration of endothelin antagonists, (b) plasma endothelin concentrations are similar in patients with and without HRS, and (c) plasma endothelin does not change after volume expansion or following resolution of HRS.

The urinary excretion of prostaglandin E2, 6-keto prostaglandin F1α (a prostacyclin metabolite) and kallikrein is decreased in patients with HRS, which is compatible with a reduced renal production of these vasodilator substances (Arroyo *et al.* 1983). Renal failure in HRS could, therefore, be the consequence of an imbalance between the activity of the systemic vasoconstrictor systems and the renal production of vasodilators. Another possibility, however, is that renal vasoconstriction could be caused primarily by overactivation of RAAS and SNS along with the reduced synthesis of prostaglandins and kallikrein as a secondary event that would contribute to renal insufficiency.

Renal hypoperfusion in HRS could also be amplified by the stimulation of intrarenal vasoconstrictors. For example, renal ischaemia increases the intrarenal generation of angiotensin-II, endothelin, and adenosine, which are renal vasoconstrictors. Adenosine also potentiates the vascular effect of angiotensin-II. The observation that dipyridamole, an inhibitor of adenosine metabolism, impairs renal perfusion in patients with cirrhosis and ascites but not in normal subjects, indicates an increased sensitivity to intrarenal vasoconstrictors in decompensated cirrhosis (Llach *et al.* 1993). Other intrarenal substances with vasoconstrictor effect implicated in HRS include leukotrienes and F2-isoprostanes.

Given that the pathogenesis of renal vasoconstriction in HRS is multifactorial, it is unlikely that it may be improved by acting on one of the renal mechanisms. This has been attempted with RAAS inhibitors, as well as with α-adrenergic, endothelin, and adenosine antagonists, or prostaglandins (Arroyo *et al.* 1981, 1999; Esler *et al.* 1992). A more rational approach is to treat the initial events of the syndrome such as the circulatory dysfunction and portal hypertension.

Patients with HRS exhibit an extremely low urinary sodium excretion, an inability to excrete free water, and hyponatraemia. Sodium retention is due to decreased filtered sodium and increased sodium reabsorption in the proximal tubule. The amount of sodium reaching the loop of Henle and distal nephron, the site of action of frusemide and spironolactone, respectively, is very low. The delivery of frusemide and spironolactone to the renal tubules is also reduced because of renal hypoperfusion. It is, therefore, not surprising that patients with HRS respond poorly to diuretics.

Clinical aspects of hepatorenal syndrome

Assessment of renal function in cirrhosis

The first step in the diagnosis of HRS is the demonstration of a reduction in renal perfusion and GFR; however, this is a challenging task in advanced cirrhosis (Arroyo 2002). In patients without cirrhosis, serum creatinine concentration is only a rough estimate of GFR. There are, however, two important points that should be kept in mind when using creatinine as a measurement of renal function in patients with cirrhosis. First, serum creatinine should be measured several days after diuretic withdrawal because diuretics are associated with mild to moderate impairment in GFR. Second, serum creatinine is not a very sensitive marker of renal function in cirrhosis because patients with moderate or even marked reduction of GFR have normal or only slightly increased serum creatinine. The low serum creatinine is explained by a low endogenous production of creatinine resulting from poor nutritional status and decreased muscle mass. The relationship between inulin clearance and serum creatinine has been evaluated in a large series of patients with ascites. The concentration of serum creatinine with a greater sensitivity and specificity for the detection of a significantly reduced GFR (inulin clearance < 50 ml/min), as assessed by receptor-operated curves, was 105 μmol/l. Although creatinine clearance can be used to assess renal perfusion in cirrhosis, it may overestimate GFR because creatinine is secreted by the renal tubules and has the additional inconvenience of requiring a very accurate 24-h urine collection. Similarly blood urea nitrogen and serum urea are lower than expected because of reduced hepatic synthesis of urea and a low dietary protein intake (Arroyo *et al.* 2002).

Another method for assessing renal perfusion in cirrhosis is the measurement of the resistive index of the renal circulation by duplex Doppler ultrasonography. The resistive index is calculated from the Doppler waveform obtained from the arcuate or interlobar arteries and provides an estimate of renal vascular resistance. Using this technique, a significant proportion of cirrhotic patients with ascites and without HRS demonstrate increased renal vascular resistance compared to patients without ascites and normal subjects, thus confirming the presence of renal vasoconstriction long before the development of HRS (Platt *et al.* 1994). Furthermore, patients with increased renal resistive index but without renal failure have a greater risk of developing HRS than do patients with normal renal perfusion; this supports the concept that in cirrhosis with ascites there is a continuum of changes in renal perfusion, and that HRS is the end of this spectrum.

Diagnosis of hepatorenal syndrome

The diagnosis of HRS is based on the demonstration of a marked reduction in GFR and exclusion of other causes of renal failure. (Arroyo *et al.* 1996; Cardenas *et al.* 2000). The key elements of diagnosis are defining the reduction of GFR and how other potential causes of renal failure can be excluded. Table 1 shows the diagnostic criteria of HRS proposed by the International Ascites Club (Arroyo *et al.* 1996). The cut-off values of serum creatinine and creatinine clearance chosen to define HRS are 132 μmol/l and 40 ml/min, respectively. Cirrhotic patients with serum creatinine greater than 132 μmol/l have a GFR, as estimated by inulin clearance, of less than 30 ml/min. Nonetheless, this cut-off may underestimate the number of patients with severe renal failure because nearly 15 per cent of cirrhotic patients with serum creatinine between 88 and 132 μmol/l have inulin clearances less than 30 ml/min (Arroyo *et al.* 2002).

Several causes of renal failure, including prerenal failure secondary to volume depletion (due to gastrointestinal fluid losses or renal fluid losses because of aggressive diuretic therapy), glomerulonephritis, acute tubular necrosis, and drug-induced renal failure, should be excluded before making the diagnosis of HRS. To exclude the possibility of an unrecognized reduction in plasma volume, renal function should be evaluated after diuretic withdrawal (5 days) and a trial of volume repletion with 1.5 l of a synthetic plasma expander or saline. In contrast to prerenal azotaemia, HRS is not reversed by administration of fluids. Shock before the development of the impairment in renal function excludes the diagnosis of HRS, because in this setting, the most common cause of renal failure is acute tubular necrosis. Likewise, the diagnosis of HRS cannot be made in patients with current or recent treatment with nephrotoxic drugs such as NSAIDs and aminoglycosides. Since patients with ongoing bacterial infections, especially spontaneous bacterial peritonitis (SBP), may develop reversible impairment of renal function during the infection (Follo *et al.* 1994), the diagnosis of HRS can only be made after its resolution. Finally, significant proteinuria (<0.5 g/day) or ultrasonographic abnormalities of the kidney exclude the diagnosis of HRS and point towards the existence of an organic cause of renal failure. In these cases a renal biopsy should be considered.

Because HRS is a functional form of renal failure, the characteristics of the urine are those of prerenal azotaemia with oliguria. Patients exhibit a low urine sodium concentration and urine to plasma osmolality ratio greater than 1. These parameters are not currently considered essential for the diagnosis of HRS because they may overlap in different types of renal failure. For example, urine volume in patients with HRS is usually less than 500 ml/day; however, there are non-oliguric forms of the syndrome (Arroyo 2002). Urinary sodium concentration is usually less than 10 mmol/l in HRS, as opposed to acute tubular necrosis, in which urine sodium is generally greater than 20 mEq/l because of impairment in the tubular reabsorption of sodium. Nonetheless, there are several documented cases of well-established HRS with urine sodium concentration greater than 20 mEq/l (Dudley *et al.* 1986). Conversely, cirrhotic patients with ascites and acute tubular necrosis usually have low urinary sodium concentration (Cabrera *et al.* 1982). Moreover, acute tubular necrosis may spontaneously develop in patients with HRS due to prolonged renal ischaemia (Mandal *et al.* 1982). The urine to plasma osmolality is greater than 1 in cirrhotic patients with HRS but also in patients with acute tubular necrosis (Cabrera *et al.* 1982). For all these reasons, the urinary indices are not currently considered important in the differential diagnosis of renal failure in cirrhosis.

Clinical types of hepatorenal syndrome

HRS is classified into two types according to the intensity and form of presentation of renal failure (Fig. 4) (Arroyo *et al.* 1996). Type-1 HRS is characterized by severe and rapidly progressive renal failure, defined as doubling of serum creatinine reaching a concentration greater than 220 μmol/l in less than 2 weeks. Although type-1 HRS may arise spontaneously, it frequently occurs in close relationship with precipitating factors such as severe bacterial infections, major surgical procedures, or acute alcoholic hepatitis superimposed on cirrhosis. The association of HRS and SBP is well documented (Follo *et al.* 1994; Navasa *et al.* 1998). Type-1 HRS develops in approximately 30 per cent of cases with SBP despite a rapid resolution of the infection with antibiotics. Patients with intense inflammatory response and high cytokine levels in plasma and ascitic fluid are more prone to develop type-1 HRS during or immediately after SBP (Navasa *et al.* 1998). Besides renal failure, patients with type-1 HRS after SBP develop liver failure (jaundice, coagulopathy, and hepatic encephalopathy) and circulatory dysfunction (arterial hypotension and very high plasma renin and norepinephrine). Type-1 HRS has a very poor prognosis with a median survival time after the onset of only 2 weeks (Fig. 5) (Ginès *et al.* 1993a).

Table 1 Diagnostic criteria of hepatorenal syndrome

Major criteria[a]

1. Low glomerular filtration rate, as indicated by serum creatinine greater than 132 μmol/l (1.5 mg/dl) or 24-h creatinine clearance lower than 40 ml/min
2. Absence of shock, ongoing bacterial infection, fluid losses and current treatment with nephrotoxic drugs
3. No sustained improvement in renal function (decrease in serum creatinine to 1.5 mg/dl or less or increase in creatinine clearance to 40 ml/min or more) following diuretic withdrawal and expansion of plasma volume with 1.5 l of a plasma expander
4. Proteinuria lower than 500 mg/day and no ultrasonographic evidence of obstructive uropathy or parenchymal renal disease

Additional criteria

1. Urine volume lower than 500 ml/day
2. Urine sodium lower than 10 mEq/l
3. Urine osmolality greater than plasma osmolality
4. Urine red blood cells less than 50 per high power field
5. Serum sodium concentration lower than 130 mEq/l

[a] Only major criteria are necessary for the diagnosis of hepatorenal syndrome.

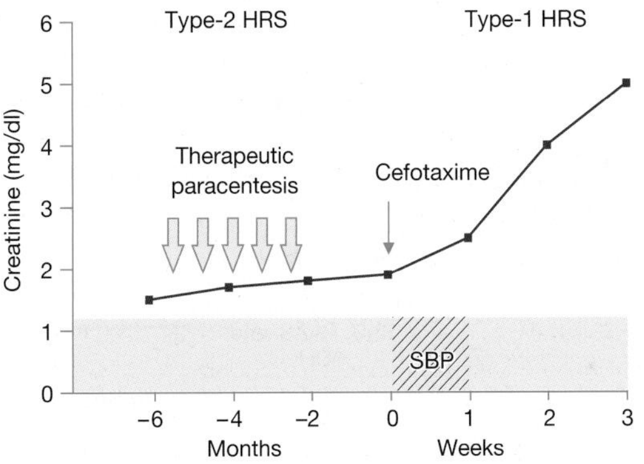

Fig. 4 Course of renal function in a cirrhotic patient admitted to hospital for the treatment of an episode of tense ascites. The patient had type-2 HRS and refractory ascites. He was treated with repeated therapeutic paracentesis. In the follow-up the patient developed signs of SBP and was treated with cefotaxime. Despite resolution of SBP a rapid deterioration of renal function (type-1 HRS) developed. The patient died 3 weeks after infection diagnosis (from Arroyo *et al.* 2002 with permission).

Type-2 HRS is characterized by a moderate and steady decrease in renal function (serum creatinine < 220 μmol/l). Patients display signs of liver failure and arterial hypotension but to a lesser degree than those with type-1 HRS. The dominant clinical feature is tense ascites with poor or no response to diuretics (refractory ascites). Patients with type-2 HRS are particularly predisposed to develop type-1 HRS either spontaneously or following infections or other precipitating events. Median survival with type-2 HRS is near 6 months, which is worse than that of cirrhotic patients with ascites without HRS (2 years).

Although the pathogenesis of both types of HRS has traditionally involved one unifying mechanism, this is probably not the case. Whereas type-2 HRS is mainly due to the deterioration of circulatory function of cirrhosis, type-1 HRS is probably related to an imbalance of intrarenal vasoactive mechanisms (Fig. 6). Renal failure is moderate and stable in type-2 HRS probably because an increased intrarenal synthesis of vasodilators diminishes the effects of systemic and intrarenal vasoconstrictors. In contrast, the rapid deterioration of renal function in type-1 HRS suggests a progressive reduction in the intrarenal synthesis of vasodilators, an increase in the intrarenal production of vasoconstrictors, or both features. An aggravation of the circulatory and renal dysfunction promoted by a precipitating factor (i.e. SBP) could trigger these intrarenal mechanisms. Type-1 HRS, could be related to the development of an intrarenal vicious circle in which hypoperfusion leads to an imbalance in intrarenal vasoactive systems, which in turn causes more vasoconstriction (Arroyo *et al.* 2002). The demonstration of a temporal dissociation between the improvement in circulatory function and increase in renal perfusion and GFR in patients with type-1 HRS treated with albumin infusion and vasoconstrictors is in keeping with this concept (Guevara *et al.* 1998a). This therapeutic approach normalizes PRA and norepinephrine concentration within 3 days. In contrast, a significant increase in renal perfusion and GFR do not occur until 1 week later. A delay in the deactivation of intrarenal mechanisms may account for this finding.

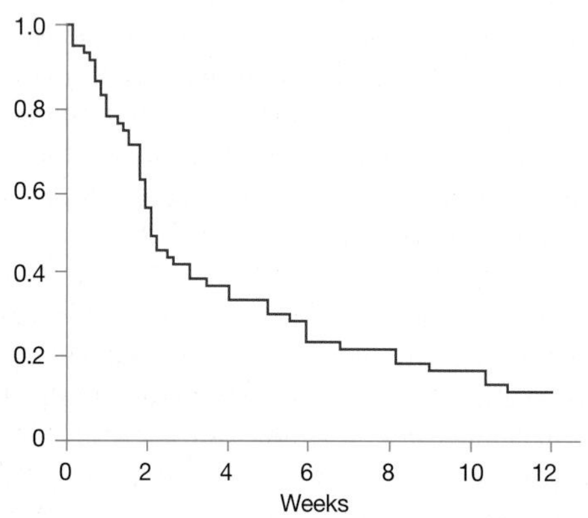

Fig. 5 Probability of survival of patients with severe HRS (from Ginès *et al.* 1993a with permission).

Treatment of hepatorenal syndrome

Over the last 20 years several vasoactive drugs (dopamine, fenoldopan, prostaglandins, misoprostol, saralasin, phentolamine, dazoxiben, norepinephrine, metaraminol, and octapressin) have been assessed as therapeutic agents for HRS (Arroyo 1999). Unfortunately, none of these produced any significant improvement in renal function. HRS was, therefore, considered an intractable terminal event of cirrhosis and there was a decreased enthusiasm for treating patients. However, in these studies, drugs were given only for a few hours or days, which is now known to be insufficient to reverse HRS. For example, some patients with HRS following a portacaval shunt placement or liver transplantation recover renal function from 1 week to 1 month after surgery (Arroyo *et al.* 1999).

With the introduction of the Le Veen shunt in 1974 (Le Veen *et al.* 1974) for the treatment of ascites and HRS there was even less enthusiasm for pursuing pharmacological treatments for HRS. For many years this was considered the effective therapy for refractory ascites and HRS based on descriptions of isolated clinical cases or small series of patients. However, several years later it was demonstrated that this

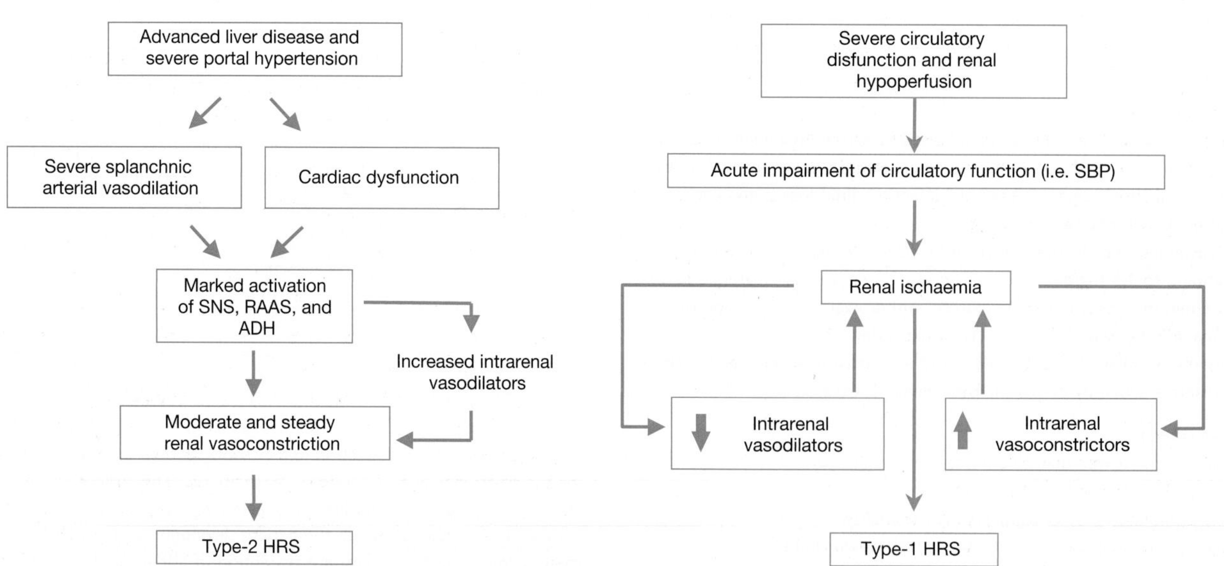

Fig. 6 Possible mechanisms of type-1 (right) and type-2 (left) HRS (from Arroyo *et al.* 2002 with permission).

shunt was actually ineffective in treating type-1 HRS (Linas *et al.* 1986). Moreover, in type-2 HRS with refractory ascites, the shunt was also shown not to be superior to therapeutic paracentesis and plasma expansion (Ginès *et al.* 1991). Moreover, Le Veen shunts are associated with severe complications such as superior vena cava thrombosis, intestinal obstruction and a high rate of obstruction requiring reoperation. These complications along with better pharmacological therapies have led to the abandonment of its use.

The concept that the majority of patients with HRS have advanced liver failure and that any improvement in renal function would have little impact on survival, also contributed to the lack of enthusiasm for attempting to improve the renal failure in these patients. However, the wider availability of liver transplantation and, particularly, the introduction of living donor transplantation for adults have changed matters. Even a small increase in early survival may allow patients to reach a transplant and increase the 10-year probability of long-term survival to near 60 per cent. This, together with a better understanding of the pathogenesis of the syndrome, has stimulated clinical investigators to assess new treatments of HRS.

Liver transplantation

Liver transplantation is the treatment of choice for patients with HRS as it offers a cure of both the hepatic failure and the circulatory and renal dysfunction (Gonwa *et al.* 1991, 1995). Immediately after transplantation, further impairment in GFR may be observed and up to 35 per cent of patients require renal support as compared with 5 per cent of patients without HRS. Because cyclosporin and tacrolimus may contribute to impairment in renal function, other drugs such as azathioprine, corticosteroids, IL-2 receptor antagonists, or anti-lymphocyte agents should be used in preference until diuresis and improvement of renal function is observed. This usually takes 48–72 h. After this initial impairment in renal function, GFR starts to improve and reaches an average of 30–40 ml/min by 1–2 months after surgery. This moderate renal failure persists during follow-up, is more marked than that observed in transplanted patients without HRS, and is probably due to the greater nephrotoxicity of cyclosporin or tacrolimus in patients with renal impairment prior to transplantation. The haemodynamic and neurohormonal abnormalities associated with HRS disappear within the first month after the operation and the majority of patients regain a normal capacity to excrete sodium and free water (Navasa *et al.* 1993).

Patients with HRS who undergo transplantation have more complications, spend more days in the intensive care unit, and have a higher in-hospital mortality rate than transplantation patients without HRS. However, the long-term survival of patients with HRS who undergo liver transplantation is good, with a 3-year probability of survival of 60 per cent (Gonwa *et al.* 1995). This survival rate is only slightly lower than that of transplantation in patients without HRS (which ranges between 70 per cent and 80 per cent).

Vasoconstrictors and plasma expansion

The use of systemic vasoconstrictors with plasma expansion seems to be the most promising approach to therapy now that several studies confirm their beneficial role in HRS. Although using vasoconstrictors in a condition characterized by renal vasoconstriction seems paradoxical, the rationale is based on the fact that the initial event in the pathogenesis of HRS is an arterial splanchnic vasodilation causing activation of endogenous vasoconstrictors. Agonists of the vasopressin V1 receptors (ornipressin and terlipressin), catecholamines, and somatostatin analogues have a predominant action on the splanchnic vessels, with little effect on the renal circulation and have been widely used in the treatment of HRS.

Initial reports more than a decade ago indicated that the short-term intravenous (IV) infusion of ornipressin in patients with HRS led to an increase in total peripheral vascular resistance, a reduction in cardiac output, marked suppression of the RAAS and SNS, and a modest but significant increase in creatinine clearance (Lenz *et al.* 1991). Based on this study and previously obtained data suggesting that volume expansion and vasoconstrictors were effective in normalizing renal sodium and water metabolism in cirrhotic patients with ascites, another study assessed the haemodynamic, neurohormonal, and renal effects of the combination of ornipressin with albumin in 16 patients with HRS (Guevara *et al.* 1998a). Eight were treated for 3 days (albumin was given at a dose of 1 g/kg on the first day and 20–60 g/day for the next 2 days; ornipressin was given IV in a stepped dose infusion of 2–6 IU/h). This short course reversed the overactivity of the RAAS and SNS. However, only a slight improvement in GFR was observed (Fig. 7). The prolonged treatment (ornipressin at 2 IU/h) for 15 days in the other eight patients resulted in a remarkable improvement in renal function, with normalization of serum creatinine, a marked increase in renal plasma flow and GFR, and suppression of the activity of vasoconstrictor systems. Albumin was given at a dose of 1 g/kg during the first day and the amount of albumin administered in the following days was adjusted according to PRA. Interestingly, in those patients in whom creatinine normalized, HRS did not recur after discontinuation of therapy. Unfortunately, in four patients treatment was stopped after 4 and 9 days due to ischaemic complications. In a subsequent study, nine patients with HRS (six with type-1 and three with type-2 HRS) were treated with terlipressin (0.5–2 mg/4 h IV) and IV albumin for 5–15 days (Uriz *et al.* 2000). Reversal of HRS was observed in seven patients (Fig. 8). There were no ischaemic complications and HRS did not recur. Five patients were candidates for liver transplantation; three were transplanted 5, 12, and 99 days after treatment, the two other patients died 30 and 121 days after starting therapy. In both studies dilutional hyponatraemia was corrected with the normalization of serum creatinine. The combined results of both studies in the 17 patients treated with ornipressin and terlipressin and IV albumin for more than 3 days are summarized in Table 2.

Other groups have also confirmed these findings. In one study of seven patients with type-1 HRS treated with ornipressin (6 IU/h), dopamine (2–3 μg/g/min), and IV albumin, HRS was reversed in four patients after 5–27 days of treatment (Gülberg *et al.* 1999). Another report of 12 patients with type-1 HRS treated with terlipressin (2 mg every 8–12 h) and albumin infusion (0.5–1 g/kg day for 5 days) demonstrated reversal of HRS in seven patients (Mulkay *et al.* 2001). In the remaining five cases, serum creatinine decreased but not to normal levels. In six patients, HRS did not recur after stopping treatment. No patient developed complications related to the treatment. Finally, a large retrospective and multicentre study reported the use of terlipressin (3.2 ± 1.3 mg/day) for 11–12 days in 99 patients with type-1 HRS (Moreau *et al.* 2002). Most patients received albumin. In this study 64 per cent of patients showed improved renal function during therapy, whereas 38 per cent did not. Thirteen patients underwent liver transplantation between 22 and 371 days after starting therapy. The median survival time was 3 weeks with survival of 60 per cent at

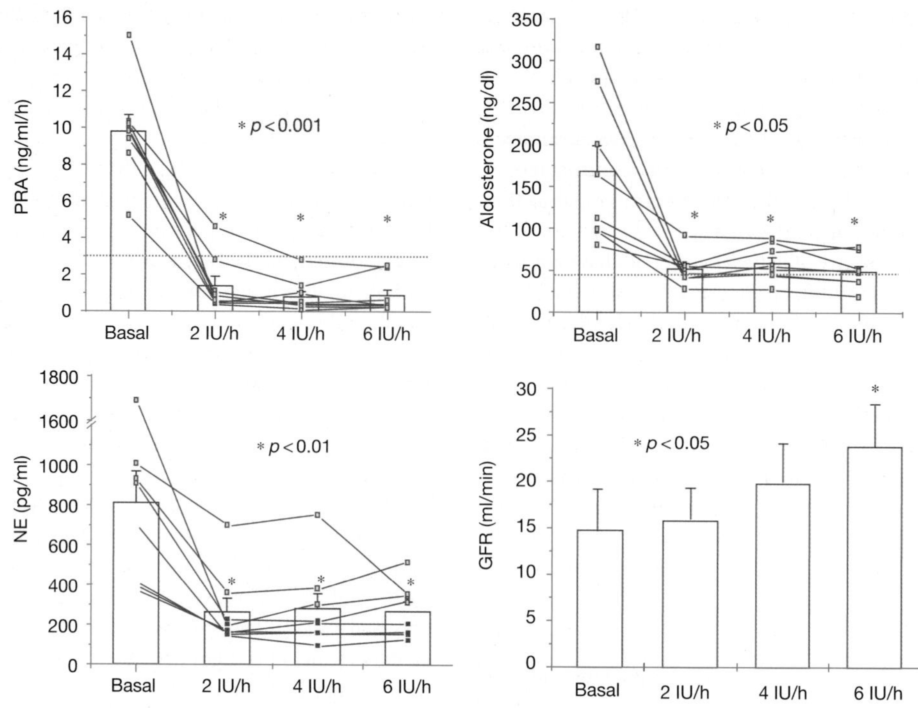

Fig. 7 Changes in plasma renin activity (PRA), plasma aldosterone and norepinephrine (NE) concentration, and GFR (inulin clearance) in patients with HRS treated with ornipressin (2 IU/h the first day, 4 IU/h the second day, and 6 IU/h the third day) plus IV albumin infusion. There was a marked suppression of the neurohormonal systems without clinically significant increase in GFR (from Guevara *et al.* 1998a with permission).

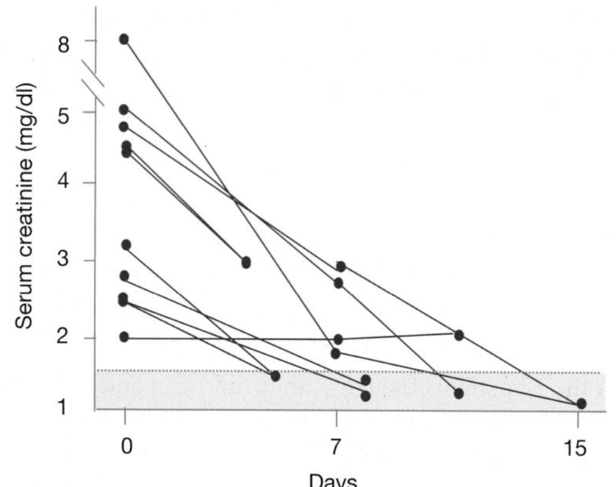

Fig. 8 Evolution of serum creatinine in patients with HRS treated by terlipressin (0.5–2 mg/4 h) and IV albumin infusion (from Uriz *et al.* 2000 with permission).

Table 2 Effect of vasoconstrictors (ornipressin and terlipressin) with volume expansion in hepatorenal syndrome

	Baseline (n = 15)	Day 3 (n = 12)	Day 7 (n = 9)	Day 14 (n = 7)
MAP (mmHg)	70 ± 8	70 ± 8	77 ± 9	79 ± 12
PRA (ng/ml/h)	15 ± 15	4 ± 2	2 ± 3	1 ± 1
NE (pg/ml)	1257 ± 938	550 ± 382	550 ± 410	316 ± 161
Creatinine (mg/dl)	3 ± 1	3 ± 1	2 ± 1	1 ± 1

Results are given as mean ± SD.

Normal values: PRA < 1.4 ng/ml/h; NE < 260 pg/ml; $p < 0.001$ for all values (analysis of variance).

MAP, mean arterial pressure; NE, norepinephrine; PRA, plasma renin activity.

Data from Guevara *et al.* (1998a) and Uriz *et al.* (2000).

2 weeks, 40 per cent at 4 weeks, 28 per cent at 8 weeks, and 19 per cent at 52 weeks. There were no significant ischaemic side effects from the therapy.

Catecholamines also seem to be an effective treatment for HRS. The use of oral midodrine (an α-adrenergic agonist), IV albumin, and subcutaneous octreotride (a somatostatin analogue) was reported in five patients with type-1 HRS (Angeli *et al.* 1999). Midodrine dosage was adjusted to increase the mean arterial pressure by 15 mmHg or more. Patients received this combination for at least 20 days initially in the hospital and then at home. In all cases there was a dramatic improvement in renal perfusion, GFR, blood urea nitrogen, serum creatinine and serum sodium concentration with suppression of PRA, aldosterone and ADH to normal or near normal levels. Two patients were transplanted 20 and 64 days after starting and while on therapy. One patient who was not a candidate for liver transplant also was alive without treatment 472 days after being discharged from the hospital. These results were compared with those obtained in eight patients with type-1 HRS treated with IV albumin plus dopamine. In all eight, a progressive deterioration in renal function was observed. Another study of 12 patients with type-1 HRS treated with IV albumin (to maintain central venous pressure over 7 mmHg) and noradrenaline (0.5–3 mg/h) for a minimum of 5 days showed significant improvement in serum creatinine in association with a marked suppression of PRA in 10 patients (Duvoux *et al.* 2002). Transient myocardial ischaemia was observed in one patient. Three patients were transplanted and three were still alive after 8 months of follow-up.

Whether albumin is necessary in the treatment of HRS with vasoconstrictors was also studied in a group of 21 patients with HRS (Ortega *et al.* 2002). The first 13 patients were treated with terlipressin (0.5–2 g/4 h) and albumin and the remaining eight received terlipressin alone. Treatment was given until normalization of serum creatinine or for a maximum of 15 days. In patients treated with terlipressin plus albumin there was a significant increase in mean arterial pressure, a marked suppression of PRA, and a decrease in serum creatinine. In contrast, no significant changes in these parameters were observed in those treated with terlipressin alone. A complete response (normalization of serum creatinine) was achieved in 10 patients treated with terlipressin plus albumin and in only two treated without albumin. Recurrence of HRS only occurred in two patients. One-month survival without transplantation was 87 per cent in those receiving terlipressin plus albumin and 13 per cent in those receiving terlipressin alone.

Several conclusions can be reached from these studies. The first is that type-1 HRS is reversible following treatment with IV albumin and splanchnic vasoconstrictors and does not recur following discontinuation of therapy. The second is that the combined use of albumin and vasoconstrictors is of pivotal importance since HRS does not reverse when vasoconstrictors or plasma volume expansion are given alone. The third is the observation that the continuous infusion of vasoconstrictors like ornipressin is associated with ischaemic complications, a feature not observed when they are given intermittently. The fourth is that there is a delay of several days between the improvement in circulatory function and the increase in GFR. Finally, reversal of HRS improves survival and a significant number of patients may survive to allow successful liver transplantation. The recommended doses and duration of vasoconstrictor therapy are summarized in Table 3.

Table 3 Recommendations for using vasoconstrictors in hepatorenal syndrome

1. Duration of therapy should be anywhere between 5 and 15 days, because improvement of renal function usually occurs slowly
2. Therapy should be aimed at reducing serum creatinine below 1.5 mg/dl
3. The recommended doses are:
   A. Terlipressin 0.5 mg intravenously every 4 h; with an increase of the dose in a stepwise fashion (i.e. every 2–3 days) to 1 mg/4 h and then up to 2 mg/4 h in cases showing no response to therapy
   B. Midodrine 7.5 mg orally three times daily with an increase to 12.5 mg three times daily if needed and octreotide 100 μg subcutaneously three times daily with an increase to 200 μg three times daily if needed
   C. Noradrenaline 0.5–3 mg/h continuous intravenous infusion
4. Concomitant intravenous albumin infusion (1 g/kg on the first day, followed by 20–40 g/day) should be administered to all patients
5. These drugs should be avoided in patients with cardiac diseases, peripheral vascular disease, and/or cerebrovascular disease, due to a likely high risk of ischaemic events

Transjugular intrahepatic portacaval shunt

Since portal hypertension is the initial event of circulatory dysfunction in cirrhosis, decrease of portal pressure by portacaval anastomosis is a rational approach for the treatment of HRS. There are several case reports showing reversal of HRS following a portacaval shunt. However, the applicability of major surgical procedures in patients with HRS carries a great risk as the majority of patients have advanced liver disease. Transjugular intrahepatic portacaval shunt (TIPS), a non-surgical method of portal decompression that acts as a side-to-side portacaval shunt, by reducing portal pressure improves sodium excretion, ascites volume, and renal function in patients with HRS. The development of TIPS has reintroduced the idea of treating HRS by reducing portal pressure.

There are four studies assessing TIPS in the management of type-1 HRS (Ochs *et al.* 1994; Alam *et al.* 1995; Guevara *et al.* 1998b; Brensing *et al.* 2000). In total, 30 patients were treated. In two series, liver transplantation was not performed. In the other two, three out of nine patients were transplanted 7, 13, and 35 days after TIPS. TIPS insertion was technically successful in all patients. Only one patient died as a consequence of the procedure. GFR improved markedly within 1–4 weeks after TIPS and stabilized thereafter. In one study, improvement in GFR and serum creatinine was related to a marked suppression of plasma renin and ADH (Guevara *et al.* 1998b). The suppression of plasma norepinephrine was lower than that of renin, a feature also observed in refractory ascites treated by TIPS. Follow-up data including hepatic function were obtained from 21 patients. *De novo* hepatic encephalopathy or deterioration of pre-existing hepatic encephalopathy occurred in nine patients. Survival rates from the 27 patients without early liver transplantation at 1, 3, and 6 months were 81, 59, and 44 per cent, respectively. These studies suggest that TIPS is useful in the management of type-1 HRS. Studies comparing TIPS with pharmacological treatment, as well as combination therapy in type-1 HRS are, therefore, needed.

Other therapeutic methods

Haemodialysis and haemofiltration are frequently used in patients with HRS, but their efficacy has not been adequately assessed (Pérez *et al.* 1996). The beneficial effect of an extracorporeal albumin dialysis system (MARS), which consists of a modified dialysis method that enables the selective removal of albumin bound substances that accumulate in liver failure, using an albumin containing dialysate was reported in patients with HRS (Mitzner *et al.* 2000). Although promising, these results require further evaluation to assess dialysis as a treatment, but more importantly as a bridge to liver transplantation.

Prevention of HRS

Two randomized controlled studies have shown that HRS can be prevented in two specific clinical settings. In patients with cirrhosis and SBP, the administration of albumin (1.5 g/kg IV at infection diagnosis and 1 g/kg IV 48 h later) together with cefotaxime markedly reduced the incidence of impairment in circulatory function and development of type-1 HRS as compared to a control group of patients receiving cefotaxime alone (10 per cent incidence of HRS in patients receiving albumin versus 33 per cent in the control group) (Sort *et al.* 1999). Moreover, the hospital mortality rate (10 versus 29 per cent) and the 3-month mortality rate (22 versus 41 per cent) were lower in patients receiving albumin. In patients with severe alcoholic hepatitis the administration of the tumour necrosis factor inhibitor, oral pentoxyfilline (400 mg t.i.d.), reduced the occurrence of HRS (8 per cent in the pentoxyfilline group versus 35 per cent in the placebo group) and hospital mortality (24 versus 46 per cent, respectively) (Akriviadis *et al.* 2000). Since bacterial infections and acute alcoholic hepatitis are two important precipitating factors of type-1 HRS, these prophylactic measures may decrease the incidence of this complication.

Drug-induced renal failure in cirrhosis

Diuretics

The use of diuretics in patients with cirrhosis and ascites carries the risk of significant side-effects such as electrolyte imbalance and volume depletion. Approximately 20 per cent of patients using diuretics (frusemide and spironolactone) may develop azotaemia due to depletion of the intravascular volume (Rodés *et al.* 1975). Diuretic-induced renal failure is usually moderate and always reversible after diuretic withdrawal. It is the consequence of an imbalance between the intravascular fluid loss caused by the diuretics and the net passage of fluid (ascites reabsorption minus ascites formation) from the peritoneal cavity into the general circulation (Shear *et al.* 1970).

Reabsorption of ascites occurs through a rich plexus of terminal lymphatics (lymphatic lacunae) on the under-surface of the diaphragm (Leak and Rahill 1978). They open directly into the peritoneal cavity by intercellular gaps and stomas. The periodic respiratory movements of the diaphragm are important in the passage of ascites into the lymphatic system and the general circulation. During inspiration, intercellular gaps and stomata close, intraperitoneal pressure is increased, and lacunae are emptied through the combined effect of local compression, and increased intra-abdominal and reduced intrathoracic pressures. During expiration, the gaps and stomas are opened and free communication is re-established (Yoffey and Courtice 1970).

Reabsorption of ascites is a rate-limited phenomenon. The average fractional reabsorption rate of radiolabelled albumin from the peritoneal cavity into the general circulation in cirrhotics with ascites has been estimated as 1.27 per cent of the intraperitoneal protein mass per hour, corresponding to a rate of ascitic fluid reabsorption of 1.4 l in 24 h (Henriksen *et al.* 1980). The rate of reabsorption of ascitic fluid varies markedly from patient to patient and may range from 0.5 to 5.5 l in 24 h (Henriksen *et al.* 1980). Although the rate of ascites formation has not been measured, these data indicate that the net passage of fluid into the intravascular compartment is very low in many patients with cirrhosis and ascites.

Patients with ascites respond well to an initial regimen of frusemide 40 mg/day and spironolactone 100 mg/day. If there is no response, diuretics may be increased in a stepwise fashion every 5 days, spironolactone up to 400 mg/day and frusemide up to 160 mg/day. Higher doses will not increase the rate of response. The goal of the treatment is to achieve a weight loss of 300–500 g/day. If diuretic therapy produces a loss of fluid greater than the net passage of ascitic fluid into the intravascular compartment, a contraction of the circulating blood volume and a concomitant decrease of GFR will occur. Interstitial fluid accumulated as oedema is more easily reabsorbed than ascites. This explains why diuretic-induced renal failure occurs less frequently in patients with both ascites and oedema than in those having only ascites (Shear *et al.* 1970).

Antibiotics

Patients with cirrhosis and ascites are at risk of developing aminoglycoside nephrotoxicity. The reported incidence is near 33 per cent, which is much higher than that found in the general patient population, which is between 3 and 11 per cent (Cabrera *et al.* 1982). Aminoglycoside nephrotoxicity in cirrhosis can lead to severe acute renal failure. Advanced liver disease and HRS are important predictive factors for the development of aminoglycoside nephrotoxicity in cirrhosis, with an incidence five times that of patients with normal pretreatment serum creatinine concentration. The diagnosis of aminoglycoside nephrotoxicity in cirrhosis with ascites and bacterial infections is challenging because these patients are at risk of developing HRS. The measurement of urinary sodium concentration, fractional sodium excretion and urine to plasma osmolality and creatinine ratios are not useful in the differentiation of HRS from acute renal failure due to aminoglycoside nephrotoxicity (Cabrera *et al.* 1982; Dudley *et al.* 1986). In contrast, the measurement of other urinary markers of tubular damage, such as β2-microglobulin and tubular enzymes, may be helpful. However, in patients with severe cholestasis or liver failure (serum bilirubin > 340 μmol/l) and marked renal dysfunction these markers are not useful (Gatta *et al.* 1981; Cabrera *et al.* 1982). Therefore, aminoglycosides should be avoided in all patients with cirrhosis and ascites.

Non-steroidal anti-inflammatory agents

Initial reports showing that patients with cirrhosis and ascites develop renal failure after cyclo-oxygenase inhibition with NSAIDs were published 20 years ago by three different groups of investigators. The first group (Boyer *et al.* 1979) showed that the oral administration of indomethacin (50 mg every 6 h for a total of four doses) produced a significant reduction of renal plasma flow and GFR in a large series of cirrhotics with ascites, but not in patients without ascites. The second group (Zipser *et al.* 1979) gave indomethacin (200 mg for 1 day) or ibuprofen (2 g for 1 day) to 12 cirrhotics with ascites and to eight normal individuals; both drugs induced a marked decrease of creatinine clearance in all cirrhotic patients whereas no change was observed in the healthy controls. The third group (Arroyo *et al.* 1983) gave an IV bolus of 450 mg lysine acetylsalicylate (equivalent to 250 mg acetylsalicylic acid) to five normal individuals, nine cirrhotics without ascites, and 19 cirrhotics with ascites. This dose did not alter renal function in normal individuals and cirrhotics without ascites, but it did reduce GFR in 11 of the 19 patients with ascites. In these three studies the degree of impairment of renal function after drug administration correlated with baseline values of urine sodium excretion and plasma renin and norepinephrine. Patients with lower sodium excretion and higher PRA and norepinephrine concentration developed greater reductions of renal plasma flow and GFR. These studies demonstrate that cirrhotics with increased activity of the RASS and SNS and marked sodium retention are particularly predisposed to develop renal failure after cyclo-oxygenase inhibition. These effects have been confirmed by other authors for indomethacin, naproxen, lysine acetylsalicylate, and sulindac. NSAIDs should, therefore, be avoided in patients with cirrhosis.

In a recent but preliminary report (Guevara *et al.* 2001), the use of the new selective inhibitors of cyclo-oxygenase-2 in patients with cirrhosis and ascites was shown not to be associated with a major derangement of renal function.

Drugs used in portal hypertension

Propranolol, the drug most extensively used to prevent variceal bleeding and rebleeding has no significant effect on renal function in patients with ascites (Rector and Reynolds 1984). The acute and chronic administration of isosorbide 5-mononitrate alone, which is also used for the primary and secondary prevention of variceal bleeding, impairs renal function in patients with cirrhosis and ascites (Salmerón *et al.* 1993). The effect of the combination of propranolol and nitrates on renal function, however, is more controversial. Some studies have shown an impairment in renal function (Vorobioff *et al.* 1993), whereas others have not (Morillas *et al.* 1994; Merkel *et al.* 1995).

Reports on the renal effects of somatostatin, a drug used for the treatment of acute variceal bleeding, are conflicting. One study showed a significant decrease in GFR, sodium excretion, and free water clearance during the acute infusion of somatostatin (Ginès *et al.* 1992), but another showed an increase in urine volume and creatinine clearance in patients with ascites who received octreotide (its synthetic analogue) (Mountokalakis *et al.* 1998). Moreover, the long-acting release form of octreotide failed to show any change in creatinine clearance or sodium excretion in cirrhotic patients with ascites (Ottesen *et al.* 2001).

Prazosin, an α-adrenergic blocker, and the new angiotensin-II receptor antagonists (losartan, irbesartan) are other drugs which have been investigated as possible treatments for portal hypertension. They reduce portal pressure by decreasing intrahepatic vascular resistance. Long-term administration of prazosin to patients with compensated cirrhosis caused vasodilation of the systemic circulation and arterial hypotension, which led to ascites formation in a significant number of patients (Albillos *et al.* 1995). These effects were not observed when prazosin was given in combination with propranolol (Albillos *et al.* 1998). In patients with ascites, angiotensin-II receptor antagonists may induce a marked decrease in arterial pressure and renal failure (Gonzales-Abraldes *et al.* 2001; Schepke *et al.* 2001).

In summary, drugs that produce arterial vasodilation (nitrates and α-adrenergic and angiotensin-II antagonists) should be given with caution to patients with cirrhosis and portal hypertension because they may impair renal function.

Renal failure in acute liver failure

The term acute liver failure is used to describe the condition in which patients develop hepatic encephalopathy less than 12 weeks after the onset of jaundice in the absence of underlying chronic liver disease. Three different subtypes of acute liver failure have been proposed by the King's College Hospital group (O'Grady *et al.* 1993): hyperacute liver failure defines those patients developing hepatic encephalopathy within 8 days, acute liver failure describes those who develop encephalopathy within 9–28 days, and subacute liver failure describes those with a development period of 4–12 weeks. Viral hepatitis is the leading cause of acute liver failure followed by drugs, toxins or chemicals (i.e. paracetamol, isoniazid, and mushroom poisoning), metabolic diseases (Wilson's disease, Reye's syndrome, and acute fatty liver of pregnancy), and cardiovascular diseases (shock liver and acute Budd–Chiari syndrome). Acute liver failure is characterized by a rapid deterioration of hepatic function, multiorgan involvement (hepatic encephalopathy, cerebral oedema, cardiovascular dysfunction, pulmonary dysfunction, renal failure, coagulopathy, pancreatitis, adrenal dysfunction), and death. Emergency liver transplantation is the treatment of choice and has postoperative survival rate of approximately 65 per cent.

Renal dysfunction is a common event in acute liver failure. The first renal function abnormalities are sodium retention and impaired free water clearance which develop in association with changes in circulatory function and compensatory stimulation of the RASS, SNS, and ADH. Subsequently, patients may develop severe renal vasoconstriction and functional renal failure. Within a few days, when renal perfusion pressure is critically reduced acute tubular necrosis may ensue. The reported prevalence of renal failure in acute liver failure is approximately 55 per cent. Renal dysfunction in the setting of acute liver failure has a similar course to that of established cirrhosis with ascites. Nonetheless, the difference is that in acute liver failure the interval between normal renal function and severe functional renal failure and/or acute tubular necrosis is a matter of days, whereas in cirrhosis with ascites it develops over months. There seems to be a higher incidence of acute tubular necrosis in acute liver failure than in cirrhosis, possibly a consequence of a more severe deterioration in circulatory function. In acute liver failure, approximately half of patients with functional renal failure progress to acute tubular necrosis. Finally, type-1 HRS is more common in patients developing acute liver failure (Ellis and O'Grady 1999).

There is a greater and earlier incidence of renal failure in patients with paracetamol hepatotoxicity than in those with other causes of acute liver failure (Ellis and O'Grady 1999). It may even occur in the absence of significant liver damage or precede other clinical manifestations of liver failure (Moore 1999), suggesting that direct paracetamol renal toxicity is an additional mechanism of injury. There are other drugs and toxins which may cause simultaneous injury to both the liver and the kidneys, that is carbon tetrachloride, chloroform, halogenated anaesthetics, sulfonamides, rifampicin, or interstitial nephritis that is phenytoin, sulfonamides, allopurinol, and penicillins. Predictors of an increased risk of renal failure in acute liver failure are paracetamol overdose, viral hepatitis, fungemia and sepsis, and stage-4 hepatic encephalopathy (Moore 1999).

Because patients with acute liver failure present with a hyperdynamic circulation due to peripheral arterial vasodilation, arterial pressure is maintained by an increase in cardiac output and stimulation of the RAAS and SNS. In patients with acute liver failure there is portal hypertension but to a lesser degree than in cirrhosis. Severe arterial hypotension is a prominent feature in patients with acute liver failure and renal failure and develops when the cardiac output is unable to increase and compensate the fall in peripheral vascular resistance. Endotoxin and NO have been implicated in the pathogenesis of the arterial vasodilation in acute liver failure.

In addition to RAAS, SNS, and ADH, intrarenal mechanisms also play a role in the pathogenesis of renal failure. The urinary excretion of prostacyclin metabolites is increased in patients with acute liver failure and preserved renal function, whereas it is reduced in those patients with renal failure (Moore 1999). In contrast, the urinary excretion of leukotrienes is increased in patients with renal failure. A shift in intrarenal cyclo-oxygenase metabolism from vasodilator prostaglandins to vasoconstrictor leukotrienes could, therefore, contribute to renal vasoconstriction in acute liver failure (Ellis and O'Grady 1999).

As in cirrhosis, renal failure in the setting of acute liver failure carries a very poor prognosis without liver transplantation. The mortality rate varies between 50 and 100 per cent depending on the underlying cause of acute liver failure. Usual indications for renal support apply in this setting. Continuous venovenous haemofiltration is the most common renal support technique (Ellis and O'Grady 1999). Preoperative renal failure is associated with higher postoperative morbidity and mortality in patients treated by liver transplantation. In patients who recover from acute liver failure, renal function can slowly be expected to return to normal.

Renal failure and jaundice

Renal failure may occur in any form of cholestatic liver disease. In patients with jaundice and renal failure, infections and toxins are mainly responsible. Leptospirosis, a spirochetal infection, may cause cholestasis and renal failure. In Weil's syndrome, the most severe form of leptospirosis, patients develop severe hyperbilirubinaemia (bilirubin levels > 1000 μmol/l) and renal dysfunction. The haemolytic–uraemic syndrome is a disease that may appear after an acute viral or *Escherichia coli (0157:H7)* infection (see Chapter 10.6.3). Patients present with fever, thrombocytopenia, hypertension, haemolytic anaemia, jaundice (from indirect hyperbilirubinaemia), renal failure, and hepatitis. Finally, patients with fulminant hepatic failure secondary to paracetamol or NSAIDs who develop severe cholestasis are at high risk of developing renal failure. Other diseases that may cause cholestasis and renal disease include amyloidosis, and sickle-cell disease. In amyloidosis the liver is frequently involved (50 per cent of those with AL amyloid and 18 per cent with AA amyloid) causing hepatomegaly and cholestasis. Patients with sickle-cell disease may also present with a sickle-cell hepatopathy with hyperbilirubinaemia and elevated transaminases as well as renal failure. Obstructive jaundice is the most common form of jaundice encountered. This is a consequence of either obstruction of the intra- or extrahepatic biliary system. Cholestatic liver disease caused by obstructing gallstones, tumours, primary sclerosing cholangitis, or primary biliary cirrhosis, can all be complicated by renal failure. The mechanisms involved include volume depletion, accumulation of bile constituents and endotoxin. Finally, postoperative jaundice carries a high risk of acute renal failure. The incidence of acute renal failure in this setting is 8 per cent, and the mortality is over 70 per cent (Fogarty 1995).

Pathogenesis of renal failure and obstructive jaundice

The pathological changes found in the kidney following the development of renal failure are non-specific and vary from subtle changes in histology to frank acute tubular necrosis, with glomerular and peritubular fibrin deposition. Although the explanation of renal dysfunction in obstructive jaundice is incomplete, a number of factors including endotoxinaemia, hyperbilirubinaemia, increased plasma bile salts, renovascular fibrin deposition, alterations in systemic and renal haemodynamics, and fluid depletion are implicated (Sitges-Serra 1999).

Endotoxinaemia

In the postoperative period, systemic endotoxinaemia can be demonstrated in at least 50 per cent of jaundiced patients, and renal impairment is rare in its absence (Bailey 1976). The effects of endotoxin are likely to be mediated by the action of several cytokines, which impair renal function by causing changes in haemodynamics and by a direct toxic action on the kidney. The direct action may be secondary to their procoagulant activity, with induction of intravascular coagulation, but they may also increase intrarenal sequestration of neutrophils, which in turn leads to a neutrophil-mediated release of cytokines.

Bile constituents

With extrahepatic obstruction, jaundice is associated with the retention of bile, of which bilirubin and bile salts constitute major components along with cholesterol and other lipids. One of the main predictive factors of postoperative renal impairment and death is the presence of hyperbilirubinaemia (Amerio *et al.* 1981). Bilirubin uncouples mitochondrial oxidative phosphorylation; an effect on renal tubular cells which may account for its toxicity. In infants hyperbilirubinaemia leads to a relative decrease in GFR and an increase in fractional sodium excretion in response to salt and water loading. Nonetheless, there is little evidence to implicate bilirubin '*per se*' in the pathogenesis of renal failure associated with obstructive jaundice.

The second most important component of bile are bile salts which seem to potentiate renal ischaemia in several experimental models (Fogarty *et al.* 1995). In rabbits for example, bile salt infusions damage aortic endothelium and the protective fibrinolytic properties of the arterial wall, thereby enhancing intravascular coagulation of renal arteries. In tubular cells, bile salts reduce sodium reabsorption affecting the renal synthesis of cyclo-oxygenase products, which are known to modulate renal sodium and water excretion by haemodynamic or direct tubular actions.

Disturbances of coagulation

Endotoxin by activating platelets, leucocytes, and complement, promotes intravascular coagulation. Endotoxin may, therefore, be responsible for the deposition of fibrin in the microvasculature in obstructive jaundice. A number of studies have demonstrated fibrinogen deposition confined exclusively to the kidney following common bile duct ligation. It has been suggested that obstructive jaundice leads to impaired clearance of endotoxin, which, in turn, causes a low grade of disseminated intravascular coagulation. Clinical studies have shown that patients with either endotoxinaemia or increased fibrin degradation products before surgery for obstructive jaundice are at greater risk of acute renal failure (Sitges-Serra 1999).

Role of prostaglandins

Prostaglandins, especially thromboxane A2, contribute to the impairment of renal function in patients with obstructive jaundice. They induce severe vasoconstriction of the afferent arteriole with a decrease of GFR, and enhance platelet aggregation with contraction of mesangial cells (Holt *et al.* 1999). Contraction of mesangial cells reduces the glomerular filtration surface and the ultrafiltration coefficient K_f with a significant reduction in GFR. Daltroban, a specific and stable TXA2/PGH2 receptor antagonist, protects GFR in experimental models of obstructive jaundice (Kramer *et al.* 1995). In addition, administration of indomethacin or other prostaglandin inhibitors impair renal function in both experimental models and patients with obstructive jaundice. These agents (NSAIDs) are a major cause of acute renal failure in patients with obstructive jaundice.

Renal endothelin system

Recent studies have demonstrated the activation of the renal endothelin system in animal models and in patients with obstructive jaundice (Kramer 1997). Endothelin, a potent vasoconstrictor, probably plays a relevant role in acute renal failure impairing renal haemodynamics and tubular functions.

Disturbances in fluid homeostasis

Studies performed in the 1960s revealed that the amount of haemorrhage required to induce hypovolaemic shock was less for jaundiced dogs than for controls. Experimental studies have demonstrated that common bile duct ligation can decrease plasma volume with associated hypodipsia, hypophagia, and inability to concentrate urine (Gillett 1971; Martinez-Rodenas *et al.* 1989). Similar findings have been confirmed in humans (Sitges-Serra *et al.* 1992). The pathogenesis of this extracellular fluid depletion in obstructive jaundice has not been completely elucidated. However, atrial natriuretic peptide (ANP), a humoral mediator released from the right atrium seems to be implicated (Valverde *et al.* 1992). ANP is well known to cause natriuresis, counterbalance the action of water- and sodium-retaining factors, inhibit the thirst mechanism, and produce peripheral vasodilation. Plasma ANP has been found to be increased in rabbits following common bile duct ligation, along with an increase in aldosterone, renin, and ADH (Valverde *et al.* 1992). These hormones are probably produced in response to a reduced extracellular volume and high levels of ANP may explain the reduced vascular reactivity in response to hypovolaemia.

Therapeutic strategies

Given that obstructive jaundice predisposes the kidney to hypoxic damage, patients with intra- or extrahepatic bile duct obstruction are especially susceptible to acute renal failure. Despite a significant amount of research into the pathogenesis of renal failure in this setting, no specific or effective therapies are available for acute renal failure in obstructive jaundice (Sitges-Serra 1999). In cases where surgery is considered to relieve obstruction, preoperative volume repletion is essential to prevent renal failure because a reduction in plasma volume is present in the majority of cases. There are, however, no studies specifically assessing the use of volume repletion in this setting (Fogarty 1995). Since patients with obstructive jaundice are often subjected to several preoperative tests that may involve fasting such as magnetic resonance cholangiopancreatography and/or endoscopic retrograde cholangiopancreatography it is very important that clinicians be aware of their volume status before these procedures. Intensive efforts should be made to correct any fluid and/or electrolyte abnormalities before surgery.

Use of antiendotoxin therapy has been attempted with bile salts and lactulose, although there are conflicting reports on the efficacy before surgery for obstructive jaundice (Pain *et al.* 1991). Sodium deoxycholate appears to be the bile salt that is most likely to confer renal protection; however, there is little data to support its use. Lactulose, a synthetic disaccharide frequently used in cirrhotic patients to prevent encephalopathy, may also prevent endotoxaemia by either reducing or altering gut flora, thereby decreasing the endotoxin pool available for absorption. Lactulose has been shown in experimental models and in humans to reduce systemic endotoxaemia in non-obstructive and obstructive jaundice (Sitges-Serra 1999). One study confirmed that the preoperative administration of oral lactulose and bile salts protected renal function and decreased mortality in patients with obstructive jaundice (Pain *et al.* 1991). Relief of biliary obstruction has also been used in the experimental and clinical setting in an effort to improve endotoxaemia in obstructive jaundice (Clements *et al.* 1993). However, there are no specific studies assessing the course of renal failure after biliary drainage, and a definitive answer about its efficacy in improving renal failure requires further controlled trials.

Although mannitol, an osmotic diuretic, has been used as a prophylatic measure against deterioration in renal function following surgery for obstructive jaundice, the results are conflicting and controversial and at present firm recommendations cannot be made.

Acute renal failure in liver transplantation

Liver transplantation has been the most important advancement for the management of endstage liver disease developed in the past two decades. The immediate outcome of orthotopic liver transplantation is dependent on several factors, including pretransplant renal function (Nair *et al.* 2002). The prevalence of renal insufficiency in patients before liver transplantation varies from 10 to 20 per cent, although many of these patients may have HRS, a potentially reversible condition. Acute renal failure is one of the most common postoperative complications of liver transplantation. The reported incidence of acute renal failure ranges from 21 to 70 per cent. This great variability reflects differences in criteria defining acute renal failure and clinical characteristics of the patients. Although between 10 and 18 per cent of patients will require dialysis after liver transplantation, their mortality rate ranges from 40 to 90 per cent (Bilbao *et al.* 1998).

The aetiology of acute renal failure after liver transplantation is multifactorial. Several preoperative, intraoperative, and postoperative factors have been identified over and above those applicable to acute and chronic liver failure. Two recent reports indicate that pretransplant renal dysfunction is an important risk factor for patient and graft survival after liver transplantation. Pretransplant renal failure increases the incidence of postoperative sepsis, number of days spent in the intensive care unit, the need for preoperative and postoperative dialysis, overall cost of liver transplantation, and short-term graft and patient survival rates (Fig. 9) (Bilbao *et al.* 1998; Nair *et al.* 2002). In addition, donor factors are not only important for the outcome of liver transplantation, but also for the risk of acute renal failure. Although liver transplantation has improved significantly during the last two decades, it remains a complex and potentially complicated surgery. Hypotension from massive blood loss, circulatory instability, duration of surgery, and many other perioperative factors are obvious risks for ischaemic renal damage. During the postoperative period, volume overload or depletion, severe infection, repeated rejection, and use of potentially nephrotoxic drugs, especially the calcineurin inhibitors and immunosuppressor agents are some of the many factors predisposing to acute renal failure (Gonwa *et al.* 2001a,b).

Prevention of acute renal failure after liver transplantation remains a challenge. Patients with HRS in the preoperative period need to be actively treated (see above). Recently, Gonwa *et al.* (2001b) showed

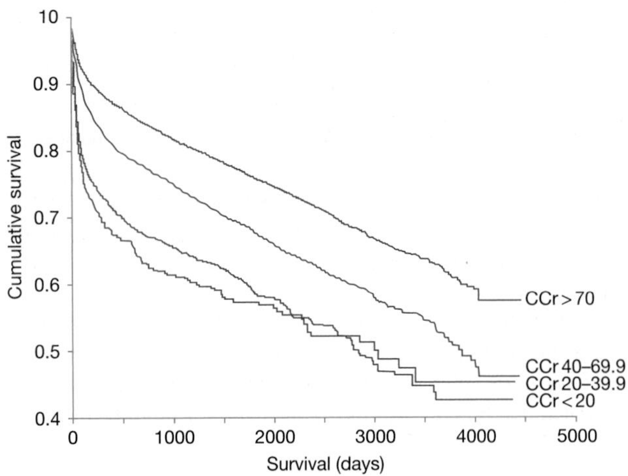

Fig. 9 Probability of survival of cirrhotic patients after liver transplantation according to preoperative creatinine clearance (from Nair *et al.* 2002 with permission).

the benefit of renal replacement therapy with continuous venovenous haemodialysis before and after liver transplantation in patients with severe renal failure. Administration of aprotinin, a powerful antifibrinolytic agent, reduced blood loss significantly during liver transplantation without any negative effect on renal function (Molenaar *et al.* 2001). A delay in the introduction of the nephrotoxic immunosuppressive drugs could be helpful in the prevention of post-transplant acute renal failure, especially in high-risk patients. Preliminary data with the use of mycophenolate mofetil or sirolimus and low doses of calcineurin inhibitors support this suggestion, but controlled studies are needed.

Glomerulonephritis in liver diseases (see Chapters 3.6 and 10.6.1)

IgA nephropathy associated with liver disease is the most frequently encountered secondary form of IgA nephropathy (Newell 1987). The pathogenesis is related to an inability to remove IgA-containing complexes by Kupffer cells in the liver, which in turn predispose to deposition of IgA in the kidney. In fact, IgA deposition in the skin and liver (hepatic sinusoids) make this hypothesis plausible. Although it is preferentially observed in patients with alcoholic liver disease it can be seen in other types of liver disease. Despite the high frequency of glomerular IgA deposits in advanced liver disease, most patients are asymptomatic. Patients may present with microscopic haematuria, mild proteinuria, and a mild degree of renal impairment. Light microscopy findings are very similar to those of patients with primary IgA nephropathy. These include mesangial hypercellularity and an increase in mesangial matrix. At present, several therapies (ace inhibitors, corticosteroids, immunosuppressive agents, IV immunoglobulin, and fish oil) have been advocated to improve the course of progressive IgA nephropathy. However, there are no specific studies assessing therapy for patients with liver disease associated IgA nephropathy.

Patients with viral hepatitis, in particular hepatitis C, are at risk of developing essential mixed cryoglobulinaemia (EMC) (Agnello *et al.* 1992) (see Chapter 4.6). The prevalence of EMC is high (41.5 per cent) in patients with chronic liver disease. When considering independent causes, HCV prevalence is higher (54.3 per cent) than HBV (15 per cent) or other causes of chronic liver disease (32 per cent), however, it is important to mention that these numbers vary according to geographical location (Lunel *et al.* 1988). EMC is a disorder in which mixed cryoglobulins (polyclonal immunoglobulin, IgG, and a monoclonal rheumatoid factor, IgM) precipitate at cool temperature and cause a constellation of clinical findings characterized by arthritis, purpura, peripheral neuropathy, weakness, glomerulonephritis, and manifestations of vasculitis. There are three types: type I, II, and III, the strongest association with viral hepatitis is with type II. The pathogenesis is complex and it is unclear why cryoglobulins are produced and which antigen triggers their production. In cases associated with hepatitis C infection, the virus RNA may be the triggering agent since it has been found in high concentrations in the cryoprecipitate (Agnello *et al.* 1992; Lunel *et al.* 1998). Another hypothesis is related to the release of a putative antigen from injured hepatocytes or its production by Kupffer cells contributing to immunoglobulin formation. In addition to increased production, a decreased clearance of cryoglobulins due to liver dysfunction may lead to cryoglobulinaemia and its subsequent deposition in the kidney, skin, and other tissues.

The diagnosis of EMC is typically made from the history, skin lesions, low complement levels, and demonstration of circulating cryoglobulins. Although the majority of patients with hepatitis C have type II associated cryoglobulinaemia, 30–40 per cent do not have detectable circulating cryoglobulins at presentation (Johnson *et al.* 1993). About 20 per cent have physical signs of chronic liver disease, 75 per cent have mild elevations of serum transaminases and in most cases liver biopsy demonstrates chronic hepatitis with or without cirrhosis (Lunel *et al.* 1998). Patients with cryoglobulinaemic glomerulonephritis usually present with proteinuria, microscopic haematuria, and mild renal insufficiency. The major clinical manifestations of EMC include palpable purpura (which is a form of vasculitis), arthralgias, lymphadenopathy, hepatosplenomegaly, constitutional symptoms, and peripheral neuropathy. Nearly 40 per cent will have signs consistent with extrarenal manifestations of cryoglobulinaemia. Approximately 20 per cent of patients have nephrotic range proteinuria and in 25 per cent of patients an acute nephritic syndrome may develop with rapid deterioration of renal function. In the majority of patients renal function will have a stable course and few will require renal replacement therapy. Laboratory features include the presence of low complement (low CH50, C4, and C3), mild elevation of serum creatinine, and presence of circulating cryoglobulins. Renal biopsy reveals a mesangiocapillary pattern of glomerulonephritis.

There are few studies that have focused specifically on the treatment of cryglobulinaemic renal disease in the setting of chronic liver disease. Since hepatitis C is the inciting event for this type of nephropathy, therapy has been directed towards eliminating the virus. In cryoglobulinaemic glomerulonephritis, patients receiving α-interferon therapy for 6 months or longer reduced proteinuria by 50 per cent, but serum creatinine did not significantly improve (Johnson *et al.* 1994). Another controlled study of α-interferon reported an improvement in serum creatinine in 60 per cent of treated patients and a better outcome was observed in those that cleared the virus; however, renal disease returned upon discontinuation of therapy (Misiani *et al.* 1994). In both studies clinical improvement occurred regardless of the fact that viraemia was suppressed or not, this might be explained by the previous duration of viraemia, the genotype of HCV or variation of the host immune response. Other treatments for hepatitis C associated renal disease have focused on treating an underlying cause when present, such as EMC. Standard treatment of EMC includes corticosteroids, cytotoxic agents, and plasmapheresis; the goal is to control the formation and deposition of cryoglobulins. Corticosteroids, although beneficial in some cases, can elevate viraemia and exacerbate hepatitis. However, if EMC is present, pulse steroid therapy may rapidly improve renal function and vasculitis. More recently, the combination of interferon and ribavirin administered to a patient with cryoglobulinaemic glomerulonephritis was successful in clearing the virus and improving renal function and extrarenal manifestations of EMC (Misiani *et al.* 1999). Although the combination of pegylated interferon and ribavirin has been very successful for treating patients with hepatitis C, no reports are available with regard to the efficacy of this combination on HCV associated renal disease.

Acknowledgements

Supported by a grant from the Fondo de Investigaciones Sanitarias de la Seguridad Social (FISS 00/0616) and from the Marató Fundació TV3 (U-2000-TV2710) and by The Clinical Investigator Training Program: Beth Israel Deaconess Medical Center—Harvard/MIT Health Sciences and Technology, in collaboration with Pfizer Inc.

References

Agnello, V. *et al.* (1992). A role for hepatitis C virus infection in type II cryoglobulinemia. *New England Journal of Medicine* **327**, 1490–1495.

Akriviadis, E. *et al.* (2000). Pentoxifylline improves short-term survival in severe acute alcoholic hepatitis: a double-blind, placebo-controlled trial. *Gastroenterology* **119**, 1637–1648.

Alam, I. *et al.* (1995). Treatment of hepatorenal syndrome with the transjugular intrahepatic shunt (TIPS) (abstract). *Gastroenterology* **108**, A1024.

Albillos, A. *et al.* (1995). Continuous prazosin administration in cirrhotic patients: effects on portal hemodynamics and on liver and renal function. *Gastroenterology* **109**, 1257–1265.

Albillos, A. *et al.* (1998). Propranolol plus prazosis compared with propranolol plus isosorbide-5-mononitrate in the treatment of portal hypertension. *Gastroenterology* **115**, 230–232.

Amerio, A. *et al.* (1981). Prognosis of acute renal failure accompanied by jaundice. *Nephron* **27**, 152–154.

Angeli, P. *et al.* (1994). Renal effects of endogenous natriuretic peptides receptors blockade in cirrhotic rats with ascites. *Hepatology* **20**, 948–954.

Angeli, P. *et al.* (1999). Reversal of type 1 hepatorenal syndrome with the administration of midodrine and octreotide. *Hepatology* **29**, 1690–1697.

Arroyo, V. Treatment of hepatorenal syndrome in cirrhosis. In *Ascites and Renal Dysfunction in Liver Disease* (ed. V. Arroyo), pp. 492–510. Malden, MA: Blackwell Science, 1999.

Arroyo, V. and Jimenez, W. (2000). Complications of cirrhosis. Renal and circulatory dysfunction lights and shadows in an important clinical problem. *Journal of Hepatology* **32** (Suppl. 1), 157–170.

Arroyo, V. *et al.* (1981). Effect of angiotensin II blockade on systemic and hepatic hemodynamics and on the renin–angiotensin–aldosterone system in cirrhosis with ascites. *European Journal of Clinical Investigation* **11**, 221–229.

Arroyo, V. *et al.* (1983). Sympathetic nervous activity, renin–angiotensin system and renal excretion of prostaglandin E2 in cirrhosis. Relationship to functional renal failure and sodium and water excretion. *European Journal of Clinical Investigation* **13**, 271–278.

Arroyo, V. *et al.* (1986). Renal function abnormalities prostaglandins and effects of nonsteroidal anti-inflammatory drugs in cirrhosis with ascites. An overview with emphasis on pathogenesis. *American Journal of Medicine* **81**, 104–122.

Arroyo, V. *et al.* (1996). Definition and diagnostic criteria of refractory ascites and hepatorenal syndrome in cirrhosis. *Hepatology* **23**, 164–176.

Arroyo, V. *et al.* (2002). Hepatorenal syndrome: pathogenesis and treatment. *Gastroenterology* **122**, 1658–1676.

Bailey, M. E. (1976). Endotoxin, bile salts and renal function in obstructive jaundice. *British Journal of Surgery* **63**, 774–778.

Bernardi, M. *et al.* The renin–angiotensin aldosterone system in cirrhosis. In *Ascites and Renal Dysfunction in Liver Disease* (ed. V. Arroyo), pp. 175–197. Malden, MA: Blackwell Science, 1999.

Bilbao, I. *et al.* (1998). Risk factors for acute renal failure requiring dialysis after liver transplantation. *Clinical Transplantation* **12**, 123–129.

Bosch, J. *et al.* (1980). Hepatic hemodynamics and the renin–angiotensin aldosterone system in cirrhosis. *Gastroenterology* **78**, 92–99.

Boyer, T. D. *et al.* (1979). Effect of indomethacin and prostaglandin A1 in renal function and plasma renin activity in alcoholic liver disease. *Gastroenterology* **77**, 215–222.

Brensing, K. A. *et al.* (2000). Long-term outcome after transjugular intrahepatic portosystemic stent-shunt in non-trasplant patients with hepatorenal syndrome: a phase II study. *Gut* **47**, 288–295.

Cabrera, J. *et al.* (1982). Aminoglycoside nephrotoxicity in cirrhosis. Value of urinary B2-microglobulin to discriminate functional renal failure form acute tubular damage. *Gastroenterology* **82**, 97–105.

Cardenas, A. *et al.* (2000). Hepatorenal syndrome. *Liver transplantation* **6** (Suppl. 1), S63–S71.

Clements, W. D. *et al.* (1993). Biliary drainage in obstructive jaundice: experimental and clinical aspects. *British Journal of Surgery* **80**, 834–842.

Dudley, F. J. *et al.* (1986). Hepatorenal syndrome without sodium retention. *Hepatology* **6**, 248–251.

Duvoux, C. *et al.* (2002). Effects of noradrenalin and albumin in patients with type I hepatorenal syndrome: a pilot study. *Hepatology* **36**, 374–380.

Ellis, A. J. and O'Grady, J. G. Clinical disorders of renal function in acute liver failure. In *Ascites and Renal Dysfunction in Liver Disease* (ed. V. Arroyo), pp. 62–78. Malden, MA: Blackwell Science, 1999.

Esler, M. *et al.* (1992). Increased sympathetic nervous activity and the effects of its inhibition with clonidine in alcoholic cirrhosis. *Annals of Internal Medicine* **116**, 446–455.

Fogarty, B. J. *et al.* (1995). Renal dysfunction in obstructive jaundice. *British Journal of Surgery* **82**, 877–884.

Follo, A. *et al.* (1994). Renal impairment following spontaneous bacterial peritonitis in cirrhosis. Incidence, clinical course, predictive factors and prognosis. *Hepatology* **20**, 1495–1501.

Gatta, A. *et al.* (1981). Evaluation of renal tubular damage in liver cirrhosis by urinary enzymes and beta-2-microglobulin excretions. *European Journal of Clinical Investigation* **11**, 239–243.

Gillett, D. J. (1971). The effect of obstructive jaundice on the blood volume in rats. *The Journal of Surgical Research* **11**, 447–449.

Ginès, P. *et al.* (1988). Atrial natriuretic factor in cirrhosis with ascites: plasma levels, cardiac release and splanchnic extraction. *Hepatology* **8**, 636–642.

Ginès, P. *et al.* (1991). Paracentesis with intravenous infusion of albumin as compared with peritoneovenous shunting in cirrhosis with refractory ascites. *New England Journal of Medicine* **325**, 829–835.

Ginès, A. *et al.* (1992). Effects of somatostatin on renal function in cirrhosis. *Gastroenterology* **103**, 1868–1874.

Ginès, A. *et al.* (1993a). Incidence, predictive factors, and prognosis of hepatorenal syndrome in cirrhosis. *Gastroenterology* **105**, 229–236.

Ginès, A. *et al.* (1993b). Oral misoprostol or intravenous prostaglandin E2 do not improve renal function in patients with cirrhosis and ascites with hyponatremia or renal failure. *Journal of Hepatology* **17**, 220–226.

Ginès, P. *et al.* (1998). Hyponatremia in cirrhosis: from pathogenesis to treatment. *Hepatology* **28**, 851–864.

Gonwa, T. A. *et al.* (1991). Long-term survival and renal function following liver transplantation in patients with and without hepatorenal syndrome—experience in 300 patients. *Transplantation* **91**, 428–430.

Gonwa, T. A. *et al.* (1995). Impact of pretransplant renal function on survival after liver transplantation. *Transplantation* **59**, 361–365.

Gonwa, T. A. *et al.* (2001a). End-stage renal disease after orthotopic liver transplantation using calcineurin-based immunotherapy: risk of development and treatment. *Transplantation* **72**, 1934–1939.

Gonwa, T. A. *et al.* (2001b). Renal replacement therapy and orthotopic liver transplantation: the role of continuous veno-venous hemodialysis. *Transplantation* **71**, 1424–1428.

Gonzalez-Abraldes, J. *et al.* (2001). Randomized comparison of long-term losartan versus propranolol in lowering portal pressure in cirrhosis. *Gastroenterology* **121**, 487–490.

Guevara, M. *et al.* (1998a). Reversibility of hepatorenal syndrome by prolonged administration of ornipressin and plasma volume expansion. *Hepatology* **27**, 35–41.

Guevara, M. *et al.* (1998b). Transjugular intrahepatic portosystemic shunt in hepatorenal syndrome: effects on renal function and vasoactive systems. *Hepatology* **28**, 416–422.

Guevara, M. *et al.* (2001). Effect of celecoxib on renal function in cirrhotic patients with ascites. A pilot study. *Hepatology* **34**, 59A.

Gülberg, V. *et al.* (1999). Long-term therapy and retreatment of hepatorenal syndrome type 1 with ornipressin and dopamine. *Hepatology* **30**, 870–875.

Henriksen, J. H. *et al.* (1980). Filtration as the main transport mechanism of protein exchange between plasma and the peritoneal cavity in hepatic cirrhosis. *Scandinavian Journal of Clinical Laboratory Investigation* **40**, 503–513.

Holt, S. *et al.* (1999). Acute cholestasis-induced renal failure: effects of antioxidants and ligands for the thromboxane A2 receptor. *Kidney International* **55**, 271–277.

Hori, N. *et al.* (1997). Role of calcitonin gene-related peptide in the vascular system on the development of the hyperdynamic circulation in conscious cirrhotic rats. *Hepatology* **26**, 111–119.

Johnson, R. J. *et al.* (1993). Membranoproliferative glomerulonephritis associated with hepatitis C virus infection. *New England Journal of Medicine* **328**, 465–470.

Johnson, R. *et al.* (1994). Hepatitis C virus-associated glomerulonephritis. Effect of alpha-interferon therapy. *Kidney International* **46**, 1700–1704.

Kramer, H. J. (1997). Impaired renal function in obstructive jaundice: roles of the thromboxane and endothelin systems. *Nephron* **77**, 1–12.

Kramer, H. J. *et al.* (1995). Impaired renal function in obstructive jaundice enhanced glomerular thromboxane synthesis and effects of thromboxane receptor blockade in bile duct-ligated rats. *Clinical Science* **88**, 39–45.

LaVilla, G. *et al.* (1992). Mineralocorticoid escape in patients with compensated cirrhosis and portal hypertension. *Gastroenterology* **102**, 2114–2119.

Le Veen, H. H. *et al.* (1974). Peritoneo-venous shunting for ascites. *Annals of Surgery* **180**, 580–590.

Leak, L. V. and Rahill, K. (1978). Permeability of the diaphrangmtic mesothelium: the ultrastructural basis for 'stomata'. *American Journal of Anatomy* **151**, 557–594.

Lenz, K. *et al.* (1991). Ornipressin in the treatment of functional renal failure in decompensated liver cirrhosis. *Gastroenterology* **101**, 1060–1067.

Linas, S. L. *et al.* (1986). Peritoneovenous shunt in the management of the hepatorenal syndrome. *Kidney International* **30**, 736–740.

Llach, J. *et al.* (1993). Effect of dipyridamole on kidney function in cirrhosis. *Hepatology* **17**, 59–64.

Lunel, F. *et al.* (1988). Hepatitis C virus infection and cryoglobulinemia. *Journal of Hepatology* **29**, 848–855.

Mandal, A. K. *et al.* (1982). Acute tubular necrosis in hepatorenal syndrome: an electron microscopy study. *American Journal of Kidney Diseases* **34**, 2363–2374.

Martinez-Rodenas, F. *et al.* (1989). Measurement of body water compartments after ligation of the common bile duct in the rabbit. *British Journal of Surgery* **76**, 461–464.

Merkel, C. *et al.* (1995). Long-term effect of nadolol or nadolol plus isosorbide-5-mononitrate on renal function and ascites formation in patients with cirrhosis. *Hepatology* **22**, 808–815.

Misiani, R. *et al.* (1994). Interferon alfa-2a therapy in cryoglobulinemia asscoiated with hepatitis C virus. *New England Journal of Medicine* **330**, 751–756.

Misiani, R. *et al.* (1999). Successful treatment of HCV-associated cryoglobulinaemic glomerulonephritis with a combination of interferon-alpha and ribavirin. *Nephrology, Dialysis, Transplantation* **14**, 1558–1560.

Mitzner, S. R. *et al.* (2000). Improvement of hepatorenal syndrome with extracorporeal albumin dialysis MARS: results of a prospective, randomized controlled clinical trial. *Liver Transplantation* **6**, 277–286.

Molenaar, I. Q. *et al.* (2001). Reduced need for vasopressors in patients receiving aprotinin during orthotopic liver transplantation. *Anesthesiology* **94**, 433–438.

Moore, K. (1999). Renal failure in acute liver failure. *European Journal of Gastroenterology and Hepatology* **11**, 967–975.

Moore, K. *et al.* (1992). Plasma endothelin immunoreactivity in liver disease and the hepatorenal syndrome. *New England Journal of Medicine* **327**, 1774–1778.

Moreau, R. *et al.* (2002). Terlipressin in patients with cirrhosis and type 1 hepatorenal syndrome: a retrospective multicenter study. *Gastroenterology* **122**, 923–930.

Morillas, R. M. *et al.* (1994). Propranolol plus isosorbide-5-mononitrate for portal hypertension in cirrhosis: long-term hemodynamic and renal effects. *Hepatology* **20**, 1502–1508.

Mountokalakis, T. *et al.* (1988). Enhancement of renal function by a long-acting somatostatin analogue in patients with decompensated cirrhosis. *Nephrology, Dialysis, Transplantation* **3**, 604–607.

Mulkay, J. P. *et al.* (2001). Long-term terlipressin administration improves renal function in cirrhotic patients with type 1 hepatorenal syndrome: a pilot study. *Acta Gastroenterológica Belga* **64**, 15–19.

Nair, S. *et al.* (2002). Pretransplant renal function predicts survival in patients undergoing orthotopic liver transplantation. *Hepatology* **35**, 1179–1185.

Navasa, M. *et al.* (1993). Hemodynamic and humoral changes after Liver transplantation in patients with cirrhosis. *Hepatology* **17**, 355–360.

Navasa, M. *et al.* (1998). Tumor necrosis factor and interleukin-6 in spontaneous bacterial peritonitis in cirrhosis: relationship with the development of renal impairment and mortality. *Hepatology* **27**, 1227–1232.

Newell, G. C. (1987). Cirrhotic glomerulonephritis: incidence, morphology, clinical features, and pathogenesis. *American Journal of Kidney Diseases* **9**, 183–190.

O'Grady, J. G. *et al.* (1993). Acute liver failure: redefining the syndrome. *Lancet* **342**, 273–275.

Ochs, A. *et al.* (1994). TIPS for hepatorenal syndrome. *Hepatology* **20**, 114A.

Ortega, R. *et al.* (2002). Terlipressin therapy with and without albumin for patients with hepatorenal syndrome: results of a prospective, nonrandomized study. *Hepatology* **36**, 941–948.

Ottensen, L. H. *et al.* (2001). Effects of a long-acting formulation of octreotide on renal function and renal sodium handling in cirrhotic patients with portal hypertension: a randomized, double-blind, controlled trial. *Hepatology* **34**, 471–477.

Pain, J. A. *et al.* (1991). Prevention of postoperative renal dysfunction in patients with obstructive jaundice: a multicentre study of bile salts and lactulose. *British Journal of Surgery* **78**, 467–469.

Pérez, G. O. *et al.* Dialysis hemofiltration, and other extracorporeal techniques in the treatment of renal complications of liver disease. In *The Kidney in Liver Disease* 4th edn. (ed. M. Epstein), pp. 517–528. Philadelphia, PA: Hanley & Belfus, 1996.

Pérez-Ayuso, R. M. *et al.* (1984a). Evidence that renal prostaglandins are involved in renal water metabolism in cirrhosis. *Kidney International* **26**, 72–80.

Pérez-Ayuso, R. M. *et al.* (1984b). Renal kallikrein excretion in cirrhotics with ascites: relationship to renal hemodynamics. *Hepatology* **4**, 247–252.

Platt, J. F. *et al.* (1994). Renal duplex Doppler ultrasonography: a noninvasive predictor of kidney dysfunction and hepatorenal failure in liver disease. *Hepatology* **20**, 362–369.

Rector, W. G. and Reynolds, T. B. (1984). Propranolol in the treatment of cirrhotic ascites. *Archives of Internal Medicine* **144**, 1761–1763.

Rodés, J. *et al.* (1975). Clinical types and drug therapy of renal impairment in cirrhosis. *Postgraduate Medicine Journal* **51**, 492–497.

Ros, J. *et al.* (1995). Role of nitric oxide and prostacyclin in the control of renal perfusion in experimental cirrhosis. *Hepatology* **22**, 915–920.

Salmerón, J. M. *et al.* (1993). Renal effects of acute isosorbide-5-mononitrate administration in cirrhosis. *Hepatology* **17**, 800–806.

Saló, J. *et al.* (1995). Effect of upright posture and physical exercise on endogenous neurohormonal systems in cirrhotic patients with sodium retention and normal plasma renin, aldosterone and norepinephrine levels. *Hepatology* **22**, 479–487.

Schepke, M. *et al.* (2001). Hemodynamic effects of the angiotensin II receptor antagonist Irbesartan in patients with cirrhosis and portal hypertension. *Gastroenterology* **121**, 389–395.

Shear, L. *et al.* (1970). Compartmentalization of ascites and edema in patients with hepatic cirrhosis. *New England Journal of Medicine* **282**, 1391–1396.

Sitges-Serra, A. Renal dysfunction and postoperative renal failure in obstructive jaundice. In *Ascitis and Renal Dysfunction in Liver Disease* (ed. V. Arroyo), pp. 79–98. Malden, MA: Blackwell Science, 1999.

Sitges-Serra, A. *et al.* (1992). Body water compartments in patients with obstructive jaundice. *British Journal of Surgery* **79**, 553–556.

Sort, P. *et al.* (1999). Effect of plasma volume expansion on renal impairment and mortality in patients with cirrhosis and spontaneous bacterial peritonitis. *New England Journal of Medicine* **341**, 403–409.

Uriz, J. *et al.* (2000). Terlipressin plus albumin infusion is an effective and safe therapy of hepatorenal syndrome. *Journal of Hepatology* **33**, 43–48.

Valverde, J. *et al.* (1992). Rapid increase in plasma levels of atrial natriuretic peptide after common bile duct ligation in the rabbit. *Annals of Surgery* **216**, 554–559.

Vorobioff, J. *et al.* (1993). Propranolol compaired with propranolol plus isosorbide dinitrate in portal hypertensive patients: long-term hemodynamic and renal effects. *Hepatology* **18**, 477–484.

Yoffey, J. M. and Courtice, F. C. Lymph flow and regional lymphatics. In *Lymphatics, Lymph and the Lymphomyeloid Complex* (ed. E. Arnold), pp. 356–443. New York, NY: Academia, 1970.

Zipser, R. D. *et al.* (1979). Prostaglandins: modulators of renal function and pressor resistance in chronic liver disease. *Journal of Clinical Endocrinology and Metabolism* **8**, 895–900.

10.6.5 Ischaemic renal disease

John S. Smyth, Paramit Chowdhury, and John E. Scoble

Introduction

Acute ischaemic nephropathy is an important cause of acute renal failure (Mayo and Swartz 1996; Haas *et al.* 2000) but differentiating acute from chronic renal ischaemia is often difficult (Chapter 9.5). Occlusion of the renal artery most often occurs in the presence of pre-existing arterial disease, but it may be a result of an embolus, *in situ* thrombosis or caused by fragments of vessel wall atheroma as in atheroembolic disease. Management in each of these cases will be different and determined by the state of the underlying kidney.

Renal collateral blood flow

The kidney can develop an extensive collateral blood supply (Fig. 1). This provides temporary supply to the kidney in the case of acute occlusion or more permanent preservation of renal function in cases of stenosis progressing to occlusion (Yune and Klatte 1976). The rate at which this can develop in man is not known. However, collateral blood flow probably explains the potential for renal recovery after acute occlusion. The converse process can also occur (Fig. 2), that is, collateral vessels proximal to the stenosis become very small after successful treatment of the renal artery stenosis. It is likely that significant collateral blood flow can be established with the same speed as it can diminish.

Renal response to ischaemia

The renal response to acute and complete occlusion of a renal artery might be expected to be infarction but experience with revascularization of acutely occluded anuric kidneys has shown that recovery is still possible. If the underlying kidney has been subjected to chronic ischaemia, infarction is less likely, although acute occlusion after long-term stenosis may be less damaging because of collateral blood flow, chronic ischaemic damage to the kidney may have already occurred. The processes within, and consequences for the kidney resulting from renal artery stenosis are complex (Chapter 9.5).

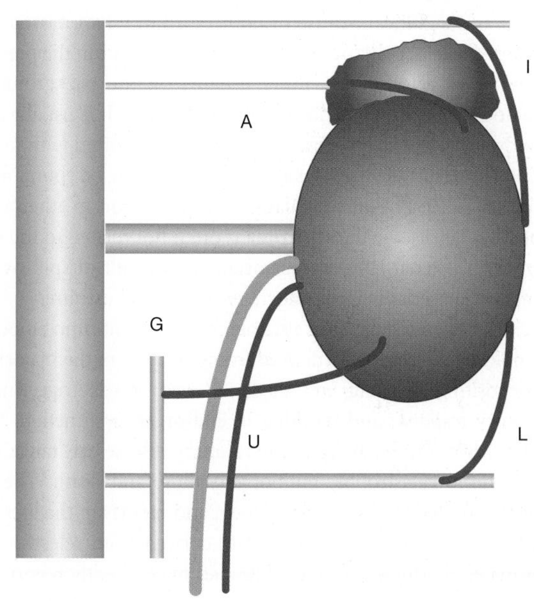

Fig. 1 Renal collateral blood supply. A, adrenal; G, gonadal; I, intercostal; L, lumbar; U, ureteric arterial anastamoses.

(a)

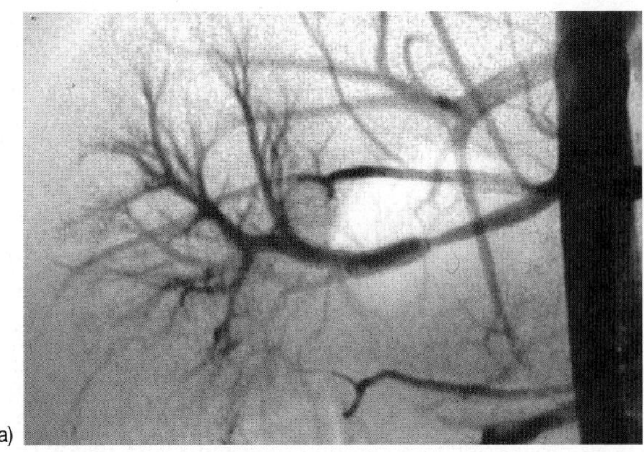

(b)

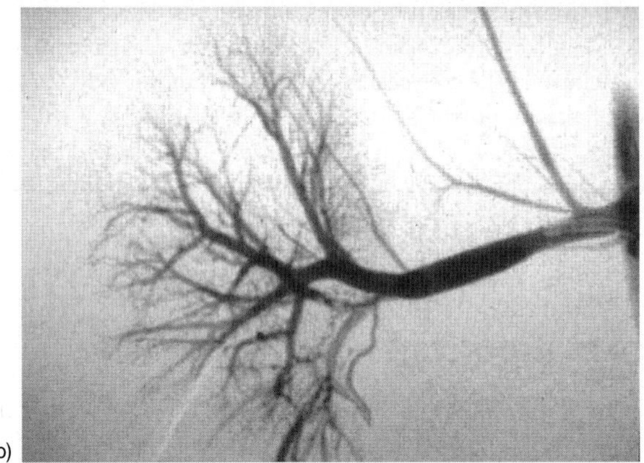

Fig. 2 Renal angiogram before and 6 months after renal angioplasty. The vessel proximal to the stenosis diminishes in size after the flow through the artery and is re-established after angioplasty. Courtesy of Dr J. Reidy.

Atheroembolic disease

Since first described by Flory (1945), atheroembolism is increasingly recognized as a significant cause of both morbidity and mortality in the developed world. Atheroembolic disease may occur in the presence of normal renal arteries but, more usually, on the background of atheromatous renal artery stenosis (Vidt *et al.* 1989). It is usually associated with severe aortic atherosclerotic disease and often with instrumentation through the atherosclerotic aorta but may be spontaneous (Belanfant *et al.* 1991). Anticoagulation is a risk factor. In atherosclerotic renovascular disease the atheroma is often not related to the renal artery *per se* but renal involvement occurs as a result of spill-over of atheromatous material from the aorta into the renal ostium.

The clinical manifestations of atheroembolism result from embolization of cholesterol rich debris (derived from the aorta in the majority of cases), depositing in small and medium sized vessels triggering an inflammatory response and resulting in end-organ dysfunction. Since almost any organ can be affected, the resulting disease can range from asymptomatic to catastrophic multiorgan failure and death. The true incidence of atheroembolism is not known and reports in the literature vary widely due to past reliance on data derived from selected post-mortem material. Moolenaar and colleagues have recently reported an incidence of 6.2 cases per million population per year (Moolenaar and Lamer 1996). In patients with established risk factors (discussed below) and a history of vascular disease, the incidence is much higher (Thurlbeck and Castleman 1957). Despite mimicking many disease states, for example, vasculitis and endocarditis, two distinct clinical syndromes have been characterized. The first comprises a disease of insidious onset presenting with fever, weight loss, and non-specific symptoms. The more classical presentation is with livedo reticularis, distal ischaemia, renal impairment, and eosinophilia. Atheroembolism predominantly affects at-risk White males older than 60 years (Moolenaar and Lamer 1996). Diabetic patients and those with a history of hypertension or vascular disease are also at increased risk (Belenfant *et al.* 1999).

Livedo reticularis is the most common cutaneous manifestation occurring in up to 50 per cent of cases. In 20 per cent of cases, distal ischaemia may lead to gangrene or ulceration. Renal involvement is present in 50 per cent with half of these patients requiring renal replacement therapy (Belenfant *et al.* 1999). Cardiac failure and severe hypertension are frequent complications and contribute to the high mortality. Coexistent renal disease, for example, vasculitis in conjunction with atheroembolism has also been described. The diagnosis requires a high index of suspicion rather than reliance on tissue examination. Tissue diagnosis is not required in patients presenting with classic signs appearing after exposure to an established risk factor (Thadhani *et al.* 1996; Belenfant *et al.* 1999). The most frequently biopsied sites are skin and kidney, which will provide an accurate diagnosis in over 75 per cent of cases. Lower limb muscle biopsy will give a sensitivity approaching 100 per cent but is not performed often. In high-risk patients, transoesophageal echocardiography and magnetic resonance imaging (MRI) can provide accurate data on the state of the ascending, thoracic, and descending aorta. Studies have reported detection of significant arteriosclerosis in 95 per cent of patients with known atheroembolism as opposed to 20 per cent of matched controls. Fundoscopy is an essential part of the examination in a patient with suspected atheroembolism as characteristic Hollenhorst plaques are seen in 10 per cent of cases (Lye *et al.* 1993).

Laboratory findings are variable and no test is specific for atheroembolism. Common findings include: normocytic anaemia, leucocytosis, thrombocytopenia, eosinophilia (80 per cent of cases), raised inflammatory markers, and transient hypocomplementaemia. The diagnosis of renal atheroembolic disease is confirmed by the presence of cholesterol clefts found on renal biopsy. These represent the sites of lodgment of cholesterol crystals although the actual cholesterol is dissolved in the slide preparation (Fig. 3). In some cases a glomerulonephritis has been reported in association with atheroembolic disease suggesting, misleadingly, a systemic vasculitis rather than atheroembolic disease (Hannedouche *et al.* 1986).

The optimal management of patients with atheroembolism is yet to be determined. Conservative management achieved the best outcome in the series of 67 patients reported by Belenfant *et al.* (1999), with a major reduction in 1-year mortality compared to previously published series. The most important step is to prevent further atheroembolism by avoiding invasive procedures and anticoagulation. Treatment of hypertension and cardiac failure with renal replacement therapy where required dramatically improved outcome. Angiotensin-converting enzyme inhibitors (ACEIs) are not contraindicated for the treatment of cardiac failure in atheroembolism, despite approximately 50 per cent of patients having coexistent renal artery stenosis. Since most patients with significant atheroembolism are malnourished, nutritional support is essential and can be provided by oral and or enteral

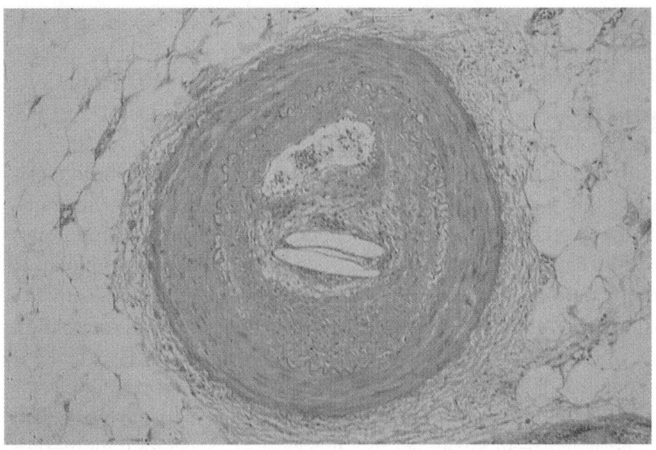

Fig. 3 Atheroembolic disease leading to cholesterol crystal deposition in the kidney. This shows the cleft left by the dissolution of the cholesterol crystal during preparation of the slide. Reproduced with permission from Dr P. O'Donnell.

means (Dahlberg *et al.* 1989). The role of corticosteroids is controversial with most data derived from case reports or small series but they may have a role in those with an acute inflammatory response and in those with gastrointestinal symptoms. Surgical intervention should only be considered as rescue therapy and or for severe atheroembolism refractory to medical management (Keen *et al.* 1995).

The effect of statins has not been prospectively studied—information is from case reports only. There are, however, good theoretical reasons why they may be of benefit: their plaque stabilizing and antiinflammatory properties may reduce the risk of recurrence of atheroembolism and modify low-grade disease (Woolfson and Lachmann 1998). There are reports advocating plasmapheresis, low-density lipoprotein (LDL) apheresis, and the use of prostaglandin analogues in the treatment of atheroembolism. None of these have shown a clear-cut benefit over standard therapy. Dialysis should be performed with minimal anticoagulation. Patients with atheroembolism have often had previous abdominal surgery and or gastrointestinal ischaemia making peritoneal dialysis impractical. The extra protein loss associated with peritoneal dialysis in already nutritionally compromised patients is another reason to prefer haemodialysis.

The overall mortality of atheroembolism is difficult to quantify because patients will inevitably be at risk of cardiovascular events. Patients with catastrophic atheroembolism leading to cardiac decompensation and renal failure have a 1-year survival of less than 50 per cent (Dahlberg *et al.* 1989). In Belenfant's (1999) series the 1-year mortality was much lower at 23 per cent. Indicators of poor prognosis are recurrent atheroembolism and gastrointestinal involvement. Up to one-third of patients presenting with significant disease will not regain independent renal function.

Occlusion in the presence of pre-existing renal artery stenosis

Acute renal artery occlusion is usually seen in patients with pre-existing long-term atherosclerotic renal artery stenosis.

Progressive occlusion of such an artery is often unrecognized. An apparent acute presentation of progression to occlusion may be the final stage in a much longer process.

Various authors have examined the progression of stenosis to occlusion and the likelihood of this is related to the pre-existing degree of stenosis (Chapter 9.5). Although acute occlusion in a normal renal artery may lead to loin pain and haematuria this does not occur after the occlusion of an already stenosed renal artery. Weibull *et al.* (1990) have shown that in patients known to have renal artery stenosis undergoing repeat angiography, progression to occlusion was only associated with a small change in plasma creatinine and without any symptoms or signs. Postma *et al.* (1989) in a small retrospective study have shown that occlusion is more likely to occur in patients with renal artery stenosis treated with an ACEI and diuretic. Although progression to bilateral occlusion may be associated with severe impairment in renal function, the only conclusive way of diagnosing progression to occlusion is by repeat angiography. Acute occlusion in a solitary functioning kidney will result in a severe decline in renal function. In atherosclerotic disease, contralateral disease is common and may occur in previously normal renal arteries (Schreiber *et al.* 1984). Although atherosclerotic renal artery disease is by far the most common cause of abnormal renal arteries, a number of other conditions may cause renal artery stenosis and occlusion. Fibromuscular dysplasia is less common than atherosclerotic disease and rarely progresses to occlusion. Renal artery aneurysms are rare and require surgical treatment as they may bleed as well as thrombose (Barth 1993).

Occlusion in the absence of pre-existing renal artery stenosis

This is relatively rare but it can present with the symptoms and signs of acute renal ischaemia or infarction (Table 1). Loin pain and haematuria in patients at risk of central arterial thrombus formation should raise the possibility of acute embolism to the renal arteries.

It may occur as the result of embolization from a central cardiac thrombus in patients with atrial fibrillation, valvular heart disease, myocardial infarction, ventricular aneurysm, or dilated cardiomyopathy. Rarely a foreign body such as a bullet following a gunshot wound (Guileyardo *et al.* 1992), may occlude the renal artery. Although the presentation may be classic, Blakely *et al.* (1994) reported a case where a nephritic urinary sediment was present similar to that seen in atheroembolic disease. Acute renal ischaemia may occur after aortic dissection or in Takayasu aortitis (Chapter 9.5). Although the renal arteries are normal in a number of cases, in each of these conditions there is a high incidence of pre-existing renal artery narrowing (Rackson *et al.* 1990; Kerr *et al.* 1994). In both cases, the other manifestations of the aortic disease will determine the outcome and renal support may be necessary.

Acute renal artery thrombosis may occur in patients with an underlying procoagulant state, for example, protein C deficiency or the nephrotic syndrome, but renal vein thrombosis is more common (Shibasaki *et al.* 1992). Renal artery occlusion has been described in a number of patients with antiphospholipid antibodies. In the case described by Ames *et al.* (1992), immune complex deposition in the renal arterial wall was also demonstrated suggesting a more complex pathogenesis than simple *in situ* clot formation due to the procoagulant state. Occlusion has even been reported spontaneously in patients with no underlying clotting disorder (Theiss *et al.* 1992).

Renal artery occlusion can occur with trauma either directly to the kidneys or through a deceleration injury. The latter occurs following a fall from a height where the patient lands on their feet. In this instance, the artery is thought to be acutely stretched on impact and occludes. There are reports of successful revascularization in such cases (Klink *et al.* 1992). Renal artery occlusion may occur in the presence of previous aortic occlusion where thrombosis occurs in the aortic stump and is potentially reversible. Reilly *et al.* (1990) have shown that this is unlikely to occur where the aortic occlusion has been achieved by surgical means. They have shown that in patients surviving more than 1 year after this procedure, no suprarenal propagation of aortic thrombosis was demonstrable. This does not apply to patients with spontaneous aortic occlusion. This is illustrated in a patient who had previously undergone axillofemoral artery anastamosis after aortic occlusion (Fig. 4). She remained well with normal renal function until presenting with acute renal failure (ARF) due to occlusion of the renal arteries (Streather *et al.* 1993). Such patients may represent a high-risk group for thrombotic renal artery occlusion. Pontremoli *et al.* (1990) have reported complete recovery of renal function after surgery for renal artery thrombosis following aortic thrombosis after 43 days of anuria in a 39-year-old patient.

Table 1 Presentations of acute renal ischaemia

Acute loin pain and haematuria
Fever
Acute renal failure
Acute-on-chronic renal failure
Acute pulmonary oedema
Associated with embolic disease elsewhere
Asymptomatic
Rash, myalgia, neurological dysfunction, and other features suggestive of a vasculitis

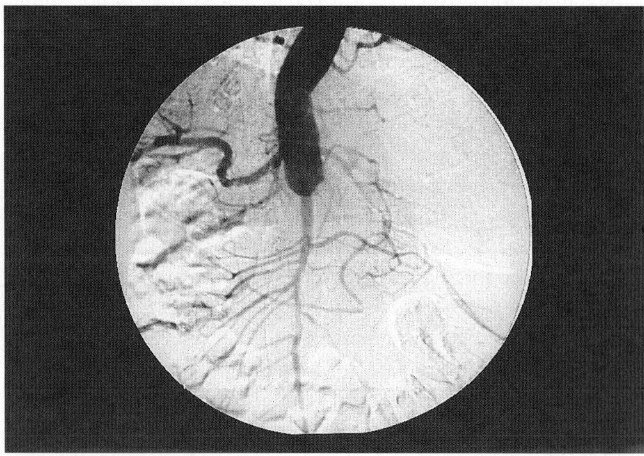

Fig. 4 Angiogram of patient presenting with ARF and known aortic occlusion. Note the absence of any renal arteries.

Acute renal failure due to the use of ACEI in the presence of pre-existing renal disease

Since the original description by Hricik *et al.* (1983) it has been recognized that the use of ACEI in the presence of renal artery stenosis may lead to a decline in function in that kidney. It is now a common cause of ARF in the United Kingdom. If a stenosed renal artery supplies all the functioning renal tissue in a patient then this can result in ARF. Although potentially reversible, as shown in Fig. 5, this renal failure may be irreversible as shown by Kalra *et al.* (1990) in a large series of patients with ARF.

The decline in renal function with the use of ACEI and renal artery stenosis has been attributed to a blockade of the efferent glomerular arteriolar tone. Under normal circumstances this is not important in maintaining filtration but when the afferent arteriolar pressure is lowered due to renal artery stenosis the increase in efferent tone is an important mechanism maintaining glomerular pressure upon which filtration depends. This efferent tone is increased by angiotensin II and

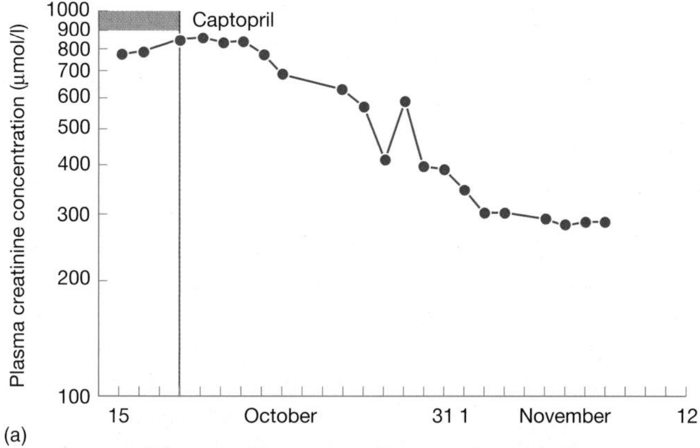

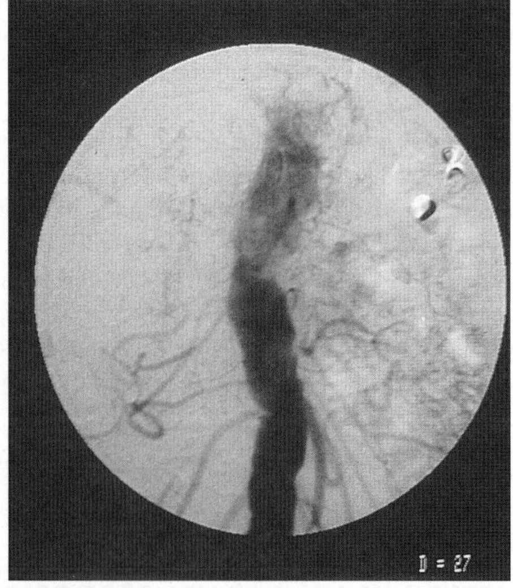

Fig. 5 ACEI-induced acute-on-chronic renal failure. (a) Creatinine concentrations in a patient presenting with ARF showing the improvement on stopping captopril. (b) Angiogram of this patient showing bilateral renal artery occlusion.

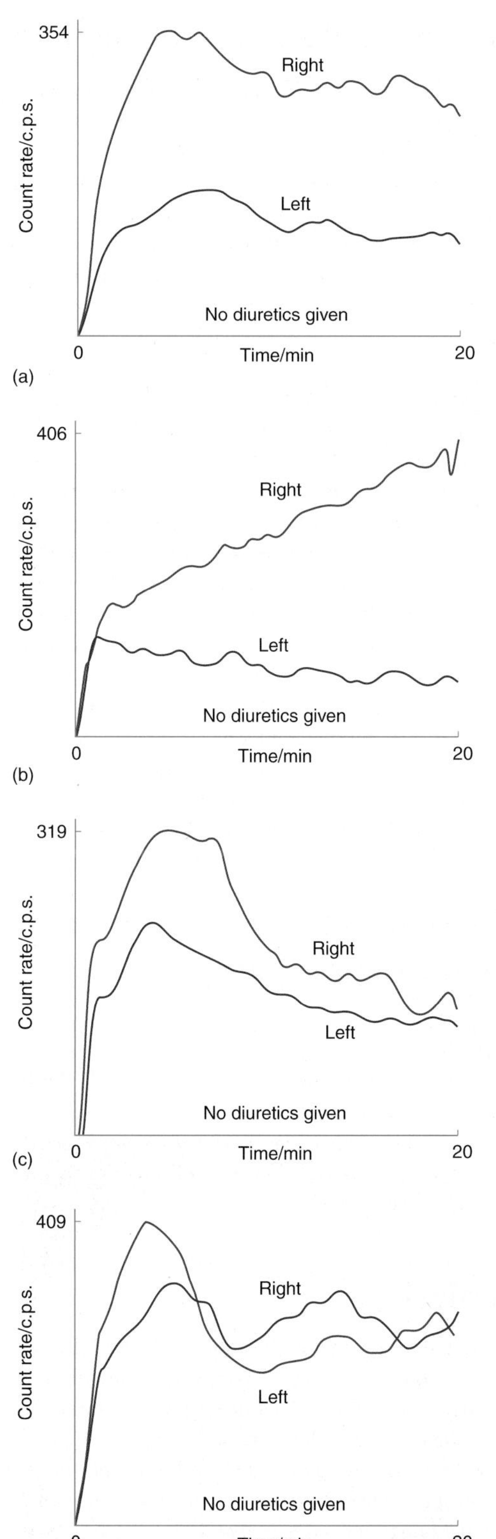

Fig. 6 Pre- and postcaptopril DTPA scans in a patient with bilateral renal artery stenosis and flash pulmonary oedema but normal renal function. (a) Baseline. (b) After captopril 25 mg. (c) Postangioplasty—baseline. (d) Postangioplasty—after captopril 25 mg. Reproduced with permission from Dr A. Hilson.

thus blocked by ACEI. The decline in filtration caused by the decrease in efferent tone (Fig. 6) should not lead to an alteration in renal blood flow; in fact it should slightly increase.

An important problem with the use of ACEI in renal artery stenosis is that the renal lesion is often asymptomatic. We have shown that 50 per cent of patients with renal failure caused by renovascular disease were on ACEI at the time of presentation (Scoble *et al.* 1989). In none of the cases was the diagnosis of ischaemic nephropathy suspected by the referring physicians. As discussed earlier, some authors have suggested a role of ACEI in acute renal artery thrombosis in the presence of renal artery stenosis (Pontremoli *et al.* 1990; Hannedouche *et al.* 1991). This may relate to a fall in systemic blood pressure as much as a change in intrarenal haemodynamics. Kalra *et al.* (1990) have found that in one-third of the 16 per cent of cases of ARF attributed by them to renovascular disease the use of ACEI contributed to the ARF. The long-term effects of ACEI in kidneys with renal artery stenosis may be profound and irreversible (Jackson *et al.* 1990).

The use of ACEI in patients with symptomatic peripheral vascular disease may be hazardous unless renal artery stenosis has been excluded.

Latrogenic renal artery occlusion

Occlusion due to dissection or thrombosis may occur during the process of renal angioplasty (Hayes *et al.* 1989). This is illustrated in Fig. 7 where attempted renal angioplasty created a false intramural passage which then thrombosed. If the dissection or thrombus is diagnosed at the time of the procedure then the use of fibrinolytic agents or stents may be useful (Salam *et al.* 1993). At the time of angioplasty there may be sufficient disruption of the arterial wall to stimulate clot formation leading to occlusion. This is probably the only time when thrombolysis is of proven use in renal artery occlusion.

The increasing use of intra-aortic stent graft placement for management of abdominal aortic aneurysms has led to an issue with these stents being placed over the renal artery ostium. Stents can be either 'uncovered' or 'covered'. 'Covered' stents have a fabric covering which lies outside the metal mesh of the expanded stent. Individual stents may be part covered and part uncovered. If the part of the stent that

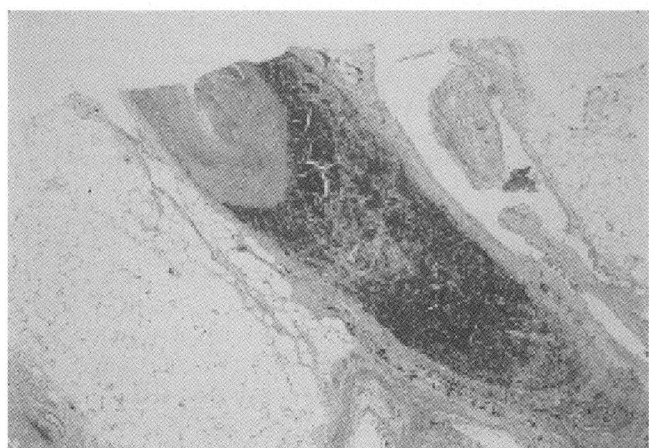

Fig. 7 Renal arterial dissection after attempted renal angioplasty. Reproduced with permission from Dr P. O'Donnell.

overlies the renal ostium is 'uncovered', that is, is just a metal mesh, then renal dysfunction does not occur.

Renal vein thrombosis

Renal vein thrombosis may lead to acute renal impairment. The classic clinical manifestations are of loin pain and haematuria. MRI may show that the incidence is higher than presently recognized.

Anatomical abnormalities of the renal veins are less well described than renal artery abnormalities. Renal vein thrombosis is more likely in the presence of clotting abnormalities. Formstone *et al.* (1996) have described a case of perinatal renal vein thrombosis associated with protein S and C mutations. The most common association is the nephrotic syndrome. An early study by Llach *et al.* (1985) showed that 22 per cent developed renal vein thrombosis. There has been much discussion as to the cause of this. It may also occur with trauma to the renal vein (Blackenship *et al.* 1997).

The investigations of renal vein thrombosis were previously dependent on renal venography. However, the advent of MRI scans has meant that renal vein imaging may be performed non-invasively (Kanagasundaram *et al.* 1998).

Treatment is with anticoagulation although there are reports of the use of thrombolytic therapy (Markowitz *et al.* 1995). These authors reviewed the 21 cases of renal vein thrombosis treated by thrombolysis. In one case, thrombolytic therapy for renal vein thrombosis resulted in a resolution of proteinuria (Morrissey *et al.* 1997).

Investigation and management of acute ischaemic nephropathy

The diagnosis of acute renal ischaemia will depend on a high clinical index of suspicion. The presence of atherosclerotic disease elsewhere will be by far the most common suggestive feature. Other factors such as the possibility of central thrombus formation or abnormal clotting state may be important as shown in Table 2. Associations of findings such as a normal renal outline on ultrasound but no function on dimethyl triethyl penta-acetic acid (DTPA) scanning or intravenous urogram suggests renal artery occlusion. Investigation will depend on what is available at the renal centre. MRI scanning is very useful but may not be able to differentiate peripheral lesions (Ghantous *et al.* 1999; Andreoni *et al.* 2002). Intra-arterial angiography is the usual method of investigation in many units but in itself may contribute to the renal dysfunction by generating atheroemboli. In a number of cases investigation of the associated disorders such as trauma or aortic dissection may be more important than the diagnosis of the cause for the acute renal ischaemia.

Table 2 Causes of acute renal ischaemia

Causes
In the presence of abnormal renal arteries
Thrombosis of a previously stenosed renal artery
Occlusion of a previously stenosed renal artery secondary to drug treatment
ARF associated with use of ACEI in the presence of renal artery stenosis
Atheroembolism
Thrombosis in a renal artery aneurysm
Latrogenic vessel damage at angioplasty of the renal artery
In the presence of normal renal arteries
Embolization from central thrombus
Aortic dissection
Takayasu aortitis
Aortic occlusion and thrombosis leading to renal artery occlusion
Trauma
Acute thrombosis caused by coagulation abnormality
Bullet embolism
Idiopathic

Management of acute ischaemic nephropathy

The management of the patient will be directed first to the most pressing clinical problem. In situations such as aortic dissection or atheroembolic disease, supportive renal replacement therapy will take priority and no direct effort to reverse the acute renal ischaemia can be made. In acute occlusion with normal renal arteries, there is unlikely to be underlying renal disease. Unless the embolization or occlusion is bilateral, the contralateral kidney should provide sufficient renal function. Management of the occlusion should be based on prevention of a reoccurrence if the contralateral kidney is intact. The need for revascularization will not be the same as in occlusion in the presence of pre-existing stenosis because collateral blood supply will not have had time to develop and the kidney is more likely to infarct.

Conservative management of acute ischaemic nephropathy

The management of ARF associated with the use of ACEI will obviously start with withdrawing the drug. This may result in a dramatic improvement of renal function as shown in Fig. 5. In this case neither renal artery was identified by angiography and the kidney relied on the collateral blood flow. This patient avoided the need for acute dialysis by stopping the ACEI. Urgent angiography should be performed in patients with ARF where renal occlusion is suspected.

Fibrinolysis

Fibrinolysis with intra-arterial recombinant tissue plasminogen activator (TPa), urokinase or streptokinase may be useful in acute occlusion. An early report showed that heparinization alone was sufficient to restore patency of an occluded renal artery in a patient with a renal embolus secondary to atrial fibrillation (Moyer *et al.* 1973). A number of cases have been reported where excellent results were obtained in terms of renal function (Kennedy *et al.* 1991). Salam *et al.* (1993) have reported fibrinolytic therapy in a larger series. The cause of occlusion included thrombosis of pre-existing stenosis, renal artery embolism, complicating renal angioplasty, and aortic occlusion. In only one of the four cases that presented with ARF was renal function restored (Salam *et al.* 1993). Although there are case reports of success, there are no large series supporting the efficacy of fibrinolytic agents. With modern radiological techniques, fibrinolysis remains a minimally invasive method of initial treatment of occlusion. Surgery in this situation can be delayed for a considerable period with an excellent outcome even in the presence of anuria. If there is evidence to suggest recent occlusion or thrombosis following renal arterial instrumentation, then fibrinolysis should be considered.

Surgery and angioplasty

The speed of intervention required will depend on whether there is significant collateral supply to the kidney present. This will, in turn, depend on whether there has been low-grade chronic renal ischaemia prior to the acute ischaemic event. Interventions such as thrombolysis are indicated in cases of embolization to previously normal renal arteries. Surgery, however, can be delayed for a considerable period in patients where occlusion has occurred after prolonged renal artery stenosis.

Angioplasty may prove useful in restoring renal function in patients presenting acutely with atherosclerotic renovascular disease but significant complications have been reported (O'Donovan *et al.* 1992). Correction of other factors will often, in the short-term, prove as important in making these patients' dialysis independent as acute angioplasty as illustrated in Fig. 5. If the initial management can improve renal function then the management of the long-standing underlying renal arterial disease can be considered without the need for immediate intervention. In some patients they may choose to have no intervention and settle for dialysis, especially if major surgery is required.

There have, however, been a number of reports of surgical treatment of acute renal artery occlusion by embolectomy or revascularization in a solitary kidney resulting in restoration of normal renal function even after a period of anuria (Baird *et al.* 1965; Perkins *et al.* 1967; Smith *et al.* 1968, 1974; Williams *et al.* 1988; Kaylor *et al.* 1989). Schonwald *et al.* (1978) reported recovery of renal function after anuria with preservation of renal function for 9 years. Surgery may be delayed for a considerable period in such cases even in the presence of anuria as shown by the case reported by Pontremoli *et al.* (1990) of resolution of function after 43 days of anuria. Surgical treatment with renal artery occlusion should be considered for patients even if prolonged periods of anuria have occurred.

Conclusion

Acute renal ischaemia due to thrombosis, embolus, or atheroembolus may present obviously with symptoms or signs of renal infarction. In more cases the presentation will be asymptomatic or with features of renal failure or systemic vasculitis. It is an important diagnosis to make as effective treatment, whether conservative, fibrinolysis, angioplasty, or surgery, may result in excellent return of renal function even after prolonged anuria. The coexisting disease will often determine the patient's longevity.

Preservation of renal function is an important goal even if it may not provide an increased lifespan to patients with acute ischaemic nephropathy.

References

Ames, P. R. J. *et al.* (1992). Bilateral renal artery occlusion in a patient with primary antiphospholipid antibody syndrome: thrombosis, vasculitis or both? *Journal of Rheumatology* **19**, 1802–1806.

Andreoni, K. A. *et al.* (2002). Incidence of donor renal fibromuscular dysplasia: does it justify routine angiography? *Transplantation* **73**, 1112–1116.

Baird, R. J., Yndt, E. R., and Firor, W. B. (1965). Anuria due to acute occlusion of the artery to a solitary kidney. *New England Journal of Medicine* **272**, 1012–1014.

Barth, R. A. (1993). Fibromuscular dysplasia with clotted renal artery aneurysm. *Pediatric Radiology* **23**, 296–297.

Belenfant, X., Meyrier, A., and Jacquot, C. (1999). Supportive treatment improves survival in multivisceral cholesterol crystal embolism. *American Journal of Kidney Diseases* **33**, 840–850.

Belenfant *et al.* (Case records) (1991). Case 2-1991. *New England Journal of Medicine* **324**, 113–120.

Blakely, P., Cosby, R. L., and McDonald, B. R. (1994). Nephritic urinary sediment in embolic renal disease. *Clinical Nephrology* **42**, 401–403.

Blakenship, B., Earls, J. P., and Talner, L. B. (1997). Renal vein thrombosis after vascular pedicle injury. *American Journal of Roentgenology* **168**, 1574.

Dahlberg, P. J., Frecentese, D. F., and Cogbill, T. H. (1989). Cholesterol embolism: experience with 22 histologically proven cases. *Surgery* **105**, 737–746.

Flory, C. M. (1945). Arterial occlusions produced by emboli from eroded aortic atheromatous plaques. *American Journal of Pathology* **21**, 549–565.

Formstone, C. J. *et al.* (1996). Severe perinatal thrombosis in double and triple heterozygous offspring of a family segregating two independent protein S mutations and a protein C mutation. *Blood* **87**, 3731–3737.

Ghantous, V. E., Eisen, T. D., Sherman, A. H., and Finkelstein, F. O. (1999). Evaluating patients with renal failure for renal artery stenosis with gadolinium-enhanced magnetic resonance angiography. *American Journal of Kidney Diseases* **33**, 36–42.

Guileyardo, J. M., Cooper, R. E., Porter, B. E., and McCorkle, J. L. (1992). Renal artery bullet embolism. *American Journal of Forensic Medicine and Pathology* **13**, 288–289.

Haas, M., Spargo, B. H., Wit, E. J. C., and Meehan, S. M. (2000). Etiologies and outcome of acute renal insufficiency in older adults: a renal biopsy study of 259 cases. *American Journal of Kidney Diseases* **35**, 433–447.

Hannedouche, T., Godin, M., Fries, D., and Fillastre, J. P. (1991). Acute renal thrombosis induced by angiotensin-converting enzyme inhibitors in patients with renovascular hypertension. *Nephron* **57**, 230–231.

Hannedouche, T. *et al.* (1986). Necrotizing glomerulonephritis and renal cholesterol embolization. *Nephron* **42**, 271–272.

Hayes, J. M. *et al.* (1989). Experience with transluminal angioplasty for renal artery stenosis at the Cleveland Clinic. *The Journal of Urology* **139**, 488–492.

Hricik, D. E., Browning, P. J., Kopelman, R., Goorno, W. E., Madias, N. E., and Dzau, V. J. (1983). Captopril-induced functional renal insufficiency in patients with bilateral renal-artery stenoses or renal-artery stenosis in a solitary kidney. *New England Journal of Medicine* **308**, 373–376.

Jackson, B., Franze, L., Sumithran, E., and Johnston, C. I. (1990). Pharmacological nephrectomy with chronic angiotensin converting enzyme inhibitor treatment in renovascular hypertension in the rat. *Journal of Laboratory and Clinical Medicine* **115**, 21–27.

Kalra, P. S., Mamtora, H., Holmes, A. M., and Waldek, S. (1990). Renovascular disease and renal complications of angiotensin-converting enzyme inhibitor therapy. *Quarterly Journal of Medicine* **282**, 1013.

Kanagasundaram, N. S., Bandopadhyay, D., Brownjohn, A. M., and Meaney, J. F. M. (1998). The diagnosis of renal vein thrombosis by magnetic resonance angiography. *Nephrology, Dialysis, Transplantation* **13**, 200–202.

Kaylor, W. M., Novick, A. C., Ziegelbaum, M., and Vidt, D. G. (1989). Reversal of end stage renal failure with surgical revascularization in patients with atherosclerotic renal artery occlusion. *Journal of Urology* **141**, 486–488.

Keen, R. R. *et al.* (1995). Surgical management of atheroembolization. *Journal of Vascular Surgery* **21**, 773–781.

Kennedy, J. S., Gerety, B. M., Silverman, R., Pattison, M. E., Siskind, M. S., and Popnd, G. D. (1991). Simultaneous renal arterial and venous thrombosis associated with idiopathic nephrotic syndrome: treatment with intra-arterial urokinase. *American Journal of Medicine* **90**, 124–127.

Kerr, G. S. *et al.* (1994). Takayasu arteritis. *Annals of Internal Medicine* **120**, 919–929.

Klink, B. K., Sutherin, S., Heyse, P., and McCarthy, M. C. (1992). Traumatic bilateral renal artery thrombosis diagnosed by computed tomography with successful revascularization. *Journal of Trauma* **32**, 259–262.

LLach, F. (1985). Hypercoaguability, renal vein thrombosis and other thrombotic complications of nephrotic syndrome. *Kidney International* **28**, 429–439.

Lye, W. C., Cheah, J. S., and Sinniah, R. (1993). Renal cholesterol embolic disease. *American Journal of Nephrology* **13**, 489–493.

Markowitz, G. S., Brignol, F., Burns, E. R., Koenigsberg, M., and Folkert, V. W. (1995). Renal vein thrombosis treated with thrombolytic therapy: case report and brief review. *American Journal of Kidney Diseases* **25**, 801–806.

Mayo, R. R. and Swartz, R. D. (1996). Redefining the incidence of clinically detectable atheroembolism. *American Journal of Medicine* **100**, 524–529.

Moolenaar, W. and Lamer, C. B. H. W. (1996). Cholesterol crystal embolisation to the alimentary tract. *Gut* **38**, 196–200.

Morrissey, E. C., McDonald, B. R., and Rabetoy, G. M. (1997). Resolution of proteinuria secondary to bilateral renal vein thrombosis after treament with systemic thrombolytic therapy. *American Journal of Kidney Diseases* **29**, 615–619.

Moyer, J. D., Rao, C. N., Widrich, W. C., and Olsson, C. A. (1973). Conservative management of renal artery embolus. *Journal of Urology* **109**, 138–143.

O'Donovan, R. M., Gutierrez, O. H., and Izzo, J. L. (1992). Preservation of renal function by percutaneous renal angioplasty in high risk elderly patients: short term outcome. *Nephron* **60**, 187–192.

Perkins, R. P., Jacobsen, D. S., Feder, F. P., Lipchik, E. O., and Fine, P. H. (1967). Return of renal function after late embolectomy. *New England Journal of Medicine* **276**, 1194–1195.

Pontremoli, R., Rampoldi, V., Morbidelli, A., Fiorini, F., Ranise, A., and Garibotto, G. (1990). Acute renal failure due to acute bilateral renal artery thrombosis: successful surgical revascularization after prolonged anuria. *Nephron* **56**, 322–324.

Postma, C. T., Hoefnagels, W. H. L., Barentsz, J. O., de Boo, T., and Thien, T. (1989). Occlusion of unilateral stenosed renal arteries—relation to medical treatment. *Journal of Human Hypertension* **3**, 185–190.

Rackson, M. E., Lossef, S. V., and Sos, T. A. (1990). Renal artery stenosis in patients with aortic dissection: increased prevalence. *Radiology* **177**, 555–558.

Reilly, L. M., Sauer, L., Weinstein, E. S., Ehrenfeld, W. K., Goldstone, J., and Stoney, R. J. (1990). Infrarenal aortic occlusion: does it threaten renal perfusion or function? *Journal of Vascular Surgery* **11**, 216–225.

Salam, T. A., Lumsden, A. B., and Martin, L. G. (1993). Local infusion of fibrinolytic agents for acute renal artery thromboembolism: report of ten cases. *Annals of Vascular Surgery* **7**, 21–26.

Schonwald, H. N., Campbell, E. W., and Galleher, E. P. (1978). Anuria secondary to renal artery obstruction in a solitary kidney: 9 year followup. *Journal of Urology* **120**, 618–619.

Schreiber, M. J., Pohl, M. A., and Novick, A. C. (1984). The natural history of atherosclerotic and fibrous renal artery disease. *Urological Clinics of North America* **11**, 383–392.

Scoble, J. E., Maher, E. R., Hamilton, G., Dick, R., Sweny, P., and Moorhead, J. F. (1989). Atherosclerotic renovascular disease causing renal impairment—a case for treatment. *Clinical Nephrology* **31**, 119–122.

Shibasaki, T., Ishimoto, F., Kodama, K., Ohno, I., and Sakai, O. (1992). Renal artery thrombosis in a patient with membranous glomerulonephritis. *Internal Medicine* **31**, 294–297.

Smith, H. T., Shapiro, F. I., and Messner, R. P. (1968). Anuria secondary to renovascular disease. *Journal of the American Medical Association* **204**, 928–930.

Smith, S. P., Hamburger, R. J., Donohue, J. P., and Grim, C. E. (1974). Occlusion of the artery to a solitary kidney. *Journal of the American Medical Association* **230**, 1306–1307.

Streather, C. *et al.* (1993). Progression of occlusive renal vascular disease and axillo-femoral bypass grafts. *Nephrology, Dialysis, Transplantation* **8**, 1186–1187.

Thadhani, R., Pascual, M., Nickeleit, V., Tolkoff-Rubin, N., and Colvin, R. (1996). Preliminary description of focal segmental glomerulosclerosis in patients with renovascular disease. *Lancet* **347**, 231–233.

Theiss, M., Wirth, M. P., Dolken, W., and Frohmuller, H. G. (1992). Spontaneous thrombosis of the renal vessels. Rare entities to be considered in differential diagnosis of patients presenting with lumbar flank pain and haematuria. *Urology International* **48**, 441–445.

Thurlbeck, W. M. and Castleman, B. (1957). Atheromatous emboli to the kidneys after aortic surgery. *The New England Journal of Medicine* **257**, 442–447.

Vidt, D. G., Eisele, G., Gephardt, G. N., Tubbs, R., and Novick, A. C. (1989). Atheroembolic renal disease: association with renal artery stenosis. *Cleveland Clinic Journal of Medicine* **56**, 407–413.

Weibull, H., Bergqvist, D., Andersson, I., Choi, D. L., Jonsson, K., and Bergentz, S. E. (1990). Symptoms and signs of thrombotic occlusion of atherosclerotic renal artery stenosis. *European Journal of Vascular Surgery* **15**, 161–165.

Williams, B., Feehally, J., Attard, A. R., and Bell, P. R. F. (1988). Recovery of renal function after delayed revascularisation of acute occlusion of the renal artery. *British Medical Journal* **296**, 1591–1592.

Woolfson, R. G. and Lachmann, H. (1998). Improvement in renal cholesterol emboli syndrome after simvastatin. *Lancet* **351**, 1331–1332.

Yune, H. Y. and Klatte, E. C. (1976). Collateral circulation to an ischemic kidney. *Radiology* **119**, 539–546.

10.6.6 Hantavirus infection

Charles van Ypersele

Viral infections induce not only glomerular but acute interstitial lesions. Several viruses, regrouped in the *Hantavirus* genus of the *Bunyaviridae* family (Table 1), are the most frequently recognized agents, responsible yearly for over 100,000 cases of infectious acute interstitial nephritis throughout Eurasia. The disease, now named haemorrhagic fever with renal syndrome (HFRS) or hantavirus disease, has a severe form, mainly in Asia, and mild forms mainly in Europe.

The hantavirus

The *Hantavirus* genus is part of the *Bunyaviridae* family. It regroups several serotypes that possess a single-stranded, three-segmented, negative-sense RNA genome (Giebel *et al.* 1989). The large (L = 8.2 kb), the medium (M = 3.6 kb), and the small (S = 1.7 kb) genome segments are enclosed in three separate nucleocapsid structures, and are surrounded by a lipid envelope containing two virus-specific glycoproteins, G1 and G2. The L segment probably encodes the viral polymerase, the S segment the nucleocapsid protein, and the M segment the G1 and G2 glycoproteins.

Hantaviruses infect various animal species worldwide: rodents and insectivores, as well as mammals such as cats (Clement *et al.* 1998).

Table 1 List of virus serotypes regrouped in the hantavirus group

Virus	Location	Reservoir	Human disease
Prospect Hill	USA	*Microtus pennsylvanicus*	None
Puumala	Europe (NW and Eastern Europe, Balkans)	*Clethrionomys glareolus*	Mild (renal)
Dobrava	Europe (Balkans)	*Apodemus flavicollis*	Severe (renal)
Seoul	Worldwide	*Rattus norvegicus*	Moderate–severe (renal)
Hantaan	Asia an S. Europe	*Apodemus agragrius*	Severe (renal)
Sin Nombre	USA	*Peromyscus maniculatus*	Severe (pulmonary)

Up to now, only rodents seem to act as a reservoir and contaminate humans who inhale aerosols of virus-containing particles excreted through lung, saliva, and urine. The virus may be lethal for sucklings, but is usually harmless for the adult rodents. Still it can be recognized by immunostaining in many organs, including the lungs where the primary target seems to be the vascular endothelium.

An increasing number of hantaviruses has been recognized, both by serotyping and by nucleotide sequencing: most of them are associated with a specific rodent reservoir. Clinical manifestations of infection depend on the type of the hantavirus. Some serotypes cause an acute renal syndrome, the topic of this section, others are responsible for a recently recognized acute respiratory distress syndrome with a poor prognosis, the so-called hantavirus pulmonary syndrome (Table 1) (Zaki *et al.* 1995).

Clinical features of hantavirus renal disease

The severity of the disease depends mainly on the hantavirus serotype (Clement *et al.* 1998), but also on genetically determined host factors (Mustonen *et al.* 1996) (Table 1). As each serotype has its own geographical distribution, the clinical picture of hantavirus disease varies worldwide. In the Americas, despite the fact that over 25 hantavirus serotypes have been identified in wild rodents and that antibodies have been observed in several subjects, only a few clinical cases of renal disease have been described (Hindrichsen *et al.* 1993; Glass *et al.* 1994). These identified serotypes are different from that responsible for the acute pulmonary syndrome. In Europe, the Puumala serotype is widely distributed. It induces a mild form of the disease. The Dobrava serotype, recognized in the Balkans, is associated with a severe hantavirus disease. In Asia, the Hantaan and the Seoul serotypes produce a severe and a moderate form of the disease, respectively.

Hantavirus disease in Europe

In Europe, hantavirus disease is mainly due to the Puumala serotype, whose animal reservoir is the red bank vole, *Clethrionomys glareolus*. It is endemic and, occasionally, epidemic in Scandinavia (where it was known as Nephropathia epidemica), western Europe, the Balkans, and the western part of the Russia (where it was known as haemorrhagic nephroso nephritis).

It affects mainly young men (male : female, 4 : 1) working in rural areas infested by rodents. Its prevalence is determined both by the growth of the infected rodent population and by the chance of contact with humans. In cold Scandinavia, prevalence peaks during the winter when rodents seek shelter in human habitats. In warmer Belgium and northern France, it peaks during the early summer, when workers are in the fields in contact with an expanding rodent population and in early winter when rodents are sheltering in barns.

The incubation period lasts between 10 and 30 days.

Clinical manifestations

The clinical manifestations of the Puumala virus infection run a two-phase course (Lahdevirta 1971; van Ypersele and Mery 1989). The first phase lasts between 4 and 14 days. It is invariably characterized by the sudden onset of fever (38–40.5°C), frequently with chills, and is rapidly associated, in most cases, with headaches, myalgias, occasionally with acute myopia and conjunctival injection or haemorrhages and more rarely with photophobia, pharyngitis, and productive cough (Table 2). Early in the development of the disease patients are often given analgesics and sometimes antibiotics which may erroneously be incriminated in the subsequent onset of renal failure.

Within an average of 2 days after the onset of fever, patients complain of loin pain occasionally associated with abdominal pain. Loin pain is sometimes unilateral (often right sided) and intense enough to mimic renal colic. The clinical picture is further complicated by nausea, occasionally culminating in profuse vomiting, and by diarrhoea. These symptoms usually subside within 10 days of the onset of fever. Central nervous system involvement manifests between days 4 and 10, not only as transient acute myopia and photophobia but also with signs of meningeal irritation. Respiratory signs have been reported in up to 24 per cent of the patients. They range from cough with auscultatory abnormalities to rare cases of acute respiratory distress syndrome requiring ventilation (Clement *et al.* 1994).

The second phase of the disease is characterized by acute renal failure. Its onset is heralded by oliguria (between days 3 and 19) or by the discovery of biochemical evidence of renal failure (usually at about day 7). Fever, loin pain, and most digestive symptoms have usually disappeared by then. The serum creatinine increases rapidly to peak values ranging from 242 to 1575 μmol/l (between days 4 and 25). Haemo- or peritoneal dialysis is required in less than 10 per cent of the patients. Renal function improves rapidly thereafter: serum creatinine returns to less than 150 μmol/l on day 18 in 50 per cent and on day 33 in over 75 per cent of the patients.

Table 2 Clinical and laboratory features (expressed as percentage of investigated patients)

	Puumala[a] virus $n = 152$	Seoul[b] virus $n = 40$	Hantaan[b] virus $n = 104$
Fever	100	100	100
White cell count			
$>8 \times 10^9$/l	79	—	—
$>10 \times 10^9$/l	—	75	91
$>30 \times 10^9$/l	—	7	20
Loin or abdominal pain	86		95
Abdominal pain	—	28	—
Headache	87	45	—
Acute myopia	17	9	52
Nausea, vomiting	48	59	—
Bradycardia	29	27	73
Conjunctival haemorrhage	18	8	—
Petechiae	—	43	95
Minor bleeding	—	18	37
Internal bleeding	—	5	34
Platelet count			
100×10^9/l	45	80	88
50×10^9/l	—	26	63
Creatinine			
>133 µmol/l	100	—	—
>884 µmol/l	—	17	42
Proteinuria	97	100	100
Microhaematuria	71	—	—
Urine output < 400 ml	63	50	53–63%
Mortality	<1%	0	3–7%

[a] Combined data from Lähdevirta (1971) and van Ypersele and Méry (1989).

[b] Personal communication from Dr J. S. Lee.

Proteinuria of variable severity (0.1–29 g/l) is virtually always present within the first 2 weeks but disappears rapidly thereafter. It is often accompanied by transient microscopic haematuria and leucocyturia.

On hospital admission (on day 7 on the average) blood pressure is often normal; but mild hypertension is recorded in one-third and hypotension in 10 per cent of the patients, a few of whom may progress to shock. Bradycardia (<60 beats/min) is noted occasionally. Enlargement of the kidneys is demonstrated clinically or by imaging techniques (ultrasound or plain X-ray of the abdomen) in most patients. Hepatomegaly and, more rarely, splenomegaly may be detected.

Thrombocytopenia is one of the most characteristic findings in the disease. It is observed in over half the patients, reaches its nadir (mean 62×10^9/l) on day 7 and returns to normal by about day 12. It is associated with a transient, usually mild, increase of serum enzymes: lactic dehydrogenases, creatine phosphokinase, and transaminases (serum glutamic oxaloacetic transaminase, serum glutamic pyruvic transaminase, and γ–glutamyl transferase). A small increase in bilirubin (maximum 40 µmol/l) is observed in less than 10 per cent of the subjects. More recently a reduction in serum cholesterol (as low as 1.4 mmol/l) and increased serum triglycerides have been observed (Colson *et al.* 1995).

An acute inflammatory reaction, present in virtually all patients, peaks during the second week and includes an elevated erythrocyte sedimentation rate, elevated fibrinogen, and a moderate leucocytosis (average 12.4×10^9/l). Mild intravascular coagulation is suggested by slightly increased fibrin degradation products observed in over one-third of the patients. Severe disseminated intravascular coagulation is present in less than 1 per cent of the cases.

This picture of hantavirus disease should not obscure the fact that the infection may be even milder: the existence of a large discrepancy between the prevalence of elevated antibody titres in the population and the reported incidence of the disease suggests that the disease is often clinically silent (van Ypersele and Méry 1989). Eventual confirmation of the diagnosis relies on the demonstration of an at least four fold increase of hantavirus antibody titres within 1–3 weeks after the onset of the disease.

Histological data

Mild mesangial proliferation may be observed but the main lesions are interstitial and comprise oedema and conspicuous mononuclear infiltrates in the medulla and, occasionally, medullary interstitial haemorrhages (Figs 1 and 2). Neither immune nor fibrin deposits are found by standard immunofluorescence techniques.

Prognosis

Fatal cases are exceptional in northern, western, or southern Europe. Renal function returns to normal with, occasionally, mild tubular lesions and hypertension (Makelä *et al.* 2000).

In eastern and central Europe and in the Balkans the mild form of the disease coexists with a more severe form characterized by a more marked haemorrhagic tendency and shock, with eventual death in a few cases. This latter clinical picture has been associated with Dobrava virus and occasionally with a Hantaan-like serotype (Clement *et al.* 1998) (Table 1). Epidemiological studies performed in the United States suggest that a mild, clinically silent, form of rat borne (Seoul-like hantavirus) HFRS may result in the late onset of hypertension (Glass *et al.* 1993), a hypothesis at variance with European studies concerning infections with the Puumala serotype (Makelä *et al.* 2000).

Diagnosis

The diagnosis rests on the serological evidence of hantavirus infection. As antibody titres remain elevated for more than 15 years, the discovery by ELISA assay of a high IgG antibody titre may not be diagnostic in an endemic area. The presence of IgM antibodies or an at least fourfold increase of the IgG antibody titre may be required. The more recently developed IgM enzyme immunoassay is now generally accepted as the serological prerequisite for confirming suspected clinical cases (Clement *et al.* 1998).

The patient should be asked about exposure to wild rodents up to 5 weeks prior to the onset of the disease. The diagnosis is suggested by the clinical picture: abrupt onset, fever, pain (abdomen, loin, headache), increased serum creatinine, proteinuria and/or haematuria, subsequent polyuria. If four or more of these six criteria are present,

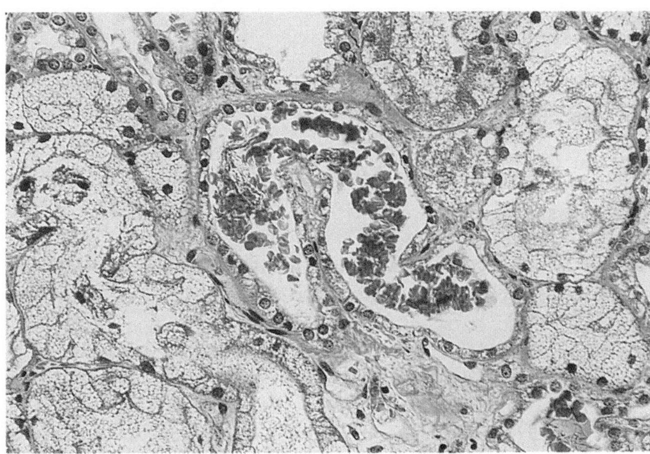

Fig. 1 Red cells within the tubule (reproduced from van Ypersele de Strihou and Méry 1989, with permission).

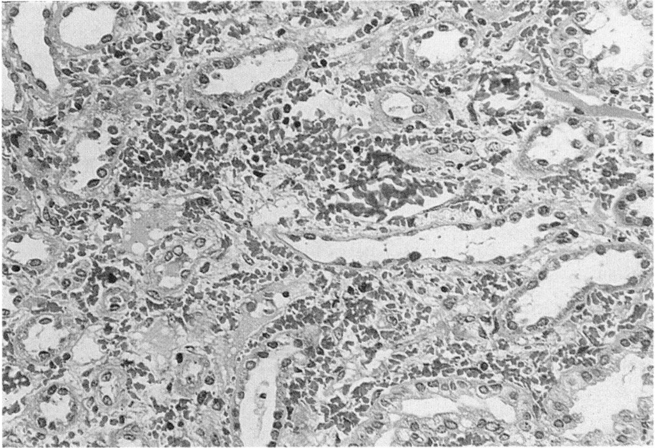

Fig. 2 Renal biopsy on the eleventh day of the disease; note the interstitial haemorrhage in the medulla (reproduced from van Ypersele de Strihou and Méry 1989, with permission).

the diagnosis can be made with a sensitivity of 97 per cent and a specificity of 93 per cent (Settergren *et al.* 1988).

Two other causes of acute interstitial nephritis should be considered in the differential diagnosis. The first is that induced by non-steroidal anti-inflammatory drugs (NSAIDs). As NSAIDs may have been taken for loin pain induced by hantavirus disease, it is important to recognize the findings which allow differentiation of the two conditions: in NSAID-induced interstitial nephritis, loin pain appears after NSAID consumption and there are neither signs of central nervous involvement nor thrombocytopenia or conjunctival haemorrhages. The second pitfall is that of leptospirosis with acute renal failure (Weil's disease). This diagnosis should be suspected if there is a history of contact with stagnant water in rural or farming environments. The patient usually presents acutely unwell and with severe jaundice, both features that are unusual in the European form of hantavirus disease (Table 3).

Treatment

Only supportive therapy is necessary.

Table 3 Differential diagnosis of hantavirus disease

	Hantavirus	NSAID	Leptospirosis (severe form)
Fever	+	−	+
CNS involvement	+	−	+
Jaundice	−	−	+
Thrombocytopenia	+	−	+
Conjunctival haemorrhages	+	−	+

Hantavirus disease in Asia

The disease is mainly due to the Hantaan virus (animal reservoir is the striped field mouse, *Apodemus agrarius*) and to the Seoul virus (animal reservoir is the urban rat, *R. norvegicus* and *Rattus rattus*). It is endemic in China (where it is known as epidemic haemorrhagic fever), Korea (where it is known as Korean haemorrhagic fever), and the eastern part of Russia. The rural form, due to the Hantaan virus is severe, affects mainly young men, farmers, and soldiers, and peaks in late spring and autumn. The urban form, caused by the Seoul virus, is less severe. It occurs throughout the year, tending to be more frequent in the autumn and early winter. The annual incidence exceeds 100,000 cases.

The clinical manifestations of the Hantaan and Seoul virus infection are much more severe than those elicited by the Puumala virus in Europe (Lee and Van der Groen 1989). They can be subdivided into five phases. The first phase lasts from 3 to 7 days and is characterized by the sudden onset of high fever, myalgias, followed by headache, severe abdominal and loin pain. Typically, there is an erythematous flush of the face, neck, and upper chest with injection of the conjunctivae, palate, and pharynx. These signs culminate in conjunctival haemorrhages and oral or cutaneous petechiae spread in the axillary pits, the upper chest, and the face. The second phase develops abruptly with severe hypotension lasting from a few hours to 2 days, progressing in some patients to a clinical state of shock with eventual death. Capillary haemorrhages are prominent when the platelet count reaches a nadir. The third phase starts with the onset of oliguria during the late shock phase. It lasts from 3 to 7 days despite the gradual return of the blood pressure to normal. Proteinuria and microscopic haematuria are present. One-third of the patients develop extensive purpura, cerebral haemorrhage, and gastrointestinal bleeding. Pulmonary oedema and central nervous system involvement predominate. About 50 per cent of the fatalities occur during this phase. The fourth phase may last a few weeks. It is heralded by the onset of diuresis followed by a striking polyuria. The last phase is that of convalescence: within 2–3 months anaemia disappears and renal function returns to normal.

Thrombocytopenia is often profound (10×10^9–20×10^9/l), associated with elevated serum fibrin degradation products (Lee *et al.* 1989). Leucocytosis is very frequent and severe. Just as in the European form, liver enzymes are elevated and an acute phase response is present (Table 2). Overall the clinical course of Hantaan virus infection is mild (i.e. without haemorrhagic phenomena) in 30 per cent, moderate in 50 per cent, and severe in 20 per cent of the patients. The clinical course of the Seoul virus infection is milder; the five phases are shorter and more difficult to recognize.

Histological data

The histological findings differ from those observed in Europe mainly in the severity of vascular congestion of the medullary vessels culminating in a haemorrhagic medulla. Occasional necrosis of the papillae has been observed.

The viral antigen (envelope glycoproteins) has been observed in the cytoplasm of tubular epithelial cells as well as in the nuclei of tubular and glomerular cells.

Prognosis

According to published series, mortality reaches 3–7 per cent. It results mainly from shock, haemorrhage, pulmonary oedema, and cerebrovascular accidents. Survivors recover usually without sequelae.

Diagnosis

The diagnosis is suspected on clinical grounds and confirmed by serology in the majority of the cases.

The differential diagnosis should take into account not only drug-induced interstitial nephropathy and leptospirosis but also other causes of haemorrhagic fever prevalent in eastern Asia, dengue, Omsk and Chikungunya haemorrhagic fever, and murine typhus.

Treatment

Supportive therapy to correct bleeding, maintain blood pressure, and manage acute renal failure is of fundamental importance. Ribavirin, given intravenously within 5 days after the onset of the disease, has been of some use in severe cases in Korea and China. Salk type vaccines, used in Korea and China, are not yet licensed by the WHO.

Laboratory outbreak of hantavirus infection

Contact with infected patients and their material carries no proven risk: the disease does not spread from person to person. By contrast, the capture of infected wild rodents and the handling of their excretions may be hazardous, as demonstrated in several laboratories in Russia, Finland, and Korea (Lee and Johnson 1982).

These accidents should be distinguished from epidemics related to infected laboratory rats whose disease was previously unsuspected. Infection has been demonstrated in laboratory rats raised not only in scientific institutes but also in commercial companies. Outbreaks of laboratory-related hantavirus infection have been described both in Asia and in Europe (Desmyter *et al.* 1983). Their clinical characteristics depend on the infecting strain. Serological evidence of previously unsuspected infection has also been obtained in subjects working in these laboratories.

The laboratory rat appears to be the only clinically relevant reservoir of the disease despite evidence that other species may be infected. Valuable rat strains have been cleared of the virus through delivery by Caesarean section and foster nursing in virus-free mothers.

Acknowledgement

The help of J. Clement in the revision of this chapter is gratefully acknowledged.

References

Clement, J., Colson, P., and McKenna, P. (1994). Hantavirus pulmonary syndrome in New England and Europe. *New England Journal of Medicine* **331**, 547–548.

Clement, J., McKenna, P., van der Groen, G., Vaheri, A., and Peters, C. J. Hantaviruses. In *Zoonoses, Biology, Clinical Practice and Public Health Control* (ed. S. R. Palmer), pp. 331–351. Oxford: Oxford University Press, 1998.

Colson, P. *et al.* (1995). Epidemie d'Lantavirose dans l'Entre Sambre et Meuse Acta Clinica Belgica **50**, 197–206.

Desmyter, J., LeDuc, J. W., Johnson, K. M., Brasseur, F., Deckers, C., and van Ypersele de Strihou, C. (1983). Laboratory rat associated outbreak of haemorrhagic fever with renal syndrome due to Hantaan-like virus in Belgium. *Lancet* **2**, 1445–1448.

Giebel, L. D., Stohwasser, R., Zoller, L., Bautz, E. K., and Darai, G. (1989). Determination of the coding capacity of the M genome segment of Nephropathia Epidemica virus strain Hällnäs B1 by molecular cloning and nucleotide sequence analysis. *Virology* **172**, 498–505.

Glass, G. E., Watson, A. J., LeDuc, J. W., Kelen, G. D., Quinn, T. C., and Childs, J. E. (1993). Infection with a ratborn hantavirus in US residents is consistently associated with hypertensive renal disease. *Journal of Infectious Diseases* **167**, 614–620.

Glass, G. E., Watson, A. J., LeDuc, J. W., and Childs, J. E. (1994). Domestic cases of hemorrhagic fever with renal syndrome in the United States. *Nephron* **68**, 48–51.

Hindrichsen, S. *et al.* (1993). Hantavirus infection in Brazilian patients from Recife with suspected leptospirosis. *Lancet*, 341–350.

Lähdevirta, J. (1971). Nephropathia Epidemica in Finland. A clinical, histological and epidemiological study. *Annals of Clinical Research* **3** (Suppl. 8), 1–154.

Lee, H. W. and Johnson, K. M. (1982). Laboratory-acquired infections with Hantaan virus, the etiologic agent of Korean hemorrhagic fever. *Journal of Infectious Diseases* **146**, 645–651.

Lee, H. W. and van der Groen, G. (1989). Hemorrhagic fever with renal syndrome. *Progress in Medical Virology* **36**, 62–102.

Lee, M. *et al.* (1989). Coagulopathy in hemorrhagic fever with renal syndrome (Korean hemorrhagic fever). *Reviews of Infectious Diseases* **11** (Suppl. 4), S877–S883.

Makelä, S. *et al.* (2000). Renal function and blood pressure five years after Puumala virus—induced nephropathy. *Kidney International* **58**, 1711–1718.

Mustonen, J. *et al.* (1996). Genetic susceptibility to severe course of nephropathia epidemica caused by Puumala hantavirus. *Kidney International* **49**, 317–321.

Settergren, B., Juto, P., Wadell, G., Trollfors, S. B., and Norrby, S. R. (1988). Incidence and geographic distribution of serologically verified cases of Nephropathia Epidemica in Sweden. *American Journal of Epidemiology* **127**, 801–807.

van Ypersele de Strihou, C. and Méry, J. P. (1989). Hantavirus-related acute interstitial nephritis in Western Europe. Expansion of a world-wide zoonosis. *Quarterly Journal of Medicine* **73**, 941–950.

Zaki, S. R. *et al.* (1995). Hantavirus pulmonary syndrome. Pathogenesis of an emerging infectious disease. *American Journal of Pathology* **146**, 552–579.

10.7 Acute renal failure in a special setting

10.7.1 Infants and children

J. Trevor Brocklebank and Maggie Fitzpatrick

Introduction

Acute renal failure (ARF) is defined as a potentially reversible decline in renal function over a period of days or weeks. In infancy and childhood it arises in a setting of physiological and anatomical maturation presenting unique difficulties both in diagnosis and management. Aspects of normal renal development must be understood so that variations due to maturation of function can be distinguished from those due to disease.

Maturation of renal function (see also Chapter 1.4)

During intrauterine life, the excretory role of the fetal kidney is minimal and the placenta performs all the excretory functions necessary for homeostasis of the fetus. The main role of the fetal kidney is to maintain the normal volume and composition of the amniotic fluid, which is composed largely of fetal urine. The amniotic fluid is ingested by the fetus and recirculated in the fetal urine. Oligohydramnios may therefore be the first indication of severe renal anomalies such as bilateral renal agenesis. In contrast, polyhydramnios may suggest fetal polyuria or abnormalities of the gastrointestinal tract such as oesophageal atresia. Furthermore, the normal development of the lungs *in utero* is dependent upon an adequate volume of amniotic fluid and major congenital renal anomalies are often accompanied by pulmonary dysplasia that may itself be fatal before the onset of the renal failure.

Fetal urine production can be detected at 9–12 weeks' gestation and nephrogenesis is completed at 36 weeks when there is the full complement of 1 million nephrons (Bard and Woolf 1992). During this period, there is an exponential relationship between postconceptual age and glomerular filtration rate (GFR). At 26 weeks it is 0.6 ml/min and doubles by 33 weeks to 1.4 ml/min. When the results are corrected for body weight the increase is linear, averaging 0.7 ml/min/kg at 26 weeks and 0.8 ml/min/kg at 33 weeks and 1 ml/min/kg at term. There is a more rapid acceleration during the first 2 weeks of extrauterine life (Guignard *et al.* 1975). Similar results have been obtained using inulin (Coulthard 1985) and creatinine clearances to measure the GFR (Al-Dahhan *et al.* 1983).

The GFR increases further during the first 2 years of life, averaging 10 ml/min at 1 month and 35 ml/min at 2 years. Thereafter, it increases linearly at a rate of approximately 8 ml/min/year of life to 80 ml/min at 12 years. Up to this age there is no difference between boys and girls, but at puberty there is a greater rate of increase in boys. Centile charts for uncorrected GFR against age have been constructed and these may prove useful in clinical practice as they avoid the difficulties caused by normalizing for differences in body size (Heilbron *et al.* 1991). It is of interest that this pattern of maturation of GFR closely parallels the height and weight centiles.

There is controversy about the correct way of normalizing the GFR to correct for differences in body size. In the neonate there are practical and theoretical reasons to correct the GFR for body weight which can be relatively easily measured and correlates with metabolic rate. In older children the body surface area correction is used, although it has physiological and theoretical limitations not least because it is a highly derived factor. When this correction is made the GFR averages 30 ml/min/1.73 m^2 at 1 month and increases to 120 ml/min/1.73 m^2 by the age of 5 years where it remains until puberty. It is important to recognize that infants and children have a reduced GFR compared with adults even when corrected for differences in body size.

Hypoxia and labour result in the stimulation of a number of endocrine systems including vasopressin, catecholamines, renin, angiotensin II, and aldosterone (Daniel and James 1983). These vasoactive substances may reduce further GFR and has led to the concept of vasomotor nephropathy as a cause of ARF in the neonate (Toth-Heyn *et al.* 2000).

Although many functions of the kidneys of newborn babies are immature, the kidney of the term infant is well adapted for the demands of normal postnatal life. In contrast, the kidneys of very low birthweight babies are even more immature and the maintenance of fluid and electrolyte balance is difficult even under normal extrauterine conditions. Plasma sodium concentrations less than 130 mmol/l has been observed in upto 43 per cent of normal babies less than 30 weeks' gestational age (Haycock and Aperia 1991). Wide ranges of urinary sodium loss as high as 21 mmol/kg/day have been observed in very low birthweight infants and this is associated with high fractional excretion of sodium up to 10 per cent in stable, 28-week gestation, preterm infants. Studies have shown a deficiency of Na^+,K^+-ATPase in the developing proximal renal tubular cells of fetal rabbits, lending support to the concept that the hyponatraemia is due to urinary sodium loss rather than excess water. In contrast, the newborn kidney has a limited ability to excrete a sodium load, mainly because of the reduced GFR and an increased reabsorption by the distal renal tubular cells due to the high plasma aldosterone concentrations (Drukker *et al.* 1980).

Table 1 Summary of urinary diagnostic indices in neonates and children

Diagnostic index	Renal failure neonate	Renal failure child	Prerenal failure neonate	Prerenal failure child
U_{Na}mmol/l	>60	>60	<30	<20
U/P Na	0.45	0.50	0.23	0.5
U/P urea	<6	<3	>30	>20
U/P creatinine	<10	<20	>30	>40
U/P Osm	<1.1	<1.1	>2	>2
FE_{Na}(%)	>3	>2	<3	<1
RFI	<3	<1	<3	<1

U, urine; *P*, plasma; Osm, osmolality; RFI (renal failure index) = $U_{Na} \times P/U_{creatinine}$.

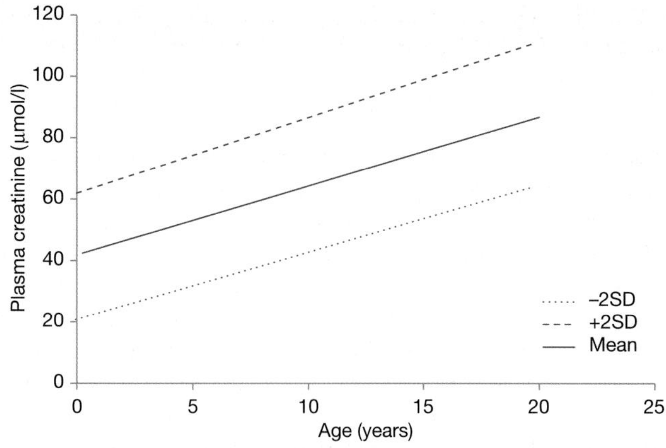

Fig. 1 Reference ranges for serum creatinine (Savory 1990).

These observations limit the value of urinary electrolyte measurements in the diagnosis of ARF in infancy (Table 1).

The newborn kidney is unable to conserve water by increasing the urine osmolality to a value greater than 600 mOsm/kg. The maximum urinary osmolality of 1200 mOsm/kg is reached at about the age of 2–3 years (Polacek *et al.* 1965). Infants void inappropriately large volumes of dilute urine even at times of increased extra renal fluid loss such as in gastroenteritis and easily become dehydrated. Polyuric ARF is well described in the neonate (Grylack *et al.* 1982). Conversely, the newborn has an impaired ability to excrete large amounts of free water (Guignard *et al.* 1976). Because of these and other immature functions of the kidney, young children are more at risk than older children and adults of developing ARF in response to the stresses imposed by illness.

Changes in plasma creatinine with age (see also Chapters 1.3 and 1.4)

At birth, the normal plasma creatinine reflects the maternal level with a large normal range of between 17 and 188 μmol/l. The mean plasma creatinine at birth is 73 μmol/l; it rises during the first 48 h when it averages 221 μmol/l in most preterm infants (Miall *et al.* 1999). It falls rapidly during the next 2 weeks of life. These large rises in creatinine after birth are probably related to the immaturity of renal tubular excretion and should not be interpreted in isolation as indicating renal failure. The normal plasma creatinine concentration and its rate of fall after birth are inversely related to gestational age. In a term infant aged 28 days it averages 35 μmol/l but at the same age the creatinine of a 28-week gestation baby is 60 μmol/l (Feldman and Guignard 1982; Rudd *et al.* 1983). Thereafter, there is a slow increase in the normal plasma creatinine with increasing age, averaging 45 μmol/l at 1 year of age and 60 μmol/l at 12 years (Fig. 1).

Because the placenta performs the excretory functions of the kidney, infants born with irreversible renal failure such as renal agenesis have a plasma creatinine within the normal range at birth and azotaemia does not become apparent until several days later.

Glomerular filtration can be estimated from the plasma creatinine in children over the age of 2 years from the formula; GFR (ml/min/1.73 m^2) = 40 × height (cm)/creatinine (μmol/l) (Morris *et al.* 1982). This relation between GFR and plasma creatinine holds only in steady-state conditions; in ARF, where there is an abrupt reduction in GFR, the plasma creatinine may not increase for up to 24 h after the onset of the renal insult and here the formula is of little value. Interpretation of a single plasma creatinine concentration in infancy is further complicated by the inaccuracy of its chemical measurement at low plasma concentrations. Furthermore, analytical interference with the Jaffe reaction by unconjugated bilirubin causes falsely low levels. Ketones and some drugs, such as the cephalosporin antibiotics, may cause falsely high levels of plasma creatinine. These problems in the measurement of creatinine create difficulties in the interpretation of a single blood test, particularly in the neonatal period (Brocklebank 1988). Repeated samples demonstrating an increasing plasma creatinine concentration are necessary for the diagnosis of renal failure.

Normal urine composition and flow rate

The onset of urine flow in term infants is variable but most will have voided urine in the first 24 h. Undetected spontaneous voiding during delivery may explain apparent anuria. True anuria suggests either an obstructive uropathy such as urethral valves or bilateral renal infarction from cortical necrosis or renal venous thrombosis. Oliguria is defined as a urine flow rate less than 0.5 ml/kg/h in the newborn infant and less than 1.0 ml/kg/h in the first year of life. In older children, oliguria is present when the urine flow rate is less than 500 ml/m^2/24 h. It is important to recognize that renal failure can occur with normal urine flow rates of between 1 and 3 ml/kg/h or with polyuria in a third of term neonates (Grylack *et al.* 1982).

Haematuria is an unusual finding in normal children, although up to 10 per cent of normal premature infants may have up to 1+ on dipstick testing. Haemoglobinuria is always abnormal and can be distinguished from haematuria by the absence of red blood cells on microscopy of the urine. Transient proteinuria up to 100 mg/dl may be present during the first week of life in the premature infant but is abnormal if it continues beyond this time. Up to 25 per cent of normal term and preterm infants have glycosuria of between a trace and 2+ on the dipstick test. Hyaline and granular casts are found in up to 10 per cent of normal urine specimens but cellular casts are always abnormal (Rhodes *et al.* 1962; Smith and Scrivens 1964).

The normal urine osmolality of the newborn infant ranges between 14 and 600 mOsm/l. There is a wide range of urinary sodium excretion up to 21 mmol/kg/day. The fractional excretion of sodium may vary from 10 to 2 per cent depending upon gestational age.

Normal blood pressure

Blood pressure measurement by sphygmomanometry is not easy in infants, especially with very low birthweight, and invasive monitoring using intra-arterial catheters is often necessary in an acutely ill newborn. In the premature infant, mean intra-aortic pressure averages 33 mmHg in the first 12 h (Versmold *et al.* 1981). A standard mercury manometer can be used in older children but it is important to use a blood pressure cuff that covers at least two-thirds of the upper arm. Using this method to measure blood pressure the mean pressure at 7 days is 73/50, at 1 year of age 94/53, and 105/65 at 12 years (Task Force on Blood Pressure Control in Children 1987). Doppler or oscillometric methods can be used. Normal blood pressure measured by oscillometry and standardized for height rather than age have been constructed (Soergel *et al.* 1997). Care should be taken when selecting an automated device for measuring blood pressure as many do not reach the recommendations of the European Society of Hypertension (O'Brien *et al.* 2001).

Renal growth measured by ultrasound

During early fetal life the kidneys are too small to identify, at 15 postmenstrual weeks only 50 per cent of normal kidneys are seen, but by 20 weeks the majority of kidneys can be visualized (Lawson and Foley 1981). Normal standards have been established for both kidney length (Schlesinger *et al.* 1987) and volume (Jean *et al.* 1982) compared with infant's weight and gestational age. The kidney of a preterm infant weighing 600 g would be expected to be between 26.4 and 35.7 mm in length, and 40.6–49.9 mm in a 2500-g infant. At birth, a normal kidney is between 4 and 6 cm in length, at 12 months 4–7 cm, and by 10 years of age 7.5–10.5 cm (Han and Babcock 1985). Normally, the kidney and liver have similar echogenicity during the first year of life. This is probably because of the increased cellularity of the immature kidney. Generalized increased echogenicity implies parenchymal disease. When the increased echogenicity is limited to the cortex, then glomerular or tubular interstitial disease is likely (Winkler and Altrogge 1985; Platt *et al.* 1991). Significant dilatation of the collecting system is said to be present in the newborn when the anterior–posterior diameter of the renal pelvis is 1.5 cm or more. Non-visualization of the bladder, particularly when the kidneys are small, suggests renal agenesis (Dubbins *et al.* 1981).

Incidence

When considering the population at risk, the newborn infant is highly susceptible to ARF, probably because of the complex nature of the associated diseases in this age group. In one study, 23 per cent of babies admitted to a neonatal intensive care unit were considered to have renal failure defined as oliguria and azotaemia. Three-fourths of these responded to a trial of volume expansion with 20 ml/kg of a saline solution with a diuresis and were classified as having prerenal renal failure. Intrinsic ARF was considered to be present in the remaining babies, who represented 6 per cent of the total admissions to the unit (Norman and Asadi 1979). Other studies have shown ARF to be present in between 1–3 per cent of total admissions to neonatal units and that 50 per cent of these respond to a fluid challenge (Mathew *et al.* 1980; Chavalier *et al.* 1984; Stapleton *et al.* 1987). ARF requiring dialysis treatment in the neonatal period occurs in ~0.2 per 1000 live births and 25 per cent of all children dialysed for ARF were newborn infants (Brocklebank 1988). These figures are almost certainly underestimates of the true incidence in the newborn period because non-oliguric renal failure is easily missed.

In the Yorkshire Region of the United Kingdom the annual incidence was 0.8 per 100,000 total population or 4 per 100,000 child population, about one-fifth of the incidence in adults. The age related yearly incidence in this population was; 19.7 per 100,000 in the first year of life; 5.9 per 100,000 in the 1–4-year age group and 1.5 in the 5–15-year group (Moghal *et al.* 1998).

Diagnosis

Prenatal diagnosis

Severely abnormal kidneys can be identified during routine antenatal ultrasonography at around 20 weeks postconceptual age. Other non-lethal anomalies may not be detected on later scans. Increased renal echogenicity is found in infants with renal dysplasia, multicystic dysplastic kidneys and infantile polycystic kidney disease. Although 20 per cent of kidneys with increased echogenicity many be normal, the finding is associated with a high mortality rate, especially when there is associated oligohydramnios (Estroff *et al.* 1991). A more common finding is bilateral hydronephrosis, which may indicate vesicoureteric reflux, or supra- or infravesical obstruction. Urethral valves, the most important treatable cause of ARF in the neonatal period, may not be apparent until scans at 30 weeks' gestation (Hutton *et al.* 1994).

The major difficulty is in identifying those fetuses with significantly impaired renal function, at a stage in pregnancy when appropriate counselling can be offered to the parents. The gestational age at presentation may be a good predictor of outcome; half of the fetuses found to have urethral valves at or before 24 weeks' gestation age had renal failure at birth compared with only 1 out of 15 detected on a later ultrasound scan (Hutton *et al.* 1994). Biochemical analysis of the fetal urine taken from the bladder at the time of amniocentesis is used in an attempt to identify those fetuses with a poor renal prognosis. High fetal urinary sodium and calcium concentrations for gestational age were found to indicate a poor renal prognosis (Nicolini *et al.* 1992; Lipitz *et al.* 1993). Other useful markers include the small molecular weight proteins β_2 microglobulin, α_1-microglobulin and retinol binding protein (Nolte *et al.* 1991; Freedman *et al.* 1997). Epidermal growth factor has also been suggested as a marker to predict the outcomes of antenatally diagnosed obstructive uropathies (Vates *et al.* 1997). Elevated levels of maternal plasma α-fetoprotein are typically found when the fetus has either congenital nephrotic syndrome or a neural-tube defect, but α-fetoprotein may also be elevated when there are minor renal anomalies, making it difficult to predict the outcome of individual pregnancies (Petrikovsky *et al.* 1991).

The majority of neonatal deaths resulting from severe fetal renal disease are due to pulmonary hypoplasia; renal failure occurring later. Thus, the most important factor, which predicts outcome is the presence of oligohydramnios. Treatment includes attempts to increase the volume of amniotic fluid by amnio-infusion. The treatment of obstructive uropathy by vesicoamniotomy has received much interest but remains controversial. These procedures carry a significant mortality and there are no clear guidelines for patient selection (Freedman *et al.* 2000).

Neonatal diagnosis (Table 2)

Prerenal failure

Dehydration is the single major cause of renal failure in the preterm and term newborn where the high insensible fluid losses due to increase skin permeability and obligate high urine water and salt losses may not be adequately replaced. In one study of 231 neonates 86 per cent had renal insufficiency due to prerenal causes, 11 per cent due to renal parenchymal causes and 3 per cent a consequence of postrenal anomalies (Hentschel *et al.* 1996). The most important cause of prerenal failure is respiratory distress syndrome that reduces both GFR and renal plasma flow. Positive pressure ventilation reduces cardiac output, which further compromises renal plasma flow. Renal function improves as the lung disease improves (Guignard *et al.* 1976).

Providing the renal under perfusion can be corrected promptly, renal failure is reversible. The correct diagnosis of prerenal failure is often difficult. Most children with prerenal failure have oliguria or anuria. If a urine sample can be obtained then comparison of the urine to plasma concentrations may be helpful as shown in Table 1. But renal immaturity creates an overlap between the abnormal and normal ranges making interpretation difficult, particularly in infants less than 29 weeks gestational age. The two most useful indices are the fractional excretion of sodium (FE_{Na}) and the renal failure index: a value of greater than 3 for either indicates parenchymal renal disease and less than 3 prerenal renal failure (Gouyon and Guignard 2000). An oliguric baby who is not fluid overloaded will probably have prerenal failure and a fluid challenge will restore renal perfusion and urine flow.

Reduced renal perfusion due to congenital heart disease or cardiac surgery accounts for most of the renal failure that occurs in this age group. Drug treatment with prostaglandin inhibitors or angiotensin-converting enzyme inhibitors may induce renal failure by further compromising renal perfusion (Mann *et al.* 1993). Furthermore, prenatal exposure to these drugs *in utero* may cause renal failure at birth. The aminoglycoside antibiotics are nephrotoxic and even their topical administration can induce nephrotoxicity in the new born because of increased permeability of the skin at this age (Bamford and Jones 1978).

Table 2 Main causes of acute renal failure

Neonates	Children
Prerenal	
Hypovolaemia	Hypovolaemia
High insensible losses	Gastroenteritis
Haemorrhage	Burns
Hypoxia	Haemorrhage
Renal	
Malformations	Acute on chronic disease
Dysplasia	Haemolytic uraemic syndrome
Polycystic kidney disease	
Vesicoureteric reflux	Glomerulonephritis
Acute tubular necrosis	Postinfectious nephritis
Sepsis	Henoch–Schönlein nephritis
Blood loss	
Hypoxia	Shunt nephritis
Pyelonephritis	Subacute bacterial endocarditis
Cortical necrosis	
Renal venous thrombosis	Mesangiocapillary GN
Drug toxicity	Goodpasture's syndrome
Tubular toxicity	Idiopathic
Interstitial nephritis	Acute pyelonephritis
	Acute tubular necrosis
	Sepsis
	Hypovolaemia/shock
	Haemorrhage
	Drug toxicity
	Tubular toxicity
	Interstitial nephritis
Postrenal	
Urethral valves	Urethral valves
Bilateral PUJ obstruction	Renal calculi
Ureterocele	Tumour lysis syndrome
Fungal urinary infection	Malignancy
Neurogenic bladder	Neurogenic bladder
Metabolic stone disease	

Parenchymal acute renal failure

Abnormal antenatal ultrasound findings should be confirmed immediately after birth. Bilateral renal dysplasia or hypoplasia is the most common finding and may also be associated with defined clinical syndromes. It is important to identify any associated anomalies that may influence the prognosis and management. Bilateral polycystic kidneys, of course, have a characteristic ultrasound appearance.

Any severe systemic infection may cause ARF. Infants with vesicoureteric reflux are at increased risk of acute pyelonephritis, which may precipitate ARF. For this reason, it is normally recommended that infants with antenatally detected reflux are treated following delivery with prophylactic antimicrobials, usually trimethoprim.

The clinical triad of renal enlargement, thrombocytopenia and a blood film showing red cell fragmentation suggestive of a microangiopathic haemolytic anaemia suggests renal venous thrombosis. Symptomatic thrombotic disease has been reported in 5 per 100,000 births and half of these involved the renal vein. Other affected veins include the superior and inferior vena cava and femoral veins. Arterial thrombosis is less frequent (Nowark-Gott *et al.* 1997). Diagnosis can be made by renal Doppler ultrasound, which may show the thrombus in the renal vein and absent intrarenal flow. Adrenal haemorrhage and adrenal failure are recognized associations (Howlett *et al.* 1997). It is bilateral in 5 per cent of cases. Predisposing factors include hereditary thrombophilia that is found in 5 per cent of affected children. It is important to measure the platelet count, the activated partial thromboplastin time, protein C, protein S, antithrombin and factor XII concentration and compare these with the normal ranges for children of similar gestation and postnatal ages. Other risk factors include maternal diabetes, dehydration, septicaemia, asphyxia, congenital heart disease and indwelling central venous catheters. Although heparin treatment (4–14 μ/kg/h) may cause haemorrhagic complications, it is recommended and requires careful control. Thrombolytic therapy has also been used but there is no consensus about treatment. Treatment does not prevent later renal complications that include hypertension, renal atrophy, and renal failure (Nuss *et al.* 1994; Schmit and Andrew 1995).

Antenatal ultrasound has made possible the early diagnosis and prompt treatment of renal anomalies. Significant dilatation of the renal pelvis without associated dilatation of the ureters or bladder suggests obstruction at the pelviureteric junction. When there is renal failure it implies severe bilateral renal disease and malformation of the contralateral kidney; multicystic dysplasia is a frequent association. Multicystic renal dysplasia may be difficult to differentiate from hydronephrosis due to obstruction at the pelviureteric junction, and DMSA and DPTA scans have very little diagnostic value in infants less than 1 month old.

Postrenal failure

When there is dilatation of both the pelvicalyceal system and ureters the obstruction is probably at or below the bladder. A micturating cysto-urethrogram with prophylactic antibiotic cover, should be done in a centre familiar with this investigation in the newborn. Urinary infection remains an important complication precipitating renal failure in an infant with vesicoureteric reflux or a partially obstructed urinary tract.

Children (Table 2)

Prerenal renal failure

Reduced renal perfusion due to congenital heart disease or cardiac surgery accounts for most of the renal failure that occurs in this age group. Drug treatment with prostaglandin inhibitors or angiotensin-converting enzyme inhibitors may induce renal failure by further compromising renal perfusion (Mann *et al.* 1993). Furthermore, prenatal exposure to these drugs *in utero* may cause renal failure at birth. The aminoglycoside antibiotics are nephrotoxic and even their topical administration can induce nephrotoxicity in the newborn because of increased permeability of the skin at this age (Bamford and Jones 1978).

Dehydration from diarrhoeal illnesses is an important cause of ARF in developing countries (Srivastava *et al.* 1990) but is uncommon in developed countries because of the routine use of oral rehydration solutions. Similarly, other prerenal causes of renal failure such as trauma and burns are now seen rarely because of improved resuscitation. Together they account for less than 1 per cent of cases requiring dialysis. Poor renal perfusion following cardiac surgery accounts for 20 per cent of cases of toddlers and 5 per cent of school age children who require dialysis for ARF. The urinary indices (Table 1) may be helpful in the diagnosis of prerenal failure in children of this age group.

Parenchymal acute renal failure

Diarrhoea-associated haemolytic uraemic syndrome (HUS) is the most common cause in Europe and North America. It is the most significant complication of infection by verocytoxin producing *Escherichia coli*—VTEC—usually of the serotype 0157 : H7 (Milford *et al.* 1990) (see Chapter 10.6.3).

HUS is characterized by the sudden onset of haemolytic anaemia with fragmentation of red blood cells, thrombocytopenia and ARF after a prodromal illness of acute gastroenteritis often with bloody diarrhoea. Oligoanuria occurs in over half of all cases and every child, unless anuric, has microscopic haematuria and proteinuria. Major neurological dysfunction occurs in third and is associated with a poor prognosis. Signs that should alert the paediatrician to HUS in a child with diarrhoea are the presence of bloody diarrhoea, decreasing urine output and the development of oedema and the sudden onset of pallor, mild jaundice, and petechiae.

Early dialysis will prevent most complications if the child is oligo-anuric. The haemoglobin should be maintained above 7–8 g/dl and early dialysis allows blood transfusions to be given with less risk of volume overload and hyperkalaemia. Studies are in progress to identify novel treatments that may halt the development of HUS in patients with VTEC, such as the use of a synthetic oligosaccharide receptor for the verotoxin but as yet there is no effective therapy (Armstrong *et al.* 1995). Antibiotics are not indicated, and probably aggravate the renal failure.

Any severe systemic infection may cause ARF. Infected ventriculo-atrial shunts and subacute bacterial endocarditis complicating congenital heart disease are important diagnoses to consider because the renal outcome is good providing treatment with the appropriate antibiotics is given early (Haffner *et al.* 1997). It should be suspected when a susceptible child has haematuria, and confirmed by a low C3 complement level and positive blood cultures. Primary glomerulonephritis is the cause of ARF in about one in five cases of children of school age but seldom requires dialysis treatment. It should be suspected when haematuria is associated with heavy proteinuria (3–4 + Albustix®) and red-cell casts are seen on urine microscopy. Acute glomerulonephritis may follow a variety of infections but poststreptococcal glomerulonephritis is still the most important cause. Streptococcal skin infections of scabies or mosquito bites are common in developing countries. However, preceding streptococcal infections may not always be apparent from the history and infection should be confirmed by the antistreptolysin-O titre that typically increases about 2 weeks after the infection and continues to rise for the next 4–6 weeks. The plasma concentration of the C3 complement may remain less than normal for up to 3 months. Children with poststreptococcal glomerulonephritis characteristically recover during the second week of the illness and failure to do so may suggest a rapidly progressive nephritis.

Rapidly progressive glomerulonephritis may also be secondary to other primary diseases such as Henoch–Schönlein disease, mesangiocapillary glomerulonephritis, lupus nephritis or Goodpasture's syndrome. Mesangiocapillary glomerulonephritis is also associated with a persistently low C3 and in this respect may mimic both lupus and poststreptococcal nephritis, but can be distinguished from these by the presence of a serum C3 nephritic factor.

Severe renal involvement occurs in 25 per cent of children with Henoch–Schönlein disease. Those with severe disease tend to be older and have more severe and prolonged systemic manifestation particularly abdominal pain (Meadow *et al.* 1972). Severe renal disease is suspected when there is heavy proteinuria as well as haematuria or hypertension. A rising plasma creatinine or nephrotic syndome require prompt investigation by renal biopsy to establish the degree of renal involvement. It is generally accepted that prompt treatment with methylprednisolone is the most appropriate treatment (Cole *et al.* 1976). Other vasculitic diseases such as lupus nephritis and Wegener's granulomatosis are less common in children and rarely present as ARF. The diagnosis of lupus nephritis requires both specific serology and biopsy to establish the degree and nature of the renal involvement.

It is always wise to scrutinize the dose and potential toxic effects of all prescribed drugs and other possible toxins. The aminoglycoside antibiotics and many of the cytotoxic drugs used in the treatment of malignant diseases are nephrotoxic. Aminoglycosides accumulate in the proximal tubular cells and the first indication of nephrotoxicity is a Fanconi-like syndrome with polyuria, hypokalaemia, hypocalcaemia, and hypomagnesaemia. Excretory renal failure with an elevated blood urea and creatinine occurs later (Bamford and Jones 1978). The nephrotoxicity of aminoglycoside antibiotics is reversible once the treatment is stopped but the ototoxicity may result in permanent deafness.

Acute interstitial nephritis following drug exposure is easily overlooked because the urine sediment is often unremarkable. It is often secondary to drugs with the penicillin nucleus, including the cephalosporin antibiotics, and may develop in patients with pre-existing renal disease causing an unexpected rapid decline in renal function. It may also occur following viral infections and mycoplasma. If acute interstitial nephritis is suspected, then the offending drug should be withdrawn and a renal biopsy performed to establish the diagnosis (Gallego *et al.* 1991).

Drugs that disturb glomerular perfusion such as the angiotensin-converting enzyme inhibitors and prostaglandin synthetase inhibitors may cause renal failure by reducing glomerular filtration. Ibuprofen is a freely available prostaglandin synthetase inhibitor used for the treatment of pain and fever in children. These drugs may cause ARF particularly in children with pre-existing renal disease (Mann *et al.* 1993) but recovery is complete once the offending drug is discontinued.

Acute obstructive uropathy

This should be considered, particularly when there is total anuria or abdominal pain. The urine output may be normal if the obstruction is partial. A renal ultrasound and abdominal radiograph will identify the presence of bilateral hydronephrosis and/or renal calculus. Renal failure implies the obstruction is below the bladder or there is bilateral disease. It is rare to find a solitary obstructed kidney as a cause of ARF. Acute renal failure due to obstruction should be identified and relieved early as delay may result in permanent renal impairment. The kidneys may be palpable and an enlarged bladder is present when there is bladder outflow obstruction such as in urethral valves. Renal stone disease is a rare cause of ARF in childhood and is usually a complication of urinary-tract infection. Metabolic stone disease is caused by disorders such as oxalosis, cystinuria, and abnormalities of purine metabolism. The radiolucent stones characteristic of disorders of purine metabolism can usually be identified by ultrasound examination. In the tumour lysis and Lesch–Nyhan syndromes there may be both intrarenal obstruction and interstitial nephropathy due to urate crystals. In ARF due to other causes the plasma urate is never more than twice normal. In the Lesch–Nyhan or tumour lysis syndromes the urate concentrations are usually several times normal. In contrast, a very low plasma urate may suggest other purine metabolic abnormalities such as xanthinuria (Simmonds *et al.* 1989). Although purine metabolic disorders are extremely rare, they are important because treatment with inhibitors of the enzyme xanthine oxidase is specific. For this reason, the plasma urate should be measured at presentation in all cases of ARF.

Acute tumour lysis syndrome is an oncological emergency. It is precipitated by the rapid lysis of cells, which may occur spontaneously, after surgery or more usually chemotherapy. The lysis of cells leads to the release of intracellular potassium and phosphate causing significant hyperkalaemia, hyperphosphataemia and secondary hypocalcaemia within 6 h of the commencement of treatment. This may cause fatal cardiac arrhythmias before renal failure develops. The cellular breakdown releases nucleic acids, which are metabolized to uric acid. Acute renal failure may occur due to urate nephropathy or nephrocalcinosis resulting from the high calcium phosphate product greater than 4.0 (Altman 2001). Aggressive early monitoring at induction of treatment and treatment with drugs aimed to lower the plasma urate such as allopurinol or uricase may prevent renal failure. Continuous haemodialysis or haemofiltration can control hyperkalaemia and its serious consequences.

Acute on chronic renal failure

Ten per cent of children presenting with ARF have an underlying chronic renal disease (Moghal *et al.* 1998). A history of recurrent urinary-tract infections may indicate reflux nephropathy. Polydipsia, polyuria, and enuresis may suggest a urinary concentrating defect indicative of chronic renal disease. Short stature and poor weight growth velocity are sensitive indicators of chronic renal failure. Signs of chronic hypertension such as left ventricular hypertrophy and hypertensive retinopathy are features of chronic disease, as are anaemia and rickets. It is not uncommon for a radiologist to make the diagnosis of renal failure when renal bone disease is recognized on the chest radiograph of a child who is acutely breathless because of acidosis and is mistakenly diagnosed as having pneumonia. Finally, a family history of renal disease such as nephronophthisis or renal stones may indicate the acute presentation of a chronic disease.

General management

A successful outcome to the treatment of children with ARF requires the cooperation of a dedicated team of paediatric nephrologists, nurses, dieticians, dialysis technicians, pharmacists, urologists, and intensivists. Early transfer of the child with renal insufficiency to a specialized centre where all these skills are available is essential for a successful outcome.

Fluid balance

The initial assessment of the child includes an estimate of the state of hydration. If the child has been weighed recently, then a change in weight is an accurate way to assess the fluid status. Dehydration can be graded clinically using the classification suggested by Winter (1973) (Table 3). Hypotension is a sign of hypovolaemia but does not always indicate severe dehydration.

Alternative methods using bioelectrical impedance techniques to measure total body water may be useful (Smye *et al.* 1994). It is important to examine the patient frequently and adjust the rate of fluid replacement to avoid the risk of overload. The volume of fluid replacement can be calculated from this initial assessment. Thus, a 20-kg child who is 10 per cent dehydrated requires $20 \times 10/100 = 2$ l of fluid to replace the water deficit. This volume is added to the daily insensible water losses (500 ml/m^2), volume of renal and other on-going losses, and the sum is the total fluid replacement for the first 24 h.

The maintenance water requirements can be calculated using average metabolic requirements as standard (Table 4). The maintenance water requirements are approximately equal to the energy consumption in calories; for each 100 cal (420 J) of energy consumed 100 ml of water is needed. Alternative methods of calculation from body surface

Table 3 Clinical assessment of dehydration (Winter 1973)

Clinical sign	Mild (5%)	Moderate (10%)	Severe (15%)
Reduced skin turgor	+	++	+++
Mucous membranes	Dry	Very dry	Parched
Skin	Pale	Grey	Mottled
Urine output	Reduced	Oliguric	Oliguria + increased urea
Heart rate	Normal	Increased	Very increased
Blood pressure	Normal	Normal +/−	Low

area can be used where the needs are 1500 ml/m^2 body surface area. This requires the estimation of the body surface area from body weight and height using a nomogram. Under normal conditions, 55 per cent of the maintenance water is lost though the kidneys, 30 per cent in perspiration, and 15 per cent through the lungs. Faecal loss is less than 5 per cent and can be ignored, as the water gained from metabolic oxidation balances it. In oliguric renal failure the urinary losses will be negligible and in patients being ventilated the pulmonary losses are nil or water may even be retained from the inspired humidified gases. It is important to recognize circumstances where calorie expenditure and water requirements are increased, such as during febrile illnesses. Here the maintenance fluid should be increased by 10 per cent for every 1°C of fever. In some hypermetabolic states such as after surgery or burns the amount of maintenance fluid may have to be increased by as much as 50 or even 75 per cent.

Where there is doubt in a child who is not fluid overloaded a fluid challenge of isotonic saline 20 ml/kg body weight may induce a diuresis. It can be repeated in an hour with frusemide 1mg/kg if there is no response. If there is still no response then it is safer to fluid restrict the child and treat for renal failure.

The clinical assessment of fluid overload is more difficult where a change in body weight is not available. The presence of detectable oedema can be taken to represent at least 5 per cent and pulmonary oedema 15 per cent excess fluid. Fluid replacement should then be restricted and a simple approach is to replace only the ongoing losses and ignore insensible losses. Measurement of the blood pressure together with the information from an accurately kept fluid-balance chart and daily measurements of the fasting body weight provide the feedback information necessary to maintain optimal fluid balance. Dialysis treatment is indicated when there is severe fluid overload with heart failure and pulmonary oedema. It is often necessary to start dialysis treatment so that fluid can be removed in order to provide the space for the infusion of essential fluids such as blood or nutrition.

Sodium

Sodium loss can be estimated from the average electrolyte concentrations of gastrointestinal fluids (Table 5) and appropriate replacement given. In polyuric renal failure it is necessary to measure the urinary sodium concentration (normally between 40 and 60 mmol/l) to ensure accurate replacement. Hyponatraemia is a common finding in children with ARF. It is usually due to water excess rather than sodium loss unless the history suggests there have been significant gastrointestinal losses. If there is doubt, then it is safer to restrict water intake until the situation becomes clearer. Although sodium is principally an extracellular fluid cation for the purposes of calculating the deficit, the sodium space is regarded as being total body water (80 per cent body weight in a neonate and 60 per cent body weight in children) because this permits correction of the sodium lost from the extracellular fluid after expansion and from other exchangeable sodium pools such as bone. Profound hyponatraemia (sodium < 120 mmol/l) may cause neurological disturbances with seizures and an encephalopathy. Brain injury may be irreversible. Correction to a level of 125–130 mmol/l should be achieved slowly at a rate of 1 mmol/h to avoid permanent brain damage (Arieff *et al.* 1992). This can be accomplished using the formula:

$$\text{Sodium required (mmol)} = 140 - \text{target plasma sodium (mmol/l)} \times \text{weight (kg)} \times K$$

where K is the volume of distribution of sodium.

In contrast, hypernatraemia (sodium > 155 mmol/l) is more likely to be due to water loss or deficiency than salt overload. Rapid cerebral dehydration in hypernatraemia can lead to rupture of the blood vessels connecting the brain to the rigid skull and the mortality is as high as 50 per cent (Lee *et al.* 1994). Very low birthweight infants nursed under radiant heaters or receiving phototherapy are at risk of hypernatraemia unless the increased insensible loss is balanced by increased water intake.

Potassium

Hyperkalaemia is an important complication of ARF and should be prevented or corrected promptly to avoid cardiac arrhythmias. The maintenance of adequate nutrition is fundamental to reduce catabolism and promote the intracellular uptake of potassium. If the serum concentration is 6 mmol/l or more, then additional emergency measures are needed (Table 6). Nebulized salbutamol, which is readily

Table 4 Energy requirements by body weight (Holliday and Segar 1957)

Body size (kg)	Energy requirements (cal/kg)
0–10	100
11–20	1000 + 50
20 or more	1500 + 20

Table 5 Electrolyte content of gastrointestinal fluids

Fluid	Na (mmol/l)	K (mmol/l)	Bicarbonate (mmol/l)	Chloride (mmol/l)
Stomach	140	15		150
Small bowel	140	15	40	15
Diarrhoea	40	40	40	40

Table 6 Strategies for the treatment of hyperkalaemia

Stabilization of the myocardium	
10% Calcium gluconate	0.5–1 ml/kg iv over 5–10 min
Shift of potassium from extracellular to intracellular compartment	
Sodium bicarbonate	1–2 mmol/kg iv (=1–2 ml/kg of 8.4% solution)
Salbutamol	2.5 mg if < 25 kg and 5 mg if >25 kg via nebulizer 4 μg/kg infused iv over 10 min
Dextrose and/or insulin	0.5–1 g/kg/h dextrose (2.5–5 ml/kg/h of 20% dextrose) with insulin 0.2 units for every gram of glucose administered
Removal of potassium from the body	
Ion exchange resins	
Calcium resonium	1 g/kg po or pr
Sodium resonium	1 g/kg po or pr

available on most paediatric wards, is an effective and prompt method of reducing the plasma potassium whilst preparations are being made for dialysis treatment (McLure *et al.* 1994). Salbutamol acts by stimulating potassium movement from the extracellular into the intracellular space. Other agents with a similar mode of action include sodium bicarbonate, and insulin with dextrose. The administration of sodium bicarbonate may be complicated by a reduction in the plasma ionized calcium with possible risk of tetany. If used repeatedly hypernatraemia, intravascular volume, overload, and hypertension may result. The administration of insulin and dextrose requires regular monitoring of blood glucose levels. Ion exchange resins remove potassium from the body by exchanging potassium for calcium or sodium, which is passed from the body in the stool. The dose can be repeated 4 hourly as necessary but the effects are not apparent for at least 24 h. Plasma potassium levels should be measured regularly once therapy for hyperkalaemia has been commenced. In the anuric or severely oliguric child the plasma potassium levels are unlikely to fall spontaneously and these measures are used to keep the potassium concentrations at a safe level whilst preparations are being made for dialysis treatment.

Urea

Urea itself is not a toxin, although the blood concentration can be used as a marker of the severity of ARF. It increases rapidly in catabolic states such as in renal failure complicating infection, trauma, surgery, or burns, when it is important to ensure adequate nutritional energy intake. Dehydration should also be suspected when the blood urea is proportionately greater than would be expected from the serum creatinine. 'Uraemia' is a clinical state that is not directly related to the blood urea concentration. There is no defined level of blood urea when dialysis treatment for ARF is needed but it should be considered when the concentration approaches 20 mmol/l.

Acidosis

The normal daily rate of acid production is 1 mmol/kg (Relman 1964) so the maintenance bicarbonate requirement is 1–2 mmol/kg/day. In oliguric ARF the inability to excrete, and the increased rate of production of hydrogen ions, result in acidosis. Good nutrition reduces the rate of endogenous acid production and is an essential part of treatment. Bicarbonate replacement can be calculated assuming the bicarbonate space is 30 per cent of body weight, and the respiratory component to the acidosis corrected by adjusting the ventilator setting where appropriate. The correct diagnosis of acid–base disorders can be made by reference to nomograms based upon the Henderson–Hasselbalch equation (Arbus 1973). A total of 1 mmol of sodium is given with each 1 mmol of bicarbonate given to correct acidosis but the resultant hypernatraemia may cause intracerebral haemorrhage, particularly in newborn infants (Lee *et al.* 1994). Acidosis ($pH < 7.2$) is an indication for dialysis.

Other biochemical abnormalities

Hypocalcaemia and hypomagnesaemia are frequent findings in ARF but rarely cause seizures because the proportion in the ionized form remains normal. Calcium and magnesium supplements are seldom required unless the child is symptomatic. This may occur due to the over correction of acidosis. Hypoglycaemic convulsions may occur in the newborn period. Hyperglycaemia due to the insulin resistance induced by uraemia is more likely, especially when high glucose-containing peritoneal dialysis solutions are prescribed. Hyperglycaemia requires treatment with insulin infusions. Untreated hyperglycaemia may lead to cerebral venous thrombosis.

Blood pressure

Hypertension may complicate ARF due to a number of causes, the commonest of which are glomerulonephritis, obstructive uropathy, renovascular disease and the haemolytic uraemic syndrome. It may be secondary to volume overload or as a consequence of medical treatment of the underlying disease. Hypertension becomes an emergency where organ damage has occurred or is imminent. The tissues susceptible to damage include the brain, the retina, heart and kidney, with the major pathological process being arteriolar fibrinoid necrosis. Often there may, even in severe hypertension, be no symptoms and when present they are predominantly neurological, including facial palsy, convulsions and hemiplegia. Hypertensive encephalopathy may present with confusion or seizures. Cardiac failure may be the first presenting feature in very young children. The principles of the management of hypertensive emergencies are as important as the drugs used (Deal 1992; Adelman *et al.* 2000). The level of renal function will influence management particularly the drugs used and dialysis or filtration may be required to achieve optimum blood pressure control. Renin dependent hypertension will influence the use of angiotensin-converting enzyme inhibitors but care must be exercised with these drugs when there is renovascular disease. Catecholamine-driven hypertension will need both α-adrenergic and β-blockade. If the blood pressure is lowered too rapidly there is risk of ischaemic damage to watershed areas of the brain, particularly the visual cortex, cerebellum, and end arteries even though the measured blood pressure may still be relatively high. Drugs used in hypertensive emergencies are shown in Table 7. The aim should be to reduce blood pressure initially by only one-third of the difference between the acute blood pressure level and the appropriate normal value. Longer acting drugs should be introduced 24 or 48 h after the pressure is satisfactorily controlled.

Frequent and reliable blood pressure monitoring is necessary. An intravenous infusion of normal saline is used if the blood pressure falls. Hypotension should be corrected promptly to ensure renal perfusion is preserved. If this fails then inotropic sympathomimetic drugs such as dobutamine and dopamine are necessary. In modest doses

Table 7 Drugs used for the emergency treatment of hypertension

Drug	Dose
Nifedipine	0.25–0.5 mg/kg sublingually
Hydralazine	1–4 mg/kg/day
Labetolol	1–4 mg/kg/h iv infusion
Diazoxide	2–5 mg/kg iv bolus
Sodium nitroprusside	0.5–8 μg/kg/min
Nicardine	1–5 μg/kg/min

(<5 μg/kg body weight/min) these drugs may have the additional benefit of increasing renal blood flow. Central venous or pulmonary-wedge pressure measurements can be used to guide blood volume replacement.

Haematological disorders

Anaemia is a common finding in children with ARF but seldom presents as an acute problem requiring immediate blood transfusion. An exception to this is the HUS when the haemolysis is rapid. Blood transfusions should be given during dialysis in an anuric patient to avoid the risk of inducing hypertension or heart failure. It is safer to administer small volumes (10 ml/kg) at regular intervals rather than to attempt to correct the haemoglobin deficit with one large infusion.

Bruising and bleeding disorders occur in the later stages. Abnormalities of platelet function and deficiencies of coagulation factors require infusion of platelets and cryoprecipitate. In HUS, bleeding due to thrombocytopenia can be a major problem and, when the platelet count is less than 20×10^9/l should be corrected before the insertion of peritoneal catheters or central venous lines, to limit the risk of bleeding during the procedures.

Prolonged prothrombin and other clotting times may be found particularly in children with associated liver failure or where there is a lupus anticoagulant. This requires more detailed investigation to identify the specific defect. Fresh frozen plasma can be given while awaiting detailed investigations.

Infection

Infections are serious complications of ARF and have a significant impact on the mortality and morbidity at any stage of the disease. Central venous lines are a common portal of entry and should be removed as soon as possible. Similarly, bladder catheters should be inserted only when there is concern about bladder drainage such as in obstruction from urethral valves. Pyelonephritis in an oliguric patient is extremely difficult to diagnose. A diagnosis of septicaemia should be considered if the clinical condition worsens at any stage of the illness, prompting cultures of urine, and blood from all venous access lines. Whenever possible the lines should be removed. The usual infecting organisms are *Staphylococcus epidermidis*, *Staphylococcus aureus*, or coliforms. Opportunistic infection, especially with *Candida albicans*, which may spread from the mouth to the oesophagus or central venous lines, requires prompt treatment. Candida urinary tract infections may be difficult to treat because the hyphae grow along the renal tubules or produce fungal balls that obstruct the urine flow and prevent the antifungal drugs from entering the urine.

The kidney excretes many drugs and as a result their half-lives are prolonged in renal failure (Trompeter 1987). Antibiotic dosage regimens should be adjusted frequently either by reducing the dose or increasing the interval between doses so that high plasma concentrations and consequent toxicity are avoided. This applies particularly to the aminoglycoside antibiotics where the ototoxicity and nephrotoxicity are related to high plasma concentrations of the drugs.

Neurological disorders

Neurological disturbances can occur at any stage during ARF. Hyponatraemia (serum sodium < 120 mmol/l), hypernatraemia (serum sodium > 155 mmol/l), hypocalcaemia, hypomagnesaemia, and hypoglycaemia can all cause convulsions. Although urea itself is not toxic, it is used as a marker of the severity of the uraemic state and seizures tend to occur when it is high (usually > 20 mmol/l). Uraemia can cause many strange neurological disorders including confusional states, transient hemiplegias, meningism, and dystonia. It is unwise to make early predictions about the neurological outcome in uraemia as an apparently severely brain-damaged child can make a full neurological recovery. The neurological disability usually improves within a few days of the start of dialysis and anticonvulsant treatment is not generally required. Phenytoin, is excreted by the liver, and can be used safely provided the blood concentrations are maintained within the therapeutic range.

Table 8 Intake of electrolytes and protein provided by milk regimens

Nutrient	Na (mmol/100 cal)	K (mmol/100 cal)	Protein (g/100 cal)
Breast milk	1	2	1.5
Cow's milk	3.5	6	5
Prepared milk	1.5	2	2
Recommended dietary intake/day	1–2	1–2	1–2

Nutrition

An adequate energy intake is fundamental and the services of an experienced paediatric dietician are needed. The patients are usually catabolic and the rate of rise of blood urea and potassium may be rapid. Dialysis treatment may be avoided or at least delayed by ensuring an adequate diet. The maintenance energy needs can be estimated from Table 4 and every effort should be made to meet them. The major constraint is the necessity to restrict fluid intake, particularly in babies, where high energy-containing supplements can be added to the normal milk formula. Cows' milk should be avoided because of its higher electrolyte and protein content, and breast milk or prepared milks are preferred (Table 8). In older children, dietary restriction is not usually necessary because they are anorexic and the dietician's skill is needed to encourage them to eat. Oral nutrition is preferred, supported by nasogastric tube feeding when necessary.

After abdominal surgery or when enteral nutrition is restricted because of vomiting, parenteral nutrition is used, but adequate nutrition can often only be achieved by allowing excess fluid intake. Here, the nutritional needs take precedence over fluid restriction and frequent dialysis treatment will compensate for the increased fluid and electrolyte intake.

Renal replacement therapy

The indications for renal replacement therapy are shown in Table 9. Initiating treatment before the onset of severe acidosis, uraemia, and resistant hyperkalaemia are present may reduce the morbidity and mortality of ARF (Gettings *et al.* 1999). Two studies (Best *et al.* 1996; Smith *et al.* 1997) of meningococcal disease reported lower mortality in the treated group compared with historical controls.

The choice of renal replacement therapy depends largely upon available resources. The choice is between acute peritoneal dialysis,

Table 9 Indications for renal replacement therapy

Persistent hyperkalaemia
Diuretic resistant volume overload ± associated hypertension and heart failure
Refractory acidosis
Severe uraemia with risk of encephalopathy and/or pericarditis
Requirement to create space for the improvement of nutritional intake
Resistant hypo- or hypernatraemia
Resistant hypocalcaemia and hyperphosphataemia
Hyperammonaemia with inborn errors of metabolism
Tumour lysis syndrome
Removal of dialysable drug or toxin
Hyperpyrexia/hypothermia

continuous venovenous haemofiltration (CVVH), continuous venovenous haemofiltration and dialysis (CVVHD), and acute haemodialysis. The advantages of peritoneal dialysis over haemodialysis or CVVH are that no special equipment or central vascular access is required and anticoagulation is not necessary. The advantages of continuous venovenous systems of haemodiafiltration over intermittent haemodialysis and peritoneal dialysis are the accurate control of ultrafiltration and solute clearance. These are preferred in critically ill infants and children (Reeves *et al.* 1994).

Peritoneal dialysis

Peritoneal dialysis is simple, safe, and effective, and can be used in children of all sizes provided the peritoneum is intact (Reznick *et al.* 1991). The peritoneal membrane of children is functionally more efficient than in adults. This difference has been attributed to the greater body surface area : weight ratio in infants than adults (Esperance and Collins 1966). The solute transport characteristics of the peritoneal membrane in children have been assessed by measurement of the mass transfer coefficients for urea, creatinine, uric acid, and glucose, and found to be similar to adult values when corrected for body surface area (Morgenstern *et al.* 1984). Ultrafiltration rate may be poor and this has been attributed to the rapid rate of glucose absorption from the dialysate. Children have relatively greater rates of fluid absorption by the peritoneal lymphatics, reducing the net ultrafiltration rate (Mactier *et al.* 1988). In the newborn, the dialysate exchange volume (Kohaut 1986) influences the ultrafiltration rate.

Peritoneal dialysis fluid contains electrolytes, an osmotic agent (glucose or icodextrin) and an acid buffer (lactate or bicarbonate). Commercially manufactured solutions in the United Kingdom are available in 1.36, 2.27, and 3.86 per cent glucose concentrations. In North America, 0.5, 1.5, 2.5, and 4.25 per cent are available. Using higher glucose concentrations in the dialysis fluid will increase the volume of fluid removed from the patient (ultrafiltration). Dialysate volumes of 10–50 ml/kg per cycle are used with dwell times varying between 20 and 60 min. Removal of solutes and water may be increased by larger cycle volume or increasing the frequency of cycles.

A Tenckhoff catheter may be inserted surgically or at the bedside by an experienced paediatric nephrologist using a peel away sheath system under sedation and local anaesthesia. When catheters are inserted at the bedside in small infants or the new born babies it is a wise precaution to insert the catheters after abdominal ultrasound has identified the positions of the abdominal organs. This reduces the risk of inadvertent organ damage. Absolute contraindications to peritoneal dialysis include an omphalocele or gastroschisis, a diaphragmatic hernia, peritonitis or other disease affecting the peritoneal membrane, and bladder extrophy. Relative contraindications include recent abdominal surgery and high levels of ventilatory support. It may be possible to anticipate ARF developing after surgical procedures such as cardiac surgery when it is advisable to insert the peritoneal catheter at the time of surgery (Shaw *et al.* 1991). Large cycle volumes may inhibit pulmonary function and cardiac output, particularly in newborn infants after cardiac surgery (Bunchman *et al.* 1992) and smaller volume cycles are then preferred; using a high glucose-containing solution to increase the ultrafiltration rate.

The major complication of peritoneal dialysis is peritonitis usually due to *S. epidermidis*. Prompt diagnosis and treatment with appropriate intraperitoneal antibiotics (vancomycin, 25 mg/l of dialysis solution) is important to preserve the peritoneal membrane as well as reduce morbidity and mortality. Hyperglycaemia may occur when high glucose solutions are used and plasma glucose concentrations should be measured at least 4 hourly. The newborn infant and small children can become dehydrated when hypertonic glucose solutions are used. Accurate fluid balance and regular measurement of body weight are essential. Conversely, peritoneal drainage may be compromised, causing fluid retention. This is usually due to a misplaced catheter or its obstruction by the omentum. Peritoneal catheters can erode the bowel of the newborn causing peritonitis. When drainage cannot be improved by replacing the catheter an alternative dialysis technique should be used.

Acute haemodialysis

Acute haemodialysis presents greater technical difficulties than peritoneal dialysis because of the higher solute fluxes and ultrafiltration and because of the difficulties of gaining vascular access. It is used less now as the continuous renal replacement therapies are preferred. It still has a place in treatment once the patient has been stabilized. The disadvantages include the need for good vascular access, anticoagulation, and for special equipment and skilled nursing staff. Relative contraindications include haemodynamic instability and coagulopathy. Rapid ultrafiltration may produce hypotension that may result in renal ischaemia prolonging the duration of renal failure. Rapid fluctuations in the concentrations of blood urea may cause disequilibrium particularly when the urea concentrations are high. Disequilibrium syndrome is complex and the pathogenesis multifactorial; symptoms include restlessness, fatigue, headache, nausea and vomiting that may progress to confusion, seizures, and coma. The correct choice of dialyser and blood flow rate aiming for a urea clearance of 1 ml/kg/min will prevent this severe complication.

Haemofiltration

There is debate about the relative merits of haemofiltration where solutes are cleared by convective mass transfer and dialysis where solute removal is predominantly by diffusive mass transfer. There are less hypotensive episodes with haemofiltration (Altieri *et al.* 2001).

An alternative method employs haemodialysers rather than filters, a technique known as slow efficient dialysis or CVVHD. Here convective and diffusive mass transfer are combined (Bradbury *et al.* 1995). A dialyser with a surface area of 0.3 m^2 can be used in children of less than 15 kg, and one of 0.5 m^2 for bigger children. The urea clearance can be adjusted by altering the blood flow or dialysate flow rates.

The major problem with continuous renal replacement therapies is gaining adequate vascular access, either arterial (for continuous arteriovenous haemofiltration) or venous (continuous venovenous haemofiltration). In most cases, a single venous puncture with a double-lumen catheter is adequate, but in small infants and the newborn the femoral or umbilical vessels can be used. The efficiency of all these methods is dependent upon the internal diameter and lengths of the intravascular catheter used (Jenkins *et al.* 1988) and consequently only slow blood-flow rates of between 4 and 6 ml/kg/min can be achieved in the newborn. The venous cannulas range from between 6.5Fg in infants less than 10 kg and 11.5Fg in children greater than 20 kg.

When the filtration rate is greater than a third of the blood flow rate the resulting haemoconcentration across the filter increases the chances of it clotting, which is a major technical problem in small infants. Here pre-dilution, where replacement fluid is infused before the filter, will permit higher flows to be achieved and reduce the risk of the filter clotting. On the other hand this dilutes the blood concentration which reduces the diffusive transport. In practice this does not seem to be a problem. Post dilution achieves greater convective solute transport but here the blood flow is limited and the filters seem to clot more easily in children (Ahrenholz *et al.* 1997).

A priming volume of the extracorporeal circuit greater than 10 per cent of the child's blood volume may lead to hypotension. This can be avoided by priming the system with blood or albumin.

A bicarbonate-based replacement solution is preferred because most ill children have a lactate acidosis. Potassium and phosphate should be replaced if plasma levels are below the normal range. This can be achieved by their addition to the haemofiltration replacement fluid in the desired physiological concentrations, that is, potassium 3–4 mmol/l and phosphate 1–2 mmol/l. Heparin remains the anticoagulant of choice in most units; a loading dose of 20 units/kg is generally given followed by an infusion prefilter of 10–30 units/kg/h to achieve an APTT 60–90 s or an ACT of 130–170 seconds. If citrate is used, then calcium should be infused through a separate line. Prostacylin may be used when heparin is contraindicated but is seldom sufficient alone, so is used with low-dose heparin.

The net fluid balance will be the sum of other fluid input (drugs, TPN, etc.) and losses (urine, nasogastric, insensible losses and ultrafiltration). It is possible to achieve high rates of ultrafiltration, but even in the most extreme states of fluid overload it is unwise to remove more than 10 per cent of the child's body weight in a single 24-h period.

Specific management

Glomerulonephritis

Renal biopsy

When the clinical features suggest a diagnosis of intrinsic renal disease a biopsy may help establish the specific diagnosis and therefore guide therapy. Histological diagnosis is particularly important in identifying rapidly progressive glomerulonephritis and tubulointerstitial nephritis. Management decisions especially those relating to the use of immunosuppressive agents depend on an accurate assessment of the histological findings and specific treatment needs to be started as early as possible to ensure a successful outcome. If there are no signs of recovery within two weeks of the onset then a renal biopsy may be necessary to predict the renal outcome.

Specific treatment

Rapidly progressive glomerulonephritis is a rare cause of ARF in children. A variety of treatments have been recommended in HSP, including corticosteroids, cytotoxic drugs, anticoagulants and plasma exchange, either singly or in combination (Oner *et al.* 1995). The lack of controlled trials, together with a spontaneous remission rate that can be as high as 50 per cent in some cases (Meadow 1978), makes it difficult to make an 'evidence based' choice of treatment. High-dose intravenous methyl prednisolone (20 mg/kg) was found to have been helpful in the treatment of rapidly progressive glomerulonephritis following Henoch–Schönlein nephritis, but not mesangiocapillary glomerulonephritis (Cole *et al.* 1976). It has the advantage of being relatively free of severe side-effects. A more aggressive combination treatment is with methyl prednisolone (30 mg/kg), cyclophosphamide (2 mg/kg), and dipyridamole but there is no evidence that it is superior to methylprednisolone alone. Plasma exchange has been used, particularly where there is a measurable antibody that can be cleared from the plasma, such as antibodies against double-stranded DNA in lupus nephritis or against glomerular basement membrane in Goodpasture's disease. It is a difficult technique in small children with renal failure and demands very close attention to fluid balance. One controlled trial in adult patients with lupus nephritis showed no benefit of plasma exchange over conventional treatment with prednisolone and cyclophosphamide (Lewis *et al.* 1992). There have been no controlled studies of plasma exchange in children.

Obstructive nephropathy

Obstructive nephropathy should be managed in cooperation with a paediatric urologist and radiologist. Treatment of the obstruction usually requires a general anaesthetic and it is a matter of careful clinical judgement whether the child is fit for surgery or requires prior treatment with dialysis. Obstruction below the bladder is easily managed by a bladder catheter and when above the bladder by percutaneous nephrostomies. The relief of obstruction is followed by a diuresis and a falling blood urea. Attention should be paid to the fluid and electrolyte balance during this recovery phase and excess losses of water, sodium, potassium, and bicarbonate should be replaced.

Prognosis

The initial results of treatment of ARF in children are determined by the cause of the renal insult. In isolated renal failure without other organ failure the immediate results of treatment are good. However, when there is evidence of other organ failure the mortality increases (Gallego *et al.* 1993). Because of this variability in outcome and the many ethical issues surrounding initiating dialysis treatment of critically ill children, scoring systems have been devised that are designed to differentiate potential survivors from likely non-survivors. The acute physiology and chronic health evaluation (APACHE 11) score, and a modification of this system and the paediatric risk of mortality score (PRISM) have both been applied to the study of children. They incorporate a series of physiological and laboratory variables from which a score is calculated to determine the probability of death. The mean score of the non-survivors was greater than the survivors when both the PRISM (Fargason and Langman 1993) and the APACHE (Bradbury *et al.* 1995) scoring systems were calculated. However, there was considerable overlap in both of the scores between the two groups, which limits their value when assessing an individual patient's chances of survival.

In a series of 22 children admitted to a paediatric intensive care unit who were treated with CVVH/D, nine survived. The survivors were less fluid overloaded than the non-survivors but there was no difference in the age, weight, PRISM score blood pressure or mean airway pressure between the survivors and non-survivors (Goldstein *et al.* 2001).

The mortality rates are greatest when there is multiple organ failure. Two-thirds of children who develop ARF after cardiac surgery die during the acute illness and the mortality is highest in the neonatal age group. Those with cyanotic heart disease have the worst outcome. At 5 years follow-up, 25 per cent of the survivors had significant renal functional abnormalities ranging from a reduced GFR to minor abnormalities of renal tubular function (Shaw *et al.* 1991).

In diarrhoea-associated HUS, in which only the kidney is usually involved, three-fourths of the children make a full recovery. Only 1–2 per cent die during the initial illness, 15 per cent fail to regain renal function and progress to long-term dialysis and subsequent renal transplantation, and ~10 per cent are left with a degree of renal insufficiency and hypertension. A small proportion of the survivors are left with neurological damage (Trompeter *et al.* 1983). Those with renal impairment or who die early have, on average, a higher polymorphonuclear leucocyte count at initial presentation than those who make a complete recovery. Unfortunately, there is a large overlap, limiting the usefulness of this measurement when considering the individual patients (Walters *et al.* 1989).

These children have been subject to many other insults including hypoxia and hypotension, as well as uraemia, and it is not surprising that some have neurodevelopmental delay. In one study, two out of six babies under 3 months of age were left with gross motor and global delay (Kohaut *et al.* 1987).

Although the treatment of ARF may have a high mortality, the long-term outcome of those who survive is generally good and justifies the effort involved in achieving a successful outcome. It is, however, important to recognize that many of the survivors have some degree of renal functional abnormality, which may not be immediately apparent. For this reason, it is important that they remain under long-term observation.

References

Adelman, R. D., Coppo, R., and Dillon, M. J. (2000). The emergency management of severe hypertension. *Pediatric Nephrology* **14** (5), 422–427.

Ahrenholz, P., Winkler, R. E., Ramlow, W., Tiess, M., and Muller, W. (1997). On-line hemodiafiltration with pre- and postdilution: a comparison of efficacy. *International Journal of Artificial Organs* **20**, 81–90.

Al-Dahhan, J., Haycock, G. B., Chantler, C., and Stimmler, L. (1983). Sodium homeostasis in term and preterm neonates. 1. Renal aspects. *Archives of Disease in Childhood*, **58**, 335–342.

Altieri, P., Sorba, G., Bolasco, P., Asproni, E., Ledebo, I., Cossu, M., Ferrara, R., Ganadu, M., Cadinu, F., Serra, G., Cabiddu, G., Sau, G., Casu, D., Passaghe, M., Bolasco, F., Pistis, R., and Ghisu, T. (2001). Predilution haemofiltration—the Second Sardinian Multicentre Study: comparisons between haemofiltration and haemodialysis during identical *Kt/V* and session times in a long-term cross-over study. *Nephrology, Dialysis, Transplantation* **16**, 1207–1213.

Altman, A. (2001). Acute tumour lysis syndrome. *Seminars in Oncology* **28**, 3–8.

Arbus, G. S. (1973). An *in vivo* acid–base nomogram for clinical use. *Canadian Medical Association Journal* **18**, 291–293.

Arieff, A. I., Ayus, J. C., and Fraser, C. L. (1992). Hyponatraemia and death or permanent brain damage in healthy children. *British Medical Journal* **4**, 51–52.

Armstrong, G. D. *et al.* (1995). A phase I study of chemically synthesized verotoxin (Shiga-like toxin) Pk-trisaccharide receptors attached to chromosorb for preventing haemolytic-uremic syndrome. *The Journal of Infectious Diseases* **171**, 1042–1045.

Bamford, M. F. and Jones, L. F. (1978). Deafness and biochemical imbalance after burns treatment with topical antibiotics in young children. Report of 6 cases. *Archives of Disease in Childhood* **53**, 326–329.

Bard, J. B. L. and Woolf, A. S. (1992). Nephrogenesis and the development of renal disease. *Nephrology, Dialysis, Transplantation* **7**, 563–572.

Best, C., Walsh, J., Sinclair, J., and Beattie, J. (1996). Early haemo-diafiltration in meningococcal septicemia. *Lancet* **347**, 202.

Bradbury, M. G., Brocklebank, J. T., Dyson, E. H., Goutcher, E., and Cohen, A. T. (1995). Volumetric control of continuous haemodialysis in multiple organ failure. *Archives of Disease in Childhood* **72**, 42–45.

Brocklebank, J. T. (1988). Renal failure in the newly born. *Archives of Disease in Childhood* **63**, 991–994.

Bunchman, T. E., Gardner, J. J., Kershaw, D. B., and Maxvold, N. J. (1994). Vascular access for haemodialysis or CVVH(D) in infants and children. *Dialysis and Transplantation* **23**, 314–318.

Bunchman, T. E., Meldrum, M. K., Meliones, J. E., Sedman, A. B., and Kershaw, D. B. (1992). Pulmonary function variation in ventilator dependent critically ill infants on peritoneal dialysis. *Advances in Peritoneal Dialysis* **8**, 75–78.

Chavalier, R. L., Campbell, F., Norman, A., and Brenbridge, A. (1984). Prognostic factors in neonatal acute renal failure. *Pediatrics* **74**, 265–272.

Cole, B. R., Brocklebank, J. T., Kimstra, R. A., Kissane, J. M., and Robson, A. M. (1976). Pulse methylprednisolone therapy in the treatment of severe glomerulonephritis. *Journal of Pediatrics* **88**, 307–314.

Coulthard, M. G. (1985). Maturation of glomerular filtration in preterm and mature babies. *Early Human Development* **11**, 281–292.

Daniel, S. S. and James, S. L. Renal response of the fetus to hypoxia. In *Neonatal Kidney and Fluid-Electrolytes*. Boston, MA: Martinus Nijhoff, 1983.

Deal, J. E. (1992). Management of hypertensive emergencies. *Archives of Disease in Childhood* **67**, 1089.

Drukker, A. *et al.* (1980). The renin angiotensin system in newborn dogs: developmental patterns and response to acute saline loading. *Pediatric Research* **14**, 303–307.

Dubbins, P. A., Kurtz, A. B., and Wapner Goldberg, B. B. (1981). Renal agenesis: spectrum of *in utero* findings. *Journal of Clinical Ultrasound* **9**, 189–193.

Esperance, M. J. and Collins, D. L. (1966). Peritoneal dialysis efficiency in relation to body weight. *Journal of Pediatric Surgery* **1**, 162–169.

Estroff, J. A., Mandell, J., and Benacerraf, B. R. (1991). Increased renal parenchymal echogenicity in the fetus: importance and clinical outcome. *Radiology* **181**, 135–139.

Fargason, C. A. and Langman, C. B. (1993). Limitations of the pediatric risk of mortality score in assessing children with acute renal failure. *Pediatric Nephrology* **7**, 703–707.

Feldman, H. and Guignard, J. P. (1982). Plasma creatinine in the first month. *Archives of Disease in Childhood* **57**, 127–130.

Freedman, A. L., Bukowski, T. P., Smith, C. A., Evans, M. I., Berry, S. M., Gonzalez, R., and Johnson, M. P. (1997). The use of urinary β_2 microglobulin to predict severe renal dysplasia in fetal obstuctive uropathy. *Fetal Diagnosis Therapy* **12**, 1–6.

Freedman, A. L., Johnson, M. P., and Gonzalez, R. (2000). Fetal therapy for obstructive uropathy: past, present, future. *Pediatric Nephrology* **14**, 167–176.

Gallego, N., Teruel, J. L., Mamposa, F., and Ortuno, J. (1991). Acute interstitial nephritis superimposed on glomerulonephritis: report of a case. *Pediatric Nephrology* **5**, 229–231.

Gallego, N., Gallego, A., Pascval, J., Liano, F., Estepa, R., and Ortuno, J. (1993). Prognosis of children with acute renal failure: a study of 138 cases. *Nephron* **64**, 399–404.

Gettings, L. G., Reynolds, H. N., and Scalea, T. (1999). Outcome in post-traumatic acute renal failure when continuous renal replacement therapy is applied early vs. late. *Intensive Care Medicine* **25**, 805–813.

Goldstein, S. L., Currier, H., Graf, J. M., Cosio, C. C., Brewer, E. D., and Sachdeva, R. (2001). Outcome in children receiving continuous veno-venous haemofiltration. *Pediatrics* **107**, 1309–1312.

Gouyon, J. R. and Guignard, J. P. (2000). Management of acute renal failure in newborns. *Pediatric Nephrology* **14**, 1037–1044.

Grylack, L. *et al.* (1982). Non oliguric acute renal failure in the newborn. *American Journal of Disease in Children* **136**, 518–520.

Guignard, J.-P., Torrado, A., Da Cunha, O., and Gautier, E. (1975). Glomerular filtration rate in the first three weeks of life. *Journal of Pediatrics* **87**, 268–272.

Guignard, J.-P., Torrado, A., Mazouni, S. M., and Gautier, E. (1976). Renal function in respiratory distress syndrome. *Journal of Pediatrics* **88**, 845–850.

Haffner, D., Schindera, F., Aschoff, A., Matthias, S., Waldher, R., and Scharer, K. (1997). The clinical spectrum of shunt nephritis. *Nephrology, Dialysis, Transplantation* **12**, 1143–1148.

Han, B. K. and Babcock, D. S. (1985). Sonographic measurements and appearance of normal kidneys in children. *American Journal of Roentgenology* **145**, 611–616.

Haycock, G. B. and Aperia, A. (1991). Salt and the newborn kidney. *Pediatric Nephrology* **5**, 65–70.

Heilbron, D. C., Holliday, M. A., Al-Dahwi, A., and Kogan, B. A. (1991). Expressing glomerular filtration rate in children. *Pediatric Nephrology* **5**, 5–11.

Hentschel, R., Lodges, B., and Bulla, M. (1996). Renal insufficiency in the neonatal period. *Clinical Nephrology* **46**, 54–58.

Holliday, M. A. and Segar, W. E. (1957). The maintenance need for water in parenteral fluid therapy. *Paediatrics* **19**, 823–832.

Howlett, H., Greenwood, K. L., MacDonald, L. M., and Saunders, A. J. (1997). The ultrasound appearances of neonatal renal vein thrombosis. *British Journal of Radiology* **70**, 1191–1194.

Hutton, K. A., Thomas, D. F., Arthur, R. J., Irving, H. C., and Smith, S. E. (1994). Prenatally detected posterior urethral valves: is gestational age at detection a predictor of outcome? *Journal of Urology* **152**, 698–701.

Jean, T. Y., Dramaix-Wilmet, M., and Glkhazen, M. (1982). Measurement of fetal kidney growth on ultrasound. *Radiology* **144**, 159–162.

Jenkins, R. D., Kuhn, R. J., and Funk, J. E. (1988). Clinical implications of catheter variability on neonatal continuous hemofiltration. *Transactions of the American Society of Artificial Internal Organs* **34**, 108–111.

Kohaut, E. C. (1986). Effect of dialysate volume on ultrafiltration in young patients treated with CAPD. *International Journal of Pediatric Nephrology* **7**, 13–16.

Kohaut, E. C., Whelchel, J., Waldo, F. B., and Diethelm, A. G. (1987). Aggressive therapy of infants with renal failure. *Pediatric Nephrology* **1**, 150–153.

Lawson, T. L. and Foley, W. D. (1981). Ultrasound evaluation of fetal kidneys. *Radiology* **138**, 153–158.

Lee, H. J., Arcinue, E., and Ross, B. D. (1994). Brief report: organic osmolytes in the brain of an infant with hypernatraemic dehydration. *New England Journal of Medicine* **331**, 439–442.

Lewis, E. J., Hunsicker, L., Lan, S.-P., Rohde, R. D., and Lachin, J. H. (1992). A controlled trial of plasmapheresis therapy in severe lupus nephritis. *New England Journal of Medicine* **326**, 1373–1379.

Lipitz, S. *et al.* (1993). Fetal urine analysis for the assessment of renal function in obstructive uropathy. *American Journal of Obstetrics and Gynecology* **168**, 174–179.

Mactier, R. A., Khanna, R., Moore, H., Russ, J., Nolph, K. D., and Groshong, T. (1988). Kinetics of peritoneal dialysis in children: role of the lymphatics. *Kidney International* **34**, 82–88.

Mann, J. F., Goerig, M., Brune, K., and Luft, F. C. (1993). Ibuprofen as an over-the-counter drug: is there a risk of renal injury. *Clinical Nephrology* **39**, 1–6 (review).

Mathew, O., Jones, A. S., James, E., Bland, H., and Groshong, T. (1980). Neonatal renal failure: usefulness of diagnostic indices. *Pediatrics* **65**, 57–60.

McLure, R. J., Prasad, V. K., and Brocklebank, J. T. (1994). Treatment of hyperkalaemia using intravenous and nebulised salbutamol. *Archives of Disease in Childhood* **70**, 126–128.

Meadow, S. R. (1978). The prognosis of Henoch–Schönlein nephritis. *Clinical Nephrology* **9**, 87–90.

Meadow, S. R., Glasgow, E. F., White, R. H. R., Moncrieff, M. W., Cameron, J. S., and Ogg, C. S. (1972). Schönlein–Henoch nephritis. *Quarterly Journal of Medicine* **163**, 241–258.

Miall, L. S., Henderson, M. J., Turner, A. J., Brownlee, K. G., Brocklebank, J. T., Newell, S., and Allgar, V. L. (1999). Plasma creatinine rises dramatically in the first 48 hours of life in preterm infants. *Pediatrics* **104** (6), 1–4.

Milford, D. V., Taylor, C. M., Guttridge, B., Hall, S. M., Rowe, B., and Kleanthous, H. (1990). Haemolytic uraemic syndrome in the British Isles 1985–1988: association with verocytotoxin producing *E. coli*. Part 1: clinical and epidemiological aspects. *Archives of Disease in Childhood* **65**, 716–721.

Moghal, N. E., Brocklebank, J. T., and Meadow, S. R. (1998). A review of acute renal failure in children: incidence, etiology and outcome. *Clinical Nephrology* **49**, 91–95.

Morgenstern, B. Z. *et al.* (1984). Transport characteristics of the pediatric peritoneal membrane. *Kidney International* **25**, 259–264.

Morris, M. C., Allanby, C. W., Toseland, P., Haycock, G. B., and Chantler, C. (1982). Evaluation of a height/creatinine formula in the measurement of glomerular filtration rate. *Archives of Disease in Childhood* **57**, 611–615.

Nicolini, U., Fisk, N. M., Rodeck, C. H., and Beacham, J. (1992). Fetal urine biochemistry: an index of renal maturation and dysfunction. *British Journal of Obstetrics and Gynaecology* **99**, 46–50.

Nolte, S., Mueller, B., and Pringsheim, W. (1991). Serum alpha 1-microglobulin and beta 2-microglobulin for the estimation of fetal glomerular renal function. *Pediatric Nephrology* **5**, 573–579.

Norman, M. E. and Asadi, F. K. (1979). A prospective study of acute renal failure in the newborn infant. *Pediatrics* **63**, 475–479.

Nowark-Gott, U., von-Kries, R., and Gobel, U. (1997). Neonatal symptomatic thromboembolism in Germany: two year survey. *Archives of Disease in Childhood* **76**, F163–F167.

Nuss, R., Hays, T., and Manco-Johnson, M. (1994). Efficacy and safety of heparin anticoagulant for neonatal renal vein thrombosis. *American Journal of Paediatric Haematology–Oncology* **16**, 127–138.

O'Brien, E., Waeber, B., Parati, G., Staessen, J., Myers, M., on behalf of the European Society of Hypertension working Group on Blood Pressure Measurement (2001). Blood pressure measuring devices: recommendations of the European Society of Hypertension. *British Medical Journal* **222**, 531–536.

Oner, A., Timaztepe, K., and Ozlem, E. (1995). The effect of triple therapy on rapidly progressive type of Henoch–Schönlein nephritis. *Pediatric Nephrology* **9**, 6–10.

Platt, J. F., Rubin, J.M., and Ellis, J. H. (1991). Acute renal failure: possible role of duplex Doppler US in distinction between acute pre-renal failure and acute tubular necrosis. *Radiology* **179**, 419–423.

Petrikovsky, B. M., Nardi, D. A., Rodis, J. F., and Hoegsberg, B. (1991). Elevated maternal serum alpha-fetoprotein and mild fetal uropathy. *Obstetrics and Gynecology* **78**, 262–264.

Polacek, E., Vocel, J., Neugebauerova, M., Sebkova, M., and Vechetova, E. (1965). The osmotic concentrating ability in healthy infants and children. *Archives of Disease in Childhood* **40**, 291–294.

Relman, A. S. (1964). Renal acidosis and renal excretion of acid in health and disease. *Advances in Internal Medicine* **12**, 295–298.

Reznick, V. M., Griswold, W. R., Peterson, M., Rodarte, A., Ferris, M. E., and Mendoza, S. A. (1991). Peritoneal dialysis for acute renal failure in children. *Pediatric Nephrology* **5**, 715–717.

Reeves, J. H. *et al.* (1994). A review of venovenous haemofiltration in seriously ill infants. *Journal of Paediatrics and Child Health* **30**, 50–54.

Rhodes, P. G., Hammel, C. L., and Berman, L. B. (1962). Urinary constituents of the newborn. *Journal of Pediatrics* **60**, 18–23.

Rudd, P. T., Hughes, E. A., and Platzek, M. M. (1983). Reference ranges for plasma creatinine during the first month of life. *Archives of Disease in Childhood* **58**, 212–215.

Savory, D. J. (1990). Reference ranges for serum creatinine in infants, children and adolescents. *Annals of Clinical Biochemistry* **27**, 99–101.

Schlesinger, A. E., Hedlund, G. L., and Pierson, W. P. (1987). Normal standards for kidney length in premature infants—determination with ultrasound. *Radiology* **164**, 127–129.

Schmit, B. and Andrew, M. (1995). Neonatal thrombosis: report of a prospective Canadian and International Registry. *Pediatrics* **96** (5), 939–943.

Shaw, N. J., Brocklebank, J. T., Dickinson, D. F., Wilson, N., and Walker, D. R. (1991). Long term outcome for children with acute renal failure following cardiac surgery. *International Journal of Cardiology* **31**, 161–166.

Simmonds, H. A., Cameron, J. S., Barratt, T. M., Dillon, M. J., Meadow, S. R., and Trompeter, R. S. (1989). Purine enzyme defects as a cause of acute renal failure in childhood. *Pediatric Nephrology* **3**, 433–437.

Smith, F. G., Jr. and Scrivens, B. (1964). Urinary protein excretion in the premature infant. *Journal of Pediatrics* **65**, 931–933.

Smith, O. P., White, B., Vaughan, D., Rafferty, M., Claffey, L., Lyons, B., Casey, W. (1997). Use of protein-C concentrate, heparin and haemodiafiltration in meningococcous-induced purpura fulminans. *Lancet* **350**, 1590–1593.

Smye, S. W., Norwood, H. M., Burr, T., Bradbury, M., and Brocklebank, J. T. (1994). Comparison of extracellular fluid volume measurement in children by ^{99}Tc-DTPA clearance and multifrequency impedance techniques. *Physiological Measurement* **15**, 251–260.

Soergel, M., Kirschstein, M., Busch, C., Danne, T., Gellermann, J., Holl, R., Krull, F., Reichet, H., Reusz, G., and Rascher, W. (1997). Oscillometric twenty-four ambulatory blood pressure values in healthy children and adolescents: a multicenter trial including 1141 subjects. *Journal of Pediatrics* **130**, 178–184.

Srivastava, R. N., Bagga, A., and Moudgil, A. (1990). Acute renal failure in North Indian children. *Indian Journal of Medical Research. Section A—Infectious Disease* **92**, 404–408.

Stapleton, F. B., Jones, D. B., and Green, R. S. (1987). Acute renal failure in neonates: incidence, etiology and outcome. *Pediatric Nephrology* **1**, 314–320.

Task Force on Blood Pressure Control in Children (1987). Report of the Second Task Force on Blood Pressure Control in Children. *Pediatrics* **79**, 1–25.

Toth-Heyn, P., Drukker, A., and Guignard, J.-P. (2000). The stressed neonatal kidney: from pathophysiology to clinical management of the neonatal vasomotor nephropathy. *Pediatric Nephrology* **14**, 227–239.

Trompeter, R. S. (1987). A review of drug prescribing in children with end-stage renal failure. *Pediatric Nephrology* **1**, 183–194.

Trompeter, R. S. *et al.* (1983). Haemolytic uraemic syndrome: an analysis of prognostic features. *Archives of Disease in Childhood* **58**, 101–105.

Vates, T. S., Johnson, M. P., Evans, M. I., and Freedman, A. L. (1997). The use of epidermal growth factor to predict outcomes in fetal obstructive uropathy. *Journal of Urology* **157**, 130A.

Versmold, H. T., Kitterman, J. A., Phipps, R. H., Gregory, G. A., and Tooley, W. H. (1981). Aortic blood pressure during the first 12 h of life in infants with birth weight 610 to 4220 grams. *Pediatrics* **67**, 607–613.

Walters, M., Matthew, I. U., Kay, R., Dillon, M. J., and Barratt, T. M. (1989). The polymorphonuclear leucocyte count in childhood haemolytic uraemic syndrome. *Pediatric Nephrology* **3**, 130–134.

Winkler, D. and Altrogge, H. (1985). Sonographic signs of nephritis in children. A comparison of renal echography with clinical evaluation, laboratory data and biopsy. *Pediatric Radiology* **15**, 231–233.

Winter, R. W. *The Body Fluids in Pediatrics*. Boston, MA: Little Brown, 1973.

10.7.2 Pregnancy

Michel Beaufils

Acute renal failure (ARF) has for decades been a life-threatening complication of pregnancy, largely a result of septic abortion, haemorrhage, and perinatal infection, although its incidence has decreased sharply in the past 20 years (but less so in developing countries). It remains a problem, mostly in the context of pre-eclampsia with or without the HELLP (haemolysis, elevated liver enzymes, low platelet count) syndrome. The mortality remains significant in the acute period, and progression to endstage renal failure is not exceptional.

Frequency

Table 1 shows the main published series of ARF in pregnancy. It can be seen that:

1. While ARF occurred in about 0.5 per 1000 pregnancies 30 years ago, its incidence is 10 times lower in the latest studies. In two series (Chapman and Legrain 1979; Lindheimer *et al.* 1983), no case of ARF was observed in 12,000 and 20,000 births, respectively. Two studies (Donohoe 1983; Stratta *et al.* 1996) document this decrease of frequency with time.
2. Complications of pregnancy accounted for 17–43 per cent of cases of ARF in the 1960s, while it now accounts for less than 10 per cent in most countries. Nevertheless, pregnancy is still responsible for 15–20 per cent of ARF in various developing countries (Naqvi *et al.* 1996; Selcuk *et al.* 1998).

The reported frequency of ARF varies depending on (a) the definition ranging from 'oliguria with azotaemia' to 'require dialysis' and (b) the population served. It is more common in poor countries, blacks, and hypertensives. It is now more useful to express the incidence in relation to births than as a proportion of all ARF. The given incidence is now ~1/20,000 births.

The mortality rate from ARF in pregnancy also varies between series, 56 per cent in old studies or in countries without access to modern medical care, compared to ~10 per cent in Europe and North America.

Aetiology

Table 2 lists the main circumstances associated with ARFs in pregnant women.

Functional renal failure (prerenal azotaemia)

Normal pregnancy is characterized by a progressive increase in plasma volume of about 50 per cent, and this expansion is a critical factor for outcome. Pregnant women are particularly sensitive to any volume depletion, which leads to functional renal failure. This is easy to recognize: the patient is oliguric, the urinary osmolarity is increased, the urine/plasma ratio for urea exceeds 10, and urinary concentration of sodium is usually less than 10 mmol/l, implying that tubular reabsorptive function is preserved, differentiating it from acute tubular necrosis. The response to restoration of the blood volume is prompt.

Water and electrolyte depletion due to hyperemesis gravidarum (now very rare) is the classical cause of functional ARF.

Table 1 Main published series of acute renal failure in pregnancy

Author	Period	*N*	Births (‰)	ARF (%)	Mortality (%)
Knapp	1951–1957	23	0.7		48
Smith	1957–1965	70			16
Barry	1958–1964	51		17	22
Silke	1959–1968	81			28
Kerr	1960s		0.2		
Smith	1960s	82			33
Harkins	1960–1971	31			22
Chugh	1965–1975	72		22	56
Silke	1969–1978	41			10
Grünfeld	1957–1979	57			14
Chapman	1970–1975	0[a]	0	0	0
Donohoe	1961–1970	20	0.34		15
	1971–1980	4	0.05		0
Lindheimer	1973–1980	0[b]	0		
Stratta	1958–1967	26		43	
	1968–1977	40	0.3	13.4	32
	1978–1987	15	0.06	2.8	
	1988–1994		0.05	0.5	0
Sibai	1977–1989	31	0.07		10
Firmat	1978–1991	27[c]		5.4	30
		134[d]		27	21
Nzerue	1986–1996	21	0.2		15
Selcuk	1980–1985			17.4	
	1985–1989			15.4	
	1989–1997			13.5	
Naqvi	1994	43		18	23

[a] No case of acute renal failure in 12,000 births.

[b] No case of acute renal failure in 20,000 births.

[c] Cases related to other pregnancy complications.

[d] Cases related to septic abortion.

Table 2 The main mechanisms of acute renal failure in pregnancy and their usual clinical context

Prerenal azotaemia
Water and electrolyte depletion: vomiting, diarrhoea, diuretics
Oedema-forming states: pre-eclampsia, nephrosis, heart failure
Haemorrhage
Obstruction
Nephrolithiasis
Gravid uterus
Tubular obstruction (uric acid)
Acute interstitial nephritis
Pyelonephritis, septicaemia
Drugs
Glomerular nephritis
Acute tubular necrosis
Pre-eclampsia, HELLP syndrome, abruptio placentae
Acute fatty liver
Haemorrhage, drugs, septic shock, haemoglobinuria, amniotic fluid embolism
Prolonged intrauterine fetal death
Microangiopathic syndromes
Haemolytic–uraemic syndrome
Thrombotic thrombocytopenic purpura
Bilateral renal cortical necrosis
Severe pre-eclampsia, abruptio placentae
Septic or haemorrhagic shock

Relative or absolute hypovolaemia is a hallmark of pregnancy-associated hypertension, and especially of pre-eclampsia (Chesley 1972; Beaufils *et al.* 1981). The latter is often associated with a decrease in renal function, but rarely meets the definition of ARF. True acute renal failure may complicate pre-eclampsia, but in virtually all cases it is accounted for by acute tubular necrosis.

Blood loss, diarrhoea, and use of diuretics may also cause (or contribute to) functional renal failure. Prompt diagnosis and correction of volume depletion is essential.

Acute pyelonephritis

The incidence of acute pyelonephritis is increased in pregnancy; it occurs in 1–2 per cent of women without previous bacteriuria, and in up to 40 per cent of patients with untreated bacteriuria (Little 1965). Acute pyelonephritis does not usually affect renal function in non-gravidas, unless there is associated obstruction. By contrast, it may be particularly severe in pregnant patients. It is often associated with a marked decline in renal function and multiorgan failure (Cunningham *et al.* 1973). The incidence of ARF is relatively low. Acute pyelonephritis accounts for 3–5 per cent of cases of ARF in pregnant women in a French study (Grünfeld *et al.* 1980), whereas it is reported as high as 45 per cent in others (Ventura *et al.* 1997). Moreover, drug nephrotoxicity may be an additional factor in such patients.

Obstruction

Urinary tract obstruction is a rare cause of ARF in pregnancy. Although the frequency of renal stones is no greater in pregnant women, nephrolithiasis, can cause ARF (Naqvi *et al.* 1996). Loin pain or gross haematuria, and urinary infection, suggest the diagnosis. Ultrasonography allows quantification of the dilatation, and often visualization of stones. When coupled with colour Doppler, it can demonstrate the interruption of ureteral flux and the absence of ureteral ejaculation (MacNeily *et al.* 1991). Intravenous pyelography is an acceptable investigation provided radiation dose is limited. Relief of obstruction by percutaneous nephrostomy, ureteric stenting, or basket extraction, is usually necessary (Thorp *et al.* 1999).

Ureteric obstruction by the gravid uterus is a rare cause of acute renal failure (Brandes *et al.* 1991; Jena and Mitch 1996). Of 14 cases reviewed by Brandes, 11 occurred in primigravidas, four had twin gestation, and four had polyhydramnios. Serum creatinine ranged from 248 to 1025 μmol/l. In eight cases, delivery (vaginal or Caesarean section) was followed by resolution of renal failure. In other cases, occurring too early in pregnancy for immediate delivery to be possible, ureteral stenting was successful and allowed delivery to be delayed for between 5 and 15 weeks; in one case, the amniotomy alone resulted in prompt diuresis (Brandes and Fritsche 1991).

Renal tubular obstruction by uric acid has been reported in a few patients. Serum uric acid exceeded 700 μmol/l and was unexplained, but dehydration contributed. Tubular deposition was attributed to an increased concentration of tubular fluid uric acid and an acidic urine. Renal failure resolved after hydration, alkalinization of the urine, and mannitol administration (Alexopoulos *et al.* 1992).

Acute tubular necrosis

Septic abortion

Septic abortion has, until recently, been the major cause of acute renal failure, and of maternal death. Mortality decreased after the availability of antibiotics. The incidence declined further when oral contraception became widely available in the 1960s. Finally, septic abortion has become rare in all countries where abortion has been legalized. The mortality in legal abortion has been estimated as 0.4 per 100,000 procedures, obviously far less than that of illegal abortion (Stubblefields and Grimes 1994).

Septic abortion remains a major health problem in developing countries. According to the World Health Organization, it accounts for 1,00,000–2,50,000 maternal deaths a year, many of them probably involving ARF.

In a study of 500 cases of ARF in Buenos Aires between 1978 and 1991 (Firmat *et al.* 1994), septic abortion accounted for more than 80 per cent of the cases related to pregnancy. Vladutiu *et al.* (1995) reported the Romanian experience during the years 1979–1989 when abortion was prohibited. More than 20 per cent of all ARF patients (131/653) had had illegal abortions. This proportion fell to 1.5 per cent after liberalization.

The ARF following septic abortion is usually associated with infection by Clostridia species. Patients present with hyperthermia (40°C or more), myalgia, vomiting, and diarrhoea. Diagnosis may be difficult at this stage if the abortion is not admitted, since vaginal bleeding is not always apparent. The patient then develops dyspnoea, hypotension, and jaundice, followed by the shock syndrome. Many patients respond well to antibiotics and volume replacement but may go on to develop ARF. The period of anuria may last 3 or more weeks, requiring dialysis and usual intensive care procedures. Although renal function often recovers completely (Firmat *et al.* 1994), bilateral cortical necrosis is a not infrequent consequence.

Pre-eclampsia

Pre-eclampsia is a clinical entity defined by the coincidence of hypertension and heavy proteinuria in the third trimester of pregnancy. It is the most dangerous form of pregnancy-related hypertension, since it is most frequently complicated by abruptio placentae, eclampsia, and/or fetal death. It occurs typically in young primigravidae, but it can complicate any pregnancy (Report of the National High Blood Pressure Education Program Working Group on High Blood Pressure in Pregnancy 2000).

Severe pre-eclampsia is associated with a virtually pathognomonic renal histological pattern, called 'glomerular endotheliosis' (Sheehan 1981). It includes large glomeruli with empty capillary lumens, endothelial cell swelling, and subendothelial 'fibrinoid' deposits (Figs 1 and 2). Endothelial and mesangial cells often contain fat vacuoles. There is no significant increase in the numbers of endothelial, mesangial, or epithelial cells. The intensity of those lesions roughly parallels the degree of proteinuria.

The classical distinction between 'pure' (of late occurrence in a primigravida) and 'superimposed' (of earlier occurrence or in a parous patient) pre-eclampsia does not make much sense. Indeed, several studies have shown that renal histological findings correlate poorly with this clinical classification. In fact, in a patient classified as 'pure pre-eclampsia', renal biopsy can reveal either the typical lesion of glomerular endotheliosis, vascular lesions, or any kind of glomerulonephritis (Delauche *et al.* 1980; Fisher *et al.* 1980).

Pre-eclampsia and its complications are now the main cause of ARF in pregnancy. While pre-eclampsia/eclampsia was reported as the cause of 10–20 per cent of cases in earlier series, it accounted for 50 per cent of cases in the series of Grünfeld *et al.* (1980). Similarly, in the

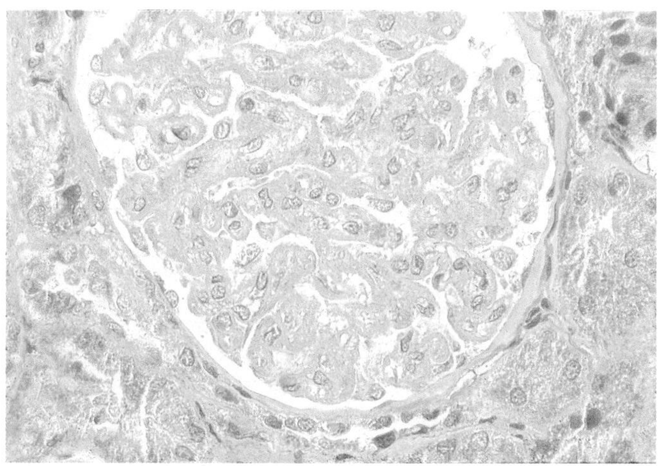

Fig. 1 Renal biopsy 8 days postpartum in a patient with pure pre-eclampsia. Thickening of capillary walls with lumens narrowed by swollen endothelial cells (Masson's trichrome 400×) (by courtesy of Dr D. Nochy).

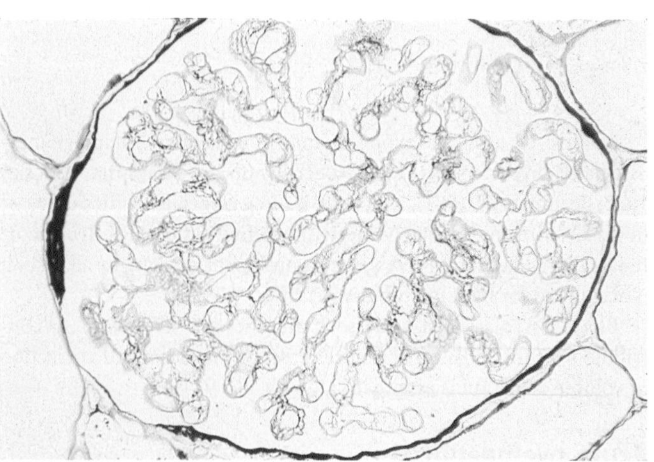

Fig. 2 Silver stain of the same glomerulus as in Fig. 1: diffuse 'double contours' of capillary walls (by courtesy of Dr D. Nochy).

report of Stratta *et al.* (1996), pre-eclampsia accounted for four of 26 cases of ARF between 1958 and 1967, and seven of 15 cases between 1978 and 1987. ARF is not related to the lesion of glomerular endotheliosis. In most cases the renal biopsy shows acute tubular necrosis. In a large cohort of 399 women with eclampsia, Mattar and Sibai (2000) reported ARF to be more frequent when eclampsia occurred before 32 weeks (9 per cent) than when it appeared later (2 per cent).

The most detailed study of ARF associated with pre-eclampsia included 30 patients (31 pregnancies), representing 1.8 per cent of patients with pre-eclampsia (Sibai *et al.* 1990). Eighteen of these patients had 'pure pre-eclampsia' defined as no known pre-existing disease (nine were nulliparous), while the remaining 12 had either pre-existing hypertension or renal disease (three were nulliparous). The onset of ARF was postpartum in all cases of 'pure pre-eclampsia', and in nine with pre-existing disease. Renal failure occurred in patients with especially severe clinical conditions: 50 per cent had abruptio placentae, 50 per cent had sepsis, and 85–93 per cent postpartum haemorrhage. The HELLP syndrome was present in 17 of 18 patients with 'pure pre-eclampsia' and three of 13 with pre-existing disease. Disseminated intravascular coagulation was diagnosed in 16 and eight patients, respectively. All patients in the 'pure pre-eclampsia' group had acute tubular necrosis. In the group with pre-existing disease, three patients had acute tubular necrosis, three had bilateral cortical necrosis, and the remaining had various forms of chronic renal disease. About half the patients in both groups required dialysis. There were three maternal deaths (10 per cent) in the period of ARF. All 16 surviving patients in the 'pure pre-eclampsia' group had reversible ARF, with normal renal function and normal urinary tests on follow-up. Nine of the 11 surviving patients in the other group required dialysis later, and four ultimately died when at end-stage renal disease. Eight of these patients had 13 subsequent pregnancies: three ended in miscarriage between 12 and 16 weeks, three were complicated by severe pre-eclampsia, and seven ended in full-term deliveries.

The pathogenesis of ARF in pre-eclamptic patients is poorly understood. The state of generalized endothelial dysfunction which will be discussed below is certainly an important component. Intense vasoconstriction and a hypovolaemic state are also common features of severe pre-eclampsia (Roberts and Redman 1993). It must also be remembered that ARF occurs in the most severe forms, associated with abruptio placentae. Disseminated intravascular coagulation is present in many of these patients (Haddad *et al.* 2000a), and haemorrhage is often superimposed. All these disorders lead to renal ischaemia and can explain tubular necrosis or bilateral cortical necrosis.

The HELLP syndrome

This syndrome was first described in 1982 (Weinstein 1982). It was originally thought to be a rare complication of severe pre-eclampsia, occurring in 4–10 per cent of these patients (Sibai 1990). More systematic attention paid to liver enzymes and platelet count showed that it is more frequent than initially believed, and that it can occur in the absence of hypertension and proteinuria (20 per cent of cases). Its significance is controversial, but it is undoubtedly associated with a poor prognosis.

The most frequent presenting symptoms are epigastric or right upper quadrant pain (65 per cent), nausea and vomiting (36 per cent), and headache (31 per cent). Visual changes, bleeding, jaundice, and diarrhoea are less frequent (Sibai *et al.* 1993). All these symptoms are relatively non-specific, so the disease may be misdiagnosed. Characteristic laboratory findings include mild haemolytic anaemia, thrombocytopenia of variable severity, a moderate increase of transaminases and lactic dehydrogenase, while alkaline phosphatase and bilirubin are most often in the normal range. This allows clear differentiation from acute fatty liver.

In a series of 442 pregnancies complicated by this syndrome, the onset was antepartum in 70 per cent and postpartum in 30 per cent. There was no pre-eclampsia in 20 per cent of cases. Disseminated intravascular coagulation occurred in 21 per cent of cases, abruptio placentae in 16 per cent, and ARF in 8 per cent (Sibai *et al.* 1993). There was a strong correlation between abruptio placentae and ARF. Perinatal death occurred in 34 per cent of cases, and maternal mortality was 1.1 per cent. Selcuk *et al.* (2000) found the HELLP syndrome associated in 36 per cent of pregnancy-related ARF.

As in pre-eclampsia, ARF occurs in the most severe cases, with multiple organ involvement (acute respiratory distress syndrome and ruptured liver haematoma), and obstetric complications such as abruptio placentae, fetal death, disseminated intravascular coagulation, postpartum haemorrhage, and sepsis (Sibai and Ramadan 1993). Maternal death occurred in 13 per cent of patients with ARF. It is not clear whether ARF is a specific component of the HELLP syndrome itself, or a complication of a particularly severe multisystem condition. Haddad *et al.* (2000) found that disseminated intravascular coagulopathy is significantly associated with abruptio placentae and ARF.

In the same series, renal histology showed acute tubular necrosis in virtually all the patients with ARF and only one showed cortical necrosis. One-third of patients required dialysis. All patients with acute tubular necrosis recovered and had normal renal function and urinary microscopy at short-term follow-up. In the long term, one patient had moderate renal failure, and another required dialysis 7 years after the pregnancy.

In subsequent pregnancies, patients who have had the HELLP syndrome have an increased risk of pregnancy complications, including pre-eclampsia, abruptio placentae, fetal growth retardation, or death. The recurrence risk of the syndrome itself is low (3–5 per cent).

Acute fatty liver

Acute fatty liver is a rare but life-threatening complication which occurs in the third trimester of pregnancy, most often in nulliparas who present with abdominal pain, vomiting, and fever, followed by progressive jaundice and hepatic failure (Kaplan 1985). Hypertension is present in 20–50 per cent of cases. Marked hyperbilirubinaemia with only minimally elevated transaminases is considered a hallmark of this disease, allowing differentiation from the HELLP syndrome and other hepatic diseases. Acute fatty liver can also occur in patients with pre-eclampsia. This association is present in up to 46 per cent of patients (Riely 1987). This syndrome may be related to a Glu474Gln mutation in long-chain hydroxyacyl-CoA dehydrogenase. The children usually have the enzymatic deficiency (Ibdah *et al.* 1999).

Pathological liver changes are characterized by microvacuolar fatty infiltration (steatosis) predominantly in the centrolobular areas (Fig. 3). Ultrasonography and computed tomography (CT) scans of the liver have been proposed as alternative diagnostic procedures. Their accuracy remains disputed.

The incidence of ARF in this condition is 60 per cent or more (Nash and Tomaszewicz 1971). Nevertheless, renal failure is usually mild and does not require dialysis. The high maternal mortality is due to hepatic failure.

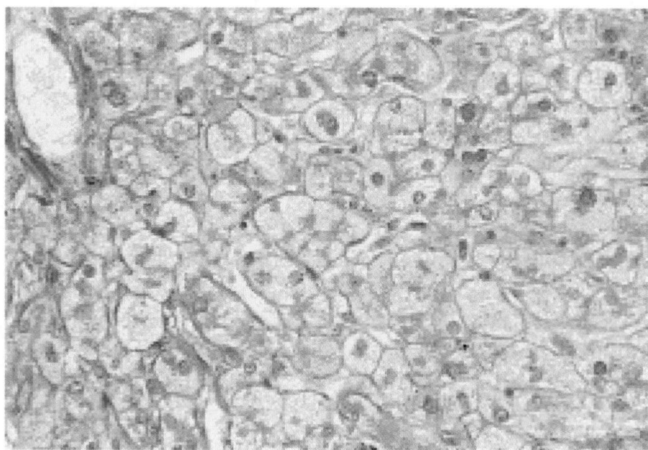

Fig. 3 Acute fatty liver of pregnancy (by courtesy of Professor P. Callard).

In the most recent series (Usta *et al.* 1994; Castro *et al.* 1999), gestational age at diagnosis ranged from 28 to 39 weeks, the disease occurring postpartum in a very few patients. Almost all patients have renal impairment, but the serum creatinine is not markedly increased, ranging from 97 to 317 μmol/l and dialysis is not required. There were no maternal deaths, in contrast with the 70–85 per cent incidence reported earlier (Kaplan 1985). Two babies died in each of the series. The recovery of renal function was complete by the seventh day in all patients. Acute fatty liver of pregnancy does not usually recur in subsequent pregnancies. No recurrence was found by Watson and Seeds (1990) in 21 patients with 25 pregnancies, but one case of recurrence was reported by Usta *et al.* (1994).

The renal histopathological findings are not consistent (Grünfeld *et al.* 1980). Kidney structure may be within normal limits, but in other cases there are focal lesions of acute tubular necrosis. Glomerular lesions or intraglomerular thrombi have occasionally been reported. A few patients have lesions quite similar to those observed in the haemolytic–uraemic syndrome.

The pathogenesis of ARF in acute fatty liver of pregnancy is unexplained. Shock is not a constant finding, nor is pancreatitis. Acute fatty liver of pregnancy exhibits some similarities with Reye's syndrome observed in children, but ARF is rare in this syndrome. Coagulation abnormalities suggestive of disseminated intravascular coagulation have often been reported. In fact, many of its features resemble the so-called 'hepatorenal syndrome' described in association with various hepatic disorders, and haemodynamic changes may play the prominent role (Grünfeld *et al.* 1980).

Haemorrhage

Uterine haemorrhage and hypotension are directly responsible for acute tubular necrosis in some cases, the frequency ranging from 7 per cent (Grünfeld *et al.* 1980) to 39 per cent in one study (Alexopoulos *et al.* 1993). However, it must be remembered that hypovolaemia due to haemorrhage is involved in many cases of ARF related to pre-eclampsia, abruptio placentae, and the HELLP syndrome (Grünfeld *et al.* 1980; Sibai *et al.* 1990). About 90 per cent of patients in Sibai's series had had postpartum haemorrhage. Therefore, this factor is more often additional than causal. In fact, patients with pre-eclampsia are more vulnerable to haemorrhage since they are already hypovolaemic, and they have an increased vasoconstrictor response (see below).

Thrombotic microangiopathies (see Chapter 10.6.4)

Haemolytic–uraemic syndrome and idiopathic postpartum renal failure

The first cases of so-called 'idiopathic postpartum renal failure' were reported in the 1960s. Since then, more than 200 cases have been described. In some series, this syndrome accounts for 5–10 per cent of pregnancy-related renal failure (Grünfeld *et al.* 1980; Stratta *et al.* 1996). In the 62 cases reviewed by Weiner (1987), only five developed before delivery. The disease occurs typically between a few hours and 8–10 weeks postpartum, but delays of several months have been reported occasionally. In most cases, pregnancy and delivery have been uneventful and most patients are multiparas. It begins with influenza-like symptoms, ARF developing after a few days. Moderate proteinuria and microscopic haematuria precede the development of anuria, which is usual. Hypertension develops in half of the cases. Microangiopathic anaemia occurs in most, but not all, cases. Numerous schizocytes are seen on the blood film; there is a high reticulocyte count, low haptoglobin concentration, and a low platelet count. The inconstancy of microangiopathic anaemia leads some authors to maintain the distinction between 'idiopathic postpartum renal failure' and the typical haemolytic–uraemic syndrome (Schoolwerth *et al.* 1976).

Apart from anaemia and thrombocytopenia, other signs of deranged clotting include prolonged thrombin time, decreased fibrinogen, and an increase in fibrin degradation products, considered diagnostic of disseminated intravascular coagulation, but intrarenal consumption and fibrinolysis have also been proposed.

Histopathological examination reveals the involvement of small arteries, afferent arterioles, and glomeruli. The changes in arteries and arterioles include intimal swelling, subintimal deposits, concentric intimal fibrosis, and fibrin thrombi. Fibrinoid necrosis is prominent in severe cases. The glomerular tufts are enlarged, with endothelial swelling and large subendothelial fibrin deposits giving a 'double contour' appearance. Deposits may lead to capillary obstruction, and occlusive thrombi are seen. The mesangial areas appear prominent. These changes are similar to those found in children with the haemolytic–uraemic syndrome.

In other patients, the lesions are more suggestive of nephrosclerosis, or even of malignant nephrosclerosis: arterial and arteriolar lesions are more severe, sometimes with necrosis; glomeruli appear ischaemic with retracted tufts and wrinkled basement membranes. It has been suggested that this histopathological heterogeneity is explained by the diversity of the disease. It is possible that ischaemic changes reflect the endpoint of an initial lesion of haemolytic–uraemic syndrome. In this respect, the timing of the renal biopsy is relevant. The predominance of chronic vascular lesions with glomerular ischaemia predicts a poor functional prognosis (Morel-Maroger *et al.* 1979; Grünfeld *et al.* 1980). The use of renal biopsy is limited because a high incidence of haemorrhagic complications has been reported repeatedly (Morel-Maroger *et al.* 1979).

Treatment

Heparin has been widely used with rather disappointing results. Fresh plasma infusion or plasma exchange, with or without antiplatelet therapy are now considered the therapy of choice (Hayslett 1985; Bueno *et al.* 1999; Elliott and Nichols 2001). Intravenous immunoglobulin has also been advocated. Treatment is more likely to be effective where glomerular lesions are active and 'fresh', and that this 'efficacy' is negligible when vascular lesions are prominent and glomerular ischaemia established, emphasizing the importance of an early aggressive treatment.

Prognosis

The clinical course is usually rapid. The maternal mortality, formerly may be as great as 50 per cent (Weiner 1987), but lower, has decreased since conservative treatment improved (Elliott and Nichols 2001). Nevertheless Egerman *et al.* (1996) reported two maternal deaths and four cases of chronic renal failure (in a series of 11 patients). There were only six live births. Renal failure was previously thought to be irreversible but Finkelstein *et al.* (1974) reported the first cases of milder and reversible renal failure, and complete or partial recovery was shown to occur in about 30 per cent of cases (Schoolwerth *et al.* 1976). Prognosis seems to be predictable from the stage of lesions seen on renal biopsy (Finkelstein *et al.* 1974; Morel-Maroger *et al.* 1979). There are anecdotal cases of subsequent pregnancies in which there has been recurrence of pre-eclampsia and microangiopathic anaemia.

Cause

The cause of idiopathic postpartum ARF remains unknown. Deficiency of a specific plasma protease responsible for the physiological degradation of von Willebrand factor seems to be involved in a very limited number of cases (Furlan *et al.* 1998), contrary to thrombotic thrombocytopenic purpura (TTP; see below). Various triggers have been described for the syndrome, pregnancy being only one of them. Endothelial damage from release of bacterial endotoxins or vasoactive amines leading to consumptive coagulopathy has been suggested. Various viral infections and drugs have also been reported as triggers (Elliott and Nichols 2001). Some patients with late postpartum ARF were found to have been taking the oral contraceptive at the time of onset. A role for such agents as triggers of the syndrome is quite possible since occurrence of the haemolytic–uraemic syndrome has also been reported in non-postpartum women patients taking the oral contraceptive (Tobon 1972; Schoolwerth *et al.* 1976). A generalized endothelial disorder is probably the key feature of this syndrome, as it is in other forms of pregnancy-related ARF (see below).

Thrombotic thrombocytopenic purpura

TTP occurs mainly in women, usually between 10 and 40 years of age (Pettit 1980). Pregnancy is a major predisposing factor for its occurrence or relapse. A few familial cases have also been reported, suggesting the possibility of a genetic predisposition (Wiznitzer *et al.* 1992; Alqadah *et al.* 1993). Unusually large forms of von Willebrand factor are usually present in plasma of patients with this disorder. The large multimers aggregate with platelets at sites where shear stress is prominent, generating thrombosis. A specific von Willebrand factor cleaving protease (a zinc metalloprotease) has been isolated from normal human plasma, and severe deficiency of this protease has been found in most patients with TTP (Furlan *et al.* 1998). Interestingly, the same deficiency is almost never observed in patients with the haemolytic–uraemic syndrome, which could be a means of differentiating these conditions. On the other hand, this deficiency is observed in conditions other than thrombotic microangiopathies (cirrhosis, chronic uraemia, acute inflammation), so it cannot be considered specific for TTP. Protease deficiency is mainly due to the presence of a circulating inhibitor, which has been reported to be an IgG antibody. In the rare congenital and familial forms, there is no inhibitor, but a constitutional deficiency of the enzyme, related to mutations in the ADAMTS13 gene (Levy *et al.* 2001).

In pregnant women, TTP occurs most often during the second or third trimester, with a mean of 23 weeks according to Weiner (1987), and its occurrence postpartum is very uncommon. The classic clinical picture is one of microangiopathic haemolytic anaemia, thrombocytopenia, neurological abnormalities, fever, and renal dysfunction. TTP has a high maternal and perinatal mortality, and the condition is not improved by delivery. This is explained by the wide distribution of vascular lesions and thrombosis. In the review by Weiner (1987), only 25 per cent of maternal–infant pairs survived when TTP occurred antepartum.

Therapeutic measures proposed for the treatment of TTP are essentially the same as for the haemolytic–uraemic syndrome (Rozdzinski *et al.* 1992; Egerman *et al.* 1996) and include plasma exchange with fresh frozen plasma. Immunosuppressive therapy has been advocated on the basis of a protease inhibitory antibody.

Bilateral cortical necrosis

Bilateral renal cortical necrosis is rare except in pregnancy when it is an associated factor in the aetiology in 60–65 per cent of the series reported (Kleinknecht *et al.* 1973; Chugh *et al.* 1994; Prakash *et al.* 1996). Bilateral renal cortical necrosis accounts for about 6 per cent of cases of ARF (Prakash *et al.* 1996) and for 20–30 per cent of pregnancy-related ARF (Grünfeld *et al.* 1980; Prakash *et al.* 1996). Patchy cortical necrosis, with complete or partial recovery of renal function, may be missed if investigations are incomplete. Bilateral cortical necrosis is most often a complication of abruptio placentae (36 per cent in the series of Chugh), and all the other conditions associated with disseminated intravascular coagulation. By contrast, it is far less frequent in pre-eclampsia (Kleinknecht *et al.* 1973; Grünfeld *et al.* 1980).

Bilateral renal cortical necrosis presents as acute renal failure in other conditions too but, unlike acute tubular necrosis, total and persistent anuria is almost constant (Kleinknecht *et al.* 1973; Chugh *et al.* 1994). Ten per cent of patients have hypertension, 36 per cent have fluid overload, and 14 per cent have hyperkalaemia (Chugh *et al.* 1994). The platelet count and plasma fibrinogen are lower in patients with cortical necrosis than in patients with acute tubular necrosis (Kleinknecht *et al.* 1973). The diagnosis can be established either by renal biopsy or, better, by selective renal angiography.

The renal lesions of cortical necrosis have been described fully in the classical work of Sheehan and Moore (1952). Renal biopsy is probably not the best diagnostic procedure because the process is patchy. However, in 14 representative (i.e. containing >15 glomeruli) renal biopsies in the series reported by Kleinknecht *et al.* (1973), renal tissue did not appear uniformly necrotic: non-necrotic areas were found in 10 of 11 specimens including juxtamedullary tissue. Extensive arterial, arteriolar, and glomerular fibrinoid thrombi were found in patients who did not survive more than 20 months without chronic dialysis.

Selective renal arteriography is the better diagnostic procedure, since it allows the best quantification of lesions, either diffuse or patchy. The kidneys are usually of normal or slightly increased size. Interlobular arteries show delayed filling and poor arborization. The cortical nephrogram appears heterogeneous, almost normal in some areas, and very poor in others, and the circulation time is prolonged.

In some cases, the cortical nephrogram is completely absent, indicating diffuse cortical necrosis. In such cases, complete anuria is to be expected (Kleinknecht *et al.* 1973).

CT scans and magnetic resonance imaging (MRI) have been more recently reported to provide strongly suggestive evidence: lack of enhancement of the renal cortex, enhancement of the medulla, and poor or absent renal excretion on CT scan. Later, cortical calcification can be seen on standard radiographs or CT scans. MRI, especially $T2$-weighted and contrast-enhanced $T1$-weighted imaging, seems also helpful in evaluating cortical necrosis (Francois *et al.* 2000).

The short-term mortality in patients with bilateral renal cortical necrosis was as high as 58 per cent in the report by Kleinknecht *et al.* (1973). This was thought to be due to inadequate dialysis before 1968. However, recent studies from developing countries again show a mortality rate of 60 per cent or more (Chugh *et al.* 1994; Prakash *et al.* 1996). Causes of death are septicaemia, pulmonary oedema, gastrointestinal bleeding, and other complications not necessarily related to renal failure or its management. A possible explanation for this high mortality rate is the high prevalence of extrarenal necrosis found at autopsy by Kleinknecht *et al.* (1973), organs involved include the adrenals, spleen, lungs, pancreas, and uterus.

In patients with bilateral renal cortical necrosis, anuria may be permanent and chronic dialysis will need to be instituted. Most often, however, patients recover some function. This improvement can take up to 3 years after onset, allowing discontinuation of dialysis. Unfortunately, renal function usually deteriorates again some months or years later, so that dialysis has to be resumed. In the series by Chugh *et al.* (1994), 19 of 113 patients were able to stop dialysis but seven of the 19 progressed to endstage renal failure over 3 months to 12 years. One patient had two successful pregnancies in the meantime.

The reason why pregnant women are especially vulnerable to bilateral renal cortical necrosis will be discussed below.

Causes unrelated to pregnancy

Occasionally, ARF may be related to acute glomerulonephritis, or bacterial endocarditis, unrelated to pregnancy. It may also be due to vasculitis, particularly lupus nephritis, which may flare up during pregnancy (see Chapters 4.5.3 and 4.7.2).

Drug toxicity may also cause ARF. ARF related to the maternal use of indomethacin and other non-steroidal anti-inflammatory drugs has been reported in many instances in newborns, and more rarely in mothers (Steiger *et al.* 1993). The main predisposing factors seem to be hypoxia, and the concomitant use of diuretics.

Pathophysiology: unifying concepts

Clinical syndromes are overlapping

The pregnancy-related ARF syndromes exhibit relatively clear distinctive features but the overlap between syndromes is considerable (Table 3). Indeed, most patients with the HELLP syndrome have pre-eclampsia, most patients with pre-eclampsia who develop acute renal failure have the HELLP syndrome, and one-half of the patients with acute fatty liver of pregnancy have pre-eclampsia. In all these cases, haemorrhage is often a triggering or aggravating factor. The haemolytic–uraemic syndrome is often preceded by hypertension and it may also develop in the context of pre-eclampsia. Conversely, microangiopathic anaemia is not uncommon in pre-eclampsia. Only a minority of patients have ARF in the setting of a 'pure' clinical situation. Acute tubular necrosis and bilateral renal cortical necrosis occur in particularly severe cases, usually including pre-eclampsia, but also in association with multiple organ involvement, abruptio placentae, disseminated intravascular coagulation, postpartum haemorrhage, and sepsis. On the contrary, the haemolytic–uraemic syndrome and TTP develop in less dramatic circumstances and pre-eclampsia is usually absent.

The pathological lesions

Pathologically, the spectrum of pregnancy-related ARF includes:

1. Acute tubular necrosis in a setting of severe pre-eclampsia and/or HELLP syndrome.

Table 3 Clinical and biological features of the main clinical syndromes leading to organic acute renal failure during pregnancy (modified from Sibai *et al.* 1994)

	PE	HELLP	Acute fatty liver of pregnancy	TTP	HUS
Typical onset	3rd trimester	3rd trimester	3rd trimester	2nd–3rd trimester	PP
PE associated		80%	46%	Rare	Possible
Hypertension	100%	80%	25–50%	Rare	50%
Low platelets	+	100%	64%	100%	50%
DIC	+	++	++	=	++
Transaminases	=	+++	+	=	=
Bilirubin	=	+	+++	+	++
Haemolytic anaemia	=	++	+	++	+++
Neurological signs	±	±	++	+++	+
Fever	=	=	+	+	+

PE, pre-eclampsia; HELLP, syndrome of haemolysis, elevated liver enzymes, and low platelet count; HUS, haemolytic–uraemic syndrome; TTP, thrombotic thrombocytopenic purpura; DIC, disseminated intravascular coagulation (modified from Sibai *et al.* 1994).

2. Microangiopathic diseases, typically idiopathic postpartum renal failure, hardly distinguishable from the haemolytic–uraemic syndrome, and from TTP.
3. Bilateral renal cortical necrosis, which may be associated with any clinical picture.

The typical lesion of glomerular endotheliosis is different from that of the haemolytic–uraemic syndrome (Droz *et al.* 2000). Nevertheless the pathological distinction between them may be difficult and the many similarities between the renal lesions seen in pre-eclampsia and 'idiopathic postpartum renal failure' have been largely emphasized. In fact, similar glomerular and vascular lesions are seen in both conditions, and they differ mainly in the extent and severity of translucent subendothelial deposits in glomeruli and of intimal proliferation and narrowing of the interlobular arteries. Both lesions may have an identical underlying mechanism. The occurrence of renal failure and the likelihood of its healing would depend on the extent of vascular lesions, and the presence of chronic ischaemia.

In such a pathological setting, superadded shock (with or without disseminated intravascular coagulation), will precipitate renal ischaemia, leading to acute tubular necrosis.

Acute tubular necrosis is related to ischaemia and/or vasoconstriction in the renal cortex, causing direct damage to proximal tubular cells. However, it has been shown recently that the medullary thick ascending limb of Henle may be more susceptible to ischaemic and/or hypoxic injury (Brezis and Rosen 1995). Tubular insult is greatly increased by prostacyclin deficiency, low nitric oxide delivery, or excess endothelin production, which are hallmarks of the pre-eclampsia syndrome.

Sheehan (1981) reported that after abruptio placentae, there is immediate renal vasoconstriction. If this lasts more than 1 h, it results in lesions of tubular necrosis, initially focal and then diffuse. If vasoconstriction persists, bilateral cortical necrosis may follow. This suggests that bilateral cortical necrosis is not a pathological, entity *per se*, but merely the final and worst result of severe and prolonged renal vasoconstriction.

The central role of endothelial dysfunction

In pre-eclampsia and related disorders, the primary phenomenon seems to be underperfusion of the placenta. In normal pregnancy, the spiral arteries perfusing the intervillous space undergo striking structural changes, which occur at 16–20 weeks. Trophoblastic invasion of these vessels results in 'physiological changes' allowing an increase in their diameter by four to six times. These vascular changes extend from the intervillous space to the inner third of myometrium. They are absent in patients who will later have pre-eclampsia or growth-retarded babies (Khong *et al.* 1986). In such patients, spiral arteries have a diameter about 40 per cent of that in normal pregnancies, and some are occluded by fibrinoid material and surrounded by foam cells. The cause of this defective trophoblastic invasion is poorly understood. Activation of NK cells and the role of HLA G have been extensively studied (Loke and King 2000). This immunological activation could precipitate apoptosis of the trophoblast, and also an inflammatory reaction (Redman *et al.* 1999). The placenta would thus release trophoblatic cells into the maternal circulation (Smarason *et al.* 1993), leading to endothelial lesions and dysfunction. Oxidative stress too could contribute to the endothelial dysfunction (Many *et al.* 2000).

When pre-eclampsia is established, generalized vasoconstriction and reduced organ perfusion appear as the predominant anomaly (Roberts and Cooper 2001). But much earlier a series of abnormalities are regularly present in women destined to have pre-eclampsia. They include:

1. A reduced stimulation of prostacyclin, with a strikingly reduced ratio of $PGI_2 : TxA_2$. This imbalance causes vasoconstriction and platelet adhesion to vascular endothelium.
2. Increased vascular reactivity to vasopressors, especially angiotensin II.
3. Increased plasma concentrations of endothelin I. The nitric oxide production may be diminished.
4. Activation of the coagulation cascade with early platelet activation, decreased concentrations of antithrombin III and increased concentrations of thrombin–antithrombin III.
5. Increased release of endothelial markers such as cellular fibronectin, von Willebrand factor, tissue plasminogen activator, and plasminogen activator inhibitor-1 in maternal plasma (Friedman *et al.* 1995). Increased mitogenic activity in the plasma.

These consistent abnormalities all point to endothelial dysfunction, and although best studied in pre-eclampsia, they are obviously common atleast to pre-eclampsia, HELLP syndrome, and the haemolytic–uraemic syndrome. Most of them are probably shared by acute fatty liver of pregnancy and TTP. In fact, the renal lesions observed in pre-eclampsia in the haemolytic–uraemic syndrome, and in TTP, are quite compatible with endothelial dysfunction being the main pathophysiological mechanism. It offers a more satisfactory explanation than disseminated intravascular coagulation (a very inconstant feature) or a Schwartzman-like reaction.

The generalized vasoconstriction observed in pre-eclampsia, as well as thromboxane excess, prostacyclin deficiency, and activation of the coagulation cascade are major predisposing factors for the development of acute tubular necrosis, and bilateral renal cortical necrosis. Such patients, especially those with abrupto placenta are especially vulnerable to exacerbated vasoconstriction and hypovolaemic shock.

Thus, the spectrum of acute renal failure in pregnant women may well reflect, more than different diseases, various facets of the same pathophysiological process, whose common pathway is generalized endothelial dysfunction. The question posed by Sibai *et al.* (1994) is pertinent. 'Are there different clinical syndromes or just different names?'

Management of acute renal failure in pregnancy

The general therapeutic measures which are mandatory in acute renal failure are essentially the same as in non-pregnant patients. However, some procedures are specific for pregnancy (Krane 1988; Maikranz and Katz 1991).

The first step is a careful search for, and treatment of, concealed uterine haemorrhage, which is frequent, and a serious triggering or aggravating factor for ARF.

The second step is to consider the possibility of immediate delivery as soon as the condition of the pregnant woman is stabilized. This option is affected by two factors:

1. If gestational age is sufficient (over 28–32 weeks, depending on fetal maturity), prompt delivery is recommended to protect both the baby and the mother.
2. The second factor is the presumed cause of ARF. If pre-eclampsia, the HELLP syndrome, or acute fatty liver are present, delivery

takes precedence, whatever the gestational age or fetal status, because it is the only means to stop the disease process, which could lead to maternal death. In other suspected diseases, and when the mother's life is not threatened, it is possible to treat both the aetiological factor and renal failure without terminating the pregnancy, thus allowing the fetus to reach a safe degree of maturity.

Both haemodialysis and peritoneal dialysis can be used safely in pregnant women (Lindheimer *et al.* 1983; Hou 1987). Dialysis should be instituted and tailored to keep the blood urea less than 20 mmol/l. Urea and other metabolites readily cross the placenta so the fetus will also be affected. Volume depletion should then be avoided to protect uteroplacental blood flow, and overload to avoid an exacerbation of hypertension. Short and frequent haemodialyses, with careful adjustments of heparin dosage, are required.

Specific measures proposed in TTP or the haemolytic–uraemic syndrome have been discussed in Chapter 10.6.4.

A renal biopsy should only be performed antepartum when its results are likely to have therapeutic implications, for example if a glomerular disease is suspected. In all other cases, renal biopsy should be postponed until after delivery.

References

Alexopoulos, E., Tampakoudis, P., Bili, H., and Mantalenakis, S. (1992). Acute uric acid nephropathy in pregnancy. *Obstetrics and Gynecology* **80**, 488–489.

Alexopoulos, E., Tampakoudis, P., Bili, H., Sakellariou, G., and Mantalenakis, S. (1993). Acute renal failure in pregnancy. *Renal Failure* **15**, 609–613.

Alqadah, F., Zebeib, M. A., and Awidi, A. S. (1993). Thrombotic thrombocytopenic purpura associated with pregnancy in two sisters. *Postgraduate Medical Journal* **69**, 229–231.

Beaufils, M., Uzan, S., Donsimoni, R., and Colau, J. C. (1981). Metabolism of uric acid in normal and pathologic pregnancy. *Contributions to Nephrology* **25**, 132–136.

Brandes, J. C. and Fritsche, C. (1991). Obstructive acute renal failure by a gravid uterus: a case report and review. *American Journal of Kidney Diseases* **XVIII**, 398–401.

Brezis, M. and Rosen, S. (1995). Hypoxia of the renal medulla—its implications for disease. *New England Journal of Medicine* **332**, 647–655.

Bueno, D., Jr., Sevigny, J., and Kaplan, A. A. (1999). Extracorporeal treatment of thrombotic microangiopathy: a ten year experience. *Therapeutic Apheresis* **3** (4), 294–297.

Castro, M. A., Fassett, M. J., Reynolds, T. B., Shaw, K. J., and Goodwin, T. M. (1999). Reversible peripartum liver failure: a new perspective on the diagnosis, treatment, and cause of acute fatty liver of pregnancy, based on 28 consecutive cases. *American Journal of Obstetrics and Gynecology* **181** (2), 389–395.

Chapman, A. and Legrain, M. Acute tubular necrosis and interstitial nephritis. In *Nephrology* (ed. J. Hamburger, J. Crosnier, and J. P. Grünfeld), pp. 383–410. New York, NY: John Wiley and Sons, 1979.

Chesley, L. C. (1972). Plasma and red cell volumes during pregnancy. *American Journal of Obstetrics and Gynecology* **112**, 440–448.

Chugh, K. S., Jha, V., Sakhuja, V., and Joshi, K. (1976). Acute renal failure of obstetric origin. *Obstetrics and Gynecology* **487**, 642–646.

Chugh, K. S. *et al.* (1994). Acute renal cortical necrosis. A study of 113 patients. *Renal Failure* **16**, 37–47.

Cunningham, F. G., Morris, G. B., and Mickal, A. (1973). Acute pyelonephritis in pregnancy: a clinical review. *Obstetrics and Gynecology* **42**, 112–117.

Delauche, M. C., Beaufils, M., Morel-Maroger, L., Leroux-Robert, C., and Richet, G. Relevance of renal biopsy to the future course of pre-eclamptic women. In *Pregnancy Hypertension* (ed. J. Bonnar, I. MacGillivray, and E. M. Symonds), pp. 221–230. Lancaster: MTP, 1980.

Donohoe, J. F. Acute bilateral cortical necrosis. In *Acute Renal Failure* (ed. B. M. Brenner and J. M. Lazarus), pp. 252–268. Philadelphia, PA: W.B. Saunders, 1983.

Droz, D., Nochy, D., Noel, L. H., Heudes, D., Nabarra, B., and Hill, G. S. (2000). Thrombotic microangiopathies: renal and extrarenal lesions. *Advances in Nephrology Necker Hospital* **30**, 235–259.

Egerman, R. S., Witlin, A. G., Friedman, S. A., and Sibai, B. M. (1996). Thrombotic thrombocytopenic purpura and hemolytic uremic syndrome in pregnancy: review of 11 cases. *American Journal of Obstetrics and Gynecology* **175** (4 Part 1), 950–956.

Elliott, M. A. and Nichols, W. L. (2001). Thrombotic thrombocytopenic purpura and hemolytic uremic syndrome. *Mayo Clinic Proceedings* **76** (11), 1154–1162.

Finkelstein, F. O., Kashgarian, M., and Hayslett, J. P. (1974). Clinical spectrum of postpartum renal failure. *American Journal of Medicine* **57**, 649–654.

Firmat, J., Zucchini, A., Martin, R., and Aguirre, C. (1994). A study of 500 cases of acute renal failure. *Renal Failure* **16**, 91–99.

Fisher, K. A., Luger, A., Spargo, B. H., and Lindheimer, M. D. A biopsy study of hypertension in pregnancy. In *Pregnancy Hypertension* (ed. J. Bonnar, T. MacGillivray, and E. M. Symonds), pp. 333–338. Lancaster: MTP, 1980.

Francois, M., Tostivint, I., Mercadal, L., Bellin, M. F., Izzedine, H., and Deray, G. (2000). MR imaging features of acute bilateral renal cortical necrosis. *American Journal of Kidney Diseases* **35** (4), 745–748.

Friedman, S. A. *et al.* (1995). Biochemical corroboration of endothelial involvement in severe preeclampsia. *American Journal of Obstetrics and Gynecology* **172**, 202–203.

Furlan, M. *et al.* (1998). von Willebrand factor-cleaving protease in thrombotic thrombocytopenic purpura and the hemolytic uremic syndrome. *New England Journal of Medicine* **339**, 1578–1584.

Grünfeld, J. P., Ganeval, D., and Bournérias, F. (1980). Acute renal failure in pregnancy. *Kidney International* **18**, 179–191.

Haddad, B., Barton, J. R., Livingston, J. C., Chahine, R., and Sibai, B. M. (2000). Risk factors for adverse maternal outcomes among women with HELLP (hemolysis, elevated liver enzymes, and low platelet count) syndrome. *American Journal of Obstetrics and Gynecology* **183** (2), 444–448.

Hayslett, J. P. (1985). Current concepts: postpartum renal failure. *New England Journal of Medicine* **312**, 1556–1559.

Hou, S. (1987). Pregnancy in women requiring dialysis for renal failure. *American Journal of Kidney Diseases* **9**, 368–373.

Ibdah, J. A., Bennett, M. J., Rinaldo, P., Zhao, Y., Gibson, B., Sims, H. F., and Strauss, A. W. (1999). A fetal fatty-acid oxidation disorder as a cause of liver disease in pregnant women. *New England Journal of Medicine* **340** (22), 1723–1731.

Jena, M. and Mitch, W. E. (1996). Rapidly reversible acute renal failure from ureteral obstruction in pregnancy. *American Journal of Kidney Diseases* **28** (3), 457–460.

Kaplan, M. M. (1985). Acute fatty liver of pregnancy. *New England Journal of Medicine* **313**, 367–370.

Khong, T. Y., De Wolf, F., Robertson, W. B., and Brosens, I. (1986). Inadequate maternal vascular response to placentation in pregnancies complicated by pre-eclampsia and by small-for-gestational-age infants. *British Journal of Obstetrics and Gynaecology* **93**, 1049–1059.

Kleinknecht, D., Grünfeld, J. P., Cia Gomez, P., Moreau, J. F., and Garcia-Torres, R. (1973). Diagnostic procedures and long-term prognosis in bilateral renal cortical necrosis. *Kidney International* **4**, 390–400.

Krane, N. K. (1988). Acute renal failure in pregnancy. *Archives of Internal Medicine* **148**, 2347–2357.

Levy, G. G. *et al.* (2001). Mutations in a member of the ADAMTS gene family cause thrombotic thrombocytopenic purpura. *Nature* **413**, 475–476.

Lindheimer, M. D. *et al.* Acute renal failure in pregnancy. In *Acute Renal Failure* (ed. B. M. Brenner and J. M. Lozarus), pp. 510–526. Philadelphia, PA: W.B. Saunders, 1983.

Little, P. J. (1965). The incidence of urinary infection in 8000 pregnant women. *Lancet* **ii**, 925–928.

Loke, Y. W. and King, A. (2000). Immunology of implantation. *Bailliere's Best Practice and Research. Clinical Obstetrics and Gynaecology* **14** (5), 827–837.

MacNeily, A. E. *et al.* (1991). Sonographic visualization of the ureter in pregnancy. *Journal of Urology* **146**, 298–301.

Maikranz, P. and Katz, A. I. (1991). Acute renal failure in pregnancy. *Obstetrics and Gynecology Clinics of North America* **18**, 333–343.

Many, A., Hubel, C. A., Fisher, S. J., Roberts, J. M., and Zhou, Y. (2000). Invasive cytotrophoblasts manifest evidence of oxidative stress in preeclampsia. *American Journal of Pathology* **156** (1), 321–331.

Mattar, F. and Sibai, B. M. (2000). Eclampsia. VIII. Risk factors for maternal morbidity. *American Journal of Obstetrics and Gynecology* **182** (2), 307–312.

Morel-Maroger, L. Kanfer, A., Solez, K., Sraer, J. D., and Richet, G. (1979). Prognostic importance of vascular lesions in acute renal failure with microangiopathic hemolytic anemia (hemolytic–uremic syndrome): clinicopathologic study in 20 adults. *Kidney International* **15**, 548–558.

Naqvi, R., Akhtar, F., Ahmed, E., Shaikh, R., Ahmed, Z., Naqvi, A., and Rizvi, A. (1996). Acute renal failure of obstetrical origin during 1994 at one center. *Renal Failure* **18** (4), 681–683.

Nash, D. T. and Tomaszewicz, T. (1971). Acute yellow atrophy of liver in pregnancy. *New York State Journal of Medicine* **71**, 458–465.

Pettit, R. M. (1980). Thrombotic thrombocytopenic purpura: a thirty year review. *Seminars in Thrombosis and Hemostasis* **6**, 350–355.

Prakash, J., Tripathi, K., Pandey, L. K., Gadela, S. R., and Usha (1996). Renal cortical necrosis in pregnancy-related acute renal failure. *Journal of Indian Medical Association* **94** (6), 227–229.

Redman, C. W., Sacks, G. P., and Sargent, I. L. (1999). Preeclampsia: an excessive maternal inflammatory response to pregnancy. *American Journal of Obstetrics and Gynecology* **180** (2 Part 1), 499–506.

Report of the National High Blood Pressure Education Program Working Group on High Blood Pressure in Pregnancy (2000). *American Journal of Obstetrics and Gynecology* **183** (1), S1–S22.

Riely, C. A. (1987). Acute fatty liver of pregnancy. *Seminars in Liver Disease* **7**, 47–54.

Roberts, J. M. and Cooper, D. W. (2001). Pathogenesis and genetics of pre-eclampsia. *Lancet* **357** (9249), 53–56.

Roberts, J. M. and Redman, C. W. G. (1993). Pre-eclampsia: more than pregnancy-induced hypertension. *Lancet* **341**, 1447–1451.

Rozdzinski, E., Herenstein, B., Schmeiser, T., Seifried, E., Kurrle, D., and Heimpel, H. (1992). Thrombotic thrombocytopenic purpura in early pregnancy with maternal and fetal survival. *Annals of Hematology* **64**, 245–248.

Schoolwerth, A. C., Sandler, R. S., Klahr, S., and Kissane, J. M. (1976). Nephrosclerosis postpartum and in women taking oral contraceptives. *Archives of Internal Medicine* **136**, 178–185.

Selcuk, N. Y., Tonbul, H. Z., San, A., and Odabas, A. R. (1998). Changes in frequency and etiology of acute renal failure in pregnancy (1980–1997). *Renal Failure* **20** (3), 513–517.

Selcuk, N. Y., Odabas, A. R., Cetinkaya, R., Tonbul, H. Z., and San, A. (2000). Outcome of pregnancies with HELLP syndrome complicated by acute renal failure (1989–1999). *Renal Failure* **22** (3), 319–327.

Sheehan, H. L. (1981). Renal morphology in preeclampsia. *Kidney International* **18**, 241–252.

Sheehan, H. L. and Moore, H. C. *Renal Cortical Necrosis and the Kidney of Concealed Accidental Haemorrhage*. Oxford: Blackwell Scientific Publications, 1952.

Sibai, B. M. and Ramadan, M. K. (1993). Acute renal failure in pregnancies complicated by hemolysis, elevated liver enzymes, and low platelets. *American Journal of Obstetrics and Gynecology* **168**, 1682–1690.

Sibai, B. M., Kustermann, L., and Velasco, J. (1994). Current understanding of severe preeclampsia, pregnancy-associated hemolytic uremic syndrome, thrombotic thrombocytopenic purpura, hemolysis, elevated liver enzymes, and low platelet syndrome, and postpartum acute renal failure: different clinical syndromes or just different names? *Current Opinion in Nephrology and Hypertension* **3**, 436–445.

Sibai, B. M., Ramadan, M. K., Usta, I., Salama, M., Mercer, B. M., and Friedman, S. A. (1993). Maternal morbidity and mortality in 442 pregnancies with hemolysis, elevated liver enzymes, and low platelets (HELLP syndrome). *American Journal of Obstetrics and Gynecology* **169**, 1000–1006.

Sibai, B. M., Villar, M. A., and Mabie, B. C. (1990). Acute renal failure in hypertensive disorders of pregnancy. *American Journal of Obstetrics and Gynecology* **162**, 777–783.

Smarason, A., Sargent, I., Starkey, P., and Redman, C. (1993). The effect of placental syncytiotrophoblast microvillous membranes from normal and pre-eclamptic women on the growth of endothelial cells *in vitro*. *British Journal of Obstetrics and Gynaecology* **100**, 943–949.

Smith, K. *et al.* (1965). Acute renal failure of obstetric origin: an analysis of 70 patients. *Lancet* **ii**, 351–354.

Steiger, R. M., Boyd, E. L., Powers, D. R., Nageotte, M. P., and Towers, C. V. (1993). Acute maternal renal insufficiency in premature labor treated with indomethacin. *American Journal of Perinatology* **10**, 381–383.

Stratta, P., Besso, L., Canavese, C., Grill, A., Todros, T., Benedetto, C., Hollo, S., and Segoloni, G. P. (1996). Is pregnancy-related acute renal failure a disappearing clinical entity? *Renal Failure* **18** (4), 575–584.

Stubblefields, P. G. and Grimes, D. A. (1994). Septic abortion. *New England Journal of Medicine* **331**, 310–313.

Thorp, J. A., Davis, B. E., and Klingele, C. (1999). Severe early onset preeclampsia secondary to bilateral ureteral obstruction reversed by stenting. *Obstetrics and Gynecology* **94** (5 Part 2), 806–807.

Tobon, H. (1972). Malignant hypertension, uremia and hemolytic anemia in a patient on oral contraceptives. *Obstetrics and Gynecology* **40**, 681–685.

Usta, I. M., Barton, J. R., Amon, E. A., Gonzalez, A., and Sibai, B. M. (1994). Acute fatty liver of pregnancy: an experience in the diagnosis and management of fourteen cases. *American Journal of Obstetrics and Gynecology* **171**, 1342–1347.

Ventura, J. E., Villa, M., Mizraji, R., and Ferreiros, R. (1997). Acute renal failure in pregnancy. *Renal Failure* **19** (2), 217–220.

Vladutiu, D. S., Spanu, C., Patiu, I. M., Neamtu, C., Gherman, M., and Manasia, M. (1995). Abortion prohibition and acute renal failure: the tragic Romanian experience. *Renal Failure* **17** (5), 605–609.

Watson, W. J. and Seeds, W. J. (1990). Acute fatty liver of pregnancy. *Obstetrical and Gynecological Survey* **45**, 585–593.

Weiner, C. P. (1987). Thrombotic microangiopathy in pregnancy and the postpartum period. *Seminars in Hematology* **24**, 119–129.

Weinstein, L. (1982). Syndrome of hemolysis, elevated liver enzymes, and low platelet count: a severe consequence of hypertension. *American Journal of Obstetrics and Gynecology* **142**, 159–167.

Wiznitzer, A., Mazor, M., Leibefinan, J. R., Bar-Levie, Y., Gurman, G., and Glezerman, M. (1992). Familial occurrence of thrombotic thrombocytopenic purpura in two sisters during pregnancy. *American Journal of Obstetrics and Gynecology* **166**, 20–21.

Recommended reading

Grünfeld, J. P. *et al.* (1980). Acute renal failure in pregnancy. *Kidney International* **18**, 179–191.

Krane, N. K. (1988). Acute renal failure in pregnancy. *Archives of Internal Medicine* **148**, 2347–2357.

Roberts, J. M. and Redman, C. W. G. (1993). Pre-eclampsia: more than pregnancy-induced hypertension. *Lancet* **341**, 1447–1451.

Sibai, B. M. *et al.* (1994). Current understanding of severe pre-eclampsia, pregnancy-associated hemolytic uremic syndrome, thrombotic thrombocytopenic purpura, hemolysis, elevated liver enzymes, and low platelet syndrome, and postpartum acute renal failure: different clinical syndromes or just different names? *Current Opinion in Nephrology and Hypertension* **3**, 436–445.

10.7.3 Acute renal failure in the tropical countries

Kirpal S. Chugh, Visith Sitprija, and Vivekanand Jha

Acute renal failure (ARF) is the most common nephrological emergency encountered in tropical countries. Reliable statistics on the pattern and prevalence of this condition amongst different populations are not available; but referral patterns to dialysis units suggest that community acquired ARF is far more common in the tropics than in Western countries with a temperate climate. In a recent study from the United States, intrinsic renal failure was responsible for azotaemia in 0.1 per cent of patients admitted to a hospital whereas data from a large referral hospital in North India showed that over a 1-year period, 1.5 per cent of all hospital admissions developed ARF (Jha *et al.* 1992).

The basic pathophysiological changes and management principles of ARF are the same whether a patient is encountered in the tropics or in a country with a temperate climate. There are however, a number of important differences in the pattern of ARF in the various geographical regions and ethnic populations of the world. Improvement in socioeconomic conditions, advancing industrialization, and expanding medical facilities in the developed countries have led to the near eradication of renal failure due to obstetric accidents but this has been replaced by more ARF following trauma due to high-speed traffic and industrial accidents, complex cardiovascular surgery, nephrotoxic drugs and chemicals, and cardiogenic shock (Chugh *et al.* 1991). In contrast, the hospitals in tropical regions continue to admit many patients with ARF secondary to diarrhoeal diseases, septic abortions, and other infections and environmental conditions specific to various regions (Table 1). Observations made in 3277 patients dialysed for ARF at our centre over the past 30 years provide useful information about the contribution of various medical, surgical, and obstetric conditions causing ARF in a tropical environment. The number of cases of severe ARF requiring dialysis has shown a steady increase from ~33 cases per year in the 1960s to ~200 per year in the 1990s. This reflects an increasing awareness of the condition in primary health centres, leading to more frequent referral to dialysis units. The proportion of obstetric ARF has declined from 22 per cent in the past to 8 per cent in recent years, whereas the surgical cases have increased from 11 per cent in the 1960s to more than 30 per cent in the 1990s. Diarrhoeal diseases, intravascular haemolysis due to glucose 6-phosphate dehydrogenase (G-6-PD) deficiency, copper sulfate poisoning, snake bites, and insect stings, which together constitute over 40 per cent of cases of ARF in India (Table 2), are rare in developed countries (Chugh *et al.* 1989).

Patients with ARF in tropical countries are relatively younger than those in the developed world, where the median age of patients with ARF has increased from 41 years in the 1950s to 60 years in 1980s (Turney *et al.* 1990). The average age of patients dialysed for ARF in India, on the other hand, was 34 years. Data from other tropical countries are similar.

Lastly, the facilities available in the tropical countries for treatment of renal failure are grossly inadequate. Intermittent peritoneal dialysis remains the mainstay of treatment. Haemodialysis is available in only a limited number of centres concentrated in the metropolitan cities. The number of dialysis centres has increased in recent years, but most are for stable endstage renal failure (ESRF) patients. ARF patients who are usually very sick, are referred to government-run teaching hospitals. As a result, the patients who often have severe renal failure with multiple complications at the time of presentation and require immediate dialysis, have a high mortality.

Medical causes of acute renal failure

Diarrhoeal diseases

Every year, diarrhoeal diseases cause 5–10 million deaths in children in developing countries. Poor socioeconomic conditions, lack of clean

Table 1 Comparative incidence of acute renal failure in tropical countries

Country	References	No. of cases	Medical (%)	Surgical (%)	Obstetric (%)
Singapore	Ku *et al.* (1975)	143	60	16	24
Argentina	Firmat and Pas (1975)	1000	58	28	14
Argentina	Firmat *et al.* (1994)	500	52	16	32
Thailand	Sitprija and Benyajati (1975)	162	61	15	24
Ghana	Adu *et al.* (1976)	50	62	24	4
India	Chugh *et al.* (1978)	325	67	22	11
India	Shah *et al.* (1985)	816	56	32	21
India	Muthusethupathi and Shivakumar (1987)	187	85	9	6
India	Chugh *et al.* (1987)	1862	60	25	15
Sri Lanka	Ramachandran (1994)	317	79	15	6
Nigeria	Bamgboye *et al.* (1993)	175	52	23	26
South Africa	Seedat and Nathoo (1993)	226	77	9	14

Table 2 Medical causes of acute renal failure in a tertiary referral centre in the tropics [data of Chugh *et al.* (1989) and unpublished (1987–1993)]

	1965–74	1975–80	1981–86	1987–93
Diarrhoeal diseases	23	12	10	5
IV Haemolysis due to glucose-6-phosphate dehydrogenase deficiency	12	12	6	4
Glomerulonephritis	11	9	9.5	11
Copper sulfate poisoning	5	2	1	0.3
Chemicals and drugs	4	5	7	13
Snake bites and insect stings	3	3	2.5	2
Sepsis	2	1	8	10
Transplant related	0	3	4	8
Miscellaneous and unknown	7	8	13	11
Percentage of total acute renal failure	67	55	61	64

All figures are in percentages.

water supply, overcrowding, and inadequate medical facilities are the factors responsible for the wide prevalence of diarrhoeal diseases. Children develop ARF more easily than adults following diarrhoea. Diarrhoea caused by viral gastroenteritis, bacillary dysentery, cholera, and food poisoning accounts for 35–50 per cent of the children dialysed for ARF in India (Pereira *et al.* 1989). The incidence increases during the summer, with maximum frequency during the rainy season. There has been an impressive decline in ARF due to diarrhoeal diseases from 23 per cent in the late 1960s to less than10 per cent in the past few years ($p < 0.001$), attributable to a general improvement in standard of living and early use of oral rehydration therapy. Gastroenteritis can be caused by a variety of organisms including viruses, for example, rotaviruses and Norwalk agent, and bacteria, namely *Escherichia coli, Campylobacter jejuni, Klebsiella pneumoniae, Shigella* species, *Salmonella enteritides*, and *Pseudomonas aeruginosa*. *Vibrio cholerae* continues to be endemic in parts of India, Bangladesh, and Myanmar.

Clinical features

The most striking feature is dehydration. When extreme, it manifests as hypotension, decreased skin turgor, and dryness of the tongue and oral mucosa. Small children present with lethargy, depression of the fontanelle, and sunken eyeballs. The severity of dehydration can be estimated by quantifying the amount of weight loss. Dehydration is classified as mild when the weight loss is less than 5 per cent, moderate when it is 5–10 per cent and severe when greater than 10 per cent. Renal failure is invariably oliguric. The urinary output improves after fluid replacement in 20–25 per cent of cases. Severe metabolic acidosis and hypokalaemia can develop as a result of loss of bicarbonate and potassium in the diarrhoeal fluid. The latter manifests as paralytic ileus and hypokalaemic paralysis.

Diagnosis

The clinical picture often provides a clue to the nature of the causative organism. Vomiting is an early feature of rotavirus infection. Loose, watery stools suggest infection with enterotoxigenic *E. coli* or *V. cholerae*. The presence of fever, cramps, tenesmus, and blood and mucus in stools suggests *Shigella, Salmonella*, or enteroinvasive *E. coli* infection. The diagnosis of cholera can be confirmed by microscopic demonstration of the highly motile vibrios in a hanging drop preparation of the stool; but stool culture is necessary for confirmation of other organisms.

Management

Early and complete fluid replacement is mandatory. In patients with mild to moderate dehydration who are not vomiting, rehydration can be achieved orally even as an outpatient. The World Health Organization (WHO) recommends a solution containing 20 g glucose, 3.5 g sodium chloride, 2.5 g sodium bicarbonate, and 1.5 g of potassium chloride dissolved in 1 l of clean preboiled and cooled water. The solution should be given *ad libitum*. Intravenous rehydration is only necessary in patients with severe dehydration, persistent vomiting, or paralytic ileus. The recommended replacement solution is Ringer's lactate in the dose of 30 ml/kg in the first hour. If no urine is passed, 10 ml/kg of Ringer's lactate, blood, or plasma is infused in the next hour. Persistence of oliguria despite these measures indicates established ARF. On the other hand, if the urine output improves, 40 ml/kg of Ringer's lactate should be given over the next 2 h, followed by 40 ml/kg of oral rehydration solution over the next 3 h. In older children and adults, the intravenous dose of Ringer's lactate is 110 ml/kg to be given over 4 h. Children with established ARF are usually treated by peritoneal dialysis as paediatric haemodialysis facilities are not available in most tropical countries.

The hypokalaemia associated with diarrhoea may worsen as the metabolic acidosis is corrected, and large amounts of potassium may be required to prevent life-threatening cardiac dysrhythmias. The commercially available peritoneal dialysis fluid does not contain any potassium, so potassium should be replaced through an intravenous or intraperitoneal route, guided by frequent estimations as the peritoneal dialysis is being performed.

Pathology

Renal histology reveals acute tubular necrosis (Fig. 1); acute cortical necrosis is occasionally seen in infants and children with severe volume depletion (Chugh *et al.* 1994).

Haemolytic–uraemic syndrome (see Chapter 10.6.3)

Haemolytic–uraemic syndrome has replaced diarrhoeal diseases as the most common cause of ARF in children in several tropical countries, and is responsible for 35–41 per cent of all cases of paediatric ARF in India (Srivastava *et al.* 1990). This condition is infrequent in adults.

Clinical features

Several important differences have been noted in the clinical presentation of haemolytic–uraemic syndrome in tropical countries compared to that seen in the temperate zones. The syndrome is principally seen in pre-school-age children. The main feature of the illness is oliguric

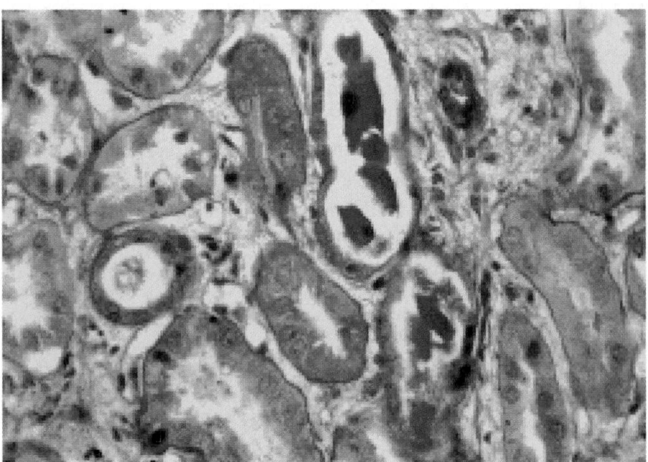

Fig. 1 Renal biopsy showing characteristic changes of acute tubular necrosis. Some of the tubules are markedly dilated with flattened epithelium. The interstitium shows areas of widening.

renal failure. Renal failure is preceded by a diarrhoeal prodrome in 70–81 per cent of patients. The prodrome is usually mild and unimpressive in comparison to the West, where it is often severe and prolonged. After an asymptomatic period ranging from 3 to 20 days, there is a decrease in urine output. Examination reveals pallor and mild jaundice. Hypertension is seen in a minority at presentation. Neurological involvement, characterized by visual disturbances, irritability, seizures, drowsiness, or coma is seen in 30–50 per cent of cases. The renal failure is usually severe and requires a prolonged period of dialysis.

Diagnosis

The diagnosis should be suspected in all children who develop oliguric ARF following a mild diarrhoeal illness. Confirmation requires demonstration of microangiopathic haemolytic anaemia, characterized by fragmented erythrocytes on the blood smear, and thrombocytopenia. The anaemia is often more severe than that predicted by the renal function, and may necessitate blood transfusions. The platelet count usually falls to ~50,000/mm^3 but is rarely severe enough to cause spontaneous bleeding. Corroborative findings include unconjugated hyperbilirubinaemia, raised plasma lactate dehydrogenase concentrations, elevated fibrin degradation products, and prolonged thrombin and reptilase times. Serum uric acid is disproportionately elevated due to haemolysis. Urinalysis shows microscopic haematuria and modest proteinuria.

Management

The treatment is mainly supportive, and includes volume replacement and control of hypertension, but children with severe renal failure are treated with peritoneal dialysis. Several specific therapies have been tried to limit vascular injury, including antiplatelet agents and anticoagulants, plasma infusions, or plasma exchange. Of these, the latter two have been used with varying success in several Western centres, but their use is limited in the tropics.

The outcome of haemolytic–uraemic syndrome in tropical countries is usually poor, with a mortality rate of about 60 per cent (Bhuyan *et al.* 1994). Of those who show some recovery of renal function, a significant proportion are left with residual dysfunction and progress to endstage renal disease over the ensuing months or years.

Pathology

The histological hallmark of this condition is thrombotic microangiopathy in the renal vasculature. Two distinct patterns of involvement are seen. Glomerular capillary lesions predominate in diarrhoea-associated haemolytic–uraemic syndrome; there is swelling of endothelial cells, widening of subendothelial regions secondary to deposition of fluffy eosinophilic material, and hypertrophy of mesangial cells. Intraluminal platelet thrombi and fibrin occlude the narrowed capillaries and arterioles. A disproportionate involvement of arterioles and small arteries with severe intimal proliferation and luminal stenosis has been reported from some tropical centers. Up to 40 per cent of these patients develop patchy or diffuse renal cortical necrosis (Srivastava *et al.* 1990).

Pathogenesis

Renal endothelial cell injury, produced by powerful exotoxins liberated by the offending organisms is considered to be the primary aetiological event. In contrast to the Western countries, where verotoxin-producing *E. coli* (O157 : H7) is the most common organism responsible for the prodromal illness, *Shigella dysenteriae* serotype I has been isolated most frequently from the stool samples of cases in the tropical countries. Other organisms include *Salmonella*, *Klebsiella*, non-verotoxin-producing strains of *E. coli*, *Shigella flexneri*, *Proteus*, and *Pseudomonas*. Haemolytic–uraemic syndrome has also been reported following non-gastrointestinal illnesses such as measles, pneumonia, and meningitis (Srivastava *et al.* 1990).

Intravascular haemolysis and glucose 6-phosphate dehydrogenase deficiency

Acute haemolysis in individuals deficient in G-6-PD, a key enzyme that protects erythrocytes from oxidant stresses, is a frequent cause of ARF in some ethnic populations in tropical countries. In India, G-6-PD deficiency is the most common cause of clinically significant intravascular haemolysis, leading to ARF in about 5–10 per cent of cases (Chugh *et al.* 1977b; Sarkar *et al.* 1993).

The prevalence of G-6-PD deficiency, which is X-linked, varies from 2.2 per cent to 20 per cent in various ethnic groups in India, Saudi Arabia, East Africa, and Nigeria. All males (hemizygotes) inherit the abnormal gene from their mothers who act as the carriers (heterozygotes). Inactivation of one of the two X chromosomes leads to two populations of red blood cells in the heterozygote females: normal and those deficient in the enzyme. As a result, female carriers do not develop clinically significant haemolysis.

Clinical features

Haemolytic crisis usually develops within hours of exposure to the oxidant stress, most commonly induced by drugs, toxins, or infections. Commonly incriminated drugs include primaquin, sulfonamides, acetylsalicylic acid, nitrofurantoin, nalidixic acid, furazolidone, niridazole, doxorubicin, and phenazopyridine. Accidental ingestion of toxic compounds such as naphthalene balls and severe metabolic acidosis of any aetiology can also precipitate haemolytic episodes. A high incidence of ARF (25.8 per cent) has been observed in G-6-PD deficient patients who developed haemolysis after ingesting fava beans. Infections that can precipitate haemolysis include viral hepatitis, rickettsia, typhoid, and urinary tract infection.

The clinical manifestations include passage of dark (cola) coloured urine and a sudden reduction in haemoglobin. In some forms of

G-6-PD deficiency, the enzyme activity is least in the senescent red blood cells, which are rapidly destroyed. The haemolysis abates following this crisis, as the residual population of young erythrocytes is able to deal with the continued oxidant stress. Patients with additional risk factors such as dehydration and septicaemia and those taking other nephrotoxic agents are more likely to develop renal dysfunction. Renal failure is oliguric in the vast majority (Sarkar *et al.* 1993), lasting from 2 to 7 days after which the patient usually enters a diuretic phase.

Diagnosis

The diagnosis should be considered when renal failure follows an acute haemolytic episode, and the patient should be thoroughly questioned about any possible exposure to oxidant agents. Haemolysis is evident from a reduction in haematocrit, an increase in plasma-free haemoglobin and unconjugated bilirubin, and a decline in plasma haptoglobin. The diagnosis can be confirmed by estimating the G-6-PD. Because the older red blood cells with the deficient enzyme are destroyed in the crisis, a misleading result may be obtained during a haemolytic episode when the red cell population consists of younger erythrocytes. The test should then be repeated after the stress is over and the patient has recovered from the acute haemolytic episode.

Pathology

Renal histology shows features of acute tubular necrosis but the tubules may contain pigmented haemoglobin casts (Fig. 2). Cortical necrosis has also been reported in rare instances (Chugh *et al.* 1994).

Pathogenesis

G-6-PD is an essential enzyme in the hexose monophosphate shunt. An increase in activity of this pathway at the time of oxidant stress leads to regeneration of reduced glutathione that protects the sulfhydryl (–SH) groups of haemoglobin and the erythrocyte membrane. Individuals deficient in this enzyme are unable to maintain an adequate level of reduced glutathione in their red blood cells. The oxidized haemoglobin precipitates within the red blood cells (forming Heinz bodies), and leads to haemolysis. A variety of mutations in the G-6-PD gene give rise to abnormal enzymes with varying degrees of activity.

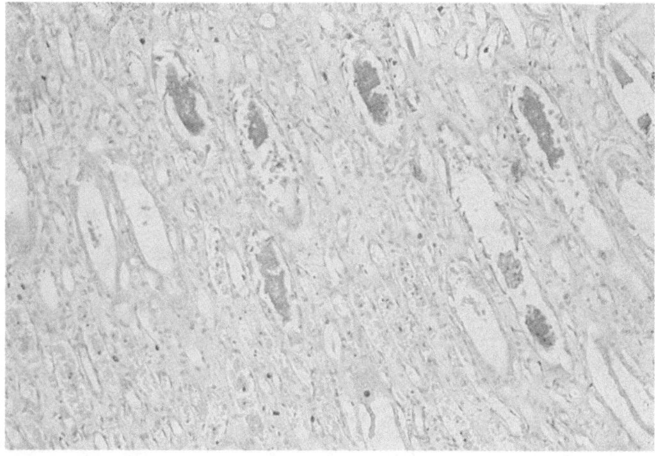

Fig. 2 Renal biopsy from a patient with glucose 6-phosphate dehydrogenase deficiency and acute renal failure following intravascular haemolysis. Necrotic tubules contain pigmented casts.

The Mediterranean variant, prevalent in the Indian population, is an unstable enzyme with very low activity, and patients with this variant exhibit chronic anaemia. The A− variant, encountered in other parts of the world, is more stable.

The mechanism of development of renal injury following haemoglobinuria is not clear. The finding of pigment casts supports the hypothesis of intratubular obstruction by local precipitation of haemoglobin in acid urine. However, the development of renal insufficiency following haemoglobinaemia is unpredictable. Early volume loading with Ringer's lactate attenuates the decline in renal blood flow and glomerular filtration rate (GFR) in the first 3–6 h. Haemoglobin is not directly nephrotoxic. However, it dissociates into nephrotoxic ferrihaemate in the acidic environment of the distal nephron. It has been postulated that other by-products of the haemolytic process, possibly the red blood cell wall or cytoplasmic constituents, could also be nephrotoxic.

Infection-related acute renal failure in the tropics

Malarial acute renal failure

Malaria is a protozoan disease caused by the *Plasmodium* parasite transmitted by the bite of the *Anopheles* mosquito. It is endemic in 103 tropical countries with a combined population of over 2.5 billion; affects 300–500 million people annually, and is responsible for 1–3 million deaths. About 90 per cent of these deaths, mostly in children, are in Africa (Breman and Steketee 1992). Of the four species of Plasmodium, *Plasmodium falciparum* predominates in sub-Saharan Africa, New Guinea, Haiti, and the Indian subcontinent and *Plasmodium vivax* is more common in Central America and the Indian subcontinent. These two protozoal infections are equally prevalent in South America, eastern Asia, and Oceania. *Plasmodium malariae* and *Plasmodium ovale* infections are rare outside Africa.

Only *P. falciparum* and *P. malariae* are associated with renal disease; *P. malariae* causes an immune-complex type glomerulonephritis, but ARF is the most important manifestation of *P. falciparum* malaria. The overall risk is less than 1 per cent, but may rise to 60 per cent in patients with severe infection. Those living in endemic areas acquire varying degrees of immunity, and the incidence amongst them is 2–5 per cent (Sitprija 1988; Barsoum 2000). Non-immune visitors to an endemic area develop severe infection and are more likely to develop renal failure; reported figures range from 25 to 30 per cent (Weber *et al.* 1991).

Clinical features

The initial symptoms are non-specific and consist of malaise, headache, fatigue, muscle aches, fever, and chills. The classic malarial paroxysms with spiking fever and rigours are rarely seen in *P. falciparum* infections (White and Breman 1994). Nausea, vomiting, and hypotension are common in non-immune individuals. Patients with severe infection may develop deep coma and seizures, non-cardiogenic pulmonary oedema, shock, and disseminated intravascular coagulation. ARF is usually seen by the end of first week and is non-oliguric in 50–75 per cent of cases (Zewdu 1994). It is usually hypercatabolic and there is a rapid rise in blood urea and serum creatinine. Hyperkalaemia is an early feature and may necessitate early dialysis. Cholestatic jaundice, characterized by elevated alkaline phosphatase concentration out of proportion to the transaminases, is seen in over 75 per cent cases of malarial ARF. Anaemia and thrombocytopenia are encountered in over two-thirds of patients. The so called 'blackwater fever', earlier believed to be a state of hypersensitivity, is now thought to be due to oxidant-stress-induced intravascular haemolysis in G-6-PD deficient subjects. Renal failure lasts from a few days to several weeks, with an average of 2 weeks.

Diagnosis

The clinical picture of severe falciparum malaria resembles other tropical infections including leptospirosis, scrub typhus, and hantavirus infection. The diagnosis is established by the demonstration of asexual forms of the parasite in peripheral blood smears stained with Giemsa stain. Staining with the fluorescent dye acridine orange allows a more rapid diagnosis (White and Breman 1994). Other laboratory features include normocytic normochromic anaemia; severe cases may have a leucocytosis, thrombocytopenia, and prolonged prothrombin and partial thromboplastin times, indicating a consumptive coagulopathy. Hyponatraemia and lactic acidosis are common.

Management

Severe falciparum malaria is a medical emergency and requires intensive care. The cinchona alkaloids (quinine or quinidine) are the mainstay of treatment because of their activity against chloroquin-resistant strains. Quinine is started intravenously at a dose of 7 mg of the salt/kg body weight, infused over 30 min, followed by 10 mg/kg body weight over 4 h. Infusion is continued at the rate of 10 mg/kg every 8 h until the patient can take oral quinine sulfate in a dose of 650 mg three times a day for a total of 7 days. Quinine therapy often causes hyperinsulinaemia, which may cause hypoglycaemia especially in pregnant women. The dose should be decreased by 30–50 per cent after the first 2 days if renal failure persists. Patients should also receive gametocidal therapy (tetracycline 250 mg four times a day for 7 days, or pyrimethamine/sulfadoxine, three tablets in a single dose). Mefloquine, halofantrine, atovaquone, artemesinin, and fansidar derivatives are alternative agents for resistant falciparum malaria. Artemisinin derivatives are the treatment of choice and are given in a dose of 10–12 mg/kg over 5–7 days in combination with tetracycline. Resistance to artemesinin has not yet been described.

Treatment of renal failure is the same as that due to other causes. Fluid should be administered cautiously especially in the absence of signs of frank dehydration, as a delayed response to water load may precipitate pulmonary oedema (Sitprija 1988). Since renal failure is hypercatabolic, frequent dialysis may be needed. The peritoneal microcirculation is impaired due to infected erythrocytes and vasoconstriction, reducing the efficacy of peritoneal dialysis. However, in practice, peritoneal dialysis is simple to perform and more easily available than haemodialysis (Trang *et al.* 1992). In a recent study, Phu *et al.* (2002) randomized patients with ARF, 69 per cent due to severe malaria, to receive pumped venovenous haemofiltration or peritoneal dialysis. Patients treated with peritoneal dialysis showed a lower rate of resolution of acidosis, a slower rate of decline in plasma creatinine, and a markedly increased risk of death (odds ratio, 5 : 1; 95% confidence interval, 1.6–16). Patients assigned to haemofiltration remained dialysis dependent for a shorter time, and resolution of acidosis and azotaemia was faster than in those receiving peritoneal dialysis. When the capital costs were excluded, haemofiltration was about 40 per cent cheaper than peritoneal dialysis. Exchange transfusion rapidly reduces the level of parasitaemia and is applied when it exceeds 10 per cent.

The mortality of malarial ARF varies between 10 and 40 per cent (Trang *et al.* 1992). The outcome is good in patients who receive early medical attention and adequate dialysis. The mortality fell from 75 to 25 per cent in one hospital after the setting up of a malarial ARF task force. Late referral, high parasitaemia, multiple organ failure, and infection in previously unimmunized subjects are associated with a poor prognosis (Trang *et al.* 1992). Younger age and absence of splenomegaly are risk factors for high mortality amongst paediatric population.

Pathology

Tubular changes may be unremarkable on light microscopy in those with mild renal failure. Severe cases reveal cloudy swelling, degeneration and necrosis of tubular cells involving predominantly the distal tubules (Fig. 3). Casts loaded with malarial pigment are often seen in the proximal tubules. The tubular cells contain haemosiderin granules. Haemoglobin casts may be seen in the lumina of the distal and collecting tubules in patients with intravascular haemolysis. Tubules and vascular endothelia show enhanced expression of TNFα, IL-1, IL-6, and GM-CSF (Rui-Mei *et al.* 1998). Varying degrees of interstitial oedema and mononuclear cell infiltrate are commonly seen.

In autopsies studies, glomerular lesions are noted in around 20 per cent of patients with falciparum malaria. They exhibit hypercellularity, mild mesangial hyperplasia, and increased mesangial matrix. The peritubular capillaries may be packed with parasitized erythrocytes in patients with heavy parasitaemia (Fig. 4). Fibrin thrombi, malarial pigment-laden macrophages, lymphocytes, and plasma cells may also be seen. The larger blood vessels are unremarkable. Immunofluorescence may show finely granular deposition of IgM and C3 in the mesangial areas and along the luminal side of the glomerular capillaries (Boonpucknavig *et al.* 1984).

Pathogenesis

Renal failure in falciparum malaria is attributed to haemodynamic alterations produced by some unique properties of this parasite which produce haemorheological changes leading to renal ischaemia. The likelihood of developing renal failure increases with increasing levels

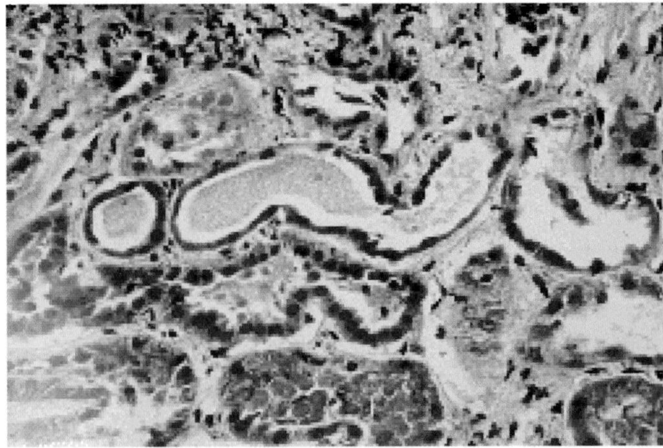

Fig. 3 Tubular necrosis in falciparum malaria.

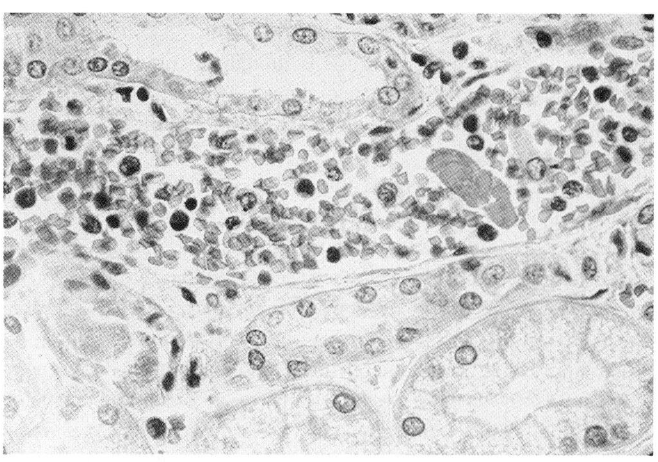

Fig. 4 Engorgement of peritubular capillary with erythrocytes and mononuclear cells in falciparum malaria. There is a mononuclear cell infiltration in the interstitium.

of parasitaemia, which exceeds 5 per cent in most patients with ARF (Sitprija 1988). The molecular mechanism involved in the pathogenesis of vascular complications of falciparum malaria are currently being unraveled. As in sepsis, there is peripheral vasodilatation with increased cardiac output and decreased renal blood flow at a later stage (Sitprija *et al.* 1996; Eiam-Ong and Sitprija 1998). Patients with severe infections often become hypovolaemic secondary to a cytokine-induced increase in capillary permeability, decreased fluid intake, and increased insensible fluid loss.

An increase in plasma viscosity secondary to an increase in plasma fibrinogen and acute phase proteins and decreased deformability of parasitized red cells have also been incriminated in the genesis of ARF. Rhabdomyolysis has also been documented in a few cases.

Leptospiral acute renal failure

Leptospirosis, the most widespread zoonosis in the world, is encountered in all continents except Antartica and is especially prevalent in the tropics. The genus *Leptospira* contains only one species, *Leptospira interrogans*, subdivided into two complexes; the pathogenic *L. interrogans* strains, and *Leptospira biflexa*, containing the saprophytic strains. Within each complex, stable antigenic variations are seen which allow classification of the organism into a number of serovars. The interrogans complex has 30 serogroups and approximately 240 serotypes.

Leptospirosis occurs in a wide range of domestic and wild animal hosts such as rats, mice, gerbils, hedgehogs, foxes, dogs, cattle, sheep, pigs, and rabbits. Even asymptomatic animals carry high number of organisms ($>10^{10}$/g) in their kidneys, and shed leptospira in urine for months to years. Pathogenic leptospira can survive outside the host for several weeks if the urine is of a neutral or alkaline pH and is shed into a moist environment which is not polluted with micro-organisms or detergents, has a low salinity, and if the ambient temperature is below 22°C (Kasi Visweswaran 1994). Human infection occurs incidentally either by direct contact with the urine or tissue of an infected animal or indirectly through contaminated water, soil, or vegetation. The usual portals of entry are abraded skin and exposed mucosae. Leptospirosis is an occupational hazard in coal miners, sewage, abattoir and farm workers, and in the aquaculture industry.

Clinical features

Leptospirosis occurs in both sexes and in all age groups, including children. The peak incidence is seen between 11 and 40 years, with a male preponderance. Although cases present throughout the year, there is a sharp increase in the incidence during or soon after the rainy season, especially following floods.

The clinical syndrome varies from subclinical infection and self-limited anicteric febrile illness to a severe and potentially fatal disease. Symptoms appear 7–13 days following exposure and are typically biphasic in character. The initial (leptospiraemic) phase is characterized by abrupt onset of high fever with chills, headache, and severe muscle aches and tenderness. About half of the patients develop anorexia, nausea, and vomiting; cough and chest pain are noted in 25–85 per cent of cases and disturbance of sensorium in 5–25 per cent. This phase lasts 4–10 days and terminates with defervescence. An asymptomatic phase of 1–3 days follows. The second or immune phase is heralded by the recurrence of fever and constitutional symptoms. An atypical pneumonia with lung haemorrhage, aseptic meningoencephalitis and myocarditis may develop. Involvement of liver and kidneys is characteristic. There is marked pain and tenderness in the right hypochondrium, along with hepatomegaly and progressive jaundice. Haemorrhagic manifestations include epistaxis, haemoptysis, gastrointestinal bleeding, haemorrhagic pneumonitis, and bleeding into the adrenal glands.

ARF occurs in 20–85 per cent of cases (Muthusethupathi *et al.* 1991; Kasi Visweswaran 1994). Renal failure is usually catabolic with rapid rises of blood urea nitrogen and serum creatinine. Oliguria is seen in 40–60 per cent. Hypotension is noted in around 22 per cent of cases and is often unresponsive to volume expansion and inotropic support. The combination of renal failure and jaundice is called Weil's syndrome. Jaundice is cholestatic with marked elevation of serum alkaline phosphatase. The survivors enter a diuretic phase by the end of the second week, which may be profound and lasts longer than that associated with other causes of ARF (Magaldi *et al.* 1992). This is accompanied by improvement in other symptoms as well. In about half the cases, renal failure is associated with polyuria and hypokalaemia along with elevated fractional excretion of potassium (Seguro *et al.* 1990). The renal failure is usually mild and non-oliguric in the anicteric patients.

Diagnosis

Diagnosis is based on either culture or serology (Sitprija and Newton 2000). The organisms can be isolated from blood during the first phase and later from urine. The growth may take up to 4 weeks in Fletcher's or Stuart's semisolid media. Antileptospira antibodies are detectable in the second phase. A single titre of greater than 1 : 400 or a four-fold increase is considered significant. The macroscopic agglutination test (MAT) or the slide test can be used as a screening test, but is not specific. The gold standard is the microscopic agglutination test but this is complex and requires maintenance of live *Leptospira* cultures (Kasi Visweswaran 1994). A single titre of greater than 1 : 800 or a four-fold increase is taken as significant. An IgM-specific dot-enzyme-linked immunosorbent assay (dot-ELISA) has been found to be specific in diagnosing leptospirosis in endemic areas (Sanford 1994). Other tests, including complement fixation, serum and salivary ELISA, rapid IgM dipstick ELISA, and gold immunoblot may be positive earlier than MAT.

Urinalysis during the leptospiraemic phase reveals mild proteinuria and hyaline and granular casts. These abnormalities disappear rapidly after the first week. The most prominent laboratory abnormality in the second phase is a conjugated hyperbilirubinaemia. In contrast to viral hepatitis, the aspartate aminotransferase (AST) concentration shows only a mild increase and the creatine phosphokinase may be increased in about 30 per cent of cases (Park, Y. K. *et al.* 1990). There is a steady increase in blood urea and serum creatinine. Hypokalaemia, secondary to increased tubular potassium excretion, is observed in 45 per cent of cases (Seguro *et al.* 1990). Neutrophil leucocytosis and elevated erythrocyte sedimentation rate are common. Thrombocytopenia is encountered in 40 per cent of cases (Winearls *et al.* 1984), and has been related to severe endotoxin injury (Yang *et al.* 2001). Haemolytic anaemia produced by leptospira haemolysins may at times be severe. The plasma levels of TNF-α, procalcitonin and soluble IL-2 receptor are elevated and are associated with the disease severity (Petros *et al.* 2000).

Management

Leptospirosis is a self-limiting disease and mild cases recover spontaneously. The emphasis is on symptomatic measures, together with correction of hypotension and fluid and electrolyte imbalance. A number of antimicrobial agents, such as penicillin, streptomycin, tetracycline congeners, chloramphanicol, erythromycin, and ciprofloxacin are effective *in vitro* and in experimental leptospiral infections. However, they do not alter the disease course unless given early. Crystalline penicillin (1.5 million units intravenously every 6 h for 7 days) or doxycycline (100 mg orally twice daily for 7 days) have shortened the duration of fever and hospital stay and hastened amelioration of leptospiruria in some studies (McClain *et al.* 1984; Watt *et al.* 1988).

Patients with renal failure need close monitoring and dialysis when necessary. Continuous venovenous haemofiltration, plasmapheresis, and blood exchange are beneficial in decreasing blood levels of cytokines and mediators (Niwattayakul *et al.* 2003; Sitprija and Chusilp 1973). Renal failure was an important cause of death in the predialysis era. With increasing availability of dialysis, death is now usually secondary to internal haemorrhage or myocarditis. Bad prognostic factors include advanced age, pulmonary complications, hyperbilirubinaemia, diarrhoea, hyperkalaemia, associated infection or underlying diseases. The long-term prognosis of ARF is good, with the GFR returning to normal within 2 months. Residual tubular dysfunction, such as a defect in the concentrating ability may be noted occasionally.

Pathology

The kidneys are typically swollen (Yang *et al.* 2001) and may be bile stained on gross examination. The main light microscopic lesions are interstitial oedema and infiltration with mononuclear cells and eosinophils. This finding is observed even in the absence of renal failure. Patients with renal failure frequently show degeneration and necrosis of tubular epithelial cells and disruption of the basement membrane, primarily affecting the proximal tubules. Bile casts and haemoglobin casts may be present in the tubular lumina. Mild and transient mesangial proliferative glomerulonephritis with deposition of C3 and IgM may be observed (Lai *et al.* 1982). Although leptospires pass through the blood vessels, vascular changes are usually not noticeable on light microscopy. Immunofluorescence may show deposition of C3 in the afferent arterioles. Electron microscopy may show dilated endoplasmic reticulum and enlargement of mitochondria in the swollen endothelial cells. The organisms may be demonstrated in renal parenchyma by staining with a silver impregnation technique.

Pathogenesis

Renal involvement in leptospirosis is thought to result from direct invasion of the renal tissue by the organism. The high blood flow rate ensures the delivery of large number of leptospira to the kidney tissue during the initial phase.

Renal damage results from the liberation of bacterial enzymes, metabolites, and endotoxins and complement-induced renal injury. Addition of leptospira endotoxin to humans macrophages induces TNF-α (Cinco *et al.* 1996). It has been suggested that the glycoprotein component of the endotoxin could inhibit the renal Na,K-ATPase, which in turn affects the apical Na–K–Cl cotransporter, leading to potassium wasting. Immunoelectron microscopic studies have shown leptospiral antigens in close proximity to the renal tubular and interstitial capillary endothelial cells (De Brito *et al.* 1992). Several leptospiral outer membrane proteins have been localized to proximal tubules and interstitium of infected animals (Barnett *et al.* 1999). The role of transcription factor NF-κB has been the subject of recent studies (Yang *et al.* 2000). An upregulation of NF-κB binding to DNA was noted after addition of outer membrane extracts from pathogenic serovars to cultured medullary thick ascending limb cells. This was accompanied by increase in the message for inducible nitric oxide synthase, monocyte chemo-attractant protein-1 and TNF-α. These changes were not observed when extract from nonpathogenic serovars were used. In addition, non-specific effects of systemic infection such as hypovolaemia, hypotension, haemoglobinuria, and myoglobinuria act as important contributory factors.

Leptospirotic guinea pigs show a number of tubular functional defects. Impaired sodium and potassium conservation are noted before the decline in GFR. This has been attributed to decreased proximal tubular reabsorption of sodium leading to an increased delivery to the distal nephron segments and insensitivity to the action of ADH (Magaldi *et al.* 1992). Both humoral and cell mediated immune responses are altered in leptospiral nephropathy. Yamashiro-Kanashiro *et al.* (1991) studied the lymphocyte subsets of patients with leptospirosis, with or without ARF, using an immunofluorescence technique. The $CD3^+$ and $CD4^+$ cells were decreased in all patients, but the number of B cells showed an increase. However, the mitogenic response to phytohaemagglutinin was depressed in patients with renal failure. The significance of these findings in the genesis of renal lesions is not clear.

As in many infectious diseases, the systemic vascular resistance is decreased while the cardiac output and renal vascular resistance are elevated. The blood volume is either normal or increased (Barsoum and Sitprija 2001). In severe leptospirosis the cardiac output is either normal or decreased and renal vascular resistance increases further. The GFR and renal blood flow are decreased, and may be of sufficient degree to cause tubular necrosis and renal failure. Non-specific effects of infection intravascular coagulation, haemolysis, rhabdomyolysis, free radical generation, jaundice and increased blood viscosity, all of which further contribute to decreased renal blood flow.

Mucormycosis

Mucormycosis is a rare opportunistic infection caused by zygomycete fungi of the order Mucorales and genera *Rhizopus, Absidia*, and *Rhizomucor*. It produces organ involvement through vascular invasion. There is thrombosis of large and small arteries (Fig. 5), with resulting infarction and necrosis of the affected organ. The major clinical modes

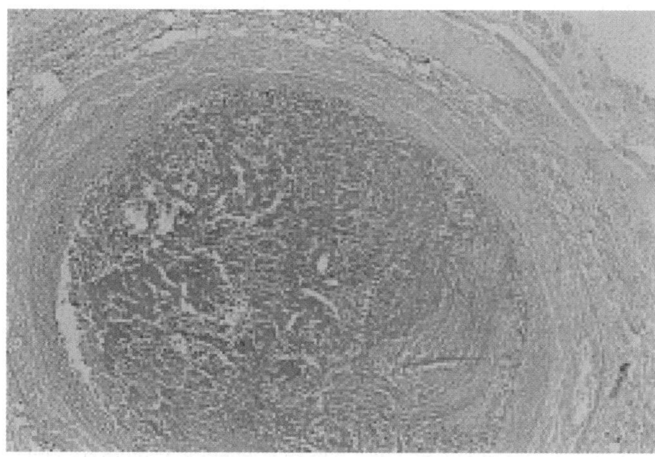

Fig. 5 H&E-stained section of a renal arteriole showing a thrombus blocking the lumen in a patient with mucormycosis involving both the kidneys. Bilateral nephrectomy was performed in this case.

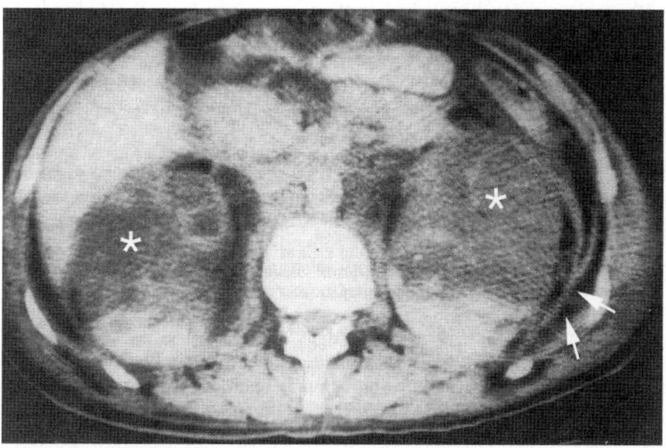

Fig. 6 A CECT scan of the abdomen showing bilateral renal involvement in mucormycosis. Enlarged globular kidneys with the absence of contrast excretion and perinephric collection are shown.

of presentation are rhinocerebral, pulmonary, gastrointestinal, and disseminated forms. Renal involvement is usually occult and detected at autopsy. Recently, a form of primary renal mucormycosis involving major renal vessels has been described. Patients with involvement of both the kidneys present with oliguric ARF. This condition should be suspected if the patient exhibits high fever, lumbar pain, and pyuria. Ultrasound and computed tomography (CT) scan reveal enlarged kidneys with evidence of perirenal collection and/or intrarenal abscesses (Chugh *et al.* 1993) (Fig. 6). A definite diagnosis requires demonstration of mucor hyphae in the material obtained by aspiration or at surgery. The only definitive treatment is extensive debridement of affected tissue, which may include bilateral nephrectomy, and systemic antifungal therapy with amphotericin B. Bilateral renal mucormycosis carries an extremely poor prognosis (Gupta *et al.* 1999). HIV serology should be obtained in all patients with this condition.

Melioidosis

Melioidosis encompasses a broad spectrum of disease processes caused by *Pseudomonas pseudomallei* and is encountered in Vietnam, Thailand, Malaysia, Central and South America, and the Caribbean islands. ARF was observed in 61 per cent of patients with acute septicaemic melioidosis in Thailand (Susaengrat *et al.* 1987). Renal involvement has not been reported from any other geographical area.

The presentation is with progressive fever, productive cough, and marked tachypnoea. Renal failure is generally oliguric and features of hypercatabolism are noted. Predisposing conditions such as diabetes mellitus or alcoholic liver disease are present in over 50 per cent of patients with renal failure (Susaengrat *et al.* 1987). Characteristic biochemical features are a high blood urea nitrogen/creatinine ratio, hyperbilirubinaemia, hyponatraemia, and hypoalbuminaemia. Multiorgan dysfunction is common and the mortality rate approaches 90 per cent. The diagnosis is established by demonstration of the organism in exudate material with methylene blue or Gram stain. Treatment requires use of parenteral ceftazidime at a dose of 120 mg/kg/day for about 30 days. Renal histology shows acute tubular necrosis and, less commonly, interstitial nephritis and microabscesses (Susaengrat *et al.* 1987).

Leprosy

ARF has been reported rarely (Singhal *et al.* 1977; Madiwale *et al.* 1994) in lepromatous leprosy. Singhal *et al.* (1977) reported three such cases. Renal histology revealed acute tubular necrosis in two of the patients. Both patients had evidence of intravascular haemolysis. The third patient showed crescentic glomerulonephritis. This lesion has also been seen in patients with erythema nodosum leprosum. Immunofluorescence shows deposition of granular IgG, C3, and fibrinogen (Madiwale *et al.* 1994). Improvement in renal function may occur if dialytic support is given in the acute phase (Singhal *et al.* 1977).

Kala-azar

Leishmania donovani causes kala-azar, a disease of the reticuloendothelial system, encountered in the tropical regions of East Africa, the Mediterranean area, Latin America, and India. It is transmitted through the bites of sandfly and manifests in the form of a febrile illness with massive hepatosplenomegaly, lymphadenopathy, and pancytopenia. ARF due to acute interstitial nephritis although rare has been described (Caravaca *et al.* 1991). The diagnosis is established by the demonstration of amastigotes in bone marrow and splenic aspirate. The renal failure recovers with successful treatment of kala-azar.

Typhoid

Typhoid is an acute systemic febrile illness caused by *Salmonella* species and is widely seen in the Indian subcontinent, Egypt, Indonesia, South Africa, and Latin America. ARF has been observed occasionally and is usually due to intravascular haemolysis in the presence of G-6-PD deficiency, myoglobinuria, or interstitial nephritis induced by ciprofloxacin, which is widely used for the treatment of this condition (Simpson *et al.* 1991). Haemolytic–uraemic syndrome has also been reported following typhoid fever. The main pathological findings are diffuse toxic damage involving tubules and localized small cell infiltration of the interstitium. The glomeruli are usually spared. Bacilli have not been demonstrated in the renal tissue. The prognosis of ARF is good.

ARF due to animal, plant, and chemical toxins

The true incidence of toxic ARF in the tropics remains uncertain because of the non-specific nature of the structural and functional abnormalities. A good history is essential for the diagnosis, and requires questions about exposure to prescription and non-prescription drugs, herbal remedies, industrial chemicals, fertilizers, paints, alcohol, or other forms of contaminated intoxicants. Traditional medicines contain nephrotoxins encountered only in developing countries. In many tribal populations, these agents are obtained from a traditional healer or a witch-doctor. The popularity of these healers is related to a combination of ignorance, poverty, lack of medical facilities, lax legislation, and a widespread belief in indigenous systems of medicine (Gold 1980; Joubert and Sebata 1982; Otieno *et al.* 1991). The indications for taking such medicines range from the frivolous like constipation, impotence, and menstrual disorders to serious diseases such as cancer and renal failure. Many preparations are well-known abortifacients. Great importance is attached to regular bowel movement in many tropical societies, and a number of these substances induce vomiting and/or diarrhoea, often to the point of producing hypotension and renal failure.

Poisoning by traditional medicines is an important cause of death in many African countries. In a Pretorian hospital in South Africa, 86.58 per cent of all deaths from acute poisoning were due to traditional medicines. At least eight remedies were associated with haematuria and renal failure (Joubert and Sebata 1982). About 25–35 per cent of all medical ARF in African hospitals develops following ingestion of herbal medications. Renal failure has also been reported following the use of tribal enemas. The enemas consist of mixture of herbs, barks, roots, leaves, and bulbs, and are administered through a truncated cow's horn or hollow reed. Increasing urbanization and industrialization has led to the use of potent chemicals, for example, paint thinners, turpentine, chloroxylenol, ginger, pepper, soap, vinegar, copper sulfate, and potassium permanganate.

Animal poisons

Snake bite

Snake bite is an occupational hazard in the rural areas of the tropics. Of the 2700 species of snakes recognized the world over, about 450 are venomous and these are distributed mainly in the tropical and subtropical regions. According to the WHO, the global annual mortality from snake bite is around 40,000, of which 23 per cent of deaths occur in West Africa, 10 per cent in India, and 20 per cent in South America.

Venomous snakes are classified into four families: (a) Viperidae, which include Russell's viper, *Echis carinatus* (saw-scaled viper), puff adder, pit viper, and rattlesnakes; (b) Elapidae, which includes kraits, cobras, mambas, and coral snakes; (c) Colubridae, of which the boomslang is an example; and (d) Hydrophidae or the sea-snakes.

ARF has been mostly reported following bites by snakes of first three of these families, with the majority following viper bites (Chugh *et al.* 1984, 1989). Snakes whose bites are known to cause renal failure include the sea-snake, Russell's viper, saw-scaled viper, puff adder, rattlesnake, tiger snake, green pit viper, *Bothrops jararaca*, boomslang, gwardar, dugite, and *Cryptophis nigrescens*.

Information on the precise incidence of snake-bite-induced ARF in different geographical regions is lacking. The incidence following *E. carinatus* or Russell's viper bites in India varies from 13 to 32 per cent (Chugh *et al.* 1984). The reported incidence from other countries varies between 1 and 27 per cent.

Clinical features

The clinical manifestations depend upon the dose of venom injected; and vary from mild local symptoms to extensive systemic manifestations. Pain and swelling of the bitten part appear within a few minutes and may be followed by blister formation and ecchymosis. Bleeding is seen in 65 per cent of cases and manifests as continuous ooze from the site of the bite, haematemesis, malena, and haematuria. Bleeding can also occur into the muscles and serosal cavities, and may be severe enough to produce shock. The blood is incoagulable in patients with severe systemic envenomation. Sea-snake bites cause myonecrosis, resulting in severe muscle pains and weakness.

The first indication of renal failure is oliguria or anuria, which develops within a few hours to as late as 96 h after the bite (Chugh *et al.* 1984). About half the cases give a history of passage of 'cola-coloured' urine. Non-oliguric renal failure is seen in less than 10 per cent of cases. Patients with severe bleeding, disseminated intravascular coagulation or secondary sepsis may present with hypotension. Life-threatening hyperkalaemia necessitating immediate dialysis may develop in those with intravascular haemolysis. Oliguria usually lasts for 4–15 days, and its persistence indicates the possibility of acute cortical necrosis (Chugh 1989).

Laboratory investigations show evidence of coagulopathy, there is severe hypofibrinogenaemia, reduction of factors V, X, and XIIIA, protein C, and antithrombin C. Depletion of factor V, X, and fibrinogen and elevation of fibrin degradation products are frequently observed. Leukocytosis and elevated haematocrit due to haemoconcentration may also be seen.

Management

Even though the basic therapeutic approach to renal failure following snake bite is the same as that for ARF due to any other cause, problems such as bleeding, shock, and sepsis complicate management. Early administration of antivenom is vital in patients with systemic envenomation. Experimental studies have shown that delay in administration results in a steep increase in the antivenom dose requirements. Indications include incoagulable blood, spontaneous systemic bleeding, intravascular haemolysis, local swelling involving more than 2 segments of the bitten limb, and a serum FDP concentration greater than 80 μg/ml in those reporting within 2 h of the bite (Warrell 1989, 1999). Knowledge of the offending snake species allows administration of monovalent antivenom wherever this is available. Immunodiagnostic techniques are helpful in the easy and rapid identification of the venom antigen. ELISA has been used extensively in the rural Thailand, but the currently available test is not quick enough for the clinicians. Precise identification of the snake is not essential for management in regions where only polyvalent antivenom is available. Indian authorities recommend initial administration of 20–100 ml, followed by a repeat dosage of 25–50 ml every 4–6 h until the effects of systemic envenoming disappear (Tariang *et al.* 1999). A simple way to monitor efficacy is by monitoring whole blood clotting time three to four times a day. Coagulability is generally restored within 6 h of an adequate dose. The test must be monitored for at least 3 more days, as delayed absorption of the venom could lead to recurrence of the coagulopathy. Immunoassays permit serial estimation of venom levels, and are useful in guiding antivenom therapy. In sea-snake envenomation, patients require from 100 to 1000 units of *Enhydrina schistosa* antivenom. Other therapeutic measures include replacement of blood loss with fresh blood or plasma, maintenance of electrolyte balance, administration of tetanus immunoglobulin, and treatment of pyogenic infection with antibiotics. The prognosis is good in patients who receive adequate doses of antivenom. The overall mortality rate is about 30 per cent (Chugh *et al.* 1984).

Pathology

The kidneys are normal or slightly enlarged, and the surface may show petechial haemorrhages. Light microscopy shows acute tubular necrosis in 70–80 per cent of patients (Chugh 1989). The tubules are lined by flattened epithelium and the lumina contain desquamated cells and hyaline or pigment casts. Varying degrees of interstitial oedema, inflammatory cell infiltration with eosinophils, mast cells and hyperplastic fibroblasts, and scattered areas of haemorrhage may be seen. Electron microscopy reveals dense intracytoplasmic bodies representing degenerated organelles in the proximal tubules, and electron-dense mesangial deposits. Acute interstitial nephritis, necrotizing vasculitis involving interlobular arteries, and crescentic glomerulonephritis may be seen occasionally (Sitprija *et al.* 1982). Acute cortical necrosis (Fig. 7) carries the worst prognosis and is seen in about 20–25 per cent of ARF cases following Russell's viper and *E. carinatus* bites (Chugh *et al.* 1984).

Pathogenesis

A number of clinical and experimental studies have provided insights into the pathogenetic mechanisms that lead to ARF in snake-bitten patients. These include direct nephrotoxicity of venom, hypovolaemia, haemolysis, myoglobinuria, and disseminated intravascular coagulation.

Renal lesions can develop as a result of direct cytotoxic effects of the snake venom on the kidney. Rats injected with the venoms of *B. jararaca, Agkistrodon piscivorus* and rattlesnake developed increased excretion of tubular enzymes and histopathological changes of acute tubular necrosis (Burdmann *et al.* 1993). Administration of Russell's viper venom leads to a dose-dependent decrease in inulin clearance in the isolated perfused rat kidney. Willinger *et al.* (1995) showed extensive destruction of the glomerular filter, lysis of vessel wall, and epithelial cell injury in all segments of the tubule following administration of Russell's viper venom to experimental animals. The structure of some of the snake venoms, including the sarapotoxin of the Israeli burrowing asp, is similar to endothelin-I, one of the most potent vasoconstrictor substances known. Vasculotoxic factors have been isolated from the venoms of several snakes, including *E. carinatus, Vipera palastinae, Agkistrodon halys, B. jararaca*, and Habu snake. Studies using the Habu snake venom have shown development of mesangiolysis.

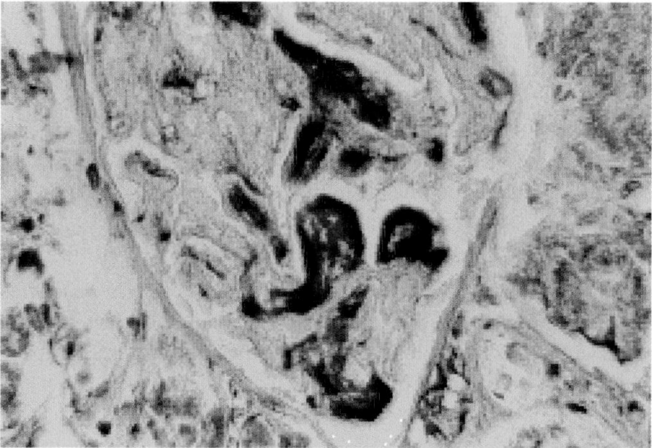

Fig. 7 Renal biopsy from a patient with acute diffuse cortical necrosis following *E. carinatus* snake bite. The section shows a single glomerulus which is structureless. Glomerular capillaries contain extensive fibrin thrombi.

Hypotension and circulatory collapse secondary to bleeding and release of kinins and depression of the medullary vasomotor centre or the myocardium play a significant pathogenetic role. Kinin-forming enzymes (kininogenases) are present in crotalid venom, *V. palastinae* depresses the medullary vasomotor centre, and *Bitis arietans* venom causes hypotension through a combination of myocardial depression, arteriolar dilatation, and increased vascular permeability.

Severe haemolysis has been observed following bites by Russell's viper and *E. carinatus* bites in humans and experimental animals. The haemolysis results from the action of phospholipase A_2, and a basic protein called 'direct lytic factor'. Phospholipase A_2 forms 70 per cent of the venom content of Russell's viper and acts on plasma lecithin, leading to the production of haemolytic lysolecithin. Microangiopathic haemolytic anaemia has been recorded following *Agkistrodon rhodostoma*, Russell's viper, puff adder, and gwardar bites. Bites by sea-snakes produce severe muscle necrosis and the resulting myoglobinuria, especially in the presence of other factors such as dehydration and acidosis, can give rise to ARF.

Disseminated intravascular coagulation has been observed in experimental animals as well as in patients bitten by viper snakes. Infusion of Russell's viper or *E. carinatus* venom into rhesus monkeys leads to disseminated intravascular coagulation (Chugh 1989). The procoagulant factors in the venom activate factors V and X, and the subsequent activation of the coagulation cascade leads to rapid thrombin formation. The fibrinolytic activity is either due to direct action of the venom or a physiological response to fibrin deposition. Phospholipase A2 also leads to platelet aggregation. The demonstration of fibrin thrombi in the renal microvasculature, both in clinical and experimental studies, confirms the role of disseminated intravascular coagulation in the genesis of renal lesions (Chugh *et al.* 1984).

Bee, wasp, and hornet stings and spider bites

Honey bees, yellow jackets, hornets, and paper wasps are stinging insects belonging to the order Hymenoptera and are found in most tropical countries. An isolated sting by these insects causes no more than a local allergic reaction, but a large dose of the venom sufficient to cause systemic symptoms may be injected upon attack by a swarm of insects (Sert *et al.* 1993). These include vomiting, diarrhoea, hypotension, loss of consciousness, and occasionally ARF. Patients with renal failure have been reported to have received from 22 to more than 1000 stings. ARF following bee or hornet stings is secondary to haemolysis, rhabdomyolysis, or both (Munoz-Arizpe *et al.* 1992; Sert *et al.* 1993), with hypotension playing a contributory role. Haemolysis results from the direct action of a basic protein fraction and melittin in these venoms, and indirectly by phospholipase A (Haberman 1977). Rhabdomyolysis has been attributed to polypeptides, histamine, serotonin, and acetylcholine present in hornet and wasp venoms. Some experimental studies have suggested a direct nephrotoxic role of these venoms. Renal biopsy invariably reveals acute tubular necrosis. In contrast to bees and wasps, a single spider bite may introduce enough venom to produce renal failure, especially in children. Venom of the spider *Sicarius* causes disseminated intravascular coagulation and renal failure.

Raw carp bile

The raw gallbladder or bile of freshwater and grass carps is used by traditional healers as an antipyretic, antitussive, antihypertensive, and to improve visual acuity, rheumatism, and general health in rural areas of South East Asia (Lim *et al.* 1993). Acute hepatic and renal failure have been reported amongst populations from these countries and in those who have migrated to the West from these countries (Park, S. K. *et al.* 1990; Lim *et al.* 1993; Lin and Lin 1999). Toxic symptoms occur 10 min–12 h following ingestion and include abdominal pain, nausea, vomiting, and watery diarrhoea. Hepatocellular jaundice and ARF occurs within 48 h of ingestion. Oliguric renal failure is observed in 54 per cent of patients, haematuria in 77 per cent, and jaundice in 62 per cent (Park, S. K. *et al.* 1990). The duration of renal failure ranges from 2 to 3 weeks. Alteration of sensorium without jaundice has been reported from Taiwan. The variation in manifestations is possibly due to differences in the varieties of carp, amount of bile ingested, and individual susceptibility. Recovery is usually complete with supportive treatment; mortality is high amongst cases presenting late.

Renal biopsies reveal tubular necrosis and interstitial oedema. The mechanism by which ARF develops is not well understood. Bile salts are known to induce haemolysis. Diuresis, excessive salt loss, and cardiac depression are noted in rats (Chen *et al.* 1984) which could lead to hypotension and contribute to renal failure. An increase in the permeability of intestinal mucosa secondary to inhibition of intestinal Na,K-ATPase leads to diarrhoea. Toxic activity has been documented in the ethanol soluble and ether-insoluble fractions of the bile. Cyprinol, a C-27 cholesterol derived bile alcohol is nephrotoxic. In an experimental study, oral administration of freeze-dried grass carp bile juice powder, 5-α cyprinol and 5-α cyprinol sulfate produced renal structural and functional abnormalities in Wistar rats (Yeh *et al.* 2002).

Other animals

Isolated instances of ARF have been reported following stings by the scorpion, jellyfish, and the giant centipede. Whereas the latter two give rise to intravascular haemolysis, renal failure following a scorpion sting is a consequence of disseminated intravascular coagulation and massive bleeding into various organs.

Plant poisons

Callilepis laureola (impila) poisoning

Callilepis laureola is a herb with tuberous rootstock, which grows in Southern and Central Africa. An extract of the tubers is used as a traditional remedy and is taken orally or as enema or douche. It is apparently used by over 50 per cent of the population in Natal, and poisoning is amongst the most common causes of ARF in the Black population of South Africa (Seedat 1993).

Clinical features

Symptoms occur in less than 24 h in 40 per cent and within a few days in about 70 per cent of the patients. The early manifestations are abdominal pain and vomiting. Hypoglycaemia is invariable and leads to alteration of consciousness and convulsions. Patients with severe poisoning may show abnormal liver function and even frank jaundice. Renal failure usually precedes hepatic dysfunction. The toxic effects are more severe in children. Treatment is supportive including correction of hypoglycaemia and volume and electrolyte replacement. The mortality rate is over 50 per cent.

Pathology and pathogenesis

The precise mechanism of renal failure is not clear but histology shows acute tubular necrosis, interstitial oedema, and dense interstitial infiltration. An alkaloid in the tuber of the plant, atractyloside, has nephrotoxic effects and inhibits oxidative phosphorylation in experimental studies (Bye *et al.* 1990). The presence of this compound can be confirmed by several assays in patients with impila poisoning (Laurens *et al.* 2001). Gastrointestinal upset leading to volume depletion resulting in renal ischaemia may also contribute to the renal dysfunction.

Djenkol bean poisoning

The djenkol (jering) trees (*Pithecolobium lobatum* and *Pithecolobium jiringa*, family mimosaceae) grow in Indonesia, Malaysia, Southern Thailand, and Myanmar. Considered a local delicacy, djenkol beans are consumed raw or in fried or roasted form. Raw djenkol beans consumed in large amounts can cause poisoning, especially if associated with low fluid intake (H'ng *et al.* 1991; Sesagothy *et al.* 1995). ARF has been reported most commonly in Java and Sumatra.

Clinical features

The symptoms of poisoning (djenkolism) may occur immediately after ingestion of beans or as late as 36 h after consumption, and include dysuria, lumbar and lower abdominal pain, hypertension, haematuria, and oligoanuria. Eiam-Ong *et al.* (1989) observed dysuria in 77 per cent, haematuria in 68 per cent, proteinuria in 45 per cent, hypertension in 36 per cent, and renal failure in 55 per cent of cases. Urinalysis reveals proteinuria and microscopy shows erythrocytes, epithelial cells, and needle-like crystals of djenkolic acid. The majority of victims recover within a few days. A great variation has been noted in individual susceptibility to the toxic effects of this bean. Toxicity may be caused by a single bean in one individual, while it may take 20 beans to cause poisoning in another.

Management

A high fluid intake and alkalinization of urine will help in dissolving the crystals. Occasional cases may need irrigation of bladder or renal pelvis with an alkaline solution. Djenkolism may be prevented by pretreatment of the beans by boiling or by liberal fluid intake.

Pathogenesis

The bean contains djenkolic acid, ($C_{11}H_{23}N_3S_3O_6$), a sulfur-rich cysteine thioacetal of formaldehyde. It forms needle-like crystals in concentrated acid urine, causing obstruction of renal tubules. The crystals may act as a nidus for stone formation. In animal experiments continuous intravenous infusion of djenkolic acid has been shown to decrease the GFR and renal plasma flow in a dose-dependent fashion (Eiam-Ong and Sitprija, unpublished data). Acute tubular necrosis is the dominant lesion in these animals, with crystals observed in only a few.

Mushroom poisoning

ARF has been observed following the ingestion of toxic mushrooms of the genera *Amanita, Galerina*, and *Cortinarius*. *Amanita phalloides* is found commonly in the tropics, and may be ingested in the mistaken belief that it is edible.

Clinical features

The toxic symptoms develop a few hours after ingestion and consist of abdominal pain, nausea, vomiting, and diarrhoea. Severe cases may develop hypotension, jaundice, fever, alteration in consciousness, and renal failure (McClain *et al.* 1989). Jaundice is hepatocellular in type. Mortality rate exceeds 50 per cent in patients with severe renal failure.

Pathogenesis

The mechanism of renal injury is not known, but volume depletion and hepatic failure contribute to the renal injury. The toxic constituent, amatoxin cyclopeptide, is thought to be directly nephrotoxic. *Cortinarius orellanus* produces a decrease in GFR, proteinuria, glycosuria, and decreased tubular reabsorption of sodium, potassium, and water within 48 h of ingestion in rats. The toxic glycoprotein of *Boletus satanas* inhibitis protein and DNA synthesis of Madin Darby canine kidney cells (Kretz *et al.* 1991).

Pathology

Histology is compatible with tubular necrosis. Degenerative changes are noted primarily in the proximal tubules. Interstitial oedema and cellular infiltration may be seen.

Marking-nut poisoning

The marking-nut tree, *Semecarpus anacardium*, found in tropical and subtropical forests, has an irritant black sap. Exposure of the skin to the sap produces painful blisters, eruption, and sloughing, resulting in deep ulceration. Accompanying symptoms include fever, dysuria, and haematuria. In severe cases the skin shows extensive erythema and bullae. Anuric renal failure may occur and may be associated with acute cortical necrosis (Mathai and Date 1979). Nephrotoxicity is due to the phenolic substance in the sap.

Other plants

Several plants are used as traditional medicines, and may cause renal failure through their indirect side-effects. These plants include *Securidaca longipedunculata, Euphorbia matabelensis*, and *Crotalaria laburnifolia*. There is no scientific evidence of a direct nephrotoxicity. Since vomiting and diarrhoea are frequently observed following consumption of these medicinal plants, ARF is attributed to volume depletion.

Chemical poisons

Copper sulfate poisoning

ARF following the ingestion of copper sulfate has been reported widely from Indian subcontinent (Chugh *et al.* 1977a). The extensive use of copper sulfate in the leather industry, coupled with low cost, and easy availability are the main reasons for its widespread usage as a mode of suicide by the poor. Its distinctive blue colour and strong metallic taste preclude its use for homicide. The incidence has shown a significant decline in the past two decades (Chugh *et al.* 1989). Another form of copper sulfate poisoning has been reported from Nigeria where ingestion of 'holy water' given by spiritual leaders was followed by intravascular haemolysis and ARF. Chemical analysis of the green water showed a very high copper content (Sontz and Schweiger 1995).

Clinical features

Symptoms appear within minutes of ingestion, and consist of a metallic taste, excessive salivation, burning retrosternal and epigastric pain, nausea, and repeated vomitings. The vomitus is blue–green in colour and turns deep blue on addition of ammonium hydroxide, allowing it to be differentiated from bile. Diarrhoea, haematemesis, and malena follow. In severe cases, jaundice, hypotension, convulsions, and coma may develop. Acute pancreatitis, myoglobinuria, and methaemoglobinaemia have also been reported (Chugh *et al.* 1977a). Renal failure is seen in 20–25 per cent of cases and is invariably oliguric. Haematuria may be seen in about 40 per cent of cases. Physical examination reveals mild icterus and extensive oropharyngeal ulceration. Death may occur in the acute phase from gastrointestinal bleeding or hepatic or renal failure. In patients who survive this phase, diuresis ensues after 7–10 days and is followed by gradual recovery.

Management

Gastric lavage should be performed using 1 per cent potassium ferrocyanide solution, which leads to formation of insoluble cupric ferrocyanide. Egg white or milk can be administered as an antidote. Emesis should not be tried. An upper gastrointestinal endoscopy is necessary to determine the degree and extent of ulceration. Volume deficit should be corrected with crystalloids and patients with haemolysis should receive blood transfusions. The hyperkalaemia is often severe and sustained because of the ongoing haemolysis and requires early and frequent dialysis. The frequency of dialysis can be reduced after the onset of the diuretic phase.

Pathology

Renal histology usually shows acute tubular necrosis. There is extensive necrosis of the proximal tubules with marked interstitial oedema. Pigmented haemoglobin casts may be noted in patients with intravascular haemolysis. Acute cortical necrosis is rare.

Pathogenesis

Direct nephrotoxicity, severe haemolysis caused by copper, and hypovolaemia secondary to fluid loss appear to be the main pathogenetic factors for development of renal failure. The fatal dose of copper sulfate is usually 30–100 g, but deaths have been reported even with doses as small as 1 g. High copper concentrations can produce considerable oxidant stress and cause haemolysis. Copper interferes with the activity of Na,K-ATPase, G-6-PD, glutathione reductase, and catalase. In experimental animals, copper sulfate produces toxic damage to the proximal tubules, leading to acute tubular necrosis.

Ethylene glycol

Di- and polyethylene glycols have been used as cheap substitutes of propylene glycol as vehicle in paediatric syrup preparations. An epidemic of diethylene glycol (DEG)-induced ARF was first reported in the 1930s amongst children in the United States who consumed sulfanilamide elixir contaminated with DEG. This prompted the passage of US Food, Drugs, and Cosmetics Act in 1938, following which there has been only one report of this kind from a Western country. This contamination continues to occur in tropical countries and epidemics have been reported from many regions including India, Bangladesh, Nigeria, South Africa, and Haiti (Pandya 1988; Hanif *et al.* 1995; Anon 1996; O'Brien *et al.* 1998; Singh *et al.* 2001). In one Indian report (Pandya 1988), 14 patients died of ARF following administration of a preparation of glycerol to lower intracranial or intraocular pressures. Analysis of this preparation showed it to be 70 per cent ethylene glycol. Renal histology at autopsy revealed acute cortical necrosis as the most frequent lesion. In other reports, several children have been affected after consuming contaminated paracetamol syrup. In one large study, 236 deaths were recorded amongst 339 children with unexplained ARF in a Children's hospital in Dhaka (Bangladesh). A total of 51 of these children were documented to have ingested a brand of paracetamol known to contain DEG, whereas 85 per cent of the remaining patients had ingested an unknown elixir for fever (Hanif *et al.* 1995).

Ethylene dibromide poisoning

Ethylene dibromide (EDB) is a pesticide fumigant used widely in the tropics, but its use has been restricted in most western countries. It is well absorbed from skin, gastrointestinal tract and intestinal mucosa. Accidental poisoning has been reported in people who were exposed to large quantities of EDB at workplace. In one instance, EDB was mistaken for ethylene bromide and administered as an anaesthetic. Suicidal poisoning has also been reported. ARF and hepatitis are the chief manifestations (Singh *et al.* 1993; Prakash *et al.* 1999). Dimercaprol has been suggested as an antidote based on the similarities in the structure of the two compounds. The mortality remains very high despite all supportive measures, and there is only one report of survival following EDB poisoning (Prakash *et al.* 1999). The mechanism of toxicity is not known. It is postulated to lead to generation of free oxygen radicals through the cytochrome P450 pathway that produce lipid peroxidation and membrane damage, resulting in hepatotoxicity and necrosis of renal tubular cells.

Chromic acid poisoning

Hexavalent chromium compounds such as chromic acid (H_2CrO_7) and its salts (chromates and bichromates) are used in the electroplating, leather tanning, and anticorrosive metal treatment industries in tropical countries. Renal lesions have been reported following acute ingestion of large quantities (Varma *et al.* 1994). Ingestion is followed by severe abdominal pain, vomiting, gastrointestinal bleed, and circulatory collapse. Renal damage manifests as ATN. Dichromate is directly nephrotoxic and produces extensive proximal tubular necrosis. Hypotension and haemolysis also contribute to tubular damage in clinical setting. Management entails gastric lavage with alkaline solutions like sodium bicarbonate to prevent further absorption and IV fluids to combat hypotension. Forced diuresis enhances renal excretion of the compound. Reducing agents like vitamin C have been shown to prevent chromic acid induced ATN in experimental animals. The prognosis following acute poisoning is usually poor.

Miscellaneous causes

Rhabdomyolysis

Myoglobinuric ARF is observed in the tropics after a variety of conditions, such as crush syndrome, burns, heat stroke, electrical injury, eclampsia, prolonged labour, poisoning with mercuric chloride, zinc or aluminum phosphide, status epilepticus, viral myositis, and status asthmaticus (Chugh *et al.* 1979; Ghosh *et al.* 1993). The diagnosis is established by the demonstration of myoglobin in urine and elevated levels of creatine phosphokinase and aldolase in the serum. Since myoglobin is a small molecule with a molecular weight of 17 kDa and binds only lightly to the plasma proteins, it escapes easily in the urine. Therefore, the urine may not contain myoglobin if the patient presents late in the course of the disease and the true incidence of myoglobinuric ARF will be underestimated. Severe hypocalcaemia and hyperuricaemia during the oliguric phase and hypercalcaemia during the diuretic phase are characteristic of this condition (Chugh *et al.* 1979). The pathogenesis of myoglobinuric ARF is similar to that following intravascular haemolysis. Renal histology shows acute tubular necrosis.

Heat stroke

Heat stroke occurs when the body thermal regulatory mechanism is unable to dissipate sufficient heat, leading to a rise in core body temperature. The incidence of heat stroke is not known. Most cases are observed in the summer months in tropical areas with high ambient temperatures and high relative humidity (Sanguangvong *et al.* 1988). The condition affects mainly elderly individuals living in poorly ventilated places, but can develop in healthy adults after heavy physical exertion in a hot and humid environment.

The characteristic features are hyperpyrexia, hyperventilation, nausea, vomiting, cramps, ataxia, incoherent speech, followed by loss of consciousness, hypotension, and vascular collapse. As the syndrome progresses, oliguric renal failure may develop. Laboratory investigations show haemoconcentration, hypernatraemia, hypocalcaemia, and elevated transaminases, aldolase, and creatine phosphokinase. Hyperkalaemia is often striking because of associated rhabdomyolysis. Haemolysis, myoglobinuria, and disseminated intravascular coagulation are seen in severe cases. Urinalysis reveals a high specific gravity, proteinuria, red blood cells with granular and erythrocyte casts. Renal function usually recovers completely.

The pathogenesis is multifactorial. Hypovolaemia, hypotension, myoglobinuria, and disseminated intravascular coagulation all contribute to the development of renal failure. Extreme hyperthermia may directly damage renal tubular cells. Management consists of rapid cooling by any method with continuous monitoring of temperature. Rehydration should be instituted with care because the fluid requirement in most patients is only 1000–1200 ml. The central venous pressure should be monitored to guide fluid therapy if hypotension persists despite successful cooling. The development of multiorgan failure indicates a poor prognosis.

Hypothermia

Hypothermia is defined as a central core temperature of 35°C or less. Hypothermia occurs mainly in the poor, homeless, and destitute during winter months. With the onset of hypothermia, there is a decrease in the oxidative tubular activity and sensitivity to ADH. These result in a reduced sodium and water reabsorption and increase in urine flow. ARF has been reported rarely (Sandhu *et al.* 1992) and probably is a consequence of hypovolaemia, hypotension, rhabdomyolysis or acute pancreatitis. Management includes the institution of adequate supportive measures and both external and core rewarming. Peritoneal or haemodialysis using warm dialysate (43–44°C) has been used successfully for this purpose even in patients without renal failure. External warming alone may precipitate hypovolaemia. Renal biopsy shows acute tubular necrosis (Sandhu *et al.* 1992).

Glomerulonephritis (see Chapter 10.6.1)

Various forms of rapidly progressive glomerulonephritis and postinfectious glomerulonephritis constitute about 10 per cent of all cases of ARF seen in the tropics. It is a particularly important cause in children.

Surgical acute renal failure

The proportion of cases of ARF attributable to surgery and its complications has increased three to five-fold in the last three decades. For example, trauma and complications of surgery were previously reported to contribute only 2–5 per cent of cases of ARF in the tropics, but in a later hospital-based study, postoperative renal failure was seen in 24 per cent of all patients with ARF and factors related to surgery were identified as the major cause in 18 per cent of cases (Jha *et al.* 1992). Obstructive uropathy constitutes a major cause of surgical ARF in certain tropical areas (Chugh *et al.* 1987). The high incidence of nephrolithiasis and misplaced faith in the efficacy of indigenous medicines in dissolving stones, with a consequent delay in surgical intervention, are the major factors contributing to this high incidence.

Obstetric acute renal failure (see Chapter 10.7.2)

Improvements in obstetric care have led to a decline in the incidence of pregnancy-related ARF from several parts of the world. At our Indian centre, the proportion of obstetric ARF cases fell from 22 per cent in the 1960s to 8 per cent in the 1990s. This followed adoption of the Medical Termination of Pregnancy Act and increased availability of medical facilities, cutting down the number of septic abortions, as well as therapeutic termination of complicated pregnancies. In other developing countries, however, obstetric complications continue to be a major cause of ARF. In Ethiopia, for example, septic abortion remains the underlying cause of ARF in 52 per cent of all patients (Zewdu 1994) and in Argentina and Nigeria, gynaecological and obstetric complications still account for 32 and 25 per cent of cases of ARF, respectively (Bamgboye *et al.* 1993; Firmat *et al.* 1994). This high incidence is mostly because of unsafe home delivery practices in rural areas and clandestine abortions conducted by untrained personnel. The abortion practices include use of sticks, insertion of abortifacient chemicals and pastes, soap solutions, and dilatation and curettage carried out under unhygienic conditions (Chugh *et al.* 1976).

Clinical features

The frequency distribution of the timing of ARF is bimodal in relation to gestation (Chugh *et al.* 1976). The first peak is seen between 8 and 16 weeks and is associated mainly with septic abortions. Pre-eclampsia, eclampsia, abruptio placentae, postpartum haemorrhage, and puerperal sepsis account for the second peak, which is seen between 34 weeks and term. These patients invariably receive their initial care at local hospitals and are referred to centres with dialysis facilities very late. The history of a clandestinely performed abortion is not often volunteered and establishing the cause of ARF is delayed until a gynaecological examination is performed. More than 85 per cent of patients are oliguric and as many as 32 per cent may be anuric at presentation (Chugh and Singhal 1981). Other findings are jaundice (34 per cent), purpura or ecchymoses (20 per cent), and neurological involvement, for example, seizures and altered sensorium (16 per cent). Firmat *et al.* (1994) noted jaundice in 84 per cent of their postabortal ARF patients.

In general, the outcome of ARF associated with pregnancy is better than that of non-obstetric ARF. However, the mortality continues to be high (35–50 per cent) in developing countries because of delay in seeking appropriate medical care, resulting in multiorgan dysfunction (Bamgboye *et al.* 1993; Zewdu 1994).

Pathology

Histology of the kidney in the majority of cases of obstetric renal failure shows the changes of acute tubular necrosis, but acute cortical necrosis has been found in more than 25 per cent of patients in certain parts of the world; comprising 19 and 38 per cent of cases of ARF in early and late pregnancy, respectively (Chugh *et al.* 1976).

Acute cortical necrosis in tropical countries

Acute renal cortical necrosis is the most catastrophic of the forms of ARF. Improvements in medical care have led to the virtual disappearance of this entity from the Western world (Madias *et al.* 1988). In India, the incidence amongst patients dialysed for ARF declined from 7.1 per cent in 1983 (Chugh *et al.* 1983) to 3.8 per cent in 1994 (Chugh *et al.* 1994).

Even though acute cortical necrosis has been observed in association with a variety of conditions, the most common antedating illness

Table 3 Aetiology of acute cortical necrosis [data from Chugh *et al.* (1994), reproduced with permission from the editor]

Category	Number	%
Obstetric	(56.6%)	
Postabortal sepsis	22	19.5
Abruptio placentae	15	13.3
Postpartum haemorrhage	12	10.5
Puerperal sepsis	7	6.2
Eclampsia	8	7.1
Non-obstetric	(43.4%)	
Snake bite	16	14.2
Haemolytic–uraemic syndrome	13	11.5
Allograft rejection	6	5.3
Pancreatitis	4	3.5
Gastroenteritis	5	4.4
Septicaemia	3	2.7
Trauma	1	0.9
Drug-induced intravascular haemolysis	1	0.9
Total	113	100

is a complication of pregnancy. In two large series of patients reported from France and India, renal cortical necrosis was due to obstetric causes in 68 and 56 per cent of patients, respectively. The aetiological factors responsible for development of acute cortical necrosis in 113 cases seen over a period of 28 years are given in Table 3.

The cardinal feature of this condition is prolonged oligoanuria. Other findings depend upon the underlying disease, with most showing evidence of severe blood loss or fulminant sepsis. Gross haematuria, loin pain, fever, and leucocytosis may be observed in some patients. Physical findings include pallor (60 per cent), purpuric spots or ecchymoses (21 per cent), jaundice (19 per cent), or hypotension (11 per cent). Hypertension not correctable by dialysis may be seen in 10 per cent of patients (Chugh *et al.* 1994).

References

Anon (1996). Fatalities associated with ingestion of diethylene glycol-contaminated glycerin used to manufacture acetaminophen syrup—Haiti, November 1995–June 1996. *Morbidity and Mortality Weekly Report* **45**, 649–650.

Adu, D., Anim-Addo, Y., Foli, A. K., Yeboah, E. D., Quartey, J. K. M., and Ribeiro, B. F. (1976). Acute renal failure in tropical Africa. *British Medical Journal* **1**, 890–2.

Bamgboye, E. L., Mabayoje, M. O., Odutola, T. A., and Mabadeje, A. F. (1993). Acute renal failure at the Lagos University Teaching Hospital—a 10-year review. *Renal Failure* **15**, 77–80.

Barsoum, R. (2000). Malarial acute renal failure. *Journal of the American Society of Nephrology* **11**, 2147–2154.

Barsoum, R. and Sitprija, V. Tropical nephrology. In *Diseases of the Kidney and Urinary Tract* (ed. R. W. Schrier), pp. 2301–2349. Philadelphia: Lippincott Williams & Wilkins, 2001.

Bhuyan, U. N., Bagga, A., and Srivastava, R. N. (1994). Acute renal failure and severe hypertension in children with renal thrombotic microangiopathy. *Nephron* **66**, 302–306.

Boonpucknavig, V., Srichaikul, T., and Punyagupta, S. Clinical pathology of malaria. In *Antimalarial Drugs: Biological Background, Experimental Methods and Drug Resistance* (ed. W. Peters and W. H. G. Richards), pp. 127–76. Berlin: Springer-Verlag, 1984.

Breman, J. G. and Steketee, R. W. Malaria. In *Maxcy—Rosenau—Last Public Health and Preventive Medicine* 13th edn. (ed. J. M. Last and R. B. Wallace), pp. 240–253. Norwalk, CT: Appleton Lange, 1992.

Burdmann, E. A. *et al.* (1993). Snake bite-induced acute renal failure: an experimental model. *American Journal of Tropical Medicine and Hygiene* **48**, 82–88.

Burnett, J. K. *et al.* (1999). Expression and distribution of leptospiral outer membrane components during renal infection of hamsters. *Infection and Immunity* **67**, 853–861.

Bye, B. N., Coetzer, T. H., and Dutton, M. F. (1990). An enzyme immunoassay for atractyloside, the nephrotoxin of *Callilepis laureola* (impila). *Toxicon* **28**, 997–1000.

Caravaca, F., Munoz, A., Pizarro, J. L., de Santamaria, J. S., and Fernandez-Alonso, J. (1991). Acute renal failure in visceral leishmaniasis. *American Journal of Nephrology* **11**, 350–352.

Case Records of the Massachusets General Hospital (1995). *New England Journal of Medicine* **332**, 1083–1089.

Chen, C. F., Yen, T. S., Chan, W. Y., Chapman, B. J., and Munday, K. A. (1984). The renal, cardiovascular and haemolytic actions in the rat of a toxic extract from the bile of the grass carp (*Ctenopharyngodon idellus*). *Toxicon* **27**, 433–439.

Chugh, K. S. (1989). Snake bite-induced acute renal failure in India. *Kidney International* **35**, 891–907.

Chugh, K. S. *et al.* (1976). Acute renal failure of obstetric origin. *Obstetrics and Gynecology* **48**, 642–646.

Chugh, K. S., Sharma, B. K., Singhal, P. C., Das, K. C., and Datta, B. N. (1977a). Acute renal failure following copper sulphate intoxication. *Postgraduate Medical Journal* **53**, 18–23.

Chugh, K. S. *et al.* (1977b). Acute renal failure due to intravascular hemolysis in North Indian patients. *American Journal of Medical Sciences* **274**, 139–146.

Chugh, K. S., Singhal, P. C., Nath, I. V. S., Pareek, S. K., Ubroi, H. S., and Sarkar, A. K. (1979). Acute renal failure due to non-traumatic rhabdomyolysis. *Postgraduate Medical Journal* **55**, 386–392.

Chugh, K. S. *et al.* (1978). Spectrum of acute renal failure in North India. *Journal of Association of Physicians of India* **26**, 147–154.

Chugh, K. S. *et al.* (1983). Spectrum of acute cortical necrosis in Indian patients. *American Journal of Medical Sciences* **286**, 10–20.

Chugh, K. S. *et al.* (1984). Acute renal failure following poisonous snake bite. *American Journal of Kidney Diseases* **4**, 30–38.

Chugh, K. S., Sakhuja, V., Malhotra, H. S., and Pereira, B. J. G. (1987). Changing trends in acute renal failure in the tropical countries. *Abstracts of the VIIth Asian Colloquium of Nephrology, No. 82, Taipei.*

Chugh, K. S., Sakhuja, V., Malhotra, H. S., and Pereira, B. J. G. (1989). Changing trends in acute renal failure in third world countries—Chandigarh study. *Quarterly Journal of Medicine* **73**, 1117–1123.

Chugh, K. S., Sakhuja, V., and Pereira, B. J. G. Acute renal failure in the tropics. In *Acute Renal Failure* (ed. K. Solez and L. C. Racusen), pp. 93–103. New York: Marcel Dekker, 1991.

Chugh, K. S. *et al.* (1993). Renal mucormycosis: computerised tomographic findings and their diagnostic significance. *American Journal of Kidney Diseases* **22**, 393–397.

Chugh, K. S., Jha, V., Sakhuja, V., and Joshi, K. (1994). Acute renal cortical necrosis—a study of 113 patients. *Renal Failure* **16**, 37–47.

Cinco, M., Vecile, E., Murgia, R., Dobrina, P., and Dobrina, A. (1996). *Leptospira interrogans* and *Leptospira peptidoglyc*ans induce the release of tumor necrosis factor alpha from human monocytes. *FEMS Microbiological Letters* **138**, 211–214.

De Brito, T. *et al.* (1992). Detection of leptospiral antigen (*L. interrogans* serovar *copenhageni* serogroup Icterohaemorrhagiae) by immunoelectron microscopy in the liver and kidney of experimentally infected guinea-pigs. *International Journal of Experimental Pathology* **73**, 633–642.

Eiam-Ong, S. and Sitprija, V. (1998). Falciparum malaria and the kidney. *American Journal of Kidney Diseases* **32**, 361–375.

Eiam-Ong, S. *et al.* (1989). Djenkol bean nephrotoxicity in southern Thailand. *Proceedings of the First Asia Pacific Congress on Animal, Plant and Microbial Toxins*, Singapore, pp. 628–632.

Firmat, J. and Pas, R. (1975). 1000 patients with acute renal failure—clinical and pathological observations. *Abstracts of Free Communications, VI International Congress of Nephrology*, No. 600.

Firmat, J., Zuccini, A., Martin, R., and Aguirre, C. (1994). A study of 500 cases of acute renal failure (1978–1991). *Renal Failure* **16**, 91–99.

Ghosh, A. K., Sakhuja, V., Joshi, K., Gupta, K. L., and Chugh, K. S. (1993). Acute myositis complicated by myoglobinuric acute renal failure. *Journal of Association of Physicians of India* **41**, 453–454.

Gold, C. H. (1980). Acute renal failure from herbal and patent remedies in Blacks. *Clinical Nephrology* **14**, 128–134.

Gupta, K. L., Joshi, K., Sud, K., Kohli, H. S., Jha, V., Radotra, B. D., and Sakhuja, V. (1999). Renal zygomycosis: an under-diagnosed cause of acute renal failure. *Nephrology, Dialysis, Transplantation* **14**, 2720–2725.

Haberman, E. (1977). Bee and wasp venoms. *Science* **177**, 314–322.

Hanif, M., Mobarak, M. R., Ronan, A., Rahman, D., Donovan, J. J., Jr., and Bennish, M. L. (1995). Fatal renal failure caused by diethylene glycol in paracetamol elixir: the Bangladesh epidemic. *British Medical Journal* **311**, 88–91.

H'ng, P. K., Nayar, S. K., Lau, W. M., and Segasothy, M. (1991). Acute renal failure following jering ingestion. *Singapore Medical Journal* **32**, 148–149.

Jha, V., Malhotra, H. S., Sakhuja, V., and Chugh, K. S. (1992). Spectrum of hospital-acquired acute renal failure in the developing countries—Chandigarh study. *Quarterly Journal of Medicine* **84**, 497–505.

Joubert, P. and Sebata, B. (1982). The role of prospective epidemiology in the establishment of a toxicology service for a developing community. *South African Medical Journal* **27**, 63–67.

Kasi Visweswaran, R. Acute renal failure due to leptospirosis. In *Asian Nephrology* (ed. K. S. Chugh), pp. 384–392. New Delhi: Oxford University Press, 1994.

Kretz, O., Creppy, E. E., and Dirheimer, G. (1991). Characterization of bolesatine, a toxic protein from the mushroom *Boletus satanas* Lenz and its effects on kidney cells. *Toxicology* **66**, 213–224.

Ku, G., Kim, C. H., Pwee, H. S., and Khoo, O. T. (1975). Review of acute renal failure in Singapore. *Annals of the Academy of Medicine of Singapore* **4** (Suppl.), 115–120.

Lai, K. N., Aarons, I., Woodroffe, A. J., and Clarkson, A. R. (1982). Renal lesion in leptospirosis. *Australian and New Zealand Journal of Medicine* **12**, 276–279.

Laurens, J. B., Bekker, L. C., Steenkamp, V., and Stewart, M. J. (2001). Gas chromatographic-mass spectrometric confirmation of atractyloside in a patient poisoned with *Callilepis laureola. Journal of Chromatography B Biomedical Sciences Application* **765**, 127–133.

Lim, P. S., Lin, J. L., Hu, S. A., and Huang, C. C. (1993). Acute renal failure due to ingestion of the gallbladder of grass carp: report of 3 cases with review of literature. *Renal Failure* **15**, 639–644.

Lin, Y. F. and Lin, S. H. (1999). Simultaneous acute renal and hepatic failure after ingesting raw carp gall bladder. *Nephrology, Dialysis, Transplantation* **14**, 2011–2012.

Madias, N. E., Donhoe, J. F., and Harrington, J. T. Postischemic acute renal failure. In *Acute Renal Failure* (ed. B. M. Brenner and F. M. Lazarus), pp. 251–278. New York: Churchill Livingstone, 1988.

Madiwale, C. V., Mittal, B. V., Dixit, M., and Acharya, V. N. (1994). Acute renal failure due to crescentic glomerulonephritis complicating leprosy. *Nephrology, Dialysis, Transplantation* **9**, 178–179.

Magaldi, A. J., Yasuda, P. N., Kudo, L. H., Seguro, A. C., and Rocha, A. S. (1992). Renal involvement in leptospirosis: a pathophysiologic study. *Nephron* **62**, 332–339.

Mathai, T. P. and Date, A. (1979). Renal cortical necrosis following exposure to sap of the marking-nut tree (*Semecarpus anacardium*). *American Journal of Tropical Medicine and Hygiene* **28**, 773–774.

McClain, J. B., Bolion, W.-R., Harrison, S. M., and Steinweg, D. L. (1984). Doxycycline therapy for leptospirosis. *Annals of Internal Medicine* **100**, 696–698.

McClain, J. L., Hause, D. W., and Clark, M. A. (1989). *Amanita phalloides* mushroom poisoning: a cluster of four fatalities. *Journal of Forensic Sciences* **34**, 83–87.

Munoz-Arizpe, R. *et al.* (1992). Africanized bee stings and pathogenesis of acute renal failure. *Nephron* **61**, 478.

Muthusethupathi, M. A. and Shivakumar, S. (1987). Acute renal failure in South India. *Journal of the Association of Physicians of India* **35**, 504–508.

Muthusethupathi, M. A., Shivakumar, S., Rajendran, S., Vijayakumar, R., and Jayakumar, M. (1991). Leptospiral renal failure in Madras City. *Indian Journal of Nephrology* **1**, 15–17.

Niwattayakul, K., Homvijitkul, J., Khow, O., and Sitprija, V. (2003) Leptospirosis in northeastern Thailand: hypotension and complication. *Southeast Asian Journal of Tropical Medicine and Public Health* (in press).

O'Brien, K. L. *et al.* (1998). Epidemic of pediatric deaths from acute renal failure caused by diethylene glycol poisoning. Acute Renal Failure Investigation Team. *Journal of American Medical Association* **279**, 1175–1180.

Otieno, L. S., McLigeyo, S. O., and Luta, M. (1991). Acute renal failure following the use of herbal remedies. *East African Medical Journal* **68**, 993–998.

Pandya, S. K. (1988). Letter from Bombay. An unmitigated tragedy. *British Medical Journal* **297**, 117–119.

Park, S. K. *et al.* (1990). Toxic acute renal failure and hepatitis after ingestion of raw carp bile. *Nephron* **56**, 188–193.

Park, Y. K., Park, S. K., Rhee, Y. K., and Kang, S. K. (1990). Leptospirosis in Chonbuk province of Korea in 1987. *Korean Journal of Internal Medicine* **5**, 34–43.

Pereira, B. J. G., Pereira, S., Gupta, A., Sakhuja, V., and Chugh, K. S. (1989). Acute renal failure in infants in the tropics. *Nephrology, Dialysis, Transplantation* **4**, 535–538.

Petros, S., Leonhardht, U., and Engelmann, L. (2000). Serum procalcitonin and proinflammatory cytokines in a patient with acute severe leptospirosis. *Scandinavian Journal of Infectious Diseases* **32**, 104–105.

Phu, N. H. *et al.* (2002). Hemofiltration and peritoneal dialysis in infection-associated acute renal failure in Vietnam. *New England Journal of Medicine* **347**, 895–902.

Prakash M. S., Sud, K., Kohli, H. S., Jha, V., Gupta, K. L., and Sakhuja, V. (1999). Ethylene dibromide poisoning with acute renal failure: first reported case with non-fatal outcome. *Renal Failure* **21**, 219–222.

Ramachandran, S. Acute renal failure in Sri Lanka. In *Asian Nephrology* (ed. K. S. Chugh), pp. 378–383. New Delhi: Oxford University Press, 1994.

Rui-Mei, L., Kara, A. U., and Sinniah, R. (1998). Dysregulation of cytokine expression in tubulointerstitial nephritis associated with murine malaria. *Kidney International* **53**, 845–852.

Sandhu, J. S., Agarwal, A., Gupta, K. L., Sakhuja, V., and Chugh, K. S. (1992). Acute renal failure in severe hypothermia. *Renal Failure* **14**, 591–594.

Sanford, J. P. Leptospirosis. In *Harrison's Principles of Internal Medicine* (ed. K. J. Isselbacher, E. Braunwald, J. D. Wilson, J. B. Martin, A. S. Fauci, and D. L. Kasper), pp. 740–743. New York: McGraw Hill, 1994.

Sanguangvong, S., Polvicha, P., Uisricoon, S., Prayoonvivat, V., and Srichikul, T. (1988). Exchange transfusion in the treatment of fatal cases of heat injury in Pramongkutkrao Hospital. *Abstracts of the Annual Scientific Meeting of Royal College of Physicians of Thailand*, Pechbury, Thailand, p. 48.

Sarkar, S. *et al.* (1993). Acute intravascular haemolysis in glucose-6-phosphate dehydrogenase deficiency. *Annals of Tropical Paediatrics* **13**, 391–394.

Seedat, Y. K. (1993). Acute renal failure in the black population in South Africa. *International Journal of Artificial Organs* **16**, 801–802.

Seedat, Y. K. and Nathoo, B. C. (1993). Acute renal failure in Blacks and Indians in South Africa—comparison after 10 years. *Nephron* **64**, 198–201.

Seguro, A. C., Lomar, A. V., and Rocha, A. S. (1990). Acute renal failure in leptospirosis: nonoliguric and hypokalemic forms. *Nephron* **55**, 146–151.

Sert, M., Tetiker, T., and Paydas, S. (1993). Rhabdomyolysis and acute renal failure due to honeybee stings as an uncommon cause. *Nephron* **65**, 647.

Sesagothy, M., Swaminathan, M., King, N. C. T., and Bennett, W. M. (1995). Djenkol bean poisoning (Djenkolism): an unusual cause of acute renal failure. *American Journal of Kidney Diseases* **25**, 63–66.

Shah, P. P., Trivedi, H. L., Sharma, R. K., Shah, P. R., and Joshi, M. N. (1985). Acute renal failure, experience of 816 patients in the tropics. *Abstracts of the XVth Annual Conference of the Indian Society of Nephrology, Bangalore*, p. 17.

Simpson, J., Watson, A. R., Mellersh, A., Nelson, C. S., and Dodd, K. (1991). Typhoid fever, ciprofloxacin and renal failure. *Archives of Diseases of Children* **66**, 1083–1084.

Singh, S., Chaudhary, D., Garg, M., and Sharma, B. K. (1993). Fatal ethylene dibromide ingestion. *Journal of Association of Physicians of India* **41**, 608.

Singh, J. *et al.* (2001). Diethylene glycol poisoning in Gurgaon, India, 1998. *Bulletin of World Health Organization* **79**, 88–95.

Singhal, P. C., Chugh, K. S., Kaur, S., and Malik, A. K. (1977). Acute renal failure in leprosy. *International Journal of Leprosy* **45**, 171–173.

Sitprija, V. (1988). Nephropathy in falciparum malaria. *Kidney International* **34**, 867–877.

Sitprija, V. and Benyajati, C. (1975). Tropical diseases and acute renal failure. *Annals of the Academy of Medicine of Singapore* **4** (Suppl.), 112–114.

Sitprija, V. and Chusilp, S. K. (1973). Renal failure and hyperbilirubinaemia in leptospirosis. Treatment with exchange transfusion. *Medical Journal of Australia* **1**, 171–172.

Sitprija, V. and Newton, P. Leptospirosis. In *Concise Oxford Textbook of Medicine* (ed. J. G. G. Ledingham and D. A. Warrell), pp. 1675–1677. Oxford: Oxford University Press, 2000.

Sitprija, V., Vongthongsri, M., Poshyachinda, V., and Arthachinta, S. (1977). Renal failure in malaria: a pathophysiologic study. *Nephron* **18**, 277–287.

Sitprija, V., Suvanpha, R., Pochngool, C., Chusil, S., and Tungsanka, K. (1982). Acute interstitial nephritis in snake bite. *American Journal of Tropical Medicine and Hygiene* **31**, 408–410.

Sitprija, V. *et al.* (1996). Renal and systemic hemodynamics, in falciparum malaria. *American Journal of Nephrology* **16**, 513–519.

Sontz, E. and Schweiger, J. (1995). The 'Green Water' syndrome: copper-induced hemolysis and subsequent acute renal failure as consequence of a religious ritual. *American Journal of Medicine* **98**, 311–315.

Srivastava, R. N., Bagga, A., and Moudgil, A. (1990). Acute renal failure in North Indian children. *Indian Journal of Medical Research* **92**, 404–408.

Susaengrat, W., Dhiensiri, T., Sinavatana, P., and Sitprija, V. (1987). Renal failure in melioidosis. *Nephron* **46**, 167–169.

Tariang, D. D. *et al.* (1999). Randomized controlled trial on the effective dose of anti-snake venom in cases of snake bite with systemic envenomantion. *Journal of Association of Physicians of India* **47**, 369–371.

Trang, T. T. *et al.* (1992). Acute renal failure in patients with severe falciparum malaria. *Clinical Infectious Diseases* **15**, 874–880.

Turney, J. H., Marshall, D. H., Brownjohn, A. M., Ellis, C. M., and Parsons, F. M. (1990). The evolution of acute renal failure, 1956–1988. *Quarterly Journal of Medicine* **74**, 83–104.

Varma, P. P., Jha, V., Ghosh, A. K., Joshi, K., and Sakhuja, V. (1994). Acute renal failure in a case of fatal chromic acid poisoning. *Renal Failure* **16**, 653–657.

Warrell, D. A. (1989). Snake venoms in science and clinical medicine 1. Russell's viper: biology, venom and treatment of bites. *Transactions of the Royal Society of Tropical Medicine and Hygiene* **83**, 732–740.

Warrell, D. A. (1999). WHO/SEARO Guidelines for the clinical management of snake bites in the Southeast Asian region. *Southeast Asian Journal of Tropical Medicine and Public Health* **30** (Suppl. 1), 1–85.

Watt, G. *et al.* (1988). Placebo-controlled trial of intravenous penicillin for severe and late leptospirosis. *Lancet* **1**, 433–435.

Weber, M. W., Boker, K., Horstman, R. D., and Ehrich, J. H. (1991). Renal failure is a common complication in non-immune Europeans with falciparum malaria. *Tropical Medicine and Parasitology* **42**, 115–118.

White, N. J. and Breman, J. G. Malaria and babesiosis. In *Harrison's Principles of Internal Medicine* (ed. K. J. Isselbacher, E. Braunwald, J. D. Wilson, J. B. Martin, A. S. Fauci, and D. L. Kasper), pp. 887–896. New York: McGraw Hill, 1994.

Willinger, G. G., Thamaree, S., Schramek, H., Gstraunthaler, G., and Pfaller, W. (1995). *In vitro* nephrotoxicity of Russell's viper venom. *Kidney International* **47**, 518–528.

Winearls, C. G., Chan, L., Coghlan, J. D., Ledingham, J. G. G., and Oliver, D. O. (1984). Acute renal failure due to leptospirosis—clinical features and outcome in-six cases. *Quarterly Journal of Medicine* **53**, 487–495.

Yamashiro-Kanashiro, E. H., Benard, G., Sato, M. N., Seguro, A. C., and Duarte, A. J. (1991). Cellular immune response analysis of patients with leptospirosis. *American Journal of Tropical Medicine and Hygiene* **45**, 138–145.

Yang, C.-W., Wu, M.-S., and Pan, M.-J. (2001). Leptospiral renal disease. *Nephrology, Dialysis, Transplantation* **16** (Suppl. 5), 73–77.

Yang, C. W., Wu, M. S., Pan, M. J., Hong, J. J., Yu, C. C., Vandewalle, A., and Huang, C. C. (2000). Leptospira outer membrane protein activates NF-kappaB and downstream genes expressed in medullary thick ascending limb cells. *Journal of the American Society of Nephrology* **11**, 2017–2026.

Yeh, Y. H., Wang, D. Y., Deng, J. F., Chen, S. K., and Hwang, D. F. (2002). Short-term toxicity of grass carp bile powder, 5alpha-cyprinol and 5alpha-cyprinol sulfate in rats. *Comparative Biochemistry and Physiology. Part C, Toxicology & Pharmacology* **131**, 1–8.

Zewdu, W. (1994). Acute renal failure in Addis Ababa, Ethiopia: a prospective study of 136 patients. *Ethiopian Medical Journal* **32**, 79–87.

10.7.4 The elderly

Norbert Hendrik Lameire, Nele Van Den Noortgate, and Raymond Camille Vanholder

Introduction

Between 1999 and 2050, demographic projections predict a major increase in the population above 65 and more particularly in the portion older than 80 years. Global life expectancy at any age has progressed in the developed world and at the age of 70 years a European man can expect to live another 12.5 years and a woman another 16 years. It is thus evident that in the next few years the practice of medicine in the Western world will be profoundly influenced by the health care needs of the rapidly enlarging elderly population.

Renal services must therefore be prepared for an increasing number of elderly patients with both acute and chronic renal failure.

The term 'elderly' changes with time and chronological age is less important than biological age which determines functional capability, although until now it cannot be accurately measured. It is likely that in the near future 75 or even 80 years of age will be the definition of 'elderly' (Akposso *et al.* 2000).

Until there is an agreed definition of 'biological age', chronological age and the cut-off point of 65 years will be used in this chapter as the definition of elderly. There are medical reasons to expect an increasing number of elderly patients with acute renal failure (ARF). First, the ageing kidney, due to structural and functional alterations, is less able to cope with rapid haemodynamic changes and with changes in water and salt balance. In particular, the glomerular reserve and capacity of renal autoregulation are diminished in the elderly kidney (Fliser *et al.* 1995).

These structural and functional alterations are described in detail elsewhere in this book. Second, an increasing number of individuals will have chronic systemic diseases, such as hypertension, diabetes mellitus, atherosclerosis, heart disease, and malignancy. Some of these diseases result in diminished renal reserve. A much more aggressive diagnostic and therapeutic approach to illness in the elderly population carries with it the risk of ARF from complications of these procedures or the subsequent therapeutic interventions. Third, the elderly population consumes twice as many medications, including nephrotoxic agents, as all other age groups combined. The marked and progressive decrease in renal function, associated with increasing age, implies that the dosage of drugs that are predominantly renally excreted should be reduced; a fact that is sometimes forgotten.

These three factors all contribute to the additional risks for the development of ARF in the elderly population and nephrologists are already now facing an increasing demand to provide renal intensive care, including acute dialysis, to very old patients.

Structural and functional alterations in the aged kidney

The main characteristic of the physiological ageing of the kidney is the limitation of the adaptive renal response to different threats to the homeostasis of the organism. Under normal circumstances, the structural and functional alterations may have no major clinical impact, since the renal functional reserve is sufficient to meet the excretory demands. However, ageing can adversely affect the course of a superimposed renal disease, and the pre-existent reduction in functional reserve in the ageing kidney may magnify the excretory defect, caused by any new insult. That such a reduction in the functional reserve exists has been suggested by an age-related impairment in renal vasodilatory response to intravenous glycine, and in postprandial hyperfiltration, following a meal in older compared to younger animals. However, it is possible that in many studies of the functional renal reserve in the elderly, confounding factors such as inadequate control of blood pressure and/or moderate cardiac dysfunction have not been excluded. In fact, healthy independent elderly individuals in good nutritional state and with regular physical activity do not show a decrease in renal functional reserve (Fliser *et al.* 1997).

Haemodynamic and neuroendocrine factors

One of the major protective adaptations of the kidney to hypotension, volume depletion, or reductions in cardiac output is the ability to autoregulate renal blood flow (RBF) and glomerular filtration rate (GFR) to a relatively constant level over a wide variety of renal perfusion pressures. It appears that in experimental states of low cardiac output or extracellular volume depletion, two situations frequently encountered in the elderly, there is a loss of autoregulation following reduction in renal perfusion pressure (Badr and Ichikawa 1988). The fall in GFR is primarily due to a failure to increase the postglomerular resistance. In addition, a displacement of the autoregulation curve of both RBF and GFR to the right has been observed in the presence of an increased sympathetic tone, present in clinical situations such as heart failure or shock. In these situations, a modest reduction in arterial blood pressure can threaten the preservation of renal haemodynamics and GFR.

Baseline and stimulated plasma norepinephrine increase with advancing age and these have been interpreted as indicating that there is a 'constant hyperadrenergic state in the elderly' (for review, see Fitz *et al.* 1992). Intrarenal vascular tone increases with age. Vasoactive factors may contribute to this increased tone although the data describing this change are complex and contradictory. For example, high basal levels of renal nerve activity, angiotensin II (A II), and endogenous endothelin contribute to vasopressor activity, but endothelin, endothelium-derived relaxing factor blockers (L-NAME and L-NMMA), and A II all produce an exaggerated vasopressor response in aged rats (Baylis *et al.* 1998). There appears to be a decreased somatic production of nitric oxide (NO) in older animals compared to younger ones (Hill *et al.* 1997). The data for basal renin and angiotensin levels remain confusing, for example, studies report both normal and low levels of renin and angiotensin in unstressed aged rats compared to younger controls. A consistently observed blunted renin response to stimulation with artificial stressors, upright posture, or sodium depletion suggests that age does affect vascular reactivity under physiological conditions. However, other data show that vasodilators, including angiotensin-converting enzyme inhibitors (ACEIs) and A II blockers, have similar effects regardless of age (Zoja *et al.* 1992). Consequently, one may surmise that a relative increase in endogenous NO activity preserves RBF and GFR but reduces the vasodilatory reserve and adaptation to superimposed haemodynamic insults.

An important role in the preservation of renal function in the presence of increased systemic vasoconstrictors and enhanced sympathetic tone is played by the intrarenal generation of vasodilating products of arachidonic acid (i.e. PGI_2). Angiotensin stimulates synthesis of PGI_2 and PGE_2 within the kidney and prostaglandins act to preserve glomerular filtration in situations such as sodium depletion, surgical stress, and reduced cardiac output. Cyclo-oxygenase-inhibition by non-steroidal anti-inflammatory drugs (NSAIDs) reduces the GFR and RBF in these conditions. With advancing age, there is a widespread decrease in prostacyclin (PGI_2)/synthesis throughout the vascular endothelium, leading to a decrease in the PGI_2/thromboxane A_2 (TXA_2) ratio, a maladaptation which is atherogenic. The ratio of urinary PGI_2 to TXA_2 also decreases in older subjects and *in vitro* studies in the rat have been shown that the TXA_2 to PGI_2 ratio is increased in glomeruli and inner and outer medulla of older kidneys (Rathaus *et al.* 1993).

How these circulatory and neuroendocrine alterations affect the autoregulatory defence and contribute to an enhanced risk for acute renal dysfunction in elderly people is not clear. Although no formal studies of autoregulation of GFR and RBF in otherwise healthy ageing human kidneys have been performed, there is enough circumstantial evidence to suggest that the kidneys of aged individuals are more vulnerable to reductions of renal perfusion pressure than younger kidneys. A disease state in which autoregulation of RBF and GFR is likely to be impaired is the atherosclerotic involvement of afferent arterioles caused by age, hypertension, or diabetes mellitus. It is conceivable that in this situation the responsiveness of these arterioles to changes in their wall tension is decreased, making renal perfusion and function vulnerable to even small fluctuations in systemic blood pressure. A prototype of human disease, common at older age, and where the kidney is forced to autoregulate is atherosclerotic renal artery stenosis. However, every disease, characterized by enhanced sympathetic tone and/or elevated levels of A II, such as heart failure or hypovolaemia, will be associated with greater difficulty in autoregulating the GFR in the presence of a decrease in renal perfusion pressure. Direct interference with the protective autoregulatoty mechanisms, either by disease or by pharmacological interventions, may precipitate acute renal insufficiency. Drugs known to impair renal autoregulation or to interfere with the renal vasodilatory capacity include ACEIs or angiotensin receptor antagonists (ARBs), loop diuretics, and prostaglandin synthesis inhibitors, like aspirin and the NSAIDs.

Other renal functional alterations in the elderly

Concentration and dilution of the urine

The impairment of renal concentration, together with the well-known deficit in thirst perception, makes the elderly particularly liable to develop dehydration and hypernatraemia (Phillips *et al.* 1993).

Maximal diluting ability also decreases with age (Choudhury *et al.* 2000) and together with the enhanced osmotic release of arginine vasopressin (AVP) leads to a high incidence of hyponatraemia.

Urinary sodium excretion

The ability of the aged kidney to conserve sodium in response to sodium deprivation is decreased (Epstein and Hollenberg 1976) and, when sodium restriction is imposed, it takes nearly twice as long for the aged kidney to decrease urinary sodium excretion compared with younger individuals. A decrease in distal tubular sodium reabsorption may be explained by ageing-induced renal interstitial scarring and decreased nephron number, increased medullary flow, and changes in hormonal levels regulating sodium excretion. Both basal and stimulated circulating plasma renin and aldosterone levels have been found to decrease with ageing in healthy elderly subjects. Lower nephron renin content, intrarenal downregulation of renin mRNA, and ACE have been demonstrated. On the other hand, the natriuretic ability of the aged kidney appears to be blunted when faced with sodium loading or volume expansion (for review, see Choudhury *et al.* 2000). The slower natriuretic response to an acute saline load has important implications for the evaluation of the urinary parameters used in distinguishing acute prerenal and renal failure (see below).

Elevated plasma atrial natriuretic peptide (ANP) has been found in healthy elderly to be 3–5 times times those of the healthy young. The metabolic clearance of ANP in the elderly is decreased in comparison to that in the young at similar low ANP infusion rates. Also the renal natriuretic response to an ANP infusion is blunted in the aged kidney (Pollack *et al.* 1997), despite a normal increase in cyclic guanosine-monophosphate (cGMP) after ANP infusion.

Acid–base balance

The decreased renin and aldosterone activity in the elderly contributes to an increased incidence of type 4 renal tubular acidosis (hyporeninaemic hypoaldosteronism) and may cause a greater propensity toward hyperkalaemia in a variety of clinical settings, such as the presence of gastrointestinal bleeding or during potassium loading, for example, potassium supplementation associated with diuretic therapy. Given possible problems with chronic potassium adaptation with ageing, medications that inhibit the renin–angiotensin system such as ACEI, heparin, cyclosporin, tacrolimus, β-blockers, and NSAIDs may increase the risk of hyperkalaemia. Similarly, sodium channel-blocking agents such as trimethoprim, pentamidine, and potassium-sparing diuretics such as amiloride, triamterene, and spironolactone can add to underlying defects in potassium excretion (Schepkens *et al.* 2001).

Experimental evidence for enhanced risk of ARF in the elderly

The evidence that all these structural and functional renal alterations represent an enhanced risk for ARF in the elderly is indirect. For example, the age-associated structural glomerular alterations might exacerbate postischaemic reductions in GFR. Aged kidneys may have fewer nephrons to recruit to support renal function, and may thereby magnify the deficit incurred by an ischaemic or nephrotoxic insult. Alternatively, ageing tubular cells may be more vulnerable to ischaemic damage because cellular antioxidant defences decline with age and oxidant injury may be a critical determinant of ischaemic ARF (Chapter 10.2).

Experimental studies in the ageing rat have provided support for an enhanced risk of developing ischaemic and toxic ARF (see for review Lameire *et al.* 1999a). In all ischaemic models, the decline in renal function in the aged rat was significantly greater than in the young rat, and the rate of recovery was much slower. Despite the substantial differences in postischaemic renal function, evaluation of tubular injury surprisingly failed to reveal any difference among the different age groups. The lack of relationship between the severity of ARF and the extent of morphological damage strongly suggests that the age-related changes had a glomerular/haemodynamic basis, rather than reflecting an intrinsic difference in tubular susceptibility to ischaemic damage. However, following graded periods of *in vitro* anoxia, renal function, as assessed by renal cortical slice uptake of *p*-aminohippurate (PAH) and tetraethylammonium, was impaired to a greater extent in old as compared to young rats. This suggests that in addition to the changes in RBF and GFR, alterations in the metabolism and biochemistry of ageing tubular cells might play a role in mediating age-related enhancement of ischaemic renal cell injury (Lameire *et al.* 1999a).

NO is another mediator that could play a role in the greater risk of ARF in the elderly. Studies have shown that NO synthesis (NOS) blockade decreases RBF, GFR, and K_f more in ageing than in young rats, suggesting that NO may play a progressively increasing and important role in controlling renal function in advancing age than in the young (Tan *et al.* 1998). NO production appears to be reduced with ageing in isolated conduit arteries (Kung and Luscher 1995) and a 40 per cent decrease in serum NOS substrate L-arginine has been found (Reckelhoff *et al.* 1994). Similar findings have been noted in ageing humans (Schmidt *et al.* 2001). It may be that renal endothelial NO production is maximized in the normal elderly to maintain stable renal function. Measurements of NO production in the face of renal ischaemia still need to be done in human subjects.

In a rat model of ARF, an increase in glomerular NO production seems to play a protective role in renal function by counteracting the vasoconstrictor substances released during ARF. When challenged with gentamicin, older animals developed a more severe renal failure than younger animals. In addition, a lower glomerular NO production in basal conditions and a markedly blunted stimulation of NO synthesis by gentamicin were found in older animals (Valdivielso *et al.* 1996). In a renal artery clamp model (Sabbatini *et al.* 1994), the basal renal dynamics were similar in old and young animals, but 1 day after ARF, the decrease in GFR was more severe in the old than in the young, due to a greater increase of renal vascular resistance in the old animals. However, the histological renal damage after ischaemia was comparable in the two groups. Five days after ARF, the recovery of renal function was slower in older rats. In two other groups of animals, two different scavengers of oxygen-free radicals, dimethylthiourea (DMTU) and superoxide dismutase (SOD), were administered at the time of arterial occlusion. DMTU had protective effects in the young but not in the old animals; in contrast, SOD was more effective in old than in young rats. To test the hypothesis that such a difference was related to the capacity of SOD to increase NO, four more groups of young and old rats were pretreated with L-arginine, a precursor of NO. No difference in renal dynamics was detected in basal conditions, but when older rats were pretreated with L-arginine in their feed 7 days before renal artery occlusion, there was a marked improvement in GFR and RPF, and a decrease in renal vascular resistance. L-NAME, an NOS inhibitor, given to older L-arginine-fed rats abolished the renal haemodynamic response seen with L-arginine and SOD (Sabbatini *et al.* 1994).

Glomerulosclerosis may not be the primary factor leading to ischaemic renal failure in ageing rats. In fact, when histological variations between young and old rats were minimized by a low protein diet, renal artery clamping still led to a significant decrease in GFR and RPF and an increase in renal vascular resistance in older versus younger rats (Sabbatini *et al.* 1994). Studies using blood oxygenation level-dependent magnetic resonance imaging in nine elderly female volunteers between 59 and 79 years of age showed a relative inability to improve medullary oxygenation with water diuresis compared with younger subjects, thus suggesting a possible predisposition to hypoxic renal injury also in older human individuals (Prasad and Epstein 1999).

Incidence of ARF in the older population

The true incidence of ARF is difficult to estimate because the definition used in the published series is not uniform. Patients with either an acute but modest increase of serum creatinine or with severe dialysis-dependent ARF are both included. Some papers include all forms of ARF while in others only acute tubular necrosis (ATN) is considered and different criteria for dividing the patients into 'young' and 'old' are applied. However, it is clear that the frequency of severe ARF is increased with advancing age.

In a prospective, 2-year study, it was found that individuals over 70 years of age comprised more than 70 per cent of all cases of ARF (Feest *et al.* 1993). The frequency of severe ARF was 17 per million population in those under 50 years of age and was increased by 56-fold (949 pmp) in those aged 80–89 years. In a large series of 748 patients with ARF in the Madrid area, it was observed that 36 per cent of these cases were older than 70 years, although this age category represented only 7 per cent of the general population in that area. In 1991 and 1992, a total number of all ARF patients attending 13 tertiary care hospitals in the Madrid area was 209 cases pmp per year, while in the patients aged over 80 years ARF was observed in 1129 cases pmp per year (Pascual and Liano 1998).

In France, the incidence of ARF in patients admitted in nephrology units was slightly more than 100 pmp per year (Chanard *et al.* 1994).

Several reports have observed a gradual increase in the mean or median age of the patients who develop ARF in different observation periods (Lameire *et al.* 1999b).

Figure 1 depicts a recent study from the Tenon Hospital in Paris (Akposso *et al.* 2000). Between October 1971 and September 1996, 381 patients older than 80 years in a total of 2111 patients suffering from ARF were admitted to the nephrology ICU. Whereas the percentage of ARF patients over 80 years of age out of the total number of patients with ARF was always less than 4 per cent before 1978, this number has grown to about 40 per cent in the period 1995–1996.

In those series in which ARF could be related to a specific causal factor (e.g. cardiopulmonary resuscitation, postcardiac surgery, aortic aneurysm surgery), the number of elderly patients also increased. In many studies, a reduced baseline renal function emerged as a strong independent risk factor (Suen *et al.* 1998; Fortescue *et al.* 2000).

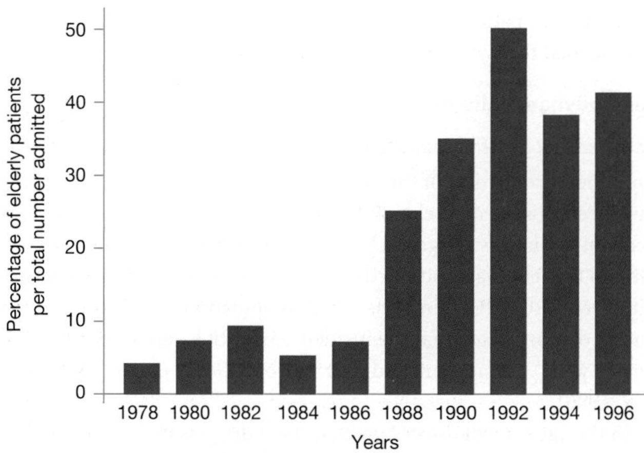

Fig. 1 Graph depicting year-wise distribution of elderly patients with ARF admitted to Tenon Hospital, Paris (Akposso *et al.* 2000).

Causes of ARF in the elderly

The aetiology of ARF is frequently multifactorial, so that any classification of ARF poses problems of definition. In many reports, the cause of ARF is defined as the most likely factor that was responsible for the deterioration in renal function.

Table 1 summarizes the distribution of all causes of ARF in elderly described in a recent series in which the aetiology was sufficiently detailed (Akposso *et al.* 2000).

Prerenal causes

A major cause of an acute deterioration in renal function in the elderly is 'prerenal failure', a decreased perfusion of the kidney, for example,

Table 1 Causes of ARF in patients older than 70 years in the Tenon Hospital (Paris) (Akposso *et al.* 2000)

Cause	Number	%
Obstructive renal failure	**85/381**	**22.3**
Prostatic adenoma	22	5.8
Prostatic cancer	19	5.0
Bladder/ureter cancer	15	3.9
Uterus/ovarian cancer	9	2.4
Colorectal cancer	5	1.3
Nephrolithiasis	5	1.3
Retroperitoneal fibrosis	8	2.1
Ureteral stenosis	1	0.3
Fecaloma	1	0.3
Prerenal failure	**92/381**	**24.1**
Dehydration	55	14.4
Heart failure	14	3.7
Dysregulation of GFR	21	5.5
Hepatorenal syndrome	2	0.5
Intrinsic renal failure	**204/381**	**53.5**
Tubulopathy		
Shock	99	26.0
Cardiogenic shock	21	5.5
Septic shock	54	14.2
Hypovolaemic shock	34	8.9
Rhabdomyolysis	20	5.2
Multiple myeloma	14	3.7
Drugs (aminoglycosides; NSAID; ACEI; iodinated contrast media)	23	6.0
Interstitial		
Pyelonephritis	8	2.1
Immunoallergic nephropathy	8	2.1
Glomerulopathies		
Goodpasture('s syndrome)	8	2.1
Wegener		
Postinfectious glomerulonephritis		
Vascular thrombosis	6	1.6
Cholesterol embol(ism)	3	0.8
Blood incompatibility	1	0.3

from a decrease in cardiac output; gastrointestinal losses caused by vomiting, diarrhoea, or bleeding; renal losses due to glycosuria; and use of diuretics (Blantz 1998).

The incidence of acute prerenal failure in the aged is difficult to estimate (Table 2). In some series, these cases are deliberately excluded from analysis, and in series where they are included, the definition of ARF is not uniform.

For example, in community-acquired ARF, prerenal azotaemia was found in 70 per cent of the patients, who had a mean age of 62.5 years. In three geriatric units, all records of patients admitted were analysed. Of a total of 273 patients with raised urea or serum creatinine on admission, 53.3 per cent had prerenal failure. This incidence increased to 70 per cent in the age group older than 85 years (McInnes *et al.* 1987). Forty-five of the 338 patients older than 70 years, hospitalized in an internal medicine unit over 1 year for a non-nephrological problem, presented with ARF. A prerenal cause was found in 20 patients (60 per cent), and was due to diuretics in 12 patients (45 per cent) (Gentric and Cledes 1991). Finally, in the Tenon study of 381 patients, 24.1 per cent of ARF patients older than 80 years were categorized as prerenal (Akposso *et al.* 2000).

Hypovolaemia

Hypovolaemia is common in the elderly and may present as either prerenal failure or, if not corrected, may progress to postischaemic ATN.

Hypovolaemia is frequently caused by dehydration and is present in approximately 1 per cent of all community hospital admissions of elderly patients (Snyder *et al.* 1987). Reduced renal water conserving capacity, reduced thirst, and reduced water intake all contribute to the genesis of dehydration in the elderly. Up to 25 per cent of non-ambulatory geriatric patients are for these reasons mildly dehydrated. Particular risk factors for dehydration in elderly nursing home residents include acute febrile illnesses, multiple drugs (especially diuretics and laxatives), age over 85 years, and being bedridden (Lavizzo-Mourey *et al.* 1988). During infections in nursing home residents, hypernatraemia, an indicator of dehydration, is seen in 25 per cent of all febrile patients. Untreated, the mortality of dehydration exceeds 50 per cent. Nursing staff documentation of impaired oral intake, in combination with an elevated serum sodium and BUN/Cr ratio, provides early clinical and laboratory evidence of dehydration in this setting (Weinberg *et al.* 1994). Hypovolaemia may also be caused by fluid redistribution from the intravascular to the interstitial space in states of cardiac failure, nephrotic syndrome, decompensated liver cirrhosis with ascites, pancreatitis, extensive burns, and malnutrition.

Table 2 Frequency of prerenal ARF in elderly subjects (%)

Author	Age				
	>85 years	>80 years	65–79 years	65–85 years	>70 years
McInnes (1987)	70				
Gentric (1991)					60
Klouche (1995)				35	
Pascual (1998)		30	28		
Akposso (2000)		24			

The diagnosis of hypovolaemic acute prerenal failure in the elderly is difficult because the clinical signs and symptoms of dehydration are often unreliable. They depend on the volume, the rate, and the nature of the fluid losses. Clinical examination will include attention to the jugular venous pressure, orthostatic changes in pulse and blood pressure, skin turgor, moisture in the axillae, and hydration of mucous membranes. Interstitial fluid loss can be detected by decreased elasticity of the skin, especially over the forehead, the sternum, and the anterior area of the thigh. These changes are difficult to interpret in the elderly in whom a loss of subcutaneous tissue elasticity is often observed. A dry tongue and oral mucosa are present with volume depletion, and also in patients breathing through their mouths. A rapid reduction in body weight indicates the volume of body fluids lost. Although prerenal failure is usually associated with oliguria, prerenal failure with preserved urine output has been observed (Miller *et al.* 1980).

The traditional urinary parameters used for differentiating prerenal from renal failure (low fractional urinary excretion of sodium and/or of urea) must be interpreted with caution, because they may merely reflect age-related disturbances in tubular handling of sodium and water. In view of the chronic reduction in urinary concentrating ability, urinary sodium and osmolality may not achieve 'prerenal' values during acute renal insults. An elevated urinary sodium concentration or FE_{Na} obtained in an elderly patient may suggest an established parenchymal injury, but prerenal hypoperfusion may still be present and should anyway be corrected. It is well known that the FE_{Na} is unreliable in sodium-retaining states such as chronic heart failure, decompensated cirrhosis, after diuretic therapy, after administration of contrast agents, in pigment-induced nephropathy, and sepsis (Vaz 1983; Zarich *et al.* 1985). In one study in which the urinary parameters of elderly and younger patients with ARF were compared, prerenal failure indices were found in 21 per cent of elderly with established ATN. The latter was defined by non-response to a trial of acute volume expansion (Lameire *et al.* 1987).

Although the vast majority of patients with prerenal ARF may be identified by clinical and urinary evaluation, there are some elderly patients whose volume status cannot be confidently assessed. In this setting, a rising central venous pressure in response to fluid therapy is a valuable guide. 'Blind' infusion of fluid should not be undertaken without haemodynamic monitoring, especially in elderly azotaemic patients with impaired heart function. As explained earlier, older hypovolaemic patients often respond slower to a challenge of an acute volume load than younger patients.

Haemodynamically mediated ARF

Non-steroidal anti-inflammatory drugs

Since the introduction of the NSAIDs, a great number of cases of ARF have been observed in elderly individuals, not only because of their frequent use in this age group but because elderly kidneys are very sensitive to the renal vasoconstriction and the sodium retention associated with these drugs (Griffin *et al.* 2000). Population-based case–control studies demonstrated that the incidence of ARF is rare (2 per 1,00,000 person years) but is increased fourfold by NSAID usage (Gutthamm *et al.* 1996).

In the age category over 60 years, these drugs were incriminated in more than 25 per cent of drug-induced ARF. In a large epidemiological study in a general internal medicine practice, renal impairment was diagnosed in 18 per cent of the patients taking ibuprofen. However, serious renal dysfunction occurred in only 0.5 per cent of the patients.

If the renal effect of the NSAID is characterized in a first phase by a functional alteration which is rapidly reversible after stopping the treatment, this can lead to ATN in the presence of prolonged renal ischaemia.

Well-known risk factors for NSAID-induced nephrotoxicity include age greater than or equal to 60 years with atherosclerotic cardiovascular disease, pre-existing chronic renal insufficiency (serum creatinine >180 μmol/l), and states of renal hypoperfusion caused by, for example, sodium depletion, diuretic use, hypotension, and sodium avid states such as cirrhosis, nephrotic syndrome, and congestive heart failure (Brater 1999). There is, however, no evidence that NSAIDs impair the renal function in otherwise healthy elderly individuals. A particular characteristic of this cause of ARF is hyperkalaemia which is sometimes out of proportion to the degree of renal impairment, especially when these patients are also treated with potassium-sparing diuretics or ACEIs. These risk factors are additive and patients with multiple risk factors are rarely included in clinical studies of these drugs.

It was originally hoped that agents with a more selective inhibition of COX-2 would not adversely affect renal function. It appears, however, that they probably have the same effects on renal function as non-selective NSAIDs (Harris and Brater 2001). It is, therefore, relevant that in elderly patients on a salt-restricted diet, the COX-2-selective inhibitor, rofecoxib, decreased GFR (iothalamate clearance) by approximately 15 per cent. In a cohort of elderly patients with decreased creatinine clearance on a low-salt diet and treated with refecoxib or indomethacin, a similar decrease in the GFR (10–12 per cent) and decreased excretion of sodium and water were found for both agents (Swan *et al.* 2000).

A post hoc analysis of the data from more than 50 clinical studies involving over 13,000 study participants treated with celecoxib for an average of 12 weeks documented a similar incidence of adverse renal effects using either celecoxib (4.3 per cent) or the non-selective NSAIDs (4.1 per cent) (Whelton *et al.* 2000). Although some studies have suggested that COX-2 inhibitors may not cause as severe a decline in renal function as compared to non-selective NSAIDs (Perazella and Eras 2000), it is premature to take comfort in these reports, because the study subjects were not at high risk of renal insufficiency. Moreover, a few cases of acute renal insufficiency caused by COX-2-selective NSAIDs have recently been reported (Perazella and Eras 2000; Wolf *et al.* 2000) and the same precautions apply thus to both the non-selective and COX-2-selective NSAIDs. In addition, most of the COX-2-selective drugs have rather long half-lives (11 h for celecoxib and 17 h for rofecoxib).

Rarely, some patients may develop an acute oligoanuric renal failure, associated with microscopic haematuria, (significant) proteinuria, and (exceptionally) eosinophilia, reflecting an allergic acute tubulointerstitial nephritis following NSAID treatment. Cure is obtained after stopping the medication. Even more exceptional is the development of a membranous nephropathy with these drugs.

Angiotensin converting enzyme inhibitors and angiotensin II receptor blockers

Several recent large clinical studies have drawn attention to the possibility of ACEIs causing ARF (The CONSENSUS Trial Study Group 1987; Pitt *et al.* 1997; Knight *et al.* 1999). Haemodynamic ARF caused by ACEIs or by A II receptor blockers develops either in patients with a stenosis of the renal artery to a solitary kidney, or with bilateral renal artery stenosis. The diagnosis of renovascular disease is frequently overlooked and its increasing prevalence is associated with age and the vascular comorbidity in the population. Renovascular disease has been found in 34 per cent of aged individuals suffering from heart failure (MacDowall *et al.* 1998), but patients with severe chronic heart failure, polycystic kidney disease, or intrarenal nephrosclerosis without renal artery stenosis are also at risk (Lameire *et al.* 1999a). ACEIs and/or A II antagonists are often indicated in these patients and the risk of haemodynamic ARF is thus not negligible. The pathophysiology of this syndrome has recently been described (Schoolwerth *et al.* 2001). The frequency of ARF induced by ACEIs in the elderly has been estimated to vary between 6 and 23 per cent in patients with bilateral renal artery stenosis and increases to 38 per cent in patients with unilateral stenosis in a single kidney.

Besides functional ARF provoked by these drugs, a possible lethal association is the development of sometimes catastrophic hyperkalaemia. We have recently described a series of 25 patients (mean age 74 years) who presented with a hyperkalaemia (mean value 7.7 mmol/l) and a mean serum creatinine level of 3.8 mg/dl (Schepkens *et al.* 2001). Fifty per cent of these patients were dehydrated and all had been treated with a combination of spironolactone and ACEIs, a regimen now recommended for heart failure.

The renal causes

Renovascular diseases (see also Chapter 10.6.6)

Acute obstruction of the renal vasculature by thrombosis of the renal artery, its intrarenal branches, by cholesterol, or non-cholesterol emboli is more common in the elderly. One important risk for intrarenal emboli is the presence of atrial fibrillation, where the relative risk for peripheral embolization (aorta, renal, pelvic, and extremities) has been calculated to be 4 in men and 5.7 in women compared to the general population (Frost *et al.* 2001).

ARF caused by complete renal artery thrombosis occurs when the occlusion is bilateral or in the case of unilateral acute occlusion, with a non-functioning contralateral kidney. Flank pain with or without low-grade fever (with an associated leucocytosis) are the most common presenting symptoms. Macroscopic or microscopic haematuria are not always present. Whereas total occlusion of both renal arteries is usually manifested by anuria, minimal output of urine may be observed and the differential diagnosis from other forms of ARF may become difficult.

The diagnostic work-up should include dimethyl triethyl pentaacetic acid (DTPA) renal scanning, demonstrating markedly diminished or absent renal perfusion, followed by aortography with delayed pictures to define reconstitution of the distal renal artery and a nephrogram.

The management of ARF due to acute renal artery thrombosis is a challenge in these patients who often have widespread vascular disease, because surgery carries a high risk. Selective infusion of streptokinase or urokinase into the occluded renal artery is the (first-line) therapy (Salam *et al.* 1993). In some patients, fibrinolytic therapy may be followed by balloon catheter angioplasty to correct residual non-ostial renal artery stenosis. If thrombolytic therapy is ineffective, surgical revascularization should be attempted promptly. Surgery may offer a better chance for renal salvage in renal artery thrombosis complicating catheter angioplasty or occurring in association with acute aortic occlusion because of the risk of distal embolization. Recovery of renal function may be expected in only 30–40 per cent of the cases (Salam *et al.* 1993).

The optimal treatment for renal infarction is uncertain, but medical therapy is generally preferred. Although surgery can restore vascular patency, it is associated with a higher mortality rate and with no better renal functional recovery than that seen with anticoagulation or thrombolytic therapy alone (Blum *et al.* 1993).

The one setting in which early surgery remains the treatment of choice is in patients with traumatic renal artery thrombosis, particularly if performed within the first few hours (Cosby *et al.* 1986).

Medical therapy will lead to improved renal function only if there is incomplete occlusion or if effective thrombolysis is initiated within 90–180 min, which represents the ischaemic tolerance of normal renal tissue (Blum *et al.* 1993). Intravenous heparin followed by oral warfarin has been the standard anticoagulant regimen in this setting. Thrombolytic therapy (with streptokinase or tissue-type plasminogen activator) can in most cases effectively lyse the occluding thrombus (Steckel *et al.* 1984). However, this option should be considered only with early diagnosis when the ischaemic renal tissue is still viable. The risk of systemic bleeding can be minimized by local intra-arterial infusion of the thrombolytic agent, rather than intravenous administration (Steckel *et al.* 1984; Blum *et al.* 1993).

Surgical revascularization can still be considered in patients with severe renal failure in whom there is no functional recovery within 4–6 weeks. Late embolectomy has led to improvement in renal function in selected patients, indicating that ischaemic atrophy can still be reversed.

The syndrome of multiple cholesterol emboli (see Chapter 10.6.6)

Recent studies suggest a much higher incidence of this syndrome than previously suspected and large series of patients suffering from multiple cholesterol emboli have been described (Belenfant *et al.* 1999). The clinical presentation and treatment of this disease has recently been summarized in an excellent review (Scolari *et al.* 2000).

Cholesterol embolization can appear either spontaneously or following an intervention such as vascular bypass, angioplasty, or arteriography and is mainly observed in elderly males suffering from generalized atheromatosis. Renal microembolization is responsible for one-third of the cases of ARF after emergency intervention for abdominal aorta aneurysm, explaining why some of these patients develop ARF without preceding hypotension. When ARF appears after an angiographic procedure, it usually presents after 2–4 weeks, which is in contrast with radiographic contrast ATN, and usually develops in a few days. In cases of cholesterol emboli, renal recovery is not observed in 30–40 per cent of the cases. Treatment with anticoagulants or streptokinase and tissue plasminogen activator are often predisposing factors. These drugs apparently destabilize the cholesterol crystals in the atheromatous plaques (Scolari *et al.* 2000).

Flank pain with or without moderate fever and leucocytosis are the initial symptoms. Micro- or macrohaematuria are not always present and accelerating hypertension, rapid deterioration of renal function, neurological symptoms, visual problems, gastrointestinal haemorrhage, or pancreatitis may be present. Ischaemic lesions at the legs or feet are frequent and present either as purpura, livedo reticularis, gangrene, or vascular ulcers. Laboratory results sometimes reveal eosinophilia, low complement, and an acute phase response. The clinical diagnosis of cholesterol emboli is confirmed by kidney biopsy in 30 per cent of the cases, muscle biopsy in 21 per cent of cases, skin biopsy in 17 per cent of the cases, or at postmortem in 22 per cent of the cases.

A recently described therapeutic protocol (Belenfant *et al.* 1999) includes complete stopping of anticoagulating drugs, forbidding any invasive intravascular procedure, prompt treatment of heart failure, and early initiation of haemodialysis associated with intense parenteral nutrition. Finally, patients who show signs of inflammation should receive corticosteroids. Peritoneal dialysis, by avoiding heparin, does not offer any advantage as was suggested in the past. With this therapeutic regimen, the authors have observed a considerable increase in the patient survival; nevertheless, 32 per cent of the patients needed permanent haemodialysis. The best results with corticosteroids have been reported by Boero *et al.* (2000). Other authors have suggested these patients be treated with statins (Woolfson and Lachmann 1998).

Acute tubular necrosis

By far the most frequent cause of ARF in young as well as in older patients is postischaemic or postnephrotoxic ATN.

In the Tenon hospital series (Akposso *et al.* 2000), organic ARF was present in 53.5 per cent of all cases and the most prominent causes of ATN were shock in 49.1 per cent, nephrotoxic drugs in 6 per cent, rhabdomyolysis in 9.8 per cent, and multiple myeloma in 6.8 per cent of the patients (Table 1).

Renal insults that characteristically cause this form of ATN include aminoglycoside nephrotoxicity, radiocontrast-induced ATN, rhabdomyolysis-induced ATN, and ATN complicating open heart surgery. In two series of ARF in the elderly the incidence of the non-oliguric form was 19 and 24.5 per cent, respectively (Lameire *et al.* 1987; Rodgers *et al.* 1990). Clearly, any insult causing oliguric ATN can also result in the non-oliguric form of the disease.

Although for didactic reasons the distinction between ischaemic and toxic ATN is often made, ATN is frequently the result of combined risk factors in any age category. Furthermore, the interaction between renal hypoperfusion and nephrotoxins is at least additive and probably synergistic. Particularly in older patients with ATN, several chronic premorbid conditions (i.e. congestive heart failure, hypertension, or diabetes mellitus) predispose to its development.

Postischaemic ATN

Postischaemic ATN accounts in tertiary care hospitals for approximately 50 per cent of all cases of ARF in the elderly (Akposso *et al.* 2000).

Postoperative ARF Complications of major surgery, including hypotension during or after surgery, postoperative fluid loss due to gastrointestinal or fistula drainage, gastrointestinal blood loss (Fiaccadori *et al.* 2001), arrhythmias, and myocardial infarction account for about 30 per cent of all cases of postischaemic ATN (Chertow *et al.* 1997). Another important factor implicated in the aetiology of postoperative ATN is sepsis, particularly arising in the abdomen.

A systematic review of 28 studies that examined preoperative risk factors for postoperative ATN found that a raised plasma creatinine or urea preoperatively were strong predictors of postoperative worsening of renal function (Novis *et al.* 1994). In some, but not all studies, advanced age and left ventricular dysfunction were also associated with a greater risk of postoperative ATN. Many of the other risk factors for ARF, including preoperative renal dysfunction, cardiac dysfunction, and vascular disease are all more common with advanced age. Since cardiac surgical interventions have become more frequent in elderly patients numerous studies have defined the risks for developing ARF in these patients (Chertow *et al.* 1998; Fortescue *et al.* 2000). Following coronary artery surgery, the three major risk factors were: old age, preoperative renal dysfunction, and postoperative haemodynamic instability, defined as the need of inotropic drugs. Although ARF occurred in 16 per cent of the patients, only 1.2 per cent required dialysis. In the latter category, the mortality was 44 per cent (Andersson *et al.* 1993).

ATN after elective or emergency operation for abdominal aortic aneurysm is particularly frequent in aged people. In patients above 70 years of age, the incidence of ATN varies between 4 and 23 per cent, depending on selection and preoperative status of the patients. Emergency intervention for ruptured aneurysm has a mortality of 50 per cent, and this result has not changed over the years (Nasim *et al.* 1995). In contrast, elective surgery is now recommended in patients in the seventies and eighties and has a mortality of 5 per cent (for review, see Olsen 1993). The most common cause of transient renal ischaemia during aortic aneurysm operation is preoperative hypotension due to hypovolaemia. However, low arterial blood pressure is not always followed by ATN. Infrarenal aortic cross-clamping causes an increase in renal vascular resistance and a decrease in RBF that may persist for hours after unclamping. The aortic clamping time is thus a major determinant of the occurrence of postoperative ATN. An important cause of renal failure after aortic clamping and unclamping is renal microembolization (see above).

Sepsis Infection and in particular Gram-negative septicaemia account for another 30 per cent of cases of ARF in the elderly (Akposso *et al.* 2000). The elderly may deviate from the classic presentation of septic shock. Acute confusional states, general weakness, or loss of appetite can be the presenting manifestations of infection and elderly patients with bacteraemia may be afebrile.

The low FE_{Na} in septic ATN, persisting during prolonged oliguria, suggesting persisting renal hypoperfusion, may give rise to confusion. It was found that the sequestration in the extracellular space of the fluid given during resuscitation in older patients is prolonged (Cheng *et al.* 1998). Volume replacement, even under Swan-Ganz monitoring, results in further fluid redistribution, with preferential sequestration of the fluid in the extracellular volume and the third space.

The multisystem organ failure syndrome The elderly have a characteristic MSOF syndrome (Wang and Fan 1990), which differs somewhat from that in young patients because of pre-existing multiple chronic organ diseases. The syndrome is most often precipitated by, in descending order of frequency, infection, metastatic carcinoma, cardiac arrhythmias, haemorrhagic shock, and acute myocardial infarction. The mortality ranges from 46 per cent when two organs have failed, to 67 per cent for three, to 80 per cent for four. ARF carries a greater than 80 per cent mortality rate in elderly patients with MSOF syndrome (Zivin *et al.* 2001).

Nephrotoxic ATN

Radiocontrast ARF Contrast nephropathy is the cause of 13 per cent of all cases of ARF and ranks third of all hospital-acquired cases of ARF (Kurnik *et al.* 1998). In general, the acute deterioration of renal function appears within 24–48 h after the contrast administration with a peak in the serum creatinine around day 3–5, followed by a return to the baseline value usually within 7–10 days in the majority of cases. A minority of patients develop further complications ranging from a prolongation of hospitalization to the need for dialysis. The mortality in these cases can be as high as 29 per cent (Kurnik *et al.* 1998). In a prospective study, 183 patients aged 70 years or older underwent 199 cardiac catheterizations and angiography (Rich and Crecelius 1990). A clinically significant increase in serum creatinine developed in 11 per cent. Multivariate analysis revealed that risk factors in these aged patients were: administration of greater than 200 ml contrast agent, a serum albumin lesser than 35 g/l, diabetes mellitus, serum sodium lesser than 135 mmol/l, and baseline serum creatinine greater than 133 μmol/l. The most important risk factors for contrast nephropathy are: a pre-existing chronic renal failure, dehydration, and diabetic nephropathy. Several studies have explored the efficacy of preventive hydration before exposure to contrast media (Rudnick *et al.* 1994; Solomon *et al.* 1994). Whereas most studies showed no differences in outcome in low-risk patients, intravenous hydration with hypotonic saline, 0.45 per cent at 1 ml/kg/h during 12 h before and after the contrast administration, significantly protects the high risk patients, including the elderly (Solomon *et al.* 1994; Ghosh 2000). This protection is explained by a reduction of the renal concentration energy at the medullary level by the hydration and the salt loading decreasing the risk of hypoxic injury in this vulnerable zone (Heyman *et al.* 1999). Until now, no study has shown that oral hydration is as effective as the parenteral route. Substances such as frusemide, mannitol, and dopamine are no longer recommended (Rudnick *et al.* 1994; Solomon *et al.* 1994) (see also Chapter 10.2). A recent placebo-controlled, prospective study has shown that the combination of hydration with the oral administration of acetylcysteine had an additional protective effect (Tepel *et al.* 2000). Although the nephrotoxicity of gadolinium is clearly lower than of the iodium-containing media, cases of ARF have been observed with this agent (Gemery *et al.* 1998).

Antibiotics Aminoglycoside antibiotics are one of the most common causes of nephrotoxic ATN in the elderly. Erroneous estimate of GFR, based on the serum creatinine concentration, may lead to inappropriate dosing. The other risk factors for aminoglycoside nephrotoxicity are the duration of the treatment, volume depletion, and concurrent cephalosporin use (Moore *et al.* 1984).

The elderly are also at significantly greater risk of the nephrotoxic effect of vancomycin. An incidence of 18.9 per cent in patients older than 60 years compared to only 7.8 per cent in younger patients was observed (Vance-Bryan *et al.* 1994). Using multivariate logistic regression models, concurrent use of loop diuretics was significantly associated with vancomycin nephrotoxicity.

Rhabdomyolysis Older people are very susceptible to rhabdomyolysis in different settings like acute immobilization, trauma, infections, cerebrovascular accidents, and hypothermia. Surgery in which there is either prolonged muscle compression due to positioning for a long procedure, or in which there is vascular occlusion because of tourniquet use in orthopaedic or vascular reconstructive surgery may lead to rhabdomyolysis (Biswas *et al.* 1997).

Most of these patients develop mild ARF, mostly not needing dialysis, and have an uneventful recovery. This cause is frequently not recognized.

Acute interstitial nephritis (see Chapter 10.6.2)

The older patient may be more at risk of AIN because of the multitude of drugs that are often prescribed to this type of patient; AIN was diagnosed in 18.6 per cent of all biopsies, performed in patients aged over 60 years (Haas *et al.* 2000). This syndrome presents as ARF with histological features of interstitial oedema and inflammation and is caused by a variety of agents, especially NSAIDs. The AIN caused by NSAIDs is clinically characterized by the combination of ARF and heavy proteinuria. Prompt recognition of AIN by renal biopsy may lead to early intervention with corticosteroids and more rapid recovery of the renal function. Without treatment, renal failure may be prolonged and even permanent.

Glomerulonephritis (see Chapter 10.6.1)

Acute glomerulonephritis is quite a common cause of ARF in the elderly. Studies of renal biopsies (Haas *et al.* 2000) show a remarkably high incidence of crescentic glomerulonephritis. Haas *et al.* (2000) recently identified all native renal biopsy specimens from patients aged 60 years or older between 1991 and 1998. Twenty-five per cent of the 4264 biopsy specimens were obtained from patients aged 60 years or older, and acute renal insufficiency was the indication for biopsy in 259 of these patients (24.3 per cent). Close to 50 per cent of the biopsies revealed glomerular diseases, 40 per cent tubulointerstitial disease, and the rest vascular diseases or multiple lesions. Among the conditions associated with rapidly progressive glomerulonephritis, both the idiopathic and anti-GBM-associated glomerulonephritis are relatively common in older patients. Any form of crescentic glomerulonephritis in the elderly has a poor prognosis.

The same principles apply to treatment of older adults with crescentic glomerular disease, but restraint should be exercised in the use of powerful immunosuppressive agents such as corticosteroids, immunosuppressive drugs, and plasmapheresis. Aggressive immunosuppression in rapidly progressive glomerulonephritis in older (>60 years) patients is associated with a relative risk of death 5.3 times higher compared to younger patients (Keller *et al.* 1994).

Diffuse proliferative glomerulonephritis, commonly occurring in association with infections, is another nephritic cause of ARF in the elderly. Clinical features of poststreptococcal glomerulonephritis in the elderly include hypertension in 82 per cent, oedema in 73 per cent, dyspnoea and pulmonary congestion in 41 per cent, and oliguria in 75 per cent of the cases. Hence, postinfectious glomerulonephritis in the elderly is easily confused with congestive heart failure. The combination of ARF, a nephritic urine sediment, and pulmonary oedema in an elderly patient must alert the clinician for this diagnosis. Poststreptococcal glomerulonephritis in the elderly seems to have a favourable short-term prognosis (Washio *et al.* 1994).

The single most common diagnosis in elderly patients suffering from ARF due to glomerulonephritis was found to be focal/segmental glomerulonephritis which, in the absence of antineutrophil antiplasmic antibodies (ANCA) testing, may include patients with undiagnosed 'vasculitis' (Davison and Johnston 1993; Haas *et al.* 2000). Compared with patients younger than age 60, the elderly have also a higher incidence of vasculitis and Wegener's granulomatosis, but the incidence of systemic lupus erythematosus is significantly lower.

Because of the potential for reversing ARF in some forms of glomerulonephritis, there should be no hesitation in performing a renal biopsy. Renal biopsy does not carry a greater risk in the older patient and adequate renal tissue can be obtained in 80–95 per cent, with a complication rate of 2.2–9 per cent (Rakowski and Winchester 1986). However, the interpretation of the histological findings may be more difficult because of additional changes in the aged kidney or intercurrent diseases as arteriosclerosis or global sclerosis.

Postrenal ARF (Klahr 2000)

Urinary obstruction is one of the important causes of ARF in the elderly. In two major series, the incidence of postrenal ARF was 7.9 and 9 per cent in patients over 70 and 65 years, respectively (Lameire *et al.* 1987). Obstructive uropathy is most frequently encountered in community- and hospital ward-associated ARF and is less common in intensive care unit-related ARF (Liano *et al.* 1998). It is, however, more common in selected patient populations such as older men with prostatic disease and patients with a single kidney or intra-abdominal cancer, particularly pelvic cancer (Feest *et al.* 1993; Bhandari *et al.* 1995). Finally, the cause of obstructive uropathy is often amenable to therapy. Thus, obstructive uropathy should be considered in each case of ARF.

ARF develops only with bilateral obstruction or obstruction in a solitary functioning kidney. This may be either intrinsic or extrinsic, and can occur at any level of the urinary tract in the elderly.

Among the causes of lower urinary tract obstruction, prostatic enlargement due either to benign prostatic hyperplasia or prostatic adenocarcinoma is the most common. Urethral stricture, iatrogenic or a result of urethral trauma, is the second most common cause of bladder outflow obstruction in males.

Benign prostatic hyperplasia affects 50 per cent of men aged 50 and increases to 90 per cent by the ninth decade of life (McConnell 1998). A small fraction of these patients develop severe obstructive ARF, which in some progresses to irreversible renal failure. Some of them may present with symptoms of advanced renal failure, rather than with prostatism. In case of prostatic carcinoma, it is usually the invasion of the uretero-vesical junctions that causes bilateral hydroureteronephrosis with progressive renal insufficiency. Rectal examination and serum prostate-specific antigen (PSA) determination are the most efficient means of excluding a prostatic malignancy.

The most common cause of postrenal failure in females is ureteral obstruction due to pelvic malignancy—in particular, invasive carcinoma of the cervix and its treatment with radiotherapy.

From all causes of retroperitoneal fibrosis, the so-called inflammatory abdominal aortic aneurysm occurs mainly in elderly men and causes radiographic demonstration of medial displacement of the ureter similar to that seen in idiopathic retroperitoneal fibrosis (Wagenknecht and Hardy 1981). Severe ureteral obstructions may be seen even with small inflammatory aneurysms. These inflammatory aneurysms are of interest because there are several reports of successful corticosteroid treatment of the ureteral obstruction when surgery was not an option (Yarger 1992). It is recommended that the ureters be placed anterior to the laterally directed iliac grafts at the time of aortoiliac aneurysm repair. If this is not done, ureteral obstruction is likely to result.

Deposition of uric acid crystals in the tubular lumen (uric acid nephropathy) may cause obstruction and its severity is directly related to the plasma uric acid. Acute uric acid nephropathy is most often seen following chemotherapy for leukaemias and lymphomas (Haas *et al.* 1999). In this setting, the liver converts the purine load generated by cytolysis into uric acid. The high filtered load of uric acid and tubular reabsorption combine to produce high tubular concentrations of soluble urate and uric acid. Acidification of tubular fluid converts urate to uric acid, which can occlude tubular lumina.

Other causes of intratubular crystalline precipitation have been recently summarized (Perazella 1999). ARF associated with calcium oxalate crystalluria can accompany ethylene glycol ingestion, administration of the anaesthetic agent methoxyflurane, and small-bowel bypass operations (Perazella 1999). High doses of methotrexate can lead to intratubular precipitation of the insoluble 7-hydroxy metabolite of methotrexate (Perazella 1999). Other crystalline substances that can potentially precipitate within renal tubules and lead to ARF include acyclovir, triamterene, sulfonamides, and protease inhibitors such as indinavir (Perazella 1999).

In patients suffering from multiple myeloma intratubular precipitation of myeloma proteins and perhaps other proteins also can lead to ARF (Moist *et al.* 1999). Dehydration with resultant high tubular water reabsorption and radiographic contrast material can facilitate myeloma protein deposition. These patients are at uniquely increased risk for ARF associated with radiocontrast administration, use of NSAIDs, and ACEIs. Less commonly, hypercalcaemia and cryoglobulinaemia can precipitate ARF. Tumour lysis syndrome is most often seen after institution of chemotherapy, but it can occur prior to any cancer treatment. Some series have documented spontaneous appearance of tumour lysis syndrome in 10–25 per cent of all cases (Maletz *et al.* 1993). These spontaneous cases should be suspected in patients with massive tumour burden with rapid turnover, such as with high-grade lymphomas. Hallmark findings include a markedly elevated uric acid concentration, associated with oligoanuric ARF. In contrast with that occurring after chemotherapy, hyperphosphataemia may not be prominent. Treatment prior to anuria consists of allopurinol, saline infusion, and loop diuretics to flush out uric acid crystals. Recognition of intratubular obstruction as a potential cause of ARF has important therapeutic implications. For example, prophylactic therapy with the xanthine oxidase inhibitor allopurinol can prevent accumulation of uric acid in tumour lysis syndrome. Moreover, forced diuresis decreases tubular salt and water reabsorption, thereby diluting tubular fluid with decreases in crystal and protein concentrations. Finally, manipulations that increase urinary pH can increase solubility of crystalline substances such as methotrexate, uric acid, and sulfonamides (Perazella 1999).

Diagnosis of postrenal ARF

Clinical

It is imperative to exclude an obstructive cause in any patient presenting with ARF, because prompt intervention may result in improvement or complete recovery of renal function. Elderly males with unexplained ARF should undergo bladder catheterization.

The presence of alternating anuria and polyuria is an uncommon but classic manifestation of urinary tract obstruction and is usually caused by fluctuating accumulation and release of urine behind a stone that changes its position. In rare cases, unilateral obstruction can lead to anuria and ARF; vascular or ureteral spasm, mediated by autonomic activation, is thought to be responsible for the loss of function in the non-obstructed kidney.

The urinary parameters in obstructive ARF are similar to those found in ATN. However, some patients may have high urinary osmolality and low urinary sodium concentrations simulating prerenal failure. Depending on the cause of the obstruction, crystalluria and haematuria may give clues to the presence of postobstructive ARF.

Important clinical sequelae are the postobstructive diuresis and hyperkalaemic renal tubular acidosis (Yarger 1992). Postobstructive diuresis, as the name implies, is the profuse diuresis (>4 l/day) that occurs after the release of the obstruction and never occurs unless both kidneys, or a single functioning kidney, are completely obstructed. The period of total obstruction is usually short, often a few days to a maximum of 1 week. Once the obstruction is relieved, the urine output generally ranges from 4 to 20 l per day. In addition to the sometimes enormous losses of water and salt, patients may also become depleted of bicarbonate, calcium, magnesium, and phosphate. The patient's volume and electrolyte status must be carefully monitored and appropriately adjusted during the diuretic phase. It is helpful to measure the total electrolyte losses in the urine. However, the phase of postobstructive polyuria can be prolonged by excessive administration of fluids. Provided the patient does not develop symptoms or signs of intravascular volume depletion, it is reasonable to infuse a daily volume somewhat less than the volume of urine passed in the preceding 24 h.

The development of hyperkalaemic, hyperchloraemic tubular acidosis can be explained by the inability to lower the urinary pH to less than 5.5 during acid loading or by an inability to secrete renin during extracellular volume contraction (hyporeninaemic hypoaldosteronism) (Klahr 2000). Although this type of hyperkalaemic tubular acidosis usually presents indolently, it tends to persist after correction of the obstruction. Patients who fail to correct their hyperkalaemia as their ARF is reversed by dealing with the obstructive lesion should be investigated for the presence of tubular acidosis.

Radiological

Ultrasonography is a safe and accessible initial investigation in the evaluation of patients with ARF. The diagnosis of obstruction is based on the finding of a dilated collecting system filled with urine. Ultrasonography exhibits a high degree of sensitivity (90–98 per cent) but a lower specificity (65–84 per cent) for detection of obstructive nephropathy (Stuck *et al.* 1987). Patients with highly distensible collecting systems or with pyelocaliectasis may be misdiagnosed as having hydronephrosis. False-negative studies have been reported in patients with very early (<8 h) obstruction (Amis *et al.* 1982; Rascoff *et al.* 1983). In many of these cases, the patients were of older age and the obstructing process, usually prostatic carcinoma or retroperitoneal fibrosis, encased the retroperitoneal ureters and renal pelvis, preventing their dilatation. In the elderly, partial obstruction may be obscured by volume depletion. When there is strong suspicion of obstruction, the ultrasonographic examination should be repeated after volume repletion.

Although intravenous pyelography and retrograde pyelography define the anatomical site and nature of the obstructive process much more accurately than renal ultrasonography, these techniques are no longer recommended as first step in the investigation of postobstructive ARF. These examinations may, however, remain necessary in the preoperative evaluation because they allow visualization of the distal point of the ureteral obstruction. This may be important when ureterolysis is envisaged in case of retroperitoneal fibrosis. Antegrade pyelography has several advantages in patients with obstructive ARF. First, if there is dilation of the renal pelvis on ultrasound, the introduction of a fine needle into the renal pelvis under ultrasonographic guidance is almost always successful. Second, if a complete obstruction is found to involve the ureters, the operator can easily proceed to a therapeutic nephrostomy. Third, this examination will demonstrate the proximal border of the ureteral obstruction. It has been shown that obstruction of the kidneys produces changes in the Doppler sonography waveform that result in an elevated resistive, or Pourcelot, index (Platt *et al.* 1989). In pathological hydronephrosis, arteriolar vasoconstriction (secondary to thromboxane production) increases the resistive index, distinguishing this disorder from kidneys that have dilated collecting systems, but are not obstructed.

Computed tomography can also be helpful in patients with an unidentified cause of obstruction in whom ultrasound has been unsatisfactory.

Although nuclear medicine imaging techniques are inferior to radiographic and ultrasonography studies in providing the diagnosis of urinary tract obstruction, they are useful for testing whether any significant degree of renal function is preserved in kidneys with severe anatomic hydronephrosis.

Treatment of the elderly patient with ARF (see Chapters 10.2 and 10.4)

In general, the non-dialytic and dialytic treatment of ARF is the same in the elderly as in other adults. Also, the drugs and other measures that might be employed to prevent ARF are the same in all age categories and have been discussed extensively in other chapters of this book. Since the selection of certain dialysis modalities may be different in the elderly compared to the younger patient population, this topic will be discussed here in greater detail.

The dialytic management (Mehta *et al.* 2001)

The indications for dialysis in the elderly are no different from those in younger adults. The selection of a given dialysis modality (haemodialysis, haemofiltration, or peritoneal dialysis) is not determined by the age of the patient itself but by a number of patient and/or disease-specific factors. These include the presence of haemodynamic instability, severe hypervolaemia, hypercatabolism, compromised pulmonary function, bleeding risk, vascular access problems and others that have been thoroughly discussed elsewhere. Dialysis therapy of ARF patients is still the subject of a number of controversies, including the role of peritoneal dialysis, the possible impact of the biocompatibility of the haemodialysis membranes, and the choice between continuous renal replacement therapies (CRRT) and the intermittent forms of haemodialysis (IHD). These controversies have always been discussed related to the ARF population as a whole (van Bommel *et al.* 1995; Lameire *et al.* 1999b) and have not focused on the elderly ARF population.

Peritoneal dialysis

The many advantages of peritoneal dialysis as a continuous dialysis technique in critically ill patients have been described (Ash and Bever 1995). Despite these theoretical advantages, there are several reasons why peritoneal dialysis is currently less frequently used in ARF patients:

1. There has been a change in the spectrum of patients developing ARF; the underlying diseases are much more serious than in the past, sepsis and hypercatabolism are often present, and ARF frequently develops quite late in the development of a multiorgan dysfunction syndrome. The lower efficiency of peritoneal dialysis in removing solute and fluid compared to extracorporeal dialysis limits its usage in patients with ARF who require significant volume and solute removal.
2. ARF often occurs in patients with intra-abdominal surgery where the insertion of an intraperitoneal catheter is not practical.
3. By increasing the intra-abdominal pressure, peritoneal dialysis may compromise lung function and is therefore inappropriate in patients with the acute respiratory distress syndrome.
4. As dextrose in the dialysate provides the osmotic gradient to achieve fluid removal, frequent exchanges with dialysate containing high dextrose is occasionally used to achieve negative balance in fluid overloaded patients. Dextrose absorption from the peritoneal cavity is frequently significant. It has been shown in five patients with ARF that high dextrose-containing dialysate resulted in a respiratory quotient greater than 1.0 consistent with net lipogenesis. Four of these five patients absorbed more than 500 g of dextrose over 24 h. As overfeeding could lead to hepatic steatosis, increased CO_2 production with worsening of respiratory failure, and hyperglycaemia, the risks of using high dextrose-containing dialysate fluids should be weighed carefully against the potential benefits (Manji *et al.* 1990).

The principles of peritoneal dialysis, its application in ARF, and the indications, contraindications, and complications have recently been described in detail (Goel *et al.* 1997; Lameire 1997).

Continuous versus intermittent haemodialysis (see Chapter 10.4)

A recent review of all clinical trials has examined the effect of dialysis-related variables on clinical outcomes in patients with ARF requiring IHD (Karsou *et al.* 2000). In particular, the role of biocompatibility of dialyser membranes and timing, intensity, and adequacy of dialysis were examined.

Direct outcome comparative studies between CRRT and IHD in elderly ARF patients are not available; however, a large prospective study comparing these different dialysis strategies on outcome of patients of all ages with ARF proved inconclusive (Mehta *et al.* 2001).

There are a number of descriptions of the application of CRRT in elderly patients with ARF (Bellomo *et al.* 1994; Gordon *et al.* 1994; Alarabi *et al.* 1997; Bent *et al.* 2001). All support aggressive renal replacement therapy in critically ill elderly ARF patients and also suggest continuous haemodiafiltration to be the preferred method. None of these studies, however, help to discern between the different treatment modalities.

Recently, 'hybrid techniques' have emerged to provide alternatives in the polarized discussion between IHD and CRRT. These 'slow, extended, daily dialysis' (SLEDD) techniques all combine the advantages of CRRT and IHD by using a dialysis monitor and water treatment module for online production of dialysate to do slow, but extended and daily, haemodialysis. Until now, no large-scale studies of SLEDD are available, but the technique is being used more and the first report was positive (Kumar *et al.* 2000).

These SLEDD modalities may be particularly appropriate in elderly, critically ill ARF patients, although comparative studies between the different dialysis modalities in this age group are not available.

It is advisable that all dialysis strategies be mastered and utilized for the appropriate indications in elderly ARF patients. However, in the old patient with ARF, daily 'slow' dialysis modalities such as peritoneal dialysis, CRRT, and SLEDD may be more appropriate than the 'classical' 4-h dialysis, even if the latter is performed daily.

Recovery and prognosis of ARF in the elderly

The recovery of renal function in elderly patients surviving ARF is usually assessed at discharge from the hospital. The cumulative results of three series, comprising a total of 296 patients (Lameire *et al.* 1996), indicated that 198 patients or 67 per cent recovered renal function completely while only 8 or 2.7 per cent did not recover sufficiently to remain independent of dialysis (Fig. 2). In at least one study

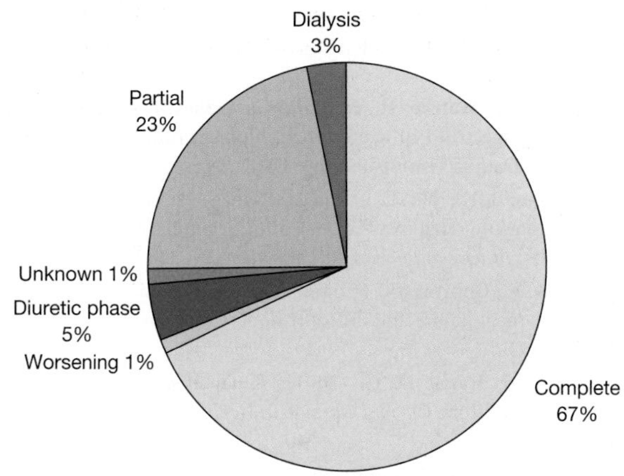

Fig. 2 Prognosis (for renal outcome) of ARF in the elderly.

(Lameire *et al.* 1987), the recovery of renal function was not different between older and younger patients.

In one study of long-term prognosis, 15 out of 35 elderly (43 per cent), surviving ARF had a normal serum creatinine at 39 months from discharge from the hospital (Gentric and Cledes 1991).

Studies in mixed ARF populations indicate that some patients will show a progressive and slow deterioration of the renal function, with age to be one determinant of long-term outcome (Bonomini *et al.* 1984).

An analysis of the long-term prognosis of elderly patients with ARF and surviving their stay in the intensive care unit revealed that 18 months after discharge from the hospital, only 10 per cent was still alive. Preliminary data suggest that most of these patients died from a cause related to their original disease responsible for the ARF (Lameire *et al.* 1996).

There is clearly no consensus whether age is an independent predictive prognostic factor. Some studies, however, concluded that it is in the elderly that outcome has actually improved (Druml *et al.* 1994).

The most recent analysis of prognosis of ARF in very old patients (>80 years old) showed that although there was a slight but significant increase in mortality when compared to an age-matched population, mortality in the elderly was no worse than the overall mortality of ARF in the literature (Akposso *et al.* 2000). However, almost half of the patients in this series suffered from either prerenal or obstruction, both known to be associated with a better chance of recovery of renal function than ATN.

Several risk models developed for critically ill patients have now been applied to patients with ARF, especially in the situation where ARF occurs as part of a multiple system organ failure (for review, see Halstenberg *et al.* 1994).

Some individual renal units, such as that in Madrid, have developed their own prognostic equations that are simpler than the risk models and can therefore be easily applied at the bedside (Liano *et al.* 1993). A recent comparative validation of several scoring systems in ARF patients revealed that the Madrid scoring system was the most accurate in predicting the prognosis of these patients (Douma *et al.* 1997).

Until a validated method of assessing the severity of disease and predicting the outcome in the individual patient with ARF is available, one cannot conclude that old age is by itself an independent indicator of a poor prognosis.

It is certainly not appropriate to deny elderly patients the full range of therapeutic options.

References

Akposso, K., Hertig, A., Couprie, R., Flahaut, A., Alberti, C., Karras, G. A., Haymann, J. P., Costa De Beauregard, M. A., Lahlou, A., Rondeau, E., and Sraer, J. D. (2000). Acute renal failure in patients over 80 years old: 25-years' experience. *Intensive Care Medicine* **26** (4), 400–406.

Alarabi, A., Nystrom, S. O., Stahle, E., and Wikstrom, B. (1997). Acute renal failure and outcome of continuous arteriovenous hemodialysis (CAVHD) and continuous hemofiltration (CAVH) in elderly patients following cardiovascular surgery. *Geriatrics Nephrology Urology* **7** (1), 45–49.

Amis, E. S., Jr., Cronan, J. J., Pfister, R. C., and Yoder, I. C. (1982). Ultrasonic inaccuracies in diagnosing renal obstruction. *Urology* **19** (1), 101–105.

Andersson, L. G., Ekroth, R., Bratteby, L. E., Hallhagen, S., and Wesslen, O. (1993). Acute renal failure after coronary surgery—a study of incidence and risk factors in 2009 consecutive patients. *Thoracic Cardiovascular Surgery* **41** (4), 237–241.

Ash, S. R. and Bever, S. L. (1995). Peritoneal dialysis for acute renal failure: the safe, effective, and low-cost modality. *Advanced in Renal Replacement Therapy* **2** (2), 160–163.

Badr, K. F. and Ichikawa, I. (1988). Prerenal failure: a deleterious shift from renal compensation to decompensation. *New England Journal of Medicine* **319** (10), 623–629.

Baylis, C., Engels, K., and Beierwaltes, W. H. (1998). Beta-adrenoceptor-stimulated renin release is blunted in old rats. *Journal of the American Society of Nephrology* **9** (7), 1318–1320.

Belenfant, X., Meyrier, A., and Jacquot, C. (1999). Supportive treatment improves survival in multivisceral cholesterol crystal embolism. *American Journal of Kidney Diseases* **33** (5), 840–850.

Bellomo, R., Farmer, M., and Boyce, N. (1994). The outcome of critically ill elderly patients with severe acute renal failure treated by continuous hemodiafiltration. *International Journal of Artificial Organs* **17** (9), 466–472.

Bent, P., Tan, H. K., Bellomo, R., Buckmaster, J., Doolan, L., Hart, G., Silvester, W., Gutteridge, G., Matalanis, G., Raman, J., Rosalion, A., and Buxton, B. F. (2001). Early and intensive continuous hemofiltration for severe renal failure after cardiac surgery. *Annals of Thoracic Surgery* **71** (3), 832–837.

Bhandari, S., Johnston, P., Fowler, R. C., Joyce, A., and Turney, J. H. (1995). Non-dilated bilateral ureteric obstruction. *Nephrology, Dialysis, Transplantation* **10** (12), 2337–2339.

Biswas, S., Gnanasekaran, I., Ivatury, R. R., Simon, R., and Patel, A. N. (1997). Exaggerated lithotomy position-related rhabdomyolysis. *American Surgery* **63** (4), 361–364.

Blantz, R. C. (1998). Pathophysiology of pre-renal azotemia. *Kidney International* **53** (2), 512–523.

Blum, U., Billmann, P., Krause, T., Gabelmann, A., Keller, E., Moser, E., and Langer, M. (1993). Effect of local low-dose thrombolysis on clinical outcome in acute embolic renal artery occlusion. *Radiology* **189** (2), 549–554.

Boero, R., Pignataro, A., Rollino, C., and Quarello, F. (2000). Do corticosteroids improve survival in acute renal failure due to cholesterol atheroembolism? *Nephrology, Dialysis, Transplantation* **15** (3), 441.

Bonomini, V., Stefoni, S., and Vangelista, A. (1984). Long-term patient and renal prognosis in acute renal failure. *Nephron* **36** (3), 169–172.

Brater, D. C. (1999). Effects of nonsteroidal anti-inflammatory drugs on renal function: focus on cyclooxygenase-2-selective inhibition. *American Journal of Medicine* **107**, 65S–70S.

Chanard, J., Wynckel, A., Canivet, E., and Jolly, D. (1994). Evaluation de la fréquence de l'insuffisance rénale aigue et de ses modalités thérapeutiques en milieu néphrologique. *Néphrologie* **15**, 13–16.

Cheng, A. T., Plank, L. D., and Hill, G. L. (1998). Prolonged overexpansion of extracellular water in elderly patients with sepsis. *Archives of Surgery* **133** (7), 745–751.

Chertow, G. M., Lazarus, J. M., Christiansen, C. L., Cook, E. F., Hammermeister, K. E., Grover, F., and Daley, J. (1997). Preoperative renal risk stratification. *Circulation* **95** (4), 878–884.

Chertow, G. M., Levy, E. M., Hammermeister, K. E., Grover, F., and Daley, J. (1998). Independent association between acute renal failure and mortality following cardiac surgery. *American Journal of Medicine* **104** (4), 343–348.

Choudhury, D., Palmer, B., and Levi, M. Renal function and dysfunction in aging. In *The Kidney—Physiology and Pathophysiology* 3rd edn. (ed. D. W. Seldin and G. Giebisch), pp. 2571–2595. Philadelphia: Lippincott Williams and Wilkins, 2000.

Cosby, R. L., Miller, P. D., and Schrier, R. W. (1986). Traumatic renal artery thrombosis. *American Journal of Medicine* **81**, 890–894.

Davison, A. M. and Johnston, P. A. (1993). Idiopathic glomerulonephritis in the elderly. *Contributions to Nephrology* **105**, 38–48.

Douma, C. E., Redekop, W. K., van der Meulen, J. H., van Olden, R. W., Haeck, J., Struijk, D. G., and Krediet, R. T. (1997). Predicting mortality in intensive care patients with acute renal failure treated with dialysis. *Journal of the American Society of Nephrology* **8** (1), 111–117.

Druml, W., Lax, F., Grimm, G., Schneeweiss, B., Lenz, K., and Laggner, A. N. (1994). Acute renal failure in the elderly 1975–1990. *Clinical Nephrology* **41** (6), 342–349.

Epstein, M. and Hollenberg, N. K. (1976). Age as a determinant of renal sodium conservation in normal man. *The Journal of Laboratory and Clinical Medicine* **87** (3), 411–417.

Feest, T. G., Round, A., and Hamad, S. (1993). Incidence of severe acute renal failure in adults: results of a community based study. *British Medical Journal* **306** (6876), 481–483.

Fiaccadori, E., Maggiore, U., Clima, B., Melfa, L., Rotelli, C., and Borghetti, A. (2001). Incidence, risk factors, and prognosis of gastrointestinal hemorrhage complicating acute renal failure. *Kidney International* **59** (4), 1510–1519.

Fitz, A. E., Kipp, U. C., and DiBona, C. A. Central and peripheral neural mechanisms regulating renal function and arterial pressure in the elderly. In *Hypertension and Renal Disease in the Elderly* (ed. M. Martinez-Maldonado), pp. 26–47. Boston: Blackwell Scientific Publications, 1992.

Fliser, D., Franek, E., Joest, M., Block, S., Mutschler, E., and Ritz, E. (1997). Renal function in the elderly: impact of hypertension and cardiac function. *Kidney International* **51** (4), 1196–1204.

Fliser, D., Ritz, E., and Franek, E. (1995). Renal reserve in the elderly. *Seminars in Nephrology* **15**, 463–467.

Fortescue, E. B., Bates, D. W., and Chertow, G. M. (2000). Predicting acute renal failure after coronary bypass surgery: cross-validation of two risk-stratification algorithms. *Kidney International* **57** (6), 2594–2602.

Frost, L., Engholm, G., Johnsen, S., Moller, H., Henneberg, E. W., and Husted, S. (2001). Incident thromboembolism in the aorta and the renal, mesenteric, pelvic, and extremity arteries after discharge from the hospital with a diagnosis of atrial fibrillation. *Archives of Internal Medicine* **161** (2), 272–276.

Gemery, J., Idelson, B., Reid, S., Yucel, E. K., Pagan-Marin, H., Ali, S., and Casserly, L. (1998). Acute renal failure after arteriography with a gadolinium-based contrast agent. *AJR. American Journal of Roentgenology* **171** (5), 1277–1278.

Gentric, A. and Cledes, J. (1991). Immediate and long-term prognosis in acute renal failure in the elderly. *Nephrology, Dialysis, Transplantation* **6**, 86–90.

Ghosh, A. K. (2000). Evidence-based nephrology: the case of contrast nephropathy. *Nephrology, Dialysis, Transplantation* **15** (3), 441–442.

Goel, S., Saran, R., and Nolph, K. D. Indications, contraindications and complications of peritoneal dialysis in the critically ill. In *Critical Care Nephrology* 1st edn. (ed. C. Ronco and R. Bellomo), pp. 1373–1381. Dordrecht: Kluwer Academic Publishers, 1997.

Gordon, A. C., Pryn, S., Collin, J., Gray, D. W., Hands, L., and Garrard, C. (1994). Outcome in patients who require renal support after surgery for ruptured abdominal aortic aneurysm. *British Journal of Surgery* **81** (6), 836–838.

Griffin, M. R., Yared, A., and Ray, W. A. (2000). Nonsteroidal antiinflammatory drugs and acute renal failure in elderly persons. *American Journal of Epidemiology* **151** (5), 488–496.

Gutthamm, S. P. *et al.* (1996). Nonsteroidal antiinflammatory drugs and the risk of hopitalisation for acute renal failure. *Archives of Internal Medicine* **156**, 2433.

Haas, M., Ohler, L., Watzke, H., Bohmig, G., Prokesch, R., and Druml, W. (1999). The spectrum of acute renal failure in tumour lysis syndrome. *Nephrology, Dialysis, Transplantation* **14** (3), 776–779.

Haas, M., Spargo, B. H., Wit, E. J., and Meehan, S. M. (2000). Etiologies and outcome of acute renal insufficiency in older adults: a renal biopsy study of 259 cases. *American Journal of Kidney Diseases* **35** (3), 433–447.

Halstenberg, W. K., Goormastic, M., and Paganini, E. P. (1994). Utility of risk models for renal failure and critically ill patients. *Seminars in Nephrology* **14** (1), 23–32.

Harris, C. J. and Brater, D. C. (2001). Renal effects of cyclooxygnease 2-selective inhibitors. *Current Opinion in Nephrology and Hypertension* **10**, 603–610.

Heyman, S. N., Reichman, J., and Brezis, M. (1999). Pathophysiology of radiocontrast nephropathy: a role for medullary hypoxia. *Investigative Radiology* **34** (11), 685–691.

Hill, C., Lateef, A. M., Engels, K., Samsell, L., and Baylis, C. (1997). Basal and stimulated nitric oxide in control of kidney function in the aging rat. *American Journal of Physiology* **272** (6 Part 2), R1747–R1753.

Karsou, S. A., Jaber, B. L., and Pereira, B. J. (2000). Impact of intermittent hemodialysis variables on clinical outcomes in acute renal failure. *American Journal of Kidney Diseases* **35** (5), 980–991.

Keller, F., Michaelis, C., Buettner, P., Bennhold, I., Schwartz, A., and Distler, A. (1994). Risk factors for long-term survival and renal function in 64 patients with rapidly progressive glomerulonephritis. *Geriatrics Nephrology Urology* **4**, 5–13.

Klahr, S. Obstructive uropathy. In *The Kidney—Physiology and Pathophysiology* 3rd edn. (ed. D. W. Seldin and G. Giebisch), pp. 2473–2512. Philadelphia: Lippincott Williams & Wilkins, 2000.

Klouche, K., Cristol, J. P., Kaaki, M., Turc-Baron, C., Canaud, B., and Beraud, J. J. (1995). Prognosis of acute renal failure in the elderly. *Nephrology, Dialysis, Transplantation* **10** (12), 2240–2243.

Knight, E. L., Glynn, R. J., McIntyre, K. M., Mogun, H., and Avorn, J. (1999). Predictors of decreased renal function in patients with heart failure during angiotensin-converting enzyme inhibitor therapy: results from the studies of left ventricular dysfunction (SOLVD). *American Heart Journal* **138** (5 Part 1), 849–855.

Kumar, V. A., Craig, M., Depner, T. A., and Yeun, J. Y. (2000). Extended daily dialysis: a new approach to renal replacement for acute renal failure in the intensive care unit. *American Journal of Kidney Diseases* **36** (2), 294–300.

Kung, C. F. and Luscher, T. F. (1995). Different mechanisms of endothelial dysfunction with aging and hypertension in rat aorta. *Hypertension* **25** (2), 194–200.

Kurnik, B. R., Allgren, R. L., Genter, F. C., Solomon, R. J., Bates, E. R., and Weisberg, L. S. (1998). Prospective study of atrial natriuretic peptide for the prevention of radiocontrast-induced nephropathy. *American Journal of Kidney Diseases* **31** (4), 674–680.

Lameire, N. Principles of peritoneal dialysis and its application in acute renal failure. In *Critical Care Nephrology* 1st edn. (ed. C. Ronco and R. Bellomo), pp. 1357–1371. Dordrecht: Kluwer Academic Publishers, 1997.

Lameire, N., Hoste, E., Van Loo, A., Dhondt, A., Bernaert, P., and Vanholder, R. (1996). Pathophysiology, causes, and prognosis of acute renal failure in the elderly. *Renal Failure* **18** (3), 333–346.

Lameire, N., Matthys, E., Vanholder, R., De Keyser, K., Pauwels, W., Nachtergaele, H., Lambrecht, L., and Ringoir, S. (1987). Causes and prognosis of acute renal failure in elderly patients. *Nephrology, Dialysis, Transplantation* **2** (5), 316–322.

Lameire, N., Nelde, A., Hoeben, H., and Vanholder, R. (1999a). Acute renal failure in the elderly. *Geriatrics Nephrology Urology* **9** (3), 153–165.

Lameire, N., Van Biesen, W., and Vanholder, R. (1999b). Dialysing the patient with acute renal failure in the ICU: the emperor's clothes? *Nephrology, Dialysis, Transplantation* **14** (11), 2570–2573.

Lavizzo-Mourey, R., Johnson, J., and Stolley, P. (1988). Risk factors for dehydration among elderly nursing home residents. *Journal of the American Geriatrics Society* **36** (3), 213–218.

Liano, F., Gallego, A., Pascual, J., Garcia-Martin, F., Teruel, J. L., Marcen, R., Orofino, L., Orte, L., Rivera, M., and Gallego, N. (1993). Prognosis of acute tubular necrosis: an extended prospectively contrasted study. *Nephron* **63** (1), 21–31.

Liano, F., Junco, E., Pascual, J., Madero, R., and Verde, E. (1998). The spectrum of acute renal failure in the intensive care unit compared with that seen in other settings. The Madrid Acute Renal Failure Study Group. *Kidney International* **66** (Suppl.), S16–S24.

MacDowall, P., Kalra, P. A., O'Donoghue, D. J., Waldek, S., Mamtora, H., and Brown, K. (1998). Risk of morbidity from renovascular disease in elderly patients with congestive cardiac failure. *Lancet* **352** (9121), 13–16.

Maletz, R., Berman, D., Peelle, K., and Bernard, D. (1993). Reflex anuria and uremia from unilateral ureteral obstruction. *American Journal of Kidney Diseases* **22**, 879–873.

Manji, S., Shikora, S., McMahon, M., Blackburn, G. L., and Bistrian, B. R. (1990). Peritoneal dialysis for acute renal failure: overfeeding resulting from dextrose absorbed during dialysis. *Critical Care Medicine* **18** (1), 29–31.

McConnell, J. D. Epidemiology, etiology, pathophysiology and diagnosis of benign prostatic hyperplasia. In *Campbell's Urology* 7th edn. (ed. P. C. Walsh *et al.*), pp. 1429–1452. Philadelphia: Saunders, 1998.

McInnes, E. G., Levy, D. W., Chaudhuri, M. D., and Bhan, G. L. (1987). Renal failure in the elderly. *Quarterly Journal of Medicine* **64** (243), 583–588.

Mehta, R. L., McDonald, B., Gabbai, F. B., Pahl, M., Pascual, M. T., Farkas, A., and Kaplan, R. M. (2001). A randomized clinical trial of continuous versus intermittent dialysis for acute renal failure. *Kidney International* **60** (3), 1154–1163.

Miller, P. D., Krebs, R. A., Neal, B. J., and McIntyre, D. O. (1980). Polyuric prerenal failure. *Archives of Internal Medicine* **140** (7), 907–909.

Moist, L., Nesrallah, G., Kortas, C., Espirtu, E., Ostbye, T., and Clark, W. F. (1999). Plasma exchange in rapidly progressive renal failure due to multiple myeloma. A retrospective case series. *American Journal of Nephrology* **19** (1), 45–50.

Moore, R. D., Smith, C. R., Lipsky, J. J., Mellits, E. D., and Lietman, P. S. (1984). Risk factors for nephrotoxicity in patients treated with aminoglycosides. *Annals of Internal Medicine* **100** (3), 352–357.

Nasim, A., Sayers, R. D., Thompson, M. M., Healey, P. A., and Bell, P. R. (1995). Trends in abdominal aortic aneurysms: a 13 year review. *European Journal of Vascular and Endovascular Surgery* **9** (2), 239–243.

Novis, B. K., Roizen, M. F., Aronson, S., and Thisted, R. A. (1994). Association of preoperative risk factors with postoperative acute renal failure. *Anesthesia Analgesia* **78** (1), 143–149.

Olsen, P. S. (1993). Renal failure after operation for abdominal aortic aneurysm in elderly patients. *Geriatrics Nephrology Urology* **3**, 87–91.

Pascual, J. and Liano, F. (1998). Causes and prognosis of acute renal failure in the very old. Madrid Acute Renal Failure Study Group. *Journal of the American Geriatric Society* **46** (6), 721–725.

Perazella, M. A. (1999). Crystal-induced acute renal failure. *American Journal of Medicine* **106** (4), 459–465.

Perazella, M. A. and Eras, J. (2000). Are selective COX-2 inhibitors nephrotoxic? *American Journal of Kidney Diseases* **35** (5), 937–940.

Phillips, P. A., Johnston, C. I., and Gray, L. (1993). Disturbed fluid and electrolyte homoeostasis following dehydration in elderly people. *Age Ageing* **22** (1), S26–S33.

Pitt, B., Segal, R., Martinez, F. A., Meurers, G., Cowley, A. J., Thomas, I., Deedwania, P. C., Ney, D. E., Snavely, D. B., and Chang, P. I. (1997). Randomised trial of losartan versus captopril in patients over 65 with heart failure (Evaluation of Losartan in the Elderly Study, ELITE). *Lancet* **349** (9054), 747–752.

Platt, J. F., Rubin, J. M., and Ellis, J. H. (1989). Distinction between obstructive and nonobstructive pyelocaliectasis with duplex Doppler sonography. *American Journal of Roentgenology* **153** (5), 997–1000.

Pollack, J. A., Skvorak, J. P., Nazian, S. J., Landon, C. S., and Dietz, J. R. (1997). Alterations in atrial natriuretic peptide (ANP) secretion and renal effects in aging. *The Journals of Gerontology: Series A* **52** (4), B196–B202.

Prasad, P. V. and Epstein, F. H. (1999). Changes in renal medullary pO_2 during water diuresis as evaluated by blood oxygenation level-dependent magnetic resonance imaging: effects of aging and cyclooxygenase inhibition. *Kidney International* **55** (1), 294–298.

Rakowski, T. A. and Winchester, J. F. Renal biopsy in the elderly patient. In *Geriatric Nephrology* (ed. M. F. Michelis and H. G. Preuss), pp. 37–39. New York: Field Rich, 1986.

Rascoff, J. H., Golden, R. A., Spinowitz, B. S., and Charytan, C. (1983). Nondilated obstructive nephropathy. *Archives of Internal Medicine* **143** (4), 696–698.

Rathaus, M. *et al.* (1993). Sodium loading and renal prostaglandins in old rats. *Prostaglandins Leukotrienes and Essential Fatty Acids* **49**, 815–819.

Reckelhoff, J. F., Kellum, J. A., Blanchard, E. J., Bacon, E. E., Wesley, A. J., and Kruckeberg, W. C. (1994). Changes in nitric oxide precursor, L-arginine, and metabolites, nitrate and nitrite, with aging. *Life Sciences* **55** (24), 1895–1902.

Rich, M. W. and Crecelius, C. A. (1990). Incidence, risk factors, and clinical course of acute renal insufficiency after cardiac catheterization in patients 70 years of age or older. A prospective study. *Archives of Internal Medicine* **150** (6), 1237–1242.

Rodgers, H., Staniland, J. R., Lipkin, G. W., and Turney, J. H. (1990). Acute renal failure: a study of elderly patients. *Age Ageing* **19** (1), 36–42.

Rudnick, M. R., Berns, J. S., Cohen, R. M., and Goldfarb, S. (1994). Nephrotoxic risks of renal angiography: contrast media-associated nephrotoxicity and atheroembolism—a critical review. *American Journal of Kidney Diseases* **24** (4), 713–727.

Sabbatini, M., Sansone, G., Uccello, F., De Nicola, L., Giliberti, A., Sepe, V., Margri, P., Conte, G., and Andreucci, V. E. (1994). Functional versus structural changes in the pathophysiology of acute ischemic renal failure in aging rats. *Kidney International* **45** (5), 1355–1361.

Salam, T. A., Lumsden, A. B., and Martin, L. G. (1993). Local infusion of fibrinolytic agents for acute renal artery thromboembolism: report of ten cases *Annals of Vascular Surgery* **7** (1), 21–26.

Schepkens, H., Vanholder, R., Billiouw, J. M., and Lameire, N. (2001). Life-threatening hyperkalemia during combined therapy with angiotensin-converting enzyme inhibitors and spironolactone: an analysis of 25 cases. *American Journal of Medicine* **110** (6), 438–441.

Schmidt, R. J., Beierwaltes, W. H., and Baylis, C. (2001). Effects of aging and alterations in dietary sodium intake on total nitric oxide production. *American Journal of Kidney Diseases* **37** (5), 900–908.

Schoolwerth, A. C., Sica, D. A., Ballermann, B. J., and Wilcox, C. S. (2001). Renal considerations in angiotensin converting enzyme inhibitor therapy: a statement for healthcare professionals from the council on the kidney in cardiovascular disease and the council for high blood pressure research of the american heart association. *Circulation* **104** (16), 1985–1991.

Scolari, F., Tardanico, R., Zani, R., Pola, A., Viola, B. F., Movilli, E., and Maiorca, R. (2000). Cholesterol crystal embolism: a recognizable cause of renal disease. *American Journal of Kidney Diseases* **36** (6), 1089–1109.

Snyder, N. A., Feigal, D. W., and Arieff, A. I. (1987). Hypernatremia in elderly patients. A heterogeneous, morbid, and iatrogenic entity. *Annals of Internal Medicine* **107** (3), 309–319.

Solomon, R., Werner, C., Mann, D., D'Elia, J., and Silva, P. (1994). Effects of saline, mannitol and furosemide to prevent acute decreases in renal function by radiocontrast agents. *New England Journal of Medicine* **331**, 1414–1416.

Steckel, A. *et al.* (1984). The use of streptokinase to treat renal artery thromboembolism. *American Journal of Kidney Diseases* **4**, 166.

Stuck, K. J., White, G. M., Granke, D. S., Ellis, J. H., and Weissfeld, J. L. (1987). Urinary obstruction in azotemic patients: detection by sonography. *American Journal of Roentgenology* **149** (6), 1191–1193.

Suen, W. S., Mok, C. K., Chiu, S. W., Cheung, K. L., Lee, W. T., Cheung, D., Das, S. R., and He, G. W. (1998). Risk factors for development of acute renal failure (ARF) requiring dialysis in patients undergoing cardiac surgery. *Angiology* **49** (10), 789–800.

Swan, S. K., Rudy, D. W., Lasseter, K. C., Ryan, C. F., Buechel, K. L., Lambrecht, L. J., Pinto, M. B., Dilzer, S. C., Obrda, O., Sundblad, K. J., Gumbs, C. P., Ebel, D. L., Quan, H., Larson, P. J., Schwartz, J. I., Musliner, T. A., Gertz, B. J., Brater, D. C., and Yao, S. L. (2000). Effect of cyclooxygenase-2 inhibition on renal function in elderly persons receiving a low salt diet. A randomized, controlled trial. *Annals of Internal Medicine* **133** (1), 1–9.

Tan, D., Cernadas, M. R., Aragoncillo, P., Castilla, M. A., Alvarez Arroyo, M. V., Lopez Farre, A. J., Casado, S., and Caramelo, C. (1998). Role of nitric oxide-related mechanisms in renal function in ageing rats. *Nephrology, Dialysis, Transplantation* **13** (3), 594–601.

Tepel, M., van der Giet, M., Schwarzfeld, C., Laufer, U., Liermann, D., and Zidek, W. (2000). Prevention of radiographic-contrast-agent-induced reductions in renal function by acetylcysteine. *New England Journal of Medicine* **343** (3), 180–184.

The CONSENSUS Trial Study Group (1987). Effects of enalapril on mortality in severe congestive heart failure: results of the Cooperative North Scandinavian Enalapril Survival Study (CONSENSUS). *New England Journal of Medicine* **316**, 1429–1435.

Valdivielso, J. M. *et al.* (1996). Increased severity of gentamicin nephrotoxicity in aging rats is mediated by a reduced glomerular nitric oxide production. *Environmental Toxicology and Pharmacology* **2** (1), 73–75.

van Bommel, E., Bouvy, N. D., So, K. L., Zietse, R., Vincent, H. H., Bruining, H. A., and Weimar, W. (1995). Acute dialytic support for the critically ill: intermittent hemodialysis versus continuous arteriovenous hemodiafiltration. *American Journal of Nephrology* **15** (3), 192–200.

Vance-Bryan, K., Rotschafer, J. C., Gilliland, S. S., Rodvold, K. A., Fitzgerald, C. M., and Guay, D. R. (1994). A comparative assessment of vancomycin associated nephrotoxicity in the young versus the elderly hospitalized patient. *The Journal of Antimicrobial Chemotherapy* **33** (4), 811–821.

Vaz, A. J. (1983). Low fractional excretion of urine sodium in acute renal failure due to sepsis. *Archives of Internal Medicine* **143** (4), 738–739.

Wagenknecht, L. V. and Hardy, J. C. (1981). Value of various treatments for retroperitoneal fibrosis. *European Urology* **7** (4), 193–200.

Wang, S. W. and Fan, L. (1990). Clinical features of multiple organ failure in the elderly. *Chinese Medical Journal (English)* **103** (9), 763–767.

Washio, M., Oh, Y., Okuda, S., Yanase, T., Miishima, C., Fujimi, S., Ohchi, N., Nanishi, F., Onoyama, K., and Fujishima, M. (1994). Clinicopathological study of poststreptococcal glomerulonephritis in the elderly. *Clinical Nephrology* **41** (5), 265–270.

Weinberg, A. D., Pals, J. K., McGlinchey-Berroth, R., and Minaker, K. L. (1994). Indices of dehydration among frail nursing home patients: highly variable but stable over time. *Journal of the American Geriatric Society* **42** (10), 1070–1073.

Whelton, A., Maurath, C. J., Verburg, K. M., and Geis, G. S. (2000). Renal safety and tolerability of celecoxib, a novel cyclooxygenase-2 inhibitor. *American Journal of Therapeutics* **7** (3), 159–175.

Wolf, G., Porth, J., and Stahl, R. A. (2000). Acute renal failure associated with rofecoxib. *Annals of Internal Medicine* **133** (5), 394 (letter).

Woolfson, R. G. and Lachmann, H. (1998). Improvement in renal cholesterol emboli syndrome after simvastatin. *Lancet* **351** (9112), 1331–1332.

Yarger, W. E. Obstructive urinary tract disease in the elderly. In *Hypertension and Renal Disease in the Elderly* (ed. M. Martinez-Maldonado), pp. 272–308. Boston: Blackwell Scientific Publications, 1992.

Zarich, S., Fang, L. S., and Diamond, J. R. (1985). Fractional excretion of sodium. Exceptions to its diagnostic value. *Archives of Internal Medicine* **145** (1), 108–112.

Zivin, J. R., Gooley, T., Zager, R. A., and Ryan, M. J. (2001). Hypocalcemia: a pervasive metabolic abnormality in the critically ill. *American Journal of Kidney Diseases* **37** (4), 689–698.

Zoja, C., Remuzzi, A., Corna, D., Perico, N., Bertani, T., and Remuzzi, G. (1992). Renal protective effect of angiotensin-converting enzyme inhibition in aging rats. *American Journal of Medicine* **92**, 60S–63S.

Index

Page numbers in **bold** refer to major sections of the text.
Page numbers in *italics* refer to pages on which tables may be found.